Textbook of Radiology & Imaging

Textbook of Radiology & Imaging

Edition 8

David Sutton

Rodney Reznek, Janet Murfitt

Volume 1

Adaptation Editor

Bharat Aggarwal

Director, Radiology Services, Max Healthcare, New Delhi, India

Adjunct Professor, Koita Centre for Digital Health (KCDH) of Indian Institute of Technology, Bombay

Associate Editors

Amit Kumar Sahu
Consultant
Department of Radiology
Max Superspeciality Hospital, Saket
New Delhi, India

Akshay D. Baheti
Professor
Department of Radiodiagnosis
Tata Memorial Center and Homi Bhabha National University
Mumbai, Maharashtra, India

Varsha Joshi
Senior Consultant Radiologist
Vijaya Diagnostic Centers
Hyderabad, Telangana, India

Section Editors

Girish Gandikota
Professor and Vice Chair of Radiology
University of Chapel Hill, North Carolina
Adjunct Professor, Radiology and Rheumatology
University of Michigan
Ann Arbor, MI, United States

Mukesh Harisinghani
Professor of Radiology
Harvard Medical School,
Massachusetts General Hospital
Boston, MA, United States

Puneet Bhargava
Professor, Director
Gastrointestinal Imaging
Abdominal Imaging Radiologist, University of Washington School of Medicine Hospitals,
Seattle, WA, United States

Sandeep S. Hedgire
Assistant Clinical Director
Cardiovascular Division, Director, Vascular Imaging
Department of Radiology, Massachusetts General Hospital, Harvard Medical School,
Boston, MA, United States

Subba R. Digumarthy
Associate Professor of Radiology
Harvard Medical School
Boston, MA, United States
Head of Thoracic Oncology Imaging
Division of Thoracic Imaging and Intervention
Massachusetts General Hospital Boston, MA, United States

Sujit Vaidya
Consultant Radiologist
The Royal London Hospital, Barts Health NHS Trust
Queen Mary University of London,
London, United Kingdom

Suresh K. Mukerji
Professor of Radiology & Radiation Oncology
University of Louisville & University of Illinois, Robert Wood Johnson Medical School, Rutgers University, New Brunswick, NJ, United States.
Faculty, Otolaryngology Head Neck Surgery, Michigan State University
National Director of Head & Neck Radiology; ProScan Imaging
Bruce Bradley Fellow; The Leapfrog Group

Suyash Mohan
Associate Professor of Radiology & Neurosurgery, Perelman School of Medicine at the University of Pennsylvania
Philadelphia, PA, United States
Formerly, Clinical Lecturer-II University of Michigan, Ann Arbor, MI, United States

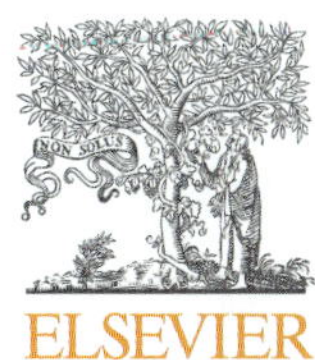

ELSEVIER

Elsevier
RELX India Pvt. Ltd.
Registered Office: 818, 8th floor, Indraprakash Building, 21, Barakhamba Road, New Delhi-110 001
Corporate Office: 14th Floor, Building No. 10B, DLF Cyber City, Phase II, Gurgaon-122 002, Haryana, India

Textbook of Radiology & Imaging, 2 Volume Set, 7e, David Sutton, Rodney Reznek, Janet Murfitt.

Publisher's note: Elsevier takes a neutral position with respect to territorial disputes or jurisdictional claims in its published content, including in maps and institutional affiliations.

ISBN: 978-0-443-07109-6

This adaptation of **Textbook of Radiology & Imaging, 2 Volume Set, 7e, by David Sutton, Rodney Reznek, Janet Murfitt** was undertaken by RELX India Private Limited and is published by arrangement with Elsevier Ltd.

Textbook of Radiology & Imaging, 2 Volume Set, 8e by David Sutton, Rodney Reznek, Janet Murfitt.
Adaptation Editor: Bharat Aggarwal

Adaptation ISBN: 978-81-312-5960-3
Adaptation e-ISBN: 978-81-312-5963-4

Set ISBN: 978-81-312-5959-7
Set e-ISBN: 978-81-312-5962-7

First Printed in India 2024, Reprinted 2025

Content Strategist: Mrinalini Bakshi
Content project Manager: Shivani Pal
Senior Production Executive: Dhan Singh
Senior Graphic Artist: Gopalakrishnan Venkatraman

Typeset by Aptara

Printed in India by Sanat Printers

Foreword

When I was a resident in the late 1980s, the only general radiology textbook we referred to was Dr. David Sutton's Textbook of Radiology. My copy was heavily underlined and annotated and dog-eared and had multiple short, "xeroxed" pages of newer information from journals stuck to the original pages by tape or gum, increasing the weight of the textbook significantly.

Even though in the later years, other textbooks became popular, Sutton was always the first book that would come to mind when we wanted residents to read up on a specific topic. In those days, with no Internet, no Pubmed, no Radiopaedia, and no other online resources, our only avenues to learn were general radiology and specialty textbooks and the popular grey and yellow journals, which in India, we would receive only about 6-9 months after publication.

Dr. Sutton died in 2002. The last (7th) edition of his book was also published in 2002. Given its immense popularity, it is no wonder that Elsevier has decided to resurrect an 8th edition of this book, in a new avatar, especially for a South Asian audience. This is no mean task. Radiology has advanced by leaps and bounds since the time Dr. Sutton updated his book. Residents, fellows, and consultants now have access to a large number of online teaching resources, some very good, many free, and some behind paywalls, but all available at the click of a mouse or the touch of a thumb. The large language models such as Chat-GPT4 are also increasing access to textual knowledge, especially for specifically structured questions. Textbooks therefore now face significant competition for eyeballs and money.

Elsevier was wise and I would say lucky to find and choose my friend Dr. Bharat Aggarwal to helm this project to bring to life this 8th edition. A third-generation radiologist, Bharat is one of the finest radiologists I have known over the last 30 years. He understands the nuances of the subject, is widely read and traveled, and hence has been able to put together an enviable roster of renowned radiologists of Indian origin, both in India and from the US and the UK, as Associate and Section Editors. His Associate Editors, Drs. Amit Sahu, Akshay Baheti, and Varsha Joshi are radiologists I have known for the last many years, all of them passionate teachers and educators. His Section Editors are all internationally renowned experts in their field. Drs. Suyash Mohan, Suresh Mukherji, Sandeep Hedgire, Mukesh Harisinghani, Sujit Vaidya, Subba Digamurthy, Girish Gandikota, and Puneet Bhargava have all put tremendous effort into their individual sections to bring the book to fruition.

It has taken about 4 years, two of which were during the challenging COVID-19 times, to make sure that each chapter in the book is as good, if not better than any online resource, with new images, algorithms, flowcharts, and tables. Some new sections have been added including Women's, Pediatric Imaging, and Interventional Radiology. It is a complete textbook that would give residents most of the information they need during their residency days and clear their examinations.

It has taken a lot of effort to maintain the flavor, language, and flow of the original book, while still ensuring that every statement of fact has been vetted and that all information is current up to the date of publication.

I congratulate Dr. Bharat Aggarwal and his team for this effort and I am sure that the book will serve as a popular and invaluable resource, not only for residents, but even for consultants, who can use this as a quick reference resource when stuck on a specific subject.

Dr Bhavin Jankharia

Preface

Radiology is a continuously evolving field. With each passing year, advancements in technology enable greater precision and improved safety. The adoption of digital tools, artificial intelligence and machine learning, coupled with a better understanding of the molecular basis of disease, has enabled the introduction of new therapies and altered decision pathways for patient care. The role of the radiologist is now central to treatment planning and disease monitoring, therefore making it vital for radiologists to not only provide diagnoses but also actively contribute to decision-making in patient care. The modern radiologist now, more than ever before, must have a strong foundational knowledge while adapting to the evolving technological advances. It is with this premise that we have adapted this new edition of Sutton's Textbook of Radiology.

It has been an honor to be invited by Elsevier to edit and update Sutton's Textbook of Radiology, the gold standard and a key reference book for practicing radiologists over multiple generations. I have attempted to share my experiences as a radiologist, a journey that began when I learned radiology from my father, Dr. Sudarshan K. Aggarwal, perhaps one of the greatest visionaries of Indian Radiology. The Diwan Chand Aggarwal Imaging Center, started by my grandfather in 1924 and taken forward by my uncle Dr. Satyapal Aggarwal, was scaled to an institution under the stewardship of my father, and managed under one core tenet—**patient first.** This created an academic environment and pushed the institute to be a teaching center from where over 100 radiology residents completed their training and are now leading radiologists across the globe. I continue to follow this philosophy of combining high-quality clinical care and academic pursuit in my ongoing tenure at Max Healthcare, one of the largest healthcare providers in India.

Despite the fact that the last revision of this book was in 2002, it has continued to be a favorite textbook among radiology residents, mainly because of the comprehensive coverage of each topic and the presentation style. We have preserved the unique style of the textbook and retained material that continues to be relevant even two decades later. This edition of Sutton is aimed at recreating an exhaustive resource and reference text for radiologists to solve diverse clinical scenarios using the latest and most appropriate technology, and develop a sound process-driven approach.

New sections on radiology physics and techniques, pediatric radiology, interventional radiology, and emergency radiology have been added to make the book comprehensive. The first section includes chapters on quality assurance, structured reporting, information technology in radiology, and a primer in artificial intelligence—knowledge of which is now extremely important to practicing radiologists. The remaining sections have been reorganized to emphasize the need for sub-specialty radiology. Chapters on nuclear medicine and dental radiology provide the practicing radiologist with an understanding of all imaging-based diagnostic techniques available today. The evolving radiology lexicons that radiologists should use in their daily practice to communicate their findings for consistent care have also been incorporated into the book.

This book was put together through the COVID-19 pandemic, the biggest medical calamity faced by our generation. I want to extend my heartfelt gratitude to all the contributors who, despite being personally and professionally impacted by COVID-19 at the frontlines during the pandemic, stood true to their commitment and contributed high-quality material that will lay the foundation for the careers of the radiologists of the future.

I acknowledge the proactivity, guidance, and support extended by the section editors, all of whom are leaders in their fields—a big thanks to Dr. Suresh Mukherji, Dr. Suyash Mohan, Dr. Girish Gandikota, Dr. Sandeep Hedgire, Dr. Mukesh Harisinghani, Dr. Sujit Vaidya, Dr. Puneet Bhargava, and Dr. Subba Digumarthy. I would also like to thank Dr. Rajesh Gothi and Dr. Shivani Khanna for editorial support, and the management of Max Healthcare for their support.

I would have been unable to complete this project without the commitment shown by my associate editors, Dr. Amit Sahu and Dr. Akshay Baheti, right from the acceptance of this challenge to its planning and smooth execution, along with Dr. Varsha Joshi.

Most importantly I thank the patient community that my family has served over almost a century, for shaping my professional career and encouraging me to be a better doctor.

There are absolutely no words to describe the encouragement and support I have received from my wife, Suman, and children, Samir and Divya, in this extended, almost four-year journey of editing Sutton and the endless personal time ungrudgingly shared.

This book is my contribution to the legacy of my family and to the specialty of Radiology.

Dr Bharat Aggarwal

Contributors

Abraham Fourie Bezuidenhout
Faculty
Department of Radiology
Beth Israel Deaconess Medical Center
Boston, MA, United States

Adriano Basso Dias
Assistant Professor
University of Toronto
Division of Abdominal Imaging, Joint Department of Medical Imaging, University Health Network Mount Sinai Hospital – Women's College Hospital, University of Toronto
Toronto, ON, Canada

Alireza B. Abadi
Resident Physician
Department of Radiology
University of Washington
Seattle, WA, United States

Alpana Joshi
Consultant & Director
Thane Ultrasound Centre
Thane, Maharashtra, India

Ameya S. Kawthalkar
Department of Radiology
KIMS Kingsway Hospital
Nagpur, Maharashtra, India

Amna Zafar
Assistant Professor of Medicine
Co-Director of Cardio-Oncology
Division of Cardiovascular Diseases and Hypertension, Rutgers Robert Wood Johnson School of Medicine
New Brunswick, NJ, United States

Amrin Israrahmed
Associate Consultant
Department of Intervention Radiology
Medanta Hospital
Gurgaon, Haryana, India

Anderson H. Kuo
Midland Memorial Hospital
Midland, TX, United States

Anisha Gehani
Junior Consultant
Tata Medical Center
Kolkata, West Bengal, India

Anto Ramesh
Founder
Chairman & Managing Director
Radblox Healthcare Services
Bengaluru, Karnataka, India

Anu Eapen
Professor
Christian Medical College
Vellore, Tamil Nadu, India

Anupam Bam
Clinical Research Medical Advisor
Novartis, Mumbai, Maharashtra, India

Anuradha Chandramohan
Professor and Clinical Lead of Abdominal Imaging Service
Department of Radiology
Christian Medical College
Vellore, Tamil Nadu, India

Aparna Katdare
Associate Professor
Department of Radiodiagnosis
Tata Memorial Hospital
Mumbai, Maharashtra, India

Argha Chatterjee
Gastroradiology
Associate Consultant
Department of Radiology
Tata Medical Center
Kolkata, West Bengal, India

Ashok Mithra
Senior Consultant Radiologist & Head of Radiology
Naruvi Hospitals
Vellore, Tamil Nadu, India

Ramandeep Singh
Clinical Fellow in Radiology
Massachusetts General Hospital
Harvard Medical School
Boston, MA, United States

Reetu John
Professor
Department of Radiology
Christian Medical College
Vellore, Tamil Nadu, India

Rohit Takhar
CARPL.ai Pvt. Ltd.
New Delhi, India

Rory L. Cochran
Massachusetts General Hospital
Harvard Medical School
Boston, MA, United States

Ruchi Rastogi
Principal Consultant
Max Superspeciality Hospital
New Delhi, India

Sachin S. Saboo
Radiologist
South Texas Radiology Group
San Antonio, TX, United States

Sandeep S. Hedgire
Assistant Clinical Director CV Division
MAS; Fellow
Cardiovascular Imaging
MAS; Clinical Fellow

Sandhya Vinu-Nair
Associate Professor
Radiology
Section Director
Emergency Radiology
University of Texas Health Science Center at San Antonio
San Antonio, TX, United States

Sangeet Ghai
Associate Professor
University of Toronto
Toronto, ON, Canada

Sanjeeva P. Kalva
Chief
Interventional Radiology
Massachusetts General Hospital
Professor of Radiology
Harvard Medical School
Boston, MA, United States

Sarv Priya
Clinical Assistant Professor
Radiology
University of Iowa Hospitals & Clinics
Iowa City, IA, United States

Satinder Singh
Professor of Radiology and Medicine (Division of CV Diseases)
University of Alabama at Birmingham Hospital (UAB)
Birmingham, AL, United States

Saugata Sen
Senior Consultant
Department of Radiology and Imaging Sciences
Tata Medical Center
Kolkata, Kolkata, West Bengal, India

Seema Kembhavi
SMO Radiology
Mackay Hospital and Health Services
Mackay, QLD, Australia

Shalini Govil
Senior Advisor Radiology Quality
Naruvi Hospital
Vellore, Tamil Nadu, India

Sharad Maheshwari
Consultant Radiologist
Kokilaben Hospital
Mumbai, Maharashtra, India

Shyamkumar N. Keshava
Professor and Head
Department of Interventional Radiology
Division of Clinical Radiology

Smita Esther Raju
Consultant Radiologist & Director of Training, Clinical Radiology
Royal Adelaide Hospital
Adelaide, SA, Australia

Somesh Singh
Consultant
Department of Radiodiagnosis
Medanta Hospital
Gurgaon, Haryana, India

Sourav Panda
Consultant Radiologist
Healthworld Hospital
Durgapur, West Bengal, India

Srinivasa R. Prasad
Professor
University of Texas MD Anderson Cancer Center
Houston, TX, United States

Subba R. Digumarthy
Associate Professor of Radiology
Harvard Medical School
Boston, MA, United States

Sumit Gupta
Instructor in Radiology
Brigham and Women's Hospital
Department of Radiology
Boston, MA, United States

Sumit Mukhopadhyay
Senior Consultant
Department of Radiology
Tata Medical Center
Kolkata, West Bengal, India

Sunaina Yadav
Imperial College London
United Kingdom

Swati Garekar
Consultant Pediatric Cardiologist
Fortis Hospital Mulund
Mumbai, Maharashtra, India

Tejas Kapadia
Consultant Paediatric Radiologist
Royal Manchester Children's Hospital
Manchester, United Kingdom

Udo Hoffmann
Chief Scientific Officer
Cleerly Inc
New York, NY, United States

Vaibhav Nichat
Pediatric Radiology Fellow
Department of Radiodiagnosis and Imaging
Postgraduate Institute of Medical Education and Research
Chandigarh, Punjab, India

Vasantha Kumar Venugopal
CARPL.ai Pvt. Ltd.
New Delhi, India

Venkat Katabathina
Associate Professor
University of Texas Health Science Center at San Antonio
San Antonio, TX, United States

Venkateswar R. Surabhi
Professor of Radiology
Department of Abdominal Imaging
Division of Diagnostic Imaging
The University of Texas MD Anderson Cancer Center
Houston, TX, United States

Vidur Mahajan
CARPL.ai Pvt. Ltd.
New Delhi, India

Viky S. Loescher
Cardiovascular-Cardiothoracic Radiologist
Mount Sinai Medical Center
Miami Beach, FL, United States

Zainab Vora
Consultant Radiologist
Apple Imaging
New Delhi, India

Contents

each other and to the direction of the wave. Electromagnetic waves travel in a straight line with the speed of light (3×10^8 m/sec in a vacuum) and require no medium to travel (i.e., they can travel in a vacuum). The velocity (c) of the wave can be calculated by the product of frequency (f) and wavelength (λ) as

$$c = f \times \lambda.$$

X-rays are made up of photons, which can behave as both waves and particles. The photon energy (E) is directly proportional to frequency ($E = h \times f$), in which h is the Plank's constant. The electromagnetic waves above the visible light of energy spectrum (ultraviolet rays, x-rays, and γ-rays) are classified as ionizing because they are capable of displacing an electron from the atom.

X-ray Units

Energy produced at source and energy deposited or absorbed by tissues is measurable (Table 1.1). *Kerma* was developed to measure the amount of kinetic energy released in matter per unit mass. *Dose is used to quantify the energy deposited or absorbed by an object.* Energy passing through a cross section (sum of energies of all photons) per unit area measured per unit time gives the energy fluence rate or *beam intensity* (signifies beam quality). Intensity is a measure of energy in a cross-section area and is mostly dependent on the number of x-ray photons (quantity).

X-ray Imaging

X-ray Tube

An X-ray tube is made up of two oppositely charged electrodes (cathode and anode) capable of producing x-rays when a current is passed through it. *When fast-moving electrons are bombarded on a metal target, the kinetic energy of the electrons is converted mainly into heat (>99%) and x-rays (<1%).* To achieve this, a large current is passed through a source, producing a large number of electrons. The source is the negatively charged cathode of the tube, which is a filament or coil usually made of tungsten. (Tungsten has a very high melting temperature and can tolerate a lot of heat.) When current is passed through the cathode, a potential difference is created in the tube across the cathode and anode. The cathode filament gets heated up to high temperatures (incandescent hot), causing violent atomic or electrical motion, and it starts emitting electrons on the surface by the process of thermionic emission. Because the electrons are negatively charged, they get repelled by the negatively charged cathode and are then accelerated at high speed toward the positively charged anode. An anode is the flat metal target and is usually made up of tungsten. The x-ray tube contains vacuum; hence, there is no hindrance to the electrons bombarding the anode target. As the electrons are accelerated toward the target because of the potential difference between the cathode and anode, they gain kinetic energy (keV). On striking the tungsten target, the electrons lose kinetic energy to produce heat and x-rays

An x-ray tube is made up of following parts (Fig. 1.2):

- Cathode: usually tungsten filament/coil embedded within a focusing cup
- Anode: target material made up of tungsten and can either be stationary or rotating. For a rotating anode, the assembly consists of an anode stem and rotor
- Tube enclosure: Pyrex glass or now made of metal and glass or metal and ceramic for longer life of the tube with vacuum inside
- Protective housing: made of heavy metal or lead with a window for the x-rays to emerge

Cathode

The filament is a coil of wire approximately 2 mm in thickness and 1 to 2 cm long. *The present radiography systems prefer two filaments of different lengths, giving two different focal spot sizes (large and small).* A small focal spot is used when better spatial resolution is required, and a large focal spot is used when imaging large body parts. The filaments are embedded in a negatively charged focusing cup (Fig. 1.2) that electrostatically limits the electron beam from spreading out and focuses on a small area of the anode. In certain scenarios such as cineradiography, digital radiography (DR), or digital subtraction angiography, x-ray tubes are used that are capable of rapidly turning on and off.

Anode

The target material at the anode end is made up of tungsten due to its high melting point and is capable of producing diagnostic quality x-rays. Tungsten has low vapor pressure (i.e., does not vaporize at the working temperatures). *The anode can be stationary or rotating.* Currently, the use of stationary anode tubes is limited

TABLE 1.1 Units of Radiation Dose

Term	Description	Conventional Unit	SI Unit
Exposure	Amount of ionization produced per unit of mass of air	Roentgen	C/kg
Kerma	Kinetic energy released in matter per unit mass	Rad	Gray (Gy) or J/kg
Dose	Energy absorbed per unit mass	Rad	Gray (Gy) or J/kg
Intensity	Number of photons × photon energy per unit area	KeV/cm²	J/m²

SI, International System of Units.

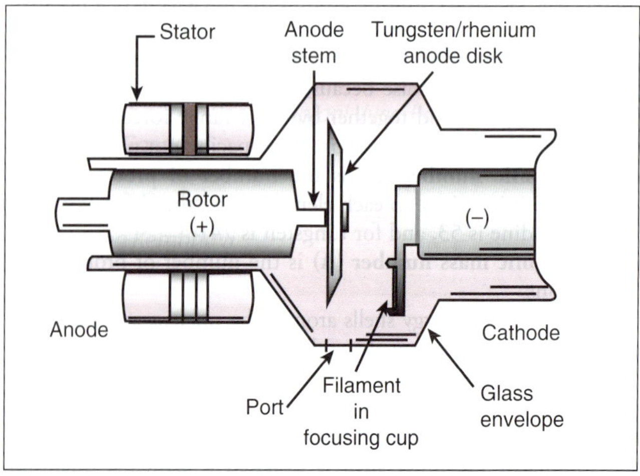

Figure 1.2 Structure of a rotating anode x-ray tube. (From: TL Fauber, *Radiographic Imaging and Exposure*, fourth ed, 15, Elsevier Mosby, May 2012, USA.)

to dental and portable radiography. Rotating anode tubes are preferred for diagnostic imaging because of their capability of avoiding high temperatures at the target surface and thus better tube life and for producing higher intensity x-rays compared with stationary tubes. The target surface of the rotating anode disc is made of tungsten and rhenium alloy. The edge of the target face is beveled and is set at an angle of 7 to 15 degrees. The beveled edge allows for use of the line-focus principle, making the apparent focus smaller than the real focus as shown in Fig. 1.2.

The line focus principle is extremely important for the rotating x-ray tube because angling the target area allows heating of the large part of target despite a small focal spot size. Thus, the *effective focal spot is much smaller than the actual focal spot.* This improves the heat capacity of the tube and improves spatial resolution.

Another important principle to remember at the anode end of the tube is the *anode heel effect*. As the electrons are bombarded on the target, the x-rays produced are emitted from the surface. But because the target is angled, some of the x-rays on the anode side of the tube have to traverse longer through the target before they are emitted, and thus their energy gets partially absorbed in the target itself. Thus, the rays on the cathode end are of higher intensity than those on the anode end. This is called the anode heel effect (Fig. 1.3). This principle is explored and is important while imaging structures of differing thicknesses. In mammography, the anode heel effect is used with the higher intensity radiation coming from the cathode end placed toward the side of chest wall, thus allowing uniform image receptor exposure.

The target material of any x-ray tube should be capable of dissipating high amount of heat quickly. The target for stationary anodes is a block made of tungsten embedded in copper. Copper is a good conductor of heat and improves the thermal conductivity of the tube. The rotating anode is made of a molybdenum disc (high thermal capacity) with graphite backing (which has higher thermal capacity), and the focal track is made of tungsten and rhenium alloy (90% tungsten and 10% rhenium). Rhenium (Z = 75, similar to tungsten with Z = 74) improves the heat capacity by reducing the effects of thermal expansion and contraction; it also adds to the mechanical strength required for high-speed rotation.

A rotating anode disc is connected to the induction motor by a molybdenum stem with a small diameter. This reduces heat conduction from the anode disc to the rotor system. The induction motor works by electromagnetic induction and has two components, the stator, which lies outside the glass–metal envelope, and the rotor, which is inside the glass–metal envelope. There are bearings between the rotor and the stator lubricated by a soft metal such as silver. The anode disc rotation in modern tubes is around 9000 rpm (rotations per minute), which allows adequate heat dissipation for short exposure times.

The tube insert containing the cathode and anode is covered by a lead lined metal housing containing oil. The oil around the tube insert acts as a coolant and as an electrical insulator.

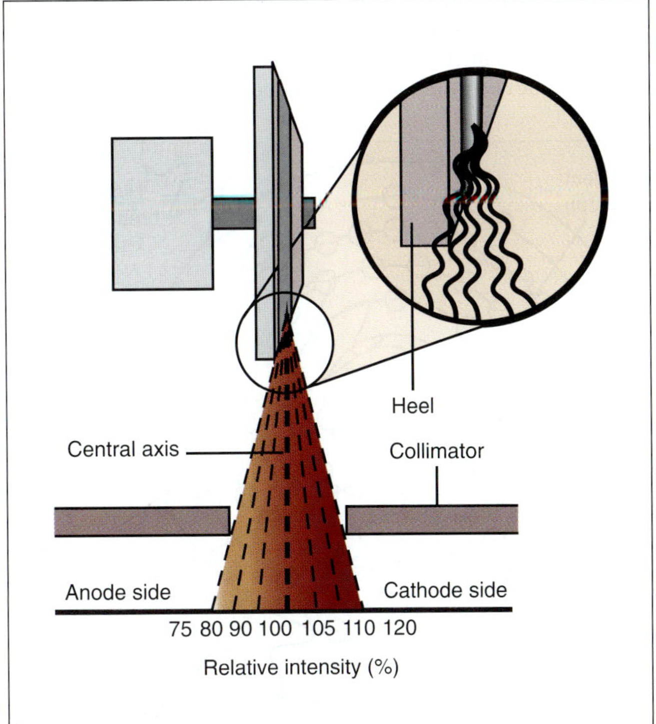

Figure 1.3 The emerging x-ray beam has reduced intensity toward the anode side of the tube because of absorption in the anode heel. (From: SC Bushong, *Radiologic Science for Technologists*, eleventh ed, 115, Elsevier, 2017, Canada.)

X-ray Tube Cooling

The heat loss from the anode can be by means of conduction, convection, or radiation.

The rotating anode disc has a high thermal capacity and is connected to the rotor by a thin molybdenum stem; thus, heat loss by conduction from the anode disc to the rotor is minimized. The anode heat is dissipated by infrared radiation to the glass or metal envelope and thus to the oil in the housing unit. Heat passes through the oil by convection and is then conducted through the shield. The heat is then removed from the shield by the surrounding air by convection currents.

Tube Rating

X-ray tube rating is exposure settings that the tube can withstand without causing damage. Each x-ray tube is provided with a set of rating charts that list the safe operating exposure factors above which irreversible damage can occur to the tube. This information is provided in the form of graphs and are called *radiographic rating charts*. These charts are important for single exposure procedures (e.g., chest radiography).

For a given anode disc rotation speed, exposure time, and kVp, only milliamperage (mA) values falling under the curve can be selected. Using mA value above this curve can cause melting of the focal tract and unacceptable tube damage. Similarly, a long exposure at a fixed low mA can melt the anode focal track. Multiple tube exposures in a short period of time can again damage the anode because of overheating. Thus, there are separate ratings charts for single and multiple exposures. Factors affecting tube rating are listed in Table 1.2.

Other ways of rating tubes are anode cooling charts and housing cooling charts. These charts provide radiographers with

TABLE 1.2 Fixed and Variable Factors Affecting X-ray Tube Rating

Fixed Factors	Selectable Factors
Anode diameter, thermal capacity of anode, anode angle	Focal spot size
Speed of anode rotation	mA
Overall tube thermal capacity	kVp
Type of rectifier and transformer	Duration of exposure

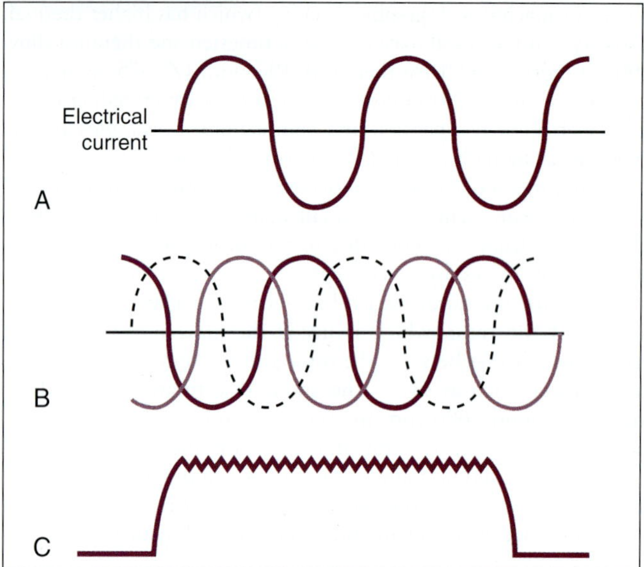

Figure 1.4 Waveforms for a single-phase (A), three-phase (B), and high-frequency generator (C). (From: TL Fauber, *Radiographic Imaging and Exposure*, fourth ed, 26, Elsevier Mosby, May 2012, USA.)

information about time intervals to be observed between two exposures to allow adequate heat dissipation.

The amount of heat generated by any exposure is called the *heat unit (HU)*. This is calculated as

$$HU = kVp \times mA \times s \times \text{generator factor}$$

The generator factor is usually 1.4 for three-phase generators. The modern x-ray units have inbuilt devices (photo diodes and temperature-sensitive resistors) that directly measure the temperature of the anode disc and oil in the housing. These data are then fed into a microprocessor chip in the tube housing that regulates exposure through activation of an error message or prevents exposure altogether.

X-ray Generators and Rectifiers

The main electrical supply to an x-ray unit is the standard AC current supply. A constant high voltage across the tube is necessary to produce x-rays of constant high intensity. For this, a rectifier is used to convert the alternating voltage to constant unidirectional high voltage, and a transformer is used to convert low to high voltage. Rectification converts the AC waveform with both positive and negative aspects to a pulsed positive waveform [2].

Three types of generators are available depending on the type of waveform and ripple they produce (Fig. 1.4).

- The single-phase generators can be half wave rectified or full wave rectified
- The three phase generators can be 6 pulse or 12 pulse; the latter produce less ripple
- High-frequency generators produce minimal ripple (~1%) and provide constant high potential

Modern x-ray equipment uses a high frequency.

X-ray Production

Electrons released from the cathode filament are focused and driven to the anode by the potential difference across the cathode and anode. As the electrons are accelerated, they carry kinetic energy (measured in kiloelectron volts or keV), which is equal to the potential difference (measured in kV) across the tube. On colliding with the target (anode) surface (0.25–0.5 mm thick), the electron may experience hundreds of interactions before being brought to rest. At the target, the electrons lose their energy by a few undermentioned defined processes:

- ***Target interactions***
  - *a. Interaction with outer-shell electron of target atom:* Tungsten (atomic number 74) has 74 electrons orbiting around its nucleus. The electron from the cathode passes through the target surface and interacts with many atoms; most of the reactions involve small deflections of the electron from its path. These interactions cause loss of kinetic energy of the electron in the form of low-energy photon, which is mostly released as heat. Unfortunately, this type of reaction makes up the majority of the interactions (99%) occurring at the target of the x-ray tube, which mainly increase the temperature of the target.
  - *b. Interaction with an inner-shell electron or nucleus of the target atom.* These are important reactions producing x-rays of diagnostic range.
    - a. The x-rays produced by interaction with target atom nuclei are called *bremsstrahlung radiation.*
    - b. The x-rays produced because of interaction with inner-shell electrons of the target atom are called *characteristic radiation.*
- ***Bremsstrahlung radiation***

Bremsstrahlung radiation literally means "braking radiation" (German). *This is the most common interaction at the target, producing x-rays in the diagnostic energy range (nearly 80%)* except for mammography tubes. When the high-velocity projectile electrons from the cathode filament are bombarded on the anode, some of them come quite close to the target atom nucleus without interacting with the orbiting electrons. When under the influence of the electric field of the nucleus, strong electrostatic forces develop between the negatively charged projectile electron and positively charged nucleus. This causes a change in the direction of the projectile electrons, slowing them down with loss of kinetic energy, deflecting the energy in the form of x-rays. The closer the projectile electron to the nucleus, the stronger the electrostatic influence, the bigger the deflection in direction, the greater the loss of kinetic energy, and the higher the energy of the x-rays produced as depicted in Fig. 1.5.

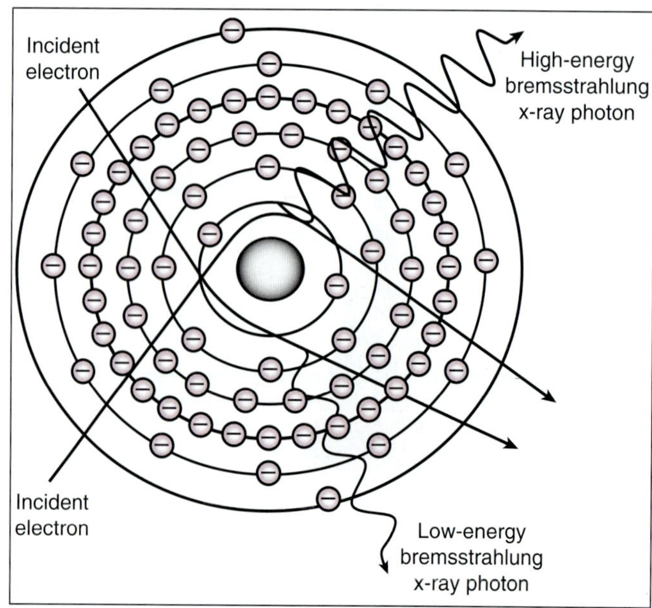

Figure 1.5 Bremsstrahlung radiation. Higher deflection angles gives higher energy emitted x-ray photon with reduced energy of the deflected electron. (From: TL Fauber, *Radiographic Imaging and Exposure*, fourth ed, 18, Elsevier Mosby, May 2012, USA.)

When a potential difference of 70 kVp is applied across the x-ray tube, the projectile electron can have kinetic energy from 0 to 70 keV. This kinetic energy is lost at the target to produce x-rays of differing energies up to a maximum of 70 keV, and they form a continuous spectrum.

- ***Characteristic radiation***

When a projectile electron collides with a K-shell electron of the target atom, it ejects the K-shell electron. For this interaction to occur, the projectile electron should have enough kinetic energy to overcome the binding energy of the K-shell electron, which in case of a tungsten target is 69.5keV. Thus, the projectile electron must possess energy equal to or above 69.5 keV to eject the K-shell electron. This creates a vacancy in the K-shell of the atom, which is filled by one of the electrons from the outer shell (this can be from any of the L, M, N, O, or P shells in the case of tungsten). In the Bohr model of the atom, the outer shells are of higher energy, and the inner shells are of low energy. An electron falling from the outer shell (high energy) to the inner shell (lower energy) loses energy in the form of x-rays called *characteristic radiation* (Fig. 1.6). The energy of the x-ray emitted is equal to the difference in the binding energies of the electrons in different shells. The x-rays emitted because of K-shell interactions are called K rays and are denoted as Kα (58 keV) for electrons falling from L shell to K shell, Kβ (67keV) for M shell to K shell, etc. The energy of the x-ray emitted in this manner is constant, and it is characteristic for the type of target material, increasing with increasing atomic number. *Compared with bremsstrahlung radiation, which has a continuous radiation spectrum, characteristic radiation has a single line spectrum with the energy dependent on the target material.*

To summarize, bremsstrahlung radiation can occur at low or high cathode electron energies, producing x-rays of variable keV (directly proportional to kVp). However, characteristic radiation (for a tungsten target with Z = 74 and K-shell binding energy of 69 keV) requires a minimum x-ray tube potential of 69 kVp. At tube potentials below 69 kVp, no useful characteristic radiation is produced (only bremsstrahlung).

- ***X-ray spectrum***

The x-ray spectrum is a graph of the number of x-rays (photons) emitted on the *y*-axis and the energy of the photons on the *x*-axis in keV. The x-ray photons emitted from the target surface are polyenergetic and have a range of low to high energies. The spectrum can have a continuous curve, which represents all the x-ray photons of different energies emitted from the target surface, or a discrete spectrum, which is represented as vertical lines on the spectrum that are of constant energy specific to the target material's electron-binding energy (Fig. 1.7).

Bremsstrahlung radiation involves x-ray photons of variable energies (low to high) and constitutes the continuous curve of the spectrum. For example, if 80-kVp potential is applied to the tube, then the energy of bremsstrahlung x-rays will range from zero to 80 keV. Most of the x-rays emitted because of bremsstrahlung radiation are of nearly one-third the kVp applied, and maximum energy is equal to the kVp applied. In Fig. 1.7, a typical spectrum of bremsstrahlung radiation is shown in which most of the x-ray photons are in the middle of the curve with very few low- or high-energy photons. Most of the low-energy photons get absorbed in the target surface itself or by the tube housing.

Characteristic radiation is the vertical lines seen on the x-ray emission spectrum, and it is not produced if the kVp applied to the tube is below the electron-binding energy of the target material (69 kVp for tungsten). In the case of a tungsten target, the characteristic radiation produced will have energy of

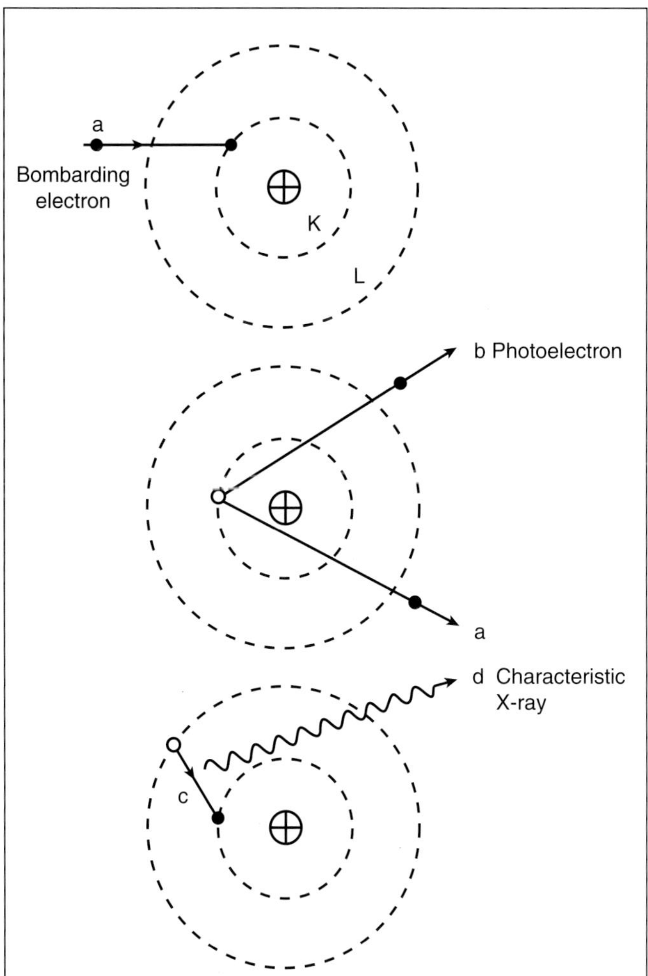

Figure 1.6 Production of characteristic radiation. a: bombarding electron collides with an electron from the K-shell of the target atom, b: photoelectron, c: outer shell electron falls in the inner shell losing energy as characteristic x-ray (d).

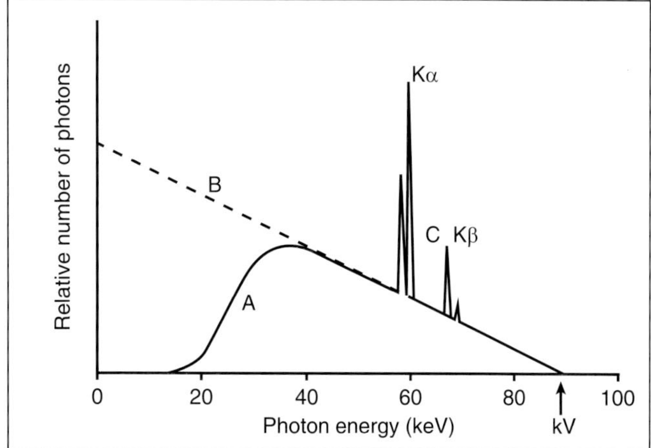

Figure 1.7 X-ray spectrum of a tungsten target at 90 kVp. *A* is the continuous curve of bremsstrahlung radiation; *C* is the linear spikes of characteristic radiation (Kα and Kβ), and *B* is the low-energy photons from bremsstrahlung radiation (*dashed line*) that get absorbed by the target surface itself and by the inherent filtration of the tube (e.g., the tube housing).

TABLE 1.3 Effect of Controllable and Constant Factors on the X-ray Emission Spectrum

Factor Affecting X-ray Spectrum	Effect on Quantity	Effect on Quality
Controllable Factors		
1. Increase in kVp	Increases the quantity of the x-ray photons produced proportional to kVp^2	Increases the energy of the x-ray photons
2. Increase in mA	Increases the quantity of x-ray photons produced proportional to mA	Does not affect the x-ray quality
Constant Factors (for the Equipment)		
1. Target material	Increase in atomic number of the target material increases the quantity of x-ray photons produced	Increase in atomic number can increase characteristic radiation with no effect on Bremsstrahlung radiation.
2. Beam filtration	Reduces the quantity of x-rays emerging from the tube; the quantity is inversely proportional to atomic number and thickness of filter used	It removes low-energy photons and thus improves x-ray beam quality
3. Voltage rectification	Tube voltage closer to constant potential increases the quantity of x-ray photons emitted	Tube voltage closer to constant potential improves x-ray beam quality

58 keV for Kα radiation (L shell to K shell), 67 keV for Kβ radiation (M shell to K shell), and 69 keV for Kγ radiation (N shell to K shell).

Thus, for lower kVp, the x-ray spectrum is from bremsstrahlung radiation. As the tube voltage is increased, characteristic radiation increases proportionally.

- ***Factors affecting the x-ray spectrum (x-ray quality and quantity)***

The total number of x-rays emitted is equal to the area under the x-ray spectrum: the larger the area under curve, the larger the number of x-rays. This gives us measure of the **quantity** of x-rays. As the curve moves to the right, more x-ray energy is emitted. This is the **quality** of the x-rays produced by the tube, and it determines the penetrability of the x-rays into matter (the higher the energy, the greater the penetrability). *The quality of the x-ray beam can be measured as air kerma (J/kg or gray in the International System of Units [SI]).*

X-ray **intensity**, as discussed previously, is number of photons × photon energy per unit area (the SI unit is J/m^2). *Intensity can be said to be a combined measure of both the quantity and the quality of the x-ray beam.* The factors affecting them individually affect the intensity of the beam. Following are the factors affecting the x-ray spectrum as described in Table 1.3.

1. **The effect of kVp on the x-ray spectrum**

As the kilovoltage applied across the tube is increased, the velocity of the electrons bombarded on the target atoms increases.

An increase in kVp increases the

- average energy of emitted x-ray photons,
- maximum energy of emitted x-ray photons,
- number of x-ray photons emitted.

Therefore, kVp affects the intensity of the x-ray beam, and the *increase in kVp grows the curve and shifts it to the right* as shown in Fig. 1.8.

2. **The effect of mA on the emission spectrum**

The milliamperage is the unit for tube current, which is the number of electrons flowing from the cathode to the anode per unit of time. Increasing the electrons bombarding the target increases the bremsstrahlung and characteristic radiation proportionally. The *milliamperage invariably increases the x-ray beam intensity and the amplitude or height of the emission but does not affect the energy of the x-ray photons and only increases the x-ray quantity.*

An increase in kVp with a constant mAs reduces differential absorption and thus reduces contrast because the beam is more penetrable. An increase in mAs increases the contrast on the image (Fig. 1.9).

3. **The effect of the target material on the emission spectrum**

Increasing the atomic number of the target material increases the x-ray beam intensity by increasing the efficiency of producing bremsstrahlung radiation and only increases the beam intensity. The choice of target material also affects the characteristic radiation because the atomic number of a material affects the K-shell binding energy (directly proportional). In the case of mammography tubes with a molybdenum target, a lower kVp is used because the binding energy of electrons in molybdenum is low (Kα characteristic radiation of 17 keV compared with 58 keV for tungsten).

4. **The effect of filtration on the emission spectrum**

The x-rays are produced from the target surface, and as they are emitted, they pass through the target itself while reaching the surface, tube glass envelope, housing oil, and housing window. This constitutes the inherent filtration of the tube, and it absorbs the low-energy x-ray photons. Additional filtration is added near the tube window to further absorb low-energy photons, which may not constitute to image formation and only increase the entrance surface dose to the patient. This is the added filtration and is usually in the form of aluminium discs of variable thickness

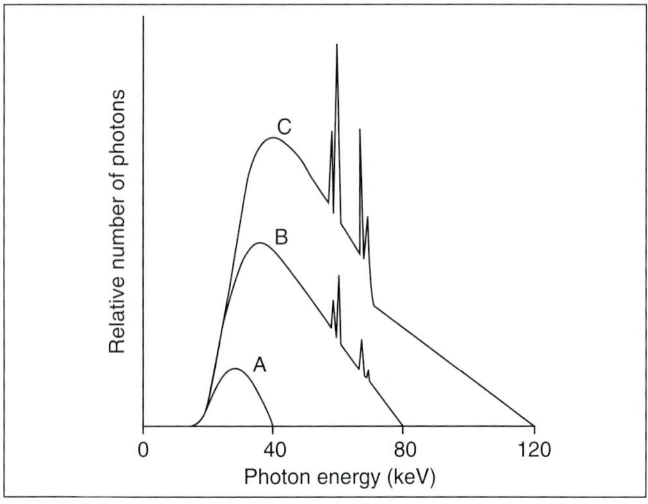

Figure 1.8 An increase in kV shifts the spectral curve to the right with an increase in amplitude of the x-ray photons, thus increasing the overall intensity of the x-ray beam. Notice that at lower kV (curve A), only bremsstrahlung radiation occurs, and the vertical characteristic radiation lines are only seen when the potential increases to more than 70 kV (curves B and C).

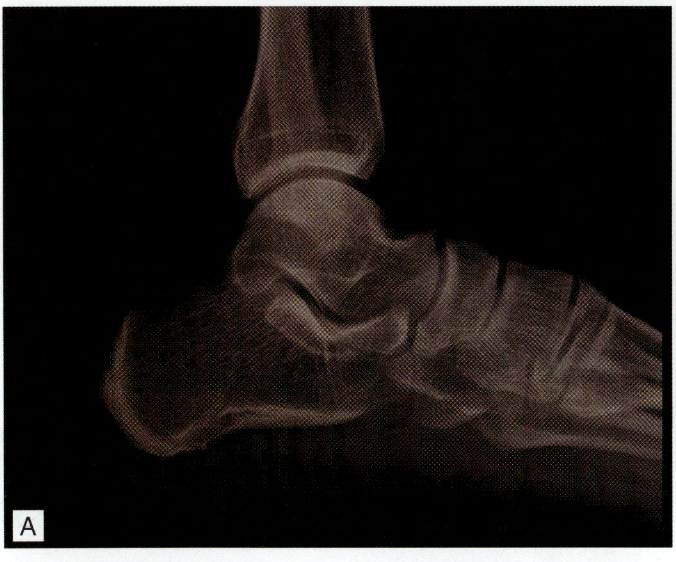

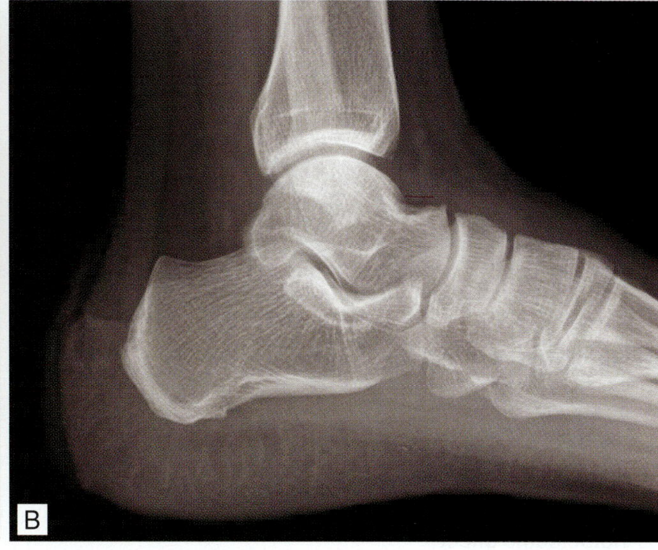

Figure 1.9 Effect of kVp and mAs on image quality. Right ankle lateral radiograph with 60 kVp and 5 mAs (A) compared with with 40 kVp and 15 mAs (B). The image contrast and resolution are better in B because of a low kVp and higher mAs technique.

(1–2 mm in thickness). Therefore, the inherent filtration is measured in terms of millimeters of aluminium equivalent.

5. **The effect of voltage rectification on the emission spectrum**

The varying voltage in single-phase generators produces x-ray photons of quite variable energy. The beam therefore contains many photons that do not contribute to image formation but increase the patient dose.

With a high-frequency generator, the x-ray intensity and beam energy are increased, with reduced low-energy photons producing constant potential to maximize intensity and minimize low-energy photons.

X-ray Interaction With Matter

The x-ray beam falling on the patient undergoes attenuation before reaching the grid–detector (or x-ray film–screen) complex. It can get absorbed, be scattered, or be transmitted through the patient.

- **Absorbed**: transfer of all the x-ray photon energy to matter
- **Scattered**: deviation of the direction of the x-ray photon with or without loss of its energy. This can emerge as secondary or scattered radiation
- **Transmitted**: unaffected and passes through the patient as primary radiation

The transmitted photons contribute to x-ray image formation as they reach the detector. The other x-rays interacting with matter (absorption or scatter) undergo multiple processes. Only two processes (photoelectric absorption and Compton scatter) are important for the purpose of radiography and are summarized in Table 1.4. The other processes are pair production and elastic scattering.

- ***X-ray attenuation***

As a monoenergetic beam passes through a medium, it eventually loses its energy because of interaction with atoms in the medium by the process of absorption or scatter; this is called *attenuation* of the beam. The attenuation of the beam depends on the probability of the interaction of the x-ray beam with an atom (electrons of the atom). This probability is proportional to the energy of the photon and the number of atoms in the material (Table 1.5).

TABLE 1.4 Summary of the Contribution of Photoelectric Effect and Compton Scattering

Attenuation Process	Interaction with Matter	Contribution to Absorption	Contribution to Scatter
Photoelectric effect (Fig. 1.10)	Incident x-ray photon collides with inner electrons of the atoms in matter and eject an electron if its energy is greater than electron-binding energy of the inner electron. The ejected electron with its reduced energy interacts with other atoms in its pathway, ultimately losing all its energy. The hole created in the inner shell is filled by electrons falling from the outer shell with release of energy in form of characteristic or secondary radiation.	Photon energy is absorbed	No photon scatter occurs
Compton scattering (Fig. 1.11)	Incident x-ray photon interacts with a loosely bound or free electron, losing some of its energy along with change in its direction. The loosely bound electron gets ejected from outer shell, taking away some of the energy of the incident photon. This energy is absorbed by material itself as the ejected electron travels only a short distance.	Some of the energy is absorbed	Major source of scatter radiation

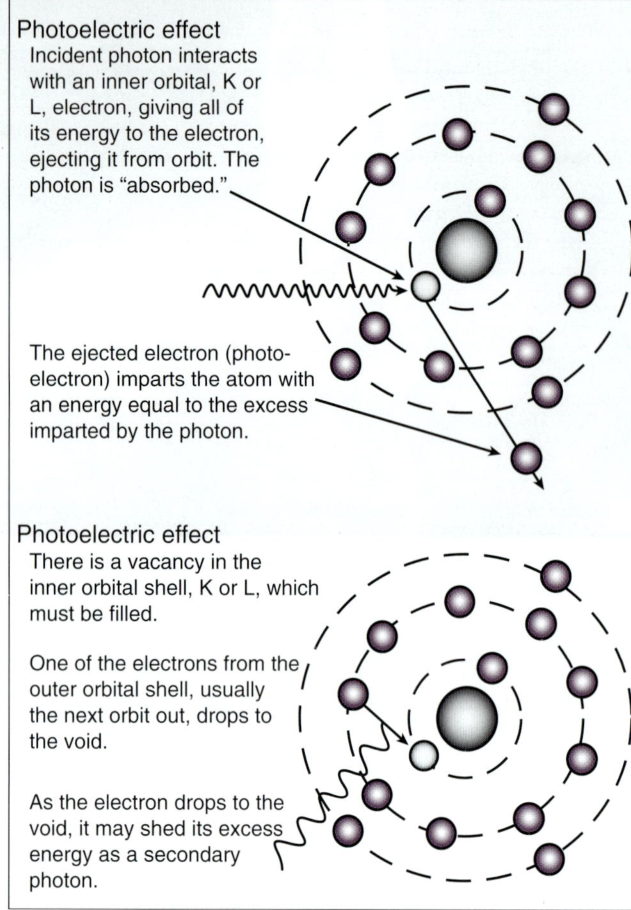

Figure 1.10 Photoelectric effect. (From: Fauber TL, *Radiographic Imaging and Exposure*, fourth ed, 45, Elsevier Mosby, May 2012, USA.)

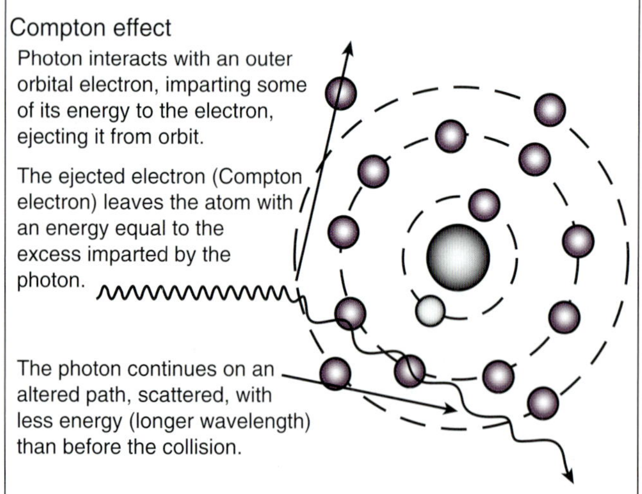

Figure 1.11 Compton scattering. (From: TL Fauber, *Radiographic Imaging and Exposure*, fourth ed, 46, Elsevier Mosby, May 2012, USA.)

- The penetrating power or effective energy of the x-ray beam can be measured by a parameter called the half-value layer (HVL). The HVL is the thickness of the material that attenuates the intensity of x-ray beam by 50% its original value
- The linear attenuation coefficient (μ) is the fraction of incident photons' energy removed from a beam per unit thickness of the attenuating medium

TABLE 1.5 Effect of Material Density, Atomic Number, and Photon Energy on Half-Value Layer and Linear Attenuation Coefficient

Half-Value Layer	Linear Attenuation Coefficient (LAC - μ)
Decreases with density of material	Increases with density of material
Decreases with atomic number of the material	Increases with atomic number of the material
Increases with photon energy of the radiation	Decreases with photon energy of radiation

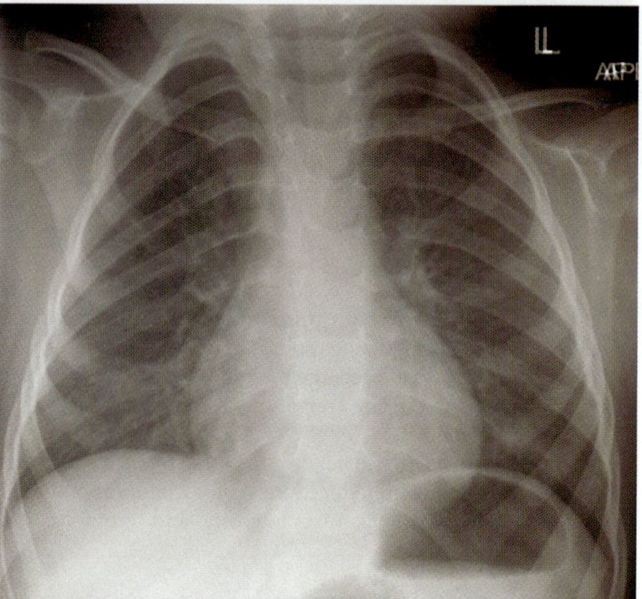

Figure 1.12 Chest radiograph. Bones show higher absorption of x-rays because of higher occurrence of photoelectric absorption and thus appear brighter on the radiograph compared with soft tissue or lung, where more x-rays are transmitted and appear darker on the radiographic image.

- ***Tissue composition***

When an x-ray beam is incident on a patient, it undergoes numerous interactions (absorption and scatter), and only 1% of the beam actually passes through the patient to fall on the receptor. The major interaction that causes absorption of the x-ray beam in the patient is by photoelectric absorption. Thus, the higher the density of the tissue (e.g., bone), the more absorption of the x-rays, and thus no x-rays reach the receptor–film in the region that appears white or **radiopaque** as it is unexposed. Similarly, the incident x-rays that directly fall on the receptor–film without passing through the patient create the darker portion of the image. Tissues that have relatively lesser density (e.g., lungs) allow more incident x-rays to pass through them and reach the receptor; thus, they appear darker, or **radiolucent**, on the image (Fig. 1.12).

Because the *photoelectric effect is directly proportional to the third power of the atomic number*, a small increase in the atomic number increases the probability of photoelectric absorption compared with the Compton effect, which is independent of atomic number. *Compton scattering is the same for higher atomic number structures such as bone (13.8) and lower atomic number structures such as soft tissue (7.4)*

Imaging With X-rays

- ***Determinants of X-ray quality***

Contrast Resolution

Contrast is the ability to distinguish two adjacent structures in an image. A high-contrast image has fewer densities but with greater differences. A low-contrast image has more densities but of fewer differences. For film-screen radiography, the image contrast largely depends on radiographic technique and exposure parameters. For computed radiography (CR) and DR, image contrast can be altered on the console after the image is acquired and is not entirely dependent on exposure factors.

Subject contrast depends on differential attenuation of x-rays in the subject. For example, in an extremity radiograph, the thicker and denser bone attenuates more x-rays compared with adjacent less dense soft tissue, giving excellent subject contrast resolution. The higher the difference in linear attenuation coefficient between tissues, the more contrast.

Effect of kV: An increase in kV (increase energy of the incident beam) reduces attenuation and thus reduces the contrast, since the incident photons are mostly of higher energy causing poor distinction of tissues of with lower densities (see Fig. 1.9).

Spatial Resolution

Spatial resolution is the ability to resolve borders between smaller objects. The sharper the edge displayed, the easier it is to distinguish the object from adjacent structures. The main factors affecting the spatial resolution are geometric unsharpness, magnification or distortion, and subject factors.

1. **Geometric Unsharpness**

There is a loss of detail caused by various factors relating to the geometry of the x-ray beam. *The geometric unsharpness or size of the penumbra depends on the size of the focal spot, object-to-receptor distance, and source-to-receptor distance.*

- The size of the focal spot is one such factor and can also be called the *focal-spot blur.* In practice, the focal spot is never a finite source of x-rays, and it is always of a rectangular shape. Thus, the same object is incident upon rays originating from different areas of the focal spot itself (Fig. 1.13). Because of this, these rays are incident upon the receptor at different points, resulting in some blurring, and this is called the *penumbra* forming the geometric unsharpness or focal spot blur. Image unsharpness caused by this phenomenon increases with the size of the focal spot
- Increasing the distance of the object from the image receptor (OID) reduces the spatial resolution by increasing the penumbra. There is also an increase in the primary and secondary scatter radiation contributing to image unsharpness
- The penumbra reduces as the source-to-image receptor distance (SID) increases, increasing the spatial resolution

2. **Magnification and distortion**

Image magnification should be maintained to minimum in radiography, however for some techniques, magnification is intentional (example magnified views in mammography).

- Magnification of image is the ratio of SID and the source-to-object distance (SOD) or can also be described at image size to object size. Magnification also depends on OID and reduces as the OID decreases (Fig. 1.14)
- Inclination of the object leads to image distortion and can cause magnification or foreshortening of part of the image depending on its position in the central x-ray beam

3. **Subject factors**

The incident x-ray beam is of uniform intensity, and the transmitted beam is of varying intensity when it reaches the receptor because of attenuation in the patient. The patient factors affecting contrast are

A. Object shape: The shape of the object affects the image quality by contributing to absorption blur, especially at the edges. Absorption blur reduces the spatial resolution and the contrast resolution of the structure imaged.

B. Movement blur (unsharpness): Patient movement during exposure can deteriorate the image quality and is a significant source of unsharpness. This can be reduced by using shorter exposure times, patient instructions (breath holding), restraining or immobilizing the patient, reducing the OID, and increasing the SID.

- ***Scatter radiation***

The image is formed by x-rays reaching the detector, which includes both the transmitted rays and scatter rays. The scatter rays are mainly from Compton interactions and form a major component of image formation. The scatter radiation contributes to

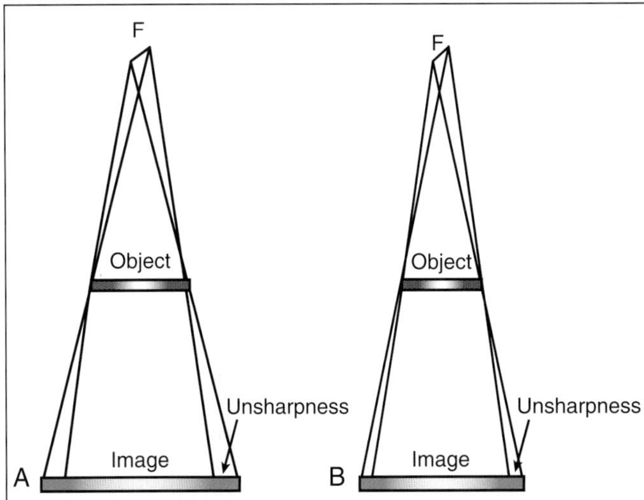

Figure 1.13 Effect of focal spot size on image unsharpness. (A) Larger focal spot size. (B) Smaller focal spot size. Note that the image unsharpness increases with size of the focal spot. (From: TL Fauber, *Radiographic Imaging and Exposure*, fourth ed, 89, Elsevier Mosby, May 2012, USA.)

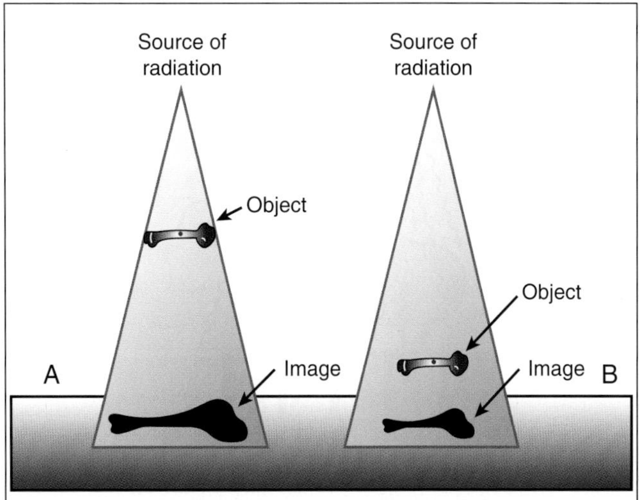

Figure 1.14 Higher magnification when the object is farther form the image (A) compared to lesser margnification when the object is closer to the image (B). (From: TL Fauber, *Radiographic Imaging and Exposure*, fourth ed, 94, Elsevier Mosby, May 2012, USA.)

patient absorbed dose and to radiation received by the staff present in the x-ray room.

The effect of scatter radiation can be reduced by limiting its formation or by preventing scatter to reach the detector.

Limiting formation of scatter radiation

This can be reduced by reducing the patient surface area to be irradiated and can be achieved by

- Using collimation in the form of a light beam diaphragm or cones or cylinders. The light beam diaphragm is integrated with the x-ray tube system in all modern equipment. Cones and cylinders are additional collimation devices that can be attached to the x-ray tube to limit the field of exposure and to image specific areas of interest (e.g., the coned view of the lumbosacral junction as part of a series of spine imaging in adults)
- Tissue compression reduces the thickness and helps in reducing scatter as well as patient dose

Limiting scatter from reaching the detector

Scatter reaching the detector can be reduced by using the use of grids or by using the air-gap technique.

Secondary radiation grid

A grid is a device placed between the patient and the image receptor to prevent scatter radiation from reaching the receptor, which reduces the scatter by 90%, thus improving image contrast (Fig. 1.15). Grids were first developed by Gustave Bucky in 1913, and 7 years later Hollis Potter developed the moving grid. Therefore, today the moving grids are called *Potter-Bucky grids*.

Grids are made of strips of high atomic number material (usually lead of 0.05–0.07mm width) sandwiched between thicker strips of low atomic number material (usually a low atomic number material, such as carbon fiber).

Only the rays passing straight through the interspace material reach the detector, and those passing obliquely are absorbed by the lead grid strips. *The transmitted incident rays usually pass the interspace material and contribute to image formation.* The scatter radiation is usually at an angle and gets absorbed by the lead strips; however, if the angle of scatter is small, it can match the angle of acceptance of the grid and can reach the image receptor, contributing to noise.

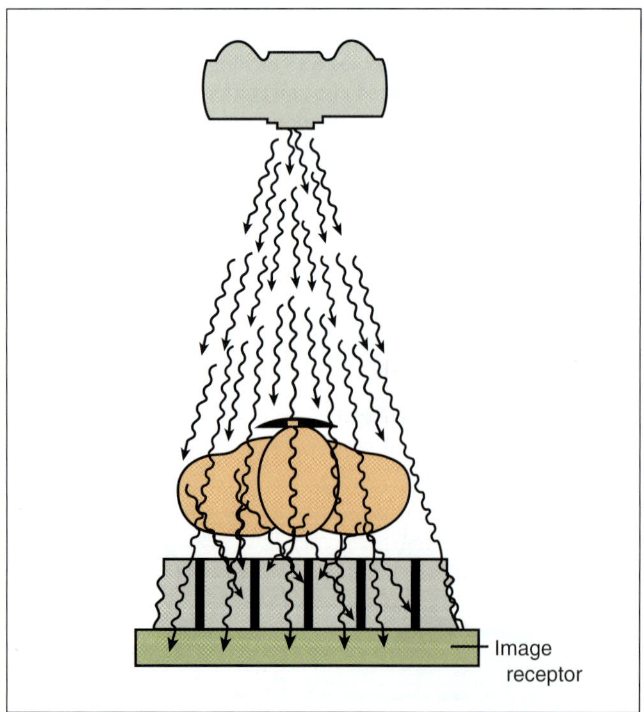

Figure 1.15 The grid interposed between the patient and the receptor absorbs about 90% of scatter radiation. (From: SC Bushong, Scatter radiation. In: *Radiologic Science for Technologists*, eleventh ed, 195, Elsevier, 2017, Canada.)

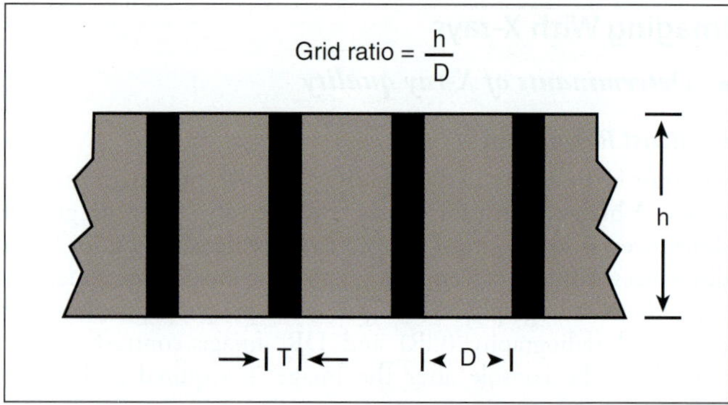

Figure 1.16 Grid ratio. *D*, thickness of the interspace material; *h*, height of the strip; *T*, thickness of the lead strip. (From: SC Bushong, Scatter radiation. In: *Radiologic Science for Technologists*, eleventh ed, 195, Elsevier, 2017, Canada.)

Grid ratio: This is an important parameter that describes the attenuation capacity of the grid. It is defined as a ratio of the height (h) of the lead strips to the width (D) between them (Fig. 1.16).

The higher the grid ratio, the better the ability to remove scatter, and it improves image contrast. But this also increases the radiation dose to the patient because it requires increasing the energy of the x-ray beam to achieve adequate exposure of the image detector.

Contrast improvement factor: This is used to calculate grid performance.

$$\text{Contrast improvement factor (K)} = \frac{\text{Radiographic contrast with grid}}{\text{Radiographic contrast without grid}}$$

A contrast improvement factor (K) of 1 indicates no improvement. Grids in use generally have K values in the range of 1.5 to 3 (usually double the contrast); this is higher for high-ratio grids.

Bucky factor: Increasing the grid ratio reduces the total amount of radiation reaching the image detector and thus can affect the image quality. To compensate, the radiation energy has to be increased, which also increases the patient dose. This increased dose to the patient can be calculated by the Bucky factor, which is a ratio of

$$\text{Bucky factor (B)} = \frac{\text{Number of x-rays incident on the grid}}{\text{Number of x-rays transmitted by the grid}} = \frac{\text{Patient dose with grid}}{\text{Patient dose without grid}}$$

The Bucky factor (patient dose) increases with an increase in grid ratio and with an increase in kVp.

Grid factor: Using a grid necessitates increasing mAs and thus increases the patient exposure. This can be measured by a parameter called the *grid factor*, which is measured as

$$\text{Grid factor} = \frac{\text{Exposure necessary with grid}}{\text{Exposure necessary without grid}}$$

The grid factor is generally in the range of 3 to 5, and this shows how much the exposure and patient dose increase because

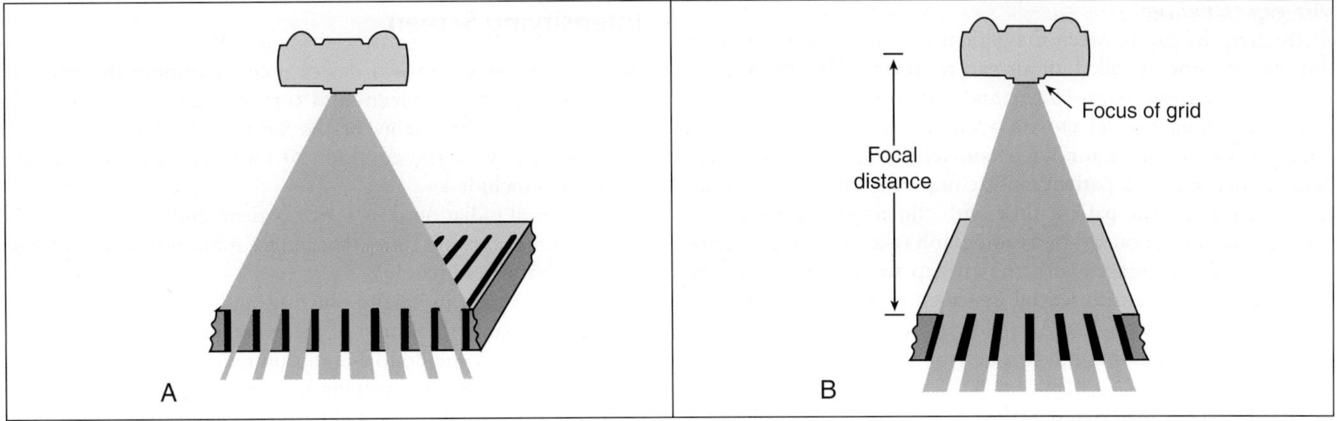

Figure 1.17 A. parallel unfocused grid (A) and a focused grid with tilted lead strips (B). (From: SC Bushong, Scatter radiation. In: *Radiologic Science for Technologists*, eleventh ed, 198, 200, Elsevier, 2017, Canada.)

of the grid. It depends on the thickness of patient, grid ratio, and the kV used.

Focused and unfocused grids

Grids with parallel orientation of the lead strips are call unfocused grids, and they tend to absorb some of the useful transmitted radiation because of divergent nature of the x-ray beams that travel obliquely at the periphery of the image (Fig. 1.17A). To counter this, focused grids were developed in which the lead strips are tilted at an angle from the center to the periphery to align toward the tube focus (Fig. 1.17B).

Moving grid

The grid can sometimes be seen on the radiographic image as grid lines. This can be negated by moving the grid at the time of exposure. Most of the newer equipment has moving grids to counter image artifacts caused by grid lines. Sometimes motion blur can occur because of the moving mechanism of the grid, but this outweighs the obvious benefits of the moving grid.

Grid cut-off

Numerous factors should be considered while using grids, and failure to follow the steps correctly can cause significant image quality compromise (Fig. 1.18). The tube needs to be at a specified distance and well centered for focused grids. The focused grid cannot be placed upside down, or the direction of its movement cannot be changed; this will lead to cut-off of the primary beam and thus significant artifacts on the image, prompting repeat imaging.

Practical aspects of using a grid

Grid greatly improves image quality by reducing scatter radiation reaching the image receptor but has a major disadvantage of necessitating an increase in patient dose.

- Grid is generally used for imaging thick body sections (e.g., the chest or abdomen) and when higher than 60 kVp is used
- For general radiology, a grid with ratio of 10:1 or 12:1 works well in balancing the patient dose and image quality
- For mammography and mobile radiography, a lower grid ratio is used
- A moving grid is part of the Bucky setup and is preferable and commonly used for body radiographs
- Stationary grids can cause artifacts on the image, appearing as grid lines, and are generally used for mobile radiography when a moving grid setup is not possible
- Moving grids are generally focused grids, and parallel or unfocused grids are used for mobile imaging and fluoroscopy

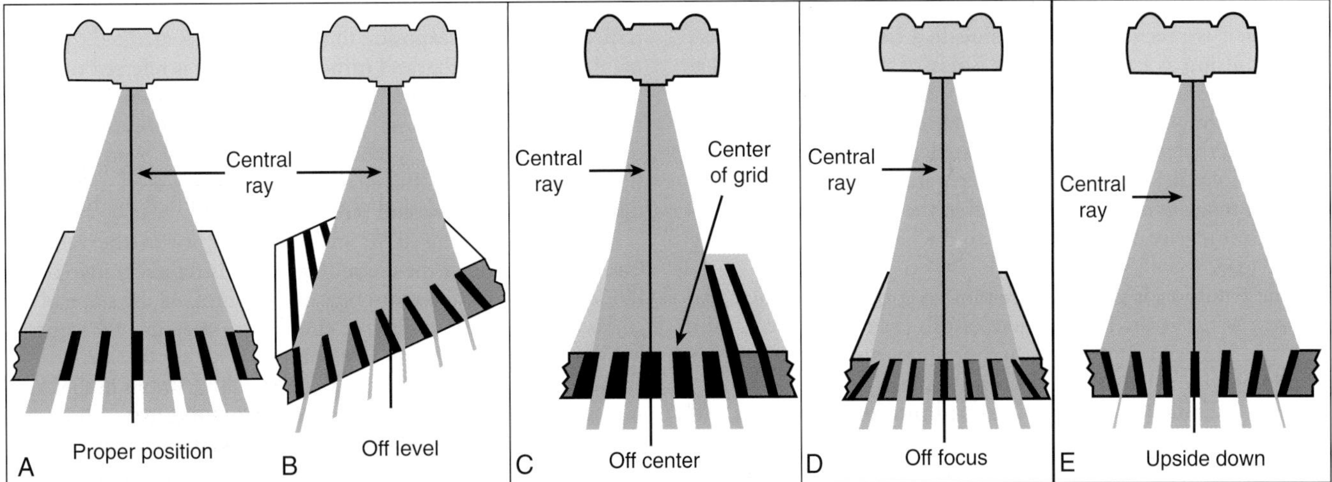

Figure 1.18 (A) Proper position of the focused grid well oriented to the focus. (B) Off-level grid. The grid is not perpendicular to the central axis (grid cut-off across the image; this is an underexposed, light image). (C) Off-center grid. This is a focused grid positioned off center (grid cut-off across the image; this is an underexposed, light image). (D) Off-focus grid (focused grid is not positioned at the focal distance required; grid cut-off toward the edge of the image). (E) Upside-down grid (severe grid cut-off toward the edge of the image). (From: SC Bushong, Scatter radiation. In: *Radiologic Science for Technologists*, eleventh ed, 202, Elsevier, 2017, Canada.)

Air-gap technique

Increasing the gap between the patient and detector without an interposing grid is called an air-gap technique. The distance is increased by about 10 to 15 cm, and this reduces the amount of scatter reaching the detector to a similar extent to that with a grid. However, the scanning parameters have to be changed, which increases the patient dose compared with a technique without a grid. The patient dose with the air-gap technique is similar to the dose caused by a radiograph taken with grid. There are a few disadvantages with the air-gap technique, including image magnification caused by increased distance (similar to a shadow cast against light). Also, air-gap technique causes some geometric blur affecting image quality.

Film-screen Radiography

Film radiography and film-screen radiography were used to capture the radiographic image for decades since the use of x-rays in medicine. Similar to the impact of digitization in photography, the use of both has drastically reduced globally with digital capture of the radiographic image almost completely replacing this technique. It will be described here briefly because it lays the foundation of currently used digital techniques in radiography.

Radiographic Film

The radiographic film is the photographic receptor used to decode the information carried by the attenuated x-ray beam, serving as the primary medium to convert the invisible radiation to an image. The radiographic film is 150 to 300 μm thick and is composed of three layers: the *base*, the *emulsion*, and the *supercoat* [3].

The *base* is a thick, translucent layer made up of *polyester*, which serves as the foundation of the radiographic film, with an intrinsic property to maintain its shape without distortion, referred to as *dimensional stability*. The *emulsion* is the most important part of the film interacting with the x-rays, contributing to the latent image formation. It is a 3- to 5-μm-thick layer composed of *silver halide crystals* dispersed in a gelatin base. The halide is 90% to 99% silver bromide (AgBr) and 1% to 10% silver iodide (AgI), forming silver iodo-bromide crystal, which is precipitated and emulsified in the crystal lattice. The emulsion is coated on both sides of the base and called *double-emulsion film* (most common). However, in a few cases such as mammography, the emulsion is coated only on one side to reduce the parallax effects, referred to as a *single-emulsion film*. The emulsion and base are separated by a thin material, referred to as *subbing or adhesive layer*, that ensures proper contact and integrity of the emulsion to the base during processing of the film.

The emulsion is covered by a thin layer of gelatin called the *overcoat or supercoat*. The functions of this layer are to protect the sensitive emulsion from scratches, pressure, and contamination and to provide suitable surface characteristics.

Radiographic films can be classified into *direct exposure* and *indirect exposure* films based on their use without or with an intensifying screen, respectively. The direct exposure films need higher exposure doses. These are mainly used for dental, extremity, and orbital radiography. The indirect exposure film (most common) is used with an intensifying screen, wherein the emulsion interacts with visible light as described in the next section.

Intensifying Screen

An intensifying screen is a device used to amplify the effect of x-rays that reach the screen–film combination. The intensifying screen converts the energy of the x-rays to visible light, which then interacts with the emulsion to form the latent image. The advantages include a

1. reduced radiation dose to the patient, and
2. shorter exposure times that reduce motion-related artifacts.

The disadvantages include

1. higher image noise and blurring, and
2. lower spatial resolution of the resultant image.

In usual practice, the double-emulsion radiographic film is sandwiched between two intensifying screens, so that the emulsion on each side is exposed to the light from its respective screen. This entire system is enclosed in a *cassette*. The intensifying screen is made up of four layers: the *base, reflective layer, protective coating*, and the heart of the intensifying screen, which is the radiographically active layer of *phosphor*.

- The *base* is the made up of an approximately 1-mm-thick layer of polyester, providing mechanical support to the active phosphor
- The *reflective layer* lies between the phosphor and the base, made up of magnesium oxide or titanium dioxide, which demonstrates isotropic emission. Isotropic Emission refers to the property of these compounds to emit light produced by the interaction of x-rays with the phosphor with equal intensity in all directions and in turn increases the efficiency of the screen–film combination
- The *protective coating* is the thin outermost transparent plastic layer of the intensifying screen, which is closest to the radiographic film. The *most important layer* of the intensifying screen is the *phosphor*, which converts the x-ray beam to light; this process is called luminescence. Originally, crystalline *calcium tungstate* ($CaWO_4$) was used as the phosphor layer, which was then replaced by *rare earth elements* such as gadolinium, lanthanum, and yttrium, which have discrete emissions near the green-yellow region and provide a higher efficiency, faster speed, and lower patient dose

Characteristic Curve

The characteristic curve is a measure of the optical density with respect to the x-ray exposure to the film. This is credited to Ferdinand Hurter and Charles Driffield and hence is referred to as the H & D curve. The characteristic curve is a graphical representation of the film's response to light and is made by plotting the optical density on the *y*-axis against the log of exposure given (log-E) on the *x*-axis. The characteristic curve is used to compare different types of films and screens.

Radiographic films have an optical density in the range of 0 to 4. The shape of the curve (Fig. 1.19) is representative of the film response to a different range of exposures. As the slope of the curve decreases, the ability of the film to measure the contrast between different exposures decreases.

At low and high radiation exposures, high variations in the exposure result in only a small change in the optical density. These portions of the curve are referred to as the toe and shoulder, respectively. The toe portion begins at the threshold and continues to the straight-line portion. It includes the base and fog density, usually up to 0.2. The point at which the curve just begins to turn up is called the threshold. It represents the first response of the material to radiation. At the middle part, or the straight line or linear portion, there is a linear relationship between density and log-exposure (log-E) of

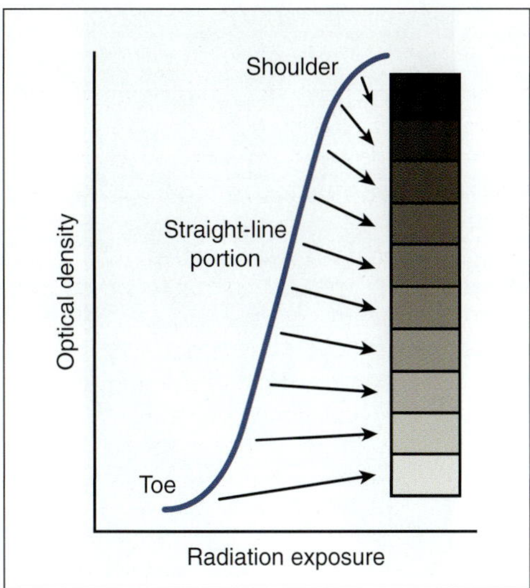

Figure 1.19 Characteristic curve showing the graphical relationship between optical density and radiation exposure. (From: SC Bushong, Scatter radiation. In: *Radiologic Science for Technologists*, eleventh ed, 312, Elsevier, 2017, Canada.)

the curve. Hence, any small changes in exposure lead to large changes in the optical density. Exposure in this area results in the best image contrast. The shoulder refers to the portion beyond the linear curve. With increasing exposure, the rate of density increase gradually declines until the maximum density is reached; beyond this point, exposure variability cannot be recorded. This maximum density is referred to as Dmax. It depends on the amount of silver halide coating and processing conditions.

The latitude is the range of exposure required to have an acceptable image. As a general rule, films with higher latitudes make the exposure less critical.

Factors determining quality of intensifying screen

The most important properties of the intensifying screen include the screen speed, intensification factor, spatial resolution, and image blur.

1. ***Screen speed***

The efficiency of the intensifying screen to convert x-rays to visible light is measured by the screen efficiency. The following properties determine the speed of the intensifying screen:

a. Phosphor material: The calcium tungstate screens are considered the reference and assigned a value of 100. The rare earth screens having higher efficiency have speeds up to 1200.

b. Thickness of phosphor layer: The higher the thickness, the higher the detective quantum efficiency and the higher the speed.

c. Reflective layer: The presence of a reflective layer increases the screen speed.

d. Crystal size: The larger individual phosphor crystals produce more light per x-ray interaction and increase the speed.

e. Concentration of phosphor crystals: A higher crystal concentration increases the screen speed.

2. ***Dyes:*** Light-absorbing dyes are added to films to control (reduce) the speed of light and improve spatial resolution.

Intensification factor

The intensification factor is defined as the ratio of the exposure required to produce the same density on a film with and without the screen.

3. ***Image noise***

An intensifying screen has many advantages, as described, but one of the major disadvantages is its contribution to the image noise and reduction of image contrast. It is higher in fast screens and high-kVp techniques. *An important concept contributing to image noise is light crossover wherein* light emitted from an intensifying screen exposes not only the adjacent film emulsion but also crosses over to the emulsion on the other side of the base.

4. ***Spatial resolution***

Another disadvantage that may be attributed to the intensifying screens is of lower spatial resolution when compared with direct-exposure radiographs. Spatial resolution is represented by the number of line pairs per millimeter (lp/mm) that may be imaged.

Operational Problems With Intensifying Screens

The intensifying screen has to be handled with utmost care because even the slightest of damage, especially from fingernails, can produce artifacts and degrade the resultant image. Dirty or damaged screens cause white spots on the image. Poor screen contact, which may be caused by worn-out contact felt, loose or broken hinges, or warped screen, results in areas of cloudy images.

Processing of Film

Production of the Latent Image

The first step in processing the film is production of latent image by the interaction of image-forming x-rays exiting the patient with the intensifying screen–film combination. During exposure of the film, photoelectrons are formed by the interaction of light photons with the bromide ions. The emulsion, as discussed previously, has various defects and impurities that provide it a crystal lattice referred to as point defects or Frankel defects, which attract these photoelectrons. The electron at the point defect then attracts a positively charged silver ion and neutralizes it to form a silver atom. This phenomenon is repeated many times over, and the result is an area of the crystal with several neutral silver atoms on the surface, which constitutes the latent image. For the latent image to be developable, 4 to 10 silver atoms must be collected at a point defect.

Development of the Latent Image

The following steps are performed for the development of the latent image. The steps are performed either in an automatic processor, which takes around 90 seconds, or the older manual processing done previously in which each film took around 10 to 15 minutes to be processed. The latent image is converted to a visible image by a reducing alkaline agent, most commonly consisting of phenidone and hydroquinone, wherein the crystals with a latent image in them allow the rest of the silver ions form a dark silver grain speck on the film while they remain crystalline and inactive. The developer contains alkali compounds such as sodium carbonate and sodium hydroxide that act as buffering agents and control the pH of the solution. Potassium bromide and potassium iodide are added as restrainers, which allow only the crystals with the latent image to be processed.

If the developing agent is too strong or the developing temperature is too high, it will develop the crystals in which no latent image is present and produces a low level of blackening called *fog*.

Fixation

After development, the film is fixed and hardened in a weakly acid solution, most commonly made of acetic acid, usually referred to as activator, which neutralizes the pH of the emulsion and stops developer action. Sodium or ammonium thiosulfate, referred to as hypo, is used as a fixing agent to remove undeveloped silver halide crystals from the emulsion. An artifact, that results from the use of the fixer is referred to as *hyporetention*, wherein fixer is retained within the emulsion, which combines with silver to form silver sulfide, which appears as yellow-brown stains.

The fixer also contains a hardener, which causes the emulsion to shrink and become more rigid. The chemicals commonly used are potassium alum, aluminum chloride, and chromium alum.

Washing and Drying

Vigorous washing of the film to remove all the chemicals from the previous step is performed. Finally, the film is dried to make it acceptable for viewing and reporting.

Screen-film Radiographic Artifacts

Artifacts are undesirable optical densities or blemishes on a medical image that may cause wrongful interpretation. These may be classified into

1. Exposure-related artifacts

   Improper screen–film matching or contact results in obscuration of the images. Patient movement can lead to blur (Fig. 1.20), and reusage of casettes lead to double exposure. These are among the most common causes of reexaminations.

2. Processing and handling artifacts

   Most of these artifacts are noted because of the defective parts of the processors. Fogging or "pi lines" (Fig. 1.21) can be seen because of stains in the rollers. Inadequate or excessive usage of chemical scan result in chemical fogging referred to as dichroic stain and curtain effect, respectively. Improper temperature or humidity can also lead to improper exposure.

Digital Radiography

Significant developments in computer technology have resulted in conventional screen-film radiography systems being replaced by DR systems, which are now the standard of care all over the world. DR is defined as the technique by which digital detectors are used to capture information produced by the interaction of x-ray photons with an object. The images are produced in a digital format that can be stored and processed on a computer. There are two types of DR systems classified based on the type of detector used: CR and direct or indirect DR.

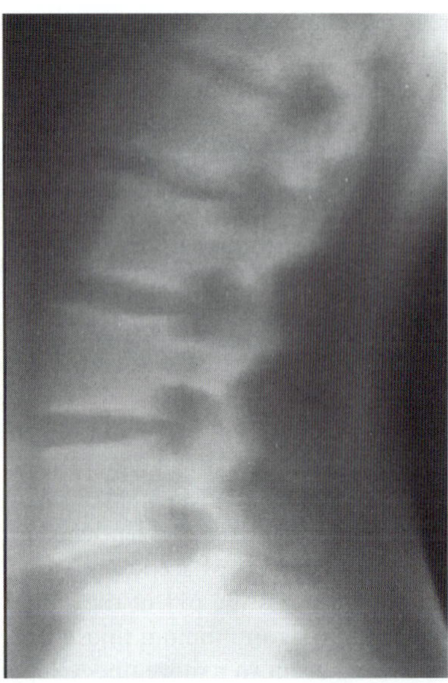

Figure 1.20 Lateral radiograph of lumbar spine shows blurring artifact caused by patient movement.

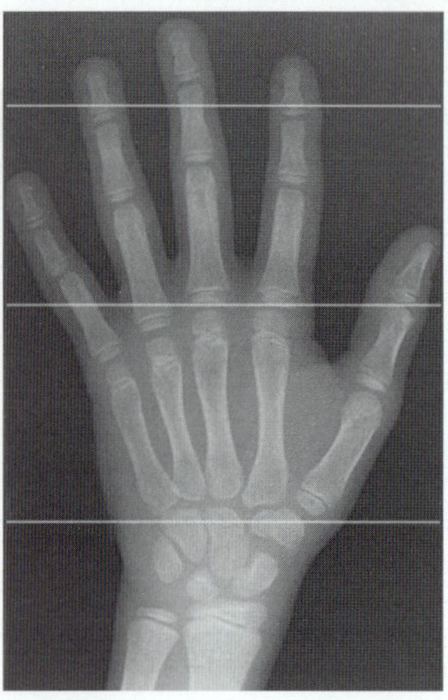

Figure 1.21 Pi lines. These are linear lines in the uniform gap in a radiograph of the hand caused by a stain in the roller.

Computed Radiography

Computed radiography uses *photostimulable phosphors (PSPs)* to capture a latent image on the imaging plate (IP). When the emission of light is delayed, allowing x-ray energy to be temporarily stored in a phosphor screen to be read-out later, it is called *phosphorescence*.

Image Receptor

The image receptor of CR, referred to as PSP, is composed of *barium fluoro-halide activated with divalent europium* (BaFX: Eu2+ in which the halide X is typically bromine or iodine) embedded in a polymer binder with a protective overcoat (Fig. 1.22). There is a black reflective layer that sends the light in a forward direction, preventing scatter of stimulating and emitted light.

- Interaction of PSP with x-ray photons results in the excitation of electrons into a metastable state. With the addition of europium, the PSP crystals develop a tiny defect called metastable sites of F centers (derived from German *Farbzentren*, or color centers). These F centers can trap the electrons for a longer time

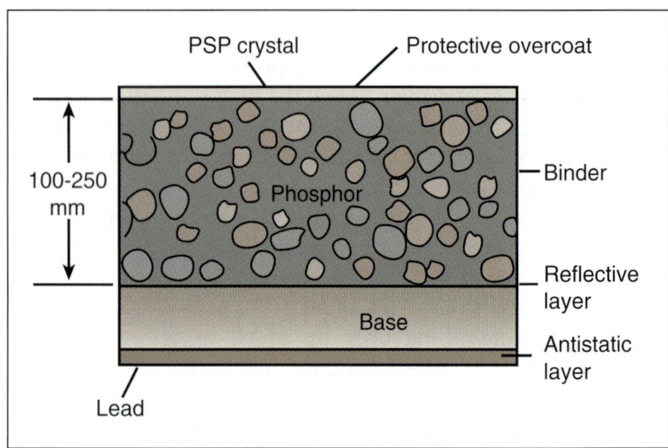

Figure 1.22 Parts of an Imaging plate in computed radiography. The image receptor is composed of barium fluorohalides activated with divalent europium embedded in a polymer binder with a protective overcoat and a reflective layer that prevents scatter of light. *PSP*, photostimulable phosphor. (From: SC Bushong, Scatter radiation. In: *Radiologic Science for Technologists*, eleventh ed, 285, Elsevier, 2017, Canada.)

- During reading out of the image, a red laser scans and exposes the IP. The photon energy of the red laser light is absorbed by the trapped electrons, which return to their ground state
- During this deexcitation, energy is released in the form of blue-green light. The intensity of the blue-green light is recorded and converted to a pixel value

The *spatial resolution* is determined by the phosphor layer thickness, diameter of the readout laser beam, and the pixel size. In contrast to film-screen radiography, which has a spatial resolution of approximately 10 lp/mm, CR has a lower spatial resolution of 2.5 to 5 lp/mm.

Computed Radiography Reader

A CR reader is a compact mechanical, optical, and computer assembly with drive mechanisms that automatically transport the IP through different processes. The time taken for scanning an IP is approximately 40 to 90 seconds depending on the PSP size, resolution desired, and dual- or single-side readout. The modern CR systems that use line scanning techniques can reduce the image readout time to as low as 20 seconds.

Image formation: The sequence of events in producing an image with CR begins with the interaction of x-ray photons with the IP.

1. *Latent image formation*

X-ray photons are absorbed by the phosphor, resulting in the excitation of electrons in a metastable state. The electrons become temporarily trapped at specific sites throughout the layer of phosphor crystals producing the latent image

2. *Stimulation with laser*

The IP is scanned with a finely focused beam of red laser. The diameter of this laser beam is an important determinant of the spatial resolution of the image. The smaller the diameter, the higher the spatial resolution.

3. *Detection of the emitted light*

Upon stimulation with a laser beam, the electrons return to the ground state with the emission of a shorter wavelength light in the blue region of the visible spectrum. The light photons are directed through a light-channeling guide onto a photocathode layer on the input side of a photomultiplier tube, which amplifies the signal from the light photons. The sampling rate of this emitted light also determines the spatial resolution of the image. The output is an analog signal that is converted digitally into an electrical signal by an analog-to-digital converter (ADC) and used to form an image that is transmitted to a computer system and transferred to a workstation for interpretation.

A picture element or pixel is a quantized value and represents the smallest area in the digital image. The CR image consists of multiple rows and columns of pixels representing at different locations.

4. *Erasing imaging plate*

To reuse an IP, all the residual excited metastable electrons need to be removed. If the residual latent image remains, it will lead to ghosting on subsequent use. This is done by flooding the PSP with very intense white light.

Recent developments in computed radiography

- **Dual-sided reading:** The CR reader is equipped with two sets of detectors that can detect and capture light from the PSP upon stimulation with a laser beam. This results in a higher signal-to-noise ratio (SNR) in these systems.
- **Solid-state semiconductor laser diodes:** These are more durable than the helium–neon gas lasers, resulting in longer shelf lives of the equipment.
- **Line scan reader:** These have a laser line source with a shaping lens that refine the beam into a fine line rather than a point fed to a charged-coupled device (CCD) photodetector array, resulting in an increased speed of processing.

Advantages of computed radiography

1. *Improved contrast resolution:* The PSP receptors in CR have an excellent linear optical density response to the intensity of x-ray, in contrast to the classic sigmoid-shaped curve of the conventional film-screen combination. The CR therefore produces good contrast over a much wider range of exposures.
2. *Dose reduction:* The wide latitude allows low radiation exposure without a drop in quality.
3. *Repeat rate reduction:* The wide dynamic range leads to reduced rates of failed x-ray exposure.
4. *Compatible with a conventional X-ray imaging system:* It can be retrofitted and used in existing x-ray systems.
5. Use in *picture archiving and communications system:* This is the biggest advantage of all forms of digital imaging over conventional film-screen radiography.

Disadvantages of computed radiography

1. *It is a time-consuming* technique because of the handling, transporting, and loading of individual IPs in the reader.
2. *Loss of latent image* happens immediately and decays with time, making it a time-bound technique.
3. *It has a lower spatial resolution* than film-screen radiography.
4. Separate read-out electronics contribute to *noise*.

Digital Radiography

Digital radiography is the technique of converting x-ray into electrical charges using combined image capture and image readout process followed by analog-to-digital conversion to produce a final digital radiograph. Unlike CR, there is no handling and processing of a cassette because the image is produced directly from the image detector and displayed on screen in a matter of seconds. This may be done by direct or indirect means.

1. Indirect DR

Indirect conversion is a two-step process for x-ray detection using scintillators that convert x-ray energy to visible light. The visible light is then converted into an electric charge using photodetectors. Thallium-doped cesium iodide (CsI) is the most commonly used phosphor material as the scintillator. Another material that some systems use is gadolinium oxysulfide or Gadox (Gd_2O_2S), which has an amorphous structure that results in the spread of light produced by x-ray absorption, leading to a poorer spatial resolution

Indirect digital radiography

X-ray → Scintillator → Stored electrons → Light photons → Photodiode → Charge → ADC

2. Direct DR

Direct-conversion is a single-step process, wherein photoconductors directly convert x-ray photons into an electric charge (Fig. 1.23).

Direct digital radiography

X-ray → Photoconductor → Charge → ADC

The photoconductor materials used commonly include amorphous selenium (a-Se) and lead iodide. A-Se is most

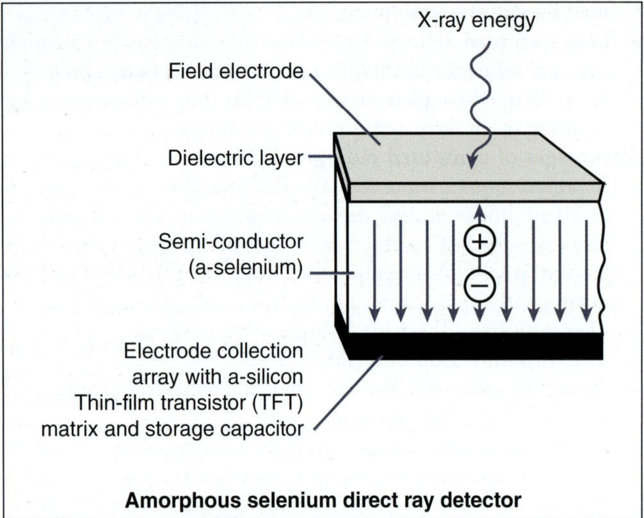

Figure 1.23 The image acquisition process of a direct capture digital radiography system. *TFT*, thin-film transistor. (From: C Carter, *Introduction to Digital Radiography and PACS*, first ed, Mosby Elsevier, 2007, Canada.)

commonly used because of its excellent x-ray detection and high intrinsic spatial resolution. Because selenium has a relatively low atomic number, which results in less x-ray absorption in the general radiography kV range, the K-edge of selenium is better suited for the diagnostic kV range used in mammography.

The readout can be done by two systems: a *selenium drum* or a *thin film transistor array*. The readout is by gating each row of thin-film transistor (TFT) switches, corresponding to 1 pixel, similar to indirect DR. The resulting electrical signal is then digitized and transferred to the system computer.

Postprocessing

Following the readout of the image in direct and indirect DR, the image data will be processed before display, and this forms the most influential final step that reflects the way a radiologist sees the end product. Postprocessing, in general, improves the image quality by optimizing contrast, reducing image noise and technical artifacts. The factor that cannot be adjusted by postprocessing is spatial resolution.

- A technique called *low-pass spatial filtering* is performed, by which a weighted average of grayscale value is stored in each pixel and the value of the neighboring pixels is generated to remove image noise. The effect smoothens the final image; however, it blurs small details or edges
- Another filter called *high-pass edge enhancement* does the opposite by adding a proportion of the difference in grayscale values between neighboring pixels to heighten the contrast resolution

Recent Developments in Digital Radiography

- **Mobile DR:** A portable DR system, allowing imaging of critical patients, is performed most commonly with a mobile 17- × 14-inch flat-panel detector (FPD)
- **Wireless DR systems:** A wireless portable DR system can transfer image data wirelessly to the monitor. This has the advantage that the cables do not interfere with surrounding machines, allowing radiography of difficult regions of the body such as trauma settings or limbs with limited mobility, axilla, the temporomandibular joint, etc.
- **Image stitching:** Automatic image reconstruction is possible after multiple sequential exposures, which is especially useful for whole-spine imaging and scannogram
- **Dual-energy imaging:** Separate generation of bones and soft tissue structures from two exposures with different kilo voltage techniques. Finds application in better characterization of pulmonary nodules, calcified pleural plaques, coronary artery calcification, etc.
- **Tomosynthesis:** Multiple low-dose exposures at various angles are taken during an arc motion of the x-ray tube with a stationary detector. Using pixel shift, many projections are created after adding these low-dose images. It is now used predominantly for mammography. It is also used for better delineation of bronchiectasis in cases of cystic fibrosis
- **Computer-aided diagnosis:** This is a useful tool that marks suspicious areas for review by the radiologist, preventing overlooking significant findings

Image Quality Determinants of Digital Radiography

The major determinants of the image quality are as follows:

1. **Spatial resolution**

Spatial resolution in DR determined by the focal spot size and pixel size. Spatial resolution is inversely proportional to the pixel size. The pixel is expressed in length and width. It is represented as line pairs per millimeters.

2. **Contrast resolution**

Contrast resolution is the measure of grayscale differentiation in an image measured dynamic range. Dynamic range, or the bit depth, is the number of possible grey shades an image can reproduce. Digital imaging systems have much better contrast resolution than conventional screen-film radiography. In digital detectors, a wide and linear dynamic range is seen, with four to five orders of magnitude. The other major advantage of digital imaging is the ability of postprocessing that allows us to exploit the complete dynamic range by windowing.

3. **Modulation transfer function**

Modulation transfer function (MTF) measures the ability of a system to modulate input signal. It takes into account both the spatial and contrast resolution. The ideal imaging system with an MTF of 1 would produce an image that appears exactly like the object.

4. **Detective quantum efficiency (DQE)**

Detective quantum efficiency (DQE) is a measure of the efficiency of x-ray absorption and represents the probability that an x-ray will interact with the image receptor. It is calculated by measuring the SNR at the detector output. It is primarily determined by the absorption coefficient of the compound in the image receptor. The DQE of DR is higher than the film-screen radiography, which contributes to a lower patient dose in the former (Fig. 1.24).

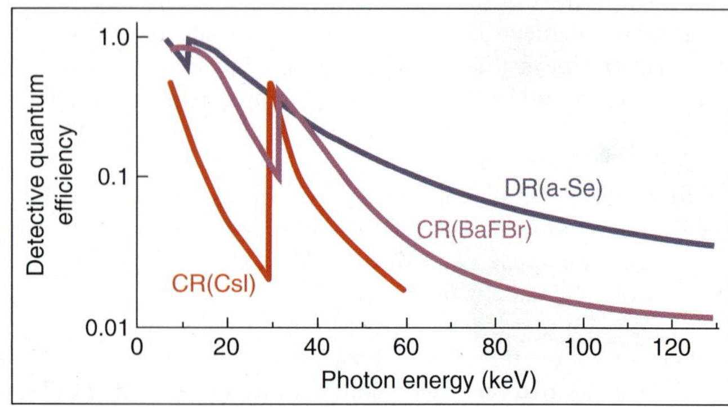

Figure 1.24 Detective quantum efficiency as a function of x-ray energy for various image receptors in computed radiography (CR) and digital radiography (DR). (From: SC Bushong, Scatter radiation. In: *Radiologic Science for Technologists*, eleventh ed, 319, Elsevier, 2017, Canada.)

Digital Radiography Artifacts

These may be classified into the following:

1. *Patient-related factors.*

Patient motion and improper positioning leading to artifacts are common to screen-film and DR. Because the IP is very sensitive to scatter radiation, primary beam collimation is of utmost important. If the image collimation is not parallel to the IP, it hampers the image quality.

2. *Image receptor–related factors.*

These are usually encountered in CR wherein incomplete erasure of the IPs results in overwriting and ghost artifacts (Fig. 1.25). Cracks resulting from aging of the IP also produce superimposed focal artifactual opacities.

3. *Software-related factors.*

Artifacts associated with image transmission errors can be caused by either communication errors or data cable malfunctioning, which will result in corrupted or incomplete images.

Fluoroscopy

Technique of Fluoroscopy

Whereas general radiography provides single, discrete images, fluoroscopy provides real-time dynamic viewing of anatomic structures. Thus, fluoroscopy is used for examination of moving internal structures and fluids.

Fluoroscopy is used for various diagnostic and interventional procedures.

I. General fluoroscopy room
   A. Any barium study such as barium swallow and upper gastrointestinal (GI) series.
   B. Iodinated studies such as hysterosalpingography and urology procedures such as micturating cystourethrography.
II. Interventional radiology.
III. Operating room (OR): during procedures for alignment of bones, surgical fixation, etc.

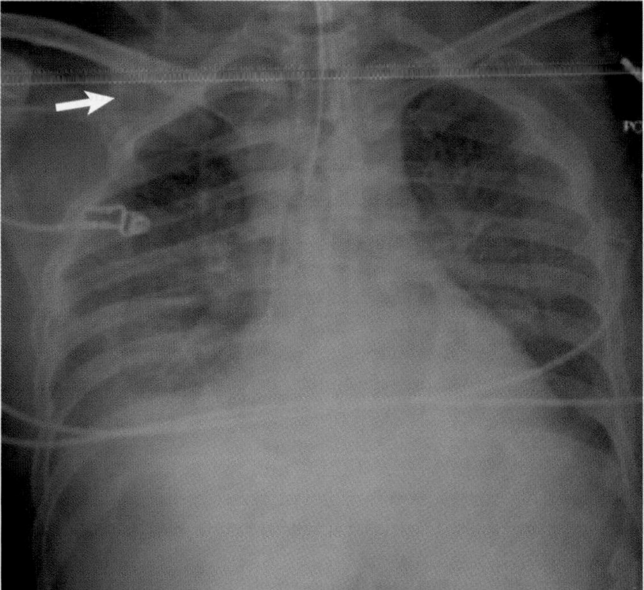

Figure 1.25 Ghost artifact. Incomplete erasure of the image from the previous exposure (*arrow*) in a chest radiograph leads to a double image. The pelvic bones from a prior exposure can be seen superimposed on the heart and upper abdomen.

Types of equipment [4]

I. *Radiography/fluoroscopy (R/F) units with under-table x-ray tubes*: The x-ray tube and collimator are mounted below the table. The image intensifier tower is mounted above the table on a carriage that can be panned over the patient.
II. *R/F units with over-table x-ray tube*: Radiography can be performed with the same x-ray tube and Bucky.
III. *Fixed C-arm positioners:* These are ceiling- or floor-mounted models. There is a floating tabletop that allows for easy patient movement.
IV. *Biplane system (two C-arm units)*: One is floor mounted, and the other is ceiling mounted. One of the two or both can be used during the examination. It carries the advantage of the ability to see two projections without delay because of C-arm movement. It is used in dedicated cardiac, neuroangiography, and interventional radiology suites.
V. *Mobile C-arm positioners*: These are useful during orthopedic and vascular surgical procedures in the OR.

Fluoroscopic Imaging Chain [4]

A typical fluoroscopic imaging chain consists of a generator, x-ray tube, collimator, filter, grid, image intensifier, and video camera system. In modern fluoroscopy systems, FPDs are replacing the image intensifier.

Fluoroscopy can be performed in a continuous manner or can be pulsed. *The advantages of pulsed fluoroscopy are improved temporal resolution (which reduces motion blur) and reduced radiation dose.* The disadvantages of pulsed fluoroscopy include an increase in noise perception, flicker effect, and reduced visibility of fine catheters and guidewires.

Fluoroscopic Detector Systems

Fluoroscope was invented by Thomas Edison in 1898 [5]. In the original fluoroscope, a fluorescent screen was placed in the x-ray beam directly above the patient. The radiologist had to stare directly into the screen, and a dark room was required because the image was dim. The image intensifier was developed in the 1950s and eliminated the need for a dark room and allowed cone vision to be used for image visualization. Fluoroscopic images are now viewed on a television or flat-panel monitor.

Image Intensifier–based Fluoroscopy Systems (Fig. 1.26)

The main function of an image intensifier is to amplify and convert incident x-rays into visible light. The important components include an input phosphor, photocathode, electrostatic focusing lenses, accelerating anodes, and output phosphor.

- The input phosphor is made up of cesium iodide and emits part of absorbed x-ray photons as a large number of light photons. Because the K-shell binding energies of Cs and I are approximately 35 keV, it efficiently absorbs x-rays
- The photocathode absorbs these light photons and converts them into photoelectrons
- The electrostatic lens focuses these photoelectrons to the output phosphor. At the same time, these photoelectrons are accelerated by an accelerating voltage of approximately 30 keV
- These energetic electrons are absorbed by the output phosphor, which converts them into large numbers of light photons. The output phosphor is made up of silver-activated ZnCdS (zinc–cadmium–sulphide)
- The output phosphor is coupled to the camera or CCD
- The light image on the output of image intensifier is several thousand times brighter than that of input phosphor. This

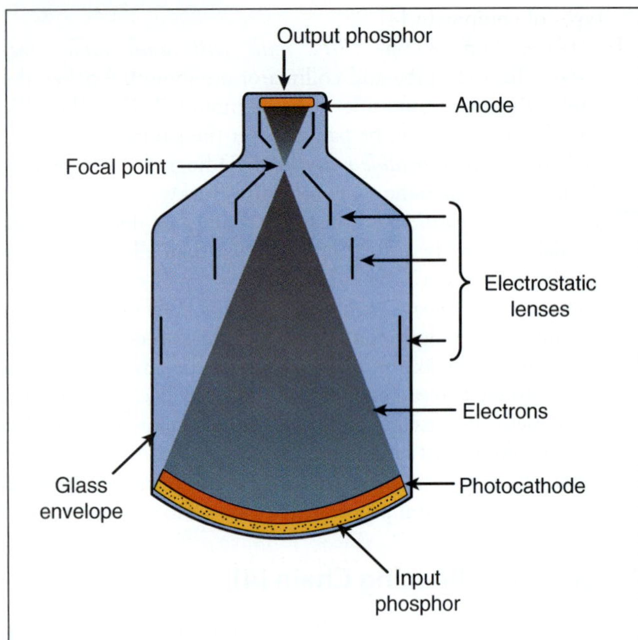

Figure 1.26 Image intensifier. (From: Bushberg, *The Essential Physics of Medical Imaging*.)

increase in brightness at the output phosphor relative to input phosphor is called brightness gain.

$$\text{Brightness gain} = \text{Minification gain} \times \text{Flux gain}$$

in which minification gain is the ratio of the area of output phosphor to input phosphor, which is equal to the square of ratio of diameters. Flux gain is the number of photons generated by the output phosphor for every photon generated by the input phosphor. Instead of brightness gain, modern systems use a "conversion factor" for expressing the intensification by an image intensifier:

$$\text{Conversion factor} = \text{output phosphor illumination (Candela/m}^2\text{)/} \\ \text{input exposure rate (milli Gray/s)}$$

Limitations of image intensifiers

1. *Lag* is transient persistence of previously acquired image caused by continued luminescence at the output phosphor even after the x-ray stimulation is stopped.
2. *Geometric distortion* occurs because of projection of a curved input phosphor to a flat output phosphor. The input phosphor is curved to allow focusing of electrons and to minimize stress from the vacuum.
3. *Pin-cushion distortion* is magnification and stretching at the periphery of an image.
4. *S-distortion* is caused by local magnetic fields.
5. *Vignetting* is fall-off of brightness at the periphery.
6. *Veiling glare* is caused by light scattered within the output phosphor, which decreases the contrast.

Digital Fluoroscopy System

To overcome the limitations of conventional fluoroscopy, digital fluoroscopy was developed.

Flat-panel detectors

One major advance in modern fluoroscopy units is the introduction of FPD arrays, similar to DR. FPD replaces the image intensifier, lens, and camera system. It directly records the real-time fluoroscopic image sequence. Unlike CCD cameras, FPD systems do not need a video system. FPD directly or indirectly converts incident x-ray photons into electronic signals, which are displayed on the monitor.

- FPD consists of TFT arrays of individual detector elements (dexels or DEL) arranged in a square or rectangle
- Each detector element has a capacitor and a transistor
- The capacitor accumulates and stores the signal as electrical charge, and the transistor functions as a switch
- Indirect x-ray conversion modes are used more commonly than direct ones in fluoroscopy. In indirect TFT, x-rays are first converted to light by phosphor, and then this light is converted into charge by photodiode
- The charge stored in capacitor is dependent on the incident x-ray flux on the detector element
- Reading the array discharges the capacitor and makes them ready for next frame acquisition

Advantages of FPDs are the smaller equipment size, thereby increasing flexibility; better dynamic range; improved coverage of corners because of a square or rectangular field (circular field in II); better stability; lower radiation dose rates because of improved DQE; and lack of glare and geometric distortions.

Disadvantages include the higher cost and lower spatial resolution with a very small or very large field of view.

The only similarity between an image intensifier and FPD is the use of a scintillator. In FPD, pixel binning (combining of adjacent pixels) can be used to reduce noise. Binning also helps in allowing fast frame rate imaging. The image distortion artifacts seen with image intensifiers are not seen with FPD.

Postprocessing techniques [6]

1. *Last image hold*: This permits visualization of the last image even when the x-ray beam is switched off. This image helps in guidance without additional radiation to the patient or medical staff.
2. *Grayscale processing* adjusts brightness and contrast depending on the region of interest.
3. *Temporal frame averaging*: Two or more successive images are averaged to form a single image with noise reduction.
4. *Measurement of distance* is possible because of digital image and calibration.

Recording fluoroscopic images

Various methods of image recording can be used during fluoroscopy: direct film recording, indirect recording, and recording motion.

Digital Subtraction Angiography

Image subtraction technique is used in digital subtraction angiography (DSA) to remove the effects of stationary anatomic structures (especially bones) from the images of contrast-enhanced blood vessels. Thus, precontrast mask image is subtracted from the postcontrast image to reveal only the contrast-enhanced vessel (Fig. 1.27). The various subtraction techniques include temporal subtraction, energy subtraction, and hybrid subtraction.

- Temporal subtraction can be done using the mask mode or time-interval difference (TID) mode. Mask mode results in successive subtraction images of contrast-filled vessels. TID mode produces subtracted images from progressive masks and following frames
- Energy subtraction is based on the abrupt change in photoelectric absorption at the K-edge of contrast media compared with that for soft tissue and bone
- Hybrid subtraction is a combination of temporal and energy subtraction

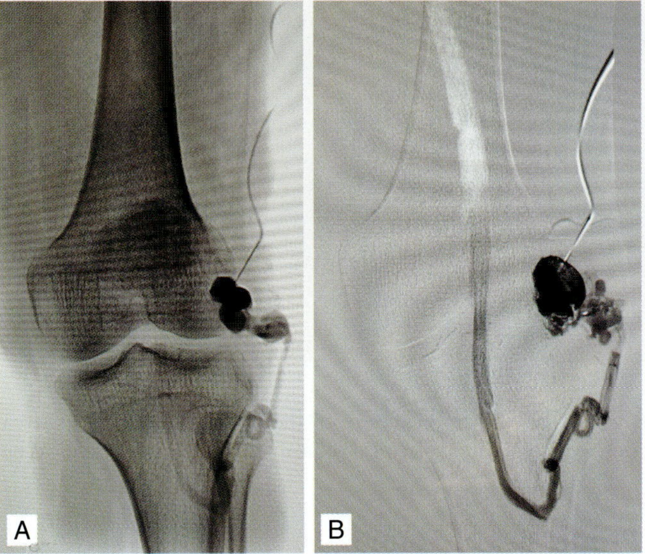

Figure 1.27 Digital subtraction angiography. (A) Postcontrast image of a venolymphatic malformation around the knee. (B) Subtracted image. The precontrast image (not provided) is subtracted from the postcontrast image to reveal only the contrast enhanced vessels. (Courtesy: Dr. Sagar Tyagi.)

A special technique used in DSA that helps in placement of catheters and guidewires is the roadmap (Fig. 1.28). Here, the mask image used is a subtracted fluoroscopic image with maximum contrast opacification of vessel. The subsequent fluoroscopic images are subtracted from this mask image, highlighting the vessel of interest [3]. Other techniques that can be used for DSA include fluoroscopy fade, stepping technique, and three-dimensional (3D) rotational angiography.

A new combined angiography/computed tomography (CT) suite has been developed that uses FPD technology and allows obtaining 3D rotational DSA or cone-beam volume CT interchangeably with the same FPD C-arm motion without patient transfer. This is especially useful in immediate detection or exclusion of intracranial complication that might have occurred during neurovascular procedures without patient transfer to the CT scanner [7].

Digital subtraction angiography is susceptible to patient motion, which can be corrected by computer manipulation of digitally stored images. This can be done by spatial displacement of mask image (mask pixel shift technique), which allows re-registration or by remasking (selecting recent image as new mask image). Other postprocessing techniques include image summation and landmarking. Summation helps in adding up frames to allow visualization of vessel as a complete structure. Landmarking allows anatomic landmarks to be added to subtraction image by adding a lesser intensity area of original image to the subtracted image.

Suggested Readings

- SC Bushong, Radiologic Science for Technologists: Physics, Biology, and Protection, 2018.
- S BA, The AAPM/RSNA physics tutorial for residents: general overview of fluoroscopic imaging. Radiographics 20 (4) (2000): 1115–1126. [Internet] [cited 2021 Aug 13]. Available from: https://pubmed.ncbi.nlm.nih.gov/10903700/.
- SC Bushong, Radiologic Science for Technologists: Physics, Biology, and Protection, 2017.

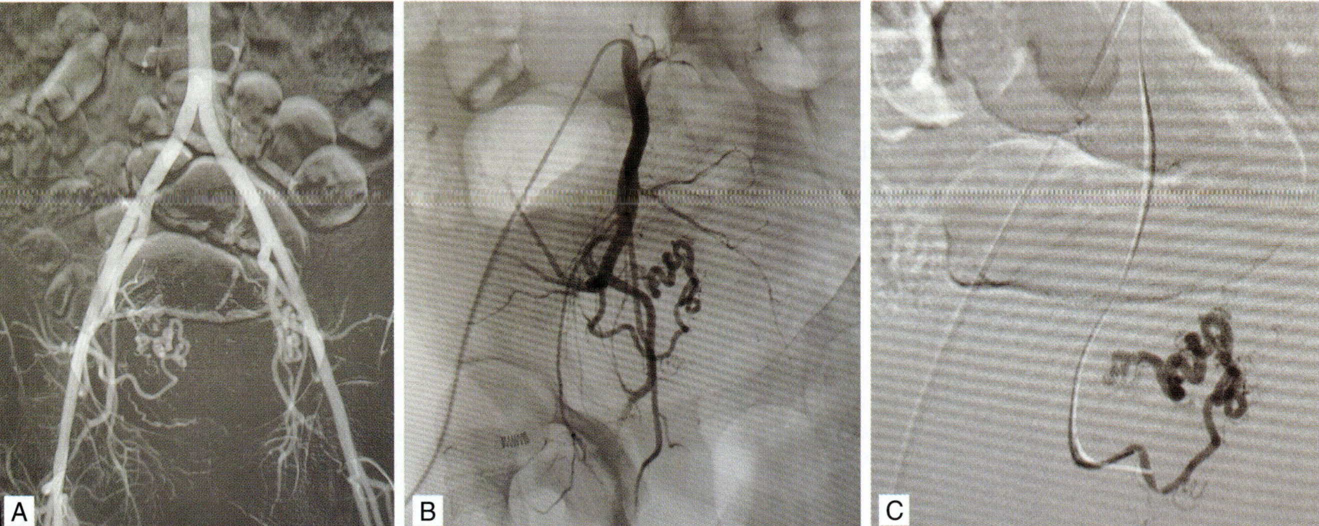

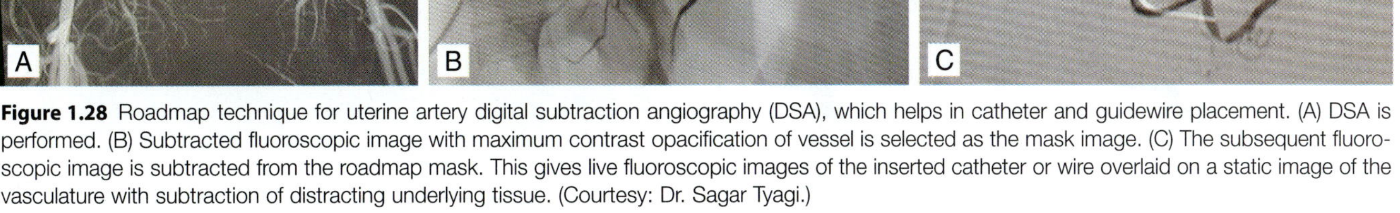

Figure 1.28 Roadmap technique for uterine artery digital subtraction angiography (DSA), which helps in catheter and guidewire placement. (A) DSA is performed. (B) Subtracted fluoroscopic image with maximum contrast opacification of vessel is selected as the mask image. (C) The subsequent fluoroscopic image is subtracted from the roadmap mask. This gives live fluoroscopic images of the inserted catheter or wire overlaid on a static image of the vasculature with subtraction of distracting underlying tissue. (Courtesy: Dr. Sagar Tyagi.)

2

Ultrasound Physics

NIKITA NANWANI, VAIBHAV NICHAT

Introduction

Ultrasound is sound waves with frequency greater than the human audible range (20–20k Hz). Ultrasound devices in medical fields use sound waves in the range of 1 to 20 MHz. Ultrasound imaging and Doppler ultrasound detect sound waves reflected from the body and display it in the form of images.

The various modes of image display in ultrasonography (USG) are A- mode, B-mode (most commonly used), M-mode, and Doppler mode. *A (amplitude) mode* is 1D representation of structures and is used in ophthalmology to measure the axial length of the eyeball. *B (brightness) mode* displays two-dimensional (2D) images in which echo amplitude is depicted as dots of different brightness. The routine grayscale ultrasound examination is a B-mode USG. *M (motion) mode* shows movement as a function of time and is used in cardiac imaging. *Doppler* mode is used to measure blood flow and velocity.

Principle of Ultrasound

Ultrasound works on the pulse echo principle (Fig. 2.1), which is facilitated by piezoelectric material in ultrasound probe crystal. When a piezoelectric crystal is electrically pulsed, it changes shape and vibrates, producing a sound beam that propagates through tissues. The reflected echoes reach the transducer causing its vibrations which produces electrical voltage comparable to returning echo.

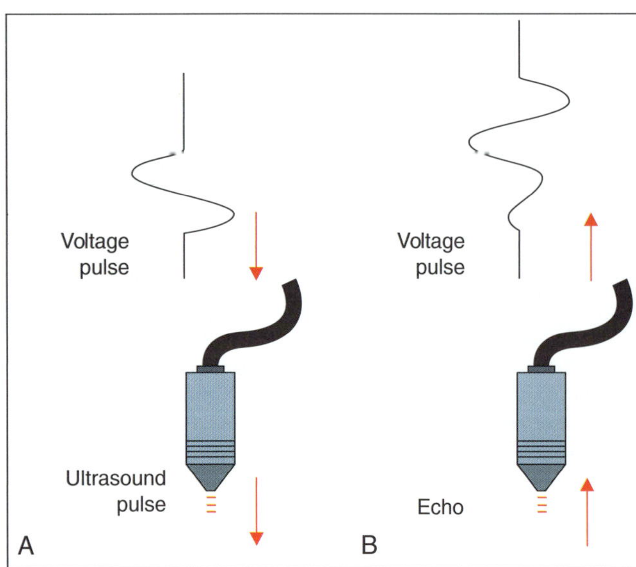

Figure 2.1 The pulse-echo principle. Piezoelectric crystal in the transducer converts electric voltage to ultrasound pulse (A) and converts received echoes (B) into electric voltage pulses.

Properties of Sound

Unlike x-rays, sound is mechanical energy, requires a medium for travel, has tissue-dependent velocity, and does not cause ionization. Sound travels as a longitudinal wave with peaks and troughs (Fig. 2.2).

The propagation velocity depends on tissue and is constant for a particular tissue (Table 2.1). It is inversely proportional to the compressibility and density of tissue and directly proportional to the stiffness of tissue. Thus, the velocity of sound is less in air (330 m/sec), which has high compressibility; in soft tissue, it is 1540 m/sec. Thus, to get the best images of soft tissues, USG machines are calibrated to this speed (1540 m/sec).

Acoustic Impedance

The resistance offered by tissues to the movement of particles caused by ultrasound waves is called the *acoustic impedance* (Z).

$$Z = \rho c,$$

in which ρ is the density of tissue and c is the speed of the ultrasound wave in the tissue.

- Unit: Rayl, which is kg/(m^{2}s)

Thus, acoustic impedance is directly proportional to the density, rigidity of tissue, and speed of sound in a material. (Analogy: A high

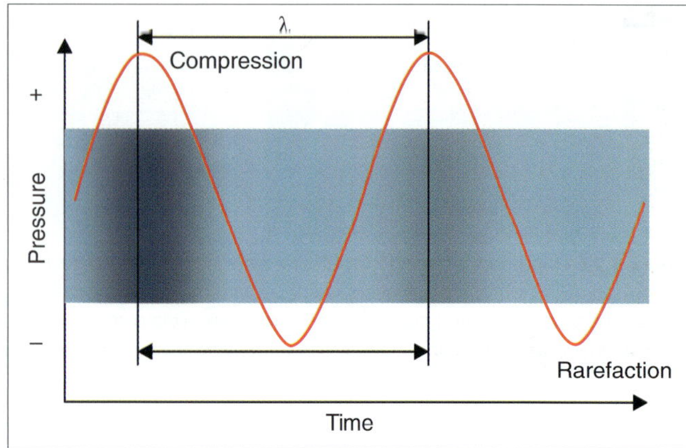

Figure 2.2 Anatomy of sound wave with areas of compression (peaks) and rarefaction (trough). Wavelength (λ) = Distance between corresponding points on the time pressure curve. Period (T) = Time (T) to complete a single cycle. Frequency (f) = Number of complete cycles in a unit of time = $1/T$.

TABLE 2.1 Ultrasound Velocities of Interest in Ultrasound Imaging [1]

Material	Speed of Sound (m/sec)
Air	330
Fat	1450
Water	1480
Soft tissue (average)	1540
Bone	4080
Piezoelectric crystal	4000

jumper landing on a foam mattress [soft and light] will find that it yields to his body much more readily than concrete [solid and heavy].) Acoustic impedance mismatch is the difference in acoustic impedance at interface of two tissues and determines the amount of energy reflected at the interface, which in turn is detected and displayed as images in ultrasound imaging. If the mismatch is high (e.g., air–bone interface), almost 100% sound is reflected back with almost no transmission. If mismatch is low (e.g., fat–muscle interface), there is better sound transmission with decreased reflection. Piezoelectric crystals at the transducer head have very high acoustic impedances compared with skin. Therefore, the matching layer is used in front of the piezoelectric crystal to reduce this difference and allow for better sound transmission into the body (discussed later under transducers).

Interaction With Tissue

There are four mechanisms by which sound can interact with tissues: absorption, reflection, refraction, and scatter.

Absorption

Major mechanism. The higher the frequency, the greater the absorption.

Reflection

The higher the acoustic impedance mismatch, the greater the reflection. Thus, to decrease the acoustic impedance mismatch and thereby allow better sound transmission between the transducer and the skin, ultrasound gel is used. Gel also decreases the amount of trapped air between the transducer and the skin. The other practical application is when examining the pelvis, the urinary bladder should be as full as possible to lift the intestine out of the way. Ultrasound reflection also depends on the size and surface features of the interface. Reflecting surfaces can be specular or diffuse (Fig. 2.3).

- A specular reflector is large and smooth like a mirror and forms an image only when the incident sound is perpendicular to the surface because with an oblique incident sound, the reflected sound is reflected away from the transducer, and no image is formed. Examples of specular reflector are the diaphragm, fetal skull, and vessel wall (see Fig. 2.3A)
- A diffuse reflector is more frequently encountered and is made up of small interfaces, each being much smaller than the incident sound wavelength. Echo is scattered in all directions with only a portion of reflected waves reaching the transducer and forming an image. The characteristic echo pattern of solid organs and tissues such as the liver (see Fig. 2.3B) is attributable to diffuse reflection

Refraction

Change in velocity and angle as beam crosses an interface.

Scatter

Small surfaces scatter sound in many directions because of reflection and refraction. Examples are the liver and kidney parenchyma. Based on the amount of scatter compared with background signal, a tissue or lesion is categorized as hyperechoic, hypoechoic, or anechoic when the amount of scatter is more, less, or no scatter at all, respectively.

The result of all interactions is sound attenuation, that is, the decrease in the intensity of the ultrasound waves as they pass through tissues, similar to sound that becomes fainter when one moves further away from it. Attenuation is measured in decibels per centimeter. Attenuation is directly related to the sound frequency. Thus, for deeper tissues, lower frequency transducers (3.5 MHz) should be used to allow adequate penetration without attenuation, but for superficial organ scanning in adults or for children, 5 MHz or greater is best.

Pulse Echo Instrumentation

Components of an ultrasound system:

1. Transducer (described later): forms the ultrasound pulse.
2. Transmitter or pulsar: energizes the transducer.

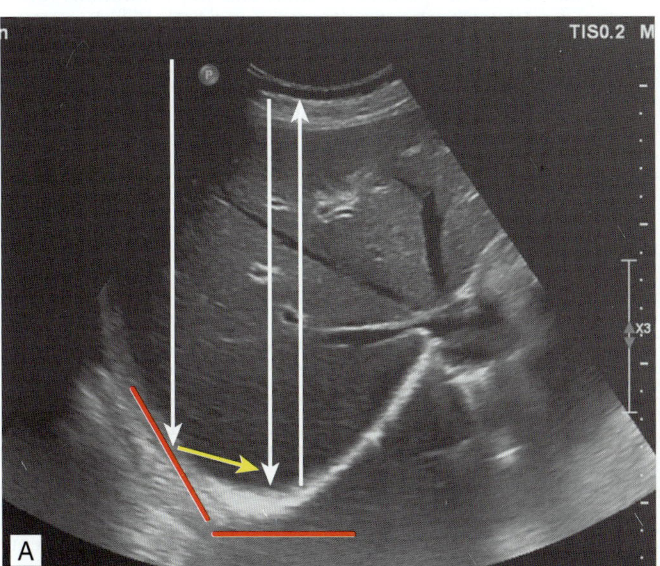

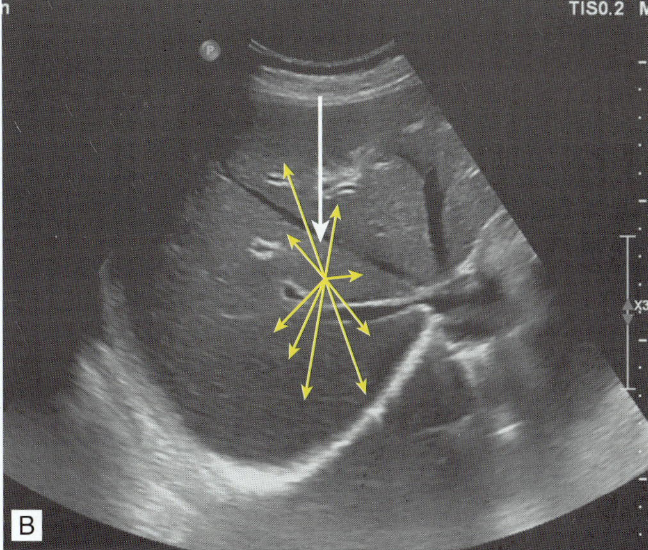

Figure 2.3 (A) The diaphragm as a specular reflector. (B) The liver parenchyma as a diffuse reflector.

3. Receiver or signal processor: performs functions of preamplification, amplification, compensation, compression, demodulation, and rejection.
4. Transmit and receive switch: ensures the electrical signals travel in the correct direction.
5. Scan converter: part of the machine that makes grayscale imaging possible and is responsible for storage of the image data. The older systems were based on analog, but the current systems are digital.
6. Display.
7. Master synchronizer: part of the machine responsible for controlling the timing of the echoes. It ensures that a new pulse is not sent out until the previous pulse has returned.

Transducer

Most clinical applications use pulsed ultrasound, in which brief bursts of acoustic energy are transmitted into the body. The source of these pulses is the ultrasound transducer. A transducer is any device that converts one form of energy to another. *In USG, the transducer with piezoelectric crystals converts electrical energy to mechanical (sound) energy and vice versa.* It acts as both a transmitter and receiver of sound. The returning echoes are represented as points of brightness in B-mode imaging.

Key Terms Related to Transducers

Bandwidth: The range of frequencies produced by a given transducer is termed its *bandwidth*. Bandwidth determines the purity of frequency emitted and pulse length. A narrow-bandwidth transducer emits relatively pure frequency sound and longer pulse length. However, the resolution is less.

Quality Factor: Quality factor describes the amount of ringing the crystals undergo when power is applied to the transducer. (Analogy: When a church bell is struck, it vibrates rapidly, and then the vibration gradually stops.) Thus, decreasing quality factor decreases ringing in the transducer and improves its performance. When the bandwidth is wide, the Q factor is low as in pulse-wave transducers. When the bandwidth is narrow, the Q factor is high as in continuous-wave transducers and therapeutic USG.

Frequency of Transducers: The resonant frequency of the transducer is determined by its thickness (inversely related). Generally, thickness (t) of crystal is equal to one-half of the wavelength (λ) (i.e., $t = \lambda/2$). Transducer frequency can vary from 2.0 MHz to 50.0 MHz and its selection is primarily based upon the patient's body habitus and the region to be scanned.

Pulse Repetition Frequency: Each pulse of a transmitter contains a transmit and a receive phase. The ultrasound pulses must be spaced with enough time between the pulses to permit the sound to travel to the depth of interest and return before the next pulse is sent. Pulse repetition frequency (PRF) is the number of pulses of ultrasound sent out by the transducer per second. It depends on the velocity of sound and depth of tissue being imaged. The deeper the tissue, the lower the PRF because the echo takes a longer time to travel.

Construction of an Ultrasound Transducer or Probe (Fig. 2.4)

1. **Crystal or piezoelectric material**
   A transducer or probe can have a single element in the form of disc or multiple elements, called as *transducer array*. The number, size, shape, and arrangement of transducer elements vary according to the transducer type and application.

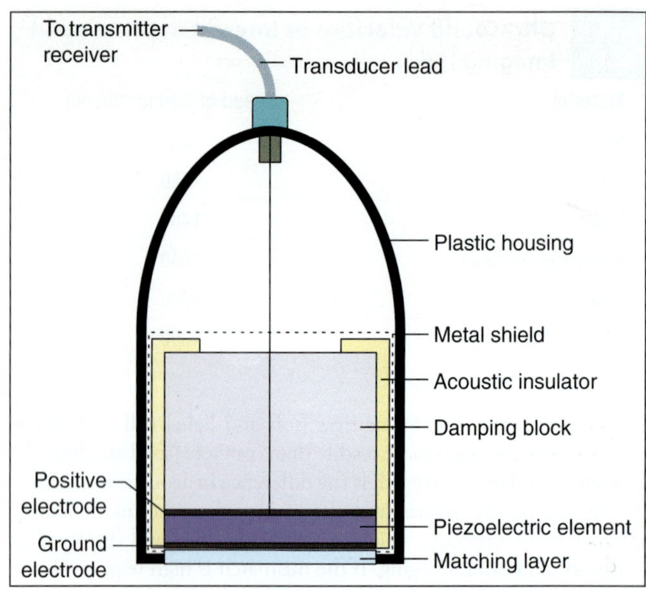

Figure 2.4 Ultrasound transducer–probe construction.

   Whereas older systems used natural piezoelectric material quartz, most used material nowadays is artificial lead (Pb) zirconate titanate (PZT). PZT is created by heating it to Curie point, which is the temperature at which an ultrasound transducer gains its piezoelectric properties. While being heated, the PZT is placed into a magnetic field, which causes dipoles in the PZT to align themselves in relation to the magnetic field. Finally, the material is cooled, and it gains its piezoelectric effect. If the transducer is heated again above Curie point, it loses its piezoelectricity. Therefore, ultrasound transducers must never be heat sterilized.
   Emerging technology for transducer material includes silicon-based capacitive micro-machined ultrasound transducers, polyvinylidene fluoride, and single-crystal technology [2].
2. **Electrodes**
   Electrodes enable electrical connection. Positive electrode is at the back of the element, and ground electrode is on the front.
3. **Damping or backing block**
   The damping or backing block is adhered to the back of the crystal behind the positive electrode and stops vibrations reverberating back into the piezoelectric material. Thus, it determines the length of the ultrasound pulse by determining how much it is dampened via the Q-value. (Analogy: If a bell is grabbed while it is ringing, it decreases the ringing time of the bell.)
   Color wave transducers do not have backing material and subsequent narrow-bandwidth, high Q-factors.
   Pulsed-wave transducers have typically low Q-factors because they need damping to make the pulse short.
4. **Matching layer**
   The matching layer is the part that comes in contact with the patient's skin and is placed in front of piezoelectric crystal. It consists of a material with acoustic impedance between the soft tissue and the transducer material. Thus, it allows close to 100% transmission of the ultrasound from the element into the tissues by decreasing the impedance mismatch. The matching layer thickness is one-fourth the wavelength of sound in that material and is referred to as quarter-wave matching [2].
5. **Housing**
   Housing is the electrical insulation and protection of element, consisting of a plastic case, metal shield, and acoustic insulator.

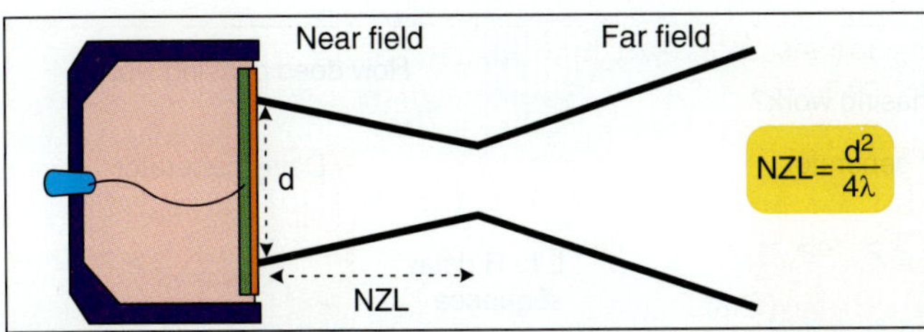

Figure 2.5 Ultrasound beam profile with near and far zones. Near zone length (NZL) = $d^2/4\lambda$, in which d = diameter of transducer and λ = wavelength.

6. **Lens**
   The lens helps in focusing the beam and is usually incorporated after the matching layer. In array transducers, it is usual for one large lens to extend across all the transducer elements. Modern transducers use electronic focusing.
7. **Wire**
   Wire is used to transfer electrical signals to and from the transducer. Modern scan heads often contain more than 100 individual transducer elements, each of which is supplied with electrical energy via a wire.

Beam Formation and Focusing

In the case of pulsed ultrasound, the term *beam* means the width of the pulse as it travels away from the transducer. According to *Huygen's principle*, the beam starts out as small wavelets at the face of the transducer. The interference of the wavelets produces a propagation sound beam. The direction in which the beam travels is perpendicular to the wavefront.

An ultrasound beam consists of near and far zones (Fig. 2.5). The *near or Fresnel zone* is the region between the transducer and the minimum beam width. This is the most useful part of the beam. The *far or Fraunhofer zone* is the region beyond the minimum beam width. *The focal length or focal distance is the distance between the transducer surface and end of near zone length (i.e., where the beam is narrowest).*

Thus, to get as long a near-zone length as possible, we would have to make the transducer wider. However, the resolution will be reduced, and the width of the whole transducer array will be much larger. To overcome this, a stepped linear array is used (discussed later).

Beam focusing improves resolution by decreasing the minimum beam width compared with that produced without focusing. However, well beyond the focal region, the width of the focused beam is greater than that of the unfocused beam. Focusing decreases the near-zone length as it moves the end of near zone toward the transducer. Various methods to achieve beam focusing are by using the lens; using curved transducer elements rather than flat elements; and electronic focusing, which is achieved by using a curved pattern of phased delays.

Types of Transducers (Fig. 2.6)

Ultrasound transducers typically consist of 128 to 512 [3] piezoelectric elements arranged in linear or curvilinear arrays. Each element is individually insulated.

Mechanical Transducers: The beam is steered mechanically by spinning or rotating element or array housed in an acoustic coupling liquid. It could be single element transducer with fixed focus that were used in early ultrasound scanners, or it could consist of annular arrays of elements with electronically controlled focus which are used in 3D USG.

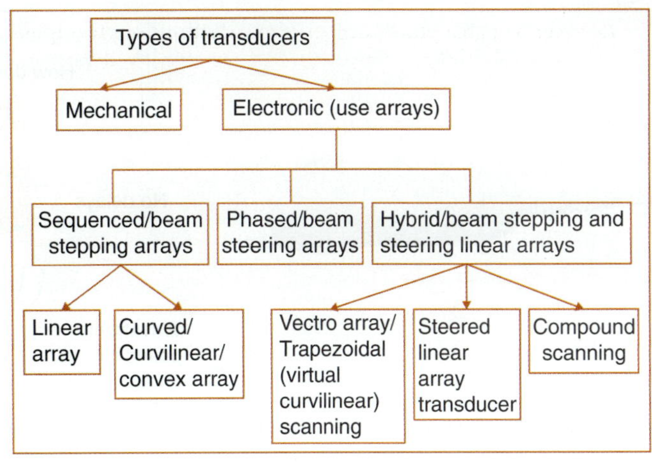

Figure 2.6 Types of transducers.

Electronic Transducers: Electronic transducers have multiple active elements that form an array. An array is formed by slicing down a single slab of PZT into multiple subelements. Each subelement has its own wire and can fire independently. Thus, the elements can be excited selectively as needed to shape and steer the beam. There are two broad types of arrays, sequenced and phased (discussed later).

Key Concepts in Understanding Working Mechanism of Different Types of Electronic Transducers

Beam Formation by Sequencing in a Linear Array (Fig. 2.7): In a linear array, elements are placed next to each other and activated as a group. The initial elements are then inactivated, and the next group of elements is activated. This moves the beam along. Thus, wide beams can be produced in a smaller space than can be produced with wide transducers activated individually. Longer near-field distance can be achieved.

Beam Focusing by Phasing in a Linear Sequenced Array: The transmitted beam can be focused to a specific point by phasing (i.e., activating outermost transducers first, then the inner two, then the innermost, etc.). Similarly, during reception of echoes, *dynamic focusing* can be done (i.e., preferentially receiving echoes from a particular depth). This is what happens when the focus is set on the ultrasound machine.

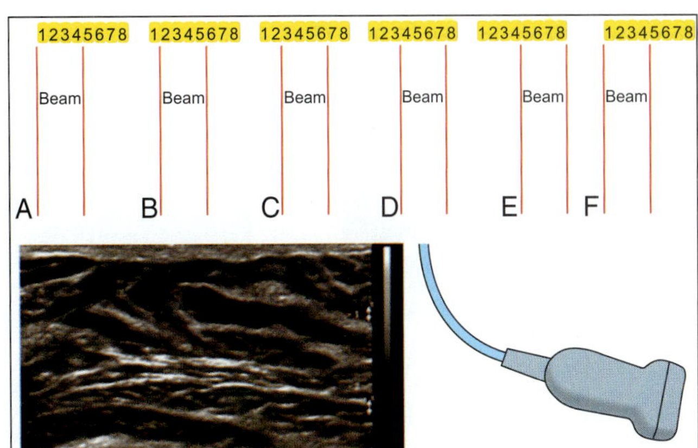

Figure 2.7 Linear sequenced array. A voltage pulse is applied simultaneously to all elements in a small group, first to elements 1 to 4 (for example) as a group (A), then to elements 2 to 5 (B), etc. across the transducer assembly (C–E). The process is then repeated (F).

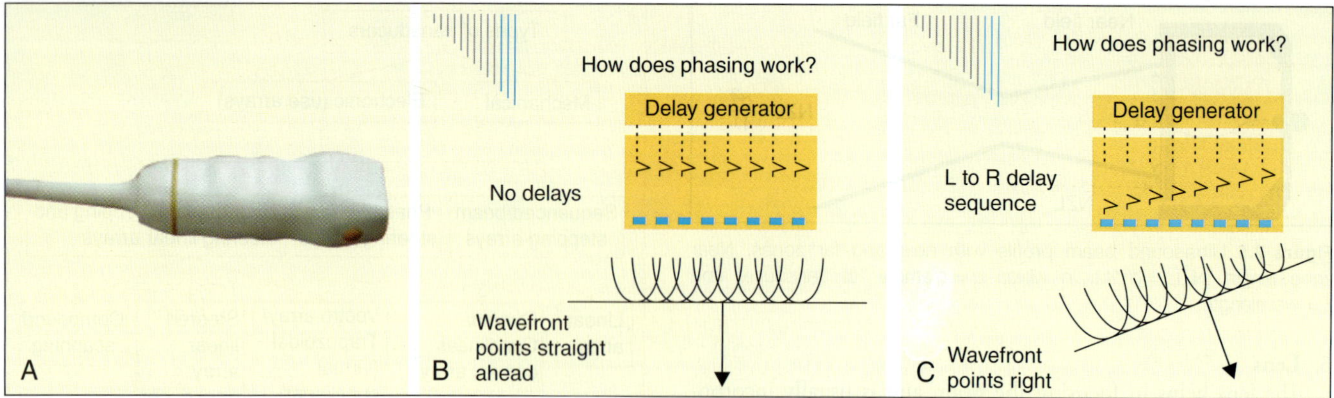

Figure 2.8 (A) Phased transducer. (B) Beam formation without phase delay. (C) Beam steering by phasing.

Beam Steering by Phasing in a Phased Array (Fig. 2.8): Phasing implies changing the timing of excitation of elements to shape and steer the beam. In contrast to linear and curved arrays, all the elements work together in a phased array (see Fig. 2.8).

Compared with a nonphased array, a phased array has smaller transducer footprint, requires a small acoustic window, and can do precise beam focusing and steering. Thus, the major advantage is that very broad image field can be visualized at larger depths that too with a narrow transducer footprint. Phased-array transducers are widely used in cardiac scanning because these transducers fit easily between the ribs. An endovaginal transducer is also a phased-array transducer.

Hybrid Beam-Stepping and Beam-Steering Transducers

These are linear arrays in which both beam stepping and beam steering are used.

Trapezoidal or Virtual Curvilinear Scanning (Fig. 2.9A): This is a linear array with the image format of a curvilinear array but with a flat top (hence, virtual curvilinear). Being a linear array, it overcomes the high pressure required for a convex array to maintain contact. The image shape is trapezoidal. This is achieved by steering the scan lines situated toward the ends of the transducer progressively outward. Thus, the image is widened in the far zone similar to a curvilinear array, giving the advantage of a large field of view.

Steered Linear-Array Transducers (Fig. 2.9B): This is a linear array with the ability to steer all transmit and receive beams to the right or left. Thus, the image is parallelogram shaped (Fig. 2.9B). It is useful in Doppler imaging and to view vessels in difficult areas, such as under the angle of the jaw.

Compound Scanning (Fig. 2.9C): Compound scanning superimposes several angled views in a single "compound" scan. The gray level of each pixel is the average of the values for that pixel in the several superimposed views. It is an extension of the steered linear array technique. It can be done using both linear and curvilinear arrays.

Table 2.2 summarizes the properties of commonly used transducers.

Three- and Four-Dimensional Transducers

These are used to create 3D image and volume scanning. Three ways to generate a 3D image are a freehand technique, an automated 3D technique using a mechanical transducer, and electronic using a 2D array or matrix array technology.

- In the *freehand or manual technique*, the operator moves the transducer steadily across the path to gather 2D slices. The 2D slices, after being converted to 3D format, may then be sliced to view coronal, sagittal, and axial planes. The limitation of this technique is the need for steady transducer movement, so it is highly operator dependent
- The *mechanical or automated 3D technique* uses a mechanical transducer. It uses sequenced array transducers mounted onto a motor that sweeps the image plane from side to side. It permits measurement on the screen of the 3D image as well as real-time 3D or four-dimensional (4D) imaging, the frame rate of which is governed by the speed of the motor
- The newest technique is electronic using latest *2D array or matrix array technology* [2]. It acquires real-time volumes using transducers containing as many as up to 10,000 elements compared with 12 to 512 elements in standard transducers [2]. The arrays could be linear or annular arrays. Whereas linear arrays allow electronic beam steering by phasing, annular arrays have to be steered mechanically. The advantages are linear arrays enable precise focusing because of use of multiple elements, and the beam can be focused in both the elevation plane and lateral plane

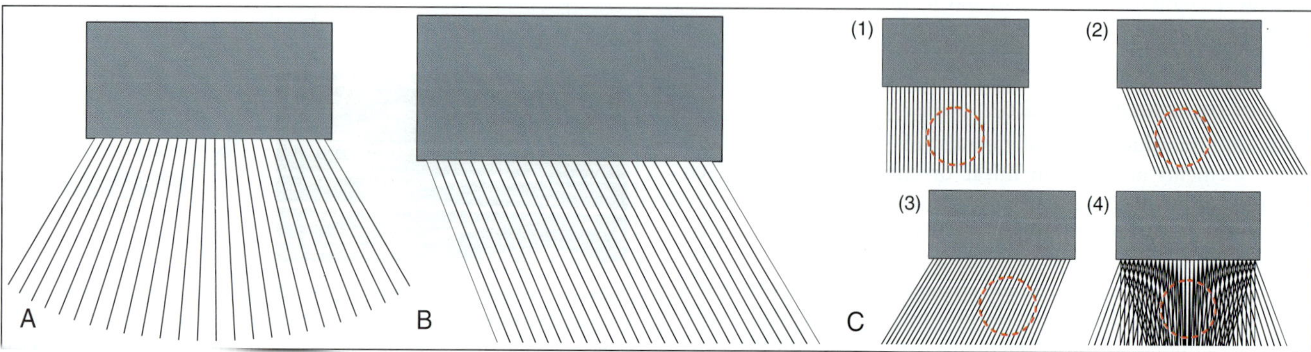

Figure 2.9 Hybrid transducers. (A) Trapezoidal transducer. (B) Steered linear array transducer. (C) Compound scanning.

TABLE 2.2 Summary of Properties and Functioning of Commonly Used Transducers

Property	Linear Transducer	Convex Transducer	Phased Transducer	Vector or Trapezoidal Transducer
Array terminology: words in parentheses are implied in abbreviated common terminology	(Phased) linear (sequenced) array	(Phased) convex (sequenced) array	(Linear) phased array	(Phased and sequenced) (linear) vector array
Category	Beam-stepping array	Beam-stepping array	Beam-steering array	Hybrid beam-stepping and beam-steering array
Shape of the image	Rectangle or parallelogram (when steered), flat top	Sector; curved top (because the elements are arranged in an arc)	Sector; pointed top	Sector; flat top
Beam scanned by	Sequencing: sequential scans of a subset of transducer elements	Sequencing	Phasing: scans of entire set of transducer elements by applying sequential electronic delays	Sequencing and phasing
Beam focused by	Phasing	Phasing	Phasing	Phasing
Use	Vascular and high-resolution imaging	Abdominal and gynecology and obstetrics imaging	Cardiac, neonatal brain, endocavitary transducers	Abdominal, cardiac, Doppler

Ultrasound Gel and Acoustic Coupling Agents [4,5]

Gel is needed to remove pockets of air between probe and the patient's skin, which would otherwise prevent sound transmission into patient's body. Thus, ultrasound gel acts as a medium to transmit sound and as a lubricant. Liquids such as water and alcohols are suitable media; however, being volatile and having low viscosity, they are inappropriate. That is why specific gels have been developed. Hydrogel is preferred over Lipogel because it can be easily removed by tissue or a towel. *Ingredients of ultrasound gel include distilled water, carbomer, ethylenediaminetetraacetic acid (EDTA), propylene glycol, glycerin, and trolamine.* Occasionally, colorant is used, usually a blue color.

In case of a patient having an open wound, a skin rash, or any other risk of infection, the transducer or patient's skin should be covered with plastic, and gel should be used on both sides of the plastic. The transducer must be cleaned after every patient.

Image Quality

The quality of an ultrasound image is determined by spatial resolution, contrast resolution, temporal resolution, and absence of certain artifacts.

Spatial Resolution

Spatial resolution is the ability to differentiate two closely situated objects as distinct structures. It is considered in three planes, with different determinants of resolution for each. Resolution along the axis of the ultrasound beam is *axial resolution* (see Fig. 2.10A), resolution in the plane perpendicular to the beam and parallel to the transducer is *lateral resolution*, and resolution in the plane perpendicular to the beam and to the transducer is *azimuth or elevational resolution or slice thickness* (see Fig. 2.10B).

- Axial resolution is the ability to separate two objects lying along the axis of the beam. It can be improved by a shorter wavelength (higher frequency) and shorter length of pulse (lower Q-value of backing material). But the problem with high-frequency transducers is poor penetration
- Lateral resolution is the ability to resolve two adjacent objects and is best achieved within the focal zone. Its key determinant is width of the ultrasound beam, which can be altered by focusing the beam, usually by electronic phasing. It can be improved by using focused transducers, adjusting focal position, and using multiple focal lengths. However, this reduces frame rate
- Azimuth, elevational resolution, and slice thickness are directly related to transducer height and are fixed for standard 2D transducers

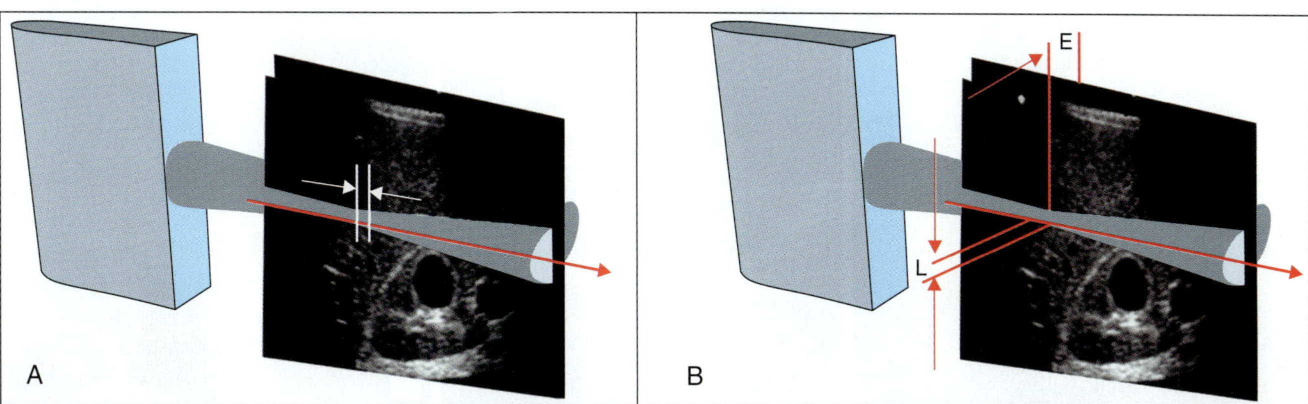

Figure 2.10 (A) Axial resolution. (B) Lateral (L) and elevation (E) resolution.

Temporal Resolution

Temporal resolution is the ability of the system to display events occurring at different times as separate images and is measured in frames per second. Factors that decrease temporal resolution include a greater number of focal zones, having Doppler on, imaging a deeper object (echo takes longer to return), and large sector width (more space to scan).

Contrast Resolution

Contrast resolution is the ability of a grayscale display to distinguish between echoes of slightly different intensities. Contrast resolution depends on the number of bits per pixel in the image memory and can be improved by increasing the number of bits per pixel (more gray shades) [6].

B-Mode Imaging Artifacts

Artifacts are incorrect representations of anatomy or function that can enhance or degrade the diagnostic value of the ultrasound image. The causes are machine and operator related, as well as intrinsic to the characteristics and interaction of ultrasound with the tissues. Remedying these potentially avoidable artifacts is important for maximizing image quality and thereby increasing diagnostic accuracy.

Assumptions in Ultrasound Imaging

Sonographic instruments are based on following assumptions, violation of which results in artifact.

1. **Velocity of sound:** Sound travels at uniform speed of 1540 m/sec throughout the tissues. Alteration in the velocity results in *propagation velocity artifact.* It is also assumed that the longer the roundtrip travel time of ultrasound wave, the deeper the object or target is situated.
2. **Attenuation of sound:** Sound waves decrease in intensity at a constant rate as they travel through tissues. If the wave travels through tissues that do not attenuate much or attenuate more, then artifacts such as *increased through transmission, enhancement, and shadowing* arise, respectively.
3. **Path of sound:** Sound waves travel in a straight line; are reflected off a reflector only once; return directly back to the probe at the same angle, exactly to the point from which they left the probe; and echo originate only from objects located along the beam axis. If the sound waves undergo more than one reflection, then artifacts such as *mirror image, reverberation, or comet-tail artifacts occur.* And if the direction of the beam or its echo is altered, *refraction or anisotropy artifact* may be produced.
4. **Beam profile:** Sound beam generated by the transducer is a narrow line. Violation results in *side lobe or grating lobe artifacts.*

Classification of Ultrasound Artifacts

We shall classify the artifacts based on these assumptions and their violation into following groups: propagation velocity artifact, attenuation errors, path of sound-related artifacts, beam profile–related artifacts, and miscellaneous.

Propagation Velocity Artifact or Misregistration Artifact

In the case of a fatty lesion, the slower speed of propagation (~1450 m/sec) means that the echo will take longer to return to the transducer; thus, the lesion is displayed deeper in the image than its true location. This can be minimized by using multibeam (spatial compounding) features and improved signal processing.

Attenuation Artifacts (Fig. 2.11)

Although most artifacts degrade the ultrasound image and impede interpretation, shadowing and enhancement are of clinical value. *Shadowing* (see Fig. 2.11A) results when there is a marked reduction in the intensity of the ultrasound deep to a strong reflector, attenuator, or refractor; consequently, no information is received from the area behind the structure. Clean, dark shadows are seen behind calcified objects when the focal zone is at or just below the structure. *Edge shadowing* (see Fig. 2.11B) is caused by excessive refraction and commonly occurs from the edges of vessels, cystic structures, and bones. Converse to shadowing is enhancement or increased through-transmission artifact. *Enhancement* (see Fig. 2.11C) is seen when then there is less attenuating object compared with

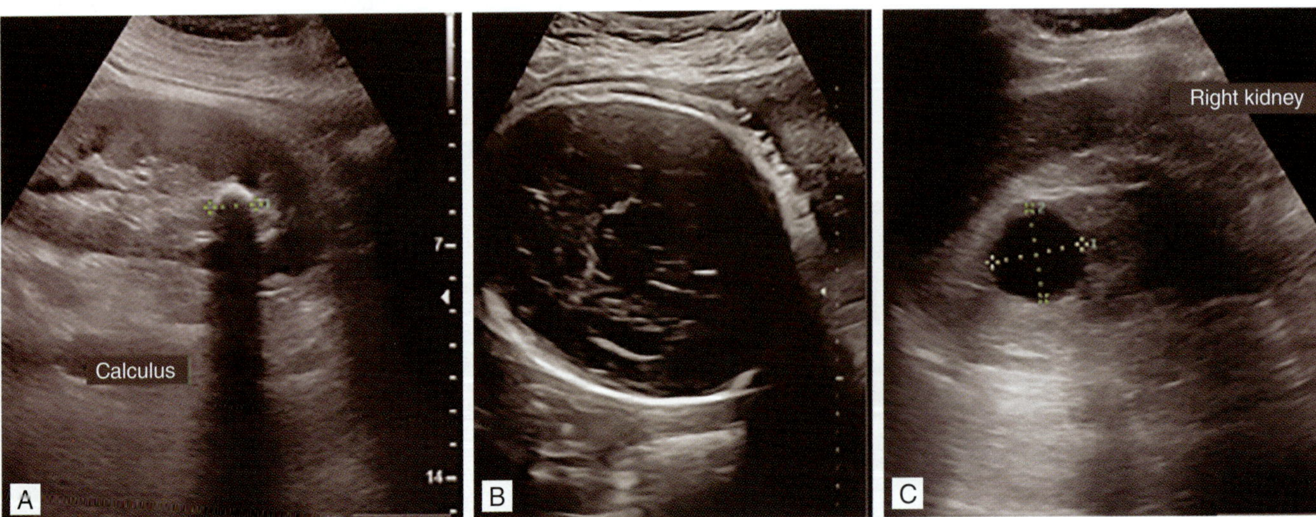

Figure 2.11 Attenuation artefacts. (A) Shadowing deep to renal calculus. (B) Edge shadowing of the fetal skull. This is caused by beam bending at a curved surface with resultant loss in intensity, producing a shadow. (C) Acoustic enhancement artifact is seen in the renal parenchyma deep to a simple renal cyst.

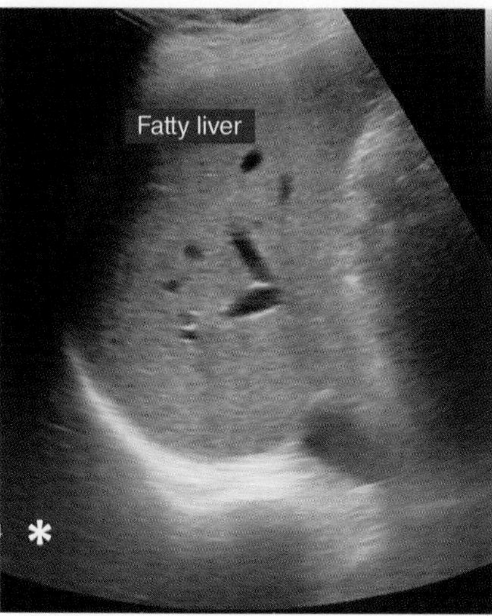

Figure 2.12 Grayscale image showing artifactual mirror image of the liver (*asterisk*) deep to the diaphragm caused by specular reflection from the diaphragm.

surrounding tissues. Consequently, increased amplitude of the beam reaches and is returned from the area deep to this object compared with surrounding tissues. Therefore, this area appears bright compared with surrounding tissues. The enhancement artifact is commonly encountered deep into fluid collections such as cysts, the urinary bladder, or ascites. Thus, it helps in confirming the fluid nature of the object. One has to be wary of misinterpretation as well. For example, kidneys scanned through ascites fluid can appear echogenic because of the enhancement artifact, raising false suspicion for medical renal disease.

Path of Sound-Related Artifacts

Mirror Image Artifacts and Multipath Artifacts: The ultrasound beam encounters a highly reflective surface. The reflected echoes then encounter another reflective structure on their way back and are reflected back toward the reflective interface before being reflected to the transducer, where they are detected. The display shows a duplicated structure equidistant but on the opposite side of the reflector, creating a mirror image. This most often happens at the diaphragm, where the liver is seen in the chest cavity because of sound waves being reflected off the diaphragm (Fig. 2.12).

Reverberation Artifacts: Reverberation artifacts arise when the ultrasound signal reflects repeatedly between highly reflective interfaces near the transducer, resulting in delayed echo return to the transducer. This appears in the image as a series of regularly spaced echoes at increasing depth. It can be reduced by changing the scanning angle or placing transducer in such a way so as to avoid the parallel interface that contribute to artifact. Reverberation may be helpful in identification of a specific type of reflector, such as a surgical clip or needle during biopsy.

Two types of reverberation artifacts are comet-tail and ring-down artifacts.

- In *comet-tail artifact*, the repetitive reflections occur within very small structures, such as tiny cysts in the case of von Meyenburg complexes and tiny crypts in the wall of the gallbladder in the case of adenomyomatosis (Fig. 2.13). Accordingly, the reverberated echoes may not be individually visible. The tapered, comet-tail appearance is caused by the decreasing amplitude of each reverberation as a result of beam attenuation
- *Ring-down artifact* occurs when the ultrasound waves cause oscillation within fluid trapped by a tetrahedron of gas bubbles

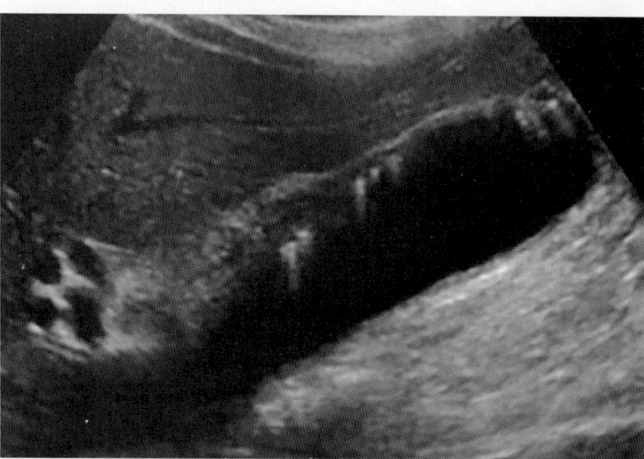

Figure 2.13 Comet-tail artifact in gallbladder adenomyomatosis.

Refraction: When an ultrasound beam is incident on a boundary between two tissues at an angle other than 90 degrees and if these tissues do not have the same speed of sound, there is a change in the direction of the ultrasound beam (refraction) This results in artifactual representation of objects on the display even when they are not truly in the scanned field of view Thus, refraction can cause *object position misregistration, duplication, or lateral defocusing* at the edge of curved structures. This artifact is most often observed in pelvic structures deep to the rectus muscles and midline fat. It can be minimized by increasing the scan angle so that sound waves travel perpendicular to the interface.

Anisotropy (Fig. 2.14): Anisotropy is an artifact caused by structures that are composed of bundles of highly reflective fibers running parallel to each other, such as tendons and ligaments. If the sound beam hits the tendon or ligament fibers perpendicular to their length, it is reflected directly back, resulting in an echogenic appearance. But if the angle of insonation is not perpendicular to the tendon fibers, the beam is reflected away from the transducer, leading to the generation of an image with artifactual hypoechogenicity within the tendon.

Beam Profile–Related Artifacts

Beam Width Artifacts and Side-lobe and Grating-lobe Artifacts (Fig. 2.15): Although most of the energy generated by a transducer is emitted in a beam along the central axis of the transducer (M in Fig. 2.15A), some energy is also emitted at the periphery of the

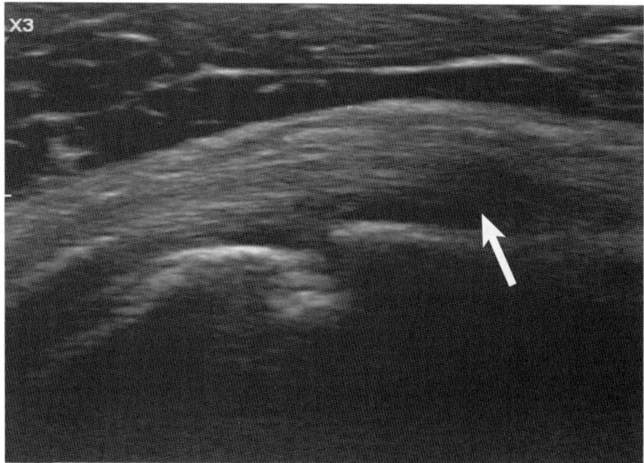

Figure 2.14 Anisotropy. Short-axis image of the supraspinatus tendon. Artifactual hypoechogenicity (*arrow*) may simulate tendinosis or a tear.

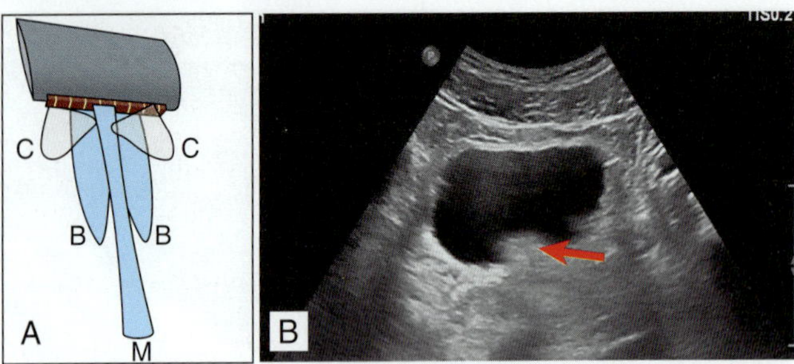

Figure 2.15 (A) Along with main central beam (M), the side lobes are also generated. (B) Side lobe artifact caused by soft tissue close to the urinary bladder wall *(red arrow)* leading to an artifactual appearance of soft tissue mass in the urinary bladder lumen.

primary beam. These are called *side lobes* (B in 14A) and *grating lobe*" (C in Fig. 2.15A) and are lower in intensity than the primary beam.

Side lobes or grating lobes may interact with strong reflectors that lie outside of the scan plane and produce artifacts that are displayed in the ultrasound image (see Fig. 2.15B). They are more evident when the misplaced echoes overlap an expected anechoic structure. They can be minimized by placing the transducer at the center of the object of interest and adjusting the focal zone to the appropriate depth.

Miscellaneous Artifacts

Speckle Artifacts: Closely spaced, very small objects or reflectors, as in solid organs such as the liver and kidney, generate echoes that cannot be resolved. This results in speckle with resultant granularity and noise in the image. Speckle can be reduced by newer imaging techniques such as spatial compounding.

Tips to Avoid Artifacts

- Know the pitfalls
- Know the anatomy
- Beware of strong reflections
- Use multiple views. Every ultrasound examination is a search and is incomplete if it does not provide 3D information about the area of interest and all the neighboring organs. Hence, do not hesitate to toggle the transducer manually, sweep the organ, and take multiple scans. If you cannot see what is needed, turn the patient over to each side, make the patient oblique, or examine the patient while she or he is standing
- Remember that artifacts are inconsistent

Doppler

Doppler ultrasound is based on *Doppler effect* (i.e., the shift or change of frequency in an ultrasound wave caused by a moving reflector, such as blood cells in the vasculature). The difference between the incident and returning frequencies is called the *Doppler shift frequency*. This is the same effect that causes a siren on a fire truck to sound high pitched as the truck approaches the listener (the wavelength is compressed) and a shift to a lower pitch sound as it passes by and continues on (the wavelength is expanded). The moving reflectors in the body are the blood cells. By comparing the incident ultrasound frequency with the reflected ultrasound frequency from the blood cells, it is possible to discern the velocity of the blood. The Doppler effect can also be used to measure tissue motion.

The relationship of the returning ultrasound frequency to the velocity of the reflector is described by the *Doppler equation,* as follows:

$$\Delta F = F_R - F_T = 2 \cdot F_T \cdot v / c$$

The Doppler frequency shift is ΔF, F_R is the frequency of sound reflected from the moving target, F_T is the frequency of sound emitted from the transducer, v is the velocity of the target toward the transducer, and c is the velocity of sound in the medium.

The Doppler frequency shift (ΔF) applies only if the target is moving directly toward or away from the transducer. In most clinical settings, the ultrasound beam usually approaches the moving target at an angle designated as the Doppler angle. In this case, ΔF is reduced in proportion to the cosine of this angle, as follows:

$$\Delta F = F_R - F_T = 2 \cdot F_T \cdot v \cdot \cos\theta / c$$

in which θ is the angle between the axis of flow and the incident ultrasound beam.

In practice, Doppler angles should be less than 60 degrees because at angles greater than 60 degrees, the cosine value changes rapidly. Because cos (90) is zero, no Doppler shift is produced when the motion is perpendicular to the sound beam. The maximum frequency shift occurs when the reflector is moving directly toward the detector (i.e., θ is equal to 0 degrees) or directly away from the detector (i.e., θ is equal to 180 degrees).

Types of Doppler

Continuous-Wave Doppler

As the term says, these transmit and receive sound waves continuously; thus, they need to contain two separate elements for transmitting and receiving. The Doppler effect is emitted as audible sound as the Doppler shift is in the audible sound range. The higher the sound pitch, the higher the velocity, and the harsher the sound, the greater the turbulence. These are usually dedicated handheld devices (e.g., cardiotocogram for the fetal heart).

- Advantages are it is cheap, easy to use, and sensitive to flow
- Limitations are the inability to objectively measure velocity, depth, and output generally is a combination of arterial and venous signals because all vessels in the beam path are insonated until the beam is attenuated and arteries and veins lie close together

Pulsed-Wave Doppler

Unlike continuous-wave doppler, in pulsed-wave Doppler, the same elements are used for transmitting and receiving, Brief pulses of ultrasound energy are emitted. Only returning echoes at specific depths can be accepted by using range gating. Duplex involves Doppler imaging overlaid over B-mode imaging.

Three types of pulsed wave Doppler are color, power, and spectral Doppler.

Color Doppler (Fig. 2.16A): Color Doppler provides a 2D visual display of moving blood. Color Doppler information is displayed on top of the B-mode image. The measured Doppler frequency shifts are encoded as colors. Colors are assigned dependent on motion toward or away from the transducer. *Red signifies motion toward the transducer, whereas blue signifies motion away from the transducer.* Turbulent flow may be displayed as green or yellow. *Color intensity varies with flow velocity.*

- Advantages are the ability to provide information in the direction and magnitude of the flow over a large region of interest, it can detect flow in vessels too small to see by imaging alone, and it allows complex blood flow to be visualized
- Disadvantages are angle dependence, aliasing, inability to display entire Doppler spectrum in the image, and artifacts caused by noise

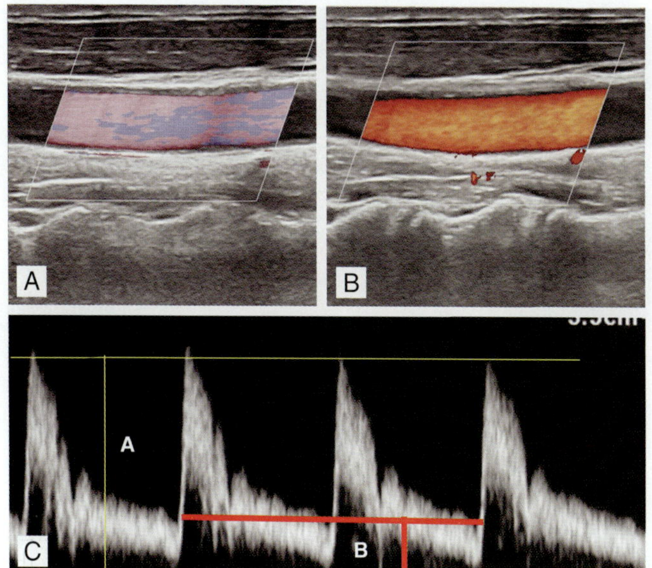

Figure 2.16 (A) Color Doppler. (B) Power doppler. (C) Spectral doppler. A, peak systolic velocity; B, end-diastolic velocity.

Power Doppler (Fig. 2.16B): Power Doppler images map only the power or amplitude of the Doppler signal without any indication of the velocity because it is based on Doppler signal strength alone without taking Doppler shift into consideration. *Unlike Color Doppler, in which positive and negative velocities of the same magnitude from a given region would be cancelled out, in power Doppler, these are summed up. Thus, in power Doppler, the main emphasis is on the quantity of blood flow.*

- Advantages are less dependence on insonation angle; very low flow rates can be detected because noise is reduced, allowing higher gain settings (vs color Doppler in which noise appears across the entire frequency spectrum); and aliasing is not a limiting factor
- Disadvantages are flow direction is not displayed and artifacts can occur because of tissue motion

Spectral Doppler (Fig. 2.16C): As the term says, spectral Doppler displays the range of Doppler frequencies or velocities returned (along the y-axis) over time (along the x-axis) in the form of a spectrum. Whereas velocities above horizontal axis suggest flow in one direction, those below horizontal axes suggest flow in the opposite direction.

Different spectral traces are produced depending on differences in vessel wall resistance. These peripheral resistances are indicated by Doppler flow indices:

1. S/D ratio = Peak systolic velocity (PSV)/End-diastolic velocity (EDV).
2. Resistive index (RI) = PSV - EDV/PSV. *RI increases with vessel narrowing and increased resistance to blood flow.*
3. Pulsatility index (PI) = Peak systolic velocity - Minimum diastolic velocity/Mean velocity. It is used to assess resistance in a pulsatile vascular system, along with RI.

High-resistance vessels such as peripheral vessels (femoral artery) show highly pulsatile spectrum with sharp upstroke and narrow range of velocities (Fig. 2.17A), but low-resistance vessels such as vital organs and blood vessels (e.g., the internal carotid artery) that need flow even during diastole show low pulsatility with a large range of velocities (Fig. 2.17B).

Doppler Artifacts

Major Sources of Doppler Imaging Artifacts

Doppler Frequency: An increase in transducer frequency increases Doppler sensitivity, but at the same time, it increases attenuation, resulting in diminished penetration.

Wall Filters: Wall filters are used to remove low-frequency signals form adjacent tissue motion. These remove signals that fall below a given frequency limit. But at the same time, this may also remove signals from low-velocity blood flow. In general, the filter should be kept at the lowest practical level, usually 50 to 100 Hz.

Pulse Repetition Frequency: As discussed earlier, PRF is dependent on depth, with lower PRF required for greater depth. If PRF is less than twice the maximum frequency shift produced by movement of the target (Nyquist limit), aliasing results. In these cases, lower frequency shifts than are actually present are displayed.

Doppler Angle: As discussed earlier, the Doppler angle should be less than 60 degrees.

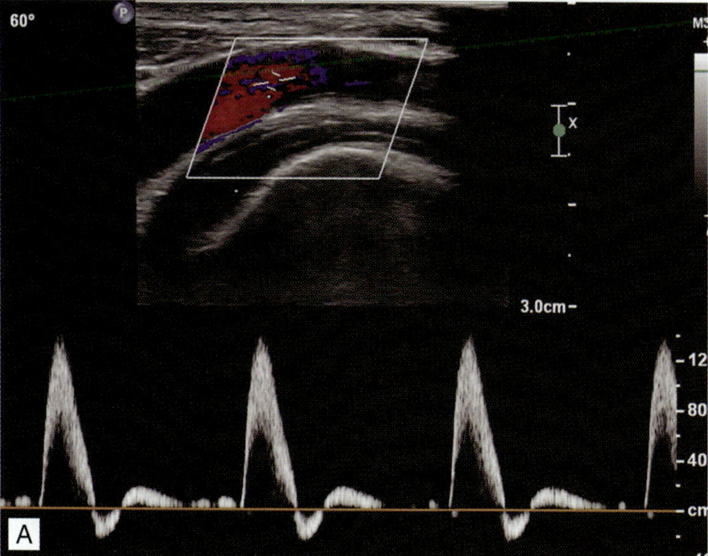

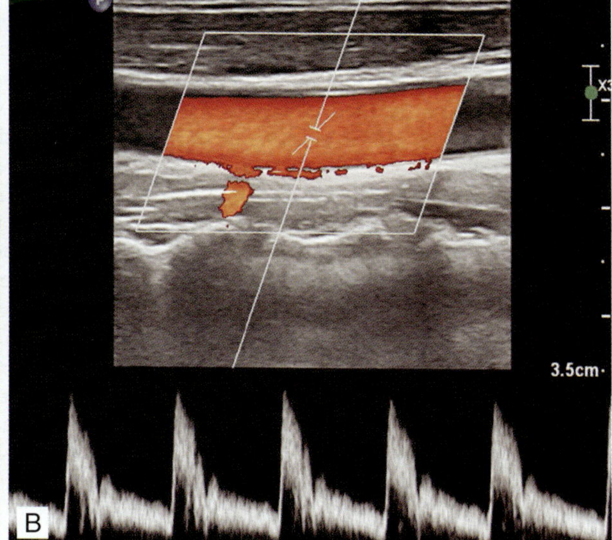

Figure 2.17 (A) High-resistance vessel femoral artery spectral Doppler showing sharp upstroke and narrow range of velocities. (B) Low-resistance vessel internal carotid artery Doppler showing low pulsatility with a large range of velocities.

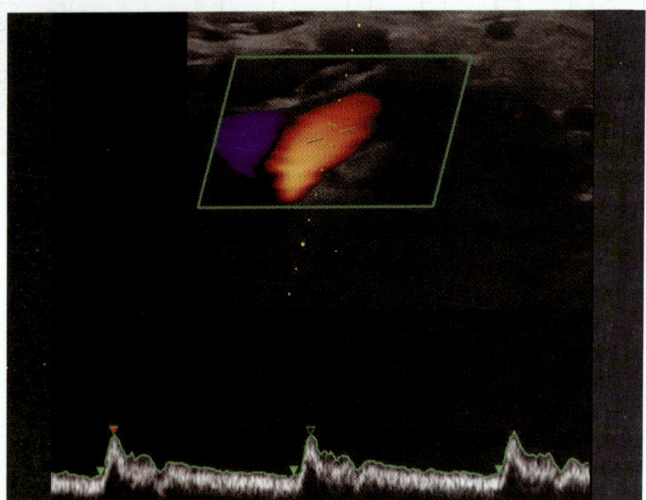

Figure 2.18 Spectral broadening in internal carotid artery Doppler caused by stenosis.

Sample Volume Size: Large sample volume increases vessel wall noise. Thus, the sample volume must be adjusted to exclude vessel walls, which lead to unwanted clutter.

Doppler Gain: An increase in gain increases the noise appearing at all frequencies. Excessive or insufficient Doppler gain results in over- or underestimation of velocity, respectively. *The right approach to setting Doppler gain is to place the sample volume in the vessel and increase Doppler gain to a level at which noise is visible in the image. Then the gain should be gradually reduced to a point at which noise first disappears completely.*

Doppler Artifacts

Spectral Broadening Artifacts (Fig. 2.18): The spectral broadening artifact occurs when there is an increase in the range of flow velocities within a sample volume, as in stenosis. Artifactual spectral broadening can occur because of improper positioning of the sample volume near the vessel wall, use of an excessively large sample volume, or excessive system gain.

Artifactual Vascular Flow (Fig. 2.19): The Doppler effect (shift) is not specific to vascular flow and occurs with movement of any reflector toward or away from the ultrasound beam. Fluid or solid tissue motion can mimic vascular flow. Transmitted pulsations, especially close to the heart or major arteries, can therefore result in artifactual appearance of flow within thrombosed veins or avascular areas. Artifactual vascular flow can also be visualized if the color gain is too high or the color-write priority is too high.

Aliasing and Velocity Scale Errors (Fig. 2.20): In Doppler imaging, the velocity scale setting in the machine is crucial for accurate signal display. When the velocity scale range is set too high, low-flow states may not be represented. Conversely, when the range is set too low, aliasing artifact occurs. Clinically, aliasing is most often encountered in abrupt transition to high-flow states such as vascular stenosis. The Nyquist limit states that the sampling frequency must be greater than twice the highest frequency of the input signal to be able to accurately represent the image Nyquist limit = PRF/2. If the velocity of the flow is greater than the Nyquist limit, the Doppler shift exceeds the scale, and "wraparound" occurs (see Fig. 2.20).

Aliasing can be avoided by increasing the velocity scale range (which also increases the pulse repetition frequency), increasing the Doppler angle, or using a lower frequency transducer.

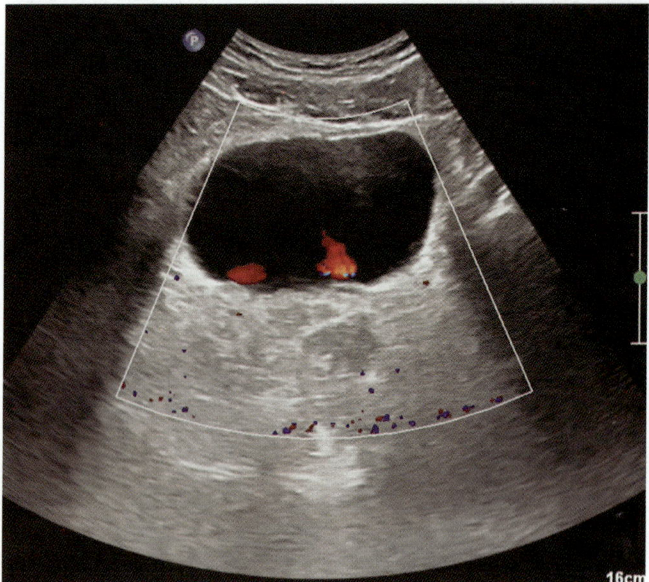

Figure 2.19 Artifactual vascular flow. This is used to advantage to show flow from each ureteric orifice in the urinary bladder, which is seen as color Doppler jets.

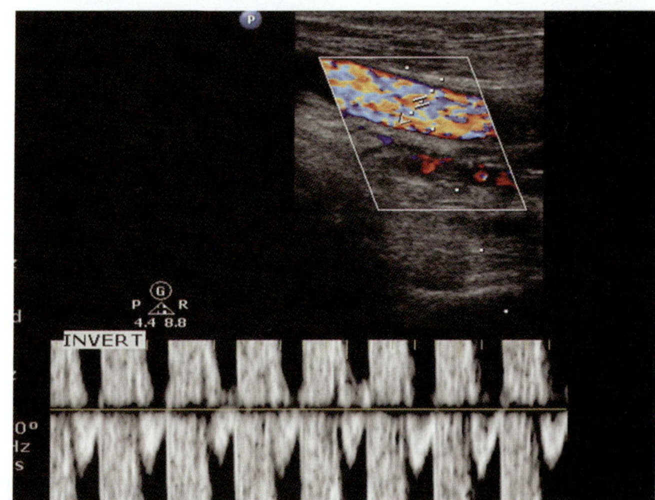

Figure 2.20 Aliasing caused by undersampling (lower pulse repetition frequency) in spectral Doppler. Aliasing is seen as a "wraparound" of the higher frequencies that are displayed below the baseline. In color Doppler, aliasing is seen as wraparound of the frequency color map from one flow direction to the opposite direction without transition of unsaturated color that is seen in true change in flow direction.

Blooming Artifacts: Blooming artifact occurs when color reaches beyond the vessel wall, making the vessels look larger than expected. It is dependent on gain, wall filter, and color overwrite. Lowering the gain and increasing the wall filter decrease the artifact.

Twinkle Artifacts (Fig. 2.21): Twinkle artifact is the artifactual depiction of color signal on crystalline materials in the body. This artifact occurs just deep to strong reflectors with rough surfaces and appears as a closely spaced band of randomly alternating Doppler signals. The spectral tracing is flat. *The twinkle artifact is quite useful clinically because it can aid in the detection of small stones, calcifications, and other crystalline material within the body.*

Direction Ambiguity Artifact: The direction ambiguity artifact is primarily caused by operator error in using the hardware. When

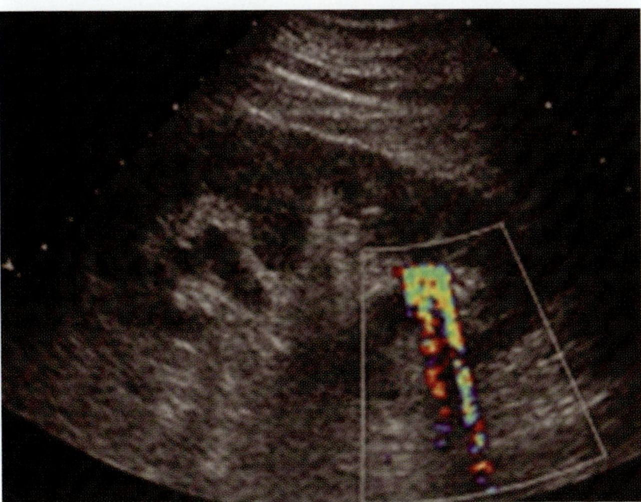

Figure 2.21 Appearance of twinkle artifact on color Doppler.

the ultrasound beam intercepts a vessel at or close to 90-degree angle, with the beam side lobes interrogating flow both upstream and downstream, the resulting signal is manifested as a spectral tracing both above and below the baseline. Clinically, this artifact is most often seen when evaluating flow in solid organs such as the liver, where the vessels can course in multiple planes and directions. Simply altering the transducer position to change the beam angle away from perpendicular will correct for the direction ambiguity. This should be distinguished from true bidirectional flow (e.g., neck of pseudoaneurysm) in which the flow is never simultaneously symmetric above and below the baseline.

Practical Tips and Image Optimization Summary

1. Select the most appropriate anatomic area presets. Application specialists can assist in the customization of presets in clinical practice.
2. Appropriate transducer selection is governed by anatomic size and location (depth). The highest frequency should be used without compromising penetration.
3. A small sector width or scan area increases the image quality and frame rate.
4. Gain: signal amplification
   a. Gain control: regulates the overall gain.
   b. Time gain compensation (TGC): Compared with gain control, TGC adjusts gain at specified depth. The bottom control adjusts gain at the bottom of the image and the top control at the top of the image. Because ultrasound lines have minimum density at the bottom of the image, TGC is increased at the bottom, and the TGC at the top of the image is generally kept at low levels. This compensates for attenuation that occurs at the depth.
5. An appropriately positioned focus and number of focal zones are generally indicated on the side of the image.
6. Use a small Doppler box because a small box means a greater frame rate, which means more real-time images.
7. Use low Doppler PRF for low flow.
8. Use an appropriate Doppler angle (<60 degrees).

Special Imaging Modes

Tissue Harmonic Imaging (Fig. 2.22)

Harmonic imaging is a technique in ultrasonography that provides images of better quality as compared with conventional ultrasound technique by tuning the receiver to the high (harmonic) frequency alone, which are produced at a depth in the patient's body because of nonlinear propagation of sound.

Advantages of tissue harmonic imaging are improved lateral resolution caused by the narrow beam; elimination of near-field artifacts (e.g., noise and reverberation) because harmonic beams do not interact with superficial structures; elimination of grating lobes; increased signal-to-noise ratio; and improved resolution in obese patients. However, it is not so useful in superficial structures, and effects are lost in very deep structures.

Spatial Compounding

In conventional sonography, tissue is insonated from a single direction. Spatial compounding combines images obtained by insonating the target from multiple angles. It reduces speckle because only the signal is reinforced, but speckle being random is not reinforced. Consequently, granularity and noise are reduced in the image. Thus, detection of interfaces is improved.

Ultrasound Elastography

Ultrasound elastography or sonoelastography is used to detect different pathologies in tissues using the differences in mechanical properties of tissues such as stiffness and elasticity. These are assessed in response to mechanical pressure on tissue using sound waves. In contrast to conventional USG, which is based on bulk modulus, elastography is based on strain modulus, which has

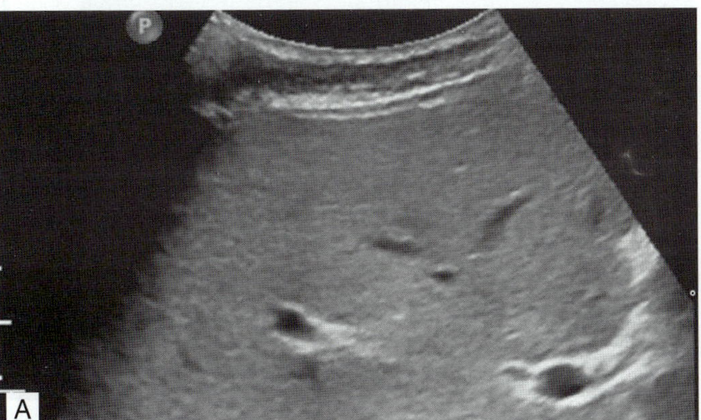

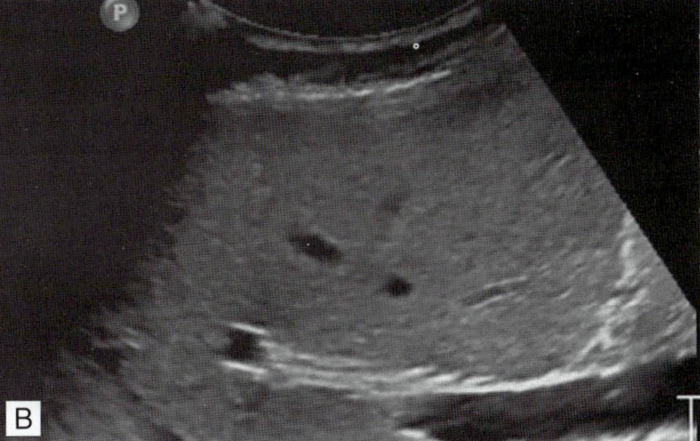

Figure 2.22 Harmonic imaging. Tissue harmonic imaging (B) reduces noise and clutter compared with a conventional image (A).

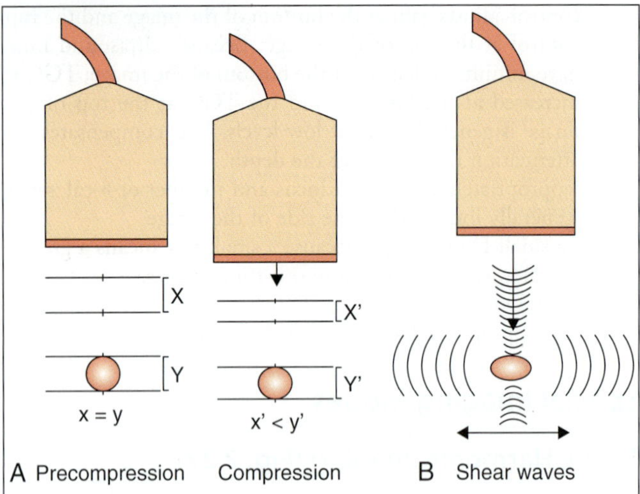

Figure 2.23 Elastography. (A) Strain elastography (SE) and (B) shear-wave elastography (SWE). The precompression frame is compared with a frame obtained after compression. In this example, the lesion is compressed much less than the surrounding tissue, indicating relative stiffness. SE is not quantitative and indicates only the relative hardness or softness of lesions compared with their surroundings. In SWE (B), high-intensity compression pulses from the transducer are focused on an area of interest, resulting in the generation of low-frequency transverse shear waves. Speckle displacement resulting from shear (transverse) waves is tracked with multiple imaging frames to estimate the shear-wave velocity. Shear-wave velocity is directly related to the Young modulus, permitting a quantitative estimate of tissue stiffness.

much higher dynamic range and thus permits much higher contrast resolution. Techniques include strain elastography (also known as static or compression elastography) and shear-wave or transient elastography (Fig. 2.23)

Strain elastography provides an indication of relative tissue stiffness (Fig. 2.24). Shear-wave elastography provides a quantitative estimate of the tissue stiffness (strain modulus) (Fig. 2.25).

Tissue stiffness or elasticity is expressed by the Young modulus—the ratio of compression pressure (stress) and the resulting deformation (strain). $E = \sigma/\varepsilon$, in which E is the Young modulus expressed in pascals (Pa); σ is the stress, expressed in Newtons; and ε is displacement expressed in meters squared (m^2).

Elastography has various applications, including (but not limited to) assessment of degree of hepatic fibrosis and characterization of liver lesions, diffuse renal parenchymal changes and characterization of renal lesions, breast mass diagnosis, prostate cancer detection, thyroid lesion characterization, and tendon imaging.

Three- and Four-Dimensional Ultrasonography

Three-dimensional USG or volume sonography converts standard 2D grayscale ultrasound images into a volumetric dataset by acquiring a large number of datasets of 2D images from patient. After acquisition, these volumetric data can be qualitatively and quantitatively assessed with the use of many analysis tools, such as surface and volume rendering, multiplanar imaging, and volume calculation techniques. It can also be postprocessed. Because of volume imaging, it is possible to display information in any orientation and any of the planes. If the 3D ultrasound is acquired and displayed over time, it is termed as *4D ultrasound, live 3D ultrasound, or real-time 3D ultrasound.*

Three-dimensional USG is particularly useful in gynecologic imaging because coronal images of the uterus can be obtained, thereby aiding in Mullerian anomaly identification (Fig. 2.26) and intrauterine contraceptive device (IUCD) position. It also helps in differentiating intrauterine pathologies such as endometrial polyps, fibroids, and adhesions.

Fusion or Hybrid Imaging

Fusion imaging enables the simultaneous display of real-time sonography and stored computed tomography (CT) or magnetic resonance imaging (MRI). A tracking system enables assessment of transducer position on the patient and automatically moves the CT or MRI image to correspond with the plane of the sonographic image. This has a combined advantage of CT/MRI and USG (i.e., better lesion detection and high resolution with improved biopsy guidance and the ability to assess relevant anatomy during tissue ablation using real-time sonography).

Intravascular Ultrasonography

In intravascular ultrasonography (IVUS), a miniature ultrasound transducer and a vascular catheter are paired. The IVUS probe is placed in the circulatory system, and the transducer analyzes the

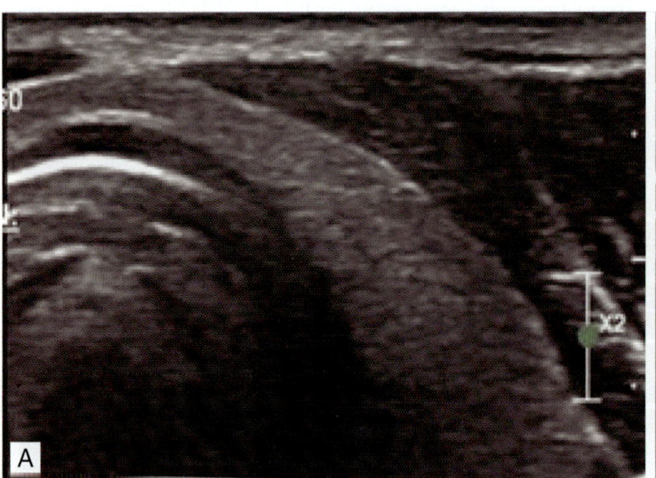

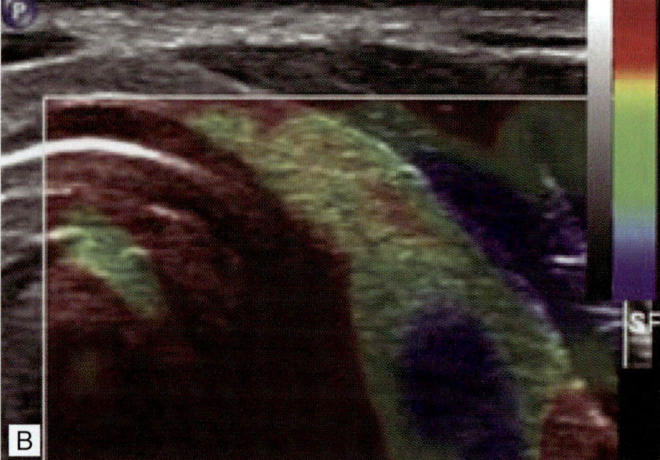

Figure 2.24 A gray-scale image (A) and strain elastogram (B) of a normal thyroid. In the elastogram, the color map displays relative stiffness with softer areas appearing as shades of red, orange, and yellow and stiffer areas as dark blue.

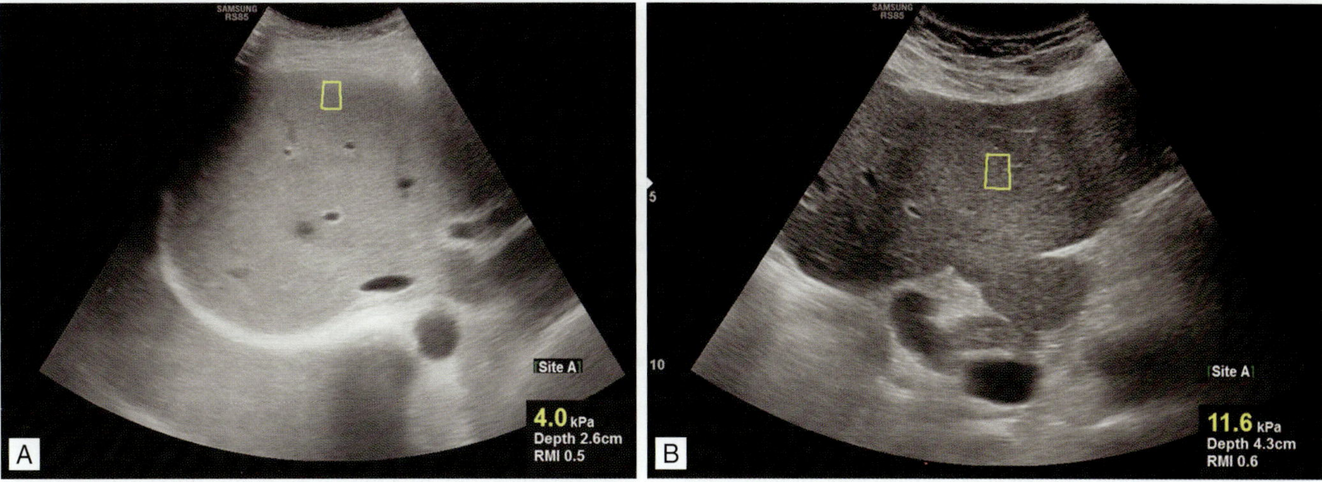

Figure 2.25 Shear-wave elastograms of a normal liver (A) and a cirrhotic liver (B). Increased tissue stiffness (Young modulus) is seen in cirrhotic liver because of hepatic fibrosis. The Young modulus measured in liver tissue samples by shear-wave elastography indicates a Young modulus of 4.0 kPa in the normal liver compared with a Young modulus of 11.6 kPa in the cirrhotic liver.

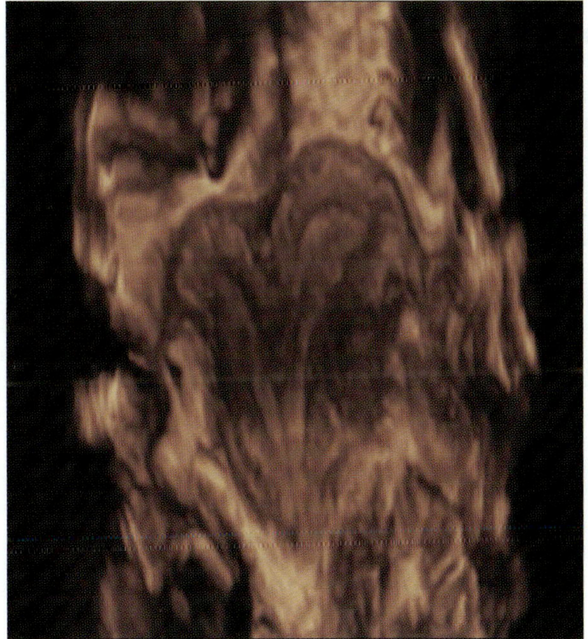

Figure 2.26 Transvaginal three-dimensional ultrasound image showing a bicornuate uterus.

vessel wall. The most important application is 2D assessment of plaque within vessels. A combination of IVUS and 3D sonography to provide improved diagnosis and enhanced treatment of otherwise difficult-to-evaluate vascular conditions holds future potential [2].

Contrast-Enhanced Ultrasonography

Ultrasound contrast agents are different from CT and MRI contrast and are encapsulated microbubbles containing air, nitrogen, or insoluble gaseous compounds such as perfluorocarbons with the majority having diameters from 3 to 5 µm. The stability of the gas is maintained by encapsulating it in a shell, such as human albumin and phospholipid. Being small in size, these microbubbles may also be used for tissue perfusion.

Contrast-enhanced ultrasonography (CEUS) is based on the large difference in acoustic impedance of these gas microbubbles and tissues, nonlinear compressibility of the gas bubbles, and the resultant shift in frequency of returning echoes that generates harmonics. The bubbles, being small compared with the wavelength of the ultrasound beam, act as a point source of sound, producing reflections in all directions.

- To fully use the properties of contrast agents, imaging techniques other than standard B-mode scans are necessary. CEUS enables visualization of exceedingly small blood vessels, even capillaries, and isoechoic tumors that would have otherwise been missed during routine sonographic imaging
- CEUS can assist in targeted delivery of drugs through a specialized outer shell and medication inside the bubble. After the microbubbles reach the area of interest, high-intensity sound waves can be used to pop the bubbles, releasing the medication contained within
- CEUS is also being used for noninvasive pressure measurements in the heart and liver [2]

The advantage of CEUS is that it can be used in patients in whom contrast-enhanced CT or contrast-enhanced MRI cannot be done because of renal failure or iodinated contrast allergy.

The major application of CEUS has been in liver lesion characterization based on contrast kinetics in these lesions. The scope has widened and includes assistance in intervention of isoechoic liver lesions; assessment of response to locoregional therapy for hepatocellular carcinoma; and evaluation of hepatic artery flow in liver transplant patients, especially when the hepatic artery is not accessible by Doppler because of postoperative edema.

The other areas where CEUS has been found useful includes the kidney, pancreas, and breast.

Nonvascular applications of CEUS include voiding sonocystourethrography for vesicoureteric reflux, sonohysterosalpingo contrast for tubal patency, CEUS-guided interventions such as percutaneous cholangiography, and delineation of abscesses and fistulae.

Therapeutic Applications of Ultrasonography

High-Intensity Focused Ultrasonography

High-intensity focused ultrasonography (HIFU) is based on three important capabilities of ultrasound, which are destruction of tissue at the focal zone using sufficiently high intensities, production of highly localized energy deposition by focusing the ultrasound beam, and the capability to control the location and size of the focal zone.

HIFU exploits thermal and cavitation bioeffects. Using HIFU at 1 to 3 MHz, high focal peak intensities of 5000 to 20,000 W/cm^2 may be achieved (routine diagnostic USG, 50–500 mW/ cm^2) [7]. With the ultrasound beam being focused on a small point several millimeters in size, rapid temperature elevation and resultant tissue coagulation can be achieved without causing damage to adjacent tissues. In general, elevation of tissue to a temperature of 60°C for 1 second is sufficient to produce coagulation necrosis [7].

HIFU is a promising tool for minimally invasive treatment of bleeding sites; uterine fibroids; and tumors in the prostate, liver, and breast. Similar to diagnostic USG, HIFU is also limited by the presence of gas or bone between the transducer and the target tissue. Unintended normal tissue heating and damage may occur along the reflected path of sound by reflection of high-energy ultrasound from strong interfaces produced by bowel gas, aerated lung, or bone.

HIFU can be done under USG or MR guidance. Advantage of USG guidance is its capability of verifying the acoustic window and sound path for the delivery of HIFU. Advantage of MR guidance is capability of monitoring temperature elevation during treatment, which is not possible with USG.

Ultrasound Safety and Bioeffects [8,9]

Although ultrasound is generally safe, there are some theoretical risks. To reduce the probability of these risks, a few values that must be monitored and kept within certain limits as follows:

- Thermal index: measures the ability of the ultrasound to heat up the local tissue
- Mechanical index: measures the maximum amplitude of the pressure pulse and indicates the risk of cavitation

Complications of Ultrasound

While complications of ultrasound are extremely rare in clinical practice, the following complications have been documented in the literature.

- Local heating: This is more with Doppler imaging because of a larger duration of pulse and high PRF are used, thereby increasing the amount of energy introduced in scanning (spectral Doppler > color Doppler > B-mode USG) [1]
- Cavitation: This is the action of an acoustic field within a fluid to generate bubbles. The pressure changes cause microbubbles in a liquid to expand increasingly and then collapse. There is an increased risk of cavitation in
  - gas-containing structures (e.g., bowel, lung),
  - low-frequency pulses (i.e., longer wavelengths),
  - higher power or intensity of pulses, and
  - use of ultrasound contrast agents.
- Mechanical damage to cell membranes

Suggested Readings

- P Hoskins, K Martin, A Thrush, Diagnostic Ultrasound: Physics and Equipment, third Edition, CRC Press, Boca Raton, FL, 2019.
- K Frederick, Sonography Principles and Instruments, Elsevier, 2022.
- M Rumack Carol, Diagnostic Ultrasound, Elsevier/Mosby, 2018.

3

Computed Tomography Physics

VAIBHAV NICHAT, NIKITA NANAWANI

Introduction

Computed tomography (CT) or computerized axial tomography was invented by Sir Godfrey Newbold Hounsfield in 1967 [1]. Hounsfield was an electric engineer with special interest in computers. While working as a senior researcher, he thought it could be possible to image an object with its internal constituents by acquiring x-rays at various angles. Later, he began working on computer software that could convert x-rays into images and eventually invented computed tomography, which was first used clinically in England in 1971. Hounsfield was felicitated with the Noble Prize in 1979 for his remarkable contribution in developing this new diagnostic technique [2]. CT technology has undergone many evolutions and advancements since then and is now one of the mainstay investigations in radiology, with approximately 75 million scans performed per year in the United States alone [3].

The standard CT attenuation value is called the Hounsfield unit (HU) in honor of its inventor. The HU value is a dimensionless universally accepted unit of CT used to express CT numbers in a standardized and convenient form [4]. HU values are derived from linear transformation of the measured attenuation coefficients and can be calculated using the following formula [5]:

$$\text{HU value} = 1000 \times (\mu^{\text{measured}} - \mu^{\text{water}})/\mu^{\text{water}}$$

[Attenuation coefficient (μ) of water is 0.192]

Hounsfield unit values of various substances and organs are listed in Table 3.1 [6].

The basic concepts of a CT scan are very similar to those of x-rays. An object essentially consists of multiple substances with different attenuation coefficients. X-rays from various angles are projected on the object. The attenuation values of the transmitted radiations are measured. Using various mathematical algorithms, a final reconstructed image is generated from these projections. Various methods of image reconstruction have been devised over a period of time to reduce image artifacts and to get a true image of an object, which will be discussed later in this chapter [5,7].

Components of a Computed Tomography Machine

Knowledge of various components of a CT machine is important to understand its functioning. Different components of CT scanners are described in Fig. 3.1. Their synchronous work generates an image spontaneously [5]. Before studying various components of a CT machine, we must know the orientation of the various axes used in CT. The *z*-axis is along the long axis of a patient lying on the tabletop, the *y*-axis is along the ground-ceiling plane, and the *x*-axis passes transversely across the patient, perpendicular to both the *y*- and *z*-axes [8].

X-ray Source

The basic design of a CT tube is similar to that of an x-ray machine. The main difference lies in the fact that the CT tube operates at a high mA and kV and a very high heat capacity (~4 MJ), with good heat dissipation. The tube voltage can fluctuate with a range of 80–140 kV, and the current can go up to 1000 mA. Power loading can reach up to a 100 kW. Cooling of the x-ray source happens by oil and air [9].

The tube rotates perpendicular to the *z*-axis of the patient. The arrangement of the x-ray tube in CT is made in such a way that anode–cathode axis lies parallel to the rotational axis to reduce the anode heel effect. Two sizes of focal spots are used in the CT x-ray tube—small for less power loading (0.6 mm for high-resolution CT scans) and large for higher power loading (~1 mm for other purposes). Depending on the movement of x-ray tube, scan time, and number of detectors, CT scanning has evolved across various generations, which are discussed subsequently [10].

TABLE 3.1 Hounsfield Unit Values of Various Substances and Organs

Substances	HU Value
Air	−1000
Lung	−500
Fat	−50 to −100
Water	0
Cerebrospinal fluid	15
Kidney	30
Blood	30–45
Muscle	10–40
Gray matter	37–45
White matter	20–30
Liver	40–60
Calcification	>80
Contrast	100–300
Cancellous bone	700
Cortical bone	3000

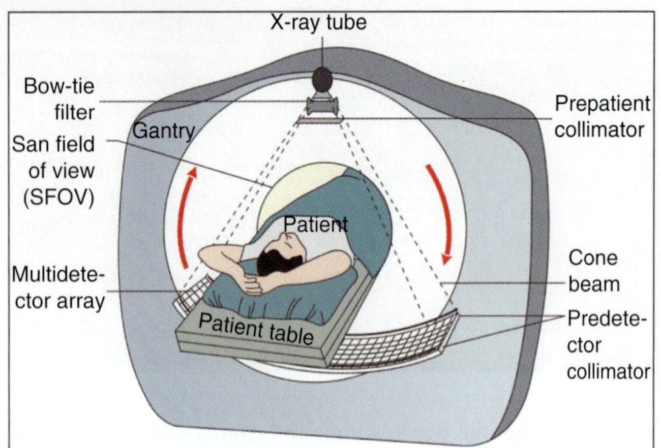

Figure 3.1 Schematic representation of a multidetector computed tomography scanner hardware and its parts.

Filter

The main purpose of the filter is to remove unwanted low-energy x-rays and reduce the direct patient dose. These low energy x-rays do not contribute to image generation. Filters also help in the formation of monochromatic beams and increase the mean energy of x-rays (beam hardening effect). A bow-tie filter is a special type of filter used in the newer generation CT scanners. It has a thinner portion in the center and a thicker portion at the periphery. The aims of this filter are to reduce unnecessary radiation dose to the periphery and make the dose evenly distributed in the center and peripheral part of the tissue [11].

Collimator

The collimator is a beam restrictor device allowing sufficient x-rays to pass through the patient to cover only the scanning area. *The purpose of the collimator is to reduce scatter radiation* [12].

Detector

Ionization chamber detectors were used previously in old CT scanners. Solid-state scintillating detectors are used in all modern CT scanners. They convert x-rays into light. Rare earth screen materials are used to improve intensification conversion factors and detector efficiency. All the detectors are mounted on an electronic array along with photomultiplier tubes, which provide power signals and simultaneously collect electronic information from them. These electronic signals are processed, amplified, and converted to digital forms and stored. Multidetectors are used in modern scanners. Slice thickness and resolution are determined by the detector size. Multiple detectors with smaller widths give better resolution. Five-millimater width detectors either give 5-mm thickness of slices or 10-mm thickness of slices [13]. *Ideal properties of the detector also include stability, noise-free response, wide dynamic range, low cost, small size, and negligible afterglow* [10].

Generator

The generator provides constant and stable power supply to the CT x-ray tube and detector array. *It helps in maintaining stable current and voltage over wide ranges, resulting in faster rotation of tube with reduction in scan time.* Because of the heavy weight of the generator, the gantry can only be tilted by up to 30 degrees [5].

Patient Table

The patient lies on the table as it moves through the gantry aperture while scanning. It is machine driven and manufactured to sustain heavy weights of greater than 200 kg in some modern scanners [10].

Console

The CT room is equipped with one to three console monitors for imaging, postprocessing of images, and viewing of images. Patient entry, details, protocol selection, optimizing technical factors, postprocessing of the images, and filming can be done on the console. It can be connected with the online software Radiology Information System (RIS) and picture archiving and communication system (PACS) network [9].

Computed Tomography Generations

Multidetector and slip-ring technology are the newest advances in CT scanners that have enabled faster acquisition of image data, allowing for diversifying the use across a number of high-end applications in different body systems [9]. In the earlier generation CT scanners, electric cables were connected from a stationary x-ray generator to a rotating x-ray tube and likewise from a rotating detector system to the reconstruction computer system. As a result, the gantry had to rotate back to prevent entanglement and overstretching of electric cables, reducing the speed of acquisition. To solve this limitation, slip-ring technology was developed to allow free movement of the x-ray tube and gantry without any coiling of electric cables. *The slip ring has two parts, a metal ring and a connector. The metal ring is mounted on the outer part of the gantry. Detector arrays are connected to this metal ring with a connector. This helps in smooth transfer of collected data from detector arrays to the metal ring with continuous, unidirectional motion of the gantry while also maintaining electrical contact with the stationary generator component* [8]. This being the basic electro-mechanical building block for modern CT led to sequential improvements in CT technology, reducing scan times and helping parallelly transmit continuous data for image reconstruction [12]. Improvement in various technologies in the CT scan led to evolution of different generations of scanners as listed in Table 3.2.

In the first- and second-generation CT scanners, the source and detector were rigidly coupled with each other; in the translate and rotate type of scanners, the source and detector were located on the opposite sides of the patient. Each projection was acquired during a translation motion, after which the source and detector assembly would have to rotate to acquire the next projection using another translate motion. Multiple such projections would then be used to create an image for that cross section. The patient table would then move to acquire the next set of projections to create the next image. The *first-generation* scanners used a pencil beam and a single detector system and had a longer scan acquisition time of approximately 30 minutes. The *second-generation* scanners reduced scan acquisition time using a thin fan beam of x-rays with multiple detectors arranged in a linear array along the x–y axis [5].

The translate–rotate scanners were replaced by the rotate–rotate type in subsequent CT generations.

The introduction of *third-generation* scanners removed the translator motion and covered the whole cross section of patient in a single rotation by mounting multiple detectors in an arc fashion, helping in continuous data acquisition [14].

In the *fourth-generation* scanners, the detector elements were removed from the rotating gantry and placed as a stationary layer

TABLE 3.2 Various Generations of Computed Tomography Scanners

First generation	■ Translate and rotate type ■ Single source and detector with fixed coupling ■ Source and detector work as an assembly. They first move together and later rotate to image a single slice. ■ Uses pencil beam x-ray ■ *Moves 1 degree at a time (to image a slice, it would take 180 degree rotation)* ■ Longer scan time (~30 min) [5]
Second generation	■ Translate and rotate type ■ Single source with multiple detectors (~30) ■ Uses a fan beam ■ Shorter scan time (~90 sec) [5]
Third generation	■ Rotate and rotate type (no translator motion) ■ *Single source with multiple detectors (~300–700)* ■ Uses a fan beam ■ Moves with more arc coverage ■ Shorter scan time (4–9 sec) ■ Better image quality [14]
Fourth generation	■ *Rotate and fixed type (rotator x-ray tube and stationary row of circular detectors)* ■ Single x-ray source and multiple detectors in range of thousands ■ Wider fan beam ■ Scan time is further shortened ■ Disadvantage: less spatial separation than third-generation computed tomography (CT) scanners [19]
Fifth generation	■ *Stationary and stationary type (source and detectors are both fixed)* ■ *Also known as ultrafast CT or electron-beam CT* ■ Used for cardiac imaging ■ Very short scan time in milliseconds [16]
Sixth generation	■ Combination of helical scanning, third- or fourth-generation scanner, and slip-ring technology ■ Allows three- and fourth-dimensional imaging protocol acquisitions in one breath hold [17]
Seventh generation	■ Multiple array of detectors ■ *Uses cone beam* ■ Disadvantage: Increased scatter radiation because of the cone beam [17]

of detectors outside the arc of the x-ray tube [15]. Fig. 3.2 illustrates the designs of first- to fourth-generation CT scanners.

Fifth-generation CT (electron-beam CT) was invented to remove the mechanical component of the CT machine, and it replaced the x-ray tube with an electron-beam scanner that was deflected around the patient onto a half-circle tungsten target to generate the x-rays, which were detected by a detector ring on the opposite side. Because of the high cost of running this equipment, it was discontinued shortly after a few years of usage [16].

The *sixth-generation* helical CT scanners allowed continuous x-ray generation because of the ability of the table to continuously rotate around the patient and allowing table movement to happen simultaneously. This created an image in a helical or spiral pattern and allowed whole-body scanning in a matter of seconds. It is the most widely used CT scanner with the basic design of a third- or fourth-generation scanner *along with the addition of slip-ring technology* [17].

The method of generation of the x-ray beam has also undergone advances with cone beam now used in modern

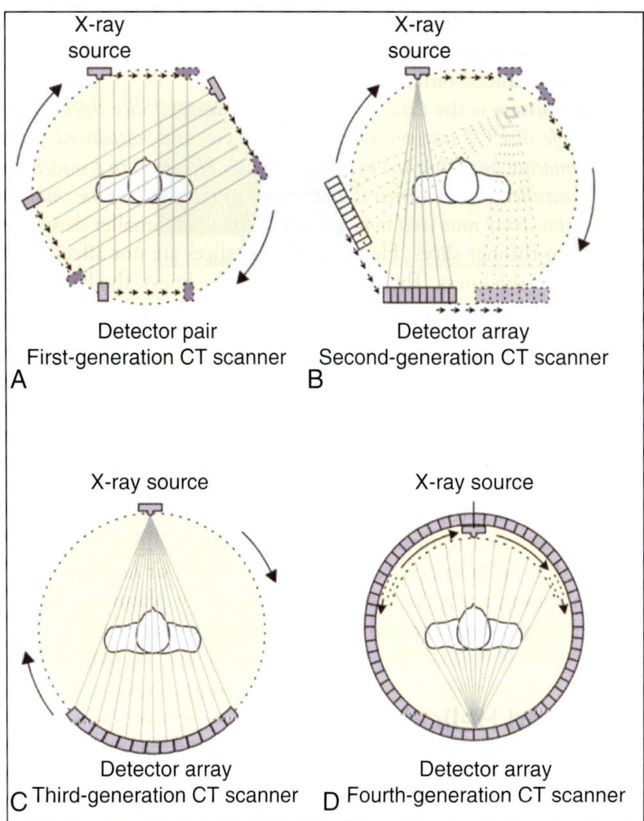

Figure 3.2 (A–D) Schematic diagrams showing various types of computed tomography generations.

seventh-generation CT scanners. This allows having multiple rows of detectors and allowing larger z-axis coverage per rotation. Dual-energy and dual-source CT scanners use the same principle of tube and detector assemblies [15,18]. *Helical scan acquisition with multiple rows of detectors is also known as multidetector CT or multislice CT.*

Parameters for Image Acquisition and Modes of Scanning

There are some basic parameters that a radiologist should be aware of that impact the quality of scanning, speed of acquisition, and radiation dose. The radiologist can modify these parameters to optimize scanning for different body areas. The manufacturers of CT equipment provide preset scanning protocols for different body areas and applications. Depending on the institution's own policies, processes, and experience, these can be modified and stored on the console as institution-specific protocols.

Rotation time *is the time taken by the x-ray tube to complete one rotation around a patient.* A faster scan helps to minimize motion artifacts with good spatial resolution [15].

Pitch *is defined as the distance traveled by the table during a single rotation divided by the total width of simultaneously acquired slices.* Pitch is an important entity that decides the scan time and resolution. There are two methods to calculate pitch in a multislice scanner [15].

- In a single-slice CT scanner, pitch is the table distance traveled in a single 360-degree rotation divided by the width of the slice
- Multislice scanner pitch (also known as beam pitch) is the table distance traveled in a single 360-degree gantry rotation divided by the total thickness of all simultaneously acquired slices

TABLE 3.4 Factors Affecting Spatial Resolution

Spatial resolution can be increased by

- **Decreasing pixel size:** Pixel size is directly proportional to the field of view (FOV) and inversely proportional to the matrix size.
- **Decreasing FOV:** A smaller FOV leads to smaller pixel size and increased spatial resolution.
- **Increasing matrix:** Pixel size decreases by increasing the matrix size.
- **Type of algorithm:** High-resolution algorithms such as bony algorithms have higher spatial resolution. Soft tissue kernels have less spatial resolution.
- **Small size of detector:** A smaller thickness of the detector means that the detector has to cover a smaller area of interest, leading to increase in spatial resolution.
- **Smaller focal spot size:** The smaller the width of the x-ray projection path, the greater the spatial resolution.
- **Increasing sampling frequency:** It gives finer resolution of an image because of increasing details of tissue acquired.
- **Decreasing slice thickness:** The thinner the section thickness, the higher the resolution. It also helps in mitigating partial-volume effects.
- **Decreasing pitch:** Resolution is increased by decreasing pitch.
- **Decreased patient motion:** Patient motion degrades spatial resolution.
- **Isometric imaging:** Increases spatial resolution in all planes.

TABLE 3.5 Factors Affecting Contrast Resolution

Contrast resolution can be increased by

- **Decreasing kV:** Increasing kV increases the mean energy of the x-ray beam, leading to increased penetrating power through tissue and decreasing contrast resolution.
- **Increasing tube current and decreasing noise:** Noise is decreased by increasing the tube current, increasing the contrast resolution.
- **Tissue characteristics:** Tissues having greater difference in linear attenuation coefficient have more contrast resolution. For example, it is very easy to differentiate between calcium and fat.
- **Contrast media:** Both oral and intravenous contrast media increase contrast resolution.

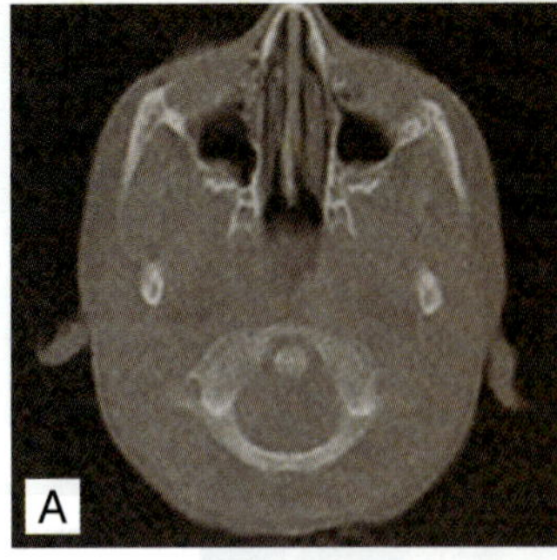

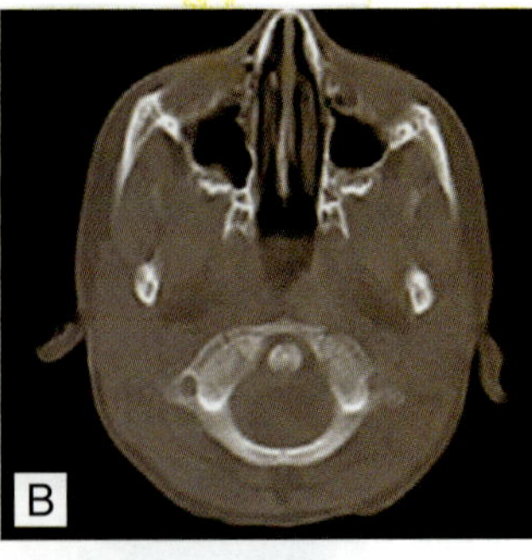

Figure 3.14 (A) An image with noise. (B) An image without noise.

Noise is decreased by increasing the number of photons, tube current, kilovoltage, rotation time of the gantry, and slice thickness and by using advanced reconstruction algorithms [34].

Artifacts

Computed tomography artifacts are deviation of HU values of tissue in the reconstructed image from their actual HU values. Artifacts deteriorate image quality and can obscure or imitate pathologies. Depending on the source of origin, they are divided into the following four types [36,37].

1. **Patient-related artifacts:** Various subtypes of patient-related artifacts, their causes, and correction techniques are discussed in Table 3.6 [36]
2. **Physics-related artifacts:** These are caused by processes involved in CT scanning and recovering data. The types of physics-related artifacts with correction techniques are discussed in Table 3.7 [36]
3. **Hardware-related artifacts:** These are the result of errors, imbalances, calibration drifts, malfunctions, and measurement inaccuracies in hardware design. They are discussed in Table 3.8 [36]

TABLE 3.6 Patient-Related Artifacts

Subtype	Causes	Correction Techniques
Motion artifact: It happens because of voluntary or involuntary movements of the patient. This can lead to misregistration of data and manifests as directional shading and streaking in reconstructed images. The streaks occur between high-contrast edges and the x-ray tube position when motion occurs (Fig. 3.15).	▪ Respiratory chest movements ▪ Cardiac pulsations ▪ Vascular pulsations ▪ Swallowing mechanism ▪ Unconscious movements	▪ Reducing scan time ▪ Helical acquisition ▪ Cardiac electrocardiographic gating ▪ Proper breath holding ▪ Proper patient instructions on the need to stay still ▪ Use of positioning supports ▪ Specialized motion correction software ▪ Sedation and immobilization may be used in pediatric and unconscious or uncooperative patients
Metallic artifact: Artifacts are more with elements that have high atomic numbers than those with low atomic numbers (Fig. 3.16).	▪ Metal objects within the region of interest ▪ Earrings ▪ Dental braces ▪ Metal clips ▪ Body implants	▪ Removing all removable metal items before scanning ▪ Angulating the gantry to avoid metal objects within the scanning field ▪ Increasing kV to increase penetration ▪ Metal artifact reduction software on newer scanners
Incomplete projection: Artifacts are produced by objects lying outside the region of interest of scanning (Fig. 3.17).	▪ Artifacts of the hands lying by the side of body in chest and abdomen scans	▪ Proper positioning so that nothing lies outside the field of the scan

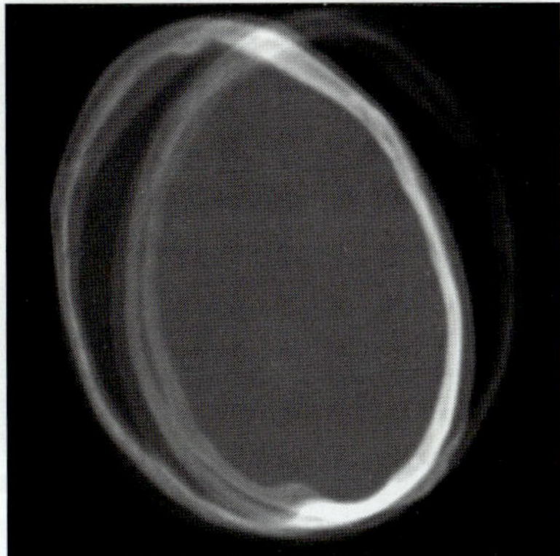

Figure 3.15 Noncontrast computed tomography head showing a motion artifact.

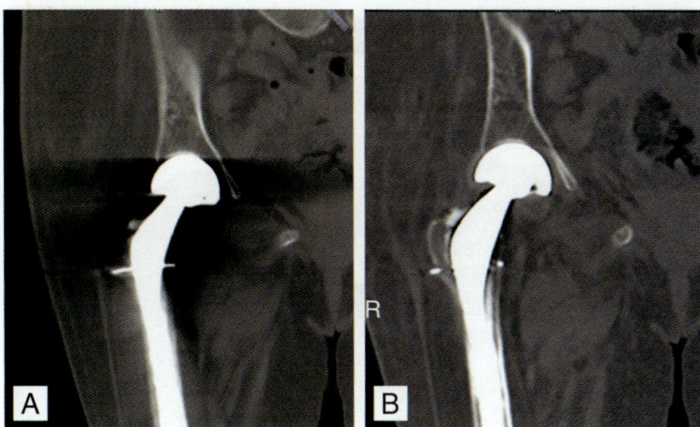

Figure 3.16 (A) Metallic artifact caused by a femur implant. (B) Neutralization of the artifact using metal artifact reduction software.

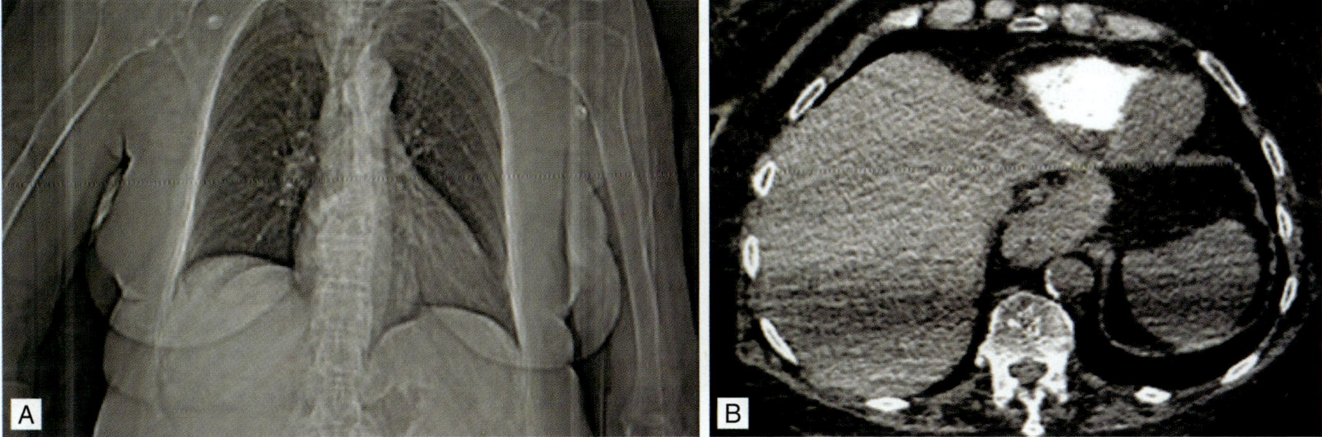

Figure 3.17 (A) CT topograph of chest showing both the arms lying by the side of body. (B) Asymmetrical linear low-density bands seen over the liver and spleen because of incomplete projection of the arms lying by the side of body, causing degradation of image quality.

TABLE 3.7 Physics-Related Artifacts

Subtype	Causes	Correction Techniques
Cupping artifact	■ When polychromatic x-rays pass through the center of the cylinder, rays get hardened more than when they pass through the peripheral part of the cylinder. When these hardened beams pass through an object, attenuation of an object gets altered compared with the original attenuation.	■ Tilting the gantry ■ Appropriate calibration ■ Use of a bow-tie filter ■ Iterative reconstruction algorithms using software correction
Steak and dark bands: It is also a type of beam-hardening artifact (Fig. 3.18).	■ When the x-ray beam passes between two dense objects, streak and dark bands are generated. ■ Artifact is seen in scans with dense bony regions or high-density intravenous contrast.	■ Beam-hardening correction software ■ Use of a prehardened beam by the filter ■ Calibration of machine
Partial volume: The CT number of a particular voxel is the average of CT numbers of all the tissue in that voxel (Fig. 3.19).	■ Blurring of image ■ Size overestimation ■ Inadequate spatial resolution	■ Thinner acquisition ■ Iterative reconstruction ■ Increased reconstruction filter ■ Increased tube potential
Photon starvation (Fig. 3.20)	■ When the x-ray beam has to pass through an area of large thickness, most of the photons get removed, and only a few photons are left to image the remaining structures, producing noise and streak like artifact caused by photon starvation.	■ Automated tube current modulation, which helps in increasing photon release when the beam has to pass through a larger thickness of tissue than a narrow portion ■ Adaptive filtration software smoothens out the image in the region of photon starvation and reduces noise.

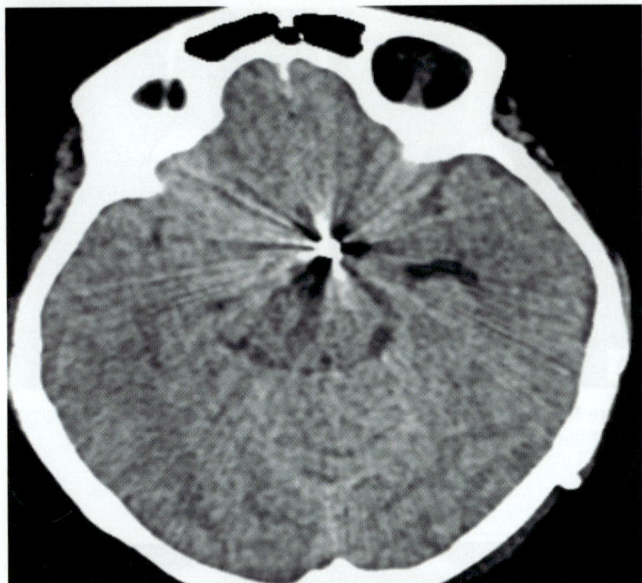

Figure 3.18 Streak and dark bands artifact. Multiple alternate hyperdense and hypodense bands are seen because of anterior communicating artery aneurysm coiling.

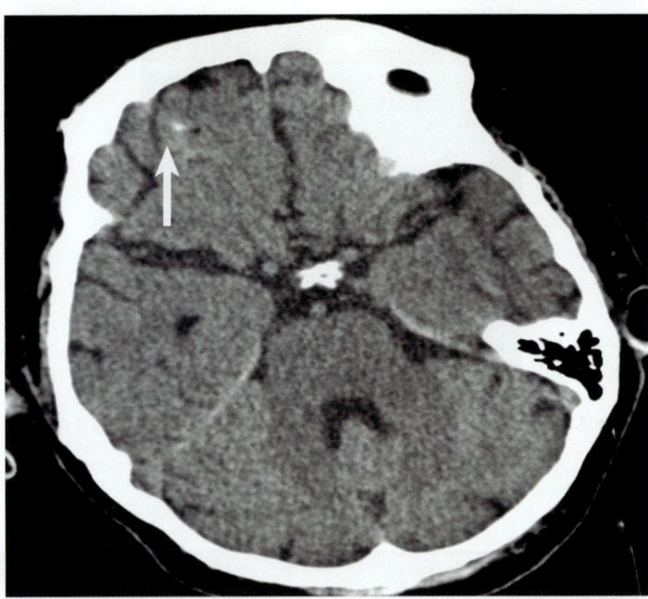

Figure 3.19 Partial-volume artifact of temporal bone seen as a calcific focus (*arrow*) in the right frontal lobe.

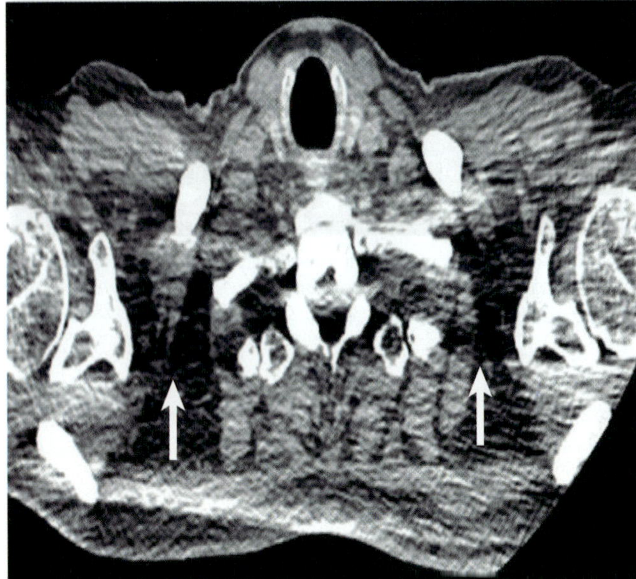

Figure 3.20 Computed tomography scan of the shoulder region shows that attenuation is much higher in the lateral direction than the anteroposterior (AP) direction. Projections in the lateral direction are "photon starved" and show higher noise than those in the AP direction, resulting in photon starvation artifact in the lateral direction (*arrows*).

4. **Helical- and multisection-related artifacts:** These arise because of reconstruction algorithms. Table 3.9 describes subtypes of helical- and multisection-related artifacts along with their causes and correction techniques [36,37]

TABLE 3.8 Hardware-Related Artifact

Subtype	Causes	Correction Techniques
Ring artifact: This artifact is more common in solid-state detectors than xenon gas detectors. They rarely simulate any pathology (Fig. 3.21).	▪ Uniform circular or semicircular artifact is produced at every rotation due to faulty detector.	▪ Repair of faulty detector ▪ Recalibration of machine ▪ Software correction

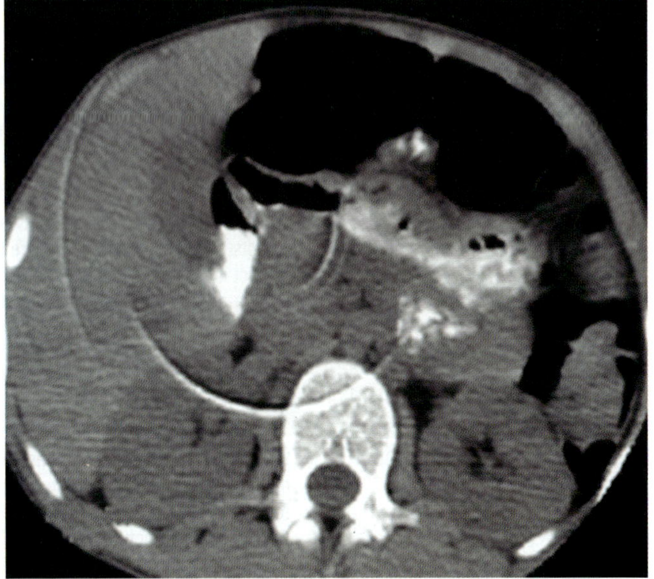

Figure 3.21 Ring artifact caused by a defective detector.

Dosimetry

Radiation originating from CT examinations is a major contributor of radiation dose to the patient population from medical purposes. There is a concern regarding radiation doses because of these examinations in both children and adults; this

TABLE 3.9 Helical- and Multisection-Related Artifacts

Subtype	Causes	Correction Techniques
Helical artifact (Fig. 3.22)	▪ Helical artifact is seen during image generation and reconstruction, causing distortion of image due to rapid anatomic change in structure along the *z*-axis when the gantry rotates around the patient.	▪ Correction software ▪ Advanced reconstruction algorithms
Cone-beam artifact	▪ Wider collimation helps in collecting larger data because of an increased number of slices per rotation in the cone beam. Artifacts are more for the outer row of detectors because of off-center positioning of objects leading to apparent elongation of data. Artifacts are more common in 64-slice scanners than 32-slice scanners.	▪ New reconstruction techniques
Stair-step artifact (Fig. 3.23)	▪ It is seen on reformatted images after scanning at wide interval in between two projections. ▪ It can be identified around the corners of the scanned object.	▪ Thin slice acquisition ▪ Overlapping image reconstructions ▪ Multidetector CT scanners eliminate this artifact
Zebra artifact	▪ It is seen caused by helical interpolation of the data process producing noise inhomogeneity along the *z*-axis. ▪ Thin dark lines are seen at regular intervals in reformatted images with helical multisection scans. ▪ Noise is generated in reformatted images that are reconstructed from helical scans.	▪ Thin collimation ▪ Longer scan duration

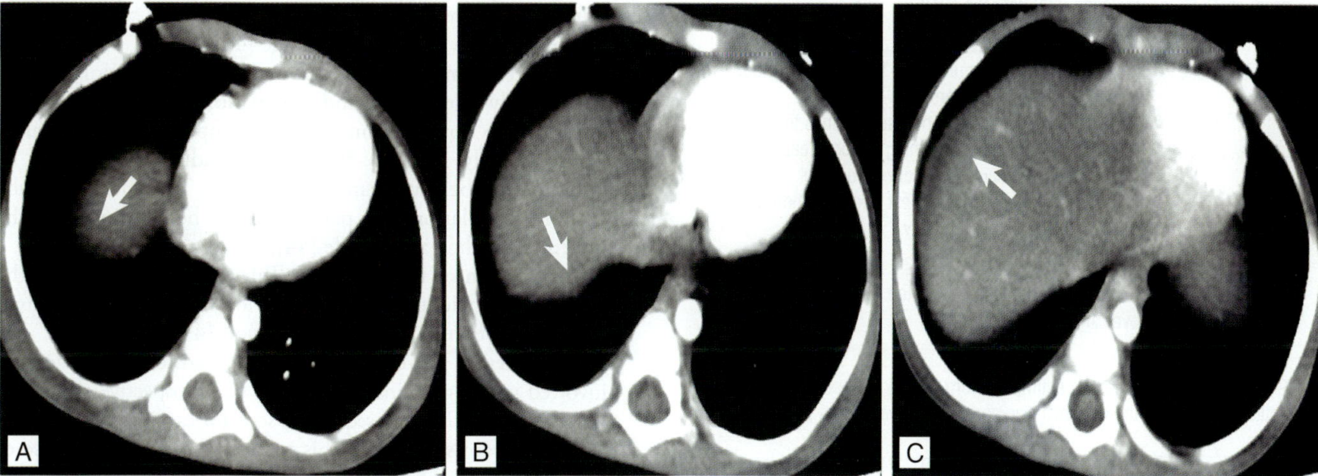

Figure 3.22 A to C, Helical artifact. Contrast-enhanced computed tomography scan of abdomen at the liver sections shows helical curved low-attenuation areas at the margins of liver as indicated by the white arrows.

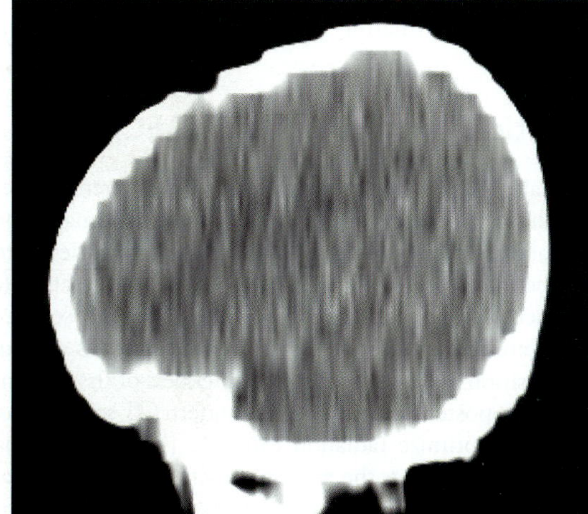

Figure 3.23 Stair-step artifact. Sagittal reformatted image of computed tomography (CT) head scanning at a 5-mm reconstruction interval. In modern imaging, these are usually seen with a lower row multidetector CT.

is discussed in more detail in Chapter 5. CT is used for diagnostic and intervention imaging as well as radiation planning, and monitoring radiation exposure is important [12].

The CT dose index is a universal standardized unit used to measure the radiation dose output of a CT scanner machine. Various dose indices have been developed over a period of time to measure radiation exposure caused by CT and are discussed in Table 3.10. These are automatically provided by CT machines for every scan [12].

Dose reference levels of various types of adult CT scans are displayed in the tabulated format in Table 3.11 [38]. Almost all the CT scanners calculate and display these values as a part of patient information at the end of scan as mentioned in Fig. 3.24 [39].

Dose Optimization and Factors Affecting Patient Dose

Computed tomography scanner manufacturers have been striving to develop various optimization techniques to reduce radiation doses to patients while at the same time generating quality images

TABLE 3.10 Computed Tomography Dose Indices

CT dose index (CTDI)	▪ It is a dose calculated from single rotation of gantry using a pencil ionization chamber. ▪ Unit: mGy [13]
$CTDI_{100}$	▪ It is the dose calculated over a length of 100 mm using a pencil ionization chamber. ▪ Unit: mGy [13]
$CTDI_w$ (weighted average)	▪ It is the weighted average dose of the central and peripheral parts of the organ covered in the scan. ▪ It is an adjusted dose for spatial variation because the dose at the periphery is more than at the center. ▪ $CTDI_w = 1/3\ CTDI_{100}$ of central part + $2/3\ CTDI_{100}$ of peripheral part ▪ Unit: mGy [40]
$CTDI_{vol}$	▪ It is the radiation dose calculated for the volume of the scanned organ. ▪ $CTDI_{vol} = CTDI_w/pitch$ ▪ To keep uniformity in radiation dose measurement, $CTDI_{vol}$ is widely used. ▪ Unit: mGy [41]
Dose-length product (DLP)	▪ DLP can be calculated by multiplying the length of the scan (cm) with the $CTDI_{vol}$. ▪ Unit: mGycm [41]
Effective dose	▪ It can be derived by multiplying the DLP with organ-specific conversion factors. ▪ Different tissues have differing sensitivities to radiation, so the tissue-weighing factor of each organ can be used to calculate the effective dose. ▪ Conversion factors for the chest and abdomen are 0.014 and 0.015, respectively. ▪ Unit: mSv [41]
Multiple-scan average dose (MSAD)	▪ It is an average dose calculated over multiple scans over an interval length [41].
Size-specific estimated dose	▪ It can be estimated from $CTDI_{vol}$, measurements of the patient's size and conversion factors [42].

TABLE 3.11 European Dose References Levels for an Adult Patient for Various Computed Tomography Scans

Dose Reference Levels	$CTDI_{vol}$ (mGy)	DLP (mGycm)	Effective Dose (mSv)
CT of the head	60	1050	2
CT of the chest	30	650	12
CT of the abdomen	35	780	13
CT of the pelvis	35	570	10

$CTDI_{vol}$, computed tomography dose index volume; *CT*, computed tomography; *DLP*, dose-length product.

for diagnosis. Radiologists should make every effort to decrease the radiation dose and follow the principle of ALARA (as low as reasonable achievable) while maintaining image quality.

- Minimizing the scan range of CT scan is a straightforward way to achieve this goal
- For multiphase CT protocols, the number of required phases should be minimized
- Noncontrast scan should be obtained only when needed

Total mAs: 2483	Total DLP: 736							
	Scan	Q.ref.mAs @120kV	kV	Q.ref. mAs	eff. mAs	CTDIvol* mGy	DLP mGycm	T rot. s
Patient Position HFS								
Topogram	100		Sn100		60 mA	0.01 L	0	
NCCT Abdomen	200	110	120	110	51	4.54 L	211	0.5
Premonitoring	300	20	100	28	6	0.24 L	0	0.5
Monitoring	405	20	100	28	6	1.22 L	1	0.5
CECT Abdomen	500	110	120	110	51	4.59 L	213	0.5
CECT Abdomen	600	110	120	110	51	4.54 L	211	0.5
CECT Abdomen	700	110	120	110	42	3.75 L	100	0.5

Figure 3.24 Triple-phase computed tomography (CT) scan of an abdomen done for gastrointestinal bleed. The dose chart shows the CT dose index and dose-length product (DLP) of various phases. The effective dose can be calculated by adding the individual DLP (total DLP, 736 mGycm) and then multiplying it with conversion factor of abdomen (0.015). The effective dose in this scan is 11.04 mSv.

- Clinical indication and protocol of CT perfusion should be determined because of the associated substantial radiation dose

Other useful dose optimizing strategies are discussed in the following section [43].

Body size–adapted CT protocols: This is a principal part of optimizing CT doses. Optimal tube voltage and current should be determined for patients of each body size to obtain a diagnostic range of images by keeping radiation doses to the minimum. To reduce image noise, higher tube current should be used along with low CT voltage [44].

Tube current modulation: Tube current modulation according to body size, shape, and attenuation parameters contributes to dose optimization without hampering image quality. Approximately 25% to 50% of the radiation dose can be reduced by tube current modulation [45]. To avoid faulty tube current modulation, the patient should be positioned at the isocenter on the gantry table [44].

Optimization of tube voltage: This is done by selecting the most dose efficient tube voltage. A lower tube voltage is used for contrast-enhanced CT examination [45].

Scan modes: A low-dose scan mode is used to reduce the dose involved in CT examinations such as in a prospective electrocardiography (ECG)-gated sequential scan for cardiac imaging [46].

Iterative reconstruction: This reduces the quantum noise of an image without hampering image quality such as spatial and temporal resolution. It uses less projection and low-dose data. This helps in reduction of radiation dose to the patient with a reduction in noise. This benefit is most apparent in low-dose CT acquisitions in which noise obscures visualization of clinically relevant information [24].

Automatic Exposure Control (AEC)

The optimal dose requirement is different for different tissues. For example, the same kV and mA are not sufficient to image both the chest and abdomen appropriately. Instead, the dose varies from slice to slice, especially in spiral acquisition. Dynamic modulation (angular adjustment) of the tube current is done by the x-ray source while spiral scans are acquired. For example, more current is used during lateral acquisition because of increased thickness of tissue compared with the anteroposterior direction. All modern CT scanners use this technology to optimize radiation exposure [47]. The mechanism behind AEC depends on the x-ray numbers and energies reaching the detectors. The detectors accordingly give feedback to the tube to modulate current according to the size and attenuation properties of the tissue being imaged. As attenuation increases, tube current also increases and vice versa. While imaging varying thickness of tissue,

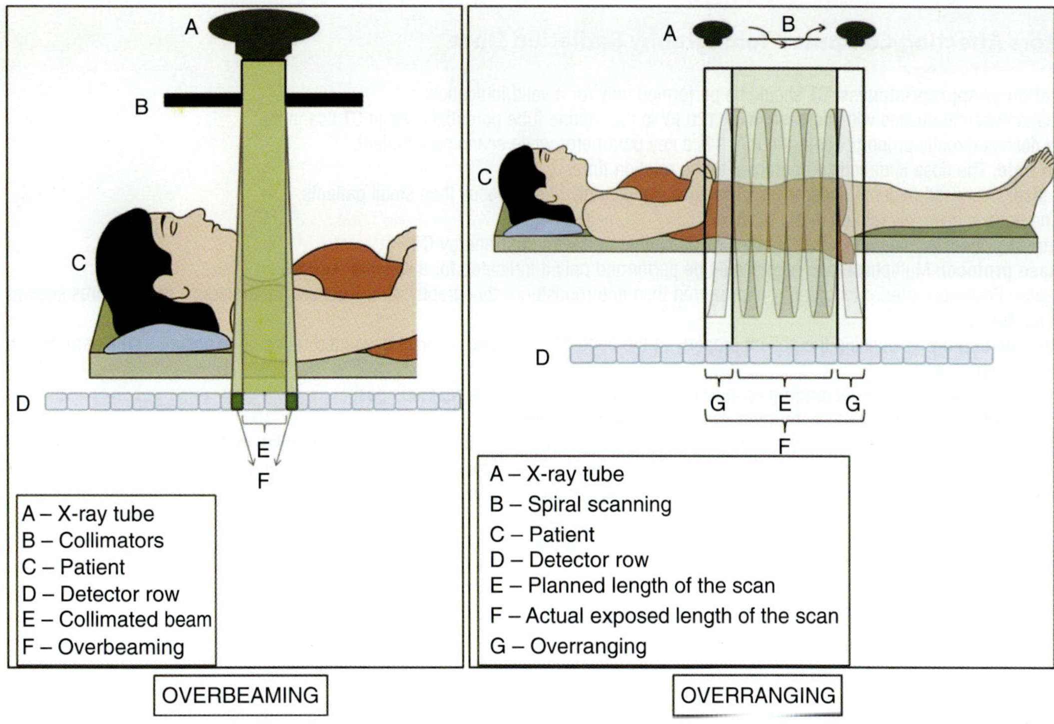

Figure 3.25 Schematic self-explanatory diagram showing the effect of overbeaming and overranging in computed tomography with adaptive collimation.

current modulation is done by the data collected during the scanogram. Up to 50% of radiation can be reduced with this technology. While imaging pediatric patients, kV should be reduced because AEC only deals with current modulation [48].

Overbeaming and Overranging

In a single-slice CT scanner, the fan beam width corresponds exactly to or less than the detector width. In a multidetector CT scanner, the width of the fan beam is always greater than the detector width because all the effective operating detectors should be covered by it. During this process, the fan beam projects outside the effective operating row of detectors, resulting in excessive radiation dose to the patient and simultaneously not contributing to image generation. This effect is known as overbeaming (Fig. 3.25). Although it may appear as a small dose over a single slice, it adds up over the length of the scan and increases the overall radiation dose to the patient [49].

Because of the need for reconstruction of images, spiral CT machines scan patients a little more at the ends of the area of interest. To interpolate the data, this extra scanning at the beginning and end of area of interest is necessary. This excessive scanning at the end of area of interest is not wasted as in overbeaming; it is used for reconstruction of images. This is called overranging (see Fig. 3.25). *Modern CT scanners use adaptive or dynamic collimation to reduce the radiation dose to patients by up to 40% at the beginning and end of scanning.* Dynamic collimators are mechanical blades that move inward and outward of the radiation field to reduce overranging [50].

The approach and techniques to reduce radiation dose are described in Table 3.12 [51,52].

Advanced Computed Tomography Applications

With a great demand to assess functional and molecular information in addition to anatomic information, multiple advances have happened in CT scanners. A few of these are discussed here in brief [53]. Readers can read more details in the individual chapters pertaining to these topics.

Cardiac Computed Tomography

It is now possible to image the heart and coronary arteries because of improved spatial and temporal resolution of CT scanners enabled by ECG gating. High-resolution cardiac images can be reconstructed at any phase because of ECG-gating and breath-hold technique. ECG gating can be prospective or retrospective. In retrospective gating, a scan is acquired during a complete cardiac cycle, and cardiac function can also be calculated. In prospective gating, the scan is specially acquired during the end diastole phase to reduce the radiation exposure to the patient [54].

Computed Tomography Perfusion

The same body part is scanned repeatedly after contrast administration over a defined period of time in perfusion CT. Different organs have different acquisition times for perfusion scanning; for example, myocardial perfusion takes around 30 seconds, and brain perfusion takes 40–60 seconds. Various parameters are calculated in perfusion studies such as mean transit time, time to peak, blood flow, and blood volume and are plotted graphically or on color-coded maps (Fig. 3.26). Radiation dose is an issue in CT perfusion caused by repeated and continuous scanning of a particular organ; the radiation dose is generally five times higher than in a routine scan. A few current and evolving applications of CT perfusion techniques are listed below [55].

- To evaluate acute stroke [56]
- To identify occult malignancies [57]
- To characterize lesions into benign and malignant [57]
- To monitor therapeutic response of various treatment regimes on tumors [57]

TABLE 3.12 Factors Affecting Computed Tomography Radiation Dose

1. **Justification or appropriateness:** CT should be performed only for a valid indication.
2. **kV:** Radiation dose increases with increase in kV. 120 kV is the routine tube potential used in CT scanners.
3. **mA:** The dose is directly proportional to the mA. It is a key parameter while scanning a patient.
4. **Rotation time:** The dose is directly proportional to the rotation time.
5. **Patient size:** Oversized patients undergoing CT receive significantly higher doses than small patients.
6. **Pitch:** The dose is inversely related to the pitch.
7. **Noncontrast phase:** Virtual noncontrast images can be generated with dual-energy CT.
8. **Multiphase protocol:** Multiphase scanning should be performed only if indicated for a specific purpose.
9. **Topography:** Posterior-anterior topography is preferred than anteroposterior topography; this reduces radiation dose to structures such as the gonads, thyroid, and breast.
10. **Isocenter positioning:** Positioning the patient properly at the center of the table reduces unwanted radiation exposure to the periphery according to the inverse square law.
11. **Reducing overbeaming and overranging** (discussed in the text) decreases the radiation dose.
12. **AEC and iterative reconstruction techniques** reduce radiation exposure.
13. **Bow-tie filters:** Beam hardening causes elimination of low-energy x-rays, which are sources of the radiation dose.
14. **Cardiac imaging:** Use of prospective gating has significantly lower radiation dose than retrospective gating.
15. **Section thickness:** An increased radiation dose is associated with thinner collimation.
16. **Scan length:** The radiation dose is directly proportional to the scan length.
17. **Dual source CT:** Dual-source CT can produce good image quality at a similar or lower radiation dose than single-source CT.

AEC, automatic exposure control.

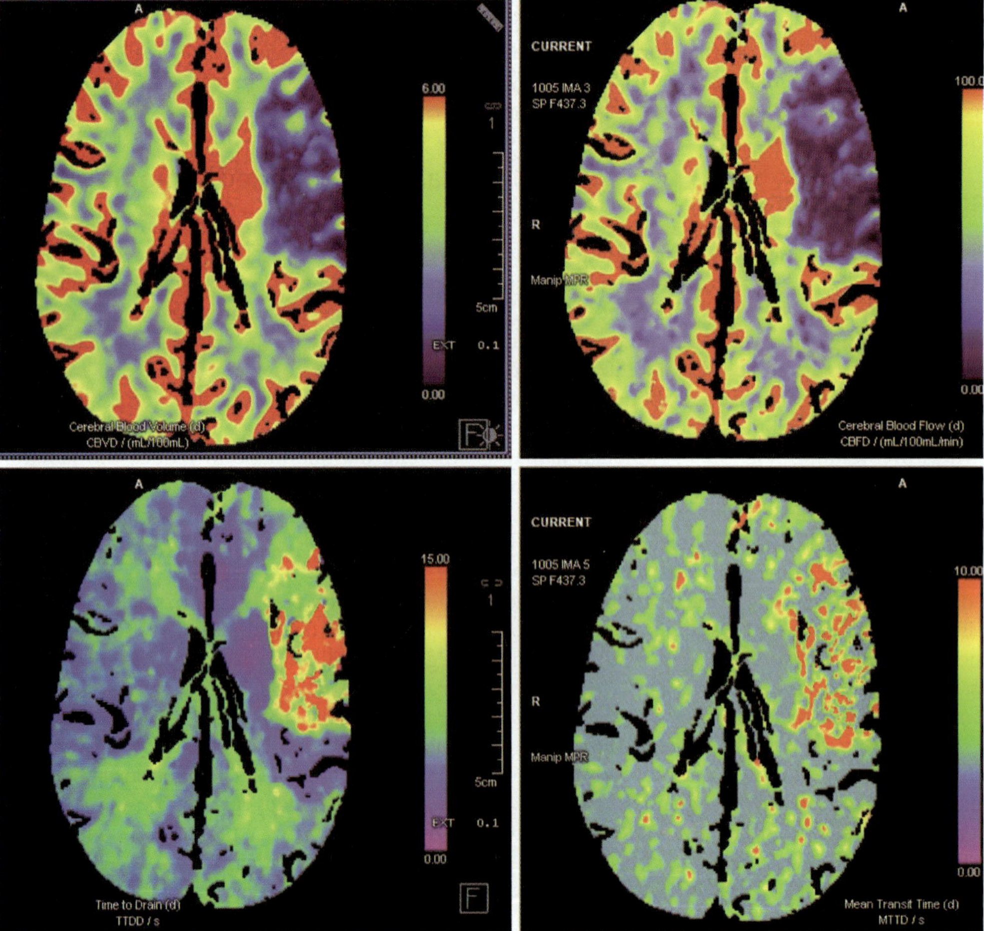

Figure 3.26 Computed tomography perfusion done in a patient with right hemiplegia. Altered perfusion parameters are seen in the left middle cerebral artery territory suggestive of infarct. Cerebral Blood Volume image shows blue color in left middle cerebral artery territory corresponding to decreased volume of blood supplied to brain parenchyma. Cerebral Blood Flow image also shows blue color suggestive of decreased volume of blood passing through a given amount of brain tissue per unit of time. Time to Drain and Mean Transit Time images show yellow/red color indicating prolonged perfusion.

Dual-Energy Computed Tomography

X-rays interact with matter via the photoelectric effect and Compton effect. The Compton effect produces the majority of the scatter radiations. The photoelectric effect deals with K-edge electrons, producing photoelectrons, positive ions, and energy. Different tissues and materials have different atomic numbers and different K-shell energies. However, one cannot separate soft tissues with similar HU values from each other on single-energy CT scans. For example, it is difficult to separate and classify iodinated contrast from other materials such as bone that have similar HU values in single-energy CT scans. These materials are, however, governed by different atomic numbers, different K-shell energies, and different linear attenuation coefficients at high- and low-energy levels [58].

Dual-energy CT is an advanced CT technique in which materials with different K-edge energy characteristics can be separated by different x-ray energy spectra. Unlike the single energy dataset produced by routine conventional single-energy CT, dual-energy CT scanners produce two energy datasets. Various materials have characteristic attenuation values at different energy levels because of their linear attenuation coefficients and can hence be identified accurately based on their appearance on the two different data sets. Dual-energy CT can thus be used to delineate and differentiate any tissue when imaged with both low- and high-energy x-ray beams. The various types of scanners used for dual-energy imaging are summarized in Table 3.13 [59].

Images in dual-energy CT's are most commonly obtained at 80 and 140 kV. Weighted average images are usually reconstructed in all dual-energy CT scanners. They represent a linear blend of data obtained from low- and high-energy spectra. Usually 20% to 30% of low-energy data and 70% to 80% of high-energy data are used to construct weighted average images. These data are similar in appearance to the data acquired by a routine 120-kVp single-energy CT scanner. Radiation exposure is similar or less than in the conventional single-energy CT because of iterative reconstruction and automated current modulation techniques.

Apart from the "regular" image set, various image reconstructions are possible with these two energy datasets, such as monoenergetic images, virtual noncontrast images, iodine concentration maps, and weighted average images (Fig. 3.27) [60]. This technique can also be used for metal artifact reduction. By acquiring CT at high- and low-energy spectra, it is possible to perform greater degree of material decomposition (separation) based on differences in attenuation at different energies. Material decomposition is used to accurately differentiate materials that have identical appearance on single-energy CT such as calcium, iodinated contrast, and hemorrhage. One such example is the use of dual-energy CT to differentiate the types of renal calculi by using the ratio of low-energy versus high-energy attenuation (Fig.3.28) [58].

Similarly, because we know that iodine attenuation is higher at 80 kVp than 120 kVp, it is possible to create virtual nonenhanced images by identifying and subtracting iodine content. This obviates the need to obtain a noncontrast phase in most patients, thus decreasing the radiation dose (Fig. 3.27B) [60]. Dual-energy CT can also be used to

TABLE 3.13 Designs of Dual-Energy Computed Tomography Scanners

Dual-Energy Dual Source	DUAL-ENERGY SINGLE SOURCE		
	Rapid kV Switching	Dual-Layer Detectors	Split-Filter Twin Beam
▪ Two x-ray sources function independently of each other and work at low-energy (80 kVp) and high = energy (140k Vp) levels (Fig. 3.31A).	▪ A single x-ray source produces rapidly alternating low- and high-energy rays (Fig. 3.31B).	▪ A single x-ray source operates at high tube kilovoltage (Fig. 3.31C).	▪ A single x-ray source operates at high tube kilovoltage (Fig. 3.31D).
▪ Two detector arrays are positioned opposite to two x-ray sources at right angles to each other.	▪ Single rapid response detector array	▪ Dual layered detector array to separate low and high energy x-ray photons. The top yttrium layer absorbs low-energy data, and the bottom gadolinium layer absorbs high-energy data.	▪ Two filters at the tube end (gold and tin) split the beam into high- and low-energy spectra before it reaches the patient.

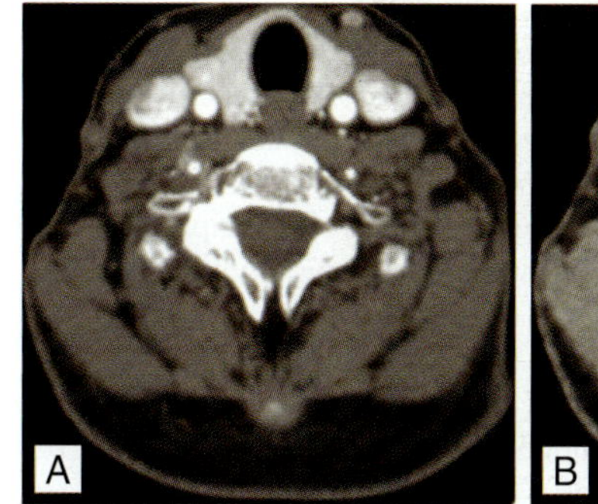

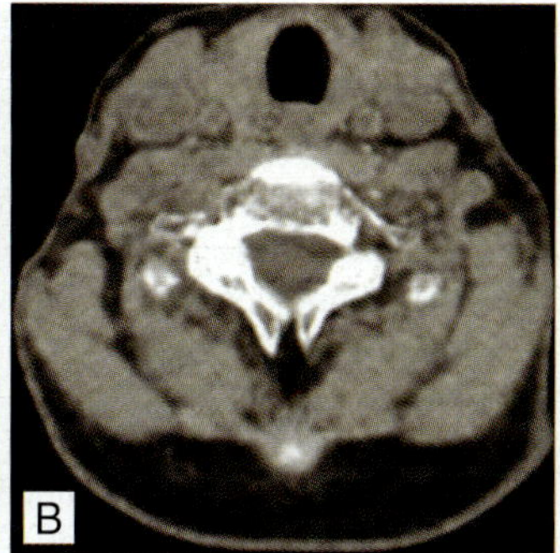

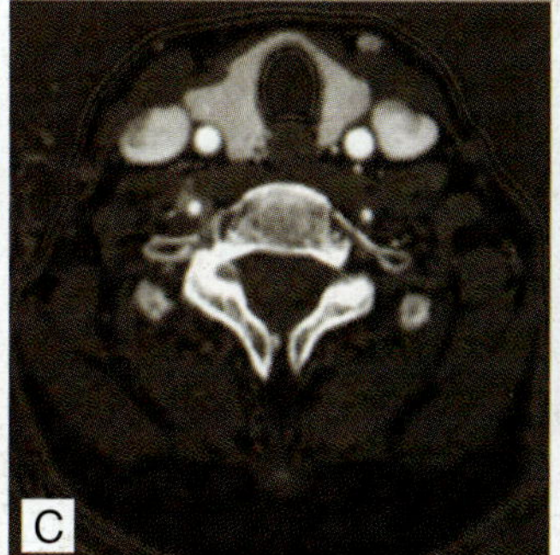

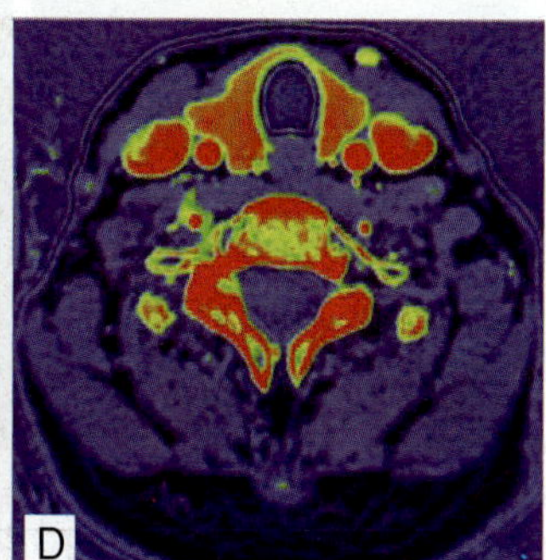

Figure 3.27 Set of images show types of image data generated with dual-energy computed tomography (CT). (A) Routine contrast-enhanced CT. (B) A virtual noncontrast image. (C) and (D) Material differentiation iodine reconstruction images on grayscale and color maps, respectively, which help in deriving quantitative and qualitative iodine uptake.

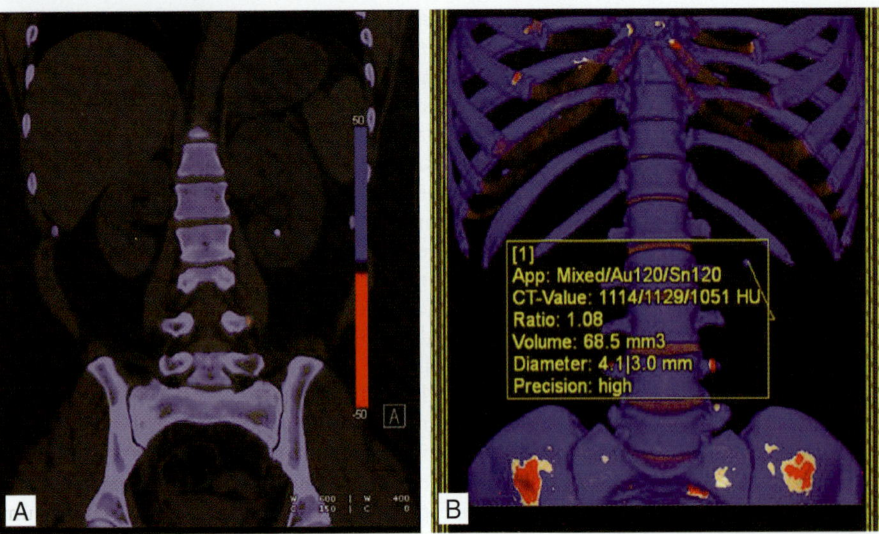

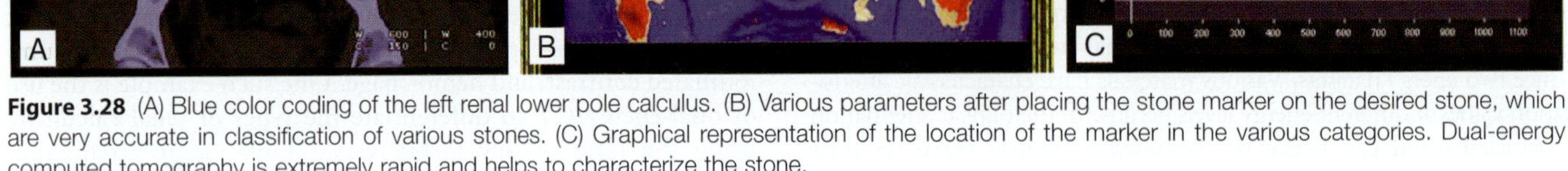

Figure 3.28 (A) Blue color coding of the left renal lower pole calculus. (B) Various parameters after placing the stone marker on the desired stone, which are very accurate in classification of various stones. (C) Graphical representation of the location of the marker in the various categories. Dual-energy computed tomography is extremely rapid and helps to characterize the stone.

remove calcium from atherosclerotic blood vessels or to reduce artifacts of metals in stents and implants [61]. Using the same principle, one can also display iodine content as a pure iodine map, quantifying the exact amount of concentration of iodine in every voxel. Iodine overlay maps that superimpose the colored iodine content on top of grayscale virtual noncontrast images can also be created [59].

A few important applications of dual-energy CT scanners are listed below.

Central Nervous System

- Calcium removal from carotid arteries in head and neck angiography along with bone removal
- Easy identification of intracranial hemorrhage using virtual noncontrast images for those who undergo CT angiography of the head
- Bone removal in CT angiography [60]

Cardiovascular System

- To assess myocardial viability and myocardial perfusion (Fig. 3.29)
- To detect myocardial iron deposition
- To evaluate coronary stents
- To characterize and remove calcified plaques from peripheral vessels and coronary arteries
- To look for aortic endoleaks after treatment [62]

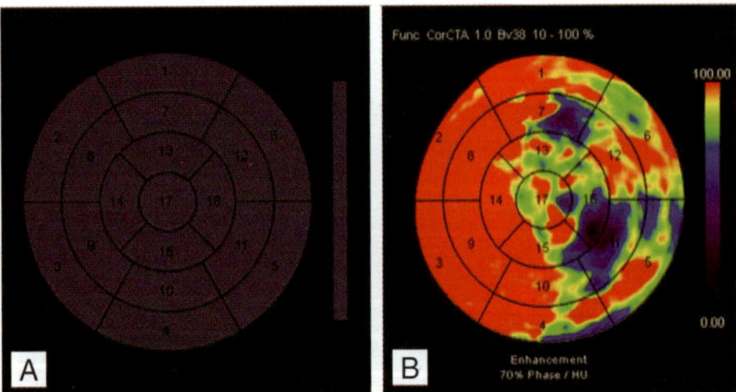

Figure 3.29 (A) The 17-segment model of heart. (B) Good perfusion of the left anterior descending artery territory and right coronary artery territory in red color. B also demonstrates that there is widespread decreased perfusion of left circumflex artery territory, giving green, blue, and yellow colors.

Thoracic System

- To perform pulmonary perfusion: to accurately diagnose subtle tiny peripheral pulmonary thromboembolism by detecting perfusion deficit and iodine maps
- To characterize solitary pulmonary nodules: Dual-energy CT quantitatively measures the degree of accumulation of iodine concentration in the solitary pulmonary nodule, which correlates with the risk of malignancy [63]

Gastrointestinal System

- CT colonography: Colonic masses and polyps enhance by 40 to 50 HU on postcontrast images; thus, iodine density maps help in distinguishing colonic masses and polyps from stools
- To detect liver steatosis: The material decomposition technique helps in generating monoenergetic fat-weighted images. Dual-energy CT accurately quantifies the amount of fat deposited in the liver using fat-weighted images
- To detect iron deposition in the liver
- To detect gallstones [59]

Urinary System

- To detect and characterize renal stones: Uric acid stones can be treated with oral medications by dissolving them. Struvite calculi are treated by lithotripsy. Calcium oxalate and cystine stones are resistant to lithotripsy
- To characterize renal cysts: Dual-energy CT helps to distinguish hyperdense cysts from enhancing cysts without acquiring noncontrast images [64]

Musculoskeletal System

- To detect gout and pseudogout crystals and to differentiate the two pathologies (Fig. 3.30)
- To reduce artifacts when imaging implants
- Dual-energy CT helps in superior differentiation of marrow

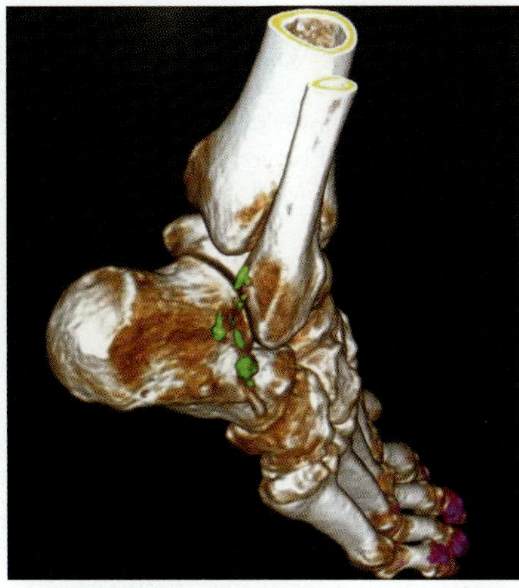

Figure 3.30 Volume-rendered image of dual-energy computed tomography of the ankle showing green color crystal posterior to the fibula suggestive of gout.

edema from trabecular bone network, leading to easy detection of fractures and marrow lesions

- To visualize tendons and ligaments: It is easier to image tendons and ligaments with dual energy than with single-energy CT. The dual-energy CT material decomposition technique is a valuable tool to display tendons and ligaments [65]

Photon-Counting Computed Tomography

Photon-counting CT is based on direct conversion technology and converts x-ray photons directly into electronic signals and was launched in end of 2021. Cadmium-based semiconductor material is used in the detectors that precisely measure the number of reaching x-ray photons and calculate the accurate energy of each photon. This mechanism helps in better signal-to-noise ratio, spatial resolution, contrast resolution, and reduced noise. Accuracy is also increased with reduction in CT artifacts by calculating the exact concentration of materials within the voxel (e.g., iodine, calcium). Photon-counting detectors have practically zero electronic noise [66].

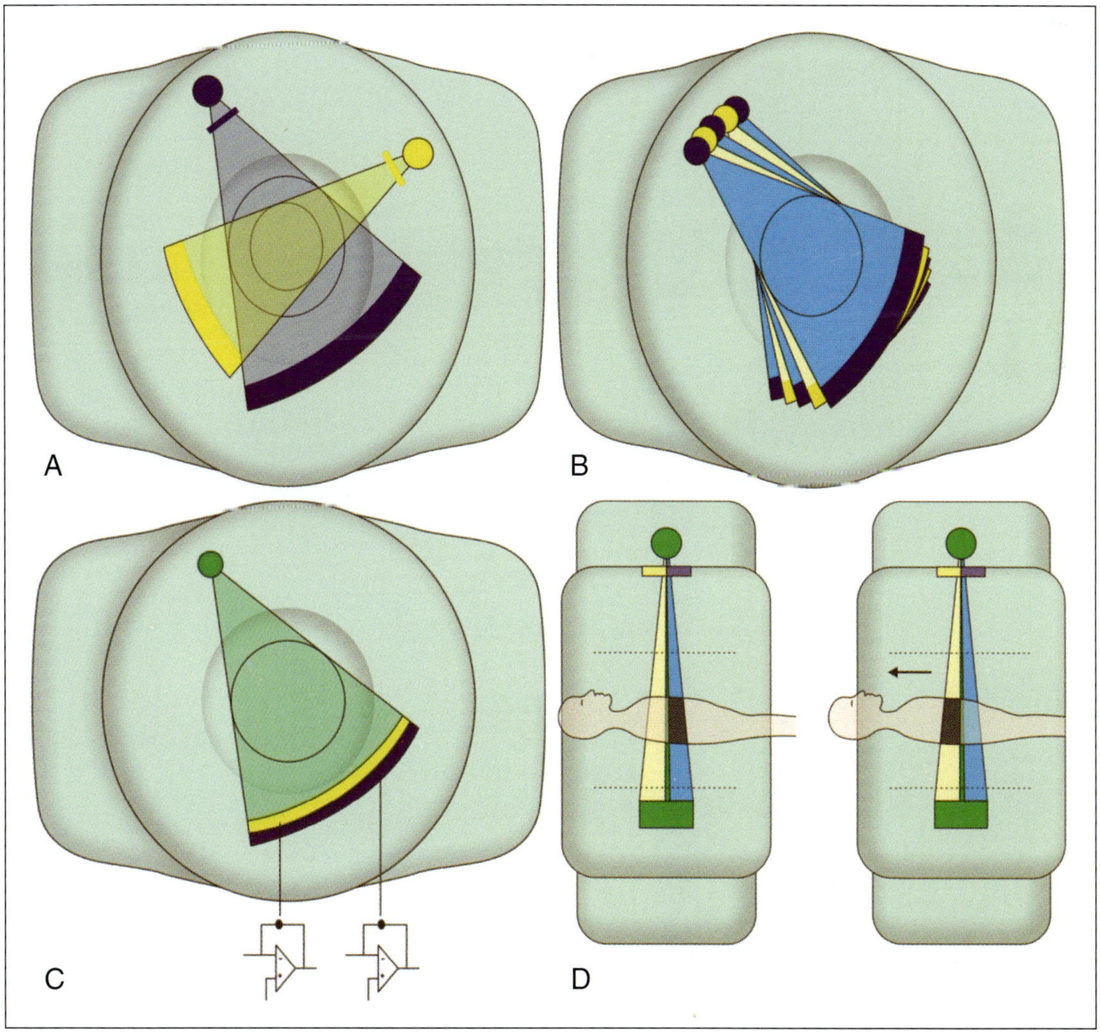

Figure 3.31 Types of dual-energy computed tomography (CT). (A) Dual-source CT scanner. (B) Single-source CT scanner with rapid kV switching technique. (C) Single-source CT scanner with dual layer detectors. (D) Single-source CT scanner with a split-filter twin beam.

Suggested Readings

- P Allisy-Roberts, J Williams, Farr's Physics for Medical Imaging, second ed., 2007, 1.
- TS Curry, JE Dowdey, RC Murry, EE Christensen, Christensen's Physics of Diagnostic Radiology, fourth ed., Lea & Febiger, Philadelphia, 1990.
- JT Bushberg, The Essential Physics of Medical Imaging, second ed., Lippincott Williams & Wilkins, Philadelphia, 2002.
- N DeMaio Daniel, Mosby's Exam Review for Computed Tomography, third ed., Elsevier, 2018.
- R Haaga John, CT and MRI of the Whole Body, fifth ed., 2-Vol. set., 2009.

4

Principles of MRI Physics

MILIND D. DHAMANKAR, JOHN E. KIRSCH

Introduction

It can be emphatically stated that radiologists have broadened their contribution to patient management due to the versatility and innovations of magnetic resonance imaging (MRI). Advances in imaging technology are expanding the capabilities of MRI to support precision medicine [1]. MRI is a prescription device that is ordered by a physician to get insights into a specific patient condition so that the radiologist can provide actionable steps for the management of the patient. Personalization of the magnetic resonance (MR) exam starts at the time of the first scan. The scanner calibrates to the patient's physiology and body condition. Better differentiation between normal and abnormal tissues can be achieved with MRI scans of various tissue contrasts. Interrogation and quantification of biochemical composition of tissues is possible with MRI. Insights into functional and pathophysiological mechanisms of the body can be achieved using MRI techniques. Multiparametric MRI [2] imaging is becoming common place where high spatial resolution scans with minimal motion artifacts are acquired along with other scans that provide additional insights about the disease and/or the body. All of this is accomplished in shorter MRI scan times and a more comfortable patient experience.

Major developments in MRI scanner hardware, image acquisition software and techniques, computational speed, postprocessing techniques, quantification, and artificial intelligence (AI) algorithms have significantly improved the quality of MR images, the diagnostic value the radiologists can glean from them, and operational workflow [3]. More recently, deep learning algorithms are being deployed to assist radiologists in reporting these increasingly larger and complex datasets.

Fundamentals of MRI

An MR image displayed on a monitor or on a film is a representation of sectional anatomy acquired by a complex cascade of events during an MR examination. Generally, a well-defined MR "protocol" is planned for the examination with respect to slice orientation, tissue contrast, and specific image parameters that need to be acquired for a diagnostic study. After "registering" the patient in the MR system software, the patient is positioned into the MRI scanner (i.e., the magnet) with an appropriate pickup coil (i.e., an antenna) for the anatomy to be examined. The technologist will run a series of MR scans known as "pulse sequences" that transmit radiofrequency (RF) waves into the patient's body for a short period of time. Simultaneously, the MR system software orchestrates coordination with various MR system hardware components to spatially encode and collect the signal emitted from the patient. This signal is then received by the coil, digitized and stored in a raw data matrix (known as "*k* space"), and later converted by reconstruction methods to produce an MR image.

It is critical for every scan performed that the technologist selects the right scan strategy (correct MR sequence/s and sequence parameters) with respect to three parameters: the total scan time to acquire the desired tissue contrast (time of acquisition, TA), the spatial resolution and the overall signal-to-noise ratio (SNR) including contrast-to-noise ratio (CNR) (Fig. 4.1). These three parameters need to be balanced for every scan to maximize scan efficiency optimizing image quality and diagnostic information.

i. TA represents the time to acquire the images of a desired contrast. TA depends on many factors that determine the speed by which the raw data matrix, or *k* space, gets sampled as well as the size of that matrix
ii. Spatial resolution is the ability to distinguish closely spaced structures. Spatial resolution is dependent on matrix size, field-of-view (FOV), and slice thickness
iii. SNR is the ratio of wanted/desired signal to background noise. CNR is the difference of SNR between adjacent structures to help differentiate normal from abnormal tissues

TA, SNR, and resolution depend on many scan parameters that will be discussed later in this chapter. Attention to those dependencies will also help the reader mitigate some image artifacts. Since these factors are all interrelated, the technologist must constantly balance among them by adjusting parameters,

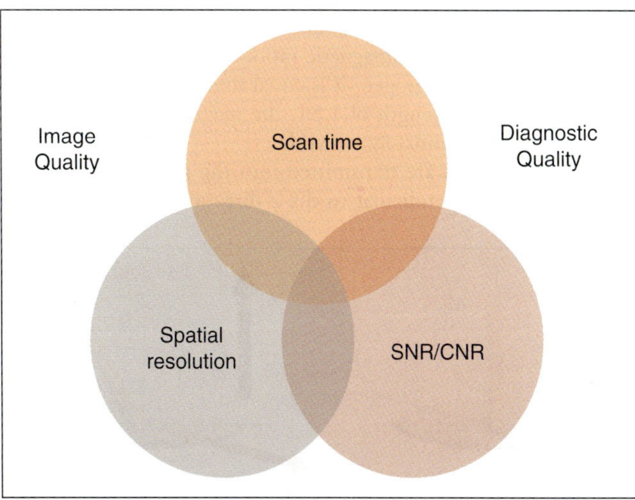

Figure 4.1 Three parameters need to be considered for every scan to maximize scan efficiency and diagnostic information: scan time, spatial resolution, and signal-to-noise ratio (SNR).

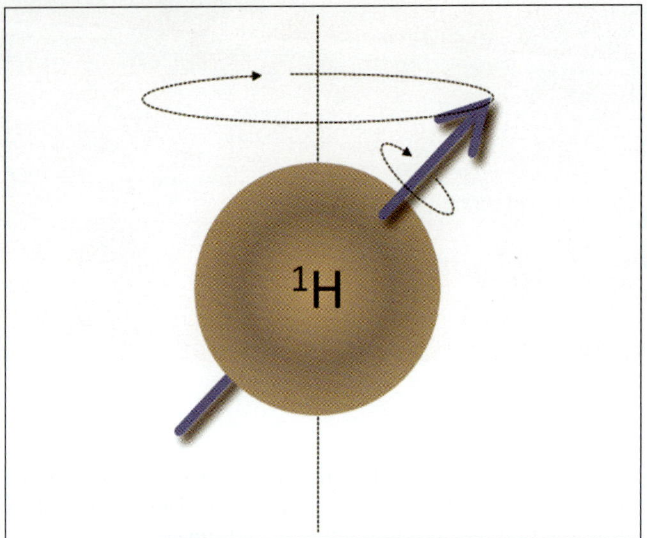

Figure 4.2 The hydrogen nucleus, which consists of a single proton, is like a little spinning magnet.

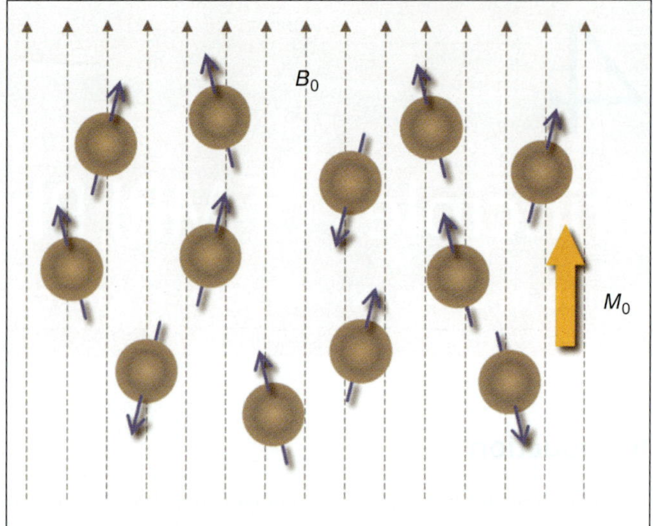

Figure 4.3 In the presence of an external magnetic field, hydrogen protons in the body align themselves either parallel or antiparallel to the field, also referred to as the static B_0 field.

personalizing them to the patient's condition to acquire diagnostic images in a reasonable time while providing the desired diagnostic information that was protocoled.

B_0, Magnetization, and RF

MRI is based on probing hydrogen protons in the body. The hydrogen nucleus, a single proton, is like a little spinning magnet (Fig. 4.2), performing a precessional motion that resembles the wobbling of a spinning top. When the patient is positioned in the magnet, the protons in the body align themselves either parallel or antiparallel (Fig. 4.3) to the external magnetic field of the magnet known as the static B_0 field. There are slightly more protons in the parallel state, collectively leading to a bulk magnetization that initially aligns in the direction of B_0 (known as the state of thermal equilibrium). Essentially, the patient's body becomes magnetized. This bulk magnetization will ultimately contribute to the MR signal.

Because the initial net *longitudinal magnetization* is parallel to the external magnetic field (conventionally known as the "z" direction), it cannot be detected. However, it spins at a characteristic rate called the Larmor frequency which is directly proportional to the magnetic field strength. The proportionality constant, known as the gyromagnetic ratio, is unique to the nucleus being probed. For hydrogen, it is equal to 42.57 MHz/T. Therefore, at a B_0 field strength of 1.5T, the magnetization spins at a frequency of approximately 64 MHz.

When RF waves are transmitted into the patient, a temporal magnetic field perpendicular to the z direction, known as B_1^+, is created (Fig. 4.4). If the frequency of this transmission matches the Larmor frequency of the magnetization (known as the resonance condition), it rotates the net magnetization out of the longitudinal z direction, creating a perpendicular component of magnetization (*transverse magnetization*) in the x–y plane that rotates at the Larmor frequency. This rotating magnetic field, known as B_1^-, induces an electric current in an antenna also referred to as an MR receiver coil (Fig. 4.5). This signal is then picked up, digitally sampled, and processed.

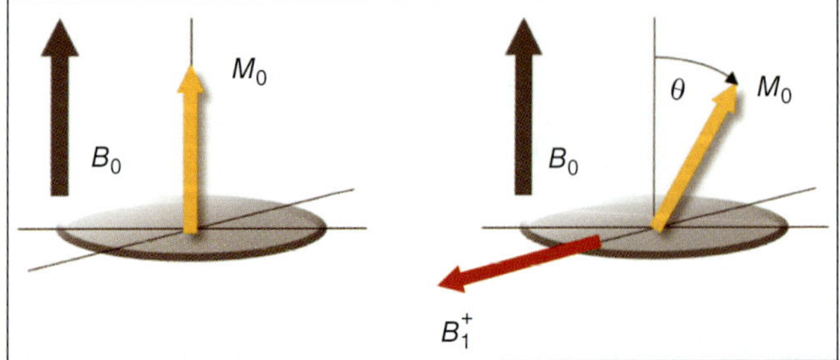

Figure 4.4 RF transmission waves create a B_1^+ field that is perpendicular to the direction of the static B_0 field. This then rotates the magnetization out of the direction of B_0 by a flip angle theta.

T1, T2, and T2* Relaxation

The moment the RF pulse is switched off, the magnetization begins to "relax" and starts returning to its original position along the longitudinal z direction of B_0. The longitudinal component of the magnetization grows back to its original magnitude at thermal equilibrium. Fig. 4.6 demonstrates the exponential growth of longitudinal magnetization over time. The characteristic time constant that represents the time it takes for the longitudinal magnetization to recover to 63% of its original value is known as T1, the longitudinal (also known as spin-lattice) relaxation time, and has a unique value associated with each type of tissue.

Simultaneously, the transverse component of magnetization decreases after the RF pulse is switched off because the

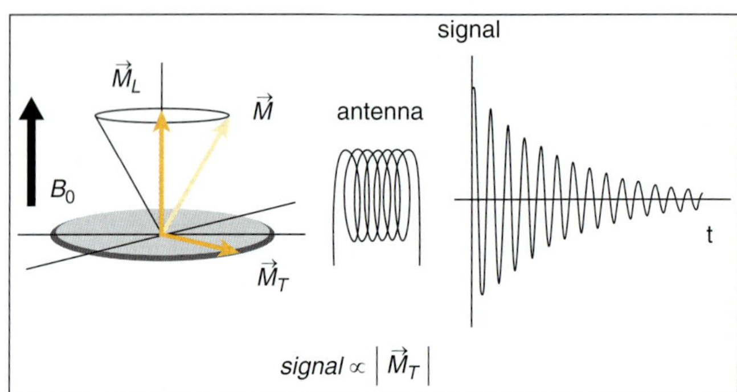

Figure 4.5 When rotated out of the direction of B_0, the net magnetization has a longitudinal (z) component and a transverse (xy) component that then can be detected by an MR receiver coil. B_1^- is related to the transverse component of the magnetization.

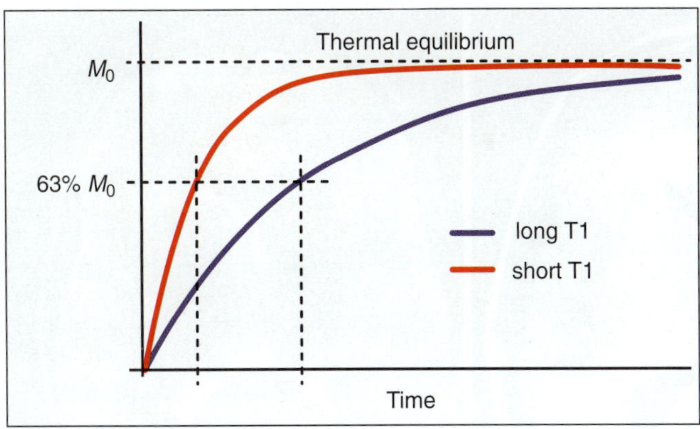

Figure 4.6 Exponential growth of longitudinal magnetization to thermal equilibrium. The rate of growth is determined by the T1 relaxation of the tissue.

magnetization loses phase coherence and the protons that comprise the magnetization collectively progress out of phase (known as "spin dephasing"). Fig. 4.7 shows the exponential decay of transverse magnetization over time. The characteristic time constant that represents the time it takes for the transverse magnetization to decay to 37% of its original value is known as T2, the transverse (also known as spin-spin) relaxation time, and has a unique value associated with each type of tissue.

In addition to the irreversible T2 relaxation process, faster decay known as T2* relaxation represents an additional but reversible dephasing process that further reduces T2 (i.e., T2* < T2). This is based on other aspects that can produce spin dephasing, including magnetic susceptibility which is not a part of the T2 process.

T1 and T2 relaxation times are unique characteristics of the various tissues in the body (Table 4.1). Water has a relatively long T1 and T2 time, while fat has a relatively short T1 and T2 time. All tissues will have unique combinations of T1, T2, and T2* relaxation, which ultimately produces the exquisite tissue contrast that is so unique to MRI. These properties are dependent on field strength where T1 tends to increase with B_0 while T2 changes to a lesser extent.

Spatial Encoding

Spatial encoding of the signal is necessary to produce the image. MRI exploits the fact that the frequency at which the transverse magnetization rotates about the x–y plane is directly proportional to the magnetic field strength according to the Larmor equation. At the main static magnetic field strength (B_0) that is spatially uniform and homogeneous there is no distinction in spatial location of the signal that would get detected. However, if a gradient magnetic field (G) is applied, superimposed on the B_0 field such that the total magnetic field varies linearly in space, then a one-to-one relation between frequency and space exists (Fig. 4.8). This forms the basis for spatial encoding in MRI.

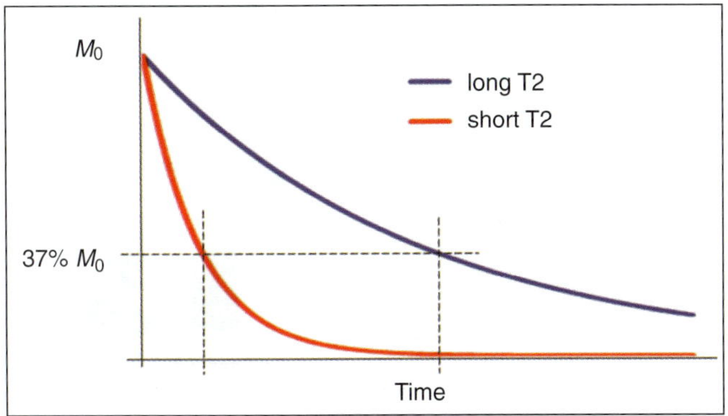

Figure 4.7 Exponential decay of transverse magnetization. The rate of decay is determined by the T2 and T2* relaxation of the tissue.

TABLE 4.1 Approximate Values of T1 and T2 at 1.5T

Tissue	T1 (ms)	T2 (ms)
Water (CSF)	4000	2000
Fat	250	70
Gray matter	900	90
Muscle	900	50
Liver	500	40

The values are "typical." Numerous papers have been published about T1 and T2, and values vary significantly at times due to methodology and statistics.
(Source: http://mriquestions.com.)

Since the signal must come from a point within the body, there are three independent G fields representing the three physical directions in space, namely X, Y, and Z axes. During the time when the RF is applied, a G field can selectively "excite" a slice at a physical location in space that rotates the magnetization out of the longitudinal z direction and creates a transverse component in the x–y plane. After this plane of excitation, a G field within that plane can then be applied to uniquely spatially encode the transverse magnetization in one direction also referred to as phase encoding. Finally, at the time the signal is detected, the third G field in the other perpendicular direction in that excited plane would be applied (referred to as frequency encoding) to complete the spatial encoding of that slice.

In summary, the complete MRI process involves applying a combination of multiple magnetic fields. A main B_0 magnetic field magnetizes the body and creates the initial bulk magnetization. A perpendicular B_1^+ magnetic field rotates that magnetization, and spatially varying G magnetic fields encode the signal that produces the image from a specific location in physical space. T1 and T2 relaxation are the two primary MRI relevant properties of the tissues. And

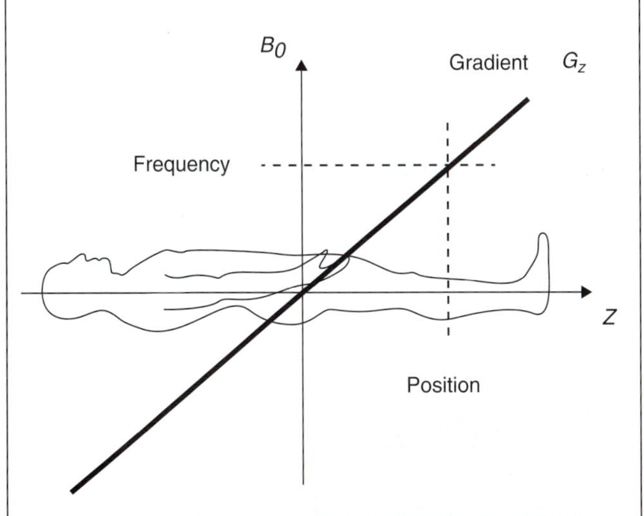

Figure 4.8 The gradient magnetic field (G). When applied, it creates spatially varying B_0 magnetic field that produces a one-to-one relation between the magnetization Larmor frequency and space, and is the basis for spatial encoding of the MRI signal.

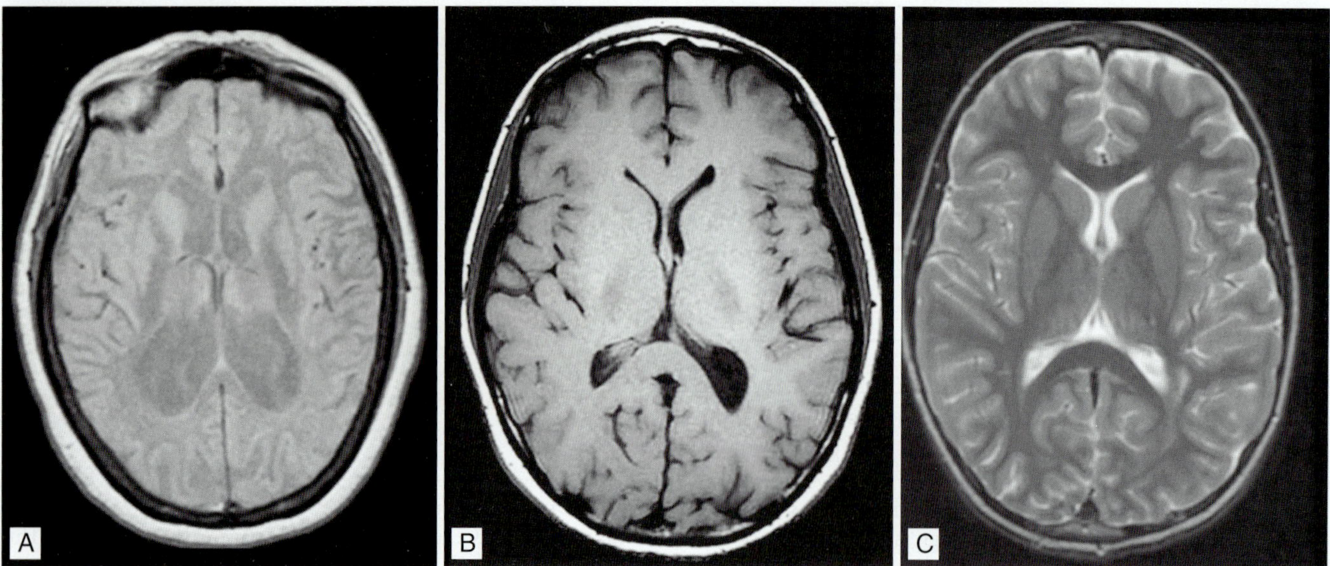

Figure 4.9 Three fundamental types of the tissue contrast in MRI that exploit tissue differences in T1 and T2 relaxation. Axial images of the brain with the tissue contrast of (A) proton density weighting (PDw), (B) T1 weighting (T1w), and (C) T2 weighting (T2w).

it is the timing of everything combined that ultimately produces the unique contrast and resolution of the MRI image (Fig. 4.9).

MRI Hardware

The clinical MRI scanner consists of the following main hardware components (Fig. 4.10B):

1. Magnet and shim coils
2. Gradient system including *X*, *Y*, and *Z* gradient coils, gradient amplifier, and electronics
3. RF system including transmit and receive coils and electronics
4. Host computer, image processor, operator console, display monitor
5. Patient table

A typical layout of an MRI system is shown in Fig. 4.10A.

The magnet or gantry is usually housed inside an RF-shielded cabin and is typically called the magnet or examination room because the patient lies on the patient table and is initially positioned in the magnet for the MR examination (Fig. 4.10B). Since the scanner usually operates in the MHz frequency range, the RF shield prevents outside interference from adulterating the MR signal and helps reduce artifacts in the image. It also prevents the emission of RF from the magnet room. A technologist operates the MR scanner from the control room at a computer console. Remaining electronics are typically located in an adjacent equipment room.

Workflow of an MRI Examination: An MR image displayed on the console monitor is a representation of anatomy after a series of events. First, the patient is reclined on the patient table and positioned inside the magnet with an appropriate receiver coil (antennae) for the anatomy to be examined (Fig. 4.10A). Second, the operator/technologist plans the exam protocol with different measurements and runs those scans on the patient. For each scan, RF waves are transmitted into the patient. *X*, *Y*, and *Z* direction gradients are switched on and off to spatially localize the signal coming from the patient, which gets picked up by the coil receiver. This is then digitized, stored, and processed to generate images of various anatomical orientations and of different tissue contrasts.

Magnets (B_0): The main role of the magnet in an MRI scanner is to provide a strong static B_0 magnetic field (typically ranging from 0.2 to 3.0 Tesla for clinical systems, with 7 Tesla systems now also introduced in some larger institutions) to essentially magnetize the body and establish the initial MR thermal equilibrium condition. It must therefore be stable over time and spatially uniform (or homogeneous) across a large volume of space so that

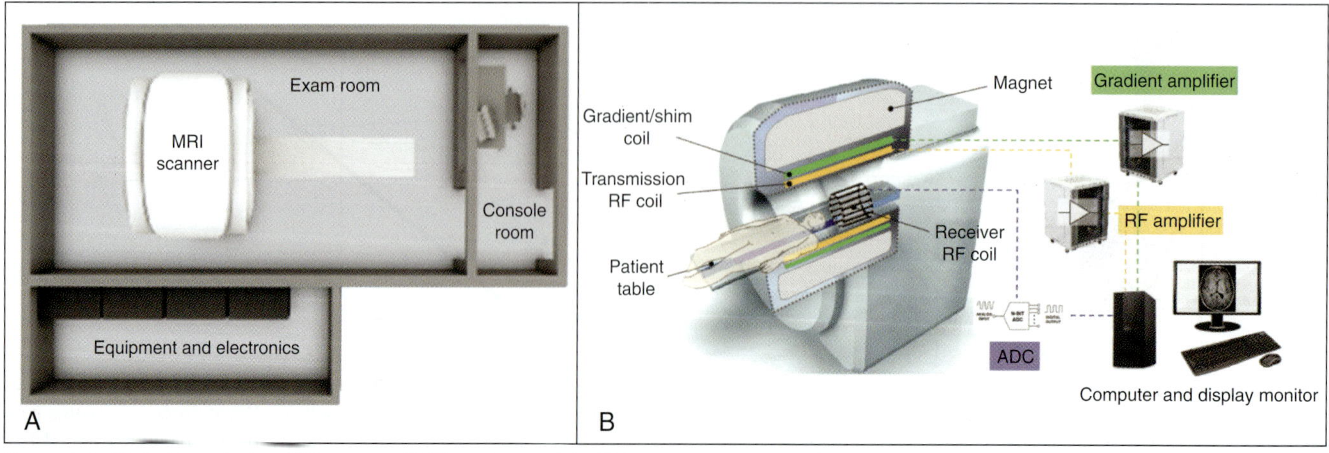

Figure 4.10 Typical layout of an MRI system. (A) The suite consists of the exam room, console room, and equipment room. (B) The system consists of the magnet, patient table, gradient coil, transmission coil, receiver coil, and computer for measurement control and image display.

good image quality can be obtained particularly for techniques that are sensitive to spatial variations in B_0, such as spectral fat suppression or spectroscopy. Contemporary *actively shielded magnets* have counterrunning coil windings surrounding the main field windings to reduce stray fields thereby producing smaller magnet footprints facilitating more compact installations.

There are three types of magnets used for MRI scanners: permanent, resistive, and superconducting.

Permanent magnets: Generally, these are used in low-field strength (<0.4T) MRI systems since it is difficult to achieve high-field strengths on the scale of a human scanner and are made from various magnetite materials. As the name suggests, the magnetic field is always present, and has comparatively minimal maintenance costs. One disadvantage is that they can be sensitive to temperature and image quality may therefore become impacted.

Resistive magnets: These magnets are made from conducting wire. A magnetic field is produced when a constant electrical current is passed through the windings. These systems must have a constant supply of electrical current which can be expensive. However, by switching off the electricity, it is easy to switch off the magnetic field in times of emergency. Their field strength can be limited (typically <0.6T).

Superconducting magnets: These magnets are the most widely used for clinical MRI systems (Fig. 4.11). They use superconducting wires that possess no electrical resistance when cooled to -270°C. These magnets are always fully energized. Current designs use only liquid helium to maintain the ultracold temperature and superconductive properties. Refill rate of helium is low compared with earlier designs. Although rare, one potential safety concern with this configuration is if the superconducting properties are lost for some reason, this leads to an irreversible event known as a *magnet quench* which results in a rapid loss of the magnetic field as well as a large and rapid release of helium gas. In contrast, a magnetic quench may also be manually induced in certain cases to demagnetize the system in a more controlled manner, as a lifesaving procedure, for example, when a person is pinned against the gantry due to a magnetic object. Every installed MR machine has a single button manual emergency

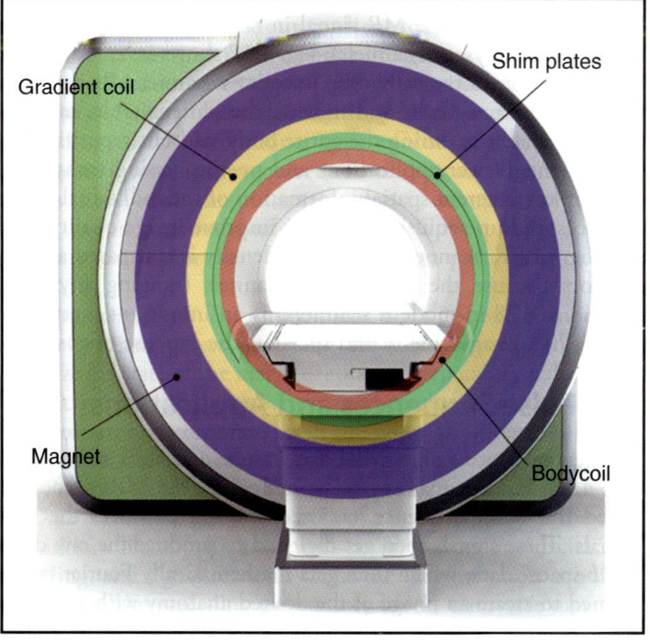

Figure 4.11 Schematic cutout of a superconducting magnet showing the primary components inside the bore.

quench system in place for this purpose, usually in the control room. Most recently, completely sealed magnets have been realized that require no recirculation system [4]; however thus far their field strength has been limited (≤1.5T).

Hybrid magnet designs also exist that combine MRI with other imaging or therapeutic technologies, as, for example, the MR-positron emission tomography (PET) system described later in this chapter.

Shimming: This is used to correct minor spatial imperfections in the main static magnetic field and achieve the best spatial uniformity or homogeneity. *Passive shimming* is a coarse method used during installation to optimize the site-specific homogeneity using iron shim plates in an empty magnet bore (Fig. 4.11). *Active shimming* is controlled by the operating software to correct subject-specific distortions of the field. When the patient is positioned in the magnet, magnetic susceptibility variations in the patient tissues distort the magnet homogeneity on the order of around 0.5–1.0 ppm. Active shimming globally corrects these errors but only to a certain extent. Spatially varying linear or first-order correction is possible by adjusting the gradient baseline DC electrical current. Spatially varying second-order shims associated with a separate shim coil in the magnet bore are additionally adjusted to optimize the field that contains the human subject. A fast MR-based scan is usually carried out to first map the B_0 field of the patient. Based on the results, required corrections are applied to the shim coils to optimize the homogeneity. This is particularly helpful for off-center imaging like shoulder imaging and applications that are sensitive to spatial B_0 variations that require good homogeneity.

Gradient (G) system: The gradients are essential for spatial encoding. By changing the main B_0 magnetic field in a predictable and controlled manner, magnetic field gradients that vary the B_0 field linearly in space enable the Larmor precessional frequency of the magnetization to become a function of their physical location which in turn allows the ability to spatially encode the MR signal. *X*, *Y*, and *Z* gradient coil sets are located within the magnet bore as shown in Fig. 4.11. These coils are driven by specially designed amplifiers at very high currents and voltages in present day systems (800 A and 2000 V are typical), which is necessary to create the rapidly pulsed gradient magnetic field and achieve rapid scanning and high spatial resolution. They are also used as well for the linear first-order shim terms described previously. Gradients play a significant and critical role in many applications like diffusion-weighted imaging (DWI) and MR angiography (MRA).

Nearly all modern scanners use actively shielded gradient coils that consist of a primary inner winding to produce the desired gradient field in the bore and a secondary outer counter winding that actively cancels the fields to prevent generation of unwanted eddy currents in surrounding conductive surfaces such as the magnet vessel cryoshields. Typically, gradient coils are composed of individual wires wrapped onto cylindrical formers made of fiberglass and embedded or coated with epoxy resin.

Gradient performance is critical to successfully execute many of the advanced MRI applications, so it is essential to understand what the important characteristics are of gradient systems. Table 4.2 lists key features of the gradient and typical maximum performance values that will help the reader to compare the technical specifications of different models and manufacturers. Most routine clinical scans do not require maximum gradient performance. However, some of the newer techniques, faster sequences, and/or tasks in a shorter time may require maximum gradient power. For such applications, investment in good state-of-the-art hardware needs to be carefully considered. In contrast, maximum gradient capabilities may also be limited by safety constraints such as peripheral nerve stimulation.

Radiofrequency system: The RF system generates RF pulses that are transmitted through a transmitter antenna coil at a specified

that will answer all diagnostic needs in all anatomical regions. Also, there are many tissue-specific properties that influence the MR signal. Hence a wide range of pulse sequences are required. Different vendors may name their sequence slightly differently and many times use acronyms for the sequences and techniques (refer to Table 4.3 for a sampling of the more common vendor nomenclatures for sequences and techniques). Newer pulse sequences are either fast and/or increase confidence in diagnosis. Designing new pulse sequences is a challenging task and demands deep knowledge of physics, hardware, software, and clinical relevance.

Basic pulse sequences: The following describes several fundamental details of the most common pulse sequence schemes used in clinical imaging and how they can be manipulated to derive the tissue contrast.

TABLE 4.3 Vendor MRI Acronyms

Sequence Type	Siemens	GE	Philips
Spin echo (SE)	T1W images depict the anatomy very well while T2W help highlight the pathology.		
Conventional SE—a 90° RF pulse followed by a 180° refocusing pulse	SE	SE	SE
Double SE—a 90° RF pulse followed by two 180° refocusing pulses	PD + T2	PD + T2	PD + T2
Turbo spin echo (TSE)/fast spin echo (FSE)	TSE group of sequences are faster sequences compared with SE and serve the same purpose		
Multiecho SE—a 90° RF pulse followed by multiple 180° refocusing pulses	Turbo SE (TSE)	Fast SE (FSE)	Turbo SE (TSE)
Single-shot TSE/FSE technique	HASTE	Single-shot FSE (ssFSE)	Single-shot TSE (ssTSE)
TSE/FSE with a 90° RF pulse driven equilibrium	RESTORE	Fast recovery FSE (FRFSE)	DRIVE
Number of echoes	Turbo factor	Echo train length (ETL)	Turbo factor
Gradient echo	An RF pulse of flip angle (FA) α° (e.g., 30°) is applied instead of the 90° RF pulse, and the 180° refocusing pulse is omitted. These sequences are faster that SE and are used for breath hold abdominal imaging. They are used for 3D acquisitions in shorter times. T1W images applied for postcontrast studies. GRE sequences are used for time-of-flight MR angiography applications		
Spoiled transverse magnetization	FLASH	SPGR	T1-FFE
Coherent rephased transverse magnetization (FID)	FISP	GRASS	FFE
Coherent: Steady state free precession (SE)	PSIF	SSFP	T2-FFE
Coherent: Fully refocused (FID+SE)	TrueFISP	FIESTA	Balanced FFE
TrueFISP dual excitation	CISS	FIESTA-C	
Multiecho data image combination	MEDIC, DESS	MERGE	M-FFE
Ultrafast GRE	TurboFLASH	Fast GRE, Fast SPGR	TFE
Ultrafast GRE 3D	MPRAGE	3D-FGRE, 3D Fast SPGR, BRAVO	3D TFE
Volume interpolated 3D GRE	VIBE	LAVA	THRIVE
Hybrid	TGSE sequence contains both TSE and GRE signals. This makes TGSE faster than both TSE and GRE sequences		
TSE + GRE	Turbo GSE (TGSE)		GRASE
Specific tissue suppression techniques	By selecting specific inversion times, signal from selective tissues (e.g., fat and white matter in STIR or water and CSF in FLAIR) can be suppressed		
Inversion recovery	IR, Turbo IR (TIR)	IR, MPIR, FastIR	IR-TSE
Short TI (80–150 ms) (should not be used in postcontrast studies)	STIR	STIR	STIR
Long TI (1500–2500 ms) (FLAIR can be used postcontrast)	Dark fluid	FLAIR	FLAIR
True inversion recovery	True IR		Real IR
EPI	Ultrafast sequence where all required data are acquired in a single excitation. Applications include diffusion, perfusion, fMRI, and real-time imaging		
Single shot (SE, GRE)	EPI	EPI	EPI

TABLE 4.3 Vendor MRI Acronyms—cont'd

Sequence Type	Siemens	GE	Philips
Multishot (readout-segmented EPI)	RESOLVE	MUSE	
Parallel imaging techniques	iPAT		
▪ Image-based algorithm	mSENSE	ASSET	SENSE
▪ *k*-space-based algorithm	GRAPPA	ARC	
Metal artifact reduction sequences (MARS)	View angle tilting (VAT) Slice encoding metal artifact compensation (SEMAC)	Multiacquisition variable resonance imaging combination (MAVRIC)	O-MAR VAT O-MAR XD
Gradient moment nulling	Flow comp/GMR	Flow comp	Flow comp, flag
Ramped RF pulse	TONE	Ramped pulse	TONE
Magnetization transfer contrast	MTC	MTC	MTC
Prep-pulse chemically	FatSat	FatSat, ChemSat	SPIR
Water excitation	Water excitation	Water excitation	Proset
Prep-pulse spatially	PreSat	SAT	REST
Moving sat pulse	Travel sat	Walking sat	Travel REST

Vendor nomenclatures for sequences and techniques are based on interpretation of available data and from a reference—W Nitz, MR imaging: acronyms and clinical applications, Eur Radiol 9 (5) (1999) 979–997.

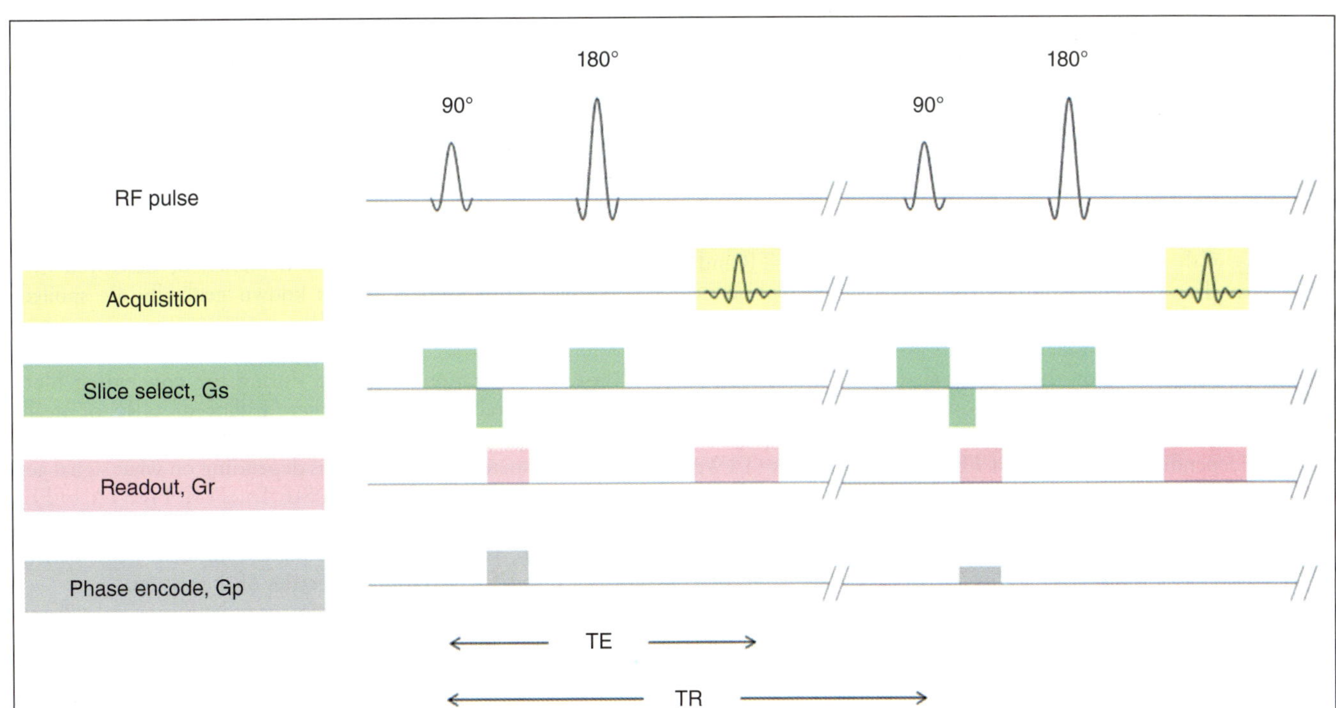

Figure 4.15 A basic 2D spin echo (SE) pulse sequence timing diagram. *Gp*, phase-encoding gradient; *Gr*, readout gradient; *Gs*, slice select gradient; *RF pulse*, radiofrequency pulse; *TE*, time of echo; *TR*, repetition time.

Spin echo sequence: Fig. 4.15 shows the pulse sequence timing diagram for a basic 2D spin echo (SE) technique during the data acquisition block described in Fig. 4.14. Timing parameters of repetition time (TR) and echo time (TE) are defined.

In the 2D SE sequence, a 90° RF pulse rotates the magnetization 90° out of the longitudinal direction. Applying the slice select gradient (Gs) simultaneously creates the transverse magnetization at a specific slice location. This then is followed by a 180° refocusing pulse. The phase-encoding gradient (Gp) and the readout gradient (Gr) are pulsed to spatially encode the signal. The SE signal that is then generated at a time TE is digitized during the readout period, also known as the "ADC on time" as shown in the acquisition timing. This digitized signal would constitute one line in the raw data *k*-space matrix. This sequence is then repeated with regular steps changing the Gp amplitude at a rate defined by TR. Once *k* space is completely filled and the 2D raw data matrix is Fourier transformed, it will generate an

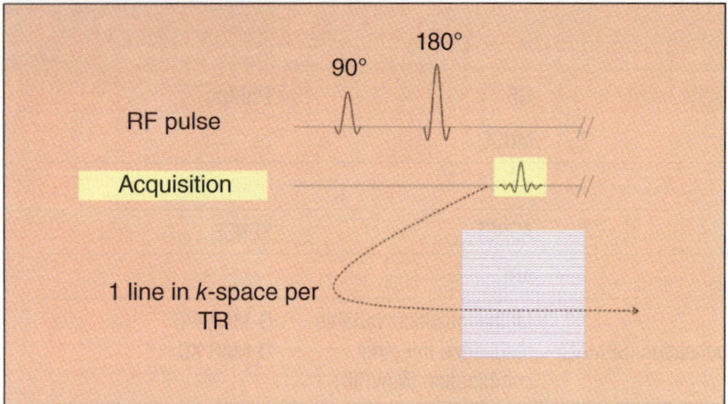

Figure 4.16 A single echo spin echo pulse sequence schematic as it relates to *k*-space encoding.

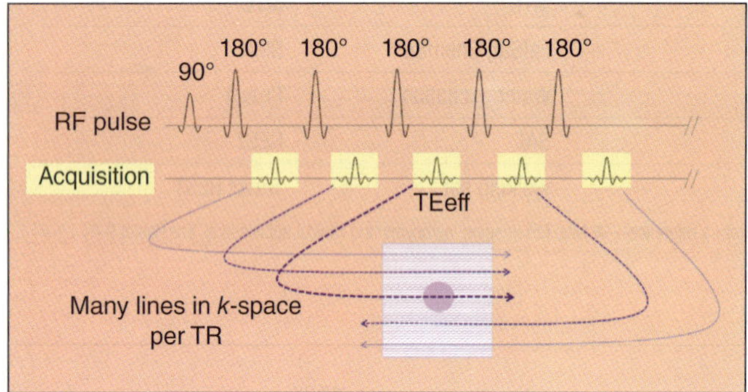

Figure 4.17 A TSE/FSE pulse sequence schematic with five sequential spin echoes as it relates to *k*-space encoding. Filling five lines of *k* space within a single TR interval reduces the scan time by a factor of 5. TEeff is the echo that fills the center of *k* space where the signal and contrast dominates the information.

MR image of that slice with a contrast determined by the TR and TE values. This sequence timing diagram classically represents the interplay of RF pulses and gradient pulses in the simplest form. The *X*, *Y*, and *Z* physical gradients assume the roles of Gs, Gp, and Gr, depending on the selected anatomical orientation.

Fig. 4.16 is a simple representation of a conventional single echo SE sequence. It depicts filling of one line in *k* space per TR interval. Depending on the TR and TE values the contrast (T1W, T2W, or PD-weighted) of the image will be produced, and the scan time will be defined by the TR and the number of lines required to fill the *k*-space matrix.

Turbo spin echo sequence (TSE) or fast spin echo (FSE) variant: Instead of filling a single *k*-space line for each TR as in a SE sequence, TSE/FSE generates multiple SEs that contribute multiple *k*-space lines for a given TR interval (Fig. 4.17). This facilitates filling of *k* space faster thus decreasing scan time proportionally (Fig. 4.17).

Gradient-echo sequence: If an RF pulse of flip angle (FA) $\alpha°$ (e.g., 30°) is applied instead of the 90° RF pulse, and the 180° refocusing pulse is omitted, this would comprise a gradient-echo GRE sequence as shown in Fig. 4.18.

By the elimination of the refocusing pulse, the readout gradient preparation pulse must be inverted so that an echo is formed during the readout of the signal. GRE sequences are typically faster than SE sequences. Use of a FA less than 90° allows for the reduction of TR while still maintaining sufficient signal levels and tissue contrast. 3D imaging in acceptable scan times is therefore possible with GRE sequences. Similar to SE, the tissue contrast of GRE sequences is determined by the TR and TE, but also now by the FA that is used.

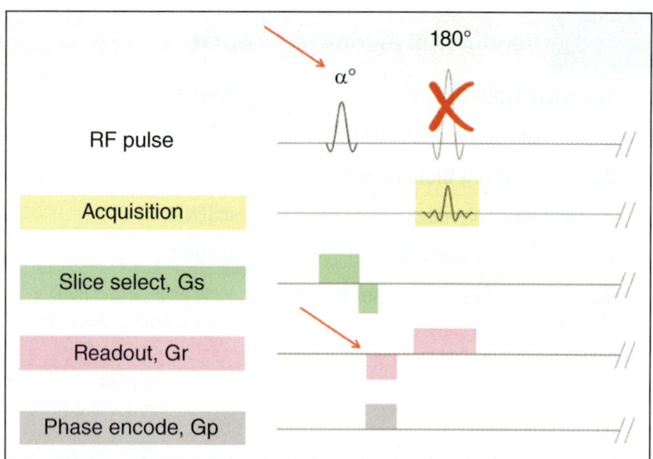

Figure 4.18 A basic 2D gradient echo (GRE) pulse sequence timing diagram and its differences relative to a SE sequence. *Gp*, phase-encoding gradient; *Gr*, readout gradient; *Gs*, slice select gradient; *RF pulse*, radiofrequency pulse.

The absence of the refocusing pulse, however, introduces T2* (instead of T2) weighting into the tissue contrast which adds additional complexity due to magnetic susceptibility differences among other factors. Additionally, with the use of short TR for 3D imaging, GRE contrast is a mixed contrast based on T1, T2, and T2* components and requires better understanding of many parameters. SE contrast in contrast provides a good basis to understand contrast from other sequences. Faster versions of SE like TSE/FSE are commonly used for T1W for good anatomical delineation and T2W images highlight the pathology better.

GRE sequences can be broadly classified into two main groups depending on what is done during the concluding block (Fig. 4.14).

- If the coherence of the residual transverse magnetization at the end of the acquisition block is dephased or destroyed by a gradient/crusher pulse, this is known generally as "spoiled" GRE (FLASH, SPGR, T1-FFE)
- Alternatively, a second type attempts to maintain the transverse magnetization coherence during the concluding block and is generally known as either "balanced" GRE or steady state free precession

There are numerous variants of this depending on what signal gets tapped into (FISP, GRASS, FFE, PSIF, TrueFISP, FIESTA, bFFE). The use of a specific GRE technique will depend on the desired tissue contrast as all these variants possess different dependencies on the T1 and T2 relaxation properties of the tissues.

Hybrid sequences: By taking advantage of hardware and software developments, modifications in existing pulse sequences have led to newer sequences with wider clinical applications, sometimes along with shorter scan times. By combining signals tapped from different evolutions of the magnetization, sequences like MEDIC/MERGE/M-FFE, DESS, and CISS/FIESTA-C are offshoots of GRE sequences, useful for specific roles such as cervical spine imaging, cartilage imaging, or heavily T2W imaging, respectively, among other uses. Hybrid techniques like TGSE/GRASE combine TSE and GRE sequences timing schemes to yield faster scan times.

Pulse Sequence Modifiers

Modifications in the preparatory block: Introducing RF during this block of the pulse sequence can change the application in various ways. By introducing a preparatory 180° RF pulse to initially invert the longitudinal magnetization, this can produce

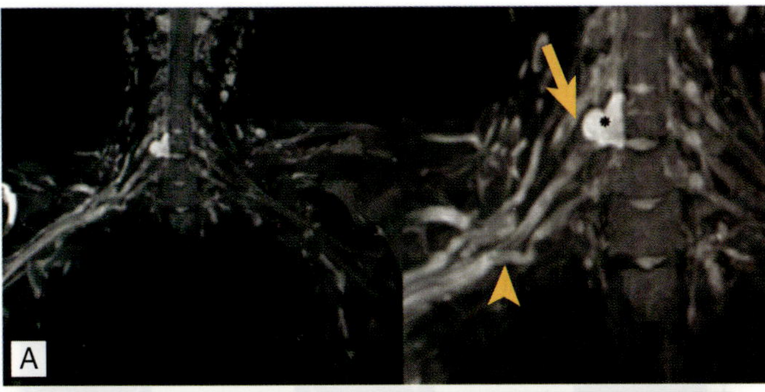

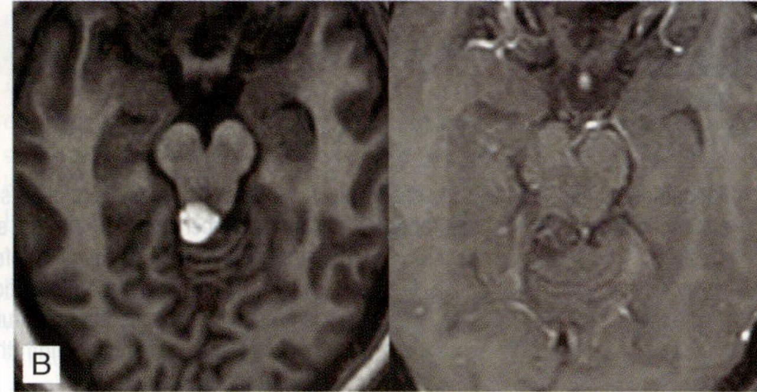

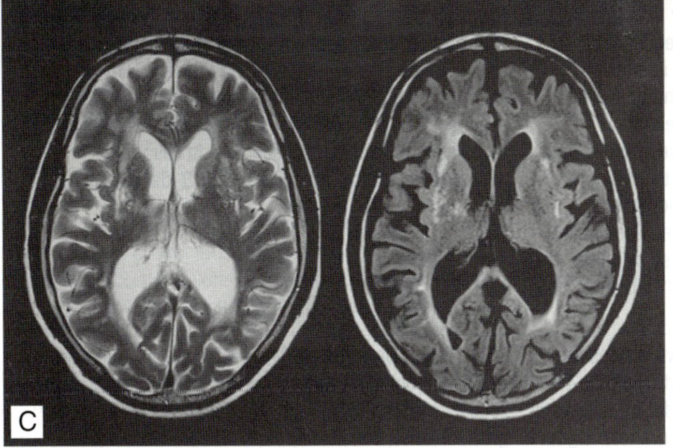

Figure 4.19 (A) Example of a 3D STIR SPACE T2W technique showing excellent fat suppression, high resolution, and contrast-to-noise ratio (CNR). Trauma: A patient with deficit in areas C5–C6 and right C7, in the context of trauma sustained 2 months prior. Results: Thickening in T2 hyperintense signal of C6 root on the right (*arrow*). Radicular avulsion of C7 root on the right with pseudomeningocele (*asterisk*). T2 hyperintense signal of C8 root on the right in the interscalene triangle (*arrowhead*). (Courtesy: Pierre Pottecher MD, Groupe IMARA, Annecy Clinique Générale GIE IRM74, Annecy, France). (B) Example of spectral fat suppression. This case of an incidental finding of a lipoma highlights the use of an MR FatSat technique to help tissue-specific diagnosis without the need for biopsy. Hyperintense signal on axial T1 SE (left), and nonenhancing lesion showing suppression of lipid signal on postcontrast axial FatSat T1 SE (right). (Courtesy: Swatee Halbe MD, Apollo Specialty Hospitals, Vanagaram, Chennai, India). (C) Fluid attenuated inversion recovery [FLAIR] (FLAIR, Dark Fluid) (right) suppresses signal from the CSF, so periventricular lesions are better delineated compared with the conventional T2W (left). (Courtesy: Wallabh Upasani, M.D., Director Sun Scan Center, Thane, India.)

fundamentally different contrasts such as inversion recovery (IR), or MPRAGE/BRAVO/3DTFE, that help to accentuate T1-weighted contrast or selectively suppress-specific tissues like fat (short tau inversion recovery [STIR] or fat saturation) (Fig. 4.19A and B) or CSF (fluid attenuated inversion recovery) (Fig. 4.19C). Preparatory RF pulses can also be used to do spectral fat suppression, blood suppression, or spatial suppression to aid in mitigating artifacts from either breathing or blood flow.

It should be especially noted that the bright signal from fat is often a hindrance to diagnosis in MR imaging. Techniques like fat saturation, water excitation (WE), STIR, and subtraction of pre- and postcontrast T1W images are commonly employed in clinical routine. These fat suppression techniques meet the requirements of a broad range of imaging protocols and clinical applications and provide greater flexibility, speed, and ease of use. The reader is referred to Table 4.4 for the different basic fat suppression techniques and their clinical applications.

2D or 3D acquisition: Most sequences can be applied as 2D slices or as a true 3D encoded volume. GRE sequences are better suited for 3D acquisitions than SE sequences because they can use very short TR while still maintaining appropriate signal levels and usable contrast in reasonable scan times. The biggest advantage of 3D imaging is that it affords higher SNR and thinner contiguous slices. Isotropic 3D encoding also enables the possibility to reconstruct images in other planes at high resolution, which can be important in knee and body imaging.

Changing sequence timing and other parameters—TR, TE, TI (inversion time), FA: These are important parameters an operator or technologist can control to change the desired contrast of the MR image. Different combinations of TR, TE, and TI can control T1 and T2 contrast weighting with SE, TSE/FSE, or IR. Fig. 4.20 illustrates the interdependence of sequence parameters like TR and TE on image contrast like T1-weighted (T1W), T2-weighted (T2W), and proton density-weighted (PD) images. With GRE, changing the FA can also alter the contrast, and for different TE values, the signals from fat and water will phase cycle, producing "in phase" (where fat and water signals add) and "opposed phase" (where fat and water signals subtract) images. With sequences like TSE/FSE/TGSE there are parameters like the number of echoes, or turbo factor that can influence the speed and shorten scan time (Fig. 4.21).

Using Different Schemes in *k*-Space Manipulations

The acquisition, detection, and digital sampling of the MR signal that fills the *k*-space matrix are necessary to generate an image. All techniques that manipulate *k*-space filling will potentially affect the acquisition time and contrast, as well as the appearance of artifacts. Subsampling of *k* space can be used to reduce artifacts or increase speed. The following are only some of the more common techniques that manipulate *k* space.

k-space trajectories: The most frequently used way of filling *k* space is row by row, known as Cartesian or rectilinear sampling. However, other trajectories filling *k* space exist. For example, although echo-planar imaging (EPI) is also Cartesian, it fills the rows in a chronologically ordered zigzag pattern. A common strategy to mitigate motion artifacts is to use a radial filling of *k* space (BLADE, PROPELLER, MultiVane) and is employed in a lot of body imaging with free breathing. Filling *k* space from the center outward either radially or spirally (UTE, ZTE) allows the ability to capture tissue signals with extremely short T2 such as lung parenchyma or cortical bone.

k-space undersampling: There is a lot of redundancy in *k*-space information. Undersampling strategies exploit this to reduce scan time with minimal compromise in either SNR or spatial resolution. In its simplest form, owing to the symmetry of information in *k*-space partial Fourier fills only part or up to half of the rows in Cartesian sampling with a proportional reduction in scan time. This

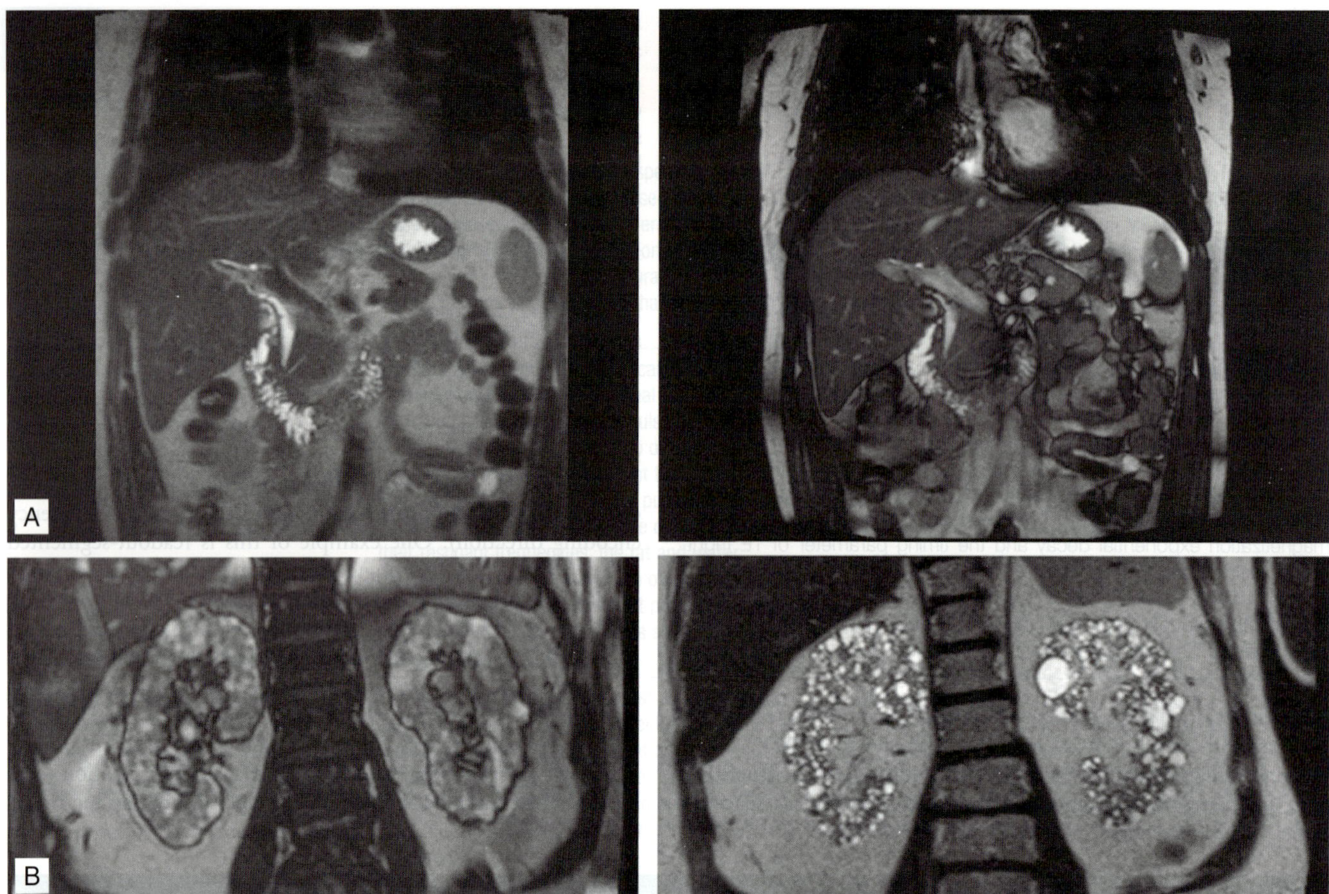

Figure 4.22 (A) HASTE (ssFSE, ssTSE) and TrueFISP (FIESTA, bFFE) sequences can be complementary to TSE/FSE in body imaging. They are motion insensitive and are rapidly acquired. HASTE (left) is good for a motion insensitive T2W. This coronal HASTE shows bright fluid in the bile duct, duodenum, and the stomach. TrueFISP (right) is good for fast anatomical overview. This coronal TrueFISP shows the portal vein, bile duct, and bowel. (B) Due to the mixed T1 and T2 weighting associated with TrueFISP, this scan (top) did not show the small renal cysts as well as the HASTE sequence (bottom) in this patient with lithium toxicity. HASTE is a heavy T2w sequence that shows multiple renal cysts in this case as bright signal. (Courtesy: Mukesh Harisinghani MD, Massachusetts General Hospital, Boston, Massachusetts, USA.)

different rates since edge definition tends to be constant over time while signal and contrast are critical to sample repetitively at high temporal resolution. Generally referred to as "keyhole" techniques (TWIST, TRICKS, etc.), they are used for interventional work and DCE. Another time-efficient strategy is to use the same *k*-space lines across different images that reflect different points in time, known as "view sharing" or "shared echo." This can be coupled with radial *k*-space filling (e.g., StarVIBE) and is also commonly used to acquire different cardiac phases with balanced GRE sequences. Finally, dynamic contrast methods may employ different *k*-space reordering schemes such as centric ordering where instead of filling *k*-space row by row from the top of the matrix down, it starts in the middle and fills *k* space from the inside out. This is effective especially with Care Bolus techniques that require precise timing of the acquisition and passage of the contrast bolus.

Using Artifact Reduction Techniques

Because there are so many different pulse sequence techniques in MRI, artifacts can manifest in a variety of ways, and various methods and approaches to minimize them have been developed over the years.

Motion reduction: Motion is a very common challenge, especially in abdominal applications. A straightforward approach is to use regional saturation bands during the preparatory sequence block to suppress signal from moving tissue like abdominal fat or in-flowing blood. Prospective navigator methods (e.g., PACE) can be integrated into pulse sequences that produce an additional MRI signal that can be tracked in real time to detect motion traits that are then used to correct the data retrospectively or modify the sequence execution prospectively. Since motion produces phase shifts in the MR signal, it is possible to use gradient pulsing to correct this phase shift (flow compensation, GMN, GMR) and is used routinely in MRA and to reduce breathing and cardiac motion. If the heart and/or breathing cycle is monitored, it is possible to use the physiological traces prospectively with triggering or gating to synchronize the pulse sequence acquisition or retrospectively to reorder *k* space to regularize the data (e.g., ROPE). Finally, one of the simplest strategies is to do multiple acquisitions (or NEX) to average out motion-related artifacts provided it is sufficiently asynchronous relative to the pulse sequence repetition rate (TR).

B_0 error reduction: MRI is fraught with B_0-related artifacts and there are some simple approaches that can be used to mitigate them. Chemical shift misregistration between fat and water can be minimized by increasing the sampling bandwidth during the ADC on time of the acquisition block of the sequence. Metal implants always pose a challenge that distort the B_0 field locally and this strategy also works well for this. Metal artifacts can

additionally be reduced by increasing the transmission bandwidth of the RF pulsing.

The clinical need to image close to implants has led to the development of specialized metal artifact reduction sequences. View angle tilting angles the spatial encoding to realign pixels that would otherwise be displaced by metal-induced distortion (in-plane distortions) but is limited and can induce blurring if applied too severely. Other techniques such as slice encoding metal artifact compensation and multiacquisition variable resonance imaging combination capture the off-resonance signal from regions of B_0 distortions and combine them together to produce the images. This corrects the in-plane as well as the through-plane distortions, however this comes typically at the expense of longer scan times.

Using CNR improving techniques: Achieving better CNR to easily distinguish the normal from the abnormal tissue is a strength of MRI and its techniques [6] (Fig. 4.19C). Some pulse sequence techniques also exist to help improve overall CNR. A general method that can be used with any pulse sequence technique is multiple repeated (also referred to as "concatenated") scans that helps to minimize the effects of slice-to-slice crosstalk improving SNR and CNR. Time sequential blocks of slices are acquired in a "gap and fill" manner, such as acquiring the odd-numbered slices in a first pass and even-numbered slices in a second pass. Although this also helps to reduce tissue heating from the RF pulsing, it comes at the expense of scan time. Specific to time-of-flight (TOF) MRA is the use of spatially varying RF FAs (e.g., TONE) which helps to increase vessel depth penetration and improve their patency and visualization. Something that is also useful for MRA and in muscle studies as well is to add a magnetization transfer (MT) pulse during the preparatory block. MT is pulsed off resonance to directly saturate bound hydrogen that is not directly observable which then transfers its magnetization to the free hydrogen that is detected in MRI. This indirectly affects the image contrast and is therefore referred to as MT contrast. It is also used in the brain with postcontrast studies because the MT pulse negligibly affects the enhancing lesion or structure but suppresses the background tissue signal thus improving the CNR. Finally, MT pulses and MT contrast can be used as an inference of bound hydrogen content.

A few selected commonly used MR applications are described in greater detail in the following.

Diffusion-Weighted Imaging and Diffusion Tensor Imaging

Fundamentals of DWI: DWI assesses random Brownian motion of tissue-free water and provides clues about the microenvironment in which the water molecules are dispersing (Fig. 4.23). Diseases may directly or indirectly change the diffusion characteristics of the underlying tissue—for example, the failure of the sodium–potassium ATP pump causes cytotoxic edema following acute brain infarction. This process shifts extracellular fluid into the intracellular space in the affected area (causing restricted Brownian motion) which shows up as restricted diffusion on DWI images compared with the unaffected brain tissue (Fig. 4.24). Ischemia can therefore become highlighted [7]. DWI thus uses the local diffusion characteristics of a tissue to generate MR contrast. In the affected brain tissue associated with cytotoxic edema, water cannot diffuse as freely in all directions compared with water in the CSF that is unrestricted (Fig. 4.25). Note that while cytotoxic edema shows restricted diffusion, vasogenic edema does not do so. Also, generally speaking, it is easier for water to diffuse along the length of a white matter fiber rather than across the fiber, because of the anatomy of the white matter tracts with nerve fibers traversing along the length of the tract. This property is known as *anisotropy*.

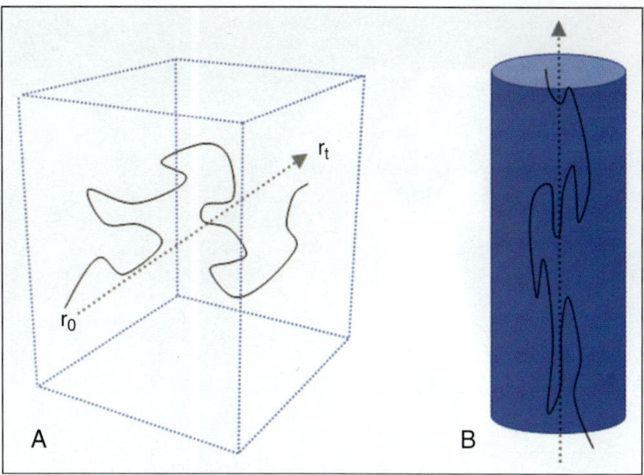

Figure 4.23 Different types of diffusion motion. (A) Brownian motion of freely moving hydrogen, (B) anisotropic motion such as along a myelin tract restricted axially but not longitudinally.

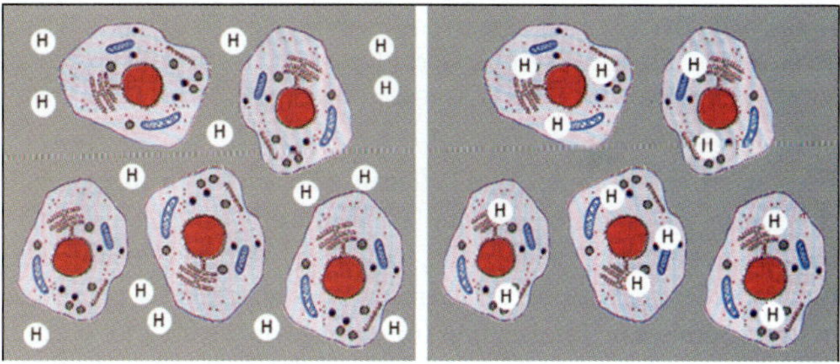

Figure 4.24 Restricted diffusion motion in the tissue. Extracellular hydrogen (H) is relatively free to move around (left) but intracellular hydrogen is restricted by the cell wall boundaries (right).

b value: Conventional DWI acquires data that are sensitized to diffusion in three orthogonal directions (typically, the *x*, *y*, and *z* axis). Three diffusion gradient pulse combinations are applied in sequential acquisitions that sensitize the magnetization to diffusion in *x*, *y*, and *z* directions, respectively. Typically, only a combined image from the source images is reviewed for diagnosis and is called the trace-weighted image. The strength of the diffusion gradient, the duration of the gradient and the time between the diffusion gradients determines the sensitivity of the sequence to diffusion and is commonly called the "*b* value." It is usually expressed in units of s/mm^2. Higher *b* value means higher sensitivity to diffusion restriction, but at the expense of loss of SNR. As the *b* value increases the signal from water molecules decreases. At high *b* values (e.g., $b = 1000$) only tissues with restricted motion of water molecules will have high signal. Fig. 4.26 illustrates the role of higher *b*-value scans where the signal from the bladder significantly drops in $b = 1000$ scan while the restricted diffusion in the area of the rectum shows comparably higher signal.

T2 shine-through and ADC: Essentially DWI is a T2W sequence. Hence structures which are normally bright on T2W such as fluid or edema will also tend to appear bright on DWI, especially the low *b*-value images, even if they do not necessarily demonstrate restricted diffusion. This is commonly referred to as "T2 shine through" and needs to be differentiated from true restriction.

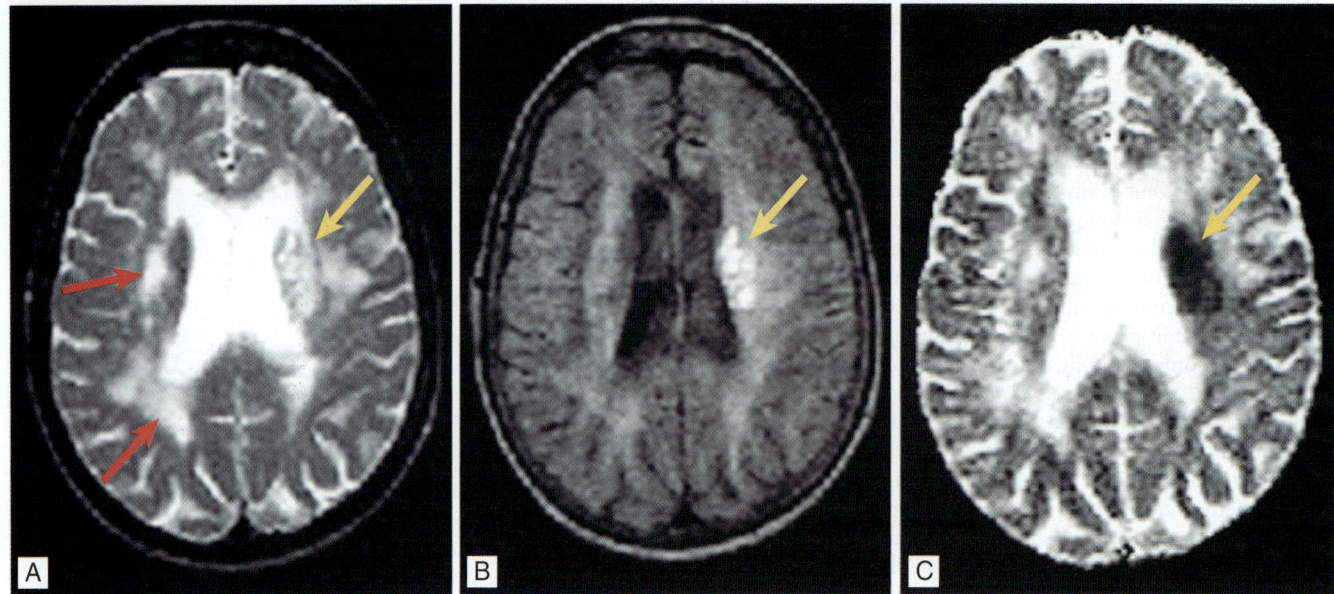

Figure 4.25 DWI helps distinguish time of strokes particularly helpful in patients with multiple lesions. (A) The T2w TSE result shows hyperintense signal from old (*red arrows*) as well as recent (*yellow arrow*) stroke that cannot be distinguished. (B) The DWI image at b = 1000, however, highlights recent stroke (*yellow arrow*). (C) The ADC map shows hypointense signal in the area of acute stroke (*yellow arrow*). (Courtesy: Alex de Crespigny, PhD.)

Because of this complexity, DWI can be difficult to interpret in conditions where the underlying T2 contrast is actually altered. A quantitative metric called ADC (apparent diffusion coefficient) helps in these situations. ADC maps are created on a pixel-wise basis by combining information from image data with and without diffusion weighting. ADC maps remove the "T2 shine through" effect, and theoretically portrays a more direct representation of the diffusion characteristics of the tissue (Fig. 4.26C). The signal intensities and appearances of DWI trace-weighted images and ADC maps are generally very different. The ADC map is a quantitative display of actual ADC values. In contrast, the signal intensity of each voxel in a diffusion-weighted image will be inversely related to its ADC value. In other words, a decrease in ADC value generally is associated with higher signal intensity on the diffusion-weighted result. Figure 4.26C in the case of rectal CA shows a lower ADC value while the b = 1000 scan has high signal intensity (Fig. 4.26B).

Diffusion tensor imaging: To obtain information about anisotropy of the underlying tissue, conventional DWI is not sufficient. Instead, a complex mathematical construct is used to model 3D anisotropy called the diffusion tensor. By applying diffusion sensitization in multiple directions (at least 6, but typically 20 or more), the directional variation in the tendency of water molecules to diffuse within a voxel is achieved using DTI. Important information about tissue connectivity is provided by DTI as it describes the diffusion along each direction and cross interactions between the directions (Fig. 4.27). Fiber tracking, or tractography, is a process of tracing the 3D course of white matter fiber tracts using DTI datasets (Fig. 4.28). This can be used to assess integrity, displacement, or involvement of white matter tracts in different clinical conditions, most commonly for presurgical planning of tumors. Modern software allows the calculation of qualitative and quantitative values with a single mouse click. Fractional anisotropy maps, ADC, volume ratio, Eigen value maps, tensor maps, and others are calculated and displayed in various grayscale and color formats for easier interpretation.

Susceptibility-Weighted Imaging

Susceptibility-weighted imaging (SWI) is a high-resolution 3D flow compensated T2*-weighted GRE sequence designed to accentuate susceptibility tissue differences. Magnetic susceptibility is a property that reflects how the B_0 magnetic field behaves within a tissue (i.e., positive susceptibility slightly increases the B_0 field while negative susceptibility slightly decreases it), and therefore provides additional

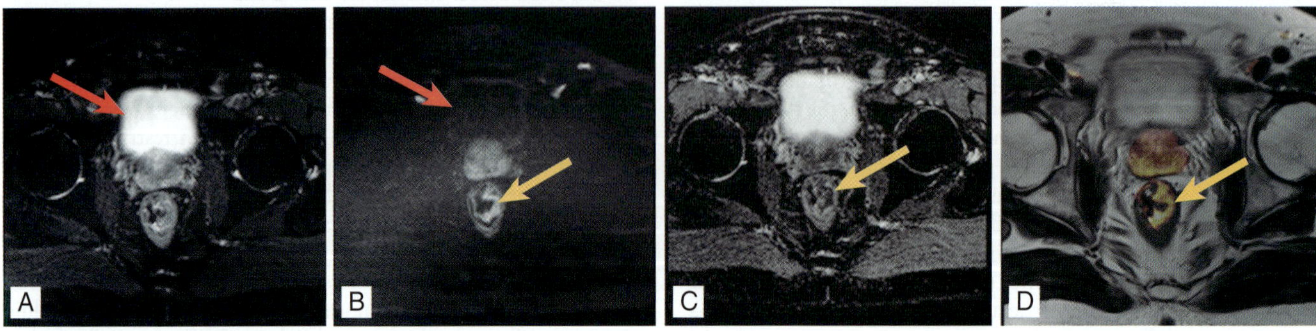

Figure 4.26 Diffusion-weighted imaging (DWI) images at 3T illustrate the role of higher b values. In this case of rectal carcinoma, the signal of fluid in the bladder (*red arrow*) is high at (A) b = 0 and low at (B) b = 1000 s/mm^2. Signal in the area of rectal carcinoma (*orange arrow*) where there is true restriction of water molecular motion decreases to a far lesser degree. The ADC map (C) shows a reduced value. A fused image of color rendered b = 1000 and T2W (D) provides for anatomical correlation and better visualization of the rectal carcinoma (*orange arrow*). (Courtesy: Thian Yee Liang, MBBS (S'pore), FRCR (UK), MMed (Diag Radiol, NUS), Head, Division of Body Imaging, National University Hospital, Singapore.)

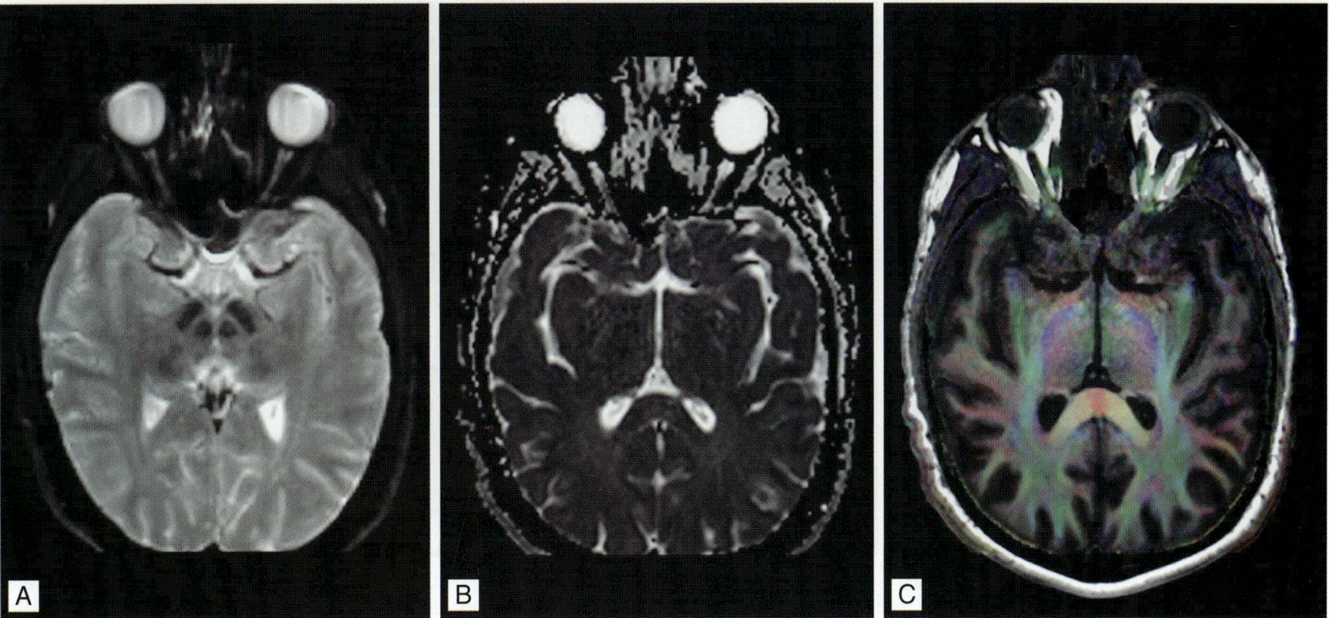

Figure 4.27 Diffusion tensor imaging (DTI) of the optic nerves in a healthy volunteer. (A) b = 0 magnitude image, (B) apparent diffusion coefficient (ADC) map, and (C) fusion of T1W and color fractional anisotropy (FA) map. (Courtesy: Siemens Healthineers.)

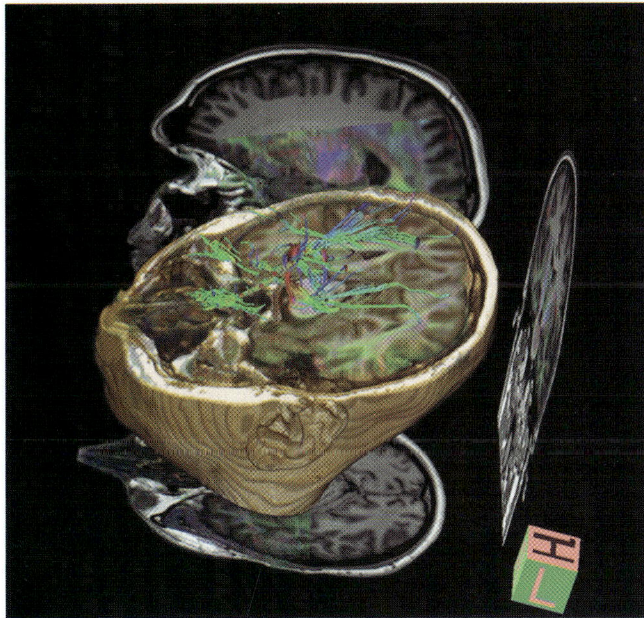

Figure 4.28 3D rendering of DTI tractography of the optic nerves in a healthy volunteer. (Courtesy: Siemens Healthineers.)

potentially useful diagnostic information. A set of four images can be available per slice position for review. A magnitude image, a phase image, a mask of the filtered phase image, and SWI image that provides contrast sensitive to venous blood, hemorrhage, iron storage, and various stages of blood products like deoxyhemoglobin, methemoglobin, and hemosiderin (as in granulomatous angiitis) [8]. In regions with higher susceptibility the signal will decrease due to the increased spin dephasing and T2* shortening, while additional sensitivity is gleaned from the signal phase changes associated with subtle differences in B_0. The susceptibility effects and hence the conspicuity of the lesions is better demonstrated by SWI compared with conventional sequences including standard GRE. Fig. 4.29 illustrates that GRE can also show small hemosiderin deposits while in T1W and TSE T2W images the deposits are not well seen. Higher magnetic field strength such as 7T accentuates the susceptibility effects [9] as shown in the clinical case in Fig. 4.30.

Its applications are numerous, most commonly related to detecting intracranial hemorrhage [10]. Following are few of the applications of SWI.

1. In diffuse axonal injury, shear stress injuries and the presence of microscopic hemorrhages can be demonstrated by SWI, particularly in the direction perpendicular to the corpus callosum with confidence. This would have even greater significance legally in a case of nonaccidental trauma
2. Tumoral calcification and peritumoral veins can be differentiated on SWI phase images [8]—hyperintensity for veins (paramagnetic) and hypointensity for calcification (diamagnetic)
3. It can detect hemorrhagic changes in arterial and venous infarcts
4. SWI helps evaluate intracranial metastatic disease for multiplicity (if hemorrhagic) that would alter treatment plans
5. SWI can identify very small lesions, particularly calcified neurocysticercosis, cortical calcifications, calcified tuberculoma, or a cavernoma
6. SWI is more sensitive in detecting vascular lesions such as venous angiomas and cavernomas, which are much more conspicuous on SWI than on conventional imaging
7. SWI can detect and depict venous sinus thrombosis in greater detail than conventional imaging and provides greater details. For example, the exact extent of the thrombus can be seen very well with SWI
8. Dementia in Alzheimer's disease is associated with the presence of amyloid plaques, which may be demonstrated using SWI on ultrahigh-field MR systems. In the vascular type of dementia associated with amyloid angiopathy, SWI demonstrates microhemorrhages in the vessel wall. The possibility of these microhemorrhages leading to dementia is currently being correlated. Hence SWI has a big role in neuroscience research including diseases like Alzheimer, MS, and dementia

Magnetic Resonance Angiography

MRA is a technique to visualize blood flow in macroscopic vessels. With appropriate sequences and analysis, the flow velocity,

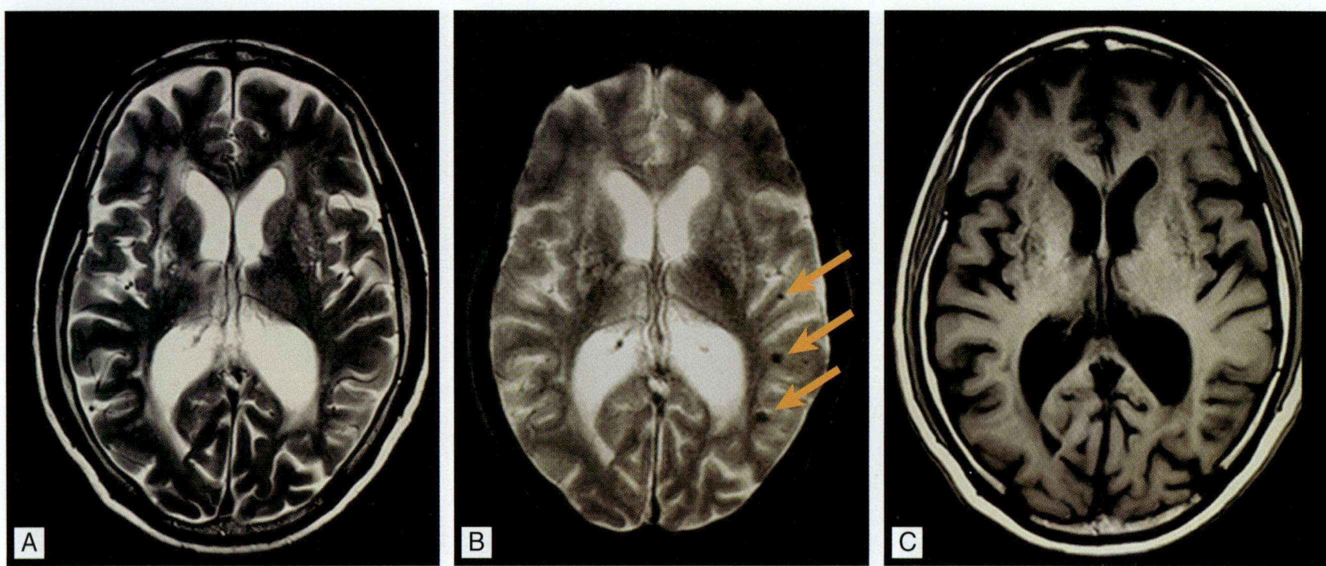

Figure 4.29 Hemosiderin deposition in the brain is not well visualized on transverse T2W (A) and T1W (C) images. However, T2*-weighted GRE that accentuate susceptibility differences (B) shows multiple small areas of hemosiderin deposits (*orange arrows*). (Courtesy: Wallabh Upasani, MD, Director Sun Scan Center, Thane, India.)

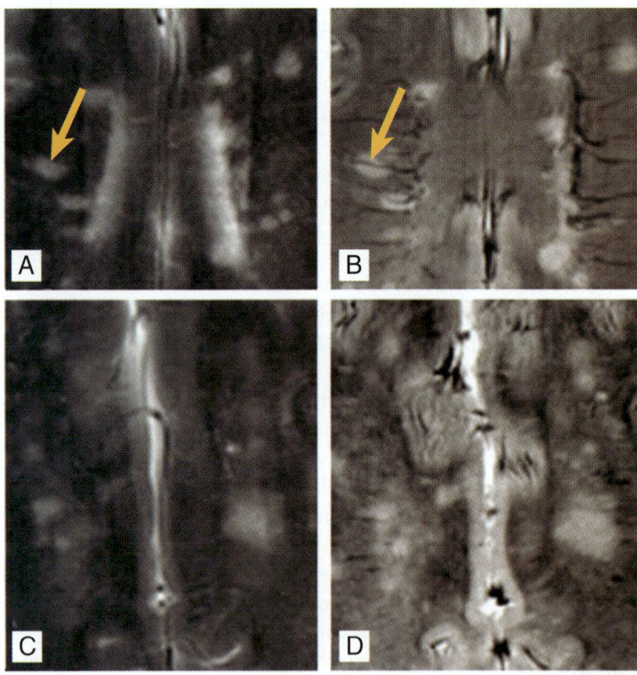

Figure 4.30 Example of clinical utility of SWI at 7T in multiple sclerosis (MS). This young patient (A, B) has a 4-year history of progressive MS, whose diagnosis is not in question. This image exemplifies a characteristic of MS well visualized with the high resolution of 7T, namely, the central vein coursing through the middle of the MS plaque. The arrows point to the same plaque on a (A) 3T T2w sequence, and a (B) 7T T2* GRE sequence. This imaging feature can be very useful in patients with lesser disease, where the diagnosis of MS is uncertain. An older patient (C, D) with cognitive issues was referred to the multiple sclerosis clinic for possible MS due to a 3T MRI. Images show a heavy burden of white matter disease, from a (C) 3T T2w sequence, and a (D) 7T T2* GRE sequence. In distinction to the MS patient of (A, B), no definitive central vein is seen at either field strength, and the diagnosis of nonspecific vasculopathy was raised. A subsequent parotid biopsy revealed underlying Sjogren's disease, whose chronic small vessel disease likely caused the findings. (Courtesy: Stephen Jones, MD, PhD, Cleveland Clinic, Cleveland, Ohio, USA.)

flow direction as well as the vascular structural information can be gathered. These advantages over other imaging techniques have made MRA a popular approach. The vascular anatomy is displayed as planar MR images ("raw" data) as well as a ray-traced projection over a 3D volume called maximum intensity projection, minimum intensity projection, cinematic rendered, or any other volume rendered methodology. Depending on the technique used, MRA can be performed with or without injecting any exogenous contrast agent.

Noncontrast MRA: For noncontrast MRA, flowing blood containing free water hydrogen acts as an intrinsic source of signal. 2D and 3D TOF and phase contrast (PC) techniques are used in routine clinical practice. With TOF, a GRE sequence is employed, and flowing blood appears bright relative to the stationary tissue when the excitation volume is perpendicular to the flow since the fresh inflow of blood is not in the steady state compared with the stationary tissue. MRA is useful to assess aneurysms, arteriovenous malformations, occlusive disease/stroke, cerebral venous disease, tumor, and other conditions [11]. Single volume or thin multislab techniques of TOF MRA are useful for the evaluation of large vessels at the base of the brain, large vessel occlusive disease or Circle of Willis aneurysms. To evaluate slower flow as in arteriovenous malformations or examination of distal arterial vasculature or peripheral aneurysms, thin multiple overlapping slabs that maximize the TOF effect is better than a single large volume. The evaluation of venous sinus thrombosis, venous disease, or evaluating draining vein of arteriovenous malformation is best performed with a stacked 2D slice sequential technique.

The PC technique takes advantage of the signal phase shift that occurs from moving spins in the presence of a spatial magnetic field gradient and is obtained from the difference in phase between the flowing blood and stationary tissue. Two sets of GRE images are acquired typically by employing flow-encoding gradients in one and no flow-encoding gradients in another as reference. With the application of flow-encoding gradients, the signal phase from flowing blood is shifted whereas the phase from the stationary background does not change. By subtracting the phase information between these two images, only the vessel phase is nonzero and visible, while the stationary tissue phase gets cancelled. 2D PC techniques are routinely used for flow quantification since the signal phase from blood flow will be directly proportional to the velocity and directionality. PC techniques can quantitate the characteristics of flow, tend to be improved at 3T due to higher SNR, but in general have long scan times. 3D TOF techniques in contrast are faster and robust for intracranial applications but cannot yield quantitative flow information.

Another noncontrast MRA technique used primarily outside of the brain is generated by subtracting two sets of images acquired with maximum and minimum flow during the cardiac cycle (NATIVE, Inhance, TRANCE). It consists of two non-ce MRA applications: a TSE/FSE-based technique is optimized for the use in peripheral angiography, and steady state free precession that is optimized for the use in thorax (e.g., thoracic aorta) and abdomen (e.g., renal arteries). An IR slab is positioned in the area of interest. When fresh arterial inflow of noninverted magnetization enters the region, data acquisition occurs during the TI period and that produces bright signal. This technique has a disadvantage that distal vessels have lower signal.

Contrast-enhanced MRA: This is a T1-weighted GRE technique that uses contrast agent injection to shorten the T1 of blood compared with surrounding tissues. The timing of the data acquisition and contrast agent bolus arrival is very critical for success of the technique. Using test bolus or automatic detection of bolus arrival has been conventionally used to align the acquisition timing. Acquired time sequentially in rapid succession, dynamic 4D MRA techniques are a more recent addition to contrast-enhanced MRA (ce-MRA). In 4D MRA, multiple fast 3D measurements provide valuable clinical information temporally as well as spatially owing to advances in hardware and software capabilities. MRA of the cerebrovascular system has advantages over other imaging techniques because the brain parenchyma and the vasculature from the aortic arch through the intracranial circulation can be studied at the same time. Fig. 4.31 shows a large FOV ce-MRA. Various time-efficient sampling methods (TRICKS, TWIST, 4D TRAK) further improve time-resolved ce-MRA providing complete full body FOV 3D datasets in as little as 2 seconds per frame. They provide the user greater flexibility in tailoring temporal and spatial resolution for dynamic MR imaging. Please refer to Table 4.5 for comparison of ce MRA and noncontrast MRA.

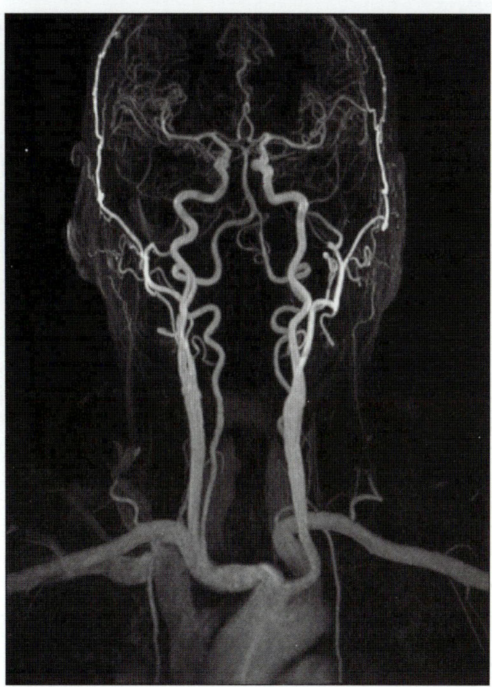

Figure 4.31 Large field-of-view (FOV) contrast-enhanced MR angiography (ce-MRA). Maximum intensity projection (MIP) of a large FoV (255 × 340 mm), subtracted dataset (pre- and postcontrast 3D ce-MRA) using a 64-channel Head/Neck array coil at 3T. Time-to-center (TTC) was 5 seconds from bolus injection. The acquisition was optimized for the image contrast enhancement by matching the contrast arrival timing with the acquisition of the central phase-encoding steps (i.e., TTC). The total scan time (21.36 seconds) is kept short within a breath-hold to suppress bulk breathing motion. (Courtesy: Department of Radiology, Centre Hospitalier Universitaire Vaudois (CHUV), Switzerland.)

MR Spectroscopy

MR spectroscopy (MRS) is a technique that provides information about metabolites in the brain [12] or in other regions like breast or prostate. For example, it can quantify the amount of lactate, lipids, or choline in a voxel. Each of these metabolites reflects specific cellular and biochemical processes in that anatomical

TABLE 4.5 Comparison of Contrast-Enhanced MR Angiography (ce-MRA) and Noncontrast MRA

Feature	ce-MRA Techniques	Noncontrast MRA Techniques
Use of gadolinium contrast agent	Required. Concerns for complications of gadolinium-based contrast media especially nephrogenic systemic fibrosis (NSF) and retention. With the use of AI algorithms, the total dose may reduce, but gadolinium is required	No gadolinium contrast required. Comparatively safe
Sequences and techniques	T1-weighted GRE 3D technique: ce-MRA 4D ce-MRA techniques TRICKS, TWIST, 4D TRAK	2D and 3D time-of-flight (TOF) and phase contrast (PC), TSE/FSE-based techniques using subtraction of two images—NATIVE, Inhance, TRANCE
Time to acquire dataset	Very fast—few seconds	Few minutes. Depends on many sequence parameters and patient's physiology if ECG trigger is used
Timing of contrast	Very crucial and needs to be synchronized with the sequence type for good CNR	Not relevant, easy to perform but can have blurry images
Temporal and spatial resolution	Excellent visualization in 4D. Good for understanding dynamic flow	Phase contrast technique is helpful but accurate determination of velocity encoding required for proper selection of sequence parameters
Flow quantification	Only relative quantification possible with perfusion studies	Possible with phase contrast techniques

location, which can have diagnostic and prognostic implications. Although multinuclear capabilities allow the opportunity to probe several different nuclei, in clinical routine hydrogen protons (^{1}H) are most commonly used due to their abundance in the tissue.

Principle: MRS exploits the concept of chemical shift. The resonant frequency of the hydrogen nucleus is altered by its chemical environment, which is called a chemical shift, the extent of which depends on the number and type of adjacent atoms and molecular structures. Fourier transformation of the MR signal (usually as a free induction decay, or FID) converts the signal into a spectral plot in the frequency domain as shown in Fig. 4.32A. The horizontal axis of this plot is usually displayed in parts per

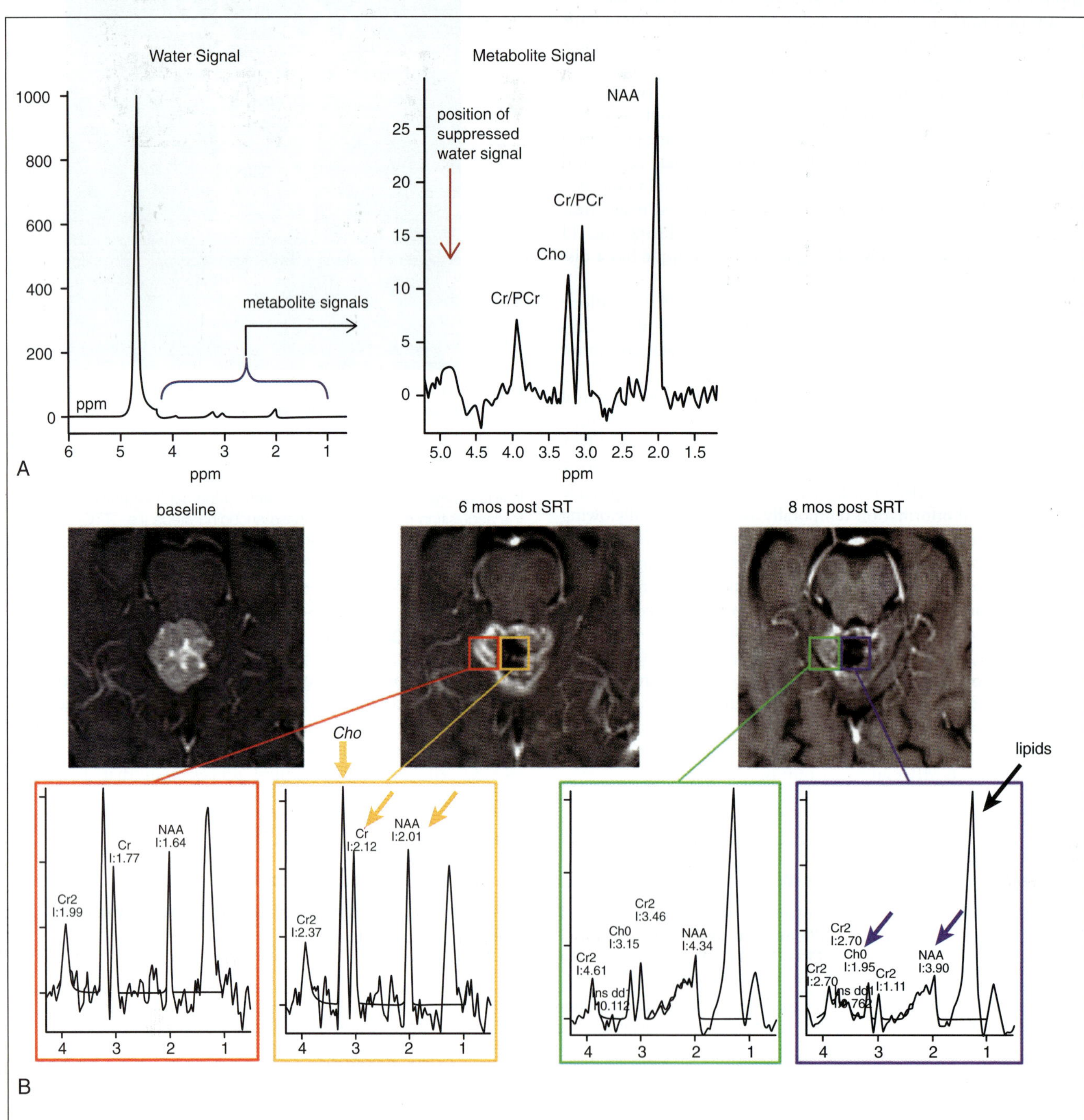

Figure 4.32 MR spectroscopy (MRS). The property of chemical shift allows the ability to assess different metabolites in the frequency domain as a spectrum. (A) The signal from a 1H MRS measurement in the human brain is the sum of a large water signal and small metabolite signals. On the left represents the Fourier transformation of the FID with prominent water signal at a chemical shift of 4.7 ppm. Metabolite peaks are hardly visible. Suppression of the water signal from the FID and subsequent FT and processing reveals the metabolite signals. This is an example of 1H MRS spectrum of a normal adult brain. (B) MRS can be complementary to many MR exams. Using multivoxel MRS over the lesion, findings on 1H MRS helps identify residual or recurrent tumor. The spectra help to differentiate residual or recurrent tumor from post-treatment abnormality (i.e., radiation necrosis). Reduced NAA, Cho, Cr (*blue arrows*), and increased levels of lipid (*black arrow*) are seen in this case of radiation necrosis following stereotactic radiosurgery (SRT) in a metastatic breast cancer patient as compared to yellow arrows. Choline is at 3.2 ppm, Creatine at 3.0 and NAA and 2.0 in all of the spectra. (Courtesy: James N. Scott, MD, MSc, FRCPC, Foothills Medical Centre, Calgary, Canada.)

TABLE 4.6 ^{1}H Proton MR Spectroscopy (MRS) of Normal Brain Metabolites

Metabolite	Peak Position (ppm)	TE
NAA	2.01, 2.60	Short and long
Cr/PCr	3.02, 3.94	Short and long
Cho	3.22	Short and long
Glucose (Glc)	3.43, 3.80	Short
Myoinositol (ml)	3.56, 4.06	Short

Note: Water is defined by convention at 4.7 ppm. Chemical shifts are from reference: T Michaelis, K Merboldt, W Hänicke, M Gyngell, H Bruhn, J Frahm. On the identification of cerebral metabolites in localized1H NMR spectra of human brain in vivo, NMR Biomed 4 (2) (1991) 90–98.

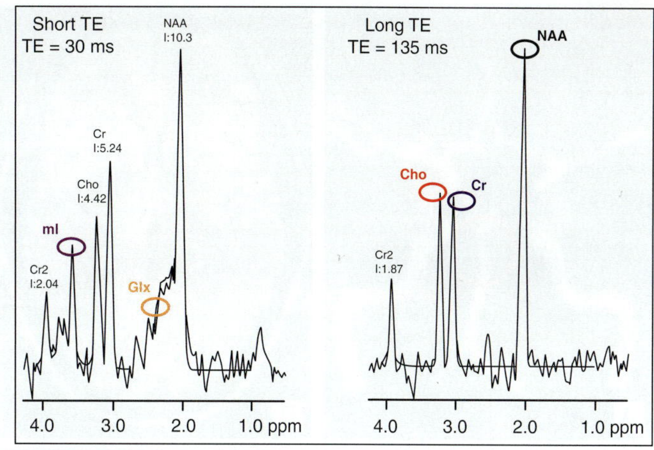

Figure 4.33 Proton (1H) MR spectroscopy (MRS) of normal brain metabolites. Water is defined by convention at 4.7 ppm and is suppressed to visualize the metabolites effectively. Short TE spectra (*left*) exhibit different metabolite distribution than longer TE spectra (*right*). (Courtesy: James N. Scott, MD, MSc, FRCPC, Foothills Medical Centre, Calgary, Canada.)

million (ppm) since this remains a constant rather than absolute frequency in Hz which will be scaled according to the magnetic field strength and is represented by specific metabolites [13] at different frequencies or chemical shifts as illustrated in Fig. 4.32A and Table 4.6. The shift is a relative property and proportionally increases in frequency with increased field strength which is why MRS is more accurate at 3T and higher fields since it is easier to resolve small shifts. Based on the MRS technique, single-voxel spectroscopy (SVS) or chemical shift imaging (CSI), sequence parameters, and postprocessing steps, each of these metabolites can reflect specific cellular and biochemical processes in that anatomical location.

- SVS produces a single spectrum from a single localized volume in one measurement. SVS is simple to use, has a better shim on a smaller voxel and has less contamination. Typically, SVS is used in well-defined lesions
- CSI in contrast combines features of imaging as well as spectroscopy. CSI collects spectroscopic data from multiple adjacent voxels covering a large VOI in a single measurement. CSI is more efficient than SVS if a larger area needs to be examined particularly diffuse lesions but typically has longer scan times

Technique: The general strategy with MRS is to obtain the spectra within a defined voxel(s) that is usually isotropically 10–20 mm in size. To localize the voxel, the MRS technique is typically a three RF pulse preparation, applying a selection gradient on all three physical axes where the intersection of each selective excitation defines the voxel to be probed. Two different methods, each with three successive selective RF pulses, are frequently used for SVS—double spin echo, SE (90-180-180-echo), or stimulated echo, STE (90-180-90-echo). Once the echo is formed in either case, the signal is sampled over a long period of time relative to an imaging technique to resolve small chemical shifts. One common challenge with MRS is that the RF pulses usually have very wide transmission bandwidths to capture all chemical shift species and can be limited by both RF hardware capabilities as well as increased RF heating.

The size and positioning of the voxel are critical for successful analysis. Conducting an MRS experiment after gadolinium contrast injection is an advantage because the lesion is better visualized, and the voxel can be better positioned. It is critical to shim the region of interest to <0.1 ppm before data acquisition, otherwise peaks become broadened and difficult to resolve [14]. The choline peak, for example, is noticeably affected and can be reduced by as much as 40% (particularly in the breast) [15], depending on the organ, degree of enhancement, and type of contrast agent used.

Metabolite assessment: Metabolites like myo-inositol (ml), glutamate and glutamine (Glx), lactate, and lipids are best analyzed with short TE (30 ms), while *N*-acetyl aspartate, choline, creatinine, and lactate are best analyzed with intermediate or long TE (135 ms or 270 ms, respectively) (Fig. 4.33). *N*-acetyl aspartate is a marker for neuronal and axonal integrity. It is decreased in conditions where there is neuronal loss or damage. Creatinine is associated with cellular ATP metabolism and is a measure of energy stores. It is a stable cerebral metabolite and is used as an internal standard to measure other peaks against. Choline is a measure of cellular proliferation and is elevated in tumors and inflammatory processes. Lactate is the end product of glycolysis and its presence indicates anaerobic metabolism. Myo-inositol is a marker for gliosis and reactive astrocytosis. Lipid peak may be present due to voxel contamination from fat (e.g., scalp) but may also indicate necrosis from infection or tumor.

Clinical applications of MRS include characterizing and grading neoplasms, differentiating recurrent tumor versus secondary necrosis due to therapy (Fig. 4.32B), or for monitoring under radio-chemotherapy. Particularly for the brain, other indications include characterizing infection, demyelination or other white matter diseases, evaluating neurodegenerative diseases, etc.

Perfusion-Weighted Imaging

Perfusion imaging involves visualization and quantification of delivered blood flow at the capillary level where exchange of nutrients and oxygen takes place. Established MRI techniques to measure perfusion include:

1. *Dynamic contrast enhancement (DCE)*: This consists of a T1-weighted 3D spoiled GRE sequence acquired temporally in a repeated manner during gadolinium contrast injection which is used to depict microcirculatory uptake. Gadolinium causes reduction in the T1 relaxation time and signal changes are seen as increased signal intensity. Typically it is evaluated as "wash-in" and "wash-out" graphs when analyzed over time. DCE scans and analysis are a direct measure of vascular permeability. In a breast lesion if there is a rapid wash-in and a fast wash-out DCE curve, this pattern may be suggestive of an aggressive cancer
2. *Dynamic susceptibility contrast*: Dynamic susceptibility contrast (DSC) is based on a T2*-weighted 2D GRE EPI sequence to acquire rapid sequential time points during contrast injection to measure bolus first pass perfusion. DSC provides a measure of vascularity, relative cerebral blood flow, microvascular density or relative cerebral blood volume, and

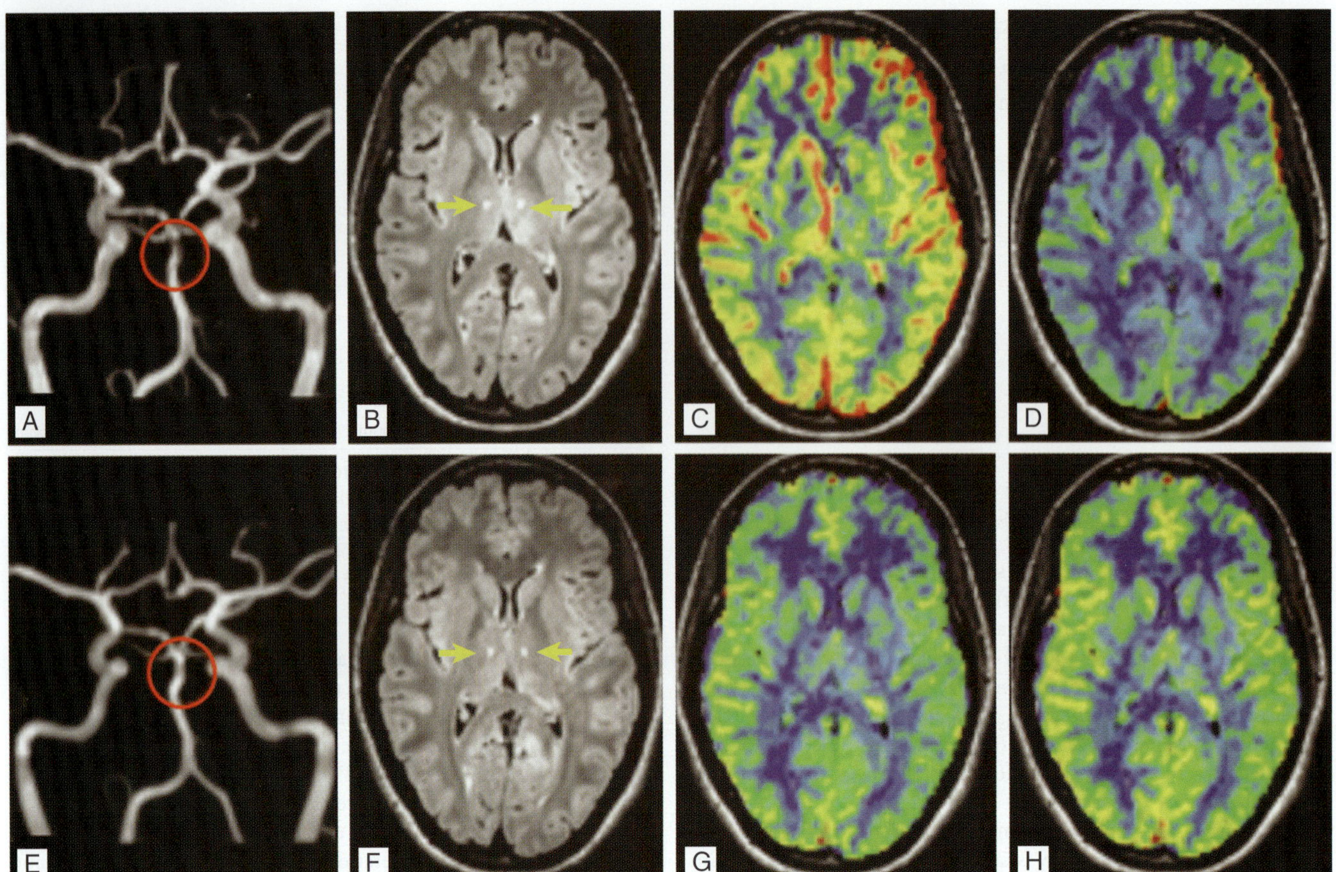

Figure 4.34 Case demonstrating the value of arterial spin labeling (ASL). A patient with a stenosis of the distal basilar artery on coronal MIP of a 3D TOF MRA (A) (*red circle*). The FLAIR image in the subacute phase (B) shows bilateral thalamic lesions (*yellow arrows*). 3D ASL shows a serpiginous, high absolute CBF close to the lesion in the right thalamus, but not in the left (C). The normalized CBF shows inhomogeneous perfusion throughout the gray matter, and relatively low perfusion in the posterior circulation territories and the right hemisphere (D). After 5 months, the basilar artery has normalized on MRA (E) (*red circle*). The thalamic lesions did not change substantially on the FLAIR image (F) (*yellow arrows*); absolute CBF from 3D ASL images shows globally reduced perfusion (G); normalized CBF shows more homogeneous perfusion throughout the gray matter (H). 3D ASL can provide significant information that cannot be easily produced with other noninvasive techniques, and might provide new insight into the functional, vascular, and neuronal changes that often coexist with an ischemic brain accident. (Courtesy: Fabrizio Esposito, PhD, Scuola Medica Salernitana University of SalernoVia, Baronissi, Italy.)

other hemodynamic metrics like mean transit time and bolus arrival time. T2*-based DSC is complementary to T1-based DCE perfusion partly due to their different temporal resolutions. DSC has better temporal resolution because it is required to measure the bolus during first pass perfusion. Both techniques require a bolus of contrast media injected into a peripheral vein preferably on the right arm

3. *Arterial spin labeling* [16]: Arterial spin labeling (ASL) is an alternative method to measure perfusion directly without the use of an exogenous contrast agent. ASL uses magnetization prepared or tagged in-flowing arterial blood as a labeled freely diffusible intrinsic tracer. ASL may show signal representing flow in collateral vessels (Fig. 4.34)

Key applications for perfusion-weighted imaging (PWI) are cerebrovascular diseases, acute stroke, transient ischemic events, hemorrhages, Moya-Moya disease, and tumor grading, to name a few. PWI is also used in assessing lesions outside the brain, as, for example, for prostate or breast cancer.

Advanced Applications

***Functional MRI (fMRI)*:** This is primarily a study of brain function [17]. It can be used clinically for presurgical planning, for example, by mapping of brain functions in relation to intracranial tumors, epileptic foci or vascular malformations before surgical excision. The goal of fMRI in this case is to maximize resection of the pathological tissue while sparing eloquent cortices, reducing surgical risk, and improving patient rehabilitation. For example, for a left frontal lobe tumor, fMRI to identify and map the Broca's speech area before surgery helps prevent inadvertent damage to it during surgery. fMRI is an adjunct for the neurological diagnosis and supports neuroscience research.

Principle of fMRI: fMRI is usually a task-based application (although nontask-based "resting state" fMRI has gained interest in more recent years) and involves the following steps: preparation of the patient and task experiment, acquisition of the MRI scan while making the patient perform specific tasks based on the functions which needs to be mapped, and then processing of the data by analyzing the difference in the task-based signal compared with the basal state of neurons. The result when overlaid on anatomy then represents macroscopic neuronal activity as a response to the task stimulus.

BOLD imaging: The fMRI signal response is based on small changes in blood flow in regions of neuronal activation and is referred to as BOLD (blood oxygen level-dependent) contrast. Blood is used as an endogenous contrast agent to detect neuronal activity. Hemoglobin delivers oxygen to the cells. Oxygenated hemoglobin is diamagnetic and does not alter the localized magnetic field homogeneity because iron molecules are surrounded by oxygen molecules shielding the susceptibility effects of the iron. Deoxygenated hemoglobin is paramagnetic and will therefore disrupt the local magnetic field. If an MR sequence like FID-based EPI is used that is sensitive to field inhomogeneities (accentuating T2* differences), then an area with relatively less deoxyhemoglobin levels present from neuronal activity will have lower field inhomogeneities (longer T2*) compared with surrounding areas and will be detected as increased signal in the image. This is the basis behind the BOLD mechanism.

Task-based paradigms: These differ depending on the area of the brain being examined. Motor, visual, auditory, or cognitive paradigms are typically used. There are two major classifications of functional paradigms, those that are "block design" and "event related." The BOLD-related signal increase in FID-EPI is very small (0.3–5% compared with basal state, depending on the activation response and magnetic field strength) so data averaging is required to gain statistical confidence. In a block design, 10–30 seconds of stimuli alternating with either resting condition or control condition is commonly used.

Typical steps for fMRI data processing include motion and physiological correction, system-dependent detrending, registration, filtering, and statistical analysis. Synchronization to external devices for controlling stimulation systems is getting easier through software user interface at the scanner that helps the delivery of the stimuli synchronous to data acquisition. Choice of the control condition is important and requires detailed knowledge of the underlying neuroscience. fMRI results can show significant intersubject variation making conclusions at times challenging.

MR fingerprinting (MRF): This is a new technique for estimating multiple quantitative parametric tissue maps simultaneously [18] in reasonable scan times. The term "fingerprinting" gets its name from the fact that these quantitative maps are derived from a unique MRI signal pattern analogous to a fingerprint where pattern matching is conducted. The acquired signal pattern is matched against "fingerprints" from a predefined dictionary of expected signal responses based on Bloch equation simulations associated with both the acquisition parameters and the tissue properties. A unique match in the pattern can therefore only be achieved by an equally unique combination of T1, T2, and other quantitative values with the complete tissue maps being generated on a pixel by pixel basis. The combination of novel acquisition techniques, pattern recognition algorithms, and a large dictionary of precomputed signal responses makes MRF an elegant, powerful, and promising tool for quantitative multiparametric analysis of normal and abnormal tissues that can provide insights to diagnose diseases based on unique fingerprint patterns. For example, 3D whole brain MRF and partial volume (PV) MRF techniques can aid detection and characterization of lesions in epilepsy patients or for brain tumors using k-means clustering of quantitative MRF results. MRF can provide new, clinically relevant information about subtle tissue changes which may not be apparent on conventional weighted MR images. Properties of component tissues, including diseased tissues in tumors, can be determined without previous knowledge by MRF.

Hepatic fat and iron quantification: These are important biomarkers [19] for various disease processes and the ability of MRI to help quantify them opens possibilities of *virtual biopsy*. Please refer to the chapters on liver and adrenal disease for additional information. To achieve accurate outcomes, there have been challenges such as different T1 weighting of the fat and water signals, T2* decay, and complex decay of fat due to its multipeak spectrum. These issues have limited accurate quantification of fat with MRI in the past. R2*-based methods have significantly improved with hardware and software developments allowing shorter TE values and more data points for better estimations. The precession frequency increases at higher field strengths, making the echo spacing required tighter at 3T for a specific phase offset between water and fat and thus needing faster acquisitions. These developments make the data less sensitive to fat and water errors. This helps the correlation of R2* estimates from MRI data to the true R2* of the tissue. Newer quantification algorithms quantify liver iron as R2* estimates and provide limits of agreement and coefficient of variation as additional inputs forming part of a wider diagnostic process.

MR fat quantification is based on measuring different chemical shift effects of hydrogen protons in water and in triglycerides of fat. MR iron quantification is based on quantifying signal decay as a function of varying TE. The effects of fat and iron on the MR signal are competing factors for one another but can be exploited by techniques of acquisition [20] and processing to simultaneously estimate and mutually correct each other. Fast multiecho GRE sequences are used along with MRS as an adjunct. System-specific quality control may be necessary to ensure quantitative accuracy to interpret the results.

One such implementation includes a regular opposed-phase/in-phase two-point Dixon protocol where water/fat separation is acquired (see Table 4.4). The Dixon method acquires two datasets at slightly different TEs, one that is "in-phase" and one that is "opposed-phase." It is then mathematically possible to separate out the fat content of the signal from the water content. Dixon technique exploits the fact that fat and water are separated in frequency by approximately 3.5 ppm which leads to phase cycling between the fat and water signals. An advantage of the Dixon technique is the potential for absolute quantification of the percentage of fat in each voxel. Because the signals of fat and water can be completely separated, it is then possible to use this information to quantitatively assess fat content.

MR elastography: Percutaneous liver biopsy and histopathological analysis are used as standard methods to confirm and classify cirrhosis or nonalcoholic steatohepatitis. Noninvasive tests such as ultrasound elastography and MR elastography (MRE) of the liver are now clinically available [21]. MRE is a technique done in addition to standard diagnostic liver imaging. Given that liver fibrosis is often spatially heterogeneous, the volume of liver sampled in MRE is an advantage compared with liver biopsy and ultrasound elastography.

As there is an external mechanical component in MRE, having an appropriate setup for an MRE examination is important (Fig. 4.35). The "paddle" (passive driver) must be correctly positioned and has good contact with the upper abdomen. It should be completely flat against the body surface. Breath holds

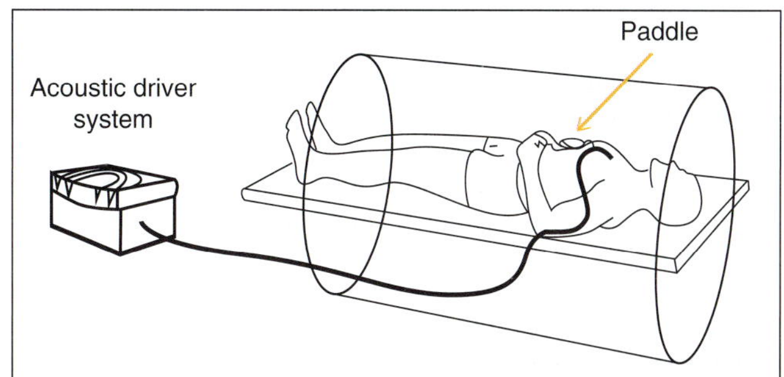

Figure 4.35 MR elastography setup. Careful placement of the mechanical paddle is necessary for good results. This is connected to an external acoustic driver system that allows control of the frequency and duration of the acoustic waves. (Courtesy: Siemens Healthineers.)

TABLE 4.8 US FDA Regulatory Classification of Computer-Aided Diagnosis (CAD) Devices

Classification	Description	Example/s
Computer-aided triage (CADt)	Software devices with AI algorithms that assist hospital networks and trained radiologists in workflow triage by flagging and communication of suspected positive findings. CADt aids in prioritizing/triaging time sensitive patient detection and diagnosis	qER from Qure.ai is a triage and notification tool that prioritizes head CT scans with critical abnormalities such as a bleed, fracture, mass effect, or midline shift on the radiology worklist for priority review. HealthPNX from Zebra Medical Vision Ltd. for pneumothorax (PNX) based on chest x-rays
Computer-aided detection (CADe)	Software devices with AI algorithms that aids in localizing/marking regions of that may reveal specific abnormalities	InferRead lung CT. AI from Beijing Infervision Technology Co., Ltd. is designed to aid the radiologist in the detection of pulmonary nodules during the review of CT examinations of the chest on an asymptomatic population
Computer-aided diagnosis (CADx)	Software devices with AI algorithms that aids in characterizing/assessing disease, disease type, severity, stage, progression	QuantX from Quantitative Insights, Inc. is a CADx software device used to assist radiologists in the assessment and characterization of breast abnormalities using MR image data
Computer-aided detection/ diagnosis (CADe/x)	These devices aid in localizing and characterizing conditions	MammoScreen from Therapixel is a software for supporting radiologists in identifying findings on screening FFDM mammography for lesions suspicious for cancer. Research AI prototypes for detecting, characterizing, and reporting prostate MR scans are showing promising results [27]
Computer-aided acquisition/ optimization (CAD a/o)	AI algorithm-based software that aids in the acquisition/optimization of images/diagnostic signals	Caption Health, Inc.'s Caption Guidance software is an accessory to uSmart 3200t Plus ultrasound system. Caption guidance is intended to assist medical professionals in the acquisition of cardiac ultrasound images

(Note: Regulatory classification of computer-aided diagnosis (CAD) devices is based on interpretation of available data on US FDA's website—https://www.accessdata.fda.gov/scripts/cdrh/cfdocs/cfpmn/pmn.cfm.)

PET-MRI

PET-MRI is a combination of an MRI scanner and a PET scanner built into one imaging device [32]. The FDA clearance of an MR-PET system was first granted in June 2011. Patient comfort regarding examination, positioning, and scanning with a combined scanner has significantly improved since then. PET-MRI measurement consists of two simultaneous acquisitions where the MR data and PET data are acquired at the same time to facilitate coregistration of the information. The initial MR acquisition also obtains data required for the attenuation correction of the PET data. Based on the scan protocol, additional MR images are typically acquired while the PET protocol is continuously running. The MR data acquisition complements PET image reconstruction with attenuation correction, motion, and volume correction. The PET acquisition in turn also supports the MR image correction. MR-PET brings imaging of morphology, function, and metabolism together.

PET-MRI uniquely allows simultaneous acquisition of MR and PET data. This enables the registration and fusion of anatomic, physiologic, functional, and metabolic information due to the precisely aligned MR and PET image coordinate systems. Depending on the region of interest, approved gadolinium contrast agents may be used. This system may also be used for imaging during interventional procedures when performed with MR compatible devices, such as MR safe biopsy needles. The PET maps and measures the distribution of PET radiopharmaceuticals in humans to aid the physician in determining various metabolic (molecular) and physiologic functions within the human body for the evaluation of diseases and disorders. The combined system utilizes the MR for radiation-free attenuation correction maps for PET studies. The system also provides inherent anatomical reference for the fused PET and MR images due to precisely aligned MR and PET image coordinate systems.

These systems are designed for whole body oncology, neurology, and cardiology examinations (Fig. 4.38). In neurology, clinical applications include imaging in neurodegenerative disorders like Parkinson's disease, Alzheimer's disease, vascular dementia, imaging in stroke for tissue viability, neuro-oncologic imaging for tumor viability, epilepsy imaging for accurate localization of epileptic foci, and to study brain development in pediatric neurology. PET-MRI is taking an emerging role in oncology imaging by providing anatomical, functional, physiological, and metabolic information to supplement data from other diagnostic and anatomical imaging techniques. Biochemical compensation, function, and viability can be assessed using MRI sequences such as diffusion, SWI, perfusion, spectroscopy, and fMRI. The system also supports the generation of quantifiable PET images, using various correction algorithms that are commercially available. In oncology imaging early stage diagnosis and better staging can be achieved by advanced lesion detectability and characterization. The ability to assess response to disease-treatment early one helps monitor therapy effectively.

MRI in Therapy

Imaging plays a critical role in treatment planning and during therapy treatment. Image-guided biopsies, image-guided interventions, and intraoperative imaging have been generally adopted in healthcare. MRI has the advantage of providing multiplanar acquisition capabilities, superior soft-tissue contrast, and probe functional and chemical composition of tissues to better characterize the lesions. It has the added benefit that it does not use ionizing radiation.

Although doing an ultrasound-guided prostate biopsy, registering previously acquired MR data has yielded better targeted biopsies. There are software applications that support the radiologist for an ultrasound-guided MRI-ultrasound fusion biopsy. Similarly, MR-guided stereotactic acquisition techniques for

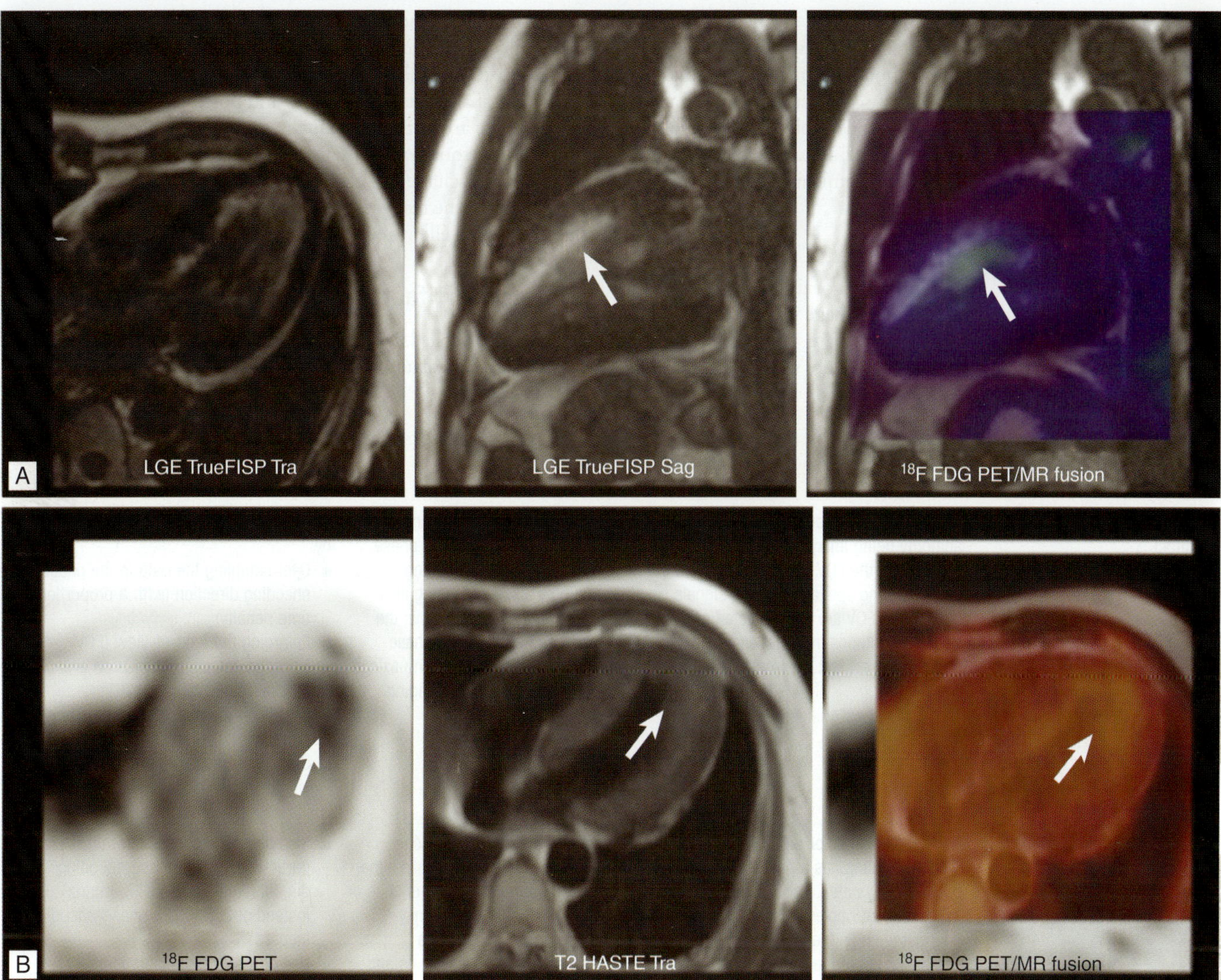

Figure 4.38 Cardiac MR/PET delineates extensive subendocardial infarction leading to acute coronary syndrome. MRI as a technique helps characterization of myocardial viability. (A) Two-chamber and four-chamber views through the left ventricle of the post-Gd TrueFISP sequence (late Gd enhancement also known as LGE) show the subendocardial contrast enhancement with increased ^{18}F FDG uptake in part of the subendocardium (*arrows*), reflecting inflammation induced by acute myocardial injury corresponding to the subendocardial infarction in the fused PET/MR images. (B) Four-chamber views of ^{18}F FDG PET, T2 HASTE, and fused PET/MR showing increased ^{18}F FDG uptake in the apical, septal, and adjacent lateral wall subendocardium (*arrows*), coregistering with the mild hyperintensity in the same myocardial region seen on the HASTE images, which reflects subendocardial inflammation secondary to acute myocardial infarction limited to the subendocardium. (Courtesy: Eunjung Kong, MD, Yeungnam University Medical Center, Daegu, South Korea.)

neurosurgical biopsy and brain tumor surgery have better patient outcomes in terms of lower morbidity and mortality rates [33]. Real-time MR imaging control, MR safe tools, needles, and MR-compatible biopsy devices support the radiologist for MRI-guided stereotactic breast and prostate biopsies.

Intensity-modulated radiation therapy planning for cancer treatment uses CT and MR data. Intensity-modulated radiation therapy contours the intensity of radiation dosage, avoiding vital structures, and thus complications arising from treatment. Since radiation shrinks the size of the tumor, anatomy can also shift due to fibrosis. MR images acquired before the next radiation cycle can then be fused with the previous CT scan to detect any shift in anatomy. This procedure (referred to as dynamic adaptation radio therapy planning) is beneficial for accurate treatment delivery and reduced complications. MR also plays a central role in radiotherapy planning, assisting in early detection of recurrence, incomplete removal, and complications to treatment.

Using operating rooms (ORs) that have an environment that is MR-compatible has enabled using MRI during the surgery. There is a patient transport mechanism (trolley) between the OR table and MRI system. Intraoperative MRI scans aid the surgeon to access local anatomical shifts due to the resection that can help them decide the next steps. After surgery, another MRI scan can then confirm if the resection is complete and helps to visualize if there were any complications due to the procedure. In some configurations, the MR magnet is mounted on the ceiling on rails and is brought to the OR table for imaging. Other hybrid OR configurations can include an MR, CT, and an angiographic system with OR-compatible tables for all techniques and a patient transport trolley system. Although such setups may have a significant investment upfront, there are potential savings due to more accurate tumor resection, lower post-op morbidity and complications, and overall better short-term and long-term patient outcomes, which need to be studied in more detail.

MR-guided high-intensity focused ultrasound ablation has gained popularity in recent years. Focused ultrasound waves heat the targeted tissue causing coagulation necrosis without affecting the surrounding tissue. During the ablation process, MRI scans that monitor the temperature of the area (*MR thermometry*) provide a colored representation of the local temperatures. This assists in real-time adjustment to the intensity and duration of the ultrasound treatment.

MR Artifacts

An artifact can be defined as any undesired or unexpected appearance in the image. Artifacts can degrade image quality and can be confused with pathology. MRI artifacts are continually being addressed by the device manufacturers who with their mature understanding of the source of artifacts are always improving on image quality through SNR optimization, speed, and artifact mitigation techniques. A general description is provided of some fundamental artifacts, their causes and possible remedial measures to reduce the artifacts. Additionally some carefully chosen artifacts that are less commonly discussed in the literature yet are quite prevalent and challenging in routine clinical practice on present day scanners. The reader is also encouraged to pursue further reading of some excellent reviews on this subject [34–36].

Common Artifacts

Please refer to Table 4.9 for details regarding various common artifacts. It is useful to systematically examine general features of the images and

TABLE 4.9 Common MRI Artifacts

Artifact	Causes	Axis	Remedies
Aliasing, or wrap around artifact 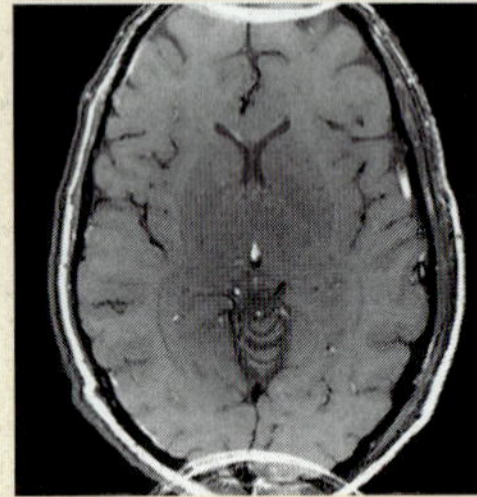	Aliasing occurs when the field-of-view (FOV) is smaller than the anatomy being imaged. The part of the body that lies beyond the edge of the FOV is projected onto the other side of the image. During spatial encoding, signals from the anatomy outside the FOV are also detected and allocated pixel positions. Hence a limitation in signal encoding appears in the image as a wraparound artifact of structures outside the FOV	Can occur in any axis of phase encoding. Aliasing also occurs in the slice phase-encoding axis in 3D imaging	Aliasing on MRI can be compensated for by: ▪ Over sampling the data in the phase-encoding direction (with a proportional time penalty) ▪ Enlarging the field-of-view (FOV) ▪ Using presaturation bands on areas outside the FOV ▪ Switching the phase and frequency directions ▪ Using a surface coil to reduce the signal outside of the area of interest
Truncation artifact or Gibbs ringing 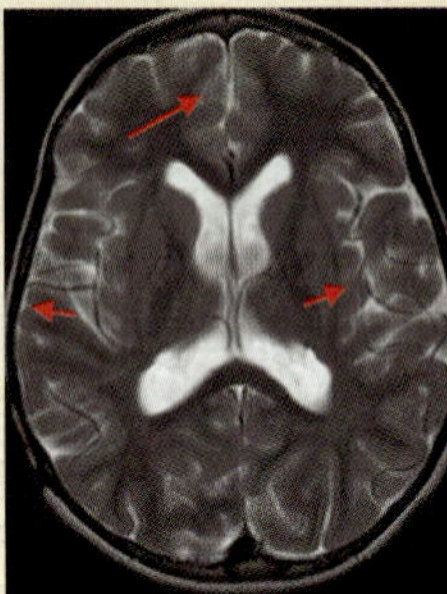 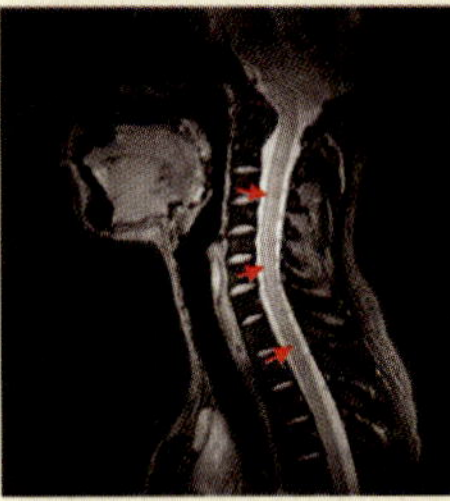	Truncation artifact or Gibbs ringing is caused by the fact that the digital sampling has a finite duration where the encoded signal becomes truncated. This manifests in the reconstructed image in the form of ripples close to tissue interfaces with high contrast such as the skull–brain interface. For example, in sagittal scans of the cervical spine, signal mimicking CSF in central canal may appear in the spinal cord and might be misinterpreted as syringomyelia	These can appear in either phase-encode or frequency-encode directions and appear close to the sharp high contrast interfaces	▪ Increasing the acquisition matrix size particularly in the phase-encoding direction (e.g., 256 × 256 matrix instead of 256 × 128 phase-encoding steps) ▪ Use of *k*-space-specific filters ▪ If fat is one of the boundaries, use fat suppression technique
Shading artifact 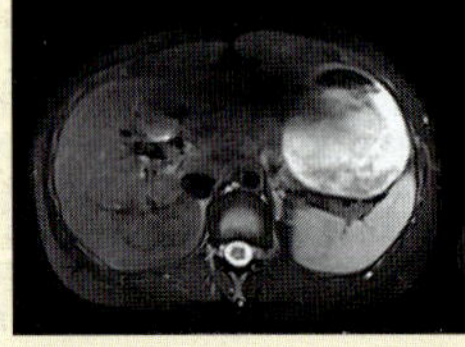	"Shading" refers to the artifactual loss of signal intensity in one regional part of the image leading to uneven brightness and/or contrast. Causes for shading are numerous, including nonuniform excitation and flip angle, abnormal loading or coupling of the coil at a point when a large patient, for example, touches one side of the coil, inhomogeneity in the magnetic field, or even voltage saturation of the analog-to-digital converter (ADC)	Not axis specific	▪ Use the proper size coil for patient size and the examined part ▪ Shimming to reduce the inhomogeneity of the magnetic field ▪ To avoid ADC overflow, use proper scanning parameters

TABLE 4.9 Common MRI Artifacts—cont'd

Artifact	Causes	Axis	Remedies
External RF interference artifact/zipper artifact 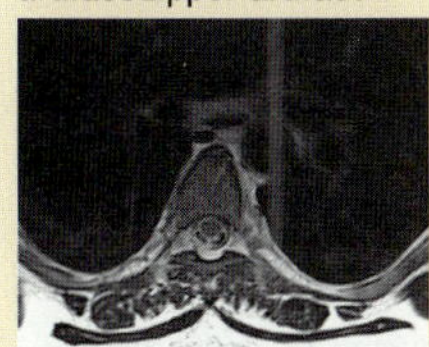	Since clinical scanners operate in the MHz frequency range, this range is transmitted by many peripheral devices in a hospital setting or clinic. Although MRI exam rooms are well shielded from these external RF sources, sometimes their signal can get picked up during the scan if the shielding is somehow compromised. Since most sources have a constant frequency, this usually will show up as vertical or horizontal lines depending on the direction of frequency encoding	Frequency encoding	▪ Make sure the MR scanner room-door is shut during imaging ▪ Remove all electronic devices from the patient before imaging ▪ If the artifact persists despite all nearby electronic equipment being turned off, it is possible that the RF shielding is compromised
Elevated noise in parallel imaging 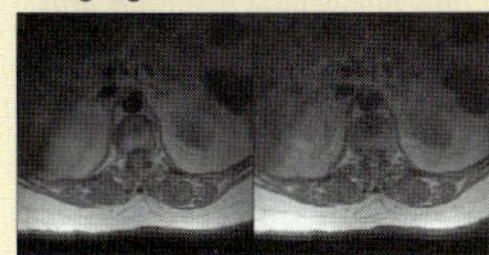	Elevation of noise in parallel imaging MRI (e.g., SENSE) is manifest as a nonuniform graininess typically in the center of the image more than the superficial tissues	Phase-encoding direction, and typically in the center of the image	▪ This artifact can be reduced using lower acceleration factor and increasing the FOV
Slice-to-slice crosstalk 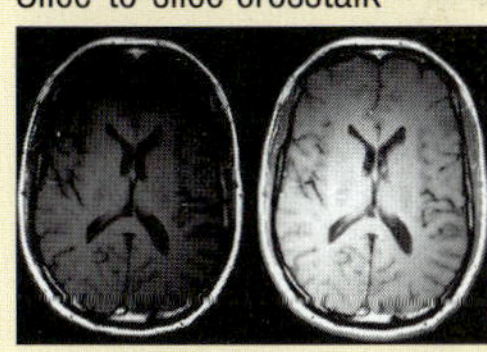	An RF excitation pulse is not precisely square in space. As a result, residual magnetization in slices adjacent to the one being excited may interfere and influence the excitation process. This can result in reduced signal intensity and tissue contrast	Slice selection direction	▪ Increase interslice gap ▪ Scanning with chronologically interleaved slices. For example, odd slice numbers 1, 3, 5, 7, ... are excited first followed by slices 2, 4, 6, 8, ... This allows magnetization from neighboring slices more time for relaxation recovery
Motion or ghosting artifact 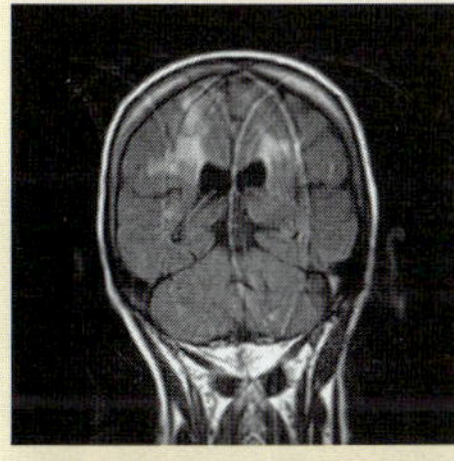	These artifacts occur due to moving of tissue or fluids during the scan. It manifests as ghosting in the direction of phase-encoding with Cartesian sampling. These artifacts may be seen across the entire FOV from periodic movements due to arterial pulsations, swallowing, breathing, or peristalsis. Nonperiodic patient movement may cause smearing of the image Note: Ghosting artifacts in EPI scanning are characteristically split by half of the FOV (referred to as "N/2" or Nyquist ghosts). They are typically not related to patient movement, but rather hardware and sequence parameters	Phase-encoding direction for Cartesian sampling Radial sampling in contrast will exhibit motion in a completely different way	▪ Cardiac/respiratory gating ▪ Spatial presaturation bands placed over moving tissues or before entry of the slice to minimize blood pulsationSwap phase and frequency directions. For example—in sagittal image of the spine with phase encoding in anterior to posterior direction pulsation of aorta causes ghosting over the spinal cord. If phase-encoding gradient is applied in head to foot direction, this artifact will not overlap over the spinal cord ▪ Choose ultrashort scan time when motion is from patient movement ▪ Apply gradient moment rephasing (GMR) or flow compensation technique
Technique-related blurring 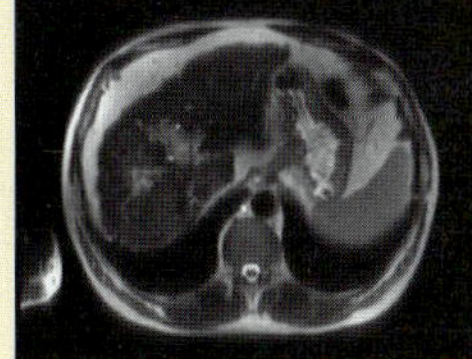	Blurring in images can be caused by low spatial resolution, excessive filtering, among other things. Blurring of images associated specifically with the FSE/TSE technique occurs due to signal decay during the signal readout. T2 relaxation and consequential signal decay will occur during the TR interval while the lines of *k* space are being filled. Each echo of the FSE/TSE readout is collected at a different point along the T2-decay curve. The lines of *k* space will therefore be weighted by the T2 decay according to how *k* space becomes filled with each echo. For example, subtle knee meniscal tears may be blurred out on proton-density-weighted FSE images. When long and short T2 tissues are juxtaposed, an interesting paradoxical phenomenon called pseudoedge enhancement may occur and is most commonly seen on axial T2-weighted FSE images of the lumbar spine as white "halos" surrounding nerve roots	Phase-encoding direction	▪ Avoid long echo train lengths ▪ Reduce echo spacing ▪ Avoid short effective TE

Continued

TABLE 4.9 Common MRI Artifacts—cont'd

Artifact	Causes	Axis	Remedies
Susceptibility artifact 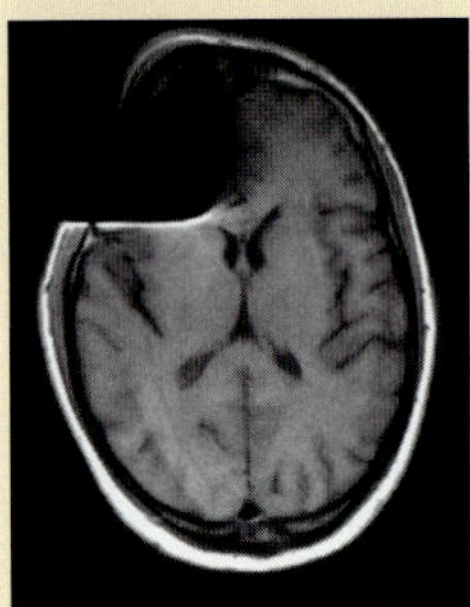	Magnetic susceptibility is a property of matter that reflects how the B_0 magnetic field behaves in and around the medium. In regions with higher susceptibility the signal will decrease due to the increased spin dephasing and T2* shortening. Susceptibility artifacts are seen near metal implants, or near hemorrhage due to higher iron content Note: This can be exploited because susceptibility effects and hence the conspicuity of the lesions is better demonstrated by SWI compared with conventional sequences. Susceptibility also forms the basis of Dynamic susceptibility contrast (DSC) MR perfusion studies and is also used to quantify myocardial and liver iron overload	Not axis specific	■ Use SE or FSE/TSE sequences because magnetic susceptibility is more prominent in GRE sequence ■ Remove/avoid metal near imaging planes ■ In cases with metal implants use newer artifact reduction techniques like MARS or by increasing sampling bandwidth, reducing TE, using thin slices and higher resolution ■ Susceptibility artifacts can also be reduced by use of parallel imaging and use of sequences with radial *k*-space sampling like BLADE/PROPELLER
Chemical shift or pixel misregistration artifact 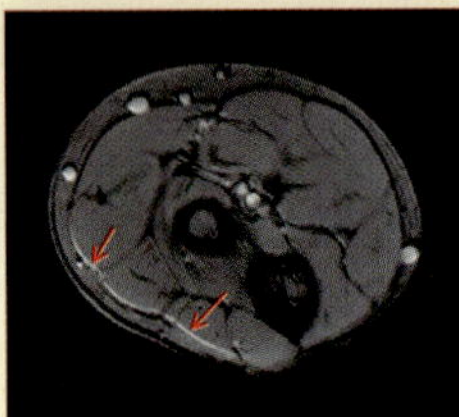	Chemical shift is due to the differences between Larmor frequencies of fat and water. This can result in a spatial misregistration of pixels of fat relative to water in the direction of frequency encoding. Note: A second type of chemical shift artifact occurs specifically with GRE techniques when a tissue is comprised of a mixture of fat and water. Fat and water signals will phase cycle with increasing TE leading to in-phase and opposed phase conditions. At TEs when fat and water are in phase, their signals add, while at TEs when fat and water are out of phase, their signals will subtract, and leads to boundary artifacts sometimes referred to as "India ink" artifact	Misregistration artifact occurs in the frequency-encoding direction	■ For chemical shift misregistration ■ Fat suppression techniques ■ Increase sampling bandwidth

the artifact to try and understand its genesis and characteristics while interpreting images with artifacts. These features include:

1. The type of sequence and protocol parameters used because certain EPI sequences, GRE sequences are prone to exhibit specific artifacts (see Table 4.9 for examples)
2. The gradient axis (mainly phase and frequency axis) because artifacts appear along one axis and that provides clues to the type of artifacts and possible remedies. Table 4.9 lists the axis for most of the artifacts to simplify that understanding
3. Presence of foreign bodies or metal implants. Artifacts result from local magnetic field inhomogeneities introduced by the metallic object(s)

For the remainder of this section, a selected group of artifacts is described. Although less commonly discussed in the artifact literature, they are nevertheless quite relevant in today's routine clinical practice.

B_1^+ Inhomogeneity

With the advent of higher field strengths in MRI where 3T is becoming the field strength of choice for clinical imaging, a prevalent artifact is image shading and spatial inhomogeneities caused by distortions of the B_1^+ magnetic field generated by RF transmission [37,38]. The origins of this are predominantly related to the tissue property of magnetic permittivity which has led to the term "dielectric effect" or "dielectric resonance" describing the characteristic appearance of this type of artifact (the ratio of the permittivity of a tissue to free space is called the dielectric constant).

The spatial wavelength of the B_1^+ field is dictated by the permittivity but is also dependent on the magnetic field strength where it becomes comparable in size to the patient's body at 3T and grows shorter at higher field strengths like 7T (Fig. 4.39A, B).

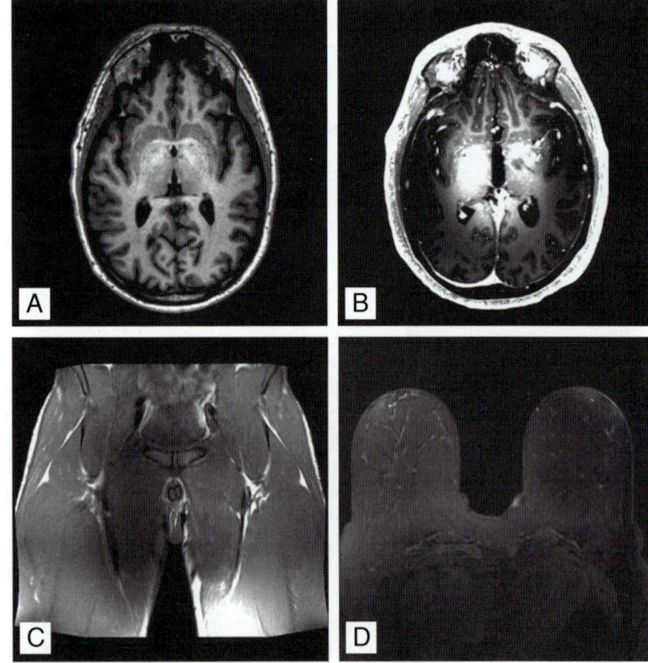

Figure 4.39 B_1^+ inhomogeneity. The spatial wavelength of the B_1^+ field is dependent on the magnetic field strength and becomes increasingly smaller at higher field strengths. Since this will be directly proportional to the RF flip angle, it results in shading and image inhomogeneities. An axial brain scan is shown at (A) 3T and at (B) 7T. Note the strong central brightening at 7T due to this effect. Large FOV imaging in the body can result in strong shading at 3T as seen in the pelvis (C) and even at 1.5T as shown in the breast (D).

Since the field strength of B_1^+ is directly proportional to the RF FA, this leads to the characteristic image inhomogeneity and shading effects. Different imaging techniques will be more (as in the case of SE and FSE/TSE) or less (as in the case of GRE) sensitive to FA variations so this artifact will also depend on the type of sequence. In addition to field strength dependence, permittivity is very tissue dependent. The relative effect depends on how different the tissue permittivity is from the surrounding air. Permittivity in fat is similar to air (the dielectric constant therefore being close to unity) while pure water is very different. The greater the difference in permittivity, the larger the degree of B_1^+ field inhomogeneity leading to more prominent shading effects (Figs. 4.39C, D.

This artifact is minimal at 1.5T, but at 3T it can be significant, and mitigation is challenging. Image filters are marginally helpful. Using techniques and RF pulsing that are less prone to the FA dependence are effective but can compromise diagnostic information. B_1 shimming has been more recently introduced but has had limited success due to the lack of the number of transmission channels necessary to shape complex field geometries. Current clinical scanners only possess two channels, while research systems have been built with up to 16 and 32 independent channels of transmission.

Incidental MT

With the dramatic improvements in MR hardware performance in recent years, scans have become increasingly faster and scan times proportionally shorter. This generally results in increased RF duty cycle for a given scan. In addition to causing higher SAR in the patient, it can lead to a lesser known subtle yet significant artifact that decreases the tissue contrast and drops the overall signal, referred to as "incidental MT" [39]. In general, MT is a process that exchanges magnetization between bound and free hydrogen. Some tissues contain bound hydrogen, for example, in long chain proteins which is not visible in MRI imaging due to its extremely short T2 relaxation. However, its presence can be inferred by exciting the bound component off resonance and observing the MT effect it has on the free hydrogen on resonance which can then be easily imaged. If exploited, MT can provide unique information about changes in the content of bound hydrogen. However, incidental effects produced by multislice imaging and high RF duty cycle can lead to degradation in image quality in the form of poor contrast and low SNR.

This artifact phenomenon is most prominent in T1-weighted brain imaging at higher field strengths using high RF duty cycle multislice scanning techniques like SE or FSE/TSE. White matter contains measurable bound hydrogen that can lead to strong incidental MT effects (Fig. 4.40). Although slice-to-slice crosstalk using small slice gaps can yield similar compromises through direct magnetization saturation (Fig. 4.40A), very large gaps that eliminate crosstalk still lead to the poor tissue contrast and low SNR from incidental MT (Fig. 440B), where the absence of incidental MT on a single slice acquisition shows markedly improved gray–white differentiation and greater SNR (Fig. 4.40C).

Incidental MT tends to be more prevalent at higher field strengths, and mitigation strategies can be difficult without tradeoffs. Lowering the RF duty cycle by decreasing the number of slices acquired per TR interval can improve things but increases overall scan time for the same slice coverage. Decreasing FAs can also help but may alter the tissue contrast and SNR. The best strategy is to increase the slice gap and use multiple measurements or concatenations. This minimizes both crosstalk and MT effects, as well as SAR, but with a proportional increase in scan time.

Dixon Pixel Swap

Fat signal can at times be a confounding factor for interpretation. Different methodologies exist to suppress fat, but one that has gained popularity in recent years is a technique first described by Dixon in 1984 [40]. When implemented successfully it offers a clear advantage over other strategies such as spectral suppression that is sensitive to spatial B_0 inhomogeneities and STIR that is sensitive to spatial B_1^+ inhomogeneities, both of which can be challenging in large FOV body applications. The Dixon method can produce highly uniform fat suppression and offers the ability to produce fat-only and water-only images which is also why it sometimes is referred to as fat-water separation imaging.

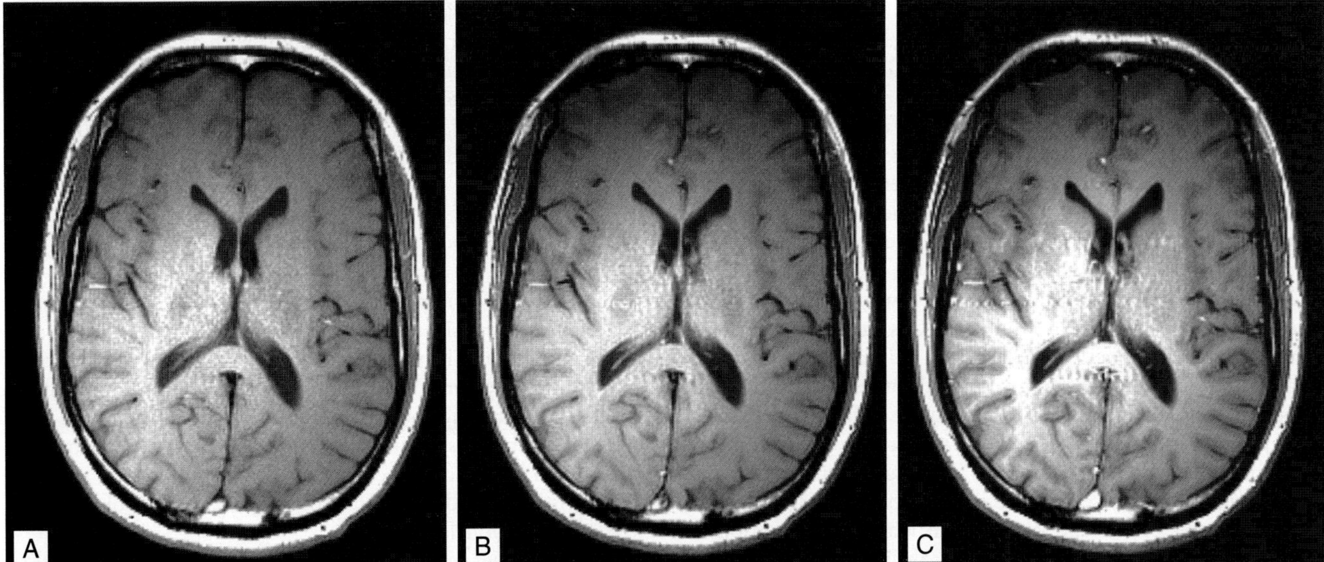

Figure 4.40 Incidental magnetization transfer (MT). Multislice 2D imaging can lead to incidental MT effects that can degrade both SNR and CNR. Direct saturation effects occur due to slice-to-slice crosstalk (A), but even when very large slice gaps are used where no crosstalk occurs, incidental MT still exists (B). In a single slice acquisition where no crosstalk or incidental MT will occur, SNR and CNR is recovered (C).

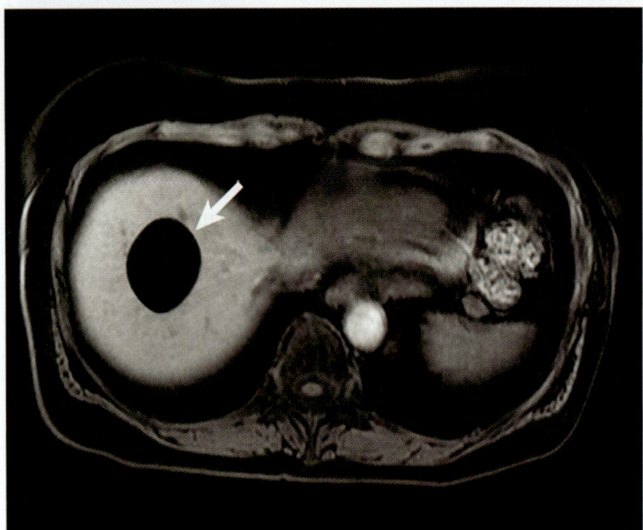

Figure 4.41 Dixon pixel swap. Breakdown in the processing to separate fat and water signals can lead to wholesale or partial pixel swap (*arrow*).

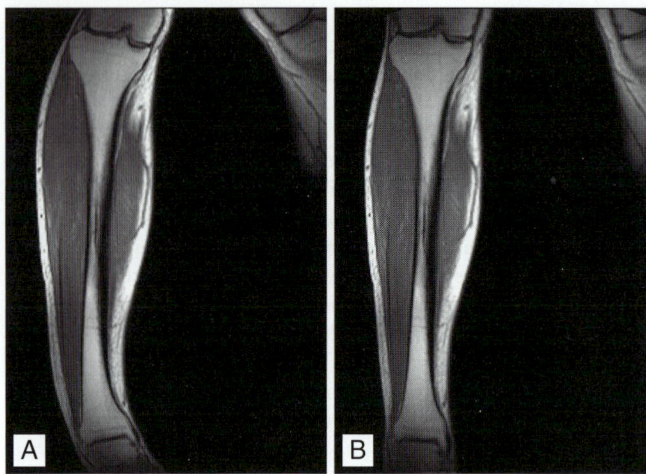

Figure 4.42 Gradient nonlinearity. Accurate spatial encoding of the MR signal depends on the spatial linearity of the gradient field. In large FOV applications the fall-off of the gradient field far from isocenter can cause visible distortions (A). However, because the nonlinearity is based on the design of the gradient coil, it can also be easily corrected in processing (B). This can be critical in applications that require a high degree of spatial accuracy such as stereotactic planning.

However, it has taken decades for it to be become accepted because the calculation of the fat-only and water-only images can at times produce an artifactual "pixel swap" where the fat and water pixels at a given position become reversed. Underlying factors that can confound the phase cycling can lead to a breakdown in this processing and cause this "pixel swap" artifact to occur. Over the years, the technique has become more robust, but this artifact can still occasionally happen.

Wholesale image swapping can occur on rare occasion where the entire fat-only image is swapped with the water-only image. However, the more concerning scenario is a partial swap where only some tissue pixels in the image get swapped. In most cases the artifact is obvious to the reader (Fig. 4.41), but at times it can be extremely difficult to detect and could in the worst case scenario potentially lead to errors in diagnosis if not recognized. It is therefore good practice to always refer back to the acquired data when there is uncertainty in interpretation.

Gradient Nonlinearity

With each incremental advance, gradient amplitude and slew rate performance keeps improving which brings faster scans and more applications to probe the human body. However, there are physiological constraints to reduce peripheral nerve stimulation and engineering constraints to keep the magnets short with ever increasing wider bore sizes, and this can lead to gradient-related spatial nonlinearities that have become more prevalent.

It is not uncommon to think of an MRI scanner like a camera that simply takes "pictures." However, MRI is based on generating a variety of magnetic fields, whether it be the main static B_0 field, or the B_1^+ transmission field, or the gradient field G for spatial encoding. And all these fields are produced with coils that have finite physical dimensions. The reality is that they all suffer from spatial distortions and nonlinearities. The B_0 and B_1^+ fields are typically unpredictable since they become distorted by the human body associated with tissue variations in magnetic susceptibility and permittivity, respectively. However, the gradient distortions are predominantly associated with the fall-off of the field toward the edges of the FOV that reflect the dimensions of the gradient coil geometry and is therefore highly reproducible and predictable. This in turn produces a spatial image distortion that at least in principle can then be corrected during the image reconstruction process.

In general, the gradient nonlinearity distortion becomes worse away from isocenter. Since it is basically a relative error, the degree of spatial distortion is independent of the scan parameters. Changing the gradient strength for spatial encoding will do nothing to change the extent of the error. The distortion will always exist to the same degree and is based on the gradient coil winding pattern. The largest distortion will typically occur along the Z axis (head to foot) which is most obvious with large FOVs in the sagittal or coronal plane as shown in Fig. 4.42A. However, much of this distortion can be corrected if the gradient field generation pattern is known (Fig. 4.42B). Gradient nonlinearity distortion correction can be of utmost importance if spatial accuracy is paramount for applications such as stereotactic planning, prosthetic modeling, or quantitative tissue segmentation.

Artifacts in MRI are numerous, but with an understanding of their origins more times than not they can be either mitigated or even completely avoided. However, this also reflects how versatile this imaging technique is and how rich the diagnostic information is that it provides.

MRI Safety

For any device or apparatus employed for use in patient care, there are safety considerations that must be defined, followed, and enforced to ensure the welfare of the patients as well as the healthcare staff. If one considers the primary hardware components of an MRI scanner, and the different aspects that make up the scan, there are safety considerations associated with each of them. This section will briefly describe the most important aspects of safety in MRI for each and will discuss them in the context of patient as well as occupational concerns.

Guidelines and governing bodies: There exist various committees and agencies in the United States as well as the world that focus on establishing standards and guidelines for MRI safety. Probably the most comprehensive of these that is generally accepted as the universal standard is the International Electrotechnical Commission

(IEC) IEC 60601-2-33 requirements for the safety of MR equipment for medical diagnosis (https://www.iec.ch/). This documentation provides details and standards about every aspect of the MRI devices and scans generated from them. The FDA of the US government provides guidelines for both MRI manufacturers and implant device manufacturers for safety and efficacy (https://www.fda.gov/). The American College of Radiology (ACR) has established the generally accepted definition for safe workflow practices and the classifications for MR safety (https://www.acr.org/). Other groups concerned with safe practices also exist such as the American Board of Magnetic Resonance Safety, and the reader is encouraged to consult these and their associated documentation for more in-depth reading.

MAGNET (B_0) and spatial gradient-related forces: The first and probably most important concern is associated with the magnet that creates the static B_0 main magnetic field establishing the thermal equilibrium of the bulk magnetization in the body. It is well known that magnets attract ferromagnetic objects with great force and can be shown to be proportional to the mass of the object, the magnetic field strength, and what is known as the spatial gradient, defined as the change in magnetic field across spatial distance. Intuitively, the larger the object mass the greater the pull, and that the larger the magnetic field the greater the pull. However, it is not so obvious that the force is also dependent on the stray field pattern of the magnetic field that emanates away from the magnet which comprises the spatial gradients. It is beyond the scope of this discussion to go into the details of this but suffice it to say that the largest spatial gradients (and therefore the pull) exists not inside the magnet but primarily at the opening of the magnet. Therefore, it is important to know that any object, whether it is a stethoscope, a wheelchair, a ventilator, or an implant such as a prosthetic device, is most sensitive to the forces of the magnet near the opening bore of the magnet and not inside the magnet where the field strength is the strongest.

In siting considerations for MRI scanners and the magnet, the ACR has defined four physical occupational zones for safety management and access control [41]. Zone 4, the most restrictive, is the actual scan room where only qualified personnel and patients may enter. Zone 1 is the least restrictive that allows total public access. One of the primary criteria used in defining and controlling these zones is the 5-gauss (500 μT) line which historically has been considered the lowest magnetic field strength threshold that can potentially adversely affect people with cardiac pacemakers. Very strict guidelines for specifying the 5-gauss line location are necessary for all MRI environments whether in a hospital or an outpatient clinic.

One other safety concern with superconducting magnets of such high-field strength is quench events. Although it is extremely rare, if a magnet loses its superconducting properties, a quench leads to an uncontrollable and irreversible sequence of events. Rapid loss of the magnetic field with a patient in the bore can lead to electrical stimulation throughout the body, and the large release of helium gas can lead to asphyxiation. Because of these dangers, manufacturers have protections in place and healthcare providers have very strict guidelines on how to handle such an event.

RF transmission (B_1^+) and SAR-related tissue heating: The second most important safety aspect is related to the RF transmission, which generates the B_1^+ magnetic field that is perpendicular to the main B_0 direction. This drives the magnetization out of the longitudinal direction so that transverse magnetization can be detected as the MRI signal. Faraday's law of induction and Maxwell's equations dictate that a changing dynamic magnetic field will generate a concurrent electric field. To invoke a change in the rotation of the magnetization, the resonance condition must be met, which means that the RF transmission must match the Larmor frequency of the magnetization. This produces a time-varying B_1^+ magnetic field which in turn produce the electric field according to Faraday's law. This electric field due to the electrical conductivity of the tissues produces eddy currents that dissipate in the form of heat leading to what is known as the specific absorption rate (SAR)—or the rate that the body absorbs the RF transmission. SAR will vary greatly depending on the type of MRI technique, where some such as TSE/FSE possess high SAR while others such a low FA GRE possess low SAR. Because it is also dependent on the tissue conductivity, SAR will tend to be greater in muscular athletic patients.

What ultimately matters, however, is not the rate of RF absorption which is related to temperature rise, but rather the total energy absorbed over time, sometimes referred to as the specific energy dose, since this will define the total temperature rise and whether this reaches a level that produces tissue damage. This will also strongly depend on internal thermal regulation in the form of blood perfusion, so patients who are compromised are more susceptible to tissue heating.

Finally, localized heating can occur with implants, especially wires and probes that are conductive, leading to potentially significant temperature increases at the tip. Therefore, care must always be taken to monitor scanning of implants according to the implant manufacturer's guidelines.

Gradients (G) and dB/dt-related peripheral nerve stimulation: Another key aspect to the MRI scan is the spatial encoding, requiring the rapid pulsing of gradient magnetic fields, *G*, superimposed on the main static magnetic field (B_0) that provides the one-to-one relation between the transverse magnetization Larmor precessional frequency and physical space. As with the B_1^+ field, the changing magnetic field associated with the gradient pulsing will induce electric fields according to Faraday's law of induction. Although heating from this is minor compared with RF transmission, the potential for inducing electrical stimulation of peripheral nerves exists. If the pulsing is sufficiently fast, this can lead to pain and even induce convulsions. Therefore, strict limits have been set by the IEC to ensure patient safety. One must also be cognizant of active implants that possess electronic controls that could malfunction due to electrical currents induced by the gradient pulsing.

Other safety concerns (acoustic noise): In addition to peripheral nerve stimulation, acoustic noise can be considerable especially on state-of-the-art scanners that can generate gradient fields at very fast rates. The noise is created by the torsional forces in the gradient windings producing pressure waves that lead to the ubiquitous knocking sounds whenever the gradients are pulsed. The IEC has set standards for acoustic noise that to be met typically requires sound mitigation for the patients in the form of ear plugs and/or some type of noise reducing device like headphones.

Implant safety: Very few scenarios currently are considered absolute contraindications with clinical MRI. It is therefore critical to provide explicit definitions to classify implants and devices to ensure patient safety during scanning. The ACR ((https://www.acr.org/)—specifically for MRI—https://www.acr.org/Clinical-Resources/Radiology-Safety/MR-Safety) along with the American Society for Testing and Materials have created three categories that have been generally accepted as the standard for this: MR Safe, MR Unsafe, and MR Conditional [42] (Fig. 4.43). Most devices fall under MR Conditional status, which basically means that based on rigorous testing according to the FDA guidelines ((https://www.fda.gov/—specifically for MRI—https://www.fda.

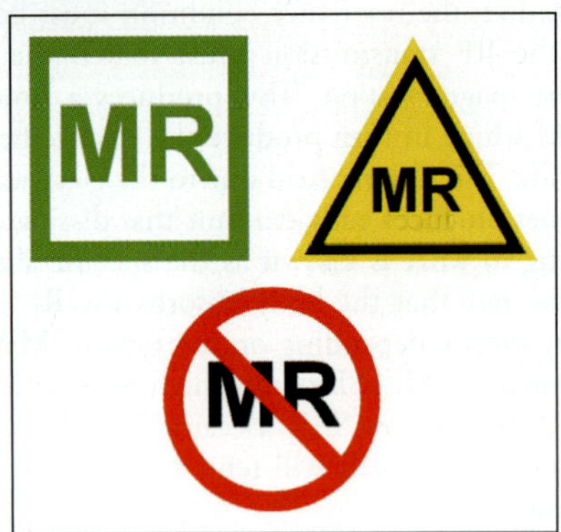

Figure 4.43 American College of Radiology (ACR) categories for implant and device safety. MR safe is depicted as a green box. MR unsafe is depicted as a red crossed out circle, and MR conditional is depicted as a yellow triangle.

gov/regulatory-information/search-fda-guidance-documents/testing-and-labeling-medical-devices-safety-magnetic-resonance-mr-environment), a device can be scanned safely at conditional levels that are at or below the levels specified by the IEC ((https://www.iec.ch)—specifically, diagnostic imaging and MRI—https://www.iec.ch/dyn/www/f?p=103:7:7079002326689::::FSP_ORG_ID,FSP_LANG_ID:1361,25). In clinical practice, it is always recommended to follow the latest MR Conditional limits set by the implant manufacturer to ensure the safety of the patient.

Suggested Readings

- T Budrys, V Veikutis, S Lukosevicius, R Gleizniene, E Monastyreckiene, I Kulakiene, Artifacts in magnetic resonance imaging: how it can really affect diagnostic image quality and confuse clinical diagnosis? J Vibroeng 20 (2) (2018) 1202–1213.
- MRI Questions & Answers; MR imaging physics & technology [Internet]. Questions and Answers in MRI. Available from: http://mriquestions.com/index.html.
- W Edelstein, G Glover, C Hardy, R Redington, The intrinsic signal-to-noise ratio in NMR imaging. Magn Reson Med 3 (4) ((1986) 604–618.
- K Kanal, A Barkovich, C Bell, J Borgstede, W Bradley, J Froelich, et al., ACR guidance document on MR safe practices: 2013, J Magn Reson Imaging 37 (3) (2013) 501–530.
- DK Jones, Diffusion MRI: Theory, Methods, and Applications. Oxford, MA: Oxford University Press, 2010.
- A Padhani, A Makris, P Gall, D Collins, N Tunariu, J de Bono, Therapy monitoring of skeletal metastases with whole-body diffusion MRI, J Magn Reson Imaging 39 (5) (2014) 1049–1078.

5

Concepts in Radiation, Contrast and Safety

AMEYA S. KAWTHALKAR, AKSHAY BAHETI

Radiation

Everything in our universe is made up of two things, either matter or energy. Radiology at its essence is the science of using energy to look at matter. Whether it is sound waves for ultrasound, electromagnetic waves of different wavelengths for radiographs and computed tomography (CT; x-rays), magnetic resonance imaging (MRI; radiofrequency waves), or nuclear medicine (gamma rays), radiology is concerned with optimizing energies to see what is invisible to the human eye. Ionizing radiation (x-rays and gamma rays) can however have adverse effects on human tissues, although recent research shows that radiation in diagnostic imaging for patients is not as harmful as previously believed [1]. This section deals with the adverse effects of ionizing radiation (x-rays and gamma rays).

Radiation doses and units: To understand the effects of radiation on human tissues, it is important to quantify the amount of radiation received. *Radiation dose* is a generic term which encompasses absorbed dose, equivalent dose, and effective dose.

Absorbed dose: This is the energy deposited by ionizing radiation into any medium per unit mass. The units of absorbed dose are "rad" (CGS unit) and "gray" (SI unit). 1 gray = 100 rad [2].

Equivalent dose: Different types of ionizing radiation deposit different amounts of energies into any medium, depending on the properties of the ionizing radiation. The absorbed dose deposited in a tissue multiplied by the radiation weighting factor of that ionizing radiation gives us the equivalent dose [2]. Thus,

$$\text{Equivalent dose} = \text{Absorbed dose} \times \text{Radiation weighting factor}$$

For x-rays, electrons (beta particles), and gamma rays, the radiation weighting factor is 1. Thus for x-rays, electrons (beta particles), and gamma rays, the equivalent dose is numerically equal to the absorbed dose. For alpha particles the radiation weighting factor is 20 and for protons it is 2.

The units of equivalent dose are "rem" (CGS unit) and "sievert" (SI unit). 1 sievert = 100 rem. For an x-ray or a CT, 1 Sv = 1 Gy, as the radiation weighting factor is 1.

Effective dose (E): Every tissue in the human body has a different sensitivity to ionizing radiation, called as the *tissue weighting factor*. The sum of equivalent doses to all tissues and organs of the body multiplied by the tissue weighting factor for each gives us the effective dose [3].

$$\text{Effective dose for the entire body} = \text{Equivalent dose} \times \text{Tissue weighting factor}\left(\text{summed for all organs of the body}\right)$$

The units of effective dose are the same as those for equivalent dose, "rem" (CGS unit) and "sievert" (SI unit). 1 sievert = 100 rem.

Thus, when we speak of dose limits to specific tissues or organs we use the equivalent dose, and when we speak of dose limits to the whole human body we use the effective dose. The equivalent dose and effective dose both deal with stochastic effects of radiation on the human body. We will discuss stochastic and determin istic effects of radiation in a later section.

A few other terms need to be understood with respect to radiation doses.

- *Collective dose*: The amount of radiation received in a given period of time by a certain population. For example, the amount of radiation received by people living in a particular region or country from background natural sources such as radioactive substances in the Earth's crust is a collective dose for the population. Another example is the amount of radiation received by people living in the vicinity of nuclear accidents such as the Chernobyl reactor explosion in the former USSR, the Fukushima Daiichi nuclear disaster, etc.
- *External dose*: The dose received from sources of radiation outside the body. For example, the radiation dose received by patients undergoing radiography, CT, and fluoroscopy where the sources of radiation are outside the body
- *Internal dose*: The dose received from radioactive substances introduced into the body. For example, the radiation dose received by patients undergoing a PET/CT or a bone scan from the radionuclides injected intravenously for these examinations
- *Dose limit*: The permissible upper boundary of radiation dose [4]
- *Activity*: The rate of disintegration or decay of radioactive material. Used in nuclear medicine rather than other conventional diagnostic radiology. The units of activity are "curie" (conventional unit) and "becquerel" (SI unit)
- *Exposure*: An old term used to express amount of ionization caused by radiation in a specified volume of air. It had the disadvantage of quantifying only the ionization in air and not the amount of radiation deposited in the human body. Roentgen was the unit of radiation exposure
- *Kerma*: It stands for "kinetic energy released to matter" and quantifies the amount of kinetic energy released by ionizing radiation into a material per unit mass. Kerma is measured by the same units as absorbed dose, "rad" (CGS unit) and "gray" (SI unit) [5]

Sources of Radiation

Human beings are living in an ocean of radiation, whether from outer space, the earth itself, or from man-made sources.

- *Natural background radiation*: This consists of radiation emitted by radioactive materials within the Earth's crust, and also radiation from outer space (cosmic radiation). It varies from region to region and country to country. The average natural background radiation, every year worldwide, is approximately 2.4 mSv/year. In India, the natural background radiation is 2.2 mSv/year. However, there are areas in Kerala (southern India) where the annual natural background radiation can be as high as 70 mSv/year [6]
- *Man-made radiation*: The most important source in current times is diagnostic medical imaging and therapeutic radiation. X-rays from radiographs, fluoroscopy, and CT scans form the bulk of this radiation. Other man-made sources are fall-out from nuclear weapons tests, nuclear discharges, and certain radioactive materials used in building constructions [7]

Effects of Radiation

The ionization caused by ionizing radiation causes both chemical and biologic changes in tissues. The effects can occur on all molecules, but biologically the most important are the effects on proteins (such as enzymes) or nucleic acids (mainly DNA). The damage caused by radiation may be direct (e.g., direct breakage of molecular bonds) or indirect (caused by free radicals produced by the radiation through ionization of water). Indirect damage through free radicals is more common.

The effects of radiation are divided into stochastic and deterministic effects [8].

a. *Stochastic effects*: These are random events of chance. They do not have a threshold (or minimum) dose for occurring. These include carcinogenesis and genetic mutations. The probability of stochastic effects occurring increases with the radiation dose. The severity of these effects is however not dose related
b. *Deterministic effects*: These effects have a threshold (or minimum) dose for occurring, and can be predicted with a degree of certainty after a known dose of radiation. The severity of the effects is dose related. These include skin erythema, cataracts, bone marrow suppression, and sterility, among others. Higher doses cause more severe deterministic effects. Usually different effects occur at different thresholds of radiation dose, and manifest varying time durations, with some being immediate (such as skin erythema), and some delayed (cataract) while effects in germinal cells may take generations to manifest. The various deterministic effects and thresholds at which they occur are enumerated in Table 5.1 [8]. It is important to note that all these effects occur in the dose range of grays, while diagnostic imaging employs radiation of the order of mGy. Therefore, deterministic effects are not seen with routine diagnostic imaging, but with therapeutic radiation and nuclear accidents, while stochastic effects and radiation-induced carcinogenesis remain a concern. We will now discuss radiation risk models to understand this better

Linear No-Threshold Model and Its Limitations

The models of radiation risk are based on epidemiologic data from high radiation exposure (minimum 100 mGy), as in the 1945 nuclear blasts or the Chernobyl disaster. The observed findings in the atomic bomb survivors demonstrated a linear relation between the degree of radiation exposure and the incidence of cancer in the survivors. In other words, the higher the degree of radiation exposure, the higher was the incidence of cancer. As data were available only in patients with higher degrees of exposure, it was hypothesized that the same linear relation would hold true for low-dose radiation as well. This model is called the linear no-threshold model [11,12]. The model states that there is no lower threshold below which the risk of radiation-induced carcinogenesis is negligible. The linear no-threshold model is the accepted model by various international bodies including the National Council on Radiation Protection and Measurements, the International Council on Radiation Protection (ICRP), and the United Nations Scientific Committee on the Effects of Atomic Radiation. Annual radiation limits for radiation workers, for example, are prescribed based on this model.

Many scientists however argue that the human body has various defense mechanisms such as DNA repair and apoptosis to take care of low-dose radiation. In fact, areas in Kerala and Iran where the annual background radiation exposure is more than 70 mGy do not demonstrate an increased incidence of cancer. Accordingly, they advocate a model with a threshold for carcinogenesis at low doses. Indeed, after over a century of use of diagnostic radiation, there is still no definitive evidence that low-dose radiation causes

TABLE 5.1 Threshold Dose for Common Deterministic Adverse Effects of Radiation and Average Time for the Effects to Manifest [9,10]

Deterministic Effect	Threshold Dose	Time to Manifest
Skin erythema	2 Gy	1–24 hours
Skin necrosis	15 Gy	4 weeks
Skin epilation	3 Gy (reversible) and 7 Gy (irreversible)	3 weeks
Cataract	2–10 Gy	Years to decades
Sterility	2.5–3.5 Gy	Days to weeks
Lung parenchymal injury	10 Gy	80–180 days
Acute radiation syndrome (consists of bone marrow syndrome, gastrointestinal (GI) syndrome, cardiovascular (CV) syndrome, and central nervous system (CNS) syndrome)	0.7–10 Gy (bone marrow syndrome/suppression)	2–4 weeks
	More than 10 Gy (GI syndrome)	2 weeks (death)
	More than 50 Gy (CV and CNS syndromes)	Less than 3 days (death)

increased cancer risk. Thus, the French Academy of Sciences and National Academy of Medicine, the Health Physics Society, and the American Association of Physicists in Medicine state that there is no evidence that radiation <100 mSv causes increased incidence of cancer [13–15].

In summary, based on the available evidence, minimizing radiation exposure for patients and radiology staff alike is a must. However, the true risk of low-dose radiation, particularly for patients who do not have continuous exposure, is likely negligible if any.

Principles of Radiation Protection

The ICRP proposed three principles of radiation protection, namely, justification, optimization, and dose limitation [8].

a. *Justification*: The benefits of using any imaging technique which involves ionizing radiation should outweigh the risks associated with its use. For example, it is important to consider whether ultrasound would suffice as a diagnostic technique for an investigation instead of CT, especially for pediatric patients
b. *Optimization*: Optimization involved the principle of *As Low As Reasonably Achievable*. This means the radiation exposure itself and the number of people exposed to it should be kept as low as feasible. For example, low-dose algorithm CTs are now widely accepted as diagnostically adequate for a range of indications including *detection of renal calculi and CT lung screening* [16]
c. *Dose limitation*: The total dose to any person from a diagnostic imaging technique should not exceed the maximum limits as per the national guidelines. Dose limits are the permissible upper boundaries of radiation doses for a particular section of the population. The approximate amount of radiation obtained from different radiological studies is as outlined in Table 5.2 [17]. The permissible dose limits for healthcare workers and general population vary from country to country, for example, the dose limits in the United Kingdom are different from those in India. There are also the global dose limits recommended by the ICRP. These dose limits are enumerated in Table 5.3. The dose limits for general public and occupational radiation workers are effective doses, as they pertain to the whole body. Dose limits for lens of eye, skin, and extremities are equivalent doses as they pertain only to select organs. Of note, the dose limit to the lens for occupational workers has been reduced by ICRP and IRR17 to 20 mSv, while the Atomic Energy Regulatory Board, India guidelines currently continue to retain the old limit of 150 mSv at the time of writing the chapter [18,19]

TABLE 5.2 Usual Effective Dose for Common Imaging Investigations [17]

Investigation	Effective Dose (in mSv)
Chest radiograph (PA view)	0.1–0.2
KUB radiograph	0.6
Lumbar spine radiograph	1.5
Extremity radiograph (hand, foot, etc.)	0.001
Barium studies with fluoroscopy	6–8
Mammography	0.4
Head CT (single phase)	2
Thorax CT	7–8
Abdomen and pelvis CT (single phase)	10
Coronary angiography	12
Bone densitometry (DEXA)	0.001
PET/CT	25

Practical Aspects of Radiation Protection

Factors of radiation protection: The three key elements on whose edifice radiation protection rests are time, distance, and shielding [20].

a. *Time*: The duration of radiation exposure should be kept as minimum as possible. An example is *using intermittent fluoroscopy* rather than continuous fluoroscopy to minimize the radiation dose to the patient and health worker
b. *Distance*: The amount of radiation exposure from a source is inversely proportional to the square of the distance from the source. So if a person is standing at 2 m from a source compared with 1 m, their radiation exposure reduces by one fourth. It is important to practice this as much as possible especially in the interventional radiology or fluoroscopy suites. When performing mobile radiography, it is important to use a 2-m control cable length to provide adequate distance for the radiography unit operator (of at least 2 m) from scatter radiation from the machine and patient
c. *Shielding*: There are many ways of shielding the health worker or patient from radiation. These include radiation protection accessories such as lead aprons, thyroid collars, lead caps, lead goggles, and gloves. Other methods of shielding are lead shields in the fluoroscopy or CT suite, using lead lined glass and lead lined walls, or using walls of a particular recommended thickness (called lead equivalent) in construction

TABLE 5.3 Effective dose Limits for General Public and Occupational Workers in Annual Equivalents (mSv/year) Recommended by International Commission on Radiation Protection (ICRP), the Atomic Energy Regulatory Board (AERB) for India, and the Ionizing Radiation Regulations 2017 (IRR17) for the United Kingdom (UK) [18,19]

Dose Limits (mSv/year)	ICRP (Global)	AERB (India)	IRR17 (UK)
General public	1	1	1
Occupational workers	20 mSv averaged over 5 years; maximum 50 mSV in a year	20 mSv averaged over 5 years; maximum 30 mSV in a year	20 mSv averaged over 5 years; maximum 50 mSV in a year
Lens of eye	20	150	20
Skin, hands, and feet	500	500	500

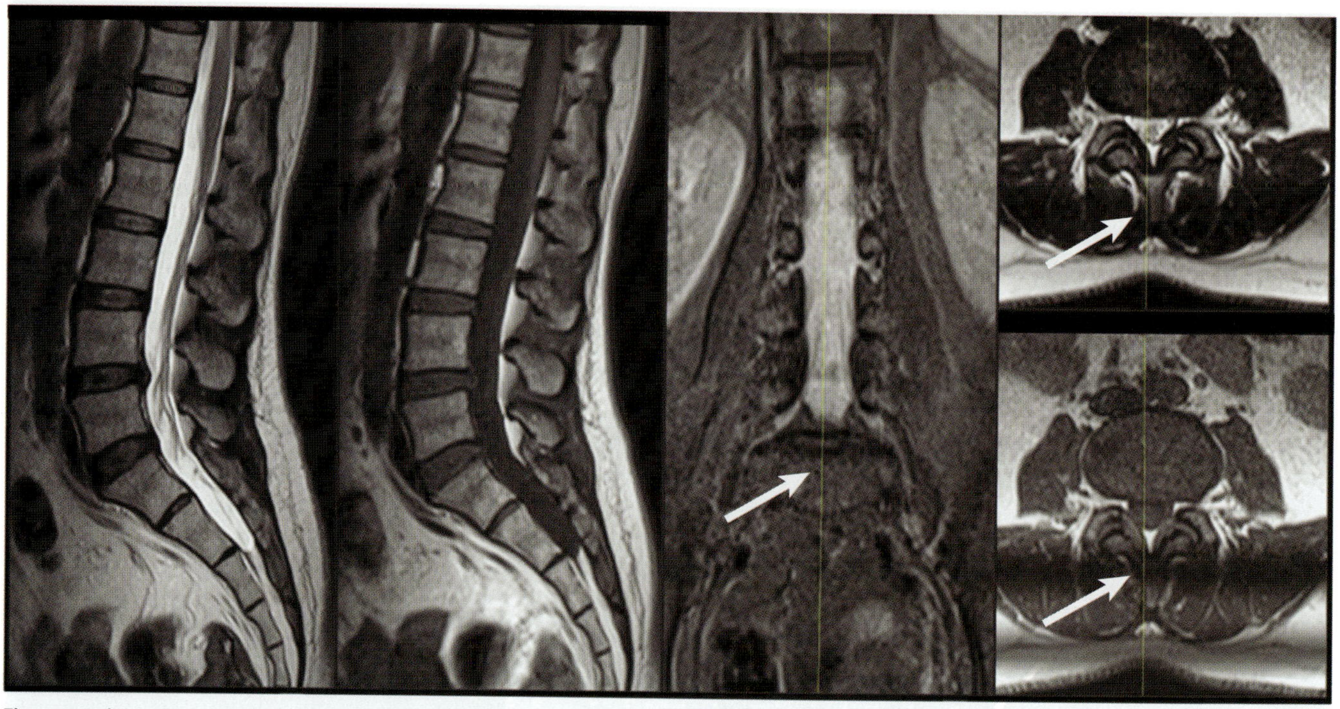

Figure 6.3 An example for a hanging protocol showing images of a lumbar spine MRI examination displaying all image series for simultaneous viewing. The *arrow* shows the reference plain of the displayed sagittal images on the coronal and axial scans.

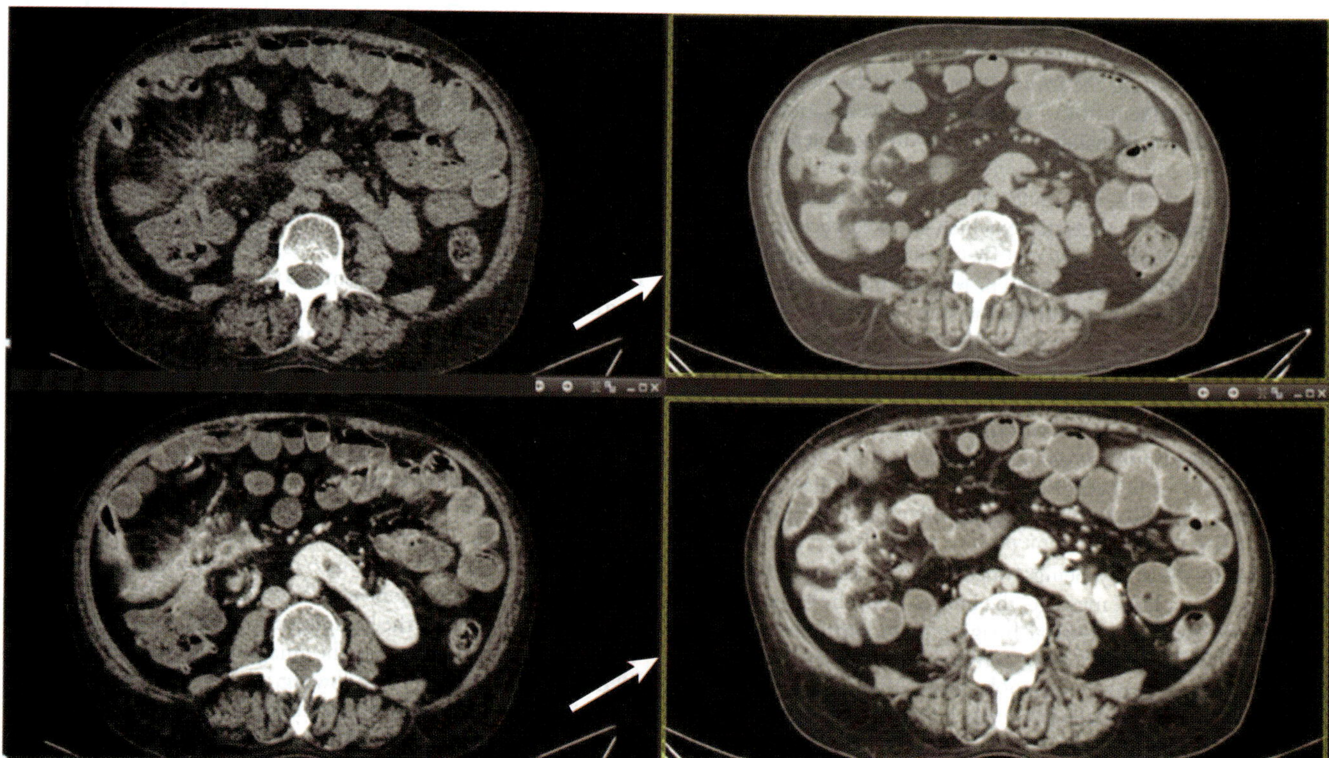

Figure 6.4 A hanging protocol for comparison of multiple series of a current and previous CT abdomen scan. The images with the yellow dotted border (*white arrows*) represent the previous scan images.

The other important component of the PACS is the *archival or storage*. Archival of data is primarily on the server and extendable using disks, tapes, and hard drives organized in clusters. The PACS servers and attached archival media can be located in-house, in external data centers or on the cloud. To ensure that the data do not get lost due to hardware or software failure, storage systems have inbuilt redundant array of independent disks to ensure that the database and image data are safe.

In a PACS solution, archival solutions allow structured storage of image data so that the images can be *retrieved* at the time of reporting by the radiologist, viewing by the referring teams at the time of consults or surgeries; for comparison or research. The capacity of storage depends on institutional and regulatory factors. Clinical imaging data are estimated to amount to 2314 exabytes (2.3 billion gigabytes) globally by 2020 (IDC 2014) [13].

Although most traditional PACS systems required the imaging departments to set up data centers with multiple racks of servers, cloud-based services are now becoming more available to reduce the capital cost of setting up a PACS solution. Various forms of archival are used depending on the need for speed in retrieval of data, which include on-line, near-line, and off-line archival, with immediate retrieval of the historical data in the on-line archival and a manual intervention required to retrieve the data from an off-line archival. With reduced cost of storage today, most imaging departments prefer on-line or near-line availability of archival data. PACS archival systems store data in DICOM format. A newer class of archival systems, vendor neutral archivals, is now available which can also store data in other formats, thereby integrating image AND document data with data from departments like cardiology, gastroenterology, dermatology, and even pathology. This acts as a gateway to the PACS and other non-DICOM data sources, thereby integrating a greater number of patient records. It also mitigates data migration issues if an imaging department changes the PACS vendor, who at times keep some proprietary tags on the archived data, even on a DICOM format.

For the IT infrastructure of the hospital and radiology department to be efficient, it is important to have high-speed network of wiring and Wi-Fi within the hospital. A high-speed, preferably dedicated, bandwidth is also necessary between different facilities and to an offsite data center/cloud solution. To ensure data security and privacy of patients, any hospital network needs to be protected from hackers by effective use of firewalls, virtual private networks, and antivirus software.

Newer PACS systems have integrated advanced postprocessing capabilities to ensure that the radiologist using a single interface to fulfill all the requirements. Depending on the budgets available the advanced postprocessing software can be available as a part of the solution across the department and hospital, instead of having stand along multimodality work stations.

It is also possible to make personalized or departmental research folders on the PACS, which are also used as teaching folders.

AI applications are now linked on PACS systems to improve the quality and productivity of radiologists. Current concepts and applications of AI have been covered in a separate chapter.

Besides all the advantages previously mentioned, the availability of PACS and RIS has also led to significant savings for imaging centers and hospitals:

- Space, which is at a premium. The PACS and other IT solutions have now replaced multiple rooms and storage facilities of the medical records department where racks of films used to be stored and carted to the department when a previous study needed to be compared
- Film cost: there is no need to print films in a digital ecosystem, saving the cost of printing multiple films, especially in cross-sectional imaging studies. With the availability of patient portals and high-speed internet, there is also a reduced demand to burn the large image datasets of CTs and MRIs on CDs and DVDs. In fact, newer computer systems do not even have in built CD or DVD readers
- Environmental impact: Reduction in use of films and CDs have also resulted in positive impact on the environment

Some RIS-PACS vendors provide a comprehensive solution of all the components whereas other vendors provide only the PACS viewer, with the advanced applications provided by companies that manufacture dedicated postprocessing software. It is also pertinent to note that a number of free-to-download DICOM viewers with basic functionality are available on the internet for personal review of imaging studies by radiologists or referring physicians. Image CDs provided to patients as a part of their medical record also have such embedded software for easy review of images.

A *Mini PACS* is a loose term that has been used to define a low cost, small-scale PACS solution usually built using open source nonpropriety software, which has limited functionality and archival options, may not have any linkage with other IT systems and is used by smaller and stand-alone imaging centers, radiologists working remotely or even for dedicated techniques like mammography viewing, postprocessing, and reporting systems [14].

An efficiency enhancing tool used with the PACS in some departments is a voice recognition software that translates voice to text. This software is specially designed and trained to identify medical terminology and can be server based, cloud based, or installed on the desk tops. Although some vendors provide dictation microphones (Fig. 6.5) others even use the cell phone or desk top microphone for dictation.

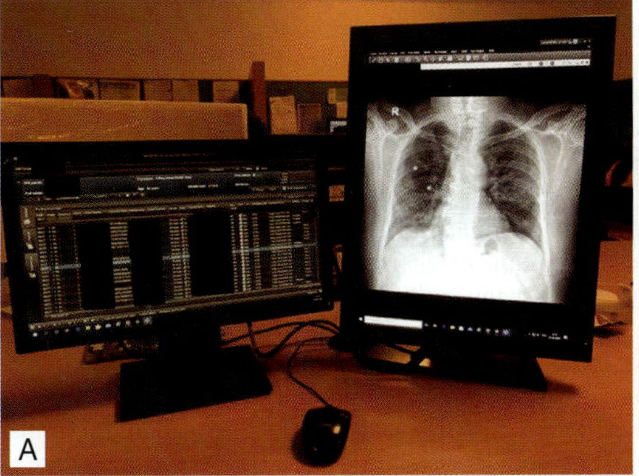

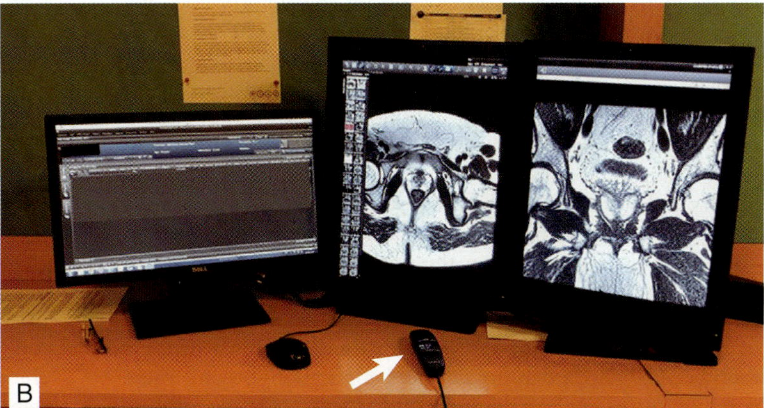

Figure. 6.5 (A) shows a standard two monitor workstation configuration with one medical grade monitor (on the right) displaying the images in the PACS and a regular monitor with RIS on the left. (B) shows two medical grade monitors on the right and in the center with a regular monitor on the left. A voice-to-text dictation microphone is seen in (B) (*arrow*).

DICOM

DICOM is the international standard used to define the format for creating, exchanging, and storing images. It is applicable for the image and all information related to the image. First published in 1993 and used in radiology, it is now used in other departments including cardiology, radiation oncology, ophthalmology, and dentistry [15]. Image files that are compliant with DICOM standard are referred as "DICOM files" and are represented as ".dcm." In contrast to other image file formats (JPEG, TIFF, etc.), the DICOM files are not recognized by Windows-based software and require the DICOM viewing software or browser to view these images on personal computers.

There are two components of a DICOM file—header and image datasets, packed in a single file. The header consists of demographic information about the patient, acquisition parameters of imaging, image dimensions, matrix size, color space, and some additional information required by the software to accurately display the image. Image dataset is a single attribute that consists of all pixel intensities. These datasets are stored as a long series of 0s and 1s, which can be reconstructed as an image.

Although DICOM images have acceptance in medical practice, there are two disadvantages—large file sizes and special software for viewing. To use these images for educational purpose or publication, they need to be converted into other compatible formats and the patient information should be removed from the images. Major disadvantage of other file formats, compared with DICOM, is that the user-determined window level and window width set at the time of creation of an image cannot be adjusted and postprocessing cannot be performed.

Postprocessing and Advanced Image Visualization

Traditionally, a radiologist would need to purchase a multimodality workstation to perform specialized postprocessing tasks. For small imaging centers with few radiologists, this continues to be purchased along with new CT or MR scanners. Most *enterprise PACS systems have in-built multimodality postprocessing tools for advanced visualization*, which is usually linked to a server-based advanced postprocessing software application. This application gets launched through the click of a mouse on an embedded link on the PACS user interface. Modern-day ultrasound, CT, and MR scanners provide dynamic and 3D datasets which allow the radiologist to process or manipulate the images to either visualize the organs and abnormalities in a different plane, orientation, or form (example being a 3D image) to improve their efficiency and diagnostic capabilities.

Basic postprocessing applications include multiplanar reconstructions, maximum intensity projections, 3D visualization, and spine labeling. More advanced applications include cardiac CT, vessel evaluation, perfusion (CT and MR), MR spectroscopy, volumetry and organ segmentation, transcatheter aortic valve implantation planning and, RECIST templates for oncology reporting, among others. Depending on the techniques available, types of referrals, research orientation, and budgets, most of these postprocessing applications are provided as options at the time of purchase of the equipments or the PACS. With time, a number of these tools become standard as the advanced applications become more common. An example of this is the cardiac postprocessing software for the evaluation of coronary arteries is now a standard software for all 64 slices and above CT scanners. This was previously a "package" that had to be purchased in addition to the scanner.

Increasing number of AI applications, which are still at a nascent stage, can also be integrated with PACS systems, wherein the postprocessed images from the AI solution is sent to the PACS as a separate series. In some instances, the PACS also launches these applications so that the radiologists can modify the results of the AI solutions. Details of the current status of AI in radiology are described in a separate chapter.

Radiology Workstations and Monitors

To be able to use all the IT tools available to them, radiologists need high end computer systems with some enhanced features and faster computing power to ensure efficiency and productivity. Since there is concurrent usage of multiple software including RIS, PACS, EMR, and even postprocessing software, a single monitor is usually not sufficient. It is also necessary to view images on specialized monitors, which adhere to certain defined standards so as to adequately visualize images from different imaging techniques without missing any abnormality due to inadequate specifications of the monitor—these are called diagnostic grade monitors. The combination of monitors usually includes at least one standard computer monitor, for viewing applications such as RIS, EMR, dictation software, medical resources, and other nonmedical software including the internet and email. In addition, radiologists use different combinations of medical grade monitors along with regular monitors, depending on the type of work and techniques being reported by them (Fig. 6.5B). Some radiologists prefer two nonimaging monitors due to the greater number of nonimage-based applications being used by them. At any given point of time, majority of radiologists have three to five applications open on nonimaging monitors [16].

The diagnostic workstations should have a high processing speed, random access memory, and storage to ensure that the processing power for medical applications is adequately supported.

Although there are multiple parameters that are characteristic for diagnostic or medical grade monitors [17], the major criteria determining the quality of monitor and which monitor is suited for reporting a particular technique include

- Luminance is the photometric measure of luminous intensity "L" and defines amount of light visually perceived by the eye. It is measured as Candela (cd). One cd is roughly the luminous intensity of one common candle. For monitors, it is measured as candelas per square meter (cd/m^2) and is a function of the backlight system of the monitor
- Contrast/brightness is calculated as luminance ratio (LR) which is the ratio between the maximum and minimum luminance. For example a maximum luminance of 450 cd/m^2 and minimum of 1 cd/m^2 would yield a LR of 450:1
- Ambient light also plays an important factor in capability to see pathologies in the darker areas of the monitor. This adds to the minimum luminance, which should be adjusted on the monitor as 1.5 times the measured ambient light for correction
- Display format defines the number of pixels and diagonal screen size. It is a multiple of the number of pixels in both the planes. Monitors are usually available in 2, 3, 5, or 10 megapixel configurations. Color monitors are less efficient, by about 50%, for passing luminance energy compared with monochrome monitors and requiring higher maximum luminance than monochrome displays. Table 6.1 lists the recommendations for display standards in primary diagnostic work by the Royal College of Radiologists [18]
- Display size determines the ability of the radiologist to view the entire image, including the periphery and is measured as

TABLE 6.1 Recommendations for Display Standards in Primary Diagnostic Work by Radiologists

Technique	Minimum Resolution	Luminance (min/max) (cd/m^2)
Plain x-ray	2048 × 1536 3 MP	1/350
CT	1600 × 1200 2 MP	1/350
MR	1600 × 1200 2 MP	1/350
Ultrasound	1600 × 1200 2 MP	0.8/250
Fluoroscopy	1600 × 1200 2 MP	0.8/250
Nuclear medicine	1600 × 1200 2 MP	0.8/250
Breast radiology	2560 × 2048 5 MP	1/400
Mobile review	1600 × 1200 2 MP	1/250

the diagonal size of the monitor. Monitor of 21 inches or 53 cm is considered optimal. A width to height ratio of 3:4 or 4:5 is ideal for a monitor. Newer wider monitors with a greater width (16:9 or 16:10) can also serve as dual monitors

Other characteristics that help in selection of workstations include quality of the graphics card, the graphic bit display, and the operating system.

With advances in resolution of mobile devices like smart phones and tablets, it is now possible to visualize the PACS images on these devices remotely and on the move. Mostly mobiles are used by the radiologist or referring physician to review images for quality, during rounds and communicating reported findings with patients, but should not be used to provide a formal report.

Teleradiology

As the name suggests, teleradiology is the practice of radiology wherein a radiologist reports imaging studies from a location which is different from where the scans are done. Teleradiology can be used in multiple ways to provide timely and expert reporting on scans anywhere in the world. The provider (radiologist) and seeker (imaging center or radiology department) can be part of the same organization in instances where there is need for night and/or emergency reporting. There are a number of teleradiology service provider companies globally covering for either shortage or radiologists or second opinions. Outsourcing by teleradiology can also serve as a conduit for reducing the cost of hiring radiologists in some instances, such as night reporting services that gave a big impetus to teleradiology in the late 1990s in the United States. Today there are cross border services available, which need to ensure that the local privacy and security laws for the region where the patient lives (and gets the imaging done) are adhered to. HIPAA and GDPR adherence is extremely important for teleradiology service providers in the United States and Europe. There is also a requirement in many states and countries, for the radiologists having a license to practice in the specific state or country of image origination; and also the location from where they report. This was formalized by the American College of Radiology as far back as in 1994 as the ACR standard for teleradiology [19].

The software for teleradiology is usually a part of the PACS and RIS systems, which can be purchased in isolation or within the larger IT infrastructure. The commercial systems were actually available in the late 1980s but had limited capability and scale [19]. To provide teleradiology services, a good internet connectivity is required, which is now accessible and affordable across most countries in the world.

In summary, it is extremely important for all radiologists to be aware of the role of various IT applications in their day-to-day lives; and to use these tools to raise the efficiency of their work, improve quality, optimize cost of delivery, and stay relevant in clinical decision making. Radiology is now truly digital.

Suggested Readings

- M Yousef, Z Hamideh, Hospital Information System (HIS): at a glance, Asian J Comput Inform Syst 1 (2) (2013) 2321–5658.
- M James, The case for RIS/PACS integration, Radiol Manage 24 (3) (2002) 24–29.
- M Napoli, M Nanni, S Cimarra, L Crisafulli, P Campioni, P Marano, et al., Picture archiving and communication in radiology, Rays 28 (1) (2003) 73–81.
- S Christopher, et al., Big data for deep learning in radiology: population-based imaging, Health Manag 18 (6) (2018).
- A Sharma, K Wang, E Siegel, Radiologist digital workspace use and preference: a survey-based study, J Digit Imaging 30 (6) (2017) 687–694.

7

Quality Assurance and Structured Reporting

SHALINI GOVIL, ANTO RAMESH, ASHOK MITHRA

Introduction

Radiology quality improvement programs (QIPs) have come of age, with most radiologists having some experience of quality assurance (QA), usually from hospital activities mandated by accrediting bodies and regulatory agencies, such as The *Joint Commission International (JCI)*. Apart from what is mandated, all radiologists desire to provide high-quality reports in a safe, efficient, and timely manner. Large departments in institutes dedicate staff, technology, and financial resources to run wide-ranging QIPs, whereas smaller practices address only the core principles of QI.

A QIP enables *safe, effective, and patient-centered care* through the systems, processes, methods, and essential components of effective quality management. The QIP team is composed of radiologists, technologists, nurses, patients, medical physicists, equipment vendors, administrators, schedulers, and the information technology team.

Despite the administrative jargon, the essence of quality care lies in the promise made when embarking on a career in medicine: that is, "*to help and do no harm.*" QI is merely an attempt to achieve this in an organized manner.

The Institute of Medicine in America defined quality as "The degree to which health services for individuals and populations increase the likelihood of desired health outcomes and are consistent with current professional knowledge" [1]. The American College of Radiology defines quality as "*doing the right thing, at the right time, in the right way, for the right person, to have the best possible results*" [2].

In radiology, quality is *consistently providing timely access to appropriate, optimal imaging, and accurately interpreted reports in a safe, efficient, and effective manner* [3,4].

Six Domains of Healthcare Quality (Institute of Medicine)

The six specific Institute of Medicine aims for improvement of the healthcare system are known as the STEEEP principles: safe, timely, effective, efficient, equitable, and patient centered [1].

1. **S**afe: Avoiding harm to patients from the care that is intended to help them.
2. **T**imely: Reducing waits and sometimes harmful delays for both those who receive and those who give care.
3. **E**ffective: Providing services based on scientific knowledge to all who could benefit and refraining from providing services to those not likely to benefit.
4. **E**fficient: Avoiding waste, including waste of equipment, supplies, ideas, and energy.
5. **E**quitable: Providing care that does not vary in quality because of personal characteristics such as gender, ethnicity, geographic location, and socioeconomic status.
6. **P**atient centered: Providing care that is respectful of and responsive to individual patient preferences, needs, and values and ensuring that patient values guide all clinical decisions.

The Quality Improvement Program

Imaging services should maintain active quality, safety, and performance improvement programs. Acquisition of relevant data is followed by analysis and priority listing of factors that cause process failure, error, or adverse events. Pilot solutions are implemented and monitored, with consistently successful solutions being implemented on a wider level (Box 7.1).

QIP requires careful, dedicated, and continuously planned effort with a number of skilled and committed team members, whose goal is do the right thing in a timely fashion for every case. The QI process can be sustained by offering rewards and celebrating successes, with all lessons learned and disseminated throughout the department/organization.

QIP "ticks many boxes." It can facilitate continuous improvement of performance, safety, and clinical outcomes; meet regulatory requirements; and reach the common goal of providing safe, effective, value-added radiology, and stay competitive within the rapidly changing healthcare environment.

BOX 7.1 Radiology Quality Improvement Program (QIP)

- Implements change
- Meets regulatory requirements
  - Patient safety
  - Image quality
  - Report quality
  - Processes
  - Customer service
  - Performance monitoring
  - On-the-job training
  - Data analysis and display

BOX 7.2 Nine Steps on The Radiology Quality Map

1. Imaging order entry:
   ordering the examination requested by the referring physician
2. Appointment scheduling:
   timeliness of scheduling affecting the outcome of patient care
3. Initial radiology encounter:
   patient engagement at arrival in the radiology department
4. Imaging protocol selection:
   choosing the appropriate imaging technique and parameters
5. Patient care:
   ensuring patient comfort
   addressing safety issues
   monitoring the effectiveness and efficiency of the process
6. Image acquisition and finalization
7. Image interpretation
8. Communication of imaging interpretation:
   - accuracy
   - timeliness
   - reliability
   - clarity
   - brevity
   - clinical relevance
9. Patient management and outcome

The Radiology Quality Map

Swensen and Johnson [5] proposed a radiology quality map that follows the path of the patient from the referring physician, through the radiology department to the final radiology report impacting patient outcome (Box 7.2). Each step has multiple processes that provide opportunities for improvement and incremental improvements at each step leads to better patient outcomes. This radiology quality map is the "product" that needs to be improved by way of QIP.

Quality Management: *Definitions and Metrics*

For most of the 20th century, the term quality control (QC) in radiology referred to equipment and image QC with standards in place for regular testing, monitoring, and maintenance that were performed and documented by a technician supervisor. Doctors, long considered noble and infallible, were exempt from "control." Although the nobility of the profession remains paramount, the emergence of healthcare as an industry has brought quality management in its wake. A glossary of common terms used in quality management is provided in Table 7.1 [6].

Quality Control Versus Quality Assurance

QC is defined as a set of processes used to monitor and improve technical performance, whereas QA is a comprehensive process that evaluates the quality of patient care and the clinical performance of all practitioners in any healthcare system, against established quality standards. QC is reactive and product oriented, looking for defects and errors after the product is built, whereas QA is proactive and process oriented, collecting and evaluating feedback from customers to improve processes.

Fig. 7.1 is a Venn diagram depicting the commonalities and differences between QC and QA. Both work toward the common goal of high-quality products and processes, customer loyalty, and fixing minor faults before they become major errors. Although QA achieves this through audit, root cause analysis (RCA), and training; whereas QC tests and verifies, identifies, and document problems before releasing the product.

In medicine, an error prevented is a life saved. In radiology, QA studies the processes and procedures between order entry and the final report to identify and address issues *before they cause*

TABLE 7.1 Glossary of Terms [6]

Term	Definition
Quality control	Processes for monitoring and improving technical performance
Quality assurance	Comprehensive process used to monitor and evaluate the quality and appropriateness of patient care (ensuring compliance with preestablished quality standards) and the clinical performance of all practitioners in any healthcare system
Quality improvement	Proactive activities aimed at improving the processes that enhance the quality of care and services
Performance improvement	Concept of improving output, efficiency, or effectiveness through implementing change on the basis of analysis and measurement of collected data
Total quality management	Umbrella under which all processes that are established to monitor and assure quality are subsumed, including the formal organizational quality infrastructure and related quality improvement activities within a department or organization
Patient safety programs	Processes used to identify actual and potential problems in medical systems and procedures
Risk management programs	Programs developed to help prevent accidents and injuries and reduce the cost of claims and the risk of other financial losses

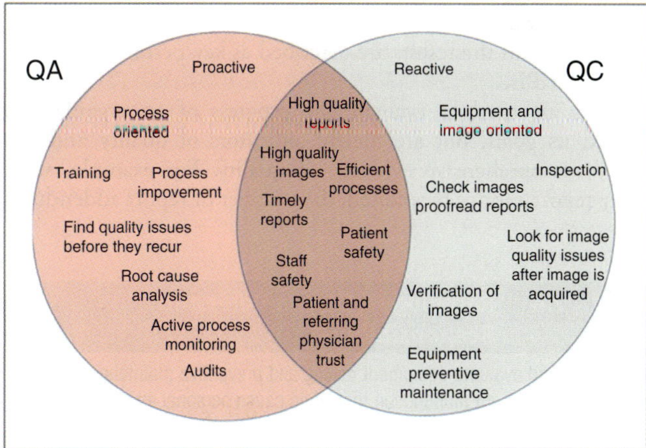

Figure 7.1 Venn diagram visually representing shared and differing goals, roles, and responsibilities of QA and QC.

BOX 7.3 Radiology QA Team Roles and Responsibilities

- Plan, develop, and implement QA policies, processes, and procedures
- Document and update SOPs and best practices
- Audit processes, procedures, and reports to meet regulations and maintain standards
- Monitor current processes to find and correct discrepancies
- Train and educate all members to ensure processes and procedures are followed
- Perform root cause analysis + implement solutions for current process and procedure flaws
- Collect and evaluate feedback from referring physicians and patients
- Ensure that documented processes comply with regulatory standards

significant error. It focuses on the prevention of error through training, structured reporting checklists, and skill-building. The QA team plans and implements best practices and defines how to build, audit, and maintain clinical excellence (Box 7.3). An example of QA in radiology is the random reviewing of images and reports to identify the errors that indicate a need for technician and radiologist re-training.

QC inspects and tests equipment and images to ascertain flaws related to equipment malfunction or technical error that can lead to diagnostic error or even injury (Box 7.4). An example of QC in radiology would be an x-ray image being rejected as soon as it is taken because of wrong technical factors.

TABLE 7.2 Radiology KPIs [6]

Dimension of Care	Performance Indicators
Patient safety	Patient falls, contrast material reactions and extravasations, minor and major procedural complications, physician compliance with hand-washing requirements, compliance with preprocedure time-outs, verification and documentation of patient identification, radiation dose reduction at CT
Effectiveness	Outcomes measures for procedures (e.g., biopsy), appropriateness of imaging studies, positive predictive rates for techniques, physician performance assessment and peer review
Efficiency	Reduction of unnecessary studies, number of technologists per scanner, scanner utilization, scanning room turnaround time, equipment downtime for maintenance
Patient-centeredness	Patient satisfaction surveys, analysis and management of customer complaints, communication and follow-up of abnormal results
Timeliness	Report turnaround time, time to next available appointment, interventional suite turnaround time, patient throughput in CT scanner, patient wait times, sample delivery times to pathology laboratory

Key Performance Indicators

"You can't manage what you can't measure" is an old saying that captures the need for measuring the level of existing quality before deciding how to improve quality. Departments, institutions, and regulatory organizations mandate-specific technical and clinical metrics be continuously monitored, analyzed, and reported to ensure performance improvement occurs through increased output, efficiency, and effectiveness. Analytic tools are used to achieve these goals and the results are described as key performance indicators or KPIs.

KPIs are used to evaluate the progress of an organization toward its goals, but are merely indicators of quality and not actual, comprehensive evidence of quality. For example, since every report cannot be audited, the number of report addendums are monitored, assuming that they are all events when an error in the original report was detected and corrected. Addendums, however, can be raised for reasons ranging from a significant laterality error to the correction of an insignificant typographical error. In addition, addendums are only raised on errors that are noticed and corrected. *The addendum rate is thus an indicative error rate and not an actual error rate.*

The main performance indicator categories include accuracy, productivity, patient safety, access to services, and customer satisfaction. Core quality metrics include critical incident reporting, expensive equipment downtime, and positivity rate of high-risk/high-cost procedures.

Table 7.2 lists some of the common KPIs used in radiology [6].

BOX 7.4 Radiology QC Team Roles and Responsibilities

- Ensure and evaluate equipment testing and preventive maintenance
- Detect equipment malfunction that could cause personal injury or compromise image quality
- Ensure equipment and images are in compliance with regulatory standards
- Document inspection reports, noting any deviations from established standards
- Identify and document image flaws before release
- Identify, document, recall images with flaws after release, for example, CT brain calibration artifact
- Work with QA team to identify areas that need improvement and training needs
- Evaluate feedback and complaints, to find solutions to issues raised
- Ensure that only high-quality images are released

Sequential Steps in The Quality Improvement Process

To achieve continuous quality improvement, the sequential steps taken for a QI project should be generic and capable of repeated cycling over a range of processes. Jonathan Kruskal in 2011 described the standard sequential steps in a generic quality improvement process, summarized in Box 7.5.

Identify and Define The Process or Problem With Information-Gathering Tools

- To run a successful QIP, data collection and analysis of the problem is as important as the solution and implementation strategies, and requires the use of information-gathering tools (Box 7.5)
- **Customer surveys** seek feedback from patients, their families and referring physicians that reveal opportunities for improvement; attending to the specific issues raised is a simple way of

BOX 7.5 QI Process—Sequential Steps

- Identify problems with information-gathering tools:
  - customer surveys
  - safety and environment-of-care walkabouts
  - process bottlenecks
  - peer review and error reporting
  - monitoring of compliance
  - brainstorming sessions
  - strength, weakness, opportunity, and threat analyses
- Display data using visual quality analysis tools:
  - flow charts, cause-and-effect diagrams "fishbone" (Fig. 7.2)
  - Pareto diagrams, check sheets, control charts (Fig. 7.3)
  - histograms
  - scatter diagrams
  - control charts (Fig. 7.4)
  - radar or "spider" charts (Fig. 7.5)
  - "spaghetti" motion diagrams (Fig. 7.6)
  - bubble charts
- Identify contributing root causes
- PDSA: the plan-do-study-act cycle

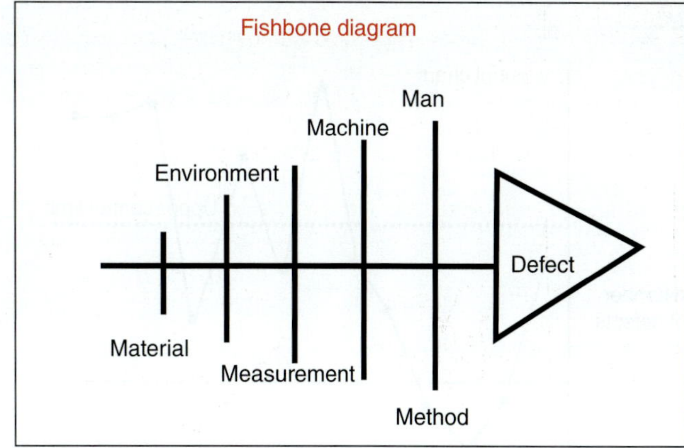

Figure 7.2 Cause-and-effect/"fishbone" or Ishikawa diagrams are a standard tool used in root cause analysis. The head of a fish is the "defect" and the bones of the fish are the causes for the defect. Categories of causes include: people, materials, methods, machines, measurement, environment, and other modified to match the problem being addressed.

bringing about change and building trust. **Safety and environment-of-care walkabouts** by trained observers help identify risks and lacunae in the facility that do not conform to recommended safety guidelines [7]. **Process bottlenecks** tend to occur at points where the demand overwhelms available resources, waxing and waning during peak and lean times [8]. **Peer review and error reporting** highlight areas requiring clinical or technical improvement [9,10], and is explained in greater detail later in this chapter. **Brainstorming** as a team of varied voices from grassroots to stakeholders is an excellent way of identifying problems and finding solutions. **Strength, weakness, opportunity, and threat analyses** identify major stressors—both internal (strengths/weaknesses) and external (threats/limitations/competition) as well as opportunities for improvement

Display Data Using Visual Quality Analysis Tools

Like scientific data, quality data should be collected, displayed, and analyzed, using scientific statistical tools such as the visual quality analysis tools listed in Box 7.5 and illustrated in Figs. 7.2–7.6 [11–15].

- **Cause-and-effect diagrams** "fishbone" or Ishikawa diagrams are a standard tool used in RCA. The head of a fish is the "defect" and a line drawn horizontally away from the head is the spine, along which causes are inserted in categories like the bones of a fish (Fig. 7.2)
- **Pareto charts** contain both bar and line graphs and highlight the most important quality issues. The bar height decreases from left to right, in decreasing order of frequency or importance
- **The Pareto principle:** For many events, ~80% of effects come from 20% of causes—that is, the vital few versus the trivial many. Identifying and focusing on this 20% will produce 80% of the desired results; the "vital few" should therefore be the area of focus to produce best results with economy of effort (Fig. 7.3) [13]

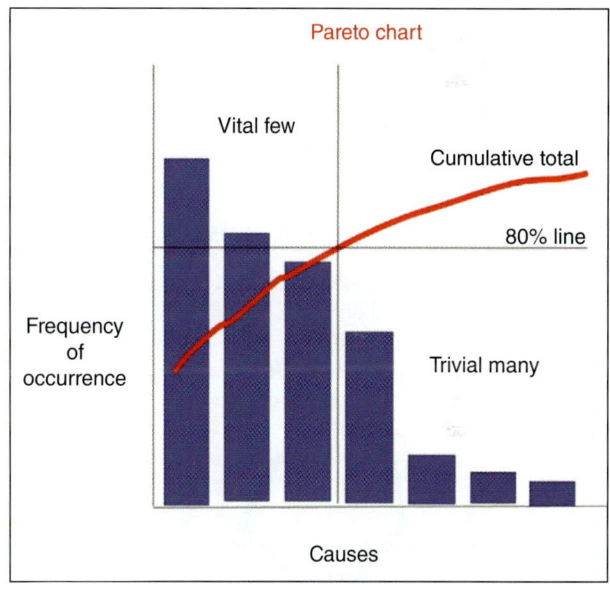

Figure 7.3 Pareto charts contain both bar and line graphs highlighting the most important quality issues. The bar height decreases from left to right, in decreasing order of frequency or importance.
The Pareto principle: "80/20": For many events, ~80% of effects come from 20% of causes—that is, the vital few versus the trivial many. The "vital few" should therefore be the area of focus to produce best results with economy of effort.

Identify Contributing Root Causes

RCA is an iterative, continuous process used to identify and correct major contributing causes of a problem. The **"5-Why?"** approach is a series of iterative questions posed to drill deeper into contributing factors; at every stage of reviewing "what happened," the question "why" is asked of every response. This can be done as part of a brainstorming session and combined with a fishbone approach and Pareto principle (Box 7.6).

The Plan-Do-Study-Act Cycle

The plan-do-study-act cycle is a series of steps where a proposed solution is tested on a small scale before changes are applied to the

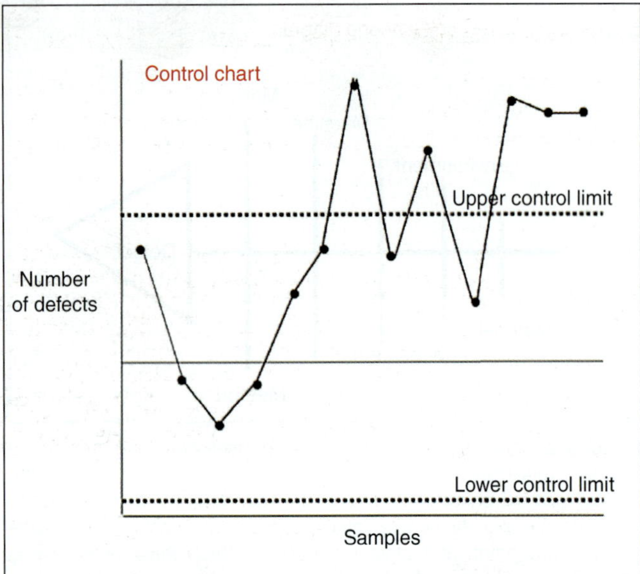

Figure 7.4 Control charts study how a process changes over time, to determine whether a process needs formal examination for quality-related problems.
Current data are either stable (within defined control limits) or unpredictable (falling above or below the control limits).
Regular analysis should be done to identify problems and correct them as they occur, and keep things "under control."

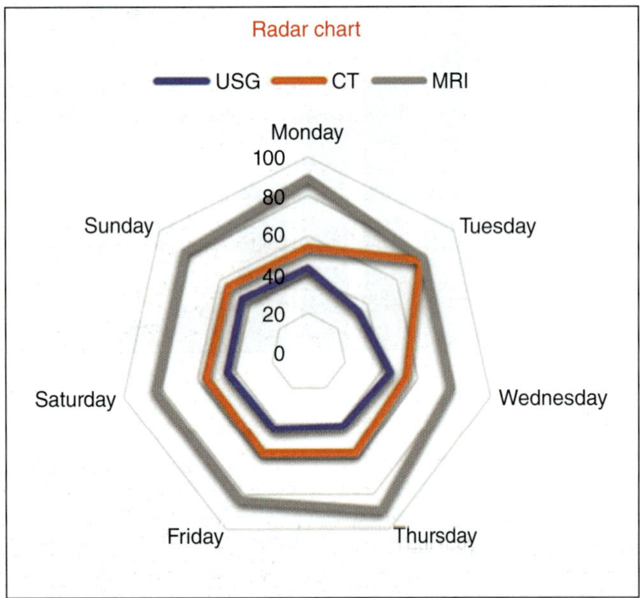

Figure 7.5 Radar charts or "spider" or "web" charts allow comparison of several variables over time, ideally suited for tracking performance metrics over time.
Radar charts highlight those variables undergoing the most or the least change.
In this example of case numbers on different days of the week, CT sees the largest increase in number and this occurs on Tuesdays.

whole system. Effects are monitored and fed back resulting in a trial-and-learning cycle that perpetuates quality improvement of the process or product.

- **Plan:** Define objective, identify team, set goals, and develop a solution

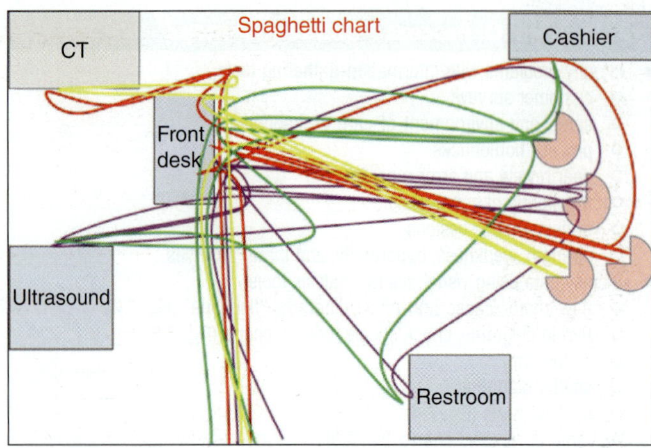

Figure 7.6 Spaghetti or workflow diagrams.
Records the actual paths of movement of people and reveals the physical bottlenecks that reduce efficiency.
In this example of the flow of patients from entry to exit through a radiology department, a bottleneck is clearly visualized at the front desk because of repeated events at the same desk.

BOX 7.6 Identify Contributing Root Causes

- Brainstorming session
- Identify contributing factors on a fishbone diagram
- Collect data
- Apply to a Pareto chart
- Pareto chart displays relative importance of each contributing factor
- Apply Pareto ("80/20") principle
- Identify 20% contributing factors responsible for 80% effects

Pareto principle identifies 20% "vital few" factors that cause the greatest problems.

- **Do:** Implement changes, choose metrics to monitor progress, identify and overcome barriers before rolling-out a wider implementation
- **Study:** Implement strategy, collect data, and identify areas needing further improvement
- **Act:** Implement interventions deemed successful after the study phase and modify or abort unsuccessful interventions before the next cycle is attempted

Essential Ingredients of a Quality Improvement Program

The framework and ingredients of a QIP will depend on the department or practice size, nature, resources, and culture of quality and safety.

Institutional Leadership

Leadership support indicates clearly that the pursuit of excellence at every level is at the core of their mission. Apart from a senior radiologist leading the QIP team as a Quality Director, the program needs a Quality Coordinator who will ensure quality metrics and KPIs are regularly measured, documented, and reported as mandated and also ensures regular meeting of interdepartmental quality forums, maintenance of adverse event reporting systems, and "walkabouts" by observer-administrators.

Just Culture of Quality and Safety

"Just Culture" is a term coined by David Marx referring to a team environment that allows members to feel comfortable confronting and revealing errors, both their own and others [16]. *A Just Culture views every failure as an opportunity to learn and welcomes monitoring and feedback.*

QIP Team

The QIP team typically consists of a Quality Director, Quality Coordinator, and a set of empanelled radiologist and technologist auditors who monitor performance metrics. In a hospital, the radiology QIP team should function within and be accountable to a Central Quality Cell. This integration facilitates interdepartmental cooperation when reviewing adverse events, enables acceptance of new hospital-wide initiatives and provides access to centrally acquired data relevant to the radiology QIP.

Fully Engaged Radiologists

- With greater penetration of regulatory mandates related to accreditations, it is easier now to achieve universal participation in quality-related processes especially when credentialing renewal depends on it. However, it is preferable to achieve a genuine "Buy-in" from radiologists who partner in the process and are not adversarial. Reinertsen et al. outlined a process that builds consensus for QIP (modified and listed in Box 7.7) [20]
- QI curves that plot incidence of undesired event against time typically show an initial increase, a plateau, and then decrease as a result of the improvement intervention [17,18]

Patient Safety and Communication

The Joint Commission requires that healthcare organizations be compliant with a set of safety goals that are upgraded each year.

BOX 7.7 Strategies for Radiologist/Technologist Engagement in QIP

- Identify common purpose: improved patient outcome and efficiency
- Renewed dedication: "correct report and image every time for all my patients"
- High-EQ QIP team: empathetic, respectful, authentic, discrete, nonjudgmental, and insightful
- Equitable and transparent QIP: universal monitoring and access to anonymized results
- Confidentiality scrupulously maintained
- Nonpunitive monitoring: "measure to improve"
- Reward for participation: *robust and comprehensive in-house training* QIP as knowledge partner:
  - discrepancy feedback with flash-learning points
  - structured procedure/disease-specific reporting templates
  - skill-based learning: reporting/technical workshops
  - on-line training modules: knowledge certifications
- Career gap analysis and "bridge-the-gap" guidance

Timeout

- Important instances of timeout include verification of patient identity, side, site, and nature of study with a timeout performed before every procedure, duly documented in the record

Critical Results

- Critical results should be communicated in a timely manner to the appropriate person and the communication documented and read back to ensure accuracy
- High volume abnormal results can prove challenging when defining what constitutes a critical result. Most institutions develop a list of critical findings for QI processes but this should serve as a supplement not substitute the radiologist's clinical assessment of criticality [19]

Radiation, Equipment, and Contrast Safety

- Regulatory standards require safety monitoring of services
- This includes protection measures for staff and patients against unnecessary or excess exposure to ionizing radiation or to risks associated with the use of medical imaging equipment, contrast media, and contact with blood and body fluids
- A radiation safety program should be in place, followed, and documented

Diagnostic Errors

- Globally, regulatory organizations mandate performance monitoring and staff participation in QIP for their institution to maintain accreditation. In the United States, diagnostic errors are the third leading cause of death with 10% of patients dying from medically preventable deaths [22–24]. It stands to reason, therefore, that the core aim of a radiology QIP should be to reduce diagnostic error

Diagnostic Error Rates

- A Mayo Clinic autopsy study in 2000 found a major diagnosis was missed during the course of medical management in 26% [25]. A 20-year literature review in 2001 found the major error rate in radiology to range from 2% to 20% [26]. The error rate in diagnostic imaging varies dependent on the method of calculation: if the denominator consists only of abnormal imaging studies, the error rate averages 30%; however, if the denominator consists of a routine blend of abnormal and normal studies, the blended error rate averages 3.5–4% [27]

Generic Factors Contributing to Reporting Error

- Radiologists use both visual perception and cognitive interpretation when reporting images. The reasons why a reporting error might occur are therefore myriad and wide ranging. Devising a classification that captures every possible reason is a challenge that needs to be approached from both radiologist-specific causes and system-specific causes
  Radiologist-specific causes of error
- Early classifications by Smith in 1967 [28] and Renfrew et al. in 1992 [29] focused on the reasons why perceptual errors occur. The Kim–Mansfield Radiologic Error Classification System expanded these earlier classifications in 2014 and

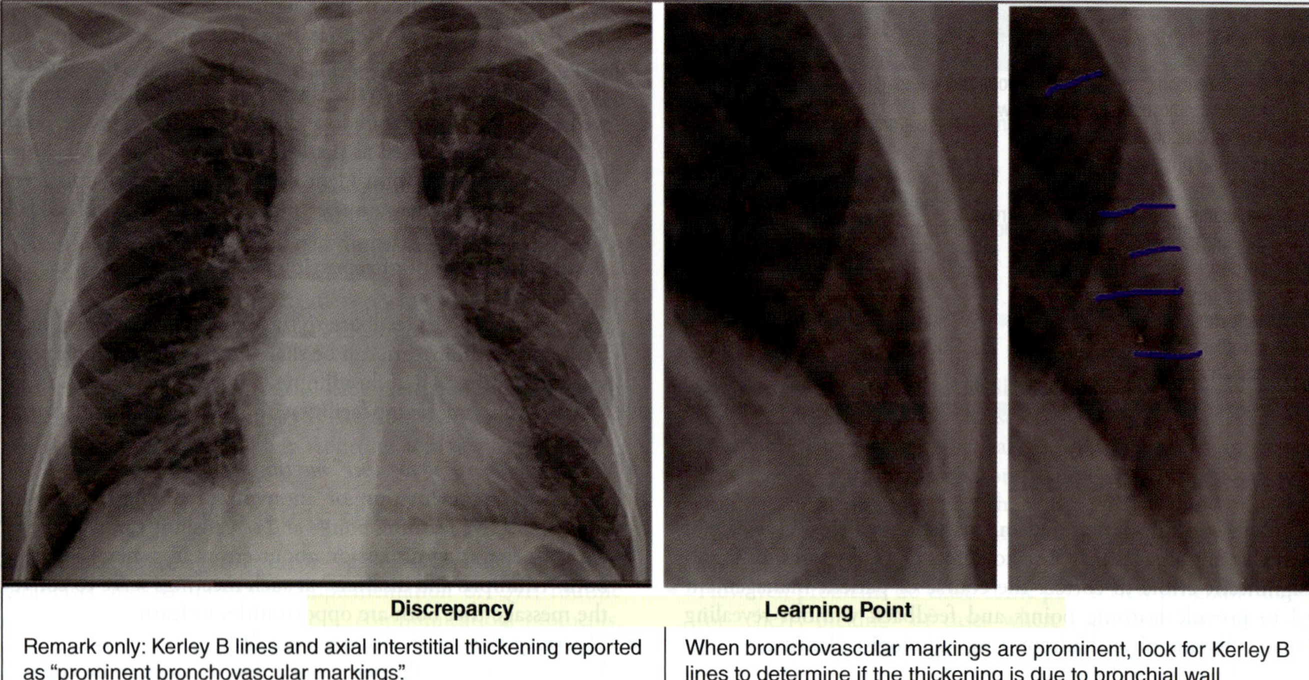

Discrepancy	Learning Point
Remark only: Kerley B lines and axial interstitial thickening reported as "prominent bronchovascular markings".	When bronchovascular markings are prominent, look for Kerley B lines to determine if the thickening is due to bronchial wall thickening alone or bronchial wall and interstitial thickening.

Figure 7.7 Feedback on report audit. Discrepancy and with annotated image illustrating the learning point.

Performance Improvement: Training "As-You-Go"

- Although performance monitoring provides information about accuracy and productivity, its primary aim should be to identify training needs. The QIP should meet these needs with robust "train-as-you-go" initiatives
- The QIP is ideally positioned to provide incremental, continuous training opportunities for the radiologist, both formally and informally, and this can begin at recruitment
- Completion of all QIP training initiatives is given credit in a radiologist scorecard (*discussed later*) at the end of the year

Recruitment Technical Assessment Feedback

- Large teleradiology practices were one of the first to institute stringent technical assessments before radiologist recruitment and found a 30% lower pass rate than the radiology qualifying board exam [32]
- A recruitment test, sometimes years after the last qualifying exam, can be a surprise for many radiologists. However, the simple act of taking the test introduces the radiologist to the concept of QA and helps recruiters identify lifelong learners who understand the need for continued training and "testing"
- Passing a stringent test can also create a sense of achievement and build a culture of quality and pride in excelling. This is a powerful learning opportunity when the cases mirror daily practice and answers are provided as each question is completed

Credentialing and Privileging

- Credentialing forms are typically filled-in at recruitment, requesting privileges for reporting/performing imaging investigations, based on the candidate's self-assessment of skill independence
- Credentialing forms can be created from core skill competencies listed in national radiology training programs within the core curriculum—for example, Fetal Medicine Foundation's nuchal translucency certification. Under each subspecialty or body system, skills can be listed by increasing complexity (Box 7.10)
- The radiologist requests either supervised or independent reporting privileges for each skill and provides information about the number of times that skill was used in the previous 5 years. The QIP Director approves requested privileges based on the information provided
- Credentialing can serve as an opportunity for training, providing radiologists with a chance to review the wide range of skills that can be acquired, understand their own skill level, document their clinical experience, make the connection between experience and skill level, articulate their strengths and limitations and objectively follow their skill improvement each year

BOX 7.10 Section of a Sample Credentialing Form

A. Breast imaging

1. Mammographic reporting of common breast diseases
2. Ultrasound of common breast diseases
3. MRI of common breast diseases
4. Performing breast biopsy and localization

B. Cardiac imaging

1. Plain x-ray reporting of cardiac disease and postoperative appearances
2. Reporting of pericardial disease as shown on CT and MRI
3. Performing and reporting 64, 128 slice CT coronary angiography, CT congenital and acquired cardiac disease, CT aortography
4. Performing and reporting cardiac MRI

- The QIP Director can use collated credentialing forms to map the range of skills as a team, identifying skill gaps and training needs

Appropriateness Criteria-Based Procedure Vetting

- Appropriate use of imaging technology should be monitored to ensure evidence-based practice, reducing duplicate or unnecessary imaging and avoid associated costs
- Before each investigation is performed, the supervising radiologist can rate the clinical indication for the imaging request against standard ACR Appropriateness Criteria, as "Usually Appropriate," "May Be Appropriate," or "Usually Not Appropriate"
- If the investigation request is rated as "Usually Not Appropriate," the case is discussed with the referring physician, a mutually agreed course of action formulated and the "Appropriateness Vetting" documented
- Appropriateness is monitored as a parameter in the accuracy audit
- Appropriateness criteria-based procedure vetting provides an opportunity for training the radiologist on appropriate indications for imaging

Reporting Templates

- Reports are best drafted using structured reporting templates to improve clarity and quality, reduce diagnostic errors, promote evidence-based medicine, provide training in real-time, and ensure consistent use of terminology across practices. Structured reporting templates, whether general or disease specific, provide an opportunity for training with the checklist style serving as a set of prompts and cues, reminding the radiologist of findings and structures to be reviewed on the image. Usage of reporting templates is monitored in the audit report

Multidisciplinary Team Meetings

- Regular multidisciplinary team meetings provide a forum for periodic interaction between referring physicians and radiologists to discuss and formulate ongoing patient care, provide feedback on previous imaging, share interesting cases, learning points, evidence-based best practice, appropriateness criteria, new protocols, new workflows, results of accuracy audits, areas of improvement, and recent advances of mutual interest
- Multidisciplinary team meetings are an effective QIP initiative that improve patient care as well as provide an opportunity for training through sharing of practical experience, theoretical updates, and the correlation of clinical, radiological features with follow-up that can include surgical and pathological final diagnosis

Monthly Continuing Medical Education

- Continuing medical education (CME) sessions held on a regular basis provide training and updates on recent advances and comprehensive knowledge on topics relevant to the practice of radiology. They foster the dissemination of evidence-based medicine throughout the group especially when there is equal participation in the CME activities
- Subspecialty lectures, quizzes, debates, panel discussions, invited lectures, clinical research projects, and "learning together" meetings provide a variety of training opportunities. Rewarding CME attendance and participation with credit points can be effective as a means of motivating busy radiologists to make time for this QIP training initiative

Group Training: Journal Club

- Journal clubs provide a forum to critically analyze current journal articles of clinical relevance to radiology and foster the principles of clinical epidemiology required to critically appraise published clinical research literature
- Journal clubs are an effective means of developing critical appraisal skills, keeping abreast of current medical literature, develop research literacy, follow evidence-based practice, stimulate academic debate, enable professional networking, and generate research ideas and publications
- Journal club is an excellent means to provide opportunities for training

Lifelong Learning: Using a Learning Management System

- Flashslides are a well-known means of offering quick-bites of image-based information on "must know," "need to know," and "nice to know" topics in a structured, multimodality, multispecialty format. Presenting knowledge in a standardized, flashcard, picture-book format (image-heavy, text-light) eases and fast-tracks learning for busy radiologists
- Uploading these flashslides and MCQs onto an LMS platform enables automated scoring and delivery of prelearning tests, learning modules, and postlearning tests
- The LMS can be set to allow multiple re-attempts until the selected answer is correct. A score of 100% on the postlearning test indicates that all flashslide images have been "tagged" to keywords and key phrases in memory
- Later, a similar image encountered, during routine reporting, will trigger "tagged" keywords for search online to confirm the diagnosis and prepare a clinically relevant, detailed report
- An in-house LMS platform accessible from any location/device can be used by the QIP to meet specific or general training needs before re-credentialing existing radiologists and to credential new recruits
- The content of a comprehensive, life-long learning set of flashslides can be created in-house by the group as an additional training activity

Reporting Workshops

- Reporting workshops can be conducted periodically when the QIP identifies reporting training needs through audit
- Based on disease-specific reporting templates, the workshop can focus on unfamiliar terminology, classification, grading, or staging systems within the template followed by a "See-one-Do-one" demonstration of cases and end with a postlearning quiz

Career Gap Analysis and Bridge-the-Gap Guidance

- Annual career gap analysis and guidance is a QI initiative that fosters the professional growth of individual radiologists as well as the whole group

- The career gap analysis is done by reviewing the radiologist's curriculum vitae alongside a benchmark for the same level of experience in an academic or referral institution
- Categories such as qualifications, awards, society memberships, subspecialization, teaching, research, publications, presentations, workshops, conferences, audit experience, and administrative experience can be scrutinized for gaps to be bridged
- A "bridge-the-gap" plan is then formulated with the radiologist and any efforts to bridge-the-gap made by the radiologist credited in their quality scorecard (*discussed later*)

Physician Scorecard and the Total Quality Score (TQS)

- Regulatory organizations and some hospitals have introduced the concept of comprehensive physician scorecards, aligned with core medical competencies
- The scorecard is a tool to evaluate performance, aligned to the needs of the organization, managed continuously, and updated regularly
- The limitation of the scorecard is it improves what is being measured to the possible detriment of what is not being measured [33–36]

Total quality score

For each radiologist, the QIP can maintain a TQS (Table 7.4) that credits general and medical competencies (Box 7.11), with data collected from the curriculum vitae, performance monitoring (accuracy, productivity), credentialed skills, service participation, and a 360-degree feedback/review.

- **Curriculum vitae score**
  Objective scoring of the curriculum vitae is a method of giving credit to qualifications and experience in a standardized fashion that provides a numerical weightage for the following: qualifications, referral hospital experience, teaching experience, subspecialization, medals and awards, presentations and publications

TABLE 7.4 Total Quality Score

Component	Score	Maximum	Scoring Method
Curriculum vitae		10	Percentage CV score × 10
QIP training		5	Percentage training module completion × 5
Productivity		25	Percentage productivity × 25
Accuracy		25	Percentage accuracy × 25
Skills		5	Percentage credentialed skills × 5
Service participation		10	Percentage participation × 10
360-degree review		20	360-degree feedback randomly sampled from juniors, peers, seniors, supervisors, front desk, technologists, nurses, patients, referring physicians
Total quality score		100	

BOX 7.11 Total Quality Scorecard

- Aligned with core medical competencies
  - Professional standing
  - Lifelong learning
  - Self-assessment
  - Cognitive expertise
  - Performance in practice
  - Core competencies:
    - Medical knowledge
    - Patient care
    - Interpersonal skills
    - Communication
    - Professionalism
    - Practice-based learning
    - Systems-based practice

- **Training score**
  The training score of the TQS credits training efforts and completion of all QIP training initiatives
- **Productivity score**
  The productivity score is based on RVUs assigned to the reports finalized by the radiologist over a year, according to a predefined RVU scoring, with the benchmark for a regular 8-hour working day set at 100 RVU of productivity
- **Accuracy score**
  The accuracy score is based on the percentage of reports that are in agreement with peer/expert auditor opinion in a minimum sample of 30 reports over 1 year
- **Skills score**
  The skills score is based on the percentage of procedures that the radiologist is credentialed to perform from a list of skills available on the credentialing form
- **Service participation score**
  The participation score is based on the radiologist's percentage participation in full-time, after-hours, flexible shift, holiday, and weekend services as well as willingness to engage in QIP training activities
- **360-degree feedback score**
  A 360-degree, multirater, multisource feedback review is a survey sampling feedback from juniors, peers, seniors, supervisors, front desk, technologists, nurses, patients, and referring physicians, ending with a self-evaluation

The TQS is the cumulative score that is a sum of all these individual components.

Accreditation by Regulatory Bodies

Need for Accreditation

Rapid changes in healthcare systems dictated the need for global and national standardization, regulatory and accrediting organizations. Accreditation programs prescribe and monitor the quality and safety standards for medical imaging services. These standards are established to provide quality service, taking into account the combined perspective of the service provider, patient, referrer, and the relevant policies of local regulatory bodies.

The Joint Commission is a US-based organization that accredits more than 22,000 US healthcare organizations and programs. The international branch, JCI accredits medical services from around the world. The Quality Council of India was established in 1997 and the National Accreditation Board for Hospitals and

Healthcare Providers, under the Quality Council of India, runs accreditation programs for healthcare organizations.

Medical imaging service standards focus on patient care and QI relevant to diagnostic imaging. The standards for accreditation are applicable to single, multiple-service providers and hospital services and all diagnostic techniques and interventional procedures, including nuclear medicine. Requirements and regulations from the Atomic Energy Regulatory Board and pertaining to the Pre-Natal Sex Determination Act are incorporated into these standards.

Medical Imaging Service Standards: A Brief Overview

- **Access, assessment, and patient care:** concerns access to imaging services, protecting patient/family rights, and enabling informed decisions and includes access to emergency imaging in keeping with local laws and regulations [37]
- **Imaging procedures and interpretation:** concerns diagnostic and interventional imaging quality with focus on best practices, policies, and guidelines
- **Facility management and safety:** concerns safety of the environment within the facility and contingency plans to handle all types of emergencies
- **Equipment, material, and medications:** concerns policies pertaining to the procurement, quality, maintenance and storage of equipment, medication, contrast media, and radiopharmaceuticals
- **Human resource management:** concerns recruitment, planning, and training of staff with focus on effectiveness and fairness and includes performance appraisal
- **Management of quality and safety:** concerns safety and protection of patients and staff from unnecessary or harmful exposure to radiation, magnetic fields, radiofrequency waves, contrast media, and the electrical and mechanical hazards associated with the use of medical imaging equipment
- **Information management systems:** concerns the use of information management systems to meet the needs of patients, healthcare providers, and stakeholders and includes policies related to confidentiality, privacy, integrity and security of records, data, and information

In all these areas, it is important to define, document, implement, monitor, and ensure compliance to all standards. Table 7.5 outlines international standards of medical imaging services as prescribed by the JCI 7th edition

Accreditation Documentation and Reporting Methods

- The QIP should maintain records of all monitoring data in an easy-to-view format for review during quality accreditation
- KPI dashboards, slide presentations, and a repository containing all raw and source data should be updated and maintained. KPI spreadsheet trackers should document KPI methodology, summaries, and raw data for scrutiny and verification
- Review of KPIs, incidents, and QI projects should be done by the QIP team on a quarterly basis to identify trends that require action and highlight training needs

Key Performance Indicators for Radiology

Most regulatory bodies recommend a minimum set of KPIs that cover professional performance, customer service, process improvement, and patient safety (Table 7.6).

TABLE 7.5 JCI Radiology and Diagnostic Imaging Services—7th Edition [44] Standards

Assessment of patients (AOP)
Standard
AOP.6.1 A qualified individual(s) is responsible for managing the radiology and diagnostic imaging services, and individuals with proper qualifications and experience perform diagnostic imaging studies, interpret the results, and report the results.
AOP.6.2 A radiation and/or diagnostic imaging safety program for patients, staff, and visitors is in place, is followed, and is compliant with applicable professional standards, laws, and regulations.
AOP.6.3 Radiology and diagnostic imaging study results are available in a timely way as defined by the hospital.
AOP.6.4 All equipment used to conduct radiology and diagnostic imaging studies is regularly inspected, maintained, and calibrated, and appropriate records are maintained for these activities.
AOP.6.5 Quality control procedures are in place, followed, validated, and documented.

TABLE 7.6 Key Performance Indicators

KPI 1	Number of interpretation errors/1000 examinations
KPI 2	Number of imaging errors/100 examinations
KPI 3	Waiting time
KPI 4	Percentage adherence to safety precautions
KPI 5	Percentage correlation of radiology reports with clinical diagnosis

KPI 1: *Performance monitoring: radiologist accuracy*
Number of interpretation errors/1000 examinations.

KPI 2: *Performance monitoring: technologist accuracy*
Methodology is identical to monitoring radiologist accuracy, with images reviewed by experts, and training provided in the form of learning points.

KPI 3: *Waiting time for diagnostics*

KPI 4: *Percentage of adherence to safety precautions*
Adherence to safety is monitored through random monthly audits by the Radiation Safety Officer, who checks for staff compliance with safety regulations regarding radiation, MRI, and contrast media (Box 7.12). The auditor provides email feedback on all points of deviation from adherence to safety.

KPI 5: *Percentage of reports correlating with clinical diagnosis*
Percentage of reports correlating with clinical diagnosis is monitored through random monthly audit of 30 mixed technique reports for correlation with the clinical provisional/differential diagnosis.
The auditor provides email feedback whenever a clinical provisional/differential diagnosis is not proved on subsequent imaging, with further adjudication by a gold standard final diagnosis, whenever available.

The New Structured Radiology Report

The radiology report translates the radiologist's interpretation of the image into words, much like a musical score translates music within the mind of a composer to the pianist. Without standard

BOX 7.12 Safety Parameters

- Radiation safety
  - Can enumerate radiation hazards
  - Uses personal protective equipment
  - Applies as low as reasonably achievable principle
  - Wears TLD badge
  - Collimates appropriately
  - Uses low-dose technique
  - Uses red light indicator
  - Closes lead door appropriately
- MRI safety
  - Can enumerate MRI hazards
  - Follows MRI safety screening precautions and practices
  - Understands MRI zones
  - Can determine medical advice and implant MRI compatibility
  - Can enumerate absolute contraindications
  - Understands MRI anesthesia protocol and maintains MRI compatible anesthesia equipment
  - Knows protocol for potential MRI emergencies
  - Maintains MRI compatible equipment and material for MRI emergency handling
  - Identifies role and lists responsibilities as staff in MRI
- Contrast media safety
  - Can enumerate contrast media reactions and grade severity
  - Follows contrast media safety screening precautions and practices
  - Understands contrast media risks
  - Can determine when benefit outweighs risk of contrast media
  - Knows how to mitigate contrast media risk
  - Can enumerate contraindications
  - Recognizes and knows how to manage intravenous contrast extravasation
  - Knows protocol for treatment of contrast media reactions
  - Maintains equipment and medication required for handling of contrast media emergency

notation to communicate rhythm and notes, much can be lost in translation. Standardization is an accepted quality initiative in medicine as can be seen in the widespread dependence on clinical guidelines. In radiology, imaging protocols and appropriateness criteria are also gaining wider acceptance.

The structured reporting template primarily arose from a need for standardization and a uniform lexicon. With the adoption of PACS, secretarial transcription of dictated reports has been supplanted by voice recognition and one-finger, "raindrop" self-typing, further driving the need for templates that minimize typing.

- For these reasons, there has been a steady, world-wide transition from conventional free-text prose to a template-based, structured radiology report, increasingly supported by radiology societies offering free templates and vendors integrating templates into reporting software
- When creating a report template, the user's freedom of choice should not be rigidly curtailed because highly rigid standards are often rejected. Adherence to standards and consequent error reduction is best when users are given a high degree of discretion at an intermediate level of standardization [38]
- Multiple studies have demonstrated referring physician preference to structured reports. Schwartz at the Memorial Sloan-Kettering Cancer Center found that structured reports received significantly higher mean ratings for clarity and content when evaluated by radiologists and referring physicians. Hawkins in 2014 reported a statistically significant reduction in the percentage of reports with nongrammatical errors from 33% to 26%. Since 2009, the RSNA (Radiological Society of North America) radiology reporting initiative has been creating a library of best-practice report templates that are available for use [39–43]

BOX 7.13 Advantages of Structured Reporting

- Quality
  - Critical quality improvement: standardization
  - Checklist: complete, answers clinical question
  - Clear communication: minimizes ambiguity
  - Standardized terminology: comparable to priors
  - Easy to read visual cue: only long sentences are abnormal
  - Improved accuracy
  - Incorporates latest guidelines and terminology
  - Effective training tool for continuous learning
  - Easy to translate and adapt in different geographies
- Data quantification
  - Radiomics
  - Automatic functions (e.g., TNM staging)
  - Integration of lab tests
    - Computer-assisted clinical decision
      - Diagnosis
      - Selection of optimal treatment
      - Prediction of risks
      - Evaluation of treatment response
      - Autoassessment: eligibility for clinical trial
  - Data sharing
    - Data registries
    - Biobanks
    - Data mining
    - Training artificial intelligence algorithms

BOX 7.14 Disadvantages of Structured Reporting

- Logical progression of prose replaced by disconnected, bulleted, prepopulated data
- Dilution of radiologists' individuality/"signature brand"
- Radiologists' resistance to change
- Learning curve: delayed TAT/reduced productivity
- Template error:
  - e.g., failure to remove the pre-populated phrase "Gallbladder: Normal" from the report of a patient who has undergone a cholecystectomy.

Boxes 7.13 and 7.14 list the advantages and disadvantages of structured reporting.

What is Structured Reporting?

- Structured reporting is a report that is organized with subheadings that categorize and classify, drilling down into increasing levels of detail

  There are three progressively structured tiers in reporting templates:

Structured Reporting Tiers

Tier 1:

Paragraphs are written in prose with generic subheadings.

Clinical information
Examination protocol
Imaging findings
Conclusion

BOX 7.15 Breast Imaging Reporting and Data System Final Assessment Categories

Category		Recommended Management
0	Need additional imaging or previous studies	Recall for additional imaging and/or await previous studies
1	Negative	Routine screening
2	Benign	Routine screening
3	Probably Benign	Short interval follow-up (6 months)
4	Suspicious	Tissue diagnosis
5	Highly suggestive of malignancy	Tissue diagnosis
6	Known biopsy proved	Surgical excision when clinically appropriate

Tier 2:

Itemized, checklist style reporting with subheadings specifying organs and structures, listed in a logical, anatomical order.

Liver
Spleen
Gallbladder
Pancreas

Tier 3:

Standard lexicon used for both normal and abnormal findings; can be examination specific or disease specific.

For example, Breast Imaging Reporting and Data System (Box 7.15)

How to write a structured report:

Structured Reporting Templates (Tier 2) will have a checklist guide of anatomical structures to be reviewed in the "Findings" section (Box 7.16).

Tier 2 guidelines:

1. Findings

If the anatomical structure is normal, enter the single word "Normal."

If the anatomical structure is abnormal:

- Describe each abnormality with bulleted points
- Keep descriptions brief and precise
- Use phrases in lieu of complete/lengthy sentences
- Do not enter negative findings in this section
- Avoid self-evident words: "noted," "measuring," "seen," etc.
- Group multiple abnormal anatomical structures and list all related abnormalities under that single group
- Check for spelling and grammatical errors

BOX 7.16 Free-text versus Structured Report

Free-text prose report
Normal and abnormal paragraphs look alike

CT abdomen and pelvis with intravenous contrast:
Clinical indication: suspected Small bowel obstruction

- A surgical wound is noted in the lower abdominal wall that is linear and enhancing. The uterus is enlarged and extends superiorly into the false pelvis. The jejunum and proximal ileum are markedly dilated down to an abrupt transition point at the superior surface of the postpartum uterus. The ileum distal to this transition point is collapsed. There is mild lower peritoneal thickening. There is no free fluid
- The liver, spleen, pancreas, both kidneys, gall bladder are normal in density, morphology, and size. There is no biliary dilatation or hydronephrosis

Impression:
Small bowel dilatation, likely distal small bowel obstruction.Enlarged uterus and surgical wound—recommend clinical correlation.

Structured report
Only the long sentences are abnormal

CT abdomen and pelvis with intravenous contrast:
Liver: normal
Spleen: normal
Portal venous system: normal
IVC, hepatic veins: normal
Biliary system and gall bladder: normal
Pancreas: normal
Adrenals: normal
Kidneys: normal
Pelvicalyceal systems: normal
Ureters: normal
Bladder: normal
Bowel, uterus, abdominal wall:

- LSCS surgical wound in the lower abdomen—linear, enhancing
- postpartum uterus enlarged into the false pelvis
- jejunum and proximal ileum markedly dilated down to an abrupt transition point at the superior surface of the postpartum uterus
- ileum distal to the transition point is collapsed

Peritoneum, omentum, mesentery: mild lower peritoneal thickening; otherwise, normal
Nodes: nil significant
Fluid: nil significant
Ovaries: normal
Visualized bones and joints: normal
Visualized lungs:
Impression: 28-year-old lady, 7 days following LSCS, now with abdominal pain, distension, and vomiting; suspected SBO.
CT abdomen and pelvis with intravenous contrast shows:

1. Jejunum and proximal ileum markedly dilated down to an abrupt transition point at the superior surface of the postpartum uterus
2. Ileum distal to the transition point collapsed
3. No evidence of bowel wall thickening, mass or volvulus
4. No evidence of bowel ischemia

Findings suggestive of high grade mid ileal obstruction, likely related to postoperative adhesions.

2. Impression
   The "Impression" is an **inference** concluded from the findings, that ideally answers the clinical question and offers a differential diagnosis.
   The "Impression" is **not a repetition** of the findings.
   - start every "Impression" with a Prologue:
     - age-sex
     - symptoms and signs
     - provisional clinical diagnosis
     - previous surgeries/treatment
     - previous imaging with dates
   - document and number salient positive findings
   - offer a differential diagnosis in order of likelihood
   - for each differential diagnosis, bracket points that favor/don't favor the diagnosis
- document pertinent negative findings
- avoid the phrase "as above"
- provide comparison with previous imaging, wherever possible *for example, "compared to previous .... dated...... there is worsening/partial resolution/complete resolution of............"*
3. Recommendations:
   - recommend follow-up/additional diagnostic studies/lab tests/HPE
   - when appropriate, to clarify or confirm the impression
   - add the phrase "if clinically indicated" at the end
   - avoid the term "recommend clinical correlation" as a general disclaimer; specify which entity needs to be correlated and why
     e.g., "Recommend correlation of these findings with the clinical possibility of TB"
4. Footnotes
   Add the following footnotes:
   - contrast reactions
   - suboptimal image quality
   - verbal communication of critical reports
   - limitations of the study

Equipment Quality Control

- Radiology report quality is dependent on the quality of the image. It is imperative therefore that a radiology **QIP** extends to cover all diagnostic imaging **equipment,** imaging **protocols** (see **KPI 1**) and **technologists** (see **KPI 2**) that produce the image
- The Joint Commission International Survey Process Guide for Hospitals, 7th, Standard AOP.6.4 mandates that all equipment used to conduct radiology and diagnostic imaging studies is regularly inspected, maintained, and calibrated; and appropriate records are maintained for these activities [44]

Selecting and Acquiring Equipment

- Choosing the right medical imaging equipment is a critical decision, given the massive financial and infrastructure costs involved. A needs assessment should be done to understand current and future operations, workload and case complexity for matching with the vendor specification that best suits the budget. Tabulation of vendor specifications eases comparison and enables ranking for use by the procurement and purchase committees

Inspecting and Testing Equipment: Calibrating, Monitoring, and Maintaining Equipment

- After installation, biomedical engineering and vendor installation teams should sign-off the equipment as being fully functional and safe, meeting standards of medical imaging safety as well as electrical safety. All technologists should be oriented and trained on functionality and safety before the equipment is used on patients
- QC should be oriented with the equipment manual and trained on preventive maintenance (PM), routine checks and calibrations that test and standardize the machine. Subsequent daily checks should be performed using a checklist approved by the vendor and any faults or operating malfunctions should be escalated immediately to biomedical engineering and documented
- To obtain maximal performance from imaging machines, regular PM, in compliance with regulatory, safety, and operating standards as recommended by the manufacturer, is critical. PM prolongs machine life and assures high-quality images at low levels of radiation exposure. Regular PM is performed by the vendor on an annual maintenance contract, organized and supervised by biomedical engineering. Documentation of PM activities should be done
- Daily equipment checklists for calibration, safety, smooth functioning, and cleanliness should be approved by the vendor and completed by the technologist operating the machine
- A **Sample** Equipment **Safety and Function Checklist** is provided at the end of this chapter

Safety

- At installation, electrical safety and equipment-specific safety related to risks from radiation, high strength magnetic fields, quench or RF should be surveyed and signed-off before using medical imaging equipment on patients
- A comprehensive radiation survey should be conducted by an external provider for all radiation producing equipment at installation and on a regular basis in accordance with regulations. Radiology QC and biomedical engineering are together responsible for radiation surveys. All details regarding the installation, calibration, maintenance and repair, and safety surveys should be recorded until the use of the equipment
- The RSO (Radiation Safety Officer) is responsible for radiation safety compliance and must ensure that patients and staff are protected from unnecessary radiation. Technologists and radiologists should follow the principle of as low as reasonably achievable and be aware of the important risks and hazards of medical imaging to patients, their families and staff (Box 7.12). Violations of regulations for radioprotection must be immediately reported to the RSO
- The QIP monitors safety by allocating one KPI for adherence to safety

Template 1: Radiology Audit Report

1. Adequacy of clinical information.
2. Appropriateness (against ACR standards of appropriateness).
3. Image quality:
   - Spatial and contrast resolution
   - Protocol adherence
   - Positioning

- o Artifacts
- o FOV

4. Accuracy of interpretation:
   - o Agree/disagree
   - o Level of discrepancy
   - o ACR categories 1–3
5. Communication clarity:
   - o Template usage
   - o Clarity of findings
   - o Critical findings reported
6. Categorization of discrepancy: Kim–Mansfield classification.
   - o Under reading: finding missed
   - o Over reading: over called
   - o Location: finding outside area of clinical interest
   - o Satisfaction of search: first abnormality found; second abnormality missed
   - o Incomplete description: insufficiently characterized
   - o Not all images read: some images left unread
   - o Faulty interpretation: attributed to wrong cause
   - o Limited differential: all possible causes not considered
   - o Normal variant: normal anatomic variant is misinterpreted as abnormal
   - o Poor communication: communication error
   - o Typographic error
   - o Erroneous report: report belongs to a different patient
   - o Erroneous recommendation
   - o Erroneous technique
   - o Physician communication: missing documentation of critical finding communication
   - o Laterality error: right–left confusion
   - o Insufficient history
   - o Previous examination: failure to review previous imaging
   - o Overreliance on previous exam: overreliance on previous findings
   - o Artifact related
7. Learning points.
8. Screenshot image of the discrepancy, duly arrowed, and labeled.
9. References for training.

Note:

This Audit Report can be sent as confidential email feedback to the individual reporting radiologist, after adding patient and examination identifiers.

Template 2: Equipment Safety and Function Checklist

Clean and disinfect

- ▪ Contact surfaces after each use of the equipment/accessories
- ▪ Spills of body fluids/contrast media/saline solution
  - o Prevent cross contamination
  - oo Avoid damage to machine hardware/electricals/electronics
- ▪ Nonpatient contact surfaces
  - o User interface screen
  - o Control room equipment
- ▪ Cleaning agent: according to vendor instructions
  - o Use nonlint cloth
  - o Vendor supplied wipe
  - o Dry cleaning for electronic components
- ▪ Ensure visible cleanliness before disinfection

X-ray equipment

- ▪ Daily check
  - o x-ray tube cables: in place
  - o x-ray tube: dust free
  - o x-ray tube rails: friction free
  - o collimator knobs/switches: friction free
- ▪ Daily warm-up exposures
  - o Before use
  - o Unit idle >2 hours
  - o Warm-up procedure
    - • Turn system on
    - • Close room door and clear room of occupants
    - • Large focal spot
    - • 70 kVp, 2 seconds, 100 mA
    - • Three exposures
    - • Wait 10 seconds between each exposure

If any unusual noise or event is observed, immediately escalate to biomedical engineer or vendor service engineer.

Ultrasound and Doppler

- ▪ Daily check and maintenance tasks
  - o Cords and wires: in place
  - o Device turned on: no warning lights or alerts
  - o Transducer check: cracks or wear points
  - o Transducer cables: wear and tear
  - o Cleaning and sterilization techniques: manufacturer recommendations
  - o NO abrasive paper products
  - o Probes: safely stored at the end of day
  - o System backup:
    - • Performed regularly
    - • Reduce recovery time in event of system failure

CT

- o Daily check and maintenance tasks
- o Deep cleaning
- o Gantry: smooth movement
- o Operating console: fully functional
- o Pressure injector: cleaned, fully functional
- o Air conditioning level: optimal, manufacturer-recommended level
- o Phantom calibration
  - • Uniform water phantom
  - • Large ROI
    - ◻ Mean CT number of water and standard deviation
    - ◻ Within established baseline and acceptable limits of variation
    - ◻ CT number for water: 0 ± 4HU
  - • Procedure
    - ◻ Manufacturer guidelines
    - ◻ Or following:
      - ▸ Attach cylindrical phantom to head holder
      - ▸ Position so that phantom water center at isocenter
  - • Axial (sequential) scans length of water phantom
  - • 5-mm reconstructed slices
  - • Brain CT acquisition parameters
  - • View central reconstructed slice
  - • Scanner analysis software
    - ◻ Draw circular ROI center of the image
      - ▸ Diameter 40% image width
  - • Water calibration: CT number of water 0 ± 4 HU
  - • Noise 10% or 0.2 HU from the baseline tests at acceptance
  - • Record acquisition parameters for repeatability
  - • Air calibration: CT number for air – 1000 ± 10 HU
- o Daily warm-up exposures
  - • Manufacturer guidelines

MRI

- ▪ Daily check and maintenance tasks

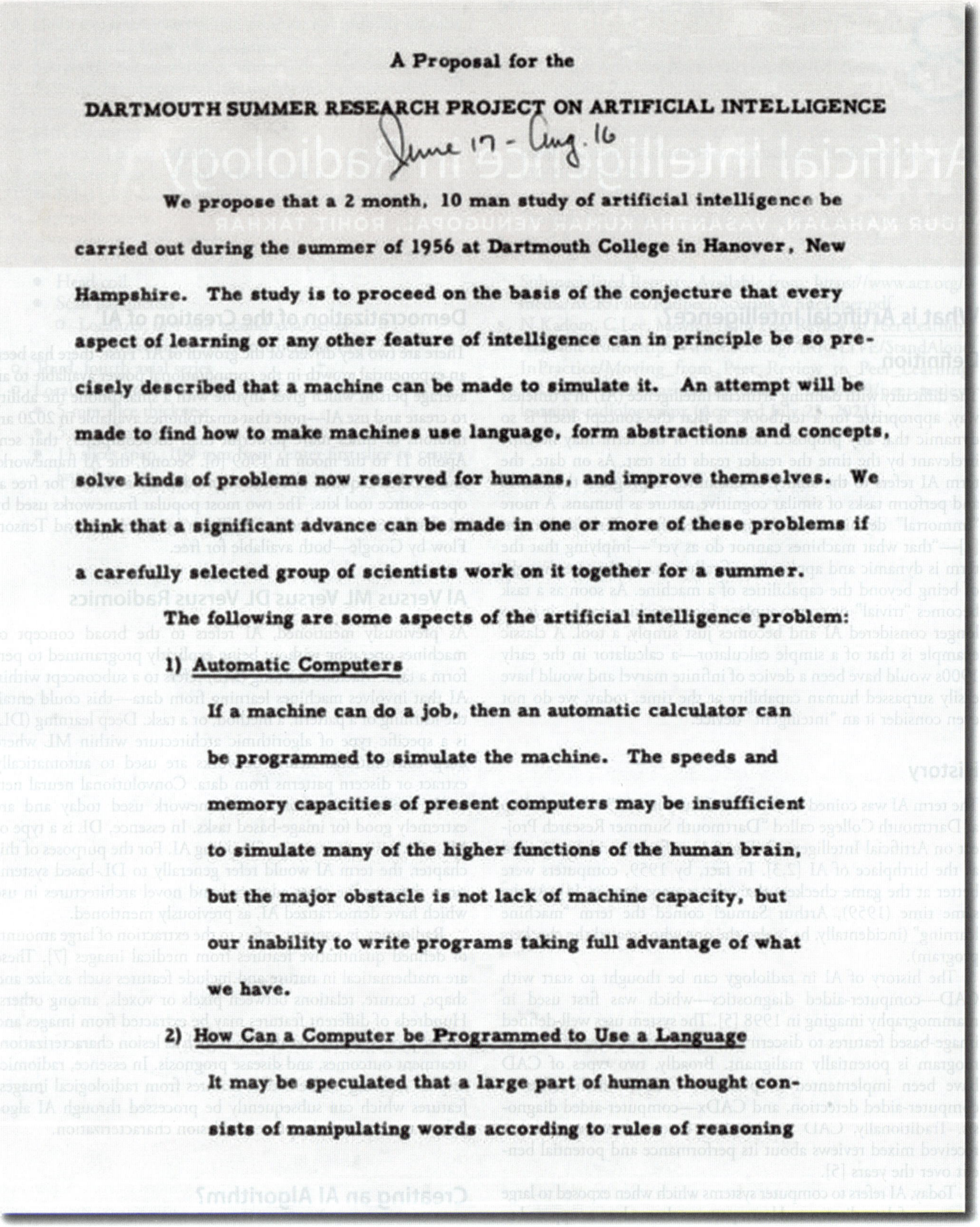

A Proposal for the

DARTMOUTH SUMMER RESEARCH PROJECT ON ARTIFICIAL INTELLIGENCE

June 17 - Aug. 16

We propose that a 2 month, 10 man study of artificial intelligence be carried out during the summer of 1956 at Dartmouth College in Hanover, New Hampshire. The study is to proceed on the basis of the conjecture that every aspect of learning or any other feature of intelligence can in principle be so precisely described that a machine can be made to simulate it. An attempt will be made to find how to make machines use language, form abstractions and concepts, solve kinds of problems now reserved for humans, and improve themselves. We think that a significant advance can be made in one or more of these problems if a carefully selected group of scientists work on it together for a summer.

The following are some aspects of the artificial intelligence problem:

1) Automatic Computers

If a machine can do a job, then an automatic calculator can be programmed to simulate the machine. The speeds and memory capacities of present computers may be insufficient to simulate many of the higher functions of the human brain, but the major obstacle is not lack of machine capacity, but our inability to write programs taking full advantage of what we have.

2) How Can a Computer be Programmed to Use a Language

It may be speculated that a large part of human thought consists of manipulating words according to rules of reasoning

Figure 8.1 The proposal for the Dartmouth Summer Research Project on artificial intelligence. (Source: J McCarthy, ML Minsky, N Rochester, CE Shannon, A proposal for the dartmouth summer research project on artificial intelligence, August 31, 1955, AI Magazine 27 (4) (2006) 12.)

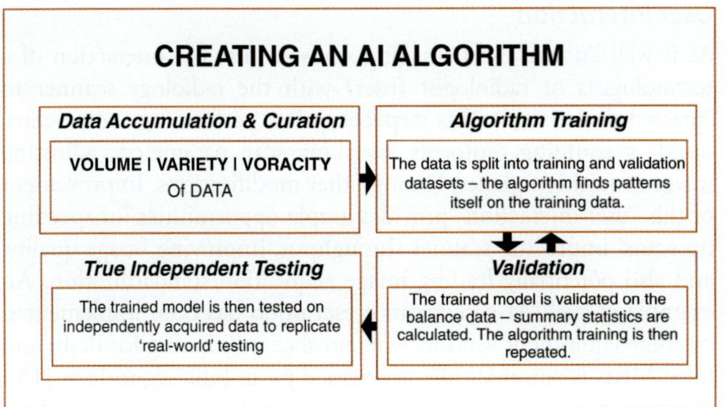

Figure 8.2 Overview of the process of creating an AI algorithm.

determine relevant patters itself. This mechanism of "creating" an AI algorithm is best described using an example—for instance, finding pneumothorax on a plain chest radiograph.

Step 1—Data Accumulation and Curation

The journey of creating an AI algorithm to automatically detect pneumothorax on a plain chest radiograph starts with data, that is, thousands of chest x-rays with and without pneumothorax need to be collected. The typical data requirement for building an AI algorithm is described by three variables—volume, variety, and veracity. Volume refers to creating an AI algorithm typically requires several thousands, if not millions, of medical imaging datasets, to reach high levels of accuracy. Variety implies that the data used to create the AI algorithm should cover as many potential presentations of the finding under study. This can include variations in shapes, sizes, number, and locations of the pneumothoraces themselves, or the presence of associated findings such as tubes/wires, effusions, and edema. Lastly, veracity refers to the confidence level of the annotation associated with the image, that is, what is the confidence level of pneumothorax being truly present in the chest radiograph. Is one simply relying on the x-ray report, or is each scan being reviewed by one (or multiple) radiologists, are the radiologists reviewing the scans thoracic subspecialists, or are they general radiologists? Are they also localizing each lesion? This is also called the "ground truth" label of the data and can vary depending on the "basis" on which one determines whether a finding is truly present in a radiograph or not. This delicate interplay between volume, variety, and veracity plays a critical part in the accuracy, and thereby success of an AI algorithm.

Step 2—Algorithm Training

Once sufficient data have been gathered and curated, it is time to "train" an AI algorithm on these data. First, the entire data are randomly divided into three separate datasets—train, test, and validate—typically in a proportion of 60%, 20%, and 20%, respectively. Subsequently, there are a series of complex mathematical models that will run through each pixel in each image in the training set and try to discern features that distinguish a plain radiograph with pneumothorax from one without pneumothorax. This is an iterative process wherein the algorithm develops a "hypothesis" around what these features are after each round of processing the training images. Then this hypothesis is tested on the test dataset—the performance feedback is then sent back into the training model wherein the mathematical models are automatically tweaked, and a new hypothesis is developed which is then again tested on the test data. This process is repeated till the model attains an acceptable level of performance (typically above 80% accuracy, but can vary depending on the clinical context) on identifying images with pneumothorax.

Step 3—Validation

Note that the current model is optimized for the test dataset since the training algorithm modulates itself for optimum performance on these data. It is therefore important to now test on the "validation" dataset, which is data that the algorithm has not "seen" before. The performance of the AI at this validation phase determines the further course of action—go back to the drawing board and try a different algorithmic approach with different data, or proceed further to true independent testing.

Step 4—True Independent Testing

Note that throughout steps 1, 2, and 3, all the data that the algorithm was exposed to, both for training and testing, were from the same initial pool of data. Hence, since the algorithm is optimized (or *tuned*) based on these data, it is bound to perform well when tested on these data. In a clinical environment, what matters is real-world performance of the AI. Hence, the last and final step in the development of any AI algorithm is testing the AI's ability to identify cases with pneumothorax at hospitals which are completely different from the ones where the initial data were obtained from. This can mean hospitals which have different equipment, different patient populations, or are in different geographies altogether—the goal is to see whether the AI performs to the expected level in an environment which is completely different from the one it was exposed to. Generally, it is seen that AI performance drops in such instances (*this is referred to as lack of generalizability of an algorithm—refer to section on generalizability*) and appropriate tweaks need to be made to the algorithm itself. Note that such drops in performance are seen more often in modalities where image acquisition parameters are more institution or operator driven such as MRI and ultrasound.

Broad Use Cases of AI

Any discussion on AI is incomplete without discussion around the "need" for AI in the first place. From a clinical perspective, AI can help improve accuracy and efficiency of radiologists, which from an economic perspective implies lower cost and/or greater accessibility of radiological services. Like the definition of AI, use cases of AI are also constantly evolving and hence need to be put into a broad framework that can survive the test of time, as the definition of AI changes. Hence, the following broad categorization is proposed.

That What Humans Can Do

These applications include tasks which radiologists have the ability to perform but can be automated by AI. This includes relatively simple tasks such autoreporting chest radiographs, discerning normal versus abnormal brain MRIs, measuring spinal canal diameters on spine MR studies, finding pulmonary nodules on chest CT scans, among others. Essentially any task that is currently done by a radiologist. The inherent advantages of automating such tasks are that simpler subtasks can be automated, speeding up the diagnostic process, and enabling radiologists to focus on more complex tasks. Classical example is that of automated reporting of normal chest x-rays [8] in out-patient settings, where ~75% scans may be normal [9], allowing radiologists to focus on the more complex task of reporting the abnormal chest x-rays, improving their accuracy and efficiency.

That What Humans Cannot Do

Tasks such as converting an MRI scan acquired using 10% contrast into a full contrast MRI image [10], determining the molecular subtype of breast malignancy using MRI [11], or even trying to derive functional information (PET) from a CT scan are tasks that human beings cannot do themselves simply because we lack the cognitive ability to process data at such levels. Radiomics, particularly texture analysis, enables a radiologist to "see" what the human eye cannot normally see. For example, Chee et al., demonstrated that it is indeed possible to predict chemotherapy response and prognosis using texture analysis of locally advanced rectal cancer on CT [12]. Such use cases, although unquestionably impactful, need to be validated stringently since it is not possible for a radiologist to simply check whether the AI is right or wrong since additional data points may be needed. A classic example of such an algorithm, as mentioned earlier, is of an AI algorithm that can produce contrast-enhanced MR images of the brain using images that contain contrast diluted to 10%.

AI in the Radiology Workflow

After taking a "task"-based view of AI to better grasp the impact and use cases associated with AI, it would be useful to take a more detailed "workflow" oriented view. Broadly, the radiology workflow can be broken into four distinct phases—prescanning, scanning (or image acquisition), postprocessing, and finally, diagnosis. AI algorithms can be placed into these four distinct phases—following are some illustrative examples.

Prescanning

Possibly the lowest hanging fruit to be impacted by AI, but the least talked about, is the prescanning phase of the radiology workflow. Curtis et al. used ML to predict patient waiting time and appointment delays before patients arrived, making the radiology workflow much more efficient [13]. In parts of the world where most population is insured, patient "no-shows" are a significant problem—Nelson et al. demonstrated that it is possible to determine whether patients will attend their scheduled hospital visits using ML techniques applied to patient demographics within the United Kingdom [14]. In essence, "prescanning" algorithms can offer direct economic benefit for radiology departments by improving operational efficiencies in a relative "low clinical impact" setting where the implications of errors made by AI may not be very grave.

Image Acquisition

Image acquisition is the phase of the radiology workflow where radiological scans are performed in patients and images are generated or acquired. From an AI perspective, this phase can be thought to comprise of two distinct components—user interaction with equipment and generation of images.

User Interaction

As is well known, most imaging scans require the interaction of a technologists or radiologist (user) with the radiology scanner to "prescribe" the scan. This step comprises performing scout scans, deciding scanning protocols, tweaking scan parameters, adjusting image acquisition planes, among other modifications. Improvement of this "user interaction" provides ample opportunities for speeding up scans, improving scanner throughput, improving image quality, and also potentially leading image acquisition standardization. An example of such AI-based scan prescription has been implemented by some equipment vendors wherein slice positioning for brain and knee MRIs is automatically performed by in-built algorithms [15]. Another example is by some ultrasound vendors wherein algorithms allow the automated selection of appropriate ultrasound slices for measurement of cranial diameter in fetal ultrasound [16]. The possibilities of such interventions that make radiologists and technologists faster and better are truly endless.

Image Generation

Mahajan et al. showed in early 2019 that it is possible to create diffusion-weighted MR images from T2-weighted images of the brain while maintaining the ability of diffusion-weighted images to differentiate acute from chronic infarcts using a technique called image-to-image translation [17]. Mardani et al. have used generative adversarial networks [18] to reconstruct high-resolution MR images from undersampled raw MR data potentially speeding up MR acquisition by several folds [19]. CT vendors have implemented DL-based iterative reconstruction for denoising of low-dose CT scan images by applying these AI techniques to raw sinogram data on their scanners [20]. All such applications of AI target the real "image generation" that is at the core of any radiology scanner—this is the intersection of physics, chemistry, and mathematical modeling and is possibly the most exciting, as yet underplayed, domain of AI in radiology (Fig. 8.3).

Postprocessing

Measurements, segmentation, anatomy tracing, or any other "non-diagnostic" task performed after image acquisition but before making a clinical diagnosis falls into the domain of image postprocessing. Detection and localization of findings can also fall into this phase of the workflow. Automated detection and segmentation of glioblastoma is one such example which has been pursued by many groups—the brain tumor segmentation challenge is an annual global challenge aiming to solve this [21]. Other applications include automated detection and segmentation of lung nodules, liver tumors, liver donor evaluation, coronary artery disease, pneumothorax, limb length, among many others. This is a vast area of application only limited by one's imagination.

Diagnosis

All these phases eventually converge into the "diagnosis"—the most cognitively demanding part of the radiology workflow. A radiologist uses images, detects, localizes, and characterizes lesions, puts them into clinical context and eventually provides a final diagnosis in the form of a clinicoradiological diagnosis. In 2017, Rajpurkar et al. published a paper demonstrating AI's capability to diagnose pneumonia on chest x-rays with comparable performance to radiologists [22]. In 2018, Chilamkurthy et al. published a paper on AI automatically detecting intracranial bleeds and other critical findings on the head CT scans [23]. Subsequently, tremendous strides have been made in using AI to diagnose

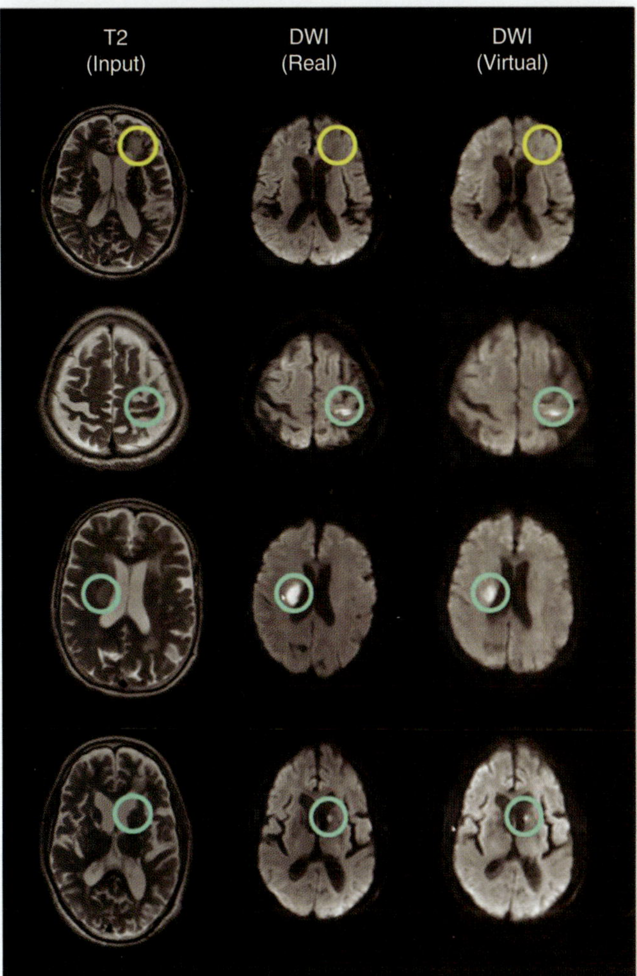

Figure 8.3 Example images of virtually generated diffusion-weighted imaging (DWI) images. Input images are T2-weighted axial MR scans.

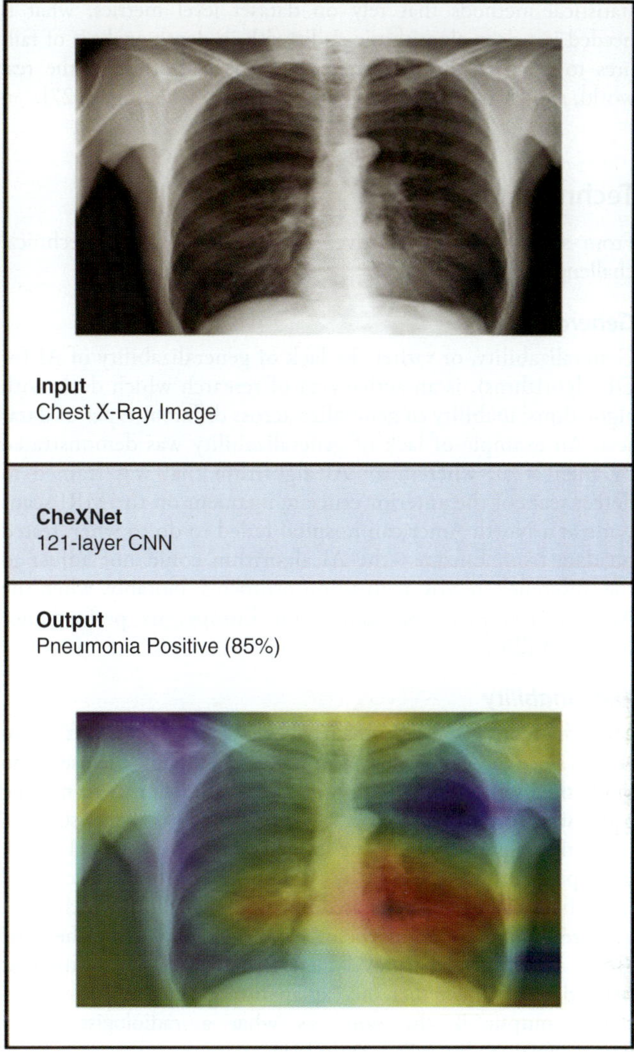

Figure 8.4 Example output from Rajpurkar et al.'s paper on radiologist level pneumonia detection on chest x-rays. The output image shows a heat map with red areas representing parts of the image, which drove the AI model toward the diagnosis of pneumonia.

tuberculosis on chest x-rays using sputum nucleic acid analysis as ground truth, as was published by Qin et al. in a comparative analysis of five different commercially available tuberculosis detection AI algorithms [24]. Such algorithms make use of AI's capability to automatically discern features after going through a high number of examples—hence, the ability to identify patients with tuberculosis simply using chest x-rays, which a radiologist may not be able to do. Additionally, AI models have been touted to be able to predict the onset of pathology before they become apparent visually, especially in the domains of breast cancer [25] and Alzheimer's disease [26]. Heat maps (Fig. 8.4) are commonly used to visualize features of medical images that the AI model has used to drive its decision of whether a particular finding/pathology is present or not in that medical image.

As on date, most diagnostic AI systems are being deployed for triaging of critical findings, screening of normals versus abnormals, or in low-resource screening settings. Triaging refers to the ability of AI algorithms to guide radiologists around which cases to read first—in a worklist of several scans, the AI can flag those which have a critical finding and hence should be read earlier by a radiologist. This happens by an integration between the AI algorithm, the radiology PACS system, and the hospital's internal IT system.

The possibilities in the future are endless, but they start becoming more difficult with increasing skill or cognitive requirement of each task.

Challenges and Limitations

Although there are thousands of research papers and hundreds of companies working on AI for radiology, the truth is that it has received limited traction in the clinical domain at the time of this chapter going to print. This is due to certain fundamental challenges with the way AI is being developed, tested, and implemented.

A brief description of these challenges is as follows.

Clinical Challenge—Implications

It is extremely important for a user or developer of AI to realize that the clinical action that is taken on the basis of an AI generated output or suggestion carries implications. These implications can be profoundly positive, as in the case of automatically diagnosing tuberculosis in a geographic area deprived of conventional testing, and as grave as wrongly predicting the onset of Alzheimer's disease in a patient who otherwise remains "normal." The general framework for AI validation and testing today relies almost entirely on statistical methods that rely on dataset level metrics, what is needed is a deep algorithmic audit with in-depth analysis of failures to evaluate the performance of the algorithm in the real world, similar to how one might "interview" a colleague [27].

Technical Challenges

From a clinicians' perspective, there are two specific technical challenges with AI today.

Generalizability

Generalizability, or rather the lack of generalizability of AI (or DL algorithms), is an active area of research which deals with algorithms' inability to generalize across different types of datasets. An example of lack of generalizability was demonstrated by Bien et al. wherein an AI algorithm that was trained to detect tears of the anterior cruciate ligament on the MRI scans done at a North American hospital failed to do so when tested on data from Europe—the AI algorithm could not adjust to the difference in MR acquisition protocols. Notably, when the AI was "retrained" on data from Europe, its performance increased [28].

Explainability

Over the years, AI algorithms have been called "black-box" algorithms since most times they are unable to "explain" themselves to guide the user (radiologist) toward the "reason" for them making a decision [29]. This is especially important for diagnostic and predictive algorithms, as mentioned earlier. Venugopal et al. attempted to "unbox AI" by attempting to find radiological insights from outputs generated by an AI algorithm which characterizes lung nodules into benign and malignant [30]. The same group also proposed a novel metric to test AI algorithms that helps determine whether the explanation given by AI for a particular output is the same as what a radiologist would give—explainability failure ratio [31].

Both generalizability and explainability are intricately linked and become extremely important in the clinical domain. They are both active areas of research and AI products that successfully incorporate both shall gain clinical traction faster than others.

Ethical and Legal Challenges

The development of AI algorithms depends heavily on access to massive amounts of data to train these algorithms. This dependency on medical data often leads to debate around access and ownership rights to medical data generated during routine process of patient care. Guidelines on use of these data vary from country to country (and within countries, state to state)—it is clear that until there are explicit legal and ethical guidelines around the use of such data, it will be very difficult for AI scientists and companies to develop products across a wide variety of applications. The other legal challenge remains that of liability—as on date, no guidelines exist for the use of unsupervised AI in clinical practice, and hence, in most instances medicolegal responsibility for the actions of AI invariably come onto the user—the radiologist. These are currently unsolved questions and hopefully the global medical technology community will come together and develop a sustainable path forward.

Suggested Readings

- P Lambin, E Rios-Velazquez, R Leijenaar, S Carvalho, RGPM van Stiphout, P Granton, et al., Radiomics: Extracting more information from medical images using advanced feature analysis, Eur J Cancer 48 (4) (2012 Mar) 441–446.
- VK Venugopal, V Mahajan, H Mahajan, Automated classification of chest x-rays as normal/abnormal using a high sensitivity deep learning algorithm. Oral Presentation at the European Congress of Radiology, Vienna, 2019.
- R Ha, S Mutasa, J Karcich, N Gupta, E Pascual Van Sant, J Nemer, et al., Predicting breast cancer molecular subtype with MRI dataset utilizing convolutional neural network algorithm, J Digit Imaging 32 (2) (2019 Apr) 276–282.
- C Curtis, C Liu, TJ Bollerman, OS Pianykh, Machine learning for predicting patient wait times and appointment delays, J Am Coll Radiol 15 (9) (2018 Sep) 1310–1316.
- Brain Tumor Segmentation (BraTS) Challenge 2020 [Internet]. Available from: http://braintumorsegmentation.org/.
- A Yala, C Lehman, T Schuster, T Portnoi, R Barzilay, A deep learning mammography-based model for improved breast cancer risk prediction, Radiology 292 (1) (2019 Jul) 60–66.

9

Introduction to Methods in Research

SUNAINA YADAV

"Today's research is tomorrows practice" [1].

Introduction

With the advent of technology and ever-changing demographics radiology is witnessing a dramatic transition from a *diagnostic science to a functional one*, capable of revealing far more than just static images of the body. Imaging data combined with deep phenotyping and functional observations hold immense potential to contribute toward improved healthcare outcomes. This is evident with applications in artificial intelligence, functional MRI studies, radiomics, imaging biomarkers, and image-guided biopsies.

The dynamic radiological landscape makes a compelling case for a change in how budding radiologists are trained for clinical practice and research careers. Clinical radiologists have a noticeable absence of knowledge regarding statistics and research methodologies crucial for pursuing an experimental practice. The focus is primarily on the tail end of the research process, that is, data interpretation and publications; however, there is little support and training provided to clinicians for planning and establishment of a research-focused practice.

Research enhances radiologists' knowledge base, resulting in active participation in impactful discourses with peers or on public platforms, a crucial aspect of clinical practice today. To achieve this, they need to be armed with an understanding of the various avenues of research.

Avenues in Radiology Research

Radiology researchers have an array of specialties to choose from. Sardanelli [2] identified 11 such areas of interest (Table 9.1). Of the proposed avenues, the explorative study of human diseases is the most popular and convenient for clinicians as they have easy access to patient data. Therefore, this chapter focuses primarily on some general considerations on this topic; however, these are not entirely exclusive and have cross-area applications.

Creating a Research Framework

Selecting an Area of Research

Doria [3] proposes the *PICO method* to formulate a feasible, novel, and relevant research question to investigate.

Patients—Who is the question about? **(Study population)**
Intervention—What interventions are of interest? **(Study variables)**
Control or comparison—What is the intervention being compared to? **(Study design)**
Outcome—What is the desired outcome? **(Final measure)**

This approach ensures that the clinicians choose a research area that is relevant and has a narrow scope to make the project achievable. A well-thought-out research area also increases the chance of attracting funding.

Choosing the Correct Study Design

Evidence-based medicine promotes a high level of evidentiary support through the amalgamation of information from literature and clinical practice to prove the efficacy of a treatment or

TABLE 9.1 Research Avenues in Radiology [2]

Areas of Interest	Implementations
Biomathematics and computer modeling	Decision support systems Reproducible simulations Predictive disease models
Contrast materials, tracers, and theranostics	Novel drugs and delivery pathways Improved patient safety Personalized medicine (dose tailoring)
Experimental models of human disease	Early detection of disease Diagnosis and staging of disease
Information technology, big data, image reconstruction, and postprocessing	Artificial intelligence Disease surveillance and trends Improved patient engagement (phone, tablets)
Imaging biomarkers, radiomics, radiogenomics, and imaging biobanks	Personalized and precision medicine Tailored therapy Re-defining new "normal" for diseases
Interventional radiology	Image-guided therapy Device and method innovation
Metabolic and functional imaging	Personalized and precision medicine Risk stratification
Methodology and statistics	Standardized descriptions and structured reports
Molecular and hybrid imaging	Personalized and precision medicine
Novel imaging methods/ techniques	Diagnostic test design (accuracy and impact) Improved performance
Radiobiology, radioprotection, and physics in radiology	Improved diagnostic performance

TABLE 9.3 Difference Between Type 1 and Type 2 Errors

Null hypothesis is…	True	False
Rejected	Type 1 error False positive	Correct conclusion True positive
Not rejected	Correct conclusion True negative	Type 2 error False negative

deeply phenotyped and imaged patient data until they reach a critical mass where the sample size has enough statistical power. A clean and richly populated dataset can fuel numerous studies and publications and is well worth the effort. A clinician with a good dataset also stands in high regard and is likely to be invited to collaborate on international projects of repute and impact.

Choice of Statistical Tests

Within a project, the statistical analysis strategy is dynamic and forever evolving. The choice of tests depends on the dataset, data quality, desired outcome measures, and software used. A detailed discussion on statistics is beyond the scope of this chapter; however, readers are directed toward *Research Methods in Radiology* by Doria [3] for a more detailed review on the use of statistics in radiology research.

Measuring Impact

Making an Impact

Research studies involve long-term planning. The outcome that most clinicians look for is a well-received publication that enhances their career goals and adds credibility to their work. Due diligence by clinician–scientists in evaluating scholarly journals for publishing their work ensures that they receive the correct readership and accolades on the excellent work done. Clinicians should not rush to publish their work in a journal of low standing, as this could severely impact the credibility and uptake of their research.

With over 80,000 peer-reviewed journals to choose from [20], it helps to know some key indicators to judge the quality of a journal. The starting point for selecting a journal could be the very journals a clinician or their colleagues frequently read and cite in their research. References within frequently read studies could also be explored. The *Google Scholar H5 index* can be referred to by researchers for identifying high-ranking journals in radiology. The recent growth in blockchain technology and cryptocurrency has also opened up new ways of publishing scientific data.

Measuring Impact

Although there are many quantitative measures of research output, three primary metrics that stand out are the impact factor (IF), H-index [21], and Altmetrics [22]. These quantitative measures become increasingly important in evaluating new hires and granting funds in a sphere of limited resources.

Impact Factor

Impact factor (IF) scores are calculated for indexed journals using the number of citations within a defined time. The IF is a well-received metric for differentiating high-quality journals from others, and researchers are routinely ranked on the cumulative impact factors garnered from their publications. However, the impact factor only measures the impact of a journal in its entirety and not the impact of individual articles or scientists.

H-Index

HI measures the productivity and impact of an individual scientist and is based on a researcher's most cited papers and the number of citations in other papers [21]. A scientist can create a profile on numerous databases such as Web of Science (WOS), Scopus, and Google Scholar to calculate their H-index.

Altmetrics

Once thought to be of no scientific purpose, social media has become an inevitable part of science. Altmetrics, also known as *article-level metrics*, analyzes scholarly impact based on various resources, including social media, mainstream media, reference managers, etc. [22]. Altmetrics does not aim to replace the traditional measures of impact such as IF and HI but complements them by re-examining the definition of impact beyond the citations.

Conclusion

Clinicians require upskilling for a more evidence-based approach to their clinical practice, including postgraduate level training in the scientific process, medical statistics, scientific writing (grants, protocols, articles), and data analysis. However, clinical research is not an individual effort and requires institutional and policy-level support. Therefore, adequate funding and proper infrastructure are vital for high-quality research coordination, data management & storage, and analysis.

The ultimate goal of clinical research is to improve patient outcomes by understanding the various parameters that govern the development, diagnosis, treatment, and prognosis of the disease.

Radiology stands at the forefront of this effort but is yet to evolve into a core research area, findings of which would underline future clinical guidelines or practice. Thus, radiology research needs to be placed in context with evolving trends, new methodologies and changing guidelines to help shape its future and drive adoption by clinicians.

Suggested Reading

• AS Doria, Research Methods in Radiology, a Practical Guide, Thieme, 2018.

10

Approach to Oncoimaging

AKSHAY BAHETI, SOMESH SINGH, AMRIN ISRARAHMED

Introduction

Cancer imaging is a rapidly evolving subspecialty of radiology. Imaging plays a central role in screening, detecting, staging, prognosticating, planning treatment, in post-treatment evaluation, and surveillance in cancer. Tremendous strides have been taken in the past few decades in understanding tumor biology, prognostication, and potential treatment mechanisms. Modern oncoimaging requires the radiologist to know basic pathophysiology and biologic behavior of various cancers (including its molecular basis), in addition to knowing about its imaging appearances. It is also essential for the radiologist to know the basic terminologies related to cancer care to contribute more meaningfully to direct patient care, especially with the now-established role of multidisciplinary teams in optimizing patient management. This chapter will highlight the basic terminologies in oncology for the reader, discuss the various roles of imaging in oncological care, focusing on response assessment criteria, and briefly discuss recent advances. Relevant radiological features and role in particular tumors have been covered in individual chapters.

Basics of Oncology

Terminologies Used in Oncology

Screening: Screening is attempting to detect cancer at an early stage where it may be asymptomatic. It also includes detection of precancerous lesions. Early detection of precancerous or cancerous lesions has the potential to save lives. The World Health Organization (WHO) has proposed 10 principles in determining the usefulness of a screening test [1]. Based on these principles, American Cancer Society has identified usefulness of imaging in screening of breast (with mammography), lung (with low-dose CT), and colon (with CT colonography) cancers.

Staging: In simple terms, staging refers to mapping of the disease to determine extent of spread [2]. Staging is immensely helpful in communicating across the various members of cancer managing team as well as to patients and their relatives, prognosticating the patient, and ensuring uniformity in management. Restaging, as its name suggests, is assessing the disease burden after treatment to evaluate response.

Different classifications are used for staging tumors include: (i) TNM staging for majority neoplasms, (ii) WHO classification for brain tumors, (iii) International Federation of Gynecologists and Obstetricians (FIGO) staging system for cancers of the female reproductive organs, (iv) Lugano classification for lymphomas, (v) French–American–British (FAB) classification for acute myeloid leukemia (AML), etc. These have been discussed in detail in the relevant chapters.

The most widely employed staging system is based on tumor (T), node (N), and metastasis (M) status of cancer: the TNM staging, espoused by AJCC–UICC (AJCC, American Joint Committee on Cancer; UICC, Union for International Cancer Control). There are periodic updates to this staging with the recent edition (8th edition) introduced in 2018 [3]. Its premise is simple—assess the tumor (T) in terms of locoregional extension, involvement of adjacent structures, involvement of vital structures, etc.; assess the involvement of locoregional and distant nodes (N), and assess for the presence or absence of metastases (M). In the case of gliomas, TNM staging cannot be applied as these show exceedingly rare nodal or metastatic spread. Instead, they are graded on histopathology: based on degree of atypia and differentiation. The grade ranges from I to IV and WHO's grading system is widely used for grading of gliomas [4]. Similarly, alternative classifications may be used for a few other malignancies as previously mentioned.

Prognosis: Prognosis is the probability of developing a particular outcome in a disease. The most important outcome is usually death versus survival when dealing with malignancies, although other outcomes like a good functional outcome are also important. Good prognosis disease means that most patients with that presentation would do well. Prognosis of each patient is multifactorial and depends on various aspects including tumor-based factors such as stage and histopathology, patient factors such as nutritional status, presence or absence of comorbidities, genetic factors, treatment availability, etc. Prognosticating the disease on case to case basis plays a very important role in deciding appropriate cancer management personalized to the individual patient. This is termed personalized medicine or personalized/precision oncology.

Neoadjuvant versus adjuvant therapy: Neoadjuvant therapy refers to any cancer-directed treatment given before the primary treatment (usually surgery), to reduce the tumor bulk or to "downstage" the tumor before surgery. This is usually in the form of chemotherapy or radiation or both. Examples of cancers where neoadjuvant treatment is commonly employed include rectal cancer, borderline resectable pancreatic cancer, ovarian cancer, and advanced breast cancer. Adjuvant therapy, in contrast, is cancer-directed treatment given after primary treatment (usually surgery) [5]. The aim of adjuvant therapy is tackle microscopic residual disease at postoperative bed as well distant micrometastases, if present. Adjuvant therapy also includes chemotherapy, radiotherapy, and hormonal therapy, often in combination.

Systemic therapy: Systemic therapy refers to treatments that target the entire body and are systemically distributed throughout the blood circulation [6]. It includes various techniques of treatment like chemotherapy, hormonal therapy, and targeted therapy or immunotherapy.

a. *Conventional chemotherapy*: This attacks cancerous (and other) cells with high mitotic rate. As it is not specific for tumor cells, there is significant treatment toxicity which can occur.
b. *Hormonal therapy*: Hormonal therapy is an effective and relatively nontoxic therapy for certain cancers, both for the treatment and for the prevention of recurrence [7]. Examples

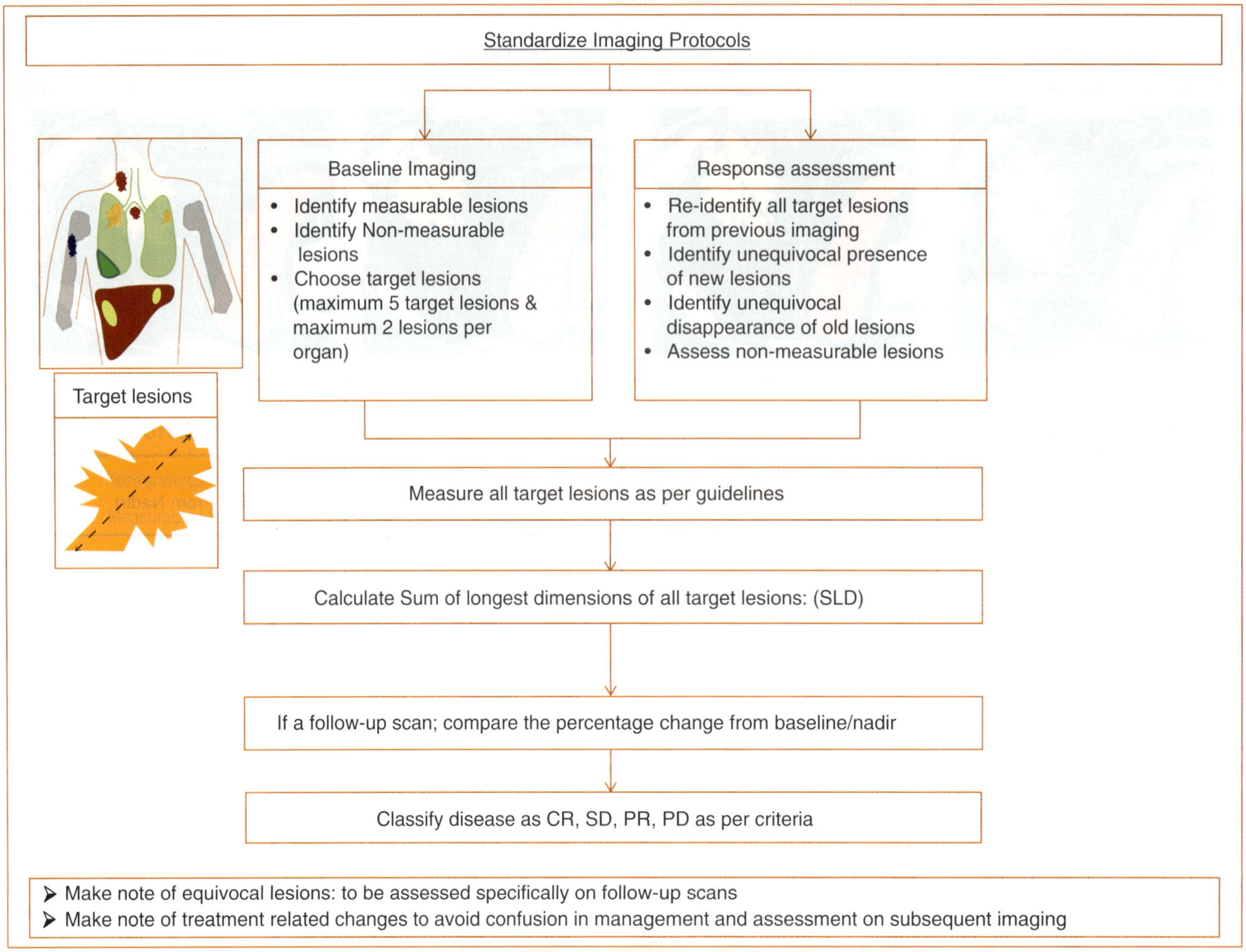

Standardize Imaging Protocols

Baseline Imaging
- Identify measurable lesions
- Identify Non-measurable lesions
- Choose target lesions (maximum 5 target lesions & maximum 2 lesions per organ)

Response assessment
- Re-identify all target lesions from previous imaging
- Identify unequivocal presence of new lesions
- Identify unequivocal disappearance of old lesions
- Assess non-measurable lesions

Target lesions

Measure all target lesions as per guidelines

Calculate Sum of longest dimensions of all target lesions: (SLD)

If a follow-up scan; compare the percentage change from baseline/nadir

Classify disease as CR, SD, PR, PD as per criteria

- Make note of equivocal lesions: to be assessed specifically on follow-up scans
- Make note of treatment related changes to avoid confusion in management and assessment on subsequent imaging

Figure 10.3 General workflow of evaluation by RECIST 1.1.

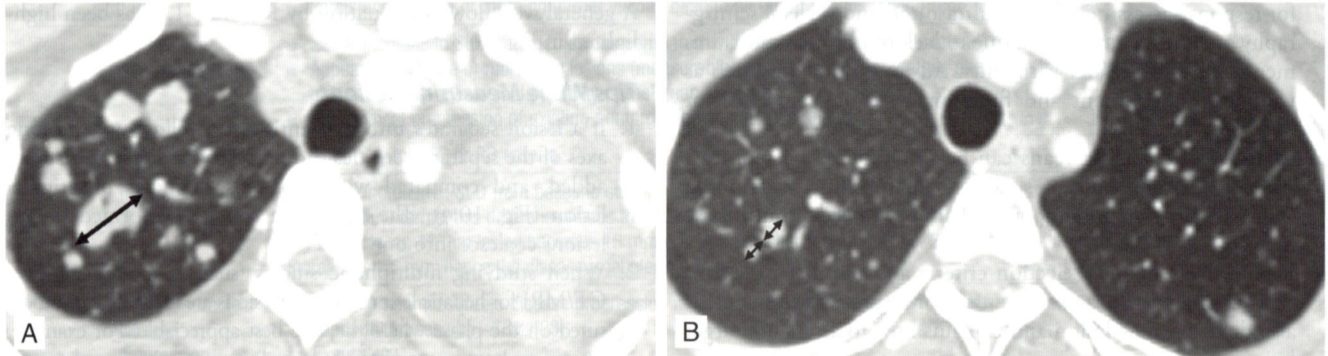

Figure 10.4 Patient of lung cancer. The baseline (A) scan shows an ill-defined left upper lobe nonmeasurable mass with effusion, and multiple right upper lobe metastatic nodules, the largest of which can be measured as a target lesion. Postchemotherapy scan (B) demonstrates substantial shrinkage of all nodules and resolution of the left effusion. The previously measured nodule has now separated into two nodules; these should be measured as shown with the individual measurements added and compared.

2. Lung nodules may respond to treatment with cavitation (Fig. 10.5); this makes measurement difficult as it is not clear whether to include the cavity in the measurement. Some nodules may also respond by becoming less solid and more ground glass in appearance (Fig. 10.6)
3. Bone metastases often respond to treatment with sclerotic changes. Development of sclerosis in a previously lytic lesion is a sign of response, but cannot be labeled so on RECIST
4. Tumors may develop cystic (Fig. 10.7) or calcific changes or hemorrhage due to chemotherapy. For example, nonseminomatous germ cell tumors with retroperitoneal adenopathy often develop cystic changes post-treatment. This is because the embryonal or yolk sac component of these mixed tumors is chemosensitive and shrinks, while the relatively benign teratomatous component is usually chemoresistant and persists as cystic changes; this is a sign of response. The teratomatous component requires surgical resection

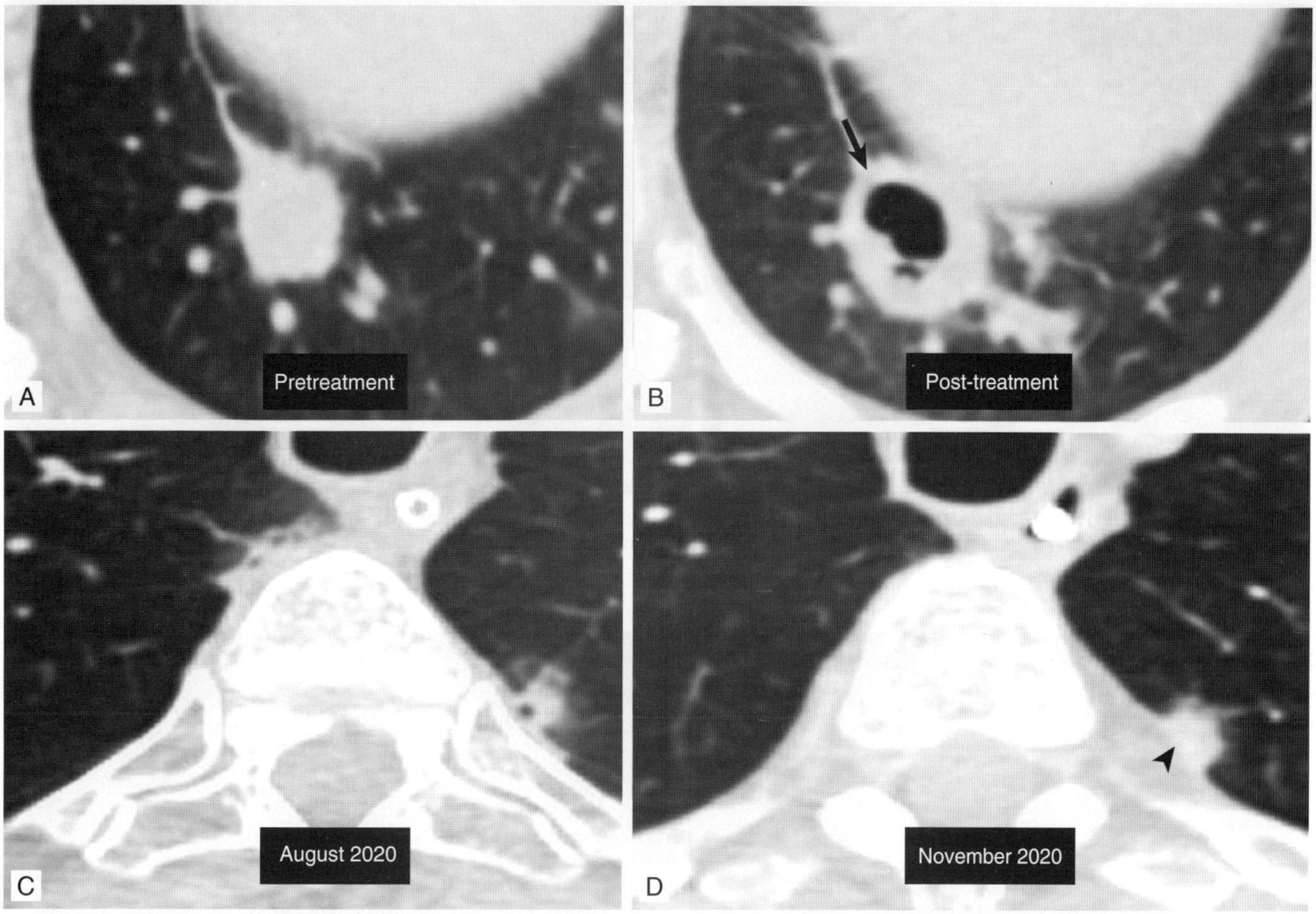

Figure 10.5 Response not considered by RECIST: cavitatory lung lesions. (A and B) Solid lung nodule (primary or metastatic) showing cavitation (*arrow*) on post-treatment scan may suggest response. Usually seen in squamous cell carcinoma, sarcomas, and antiangiogenic treatments such colorectal cancers being treated with panitumumab. (C and D) A cavitatory lung nodule showing filling in (*arrowheads*) on follow-up imaging may suggest progression.

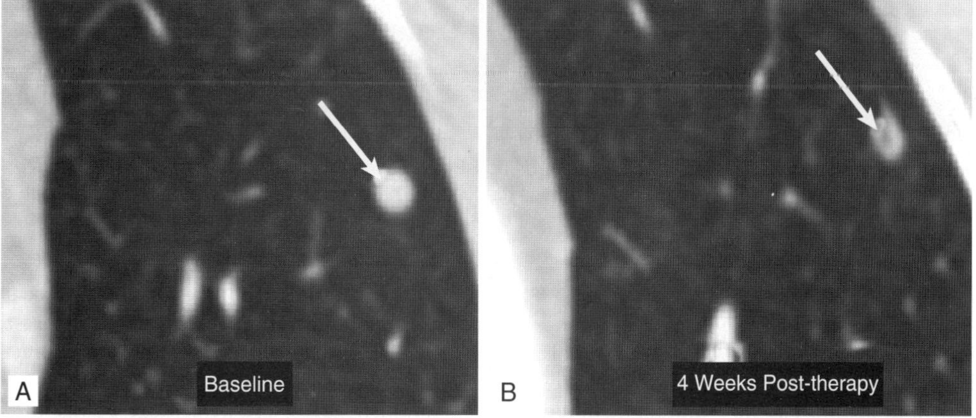

Figure 10.6 Response not considered by RECIST: change in attenuation. A solid lung nodule (*arrow*) showing decrease in attenuation and becoming more "ground glass" may suggest a response. Similarly, a ground glass or part solid nodule becoming more solid may suggest progression. These changes should be confirmed on thin sections as 5 mm slice can produce volume averaging.

5. Desmoid tumor (fibromatosis) may not show any significant change in size after treatment. However, it becomes more fibrotic with increase in the T2 hypointense component. Similarly, rectal cancers may also respond with T2 hypointense fibrosis or T2 hyperintense mucinous changes after neoadjuvant therapy (Fig. 10.8).

These limitations have led to the development of many alternate response assessment criteria, some of which are discussed ahead. Many morphology changes like cavitation or development of fibrosis continue to not have objective criteria for assessment, and need to be interpreted appropriately by the radiologist in the given clinical context

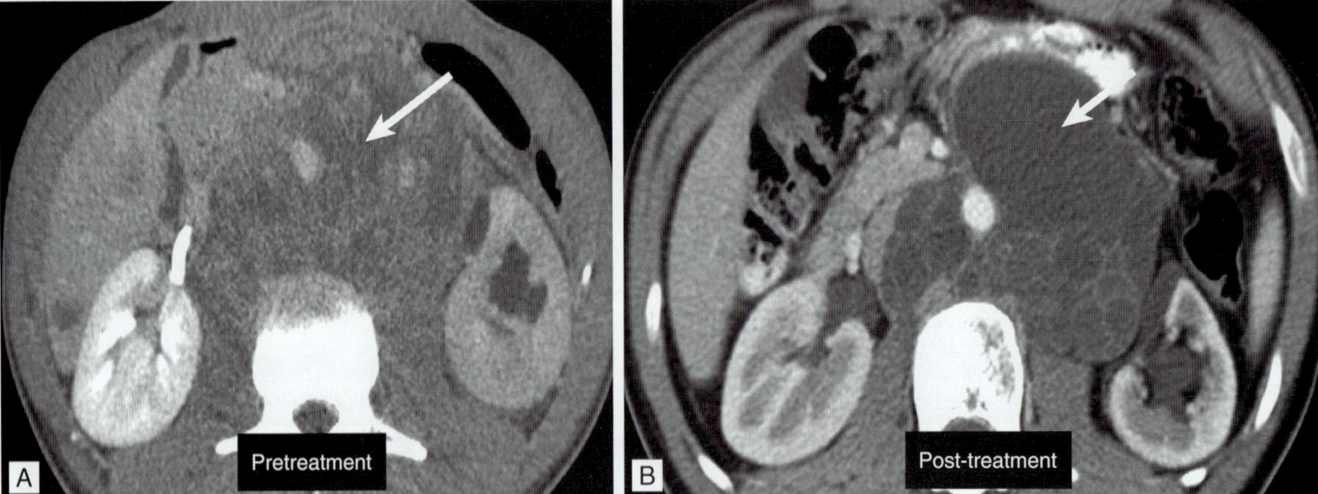

Figure 10.7 Responses not considered by RECIST: nonseminomatous germ cell tumors (NSGCT). (A and B) Development of cystic changes (*arrows*). In this case a large retroperitoneal nodal mass post-treatment shows cystic changes with enhancing septations. No solid components seen. The tumor markers had returned to normal levels.

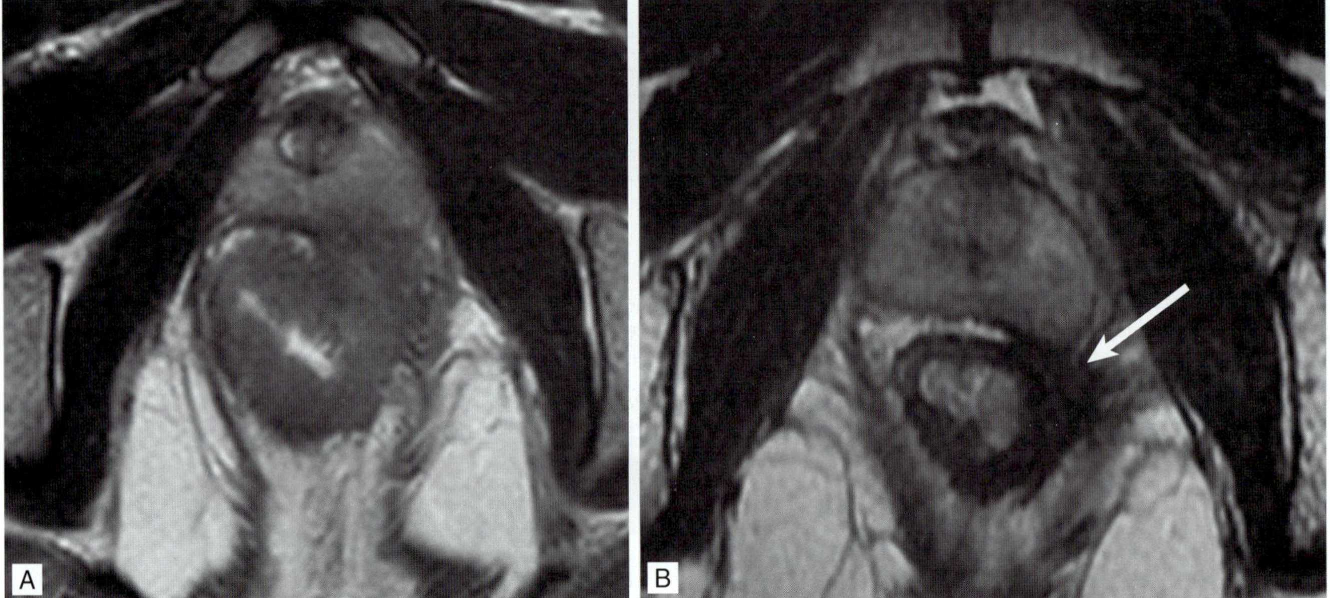

Figure 10.8 Patient with rectal cancer. Baseline axial T2W image (A) demonstrates T2 intermediate tumor involving the prostate. The patient received neoadjuvant chemoradiation. The post-treatment scan (B) demonstrates the tumor to have responded well (*arrow*), with development of T2 hypointense fibrosis (*arrow*).

RECIST in Clinical Practice

In summary, it is important to note that RECIST is an important tool in clinical trials and research where it needs to be followed stringently. The principles behind RECIST although should be applied in everyday reporting as well, as it standardizes reporting and allows for a more meaningful communication. However, one can avoid dogmatically following RECIST in a detailed manner in routine clinical practice. A few take-home messages in this regard are as follows:

1. It is important to evaluate the patient holistically based on tumor size, morphology, site, pathology, and treatment given, and not just based on size. It is important to be aware of the patient's clinical condition, tumor marker status (if relevant), and treatment to accurately assess response
2. Most institutes report lesions in two axial dimensions (long axis and short axis). One need not measure only the single longest dimension in routine clinical practice, but do ensure that the longest dimension is included in the measurement. Similarly, SLD and percentage change need not be calculated and reported in routine patients
3. Apply the RECIST principles while interpreting scans. For example, one should measure only a few well-delineated lesions. Too small to characterize lesions such as 3–4-mm lung nodules should not be considered metastatic (these are not "measurable" lesions and are statistically most commonly benign) [24]. Lymph nodes enlargement should be based on short-axis measurement rather than long axis
4. Marginal changes in tumor size should not be considered as progression or response. A disease should be labeled as PD

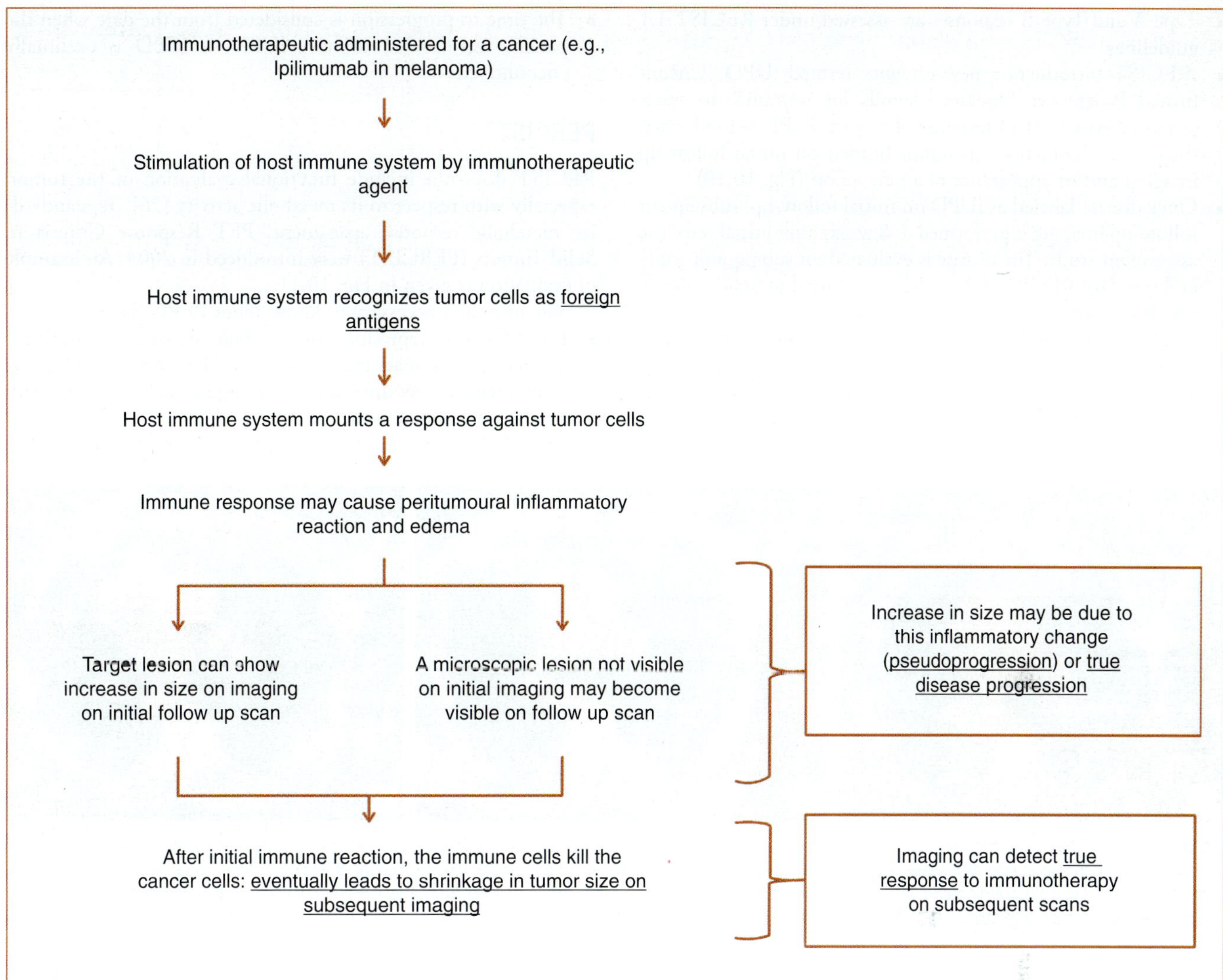

Figure 10.9 Overview of immunotherapy and its response.

only when there is categorical increase, given that RECIST also needs an at least 20% increase for categorizing PD

5. The authors prefer not to use the terminologies of RECIST such as CR, SD, PR, PD in routine reporting given that it is not a trial setting and SLD is not routinely calculated. This gives the oncologist some flexibility in ensuring holistic treatment as the patient's clinical status and tumor markers may not always be available while reporting the scan. Alternative terms are instead used to describe responses such as "stable disease burden" (equivalent to SD) or "increased disease burden" (equivalent to PD). For patients with marginal increase in size not amounting to PD, terms like "marginally increased disease burden" may be used. It is important to have the oncologist on the same page with regards the terminology used
6. Radiologists must reviews all previous serial imaging instead of only one or two previous studies. As progression is determined from Nadir, this is extremely important to evaluate for accurate response assessment
7. Finally and most importantly, given the complexity of cancer treatment, it will be common to encounter situations when there is a query or doubt regarding the patient's scan or treatment. At such instances, the best thing you can do is discuss the findings directly with the referring oncologist so as to completely understand the clinical context and implication before finalizing the report

iRECIST

Immunotherapy has a completely different mechanism of action compared with cytotoxic/cytostatic chemotherapy, for which the size-based RECIST criteria were introduced. An overview of immunotherapy has been depicted in Fig. 10.9. iRECIST criteria have been introduced to overcome the shortcomings of RECIST and standardize immunotherapy response assessment criteria [21]. Few salient points of iRECIST are listed later [25]. The definitions of measurable, nonmeasurable, target lesion as well as rules of measurement remain the same as RECIST 1.1. Patients on immunotherapy can demonstrate four types of responses:

Type A: Decrease in tumor size. No new lesions.

Type B: Stable disease. On subsequent imaging, it may remain stable or decrease in size.

Type C: Increase in size on initial follow-up with subsequent reduction in size.

Type D: Decrease in size of target lesions despite appearance of new lesions.

- Type A and Type B responses are assessed under RECIST 1.1 guidelines
- iRECIST introduces a new category termed iUPD (Unconfirmed Progressive Disease; i stands for immune) to assess potential type C or D response. The term iUPD is used when there is ≥20% increase in tumor burden on initial follow-up imaging and/or appearance of a new lesion (Fig. 10.10)
- Once disease labeled as iUPD on initial follow-up, subsequent follow-up imaging is performed 4–8 weeks after initial response assessment study. The disease is evaluated on subsequent study and standard RECIST 1.1 guidelines are used to finally classify the disease as:
  - *iPR, iSD, or iCR* when there is partial response, stable disease, or complete response, respectively; or
  - *iCPD (confirmed progressive disease)* when there is unequivocal progression in terms of increase in tumor burden or appearance of new lesions.
- The time to progression is considered from the date when the patient was labeled to have iUPD, if iCPD is eventually encountered

PERCIST

RECIST does not include functional evaluation of the tumor, especially with respect to its metabolic activity [26]. To standardize metabolic response assessment, PET Response Criteria in Solid Tumors (PERCIST) were introduced in 2009. An example of evaluation is given in Fig. 10.11.

Salient points necessary to know about PERCIST are:

- It is difficult to reproduce the metabolic status due to multiple factors such as machine calibration, FDG dose, and uptake time. Hence, it requires serial imaging on same machine with similar dose and activity
- PERCIST complements rather than replaces RECIST

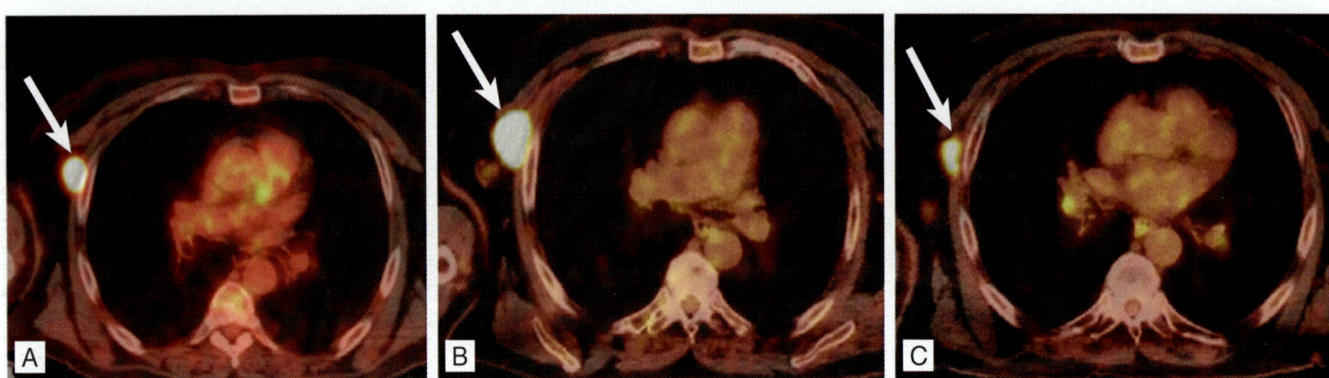

Figure 10.10 iUPD in a patient with metastatic malignant melanoma on Ipilimumab. Baseline FDG PET/CT (A) shows a right chest wall metastasis, which demonstrated increase in size at 5-week follow-up study (B), labelled as iUPD. Another 5-week follow-up scan (C) shows decrease in the lesion size, consistent with partial response (iPR) rather than progression. Other sites of metastases followed a similar pattern. (Printed with permission from: UR Lalchandani, V Sahai, K Hersberger, IR Francis, AP Wasnik, A radiologist's guide to response evaluation criteria in solid tumors, Curr Probl Diagn Radiol 48 (6) (2019) 576–585, Fig. 8. doi:10.1067/j.cpradiol.2018.07.016.)

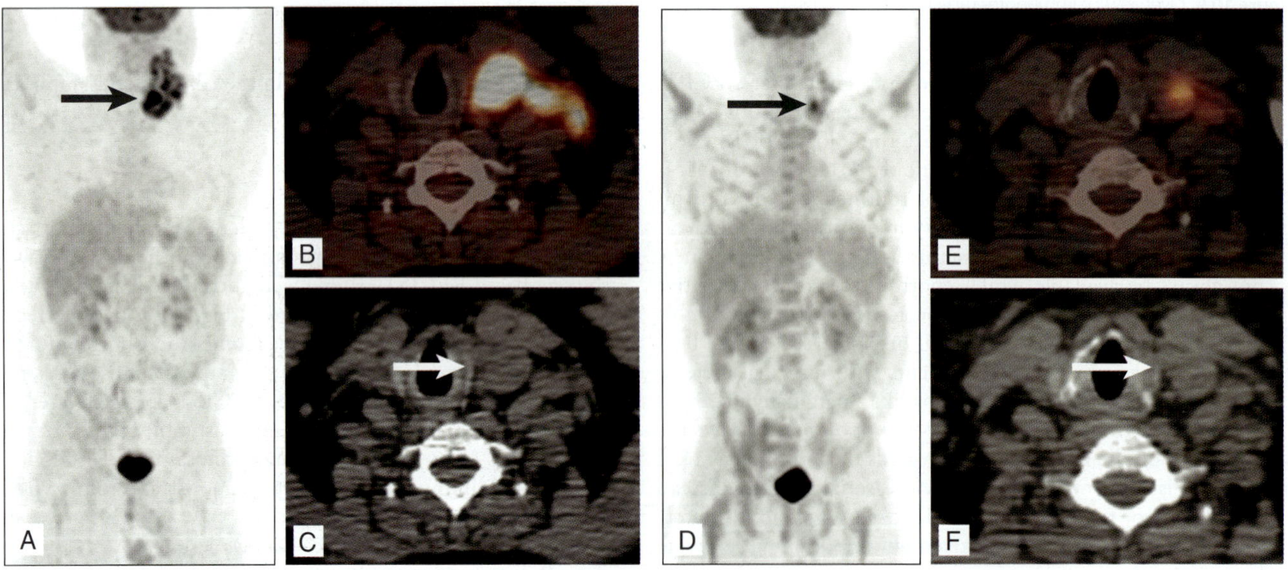

Figure 10.11 Case of carcinoma of unknown primary (CUP). (A) Maximum intensity projection (MIP) shows FDG avid left cervical nodal mass (*black arrow*). (B) and (C) images show large left cervical level IV node on fused transverse and axial CT, respectively (*white arrow*). SUV_{max} 27.7, SUL 19.9 (*SUL*, standardized uptake value corrected for lean body mass). Response assessment scan of same patient post 2# chemotherapy. (D) MIP showing focal FDG uptake in left cervical region (*black arrow*). (E) and (F) show reduction in FDG uptake and size of left level IV cervical node (*white arrow*) with residual disease suggestive of partial response. SUV_{max} 8.8, SUL 6.33. (Courtesy: Ameya Puranik, Department of Nuclear Medicine and Molecular Imaging, Tata Memorial Hospital.)

TABLE 10.2 PERCIST Response Criteria

Response	Criteria
Complete response (CR)	■ Visual disappearance of all metabolically active lesions: ○ SUL_{peak} normalizes to <liver SUL_{peak}. ○ SUL_{peak} is equal to SUL_{peak} of normal surrounding tissue.
Partial response (PR)	■ >30% and 0.8 Unit decline in SUL_{peak} between the most FDG avid lesions of two scans (not necessarily the same lesion)
Progressive disease (PD)	■ >30% and 0.8 Unit increase in SUL_{peak} between the most FDG avid lesions of two scans (not necessarily the same lesion) OR ■ Appearance of new lesions ■ >75% *increase* in total lesion glycolysis is also proposed as a criteria for PD.
Stable disease (SD)	■ Not meeting any of the criteria described earlier

- Routine clinical PET-CT heavily involves SUV_{max} (maximum standardized uptake value). To make the results more uniform, PERCIST employs SUL_{peak} (peak standardized uptake value normalized to lean body mass) instead of SUV_{max}
- Metabolic activity is mentioned as complete metabolic response (CMR), partial metabolic response (PMR), stable metabolic disease (SMD), and progressive metabolic disease (PMD)
- Validation of PERCIST is still awaited. Hence, routinely, up to five lesions may also be measured similar to RECIST
- Response criteria for PERCIST have been summarized in Table 10.2

RANO

The RANO criteria were developed in 2010 [17] as an objective response assessment tool of gliomas after chemo/radiotherapy. Conventionally, McDonald's criteria [17] and RECIST were employed for gliomas but they had several limitations. There were no clear guidelines nonenhancing tumor progressions (as in low-grade gliomas), they did not account for the heterogeneity of gliomas, had no guidance on pseudoprogression and pseudoresponse. RANO was introduced to delineate objective end points of response assessment of brain tumors [17,27].

RANO lays down guidelines of minimal essential MRI protocol required to assess gliomas: at baseline and post-treatment. Advanced imaging techniques like perfusion MR imaging, MR spectroscopy, diffusion-weighted imaging, and amino acid PET/CT ^{11}C-methionine (MET), [^{18}F] fluoroethyl tyrosine, and [^{18}F] dihydroxyphenylalanine) are not included in RANO criteria [28].

It states that postoperative and prechemoradiation "baseline imaging" should be obtained within 48 hours of surgery; as after this window period, distinguishing postoperative changes from true residual disease becomes difficult. Essential definitions of RANO different from RECIST criteria are summarized in Table 10.3. Details regarding pseudoprogression, pseudoresponse, and radiation necrosis are discussed in detail in the chapter on brain tumors, Chapter 62. Disease end points as defined by RANO have been summarized in Table 10.4. RANO also has a separate criterion for low-grade gliomas, with an addition of "minor response criteria" which corresponds to 25–50% decrease in total tumor burden on T2/FLAIR images. An immunotherapy criterion called the iRANO has also been proposed [27].

Few salient points which need to be noted are:

- Post-treatment effects can mimic progression for up to 12 weeks postradiation treatment (RT). Any enhancement in follow-up imaging occurring within 12 weeks of RT, which is seen outside the radiation field; can be termed as true progression

TABLE 10.3 Important Definitions of RANO on MRI Imaging

Sl. No.	Terminology	Definition
1.	Measurable lesion	■ Discrete lesions with clear margins, visible on at least ≥2 subsequent axial sections ■ Enhancing lesions on contrast-enhanced images ■ Measurable in two dimensions perpendicular to each other in long and short axis with both measurements ≥10 mm, respectively
2.	Nonmeasurable lesion	■ Nonenhancing T2/FLAIR hyperintense lesions with indistinct margins ■ Discrete lesion <10 mm in diameter on long axis or short axis on MRI ■ Measurable in only one dimension (usually along the margins of surgical cavity)
3.	Target/nontarget lesion	■ In the case of multiple lesions, two lesions are selected, preferably the larger one representing tumor burden with good reproducibility on follow-up imaging. These are termed as target lesions. ■ All the other lesions in brain are called nontarget lesions. ■ The sum of the products of the perpendicular diameters (SPPD) of the target lesions is calculated (unlike sum of longest dimensions in RECIST). For example, if lesion A in right parietal lobe measures 15 × 10 mm (150 mm^2) and lesion B in left parietal lobe measures 20 × 10 mm (200 mm^2); the SPPD is 150 + 200 = 350 mm^2

TABLE 10.4 Summary of RANO Criteria for End Points

	CR[a]	PR	SD	PD[b]
T1 + C pattern of target lesions	None	≥50% ↓	<50% ↓ or < 25% ↑	≥25% ↑
T2/FLAIR component of nonenhancing lesions (nonmeasurable lesions)	Stable or ↓	Stable or ↓	Stable or ↓	↑
New lesions	No	No	No	Yes
Clinical status	Stable or improved	Stable or improved	Stable or improved	Deteriorated
Corticosteroid requirement	None/physiological replacement dose	Stable or ↓	Stable or ↓	↑ Along with clinical deterioration

[a]*Findings should be sustained for at least 4 weeks. Patients having "only nonmeasurable disease" cannot achieve CR; the best response possible in these patients is SD.*
[b]*Failure to return for follow-up due to death or deteriorating condition, or unequivocal progression of nonmeasurable/nontarget lesions are all PD.*

- Lesions abutting a cyst or surgical cavity should be labeled as nonmeasurable lesions, unless there is enhancing component fitting the measurable disease criteria. Do not measure the cyst or surgical cavity for response assessment
- Lesions with large central necrosis should preferably be labeled as nontarget lesions, unless they are the only lesions present, in which case they can be considered as target lesions
- In case the findings are "equivocal of PD," then RANO permits for continuation of ongoing treatment, but if the subsequent scan after 3 months confirms PD; then the date of PD is backdated to the scan with "equivocal PD"

Choi Criteria

- The Choi criteria were first described in 2008 for response evaluation of patients with GISTs on Imatinib [18]. Imatinib is a selective tyrosine-kinase inhibitor and causes reduction in the enhancement and heterogeneity of GIST rather than of size. GIST lesions on Imatinib become homogeneous and hypoattenuating, often appearing almost cystic. In addition, the lesions become better defined. The lesions also show significantly reduced metabolism on functional imaging such as PET after therapy. This unique response was not adequately assessed by the size-based RECIST criteria. Choi criteria addresses this and incorporates changes in lesion enhancement for response assessment (Table 10.5)
- The size measurement rules are the same as RECIST, but the cutoff for PR and PD is different. However, tumor enhancement is additionally measured as mean HU value of the enhancing component (Fig. 10.12)
- Note that on occasion, a previously isoenhancing lesion which was not appreciable on the baseline scan may become newly apparent as a hypodense focus post-treatment (pseudoprogression). This should not be considered PD; obvious response in the other lesions gives a clue to this diagnosis
- In a similar fashion, development of resistance to Imatinib may manifest by development of enhancing foci in a cystic appearing lesion without increased size (nodule-in-cyst appearance)

Response Assessment Criteria for Hepatocellular Carcinoma

HCC is treated with various techniques: ablative therapies, endovascular approaches as well as targeted therapy (sorafenib). These produce varied responses including decrease in the hypervascular component and increase in the necrotic component, often without a change in size. Size-based RECIST criteria are again not sufficient for assessment. Originally proposed by the EASL (European Association for the Study of the Liver) as the EASL criteria [29], these were subsequently adopted as mRECIST criteria [30]. Liver Imaging Reporting and Data System (LI-RADS) also provides a basic framework for response assessment (LR-TR: treatment response), further discussed in the chapter on cirrhotic liver.

Modified RECIST

- As per mRECIST, only the enhancing component is measured in its longest dimension rather than the entire lesion (Fig. 10.13

TABLE 10.5 Choi Response Assessment Criteria

Response	Criteria
Complete response (CR)	▪ Disappearance of all lesions, AND ▪ No new lesions
Partial response (PR)	▪ ≥10% *decrease* in tumor size, OR ▪ ≥15% *decrease* in tumor HU (attenuation), AND ▪ No new lesions, AND ▪ No unequivocal progression of nonmeasurable disease
Stable disease (SD)	▪ Neither of the criteria defined for CR, PR, or SD
Progressive disease (PD)	▪ ≥10% *increase* in tumor size, AND ▪ Not meeting the criteria of attenuation (HU) change for partial response, OR ▪ Appearance of new lesions, OR ▪ Appearance of new nodular enhancing areas in pre-existing lesions, OR ▪ Unequivocal progression of nonmeasurable disease

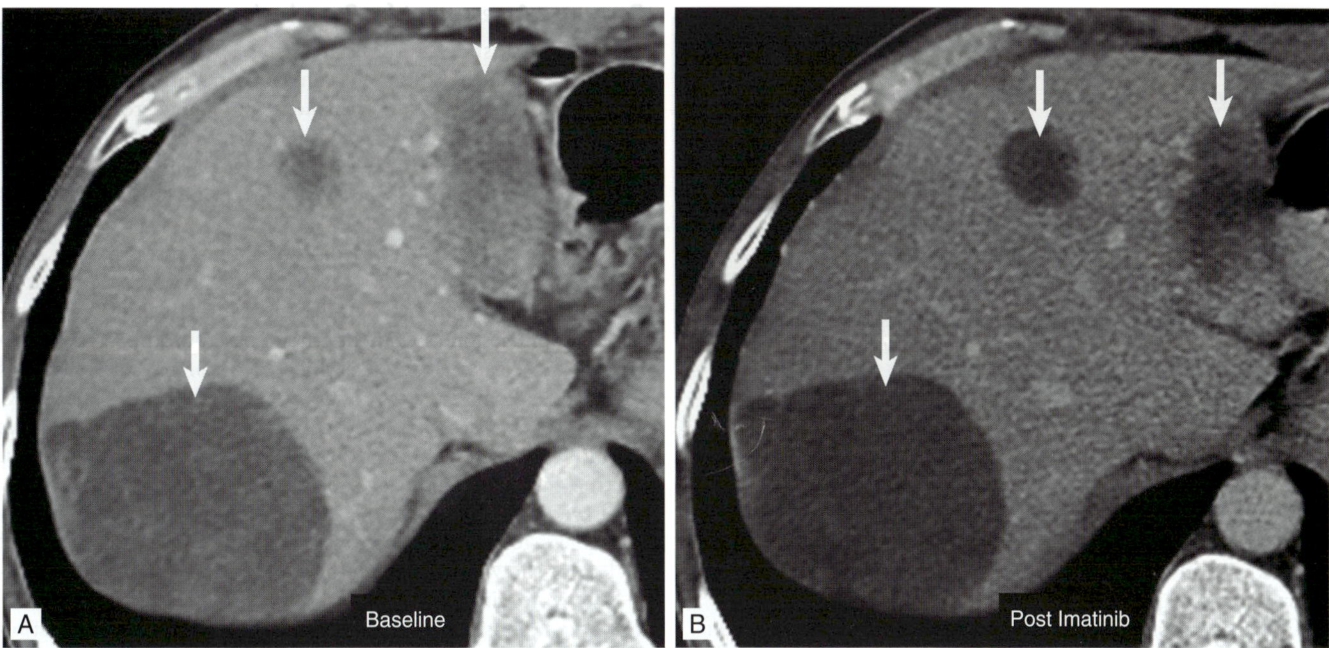

Figure 10.12 Choi criteria. Case of metastatic GIST on Imatinib. On baseline study large lesions are seen in both lobes of liver (*arrows*) showing heterogeneous enhancement and ill-defined margins. Post-Imatinib, the lesions have become homogeneous and hypoattenuating (appearing almost cystic) and are better defined. The fall in HU is >15%: suggestive of response. *GIST*, gastrointestinal stromal tumor; *HU*, Hounsfield unit.

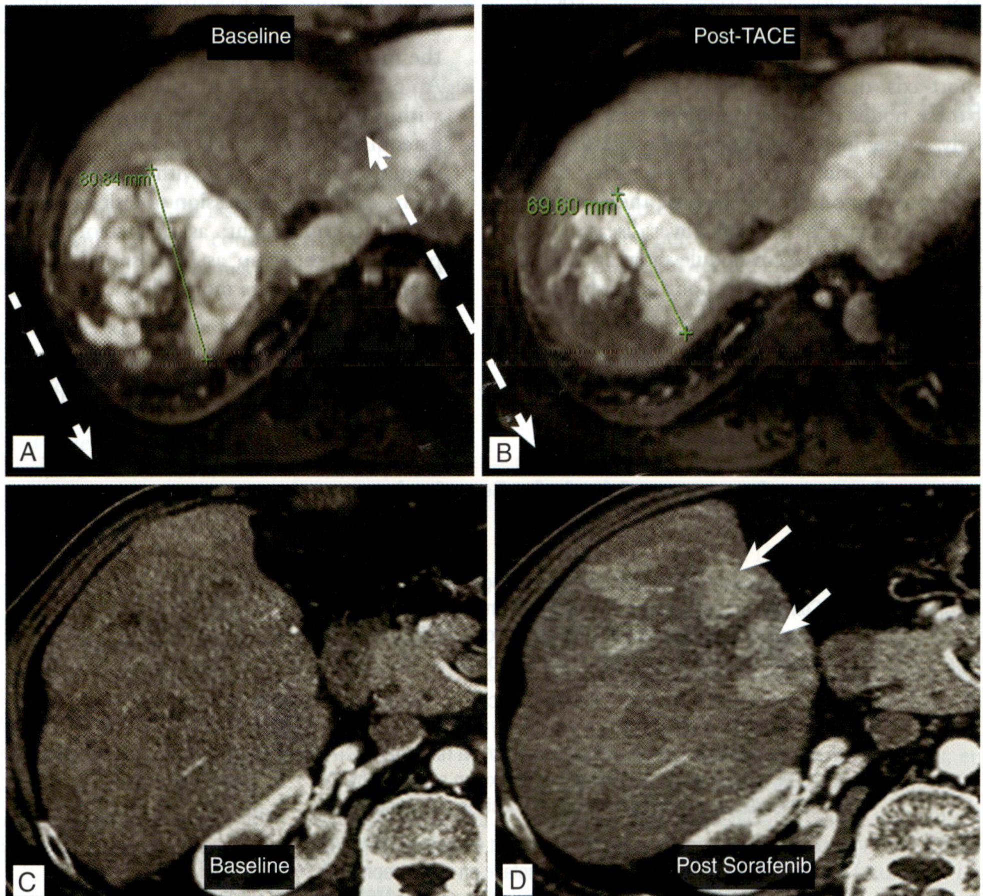

Figure 10.13 mRECIST and LI-RADS tumor response assessment. (A and B) Response in HCC. There is reduction in longest dimension of enhancing component on post-TACE imaging with increase of necrotic areas. (C and D) Progression in HCC. Appearance of new arterially enhancing foci (*arrows*) in a patient on sorafenib suggests progressive disease. *TACE*, trans arterial chemoembolization.

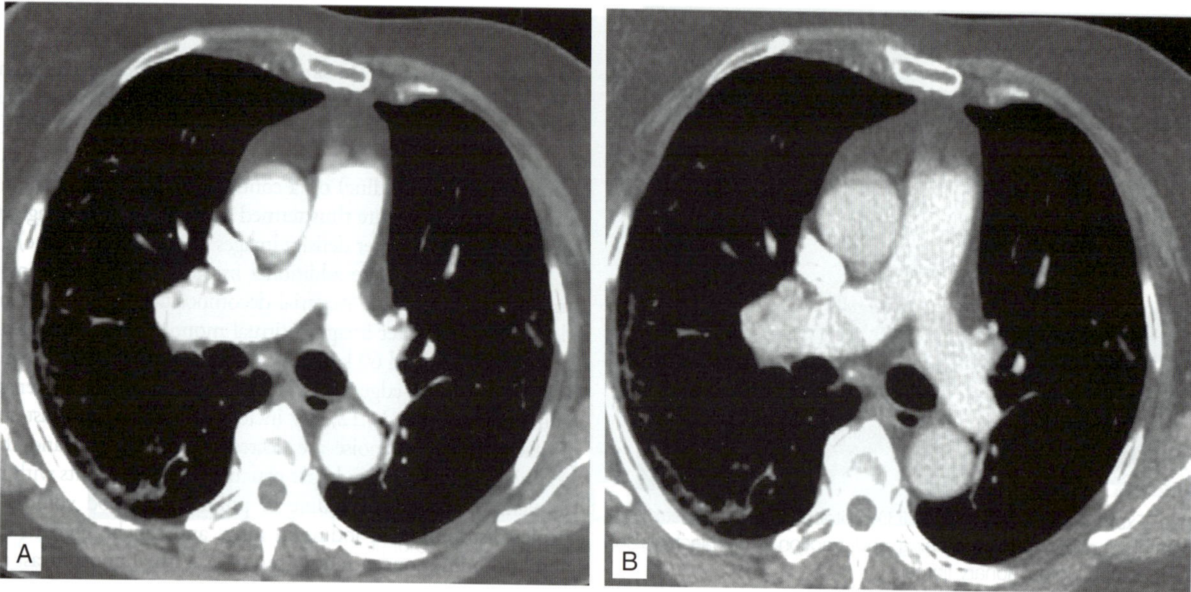

Figure 11.12 Example of improved contrast enhancement of the pulmonary arteries between a 60 kV monoenergetic image (A) and a 140 kV monoenergetic image (B) in the same patient using the same soft tissue window.

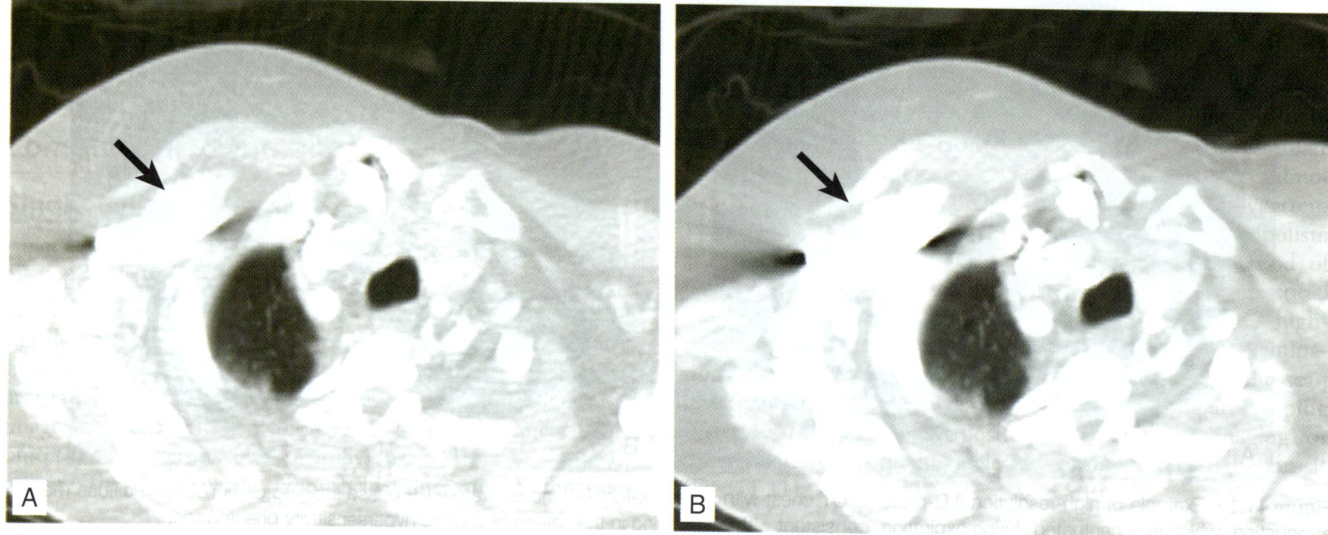

Figure 11.13 Example of decreasing contrast streak artifact within the right subclavian artery (*arrows*) between a 60 kV monoenergetic image (A) and a 140 kV monoenergetic image (B) in the same patient using the same lung window.

images can help differentiate hemorrhage, high protein content, and calcium from iodinated contrast medium [16,18]. The common types of images generated from DECT are detailed in Table 11.1.

Clinical Applications of DECT

DECT pulmonary angiography shows better pulmonary arterial contrast opacification, even at lower iodine volumes in comparison to single-energy CT performed at higher kV >100 kV (Fig. 11.14) [15,17,18]. *Additionally, DECT iodine images can help in subjective detection of areas of abnormal perfusion corresponding to perfusion defect and/or pulmonary infarct.* Since impaired pulmonary parenchymal perfusion is an independent predictor of mortality and morbidity, early detection and clinical intervention in cases with perfusion defects can significantly alter the clinical course for PE (Fig. 11.15). As mentioned in the literature, dual-source DECT images are clearly advantageous over rapid kV switching in this regard [17,18]. Similarly, DECT can also help in the assessment of

TABLE 11.1 Description of Common Image Types in DECT

Image Type	Explanation
Virtual monochromatic (keV)	Appear just like conventional CT images; at lower keV contrast enhancement is better, at higher keV noise and artifacts are reduced
Material decomposition (iodine or blood volume)	For pulmonary parenchymal enhancement
Material decomposition (water or virtual noncontrast)	For differentiating calcium or blood from iodine
Quality check images (GE)	Initial high kV images
High and low kV (Siemens)	Original low and high kV images
Blended images (Siemens)	Less noisy blended low and high kV images

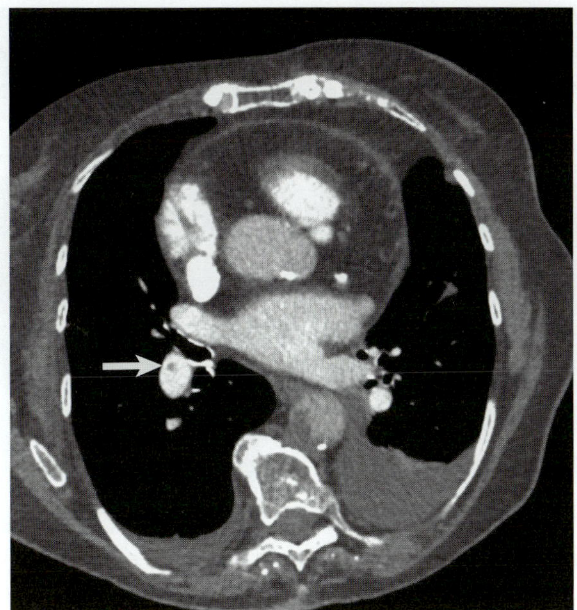

Figure 11.14 Example of a low iodine volume CT PE using only 36 cc of iodinated contrast material with satisfactory detection of pulmonary embolic disease in the right interlobar artery (*arrow*).

chronic pulmonary thromboembolic pulmonary hypertension (Fig. 11.16). It is important to consider artifacts and underlying airways-disease-related air trapping while evaluating iodine images. Other applications such as lesion and nodule characterization, cancer treatment response, and quantification of emphysema remain under investigation for proved clinical use [17,18].

Chest CT Protocols

To optimize the use of CT technology for different clinical indications, different specific protocols are typically used [19]. Chest CT is mostly performed at an end inspiratory breath-hold. Since motion artifacts and incorrect scan phase can impair optimum radiological interpretation, appropriate breath-hold is critical for contrast enhancement such as in CT pulmonary angiography.

Routine Chest CT Protocol

The most used chest protocol is routine chest CT and can be performed with or without IV contrast administration. The scan for a routine chest CT extends from lung apices to adrenal glands in an inspiratory breath-hold. CT images are typically reconstructed at slice thickness of 1.0–1.5 mm for lungs and 2.5–3.0 mm for mediastinum [19]. Additional reconstructions with multiplanar reformatting for coronal and sagittal, maximum

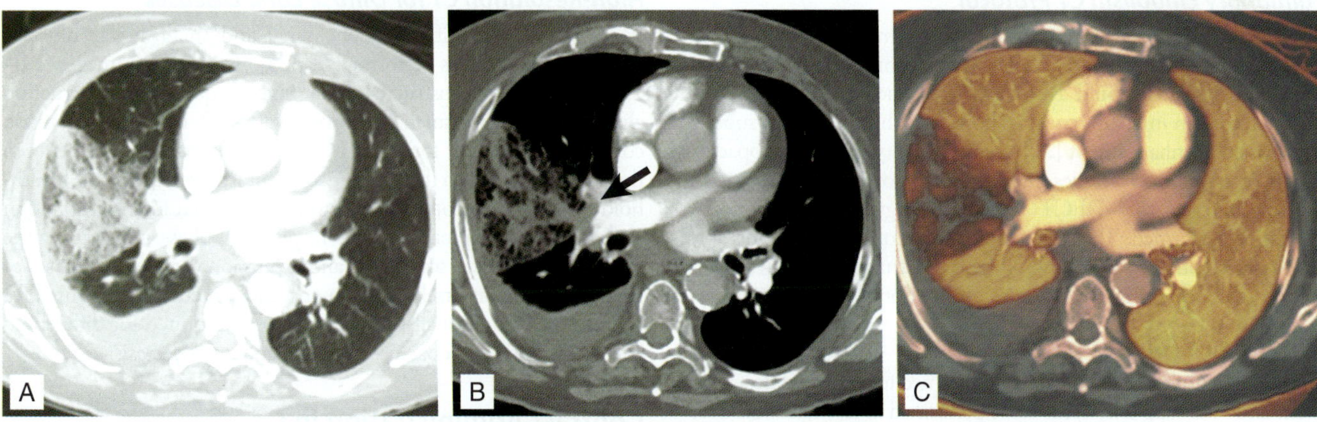

Figure 11.15 Example of a large right interlobar pulmonary embolus (*arrow*) with associated large abnormal perfusion defect on iodine images (C). Image A and B show the findings in lung and soft tissue window settings, respectively.

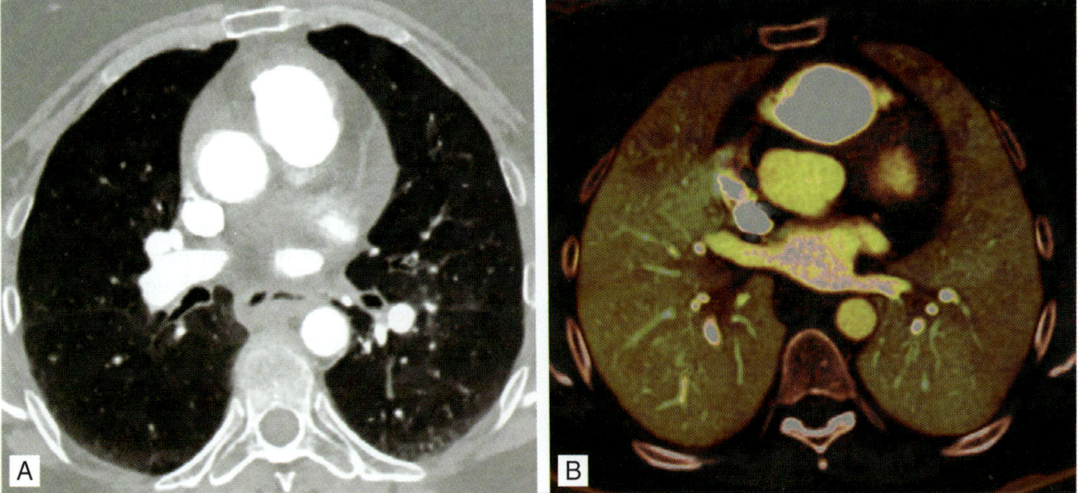

Figure 11.16 Example of CTEPH on dual-energy CT PE. Note the mosaic attenuation on lung window (A) and multifocal peripheral hypoattenuation seen on iodine perfusion (B), corresponding to chronic thromboembolic disease.

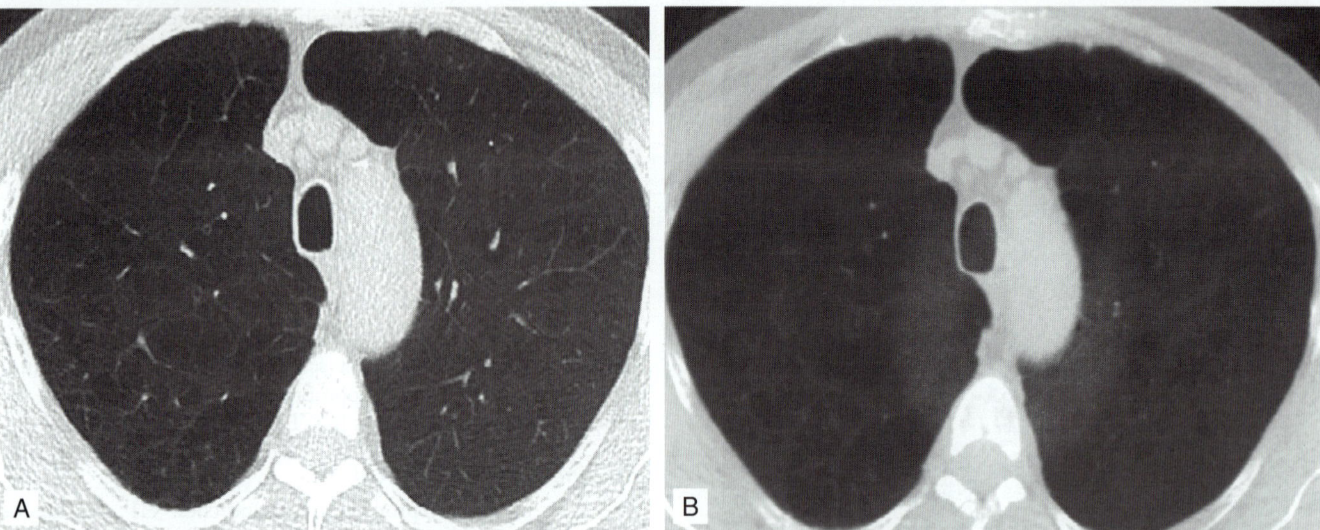

Figure 11.17 Comparison between standard CT chest (A) and minimum intensity projection CT (B). Note the increased detection of emphysema and other low-attenuation structures using minimum intensity projection.

intensity projection for nodule detection, and minimum intensity projection for emphysema detection (Fig. 11.17).

Pulmonary Embolism CT Protocol

Chest CT for PE evaluation needs to be performed with attention to several details [19]. For a good quality scan, contrast bolus should be timed and patients should avoid Valsalva maneuver during breath-hold since it can interrupt contrast bolus and thereby lead to suboptimal vascular enhancement [20]. A good quality scan shows opacification of pulmonary arteries and veins and some enhancement of thoracic aorta. Either DECT or single-energy CT at <100 kVs should be performed. The scan should be performed from lung apices to bases. Finally, images should be reconstructed at 1.0–1.5 mm section thickness using soft tissue reconstruction algorithm.

Lung Nodule Follow-Up CT Protocol

Substantial number of chest CT are performed for lung nodule assessment and follow-up and needs to be performed at low radiation dose (Fig. 11.18) [19]. *As shown in recent studies, lung nodule follow-up CT can be performed at less than 1-mSv radiation dose using iterative reconstruction or deep learning-based image reconstruction techniques* [21]. Since abdominal structures are not evaluated well at low radiation dose, the scan should be performed from lung apices to bases.

Low-Dose CT for Lung Cancer Screening

Lung cancer screening CT is also performed at low radiation dose, similar to lung nodule follow-up CT. As per the American College of Radiology guidelines, *the minimum MDCT configuration should be a four-slice CT scanner and radiation dose should be 3.0 mGy or less* [22,23]. With better reconstruction techniques such as iterative reconstruction, radiation doses can be lowered up to 0.1 mSv without compromising the image quality.

Tracheal or Airway Protocol

For assessing pathologies such as tracheal stenosis, tracheal neoplasms, and tracheobronchomalacia (Fig. 11.19), tracheal protocol is used [19,24]. The images are acquired in an end inspiratory breath-hold and include both neck and chest. Forceful expiration should be performed for acquiring expiratory phase images to detect airway collapsibility [24]. With wide detectors (16 cm), continuous scanning can be performed during the inspiratory and expiratory phase of respiration. The radiation dose for this protocol is lower than routine CT as the intent is only to evaluate airways [19].

High-Resolution CT for Diffuse Lung Diseases

For assessment of diffuse parenchymal and small airway diseases, high-resolution CT is performed [19,25]. Thin section images (1.0–1.25 mm) are reconstructed with high frequency reconstruction algorithms using a small field-of-view (FOV) including rib-to-rib coverage. The reason for small FOV is the inverse relation between the image pixel size to the FOV at constant image matrix. The breath-hold for this scan protocol needs to be performed in end inspiration and then end expiration. The inspiratory phase images can be acquired with helical scan mode and expiration with a step-and-shoot method [25]. Conversely, the step-and-shoot method can be used for both phases. Additionally, prone images are acquired for differentiation of ground glass opacities from dependent atelectasis.

Contrast Administration in CT

Save for routine chest CT and CT pulmonary angiography, other scan protocols are typically performed without the use of IV contrast [19,26]. Routine chest CT can be performed both with and without IV contrast. The iodinated contrast is injected at a rate of 2.5–3.0 mL/s using 60–80 mL of contrast. DECT can be performed using as low as 25 mL of contrast. A fixed time delay following contrast administration can alter contrast opacification due to differing injection rate, volume, patient size, and cardiac output. Thus, bolus tracking is indicated to time the scan delay for best contrast enhancement (Fig. 11.20). In this technique, a region of interest is drawn in the pulmonary trunk or aorta with a set Hounsfield unit threshold beyond which the scan is triggered. In split-bolus injection technique, an initial slower rate of contrast injection (1 cc/s) is followed by higher rate (2 cc/s) for both aorta and pulmonary artery enhancement, respectively [19,26]. This method can avoid the need for bolus tracking.

PET-CT and PET-MRI

PET

Over the last two decades, PET has become an important imaging tool in thoracic oncology (Fig. 11.21) for diagnosis, staging, and

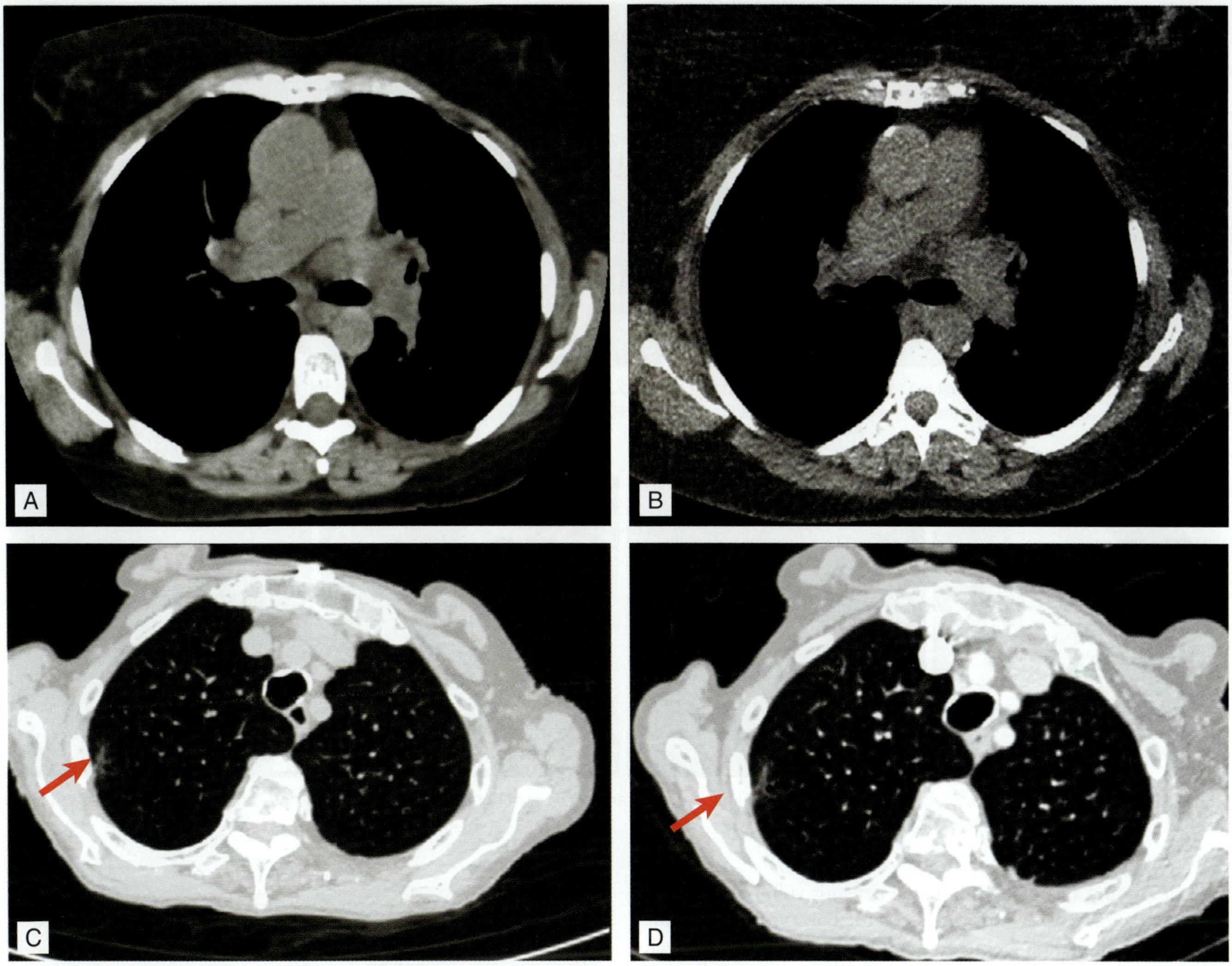

Figure 11.18 Standard-dose (A) versus low-dose (B) CT chest. Note the increased image noise and graininess of the low-dose acquisition, although images remain diagnostic for lung cancer screening. Another example case from chest CT of a 60-year-old male conducted at two different time points shows the lung nodule in the right upper lobe (*red arrows*) on low-dose CT (C) and standard-dose CT (D) images.

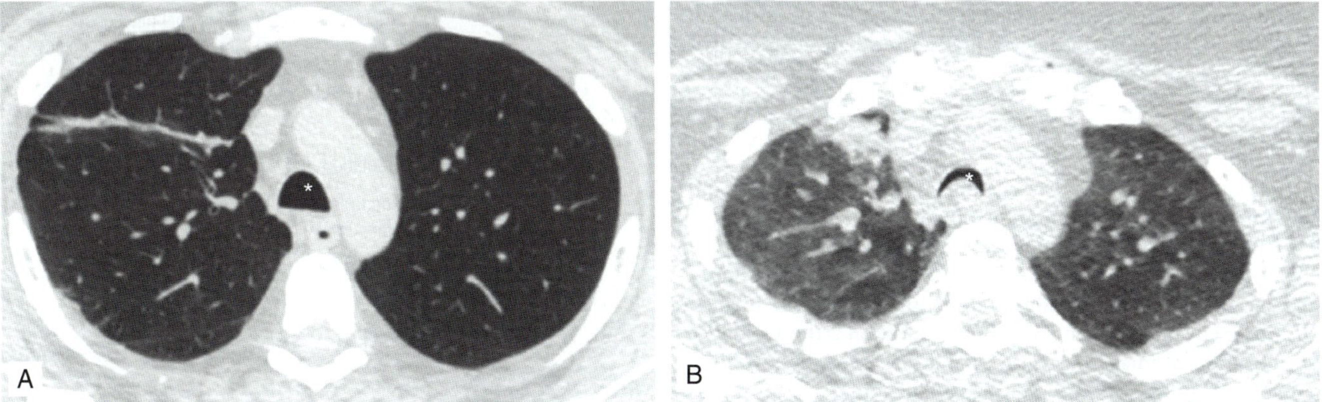

Figure 11.19 Example of tracheobronchomalacia and dynamic tracheal collapse on CT with an inspiratory (A) and expiratory (B) phase imaging. Note the significant (>50%) reduction of anterior–posterior diameter of the mid trachea during expiration with formation of a crescentic shape on the axial plane.

assessing treatment response, and in diagnosis of nononcologic processes such as inflammation [27–29]. PET integration with CT and MR has improved its diagnostic accuracy.

PET imaging is based on production of positrons from radionuclide decay. Due to its most convenient half-life of 110 minutes, ^{18}F is commonly used. It is coupled with a biologically active molecule, usually glucose, to form 2-deoxy-2-fluoro-D-glucose (^{18}F-FDG), which interacts with the membrane transporters for cellular uptake. The quantification of ^{18}F-FDG uptake is done with standardized uptake value (SUV), defined as

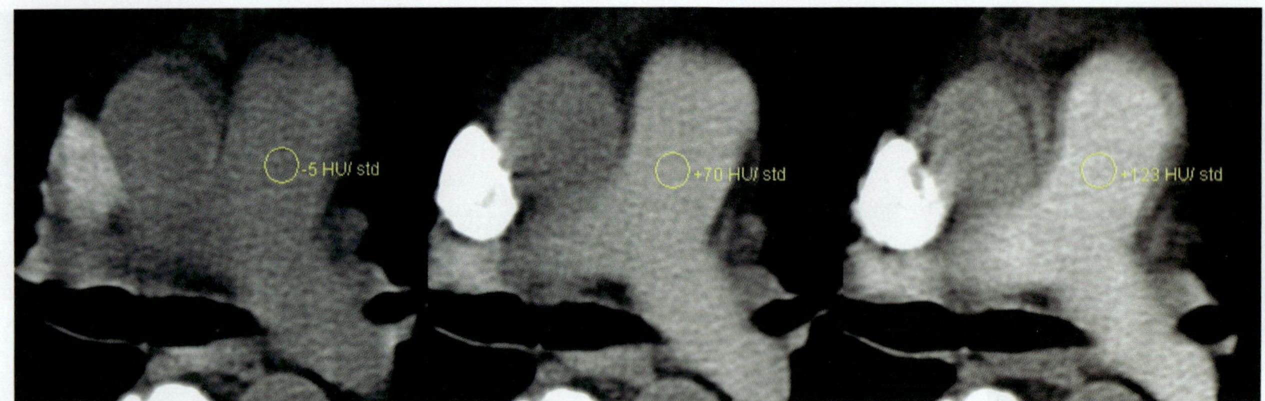

Figure 11.20 Example of bolus tracking for CT pulmonary embolus protocol. The region of interest is placed in the main pulmonary artery. The scanner initiates as soon as the contrast attenuation reaches threshold (here set at 100 HU).

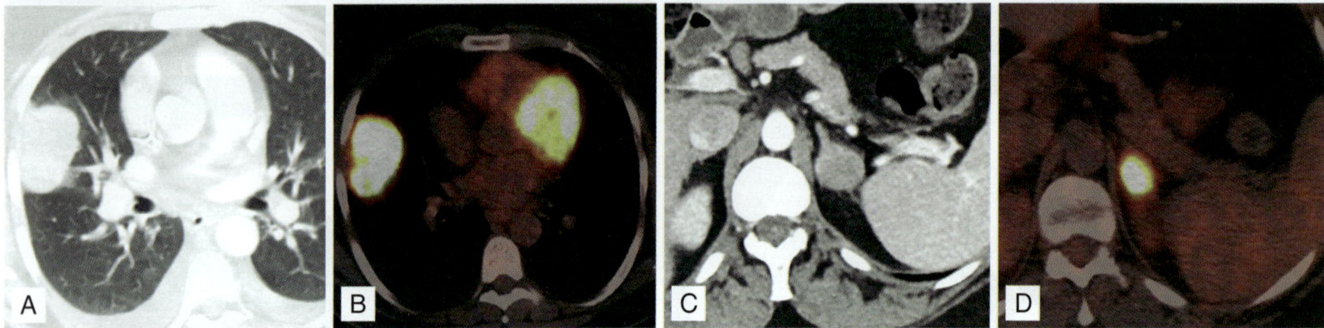

Figure 11.21 PET-CT staging for metastatic stage 4 primary lung cancer. Large FDG-avid right upper lobe mass is noted on PET-CT chest (A and B) and FDG-avid left adrenal metastasis (C and D).

ratio of amount of uptake in a tissue per unit volume, and normalizing factor. An SUV of 2.5 is regarded as a threshold value to differentiate pathologic process and normal uptake. However, there is a significant overlap of SUV for differentiating benign and malignant pathological processes [28,29]. Thus, subjective assessment of ^{18}F-FDG uptake in thoracic lesions and comparison with mediastinal blood pool is useful. If the ^{18}F-FDG uptake in the lesion is less than mediastinal blood pool, it is considered negative, and if it is equal to mediastinal blood, it is equivocal. If the ^{18}F-FDG uptake in the lesion is greater than the mediastinum, it is considered positive.

PET-CT

Integration of PET with cross-sectional imaging such as CT and MR can overcome the limitation of poor spatial resolution of PET, and also allow for anatomic and functional correlation [29]. The most common method of PET-CT integration is using a single scanner that sequentially obtains both CT and PET images. The major advantage of single scanner acquisition is the avoidance or mitigation of image misregistration artifacts, besides avoiding repeat patient visit [30]. To avoid for attenuation correction artifacts, the obtained CT images can be of lower diagnostic quality or may otherwise be of full diagnostic quality.

PET-MR

In PET-MR, MR and PET images can be either obtained concurrently using a single combined gantry or sequentially with individual machines adjacent to each other during the same examination [31,32]. Usually, a single short MR sequence is obtained for both anatomic correlation and PET attenuation correction, although additional sequences such as diffusion-weighted imaging, perfusion-weighted imaging, MR spectroscopy, and functional imaging can be performed [32].

The advantages and disadvantages of PET-CT and PET-MR are summarized in Table 11.2. The pitfalls of these techniques are summarized in Table 11.3.

TABLE 11.2 Advantages and Disadvantages of PET-CT and PET-MR

	PET-CT	PET-MR
Advantages	Widely available Quick imaging Better pulmonary spatial resolution	Lesser radiation risk Multiplanar imaging Better soft tissue resolution Additional functional imaging available such as diffusion-weighted imaging, MR spectroscopy, perfusion imaging
Disadvantages	Higher radiation risk Diminished resolution for pathologies in pleura, heart, liver, brain, bone marrow	Higher cost of equipment Standard contraindications to MRI examination apply to PET-MR

TABLE 11.3 Pitfalls of PET-CT and PET-MR

	PITFALLS	
Result	**Pulmonary Conditions**	**Extrapulmonary Conditions**
False-positive PET-CT and PET-MR	Infections TB and non-TB mycobacteria Histoplasmosis *Pneumocystis jiroveci* Sarcoidosis Pneumonitis: radiation or aspiration or drug induced Pulmonary fibrosis: active or progressive massive Postsurgical changes Connective tissue diseases Image misregistration artifacts	Infections TB and non-TB mycobacteria Histoplasmosis Sarcoidosis Silicone granuloma Normal mediastinal uptake Iatrogenic metal or talc Thymic hyperplasia Reactive lymph nodes Image misregistration artifacts
False-negative PET-CT and PET-MR	Pulmonary nodules <1 cm Carcinoid tumor Adenocarcinoma in situ Metastasis from mucinous adenocarcinoma and renal cell carcinoma Image misregistration artifacts Hyperglycemia	Normal mediastinal uptake Image misregistration artifacts Hyperglycemia

MRI

The applications of MRI in chest include assessment of mediastinal and pleural pathologies (Fig. 11.22), delineation of lung cancer from adjacent postobstructive atelectasis, cystic fibrosis follow-up, and characterization of pulmonary nodules more than 1 cm in size. Additionally, MRI is increasingly used for screening of hematologic disorders such as chronic lymphocytic leukemia and lymphoma, paragangliomas, teratomas, carcinoid tumors, and endometriosis [33,34].

Technical Considerations

Breath Holding

Respiratory motion artifacts affect the image quality of MRI chest study, which can be diminished by either respiratory gating or optimum breath holding [33,34]. Ideally, breath holding should not be exceeded above 20 seconds. In patients with difficulty in breath holding, 2 L nasal cannula oxygen can be used.

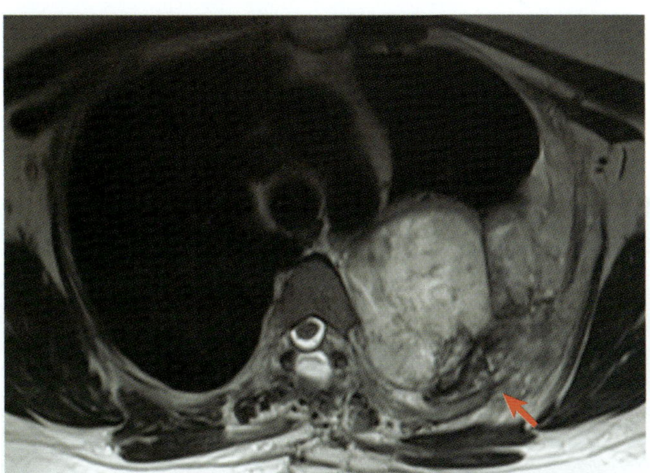

Figure 11.22 Askin's tumor. T2-weighted axial MRI image shows a large lobulated heterogenous chest wall lesion causing rib destruction (*arrow*). It shows both intra thoracic and extra thoracic extension.

Free Breathing

With the availability of sequences such as steady state-free precession, free breathing can be permitted and images can be acquired in coronal and sagittal planes.

Cardiac Gating

Cardiac gating can be performed as an Electrocardiogram (ECG) gating or peripheral gating [33,34]. With ECG gating, MR-compatible ECG leads are placed on the chest of patient previous to imaging. In peripheral gating, photosensors are placed on the patient's finger for pulse detection. Although requiring more time, ECG gating enables image acquisition during specific cardiac cycle phase, and is thus regarded superior to peripheral gating. ECG gating allows for the minimization of motion artifact due to cardiac contraction motion.

Slice Thickness

Typically, a slice thickness of equal to or more than 4 mm is preferred for thoracic MRI [33,34]. The only exception is breath-hold 3D ultrafast gradient-echo T1-weighted images, which can be obtained at 3-mm thickness.

MRI Sequences

T1-Weighted Imaging

Primary T1W sequence for thoracic MRI is breath-hold dual-echo in- and out-of-phase GRE or chemical shift MRI and usually takes about 20 seconds to image [33–35]. If a better signal quality is desired, a breath-hold ECG-gated double IR T1-weighted sequence can be performed. Chemical shift T1WI can additionally detect microscopic fat.

T2-Weighted Imaging

Breath-hold EKG-gated double IR T2-weighted pulse sequence is preferred for T2WI [35]. The limitation with this sequence is slower imaging as it acquires only one slice per 20 seconds.

Respiratory-triggered, multishot fast spin-echo T2WI is performed to assess larger lesions.

Dynamic Contrast-Enhanced Imaging

To assess the pattern and rate of contrast enhancement, dynamic contrast-enhanced (DCE) imaging is useful [33,35]. Previous to DCE, precontrast images are performed in the specific planes of desired postcontrast imaging with different timings, ranging from 20 to 30 seconds postgadolinium injection, to delayed imaging at 5 minutes or more postgadolinium injection.

Optional Sequences

Depending upon the lesion characterization, additional sequences can be acquired such as diffusion-weighted imaging, breath-hold or respiratory-triggered STIR sequences, ECG-gated double IR T1-weighted imaging [33,35].

Tissue Characterization with MRI in Chest

Cystic Lesions and Fluid Collections

Most nonhemorrhagic cystic lesions and fluid collections are hyperintense on T2WI. On postcontrast scans, these are nonenhancing or may show rim enhancement, with the exception being certain lymphangiomatous lesions [33,36]. Any evidence of irregular, nodular or asymmetric wall enhancement suggests multilocular lesions or neoplasms. Based on the proteinaceous content, the T1 signal can be hypointense for serous, and iso-to-hyperintense for proteinaceous fluid.

Blood and Blood Products

Depending upon the time since hemorrhage, blood will show variability in signal intensity. On T1WI, methemoglobin shows hyperintense signal, on T2WI, it is hypointense if intracellular, and hyperintense if extracellular. When there is chronic recurrent hemorrhage, it appears as T2-hypointense or as T2 shading. Hemosiderin is hypointense on both T1 and T2WI [34,36].

Fat

MRI can detect macroscopic fat on T1 and T2WI and confirmed on fat suppression sequences [34,35]. For microscopic fat, chemical shift MRI or in and opposed phase sequences are useful, wherein the presence of microscopic fat the signal drops on opposed phase sequences.

Other Tissues

The presence of cartilaginous tissue gives higher signal on T2WI and low signal on T1WI due to higher water content [34,35]. Smooth muscle and fibrous tissues are T2 hypointense. Lesion vascularity determined by blood vessels can be better evaluated at DCE imaging.

MRI versus CT: Benefits and Pitfalls

Although CT is a faster scanning technique and offers better evaluation of pulmonary pathologies compared with MRI, MRI has proved useful due to lack of ionizing radiation, and better tissue characterization [33]. The advantages of MRI are summarized as follows:

1. Evaluation of contents of cystic and solid lesions such as blood, fluid, protein, or fat (microscopic or macroscopic)
2. Delineation of lesion complexity such as nodular component, septations, wall irregularities
3. Better tissue characterization of muscles, cartilage, tendons, ligaments, blood vessels and nerves, and thus increasing accuracy of staging malignant tumors when involving the nerves, vessels, esophagus, or chest wall

Ultrasound

Transthoracic ultrasound (USG) of the chest is useful to evaluate diseases of the peripheral parenchymal, pleura, and chest wall. With the availability of cross-sectional imaging techniques including CT and MRI the role of USG in image guided interventional procedures of the chest and pleural space, has superseded its diagnostic utility (Fig. 11.23). Additional role of USG is for bedside imaging in the intensive care unit, where the obtained chest radiographs may be diagnostically suboptimal. Although performing USG, a 2–5-MHz curvilinear probe helps visualize deeper structures with a wider field of view and a high-resolution 7.5–10-MHz linear probe is useful for greater detail of chest wall, pleural, or peripheral lung. The normal chest wall appearance is of echogenic layers of soft tissues which correspond to muscle layers and fascial planes. The ribs are echogenic structures with distal acoustic shadowing. The visceral and parietal portions of the pleura appear as two echogenic lines deep to the ribs which slide over each other. *The normal movement of the lung relative to the chest wall has been described as the "lung sliding" sign.* Limited use of both grayscale and color Doppler imaging help in abnormality assessment for pleural diseases (pleural effusion, mesothelioma, pneumothorax), parenchymal diseases (pneumonia, neoplasms), and chest wall abnormalities (masses, rib fracture).

Anatomy

Trachea and Bronchi

The trachea is a midline tubular structure, which extends from cricoid cartilage to carina and allows the passage of air from the larynx to the bronchi of the lungs (Fig. 11.24). It is composed

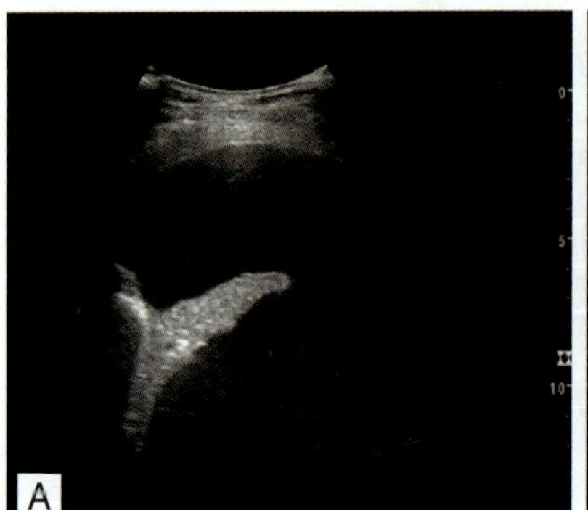

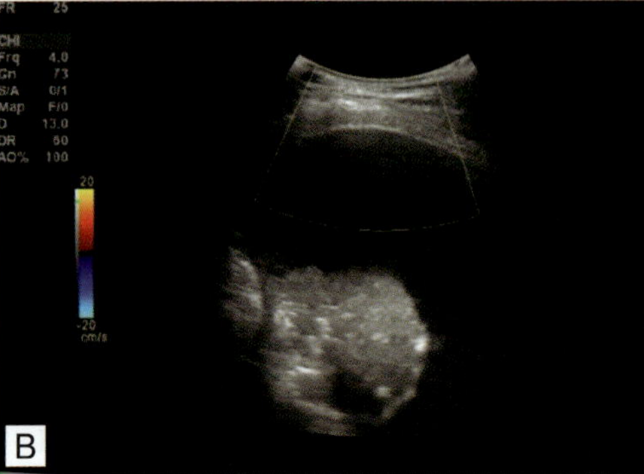

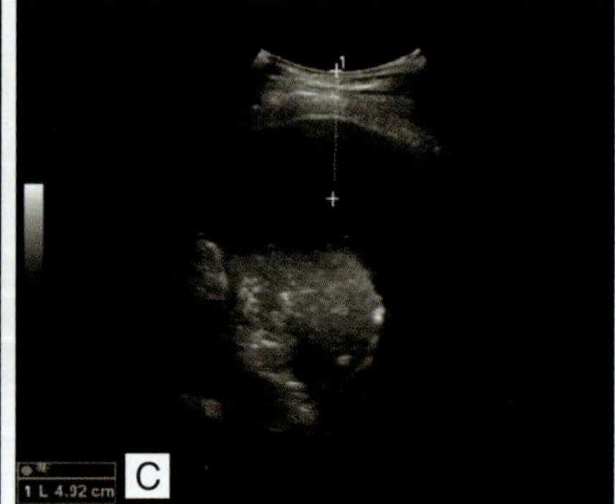

Figure 11.23 Pleural effusion as visualized in grayscale (A) and Doppler (B) ultrasound. Image C shows the calipers before thoracentesis.

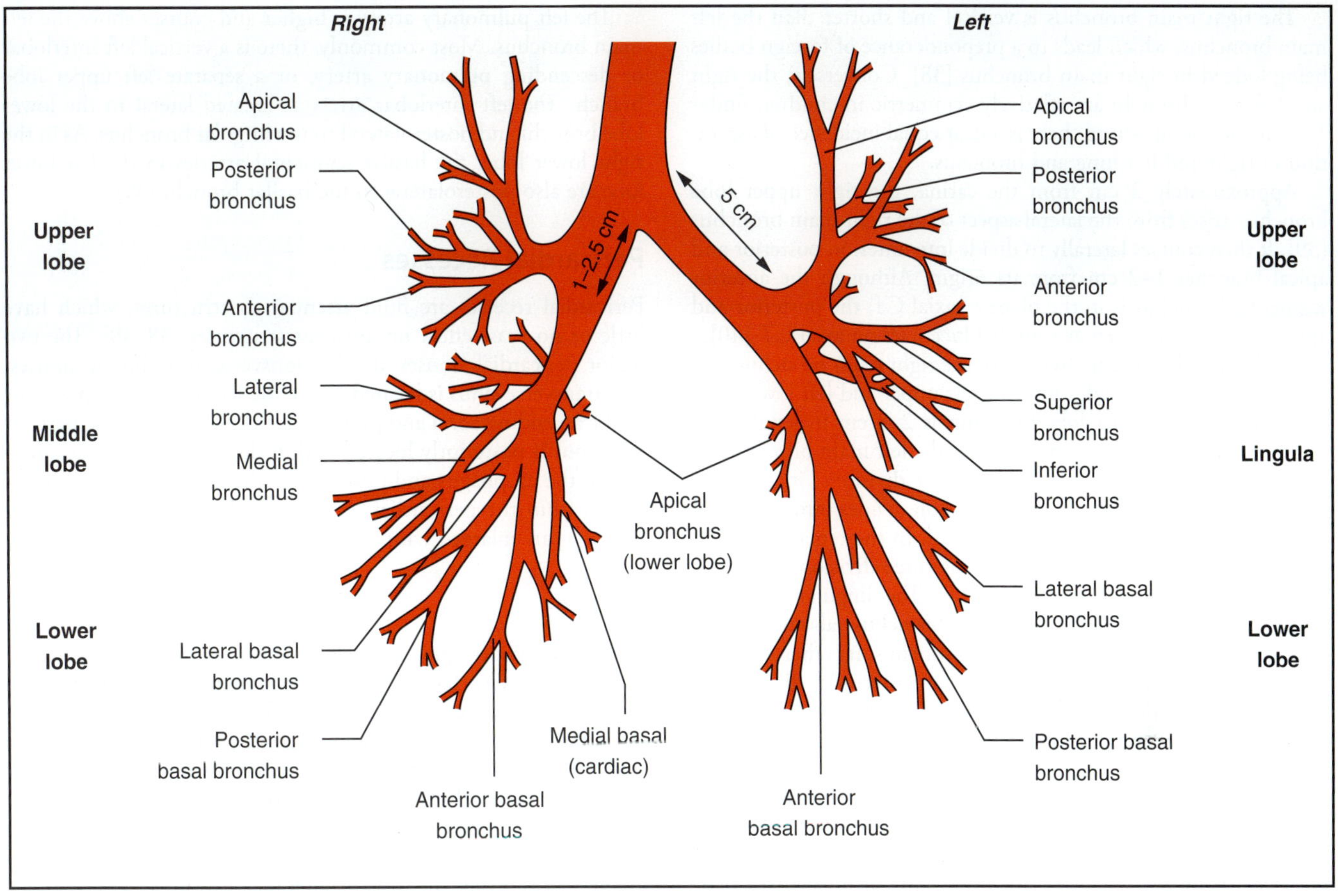

Right
Left
Upper lobe
Apical bronchus
Posterior bronchus
Anterior bronchus
Middle lobe
Lateral bronchus
Medial bronchus
Lower lobe
Lateral basal bronchus
Posterior basal bronchus
Anterior basal bronchus
Medial basal (cardiac)
1–2.5 cm
5 cm
Apical bronchus (lower lobe)
Apical bronchus
Posterior bronchus
Upper lobe
Anterior bronchus
Superior bronchus
Inferior bronchus
Lingula
Lateral basal bronchus
Lower lobe
Posterior basal bronchus
Anterior basal bronchus

Figure 11.24 Illustration showing tracheo-bronchial tree.

of cartilaginous and fibromuscular tissue and measures 6–9 cm in length. The tracheal wall contains 16–22 horseshoe-shaped cartilage rings connected by annular ligaments [37,38]. Transverse smooth muscle fibers form the posterior membranous wall of trachea. The trachea is innervated by the recurrent laryngeal nerve, the vagus nerve, and sympathetic trunks. The left recurrent laryngeal nerve loops at the arch of aorta and runs within the tracheoesophageal groove [39]. Blood supply to trachea is from branches of inferior thyroidal, intercostal, and bronchial arteries.

The trachea divides into right and left main bronchi at carina forming an angle called the interbronchial angle, which measures between 45 and 90 (usually 60) degrees [37]. The interbronchial or carinal angle can be widened by various pathologies such as left atrial enlargement (Fig. 11.25), subcarinal lymphadenopathy, lobar collapse, and large pericardial effusion.

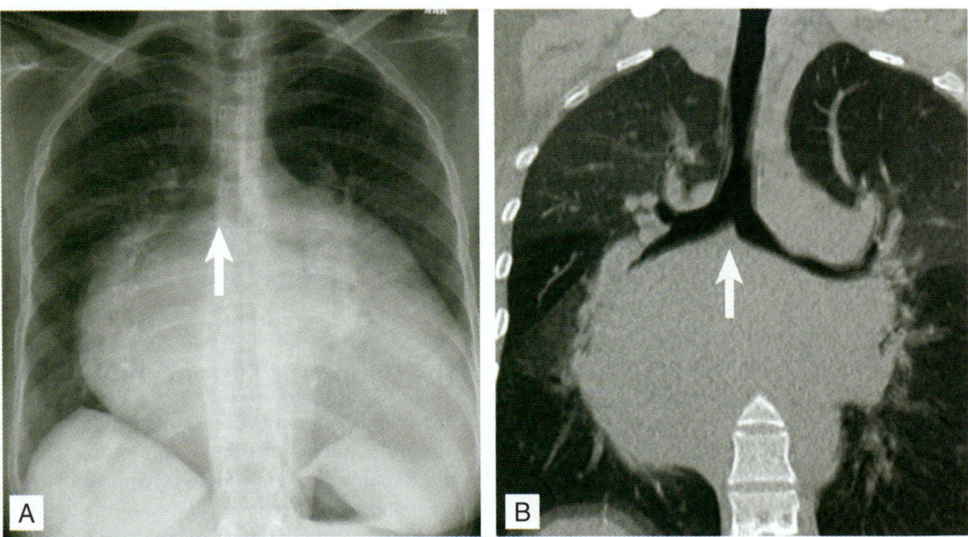

Figure 11.25 PA chest radiograph (A) demonstrating splaying of the carina secondary to left atrial enlargement (*arrow*) as demonstrated on corresponding CT chest (B).

The right main bronchus is vertical and shorter than the left main bronchus, which leads to a preponderance of foreign bodies being lodged in right main bronchus [38]. Conversely, the right and left main bronchi are relatively symmetric in children under 15 years of age, in whom there is a near equal incidence of aspiration in right and left lung and bronchus.

Approximately 2 cm from the carina, the right upper lobe bronchus arises from the lateral aspect of the right main bronchus [39]. It then courses laterally to divide into anterior, posterior and apical branches 1–2 cm from its origin. Although the anterior segmental bronchus is in the plane of axial CT, the posterior and apical bronchus are seen as rounded lucencies on axial CT [40].

At the level below the division of the right main bronchus, the left main bronchus divides into the left upper and left lower lobe bronchi. The left upper lobe bronchus is 2–3 cm in length and origins from the anterolateral aspect of the left main bronchus. It then bifurcates into superior and inferior divisions, in approximately 75% of cases. The superior division divides into the apical posterior and anterior segmental bronchi. In the remaining 25% cases, the left upper lobe bronchus has three divisions: anterior, apical posterior, and lingular bronchi. The lingular bronchus arises from the distal left upper lobe bronchus, about 1–2-cm inferior to origin of right middle lobe bronchus. It is then directed anteroinferiorly and obliquely for about 2–3 cm to divide into superior and inferior segmental bronchi [38–40]. The left lower lobe superior segmental bronchus arises within 1 cm of left lower lobe bronchus origin and then courses posteriorly and laterally. The truncus basalis arises inferior to the superior segmental bronchus. From the truncus, the basal segmental bronchi of the left lower lobe arises, which comprises the anteromedial, lateral, and posterior segments. There are many variants of normal tracheobronchial tree. The *tracheal bronchus*, found in 0.1–2% of the population, is a right upper lobe bronchus originating from the trachea. Most of these are on the right and represent displaced or supernumerary bronchi. The *accessory cardiac bronchus*, seen in 0.1% of individuals, arises from the medial aspect of bronchus intermedius or from right main bronchus. It then courses inferiorly for 1–5 cm toward heart or mediastinum [37,38]. Most of the accessory cardiac bronchi are blind-ending or may end in small bronchioles.

Pulmonary Vessels

The main pulmonary artery originates from the pulmonary valve to course posterosuperior and leftward to divide into left and right main pulmonary arteries. The right main pulmonary artery is longer and courses to the right. Posterior to ascending aorta, the right main pulmonary artery divides into the right upper lobe (truncus anterior) pulmonary anterior to right upper lobe bronchus, and the descending (interlobar) pulmonary artery. The truncus anterior divides into the segmental branches to right upper lobe [37,38]. As an anatomical variant, a separate branch originating from the interlobar artery can supply a portion of the right upper lobe posterior segment.

Anterolateral to the bronchus intermedius and posterior to right superior pulmonary artery is the right interlobar artery, originating from right main pulmonary artery. The right middle lobe pulmonary artery arises from the interlobar artery and courses laterally, parallel to the right middle lobe bronchus [39,40]. The right lower lobe pulmonary artery courses perpendicular to the axial scan plane and is visible as an ovoid structure at the level of origin of right middle lobe artery. Posterolateral to the basilar segmental bronchi are the basilar segmental pulmonary arteries.

The left pulmonary artery is higher and courses above the left main bronchus. Most commonly, there is a vertical left interlobar or descending pulmonary artery, or a separate left upper lobe branch. The left interlobar artery is located lateral to the lower lobe bronchi and posterolateral to the lingular bronchus. As in the right lower lobe, the basilar segmental arteries in the left lower lobe are also posterolateral to the basilar bronchi [39].

Pericardial Recesses

Pericardial recesses are fluid attenuation structures, which have little or no mass effect on adjacent structures [38–40]. The two major pericardial sinuses are the transverse and oblique sinuses. The transverse sinus is located above the left atrium and posterior to the ascending aorta and pulmonary trunk. The oblique pericardial sinus is posteriorly located within the pericardial space, anterior to the esophagus and posterior to the left atrium. Significant fluid within the pericardial recesses can be sometimes misinterpreted as an enlarged lymph node or a cystic lesion.

Fissures

Fissures are viscera pleural-lined thin structures that separate the lobes of the lungs (Fig. 11.26) [37,38]. Frequently, the fissures are incomplete. The *major fissures* courses from the fifth thoracic vertebra superiorly, to the diaphragm inferiorly, roughly paralleling the sixth rib. The medial portions of the major fissures are more anteriorly, above the level of hila. Conversely, the lateral portions of the major fissures lie more anteriorly, below the hila. The major fissure is visible on lateral radiograph but is not seen on a frontal radiograph. Occasionally, the superolateral major fissure can be seen as a curved line near the hilum when extrapleural fat enters the edge of the fissure to contact the posterior chest wall [40]. The *minor fissure*, which separates the anterior segment of the right upper lobe from the middle lobe, extends anteriorly and laterally from the right hilum to the lateral chest wall. In at least 50% patients, it is visible on frontal radiograph [39].

Accessory fissures are present in up to 30% of patients. The common accessory fissures include the azygos fissure, the superior accessory fissure, the inferior accessory fissure, and the left minor fissure [37–39]. The azygos fissure is formed by the downward invagination of the azygos vein through the apical right upper lobe (Fig. 11.27). It creates a curvilinear reflection that extends obliquely from the upper aspect of the right lung to terminate in a teardrop azygos vein shadow. The portion of the lung medial to this fissure is the azygos lobe. The inferior accessory fissure seen in up to 16% patients, can be seen on right or left and separates the medial basal segment from the remaining lower lobe segments. It extends superomedial from the inner third of the hemidiaphragm [39,40]. The superior accessory fissure divides the superior segment from the basal segments of lower lobe. It is horizontal and more commonly seen on the right. The left minor fissure divides the lingua from the superior division of the left upper lobe.

The Lymphatic System and Lymph Node Stations

The lymphatics remove interstitial fluid and foreign particles. They run in the interlobular septa, connecting with subpleural lymphatics and draining through the deep lymphatics to the hilum, with valves controlling the direction of flow. Normal lymphatics are not seen but thickening of the lymphatics and surrounding connective tissue produces Kerley lines, which may be transient or persistent.

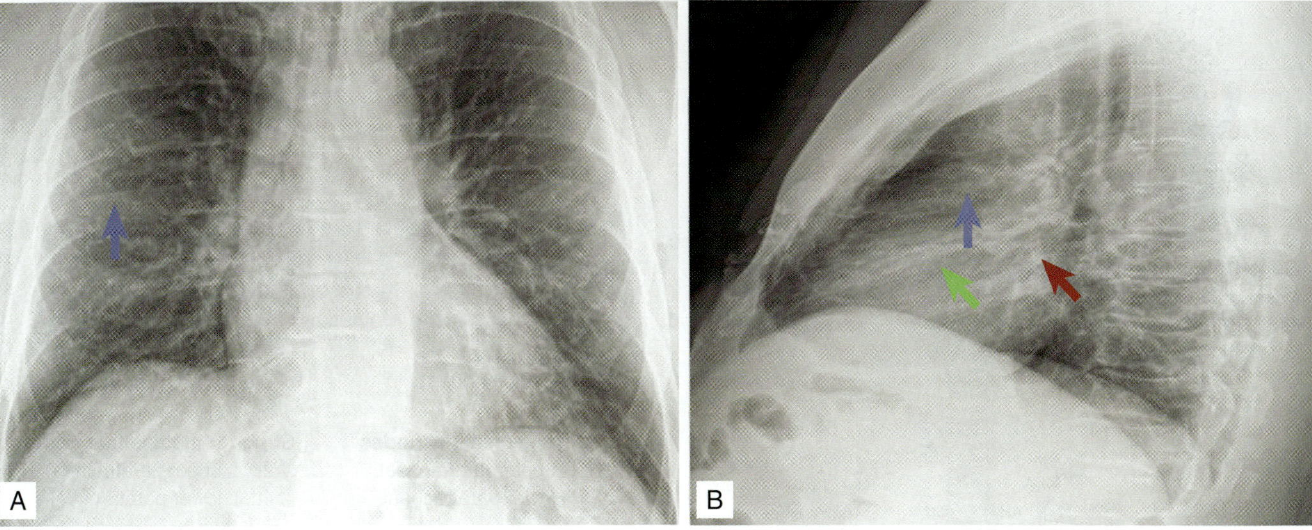

Figure 11.26 Example of the right minor fissure (*blue arrows*), right major fissure (*green arrow*), and left major fissure (*red arrow*) on PA (A) and lateral (B) chest radiographs.

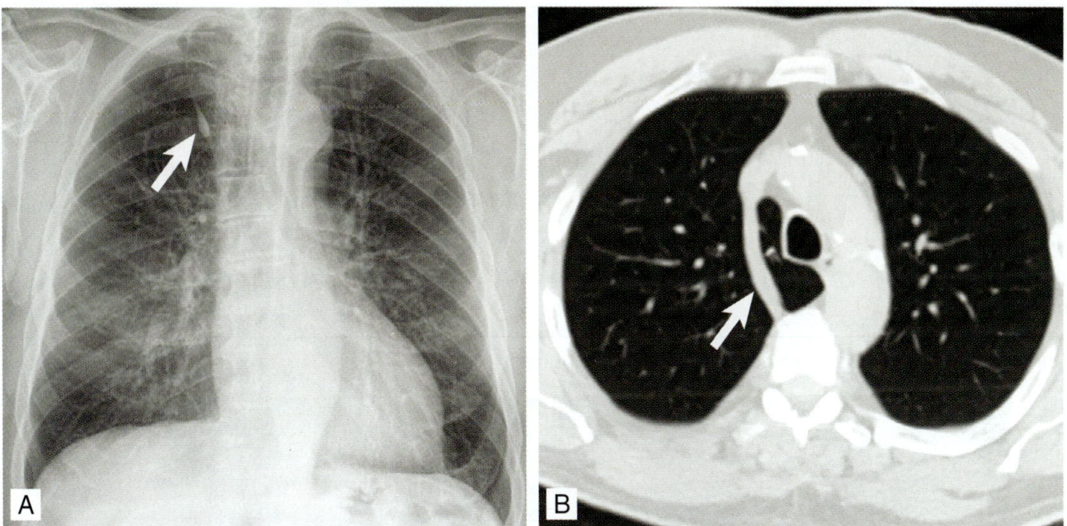

Figure 11.27 Example of an accessory azygos fissure on chest radiograph (A) and CT chest (B).

The intrapulmonary lymphatics drain directly to the bronchopulmonary nodes and this group is the first to be involved by spread from a peripheral tumor. The node map according to International Association for the Study of Lung Cancer is illustrated in Fig. 11.28. Extensive intercommunications exist between the groups but the pattern of nodal involvement can sometimes indicate the site of the primary tumor. Mediastinal nodes may be involved by tumors both above and below the diaphragm.

The Diaphragm

The diaphragm is a muscular tendinous sheath that separates the thoracic and abdominal cavities [37,39]. The right hemidiaphragm is usually found at the level of anterior right sixth rib. Usually, the right hemidiaphragm is higher by 1.5–2.5 cm or about one-half intercostal space than the left hemidiaphragm. There are three openings or hiatuses within the diaphragm to allow passage of structures between the abdomen and thorax. The first opening at T8 level contains the inferior vena cava and right phrenic nerve branches. At the T10 level pass the esophagus, vagus nerve, and sympathetic nerve branches. At the T12 level, the retrocrural aortic hiatus contains the descending aorta, azygos vein, hemiazygos vein, and thoracic duct [39,40].

Chest Radiograph

Frontal Projection

Mediastinal Contours

From cephalad to caudad, the structures forming the right mediastinal border are right brachiocephalic vein, SVC, azygos vein, and right atrium (Fig. 11.29) [11,12,41]. On the left, the subclavian artery and aortic knob forms the lateral margin of superior mediastinum.

Azygos Vein

The azygos vein runs anteriorly and inferiorly along the posterior tracheal wall at the T4-T5 vertebral level, and then laterally over the right main bronchus to terminate into SVC [11,41]. Thus, it forms an azygos arch bordered medially by air within the trachea and laterally by the aerated right upper lobe and is visualized as an ovoid density measuring less than 10 mm at the inferior aspect of right paratracheal stripe.

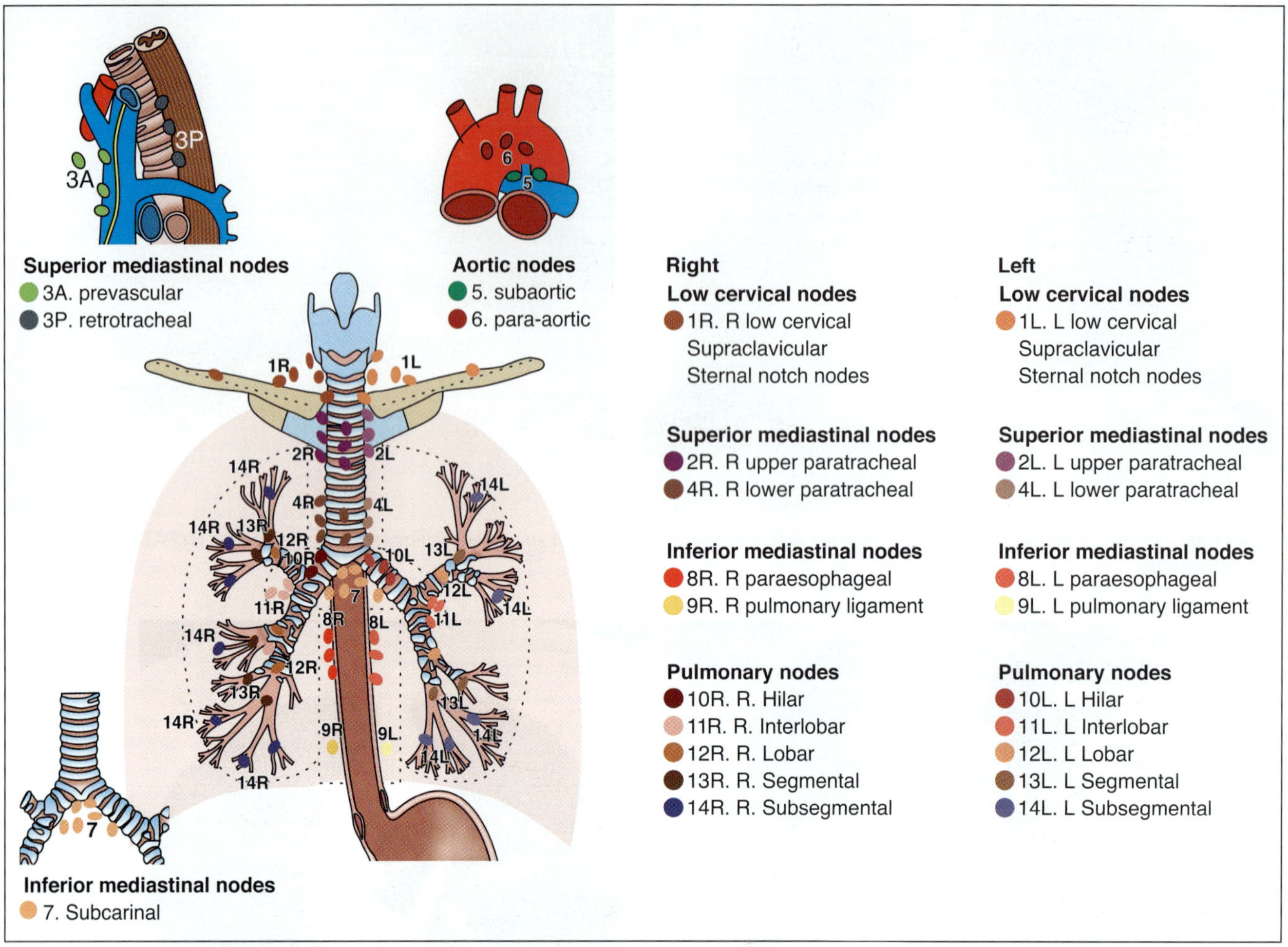

3A
3P
6
5
Superior mediastinal nodes
3A. prevascular
3P. retrotracheal
Aortic nodes
5. subaortic
6. para-aortic
1R
1L
2R
2L
4R
4L
10R
10L
11R
11L
12R
12L
13R
13L
14R
14L
7
8R
8L
9R
9L
Inferior mediastinal nodes
7. Subcarinal
Right
Low cervical nodes
1R. R low cervical
Supraclavicular
Sternal notch nodes
Superior mediastinal nodes
2R. R upper paratracheal
4R. R lower paratracheal
Inferior mediastinal nodes
8R. R paraesophageal
9R. R pulmonary ligament
Pulmonary nodes
10R. R. Hilar
11R. R. Interlobar
12R. R. Lobar
13R. R. Segmental
14R. R. Subsegmental
Left
Low cervical nodes
1L. L low cervical
Supraclavicular
Sternal notch nodes
Superior mediastinal nodes
2L. L upper paratracheal
4L. L lower paratracheal
Inferior mediastinal nodes
8L. L paraesophageal
9L. L pulmonary ligament
Pulmonary nodes
10L. L Hilar
11L. L Interlobar
12L. L Lobar
13L. L Segmental
14L. L Subsegmental

Figure 11.28 Illustration shows the IASLC lymph node map. *L.* = left, *R.* = right.

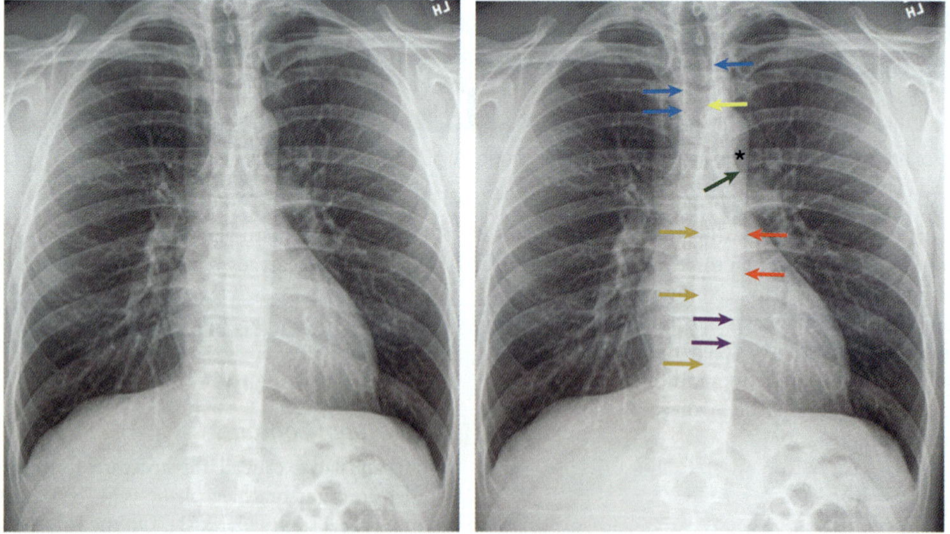

Figure 11.29 Example of normal PA chest radiograph with demonstration of the right and left paratracheal stripes (*blue arrows*), the anterior junction line (*yellow arrow*), the aortopulmonary window (*asterisk*), the aortopulmonary stripe (*green arrow*), the descending thoracic aorta (*red arrows*), the left paraspinal stripe (*purple arrows*), and the azygoesophageal recess (*brown arrows*). Note the oblique orientation of the anterior junction line from right to left over the superior two thirds of the sternum.

Paratracheal Stripes

The right paratracheal stripe is formed by visceral and parietal pleura of right upper lobe and is smooth, vertical line along the right brachiocephalic vein, and SVC measuring <4mm in thickness [11,41]. Superiorly, it extends up to the clavicle and inferiorly, it extends up to the level of azygos arch. It can be widened in paratracheal lymphadenopathy, mediastinal mass or inflammation, pleural pathologies, or malignant lesions of trachea, thyroid gland or parathyroid gland. In a minority of individuals, the left paratracheal stripe is formed by the interface between left upper lobe and left lateral tracheal wall or adjacent mediastinal fat [12]. Superior to inferior, it extends from the reflection of the left subclavian artery to the aortic arch.

Lines and Stripes

The anterior junctional line or stripe is formed by the approximation of visceral and parietal pleura of the anterior both lungs [12,41]. It is thus composed of four pleural layers and often a small amount of retrosternal fat or thymus gland is interposed in between the pleural reflections. It has an oblique course from right to left. The normal thickness of the anterior junction line is 1–3 mm. This line can be displaced by pathological changes in lung volume such as collapse or emphysema.

The posterior junction line or stripe is formed by the visceral and parietal pleural reflections of the right and left lungs anterior to the thoracic vertebral bodies, and posterior to the esophagus [41]. It is also therefore composed of four pleural layers and often some mediastinal fat. It is typically seen as a vertical line extending from the lung apices to the aortic arch. It is normally <1-cm thick.

The azygoesophageal line runs in a slight reverse-S– or reverse-C–shaped course and is formed by the contact of right lower lobe with the right wall of the esophagus and the azygos vein [41]. It is located anterior to vertebrae and posterolateral to the esophagus.

Aortic nipple is a round or triangular opacity sometimes visualized projecting from the lateral aspect of the aortic arch (Fig. 11.30) [11]. It is formed by the left superior intercostal vein as it arches anteriorly along the aortic arch to drain into left brachiocephalic vein, and measures less than 4.5 mm in diameter. It can be prominently seen when dilated, for example, in a setting of SVC or left brachiocephalic vein obstruction to provide collateral flow to hemiazygos and azygos veins [12].

The aortic-pulmonary reflection or aortic-pulmonary stripe is formed by the interface of mediastinal fat between the left lung laterally and main pulmonary artery and aorta medially [12,41]. It may be either straight or minimally curved at the lateral aspect.

Inferior to the aortopulmonary stripe, the left border of mediastinum is formed by the main pulmonary artery and the heart. The preaortic line is formed by the left lower lobe protruding anterior to the descending aorta and posterior to the heart. The left paraaortic interface is formed by the contact of lateral aspect of the descending thoracic aorta and the left lung [11].

Recesses

The azygoesophageal recess extends from the subcarinal space superiorly to the aortic hiatus inferiorly [41].

The supraaortic area is located in the left side of mediastinum, posterior to the anterior mediastinum [11,12]. Craniocaudally, it extends from thoracic inlet to aortic arch. The contents of this area include the left subclavian artery, left superior intercostal vein, left lateral tracheal wall, and mediastinal fat.

The aortopulmonary window (AP window) is a mediastinal space bounded by the aortic arch superiorly, left pulmonary artery inferiorly, ductus ligament medially, and parietal pleura and visceral pleura of left upper lobe laterally [12,41]. It contains mediastinal fat, left recurrent laryngeal nerve, left bronchial arteries, and lymph nodes. Normally, it is concave or straight on the left lateral aspect. Any convexity of AP window can be seen with the presence of a mediastinal pathology such as lymphadenopathy or focal saccular thoracic aortic aneurysm.

Hila

The hila can be divided into upper and lower zones. The upper portion of the right hilum is formed by the truncus anterior branch of the right pulmonary artery and the right superior pulmonary vein. The lower portion of the right hilum is formed by the right interlobar artery, the right superior pulmonary vein, and their branches. Medial to the right interlobar artery is the bronchus intermedius. Medial to the hilum is the right inferior pulmonary vein [11,12].

Inferior to the aortic arch and superior to the left main bronchus is the main pulmonary artery. The *upper portion of the left hilar opacity* is formed by the distal left pulmonary artery, the proximal left interlobar artery, the left superior pulmonary vein, and their branches. The upper left hilum may be partially obscured by adjacent mediastinal fat and cardiac silhouette [11,12]. The lower portion of the left hilum is formed by distal left interlobar artery and lingular artery and vein, and the left inferior pulmonary vein.

Enlarged pulmonary artery can cause hilar enlargement with central convergence of the pulmonary vasculature, named the hilar convergence sign (Fig. 11.31). Conversely in the presence of hilar mass or enlarged lymph node, there could be increased hilar density or prominent nodular contour.

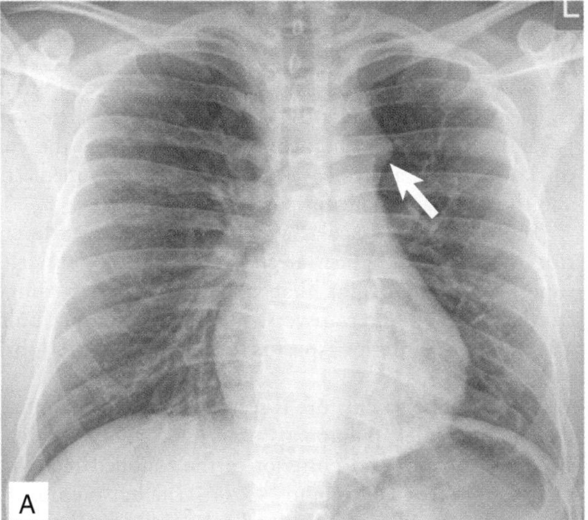

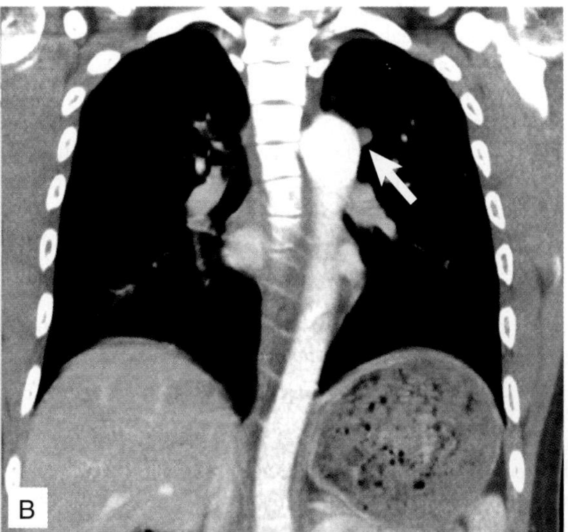

Figure 11.30 Example of a prominent aortic nipple on chest radiograph (A) corresponding to the left superior intercostal vein (B).

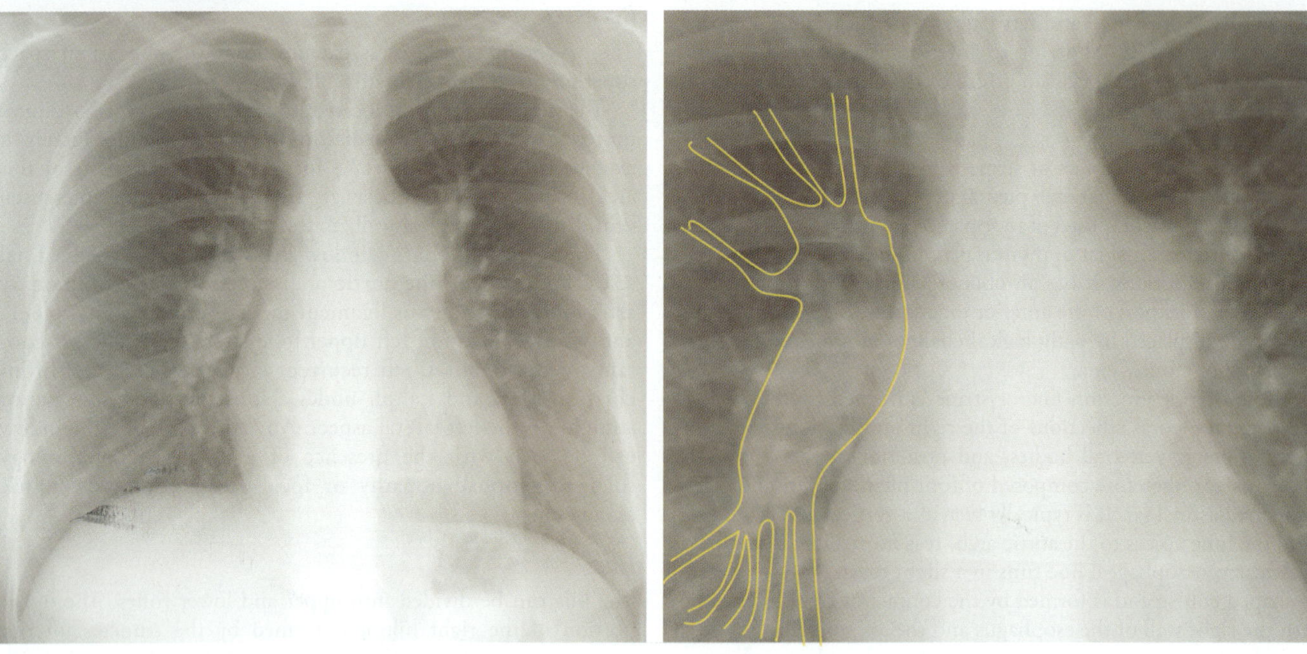

Figure 11.31 Example of hilar convergence sign with schematic drawing in setting of pulmonary artery enlargement and hypertension.

Lateral Projection

The following radiographic signs [42–44] can identify the right and left diaphragm on a lateral radiograph:

1. Magnified right ribs appear larger and more posteriorly located
2. Air-filled gastric bubble localizes the left diaphragm
3. Unlike the right diaphragm visible along its entire course, the anterior left hemidiaphragm is frequently obscured by the cardiac silhouette
4. Left diaphragm is slightly lower than the right

Mediastinal Contours on Lateral Projection

The trachea projects inferiorly and posteriorly in a vertical orientation on a lateral chest radiograph (Fig. 11.32). The anterior tracheal wall is obscured by the mediastinal fat and vessels, but the posterior tracheal stripe is formed by the interface of the right upper lobe with the trachea [44]. With variable mediastinal fat, sometimes, a thicker interface of anterior esophageal wall with the posterior tracheal wall and adjacent mediastinal fat, can be projected as tracheoesophageal stripe. Thus, the thickness of this stripe can be variable and can be up to 5.5 mm.

The most anteriorly positioned structures on a lateral view are the right ventricle and right ventricular outflow tract. The retrosternal stripe is the interface between the anterior lungs and the retrosternal soft tissues and contains fat and internal mammary vessels. It measures 7 mm or less in thickness. Inferiorly, its thickness is variable and can increase due to epicardial fat pad and adjacent cardiac apex, known as cardiac incisura [43].

Anterior to the right ventricle, main pulmonary artery, and ascending aorta, and posterior to the sternum is the retrosternal clear space. Any opacity in the retrosternal clear space may be indicative of a mediastinal pathology [42].

The radiolucent area posterior to the trachea and anterior to vertebral bodies is the retrotracheal or Raider triangle. Craniocaudally, it extends from the thoracic inlet to the aortic arch. It contains the thoracic duct, esophagus, left recurrent laryngeal nerve, mediastinal lymph nodes, and lungs [42,44]. The pathologies affecting this space are usually vascular, for example, an aberrant right subclavian artery (Fig. 11.33).

Hila on Lateral Projection

On the lateral view there is superimposition of the left and right hilar structures. At the level of the fourth or fifth thoracic vertebra is the carina [42,44]. Due to adjacent vascular structures, the right upper lobe bronchus is usually less well circumscribed as compared with the left upper lobe bronchus, and is seen as a rounded lucency along the anterior and superior aspect of the intermediate stem line. The intermediate stem line is formed by the posterior wall of the right main and intermediate bronchi and terminates at the level of termination of right lower lobe superior segmental bronchus. It measures up to 3 mm [43,44]. The distal left main bronchus is seen as a rounded lucency at the level of termination of tracheal air column inferiorly. It is continuous with the orifice of left upper bronchus and termed as the left main–upper lobe continuum [42–44].

The left retrobronchial line is formed by the approximation of posterior wall of the left main bronchus and proximal left lower lobe bronchus. It normally measures up to 3 mm in thickness and terminates at the left lower lobe superior segmental bronchus. It is located more posteriorly than the intermediate stem line [42,44]. The left retrobronchial stripe represents the combined thickness of the anterior wall of the esophagus, mediastinal fat, and the left main bronchus posterior wall.

The right hilar vascular opacity is formed by truncus anterior, the right pulmonary artery, and the interlobar artery. The superior aspect of right hilar vascular opacity is composed of truncus anterior and transverse portion of the right pulmonary artery, and the inferior aspect is formed by the interlobar artery [44].

The left hilar vasculature is seen posterior to the intermediate stem line. The left pulmonary artery is seen as a comma-shaped structure superior and posterior to the rounded radiolucent left main–upper lobe continuum [43,44]. The left pulmonary artery appears as a small aortic arch and is bordered by lung superiorly,

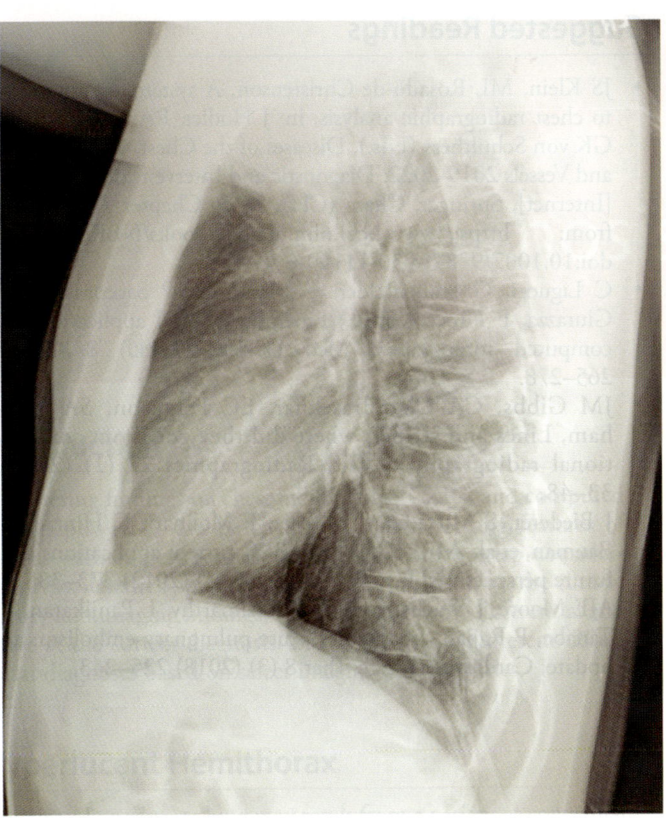

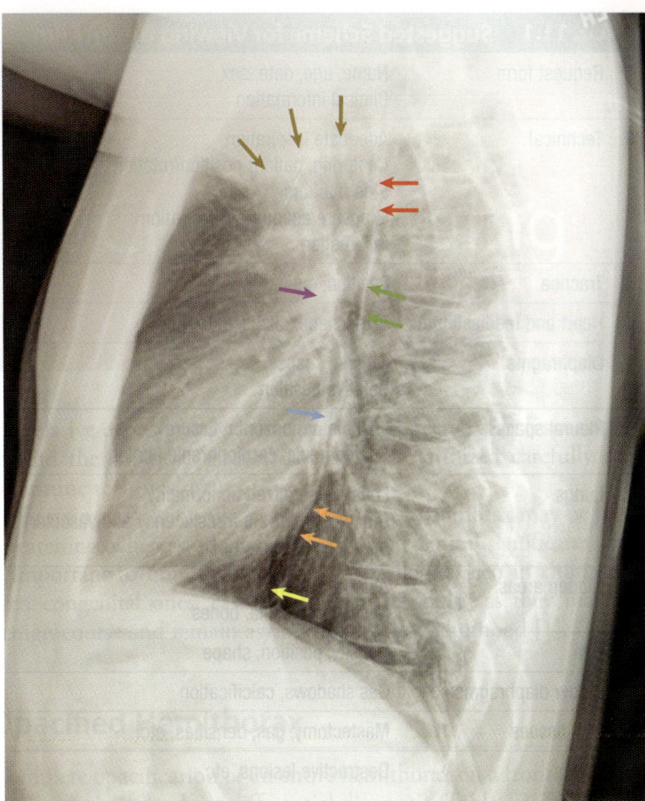

Figure 11.32 Example of normal lateral chest radiograph with demonstration of the posterior tracheal stripe (*red arrows*), the posterior wall of the bronchus intermedius (*green arrows*), the right pulmonary artery (*purple arrow*), the aortic arch (*brown arrows*), the pulmonary veins (*blue arrow*), the border of the left atrium (*orange arrows*), and the inferior vena cava (*yellow arrow*).

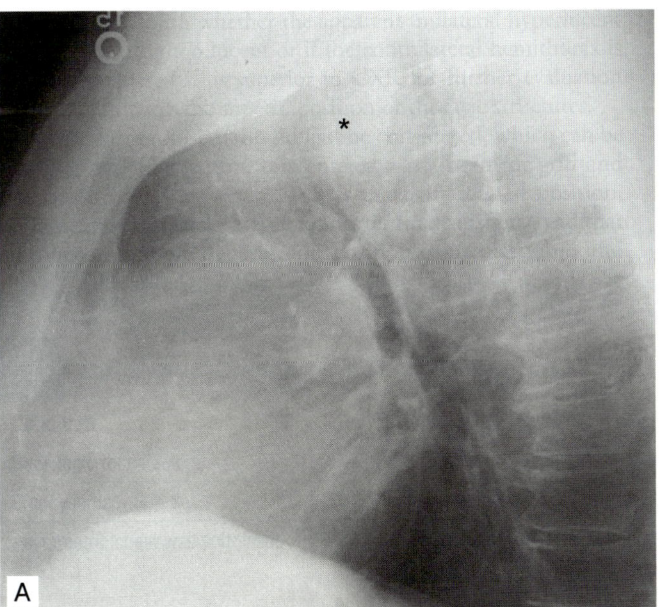

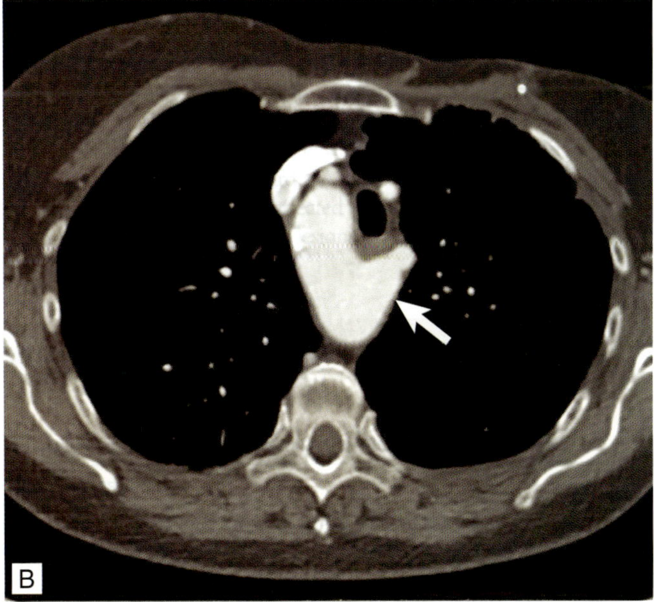

Figure 11.33 Example of aberrant left subclavian artery, which on lateral chest radiograph (A) appears as an opacity within the Raider triangle (*asterisk*). Accompanying CT chest (B) demonstrating the aberrant retroesophageal course of the left subclavian artery.

The left superior pulmonary vein does not contribute to the hilar contour on the lateral radiograph.

Inferior hilar window is the avascular region located below the right hilar vascular opacity and anterior to the comma-shaped left pulmonary artery. It is bounded by the right middle lobe bronchus anteriorly and the left lower lobe bronchus posteriorly [43,44]. A nodular opacity more than 1 cm in the inferior hilar window can be suspicious for a mass or enlarged lymph node.

Summary

Box 11.1 suggests the schematic assessment of a chest radiograph.

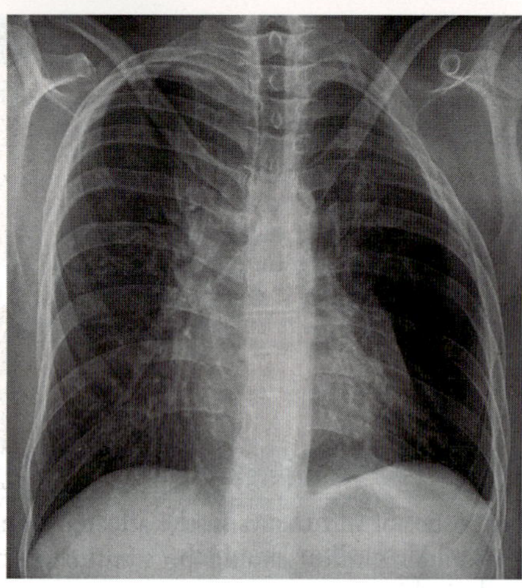

Figure 12.1 Frontal chest radiograph of a 38-year-old male with Poland syndrome shows a hyperlucent left hemithorax with left upper chest wall deformity.

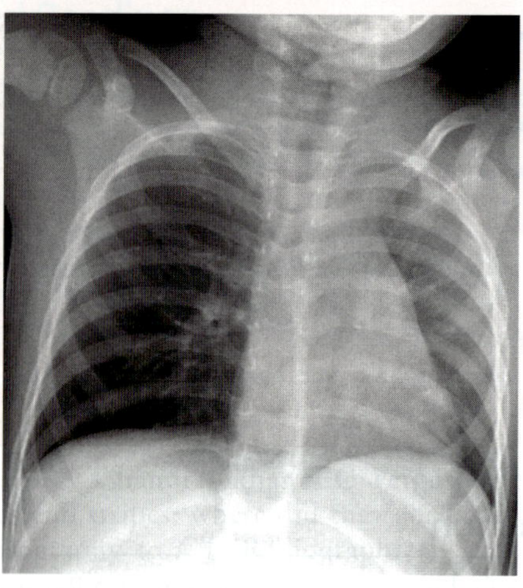

Figure 12.2 Frontal chest radiograph of a 2-year-old female with acute dyspnea demonstrates hyperlucent and expanded right hemithorax with mediastinal shift to the left. Bronchoscopy reveals an obstructing foreign body in the right main bronchus.

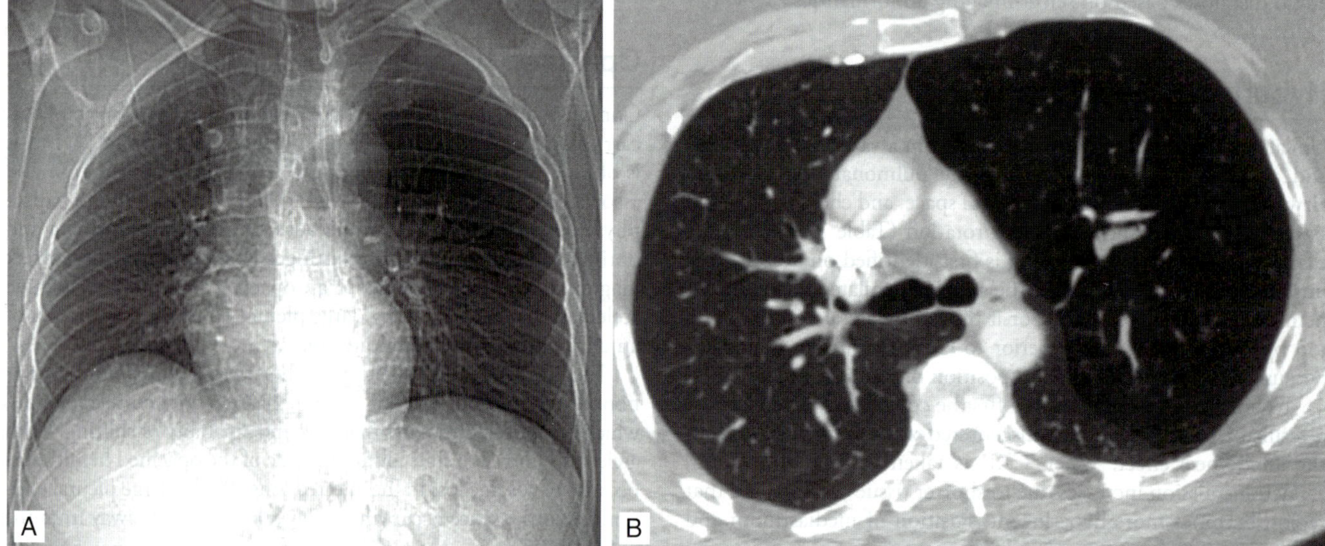

Figure 12.3 Chest CT images of a 49-year-old male show a hyperlucent left hemithorax on the scout image (A), which corresponds to hyperinflation and lucency of apicoposterior left upper lobe associated with an atretic segmental bronchus shown on axial CT image (B), consistent with congenital lobar hyperinflation and bronchial atresia.

TABLE 12.2 Differential Diagnoses in Those Presenting With an Opacified Hemithorax on Chest Radiograph

Condition	Distinguishing Features
Atelectasis of entire lung	Ipsilateral mediastinal shift and elevated hemidiaphragm; underlying cause often main stem endobronchial lesion (Fig. 12.4)
Large pleural effusion	Contralateral mediastinal shift
Pneumonia of an entire lung	No significant mediastinal shift; air bronchogram may be present
Postpneumonectomy appearance (Fig. 12.5)	Evidence of surgery (surgical clips and thoracotomy); ipsilateral mediastinal shift
Large pulmonary, pleural, or chest wall mass	Examples include mesothelioma and Ewing sarcoma; no significant mediastinal shift or mild contralateral shift
Pulmonary hypoplasia or agenesis (Fig. 12.6)	Ipsilateral mediastinal shift

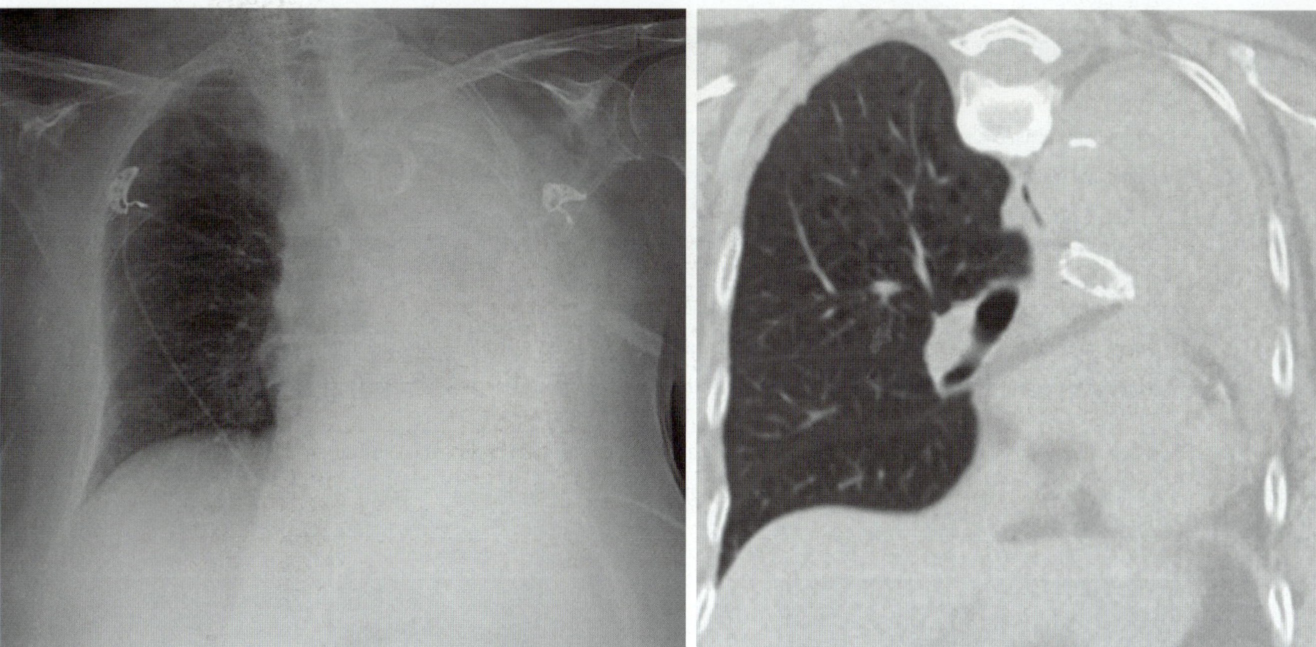

Figure 12.4 Frontal chest radiograph (A) and CT scan (B) of a 77-year-old female with known lung cancer show complete atelectasis of the left lung secondary to tumor occlusion of left mainstem bronchus.

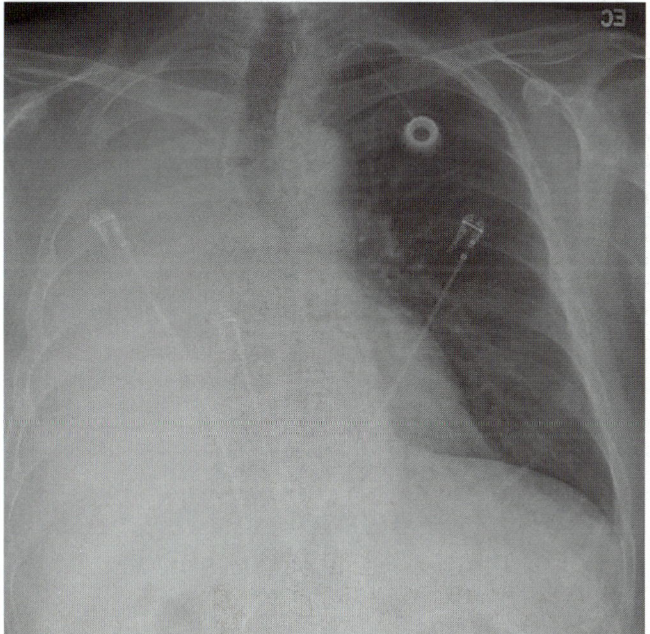

Figure 12.5 Frontal chest radiograph of a 65-year-old female status after right pneumonectomy shows expected complete opacification of the right hemithorax.

side of opacification due to the mass effect exerted by the large pleural effusion. With pneumonia of most or the entire lung, there is usually no significant shift, but air bronchograms may be present. In the postpneumonectomy patient, there is eventually volume loss on the side from which the lung has been removed.

Elevated Hemidiaphragm

When both diaphragms are elevated, the cause is usually diminished lung volumes or symmetric intra-abdominal disease.

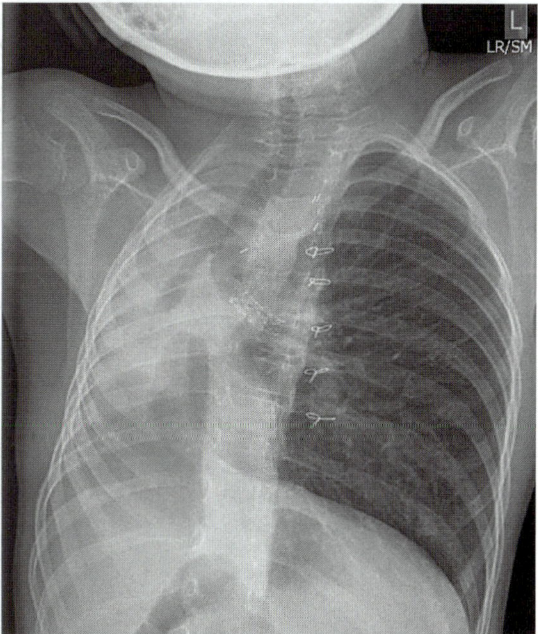

Figure 12.6 Frontal chest radiograph of an 8-year-old female with right pulmonary agenesis shows opacification of small right hemithorax with mediastinal shift to the right. The left lung is well-inflated.

An elevated hemidiaphragm has a more specific differential diagnosis (Table 12.3). A subpulmonary effusion can also mimic hemidiaphragmatic elevation (Fig. 12.7).

Widened Superior Mediastinum

Superior mediastinal widening is a common observation on CXRs. It is more difficult to identify confidently on a supine AP view because of magnification and crowding of normal vascular structures. In addition, a lordotic projection distorts and

TABLE 12.3 Differential Diagnoses in Those Presenting With Apparent Hemidiaphragmatic Elevation

	Condition	Distinguishing Features
Above	Diminished lung volume	Atelectasis or pulmonary hypoplasia; previous lobectomy recognized by rib defects and surgical clips
	Subpulmonary pleural effusion	Represents only apparent (not actual) diaphragm elevation; dome of the diaphragm more lateral than normal; ipsilateral decubitus positioning can confirm diagnosis
Diaphragm	Phrenic nerve paralysis	Causes include mediastinal masses including lung cancer (Fig. 12.8), or iatrogenesis; fluoroscopy demonstrates paradoxic motion (*positive sniff test*)
	Diaphragmatic hernia	May be due to Morgagni or Bochdalek hernia
	Diaphragmatic tumor	Consider mesothelioma, lipoma, and fibroma; serial radiographs may show growth with time
	Traumatic diaphragmatic rupture (Fig. 12.9)	Other signs of chest and/or abdominal trauma are evident; liver herniation may simulate elevated right hemidiaphragm
	Diaphragmatic eventration	Weakness and thinning of the diaphragm; no paradoxic motion on fluoroscopy (*negative sniff test*)
Below	Abdominal disease	Consider subphrenic abscess or mass and Chilaiditi syndrome; ultrasound best test for confirming subphrenic abscess

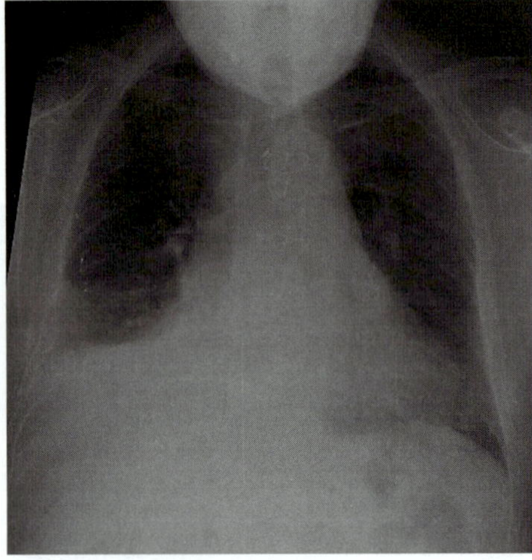

Figure 12.7 Frontal chest radiograph of a 70-year-old male with congestive heart failure shows a moderate right subpulmonary pleural effusion mimicking elevation of the right hemidiaphragm.

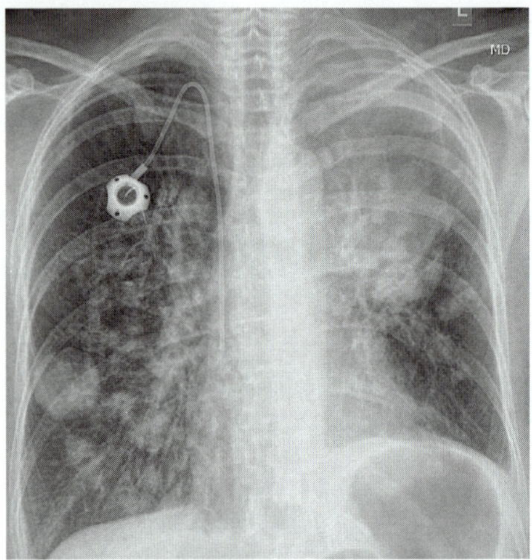

Figure 12.8 Frontal chest radiograph of a 61-year-old female with metastatic left upper lobe lung cancer shows elevated left hemidiaphragm, consistent with phrenic nerve paralysis secondary to tumor invasion.

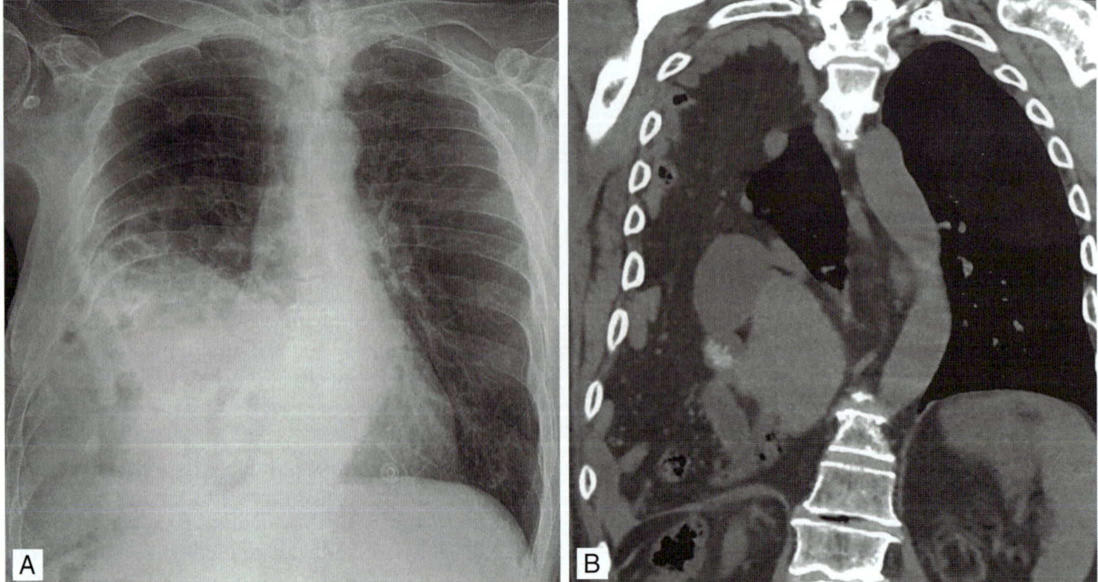

Figure 12.9 Frontal chest radiograph (A) and CT scan (B) of a 68-year-old male with history of trauma show a large right diaphragmatic hernia containing portions of the liver, gallbladder with stones, gastric antrum, duodenum, and hepatic flexure.

TABLE 12.4 Differential Diagnoses in Those Presenting With Apparent Superior Mediastinal Widening

Condition	Distinguishing Features
Radiographic technique	Magnification (anteroposterior supine chest radiograph, low-volume inspiration); lordotic position
Adenopathy	Neoplasms (lymphoma, small cell lung cancer [Fig. 12.10], metastases); infection (*Mycobacterium avium-intracellulare*, tuberculosis, coccidioidomycosis, sarcoidosis)
Traumatic vascular injury/hematoma	Traumatic vascular injuries include aortic injury, venous and arterial tears, postoperative bleeding, malposition of vascular catheters; traumatic hematomas caused by sternal or vertebral fractures
Nontraumatic vascular etiology	Tortuous atherosclerotic dilation of aorta, aneurysm (Fig. 12.11), aortic dissection, or coarctation of aorta
Mediastinitis	Causes include perforated esophagus, tracheobronchial rupture, iatrogenic (postoperative, endoscopic), fibrosing or sclerosing mediastinitis, extension of extrathoracic infections
Lipomatosis	Cushing syndrome, corticosteroid therapy, obesity

magnifies the superior mediastinum. Widening of the mediastinum is a common observation that may be related to patient body habitus or atherosclerotic dilatation of the aorta and great vessels, but there may also be urgent causes such as aortic dissection or traumatic aortic injury. Less urgent but serious conditions that widen the mediastinum include acute mediastinitis, fibrosing mediastinitis, and tumors, including lymphoma and metastases (Table 12.4).

Hilar Enlargement

In the evaluation of hilar enlargement, the first step is to differentiate vascular enlargement from hilar masses. The normal hilar contours are formed by the pulmonary arteries. In cases with bilateral hilar enlargement, it may be difficult to distinguish vascular enlargement from masses. Unilateral hilar enlargement also requires careful evaluation but is more suggestive of a mass [2] (Table 12.5).

The *hilum overlay sign* (Fig. 12.12) is useful in differentiating whether an opacity on a frontal CXR in the region of the hilum is located within the hilum versus anterior or posterior to it. *When the borders of the pulmonary arteries are clearly identifiable, it is assumed that the mass is discrete and either anterior or posterior to the hilum. If the cause of the opacity arises from the hilum, the silhouette of the normal pulmonary vessels is obliterated.* This sign should be contrasted with the *hilum convergence sign* (Fig. 12.13). The latter aids in differentiating an enlarged pulmonary artery from a juxta-hilar mediastinal mass. *If the pulmonary artery branches converge toward the apparent mass, this suggests the presence of an enlarged pulmonary artery. In contrast, if the pulmonary artery branches converge more inferiorly toward the heart, then a juxta-hilar mass is likely present.*

Airways

Focal Airway Lesions

Although patients might have significant symptoms, airway abnormalities are frequently not apparent or are overlooked on the CXR. If there is a clinical suspicion of a tracheobronchial

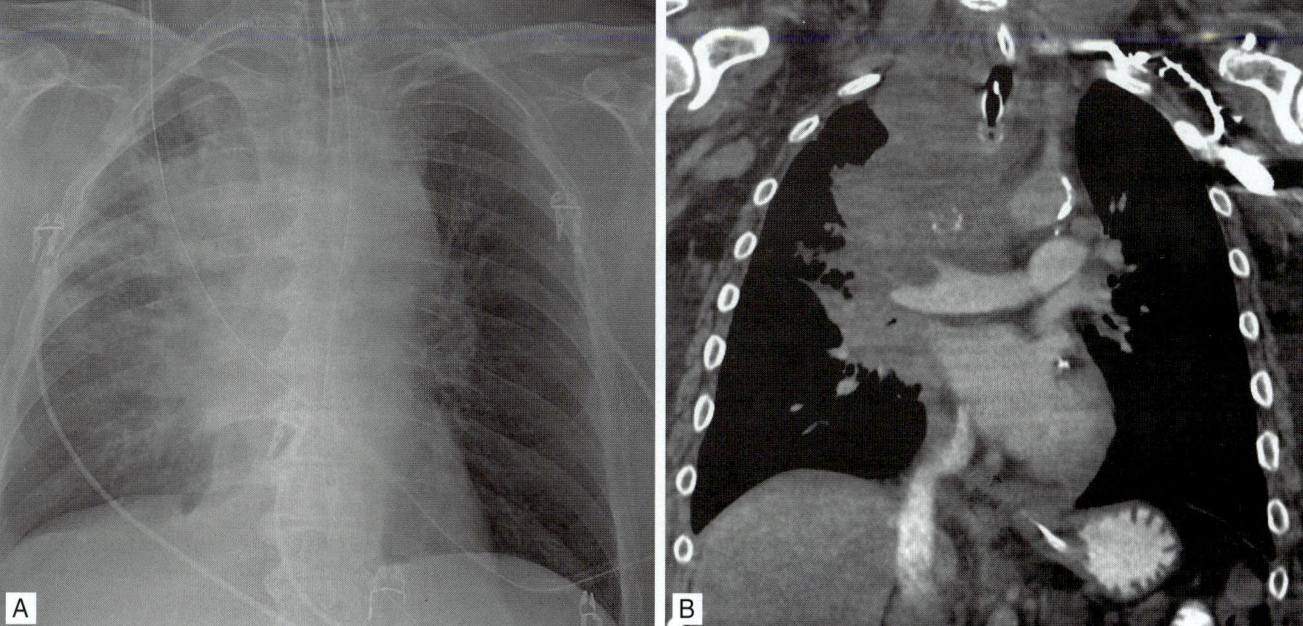

Figure 12.10 Frontal chest radiograph (A) and CT scan (B) of a 58-year-old male with small cell lung cancer show a large mass in the right paratracheal and hilar region causing widened superior mediastinum on radiograph.

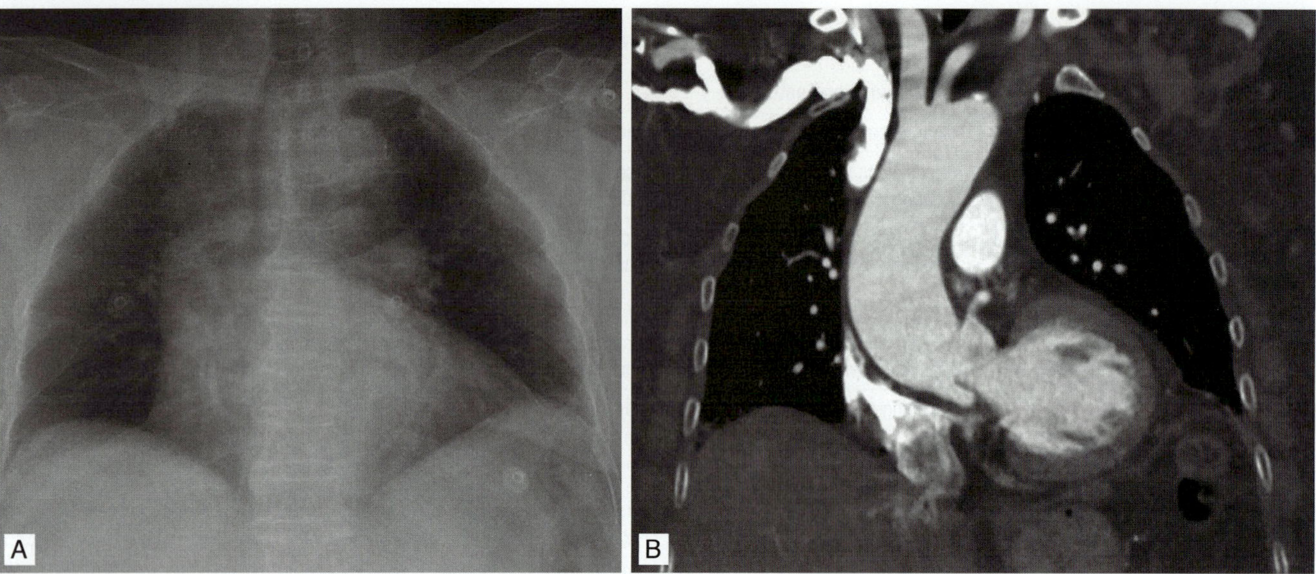

Figure 12.11 Frontal chest radiograph (A) and CT scan (B) of a 95-year-old female show widened superior mediastinum corresponding to an ascending aortic aneurysm.

TABLE 12.5 Differential Diagnoses in Those Presenting With Hilar Enlargement

Location	Conditions
Large pulmonary arteries	Pulmonary arterial hypertension, pulmonary artery aneurysms (septic emboli, Takayasu disease, Behçet disease)
Unilateral hilar mass	Lung cancer, bronchial carcinoid, metastasis, lymphoma, inflammation/infection including tuberculosis, nontuberculous mycobacteria, fungal infection, sarcoidosis (infrequent)
Bilateral hilar masses	Neoplasm (lymphoma, leukemia, metastases), inflammation/infection (Castleman disease, sarcoidosis, occupational diseases, inhalational anthrax), collagen vascular diseases (lupus, polyarteritis nodosa)

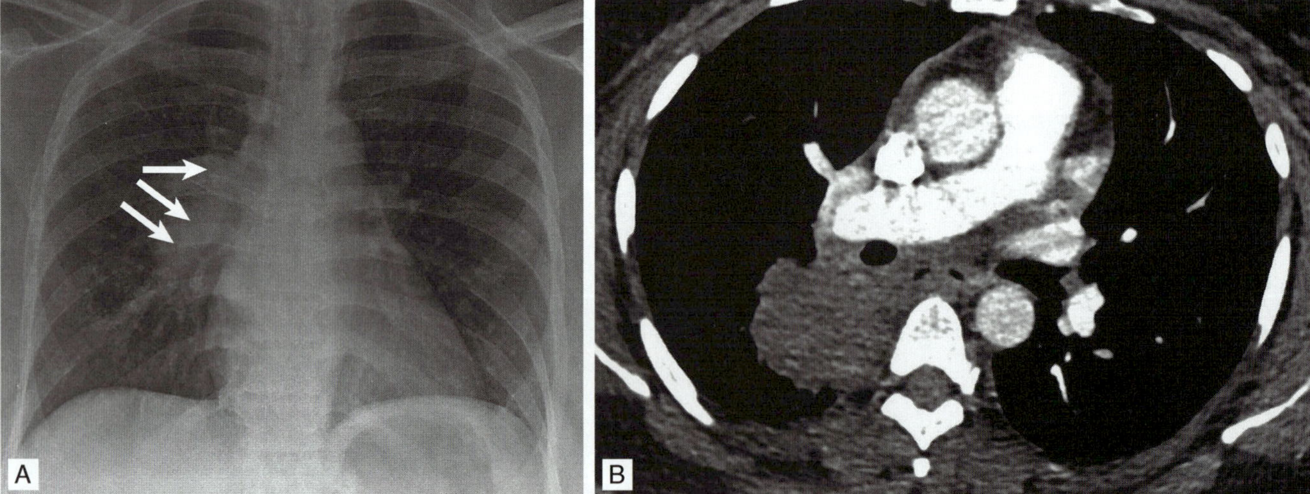

Figure 12.12 Frontal chest radiograph (A) of a 40-year-old female shows an opacity in the region of the right hilum with identifiable borders of the pulmonary arteries (hilum overlay sign, *white arrows*), corresponding to a right lower lobe mass demonstrated on chest CT (B).

abnormality, further evaluation by CT is warranted. There are several steps that help in formulating an appropriate differential diagnosis in the setting of an airway lesion.

- The first step is to determine whether the lesion is focal or diffuse. A focal lesion is one in which a single, short section of airway is affected. Most focal lesions of the large airways are tumors, whereas most diffuse lesions are tumor-like conditions
- The second step is to determine which airways are involved. Lesions that predominantly affect the trachea differ from those that are centered within bronchi. Although tumors can be benign or malignant, most central airway tumors are malignant
- The third step is to narrow the differential diagnosis using specific imaging features of the lesion and the clinical context (Table 12.6)

See Chapter 17 for a more detailed discussion of airway lesions.

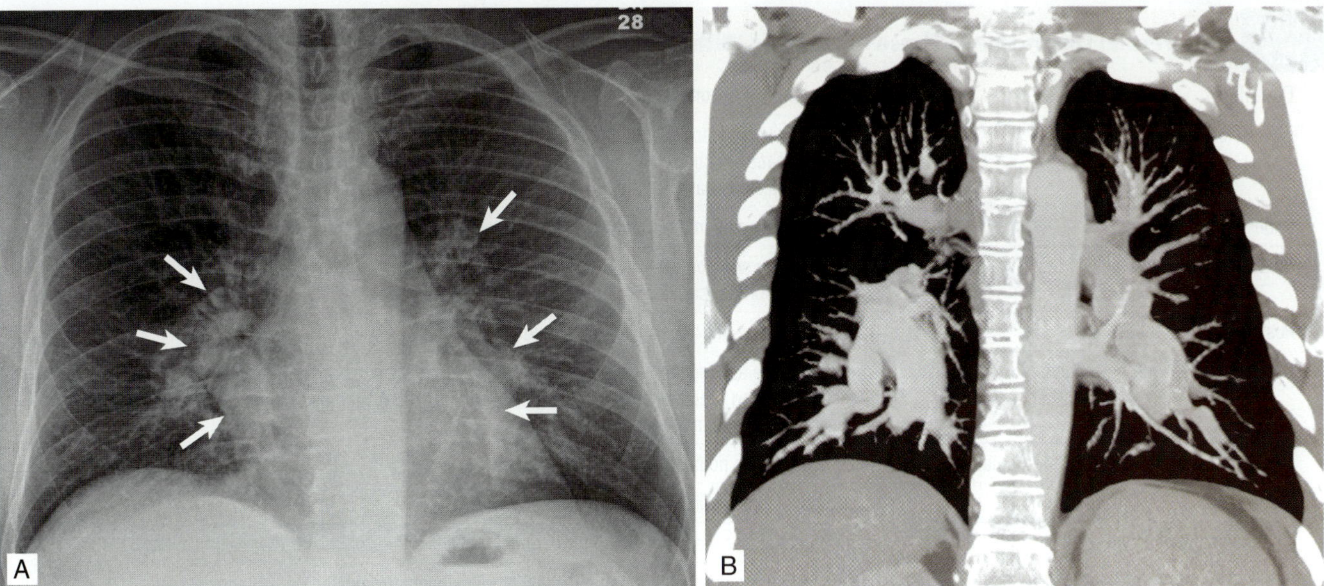

Figure 12.13 Frontal chest radiograph (A) and CT chest (B) of a 55-year-old man with IgG4-related vasculitis and pulmonary artery aneurysms show enlarged bilateral hila with enlarged pulmonary vessels converging toward the hila (hilum convergence sign, *white arrows*).

TABLE 12.6 Differential Diagnoses in Those Presenting With Focal Airway Lesions

	Condition	Distinguishing Features
Benign neoplasms	Papilloma	Nodules arising from the mucosal surface, with intraluminal growth; may be single or multiple and may cause atelectasis of the underlying lung; can rarely spread to the lungs, with multiple pulmonary nodules and air trapping
	Hamartoma	Combination of fat attenuation areas and popcorn calcifications; bronchial hamartomas tend to have more fat than pulmonary hamartomas because the bronchial wall is rich in fat; popcorn calcification helps to differentiate hamartomas from malignant tumors
	Carcinoid	Mostly in the central bronchus, while tracheal carcinoids are extremely rare; well-defined spherical or ovoid nodule with avid enhancement; carcinoids tend to produce different degrees of bronchial obstruction; "Iceberg tumor," with a small intraluminal lesion, undetectable even by direct bronchoscopy, and a large extraluminal component, easily detected by CT
Malignant neoplasms	Squamous cell carcinoma	Most common primary tracheobronchial tumor; polypoid intraluminal mass with irregular, smooth, or lobulated contours in the lower third of the trachea; can also present as an eccentric narrowing of the airway or as circumferential wall thickening; mediastinal adenopathies or pulmonary metastases in 1/3 of patients at the time of diagnosis
	Adenoid cystic carcinoma	Second most common tracheal malignancy; most frequently in the lower trachea and main bronchi with predominantly submucosal extension; CT shows a smooth mass with endoluminal and extraluminal growth, usually involving more than 180° of the airway circumference; the longitudinal axis of the tumor is classically greater than its axial extent
	Other neoplastic malignancies	Hemangiopericytoma or lymphoma, with nonspecific imaging features
	Metastasis	Indistinguishable from primary tumors by imaging and may present as a solitary tumor or multiple lesions
Non-neoplastic lesions	Tracheobronchial tuberculosis	Some degree of airway stenosis occurs in up to 90% of patients with endobronchial tuberculosis; caused by infectious necrosis and ulceration of the bronchial mucosa that leads to granulation and scarring; on CT, irregular wall narrowing, with heterogeneous contrast enhancement; tends to be multifocal, usually with a normal airway between strictures; affects the left main bronchus and distal trachea
	Postintubation stenosis	Luminal stenosis of the upper trachea; concentric narrowing with an hourglass shape, located in the subglottic area and measuring less than 2 cm
	Idiopathic tracheal stenosis	Rare inflammatory cicatricial stenosis of the upper trachea, without known cause; CT shows focal stenosis in the subglottic trachea, similar to postintubation stenosis
	Inflammatory pseudotumor	Inflammatory mass composed of a polymorphous inflammatory cell infiltrate and variable amounts of fibrosis, necrosis, and granulomatous reaction; CT shows a rounded, well-defined endoluminal lesion in the trachea or main bronchi, with smooth contours that may have calcifications, with a tendency for delayed enhancement due to the fibrotic nature
	Foreign body aspiration	Common and usually self-inflicted in children; rare and generally iatrogenic or traumatic in adults

TABLE 12.7 Differential Diagnoses in Those Presenting With Diffuse Tracheal Pathology

Condition	Distinguishing Features
Rhinoscleromatosis	Chronic, slowly progressive inflammatory disease of the upper respiratory tract, secondary to *Klebsiella rhinoscleromatis* infection; nodular concentric narrowing of the trachea, which may extend to the main bronchi. The lesions have soft tissue attenuation, classically without calcifications
Saber-sheath trachea	Fixed narrowing only in the transverse dimension; in men with chronic obstructive pulmonary disease
Relapsing polychondritis	Airway collapse seen on expiration (tracheomalacia); smooth tracheal wall thickening, sparing the posterior membrane; cartilage of nose and ears also affected
Postinfectious stricture	Granulation tissue and fibrosis is a response to infection
Granulomatosis with polyangitis	Formerly known as Wegener granulomatosis; classic triad includes upper airway disease (circumferential tracheal narrowing predominantly affecting subglottic trachea), lung involvement (cavitary pulmonary nodules and masses), and glomerulonephritis
Tracheobronchopathiaosteochondroplastica	Osteocartilaginous nodules spare posterior trachea
Sarcoidosis	Affects upper trachea in 1–3% of sarcoidosis patients
Tracheobronchial amyloidosis	Circumferential tracheal narrowing; intraluminal nodules and/or diffuse airway calcification
Extrinsic compression	Causes include enlarged thyroid, mediastinal lymphadenopathy, dilated or tortuous vessels

Diffuse Tracheal Stenosis and Wall Thickening

Causes for diffuse tracheal stenosis and wall thickening include rhinoscleromatosis, granulomatous bronchitis, amyloidosis, sarcoidosis, granulomatosis with polyangitis, relapsing polychondritis, and tracheobronchopathiaosteochondroplastica (Table 12.7). See Chapter 17 for a more detailed discussion of airway lesions.

Bronchiectasis

Bronchiectasis is an abnormal permanent dilatation of the airways, with or without thickening of the walls of the airways. In the normal state, the internal diameter of the airway is roughly equal to the transverse diameter of the accompanying pulmonary artery; *a bronchoarterial ratio greater than 1 should generally be regarded as abnormal.* There are several disease categories that may result in bronchiectasis (Table 12.8). See Chapter 17 for a more detailed discussion of bronchiectasis.

Pulmonary Nodules

Solitary Pulmonary Nodules

A pulmonary nodule is defined as any pulmonary lesion that is well-defined, discrete, approximately circular, and 3 cm or less in diameter. The term mass is used for lesions greater than 3 cm in diameter. The differential diagnosis of a nodule or mass detected on a radiograph or CT is very broad (Table 12.9). However, more than 95% fall into one of three groups: malignant neoplasms (primary or metastatic), infectious granulomas (tuberculosis or endemic fungi), or less commonly, benign tumors. Nodule size, shape, density, calcification pattern, degree of contrast enhancement, fluorodeoxyglucose avidity, and rate of growth are key imaging characteristics that when combined with clinical factors (e.g., patient age, immune status, and clinical history) help narrow the differential diagnosis [3].

Benign patterns of calcification within a solitary pulmonary nodule are one of the most reliable signs that a lesion is benign. Four patterns of calcification are characteristically associated with benign lesions: diffuse, laminated, central, and popcorn. Calcification in malignant tumors may be seen in a peripheral primary carcinoma engulfing a calcified granuloma, in which case the calcification is usually eccentric, solitary metastasis of osteogenic sarcoma or chondrosarcoma, primary pulmonary carcinoid tumors, or calcification in pulmonary carcinomas larger than 3 cm.

Multiple Noncavitary Pulmonary Nodules

Centrilobular Nodules

Centrilobular nodules are anatomically located centrally within the secondary pulmonary lobules, usually evenly spaced and several millimeters away from the pleural surfaces, interlobar fissures, and

TABLE 12.8 Differential Diagnoses in Those Presenting With Bronchiectasis

Condition	Distinguishing Features
Postinfectious bronchiectasis	Often focal in recurrent aspiration and/or pneumonia; mycobacterial infection a common cause
Postobstructive bronchiectasis	Cause may be endobronchial tumor or foreign body
Cystic fibrosis	Upper lung bronchiectasis
Asthma	Cylindric bronchiectasis, with air trapping
Allergic bronchopulmonary aspergillosis	Central cystic bronchiectasis with dense mucus plugging; finger-in-glove or tube-like opacities corresponding to mucus or hyphal plugs
Immotile cilia syndrome	Middle and lower lobe bronchiectasis; situs inversus seen in 50% of cases
Congenital causes	Williams-Campbell syndrome and Mounier–Kuhn syndrome; yellow nail syndrome in patients with discolored nails
Traction bronchiectasis	Results from fibrotic lung surrounding an airway; may be seen in fibrotic sarcoidosis, radiation fibrosis, idiopathic pulmonary fibrosis

TABLE 12.9 Differential Diagnoses in Those Presenting With Solitary Nodule/Mass

Condition	Distinguishing Features
Granuloma (Fig. 12.14)	May be other calcified granulomas or calcified lymph nodes; likelihood dependent on where patient has lived (far more common in Midwestern United States)
Lung cancer (Fig. 12.15)	Calcification seen in 6–7%; most lung cancers double in volume every 1–18 months
Metastasis	Patients with melanoma, testicular cancer, or sarcoma more likely to have a solitary metastasis than primary lung cancer
Intrapulmonary lymph node	Often found along fissures or in a subpleural location; morphology may be triangular, oval, round, or trapezoidal
Pulmonary nodule mimic	Consider clothing artifact (button), nipple shadow, skin or chest wall lesion, healing rib fracture, and enostosis in a rib
Hamartoma	Fat within a nodule nearly pathognomonic; popcorn calcification sometimes present
Pulmonary carcinoid (Fig. 12.16)	Location generally more central; can enhance avidly; high false-negative rate on FDG PET imaging
Infection (nongranulomatous)	Round pneumonia, septic embolus, or abscess
Mesenchymal or neural tumor	Consider fibroma, chondroma, lipoma, or neurofibroma
Arteriovenous malformation	Feeding artery and draining vein; multiple in hereditary hemorrhagic telangiectasia
Inflammatory nodule	Rheumatoid nodule or granulomatosis with polyangitis

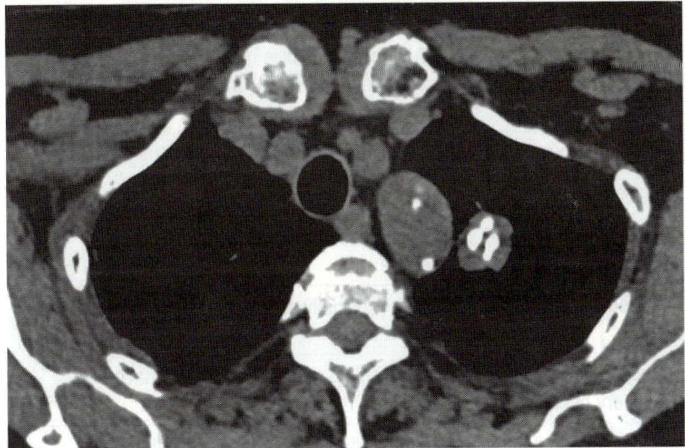

Figure 12.14 Chest CT scan of a 73-year-old male shows a lobulated nodule in left upper lobe with coarse popcorn: central calcifications. There is an adjacent enlarged partially calcified lymph node. Findings are consistent with a granuloma

interlobular septa. They reflect the presence of bronchiolocentric lung disease or bronchiolitis. The tree-in-bud pattern is branching centrilobular nodules, with a V or Y shape, usually reflecting the presence of dilated centrilobular bronchioles, their lumina impacted with mucus, fluid, or pus, and often associated with peribronchiolar inflammation. It is usually associated with aspiration (Fig. 12.17) or infection of the small airways, the most common causes being infectious bronchiolitis, bronchopneumonia, and endobronchial spread of tuberculosis or *M. avium-intracellulare* (Table 12.10).

Perilymphatic Nodules

Perilymphatic pulmonary nodules follow perilymphatic channels and are typically subpleural, occur along fissures, interlobular septa, and adjacent to the bronchovascular bundles. Unlike centrilobular nodules, nodules with a perilymphatic distribution are generally unevenly spaced from one another. This pattern is most common in sarcoidosis, lymphangitic carcinomatosis, silicosis, and other conditions as outlined in Table 12.11.

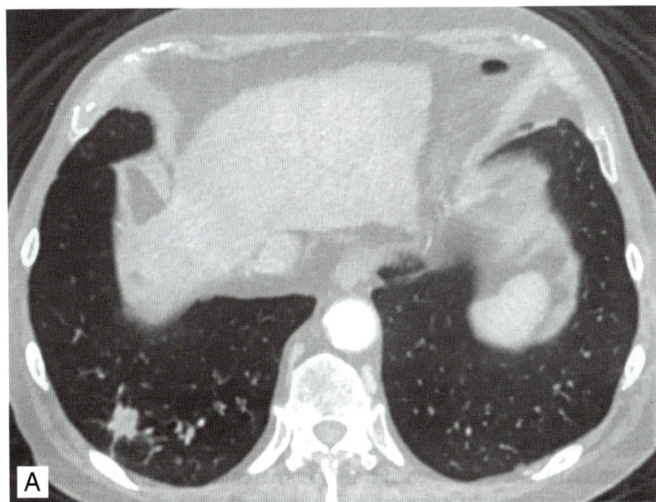

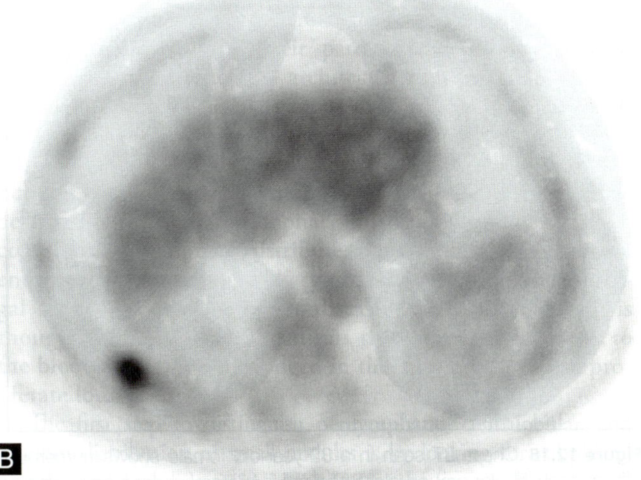

Figure 12.15 Chest CT (A) in a 75-year-old male shows a solitary spiculated right lower lobe nodule with intense FDG uptake on PET (B), which was proved to be an adenocarcinoma after resection.

TABLE 12.14 Differential Diagnoses in Those Presenting With Acute Consolidations

Condition	Distinguishing Features
Pneumonia (Fig. 12.28)	Alveoli are filled with pus or inflammatory fluid; lobar (nonsegmental) consolidation and segmental consolidation (bronchopneumonia)
Alveolar pulmonary edema	Septal thickening and ground-glass opacities; perihilar and gravitational distribution; associated with pleural effusions and cardiomegaly
Pulmonary hemorrhage (Fig. 12.29)	Patchy or confluent areas of consolidation or ground-glass opacities; interlobular septal thickening and poorly defined centrilobular nodular opacities as the hemorrhage resolves
Pulmonary infarction (Fig. 12.30)	Associated with pulmonary embolism; peripheral and lower lobe predominant consolidations

Upper Lung Predominant Disease

Alterations in ventilation and perfusion, lymphatic flow, metabolism, and mechanics predispose certain diseases to have a predilection to affect the upper lungs preferentially. Several diseases and conditions that produce an upper lung distribution are listed in Table 12.16 [5].

Lower Lung Predominant Disease

In upright individuals, the differences in perfusion and ventilation influenced by gravity result in relative overventilation of the lung apices and overperfusion of the lung bases. The combination of gravity and relative overperfusion of the lung bases leads some entities to predominantly involve the lower lung (Table 12.17) [6].

Cystic Lung Disease

Lung cysts appear as round parenchymal lucencies or low-attenuating areas with a well-defined thin wall surrounded by normal

Figure 12.28 Chest CT image in a 64-year-old male with cough and fevers shows consolidation in the right middle lobe with air bronchogram, compatible with acute lobar pneumonia.

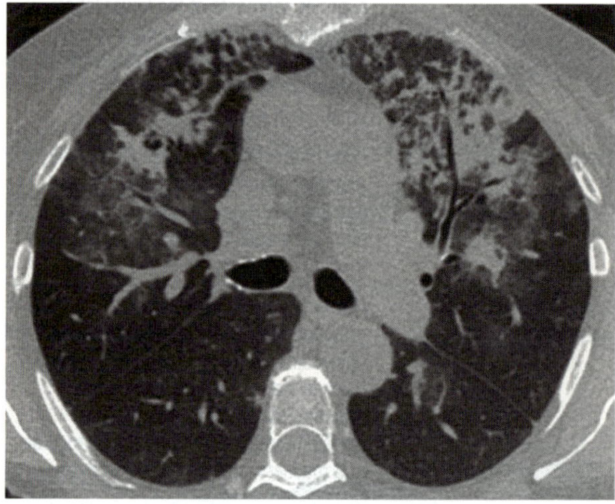

Figure 12.29 CT chest scan in a 58-year-old female with Goodpasture syndrome shows symmetric peribronchovascular consolidative and ground-glass opacities, consistent with pulmonary hemorrhage.

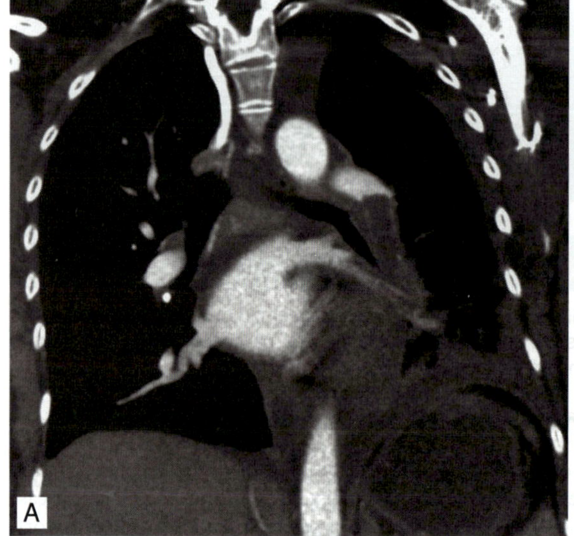

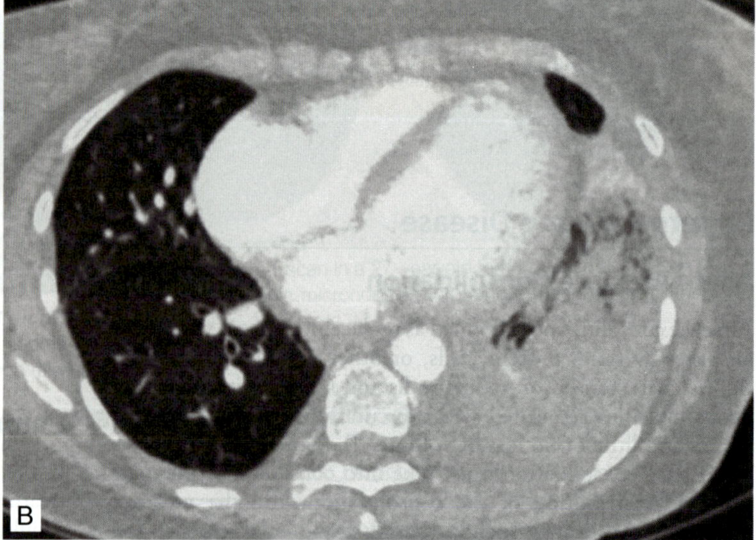

Figure 12.30 Chest CT images of a 53-year-old female show large occlusive pulmonary emboli within the left lower lobar pulmonary artery (A) with consolidation in the left lower lobe (B), consistent with large pulmonary infarct.

TABLE 12.15 Differential Diagnoses in Those Presenting With Chronic Consolidations

Condition	Distinguishing Features
Organizing pneumonia (Fig. 12.31)	Granulation tissue within the alveolar ducts and airspaces; causes include idiopathic, infection, drug reaction, radiation therapy, collagen vascular disease, or inhalation of toxic fumes; patchy bilateral consolidation, peribronchial, or subpleural in distribution; "reversed halo sign"
Eosinophilic lung disease	Elevated eosinophils in bronchoalveolar lavage fluid and peripheral blood; upper lobe and periphery predominant consolidation; typically responds to steroid therapy
Lipoid pneumonia	Aspiration of mineral, vegetable, or animal oil; single or multiple nodules or masses and localized or confluent areas of consolidation; areas of fat attenuation
Adenocarcinoma (Fig. 12.32)	Solitary nodule or mass, patchy, or confluent areas of ground-glass opacity or consolidation, or, less commonly, as numerous ground-glass and soft tissue nodules
Lymphoma	Secondary pulmonary lymphoma is much more common than primary pulmonary lymphoma; mass or mass-like consolidation with or without cavitation; air bronchograms may be seen
Sarcoidosis	Confluent granulomatous nodules may mimic consolidation; bilateral hilar lymphadenopathy with or without right paratracheal lymphadenopathy

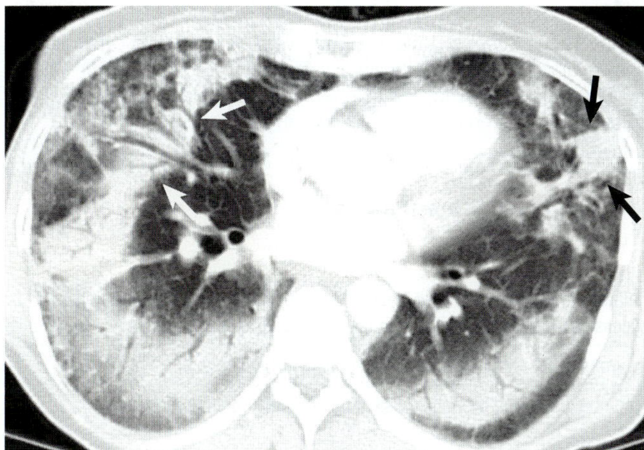

Figure 12.31 Chest CT scan in a 62-year-old female with organizing pneumonia shows chronic peribronchovascular (*white arrows*) and peripheral consolidations (*black arrows*) bilaterally.

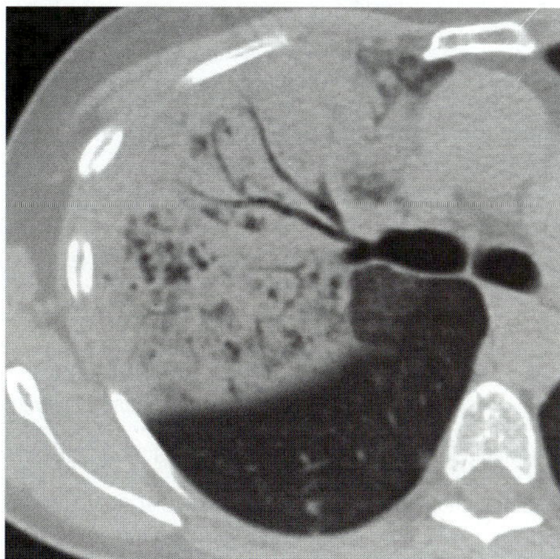

Figure 12.32 Chest CT scan in a 52-year-old female with persistent non-resolving consolidation, which was determined to represent mucinous adenocarcinoma of biopsy.

TABLE 12.16 Differential Diagnoses in Those Presenting With Upper Lung Predominant Disease

Condition	Distinguishing Features
Inhaled injurious gases	Bronchial wall thickening, diffuse bilateral consolidation, and tree-in-bud pattern that develop within a few hours after exposure
Centrilobular emphysema (Fig. 12.33)	Permanent abnormal enlargement of airspaces distal to terminal bronchioles; upper lobe predominance and is associated with cigarette smoking
Cystic fibrosis (Fig. 12.34)	Autosomal recessive genetic disorder with abnormally thick mucus, resulting in mucous plugging in small and large airways and subsequent bacterial infection; hyperinflation, bronchial wall thickening, bronchiectasis, and mucous impaction, usually in the upper lobes
Pneumoconioses	Particularly silicosis and coal workers' pneumoconiosis; small nodules that may calcify and predominantly involve the posterior portions of the upper lobes or superior segments of the lower lobes; hilar and mediastinal lymphadenopathy with peripheral eggshell calcification; progressive massive fibrosis
Hypersensitivity pneumonitis	Ill-defined centrilobular nodules and bilateral airspace consolidations with a mid and upper zone distribution; mosaic attenuation with air trapping
Tuberculosis	Apical and posterior segments of the upper lobes and the superior segments of the lower lobes; cavitary nodules and asymmetric adenopathy common
Sarcoidosis	Mid to upper lung zone; confluent granulomatous nodules may mimic consolidation; bilateral hilar lymphadenopathy with or without right paratracheal lymphadenopathy
Langerhans cell histiocytosis	Diffuse symmetric nodular opacities and irregular cysts, with upper lobe predominance; exclusively in smokers

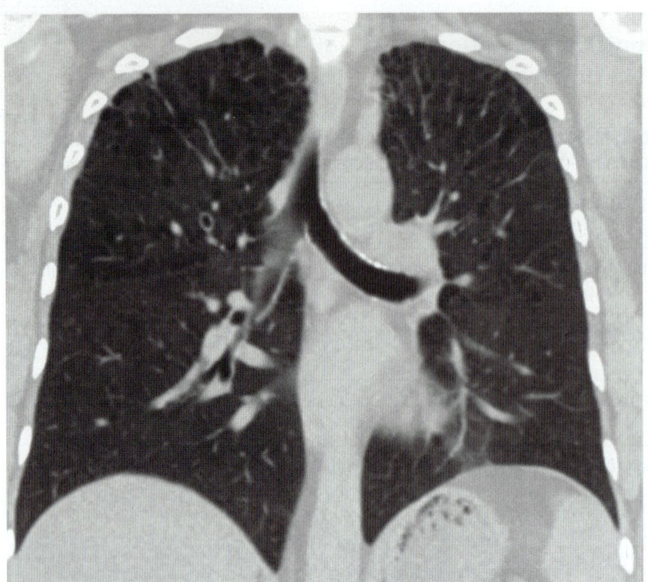

Figure 12.33 Chest CT images in a 58-year-old female smoker show upper zone predominant centrilobular and paraseptal emphysema.

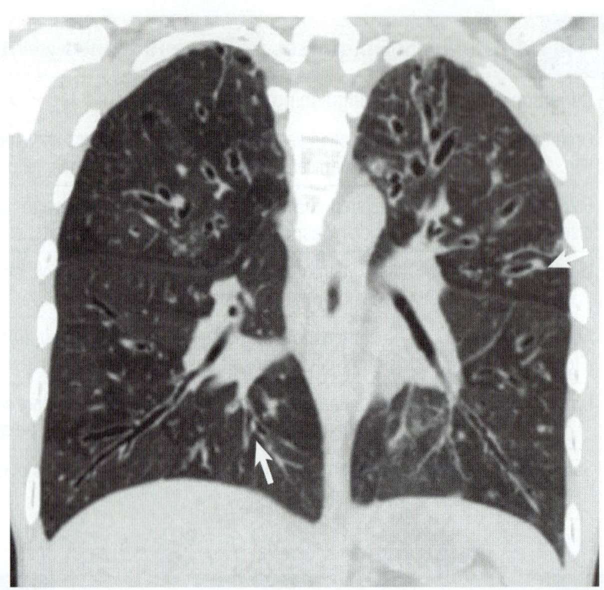

Figure 12.34 Chest CT image in a 23-year-old male with cystic fibrosis shows upper lobe predominant cystic and cylindrical bronchiectasis, bronchial wall thickening, and patchy mucous plugging (*white arrows*) with diffuse mosaic attenuation in keeping with air trapping.

TABLE 12.17 Differential Diagnoses in Those Presenting With Lower Lung Predominant Disease

Condition	Distinguishing Features
Aspiration	In recumbent patients, the posterior upper lobes and the apical lower lobes are most often involved; in erect patients, the posterobasilar lungs are more frequently involved; scattered heterogeneous opacities are more common than lobar airspace consolidation
Lipoid pneumonia (Fig. 12.35)	Bilateral opacities predominantly in the lower lobes; areas of fat attenuation within the opacities is diagnostic
Usual interstitial pneumonia (Fig. 12.36)	Subpleural reticular opacities with prominent honeycombing, traction bronchiectasis, and architectural distortion, with an apicobasilar gradient
Nonspecific interstitial pneumonia	Frequently occurs in association with connective tissue diseases (systemic sclerosis, rheumatoid arthritis, Sjögren syndrome) or drug exposure; subpleural and symmetric distribution of ground-glass opacities combined with fine reticular opacities and micronodules; lower lung zones are more affected
Lymphoid interstitial pneumonia (Fig. 12.37)	Associated with HIV infection, and Sjögren syndrome; round-glass opacities in combination with thin-walled perivascular cysts, both of which have a lower lung predominance
Hematogenous metastases	Cancers of the breast, kidney, colon, and thyroid and melanoma; round nodules of variable size that are scattered throughout both lungs and predominantly involve the lower lung
Septic embolism	Predisposing factors include tricuspid valve endocarditis, drug addiction, alcoholism, skin infection, immunologic deficiencies, and infected indwelling catheters or pacemaker wires; nodules with varying degrees of cavitation and subpleural wedge-shaped opacities with rim-like peripheral enhancement, all of which predominantly involve the lower lobes
Asbestos-related pleural disease	Pleural effusion is the earliest imaging finding of asbestos-related pleural disease, and pleural plaques, which may calcify, are the most common manifestation of pleural disease; asbestosis, which refers to the lung fibrosis caused by asbestos fibers, predominantly affects the subpleural portions of the lower lung

lung parenchyma. It is important to differentiate true lung cysts from other air-filled lung lesions such as emphysema, bullous change, and honeycombing. Diseases or conditions presenting with lung cysts occupy a broad spectrum, and cystic lung diseases are a heterogeneous group of pathologies (Table 12.18) [7]. See Chapter 18 for detailed discussion of cystic lung diseases.

Mediastinum

Prevascular Mediastinal Masses

The prevascular compartment is bordered anteriorly by the posterior aspect of the sternum, posteriorly by the ventral aspect of the pericardium, cranially by the thoracic outlet, and caudally by the diaphragm. The differential diagnosis of mediastinal masses, in general, is primarily based on the location of the mass, its tissue composition (i.e., fat content and calcifications) and the age of the patient. The most common masses arising in the prevascular mediastinum are outlined in Table 12.19 [8]. See Chapter 13 for a more detailed discussion of the mediastinum and mediastinal pathologies.

Visceral (Middle) Mediastinal Masses

The visceral compartment is bounded superiorly by the thoracic inlet, inferiorly by the diaphragm, anteriorly by the posterior

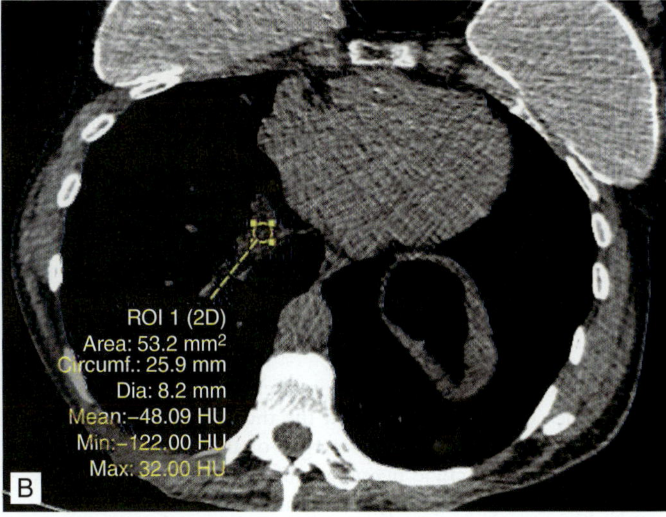

Figure 12.35 Chest CT images of a 62-year-old female show a right lower lobe consolidation with additional ground glass and tree-in-bud nodules in the left lower lobe (A). The consolidation has fat attenuation consistent with lipoid pneumonia.

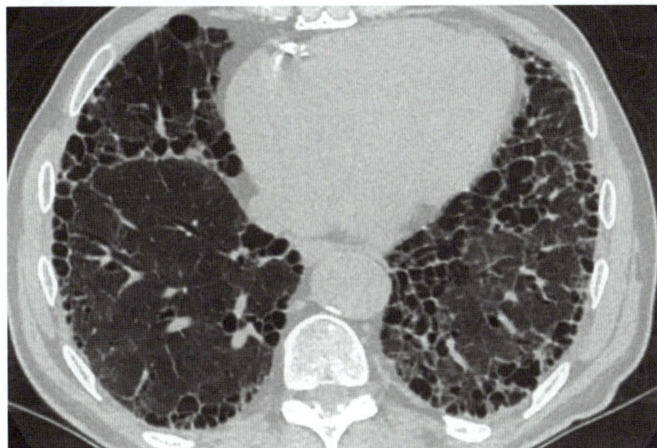

Figure 12.36 Chest CT image in a 79-year-old male shows basilar predominant fibrosis with traction bronchiectasis, bronchiolectasis, and honeycombing, consistent with usual interstitial pneumonia.

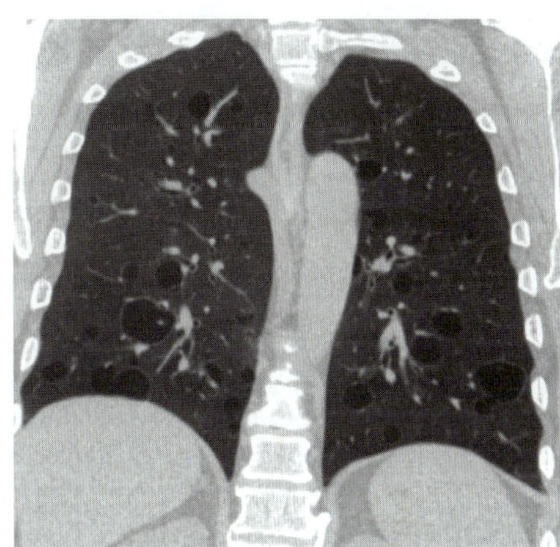

Figure 12.37 Chest CT images in a 62-year-old male with Sjögren's syndrome show lower lobe predominant variable sized thin-walled cyst in a perilymphatic distribution, consistent with lymphocytic interstitial pneumonia.

TABLE 12.18 Differential Diagnoses in Those Presenting With Cystic Lung Disease

Condition	Distinguishing Features
Lymphangioleiomyomatosis	Women of childbearing age; can occur sporadically, but more common in patients with tuberous sclerosis complex; numerous, thin-walled, well-circumscribed cysts diffusely and symmetrically distributed throughout the lungs without lobar predominance
Birt-Hogg-Dubé syndrome	Multiorgan systemic condition characterized by fibrofolliculomas, pulmonary cysts, and renal neoplasms; multiple thin-walled lung cysts predominantly in lower, peripheral lung zones, and along the mediastinum
Pulmonary Langerhans cell histiocytosis	Associated with cigarette smoking; irregularly shaped nodules in a symmetric pattern with upper-middle lung dominance. As the disease progresses, cystic degeneration appears as round or oval to bizarre with thin-wall and associated nodules
Cystic metastasis	Angiosarcoma or squamous cell carcinoma mainly in the head and neck; multiple solid nodules and multiple thin-walled cysts, often admixed with hemorrhagic change
Lymphoid interstitial pneumonia	Associated with HIV infection, and Sjögren syndrome; round-glass opacities in combination with thin-walled perivascular cysts, both of which have a lower lung predominance
Amyloidosis	Extracellular deposition of abnormal insoluble proteins; numerous peribronchovascular or subpleural cysts, frequently associated with nodular lesions that are often calcified
Neurofibromatosis	Numerous upper lobe predominant cysts bilaterally
Pneumocystis jirovecii pneumonia	Extensive ground-glass opacities or dense consolidation in the central and perihilar distribution, along with septal wall thickening; cysts are multiple, with upper lobe predominance and variations in size, shape, and wall thickness

TABLE 12.19 Differential Diagnoses in Those Presenting With A Prevascular Mediastinal Mass

Condition	Distinguishing Features
Thyroid masses	Substernal thyroid goiter manifests as heterogeneous prevascular mediastinal mass that demonstrates continuity with the cervical thyroid gland; thyroid adenoma and carcinoma less common
Germ cell tumors	Affect young patients; varying amounts of fat, fluid, calcification, and soft tissue; fat-fluid levels are highly specific for mature teratoma
Thymic masses	Thymoma, thymic carcinoma, thymolipoma, thymic cyst; rarely, thymic carcinoid or thymic lymphoma
Lymphoma or lymphadenopathy	More common in younger patients; 50–70% are Hodgkin's lymphomas; large homogenous lobulated or nodular mass that may encircle vascular structures, but does not infiltrate them

boundaries of the prevascular compartment, and posteriorly by a vertical line connecting a point on the thoracic vertebral bodies 1-cm posterior to the anterior margin of the spine. The most significant lesions include neoplasms of the airways, esophagus, and lymph nodes; enhancing masses; and non-neoplastic abnormalities such as bronchogenic and esophageal duplication cysts, as outlined in Table 12.20 [9]. See Chapter 13 for a more detailed discussion of the mediastinum and mediastinal pathologies.

Paravertebral Mediastinal Masses

The paravertebral mediastinal compartment is bounded superiorly by the thoracic inlet, inferiorly by the diaphragm, anteriorly by the posterior boundaries of the visceral compartment, and posterolaterally by a vertical line along the posterior margin of the chest wall at the lateral aspect of the transverse processes. Since the paravertebral compartment includes the thoracic spine and paravertebral soft tissues, most common masses are neurogenic neoplasms, non-neurogenic tumors, and a wide variety of miscellaneous lesions related to other underlying conditions (such as extramedullary hematopoiesis) as outlined in Table 12.21 [10]. See Chapter 13 for a more detailed discussion of the mediastinum and mediastinal pathologies.

Lymphadenopathy

Hyperenhancing Lymphadenopathy

Almost all conditions resulting in lymphadenopathy cause some degree of postcontrast enhancement. Of these, only few conditions cause intense enhancement in thoracic lymphadenopathy as described in Table 12.22.

Low-Attenuation Lymphadenopathy

Low-attenuation thoracic lymphadenopathy indicates underlying intranodal necrosis or cystic degeneration, which can be seen with several diagnoses as outlined in Table 12.23.

Calcified Lymphadenopathy

Calcified lymphadenopathy is common following tuberculosis and fungal infection, and is occasionally seen with other infections, as well as other conditions such as sarcoidosis, silicosis, and amyloidosis (Table 12.24).

Pleura

Masses

The pleura may be affected by primary neoplasms or become involved by secondary spread of intrathoracic or extrathoracic tumors. Primary pleural tumors account for approximately 10% of all pleural neoplasms, whereas secondary neoplasms account for approximately 90% of pleural tumors [11]. Common diagnoses of pleural masses are listed in Table 12.25. See Chapter 14 for detailed discussion of pleural pathologies.

Pleural Effusions

Pleural effusion is the accumulation of fluid in the pleural space when the rate of pleural fluid production outpaces the rate of absorption resulting from disruption of the homeostatic forces responsible for the movement of pleural fluid [12]. Pleural effusions may result from pleural, parenchymal, or extrapulmonary disease (Table 12.26).

TABLE 12.20 Differential Diagnoses in Those Presenting With A Visceral (Middle) Mediastinal Mass

Condition	Distinguishing Features
Hiatal hernia	Include sliding, paraesophageal, or mixed hernia; retrocardiac air-fluid level on chest radiography
Lymphadenopathy	Most common cause of visceral mediastinal mass; neoplastic (lymphoproliferative and metastatic), infectious, and inflammatory entities; multiple well-circumscribed nodules or masses at several lymph nodal stations
Congenital-developmental cysts	Include foregut duplication cysts (e.g., bronchogenic cysts and esophageal duplication cysts) and pleuropericardial or mesothelial cysts; well-demarcated round or oval cystic lesions of variable but typically homogeneous attenuation, with smooth, thin, or imperceptible walls
Esophageal lesions	Include achalasia, esophageal diverticula, esophageal varices, leiomyomas, and esophageal cancer
Tracheal lesions	Include intrinsic and extrinsic tracheal lesions
Neurogenic tumors	Arise from vagus, phrenic, or left recurrent laryngeal nerve
Pulmonary artery enlargement	Seen in pulmonary stenosis or pulmonary artery hypertension
Thoracic aortic aneurysm	Should be suspected on radiograph whenever a mediastinal mass is in the vicinity of the aorta and particularly when the border of the mass is indistinguishable from the aortic contour

TABLE 12.21 Differential Diagnoses in Those Presenting With A Paravertebral Mediastinal Mass

Condition	Distinguishing Features
Peripheral nerve sheath tumors	Most common paravertebral mass; include schwannoma, neurofibroma, and malignant peripheral nerve sheath tumor; "dumbbell" or "hourglass" configuration when involving an intervertebral neural foramen
Sympathetic ganglion tumors	Less common neurogenic tumors; include ganglioneuroma, ganglioneuroblastoma, and neuroblastoma; more fusiform than round and more vertical in orientation than peripheral nerve sheath tumors
Paragangliomas	Rare neurogenic tumors of chromaffin cell origin; most common locations in the mediastinum are along the great vessels and base of the heart (aortopulmonary paraganglia) and along the sympathetic chain in the paravertebral mediastinum; intense contrast enhancement, very high T2 signal intensity, "salt and pepper" appearance on T1-weighted images
Neuroenteric cysts	Rare subtype of foregut duplication cyst; often have a fibrous or CSF-containing connection to the intradural extramedullary space; well-circumscribed paravertebral mediastinal masses, similar to that of other foregut duplication cysts
Meningoceles	Associated with neurofibromatosis type 1; well-marginated paravertebral mediastinal masses; smooth, well-corticated pressure erosion, and scalloping of the adjacent vertebrae and ribs; direct relation to the CSF space, internal CSF attenuation, and signal intensity
Extramedullary hematopoiesis	Rare and represents paravertebral bone marrow expansion in the setting of severe anemia; multiple, bilateral, lobulated paravertebral masses
Paraspinal abscess	Bacterial, fungal, or tuberculous cause most common

TABLE 12.22 Differential Diagnoses in Those Presenting With Hyperenhancing Lymphadenopathy

Condition	Distinguishing Features
Hypervascular metastatic lesions	Include papillary thyroid carcinoma, renal cell carcinoma, neuroendocrine tumor, and melanoma
Kaposi sarcoma	Flame-shaped nodular opacities with perilymphatic and peribronchovascular distribution; hyperenhancing lymphadenopathy
Castleman disease	Uncommon benign lymphoproliferative disorder; hyaline vascular subtype shows intense homogeneous enhancement; plasma cell subtype is multicentric and less enhancing

TABLE 12.23 Differential Diagnoses in Those Presenting With Low-Attenuation Lymphadenopathy

Condition	Distinguishing Features
Metastatic disease	Often of squamous cell histology including lung, testicular, or ovarian primary tumor
Infectious lymphadenopathy	More common in mycobacterial and fungal infection
Whipple disease	Small bowel involvement nearly always present; lung involvement in 35–50% of cases
Lymphoma	Rarely results in low-attenuation lymphadenopathy

TABLE 12.24 Differential Diagnoses in Those Presenting With Calcified Lymph Nodes

Condition	Distinguishing Features
Granulomatous infections	Usually tuberculosis or histoplasmosis; calcifications often complete rather than focal
Sarcoidosis	Bilateral, symmetrical hilar, and paratracheal lymphadenopathy; calcified lymph nodes rarely in eggshell pattern; may even be relatively light with homogeneous representation, the so-called "icing sugar" pattern
Silicosis	History of silica-exposure; "eggshell calcification" pattern seen in 3–6%
Treated lymphoma	Usually 1–9 years following treatment
Metastases	Include osteosarcoma, chondrosarcoma, mucinous colorectal, and ovarian cancer
Amyloidosis	Third most common thoracic manifestation of amyloidosis after airway disease and nodular parenchymal disease; a variety of patterns of calcifications including punctate, diffuse, or eggshell

TABLE 12.25 Differential Diagnoses of Pleural Masses

Condition	Distinguishing Features
Solitary fibrous tumors of the pleura	Most are low-grade neoplasms, while 20–30% are malignant; associated with hypertrophic osteoarthropathy, clubbing and episodic hypoglycemia; well-circumscribed, form acute angles with the pleural surface, may enhance heterogeneously, calcifications in up to 25%
Pleural lipomas	Most common benign tumor of the pleura; diagnostic when the lesion is well-circumscribed and uniformly fatty; the presence of an enhancing soft tissue component should raise suspicion for liposarcoma
Pleural metastases	Most common malignancies include lung, breast, and gastrointestinal and genitourinary malignancies; invasive thymoma can also cause pleural metastases; layering or loculated pleural effusion, diffuse pleural thickening, or focal pleural nodules and masses; malignant pleural effusion is the most common manifestation of metastatic pleural involvement by imaging
Mesothelioma	Primary pleural neoplasm strongly associated with asbestos exposure; 20- to 40-year latency period between presentation and initial exposure; mediastinal pleural involvement, diffuse and often circumferential pleural thickening, thickening of the interlobar fissures, and pleural effusion, chest wall invasion, diaphragmatic invasion, and metastatic involvement of hilar and mediastinal lymph nodes
Pleural lymphoma	Primary or secondary; can mimic the appearance of mesothelioma, with diffuse pleural thickening and a pleural effusion; more often associated with pronounced mediastinal lymphadenopathy than mesothelioma

TABLE 12.26 Differential Diagnoses in Those Presenting With Pleural Effusions/Fluid

Condition	Distinguishing Features
Freely layering pleural effusion	More commonly transudative than exudative; blunting of the costophrenic angles, with concave–upward interface known as the "meniscus sign" on upright CXR; may track into the fissures and the lung apex (apical cap)
Subpulmonary pleural effusion	Fluid accumulates between the inferior surface of the lung and the hemidiaphragmatic pleura; mimics elevation of the ipsilateral hemidiaphragm (pseudodiaphragm sign)
Loculated pleural effusion	Undulating, lobulated, or other gravity-defying contour, whether located dependently or nondependently within the thorax; may accumulate within a fissure mimicking a mass
Hydropneumothorax	The presence of air and fluid in the pleural space; air-fluid level in the pleural space on an upright CXR
Empyema	Exudative pleural effusion with frank pus; caused by complications of bacterial pneumonia, or adjacent lung abscess; manifests as enhancing, separated, and thickened leaves of visceral and parietal pleura encompassing a bulging, lenticular collection of pleural fluid (split pleura sign)
Hemothorax	Blood within the pleural space, most commonly caused by chest trauma, neoplasm, infarction, infections such as TB, and coagulopathies; may not be distinguishable from a free-flowing or loculated pleural effusion on CXR; hyperattenuating fluid on CT and T1 hyperintensity on MRI suggest recent pleural hemorrhage; different densities of layering blood products result in a fluid-fluid level (hematocrit level)
Chylothorax	Disruption of the major lymphatic channels, such as the thoracic duct, results in a chylothorax; common causes include neoplasms (lymphoma), trauma, and infection (TB); CT attenuation is usually close to that of water despite the fat content; on MRI, chylothorax is T1-hyperintense and may drop out in signal on opposed-phase chemical shift sequence

Miscellaneous

Mosaic Attenuation

Mosaic attenuation is defined as variable lung attenuation that results in a heterogeneous appearance of the parenchyma. It often has a well-defined geographic distribution that follows the boundaries of secondary pulmonary lobules [13]. Expiratory CT is helpful to demonstrate air trapping, which suggests airway disease. Mosaic attenuation most commonly occurs in diseases that affect the small airways, pulmonary vasculature, alveoli, and interstitium, alone or in combination (Table 12.27).

Interlobular Septal Thickening

Interlobular septal thickening is defined as well-defined polygonal-shaped thickened outlines of secondary pulmonary lobules. Coronal reformatted images are often helpful in confirming the presence of interlobular septal thickening. Septal thickening may be smooth, nodular, or irregular. The common causes of septal thickening are outlined in Table 12.28.

Crazy Paving

Crazy paving pattern is defined as patchy or diffuse ground-glass opacities with superimposed interlobular septal thickening and intralobular lines [14]. It is a nonspecific finding that can be seen in several conditions (Table 12.29).

Halo Sign

The halo sign refers to the presence of ground-glass opacity surrounding a pulmonary nodule. This finding, first reported in immunocompromised patients with angioinvasive aspergillosis, can also be seen in various other disease entities [15] (Table 12.30).

TABLE 12.27 Differential Diagnoses in Those Presenting With Mosaic Lung Attenuation

Condition	Distinguishing Features
Occlusive vascular disease and vasculitis	Low-attenuation areas are abnormal and reflect relative oligemia; vessels are decreased in size and number in areas or low attenuation; no air trapping; common diagnoses include chronic pulmonary embolism, chronic thromboembolic pulmonary hypertension (Fig. 12.38)
Obstructive airway disease	Low-attenuation regions are abnormal reflecting air trapping in areas with obstructive small airways disease, and reduced perfusion in these affected areas secondary to vasoconstriction with relative hyperemia in adjacent healthy lungs; air trapping at expiratory CT; common diagnoses include bronchiectasis, cystic fibrosis (Fig. 12.34), constrictive bronchiolitis. Diffuse idiopathic neuroendocrine hyperplasia (DIPNECH) is a rare disease that can also present with multiple nodules (carcinoid tumors and tumorlets) that result in airway obstruction (Fig. 12.39)
Infiltrative lung parenchymal disease	The high-attenuation (ground glass) areas are abnormal; vessels are normal in size and number; no air trapping; differential diagnoses are broad including pulmonary edema, hemorrhage, and infections

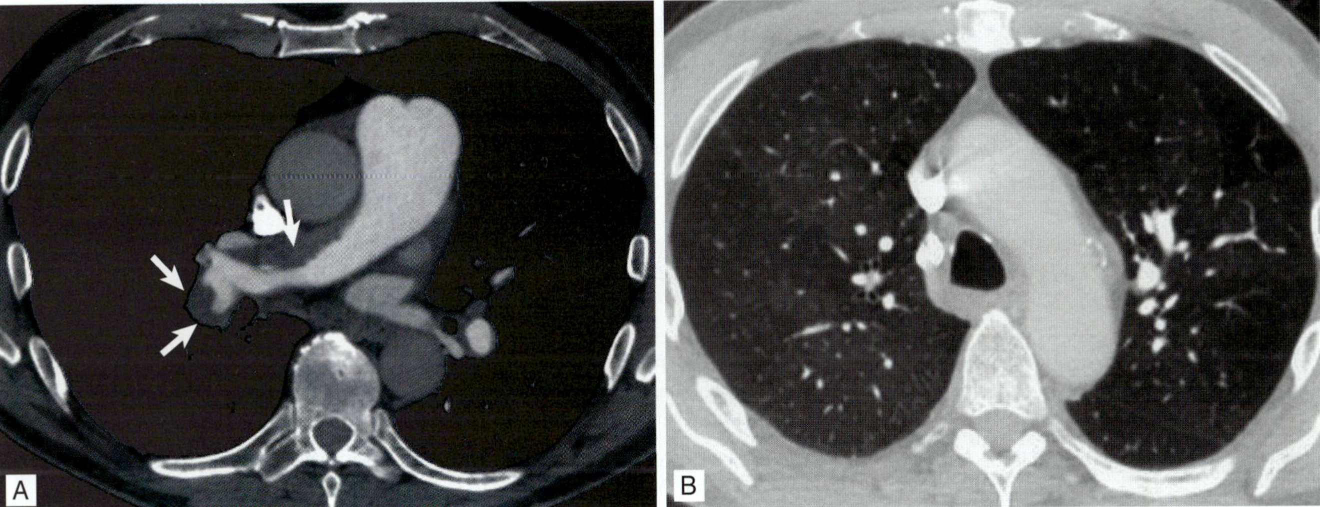

Figure 12.38 CT chest scan of a 64-year-old male with chronic thromboembolic pulmonary hypertension shows chronic eccentric filling defects within the central pulmonary arteries (A, *white arrows*) and mosaic attenuation of the lung parenchyma (B) consistent with small vessels disease.

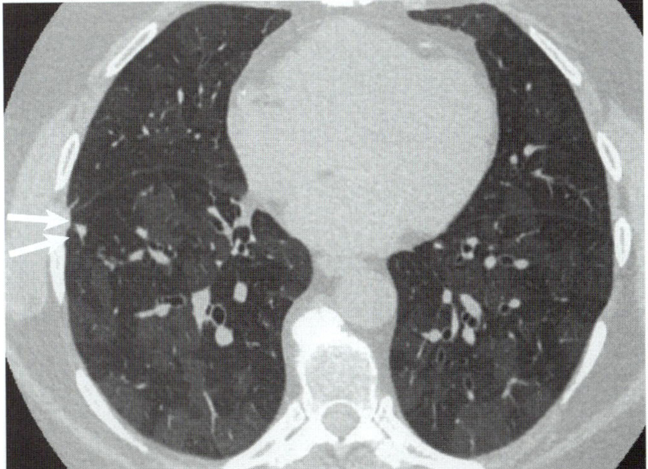

Figure 12.39 Chest CT images of a 70-year-old female show diffuse air trapping and numerous bilateral pulmonary nodules (*arrows*), consistent with biopsy-proved diffuse idiopathic neuroendocrine cell hyperplasia (DIPNECH).

TABLE 12.28 Differential Diagnoses in Those Presenting With Interlobular Septal Thickening

Condition	Distinguishing Features
Pulmonary edema	Most common cause of smooth septal thickening as the predominant or only pattern; usually bilateral and symmetric; ground-glass opacification; pleural effusions are common in cardiogenic/hydrostatic pulmonary edema (Fig. 12.40)
Lymphangitic carcinomatosis	Most often nodular and irregular; can be diffuse or asymmetric; hilar and mediastinal nodal enlargement is common (Fig. 12.41)
Sarcoidosis	Perilymphatic micronodules with symmetric hilar and mediastinal lymphadenopathy
Pulmonary hemorrhage	Ground-glass opacification with interlobular septal thickening; can be diffuse or focal
Lymphoproliferative disorders	Include lymphocytic interstitial pneumonia (LIP) and lymphoma; LIP is associated with lower lung predominant ground-glass opacity and perivascular cysts

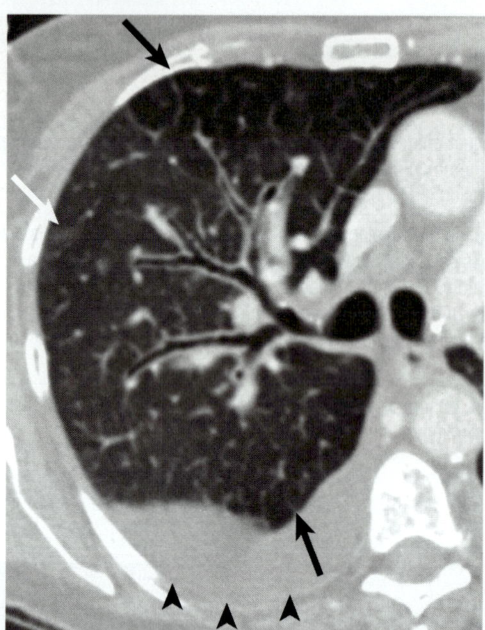

Figure 12.40 Chest CT image in a 75-year-old female with congestive heart failure shows smooth interlobular septal thickening (*black arrows*) with ground-glass opacities (*white arrow*) and pleural effusion (*black arrowheads*) consistent with pulmonary edema.

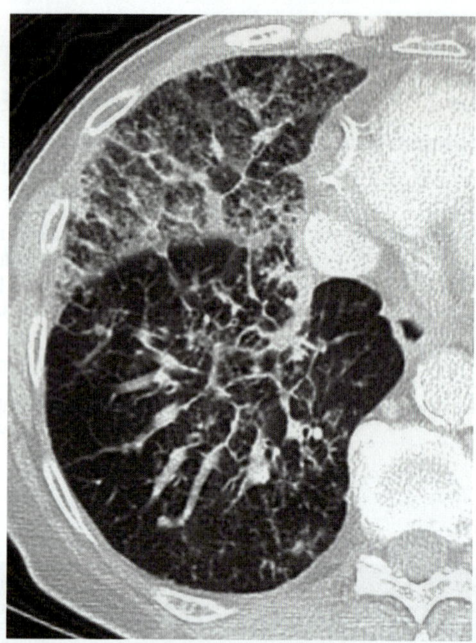

Figure 12.41 Chest CT images in an 85-year-old female with metastatic lung cancer show irregular nodular interlobular septal thickening, consistent with lymphangitic carcinomatosis.

TABLE 12.29 Differential Diagnoses in Those Presenting With Crazy Paving

Condition	Distinguishing Features
Pulmonary alveolar proteinosis (PAP)	Crazy paving was first described in PAP which is characterized by an abnormal intra-alveolar accumulation of surfactant-derived lipoproteinaceous material; ground-glass opacity typically resolves after bronchoalveolar lavage, although septal thickening may persist (Fig. 12.42)
Acute respiratory distress syndrome (ARDS)	Acute lung injury as a result of a severe pulmonary injury that causes alveolar damage heterogeneously throughout the lungs; findings resemble those of typical pulmonary edema or pulmonary hemorrhage
Acute interstitial pneumonitis (AIP)	Idiopathic extensive diffuse alveolar damage; similar to ARDS in the acute phase
Pulmonary edema	Usually bilateral and symmetric; pleural effusions are common in cardiogenic/hydrostatic pulmonary edema
Pulmonary hemorrhage	Ground-glass opacification with interlobular septal thickening (Fig. 12.43); can be diffuse or focal

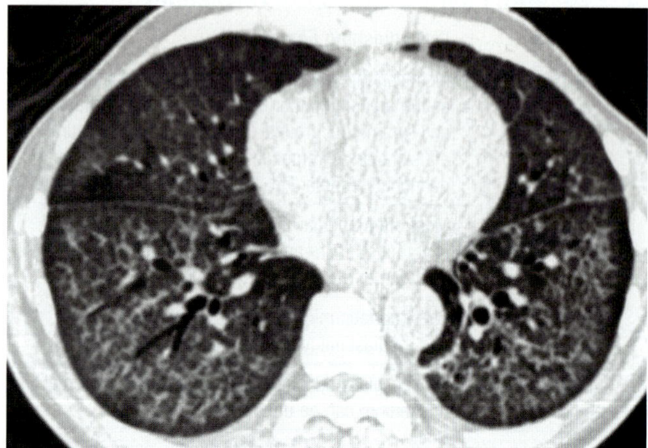

Figure 12.42 CT chest scan of a 62-year-old male shows diffuse ground-glass opacities with inter- and intralobular septal thickening. Bronchoalveolar lavage confirmed pulmonary alveolar proteinosis.

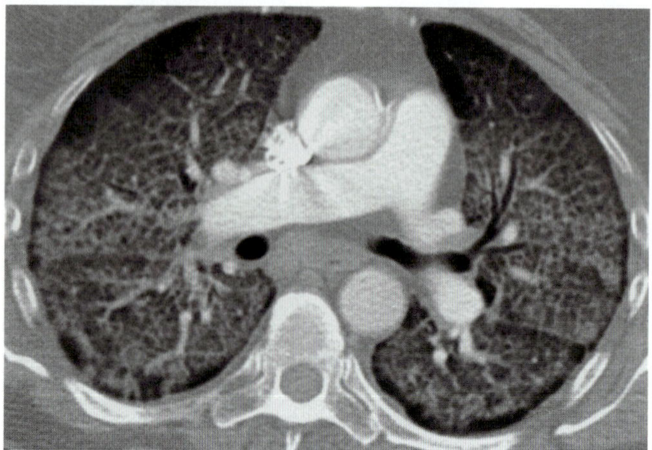

Figure 12.43 Chest CT images of a 59-year-old female presenting with hemoptysis show extensive ground-glass opacity throughout both lungs with interlobular septal thickening in a crazy paving pattern consistent with pulmonary alveolar hemorrhage.

TABLE 12.30 Differential Diagnoses in Those Presenting With Halo Sign

Condition	Distinguishing Features
Angioinvasive aspergillosis (Fig. 12.44)	Febrile neutropenic patient; pulmonary infarction, necrosis, and hemorrhage
Candidiasis	Severely immunocompromised patient
Cytomegalovirus	Most commonly 1 month or longer after transplantation
Malignancy (primary lung and metastases)	Ground-glass halo represents tumor infiltration or hemorrhage in hypervascular lesions (Fig. 12.45)
Granulomatosis with polyangitis	Multiple bilateral nodules or masses that may cavitate; tracheal stenosis or sinusitis
Organizing pneumonia	Bilateral focal consolidation or nodules; peripheral or peribronchial

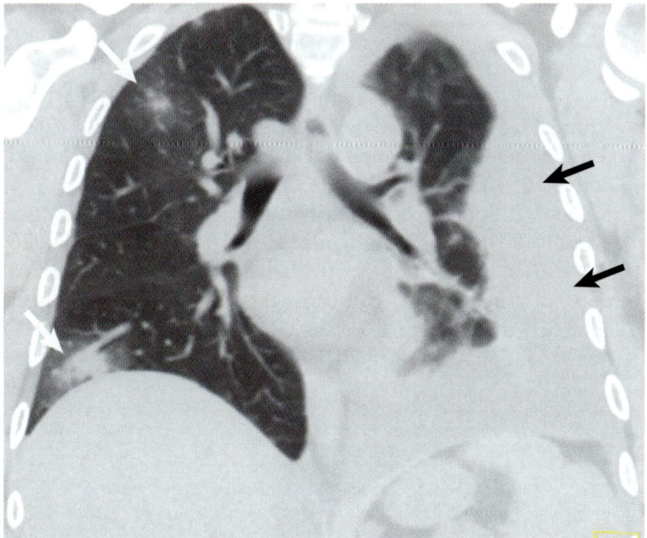

Figure 12.44 Chest CT image of a 33-year-old immunocompromised male with angioinvasive aspergillosis shows several consolidative nodules with peripheral ground-glass opacity (*white arrows*) in the right lung consistent with the halo sign, as well as a large left pleural effusion (*black arrows*).

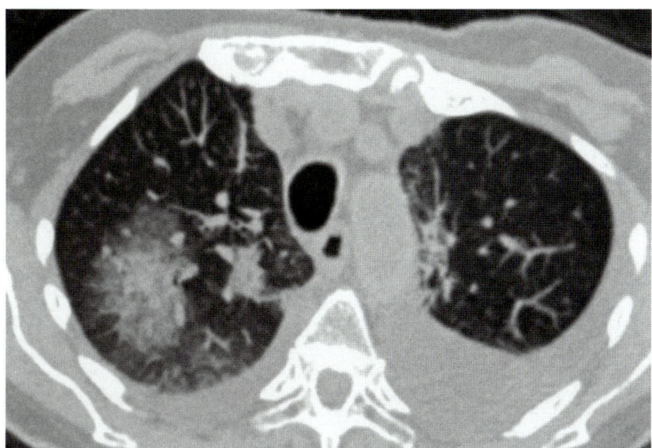

Figure 12.45 Chest CT scan of a 75-year-old female with metastatic endometrioid adenocarcinoma shows a consolidative mass with peripheral ground glass (halo sign) in the right upper lobe.

Reverse Halo Sign

The reverse halo sign, also known as the atoll sign, refers to a central area of ground-glass attenuation surrounded by denser consolidation that forms a crescentic or circular perimeter [16]. It was initially reported in cryptogenic organizing pneumonia but was later found to be present in several other diseases as outlined in Table 12.31.

TABLE 12.31 Differential Diagnoses in Those Presenting With Reverse Halo Sign

Condition	Distinguishing Features
Cryptogenic organizing pneumonia (Fig. 12.46)	Subacute to chronic pulmonary nodule and consolidation; peribronchovascular or peripheral; affect all lung zones; perilobular pattern (arcade-like sign)
Opportunistic fungal pneumonia	Consider invasive aspergillosis (Fig. 12.47) or mucormycosis
Granulomatosis with polyangitis	Bilateral nodules that may cavitate; tracheal abnormalities and sinusitis
Pulmonary infarction (Fig. 12.48)	Peripheral wedge-shaped pulmonary consolidations
Sarcoidosis	Ring-shaped consolidation histopathologically related to multiple granulomas; symmetric hilar and mediastinal lymphadenopathy; perilymphatic nodules
Lymphomatoid granulomatosis	Central ground glass consists of alveolar septal inflammatory infiltrates; peribronchovascular nodules that may cavitate; association with Epstein-Barr virus infection

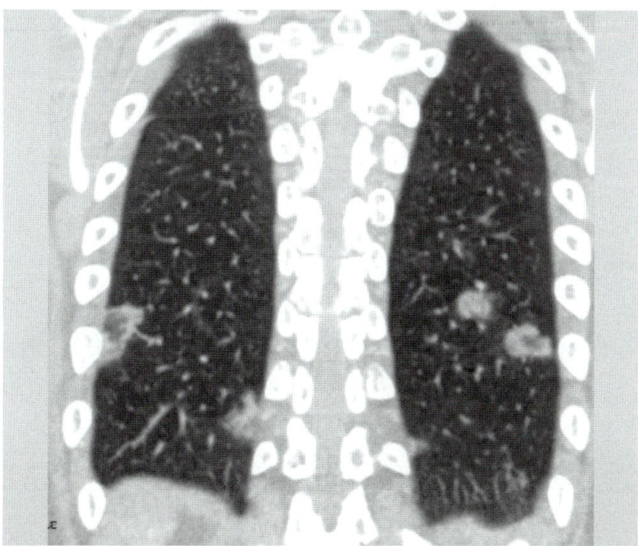

Figure 12.46 CT chest scan of a 28-year-old male with cryptogenic organizing pneumonia shows lower lobe predominant subpleural ground-glass opacities with peripheral consolidation in a reverse halo pattern.

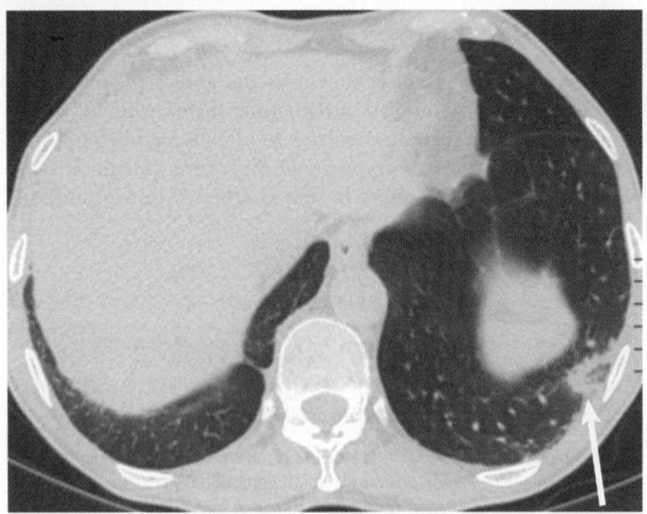

Figure 12.47 Chest CT image of a 59-year-old male with angioinvasive aspergillosis shows a peripheral consolidation with central ground glass in a reverse halo pattern.

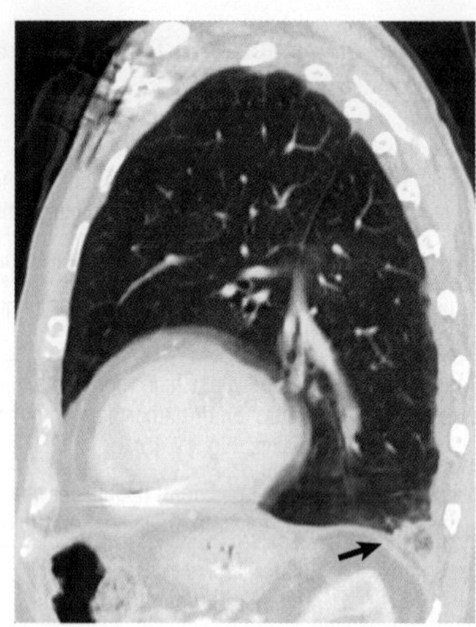

Figure 12.48 Chest CT scan of an 83-year-old man with known pulmonary embolism (not shown) shows peripheral consolidation in the left lung base with reverse halo sign (*arrow*), consistent with pulmonary infarction.

Suggested Readings

- CR Whitten, S Khan, GJ Munneke, S Grubnic, Abnormalities, Radiographics 27 (3) (2007) 657–671. doi:10.1148/rg.273065136.
- MT Truong, JP Ko, SE Rossi, et al., Update in the evaluation of the solitary pulmonary nodule, Radiogr Rev Publ Radiol Soc N Am Inc 34 (6) (2014) 1658–1679. doi:10.1148/rg.346130092.
- J Ahuja, GS Shroff, Y Mawlawi, MT Truong, Chronic airspace diseases, Semin Ultrasound CT MR 40 (3) (2019) 175–186. doi:10.1053/j.sult.2018.11.001.
- S Raoof, P Bondalapati, R Vydyula, et al., Cystic lung diseases, Chest 150 (4) (2016) 945–965. doi:10.1016/j.chest.2016.04.026.
- BW Carter, MF Benveniste, R Madan, et al., ITMIG classification of mediastinal compartments and multidisciplinary approach to mediastinal masses, Radiographics 37 (2) (2017) 413–436. doi:10.1148/rg.2017160095.

13

Mediastinum

ERIC W. ZHANG, SUBBA R. DIGUMARTHY

Anatomy

The thoracic mediastinum is defined anatomically as the compartment running between the pleural surfaces of the lungs and occupying the center of the thoracic cavity [1,2]. It runs longitudinally from the thoracic inlet superiorly to the central tendon of the diaphragm inferiorly, with the sternum, thoracic spine, and parietal pleura defining the anterior, posterior, and lateral margins, respectively. Many vital structures are housed and protected within the mediastinum, including the heart, trachea, and great vessels [3]. The mediastinum also contains structures traversing from the neck into the abdomen, such as the nerves, thoracic aorta, and esophagus.

When discussing the mediastinum, it has traditionally been useful from a radiographic point of view to subdivide the space into three parts: the anterior, middle, and posterior compartments (Fig. 13.1). *On the lateral radiograph, the anterior and middle compartments are separated by a line anterior to the trachea and posterior to the inferior vena cava. The middle and posterior compartments are separated by a line 1-cm posterior to the anterior thoracic vertebral bodies.* The main advantages of a three-compartment model are the similarities with anatomic, radiologic, and clinical models that have long been established based on true anatomic or fascial planes that exist to define these boundaries [1,4]. Subsequent four-division models have included the superior mediastinum compartment as a separate subdivision, which allows for a more specific categorization of pathologies typically found in the superior mediastinum such as those related to the thyroid gland. However, disadvantages of the four-compartment model include the increased relative complexity compared with the established three-compartment model as well as ambiguity relating to the artificial nonanatomic boundaries dividing the superior and inferior compartments.

The three-compartment model of the mediastinum has more recently been established as the new standard on cross-sectional imaging by the International Thymic Malignancy Interest Group [1]. This three-compartment method comprises the prevascular (anterior), visceral (middle), and paravertebral (posterior) compartments based upon readily identifiable landmarks and boundaries on multidetector computed tomography (CT) (Fig. 13.2). All three compartments are defined superiorly by the thoracic inlet and inferiorly by the diaphragm. The prevascular or anterior mediastinum is defined anteriorly by the sternum and posteriorly by the anterior pericardium, which wraps around the heart in a curvilinear pattern. Its major contents include the thymus, lymph nodes, fat, and left brachiocephalic vein. The visceral or middle mediastinum is defined anteriorly by the posterior boundaries of the prevascular space including the trachea and posteriorly by a vertical line connecting each thoracic vertebral body 1-cm posterior to the anterior margin of the vertebral body. Its major nonvascular contents include the trachea, carina, esophagus, and lymph nodes. Its major vascular contents include the heart, aorta (including ascending, arch, and descending portions), superior vena cava, intrapericardial pulmonary arteries, and thoracic duct. The paravertebral or posterior compartment is defined anteriorly by the posterior boundaries of the visceral compartment and posterolaterally by a vertical line outlining the posterior margin of the chest wall at the lateral margin of the transverse process of the thoracic vertebral bodies. Its major contents include the thoracic spine, paravertebral nerves, and paravertebral soft tissues. A summary of the boundaries and contents of the mediastinal compartments are listed in Table 13.1. Common and rare pathologies in each compartment are listed in Table 13.2.

Clinical Presentation of Mediastinal Disease

Initial evaluation of a patient with suspected mediastinal disease involves a thorough history and physical examination and is often supplemented by imaging and laboratory studies [2]. Mediastinal masses can be incidental findings in patients with routine chest radiographs or cross-sectional imaging. The clinical presentation of mediastinal pathology is varied, ranging from a completely

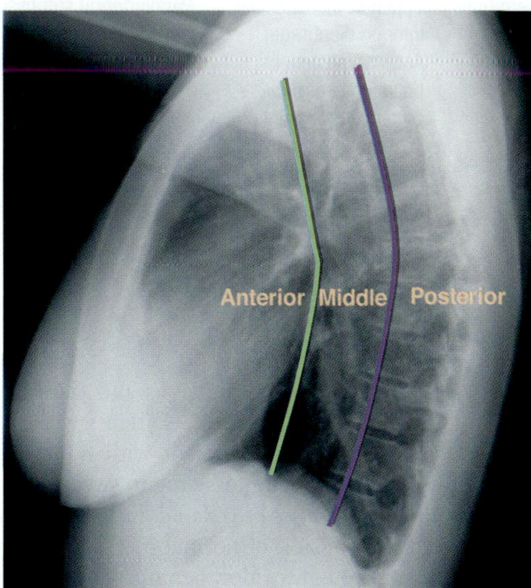

Figure 13.1 Radiographic subdivision of mediastinal compartments. The anterior and middle compartments are separated by a line anterior to the trachea and posterior to the inferior vena cava. The middle and posterior compartments are separated by a line 1-cm posterior to the anterior thoracic vertebral bodies.

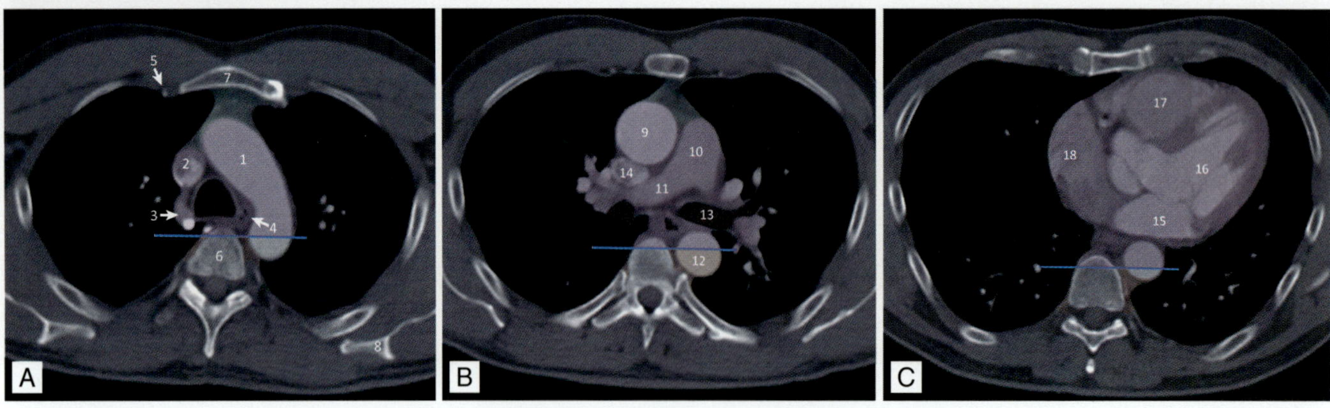

Figure 13.2 ITMIG boundaries defining the prevascular (*green*), visceral (*purple*), and paravertebral (*orange*) compartments at the level of (A) the aortic arch, (B) the main pulmonary artery, and (C) the heart chambers. 1 = aortic arch; 2 = superior vena cava; 3 = azygos vein; 4 = esophagus; 5 = right internal mammary artery; 6 = vertebral body; 7 = sternum; 8 = left scapula; 9 = ascending thoracic aorta; 10 = main pulmonary artery; 11 = right main pulmonary artery; 12 = descending thoracic aorta; 13 = left main stem bronchus; 14 = superior vena cava; 15 = left atrium; 16 = left ventricle; 17 = right ventricle; 18 = right atrium.

TABLE 13.1 Boundaries and Major Contents of Mediastinal Compartments

Compartments	Boundaries	Major Contents
Prevascular/ anterior	Superior: thoracic inlet Inferior: diaphragm Anterior: sternum Posterior: anterior pericardium Lateral: parietal pleura	Lymph nodes Fat Thymus Left brachiocephalic vein
Visceral/middle	Superior: thoracic inlet Inferior: diaphragm Anterior: anterior pericardium Posterior: vertical line 1 cm behind the anterior margin of the thoracic vertebral bodies Lateral: parietal pleura	Heart Ascending, arch, descending aorta Superior vena cava Intrapericardial arteries Thoracic duct Trachea, carina Esophagus Lymph nodes
Paravertebral/ posterior	Superior: thoracic inlet Inferior: diaphragm Anterior: posterior boundaries of the visceral compartment Posterior: vertical line delineated by the lateral margin of the transverse process of the thoracic spine and posterior margin of the chest wall	Paravertebral soft tissues Nerves Thoracic spine and ribs

TABLE 13.2 Common and Rare Lesions Encountered in Each Mediastinal Compartment

Compartments	Common Lesions	Rare Lesions
Prevascular/ anterior	Mediastinal thyroid goiters Fat deposition Epicardial fat pad Lymphadenopathy (including metastasis) Tortuous vessels Aortic aneurysms Thymoma Germ cell tumor	Lymphangioma Parathyroid adenoma Ectopic thyroid tissue Innominate artery aneurysm Sarcomas
Visceral/middle	Lymphadenopathy (including metastasis) Aortic aneurysms Pulmonary artery enlargement Dilated superior vena cava Bronchogenic cyst	Tracheal pathology Cardiac neoplasm Esophageal neoplasm Sarcomas
Paravertebral/ posterior	Neurogenic tumor Hiatal hernia Aortic aneurysms Dilated azygos vein Esophageal dilatation Osteomyelitis Metastasis	Extramedullary hematopoiesis Primary osseous neoplasm Sarcomas

asymptomatic presentation to specific signs and symptoms that may point to an intrathoracic pathology. Patients with mediastinal masses and malignancies may present with nonspecific systemic symptoms such as weight loss, night sweats, and fever. However, symptoms may also be related to mediastinal mass effects, with direct compression of normal mediastinal structures [5]. Symptoms such as cough, stridor, hemoptysis, and dysphagia may point toward specific disease processes involving the trachea and esophagus. Facial and/or upper extremity swelling suggests vascular compression on the superior vena cava and brachiocephalic veins. Hypotension and jugular vein distention may point toward tamponade physiology or cardiac compression. Horner's syndrome or hoarseness could imply a sympathetic chain or recurrent laryngeal nerve involvement. Specific signs such as muscle weakness from myasthenia gravis may prompt the search for an occult thymoma using CT or magentic resonance (MR).

Imaging Workup of Mediastinal Disease

Chest Radiography

Chest radiography is often the first technique used for the workup of suspected mediastinal processes and is often implicated in the incidental detection of mediastinal masses. An understanding of normal

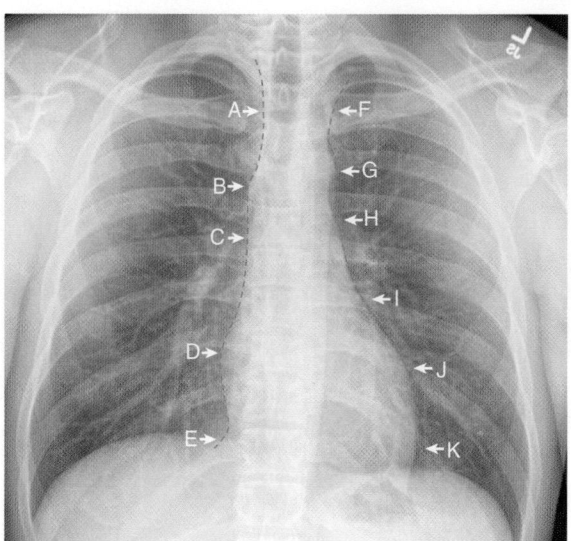

Figure 13.3 Normal frontal chest radiograph contours. A = right paratracheal stripe/great vessels; B = azygos vein; C = superior vena cava; D = right atrium; E = inferior vena cava; F = left paratracheal stripe/great vessels; G = aortic arch; H = main pulmonary artery; I = left atrial appendage; J = left ventricle; K = pericardial fat pad.

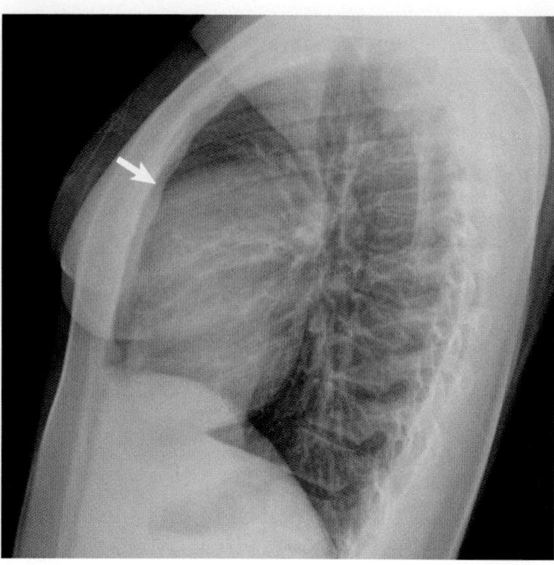

Figure 13.5 Lateral radiograph in a 34-year-old man demonstrating a rounded opacity occupying the prevascular mediastinum, obliterating the retrosternal clear space. Subsequent workup revealed a mature teratoma.

chest radiograph anatomy (Fig. 13.3), including stripes, lines, and interfaces, is critical in the detection of subtle mediastinal abnormalities [2]. Mediastinal abnormalities are detected by observing changes in normal radiographic anatomy on chest adiograph, including opacification of anatomically lucent regions, displacement or compression of mediastinal structures, and obliteration or displacement of normal mediastinal stripes and lines [4,6]. The Silhouette sign, also known as loss of silhouette sign, refers to the loss of normal silhouette seen on chest radiographs and can be used to localize atelectasis, airspace processes, and masses within the chest. Right upper lobe and right upper mediastinal pathologies can result in loss of the right paratracheal stripe (Fig. 13.4). Obscuration of the normal right heart border can indicate a pathology within the right middle lobe, medial right lower lobe, or mediastinum. Loss of the normal right hemidiaphragm can indicate a pathology within the right lower lobe. Similarly, obscuration of normal aortic knob can indicate a pathology within the left upper lobe or left upper mediastinum. Loss of the left heart border usually indicates lingular pathology. Loss of the left hemidiaphragm or descending aorta can indicate pathology within the left lower lobe or left lower mediastinum. Anterior mediastinal masses often present with a displaced anterior junction line, obliteration of the retrosternal clear space, effacement of the ascending aorta, and obliteration of the cardiophrenic angles (Fig. 13.5). Obliteration of the retrosternal clear space is less useful in large obese patients, where the retrosternal space can be filled with fat. Middle mediastinal masses can be detected by the widening of paratracheal stripes, the presence of an abnormal opacity in the aortopulmonary window, the displacement of azygoesophageal recess on the right, and the presence of a pseudoparavertebral line on the left (Fig. 13.6). On lateral projections, useful signs to look for including the "doughnut," which is formed by a lobulated mass surrounding the right bronchus forming the hole in the middle (Fig. 13.7). The hilum overlay sign is useful for distinguishing between middle mediastinal masses and anterior or posterior mediastinal masses. If hilar vessels are visible through the mass on the frontal chest radiograph, then the mass does not arise from the hilum. In most cases, due to the geometry of the mediastinum, these masses will arise from the anterior mediastinum (Fig. 13.8). Posterior mediastinal masses can be detected on radiographs through the widening of paravertebral stripes (Fig. 13.9). The cervicothoracic sign can be used to locate posterior mediastinal masses. At the level of the thoracic inlet, the posterior part of the lung extends superiorly to the clavicle compared to the anterior part; hence, any mass when situated in the posterior mediastinum, is completely surrounded by the lung tissue from all sides. This leads to a well-defined cephalic border seen above the clavicle. In contrast, anterior mediastinal masses have ill-defined cephalic margins due to their anatomical contact with the soft tissues of the neck, either at or below the clavicle indicating a cervicothoracic lesion. (Fig. 13.10).

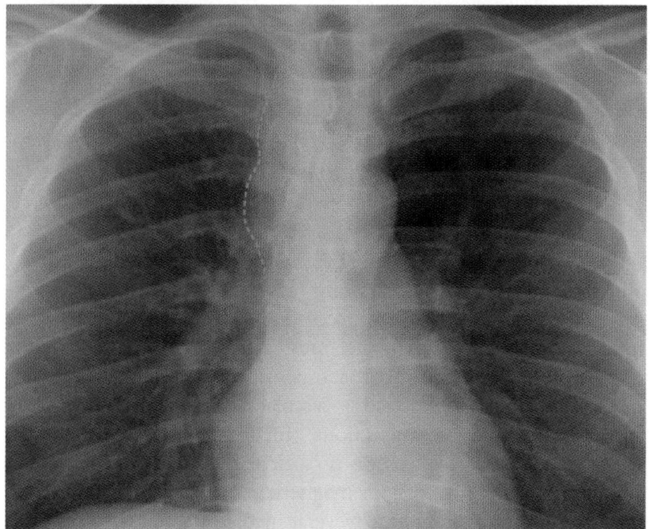

Figure 13.4 A 54-year-old man with tuberculosis presenting with right paratracheal lymphadenopathy widening the normally thin right paratracheal stripe.

Computed Tomography Imaging

CT imaging is the workhorse for the workup of mediastinal abnormalities, owing to the versatility, accuracy, speed, and availability of the technology [2,7]. Oftentimes, an abnormality

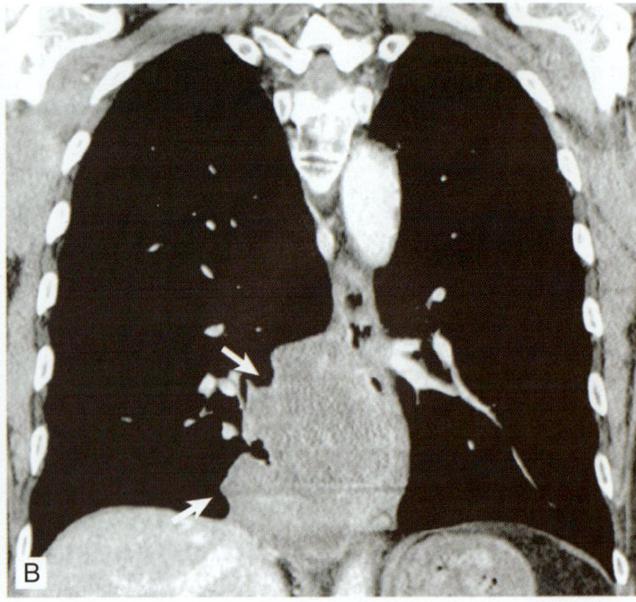

Figure 13.6 Frontal radiograph (A) in a 63-year-old man demonstrating an irregular opacity with apparent central lucency (*arrows*) displacing the azygoesophageal recess (*dotted outline*). Corresponding CT chest coronal reformats (B) demonstrating an irregular hypoattenuating likely necrotic mass (*arrows*) abutting the esophagus occupying the azygoesophageal recess, later biopsied to be metastatic renal cell carcinoma.

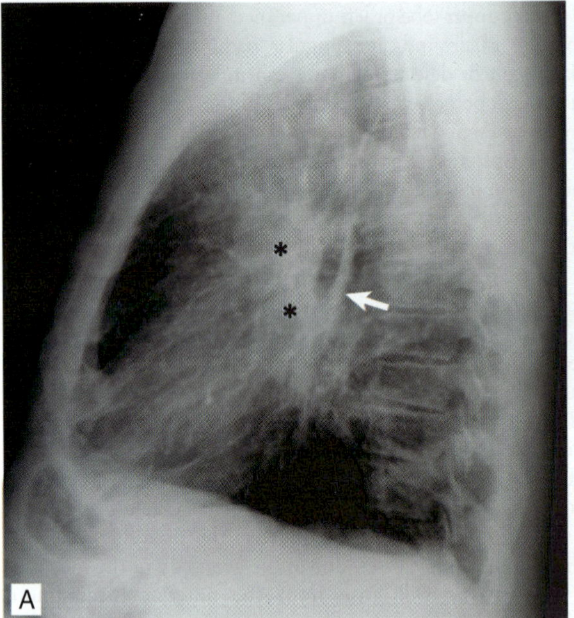

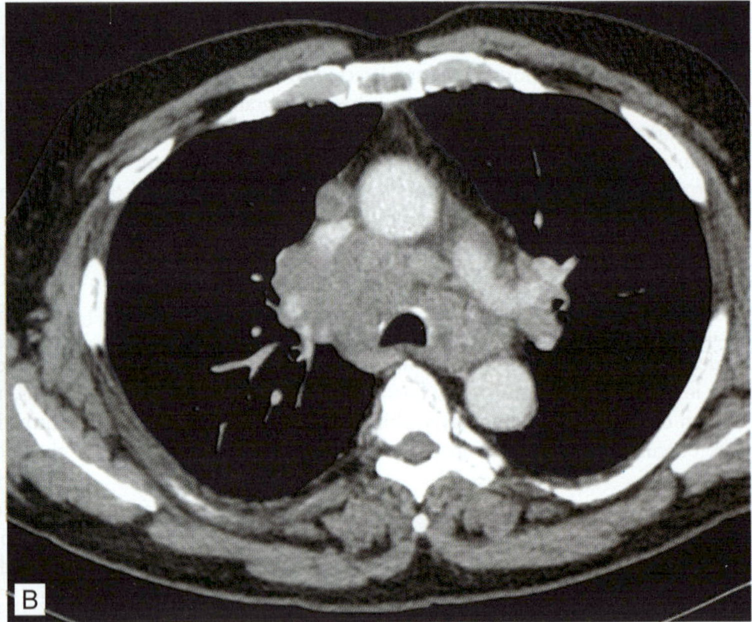

Figure 13.7 Lateral radiograph (A) in a 58-year-old man demonstrating rounded opacities (*asterisks*) anterior to the lower trachea and carina, likely involving the mediastinum and hila. There is thickening of the posterior wall of the bronchus intermedius (*arrow*). Corresponding axial CT chest (B) demonstrates extensive bilateral mediastinal and hilar lymphadenopathy, later worked up to represent nodal metastasis from lung adenocarcinoma.

spotted on a chest radiograph will be further investigated using CT imaging. Indications for use include

- investigation of a mediastinal mass detected clinically or radiographically;
- investigation of the widened mediastinum or abnormal hilum;
- investigation of suspected pneumomediastinum and/or pneumopericardium;
- staging and surveillance of malignancies;
- detection and follow-up of vascular anomalies;
- detection of clinically suspected occult mediastinal process

Compared with chest radiograph, CT imaging offers superior tissue contrast and spatial resolution, allowing for the precise characterization and localization of mediastinal processes. Fluid, fat, air, and calcification can be easily differentiated on CT, owing to detectable differences in CT attenuation measured in Hounsfield units (HU). Tissue contrast differentiation is further improved with the usage of iodinated contrast medium [2,7]. Dynamic contrast-enhanced CT is also an excellent method for assessing vascular pathology in the mediastinum, including aortic dissections, aneurysms, pseudoaneurysms, and extravasation. Calcification is particularly well demonstrated by CT, especially compared with magnetic resonance imaging (MRI), and is useful in differentiating several mediastinal lesions. However, CT characterization of soft-tissue attenuation is limited, and it is often difficult to differentiate hyperattenuating hemorrhage or

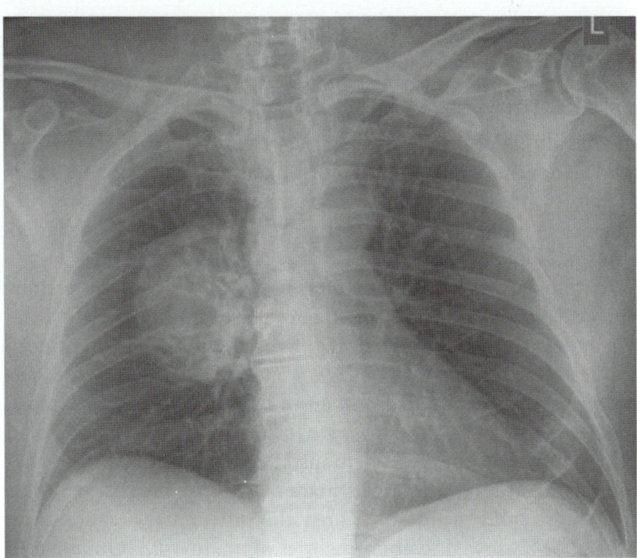

Figure 13.8 Example of hilar overlay sign in a 42-year-old man with a large anterior mediastinal mass. Notice the hilar vessels are visible and easily traceable through the mass.

proteinaceous fluid from a soft-tissue mass due to overlapping CT numbers. In contrast, CT imaging offers excellent spatial resolution. Modern high-resolution CT scanners can readily determine the location of a mass or abnormality down to 0.25-mm in-plane spatial resolution.

Magnetic Resonance Imaging

MRI offers superior soft-tissue contrast compared with CT, making it a useful adjunct and troubleshooting tool in characterizing indeterminate mediastinal masses [8,9]. By leveraging differences in T1 and T2 relaxation times between different body composition materials, smooth muscle, fibrosis, microscopic and macroscopic fat, cartilage, hemorrhage, and proteinaceous fluid can be readily distinguished. However, MRI struggles with characterization of calcium, which appears with various signal intensities on conventional spin-echo T1- and T2-weighted images. Characterization of soft tissues is further improved through the usage of dynamic contrast-enhanced MRI, which involves the injection of gadolinium contrast agents. Gadolinium molecules shorten the T1 relaxation time of voxels in which they are present and thus produce a brighter signal. Dynamic contrast-enhanced MRI has used in the characterization of neoplasms, detection of abscesses, as well as imaging of vessels and perfusion. Diffusion-weighted MRI with apparent diffusion coefficient mapping measures the random Brownian motion of water molecules in a voxel and can be utilized to assess highly cellular neoplasms including high-risk thymic malignancies and lymphoma. Diffusion-weighted MRI can also help distinguish abscesses and hematomas, which may also restrict the motion of water molecules [8,9]. Chemical shift imaging with in-and-out of phase imaging is useful for detecting microscopic fat and in the characterization of thymic lesions. Additional advantages of MRI images include increased delineation of different anatomical components, including the boundaries of the pericardium, pleura, and musculature, as well as provide a more sensitive assessment of bone marrow, paravertebral soft tissues, and spinal cord.

Positron Emission Tomography

Positron emission tomography (PET) imaging using isotope 18-fluorodeoxyglucose (^{18}FDG) has primarily been used in the mediastinum for the staging of malignancies, primarily non–small-cell lung cancer and lymphoma [10,11]. PET is often performed in combination with CT imaging or MRI to increase spatial resolution and diagnostic accuracy. PET-CT has been

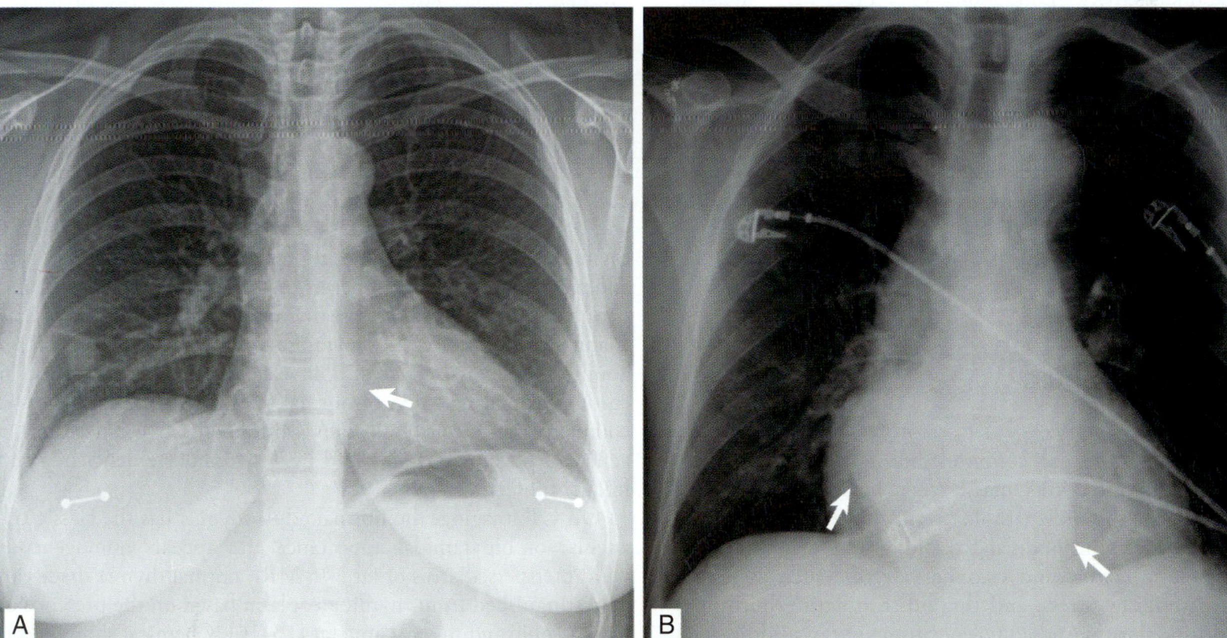

Figure 13.9 Frontal chest radiograph in a 52-year-old female (A) with a focal rounded bulge in the left inferior paravertebral stripe (*arrow*) corresponding to a paravertebral neurogenic tumor. There is an incidental known hamartoma in the right lower lung zone. Frontal chest radiograph in a 38-year-old male (B) with beta-thalassemia demonstrating bilateral paravertebral opacities (*arrows*) corresponding to extramedullary hematopoiesis.

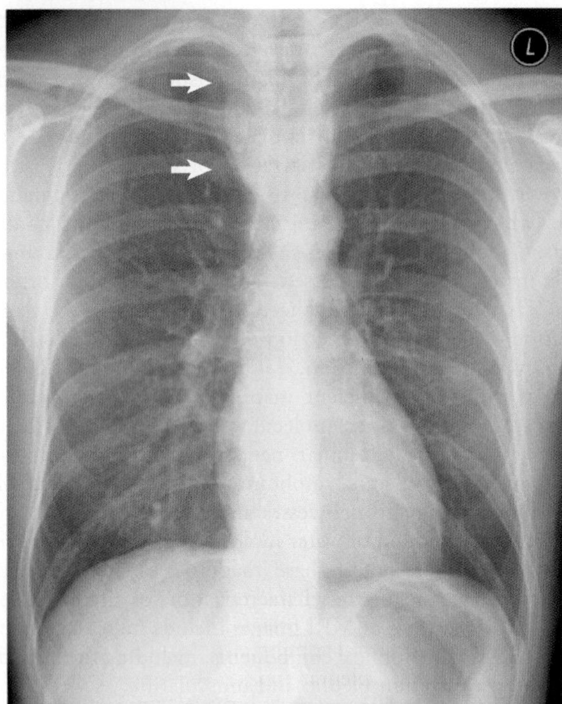

Figure 13.10 Frontal chest radiograph in a 57-year-old male with a rounded opacity in the upper paratracheal region extending above the level of the clavicles merging into the soft tissues of the neck and showing an indistinct superior border, corresponding to a mediastinal thyroid goiter.

shown to have greater accuracy for determining local tumor margins, nodal metastasis, and distant metastasis than PET or CT alone. In particular, PET-CT is useful in detecting nodal metastases below the 1-cm threshold used in CT imaging alone. Conversely, PET-CT can also help decrease false positives in reactive lymph nodes above the 1-cm threshold but without corresponding metabolic activity. Limitations of ^{18}FDG-PET imaging include false positives created by inflammatory processes unrelated to malignancies such as sarcoidosis, tuberculosis, histoplasmosis, and other chronic infections. ^{18}FDG-PET imaging is also limited for the evaluation of thymic masses, owing to overlap in standardized uptake values between normal thymus, thymic hyperplasia, and thymic malignancies. In such circumstances, a surgical or imaging-guided histopathologic biopsy is required for diagnostic confirmation.

Clinical Applications

Anterior Mediastinum

Thyroid Lesions

Thyroid abnormalities are common and account for a large percentage of thoracic inlet masses seen in adults. The most commonly seen thyroid pathology in the mediastinum is enlarged nontoxic multinodular thyroid goiters, which are the result of genetic factors and secondary factors such as iodine deficiency, smoking, stress, and thyroid-stimulating hormones [12]. Multinodular thyroid goiters occur mainly in middle-aged or older women. There are multiple other rarer causes of thyroid gland enlargement, including thyrotoxicosis, Hashimoto's thyroiditis, thyroid adenoma, thyroid carcinoma, and lymphoma. Although thyroid enlargement is relatively common, less than 5% of enlarged thyroid glands extend into the mediastinum to produce a retrosternal goiter. Most retrosternal goiters are asymptomatic. A minority of retrosternal goiters can produce symptoms based on compression of local structures such as dysphagia and stridor. The presence of pain in the goiter, the development of vocal cord paralysis, or facial and upper extremity swelling in the setting of superior vena cava obstruction are red flags, possibly alerting to the presence of an underlying malignancy.

On imaging, retrosternal goiters usually appear as well-circumscribed rounded or ovoid soft-tissue masses in the superior anterior mediastinum, sometimes involving the middle mediastinum and retrotracheal space as well. *In up to a quarter of cases, retrosternal goiters can extend posterior to the trachea and occupy the retrotracheal clear space or Raider triangle* (Fig. 13.11). These masses can calcify internally and will demonstrate continuity with the thyroid gland. If a connection is made between a mediastinal mass and the thyroid gland superiorly, the differential diagnosis can usually be narrowed to abnormalities of the thyroid. On noncontrast CT, thyroid masses may demonstrate higher attenuation than muscle, owing to high inherent iodine content. Depending on the aggressivity and rate of growth of the mass, internal foci of cystic or necrotic degeneration can be seen, manifesting as areas of low or fluid attenuation. The presence of adjacent lymphadenopathy should alert to the presence of underlying thyroid malignancy. In rare circumstances, heterotopic thyroid gland can develop in the mediastinum. Thyroid tissue will be isodense to the thyroid on CT and follow the signal intensity of the thyroid gland across all sequences on MRI. Nuclear medicine scans, including ^{123}I-sodium iodide and Tc-99m-sodium pertechnetate scans, can also be useful in distinguishing ectopic or retrosternal thyroid tissues by demonstrating unusual areas of increased activity.

Thymic Lesions

Normal Thymus: The thymus gland is a specialized lymphoid organ implicated in the development of adaptive immunity through the maturation of T cell lymphocytes. The thymus is disproportionately large at birth and throughout infancy and childhood. It is the most common cause of mediastinal abnormality seen in the pediatric population, usually manifesting as a triangular-shaped sail-like mass projecting in the right mediastinum on chest radiograph (Fig. 13.12). After reaching a maximum weight in adolescence, the thymus gradually involutes and undergoes fatty atrophy in adulthood. The thymus becomes largely fatty and imperceptible in the fifth to sixth decade of life [13]. Normal thymic tissue is usually found in the upper anterior mediastinum and may be found anterosuperior to the left innominate vein and neck base. In young adults, the thymus usually has a characteristic triangular, bilobed, and bipyramidal appearance (Fig. 13.13). Young adults between 20 and 30 years of age can have up to 1.6 cm in maximal thickness of normal thymic tissue. The thymus is completely absent in DiGeorge's syndrome (22q11.2 deletion), a genetic syndrome characterized by T lymphocyte deficiency and frequent infections.

On CT imaging, the normal adult thymus has the classic triangular or bipyramidal appearance and appears homogeneous with interspersed areas of fat. On MRI, normal thymic tissue can be distinguished from thymic neoplasm based on the presence of macroscopic and microscopic fat [13–16]. Chemical shift MRI is key in assessing the presence of microscopic fat and includes the calculation of the chemical shift ratio (CSR) or signal intensity index (SII). Dropping signal intensities within the thymic lesion on out-of-phase (OOP) images compared with in-phase (IP)

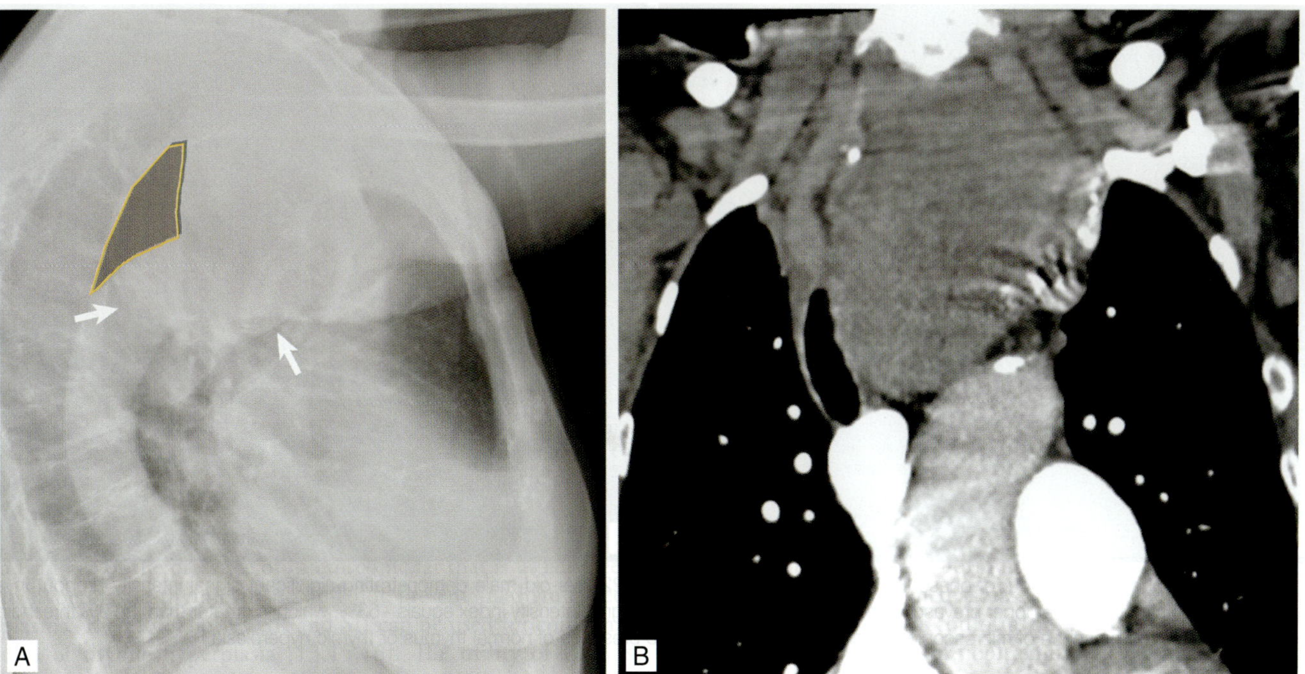

Figure 13.11 Lateral chest radiograph (A) in a 78-year-old female demonstrating a rounded circumscribed opacity (*arrows*) occupying the retrotracheal or Raider triangle (*orange*), corresponding to a large retrosternal goiter on corresponding CT chest in coronal reformat (B). Notice the significant rightward displacement of the trachea and the extension of the mass into the lower neck. The Raider triangle is bounded by the thoracic vertebral bodies posteriorly, the aortic arch inferiorly, and the posterior tracheal stripe anteriorly.

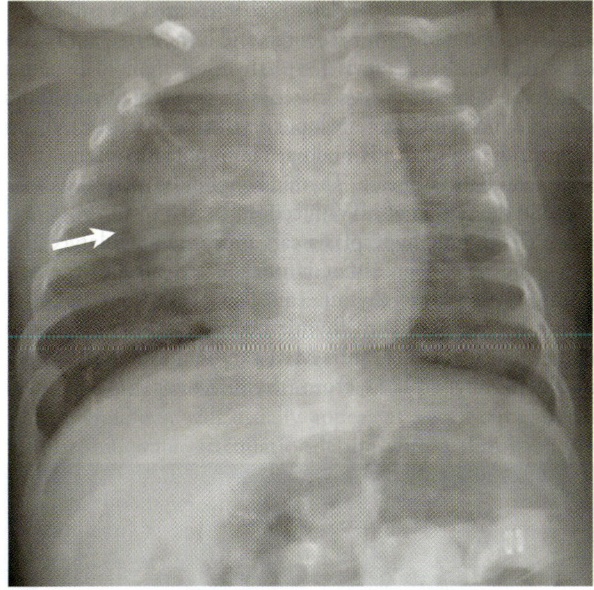

Figure 13.12 Frontal chest radiograph in a 3-month-old infant demonstrating the characteristic triangular sail-shaped opacity projecting into the right mediastinum corresponding to the normal thymus gland.

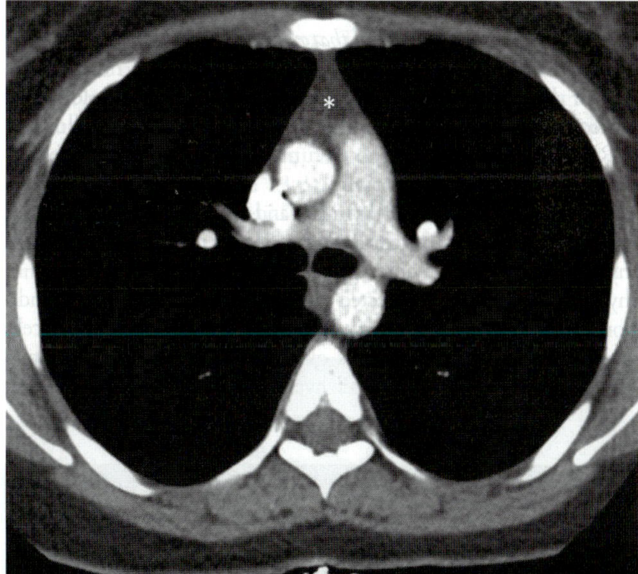

Figure 13.13 Axial CT chest in a 23-year-old healthy female with typical triangular soft-tissue density noted in the anterior mediastinum without irregular nodularity or calcification and interspersed fat density (*asterisk*), compatible with normal thymic tissue.

images indicate the presence of microscopic fat and exclude underlying tumors. The exception to this rule is cases of teratomas or dermoid tumors, in which the presence of intralesional fat should not be confused with benign thymic tissue.

The CSR is calculated by comparing the signal intensities of OOP images in the thymus and surrounding paraspinal musculature with thymic and paraspinal muscle signal intensities of IP images. A CSR ≤0.7 is compatible with normal or hyperplasic thymus. A CSR >1.0 usually indicates thymic neoplasm. A CSR > = 0.8 to < = 0.9 is indeterminate [13,15].

$$\text{CSR} = \frac{\text{OOP thymic signal intensity / OOP paraspinal muscle signal intensity}}{\text{IP thymic signal intensity/IP paraspinal muscle signal intensity}}.$$

The SII involves comparing only signal intensity dropout in the thymus between OOP and IP images (Fig. 13.14). SII >9% has

TABLE 13.3 World Health Organization Histopathological Classification of Thymic Epithelial Tumors

Type	Pathological Features	Invasiveness (%)	Ten-year Disease-free Survival (%)
Type A thymoma	▪ Spindle or polygonal cell without atypia ▪ Paucity of immature thymocytes	10–40	100
Type AB thymoma	▪ Contains both type A (lymphocyte-poor) and type B (lymphocyte-rich) cells	30–40	100
Type B1 thymoma	▪ Thymoma resembling cortical thymus	45–50	100
Type B2 thymoma	▪ Increasing epithelial/ lymphocyte ratio and atypia	65–70	85
Type B3 thymoma	▪ Increasing epithelial/ lymphocyte ratio and atypia ▪ Mature lymphocytes	85–90	35
Thymic carcinoma	▪ Epithelial cell atypia and infiltration ▪ Absence of immature lymphocytes ▪ CD5/KIT expression	90–95	15

tumor can be composed of different types of thymomas, which can lead to undersampling with percutaneous biopsies. The Masaoka–Koga staging system, based on surgical findings, is often used to predict prognosis and dictate the treatment approach (Table 13.4).

Thymomas are the most common primary neoplasms of the anterior mediastinum, with the majority arising from the upper anterior mediastinum near the ascending aorta and pulmonary artery. They are typically seen in adulthood and are rarely found in children. Although often asymptomatic, thymomas can be associated with myasthenia gravis, hypogammaglobulinemia, and aplastic anemia.

TABLE 13.4 Masaoka–Koga International Thymic Malignancy Interest Group Staging System for Thymoma

Stage	Findings
1	▪ Completely encapsulated
2	▪ Invasion of tumor capsule
3	▪ Invasion of neighboring organs
4A	▪ Pleural or pericardial implants
4B	▪ Distant (extrathoracic) hematogenous or lymphogenous metastasis

About 25–50% of patients with thymoma have myasthenia gravis while 10–25% of patients with myasthenia have a thymoma.

Many thymomas can be seen on chest radiograph, usually manifesting as a lobulated or ovoid circumscribed mass projecting unilaterally in the mediastinum [21,22]. However, depending on the size and location of the tumor, chest radiographs can also be normal or have very subtle distortions of the anterior junction line. Thickening of the anterior junction line usually indicates the presence of an anterior mediastinal mass. The lateral radiograph can also help detect the presence of thymomas in the retrosternal space.

CT imaging has increased sensitivity for detecting thymomas and help assess local invasion and aid surgical planning [19,21,22,24]. Thymomas usually appear as well-defined round or oval soft-tissue density masses on CT, usually projecting on one side of the anterior mediastinum (Fig. 13.18). Thymomas may contain curvilinear or nodular calcification and are usually homogeneous, enhancing with intravenous contrast. Nonetheless, some thymomas can present as more heterogeneous masses with cystic, necrotic, and hemorrhagic areas. Heterogeneity of tumors is associated with higher tumor grade and is often seen in thymic carcinomas, but this feature alone is not specific for a degree of invasiveness, as low-grade tumors may also demonstrate heterogeneity. Intravenous contrast is useful in delineating vascular encasement and invasion of neighboring organs. CT is also helpful in detecting the presence of intra- and extrathoracic metastasis, which if found, will upstage a patient and change management. Unlike lung cancer, thymomas rarely present with

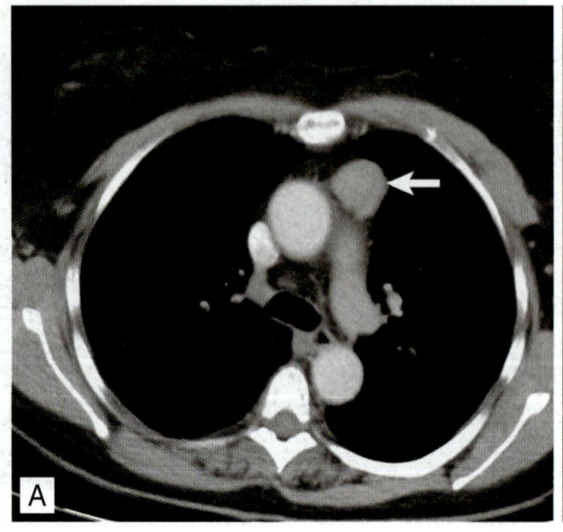

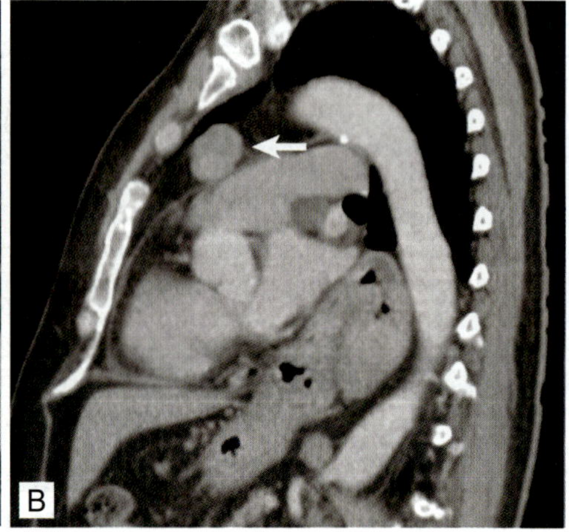

Figure 13.18 Biopsy-proved AB-type thymoma. Enhanced CT chest in axial (A) and sagittal (B) views demonstrating a round prevascular mass with mildly heterogeneous attenuation adjacent to the pericardium. No local metastases at the time of the scan.

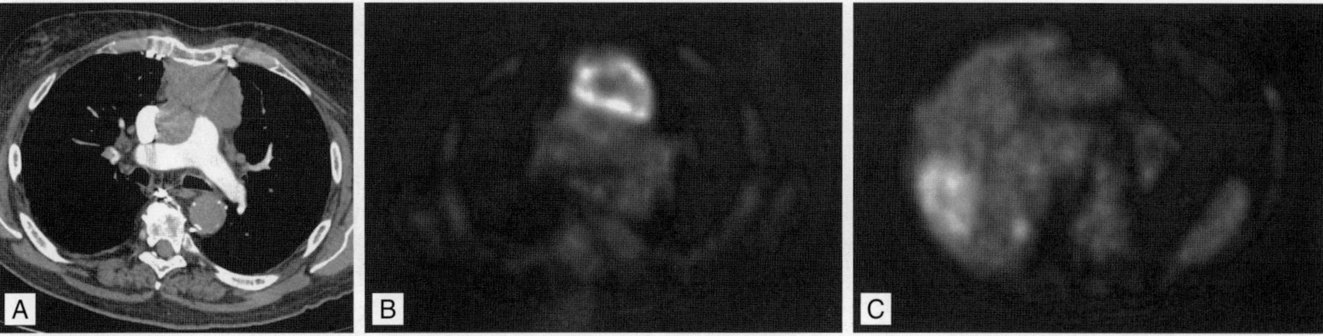

Figure 13.19 Biopsy-proved high-grade thymic carcinoma. Enhanced axial CT chest (A) demonstrating an irregular heterogeneous mass in the prevascular mediastinum. Accompanying ^{18}F-FDG PET at the same level (B) shows peripheral intense radiotracer uptake within the mass, which has a central necrotic core. At the level of the upper abdomen (C), there are several areas of intense radiotracer uptake, concerning distant metastases.

lymphadenopathy, pleural effusion, and pulmonary metastases. In contrast, thymic carcinomas will exhibit more aggressive behavior and can often present with both intra- and extrathoracic metastases (Fig. 13.19). Common areas for intrathoracic metastatic involvement in thymic carcinomas include pleural drop metastasis and invasion of contiguous mediastinal structures such as pericardium and great vessels.

On MRI, thymomas are nonspecific and can have intermediate T1 signal and hyperintense T2 signal (Fig. 13.20). *Unlike thymic hyperplasia, thymomas will not demonstrate evidence of microscopic fat on OOP images.* Dynamic enhancement MRI cannot accurately differentiate a thymoma from other anterior mediastinal masses including thymic carcinoma, lymphoma, or germ cell tumors. Furthermore, heterogeneity by itself is not an accurate assessment of the invasiveness of thymoma. MRI can help differentiate a proteinaceous and hemorrhagic thymic cyst from a solid mass.

Germ Cell Tumors

Germ cell tumors in the anterior mediastinum derive from primordial germ cell rests left behind during their embryological migration to the urogenital ridge [17,18,25]. Germ cell tumors are usually found along the median line of the body and the anterior mediastinum is the most common location for extragonadal germ cell tumors. Other common areas where germ cell tumors can be found include the pineal gland, the sacrum/coccyx, and the neurohypophysis. Most germ cell tumors, including dermoid cysts or mature teratomas, are benign. However, as many as 30% of germ cell tumors are malignant and include entities such as seminoma, choriocarcinoma, yolk sac tumors, and embryonal cell carcinoma. The World Health Organization classifies germ cell tumors into either seminomas or nonseminomatous tumors. Nonseminomatous germ cell tumors include teratomas, embryonal carcinoma, yolk sac carcinoma, and choriocarcinoma. Mixed tumors have features of more than one histologic subtype. Germ cell tumors are classically discovered incidentally on chest radiograph and usually seen in young male adults. Although many tumors are asymptomatic, some can produce cough, chest pain, and dyspnea.

Teratomas are tumors containing elements of all three germ cell layers including the ectoderm, mesoderm, and ectoderm [17,18,25]. Teratomas can be either mature or immature and are the most common mediastinal germ cell tumors. Mature teratomas are benign, well-circumscribed, predominantly cystic masses. The majority of mature teratomas contain sebaceous fat. Calcification is another characteristic of mature teratomas, seen in about half of mature teratomas. Mature teratomas contain solid components of different histologic elements called Rokitansky protuberances. Diagnosis can be confirmed by CT or MRI by the presence of a cystic mass containing macroscopic fat, calcification, and soft-tissue components (Fig. 13.21). MRI is particularly useful in

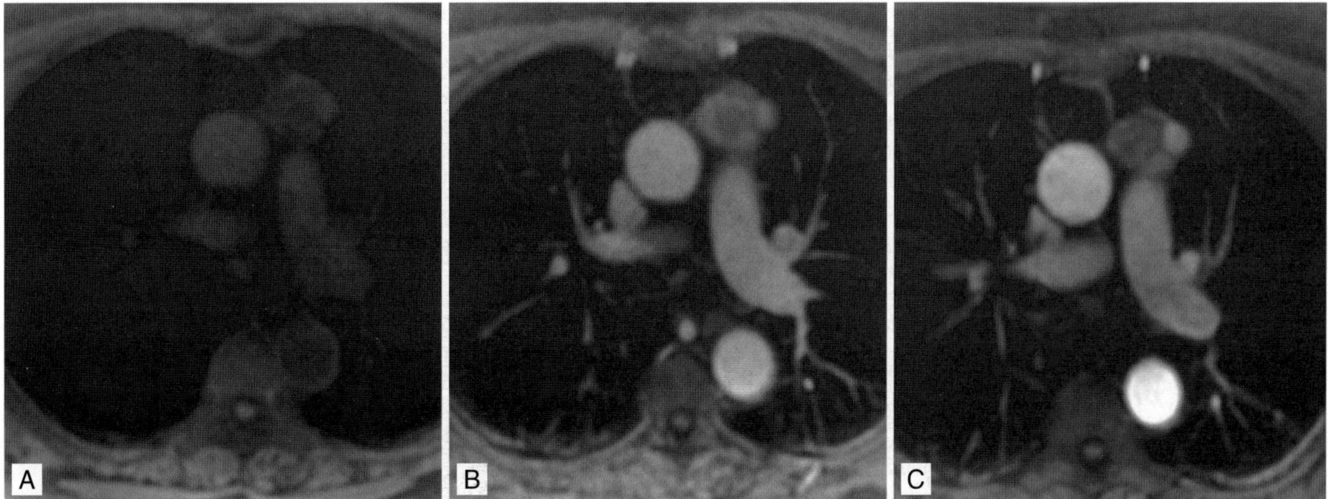

Figure 13.20 Biopsy-proved AB-type thymoma. Fat-saturated T1-weighted MRI chest pre- (A), 1 minute (B), and 5 minutes (C) postgadolinium injection demonstrating asymmetric nodular enhancement.

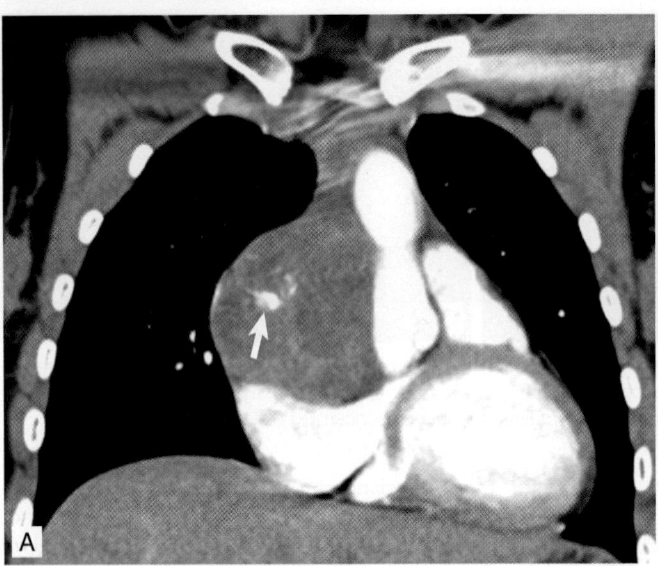

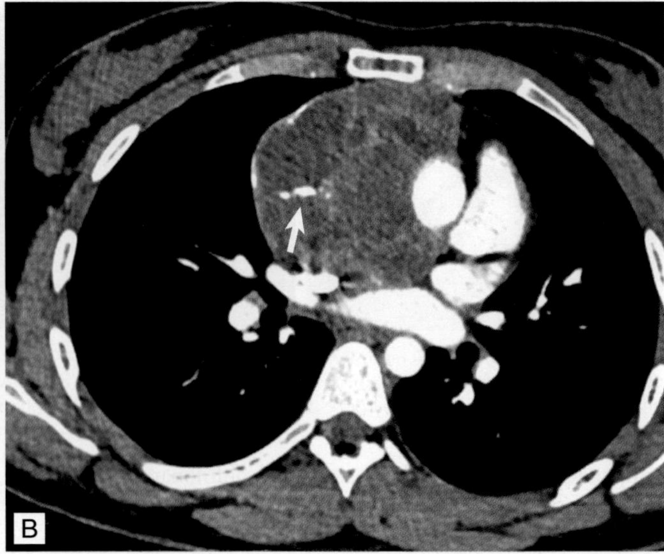

Figure 13.21 Surgically removed mediastinal mature teratoma. Enhanced CT chest in coronal (A) and axial (B) views demonstrating a well-delineated predominantly cystic mass in the prevascular mediastinum with internal soft-tissue attenuation septations of varying thickness and high-attenuation foci of calcification (*arrows*).

delineating the presence of fat, which is hyperintense on T1-weighted images and creates a chemical shift between cystic and fatty components of the tumor. Fat-fluid levels can be delineated within mature teratomas and is a specific feature for mature teratomas. Rokitansky protuberances can also sometimes be seen on MRI, manifesting as layering palm tree-like protrusions.

In comparison, immature teratomas are predominantly solid tumors containing immature neural elements. Whereas mature teratomas are benign and are surgically curative, immature teratomas can recur and have malignant potential. Distinguishing immature from mature teratomas can be difficult on imaging, as immature teratomas can also contain fat and calcification. The presence of significant solid components can suggest immature teratoma, although mature teratomas can contain solid components as well. Increased serum alpha-fetoprotein levels are also more associated with immature teratomas.

Unlike teratomas, malignant germ cell tumors including seminomas and nonseminomatous tumors do not contain macroscopic fat [17,18,25]. Seminomas usually present as lobulated well-circumscribed homogeneous masses on CT and MR images. A minority of mediastinal seminomas demonstrate high levels of B-human chorionic gonadotropin. On MRI, seminomas can demonstrate T2-hypointense fibrovascular septa, and calcification or cystic components are rare. In contrast, nonseminomatous germ cell tumors, such as yolk sac tumors or choriocarcinomas, are usually more heterogeneous with more frequently seen internal necrosis or hemorrhage. Other features of malignancy can be seen including lymphadenopathy and metastatic disease.

Lymphangioma

Lymphangiomas are rare and benign fluid-filled congenital malformations related to the failure of communication between the lymphatic system with the venous system during embryological development [17,18,26]. The classification of lymphangiomas is based upon the size of lymphatic channels. Small lymphatic channel lesions are termed simple-capillary malformations, cavernous malformations have dilated lymphatic channels, and cystic lymphangiomas (otherwise known as cystic hygromas) demonstrate the presence of cystic lymphatic collections. Lymphangiomas are primarily seen in children under the age of 2 years and are usually found in the cervical and axillary regions, with or without mediastinal extension. Less than 1% of lymphangiomas are found isolated in the mediastinum and these are often discovered incidentally on chest radiographs in children. Lymphangiomas are not confined to the anterior mediastinum and can be found in the posterior mediastinum as well. Large mediastinal lymphangiomas can cause symptoms based on the mass effect on adjacent anatomy. Lymphangiomas can be complicated by hemorrhage, infection, and rupture with chylothorax or chylopericardium.

Lymphangiomas are well-defined lobulated masses on chest radiographs with distortion of normal radiographic anatomy and are sometimes associated with chylous pleural effusions [17,18,26]. On CT, lymphangiomas appear as thin-walled cystic lobulated masses of varying size, with low-attenuation fluid (0–20 HU) and thin internal septae (Fig. 13.22). These features can also be well seen on MRI, where lymphangiomas demonstrate high T2 signal intensity in keeping with cystic fluid content. It is uncommon for lymphangiomas to calcify and there is usually no enhancing component. Large lymphangiomas tend to conform or mold around adjacent structures such as the heart and trachea. If complicated by hemorrhage, the internal fluid will demonstrate higher density on CT and can be difficult to distinguish from solid masses. In cases when lesions are equivocal on CT, dynamic-enhanced MRI with subtraction is useful to confirm the presence of hemorrhage or proteinaceous fluid (variable T1-weighted signal), without internal enhancing solid component.

Pleuropericardial Cyst

Pleuropericardial cysts are benign congenital thin-walled mesothelial cysts containing simple fluid [17,18]. They are usually seen in the anterior mediastinum at the right cardiophrenic angle, although a minority can also be found in the left anterior cardiophrenic angle or middle mediastinum. Most patients are asymptomatic, and they are often discovered incidentally on chest radiographs in adult patients. They are usually seen as a well-circumscribed, oval, or round mass, which can deform and change shape during the respiratory cycle (Fig. 13.23). *The presence of low-attenuation fluid on CT (0–20 HU) or high-signal*

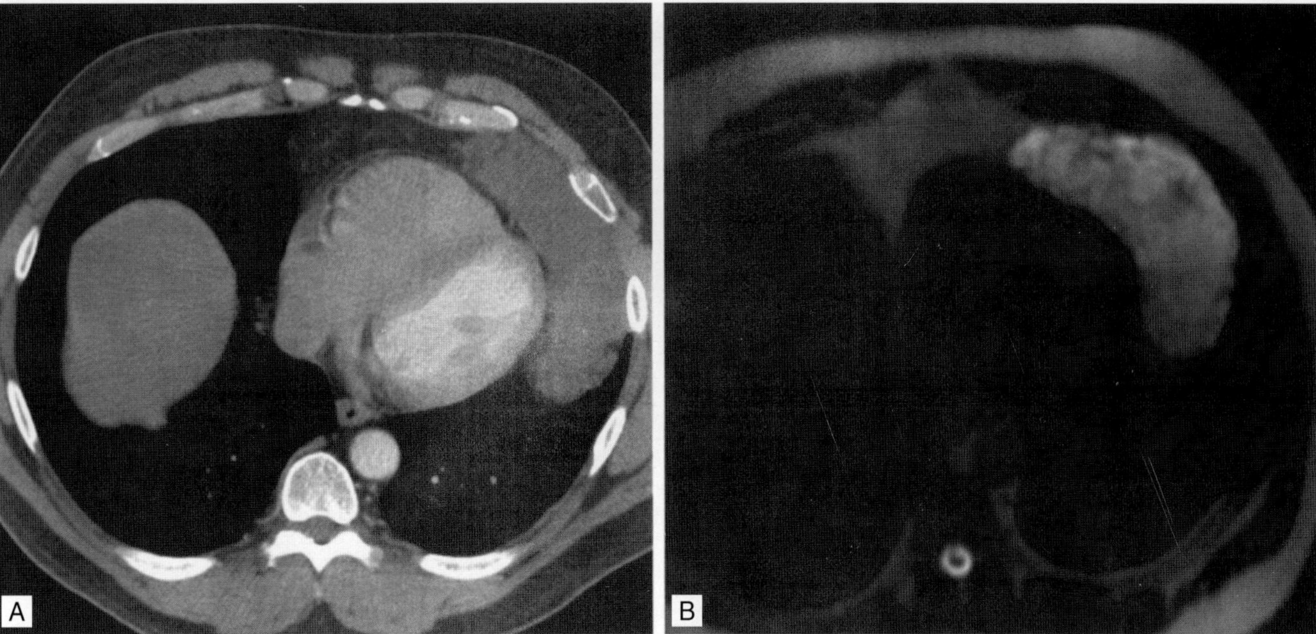

Figure 13.22 Surgically removed mediastinal lymphangioma. Enhanced axial CT chest (A) demonstrating a well-defined lobulated low-attenuation mass invaginating around the heart. On the corresponding T2-weighted MRI chest (B), the mass is uniformly hyperintense with thin internal septae.

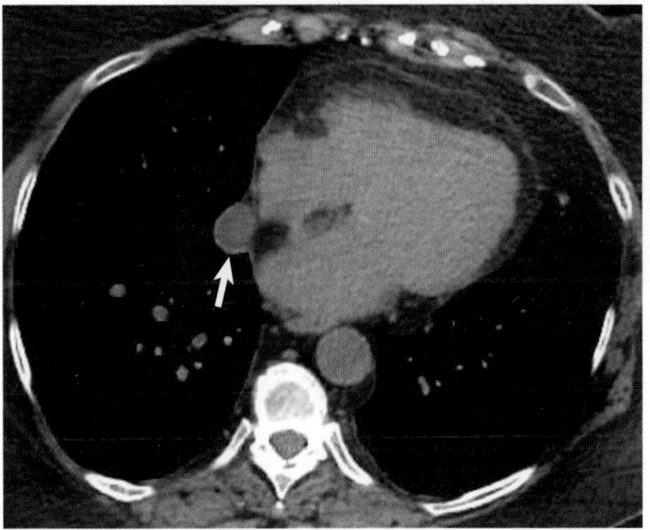

Figure 13.23 Axial-unenhanced CT chest demonstrating a round circumscribed low-attenuation cystic lesion adjacent to the right pericardium with thin imperceptible wall, likely a small pericardial cyst.

intensity of T2-weighted MRI is usually confirmatory of the diagnosis.

Lipomatous Lesions

Lipoma: Lipomas are rare mesenchymal tumors, which usually occur in the anterior mediastinum adjacent to the diaphragm [27,28]. Lipomas can also be found in other mediastinal compartments. Histologically, lipomas are composed of mature adipocytes that resemble normal fat. Most lipomas are encapsulated. They are considered benign tumors, although there are extremely rare reports of malignant degeneration in the literature. Radiographically, lipomas are usually found incidentally as a mass in the anterior mediastinum. CT imaging (Fig. 13.24) demonstrates a characteristic well-defined round or oval mass with homogeneous fat attenuation (–50 to –130 HU), no soft-tissue nodularity, and no internal contrast enhancement, although thin (<2 mm) internal septa can be seen.

Liposarcoma: Liposarcomas are malignant fatty differentiated mesenchymal tumors, very rarely seen in the mediastinum [27,28]. Liposarcomas are most commonly seen in the extremities and retroperitoneum and represent the second most common type of soft-tissue sarcoma. Liposarcomas are found almost exclusively in adults, usually in the sixth to seventh decade of life. Most liposarcomas are clinically silent and can grow to be quite large on presentation, where it can produce focal symptoms based on compression of adjacent structures. Imaging characteristics of liposarcomas on CT and MRI can be variable, depending on the degree of tissue differentiation (Fig. 13.25). A well-differentiated liposarcoma can appear almost entirely fatty, with strands of internal septa and small foci of enhancing soft-tissue components. Dedifferentiated liposarcoma can appear as an entirely solid mass with varying levels of internal cystic or necrotic degeneration. Well-differentiated liposarcoma can be distinguished from lipomas by the presence of thickened septa (>2 mm), nonlipomatous soft-tissue components, and marked septal enhancement.

Epipericardial Fat Necrosis: Epipericardial fat necrosis is an underrecognized and uncommon benign, self-limited condition, which usually presents as an acute pleuritic chest pain in otherwise healthy individuals [29]. Given the symptoms, it is often confused with acute myocardial infarction, pericarditis, or pulmonary embolism and is usually discovered incidentally on CT imaging. Epipericardial fat necrosis is characterized by focal inflammation and necrosis of the epipericardial fat, which connects the pericardium to the anterior chest wall. The condition is idiopathic and analogous to epiploic appendagitis seen in the abdomen. Radiographically, the findings are nonspecific, sometimes normal, and other times demonstrating an ill-defined opacity near the cardiophrenic angle, with or without unilateral pleural effusion. CT demonstrates accurately the presence of a round, encapsulated fatty lesion with surrounding fat stranding in the anterior mediastinum with thickening of the adjacent pericardium and pleural

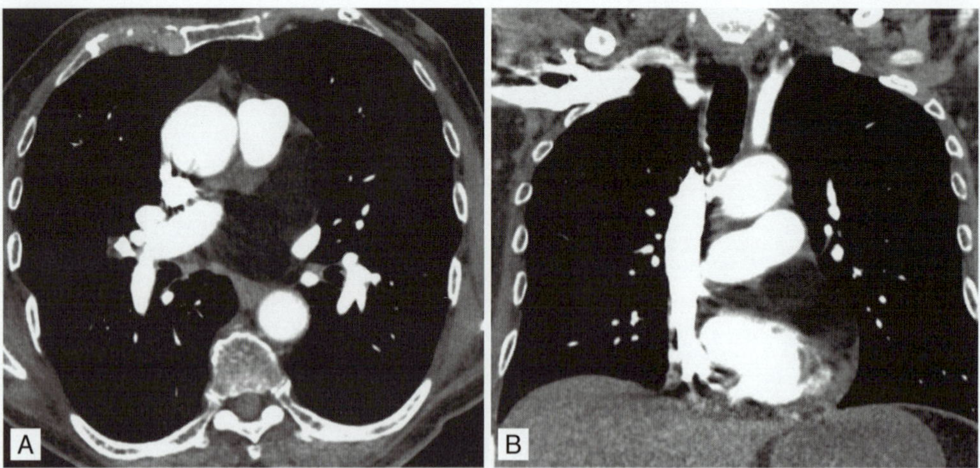

Figure 13.24 Example of a mediastinal lipoma in a 43-year-old male. Enhanced axial (A) and coronal (B) CT chest demonstrating a well-encapsulated intrapericardial mass within the visceral mediastinum with a homogenous fat attenuation with no soft-tissue septae or nodular component.

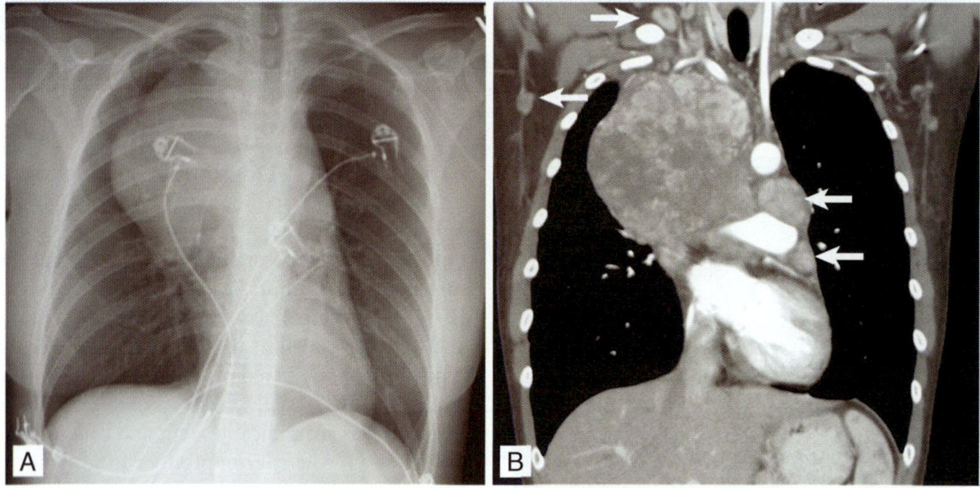

Figure 13.25 Example of a de-differentiated liposarcoma in a 45-year-old female. Frontal chest radiograph (A) and corresponding coronal-enhanced CT chest (B) demonstrating a bulky and heterogeneous mediastinal mass exerting mass effect on the adjacent structures. Multiple lymphadenopathies (*arrows*) are noted in the AP window, right axilla, and lower neck in keeping with nodal metastases.

effusions in many cases (Fig. 13.26). Given this condition is self-limited, treatment is conservative and entails usually symptomatic relief with nonsteroidal anti-inflammatory drugs.

Pericardial/Epicardial Fat Pad: Prominent pericardial fat pad is an incidental finding commonly seen at the cardiophrenic angles on chest radiographs, related to fat deposition in between the parietal pericardium and parietal pleura [30]. Enlargement of pericardial fat pads can be seen in normal individuals, as well as in obesity, Cushing's syndrome, and chronic steroid use. Radiographically, it can often be mistaken for an anterior mediastinal mass or focal pneumonia, although they are usually more radiographically lucent than real masses (Fig. 13.27). Pericardial fat pads can easily be distinguished on CT and MRI as nonencapsulated fat deposition in the anterior mediastinum adjacent to the heart and hemidiaphragm. Serial follow-up radiographs will demonstrate stability over time, providing evidence for the presence of a benign pericardial fat pad.

Mediastinal Lipomatosis: Mediastinal lipomatosis involves excessive accumulation of fatty tissue within the mediastinum [28]. It is usually seen in the setting of obesity or exogenous steroid use. High

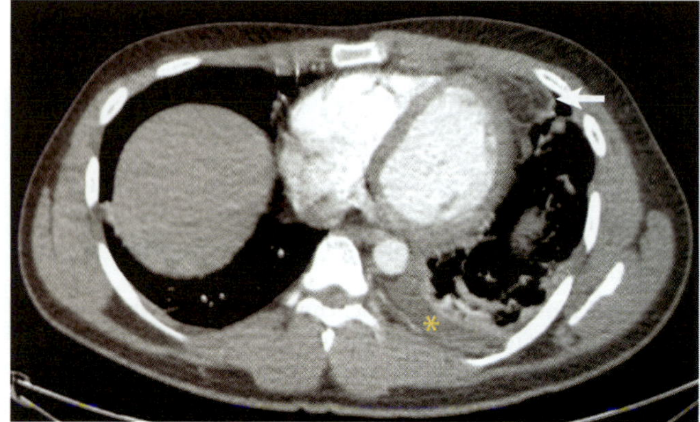

Figure 13.26 Example of epipericardial fat necrosis in a 38-year-old previously healthy male presenting with acute chest pain. Note the round, encapsulated fatty lesion in the prevascular mediastinum with surrounding fat stranding (*arrow*) and the unilateral left pleural effusion (*asterisk*). The patient was treated conservatively with NSAIDs and recovered with no complication.

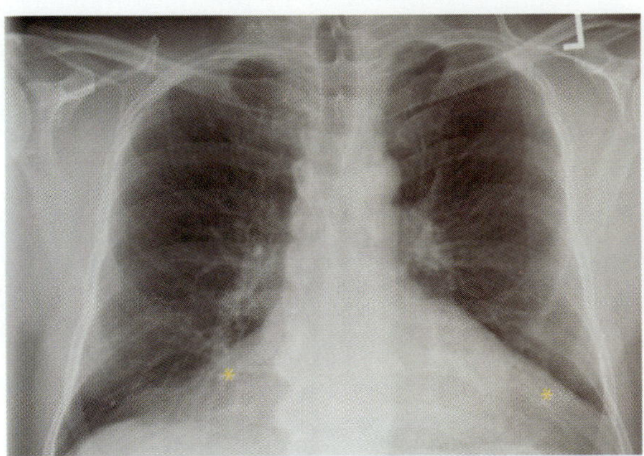

Figure 13.27 Example of prominent pericardial fat pads on frontal chest radiograph. Note the smooth contours and relative lucency of the opacities noted at the bilateral cardiophrenic angles.

levels of endogenous steroids such as in Cushing syndrome can also lead to increased fat deposition in the mediastinum. Importantly, lipomatosis involves the deposition of unencapsulated fat, which symmetrically accumulates in the upper anterior compartment and may simulate a mass on the radiograph (Fig. 13.28). CT imaging and MRI will demonstrate increased fat deposition around normal anatomic structures without evidence of compression or invasion. *Unlike lipomatous tumors, no capsule, internal septation, soft-tissue component, or contrast enhancement is noted.*

Herniation

Omental herniation into the anterior mediastinum can occur through the Morgagni foramen or through an acquired postsurgical or post-traumatic defect [31]. The foramen of Morgagni is a persistent developmental defect in the anterior diaphragm. Omental herniation is usually discovered incidentally as a mass in the anterior mediastinum on a chest radiograph. In rare cases, symptoms can occur related to the infarction of herniated fat, compression of the lungs, and intestinal obstruction/strangulation. Radiographically, most Morgagni hernias are usually located in the right anterior cardiophrenic angle. Larger hernias can contain gas-filled loops of bowel (Fig. 13.29). The diagnosis can be confirmed on CT and MRI by demonstrating the presence of omental fat, colon, and other upper abdominal organs herniating through an anterior diaphragmatic defect.

Middle Mediastinum

Congenital Mediastinal Cysts

Congenital cysts arising from the middle mediastinum encompasses foregut duplication cysts comprising of bronchogenic and esophageal duplication cysts [17,18]. Bronchogenic cysts derive from abnormal budding of the tracheobronchial tree during embryological development and are lined by respiratory ciliated pseudostratified columnar epithelial cells. They may contain clear serous fluid or thick mucoid material. Bronchogenic cysts are uncommonly associated with other congenital pulmonary malformations such as lobar emphysema or sequestration. Bronchogenic cysts can be complicated by hemorrhage or infection and expand rapidly in size. However, most bronchogenic cysts are asymptomatic, producing occasional symptoms from compression of adjacent structures. Radiographically, bronchogenic cysts appear usually as a well-defined solitary mass located inferior and on either side of the carina. On CT, they appear usually as nonenhancing, unilocular cystic lesions with thin imperceptible walls and homogeneous internal attenuation ranging from simple fluid (0–20 HU) to as high as 100 HU in a setting of hemorrhage or proteinaceous fluid (Fig. 13.30). T2-weighted MRI will demonstrate high signal with variable T1-weighted signal related to internal fluid content and without enhancement after IV gadolinium.

Esophageal duplication cysts are uncommon developmental foregut cysts that are most commonly found in infants and children [17,18]. As with bronchogenic cysts, they may also hemorrhage or become superinfected. Their imaging appearance is usually undiscernible from bronchogenic cysts, although some may demonstrate a thicker wall related to underlying mural smooth muscle. Unlike bronchogenic cysts, esophageal duplication cysts will occur along the esophagus (Fig. 13.31). Tc-99m sodium pertechnetate scan can be useful in highlighting the presence of ectopic gastric mucosa, which is present in up to 50% of thoracic duplication cysts.

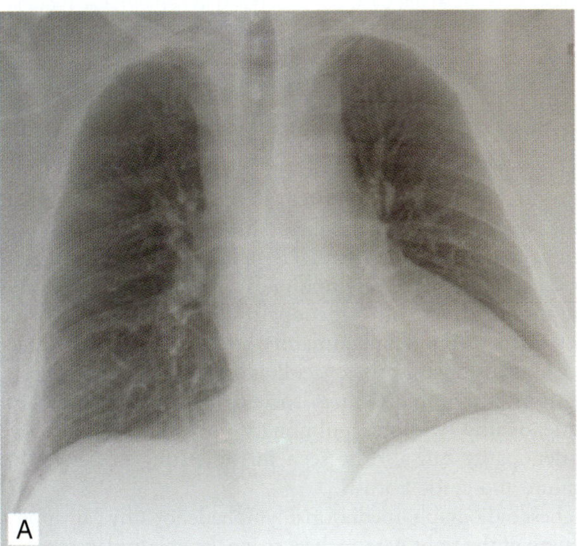

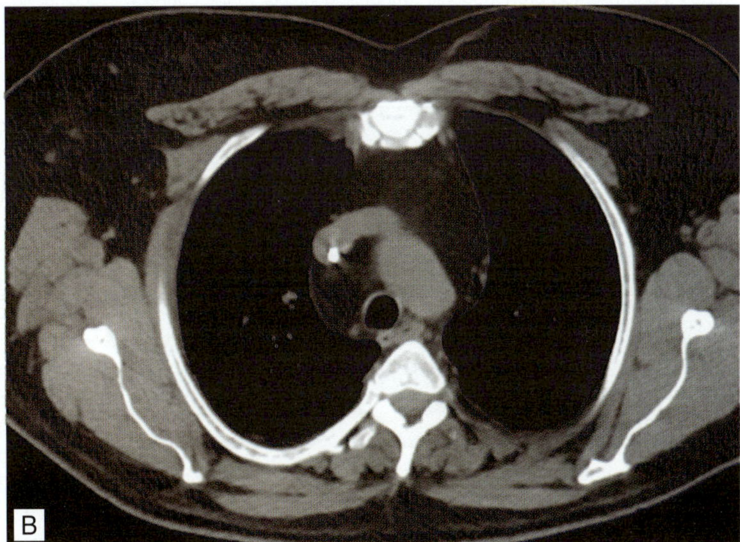

Figure 13.28 Example of mediastinal lipomatosis. Frontal chest radiograph (A) demonstrating relatively symmetric and smooth widening of the upper mediastinum. Corresponding unenhanced axial CT chest (B) revealing increased unencapsulated fat attenuation throughout the upper mediastinum.

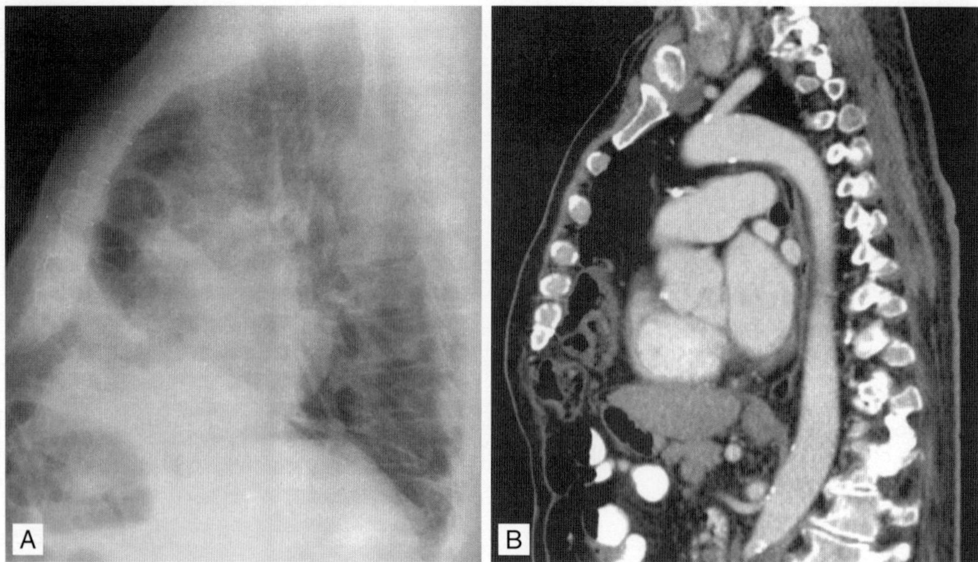

Figure 13.29 Example of a Morgagni hernia. Lateral chest radiograph (A) and corresponding enhanced coronal CT chest (B) demonstrating a focal defect in the anterior mediastinum with herniation of air-filled bowel loops in the thoracic cavity.

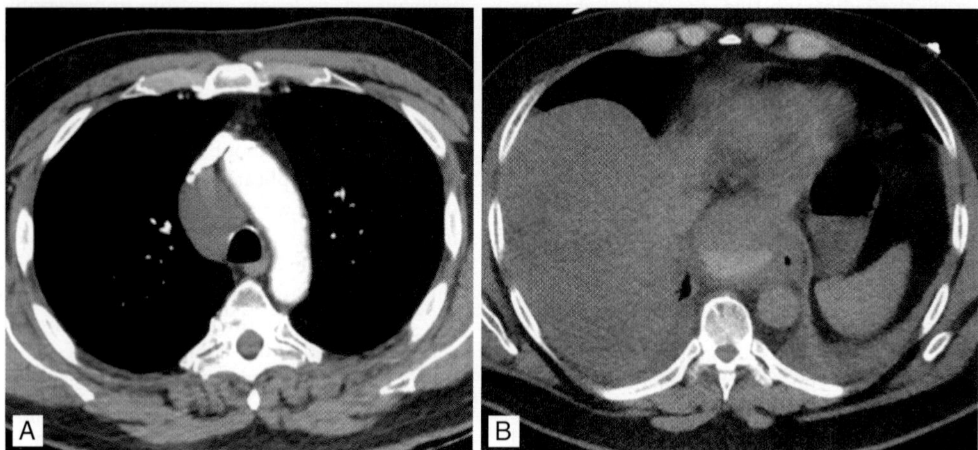

Figure 13.30 Examples of bronchogenic cysts. Enhanced axial CT chest (A) demonstrates a simple bronchogenic cyst arising in the paratracheal region with a thin imperceptible wall and homogeneous internal fluid attenuation. In contrast, an unenhanced axial CT chest (B) in a separate patient demonstrates a complicated bronchogenic cyst arising inferior to the carina with a clear fluid–fluid level within the cyst, corresponding to hemorrhagic material. Note the walls of the cyst are thicker and more ill-defined secondary to inflammatory changes.

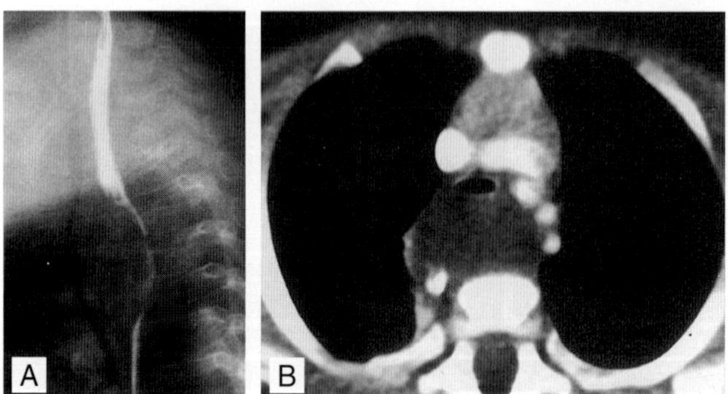

Figure 13.31 Esophageal duplication cyst. (A) Barium swallow showing smooth indentation and narrowing of esophagus. (B) Contrast CT image shows well circumscribed simple cystic lesion adjacent to the esophagus with a thin imperceptible wall.

Mediastinal Lymphadenopathy

Lymphadenopathy can be found in all compartments of the mediastinum but is most often occur in the middle compartment along the paratracheal, subcarinal, and hilar stations [2,5,33]. The differential diagnosis of mediastinal lymphadenopathy is vast, and includes metastatic disease, lymphoma, sarcoidosis, silicosis, and tuberculosis. Reactive lymphadenopathy can be seen in a wide range of infections and inflammatory conditions. Fungal infections such as histoplasmosis, coccidioidomycosis, actinomycosis, and blastomycosis can produce isolated hilar and paratracheal lymphadenopathy without pulmonary involvement. Reactive lymphadenopathy can also be seen in the setting of congestive heart failure and cystic fibrosis.

On chest radiograph, mediastinal lymphadenopathy can appear as widening of the right paratracheal stripe, lateral displacement of

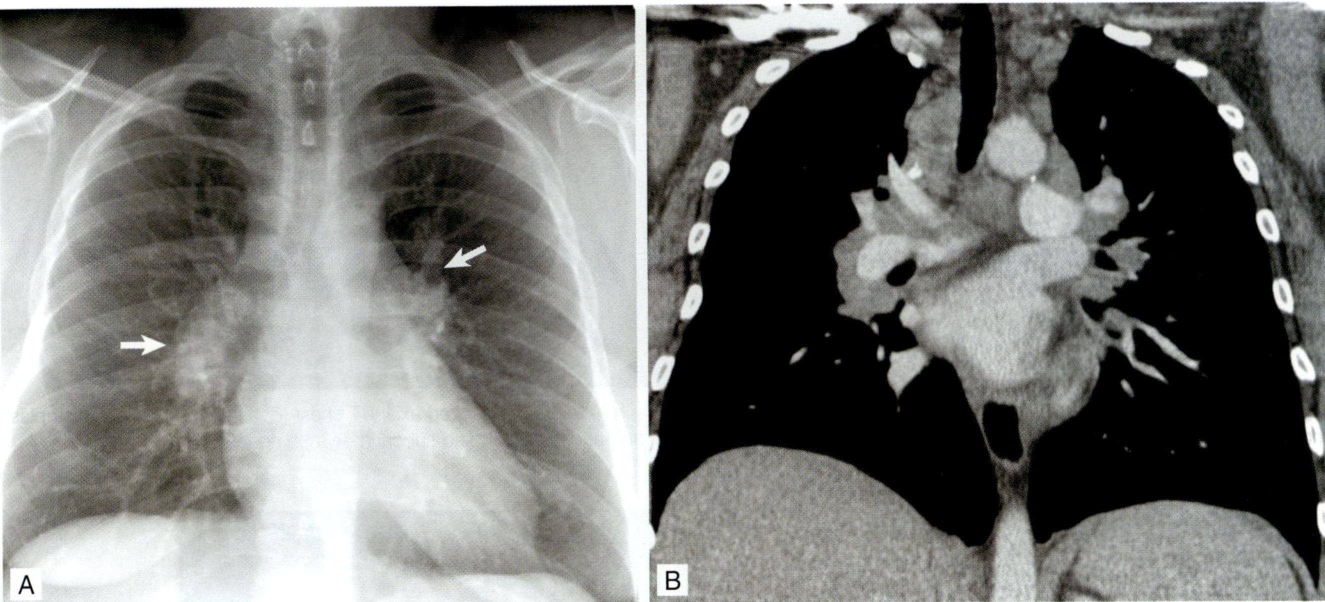

Figure 13.32 Examples of sarcoidosis in a 28-year-old female. Frontal chest radiograph (A) demonstrates bilateral perihilar and paratracheal opacities corresponding to extensive bilateral hilar (*white arrows*) and mediastinal lymphadenopathy on coronal-enhanced CT chest (B). Note the relative symmetric distribution of the lymphadenopathy.

the azygoesophageal recess, irregular widening of the mediastinal, lobulated mass in the hilar region, and as a mass in the aortopulmonary window (Fig. 13.32). Calcified lymphadenopathy can be noted as increased radiodensity on chest radiographs and can be noted in many different conditions (Table 13.5) [32]. Peripheral calcification, also known as eggshell calcification, can be seen in sarcoidosis, silicosis, amyloidosis, treated lymphoma, scleroderma, coal worker's pneumoconiosis, and histoplasmosis (Fig. 13.33).

Diagnosis of mediastinal lymphadenopathy is easily confirmed on CT imaging, which demonstrates the presence of multiple soft-tissue masses in the mediastinum [33]. In general, 10-mm short-axis diameter is considered the upper limit of normal on CT. Unlike normal lymph nodes, abnormal lymphadenopathy will usually be round or irregular in shape and not demonstrate a fatty hilum (Fig. 13.34). On MRI, lymphadenopathy is usually seen as intermediate signal intensity on T1-weighted imaging with variable enhancement and usually missing normal fatty hilum.

TABLE 13.5 Causes of Calcified Lymphadenopathy

Causes of Calcified Lymphadenopathy
Tuberculosis
Sarcoidosis
Silicosis and other pneumoconiosis
Histoplasmosis
Postradiation lymphoma
Metastasis: mucin-secreting adenocarcinoma; papillary and medullary thyroid carcinoma; osteogenic sarcoma
Scleroderma
Amyloidosis
Castleman's disease

Lymphadenopathy can be necrotic or cystic, which manifests as low internal attenuation on CT and high T2-weighted signal on MRI. Low-attenuation lymphadenopathy can be seen in a variety of conditions including tuberculosis, nontuberculous mycobacterial infection, histoplasmosis, treated lymphoma, Whipple disease, and metastases including testicular cancer and squamous cell carcinoma. Castleman's disease is an idiopathic benign lymphoproliferative condition characterized by avidly enhancing mediastinal lymphadenopathy on CT and MRI (Fig. 13.35). Other causes for hypervascular lymphadenopathy include metastasis from hypervascular tumors such as renal cell carcinoma, melanoma, Kaposi sarcoma, and thyroid carcinoma.

Esophageal Pathologies

Esophagitis: Inflammation of the esophagus can occur from a range of infectious (HIV, CMV, *Candida*, *Herpes*) and noninfectious causes (gastroesophageal reflux, caustic ingestion, medication-induced, radiation-induced) [34,35]. Double-contrast esophagography and endoscopy are the primary diagnostic techniques for evaluating the esophagus. On CT imaging and MRI esophagitis usually manifests as focal or segmental circumferential wall thickening and mural enhancement and edema. Esophagitis can also appear as a target sign on CT, which is caused by a combination of mucosal enhancement and edematous hypodense submucosa. Nonetheless, cross-sectional imaging is limited by underdistension of the esophagus, which can mimic wall thickening and a lack of specificity.

Esophageal Dysmotility: Esophageal dysmotility encompasses a wide range of pathologies, which involve the disruption of normal movement of the esophagus in transporting food from the oropharynx to the stomach [35]. Achalasia a primary form of esophageal dysmotility defined by the failure of organized peristalsis caused by impaired relaxation of the lower esophageal sphincter. Radiographically, achalasia (Fig. 13.36) can be seen as a convex opacity overlapping the right mediastinum indicating the presence

cross-sectional imaging is for accurate staging of disease, including regional and distant metastases. CT and MRI imaging cannot reliably delineate the involvement of the individual layers of the esophageal wall. However, CT and MRI are useful for assessing for invasion into the adjacent periesophageal fat and mediastinum as well as lymphadenopathy.

Fibrosing Mediastinitis

Fibrosing mediastinitis is a rare and benign condition characterized by the proliferation of fibrotic tissue in the mediastinum [37]. Fibrosing mediastinitis can be focal or diffuse. The focal form of the disease is the most common and often associated with granulomatous infections such as histoplasmosis and tuberculosis. Diffuse fibrosing mediastinitis can be idiopathic or associated with autoimmune diseases such as sarcoidosis, SLE, rheumatoid arthritis, IgG-4-related diseases, and Behcet's disease. Diffuse nongranulomatous fibrosing mediastinitis can also be seen after radiation therapy or as a complication of methysergide treatment.

Radiographically, fibrosing mediastinitis will present as abnormal widening of the mediastinum [37]. The presence of calcification can be observed. Due to fibrosis and compression of bronchovascular structures, there can often be findings of secondary volume loss and venous congestion. On CT and MRI, an irregular infiltrating soft-tissue mass can often be seen in focal granulomatous fibrosing mediastinitis, often with calcifications (Fig. 13.39). In the nongranulomatous diffuse variant of the disease, there is a more widespread extent of the infiltrative soft tissue throughout the mediastinum (Fig. 13.40). In both variants, there is often compression, encasement, and sometimes obliteration of the mediastinal and hilar bronchovascular structures. Positron emission tomography (PET)/CT is not a reliable technique for assessing fibrosing mediastinitis, which can demonstrate variable FDG avidity.

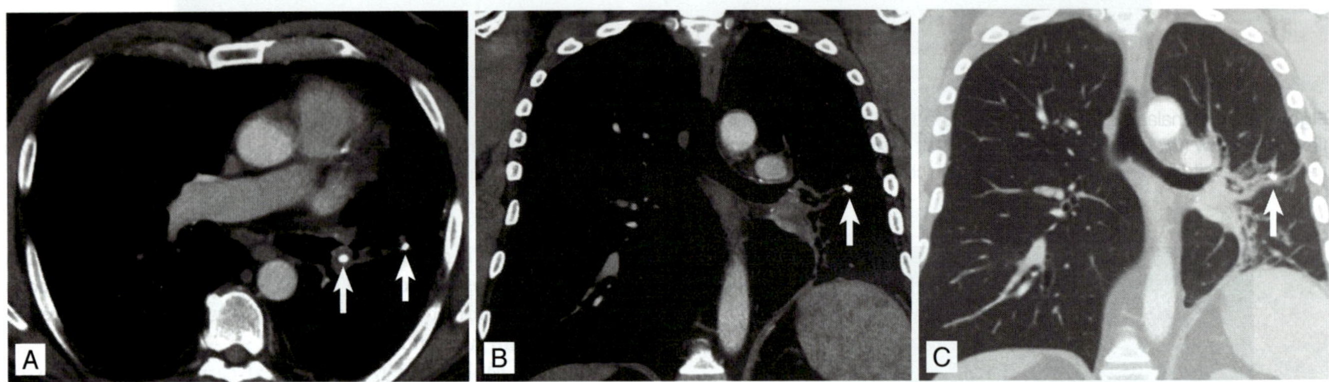

Figure 13.39 Example of focal fibrosing mediastinitis on enhanced axial (A) and coronal CT chest in soft-tissue (B) and lung (C) windows. Note the irregular soft-tissue mass infiltrating the left hilum, which is narrowing the left-sided bronchovasculature with significant linear scarring and volume in the left lower lung. Multiple high-attenuation calcifications are noted throughout (*arrows*).

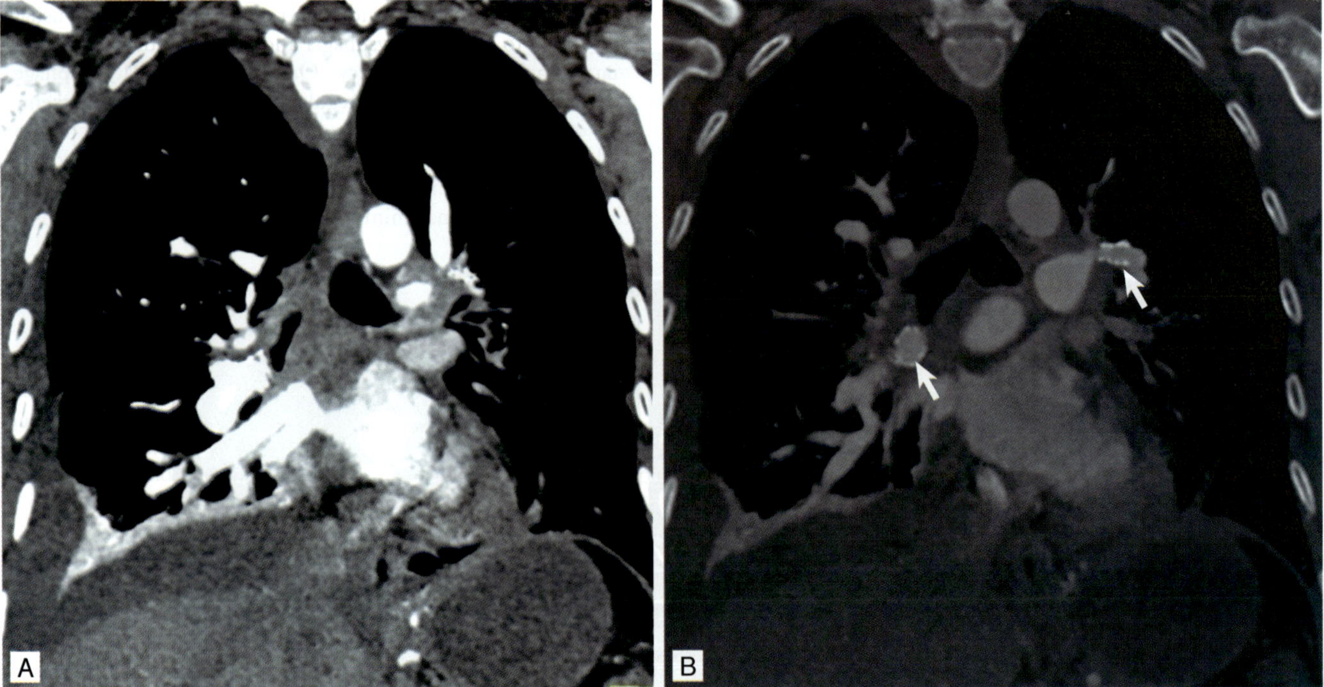

Figure 13.40 Example of diffuse fibrosing mediastinitis on enhanced coronal CT chest in soft-tissue (A) and bone (B) windows. Note the irregular soft-tissue attenuation infiltrating the entire mediastinum and bilateral hilum. Due to the fibrotic encasement and narrowing of the segmental pulmonary arteries, vascular stents were placed to keep the vasculature open (*arrows*). A right pleural effusion is also noted, likely related to congestion on the pulmonary venous blood return.

Acute Mediastinitis

Acute mediastinitis results from infection of the mediastinum and can be devastating for patients with high morbidity and mortality [38,39]. They can happen spontaneously or be associated with other infections such as pharyngitis, pneumonia, epiglottis, or bronchitis. Primary cases of acute mediastinitis are rare and the vast majority of acute mediastinitis arise secondarily from head and neck infections, iatrogenic procedures, esophageal perforations, or postoperatively. Classically, infection within the head and neck can move through the prevascular space or can break through the alar fascia and enter the retrovisceral space (also known as the danger space) to reach the mediastinum. Clinically, patients with acute mediastinitis are septic and will present with dyspnea, pain, high-grade fevers, and leukocytosis.

Radiographically, acute mediastinitis can demonstrate widening and poor definition of the superior mediastinal borders [38,39]. In advanced cases, pneumomediastinum and subcutaneous air within the soft tissues of the neck can sometimes be seen. Nonetheless, CT imaging is recommended technique for assessing acute mediastinitis owing to its superior spatial resolution and ability to detect the presence of a mediastinal abscess (Fig. 13.41). On CT, it is common to find inflammatory fat stranding, loculated fluid collections or abscesses, pneumomediastinum, as well as pleural effusions and/or empyema. In the event of an esophageal perforation, a large perforation can often be identified. In the postoperative period, CT imaging is also helpful for assessing postoperative changes, hematoma formation, and sternal dehiscence. Percutaneous aspiration or drainages can also be done under CT guidance.

Vascular Anomalies

Vascular disease is common in mediastinum and includes arterial and venous causes. Common arterial causes are thoracic aorta aneurysm, aortic dissection, tortuous innominate artery, dilatation of the main pulmonary artery, and coarctation of aorta. The mediastinal venous abnormalities include dilated superior vena cava, persistent left-sided superior vena cava, superior vena cava obstruction, and dilated azygos vein.

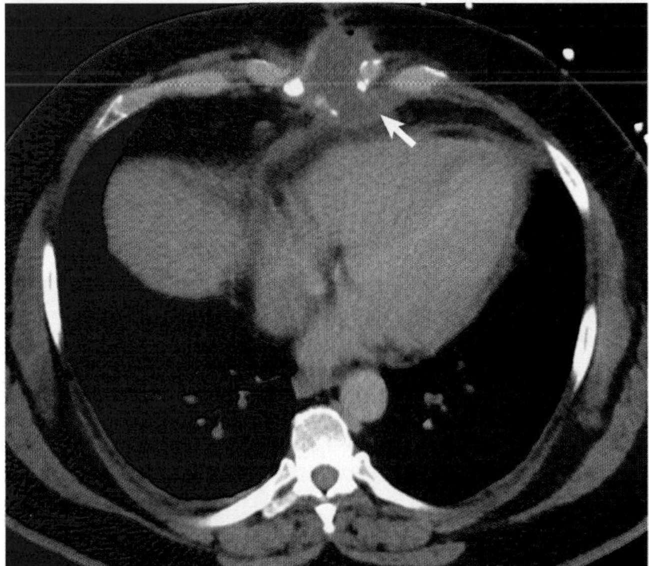

Figure 13.41 Example of acute mediastinitis and mediastinal abscess formation (*arrow*) on axial-enhanced CT chest in a patient status—after median sternotomy. The abscess is extending from the site of sternal dehiscence to the anterior mediastinum. Note the small locule of free air within the abscess and the surrounding fat stranding.

Tracheal Pathology

Lesions in the trachea usually present with either cough or dyspnea due to recurrent chest infections or stridor in children and adult patients. Tracheal lesions can produce narrowing or widening of the trachea or a mass within its lumen on the chest radiograph.

Malignant tracheal tumors such as squamous cell carcinoma and adenoid cystic carcinoma or cylindroma, benign tracheal tumors such as hamartoma and chondroma, and other lesions such as tracheobronchial papillomatosis and amyloidosis can produce a soft-tissue mass in the trachea.

Widening of the trachea is seen in tracheobronchiomegaly or the Mounier–Kuhn syndrome, which is associated with the Ehlers–Danlos syndrome. Narrowing of the trachea is seen in the sabre sheath trachea of chronic obstructive pulmonary disease, relapsing polychondritis, Wegener's granuloma, sarcoidosis, tuberculosis, trauma, tracheopathia osteochondroplastica, and tracheomalacia. The diagnosis of all tracheal lesions is confirmed by CT which shows the narrowed or widened trachea, intraluminal soft-tissue masses, a thick-walled trachea or extrinsic mediastinal disease. Tracheal lesions are discussed in more detail in Chapter 17.

Posterior Mediastinum

Neurenteric Cyst

Neurenteric cysts are rare congenital cysts along the spinal axis, made up of heterotopic endodermal tissue [40]. Patients are usually diagnosed during the second and third decades of life. Depending on the size and location of the lesion, neurenteric cysts can present with progressive focal spinal pain, radicular symptoms, paresthesia, or focal weakness. Radiographically, neurenteric cysts present as a space-occupying mass along the posterior mediastinum distorting the paraspinal lines. MRI provides superior delineation of the anatomic relation of the cyst with the spinal cord compared with CT. Nonetheless, CT imaging is useful in evaluating adjacent associated osseous malformations. On CT, neurenteric cysts appear usually as a solitary well-defined cyst with a thin imperceptible wall. On MRI, neurenteric cysts are nonenhancing lesions, which are hyperintense on T2-weighted images and hypo-to-isointense on T1-weighted images. Similar to other congenital mediastinal cysts, neurenteric cysts do not have enhancing mural nodules, which helps differentiate these cysts from spinal neoplasms.

Meningoceles

Thoracic meningoceles arise from focal protrusions of the meninges in the spine and may be congenital or iatrogenic in nature [40]. Lateral thoracic meningoceles are most often associated with neurofibromatosis type 1. Iatrogenic meningoceles can result from trauma or as a complication from spinal surgeries. Radiographically, meningoceles are seen as well-delineated paraspinal masses along the posterior mediastinum, often with smooth scalloping of the adjacent osseous structures. CT and MRI will demonstrate a well-circumscribed homogenous mass of fluid attenuation and intensity with a thin wall and no mural nodularity. Meningoceles will demonstrate a connection with the spinal subarachnoid space and the fluid they contain will follow the attenuation and intensity of cerebrospinal fluid.

Neurogenic Tumors

Neurogenic tumors are among the most common tumors found in the posterior mediastinum and encompasses nerve sheath tumors, autonomic ganglion tumors, and paragangliomas [41]. Nerve sheath tumors include benign tumors such as schwannomas and neurofibromas, as well as malignant peripheral nerve sheath tumors (MPNSTs). Tumors of the autonomic ganglion include a histopathologic continuum ranging from low-grade ganglioneuromas, intermediate-grade ganglioneuroblastomas, and highly malignant neuroblastomas. Paragangliomas are rare neuroectodermal tumors arising from the sympathetic or parasympathetic chain. Differentiation of the different neurogenic tumors involves the integration of demographics, clinical information, and imaging features.

Ganglioneuroma: Ganglioneuromas are low-grade tumors made up of well-differentiated large ganglion cells, Schwann cells, and nerve fibers [41]. They are usually slow-growing tumors, discovered commonly in children older than 10 years of age and found more commonly in males than females. Given their origin, they are usually attached to an intercoastal or sympathetic nerve. On CT, ganglioneuromas usually are circumscribed elongated masses with low internal attenuation compared with muscle, related to an abundance of myxoid content. On MRI, ganglioneuromas usually have homogenous intermediate signal on all sequences and demonstrate enhancement. On occasion, low-signal intensity curvilinear or nodular bands can be seen on T1- and T2-weighted imaging.

Ganglioneuroblastoma: Ganglioneuroblastoma makes an intermediate-grade tumor in between more benign ganglioneuromas and more malignant neuroblastomas [41]. They are usually discovered in children younger than 10 years of age with equal sex predominance. On imaging, these tumors are usually encapsulated and range in appearance from well-circumscribed enhancing solid masses to more irregular and cystic heterogeneous masses. Local invasion and metastasis at the time of diagnosis are not uncommon.

Neuroblastoma: Neuroblastomas are most commonly seen in young children under the age of 3 years. They comprise the most common extracranial solid malignancy of childhood [41]. Histologically, neuroblastomas are made up of small round cells with little stroma and no capsule. Given they are often associated with hemorrhage and necrotic degeneration; they can appear as irregular masses with internal low-attenuation and heterogeneity. Radiographically, neuroblastomas can present as a paravertebral mass with or without internal calcification. Local invasion and metastatic disease can be noted on imaging. On CT, half of neuroblastomas will demonstrate internal stippled or curvilinear calcifications. Enhancement can be homogeneous or heterogeneous, depending on the degree of necrosis (Fig. 13.42). MRI is preferable to CT in assessing the extent of tumor involvement and metastatic disease in the bone marrow and liver, to avoid radiation.

Schwannoma: Schwannomas are the most common nerve sheath tumors, frequently found associated with an intercostal nerve or spinal nerve root [41]. Most schwannomas are solitary and sporadic (Fig. 13.43), although multiple schwannomas can

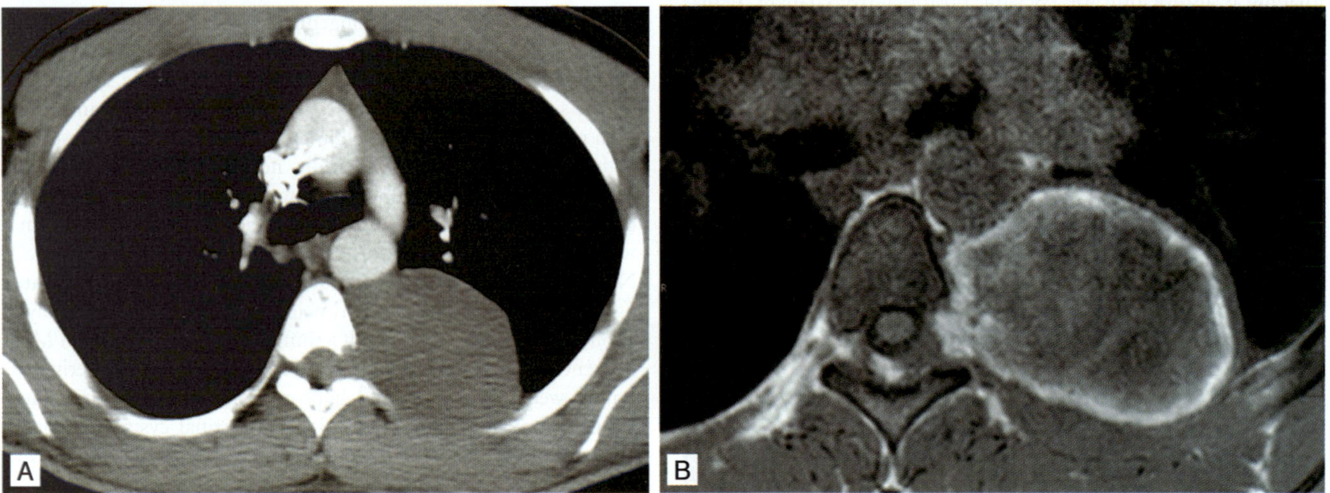

Figure 13.42 Example of biopsy-proved neuroblastoma on axial-enhanced CT chest (A) and corresponding postgadolinium-enhanced T1-weighted MRI chest (B). Note the heterogeneity of the mass on the MRI with avidly enhancing peripheral components and necrotic degeneration in the center. Also, note the component widening the left neuroforamen and eroding the adjacent vertebral body.

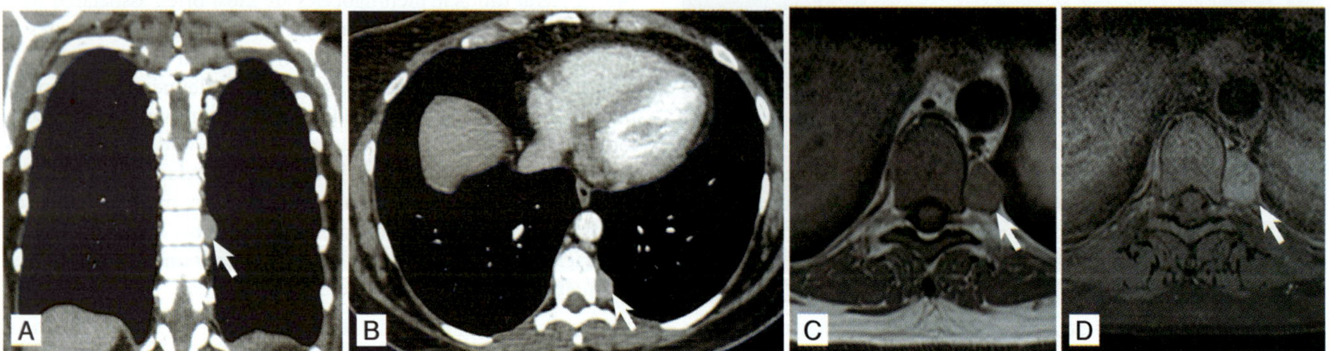

Figure 13.43 Example of peripheral nerve sheath tumor (schwannoma). On coronal (A) and axial (B) CT chest, note the well-defined ovoid noncalcified paraspinal mass (*arrows*) centered at the expected location of the left intercostal neurovascular bundle. On corresponding T1-weighted nonfat-saturated (C) and T1-weighted fat-saturated postcontrast (D) MRI chest, note the smooth encapsulated mass with relatively homogeneous and avid enhancement. The adjacent bone marrow signal is normal.

be found associated with neurofibromatosis type 2. Radiographically, schwannomas appear as well-circumscribed ovoid paraspinal mass. On CT, schwannomas are well-defined, noninfiltrating masses, which can displace the surrounding fat (termed "split fat" sign). Schwannomas are uncommonly calcified. Although not invasive, schwannomas can cause smooth erosion of adjacent bony structures over time. On MRI, schwannomas are hypo-to-isointense on T1-weighted images, hyperintense on T2-weighted images, and demonstrate avid enhancement of solid components. Large schwannomas can have cystic degeneration and hemorrhage and will appear more heterogeneous.

Neurofibroma: Neurofibromas [41] are usually found in adulthood, between the third and fifth decades. The presence of plexiform neurofibromas is considered pathognomonic with neurofibromatosis type 1. On CT, neurofibromas appear as smooth well-delineated homogeneous masses, sometimes with a split fat sign. *Unlike schwannomas, cystic degeneration is uncommon and calcifications and bony changes are also more frequently associated with neurofibromas.* On MRI, neurofibromas are low to intermediate signal on T1-weighted images and usually demonstrate homogeneous enhancement. On T2-weighted MRI, neurofibromas can demonstrate lower central intensity and higher peripheral zone intensity, termed "target" sign (Fig. 13.44).

Malignant Peripheral Nerve Sheath Tumor: MPNSTs are aggressive peripheral nerve sheath tumors characterized by large size (greater than 5 cm), irregular borders, and fast rate growth [41]. Most tumors are solitary and sporadic, although 20–30% are associated with neurofibromatosis type 1. MPNSTs usually present in the fourth to fifth decades of life and without gender predisposition. A rapidly enlarging mass in the posterior mediastinum with associated pain and neurologic deficits raise the suspicion of an MPNST. Histologically, MPNSTs demonstrate spindle cells with nuclear atypia, increased mitosis, and areas of necrosis. On imaging, they appear as large heterogeneous soft-tissue masses with an invasion of adjacent structures including bone, muscle, and pleura. CT and MRI appearance depend on the degree of internal cysts, necrosis, and hemorrhage.

Paraganglioma: Thoracic paragangliomas are rare highly vascular tumors of the mediastinum, mostly arising in adulthood between 40 and 50 years of age [41]. They may be associated with syndromes including multiple endocrine neoplasias and von Hippel–Lindau disease. Paragangliomas arise from chemoreceptor paraganglionic cells and, when active, can secrete catecholamines and cause hypertension, headaches, and blushing. Paragangliomas are not confined to the posterior mediastinum and can be found in any of the three mediastinal compartments. Paragangliomas can be found in the paravertebral space, aortic arch, along the sympathetic nerve chain, along the pericardium, along the vagus nerve, and within the interatrial septum. Radiographically, paragangliomas appear as nonspecific mediastinal masses. On CT and MRI, thoracic paragangliomas present as avidly enhancing soft-tissue masses, some with extensive hemorrhagic or cystic degeneration. Paragangliomas are usually intermediate intensity on T1-weighted images and hyperintense on T2-weighted images. Large masses are usually supplied by multiple feeding vessels and demonstrate a salt-and-pepper appearance on T2-weighted MRI, owing to the presence of vessel signal flow void amidst the hyperintense mass.

Bochdalek Hernia

Bochdalek hernia arises from herniation of abdominal contents through the foramen of Bochdalek, a persistent congenital defect in the posterior diaphragm [31]. In most cases, Bochdalek hernia is asymptomatic, although rarely strangulation of herniating bowel can occur. Most commonly Bochdalek hernias are found in the left hemidiaphragm, given the presence of the liver on the right. Small hernias can appear on the chest radiograph as a focal opacity in the posterior costophrenic angle. Large hernias containing small bowel and colon can appear as gas-filled structures in the left hemithorax and those containing solid viscera such as kidneys are of soft-tissue density. CT imaging is usually confirmatory, demonstrating the presence of the congenital defect in the posterior diaphragm (Fig. 13.45).

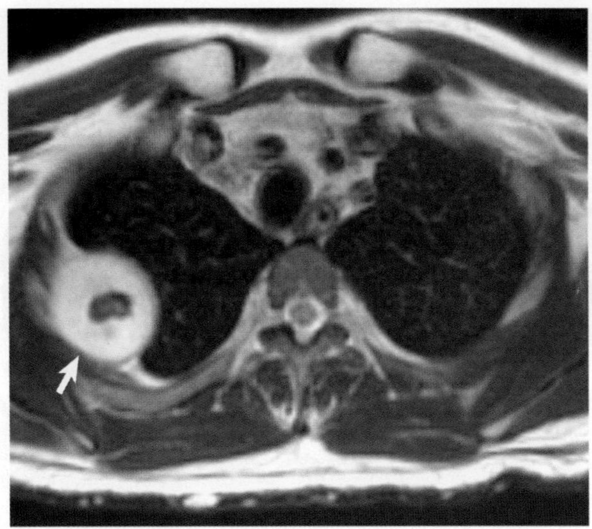

Figure 13.44 Example of a neurofibroma on axial T2-weighted image of the chest demonstrating well-circumscribed, mildly lobulated mass with internal areas of T2 hypointensity (target sign) centered within the extrapleural fat of the right lateral chest wall.

Extramedullary Hematopoiesis

Extramedullary hematopoiesis are rare centers of hemopoiesis occurring outside of the principal sites of hemopoiesis such as the long bones, ribs, and vertebral bodies [42]. This condition

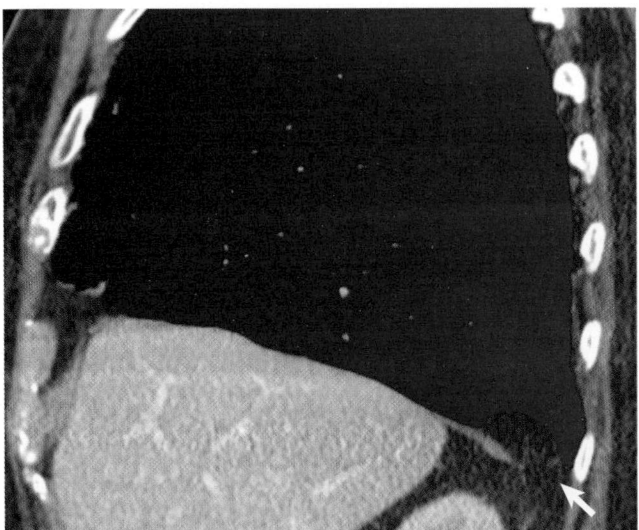

Figure 13.45 Sagittal-enhanced CT chest demonstrating example of a small right Bochdalek hernia with protrusion of fat into the thoracic cavity.

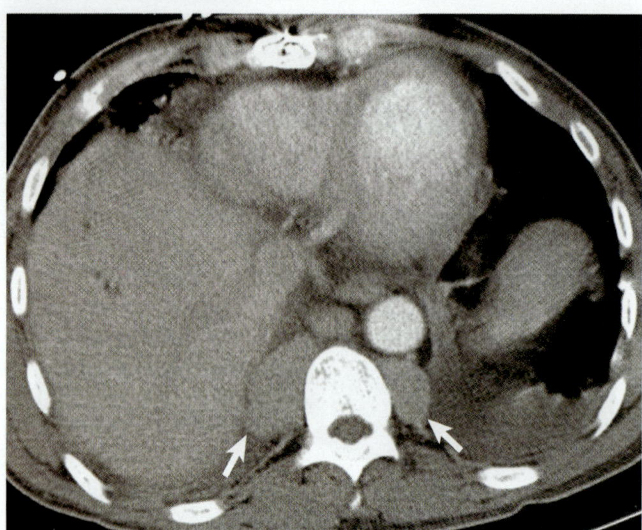

Figure 13.46 Example of biopsy-proved extramedullary hematopoiesis in a 59-year-old male with beta-thalassemia. Axial-enhanced CT chest demonstrates bilateral ovoid smoothly marginated and homogeneous soft-tissue masses in the paravertebral space.

is associated with diseases such as myelofibrosis, where the primary sites of hemopoiesis fail or are destroyed, and in hemoglobinopathies such as sickle cell disease and thalassemia. In the thorax, extramedullary hematopoiesis appears as oval circumscribed paravertebral masses along with an expansion of ribs. Extramedullary hematopoiesis can also occur in other areas of the body, including in the liver, spleen, perirenal space, and retroperitoneum. Imaging features on CT and MRI are nonspecific (Fig. 13.46). Although usually bilateral, extramedullary hematopoiesis can sometimes be unilateral. The presence of macroscopic fat can suggest a diagnosis of extramedullary hematopoiesis. However, many of these soft-tissue masses do not contain fat, making the diagnosis difficult, and often requiring biopsy for confirmation.

Suggested Readings

- BW Carter, MF Benveniste, R Madan, MC Godoy, PM de Groot, MT Truong, et al., ITMIG classification of mediastinal compartments and multidisciplinary approach to mediastinal masses, Radiographics 37 (2) (2017) 413–436.
- MY Jeung, B Gasser, A Gangi, A Bogorin, D Charneau, JM Wihlm, et al., Imaging of cystic masses of the mediastinum, Radiographics 22 (Spec No) (2002) S79–S93.
- CS Nin, VV de Souza, RH do Amaral, NR Schuhmacher, GR Alves, E Marchiori, et al., Thoracic lymphadenopathy in benign diseases: A state of the art review, Respir Med 112 (2016) 10–17.
- JD Pavlus, BW Carter, MD Tolley, ES Keung, L Khorashadi, JP Lichtenberger, 3rd, Imaging of thoracic neurogenic tumors, AJR Am J Roentgenol 207 (3) (2016) 552–561.
- AS Roberts, AS Shetty, VM Mellnick, PJ Pickhardt, S Bhalla, CO Menias, Extramedullary haematopoiesis: radiological imaging features, Clin Radiol 71 (9) (2016) 807–814.

14

Pleura, Diaphragm, and Chest Wall

DHIRAJ BARUAH, SACHIN S. SABOO, KIRAN BATRA

Anatomy

Pleura is a thin membrane of fibrous tissue lined by the mesothelium which covers the lung surface (visceral pleura) and lines inner surface of the chest wall (parietal pleura) [1]. The visceral pleura is along the lung surface and fissures. Pulmonary arteries and veins supply the visceral pleura and systemic vasculatures are for the parietal pleura. There are four parts of the parietal pleura—along the ribs and intercostal spaces is "costal part," along hemidiaphragm is "diaphragmatic part," along mediastinum is "mediastinal part," and along the cervical extension is "cervical part." Mediastinal part of the parietal pleura is continuous with the visceral pleura and extends inferiorly to form the inferior pulmonary ligament.

Pleural cavity is the potential space between visceral and parietal pleura and is lined by a thin layer of approximately 5 mL lubricating physiologic fluid. The pleural cavity is developed between the fourth and seventh weeks of the embryonic life. Pleura is permeable to both air and fluid; however, no air is normally seen in the pleural space. Pleural fluid is dynamic with approximately 100 mL of fluid produced per hour and is absorbed by the lymphatic system in the parietal pleura draining ultimately into the thoracic duct [1].

The diaphragm is a dome-shaped muscular septum surrounding a central tendon which is a physical barrier between the thoracic and abdominal cavities. Phrenic nerves are the primary innervation of the diaphragm; however, some part of the lateral diaphragm is often supplied by intercostal nerves. Third to fifth cervical roots contribute to the phrenic nerves and the nerve passes along the lateral pericardial border to reach the diaphragm [2].

The bony rib cage is supported by chest wall musculatures and provides a protective barrier for internal vital organs and also takes part in the respiration.

Physiology

Mechanical coupling between the lung and chest wall helps maintaining lung inflation [3]. As the lung has a natural tendency to collapse toward its hilum, similar magnitude of chest wall force is required to keep it expanded. With accumulation of abnormal amount of fluid (pleural effusion/empyema/hemothorax) or air (pneumothorax) in the pleural space this outward force decreases leading to collapse of a part of or whole lung depending on amount of collection. This passive collapse also depends on underlying condition of the lung and presence or absence of pleural adhesions. Sometimes, the lung may not completely collapse (e.g., fibrosis, emphysema, and consolidation) and with adhesions in the pleural space distribution of air and fluid may vary. Pleural fluid and air distribution can also vary in double lung transplant patients where a single pleural layer is used to cover both lungs.

Primary function of diaphragm and chest wall musculatures is to help in respiration with the diaphragm being the primary muscle of respiration and accessory muscles of respiration are external intercostal, sternocleidomastoid, and scalene muscles. Contraction of diaphragm along with accessory muscles of respiration expands the thoracic cavity which decreases intrathoracic pressure and draws air into the airways and lungs. In expiration, elastic recoil of the lungs during diaphragmatic relaxation pushes air out from the lung. During inspiration, the diaphragm closes the gastroesophageal junction preventing reflux and enlarges inferior vena cava (IVC) hiatus pumping deoxygenated blood to the right atrium. By increasing intra-abdominal pressure the diaphragm also helps in emesis, urination, and defecation.

Imaging Appearance of Normal Pleura, Diaphragm, and Chest Wall

Pleura is not visible normally on radiographs, however, it is often visible where two layers of pleura are outlined by the aerated lung. These places are horizontal fissure of the right lung which is often seen on a frontal radiograph and oblique fissures in both lungs often seen on the lateral radiograph (Fig. 14.1). Some common accessory fissures are inferior accessory fissure of the right lower lobe and azygos fissure (Fig. 14.2).

On a plain radiograph, diaphragmatic outline is visible between the air containing lung and opaque abdomen. Normally, the right hemidiaphragm is higher than the left because of the liver in the right upper quadrant of the abdomen (Fig. 14.3). Posterior and lateral portions of the diaphragm are usually lower than the anterior and medial portions. Motion of the diaphragm with respiration is commonly assessed using dynamic imaging like fluoroscopy, ultrasound, or magnetic resonance imaging (MRI). There are openings in the diaphragm that allow structures to pass between the chest and abdominal cavities and these openings can be seen in cross-sectional imaging. These openings are called diaphragmatic hiatuses and there are three important hiatuses (Fig. 14.4A). In the midportion of the central tendon is the hiatus for IVC, which is at the T8 vertebral level and contains IVC and right phrenic nerve (Fig. 14.4B). At the T10 vertebral level is the esophageal hiatus which allows passage of esophagus along with vagus nerve and sympathetic nerve branches (Fig. 14.4C). The third important hiatus is the aortic hiatus at T12 vertebral level which contains descending thoracic aorta along with thoracic duct, hemiazygos, and azygos veins (Fig. 14.4D).

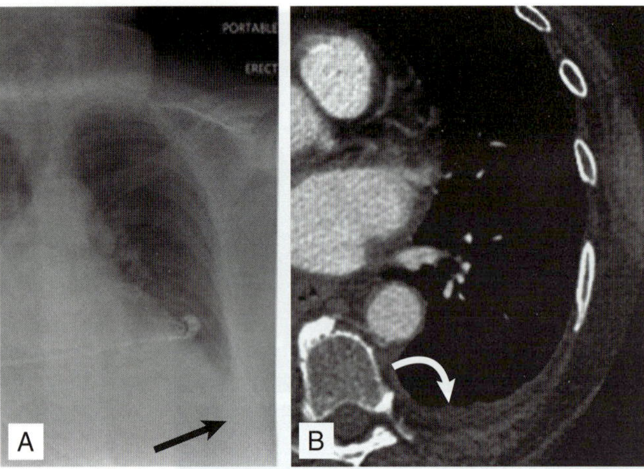

Figure 14.5 Tiny left pleural effusion. There is slight blunting of the left lateral costophrenic angle (*arrow* in A) and a small amount of fluid is seen in the CT image (*curved arrow* in B).

lupus erythematosus and rheumatoid arthritis), nonbacterial pneumonias, postmyocardial infarction syndrome, acute pancreatitis, abdominal infection, and mesothelioma.

Most common cause of hemothorax is trauma, including open or closed chest trauma. Other conditions with bleeding tendencies (including hemophilia and excessive anticoagulation) can rarely lead to hemothorax. Iatrogenic bleeding into the pleural space can occur in lung biopsy or interventional procedures. Pulmonary infarction, lung cancer, and pleural metastasis can also lead to blood stained pleural fluid.

Chylothorax is due to accumulation of a milky fluid (containing fat and fatty acids) mostly due to injury or obstruction to the thoracic lymphatic channels. Iatrogenic trauma during surgery is a common cause. Other etiologies include nonsurgical trauma, lung cancer, lymphoma, filariasis, and rarely lymphangiomyomatosis.

Imaging Appearance of Pleural Fluid

Free Fluid

Pleural fluid appears as a homogenous opacity on plain radiograph [4,5]. Location of this opacity depends on position of the patient, presence or absence of pleural adhesions, and radiographic technique. Pleural fluid initially accumulates in the posterior costophrenic angle, which is the most dependent pleural recess and can be seen as blunting of this angle on frontal radiograph (Fig. 14.5). *At least 50 mL of pleural fluid is necessary for blunting of the posterior costophrenic angle.* Approximately 100–200 mL of fluid is needed to fill this recess to be able to see the fluid above the diaphragm on frontal radiograph (Fig. 14.6). A very small effusion can be seen with decubitus view (placing the abnormal side dependent), ultrasound, CT, or MRI (Fig. 14.7). At least 10 mL of fluid is minimum to be detected on a decubitus view. With increasing pleural fluid lateral costophrenic angle on the frontal radiograph opacifies and gradually obscures the hemidiaphragm and lung base and often tracks along the fissures. On cross-sectional imaging, pleural effusion occupying less than one fourth of anteroposterior dimension of the hemithorax in the midclavicular line corresponds to less than 300 mL of pleural fluid. Pleural effusions occupying more than half of the hemithorax on cross-sectional imaging have more than 1 L of pleural fluid. Complete opacification of a hemithorax can be seen with a massive pleural effusion. Mass effect due to massive effusion can displace the mediastinum toward the contralateral side. Mediastinal deviation may be absent if the underlying lung is completely collapsed.

Distribution of pleural fluid is often atypical leading to different appearances on conventional chest radiographs. A significant amount of pleural fluid may be hidden between the lung and the hemidiaphragm (subpulmonic effusion) leading to inadequate quantification on chest radiographs compared to ultrasound and CT. Subpulmonic effusion can appear as elevated hemidiaphragm on a chest radiograph (Fig. 14.8). Some useful hint to indicate subpulmonic effusion is apex of the "apparent" elevated hemidiaphragm

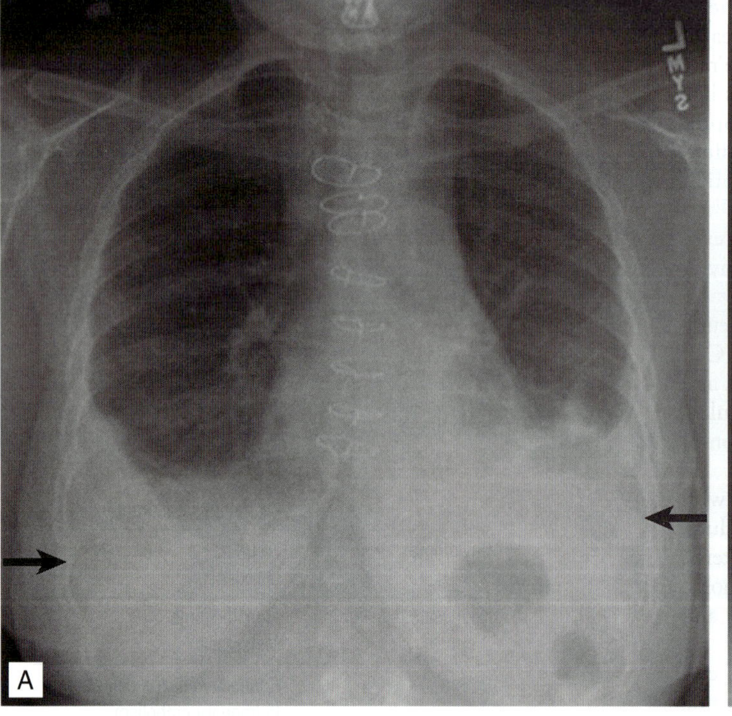

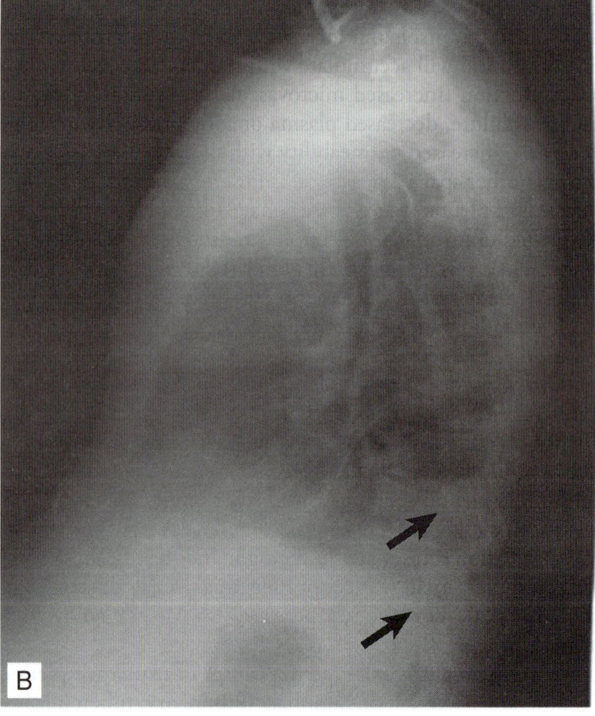

Figure 14.6 Bilateral pleural effusions. Frontal and lateral radiographs showing homogeneous opacification blunting the lateral (*arrows* in A) and posterior costophrenic angles (*arrows* in B).

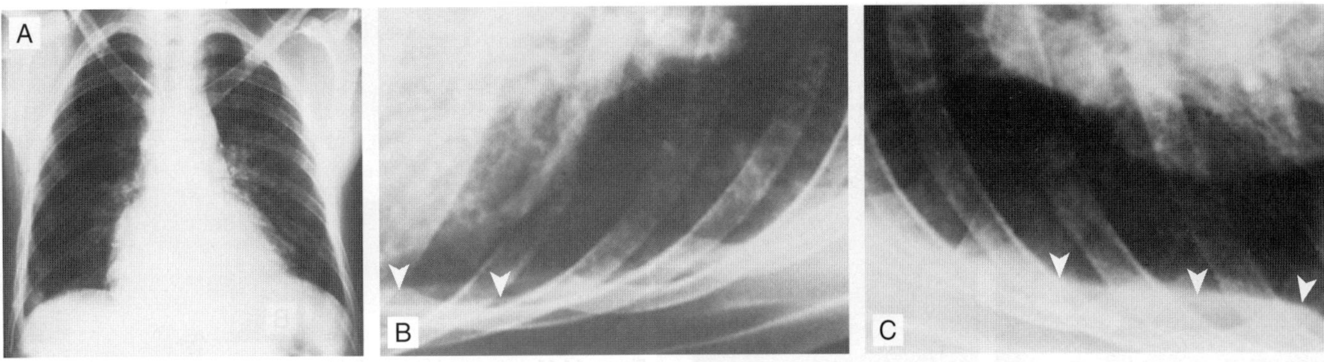

Figure 14.7 Small bilateral pleural effusions. Man aged 34, renal transplant patient with cytomegalovirus pneumonia. The effusions probably relate to renal failure rather than the pneumonia. Posterior anterior (PA) film shows subtle filling in of both costophrenic angles (A). Horizontal-beam right and left lateral decubitus films show obvious free pleural effusions collecting along the dependent lateral costal margins (*arrowheads* in B and C).

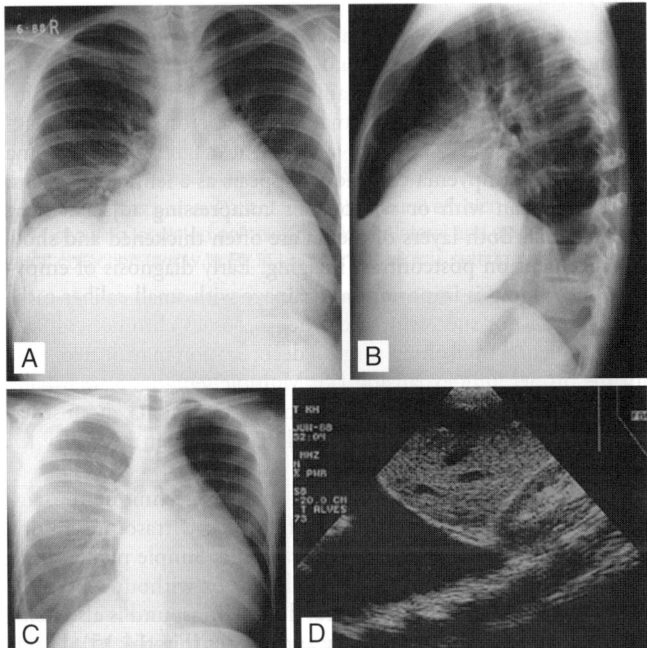

Figure 14.8 A 15-year-old male with Adriamycin-induced cardiomyopathy and recently increasing shortness of breath. Erect PA film shows a large heart and apparent elevation of the right hemidiaphragm due to a large subpulmonic effusion (A). Lateral film shows fluid tracking up the posterior chest wall and blunting the posterior costophrenic recess (B). Supine chest radiograph obtained shortly afterward showing redistribution of pleural fluid (C). The appearances are now typical of a large supine pleural effusion with increased density of the right hemithorax. Ultrasound of the right lung base reveals a large anechoic space consistent with an uncomplicated pleural effusion (D).

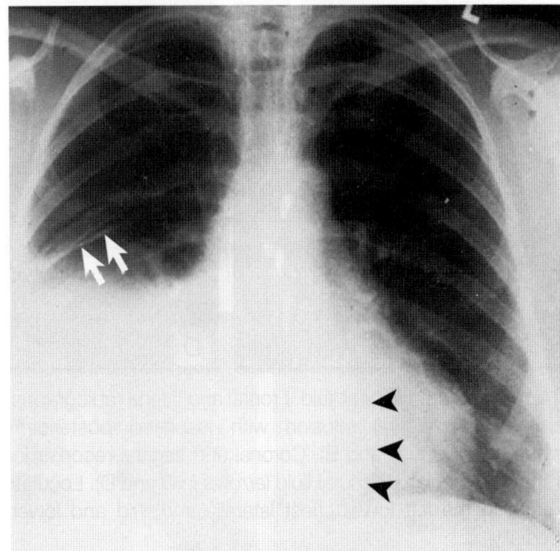

Figure 14.9 Moderate-size pleural effusion in a 56-year-old woman. Effusion of unknown etiology. PA film demonstrates typical pleural opacity with concave upper border, slightly higher laterally, and obscuring the diaphragm and underlying lung. Fluid is extending into the fissure (*arrows*) and also into the azygoesophageal recess, producing a retrocardiac opacity (*arrowheads*).

is more lateral than usual, and usually there is associated blunting of the costophrenic angle and often thickened fissure indicating fluid tracking along the fissure. Pleural fluid can collect between the lung surface and visceral pleura sparing the costophrenic angle, known as the lamellar effusion [4]. *Sometimes a significant amount of pleural fluid can collect in the azygoesophageal recess mimicking a retrocardiac mass* (Fig. 14.9).

Loculated Fluid

Loculation of pleural fluid can be seen when there is a fusion of parietal and visceral pleural layers mostly due to old pleural processes. A few diagnostic features can help in differentiating loculated pleural fluid from lung parenchymal abnormality, extrapleural opacity, and mediastinal mass [6]. Loculated pleural fluid is often associated with free fluid along the costophrenic angle or the fissure (Fig. 14.10A, B). Encapsulated pleural fluid appears like a "biconvex lens" with comparatively little depth and considerable width and the appearance varies with radiographic projections. Sharp outline helps to identify opacity outside the pleura (extrapleural) often with tapered, sometimes concave edges at the point of chest wall contact [7,8]. *An air bronchogram helps to differentiate peripheral lung abnormality from pleural fluid.* Often, cross-sectional imaging is needed to differentiate loculated pleural fluid from other conditions (Fig. 14.10C, D). Sometimes it may be difficult to differentiate loculated from free pleural fluid on CT and imaging in a different position (prone or decubitus) or with ultrasound can help solving the problem.

Pleural fluid can be loculated in the fissures and can be seen in patients with heart failure. Radiographic appearance depends on location and amount of loculated fissural fluid. Small amount of fluid in the fissures appear as fissural thickening. Loculated fluid in the horizontal fissure appears as a well-defined lenticular opacity in both frontal and lateral radiographs. Loculated fluid in the oblique fissure is often poorly defined on frontal radiograph and

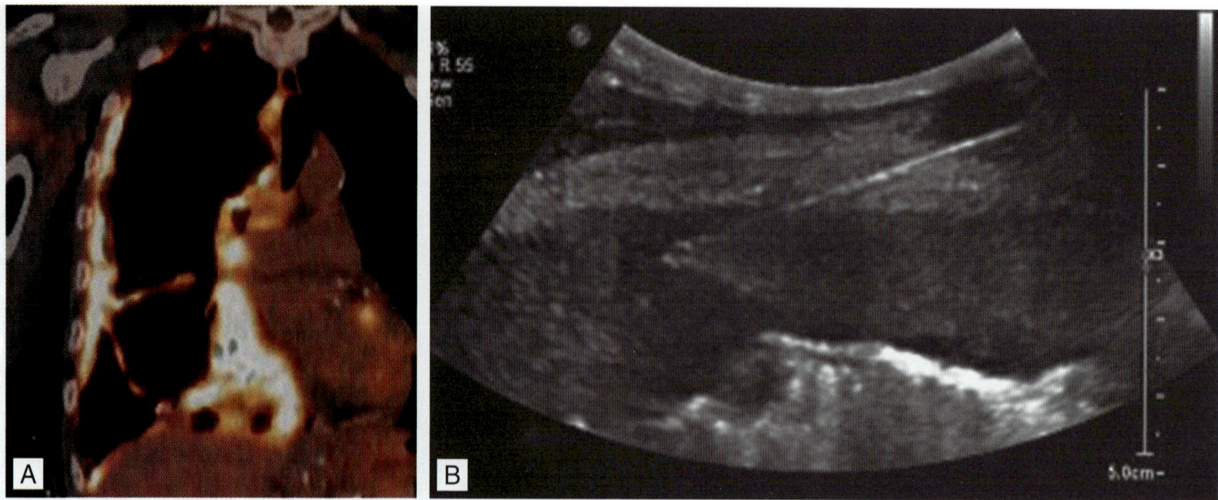

Figure 14.16 Usefulness of ultrasound in detecting pleural mass and guiding needle for biopsy. Positron emission tomography computed tomography image showing intense uptake of diffuse pleural nodularity/masses (A). Ultrasound-guided needle placement for biopsy—note the linear echogenic needle within the soft-tissue pleural mass (B).

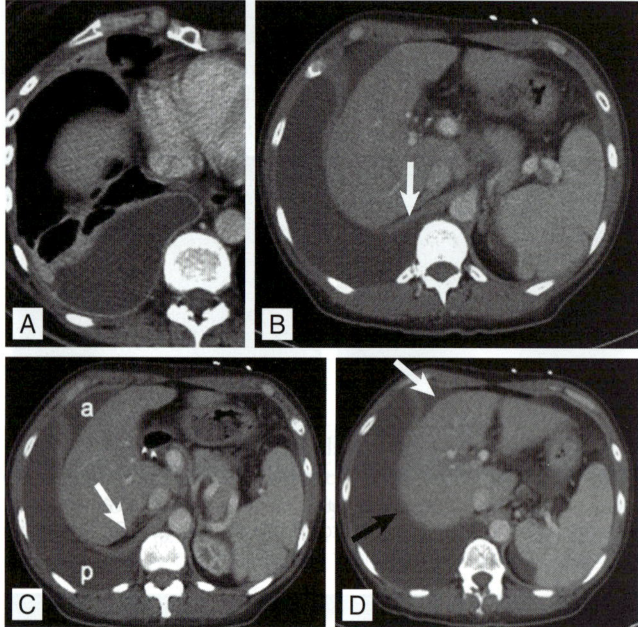

Figure 14.17 CT signs which may help diagnosing pleural effusion from peripheral lung abscess or ascites. Split pleura sign: Pleural fluid separates parietal and visceral pleura and this differentiates pleural fluid from peripheral lung abscess (A). Displaced crus sign: The right pleural effusion collects posterior to the right crus of the diaphragm (*arrows*) and displaces it anteriorly (B). Diaphragm sign: The pleural fluid (p) is over the outer surface of the dome of the diaphragm, whereas the ascitic fluid (a) is within the dome (C). Interface sign: The interface (*white arrow*) between the liver and ascites is usually sharper than between liver and pleural fluid (*black arrow* in D) (D). Bare area sign: Peritoneal reflections prevent ascitic fluid from extending over the entire posterior surface of the liver (*white arrow* in C), in contrast with pleural fluid in the posterior costophrenic recess (p in C).

or even ascites. A few signs can help suggesting pleural fluid on CT as described below [5,6,10–12].

- *Split pleura sign*: pleural fluid displaces both visceral and parietal pleura and this helps differentiating pleural fluid collection from peripheral lung abscess (Fig. 14.17A)
- *Displaced crus sign*: pleural fluid collect posterior to the diaphragmatic crus and displaces it anteriorly and ascites collects anterior to the crus and displaces it posteriorly (Fig. 14.17B)
- *Diaphragm sign*: fluid exterior to the dome of the diaphragm is in the pleura and that is within the dome is ascitic fluid (Fig. 14.17C)
- *Interface sign*: ascites being in close contact with liver and spleen will have a sharp interface with these organs as compared to pleural fluid (Fig. 14.17D)
- *Bare area sign*: ascitic fluid cannot extend to the bare area of the liver which is bounded by coronary ligament. So, fluid over the posterior surface of the liver is usually pleural fluid than ascites (Fig. 14.17C)

Pneumothorax

Collection of air in the pleural cavity is pneumothorax. Pneumothorax can occur when air enters the pleural space through a defect in the parietal or visceral pleura. There are different etiologies of pneumothorax including trauma, spontaneous, iatrogenic, etc. As pleural effusion, pneumothorax maybe localized if there are pleural adhesions. If free pleural air moves in and out with breathing it is called an *open pneumothorax*. When air enters in inspiration and remains there in expiration it is called a *valvular pneumothorax*. Increase in intrapleural pressure in a valvular pneumothorax leads to *tension pneumothorax* [5–8].

Etiology

Most common pneumothorax is spontaneous pneumothorax, usually occurs in young tall men and due to rupture of apical congenital pleural blebs. Paraseptal emphysematous bullous lesions are common factor in older individual. Other causes of spontaneous pneumothorax include chronic bronchitis, asthma, rupture of air containing lung cyst or cavity (tuberculosis, staphylococcal pneumonia, and malignancy), and interstitial pulmonary fibrosis (cystic fibrosis, histiocytosis, tuberous sclerosis, sarcoidosis, and pneumoconiosis).

Both blunt and penetrating trauma can lead to pneumothorax. Usual traumatic causes of pneumothorax are penetrating trauma, closed chest trauma (mostly due to bronchial rupture), rib fracture, pleural/lung interventional procedure, bronchoscopy, positive pressure ventilation, and thoracic surgery. Diagnostic pneumothorax to diagnose pleural condition and artificial pneumothorax to treat pulmonary tuberculosis are of historical interest only.

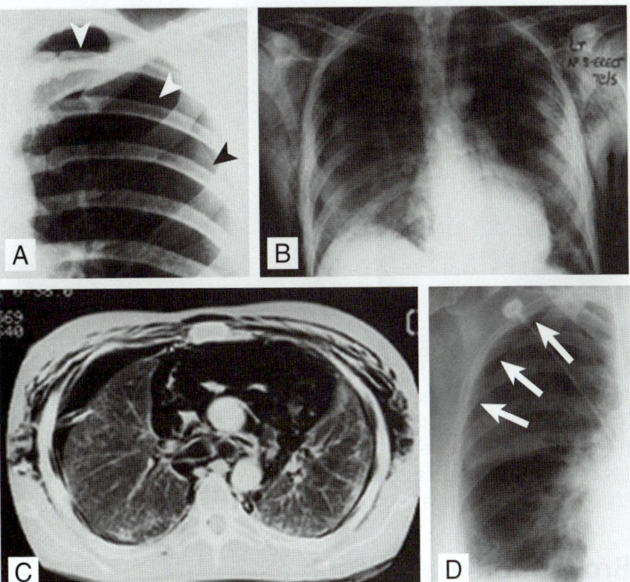

Figure 14.18 Woman aged 22 with a spontaneous pneumothorax. PA radiograph showing apical pneumothorax. The visceral pleura (*arrowheads*) separates aerated lung from the radiolucent pleural space (A). AP chest radiograph and CT scan in a patient with *Pneumocystis carinii* pneumonia complicated by bilateral pneumothoraces and extensive mediastinal and surgical emphysema (B and C). Supine chest radiograph of an intubated patient. There is a skin fold projected over the right lung apex simulating a pneumothorax (*arrows*). Close inspection reveals lung markings extending beyond the skin fold, and no fine pleural line that should be visible with a genuine pneumothorax (D).

However, artificial pneumothorax can help gaining access in some chest biopsies including biopsy of mediastinal lesions.

Imaging Appearance of Pneumothorax

A small free pneumothorax in an erect patient tends to collect in the apex [6,7]. Lung adjacent to the pneumothorax retracts toward the hilum and on a frontal radiograph a sharp radiopaque line of the visceral pleura separates air containing radiolucent avascular pleural space from lucent lung parenchyma with lung markings (Fig. 14.18A–C). A skin fold can often appear as a pneumothorax, however, unlike pneumothorax the line due to skinfold often does not follow the expected course of visceral pleura, the line is usually a thick white line compared to thin visceral pleural line and lung markings are visible outside the curvilinear shadow (Fig. 14.18D).

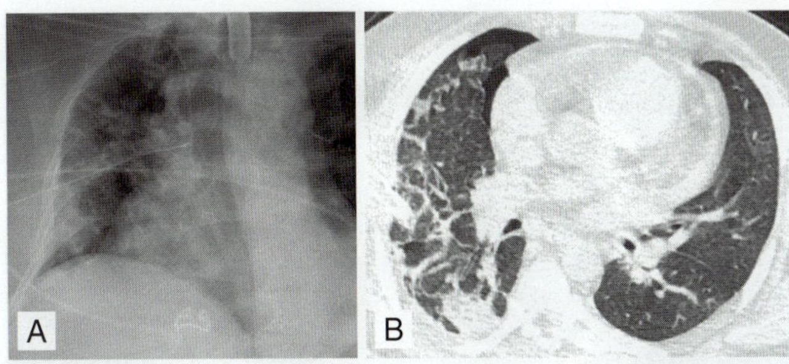

Figure 14.19 Anteromedial pneumothorax. AP radiograph in an intubated patient showing pneumothorax anteromedially (A). The pneumothorax is seen anteromedially on same day CT (B).

A small pneumothorax may be easily missed, and it is important to look for it carefully and with image magnification. In closed pneumothorax, pleural air volume is not changed in respiration and an expiratory radiograph will make it easier to see due to decrease in lung volume. A lateral decubitus radiograph with the nondependent abnormal side can help detecting small pleural air. This is particularly helpful in AP radiographs in infants and patients in the intensive care unit where a small pneumothorax is often difficult to visualize due to its accumulation anteriorly and medially (Fig. 14.19A, B) [13]. Another technique is horizontal beam "shoot-through" lateral radiograph which might help identifying anterior pneumothorax in a supine patient. With pneumothorax, a small amount of normal pleural fluid may cause blunting of the costophrenic angle. With hydropneumothorax, a horizontal fluid level is noted separating dependent fluid and nondependent air (Fig. 14.20). In patients with double lung transplant using a single pleural covering pleural effusion or pneumothorax can shift from one side to the other depending on patients position and can extend along the midline (Fig. 14.21).

Amount of collapse of the lung due to pneumothorax depends on amount of air, rapidity of development, and underlying lung condition. A large pneumothorax can lead to complete lung relaxation toward the hilum with mediastinal shift to contralateral side, which increases in expiration.

Tension Pneumothorax

Large or rapid accumulation of pleural air can lead to significant displacement of mediastinum with kinking of the great veins and acute cardiorespiratory decompensation [4]. On plain radiographs, the signs of tension pneumothorax are significant contralateral mediastinal deviation, collapsed lung maybe squashed

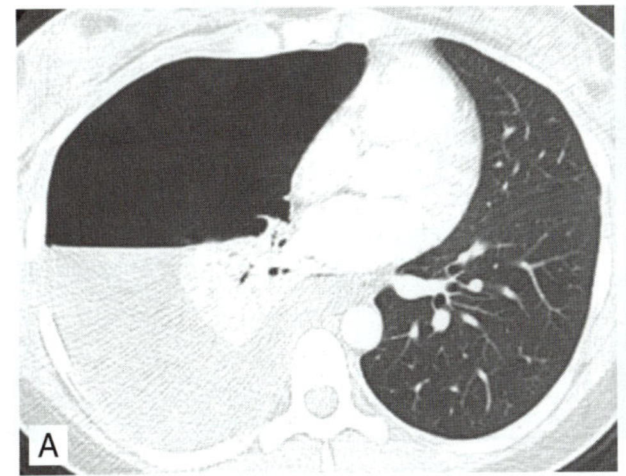

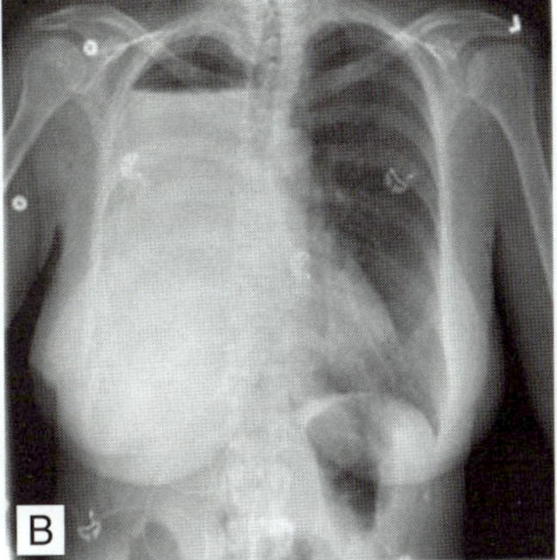

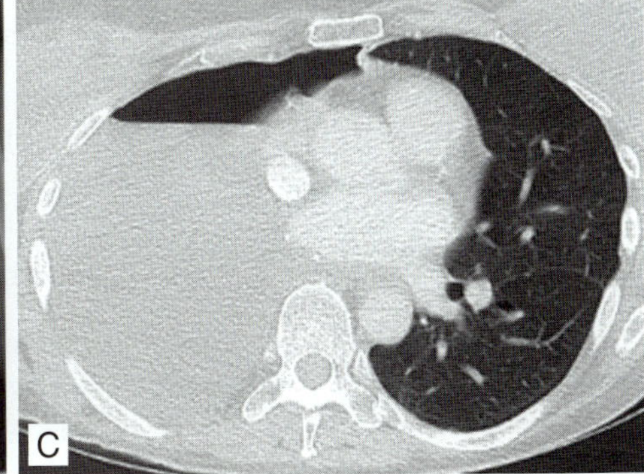

Figure 14.20 Air–fluid level. Horizontal air–fluid level separating dependent fluid and nondependent air in hydropneumothorax (A). Plain radiograph and CT showing horizontal air–fluid level in a patient postpneumonectomy (B and C).

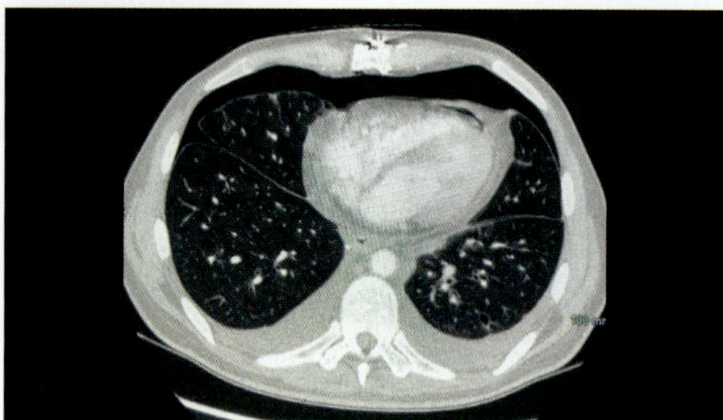

Figure 14.21 Pneumothorax in double lung transplant. Pneumothorax extending along the midline in a patient with double lung transplant with single pleural covering, also known as buffalo chest.

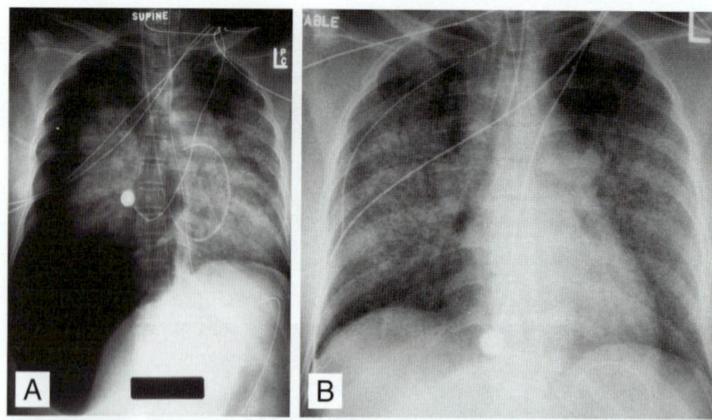

Figure 14.22 Tension pneumothorax following a transbronchial lung biopsy. There is inversion of the right hemidiaphragm, and deviation of the mediastinum to the opposite side (A). Following insertion of a right-sided chest drain the diaphragm and mediastinum have returned to a normal position (B). The diffuse bilateral infiltrate is due to pre-existing pulmonary hemorrhage.

against the mediastinum or displaced toward contralateral side and depression of ipsilateral hemidiaphragm (Fig. 14.22). Fluoroscopy can show contralateral mediastinal displacement greatest on inspiration, differentiating tension pneumothorax from large pneumothorax without tension.

Loculated Pneumothorax

Similar to loculated pleural effusion, pleural adhesions can also lead to loculated or encysted pneumothorax [7]. Loculated pneumothorax appears as an ovoid air collection close to the chest wall and may be difficult to differentiate from thin-walled subpleural lung cavity, cyst, or bulla radiographically.

Pleural adhesions extend between two pleural layers and appear as a line shadow (Fig. 14.23). Rupture of an adhesion can lead to hemopneumothorax and discharge from an underlying infected subpleural lesion can lead to pyopneumothorax.

Re-expansion Pulmonary Edema

Rapid re-expansion of a lung following drainage of a large pleural effusion or pneumothorax may be associated with a condition called re-expansion pulmonary edema with development of extensive consolidative opacities in the ipsilateral lung (Fig. 14.24) [14]. Re-expansion edema usually resolves within a day or two.

Bronchopleural Fistula

A communication between the airway and pleural space is called bronchopleural fistula (Fig. 14.25). This is a known complication following complete or partial pneumonectomy and is discussed in detail in the chapter describing postoperative complication. Other causes include bronchial carcinoma, ruptured lung abscess, and trauma. A nonresolving pneumothorax or hydropneumothorax in appropriate clinical situation raises possibility of bronchopleural fistula.

Pleural Thickening

Localized pleural thickening commonly results in bilateral apical opacification and blunting of costophrenic angle [15]. Localized pleural thickening usually results from a previous pleuritis, which is often subclinical. In the asymptomatic patient without any other radiological abnormality blunting of the costophrenic angle due to pleural thickening is of no significance. However, this may mimic a small pleural effusion and comparison with old radiographs is helpful. Otherwise, a lateral decubitus radiograph or ultrasound correlation is necessary to rule out a small amount of pleural fluid depending on clinical presentation.

Biapical pleural thickening is also a common finding, often seen in elderly and not always due to tuberculosis. Symmetrical

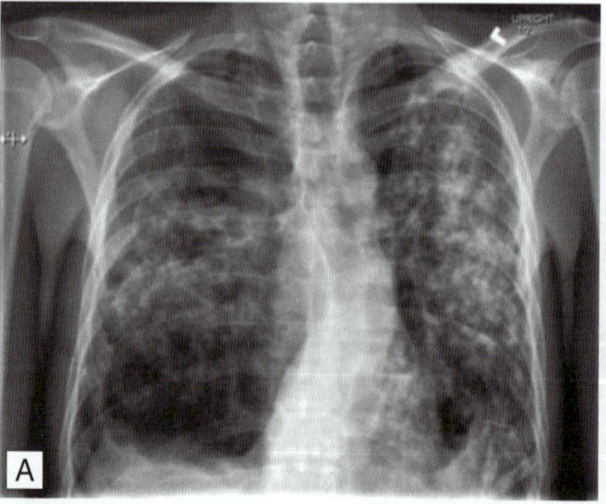

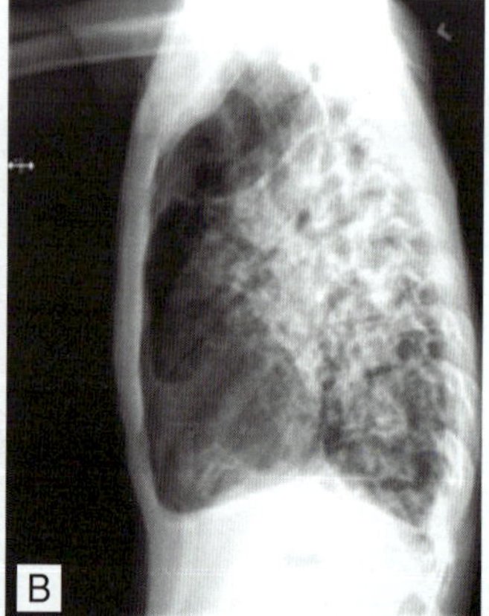

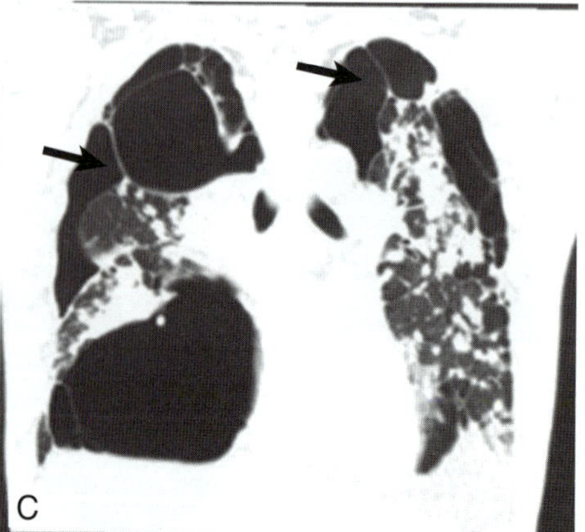

Figure 14.23 Septation in loculated pneumothorax. A 29-year-old male with known lacrimal gland cancer with multiple bilateral lung metastasis. Bilateral loculated pneumothoraces seen on frontal and lateral plain radiographs (A and B) and on coronal reformatted CT (C). Septations are nicely seen on CT (*black arrows*).

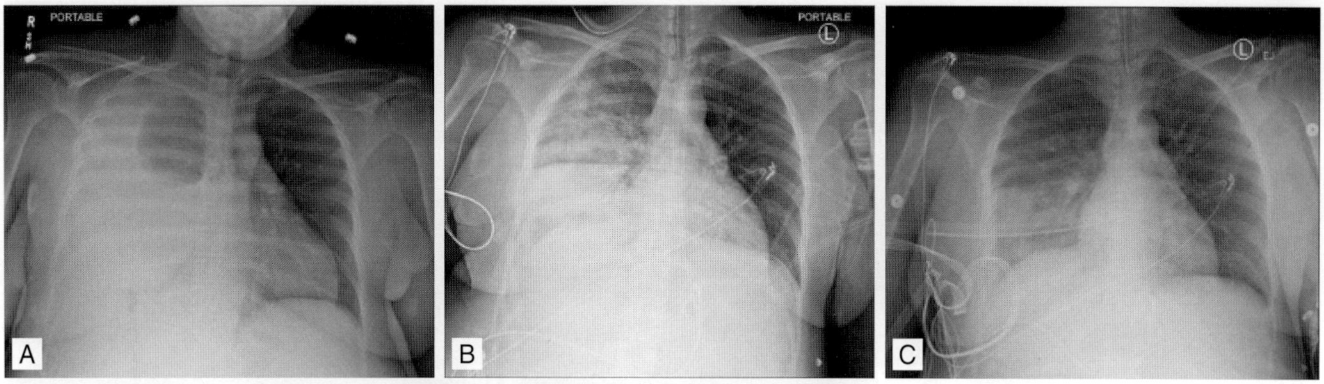

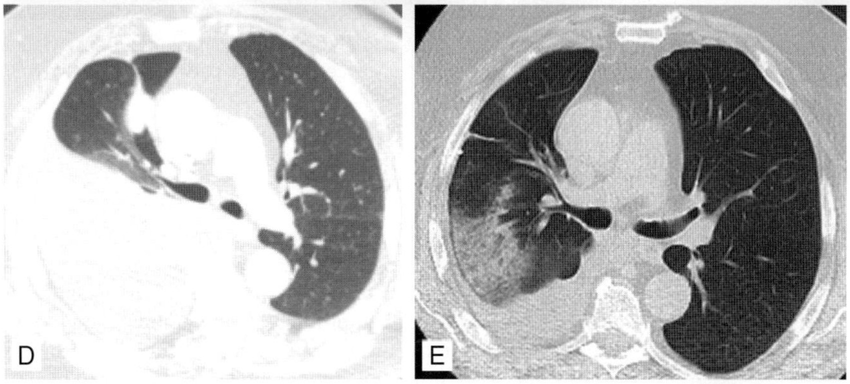

Figure 14.24 Re-expansion edema. Initial frontal radiograph in this 36-year-old female showing large right pleural effusion with underlying collapse and mediastinal deviation toward left (A). Radiograph after pleural fluid drainage showing opacification of right lung likely representing re-expansion edema (B) which was improving gradually (C). Large right pleural effusion on another patient (D). Right lung ground glass opacities after drainage of pleural fluid is likely due to re-expansion edema (E).

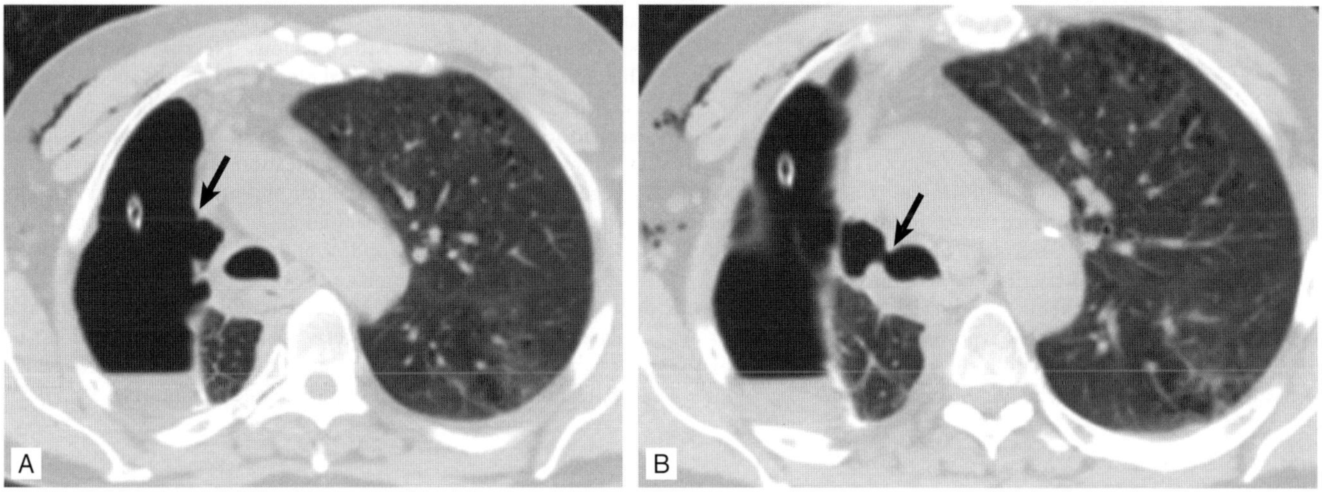

Figure 14.25 Bronchopleural fistula. A wide fistulous tract is seen connecting the pleural cavity (*arrow* in A) with the central airway (*arrow* in B). Note persistence of right pneumothorax even with a chest tube in place.

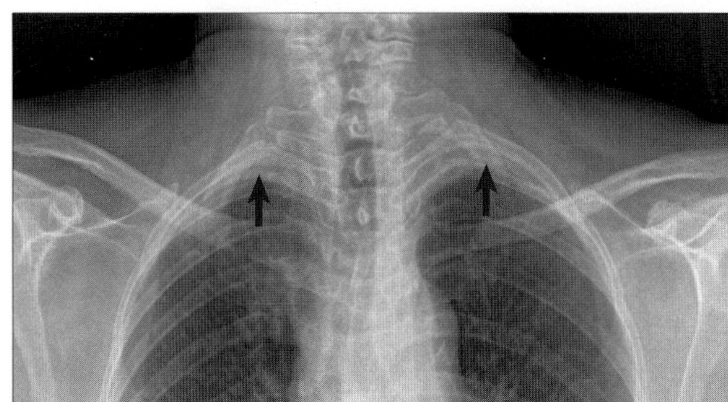

Figure 14.26 Bilateral apical pleural thickening. The apical pleural shadowing (*arrows*) is symmetrical with well-defined edges.

apical homogenous opacities on plain radiographs are due to benign pleural thickening or prominent extrapleural fat (Fig. 14.26). Asymmetrical or unilateral apical pleural thickening maybe of a pathological significance if associated with symptoms like pain. *Pancoast tumor can appear as unilateral apical thickening and it is important to look at adjacent ribs and spine for any evidence of malignant destruction* (Fig. 14.27). As bony destruction almost always suggest malignancy, these patients were evaluated with penetrated radiographs and tomography in earlier days and now with CT. Apical pleural thickening can also be seen with postradiation treatment, particularly for head and neck malignancies.

Both benign and malignant causes can lead to extensive unilateral pleural thickening. Previous thoracotomy, complicated pleural effusion and rarely chronic pneumothorax can lead to

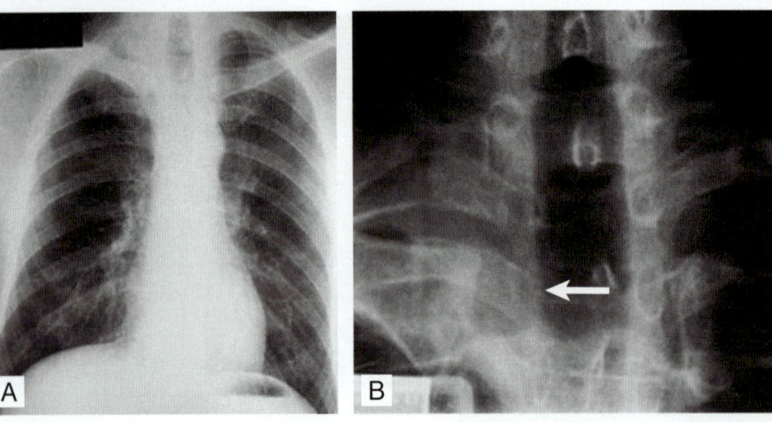

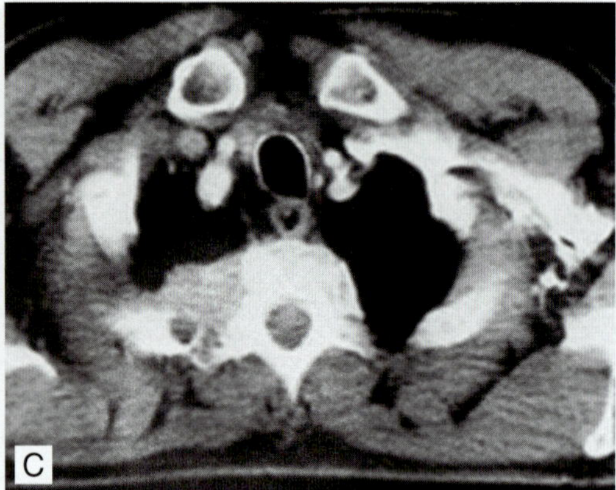

Figure 14.27 Unilateral apical pleural thickening on plain radiograph. Man aged 46 with pain in the right side of the neck and right arm. Dense pleural shadowing is present at the right (A). The left apex is clear. An AP view of the cervical spine demonstrates absence of the right pedicle of T3 (*arrow* in B). CT demonstrates a right apical mass infiltrating the third thoracic vertebra (C). Histology: anaplastic carcinoma.

TABLE 14.2 Causes of Pleural Calcifications

- Asbestos related
- Prior hemothorax
- Prior empyema
- Tuberculosis
- Radiation
- Chronic renal failure
- Prior chest surgery
- Rheumatoid arthritis
- Calcifying fibrous pseudotumor

unilateral pleural thickening. Fibrothorax is a condition when the entire lung is surrounded by a fibrotic pleura. Surgical decortication may be necessary in fibrothorax when it causes significant ventilatory restriction of the affected lung.

Bilateral pleural thickening and calcification are common manifestations of prior asbestos exposure [16]. The term asbestosis is only used if pulmonary fibrosis is present in a patient with asbestos-related pleural thickening or calcification.

Pleural Calcification

Pleural calcifications are usually due to benign etiologies and conditions causing pleural thickening can also lead to pleural calcification (Table 14.2). Unilateral pleural calcification can be seen with previous empyema, hemothorax, pleurisy, and postradiation treatment. Bilateral calcifications typically occur after asbestos exposure and some other pneumoconiosis [16]. Similar to pleural thickening pleural calcification may be incidental and patient may not remember any previous chest disease.

Pleural calcification with previous pleurisy, empyema, or hemothorax involves the visceral pleura and almost always there is associated pleural thickening. The pleural calcification in this scenario may appear as continuous sheet or in discrete plaques. On imaging, visceral pleural calcification produces dense, coarse, irregular opacities, which is often sharply demarcated laterally (Fig. 14.28). If a plaque is viewed en face on plain radiograph, it may mimic a pulmonary nodule and often radiograph in another projection helps localizing it to the pleura.

Asbestos-related pleural calcification is usually more delicate and bilateral and involves the parietal pleura. Common locations are along the diaphragm and adjacent to the axillae. CT is most sensitive technique for detection of pleural calcification (Fig. 14.29).

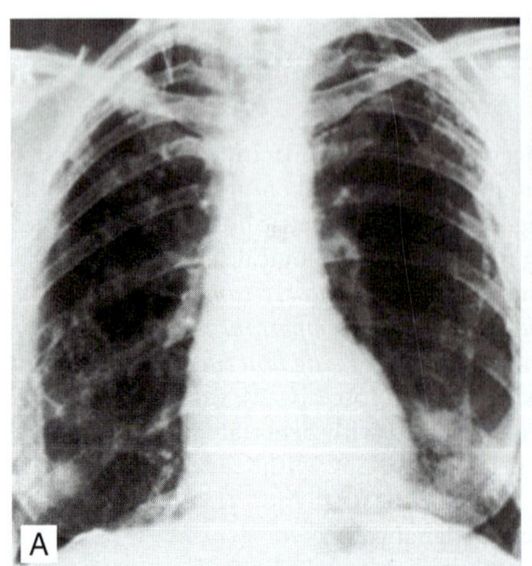

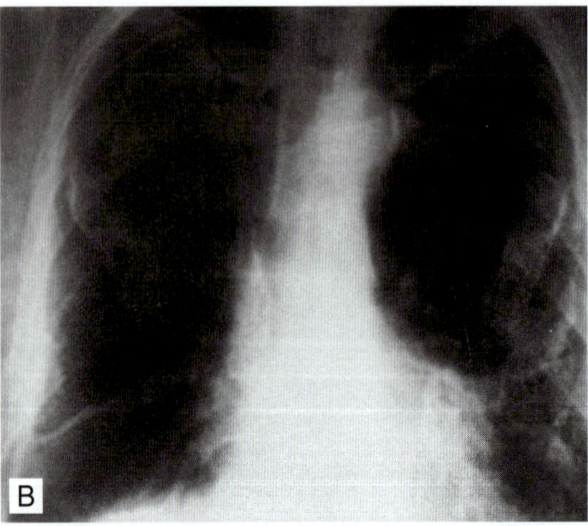

Figure 14.28 Pleural calcification in a middle-aged woman with a history of recurrent episodes of pleurisy, presumed to be tuberculosis. Extensive plaques of pleural calcification surround both lungs (A). Bilateral calcified pleural plaques seen in face over both lungs due to exposure to asbestos (B).

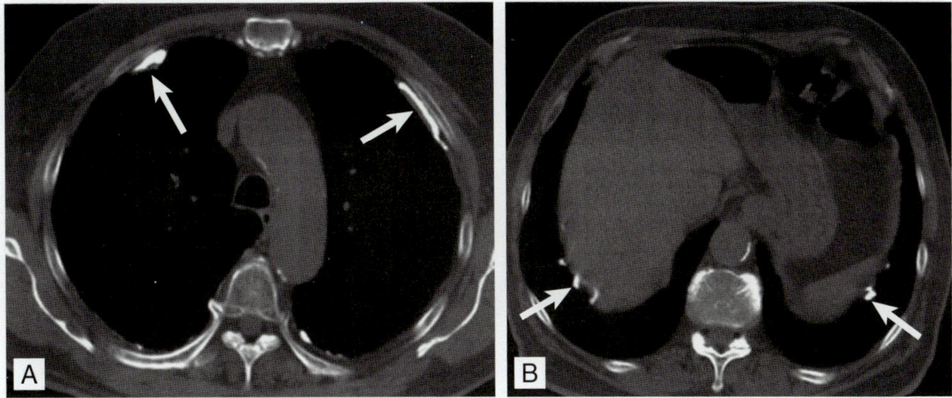

Figure 14.29 Asbestos-related pleural calcification. CT is helpful for detecting small pleural plaque. Axial CT images showing classic distribution of pleural plaques along 3 and 9 o'clock positions and along the hemidiaphragms (*arrows*).

Pleural Tumors

Pleural tumors are relatively rare compared to lung and mediastinum. Common benign pleural tumors include localized fibrous tumor (fibroma) and lipoma. Commonest malignant pleural tumor is metastasis (Fig. 14.30) with most frequent primary sites being the lung and breast. Primary malignant tumor or the pleura (malignant mesothelioma) is usually associated with prior asbestos exposure. On plain radiographs, loculated pleural fluid in the fissure can appear as a mass lesion, known as pseudotumor (Fig. 14.12A, B).

Pleural fibromas are often incidental on a chest radiograph in an asymptomatic patient. Paraneoplastic conditions associated with pleural fibroma are finger clubbing, hypertrophic osteoarthropathy, and hypoglycemia. They are slow growing tumors and usually benign, but malignant features can also be seen. On a plain radiograph, they appear as well-defined lobulated mass adjacent to the chest wall, mediastinum, diaphragm, or along the fissures (Fig. 14.31A, B). Size may be small or large enough to occupy the entire hemithorax. When small, cross-sectional imaging shows homogenously enhancing pleural tumor and with large tumor there are often nonenhancing areas suggesting intratumoral necrosis [17]. Cross-sectional imaging including CT and MRI is helpful in characterizing the tumor and showing the extent (Fig. 14.31C–F).

Subpleural or pleural lipomas appear as well-defined rounded peripheral masses on a plain radiograph. As they are soft tumors, they can change their shape with breathing. CT and MRI are diagnostic detecting fat within these tumors (Fig. 14.32).

Malignant mesothelioma is usually due to a long-term exposure to asbestos particles, particularly the crocidolite with a latent period from exposure to asbestos and development of mesothelioma is typically 20–40 years. Patients usually present with nonspecific mild chest symptoms with significant disease on imaging. Symptoms include chest pain, cough, hoarseness, dyspnea, night sweats, fatigue, weight loss, etc. On imaging, malignant mesothelioma appears as nodular pleural thickening around all or part of the lung (Fig. 14.33) often with hemorrhagic pleural effusion. Lung changes of asbestosis are not always present. Associated pleural effusion may obscure the underlying mass on a plain radiograph or noncontrast-enhanced CT. Though rib destruction can be seen with mesothelioma, *most common cause of pleural mass with adjacent rib destruction is metastatic or primary tumor involving the bone.* Cross-sectional imagings including CT, MRI, or PET are necessary for treatment planning of malignant mesothelioma [18–20]. Although all patients with mesothelioma receive some form of chemotherapy, staging helps in identifying patients who can benefit from surgery. Clinical staging with imaging is performed first which often underestimates disease burden. Surgical staging is performed after clinical staging if patient is eligible for surgery after clinical staging. There are multiple staging systems for mesothelioma and most commonly used staging system is eighth edition of the TNM (tumor, node, metastasis) system. Early-stage disease (Stage I and II) involves pleura and may involve lung parenchyma or diaphragmatic muscle, however without involvement of lymph nodes or distant organs. In this eighth edition locally advanced disease is included in the Stage III. Stage IV includes only patients with distant metastasis. *Features suggesting malignant versus benign pleural thickening are nodularity, thickening extending along the mediastinal surface or fissures, lung encasement, and loss of ipsilateral lung volume.* MRI is superior to CT for detecting mediastinal and

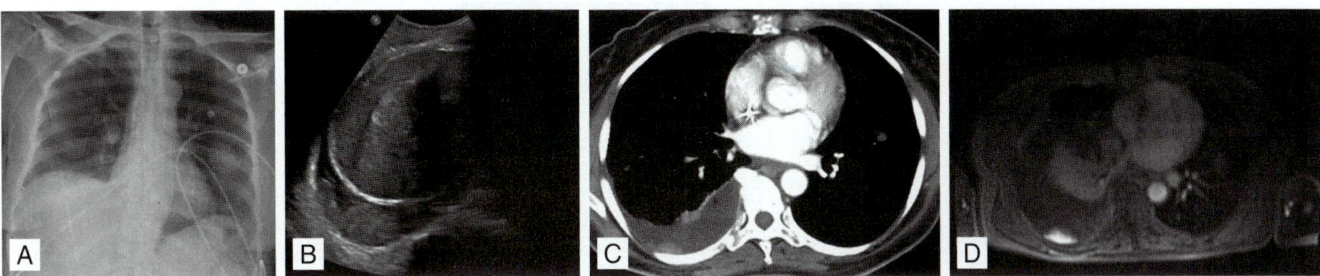

Figure 14.30 Pleural metastasis. Plain radiograph showing bilateral nodular lung metastasis with elevated right hemidiaphragm likely due to subpulmonic effusion (A). Ultrasound showing right pleural effusion with soft-tissue nodule (B). Axial contrast-enhanced CT and fat-saturated contrast-enhanced MRI showing right pleural effusion with enhancing nodule (C and D).

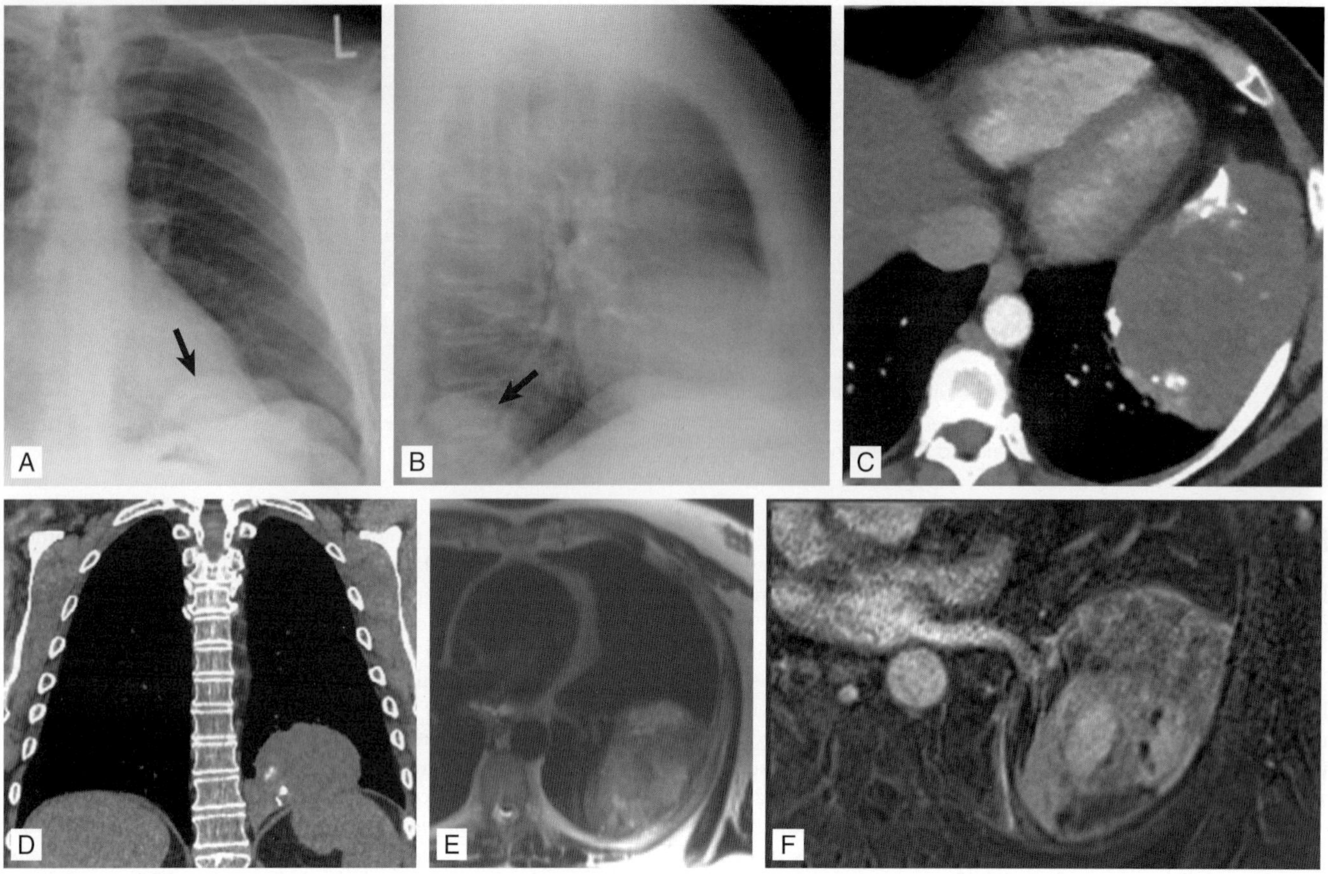

Figure14.31. Solitary fibrous tumor of the pleura. Frontal and lateral plain radiographs showing lobulated mass along the posterior left hemidiaphragm (*arrows* in A and B). Axial and coronal CT images showing homogeneous pleural mass lesion with foci of calcification (C and D). T2 and fat-saturated postcontrast T1-weighted MRI showing heterogenous tumor with multiple areas of heterogenous enhancement (E and F).

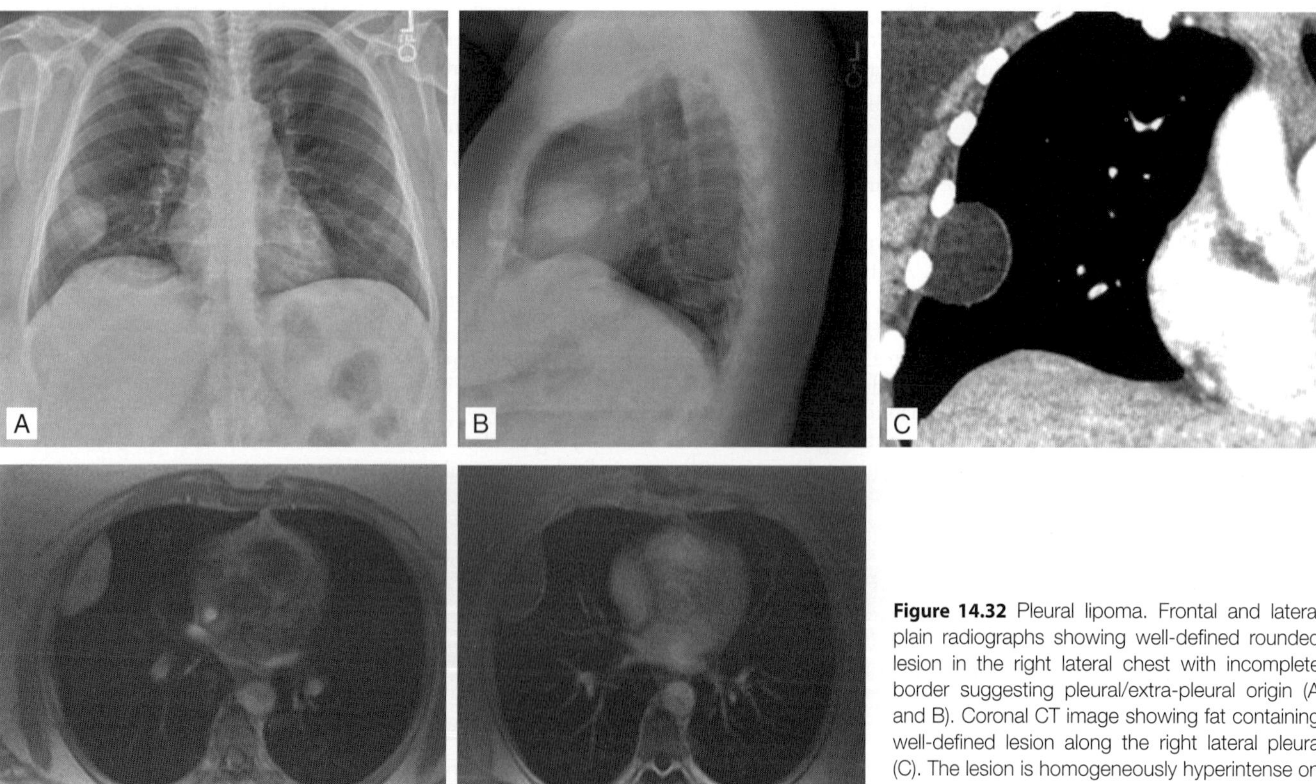

Figure 14.32 Pleural lipoma. Frontal and lateral plain radiographs showing well-defined rounded lesion in the right lateral chest with incomplete border suggesting pleural/extra-pleural origin (A and B). Coronal CT image showing fat containing well-defined lesion along the right lateral pleura (C). The lesion is homogeneously hyperintense on nonfat-saturated MRI image (D) and hypointense on fat-saturated image (E).

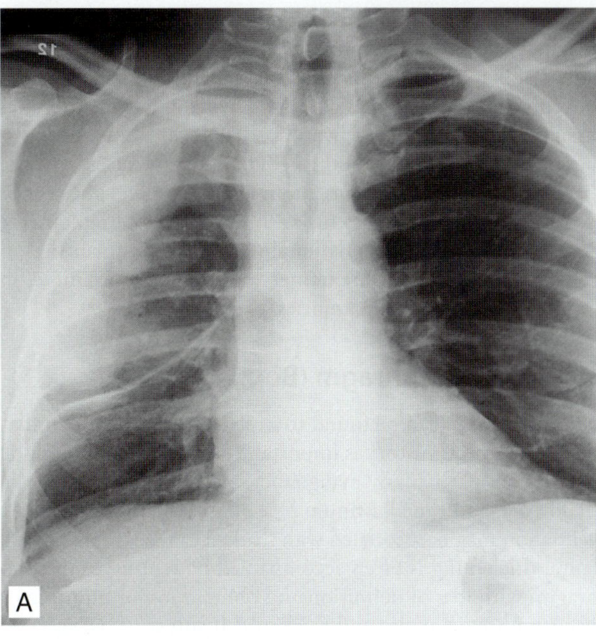

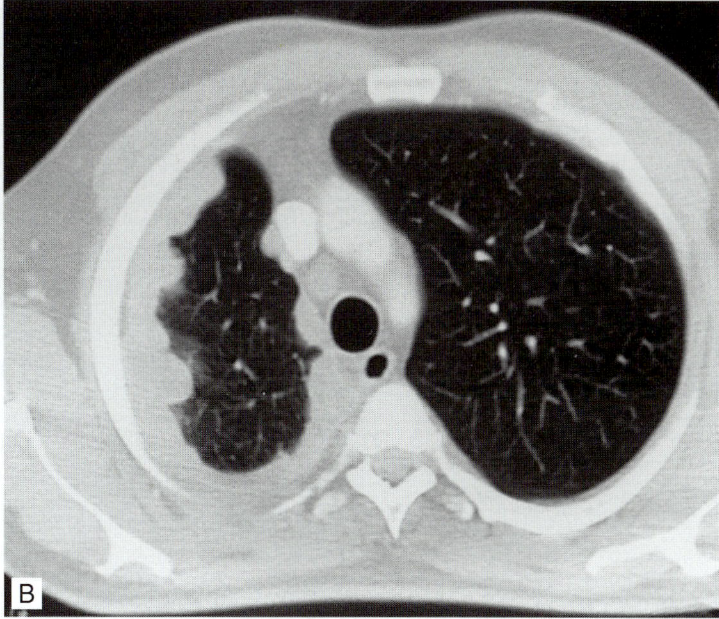

Figure 14.33 Mesothelioma. Abnormal chest radiograph shows lobulated right pleural opacities (A). CT scan through the mid thorax demonstrates encasement of the right lung by nodular pleural tumor (B).

chest wall extension and involvement of cardiovascular structures. Percutaneous or surgical needle biopsy is necessary to make a final diagnosis. Tumor seeding of malignant mesothelioma is reported along the biopsy or chest drainage tracts (Fig. 14.34). Lymphoma can also involve pleura, usually with systemic disease and isolated pleural involvement is rare. Another rare tumor that can arise from pleura is a neuroectodermal tumor called the Askin tumor.

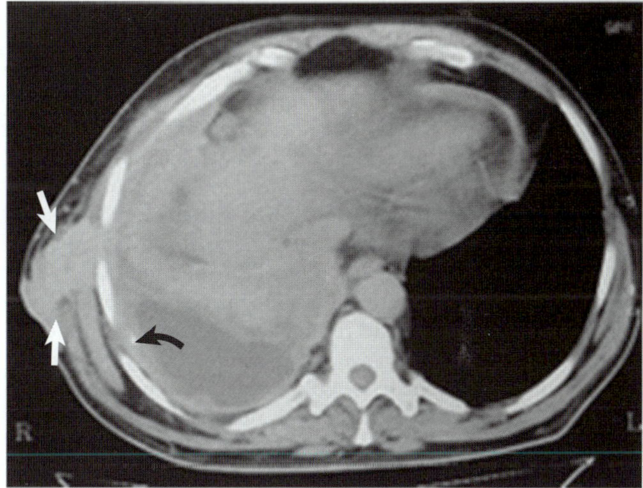

Figure 14.34 CT scan through the lower thorax of a patient with malignant mesothelioma. There is metastatic tumor seeding along the biopsy tract (*white arrows*). Note the fleck of pleural calcification (*curved arrow*).

The Diaphragm

The normal diaphragm is 2–3 mm thick [21]. On the left side where the gastric bubble lies beneath the diaphragm, the stomach wall and diaphragm form a linear density 5–8 mm thick. However on the right side thickness cannot be assessed unless the inferior surface is outlined by free intraperitoneal gas. Thickening may be a normal variant but occurs with tumors of the diaphragm, stomach and pleura, subpulmonary fluid, diaphragm humps, and abdominal lesions including subphrenic abscess, hepatomegaly, and splenomegaly.

Normal Variants

- *Scalloping* (Fig. 14.35): short curves of diaphragm convex upward are seen and this occurs predominantly on the right side
- *Muscle slips* (Fig. 14.35): these are most commonly seen in tall, thin patients, and in those with emphysema. They appear as small curved lines, concave upward, and are more common on the right side [21]
- *Diaphragm humps and dromedary diaphragm* (Fig. 14.35): these variants are probably mild forms of eventration with incomplete muscularization of the hemidiaphragm but no muscle defect. They arise anteriorly and are usually right sided, containing liver. There is no diaphragm defect. On the PA film the hump appears as a shadow in the right cardiophrenic angle and must be distinguished from a fat pad, lipoma, pericardial cyst, and Morgagni hernia. On the lateral film the hump overlies the cardiac shadow and should not be confused with middle lobe consolidation. The dromedary diaphragm is a more severe form of diaphragm hump appearing as a double contour on the PA view
- *Accessory diaphragm*: this rare condition is asymptomatic and usually right sided. The hemithorax is partitioned by the accessory diaphragm running parallel to the oblique fissure and resembling a thickened fissure. Its blood supply is often anomalous. Reported associations are other congenital lesions of the lungs such as anomalous venous drainage and lobar hypoplasia

Diaphragmatic Dysfunction

It is more commonly being unilateral and often presents on a chest radiograph as an elevation of one of the hemidiaphragm. Patients with unilateral diaphragmatic dysfunction are often asymptomatic and detected incidentally and symptomatic patients' usual clinical presentations are dyspnea on exertion and orthopnea. Eventration is the term used when a portion of the diaphragm is elevated due

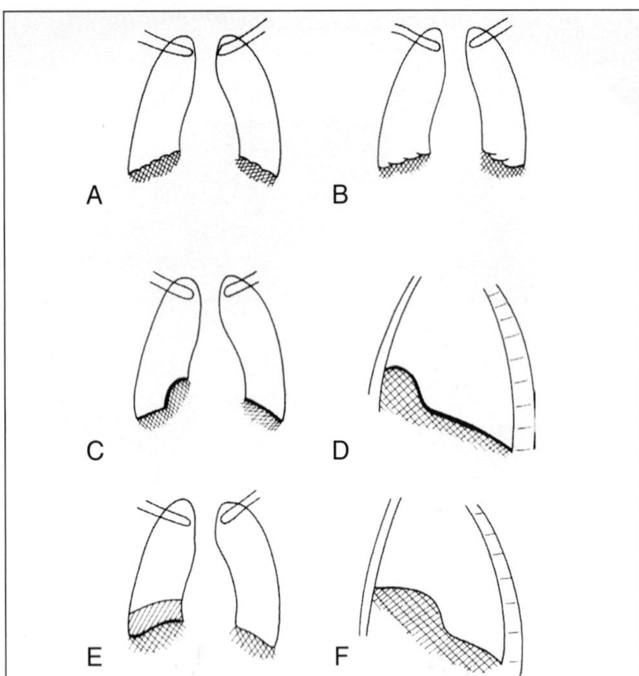

Figure 14.35 Normal variants of the diaphragm. (A) Scalloping (B) Muscle slips (C–F) Diaphragm hump.

to congenital thinning (Fig. 14.36). *Anteromedial portion of the right hemidiaphragm is the commonest location of diaphragmatic eventration* [21]. Focal bulge due to eventration can be diagnosed on plain radiograph or CT and differential includes focal diaphragmatic hernia (see below). Functional evaluation of diaphragmatic movement is commonly performed with fluoroscopic "sniff" test. Both hemidiaphragms normally move downward in deep inspiration and normal excursion is at least one intercostal space width in adults. In patients with diaphragmatic paralysis, this normal movement is absent and there may be paradoxical motion in inspiration which is more obvious with sniffing (Fig. 14.37). However paradoxical movement is also seen in a small number of normal subjects. Reduced excursion of the diaphragm frequently occurs with inflammatory processes either above or below the diaphragm; examples are subphrenic abscess and basal pneumonia. Treatment of diaphragmatic dysfunction depends on clinical severity and etiology. Asymptomatic patients with unilateral dysfunction are managed conservatively and patients with respiratory distress due to paralysis of both hemidiaphragm often require long-term positive pressure ventilation. Diaphragmatic plication is reserved for symptomatic patients with irreversible phrenic nerve damage. Phrenic nerve stimulation by surgically implanting an electrode is helpful when phrenic nerve is intact, for example, in cases with high cervical spine injuries.

The Elevated Diaphragm (Box 14.1)

Frequently no cause can be found to explain an elevated hemidiaphragm. The clinical history is important. It is essential to exclude an active lesion, particularly malignancy, by carefully assessing the lung fields, hila, and mediastinum.

- Eventration may be associated with marked cardiac displacement
- Pleural thickening is often accompanied by tenting of the diaphragm, with loss of definition and obliteration or blunting of the costophrenic angles and thickened fissures
- Subpulmonary fluid may be difficult to distinguish from an elevated diaphragm. Typically it has a straighter upper border and will change shape with patient position if it is not loculated
- Loculated subpulmonary effusions are very difficult to distinguish from a high diaphragm on plain films. Ultrasound is the definitive diagnostic investigation
- Splinting of the diaphragm occurs with upper abdominal inflammatory processes, basal pneumonia, and embolism

Determining whether diaphragm elevation is due to paralysis or an abdominal mass elevating the diaphragm may be difficult on the plain film. The position of the liver edge should be noted. If the liver edge is low then there is probably a mass within or between the liver and diaphragm, whereas a normally positioned or high liver edge favors paralysis as a cause. On the left side the gastric bubble is assessed using the same principles.

A depressed diaphragm is seen with pulmonary hyperinflation and large pleural effusions.

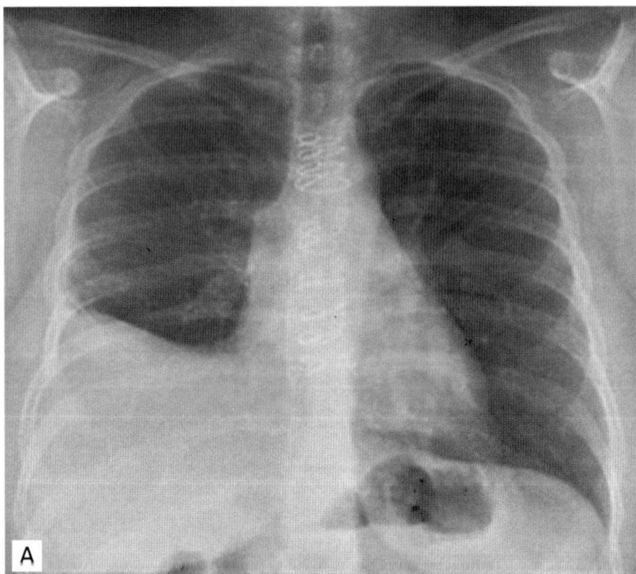

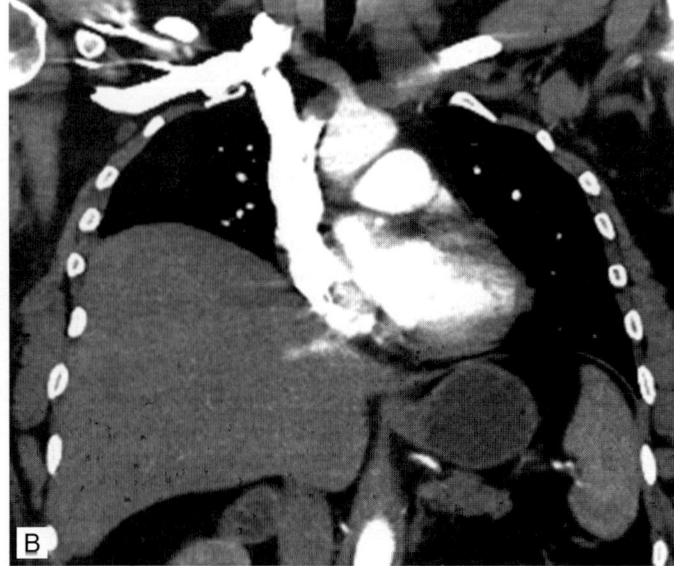

Figure 14.36 Plain radiograph (A) and coronal reconstructed CT (B) images of a patient with eventration of right hemidiaphragm.

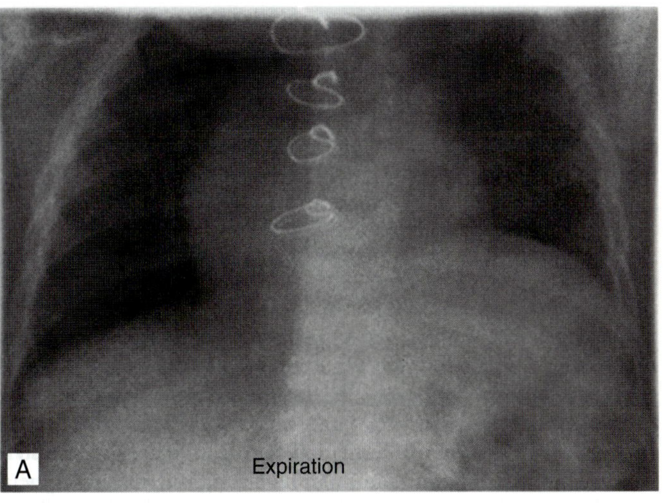

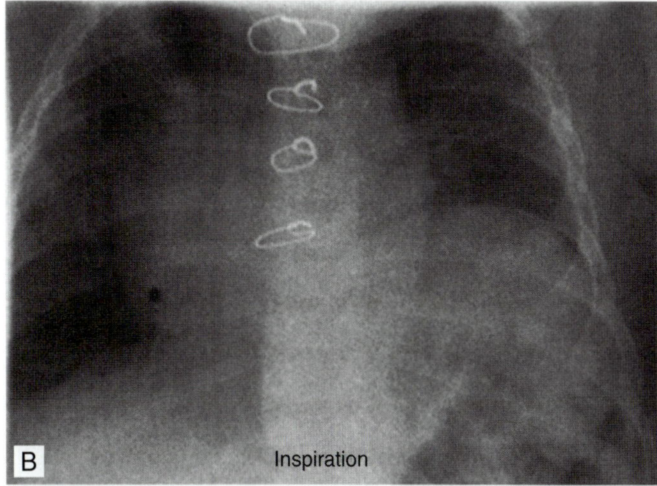

Figure 14.37 Left diaphragmatic paralysis. A 7-year-old male with prior history of cardiac surgery and left phrenic nerve injury showing paradoxical motion of the left hemidiaphragm (elevation during inspiration and depression during expiration). Normal motion of the right hemidiaphragm.

Subphrenic Abscess

These are often associated with recent surgery or sepsis. A subphrenic abscess is more common on the right than the left side. Ultrasound and CT are the investigations of choice with percutaneous drainage if appropriate.

Plain film signs of a subphrenic abscess include:

- Ipsilateral basal atelectasis and pleural effusion
- Elevated hemidiaphragm with paradoxical or decreased movement
- Abnormal gas shadow beneath the diaphragm due to infection with gas-forming organisms (Fig. 14.38); horizontal beam films improve visualization of the abscess cavity
- Depression of the liver edge or gastric fundus

Tumors of the Diaphragm

Tumors of the diaphragm are rare. Benign lesions include lipomas, neurofibromas, fibromas, and cysts. Sarcomas commonly present with a pleural effusion. Diaphragm tumors may appear as smooth or lobulated masses and need to be differentiated from lung and liver masses, hernias, and diaphragm humps. CT is the most helpful investigation.

Hernias of the Diaphragm

The classic appearance of a hiatus hernia, with a fluid level superimposed on the cardiac shadow on the PA film, is well known (Fig. 14.39). A *Bochdalek hernia* (Fig. 14.40) arises posterolaterally through the pleuroperitoneal canal and is usually congenital, presenting at birth as respiratory distress. Ninety percent are left sided. The hernia may contain omentum, fat, spleen, kidney, and bowel, in which case a gas shadow is seen within the mass. The ipsilateral lung is invariably hypoplastic with deviation of the mediastinum away from the side of the hernia. In the neonate, this condition needs to be distinguished from cystic adenomatoid malformation of the lung.

BOX 14.1 Causes of Elevation of the Diaphragm

Bilateral

Reduced pulmonary compliance, e.g., fibrosing alveolitis, lymphangitis, carcinomatosis

Technical
- Supine film, expiratory film
- Postoperative pain

Subdiaphragmatic
- Ascites, obesity
- Abdominal mass, pregnancy
- Bowel distension

Unilateral

Paralysis
- Surgery and trauma
- Idiopathic
- Radiotherapy
- Neoplastic
- Diabetes mellitus
- Infections, TB glands, herpes zoster

Congenital
- Eventration and humps

Pulmonary
- Pulmonary and lobar collapse
- Pulmonary hypoplasia
- Pneumonectomy
- Pulmonary embolism
- Basal pneumonia

Pleural
- Thickening
- Pleurisy
- Subpulmonary effusion

Bony
- Scoliosis
- Rib fractures

Subdiaphragmatic
- Gas-distended viscus
- Subphrenic abscess
- Pancreatitis
- Abdominal mass
- Hepatomegaly
- Splenomegaly

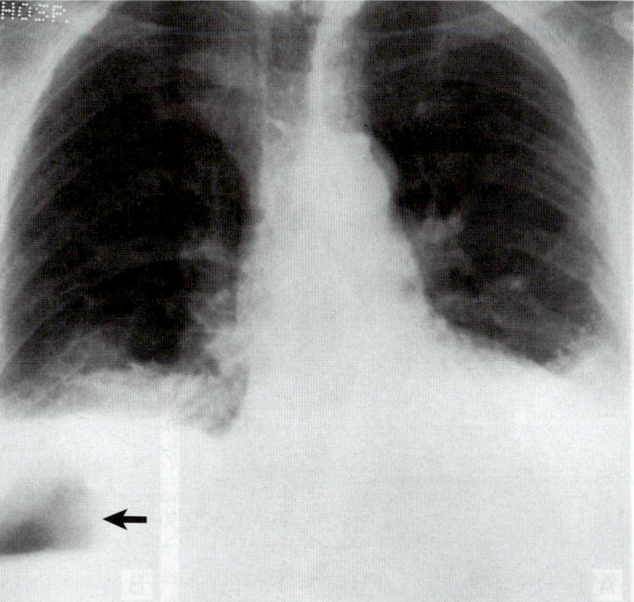

Figure 14.38 Right subphrenic abscess following cholecystectomy. A large gas shadow with an air–fluid level is seen below the right hemidiaphragm (*arrow*). There are bilateral effusions with patchy shadowing at the right base.

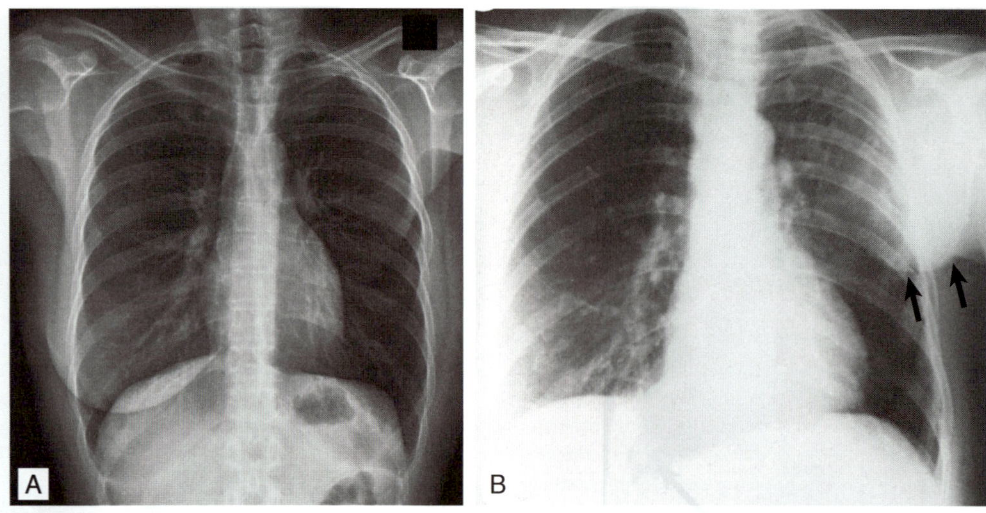

Figure 14.50 Left mastectomy in two different patients. (A) Left breast shadow is absent and the left lung is hypertransradiant. (B) Left mastectomy. Note the abnormal left axillary fold passing cranially (*arrows*). The left lung is hypertransradiant at its base. Note radiation necrosis of the upper ribs and soft-tissue calcification.

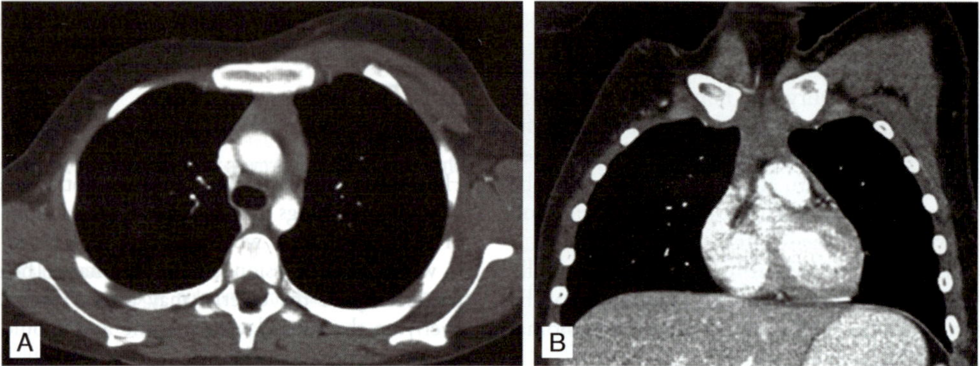

Figure 14.51 Poland syndrome. Axial (A) and coronal (B) CT images of this 11-year-old male showing absence of right pectoralis major muscle.

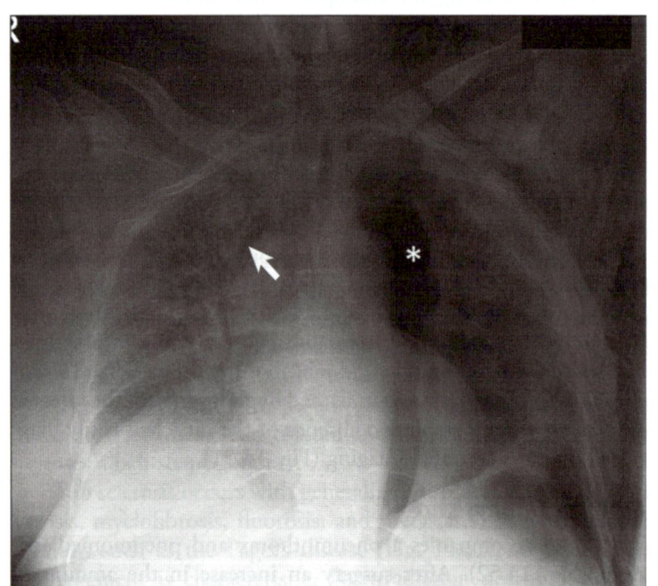

Figure 14.52 Surgical emphysema in a patient of COVID-19 infection. Note the presence of left side pneumothorax (*asterisk*) and pneumomediastinum (*arrow*).

Suggested Readings

- C Charalampos, Y Andrianna, L George, et al., Pleura space anatomy, J Thorac Dis 7(Suppl 1), (2015) S27–S32. doi:10.3978/j.issn.2072-1439.2015.01.48.
- DM Hansell, DA Lynch, HP McAdams, AA Bankier, Imaging of Diseases of the Chest, fifth ed., Mosby, 2009.
- LR Goodman, Felson's Principles of Chest Roentgenology, A Programmed Text, Elsevier, fifth edition, 2020.
- AN Leung, NL Müller, RR Miller, CT in differential diagnosis of diffuse pleural disease, Am J Roentgenol 154 (1990) 487–492.

15

Pulmonary Infections

NEERAJ KAUR, PRASHANT NAGPAL, SACHIN S. SABOO

Introduction

Inflammatory disease of the lung may be referred to as either pneumonia or pneumonitis. Although these terms are interchangeable, *pneumonia* usually implies an infection by pathogenic organisms resulting in consolidation of lung, whereas *pneumonitis* tends to refer to those inflammatory processes that primarily involve the alveolar wall, for example, fibrosing alveolitis in the United Kingdom or usual interstitial pneumonia in the United States. Typically, pneumonia is characterized by a newly recognized lung infiltrate on chest imaging together with fever, cough, sputum production, shortness of breath, physical findings of consolidation, and leukocytosis [1].

Role of Radiological Techniques in Pulmonary Infection

Radiograph

Chest radiograph (CXR) is the initial screening technique for any patient presenting with chest complaints. Standard 2 view radiographs include frontal and lateral radiographs. CXR define the extent of pneumonia, laterality of the infection, detect complications such as pleural effusion, pneumothorax, empyema, lung abscess, and identify alternative diagnosis such as underlying malignancy. Common radiographic features of pulmonary infection include consolidative opacities, ground-glass opacity (GGO) or reticulonodular opacity. Less commonly seen radiographic findings include lymphadenopathy (hilar or mediastinal), pleural effusion, cavitation, or pneumatoceles [2]. CXR are sufficiently accurate to diagnose community-acquired pneumonia (CAP) in most immunocompetent patients; however, accuracy is diminished in patients with chronic obstructive pulmonary disease, atelectasis, or congestive heart failure. The pace of radiographic improvement is related to patient age as well as initial pneumonia extent and it often lacks the clinical improvement. The accuracy of CXR for the detection of hospital-acquired pneumonia (HAP) and ventilator-acquired pneumonia (VAP) is less than that for CAP, because of confounding opacities caused by atelectasis and pleural effusions [3–6].

Computed Tomography

Three major computed tomography (CT) techniques are used for the imaging of the chest: spiral CT, high-resolution CT (HRCT), and CT angiography (CTA).

CT is the imaging technique of choice for assessing patients with suspected pulmonary infections [7] and volumetric thin-section spiral CT with thin detectors (0.5–0.625 mm) has become the routine in many institutions in evaluation of patients with clinical suspicion of infection and normal or nonspecific radiographic appearance [8].

HRCT is typically used for the assessment of interstitial lung diseases and is useful in the detection of subtle pulmonary infectious abnormalities. CT leads to early detection of the pulmonary infections compared with CXR by a lead time of at least 5 days and helps in differential diagnosis. CT can be helpful in differentiating atelectasis or cardiogenic pulmonary edema from pneumonia and detecting radiographically occult infectious bronchiolitis [4]. CT plays a major role in the identification of complications such as cavitation, abscess, empyema, chest wall, and other thoracic and upper abdominal organ extension of the infection.

CTA chest helps to delineate the vascular structures and is needed for the evaluation of the pulmonary and bronchial vasculature in the pulmonary infections. This is particularly useful for the assessment of the bronchial arteries before embolization in a patient presenting with clinical symptoms of hemoptysis.

Nuclear medicine imaging: Nuclear medicine imaging is used sometimes for the pulmonary infections such as pneumocystis jirovecii pneumonia (PJP) in the acquired immunodeficiency syndrome (AIDS) patients. The combination of a positive thallium-201 scan and a negative gallium-67 scan can be specific for the diagnosis of Kaposi sarcoma [9].

Pneumonias can be classified based on the clinical presentation, imaging morphological appearance, and etiology.

Clinical Classification

Community-Acquired Pneumonia

CAP indicates acute lung infection in patients who do not satisfy the criteria for HAP or healthcare-associated pneumonia (HCAP), and it is associated with at least some symptoms of acute lung infection, along with the presence of an acute lung opacity on a chest imaging (Fig. 15.1) [10–12]. Pulmonary opacities are radiographically seen within 12 hours of the onset of symptoms.

The common pathogens are *Streptococcus pneumonia*, *Haemophilus influenzae*, *Staphylococcus aureus*, *Moraxella catarrhalis*, *Pseudomonas aeruginosa*, atypical organisms (mycoplasma, viral, chlamydia), *Legionella*, *Klebsiella*, and other gram-negative bacteria. Recently, new pathogens such as avian influenza A viruses (H5N1), coronavirus associated with severe acute respiratory syndrome (SARS), Middle-East respiratory syndrome (MERS), swine flu (H1N1), and COVID-19 are increasingly recognized as a cause for CAP. Despite exhaustive testing, no organism is found in about 30–65% of cases. *CAP is the most common type of pneumonia, whereas the VAP is the least common* [1,12,13]. Disease severity in CAP is used to indicate prognosis and to guide management and the most commonly used scores for such assessment are pneumonia severity index, the CURB-65, the SMART-COP score, the major and minor criteria recommended by the American Thoracic Society/Infectious Disease

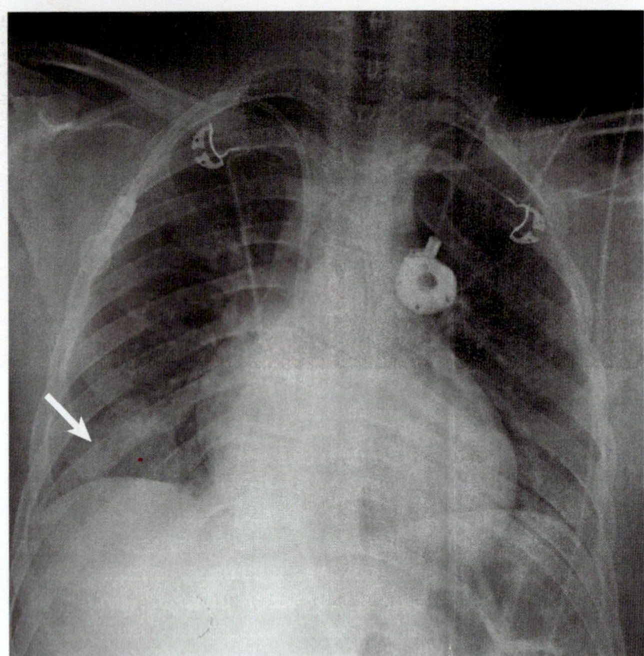

Figure 15.1 Community-acquired streptococcal pneumonia-related acute chest syndrome in sickle cell disease with worsened anemia and acute chest syndrome (ACS). There is a right lower lobe round consolidative opacity (*arrow*) suggestive of a round pneumonia. There is cardiomegaly due to hyperdynamic circulation.

Society of America and quick Sepsis Organ Failure score. Pleural effusion, multilobar involvement, and empyema are the most frequent pulmonary complications in CAP [14].

Hospital-Acquired Pneumonia

HAP is pneumonia acquired after admission to the hospital, with infection neither present nor in the incubation period at the time of the hospital admission.

Nosocomial or HAP leads the cause of death from hospital-acquired infections. This is seen in intensive care patients and those requiring mechanical ventilation. The most common organisms implicated are *Pseudomonas* and *S. aureus* [10,12,15].

Healthcare-Associated Pneumonia

HCAP is pneumonia related to risk from healthcare-related risk factors of recent hospitalization for 20 or more days in the past 90 days of infection, dialysis, nursing home residents, residents of long-term care facilities, and immunocompromised states. Pathological organisms are similar to the HAP including *Pseudomonas* and *S. aureus*. The use of the term HCAP was discontinued in the latest management guidelines [10,12,16].

Ventilator-Associated Pneumonia

Pneumonia within 2–3 days after recent endotracheal intubation-related ventilation. VAPs are typically caused by *Staphylococcus aureus*, *Pseudomonas aeruginosa*, and *Enterobacteriaceae* [10,12].

Pneumonia in the Immunocompromised Patient

All of the previously mentioned pneumonias can occur in an immunocompromised individual. However, certain infections are specifically seen in the immunocompromised states and thus are referred to as opportunistic infections. *These include fungal infections such as Aspergillus, Nocardia, and viral pathogens such as CMV, HHV 8, and parasitic infection such as pneumocystis jirovecii*, etc. [12,17].

Patterns of Pulmonary Infections

Pulmonary infections can be broadly divided into three types:

- affecting the pulmonary parenchyma called as pneumonia,
- affecting the small airways called as bronchiolitis,
- affecting the center airways called as tracheobronchitis.

Pneumonia further can be characterized into lobar pneumonia, bronchopneumonia, and interstitial pneumonia; however, it should be remembered that differentiation among different patterns is often difficult and unreliable in suggesting a particular pathogen.

Radiographic and CT Imaging of CAP

The radiographic and CT patterns of CAP can be traced to the causative agent. The lower respiratory tract (LRT) infection/pneumonia acquired by way of the airways and confined to the lung parenchyma and airways manifests radiographically and on CT through either of the three patterns:

1. Focal nonsegmental or lobar pneumonia
2. Multifocal bronchopneumonia or lobular pneumonia
3. Focal or diffuse "interstitial" pneumonia [2,18]

Lobar Pneumonia

Lobar pneumonia refers to the consolidation of partial or complete segments of lung or less commonly an entire lobe. This is the most common presentation of the CAPs and is often bacterial in origin. *Common causes of lobar consolidation are Legionella species, Streptococcus pneumoniae* (Fig. 15.2)**,** *Klebsiella pneumonia, and Mycoplasma pneumoniae* [11]. Specific radiological signs include air

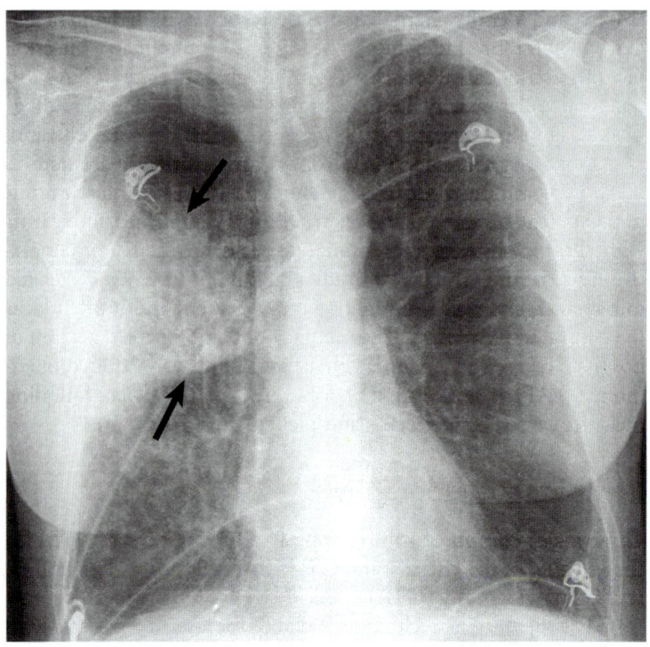

Figure 15.2 *Streptococcus pneumonia*. Frontal radiograph of the chest in a middle-aged man with COPD presenting with cough, fever, chills and underlying reveals right upper lobe pneumonia-related consolidation bound inferiorly by the minor fissure (*arrows*) along with multifocal airspace opacities in the right middle and lower lobe due to bronchopneumonia.

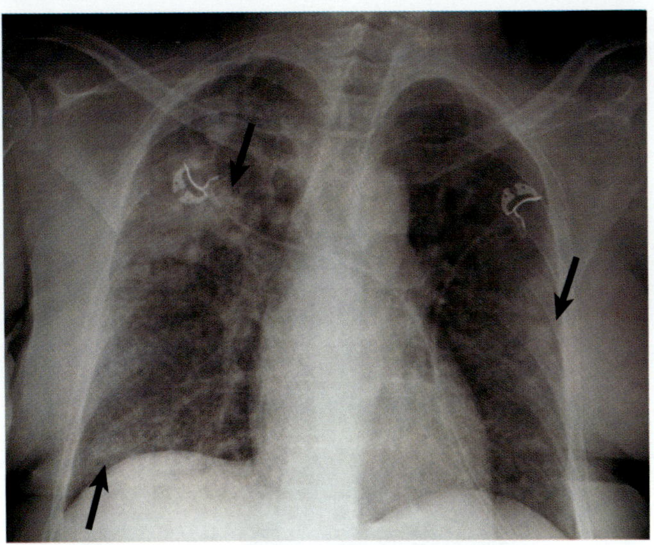

Figure 15.3 Bronchopneumonia. Frontal chest radiograph shows extensive, bilateral, diffusely distributed ill-defined nodular solid and ground-glass opacities (*arrows*) in both lungs representing bronchopneumonia pattern, which in this case was due to bacterial etiology. An area of confluence is seen in the right upper lobe.

bronchogram sign (due to the patency of the larger bronchioles), *bulging fissure sign (typically seen in the Klebsiella pneumonia)*, and no significant volume loss of the involved segment or lobe [2,11].

Bronchopneumonia (Lobular Pneumonia)

Bronchopneumonia is defined by the peribronchiolar inflammation and characterized radiologically as poorly marginated airspace nodules. Unlike lobar consolidation, air bronchograms are absent. On radiographs, these cause a typical patchy distribution of large heterogeneous scattered poorly defined airspace opacities which become more homogeneous with progression of disease (Fig. 15.3). *Most common organisms causing this pattern of disease are S. aureus, H. influenzae, P. aeruginosa, anaerobic bacteria, and fungi.* CT shows poorly defined centrilobular nodules, airspace nodules, linear, branching airspace opacities, and multifocal lobular areas of consolidation [2,11]. Infectious disease-related cellular bronchiolitis and centrilobular nodules can be seen on CT with endobronchial spread of tuberculosis (TB) and nontuberculous mycobacteria (NTMB), viral bronchiolitis, bacterial and fungal pneumonia, and allergic bronchopulmonary aspergillosis (ABPA) [8].

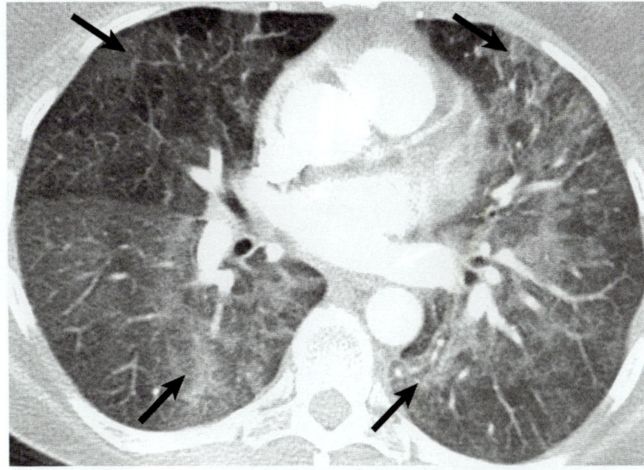

Figure 15.4 Pneumocystis jirovecii pneumonia (PJP). Axial lung window chest CT image in a 45-year-old woman with shortness of breath after chemotherapy for breast malignancy shows diffuse multifocal patchy ground-glass opacities (*arrows*) in both lungs which were confirmed to be due to PJP on bronchoalveolar lavage (BAL).

Interstitial Pneumonia/Atypical Pneumonia

Interstitial pneumonia is secondary to the infection of the peribronchial tissue and interstitial tissues and manifests radiologically as heterogeneous opacities, best described as extensive peribronchial thickening, reticular, or reticulonodular opacities distributed in a focal or diffuse distribution on radiograph. These correlate with bronchial wall thickening and bronchiolitis (centrilobular nodules) appearance on CT. These can be associated with patchy subsegmental or plate-like atelectasis. It is commonly caused by viral and atypical organisms such as mycoplasma, chlamydia, or PJP (Fig. 15.4) [2,11].

Round Pneumonia

Round pneumonia is seen typically in children, can occur in adults and is believed to be due to the incomplete development of

TABLE 15.1 CT Patterns Caused by Infectious Etiologies and Its Noninfectious Mimics in an Immunocompetent Host

CT Appearance	Pulmonary Infection	Pulmonary Noninfection Cause
Linear and ground-glass opacities	Uncommon (interstitial pneumonia)	Interstitial pulmonary edema, pulmonary hemorrhage, hypersensitivity pneumonitis, organizing pneumonia, alveolar proteinosis, and drug reaction
Centrilobular nodules	Common (bronchopneumonia)	Respiratory bronchiolitis, acute hypersensitivity pneumonitis (HP)
Tree-in-bud nodules	Common (endobronchial spread of infection)	Aspiration, pulmonary artery metastasis (rare)
Random nodules	Uncommon (ex: disseminated fungal infections and miliary TB)	Metastases
Lobular GGO or consolidation	Common	Pulmonary edema, pulmonary hemorrhage, chronic infiltrative lung diseases, drug toxicity
Nonsegmental consolidation	Common	Atelectasis
Segmental consolidation	Common	Pulmonary infarction

Ex, example.

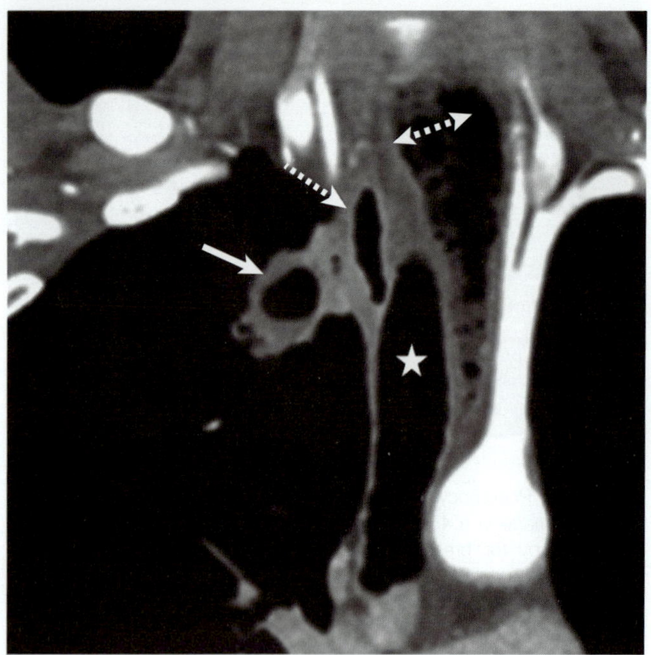

Figure 15.5 Complicated pyogenic lung abscess. Coronal chest soft-tissue window image in a 48-year-old man with history of achalasia cardia presenting with fever and difficulty swallowing shows right upper lobe pyogenic lung abscess with air–fluid level (*bold arrow*) as a sequelae of aspiration. There is adjacent focal mediastinal pleural thickening with air-filled outpouching extending into the adjacent mediastinum (*dotted arrow*), consistent with fistula of the lung abscess with adjacent mediastinum and focal mediastinitis. Note the dilated, food, and air-filled esophagus (*double arrow*) due to achalasia cardia. Star denotes trachea.

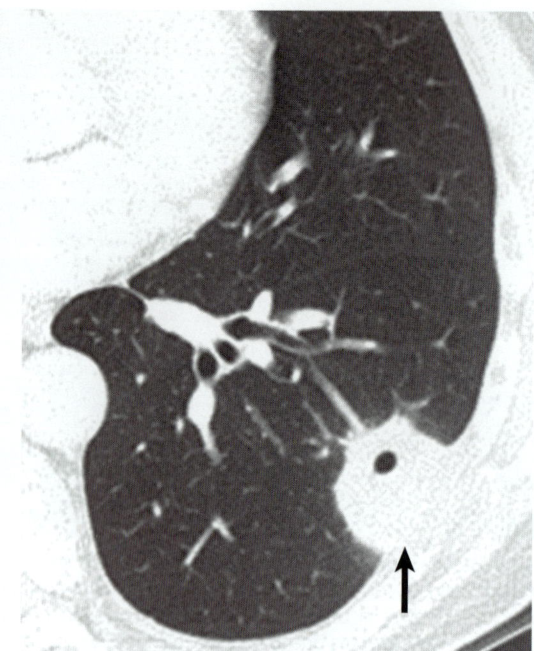

Figure 15.6 Organizing pneumonia due to *Fusobacterium necrophorum* Axial chest CT lung window image in a 58-year-old woman with high fever, weakness, and cough for 2 months shows a peripheral pleural-based cavitary nodular opacity in the left lower lobe (*arrow*).

pores of Kohn. This leads to the confinement of the infection and presents as a rounded mass-like opacity. The common causative organism is *Streptococcus pneumoniae* (Fig. 15.1) [2,11].

Table 15.1 lists differential diagnosis and approach to common CT-based signs of lung infection from other important noninfectious causes.

Some signs common to lung infections and noninfective etiologies are as follows:

- **Halo sign**, typical of early invasive fungal infection in immunosuppressed host, can also be seen with hemorrhagic metastasis in an immunocompetent host
- **Reverse halo sign** indicative of early invasive fungal infection in immunosuppressed host, can also be seen with pulmonary infarct and organizing pneumonia in an immunocompetent host
- **Crescent sign** suggests resolving invasive fungus infection with overall normal underlying lung in immunosuppressed host while this sign is suggestive of aspergilloma colonizing preexisting cavity in an immunocompetent host [3,4]

Lung Necrosis, Lung Abscess, and Cavity

On radiograph, **lung necrosis** appears as focal lucency within an area of consolidation typically later in the course of the disease. On CT, lung necrosis appears as geographic areas of nonenhancing lung parenchyma, some of which progress to discrete lung abscesses. **Lung abscess** is defined as an inflammatory mass within the lung parenchyma, the central part of which has undergone purulent liquefaction, necrosis, and pus-filled cavitation secondary to infection by pyogenic bacteria. CT shows air–fluid levels in three-fourth of cases and adjacent parenchymal consolidation in half of the cases (Fig. 15.5) [11]. A variety of organisms may be responsible, and anaerobic bacteria (most commonly *Fusobacterium nucleatum* [Fig. 15.6] and *Bacteroides* species), *S. aureus*, *P. aeruginosa*, and *K. pneumoniae* are the common causes. Other causes include septic pulmonary emboli, mycobacteria, fungi, parasites, trauma, and rarely, viral infections. Suppuration and necrosis of pulmonary tissue with secondary abscess may also occur due to malignant tumor and infected cysts [3,4].

- On radiograph, an abscess appears as irregular masses with the ill-defined outer aspect. Appearance of an air–fluid level indicates that a communication with the airways has developed [19]. The wall of the abscess may be thick at first, but with further necrosis and coughing up of infected material it becomes thinner
- On CT, lung abscess is typically round or oval, low fluid attenuation lesion (Fig. 15.7), forming acute angles with adjacent pleura, have irregular densely enhancing inner wall contour in acute stage with varying wall thickness (Fig. 15.5). This needs to be differentiated from empyema which typically has smooth inner wall contour with uniform wall thickness (Fig. 15.8). Lung abscess typically cause truncation of adjacent bronchi and pulmonary vessels which may also be seen entering an abscess wall [3,4]. Treatment-related healing of lung abscess result in thinning and more sharply defined wall of an abscess along with reduction in the size and fluid contents of the abscess

Lung cavity is an air-filled space, appearing as a lucency or low-attenuation area, within a nodule, mass, or area of parenchymal consolidation with clearly defined wall >4-mm thick. Cavities can be classified into acute and subacute cavities if they are <12 weeks old (based on previous imaging or duration of symptoms), and chronic cavities if >12 weeks old. Acute and subacute cavities are typically due to acute infection (lung abscess, necrotizing pneumonia, septic emboli, fungal infection, and nocardia), whereas chronic or indolent evolution of cavities suggests chronic infections (TB,

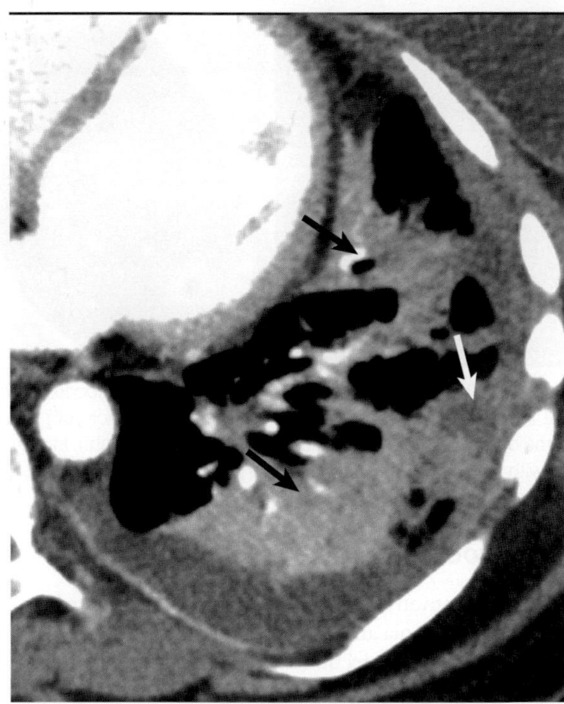

Figure 15.7 Mycoplasma pneumonia complicated by lung abscess and pleural effusion. Axial soft-tissue window in a 26 year-old woman with mycoplasma pneumonia-related partial collapse and consolidation of the left lower lobe and lingula (*black arrows*) complicated by focal left lower lobe lung abscess (*white arrow*). There is secondary left parapneumonic effusion and inflammatory mild linear enhancing left pleural thickening. Multifocal ground-glass opacities were seen in both lungs (not shown).

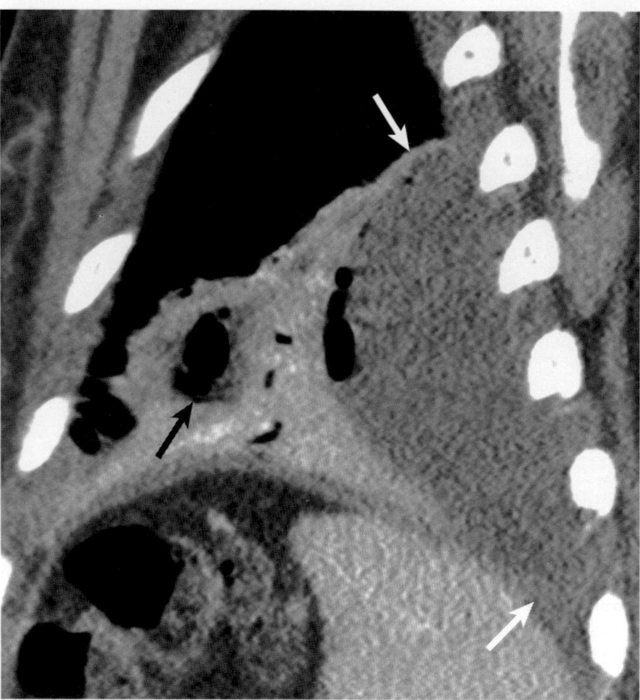

Figure 15.8 *Klebsiella* pneumonia complicated by lung abscess and empyema. Sagittal soft-tissue window chest CT image in a 43-year-old diabetic woman with new onset hemoptysis, cough, left-sided rib pain. Partially enhancing moderate to large left lower empyema (*white arrows*) containing scattered foci of air. There is a small thick-walled lung abscess along the lateral inferior lingular lobe (*black arrow*). Note pneumonia-related heterogeneously enhancing consolidative opacities involving most of the left lower lobe, with associated volume loss.

NTMB, fungal, parasitic, and viral), autoimmune conditions (rheumatoid arthritis, granulomatosis with polyangiitis), or malignancy (primary lung cancer, metastatic lung disease) [20].

Aspiration Pneumonias

Aspiration of particulate or liquid foreign material into the lungs can result in mechanical bronchial obstruction and inflammation. When the cough reflex is suppressed by stupor, alcohol, or drugs; aspiration of food from the stomach during vomiting is likely to occur. The inflammatory response excited by vegetable matter is intense and commonly followed by secondary infection with commensals and anaerobic organisms. Aspiration of infected material from nasal and oral sepsis is a common cause of lung abscess.

Radiologically, this aspiration manifests as atelectasis or suppurative bronchitis and pneumonia (Fig. 15.9). Metallic or inorganic particles typically cause mechanical effects of uncomplicated atelectasis or obstructive emphysema and they may remain undetected for long periods. Aspiration of bland substances such as water, blood, or neutralized gastric contents result in little inflammation manifesting radiologically with consolidation in dependent portions of lung while inflammatory pulmonary edema result from aspiration of acidic gastric contents. Pleural effusion is uncommon with aspiration unless complicated by pneumonia (Fig. 15.9).

Exogenous lipoid pneumonia develops when lipid-containing substances of mineral, animal, or vegetable origin travel to the LRT, most commonly through aspiration of nasally applied or ingested material, or less commonly, through inhalation. The prolonged use of liquid paraffin for constipation is the usual cause and a precipitating factor is chronic esophageal obstruction. The oil is almost inert and the reaction is indolent, granulomatous, and fibrotic; any lung damage is permanent.

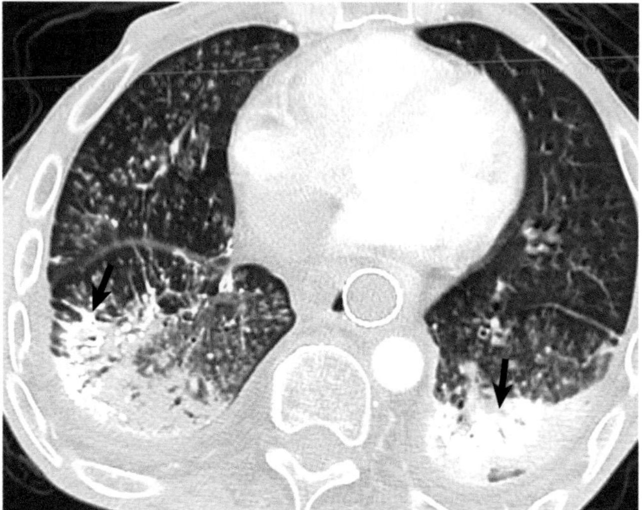

Figure 15.9 Aspiration pneumonia. Diffuse bilateral centrilobular ground-glass nodules and tree-in-bud opacities in the right middle lobe and bilateral lower lobes with peripheral consolidation, due to aspiration pneumonia. The high-density opacities, favored to represent aspirated barium contrast (*arrows*) from recent upper GI study. Note esophageal stent in the mid to lower thoracic esophagus placed for the treatment of broncho-esophageal fistula to the right lower lobe bronchus.

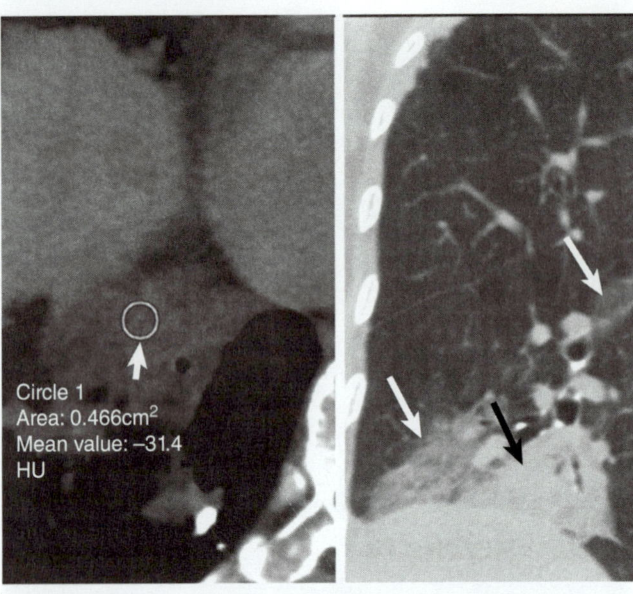

Figure 15.10 Lipoid pneumonia. Axial soft-tissue window (left) and coronal lung window (right) chest CT images in a 67-year-old man with cough, mild fever, and chest discomfort shows mixed consolidative (*black arrow*) and ground-glass (*white arrows*) opacities in the right lower lobe with some areas demonstrating fat component with mean attenuation of –31.4 HU (left image) consistent with lipoid pneumonia due to acute on chronic mineral oil aspiration.

Radiographically, there are dense well-defined tumor-like masses or an extensive bilateral opacity spreading outward from the hilar regions. On CT, bilateral consolidative and GGOs, crazy-paving pattern are the most common radiologic findings, with fatty attenuation of lesions (Fig. 15.10) in less than 50% of patients. Bronchiectasis and fibrosis result with chronicity [21]. Vegetable oils and animal fats such as milk induce a greater inflammatory response and the opacities are ill defined and bronchopneumonic [22].

Influenced by gravity, the lesions of aspiration and inhalation are found predominantly in the posterior parts of the lungs. Small aspirates are common in the elderly from incompetence of the closing mechanism of the larynx. These recurrent aspirations produce coarse peribronchial thickening, small patches of pneumonia, and eventually fibrosis and bronchiectasis.

Bacterial Pneumonias

Streptococcus Pneumoniae

Streptococcus pneumoniae/pneumococcus is the most commonly identified cause of CAP, however, its frequency has declined, and it is now detected in only about 10–15% of inpatient cases in the United States [1]. It is also responsible for most of the pneumonia in all age groups. *Classic radiographic and CT feature of acute pneumococcal pneumonia consists of a homogeneous nonsegmental consolidation that can evolve into lobar pneumonia.* The lobar pattern can mimic *Klebsiella* pneumonia except that volume of the consolidated lung remains normal. It can also present with bronchopneumonia pattern-related patchy, multifocal GGO, and consolidative opacity (Fig. 15.2). Rarely, it can appear as a spherical focal mass-like consolidation/round pneumonia (Fig. 15.1). Pleural effusion is common. Resolution is usually complete and complications like cavitation and abscess formation are unusual if treated immediately [10,11,13,23].

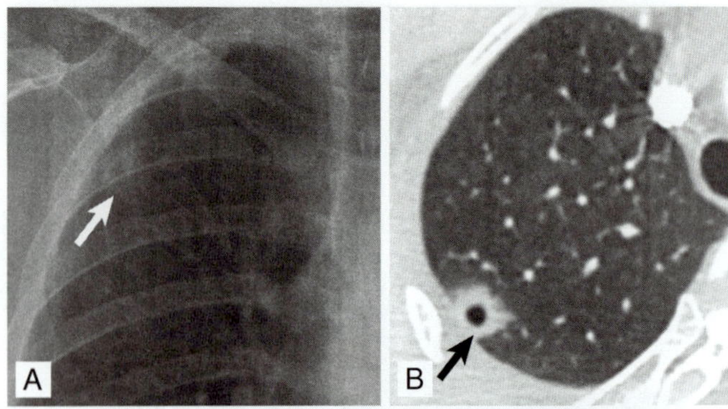

Figure 15.11 Pulmonary methicillin-resistant *Staphylococcus aureus* (MRSA) infection. A composite image with posteroanterior (left) zoomed chest radiograph and axial CT lung window image (right) in a young patient with left thumb abscess after injury, reveals right upper lobe partly cavitary peripheral nodular opacity in the right upper lobe (*arrow*).

Staphylococcus Aureus

S. aureus is a common cause of pneumonia. In debilitated patients, nosocomial pneumonia and may also cause superinfection in influenza. Hematogenous infection of *S. aureus* to the lungs/septic emboli is a common complication of intravenous drug abuse and bacterial tricuspid valve endocarditis which appears as multiple poorly defined rounded solid pulmonary nodules that cavitate (Fig. 15.11) over a period of several days and are usually peripherally located and predominate in the lower lobes. Wedge-shaped areas of peripheral consolidation are common with septic embolization.

Infection may also result from inhalation, typically leading to bronchopneumonia which appears on CT as bilateral patchy often multifocal consolidative opacities, often associated with centrilobular nodules or tree-in-bud opacity.

The "feeding vessel sign," due to hematogenously disseminated of disease to the lung, can be seen with septic emboli (Fig. 15.12). Other features are areas of atelectasis, cavitation, abscess formation pneumatoceles, pleural effusions, empyema, spontaneous

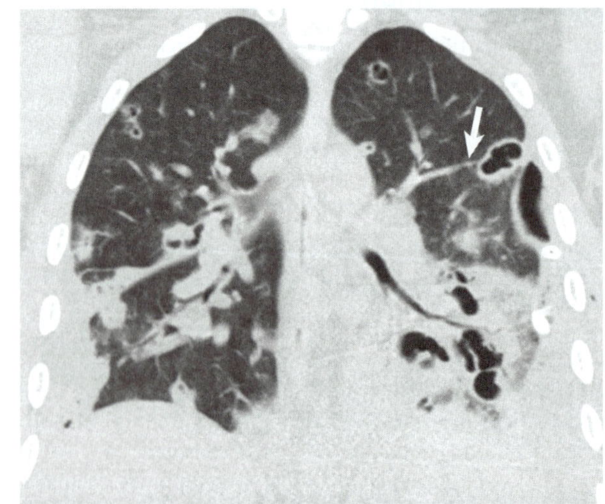

Figure 15.12 Pulmonary methicillin sensitive *Staphylococcus aureus* (MSSA) bacteremia. Coronal CT lung window image in MSSA bacteremia with sepsis associated with catheter line infection presenting with hypoxic respiratory failure shows multifocal pneumonia in the form of solid and cavitary pulmonary nodules in the predominant peripheral and peribronchial distribution, many manifesting the feeding vessel sign (*arrow*) (nodules are often closely associated with pulmonary vasculature) due to septic emboli. Also noted are bilateral loculated pleural effusions.

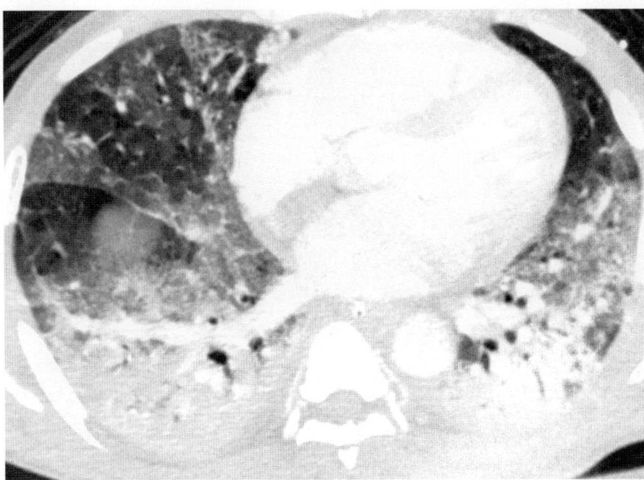

Figure 15.13 Acute interstitial pneumonia (AIP)/diffuse alveolar damage due to MRSA. Axial chest CT lung window image in a 50-year-old man presenting with shortness of breath shows multifocal patchy and geographic interstitial and airspace ground-glass and consolidative opacities with crazy-paving appearance in both lungs and gradient in the bilateral lower lobes from anterior to posterior portion. The anterior portions revealing ground-glass changes and posterior portion revealing consolidation consistent with acute interstitial pneumonia which in this case was related to MRSA.

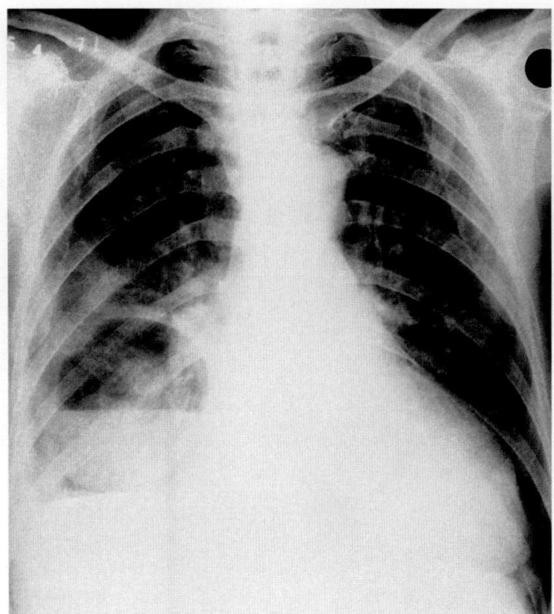

Figure 15.14 *Klebsiella* pneumonia. There is a large cavity in the right lower lobe after cavitation of pneumonic consolidation. An aortic valve replacement is present.

pneumothorax, and progression to diffuse alveolar damage (Fig. 15.13) [10,11,13,23].

Klebsiella Pneumonia

K. pneumoniae is the cause and usually occurs in elderly debilitated men. It usually causes lobar consolidation with air bronchograms, causing the volume of the affected lobe to be maintained or increased (bulging fissure sign). This frequently involves upper lobe and more often on right side. CT shows GGOs, consolidation, and intralobular reticular opacity and sharp margins of the advancing border of the pneumonic opacities. A bronchopneumonic pattern may occur. Complications of cavitation (Fig. 15.14), pulmonary abscess, pleural effusion, and empyema (Fig. 15.8) are common. Healing with fibrosis can mimic chronic fibrocavitory form of TB [11,23].

Legionnaire's Disease

Since first identified in early 1977, *Legionella pneumophila* bacteria are recognized as a common cause of CAP. The organism is ubiquitous in water, multiplying in water coolers, air conditioners and showers, and infection takes place from inhalation of an aerosol mist. It is prone to attack smokers, the debilitated and older men.

Radiographically, it presents as spreading peripheral focal consolidation like *S. pneumoniae* pneumonia, and although it may be confined to one lobe (lobar pneumonia) initially, it soon extends to several lobes (Fig. 15.15), to the opposite lung and in severe cases results in respiratory failure with diffuse alveolar damage. Cavitation occurs frequently in immunocompromised patients. Small pleural effusions are common; abscess and pneumatocele formation are rare [24]. *A characteristic feature is the slow radiographic resolution over several weeks compared with other bacterial pneumonias*, but this is usually complete [25].

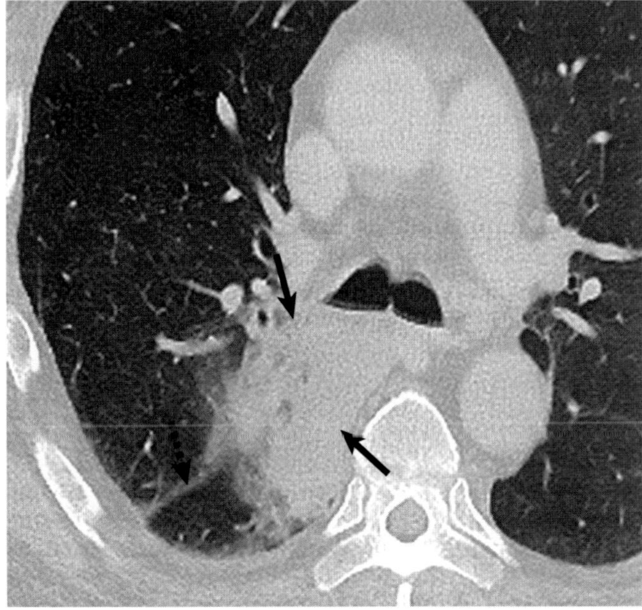

Figure 15.15 *Legionella* pneumonia. Axial chest CT image in a 60-year-old man with alcohol abuse with high-grade fever and chills shows right lower lobe consolidation with mild surrounding ground-glass opacities (*arrows*) crossing the fissure (*dotted arrow*) extending into the posterior segment of the right upper lobe suggesting aggressive infection and was proved to be *Legionella* pneumonia on positive urine test.

Haemophilus Influenzae

H. influenzae pneumonia is predisposed by immunodeficiency and debilitated status. CXR and CT usually show nonspecific bronchopneumonic pattern of multifocal, multilobar patchy with segmental, lobar or bilateral consolidation. Centrilobular nodules or tree-in-bud nodules can be seen on CT. Pleural effusions is common; however, cavitation and empyema are uncommon [26,27].

Gram-Negative Bacilli Pneumonia

The main causes of gram-negative pneumonias are *Klebsiella pneumoniae*, *Enterobacter* sp., *Serratiamarcescens*, *Escherichia coli*,

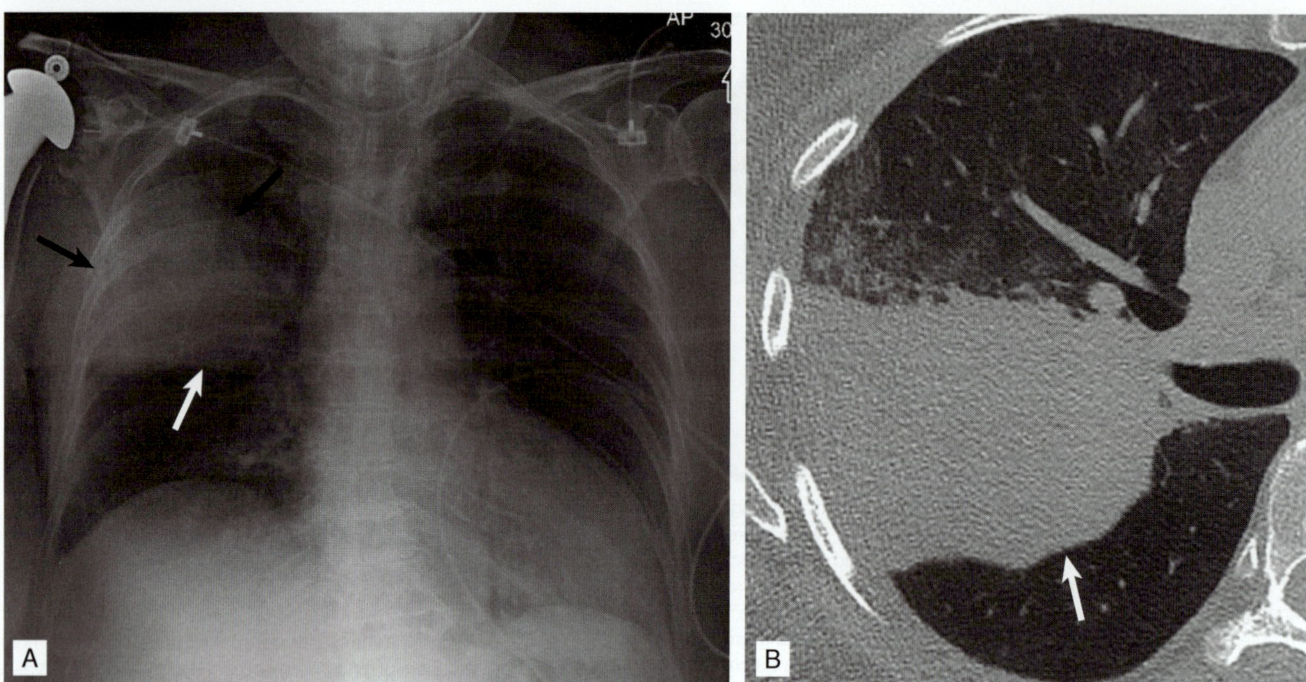

Figure 15.16 Pseudomonal pneumonia. Frontal radiograph of the chest and axial chest CT image in a middle-aged man on immunomodulator therapy for Crohn's disease and DM reveals large right upper lobe consolidation (*black arrows*) with bulging right transverse fissure (*white arrow*) on x-ray and major fissure on CT.

Proteus sp., and *Pseudomonas aeruginosa*. Patients typically have underlying debilitating chronic medical or pulmonary condition and pneumonia normally results from inhalation but may also be hematogenous in origin. They have lower lobes predominance of affection. The radiographic and CT appearances are bronchopneumonia pattern with cavitation, pleural effusions, and empyema formation like that seen with *S. aureus* infections in adults. *Escherichia coli* accounts for 4% of cases of CAP and 5–20% of cases of HAP or HCAP. *Pseudomonas aeruginosa* is the most common cause of nosocomial pulmonary infection that causes confluent (Fig. 15.16) and extensive bronchopneumonia with frequent cavitation.

Melioidosis

Melioidosis, a disease of tropical countries of the East, is caused by *Pseudomonas pseudomallei*. It may manifest years after the patient has left an endemic area. It can present with a septicemic disseminate infection with necrotizing lesions, a chronic apical pneumonia which breaks down to form a thin-walled cavity [28], lobulated heterogeneously enhancing anterior mediastinal lymph nodal mass [29] or as lung consolidative mass with pleural and pericardial effusion, and mediastinal lymph node thus can mimic lung cancer [30].

Tularemia

Infection is usually acquired by contact with infected animals with aerobic gram-negative bacillus *Francisella tularensis* and occurs through inhalation, intradermal injection, or oral ingestion. A nonspecific airspace multifocal unilateral or bilateral consolidative opacity due to pneumonia is most common finding in patients with tularemia and occurs typically in rural settings. Pleural effusion and hilar or mediastinal lymphadenopathy due to granulomatous lymphadenitis are seen in 50–90% of affected patients [31].

Atypical Pneumonia

The term "atypical pneumonia" is imprecise and arguably outdated; however, the concept of atypical pathogens is still accepted. Atypical pneumonia term was originally characterized by initial mild symptoms and scant sputum production, with progression to an illness of varying severity, extrapulmonary systemic involvement, and lack of response to penicillin therapy. "Atypical" denotes acute febrile illness characterized by acute inflammatory changes centered within the alveolar walls and interstitium and the lack of the alveolar exudate evident in most pneumonic infections [32].

The lack of typical findings of lobar consolidation on CXRs and failure to isolate a pathogen using routine bacteriologic testing methods are also common features of this group of microorganisms. Infections with *Mycoplasma pneumoniae*, *C. pneumoniae*, *Legionella pneumoniae* are the most common nonzoonotic causes, while the most common zoonotic bacteria that cause atypical pneumonias are *Chlamydia psittaci* (psittacosis), *F. tularensis*, and *Coxiella burnetti* (Q fever). Influenza virus types A and B, parainfluenza virus, respiratory syncytial virus (RSV), adenovirus, and human metapneumovirus are among the most common viruses causing atypical pneumonia and responsible for CAP in humans [33]. *The term atypical pneumonia in the radiologic reports should be carefully used by providing mention in the report if the radiographic pattern observed is commonly seen with certain infections or if it raises the possibility of alternative diagnosis* [33].

Mycoplasma Pneumoniae

This is the only member of the mycoplasma group that is commonly pathogenic in man. Although classed as bacteria these organisms are unlike other common bacterial species, being smaller and lacking rigid cell walls containing peptidoglycan. *Patients with M. pneumoniae can develop neurologic syndromes, venous thrombosis, pericarditis, and myocarditis.*

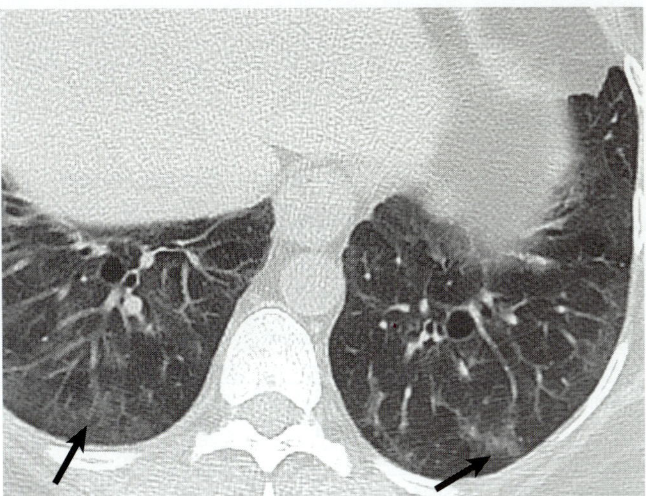

Figure 15.17 Mycoplasma pulmonary infection. Axial lung window chest CT image in a 56-year-old man with antisynthetase syndrome shows multifocal patchy diffuse ground-glass opacities and streaky linear opacities related to atypical mycoplasma pulmonary infection along with few lung cysts.

The earliest chest radiographic signs are interstitial opacities in the form off-line reticular or nodular shadows followed by the consolidation pattern, which may be segmental or lobar. CT typically shows consolidation in patchy, segmental, and lobular pattern, centrilobular nodules, or GGOs (Fig. 15.17). Cavitation, lymph node enlargement and pleural effusion are uncommon (Fig. 15.7). Mosaic attenuation and air trapping may be seen due to small airway obstruction. Adults may be more likely to present with this bronchiolitis–bronchopneumonia pattern than children in whom segmental and lobar pneumonia may be more common similar to that of bacterial lobar pneumonia [34].

Viral Pneumonias

Viral pneumonia is traditionally uncommon in adults, unless the patient is immunocompromised. Most pneumonia that complicate viral infections in adults are due to bacterial superinfection. However, viral pneumonias are not rare in infants and children. CT is currently the imaging technique of choice for the evaluation of pulmonary viral infections even though its features are usually nonspecific [8]. *Clinically, viral pneumonia in adults can be divided into atypical pneumonia in an immunocompetent hosts and viral pneumonia in immunocompromised hosts.* Influenza virus types A and B account for most viral pneumonias in immunocompetent adults [35]. Viral pneumonia usually commences in distal bronchi and bronchioles as an interstitial process with destruction of the epithelium, edema, and lymphocytic infiltration. There may also be focal inflammation of the terminal bronchioles and alveoli and progression to hemorrhagic pulmonary edema. The radiographic appearances of a viral pneumonia are very varied, but often include peribronchial opacities, reticulonodular opacities, and patchy or extensive consolidation.

CT appearances reflect various histopathologic features seen in viral pneumonia such as diffuse alveolar damage, intra-alveolar hemorrhage, and interstitial intrapulmonary or airway inflammation. CT appearances of various viral pneumonias have been summarized in Table 15.2 [36].

Influenza Virus

Influenza outbreaks occur typically in winters due to influenza type A virus.

- Pneumonia as a complication of influenza is normally due to secondary bacterial infection, often *Staphylococcus aureus*, *Streptococcus pneumoniae*, or *Haemophilus* in which case changing pattern of radiographic findings and lobar consolidation are helpful in the diagnosis of bacterial-superimposed infection
- Adolescents, elderly, and debilitated patients may develop a primary viral influenza pneumonia-related tracheobronchitis and bronchopneumonia which appear on radiograph as lower lobe predominant bilateral reticulonodular opacities and/or multifocal consolidations
- Ill-defined patchy or nodular consolidations on radiograph and CT that become confluent are also seen secondary to diffuse alveolar damage or superinfection that typically subside in 3 weeks
- Ill-defined small nodules and patchy GGOs due to influenza are reported in patients with underlying hematological malignancies [37]

Patients can progress to hemorrhagic pneumonia, acute respiratory distress syndrome, or organizing pneumonia. If the patient survives, extensive pulmonary fibrosis may develop. The swine-origin influenza A (H1N1) virus emerged in Mexico in April 2009 and become global pandemic with the dominant CT findings being GGOs, patchy consolidation, or a mixed pattern of GGOs and areas of consolidation, frequently in bilateral, peripheral subpleural, and peribronchovascular distribution [38]. Avian flu is caused by H5N1 subtype of influenza type A through contacts with birds and can show additional findings of centrilobular nodules, pneumatocele, pseudocavitation, and lymphadenopathy on CT [38,39].

Herpes Varicella Zoster

Varicella pneumonia/chickenpox occurs more often in adults than in children.

- In the acute phase of infection, the CXR and CT may show widespread random distribution multiple ill-defined, confluent nodular opacities up to 1 cm in diameter with halo sign due to multicentric hemorrhage and necrosis centered on airways, and clinically the pneumonia will be concurrent with the typical skin rash
- After recovery a small proportion of these nodules calcify and may produce a characteristic radiographic and CT appearance of randomly distributed 2–3 mm densely calcified nodules (Fig. 15.18) [40]

Disseminated varicella zoster virus infection is seen with underlying immunocompromised status [8].

Measles Giant Cell Pneumonia

Measles virus infections are frequently reported in adults and children and severe cases present with pneumonia, gastroenteritis and encephalitis especially in pregnant females and immunocompromised patients.

Bronchitis and/or bronchiolitis and interstitial pneumonia due to measles manifest radiologically with reticular nodular opacities, interlobular septal thickening, and peribronchial nodular opacities as well as mediastinal and hilar lymphadenopathy and pleural effusion while CT additionally shows centrilobular nodules and GGOs.

Remarkably swift resolution can take place, over the course of a few days however follow-up CT may demonstrate residual fibrosis [41].

EBV Pneumonia

Epstein-Barr virus (EBV) causes intrathoracic lymphadenopathy and splenomegaly as a manifestation of infectious mononucleosis and pneumonia is rare manifestation.

TABLE 15.2 CT Findings in Viral Pneumonia

Etiology of Viral Pneumonia	Pulmonary Ground-Glass Opacities and Consolidation	Pulmonary Nodules, Micronodules, and Tree-In-Bud Opacities	Interlobular Septal Thickening	Bronchial and Bronchiolar Wall Thickening	Miscellaneous Findings	Systemic Findings
Adenovirus	+++	None	None	+++	Sequalae: bronchiectasis, bronchiolitis obliterans, and unilateral hyperlucent lung	
Herpes simplex virus	+++	++	None	None	Solid lung nodules with halo sign	Gingivostomatitis, pharyngitis
Varicella	+++	+++	None	None	Solid lung nodules with halo sign, nodule calcification	
CMV (Fig. 15.19)	+++	++	None	None	Solid lung nodules with halo sign	
EBV	+++	+	+	None	Solid lung nodules with halo sign	Infectious mononucleosis Mediastinal lymphadenopathy
Influenza A	+++	+++	None	++	DAD	Avian flu (H5N1): pneumatocele, pleural effusion
Parainfluenza 1–4	+++	+++	None	None		
RSV	+++	+++	None	++	Centrilobular nodules	
HMPV	+++	+++	None	++	Centrilobular nodules	
Measles	+++	+++	++	++	Centrilobular nodules, pleural effusion, lymphadenopathy	Gastroenteritis
Hantavirus (HCPS)	+++	++	+++	None	Pulmonary edema	Shock
Coronavirus (SARS-CoV-2, SARS-CoV-1, MERS-CoV	+++	Rare	+++	Uncommon	Peripheral, multifocal opacities, crazy-paving lung pattern Pleural effusion rare	
HPIV	+	+	None	++		
Mumps	++	None	None	Rare		Parotid gland involved
Rhinovirus (Fig. 15.66)	++	+	None	Uncommon		

DAD, diffuse alveolar damage; *GGO*, ground-glass opacity; *HCPS*, Hantavirus cardiopulmonary syndrome; plus signs indicate the relative frequency of the findings from lowest (+) to highest (+++); *HMPV*, human metapneumovirus; *HSV*, herpes simplex virus; *MERS-CoV*, Middle East respiratory syndrome coronavirus; *RSV*, respiratory syncytial virus; *SARS-CoV*, severe acute respiratory syndrome coronavirus.

The CT manifestations of EBV pneumonia are similar to those of other viral pneumonias producing lobar consolidation, parenchymal diffuse and focal hazy opacities, reticular opacities, and miliary nodules or halo sign [42].

Coronaviridae

SARS-CoV-1, MERS Coronavirus, and SARS-CoV-2

Human coronaviruses can cause upper and LRT infections (pneumonia and bronchiolitis) with a potential to progress to acute respiratory distress syndrome, multiorgan failure, and death. A worldwide outbreak of SARS coronavirus (SARS-CoV-1), occurred in 2002–2003 with origin of the outbreak traced to the Guangdong Province of China and mortality close to 50% for patients older than 60. The animal hosts were the masked palm civet, raccoon dogs, and the Chinese ferret-badger. Another corona virus named MERS coronavirus was first identified in September 2012, in Riyadh, Saudi Arabia in Dromedary camels and bats.

A new coronavirus, novel coronavirus (2019-nCoV)/SARS coronavirus 2 (SARS-CoV-2) responsible for coronavirus disease 2019 (COVID-19) was initially identified in Wuhan, Hubei Province, China, in early December 2019, with the mortality rate of 3 to 5–10%. About 754 million cases and 6.83 million deaths of COVID-19 have been reported worldwide as of February 8th, 2023 (https://covid19.who.int/). Angiotensin-converting enzyme 2 is a potential SARS virus receptor; and immunopathologic mechanism, endothelial damage, and thromboinflammation may be responsible for the progression of disease severity and involvement

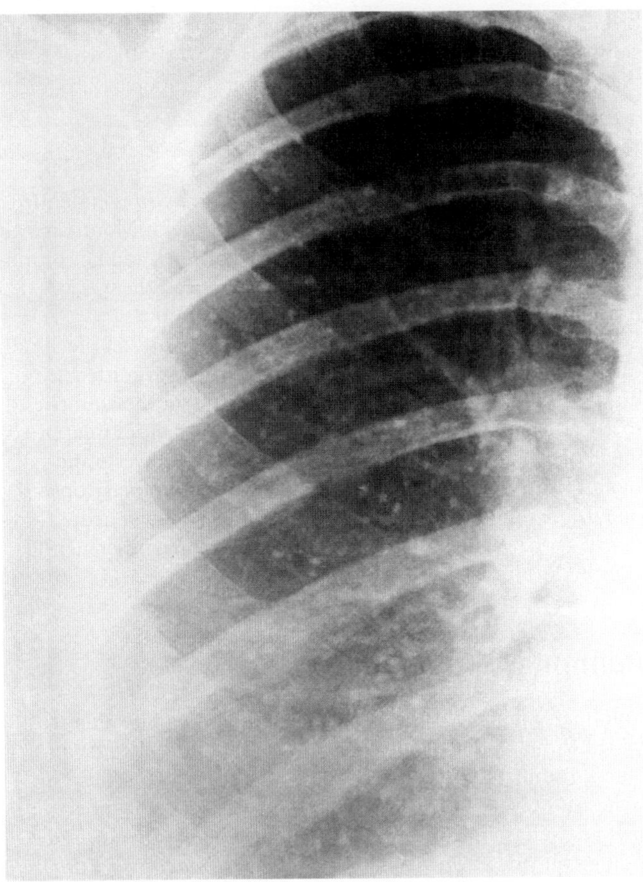

Figure 15.18 Multiple calcified varicella scars.

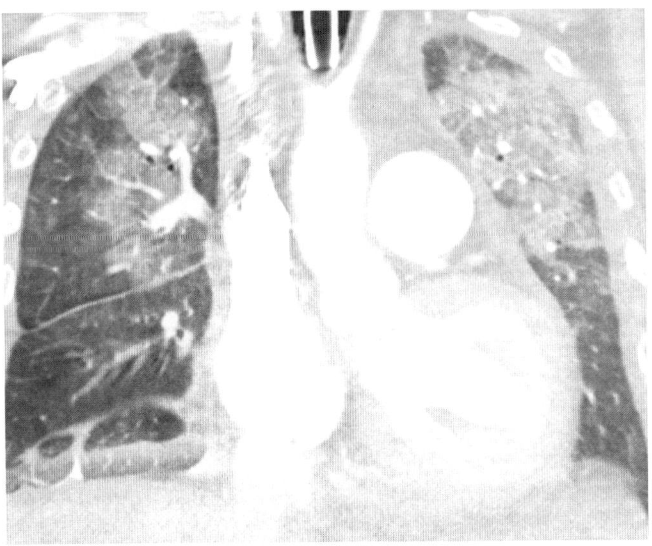

Figure 15.19 Cytomegalovirus (CMV) pulmonary infection. Coronal chest CT lung window image in a young man presenting with acute hypoxemic respiratory failure shows multifocal ground-glass opacities with areas of crazy-paving appearance in both upper lobes proved on PCR to be due to CMV.

of multiple body systems. The main modes of disease transmission were droplet and contact transmission with possible occasional airborne transmission. A diagnosis is made based by the positive reverse transcription-polymerase chain reaction test of an upper respiratory tract specimen [43].

Patient with mild symptoms of COVID-19 does not require chest CT examination. However, after confirming SARS-CoV-2 infection, chest CT may be used in moderate to severe cases to evaluate disease severity, and establishing the next management strategies. CT severity score is a semiquantitative scoring system to quantitatively estimate the pulmonary involvement by COVID-19 on the basis of the area involved. Each of the five lung lobes are visually scored on a scale of 0–5, with 0 indicating no involvement; 1, less than 5% involvement; 2, 5–25% involvement; 3, 26–49% involvement; 4, 50–75% involvement; and 5, more than 75% involvement. The total CT score is the sum of the individual lobar scores and ranges from 0 (no involvement) to 25 (maximum involvement) [44].

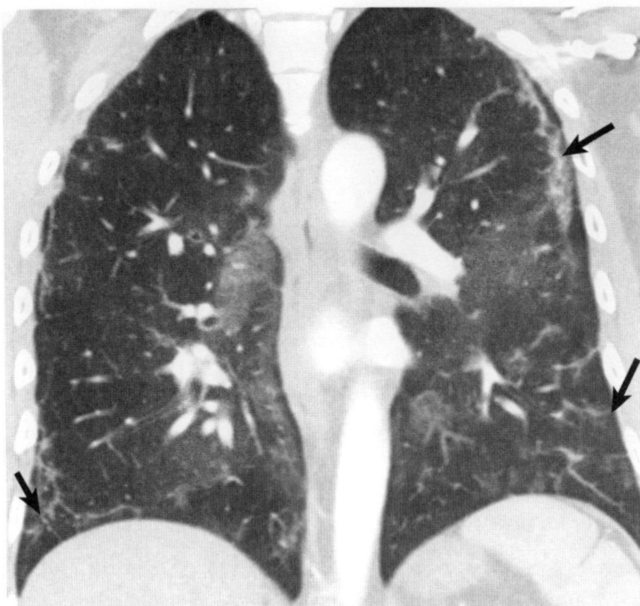

Figure 15.20 SARS-CoV-2/COVID-19 acute pulmonary infection. Coronal CT lung window image shows extensive predominantly peripheral and peri-lobular ground-glass opacities (*arrows*) in both lungs due to SARS-CoV-2.

The initial CXRs may be normal or nonspecific pulmonary opacities with rapid progression to multifocal airspace opacities predominantly in the peripheral lower lung zones.

- Normal chest CT can be seen up to 2 days after onset of flu-like symptoms in up to 50% of patients with COVID-19 infection. CT may show lung abnormalities even with an initially negative reverse transcription-polymerase chain reaction
- CT pulmonary findings caused by SARS-CoV-2 are similar to those findings of other human coronaviruses. *The most common CT finding for SARS-CoV-2 pneumonia is GGO followed by consolidation*
- The most common CT features are bilateral peripheral subpleural multifocal posterior, and diffuse or lower lobe predominant GGOs (Fig. 15.20), consolidation and reticulations related to organizing pneumonia or capillary permeability pulmonary edema-related mechanism of lung injury. The round morphology or a reversed halo or atoll sign of opacities resemble the organizing pneumonia [45]
- A reversed halo sign, halo sign, reticulation, or nodules are rare and usually manifest later in the disease course. Less commonly seen atypical findings are cavitation, isolated lobar, or segmental consolidation without GGOs lymphadenopathy, spontaneous pneumothorax, pneumomediastinum (Fig. 15.21), and pleural effusions. On CT, fine reticular opacity and pulmonary artery enlargement/thick vessel sign within pulmonary opacities and regional mosaic perfusion patterns are also commonly found in COVID-19 pneumonia compared with other viral pneumonia

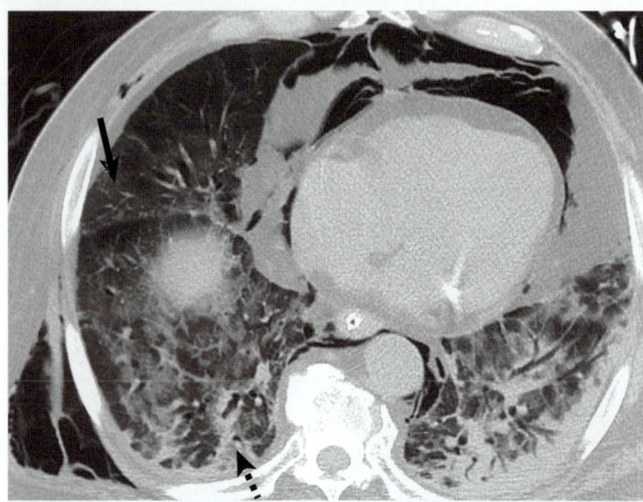

Figure 15.21 SARS-CoV-2/COVID-19 pulmonary infection complicated by pneumomediastinum and subcutaneous emphysema. Axial chest CT lung window image shows diffuse ground-glass opacities (*bold arrow*) in both lungs with bilateral lower lobe peribronchovascular and peripheral consolidative opacities (*dotted arrow*) due to COVID pneumonia with large pneumomediastinum and right subcutaneous emphysema. Note that patients with COVID-19 who require mechanical ventilation are at increased risk of barotrauma compared with ARDS alone.

- Peak pulmonary disease manifests as crazy-paving, new or worsening lung consolidative opacities, and higher rates of multilobar and bilateral involvement (Fig. 15.21)

Resolution of the lung findings may take close to a month or so. Follow-up CT obtained during recovery after 2 weeks from initial symptom onset showed a gradual decrease in consolidation, with residual GGOs [8,36,46]. Interstitial lung fibrosis can remain after the recovery in some of these patients based on the initial severity of disease with lung fibrotic changes in more than one-third of patients who survived COVID-19 pneumonia [47,48]. *Hypercoagulable state in COVID-19 disease is multifactorial in nature and result in both venous and arterial thromboembolism and result in deep venous thrombosis, PE, limb ischemia, stroke, and myocardial infarction* [43].

Chlamydial and Rickettsial Pneumonias

Psittacosis/Ornithosis

Psittacosis is a systemic disease that can cause an atypical pneumonia. This infection is due to *Chlamydia psittaci* and usually acquired by contact with sick parrots or pet birds and poultry. The pneumonia usually presents as patchy or lobar consolidation, although nodular shadows may be seen. There is often hilar lymphadenopathy. The radiographic changes may take several weeks to resolve [49].

Q Fever

This rickettsial gram-negative aerobic bacterial pneumonia is usually acquired by contact with farm livestock, cattle, or sheep and is due to *Coxiella burnetii*. The pneumonia presents on CXRs and CT as rounded areas multifocal, peripheral predominant areas of consolidation in both lungs due to interstitial and alveolar inflammation. In the early stages of the disease, CXRs might be normal. Single or multiple irregular nodules with halo sign, consolidation in patchy, segmental, or lobar distribution, necrotizing pneumonia or linear atelectasis are also known imaging findings. Pleural effusion or lymph node enlargement is not known [50]. The radiographic changes may take a month or more to resolve [2,51].

Rocky Mountain Spotted Fever

This tick-borne disease caused by *Rickettsia rickettsii* is endemic to the southern United States as well as the Rocky Mountains. It may cause patchy consolidation, pleural effusions, and be complicated by secondary bacterial pneumonia. Overall there is a 3–4% mortality and has reduced due to antibiotics [52].

Scrub typhus: This rickettsial disease is an acute febrile illness caused by the *Orientia tsugamushi*, which is transmitted by the bites of infected chigger mites and is endemic in the countries of the Asia-Pacific, and causes pulmonary abnormalities in approximately 10% of cases. The radiographic pattern is diverse and takes the form of interstitial, lobar, or widespread pulmonary opacities due to pneumonia and can develop complications of acute respiratory distress syndrome, acute kidney injury, hepatitis, meningo-encephalitis, myocarditis, and shock [53].

Pulmonary Tuberculosis

Pulmonary tuberculosis (PTB) is a common lung infection worldwide, with heterogeneous incidence geographically. The prevalence of tuberculosis has continued to decline in the United States, however, with relatively higher prevalence of tuberculosis in some states and in certain immigrant populations from developing countries from Asia and Africa. ***Mycobacterium tuberculosis*** (MTB) is the most common cause of tuberculosis; less than 5% of cases are caused by atypical mycobacteria.

Normally, infection occurs by inhalation of organisms from open case of the disease. Transmission is by droplet inhalation. Other factors that predispose to PTB are poor nutrition, alcoholism, silicosis, diabetes, pregnancy, old age, malignancy, and immunosuppression, especially by the human immunodeficiency virus (HIV) infection. In general, the occupational risk of hospital personnel is minimal and only a pre-employment CXR is needed.

Reactivation of previous infected foci is a cause in most cases of postprimary infection, and it often appears many years after first infection. Rarely, a primary infection progresses into the postprimary phase, without a latent period of intervention. Radiologically, it can be difficult to differentiate primary from postprimary tuberculosis due to their overlapping manifestations [54].

Primary Pulmonary Tuberculosis

Primary PTB occurs due to a first-time exposure to MTB and is typically seen in infants and children. Its frequency is increasing in adulthood and represents about 23–34% of all adult cases of TB [2,54]. Although CXRs are commonly used in diagnosis, they may be normal in 15% of cases of primary PTB. The four imaging manifestations of primary PTB include:

1. Lymphadenopathy
2. Parenchymal disease
3. Pleural effusion
4. Miliary disease [9]

- Lymphadenopathy is the most common manifestation of PTB in children and can present with or without pneumonia. In adults hilar or mediastinal lymphadenopathy is less common. The most common sites of nodal involvement include right paratracheal and hilar lymph nodes (Figs. 15.22 and 15.23) with CT being more sensitive than CXR. These nodes are often larger

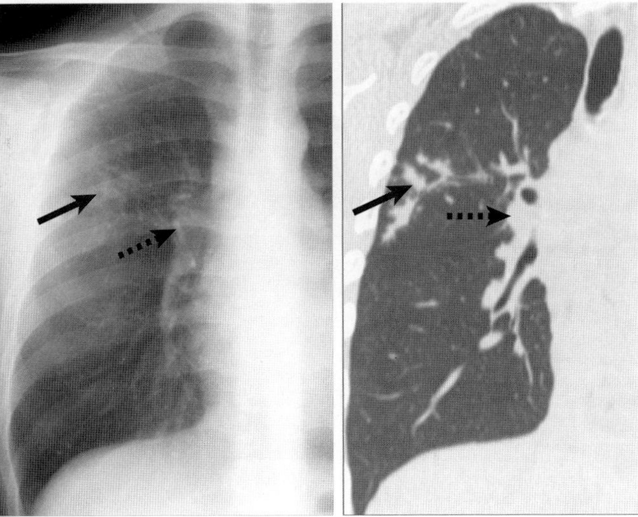

Figure 15.22 Primary pulmonary *Mycobacterium* TB (MTB) infection. A composite image with posteroanterior chest radiograph (left) and coronal CT lung window image (right) in an asymptomatic 12-year-old boy reveals right upper lobe peribronchial nodular opacities and thickening (Ghon's focus) with right hilar lymphadenopathy. The combination of the lung parenchymal infection (Ghon's focus) and lymph node MTB infection has been termed the Ranke complex.

than 2 cm, with characteristic "rim sign" due to low-density center related to caseous necrosis, and peripheral enhancing rim from granulomatous inflammation [55]. After healing the nodes involved can calcify. Lymphadenopathy is usually unilateral but may be bilateral, in which case the differential diagnosis includes sarcoidosis and lymphoma. Adjacent airways may get pressed by enlarged lymph nodes (Fig. 15.23), which cause pulmonary collapse or air trapping with hyperinflation. Caseating nodes may also erode into vessels causing miliary infection and into airways, causing bronchopneumonia [55]. Cavitation is uncommon, occurring mainly with progression of the disease

- Nonspecific focal or lobar dense and homogeneous consolidation as a manifestation of parenchymal involvement involves in any part of the lung, with predominance in the lower and middle lobes typically in adults [54,56,57]. This can be differentiated from bacterial pneumonia based on the presence of lymphadenopathy and the lack of response to conventional antibiotics
- Infection can also appear as a well-defined nodule or nodules. Healing is often complete in approximately two-thirds of cases without any sequelae on the CXR although fibrosis and calcification may occur in the remaining cases. Less than 10% of cases might have residual mass-like opacities due to tuberculomas [54,56,57]. *Ranke complex is commonly the only imaging evidence to suggest previous PTB and consists of the combination of a calcified or noncalcified lung parenchymal scarring (Ghon lesion;* Fig. 15.22) *and calcified hilar and/or paratracheal lymph nodes* [54,56,57]. These lesions may contain dormant bacilli, which might convert into postprimary TB. In rare cases of primary uncontrolled PTB, a progressive disease with multilobar involvement and cavitation may develop [58]
- Pleural effusion can be sole finding in teenagers and young adults [2,54]. The effusion may be large and relatively asymptomatic. The effusion is typically unilateral, and its complications such as empyema formation, fistulization, and rib osteomyelitis are uncommon. Ultrasonography often reveals a complex septated pleural effusion. It resolves with treatment without complication. Residual pleural thickening and calcification can remain [54,56,57]
- Miliary tuberculosis is due to hematogenous spread of infection and can be found in both primary and postprimary PTB. Clinically significant miliary disease affects between 1% and 7% of patients with all forms of tuberculosis. In primary TB, the patient is often a child, and in the postprimary cases the patients are often elderly, debilitated, or immunocompromised
  - At first, the CXR may be normal, and hyperinflation may be the earliest feature
  - Subsequently typical radiographic findings of small, discrete nodules of 1–2 mm in diameter, become apparent, evenly distributed throughout; both lungs are seen (Fig. 15.24).

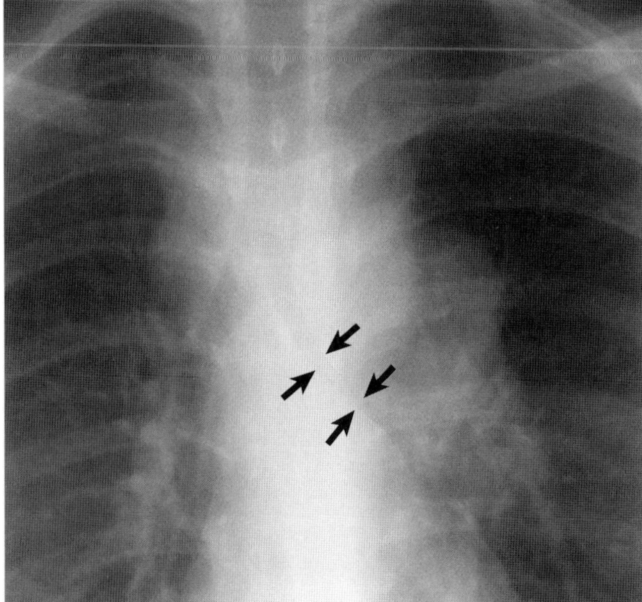

Figure 15.23 Tuberculous lymphadenopathy. There is mediastinal and left hilar lymph node enlargement causing severe narrowing of the left main bronchus (*arrows*).

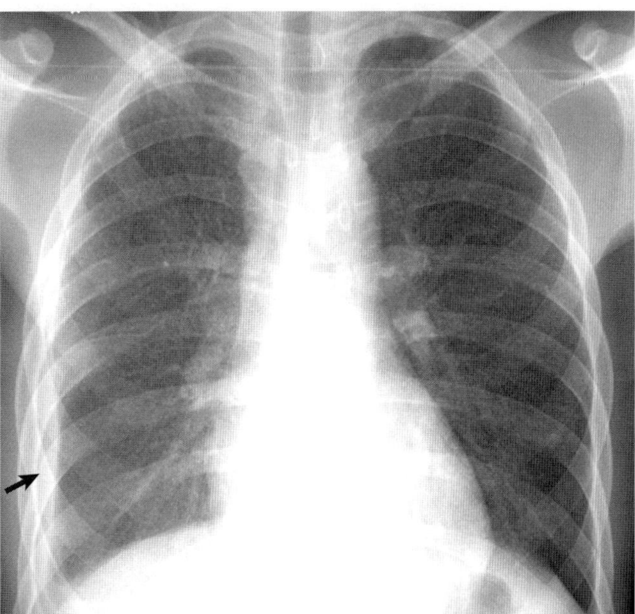

Figure 15.24 Miliary spread of *Mycobacterium tuberculosis* infection. Frontal chest radiograph shows innumerable, bilateral, diffusely distributed small nodules representing miliary hematogenous spread of MTB infection. Note small right pleural effusion (*arrow*).

Contrarily, tree-in-bud nodules are poorly defined and have a patchy distribution

- Chest CT is more sensitive than radiographs and reveals the random distribution of these tiny miliary pulmonary nodules. These nodules may enlarge and coalesce to form focal or diffuse consolidation, but they slowly resolve within 2–6 months with adequate treatment without scarring or calcification [54,57,59]

A tuberculoma is a localized granuloma/localized parenchymal disease that alternately activates and heals and may occur in the setting of primary or postprimary PTB. It is a well-defined, solitary nodule, with a diameter of up to 5 cm. It frequently remains stable for years with calcification being common, but cavitation is rare.

Postprimary Pulmonary Tuberculosis (Postprimary-PTB)/(Reactivation, Secondary, or Adulthood PT)

Postprimary-PTB typically occurs in adolescence and adulthood and most cases are due to reactivation of quiescent lesions, but occasionally due to new TB infection from an exogenous source. Primary tuberculosis is usually self-limiting, whereas postprimary PTB is progressive, with cavitation as its characteristics finding, which can result in hematogenous dissemination and endobronchial spread of TB leading to the CT features of tree-in-bud opacities. Although the imaging manifestations of primary and postprimary PTB might overlap; the differentiating features of postprimary PTB include a predilection for the upper lobes and the presence of cavitation. Lymphadenopathy is often seen in the Indian population. The three radiological manifestations include parenchymal disease, airway involvement, and pleural extension [54,56,57,59].

Parenchymal Changes

- Parenchymal disease manifests early with patchy, ill-defined, and nodular consolidation, particularly in the apical and posterior segments of the upper lobes or superior segment of the lower lobe (Fig. 15.25A). Bilateral disease seen in one-third to two-thirds of cases. Progressive infection is indicated by the extension and coalescence of consolidation areas, and cavity development (Fig. 15.26). The typical pulmonary cavities have thick, irregular walls, which evolve into smooth and thin as a response to treatment. Cavities are typically multiple and occur within regions of consolidation (Fig. 15.26). Tuberculous bronchopneumonia may occur in both primary and postprimary infection, causing patchy, often nodular, areas of consolidation. Cavitary superinfection by other bacteria should be suspected when the air–fluid level is considerable
- After antituberculous treatment healing leads to fibrosis and calcification. Resolution of pulmonary abnormalities is achieved

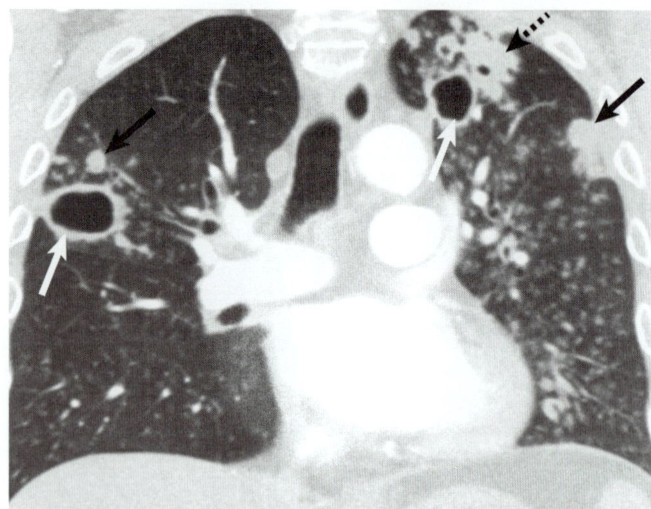

Figure 15.26 Postprimary pulmonary tuberculosis (PTB). Coronal chest CT lung window image in a 50-year-old man presenting with shortness of breath shows innumerable bilateral solid pulmonary nodular opacities (*bold black arrows*), centrilobular nodules and tree-in-bud opacities involving all the lobes of both lungs as well as a few areas of consolidative opacity most prominent in the left upper lobe (*dotted arrows*) and both upper lobe predominant thick-walled pulmonary cavities (*white arrow*) consistent with endobronchial spread of tuberculosis.

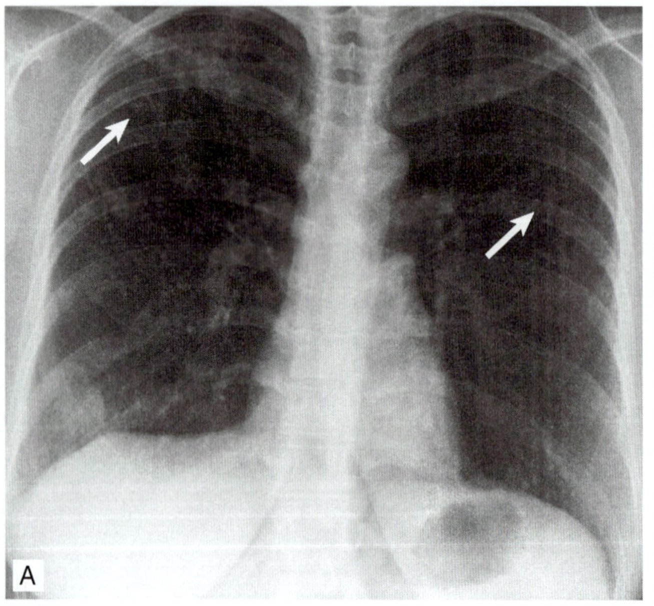

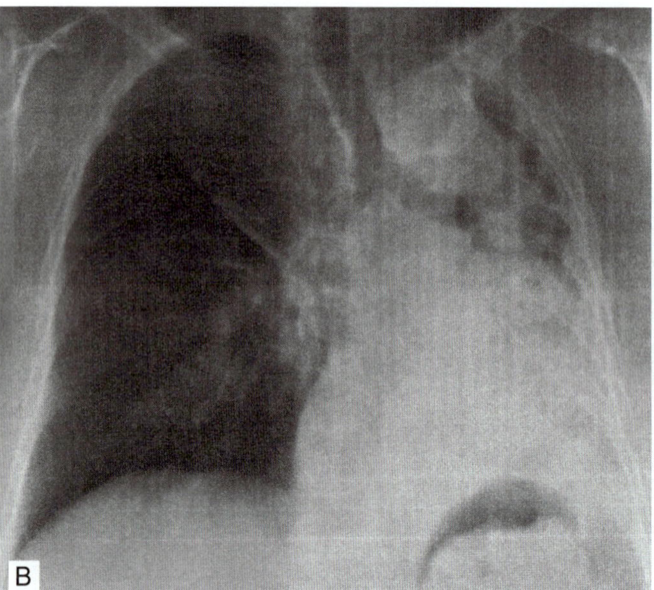

Figure 15.25 (A) Pulmonary tuberculosis (PTB) showing typical nodular opacities in the upper and mid zones of both lungs (*white arrows*) with areas of fibrosis. Another patient (B) with more long-standing disease shows collapse of the left lung, with bronchiectatic cavities within the collapsed lung. There is ipsilateral mediastinal shift and elevation of the left dome inferred by a higher position of the gastric fundus air shadow. Fibrotic changes and volume loss are also seen in the right upper lobe.

after 3 months of treatment in most cases [58]. Fibrosis and volume loss may occur at the same time as consolidation, indicating healing. Fluid levels can sometimes be seen in cavities which can indicate the presence of superinfection. With fibrosis, cavities are often obliterated. Moreover, larger cavities may persist, and areas of bronchiectasis and emphysema can occur. Healed lesions mostly calcify. Often there is evidence of severe volume loss and pleural thickening, trachea being pulled away from the midline, elevation of the hila and distortion of the lung parenchyma (Fig. 15.25B)

- *Aspergillus* and other fungi often colonize the chronic cavities, and mycetomas may develop. *Progression of disease is monitored by periodic radiographs, with the formation of new lesions or the extension of old ones indicating continued activity, whereas the contraction indicating response to treatment* [54,56,57,59]. Once the radiographic signs have stabilized, any subsequent size or density changes should raise concern for complication of reactivation, fungal invasion, or neoplasm. Lymphadenopathy and pneumothorax are seen in only about 5% of patients [57]. Other rare complications include broncholithiasis

Pleural Changes

Pleural effusion complicating primary PTB may be large and relatively asymptomatic, but they are generally small and associated with parenchymal disease in cases of postprimary PTB. The effusions are usually septated. CT shows fluid in the pleural cavity and with enhancement of the pleural layers after contrast administration. Effusion frequently transforms to empyema with thickened enhancing pleura and complex pleural effusion. Healing leads to residual pleural thickening and often calcification. *Complications of tuberculous empyema are pleurocutaneous fistula, bronchopleural fistula, and osteitis of a rib.* Secondary infection is rare. Previous thoracoplasty can also make the radiographic appearance more complicated. Apical tuberculosis is associated with the apical pleural thickening/apical cap due to chronic pleural inflammation on radiographs. CT can reveal it to be mainly due to thickened layer of extrapleural fat. *Pneumothorax* may complicate subpleural cavitary disease [54,56,57,59]. Empyema necessitates is an uncommon late complication of TB empyema in which pleura collection spontaneously erodes into chest wall resulting in abscess in the chest wall (Fig. 15.27) [58].

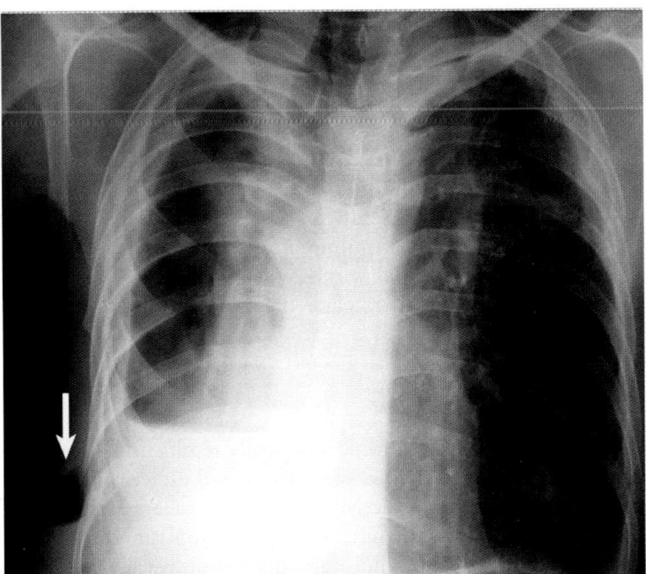

Figure 15.27 Empyema necessitans due to TB. Frontal chest radiograph shows right-sided pyopneumothorax with extension of the air (*arrow*) and fluid (not perceptible on radiograph) beyond the right lower ribs, indicating chest wall extension and is called empyema necessitans. Note sequealae of TB with the left upper lobe reticulonodular fibrotic opacities and variable volume loss bilaterally. (Courtesy: Dr Amy Mumbower.)

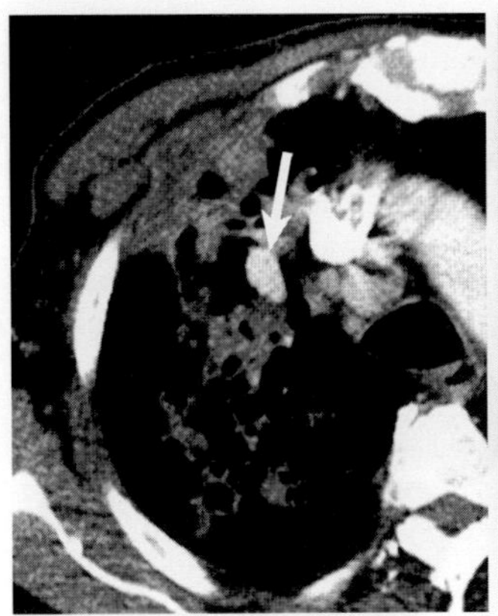

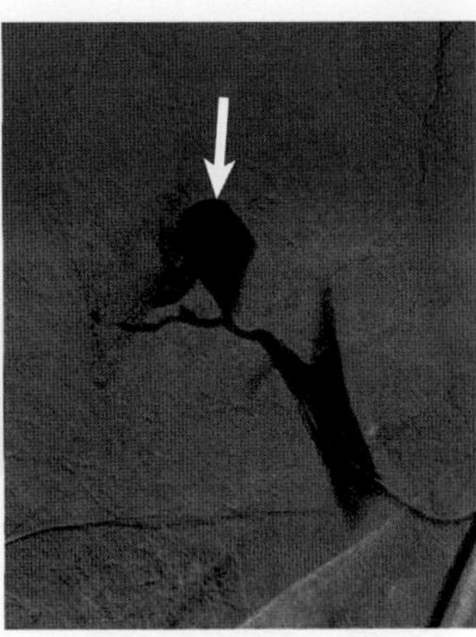

Figure 15.28 Pulmonary tuberculosis (PTB) complicated by ***Rasmussen*** pseudoaneurysm. A composite image with axial contrast-enhanced chest CT soft-tissue window (left) and coronal pulmonary artery catheter image (right) in a young patient reveals pulmonary artery enhancing pseudoaneurysm (*arrows*) along right upper lobe segmental pulmonary artery related to right upper lobe cavitary consolidative opacities due to pulmonary tuberculosis. Note enlarged enhancing mediastinal lymph nodes due to TB. (Courtesy: Dr Amy Mumbower.)

Airway Involvement

Airway involvement could be secondary to lymphadenopathy or endobronchial infection, therefore may complicate both primary and postprimary disease. Central airways compressed by enlarged nodes (Fig. 15.23) may cause pulmonary collapse or hyperinflation related to air trapping, obstructive pneumonia, and mucoid impaction. Bronchial stenosis is seen in up to 40% of patients with active tuberculosis [60] and appears on CT as long segment irregular wall thickening and luminal narrowing, luminal obstruction, and extrinsic compression. Endobronchial infection results in tree-in-bud opacities as well as traction bronchiectasis, particularly of the upper lobes.

A Rasmussen aneurysm (Fig. 15.28) is a rare deadly complication of cavitary tuberculosis caused by granulomatous weakening of a pulmonary arterial wall [58]. Fibrosing mediastinitis is a late sequela of tuberculosis, manifest on CT as localized mediastinal soft-tissue mass with calcification.

Active Versus Inactive PTB

Postprimary TB heals with parenchymal scarring and nodules and CXRs can determine the stability of the lesion, but stable lesions can contain active bacilli. CT features can help to differentiate active from inactive PTB.

Active PTB typically presents with centrilobular nodules, tree-in-bud opacities, thick-walled cavities, consolidation, miliary nodules, pleural effusions, or necrotic lymphadenopathy [54,56]. Inactive PTB can reveal conversion of thick-walled cavities into thin-walled relatively smaller smooth cavities, the development of pulmonary fibrotic opacities, and parenchymal, nodal, or pleural calcifications [54,56]. Active disease on CT must be confirmed by analysis of sputum for the presence of bacilli [58].

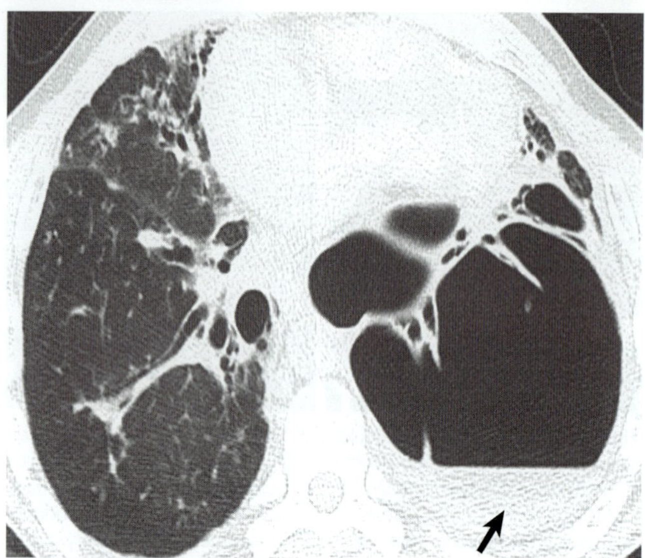

Figure 15.29 Pulmonary nontuberculous *Mycobacterium avium* infection (non-TB-MAI). Axial chest lung window image in a 43-year-old man shows layering fluid/debris in the large septated cyst in the left lower lobe (*arrow*) consistent with Bullaitis. Extensive bronchiectasis, bronchial wall thickening with tree-in-bud opacities and architectural distortion particularly in the right middle lobe, lingula, and both lower lobes due to endobronchial spread of non-TB-MAI.

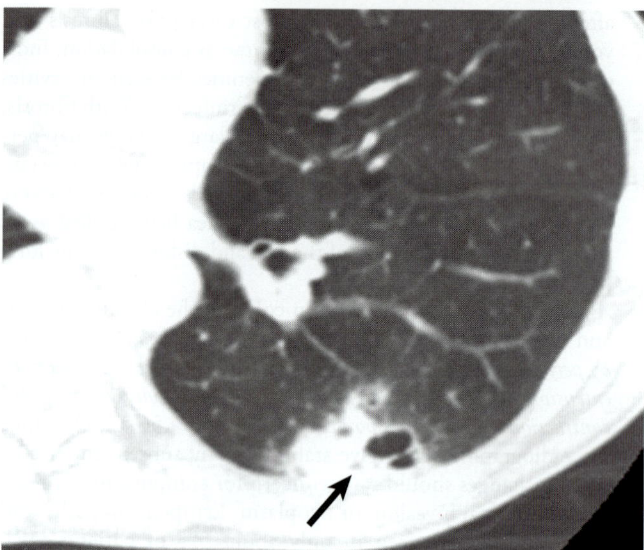

Figure 15.30 Pulmonary *Nocardia* infection. Axial CT lung window image shows nodular consolidation with areas of cavitation and surrounding ground-glass opacities (*arrow*) in the left lower lobe related to *Nocardia* infection.

Nontuberculous Mycobacteria/Atypical Mycobacteria

NTMB include at least 20 organisms that potentially cause human disease of which the most common cause of human pulmonary disease are *Mycobacterium avium*-intracellulare complex (mac), *M. kansasii, and* mycobacterium abscessus. Most NTMB are inhabitants of natural water sources. Many patients who develop NTMB infections are chronically ill and older with risk factors include chronic obstructive pulmonary disease, bronchiectasis, silicosis, cystic fibrosis, and AIDS. The pathologic patterns of most NTMB infections are similar to that of MTB infection. The most common chest CT findings of NTMB pulmonary infection irrespective of the specific species are bilateral small pulmonary nodules, cylindrical bronchiectasis, and branching centrilobular nodules (Fig. 15.29) [61]. Four imaging patterns of NTMB include:

1. Apical fibrocavitary pattern/classic pattern similar to postprimary MTB causing upper lobe consolidation, cavitation, fibrosis, apical pleural thickening, and endobronchial spread of infection-related small nodules
2. Bronchiectasis and centrilobular nodules with predominance in the right middle lobe and lingula
3. Findings mimicking hypersensitivity pneumonitis, with poorly defined ground-glass centrilobular nodules, and air trapping
4. Asymptomatic single or multiple pulmonary nodules without distant satellite nodules

Pleural effusion, lymph node enlargement, and miliary disease are rare in NTMB. However, in an individual case, these differences are not sufficient to distinguish NTMB from *M. tuberculosis* infections [62].

Actinomyces

The actinomyces (nocardia and actinomyces) are fungi morphologically, however, they respond to antibiotics as they are appropriately considered bacteria.

Actinomycosis: *Actinomyces israelii* is a commensal of the oropharynx and may rarely cause pulmonary infection by aspiration or direct extension from mediastinum or esophagus. Pulmonary actinomycosis has peak incidence in the fourth and fifth decades and CT is better at evaluating extent. Classically, it causes lower lobe peripheral airspace consolidation with areas of low attenuation, abscess formation, pleural invasion with pleural thickening, pleural effusions, and osteomyelitis of ribs, sinuses to the chest wall. Apical disease may mimic tuberculosis, and patchy pneumonia can develop occasionally. The mass-like consolidation with cavitation may even resemble lung cancer [63].

Nocardiosis: *Nocardia asteroides* is a saprophyte found worldwide in soil and infection usually occurs through inhalation of the organism particularly in debilitated immunosuppressed individuals but may occur in otherwise healthy individuals. *Nocardia asteroides* infection may complicate alveolar proteinosis. CXR and CT most commonly show nonsegmental, cavitating consolidative pneumonia (Fig. 15.30), bronchopneumonia (Fig. 15.31), often with empyema or pleural effusion. It may also present as a solitary pulmonary nodule, with or without cavitation, and sometimes with hilar lymphadenopathy. Multiple nodules may be seen, particularly in immunosuppressed patients [64].

Histoplasmosis

Histoplasma capsulatum infection normally results from inhalation of soil or dust contaminated with bat or bird excreta and is most commonly seen in Ohio and Mississippi River valleys of the United States. The radiologic manifestations of histoplasmosis occur in parallel with the clinical syndromes. Infection is usually subclinical and heals spontaneously, sometimes leaving small, calcified pulmonary nodules and calcified mediastinal nodes or hilar nodes.

- CXR appears normal in most of the patients with histoplasma capsulatum infection
- On imaging in acute disease, smaller or larger pulmonary nodules (Figs. 15.32–15.34) will be seen

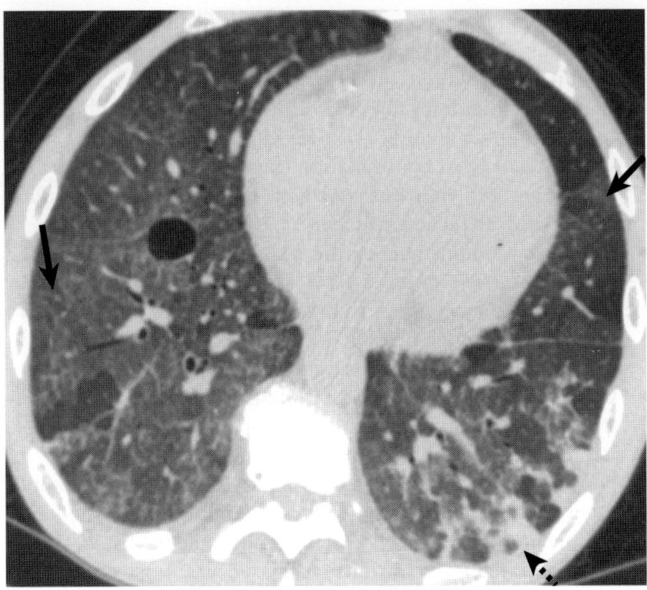

Figure 15.31 Disseminated *Nocardia* pulmonary infection. Axial lung window CT image shows multifocal diffuse ground-glass (*bold arrows*) and peripheral consolidative opacities (*dotted arrow*) in both lungs with areas of crazy-paving appearance due to disseminated nocardia infection proved with BAL fluid analysis.

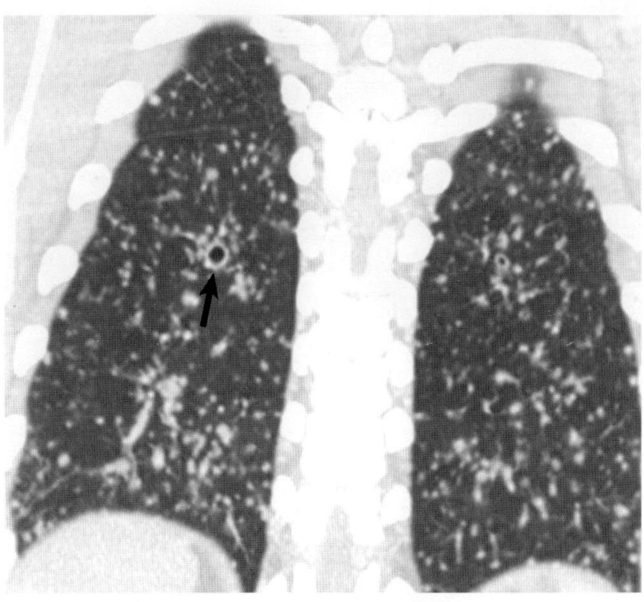

Figure 15.33 Pulmonary histoplasmosis. Coronal chest lung window image in a 45-year-old man with cough and dyspnea on exertion shows numerous small, sharply defined, random solid diffuse, and uniform in distribution miliary nodules with few thick-walled pulmonary cavities (*arrow*). Differential diagnosis of military nodules includes metastases, miliary tuberculosis, fungal infection, sarcoidosis, Langerhans histiocytosis, silicosis, and coal worker's pneumoconiosis.

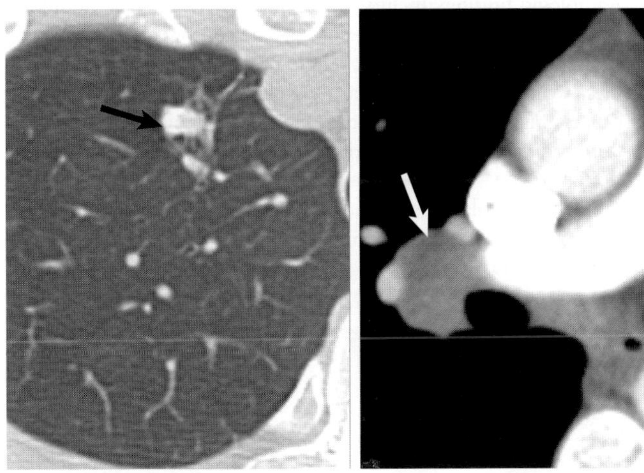

Figure 15.32 Acute histoplasmosis. Axial lung window (left image) and soft-tissue window (right image) chest CT images in a 23-year-old woman with recent history of travel currently presenting with fever and cough show clustered right upper lobe peribronchial dominant soft-tissue nodule (*black arrow*) and associated ipsilateral right hilar lymphadenopathy (*white arrow*). Differential diagnosis for such pattern includes tuberculosis, sarcoidosis, and other fungal infections. Follow-up 6-month CT chest showed development of diffuse amorphous calcification within the same right hilar node (not shown) due to post-treatment healing changes. (Courtesy: Dr Carlos S Restrepo.)

- Disseminated disease may show a miliary or diffuse reticulonodular pattern/bronchopenumonia pattern that rapidly progresses to diffuse airspace opacification. When many nodules are scattered throughout the lungs (Fig. 15.33), they closely resemble the nodules of varicella pneumonia or miliary tuberculosis except they tend to be slightly more variable

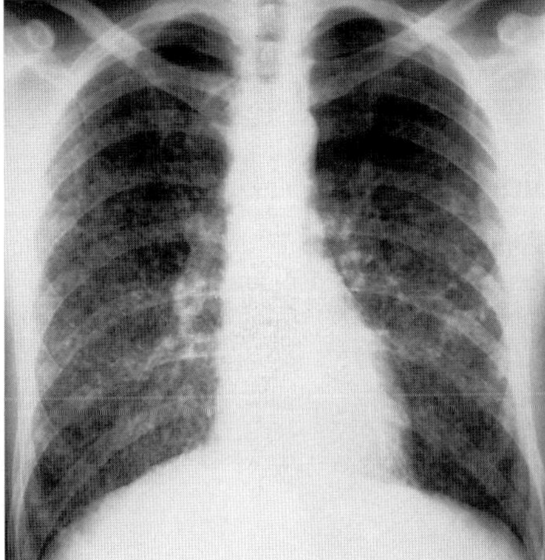

Figure 15.34 Acute histoplasmosis after massive exposure while visiting a bat-infested cave. There are widespread bilateral well-defined 3–5-mm nodules.

- Hilar node enlargement is common and sometimes may be the only visible manifestation (Figs. 15.32 and 15.35)
- In chronic state, fibrosis and cavitation with focally distorted lung in the apicoposterior distribution is seen on imaging with similar appearance to postprimary tuberculosis [65,66]
- A histoplasma may resemble a tuberculoma, being round, usually well circumscribed up to 3-cm nodule and often with central calcification. Adjacent satellite nodules can be present
- Hematogenous spread and pleural disease are rare
- ***Fibrosing mediastinitis*** is an uncommon late manifestation of mediastinal histoplasmosis due to nodal fibrosis which can cause stenosis of the superior vena cava, esophagus, trachea, bronchi, or pulmonary arteries or veins. The CXR reveals

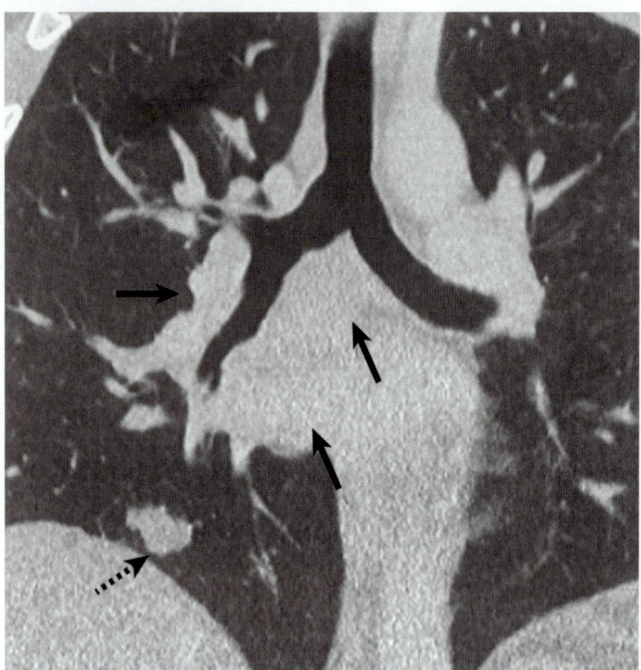

Figure 15.35 Coronal chest CT image in a 38-year-old nonsmoker man from endemic histoplasma region presenting with fever and SOB shows a lobulated right lower lobe solid nodule (*dotted arrow*) with enlarged hilar and subcarinal lymph nodes (*bold arrows*) mimicking lung cancer.

widened mediastinum along with large hilar opacities extending into the lungs along with interstitial opacities, whereas chest CT reveals soft-tissue or calcified masses (Fig. 15.36) in the distribution of lymph node locations [65,66]

Coccidioidomycosis

Coccidioides immitis causes endemic disease in parts of the south west United States, Northern Mexico, and areas of Central and South America. Approximately 60% of infections are asymptomatic with the most common radiographic feature is a nodule which calcifies with healing. The radiologic manifestations of coccidioidomycosis occur in parallel with the clinical syndromes.

- Acute coccidioidomycosis may cause a pneumonic illness and manifests on CXR and CT, as multifocal nodules (Fig. 15.37), segmental or lobar consolidation (Fig. 15.38), or peribronchial thickening and may be associated with hilar or mediastinal adenopathy or pleural effusion
- Pulmonary nodules up to the size of 3 cm in diameter can occur, and these nodules have a tendency to form thin- or thick-walled cavities (Fig. 15.39) with persistent primary infection. Although healing of lung lesion may result in a solitary nodule or coccidioidomycoma [65,66]
- Chronic coccidioidomycosis manifests as persistent or progressive consolidation, cavitation, adenopathy, effusion, multiple nodules, fibrosis, or bronchiectasis (Fig. 15.40) similar to postprimary tuberculosis. Coccidioidal cavities can be complicated by rupture into the pleural space, resulting in a spontaneous pneumothorax or a persistent bronchopleural fistula
- Disseminated coccidioidomycosis occurs most commonly in immunocompromised patients with a miliary pattern on chest imaging, usually accompanied by hilar or mediastinal lymphadenopathy and extrathoracic spread [65,66]

North American Blastomycosis

Pulmonary blastomycosis refers to respiratory infection due to *Blastomyces dermatitidis and is found in parts of the central and south east United States.*

- Radiologic findings include an asymptomatic solitary nodule, a pneumonic illness with acute or chronic consolidation in focal or bronchopneumonia pattern, single or multiple pulmonary nodules, lymphadenopathy, focal mass-like opacity mimicking lung cancer (Fig. 15.41) with satellite nodules, or miliary disease with fibronodular disease. Cavitation is occasionally seen, but calcification is rare
- Unlike histoplasmosis and coccidioidomycosis, fibrosis is uncommon, and once lesions have healed, scars are frequently inconspicuous [65,66]

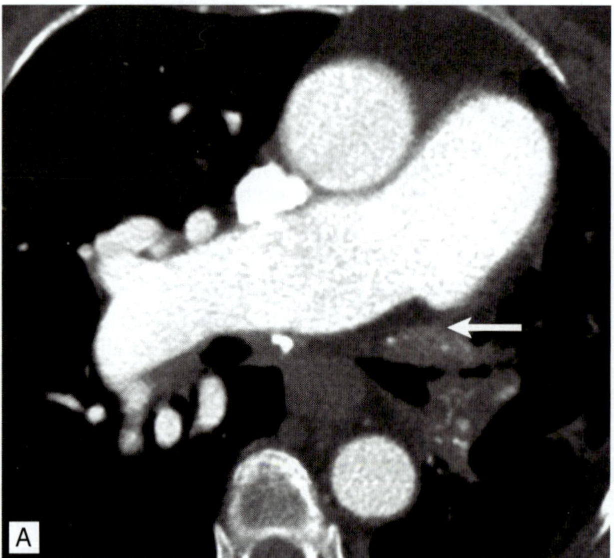

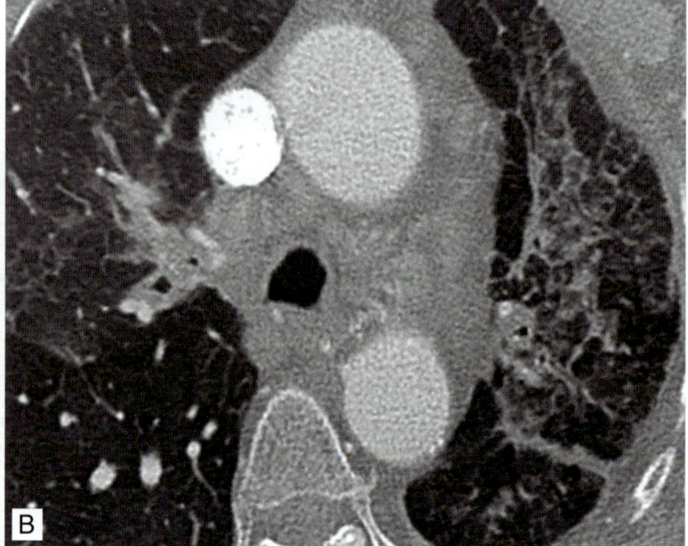

Figure 15.36 Histoplasmosis-related fibrosing mediastinitis. Axial soft tissue and lung window chest CT images in a middle age man with hemoptysis showing partly calcified left hilar ill-defined soft tissue with near complete occlusion of the pulmonary artery, bronchus, and pulmonary vein on the left side with resultant interstitial thickening in the upper lung lobe and severe pulmonary hypertension-related main pulmonary artery dilation.

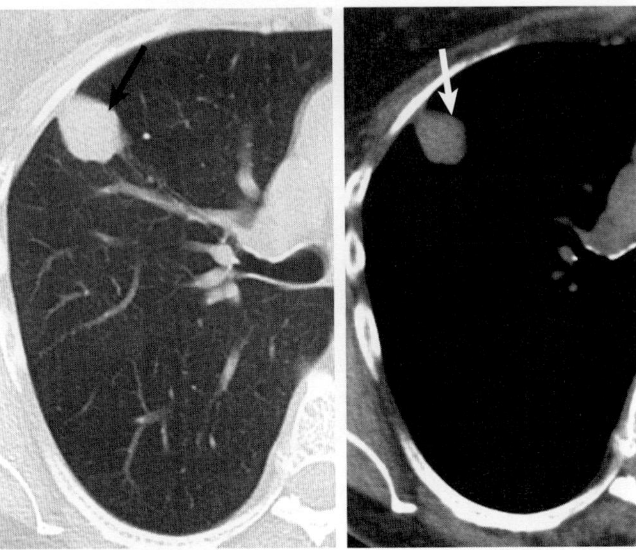

Figure 15.37 Coccidioidomycosis. Axial lung window (left) and axial soft-tissue window (right) in an 81-year-old woman with incidentally identified right upper lobe noncavitary, noncalcified peripheral soft-tissue nodule (*arrow*) closely abutting the pleura.

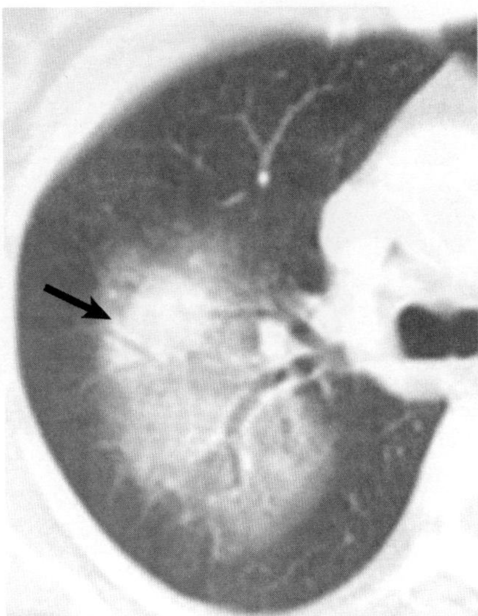

Figure 15.38 Acute coccidioidal consolidative infection. Axial CT lung window image shows confluent mixed consolidative and ground-glass opacity within the right upper lobe in a central peribronchovascular distribution (*arrow*). (Courtesy: Dr Carlos S Restrepo.)

Radiologic Features to Differentiate Endemic Fungi on Imaging

The radiologic findings of an acute fungal pneumonia due to these organisms are usually nonspecific.

- Acute blastomycosis and coccidioidomycosis are more likely than acute histoplasmosis to present as a lobar consolidation
- Cavitary consolidation is suggestive of acute coccidioidomycosis
- Although hilar adenopathy is common in all, but mediastinal adenopathy is rare except in acute coccidioidomycosis
- Pleural effusions are overall uncommon
- Persistent nodules are most common due to previous histoplasmosis or coccidioidomycosis
- Calcification is suggestive of previous *H. capsulatum* infection
- Chronic infection with these organisms typically mimics postprimary tuberculosis both clinically and radiologically in the form of upper lobe fibrocavitary disease, satellite nodules, fibrosis, and bronchiectasis [65,66]. Fibrosis is uncommon in blastomycosis

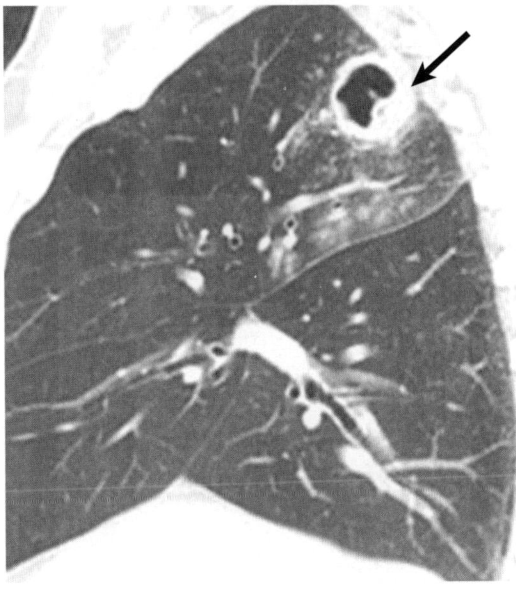

Figure 15.39 Acute coccidioidal cavitary infection. Sagittal CT lung window image shows a thick-walled cavity (*arrow*) in the posterior segment of the right upper lobe with surrounding ground-glass nodules and opacities.

Cryptococcosis (Torulosis)

Cryptococcus neoformans is a yeast form of fungus found worldwide in soil, particularly abundant in pigeon excreta and is the most common etiologic agent resulting in cryptococcosis. Infection is mostly subclinical, but is important in debilitated patients. In an otherwise healthy individual, cryptococcal pulmonary infection usually manifests as single lung mass (mimicking lung cancer) or multiple peripheral pulmonary nodules, generally without cavitation (Fig. 15.42), and uncommonly with consolidation. In patients with AIDS, diffuse interstitial opacities or bronchopneumonia pattern can be seen. Miliary nodules, single or multiple pulmonary nodules, occasionally with cavitation can also be seen. Lymphadenopathy and pleural effusion are rare. Systemic spread particularly to brain and meninges is common in AIDS and immunocompromised patients [4,17,65–68].

Candidiasis

Candida albicans is a normal mouth commensal and is rarely invasive unless the patient is immunocompromised. Pulmonary candida infection occurs most commonly from hematogenous spread with multiorgan involvement in the setting of immunosuppression, where it manifests with miliary nodules or multiple larger nodules in a centrilobular or random distribution. The second uncommon form results from aspiration of contaminated oropharyngeal secretions and results in bronchopneumonia with patchy bilateral consolidation in a peribronchovascular distribution.

In immunosuppressed patients, the CXR and CT findings of pulmonary candidiasis are small or large diffuse multiple

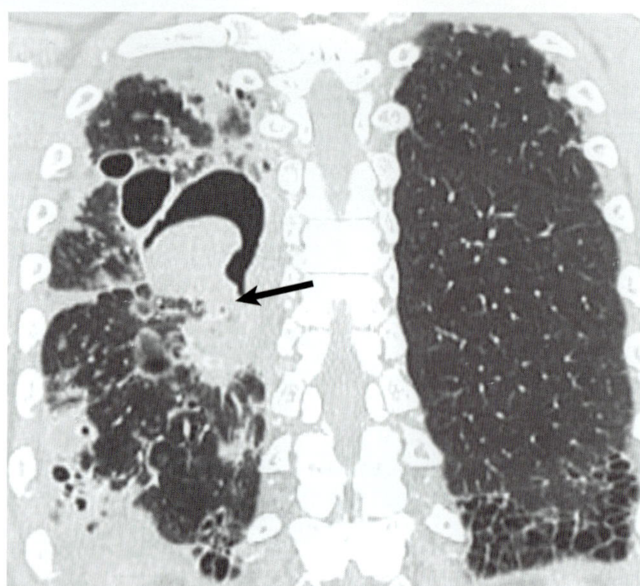

Figure 15.40 Chronic coccidioidal fibrocavitary infection. Coronal CT lung window image shows multifocal thick-walled cavitary lesions (*arrow*), peribronchovascular nodules, tree-in-bud opacities, and irregular fibrosis throughout the right lung, most pronounced within the right upper lobe due to chronic coccidioidal infection. Dominant cavity within the medial aspect of the right lung extending between the right upper and lower lobes with internal rounded soft tissue related to complication from mycetoma formation (*arrow*). Note honeycombing in basal segments of both lungs due to underlying UIP pattern of pulmonary fibrosis.

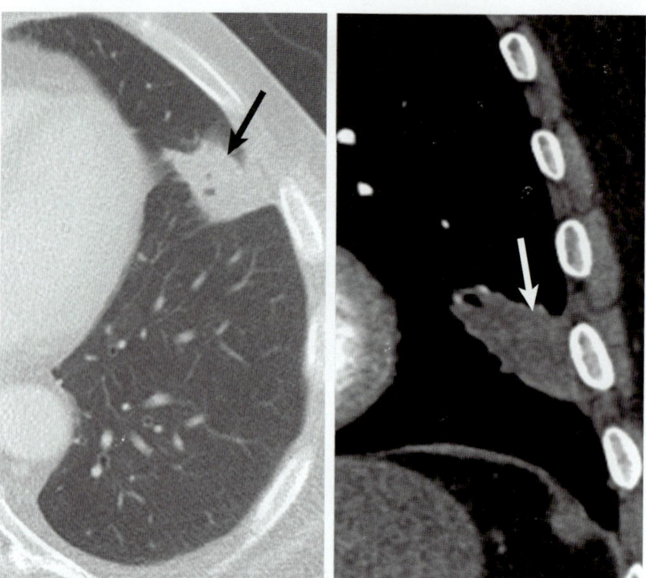

Figure 15.41 Pulmonary blastomycosis. Axial lung window (left) and coronal soft-tissue window (right) in a 67-year-old man with fever and weight loss shows peripheral lingular lobe lobular mass-like consolidation. Lung cancer was suspected, and patient underwent FNAC which showed blastomycosis. ***Differential diagnosis includes lung cancer:*** Can be difficult to differentiate as in the index case; ***Pneumonia:*** No response to conventional antibiotic therapy should raise possibility of atypical infections in endemic areas; and ***Rounded atelectasis:*** Mass-like appearance, comet-tail appearance, and adjacent pleural thickening.

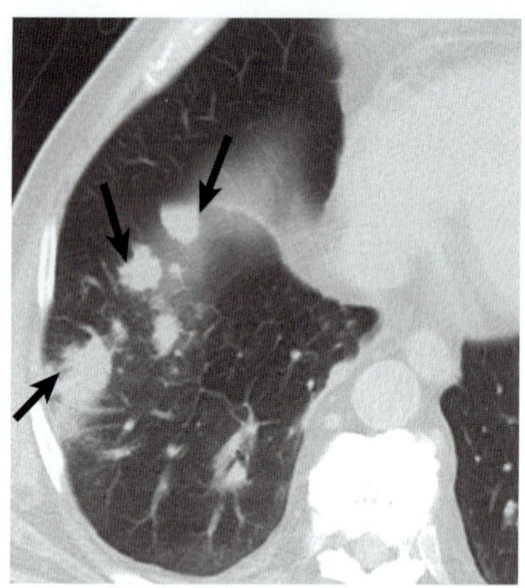

Figure 15.42 Cryptococcosis. Axial lung window chest CT image in a 76-year-old man with Hodgkin lymphoma on chemotherapy currently presenting with fever and chest pain shows multiple ill-defined soft-tissue nodular opacities in the right lower lobe (*arrows*) with minimal surrounding ground-glass opacities.

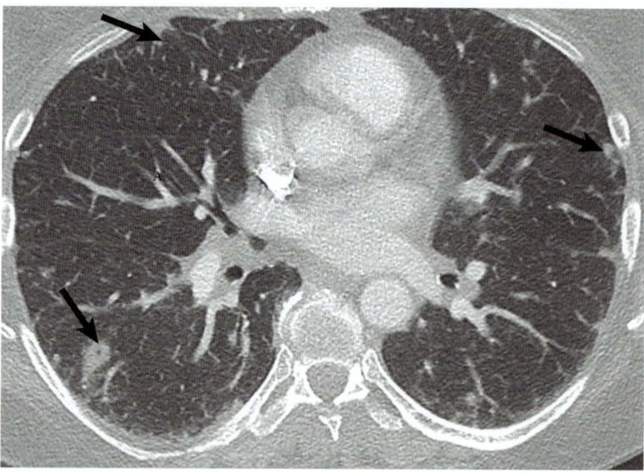

Figure 15.43 Candida fungemia. Axial chest CT image in a 36-year-old man with diabetes mellitus, fever, and chills shows multiple predominantly peripherally distributed solid pulmonary nodules (*arrows*) with some nodules showing cavitation (*arrow* in right lower lobe).

pulmonary nodules (Figs. 15.43 and 15.44) with our without "CT halo sign" along with GGOs and nonspecific focal or multilobar patchy consolidation (Fig. 15.44). Pleural effusion, cavitation (Fig. 15.43), and lymphadenopathy are uncommon.

The infectious causes of CT halo sign include fungal infections such as candida, mucormycosis, actinomycosis, bacterial infections such as *Pseudomonas* and *Legionella* and viral infections such as herpes simplex virus and cytomegalovirus [17, 69–71].

Mucormycosis/Mucor Infection

Pulmonary mucormycosis (PM) is rare fatal fungal infection caused by members of the genus *Rhizopus* or *Mucor* due to inhalation of infected spores, most often seen in immunocompromised patients, and can progress rapidly in neutropenic patients.

- Lobar and segmental consolidation (Figs. 15.45–15.47) is the most common finding on CXR with multilobar and bilateral distribution in some patients. Single or multiple nodules and masses are common

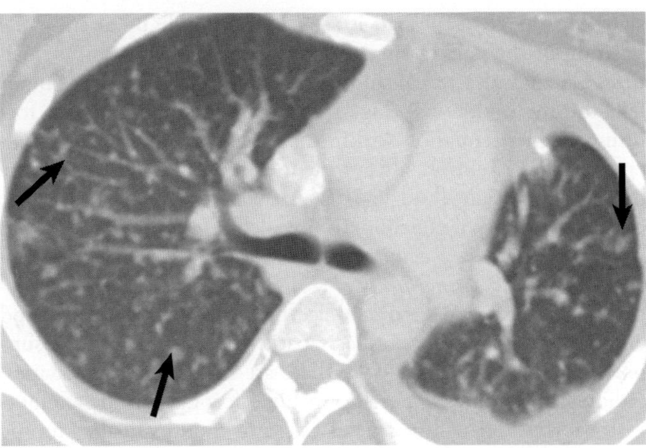

Figure 15.44 Disseminated candidiasis. Axial lung window chest CT image in a 10-year-old child with acute lymphocytic leukemia on chemotherapy with febrile neutropenia. CT shows innumerable tiny bilateral solid pulmonary nodules (*arrows*), focal consolidation, and small left pleural effusion.

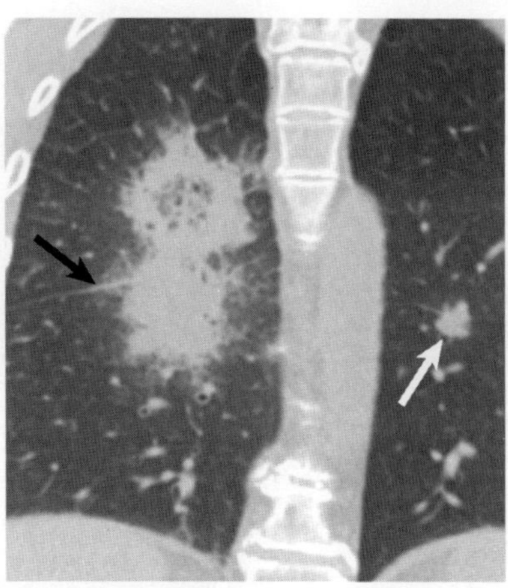

Figure 15.45 Acute mucor infection. Coronal lung window chest CT image in a 58-year-old man with AML on chemotherapy shows aggressive consolidation containing mottled ground glass in center and rim of consolidation in right lung ("reverse halo sign") crossing the transverse fissure (*black arrow*) with in right lung. Note left lower lobe solid nodule also due to mucor infection.

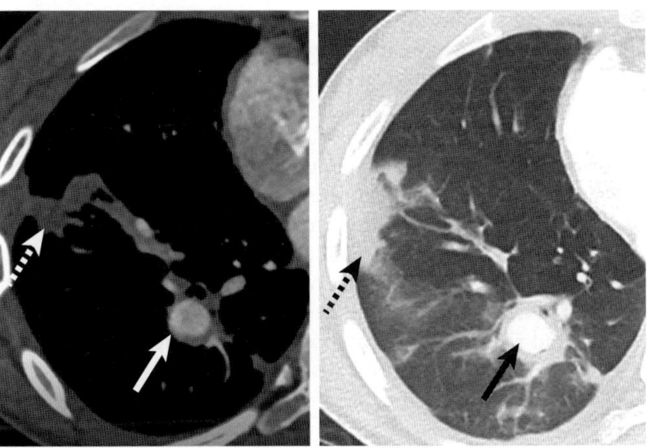

Figure 15.46 Mucormycosis pneumonia complicated by pulmonary artery pseudoaneurysm. A composite image with axial soft-tissue window (left) and axial CT lung window image (right) in a young patient reveals mycotic pulmonary artery enhancing pseudoaneurysm (*bold arrows*) along right lower lobe segmental pulmonary artery related to right lower lobe consolidative opacities due to mucor pneumonia (*dotted arrows*).

- CT shows nonspecific findings of peribronchial GGO in early phase while disease progression reveals consolidation, nodules, or masses with ground-glass halo (Fig. 15.45). Pseudoaneurysm formation (Fig. 15.46) and abrupt termination of a pulmonary artery branch/vascular cut-off sign are known with PM. The reverse halo sign (Fig. 15.47), pleural effusions and more than 10 nodules, is more common in PM than with invasive pulmonary aspergillosis (IPA). PM can involve pleura (pleural thickening or effusion), chest wall (air in the intercostal space or subcutaneous soft tissues), mediastinum, and diaphragm. *The reverse halo sign differential diagnosis includes organizing pneumonia, bland pulmonary infarct, and lung cancer* [72]

Aspergillosis

Aspergillus fumigatus is widespread in the atmosphere and it is inevitable that man inhales the spores from time to time. It can multiply when conditions are favorable in the air passages. The pulmonary manifestations are grouped into following categories [73]:

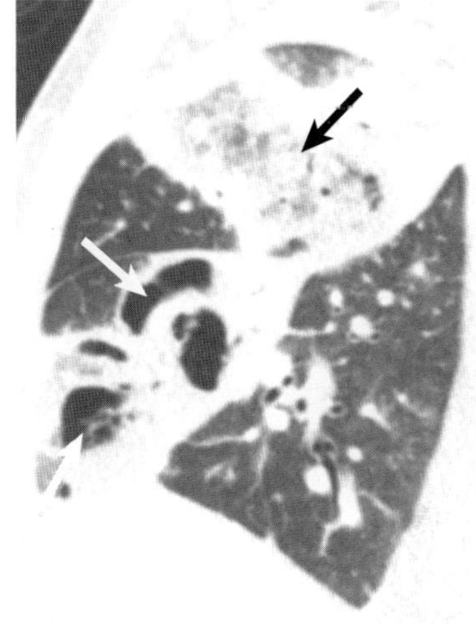

Figure 15.47 Pulmonary mucormycosis. Sagittal chest CT lung window image in a middle-aged man presenting with nonresponding fever shows right middle lobe necrotizing consolidation with cavity formation with lack of parenchymal normal vascularity. The right upper lobe reveals reverse halo sign/atoll sign characterized by central heterogeneous mixed ground-glass and consolidative opacification, crazy-paving appearance, and peripheral consolidative rim due to angioinvasive mucormycosis. This was proved on lung lobectomy specimen.

1. Aspergilloma
2. Allergic bronchopulmonary aspergillosis
3. Invasive aspergillosis:
   a) Angioinvasive
   b) Airway invasive aspergillosis (*Aspergillus* bronchopneumonia)
   c) Acute tracheobronchitis
4. Subacute invasive pulmonary aspergillosis (formerly called chronic necrotizing pulmonary aspergillosis) [2,4,20,23,69, 74–76]

Aspergilloma/Mycetoma

Any chronic pulmonary cavity may be colonized by this fungus. Such cavities are mostly secondary to tuberculosis, histoplasmosis, sarcoidosis, with rare causes including bullae, abscesses, and bronchiectasis. These are, therefore, typically found in the upper lobes. The

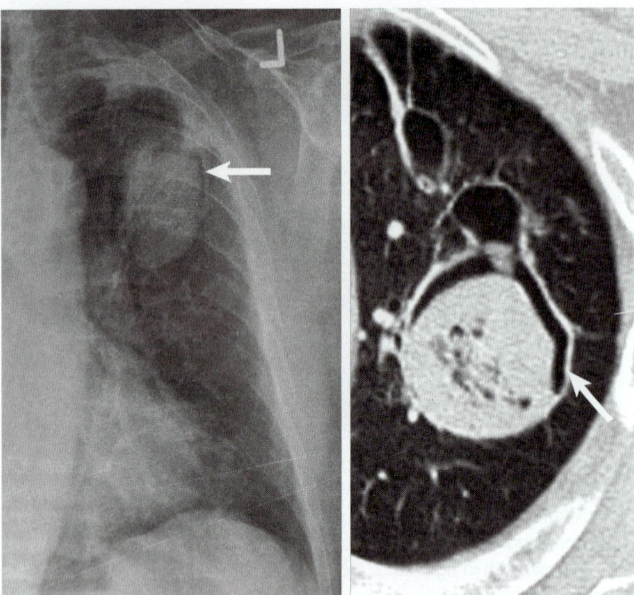

Figure 15.48 Aspergilloma of lung. Composite image of left upper hemithorax chest radiograph (left) and axial lung window (right) in a 34-year-old man with chronic asthma on steroids shows soft-tissue nodule in the dilated left upper lobe bronchus with peripheral air lucency related to air crescent sign (*arrows*) and associated adjacent pleural thickening.

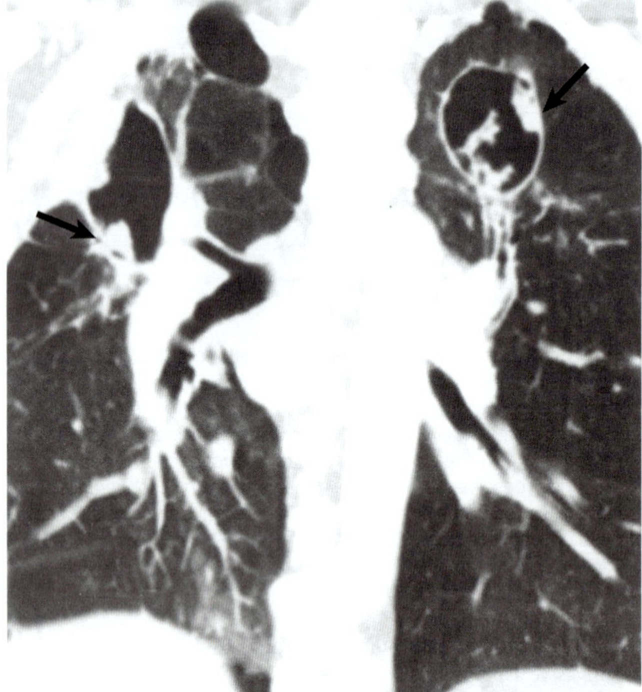

Figure 15.49 Pulmonary aspergillomas. Coronal chest CT lung window image in a 48-year-old man presenting with hemoptysis and previous granulomatous disease shows two dominant both upper lobe cavitary lesions with intracavitary lobulated soft tissue (*arrows*) due to mycetomas which was related to aspergillomas. Note cylindrical bronchiectasis and multifocal scarring in both upper lobes.

fungal hyphae form a ball or mycetoma that lies free in the cavity and patients with mycetoma generally have normal immunity.

The *CXR* and CT could show a round or oval mass surrounded by air within a cavity producing the typical air crescent sign (Fig. 15.48). The ball is seen to be mobile by altering the position of the patient on radiograph or CT to decubitus position. CT may also reveal thin fungal strands bridging the fungus ball and the cavity wall (Fig. 15.49) as well as demonstrate foci of increased attenuation within the fungal ball likely due to calcium. There is almost always pleural thickening related to the mycetoma. An air–fluid level is usually not present within the cavity. The cavity is generally thin walled. *The differential diagnosis of a mycetoma in a cavity includes lung abscess, blood clot, hydatid cyst, and cavitating tumor.*

The "air crescent" sign can also be seen in angioinvasive and chronic necrotizing aspergillosis patients who are immunosuppressed patient in which case, there are no pre-existing cavities; radiological findings appearing within a few days in the angioinvasive forms and within several weeks or months in the chronic necrotizing forms of *Aspergillus* infection.

Mycetomas are associated with the development of vascular granulation tissue in the cavity wall, which may bleed [2,4,20,23, 69,74–76].

Allergic Bronchopulmonary Aspergillosis

ABPA occurs due to Type III hypersensitivity to *Aspergillus fumigatus* and typically always affects patients with asthma or cystic fibrosis in whom the fungus has colonized the segmental and lobar central airways causing bronchial dilatation with predominance in the upper lung.

- The CXR in the acute phase shows patchy consolidation, often in the upper zones. With appropriate treatment, the appearances will return back to normal. Nodules, tram-track opacities, toothpaste/finger-in-glove opacities (Fig. 15.50A) due to dilated mucus-filled bronchi, lobar collapse and migrating opacities, and large lung volumes may be seen in long-standing cases. Pleuropulmonary fibrosis and bronchiectasis (parallel line and ring shadows) can occur with repeated attacks
- CT typically reveals bronchial wall thickening, central bronchiectasis, filled by mucoid impactions with a Y- or V-shaped finger-in-glove opacities, usually involving segmental or subsegmental bronchi (Fig. 15.50B). *High attenuation of impacted mucus (typically >100 HU) with density greater than that of paraspinal muscles is a pathognomonic finding of ABPA* (Fig. 15.50C and D). Hyperattenuating mucus is due to calcium, iron, and manganese metals or desiccated mucus similar to seen in sinusitis
- Mosaic perfusion and air trapping may be seen
- Rarely lobar or segmental atelectasis, pleural effusion, or spontaneous pneumothorax can be seen

Eventually, fibrosis can cause volume loss, cavitation, bullae, focal emphysema, and eventually end-stage upper lobe fibrosis thus may mimic previous chronic pulmonary infection including tuberculosis [2–4,7,17,23,65,66,69,70,73,75,76].

Invasive Aspergillosis

Due to underlying neutropenia in immunosuppressed individuals, *Aspergillus* may cause primary infection of the lung and airways.

a) Angioinvasive aspergillosis accounts for majority of cases of invasive aspergillosis causing pulmonary vasculature thrombosis, pulmonary hemorrhage, and infarction. This may be in the form of multiple nodules, or lobar consolidation. *On CT, a highly suggestive finding of AIA is a halo of GGO surrounding a denser central nodule (halo sign)* (Fig. 15.51), which corresponds to hemorrhagic inflammation surrounding a region of septic infarction/necrosis.

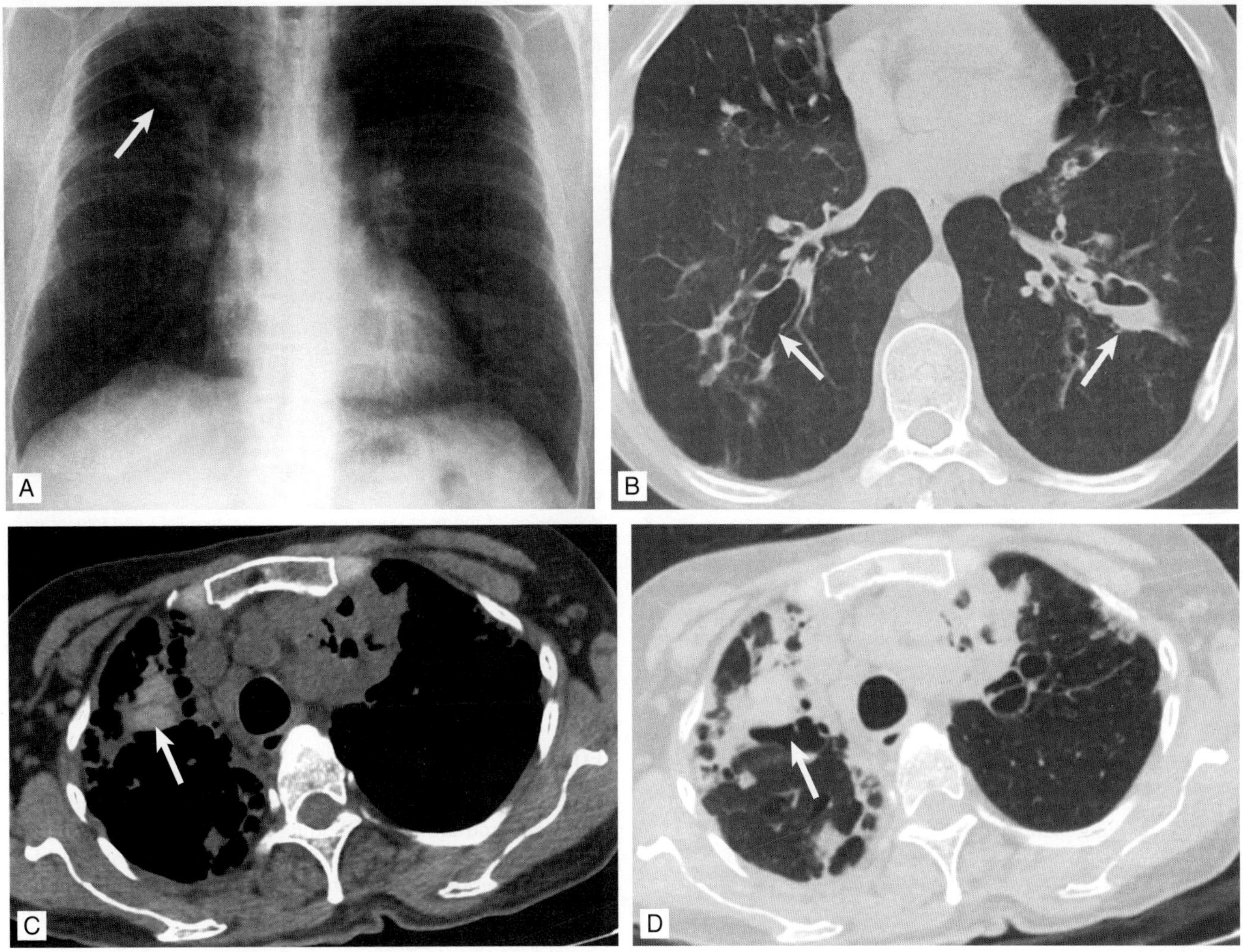

Figure 15.50 Allergic bronchopulmonary aspergillosis (ABPA). Frontal radiograph (A) shows typical finger-in-glove opacities due to mucus-filled dilated bronchi in the right upper lobe (*arrow*). Axial lung window chest CT images (B) in another 36-year-old steroid-dependent asthmatic patient with cough and shortness of breath shows extensive cylindrical bronchiectasis (*arrows*) with patchy areas of mucoid impaction and scattered centrilobular and tree-in-bud nodules due to endobronchial spread of infection. Axial mediastinal (C) and lung window (D) of a different patient with ABPA show hyperdense impacted mucus (*arrow* in C) within the dilated bronchi (*arrow* in D).

Candida, herpes simplex, and cytomegalovirus infections; Wegener granulomatosis, hemorrhagic metastases, and Kaposi sarcoma should be considered in the differential diagnoses of "halo sign" in neutropenic patients [2–4,7,17,23,65,66,69,70,73,75,76].

Cavitation (crescent sign) of such pulmonary lesions (retracted, infarcted lung/mycotic lung sequestrum), and is seen in immunocompromised patients, is normal and often happens when the white blood cell count recovers about 2 weeks after the onset of invasive aspergillosis infection and thus mimic an intracavitatory mycetoma.

b) Airway invasive *Aspergillus* appears on radiographs and CT as nonspecific bronchopneumonia pattern with patchy airspace opacities and small nodules in peribronchiolar distribution and also as bronchiolitis pattern with patchy centrilobular nodules with tree-in-bud appearance.

c) *Aspergillus* acute tracheobronchitis is rare and appears on CT as tracheal or bronchial irregular multifocal wall thickening, which are occasionally high in attenuation due to the ability of *Aspergillus* to fix calcium [2–4,7,17,23,65,66,69,70,73,75, 76].

Subacute IPA (formerly called chronic necrotizing pulmonary aspergillosis): It is uncommon and poorly understood form of

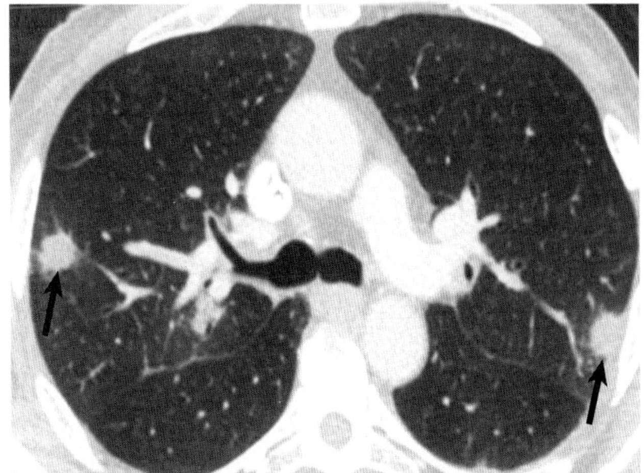

Figure 15.51 Invasive pulmonary aspergillosis. Axial lung window chest CT image in a 54-year-old man with AML, status after stem cell transplant 1 year ago currently presenting with febrile neutropenia shows solid pulmonary nodules with surrounding ground-glass opacities (halo sign) *arrow* in both upper lobes. Surrounding ground-glass opacities usually represent alveolar hemorrhage due to fungal invasion of small vessels.

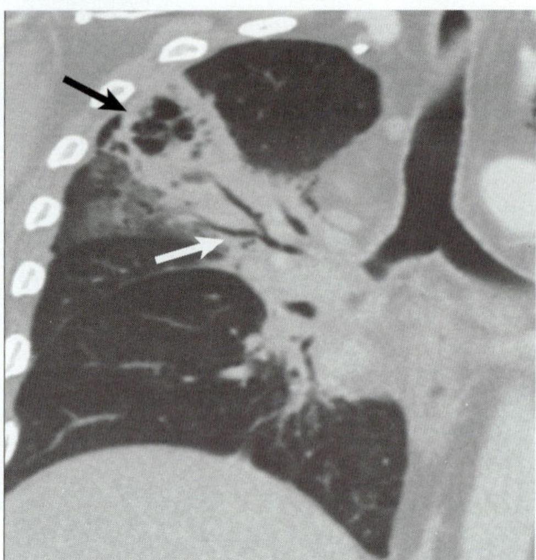

Figure 15.52 Chronic necrotizing aspergillosis/*Aspergillus* pneumonia. Coronal lung window chest CT image in a 57-year-old man with small cell carcinoma in the right perihilar region, status after chemotherapy and on steroids presenting with SOB shows cavitary consolidation (*black arrow*) in periphery, consolidation containing air bronchogram in the central right upper lobe (*white arrow*) along with surrounding ground-glass opacities in the right upper lobe which was confirmed to be *Aspergillus* pneumonia on FNAC.

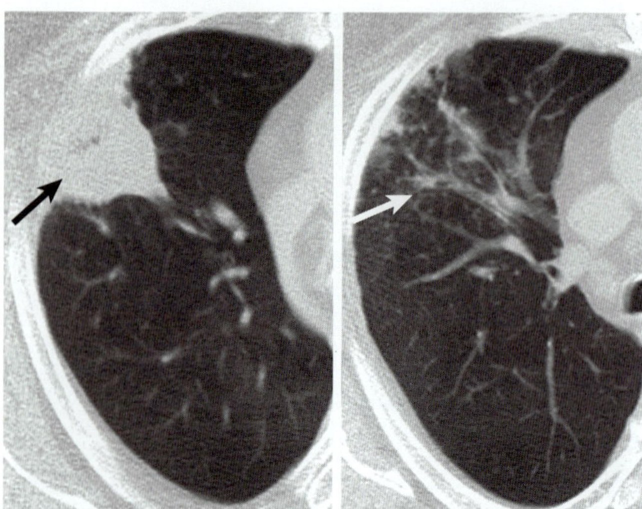

Figure 15.53 Semi-invasive aspergillosis. Composite CT axial lung window image of the right upper lobe at its superior (left) and inferior (right) aspect in a 70-year-old man with myelodysplastic syndrome and fever. Initial CT showed partly necrotic consolidation (*black arrow*) with surrounding subcentimeter peribronchial nodularity (*white arrow*) in the right upper lobe which did not resolve after course of antibiotics. Note that nonresolving pneumonia in immunosuppressed patient should raise concern for atypical infections such as fungal pneumonia besides malignancy.

locally invasive aspergillosis, which typically occurs in patients with moderately immunocompromised status and in patients with chronic lung pathology, is a more rapidly progressive infection (<3 months) usually found in moderately immunocompromised patients [77]. These should be managed as invasive aspergillosis.

On imaging, subacute IPA presents with irregular upper lobe consolidation and pleural thickening that slowly progresses to cavitation (Fig. 15.52) over months ("air crescent sign") thus mimicking chronic pulmonary infections such as histoplasmosis or TB. These cavities can show internal opacity due to fungus ("fungal ball") due to the parenchymal destruction by the fungus and thus mimicking an aspergilloma. Rarely, foci of high attenuation within the cavity due to calcification in the fungus can be seen.

The most common form of chronic pulmonary aspergillosis (CPA) is chronic cavitary pulmonary aspergillosis (CCPA), which untreated may progress to chronic fibrosing pulmonary aspergillosis. Uncommon manifestations of CPA are *Aspergillus* nodule and single aspergilloma. All these entities are found in nonimmunocompromised patients with previous or current lung disease.

CCPA shows new and progressive lung cavity in the region of chronic cavitary disease, whereas subacute IPA shows slow (over months) hyphal invasion of cavity wall.

Denning's criteria [77] for CPA on imaging consist of one or more cavitary pulmonary lesion possibly containing one or more aspergillomas or irregular intraluminal material on imaging, with serological or microbiological evidence implicating *Aspergillus* infection or an immunological response to *Aspergillus* species and exclusion of alternative diagnoses. All these are present for at least 3 months while CCPA in addition require evidence of paracavitary infiltrates (Fig. 15.53), new pulmonary cavity formation, or expansion of cavity size over at least 3 months of observation [2–4,7,17,23,65,66,69,70,73,75,76].

Fusarium

Fusarium species are fungal organisms commonly found in soil and water and are second leading cause of fungal infections in immunosuppressed patients [78]. Apart from onychomycosis and keratitis, fusariosis is uncommon in the immunocompetent host. Fusarial pneumonia occurs almost exclusively in severely immunocompromised patients in which invasive fusariosis is usually systemically disseminated, and pneumonia is common.

Scedosporium and Pseudallescheria Boydii

Scedosporium spp. fungi can be colonizers of previously damaged bronchopulmonary trees and can result in allergic bronchopulmonary reaction, invasive localized disease, and at times disseminated disease. *Scedosporium* infections typically affect severely immunosuppressed patients. Radiologic manifestations of pulmonary scedosporiosis are nonspecific and include progressive, multifocal, often bilateral nodular consolidative opacities (Fig. 15.54) with or without cavitation and rarely mycetomas. Bronchopneumonia pattern causing airway thickening, tree-in-bud opacities, patchy areas of GGO, and mediastinal lymphadenopathy due to *P. boydii* pulmonary infection are seen in lung transplanted patients [79].

Pneumocystis

This is discussed under "Acquired immune deficiency syndrome."

Parasitic Infestations

Parasitic infections are seen worldwide and are mostly seen in the tropical and semitropical countries [80]. Thoracic disease is seen in majority of the parasitic infections. Most of the parasitic infections have nonspecific features, although correlation with the clinical, imaging findings, and epidemiology helps in reaching a correct diagnosis [81].

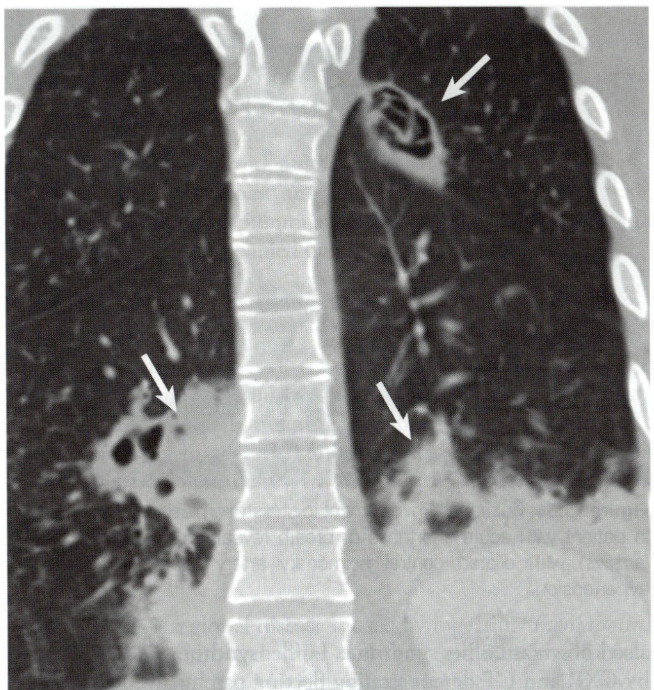

Figure 15.54 *Scedosporium fungal infection.* Coronal lung window in a 56-year-old man with AML on chemotherapy presenting with nonresponding high-grade fever to wide spectrum of antibiotics and antifungal shows a nodular-walled cavitary lesion (*white arrow*) in the left upper lobe with worsening partially cavitary consolidative opacities in both lower lobes (*white arrows*) in keeping with necrotizing pneumonitis. Follow-up CT (not shown) showed new large left pneumothorax due to rupture of cavitary lesion as well as progressive consolidation and patient subsequently expired. Autopsy revealed *Scedosporium fungal lung infection*.

Refer to Table 15.3 for common radiological findings in thoracic parasitic diseases.

Toxoplasmosis

T. gondii protozoal disease is common in developing countries. It is commonly found in mammals and birds; cats or uncooked meat are the means for human acquisition. Pulmonary involvement is typically seen in the immunocompromised humans only. On CXR and CT, bilateral interstitial opacities, ground-glass attenuation, and nodular pulmonary opacities can be seen [80,81].

Entamoeba Histolytica/Amebiasis

This protozoal infection is caused by the *Entamoeba histolytica* and is typically seen in lower socioeconomic classes in tropical and subtropical developing countries located in Central America, South America, Africa, and Asia. After malaria and schistosomiasis, amebiasis is the third most common cause of mortality due to the parasites. The mode of transmission is the feco-oral route. Contiguous spread of the infection from the liver abscess into the right pleural cavity or right lower and middle lobes parenchyma is more common route of spread.

Radiographic and CT features include elevation of the hemidiaphragm (secondary to underlying liver abscess), pleural effusion, airspace consolidation, air–fluid levels within the lung parenchyma (secondary to underlying lung abscess) and/or empyema [80,81]. Pleural effusion can be reactive and sterile in the early stages and later on classic "anchovy sauce" contents due to empyema from the rupture of the hepatic abscess through the diaphragm (Fig. 15.55) [82,83]. Ultrasound scan may reveal liver abscesses and allows assessment of the diaphragm and pleural spaces.

Simple Pulmonary Eosinophilia (Löffler's Syndrome)

This may be caused by many parasitic worms, including *Ascaris*, *Taenia*, *Ankylostoma*, and *Strongyloides*, all of which may lodge in or migrate through the lungs at some stage [80,81]. *The term Loeffler's syndrome is now applied to almost any transient migratory pulmonary opacities/focal areas of consolidation of a predominantly eosinophilic histology associated with a blood eosinophilia* [84].

Schistosomiasis

Pulmonary infection in schistosomiasis is caused typically by *S. mansoni* and *S. japonicum and exposure occurs through*

TABLE 15.3 Common Radiological Findings in Thoracic Parasitic Diseases

Malaria	Chagas	Toxoplasmosis	Amoebiasis	Ascariasis	Toxocariasis	Echinococcosis
Septal thickening (pulmonary edema and ARDS pattern) Consolidation Pleural effusion	Cardiomegaly achalasia Megaesophagus Tracheomegaly Bronchiectasis	Interstitial and ground-glass opacities Pulmonary nodules	Right pleural effusion from Liver abscess Consolidation Right diaphragm elevation Lung Abscess Pulmonary cavitation	Ground-glass opacity: Migratory, transient, and patchy opacities. Consolidation Pulmonary nodules Pneumothorax	Subpleural bilateral lower lobes Ground-glass opacity Consolidation Pulmonary nodules Linear opacities	Pulmonary cysts/ nodular opacities Pleural effusion Pneumothorax Pulmonary cavitation
Strongyloidiasis	**Dirofilariasis**	**Cysticercosis**	**Schistosomiasis**	**Paragonimiasis**		
Ground-glass opacity (patchy migratory consolidations) Septal thickening Consolidation	Solitary pulmonary nodule Predominating in right lung and lower lobes May be pulmonary infarction	Small soft-tissue calcified nodules Multiple random pulmonary nodules	Pulmonary nodules Septal thickening Ground-glass opacity Fibrosis Pulmonary hypertension	Pulmonary nodules Consolidation Pulmonary cysts Atelectasis Pneumothorax Pleural effusion Linear opacities in lung		

- **Alveolar echinococcosis and polycystic echinococcosis**: Alveolar echinococcosis is caused by *E. multilocularis*. Polycystic echinococcosis is caused by *E. vogeli*. Pulmonary disease is seen as a fibrotic mass containing cavities of varying sizes with necrosis and calcifications. CT and MRI help in characterizing the location and extent of the pulmonary infection, which frequently coexistent with liver infection. As the disease progresses, calcifications are seen. Direct extension into the lung parenchyma and chest wall invasion may resemble a metastatic tumor [82,83]

Pulmonary Infections in Congenital Disorders, Genetic Disorders, and Primary Immunodeficiency Disorders

Cystic Fibrosis (CF)

CF is an autosomal recessive condition and produces a generalized disease of exocrine glands and mucous glands resulting in abnormally viscous mucus thereby impairing mucociliary function, frequent chest infections, and development of bronchiectasis. It is now relatively common for patients to survive into adulthood, but overall the prognosis remains poor, with most deaths being a direct result of respiratory complications. *Pseudomonas aeruginosa*, *Staphylococcus aureus*, *Aspergillus*, *Haemophilus influenzae*, and *Klebsiella* species are frequent causes.

- The early radiographic changes may be limited to hyperexpansion, but eventually after repeated episodes of infection, a combination of bronchial wall thickening and bronchiectasis (Fig. 15.60) with central lung predominance, atelectasis, scarring, and multiple cystic spaces
- Clusters of ring shadows and air–fluid levels which usually indicate superadded infection
- In addition, CT findings include mucus plugging, tree-in-bud opacities, large lung volumes, mosaic perfusion and air trapping on expiratory images and hilar enlargement due to lymphadenopathy or pulmonary hypertension
- Repeated pneumothoraces, often resistant to tube drainage, are a further potentially fatal complication

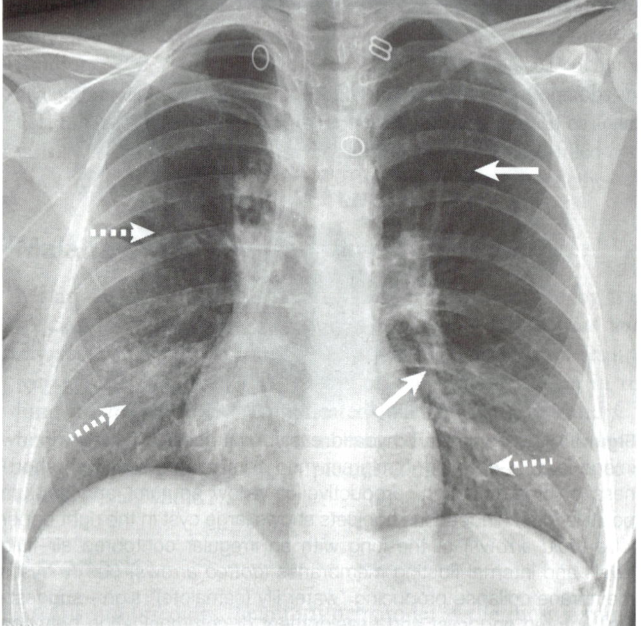

Figure 15.60 Cystic fibrosis-related acute chest syndrome. Frontal chest radiograph shows cystic fibrosis-related diffuse bilateral inflammatory bronchial wall thickening, bronchiectasis (*bold arrows*), mild right upper lobe volume loss, and peribronchial multifocal patchy opacities (*dotted arrows*).

Table 15.4 lists thoracic imaging manifestations of primary immunodeficiency disorders [86,87].

Miscellaneous Conditions with Secondary Lung Infections

Congenital Dyskinetic Ciliary Syndromes

This genetic abnormality encompasses a heterogeneous mixture of structural and functional abnormalities of cilia resulting in bronchiectasis and sinusitis as common manifestations. About 50% of these patients will have situs inversus. Sperm tails are also cilia, and males with the condition will be infertile, hence explaining the *combination of bronchiectasis, situs inversus, and male infertility in Kartagener's syndrome* (Fig. 15.61). Impairment of mucociliary clearance renders the lungs more susceptible to bronchopulmonary infections, but this is only a serious problem if the infections are repeated and severe. The radiographic signs are those of bronchiectasis with a lower or middle lobe predominance, atelectasis, and chronic obstructive airways disease [88].

Young's Syndrome

This is a combination of *obstructive azoospermia, sinusitis, and chronic pulmonary infections*. The latter begin in childhood and eventually most patients develop bronchiectasis [89].

Congenital Pulmonary Sequestration

This is a portion of disorganized pulmonary parenchyma which develops separated from the normal airways and pulmonary vessels. The blood supply is derived from the descending aorta. Sequestrated segments are situated basally in contact with the diaphragm, and appear solid when uncomplicated. *They may become infected and develop a communication with the bronchial tree, after which they may cavitate and show a fluid level.* A sequestration can closely mimic lung abscess in the presence of mucous or fluid-filled cysts with air–fluid levels which can be seen with or without infection [90].

Other Systemic Conditions for Pulmonary Infection

Systemic conditions that are associated with decreased immunity include old age, poor nutrition, diabetes, alcoholism, connective tissue disorders, many malignant diseases, and AIDS. *Pulmonary abnormalities* that predispose to chest infections include bronchiectasis and chronic bronchitis. In addition general anesthesia, especially if prolonged, may be associated with pneumonia. *Iatrogenic causes* include cancer chemotherapy, steroids, immunosuppression after organ transplantation, and radiotherapy. *Chronic infection of the paranasal sinuses* and *esophageal obstruction* may cause pneumonia or lung abscesses due to aspiration.

Pulmonary Infections in Immunocompromised Patients

Pulmonary opportunistic infections are a common complication in immunocompromised patients. The radiographic appearances are often nonspecific, and despite the high morbidity and

TABLE 15.4 Primary Immunodeficiency Disorder-Related Intrathoracic Imaging Findings

	Consolidative Lung Opacities	Bronchiectasis	Cavitation	Pulmonary Hemorrhage	Pneumatocele	Empyema	ILD	GLI-LD	Thymoma	Thymic Aplasia	Lymphoma
Chronic granulomatous disease	++	+	+++	-	-	-	++	-	-	-	-
X-linked agammaglobu-linemia	++	++	-		-	-	++	-	-	-	-
Common variable immune deficiency	++	++	-	-	-	-	+++	+++	-	-	++
Hyper-IgM syndrome	++	++	-	-	-	-	+	-	-	-	+
Hyper-IgE syndrome	++	++	+++	-	+++	+++	-	-	-	-	-
Selective IgA syndrome	+	+	-	-	-	-	+	-	-	-	+
Wiskott–Aldrich syndrome	++	-	-	+++	-	-	+	-	-	-	++
Ataxia telangiectasia	++	++	-	-	-	-	-	-	-	-	++
Good syndrome	++	++	-	-	-	-	+	-	+++	-	+
Severe com-bined immuno-deficiency	+++	+++	-	-	-	-	++	-	-	++	++
Digeorge syndrome	++	+	-	-	-	-	-	-	-	+++	-

CGD, chronic granulomatous disease; *GLILD*, granulomatous lymphocytic ILD; *IgA*, immunoglobulin A; *IgE*, immunoglobulin E; *IgM*, immunoglobulin M; *ILD*, interstitial lung disease; *PID*, primary immunodeficiency disorder; *SCID*, severe combined immunodeficiency; *WAS*, Wiskott–Aldrich syndrome. – means no association; + means not characteristic; ++ means characteristic; +++ means very characteristic.

mortality associated with chest infection in these patients a definitive diagnosis may be difficult to reach. *In order for the radiologist to have a meaningful input into the assessment of the immunocompromised patient with acute chest symptoms, the underlying cause of immunodeficiency, type of immunosuppressive therapy, white blood cell count, and overall medical status of the patient must be known.*

Although the role of the radiologist in these patients has primarily been one of detection and monitoring of pulmonary abnormalities, the introduction of HRCT now makes it possible to offer earlier and more specific diagnostic information. HRCT can detect findings suggestive of pneumonia about 5 days earlier than chest radiography. Furthermore, HRCT allows prediction of the relative chances of obtaining a positive diagnosis from transbronchial versus percutaneous biopsy, particularly when other techniques have proved nondiagnostic.

- Immunodeficiency may occur as a result of impaired cell-mediated immunity (CD4+ T-lymphocyte cells), for example, in patients with lymphoma, on immunosuppressants, intensive chemotherapy, AIDS, Digeorge syndrome, lymphoma, leukemia, and corticosteroids. This predisposes them for higher risk of infection with *Legionella*, nocardia, mycobacteria, fungi, viruses, PJP, and parasites
- Reduced humoral immunity (B-lymphocyte and complement) is most commonly seen in patients with myeloma, chronic lymphocytic leukemia, common variable immunodeficiency, splenectomy predisposing them for higher risk of infection with encapsulated bacteria like *Haemophilus* influenza, *Streptococcus* pneumonia, and *S. aureus*
- Immunodeficiency may occur as a result of reduced phagocytosis (mononuclear cell and neutrophil) can occur in the setting of hematological malignancy, intensive chemotherapy, hematopoietic stem cell transplant (HSCT), chronic granulomatous disease, diabetes, AIDS. This predisposes them for higher risk of infection with gram-negative bacteria, *Staphylococcus aureus*, *Nocardia*, *Candida*, and *Aspergillus* [91]

Hematopoietic Stem Cell Transplant

Pulmonary complications after HSCT present in a typical temporal sequence (Table 15.5). Idiopathic pneumonia syndrome is

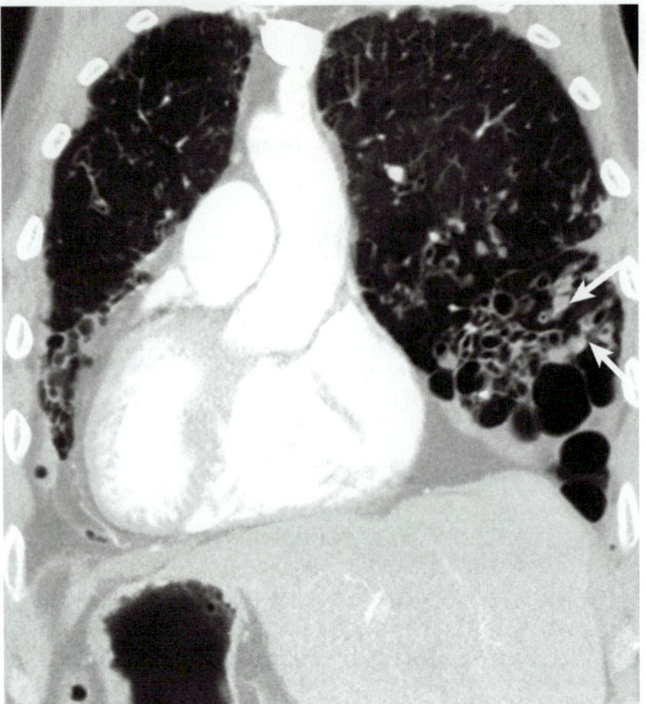

Figure 15.61 Kartagener syndrome with acute *Pseudomonas* infection. Coronal chest CT lung window image in a middle-aged man presenting with hypoxemia due to acute on chronic respiratory failure. Diffuse lower lobe predominant cystic, cylindrical and varicose bronchiectasis (*arrows*), diffuse tree-in-bud nodularity, innumerable nodular opacities in the bilateral lower lobes with new nodular opacities in the bilateral lower lobes related to pseudomonas infection on sputum culture in a patient with situs inversus. The combination of bronchiectasis, sinusitis, and situs inversus is called Kartagener's syndrome.

a diagnosis of exclusion and manifest as diffuse bilateral lung capacities on imaging with respiratory failure and diffuse alveolar damage (Fig. 15.13) [92]. *Aspergillus* spp. are the most frequent cause of fungal pneumonia during therapy for hematologic malignancies. Invasive aspergillosis is cause up to 70–90% of all fungal pneumonias followed by mucorales species [7]. Refer to Table 15.5 for HSCT and pulmonary complications.

Solid Organ Transplant Recipients and Pulmonary Infections

Patients with lung transplantation show the highest susceptibility to pneumonia among all solid organ transplant (SOT) patients [17]. Patterns of lung infections after SOT are summarized in Table 15.6.

AIDS and Pulmonary Infections

AIDS is due to infection by the HIV, and classically exposes the patient to infections normally resisted by cell-mediated immunity. Normal CXRs are common in HIV patients and hence chest CT should be considered for symptomatic HIV patients with a normal CXR [17]. The respiratory tract is the most common site of infection in patients infected with HIV (Table 15.7).

Refer to Table 15.8 for CT-based differential diagnosis of imaging findings in immunocompromised patients related to the AIDS and non-AIDS conditions.

Pneumocystis Jirovecii/Pneumocystis Carinii Pneumonia

All groups of immunocompromised patients with reduced cell-mediated immunity can get infected by *Pneumocystis carinii* protozoal infection. It is notably common in the AIDS patients and remains the most common opportunistic infection as well as the most frequent AIDS-defining diagnosis in the United States. In recent years, the rate of PJP has changed significantly in the west, with PJP becoming relatively less common as antibiotic prophylaxis was early used and wide availability of retroviral therapy [9].

Symptomatically, patients present with shortness of breath and dry cough, frequently accompanied by a pyrexia. In AIDS, although radiographic appearance can be common for up to 10% of patients early in the disease and the degree of dyspnea may precede the radiographic changes.

- Most patients will develop mid perihilar and upper zone bilateral reticular or interstitial or GGOs. This may rapidly progress to involve the entire lung
- On CT the characteristic appearances are of a GGO extending from the perihilar regions into the surrounding lung (Fig. 15.4), sporadically demonstrating a geographical pattern

TABLE 15.5 Hematopoietic Stem Cell Transplant (HSCT) and Pulmonary Complications

Time Elapsed Since Transplantation	0–30 Days (Neutropenic Phase/ Pre-Engraftment Period)	31–100 Days (Early Phase)	After 100 Days (Late Phase)
Immunity state	Severe neutropenia	Cellular and humoral immunity severely impaired	Immunosuppression recovery
Types of infection	Fungi (usually *Aspergillus*, candida, mucor): most common Bacteria: less common	CMV, RSV Fungi (*Aspergillus* and mucor) IPS PJP (uncommon)	Noninfection complications typically IPS BO OP GVHD: predisposing to bacterial infections, *Aspergillus*, mucor, and viral infection

BO, bronchiolitis obliterans; *CMV*, cytomegalovirus; *IPS*, idiopathic pneumonia syndrome; *PJP*, pneumocystis jirovecii; *OP*, organizing pneumonia.

TABLE 15.6 Solid Organ Transplant Recipients and Pulmonary Infections

Time Elapsed Since Transplantation	First Month	1–6 Months	After 6 Months
Immunity state	Effects of immunosuppression have not started	Significant impairment of the cellular immunity	Recovery of the immunosuppressed state
Causative organism or type of infection	**Nosocomial infection** (usually bacterial) Postoperative infection Aspiration pneumonia Ventilator-associated pneumonia Wound infection Catheter infection	**Opportunistic infections** Nocardia Viruses (particularly CMV) TB Fungi (*Aspergillus* and mucor) PJP IPS	Community-acquired pneumonia (usually bacterial)

CMV, cytomegalovirus; *IPS*, idiopathic pneumonia syndrome.

TABLE 15.7 Pulmonary Infections Seen In Acquired Immunodeficiency Syndrome (AIDS)/Human Immunodeficiency Virus

CD4 Lymphocyte Count	>200 Cells/mm^3	<200 Cells/mm^3	<100 Cells/mm^3
Type of infection, causative agents, or other diseases	MTB of lungs **Bacterial infections** *Streptococcus pneumoniae* *Haemophilus influenzae* *Staphylococcus aureus* *Pseudomonas aeruginosa* *Nocardia* Kaposi sarcoma	PJP *Toxoplasma gondii* Disseminated MTB	CMV (with <50 cells/mm^3) NTM (with <50 cells/mm^3) *Aspergillus* Cryptococcus Histoplasma *Toxoplasma gondii* Coccidioidomycosis, blastomycosis

CMV, cytomegalovirus; *MTB*, Mycobacterium tuberculosis; *NTM*, nontuberculous mycobacterial infections.

TABLE 15.8 CT-Based Differential Diagnosis of Imaging Findings In Immunocompromised (IC) Patients Related to AIDS, Non-AIDS Conditions

	INFECTIOUS DISEASES		NON-INFECTIOUS DISEASES	
CT Findings	AIDS	IC non-AIDS	AIDS	IC non-AIDS
Focal consolidative opacities	Bacterial pneumonia TB Fungal infection (particularly cryptococcosis)	Bacterial pneumonia TB Fungal infection	Lymphoma Kaposi sarcoma	Leukemia Lymphoma PTLD OP
Nodules or masses	Fungal infection (particularly cryptococcosis) Nocardiosis Septic emboli	Fungal infection Nocardiosis Septic emboli	Lymphoma Kaposi sarcoma	Leukemia Lymphoma PTLD
Small nodules/micronodules	Miliary TB Histoplasmosis	Miliary TB Viral pneumonia Candidiasis		Hematogenous metastasis
Diffuse ground-glass opacities/diffuse consolidation	PJP CMV pneumonia (in late stage)	PJP Viral pneumonia (particularly CMV)	Pulmonary edema	Pulmonary edema DAH Drug toxicity IPS

CMV, cytomegalovirus; *DAH*, diffuse alveolar hemorrhage; *GGO*, ground-glass opacity; *IPS*, idiopathic pneumonia syndrome; *PJP*, pneumocystis pneumonia; *PTLD*, post-transplant lymphoproliferative disorder; *TB*, tuberculosis.

- Diffuse GGO with an upper lobe distribution along with GGO with a mosaic attenuation pattern and crazy-paving pattern is also common [93]. GGOs are often more extensive and consolidation is more common in the non-AIDS immunocompromised patients compared with the AIDS patients [93]
- DAD is the next most common pathologic feature of *Pneumocystis carinii* pneumonia, particularly in the non-AIDS patients
- Pneumatocele/cyst are actually thin walled, but occasionally variable in size, shape, and wall thickness (Fig. 15.62) and can occur in one-third of cases [17]

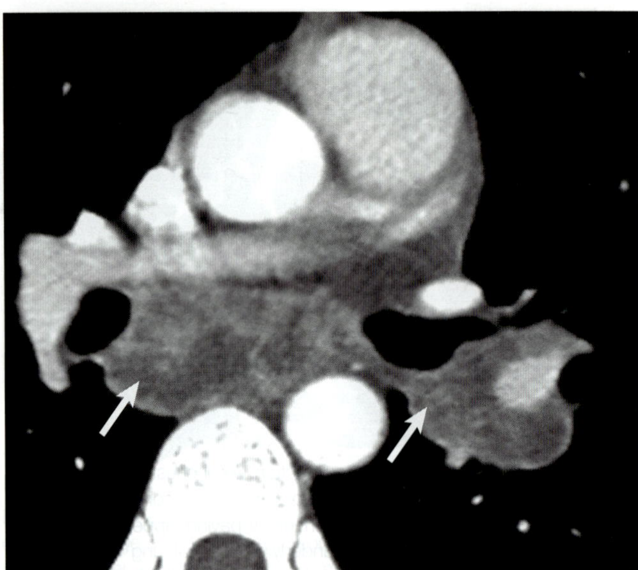

Figure 15.67 Immune reconstitution syndrome related to TB. Axial soft-tissue window chest CT image in a 38-year-old HIV-positive man with sputum cultures positive tuberculosis receiving therapy for both tuberculosis therapy and HARRT and increasing neck swelling and tenderness reveals multiple enlarged, necrotic, and confluent mediastinal and bilateral hilar lymph nodes. These findings are consistent with immune reconstitution inflammatory syndrome to tuberculosis.

Immune Reconstitution Inflammatory Syndrome (IRIS)

IRIS has feature of acute exacerbation of symptoms or paradoxical worsening of treated infections or initial expression of untreated infections during the initial months of highly active antiretroviral therapy due to inflammatory response to opportunistic pathogens. IRIS typically occurs in *Mycobacterium avium* complex infection which typically manifests as focal lymphadenitis without pulmonary lesions (Fig. 15.67). However, manifestations of IRIS may vary depending on the underlying opportunistic infection such as tuberculosis, nontuberculous mycobacteria infection, PJP, CMV, or herpes simplex virus [7,66,99].

Differential Diagnosis and Radiologic Approach to Infection-Related Various Nodules Based on the Type of Immunosuppression (AIDS versus Hematological Cell Transplant)

- Macronodules are typically related to TB, Cryptococcus, or *Nocardia* in AIDS while they are typically related to *Aspergillus* and mucormycosis in hematological cell transplant (HCT)
- Predominantly GGOs occur due to PJP pneumonia in AIDS while CMV is typical cause in HCT
- Tree-in-bud nodules typically occur due to bacterial infections and TB in AIDS while viruses such as RSV (Fig. 15.64) and parainfluenza are typical causes in HCT
- Perilymphatic nodules are typically seen due to Kaposi sarcoma and sarcoidosis in AIDS while these are rare in patients with HCT [3,4]

Suggested Readings

- P Armstrong, AG Wilson, P Dee, DM Hansell, AIDS and other forms of immunocompromise, in: Imaging of Diseases of the Chest, third ed., St Louis, Mosby–Year Book, 2000, pp. 255–304.
- P Armstrong, AG Wilson, P Dee, DM Hansell, Infections of the lung and pleural, in: Imaging of Diseases of the Chest, third ed., St Louis, Mosby–Year Book, 2000, pp. 163–254.
- YM Berkmen, Aspiration and inhalation pneumonias, Semin Roentgenol 15 (1980) 73–84.
- YM Berkmen, Uncommon acute bacterial pneumonias, Semin Roentgenol 15 (1980) 17–24.
- PC Goodman, Tuberculosis and AIDS, Radiol Clin North Am 33 (1995) 707–717.
- LR Goodman, CE Putman, Diagnostic imaging in acute cardiopulmonary disease, Clin Chest Med 5 (1984) 247–264.
- LB Haramati, ER Jenny-Avital, Approach to the diagnosis of pulmonary disease in patients infected with the human immunodeficiency virus, J Thorac Imag 13 (1998) 247–260.
- JE Kuhlman, Imaging pulmonary disease in AIDS: state of the art, Eur Radiol 9 (1999) 395–408.
- DD Maki, Pulmonary infections in HIV/AIDS, Semin Roentgenol 35 (2000) 124–139.
- PE Marik, Aspiration pneumonitis and aspiration pneumonia, New Engl J Med 344 (2001) 665–667.
- WF Dahnert, Radiology Review Manual, LWW, Wolters Kluwer N.V., 2017.
- S Digumarthy, S Abbara, J Chung, Problem Solving in Chest maging, Elsevier, 2019.
- WR Webb, CB Higgins, Thoracic Imaging: Pulmonary and Cardiovascular Radiology, Wolters Kluwer N.V., 2016.
- D Hansell, D Lynch, HP McAdams, A Bankier, Imaging of Diseases of the Chest, Mosby Elsevier, 2009.
- T Franquet, Imaging of community-acquired pneumonia, J Thorac Imaging, 33 (5) (2018) 282–294. doi: 10.1097/RTI.0000000000000347.
- G Mackenzie, The definition and classification of pneumonia. Pneumonia (Nathan) 8 (2016) 14. doi: 10.1186/s41479-016-0012-z.
- N Johansson, M Kalin, A Tiveljung-Lindell, CG Giske, J Hedlund, Etiology of community-acquired pneumonia: increased microbiological yield with new diagnostic methods, Clin Infect Dis 50 (2) (2010) 202–209. doi: 10.1086/648678.
- AM Gharib, EJ Stern, Radiology of pneumonia, Med Clin North Am 85 (6) (2001) 1461–1491, x. doi: 10.1016/s0025-7125 (05)70391-6.
- T Franquet, JH Chung, J Hodler, RA Kubik-Huch, GK von Schulthess, Imaging of pulmonary infection, in: Diseases of the Chest, Breast, Heart and Vessels 2019–2022: Diagnostic and Interventional Imaging [Internet], Cham, CH, Springer, 2019, Chapter 7.

16 Lung Tumors

BOJAN KOVACINA

Introduction

There are a large number of lung tumors. Although the great majority can be classified as benign or malignant, there are also tumors that remain indeterminate and premalignant. The diversity of lung neoplasms is due to many cell types located in lung parenchyma and airways.

Benign Lung Tumors

Hamartoma

Pathophysiology and clinical presentation: Hamartoma is the commonest benign tumor of the lung, representing three quarters of all benign lung neoplasms (Table 16.1). It consists of normal lung tissue, which has grown in a disorganized manner. Histologically, a hamartoma contains variable amount of cartilage, fat, smooth muscle, fibrous, and connective tissue. This tumor is rare in children and is commonly discovered in adults older than 50 years of age.

Hamartomas are generally asymptomatic, discovered incidentally and located in the periphery of the lung. However, 5–15% of hamartomas are endobronchial in location, and may cause symptoms due to bronchial obstruction, such as cough and shortness of breath.

Imaging features: Radiographically, a large percentage of hamartomas

- present as solitary peripheral pulmonary nodule or masse;
- typically range in size from 1 to 4 cm [1,2];
- are well circumscribed, round or oval in shape;
- have smooth or lobulated margins.

Internal calcification (usually of "popcorn" appearance) can be seen in 15–30% of cases on radiographs due to the presence of cartilage, seen more often on computed tomography (CT) scans (Fig. 16.1). *The CT scan also allows more effective detection of internal fat, which is considered pathognomonic for hamartoma.* Hamartomas may be multiple and usually grow slowly. They do not cavitate nor invade adjacent structures.

Chondroma

Pathophysiology and clinical presentation: Chondroma is another benign mesenchymal tumor and, by definition, purely consists of cartilage. Chondrosarcoma, its malignant counterpart, is extremely rare in the lungs. Chondroma may present as an endobronchial lesion and typically is asymptomatic. This entity is part of "Carney's triad," which consists of multiple lung chondromas, gastrointestinal stromal tumor, and extra-adrenal paraganglioma.

Imaging features: Radiologically, a chondroma may be difficult to differentiate from a hamartoma. It classically manifests as a small well-circumscribed nodule or mass, which may be peripheral or central/endobronchial in location [3]. Internal calcifications are seen in majority of cases and more commonly are smaller, punctate, and scaly in contrast to coarser calcifications of a hamartoma.

Lipoma

Pathophysiology and clinical presentation: Lipoma is a rare tumor consisting of adipose tissue. It is believed to originate from cells in central airways, and, therefore, commonly presents as a central endobronchial lesion. Lipoma occurs at any age. Its malignant counterpart, liposarcoma, is exceedingly rare. Given its common endobronchial location, a lipoma may cause obstructive signs and symptoms when symptomatic.

Imaging features: Lipoma is usually homogeneous in appearance and should not contain internal calcification or cavitation. The commonest radiological presentation consists of fat-density, well-circumscribed, central, or endobronchial lesion [2]. It may present with associated postobstructive pneumonitis, atelectasis, and bronchiectasis if large enough to cause airway obstruction.

TABLE 16.1 Benign Lung Tumors
Hamartoma
Chondroma
Lipoma
Leiomyoma
Papilloma
Pulmonary inflammatory pseudotumor
Adenoma
Fibroma
Myxoma
Benign clear cell tumor
Glomus tumor
Neurogenic tumor
Hemangiopericytoma
Lymphangioma
Bronchogenic cyst

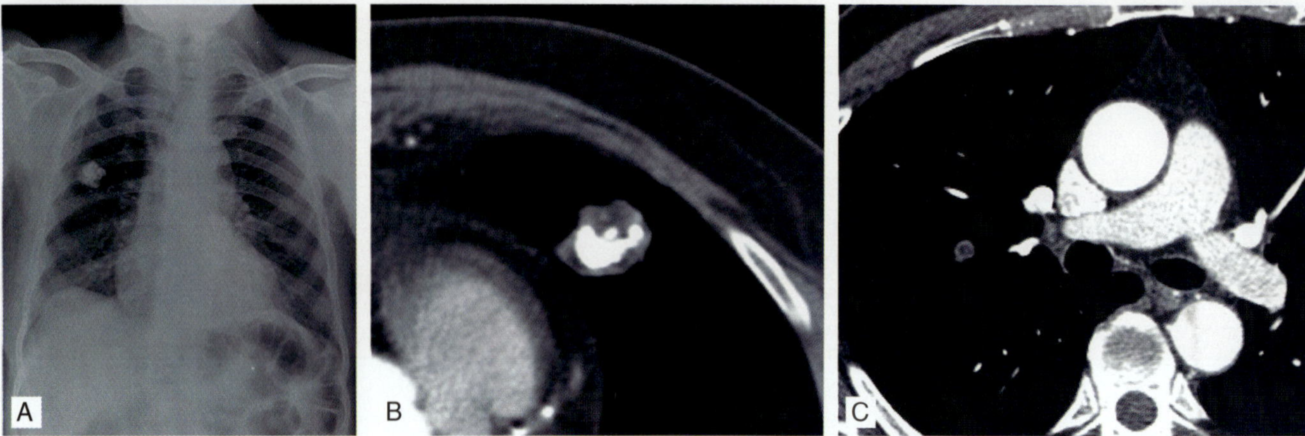

Figure 16.1 Chest radiograph (A) demonstrates well-defined right mid zone nodule with popcorn calcifications, consistent with pulmonary hamartoma. The CT scans of two different patients showing lobulated well-circumscribed 2.3-cm nodule in the lingula containing popcorn-like calcification (B) and well-circumscribed 9-mm nodule in the RUL (C) containing internal fat.

Leiomyoma

Pathophysiology and clinical presentation: Leiomyoma is a tumor of smooth muscle, and is believed to originate in the wall of peripheral airways or vessels. Parenchymal leiomyoma is usually peripheral in location and asymptomatic. In women with known uterine smooth muscle tumor, multiple scattered pulmonary leiomyomas can be seen. In this context, these are commonly called metastases, even if uterine tumor is considered benign (so-called "benign metastasizing fibroid/leiomyoma") [4].

Imaging features: Radiologically, leiomyomas present as round, small (less than 2 cm) well-circumscribed peripheral nodules, which do not cavitate and rarely calcify. When central and endobronchial in location, they may cause obstructive pneumonitis or atelectasis.

Papilloma

Pathophysiology and clinical presentation: Papilloma is caused by excessive and abnormal proliferation of stratified squamous cells. It usually presents with polypoid nodule or mass in the airway lumen. The most common locations are the larynx and upper trachea. Involvement of main bronchi and distal airways is rare (1–5%) and, if present, usually is multifocal, called laryngotracheobronchial papillomatosis. Distal disseminated parenchymal papillomas tend to be asymptomatic and require no specific treatment. Laryngeal and tracheal papilloma

- is commonly caused by subtypes of human papillomavirus;
- causes symptoms due to airway obstruction, such as wheezing, stridor, and cough;
- may present with hemoptysis;
- needs to be endoscopically resected if large;
- has propensity to reoccur;
- has a small risk of malignant transformation to squamous cell carcinoma.

Imaging features: Radiologically, laryngeal and tracheobronchial papillomas present as polypoid endoluminal nodules or masses [5]. Papillomatosis manifests as diffuse 1–5 mm nodules along the airway walls and scattered parenchymal nodules of variable size [6]. Nodules commonly demonstrate internal cavitation and can grow to become thin- or thick-walled cysts and irregular cavities (Fig. 16.2). Infrequently, these lesions may contain air-fluid levels if superinfected.

Pulmonary Inflammatory Pseudotumor

Pathophysiology and clinical presentation: Pulmonary pseudotumor encompasses a variety of pathological processes, explaining different names given to this entity in the literature. Such processes include

- plasma cell granuloma;
- mast cell granuloma;
- inflammatory myofibroblastic tumor;
- xanthoma;
- histiocytoma.

Pseudotumor is more common in adolescents, and usually is unifocal. Previous infection, trauma, and inflammation are believed to act as precipitating factors in some cases. Patients are typically asymptomatic. If endobronchial, a pseudotumor may cause symptoms of airway obstruction. Given that differential diagnosis includes more aggressive neoplasms, histological correlation is

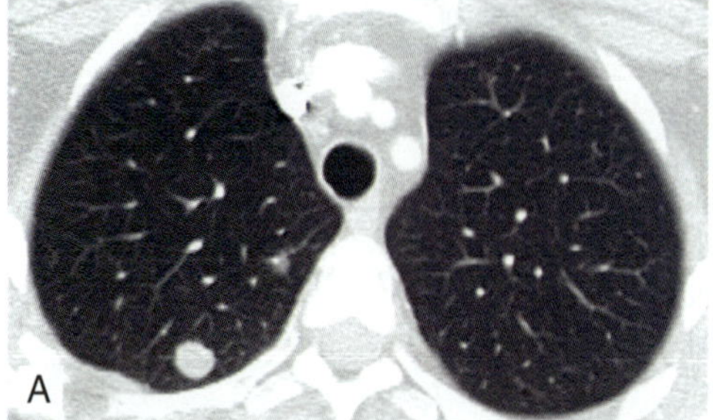

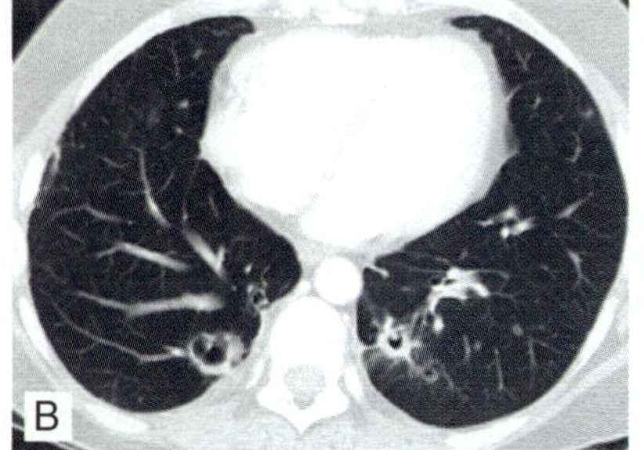

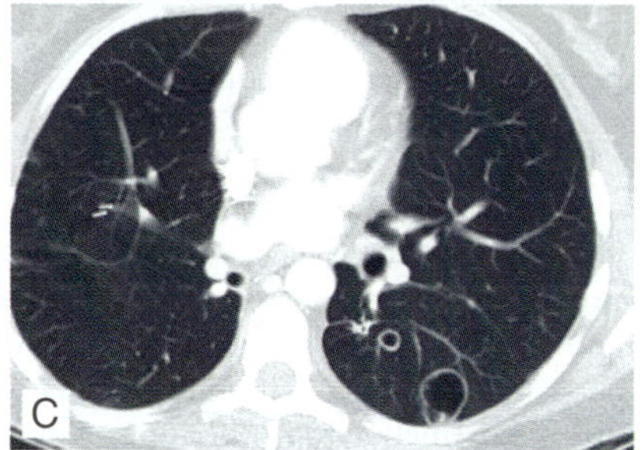

Figure 16.2 Papillomatosis. Three CT images (A, B, and C) demonstrate scattered bilateral pulmonary solid and cavitary nodules in a patient with known laryngeal papilloma (not shown).

usually required. Surgical excision is performed for large or symptomatic lesions.

Imaging features: Radiographically, pulmonary pseudotumor primarily presents as a single nodule of variable size, with slight lower lobe predilection [7]. The CT scan may additionally detect internal calcifications in about 20% of cases. Calcifications may be amorphous, mixed, fine, or dystrophic. Although commonly well defined, pseudotumors may demonstrate irregular or spiculated borders due to adjacent inflammation, which renders its differentiation from a malignant process more difficult.

Other Benign Tumors of the Lung

Other rarer benign tumors encountered in the lung typically present as nonspecific small parenchymal nodule. These include: adenoma, fibroma, myxoma, benign clear cell tumor, neurogenic tumor, glomus tumor, hemangiopericytoma, lymphangioma, and bronchogenic cyst. The last two entities may demonstrate detectable homogeneous fluid density on the CT scan if large enough, which helps differentiating them from solid entities [8].

Approach to Pulmonary Nodule

Pulmonary nodule is characterized as a focal well defined, oval, or round opacity measuring less than 3 cm in size. It represents a common challenging clinical problem because

1. it is usually discovered incidentally, and
2. its nature cannot be often definitely determined at the time of imaging presentation.

The main challenge usually is to differentiate benign versus malignant (primary lung cancer or metastasis) nature of the nodule. Some clinical parameters may help in this task, particularly age and known risk factors. For example, small well-circumscribed nodules in patients younger than 35 years without history of malignancy are commonly considered as benign and require no further investigation. Small nodules (less than 6 mm in size) also do not require further follow-up or investigation in patients without known malignancy and without risk factors for lung cancer [9]. *Several imaging characteristics are used to further attempt resolving this clinical dilemma. These include:*

- Growth rate: absolute stability in size for over 2 years and rapid doubling in size (in less than 3 weeks) are diagnostic of benign process [10]
- Internal calcifications: diffuse, central, popcorn, and laminar calcifications are considered benign patterns of calcifications in a nodule. In contrast, stippled and eccentric calcifications raise a concern for malignancy
- Internal fat: the presence of identifiable internal fat usually suggests benign process
- Shape and contour: irregular shape and spiculated contour are usually seen with primary malignant nodule. Triangular or lentiform nodule with smooth contours in perifissural/subpleural location is diagnostic of benign intrapulmonary lymph node
- Density: Solitary pulmonary nodule can be of solid, part-solid, and pure groundglass density. Persistent part-solid/part-groundglass nodule is almost invariably within the spectrum of primary adenocarcinoma, as described in following sections. Pure groundglass nodule is considered benign if less than 6 mm

The vast majority of incidentally found pulmonary nodules are discovered on CT scans. Several guidelines have been issued to render their diagnostic workup the most efficient and least costly possible. *The most widely used such guidelines are Fleischner Society guidelines for follow-up and investigation of solid, partly solid, and groundglass nodules* [11,12] (Table 16.2). These can be applied to all individuals except those <35 years of age or immunocompromised patients or those with a known or suspected malignancy. These guidelines also recommend that the follow-up CT scans are obtained with thin slices (less than 1.5 mm) to optimize comparison and interval growth detection.

Malignant Lung Tumors

Lung Cancer

Epidemiology

Lung cancer is the commonest cancer in men and the second commonest cancer in women (after breast cancer). Despite recent advances in prevention, detection, and management, it remains the commonest cause of death from cancer in both men and women. Most cases occur between fourth and seventh decades of life.

TABLE 16.2 Fleischner Society Guidelines for Management of Incidentally Detected Pulmonary Nodules

	SINGLE		MULTIPLE		COMMENTS
Solid Nodules	**Low Risk**	**High Risk**	**Low Risk**	**High Risk**	
< 6 mm	None	Consider 6–12 month	None	consider 6–12 month	If suspicious morphology or in upper lobes then 12 month
6–8 mm	6–12 month, then consider 18–24 month	6–12 month + 18–24 month	3–6 month, then consider 18–24 month	3–6 month + 18–24 month	When multiple, the most suspicious nodule guides the management
> 8 mm	Consider 3 month or Positron emission tomography (PET)/CT or biopsy	Consider 3 month or PET/CT or biopsy	3–6 month, then consider 18–24 month	3–6 month + 18–24 month	
	SINGLE		MULTIPLE		COMMENTS
Subsolid Nodules	**Groundglass**	**Partly Solid**			
< 6 mm	None	None	3–6 month; if stable consider every 2 yrs		If suspicious morphology of GG nodule < 6 mm, consider follow-up in 2 and 4 yrs
> 6 mm	6–12 month; if persistent then every 2 yrs	3–6 month; if stable then every 1 yr	3–6 month + based on the most suspicious		Highly suspicious if persistent and solid component >6 mm

Modified from: H MacMahon, D Naidich, J Goo, et al., Guidelines for management of incidental pulmonary nodules detected on CT images: from the Fleischner Society 2017, Radiology 284 (1) (2017) 228–243.

TABLE 16.3 Risk Factors for Lung Cancer

Risk Factors for Lung Cancer
Age
Tobacco
Occupational exposure
Asbestos
Arsenic
Nickel
Beryllium
Mustard gas
Radon
Chromium
Pesticides
Underlying lung disease
Emphysema
Idiopathic pulmonary fibrosis
Scleroderma
Genetic mutations
EGFR
ALK
ROS1
BRAF

In addition to increasing age, several other risk factors for lung cancer have been identified over the years (Table 16.3). The most important independent factor is cigarette smoking. A few underlying lung diseases have been proved to be associated with higher risk for lung cancer, including focal or diffuse fibrotic interstitial lung disease, and chronic obstructive pulmonary disease/emphysema. Occupational exposure to various substances and chemicals is another recognized independent risk factor, with asbestos being the commonest one. Other occupational agents that increase the risk of lung cancer include: arsenic, nickel, chromium, mustard gas, pesticides, and radon. Exposure to radioactivity is a known environmental risk factor. Finally, genetic predispositions have recently been associated with increased risk of lung cancer, particularly some specific oncogenes, enzyme defects, and Human Leucocyte antigen (HLA) antigens.

TABLE 16.4 Classification of Lung Cancers

Classification of Lung Cancers
Small-cell carcinoma
Non–small-cell carcinoma
Squamous cell carcinoma
Adenocarcinoma
Large-cell carcinoma
Adenosquamous carcinoma
Carcinosarcoma
Spindle cell carcinoma

Pathological Types

Lung cancer is divided into small-cell lung cancer (SCLC) and non–small-cell lung cancer (NCSLC) (Table 16.4). These two groups tend to have different behavior, treatment, and prognosis.

- SCLC is considered to originate from neuroendocrine cells in airways and has the strongest relation to smoking among all lung cancers. *It is typically aggressive, centrally located, associated with intrathoracic lymphadenopathy, and has propensity for early metastasis.* SCLC is radiosensitive and usually is treated with combined chemo-radiotherapy (Fig. 16.3)
- NSCLC is considered less aggressive than SCLC and is typically treated with surgical excision in early stages (Fig. 16.4 and 16.5). It accounts for 75–80% of all lung cancers [13]. NSCLC consists of three main types: squamous cell carcinoma, adenocarcinoma, and large-cell carcinoma. Some rare lung cancers have a mixed pattern/appearance, such as adenosquamous carcinomas and carcinomas with sarcomatoid features
  - Squamous cells carcinoma is strongly related to smoking and tends to be more central in location. It demonstrates internal cavitation more often than other NSCLC types. Although it can be locally invasive, it tends to metastasize relatively late in its course (Fig. 16.6)

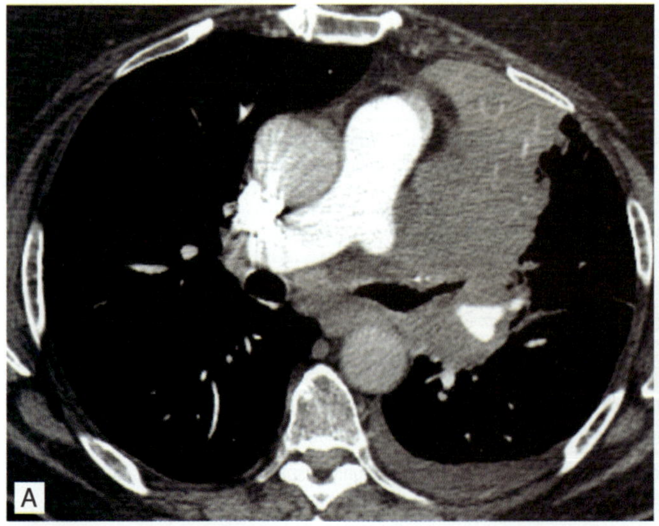

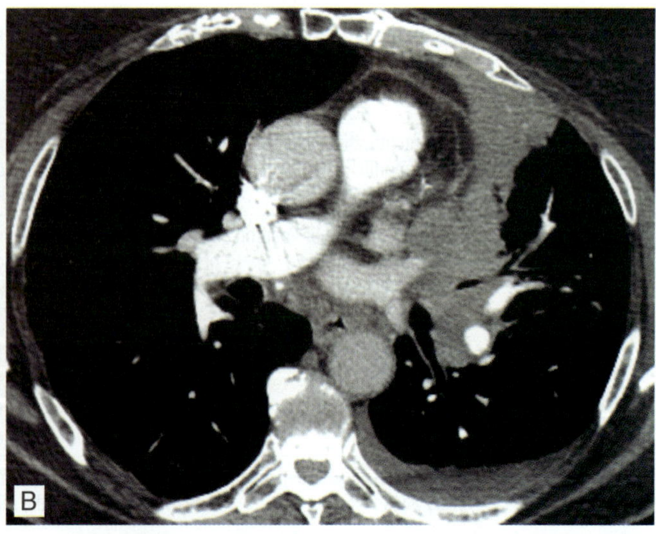

Figure 16.3 Small-cell lung cancer. Two CT images of the same patient (A and B) demonstrate a left hilar mass that is confluent with hilar lymphadenopathy, causing occlusion of the left upper lobar bronchus and complete collapse of the LUL. Additional encasement of the left pulmonary artery and malignant left pleural effusion.

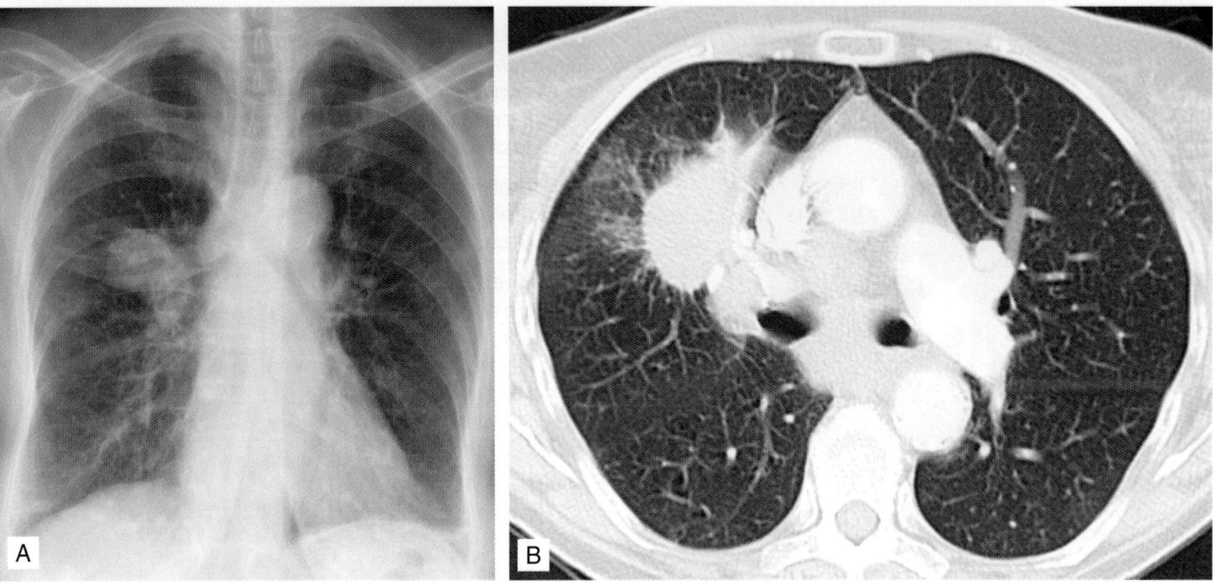

Figure 16.4 Non–small-cell lung cancer. Chest radiograph (A) and CT image (B) of the same patient demonstrate an irregular mass with spiculated contours in perihilar region of the right upper lobe.

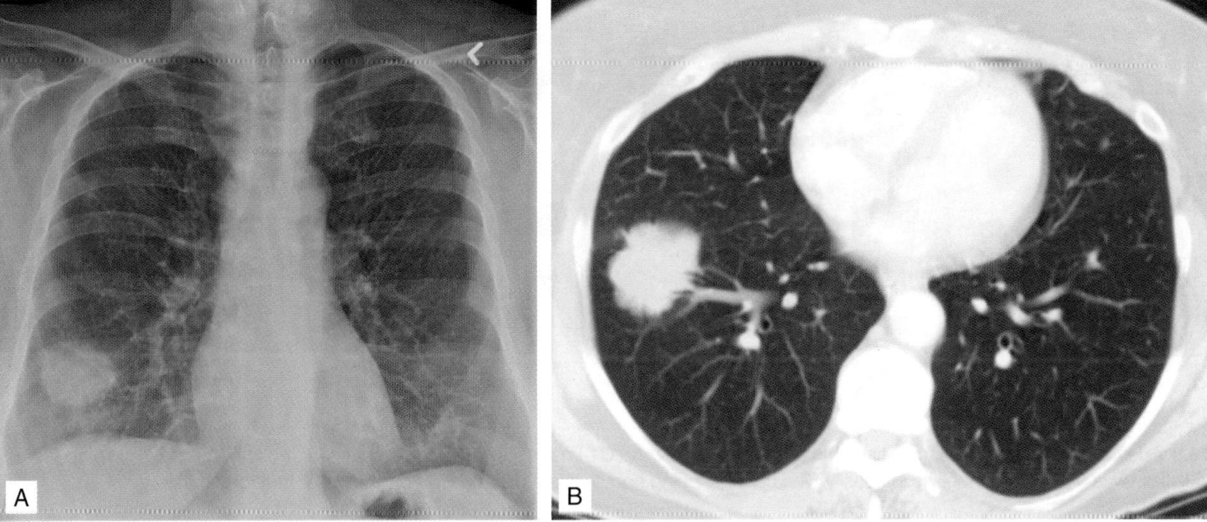

Figure 16.5 Non–small-cell lung cancer. Lobulated irregular mass in the anterior segment of the right lower lobe.

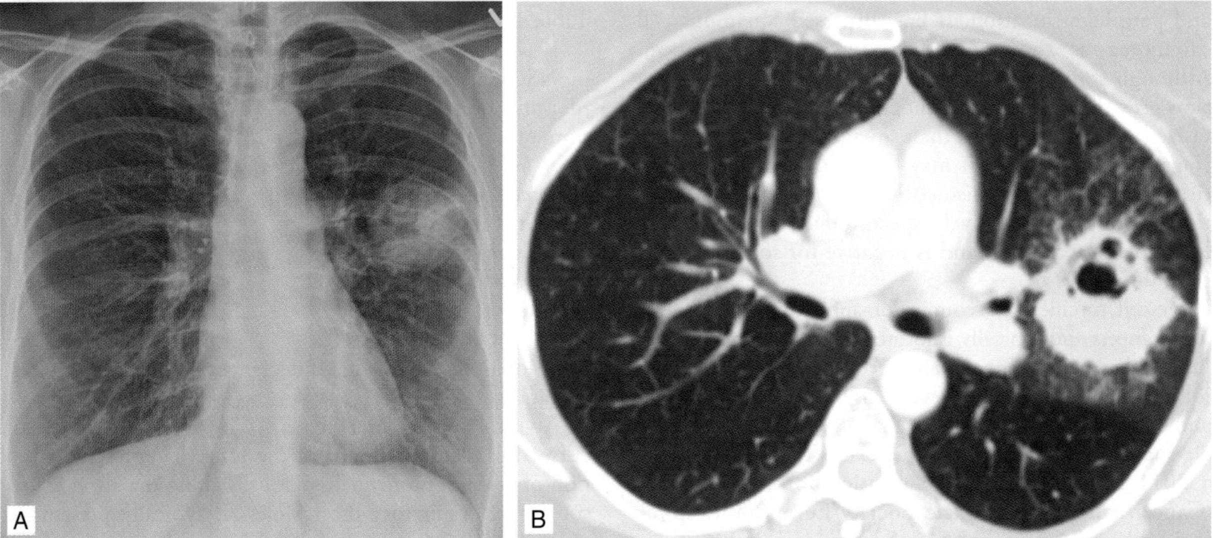

Figure 16.6 Squamous cell carcinoma. Chest radiograph (A) and CT image (B) show a large irregular mass with internal cavitation in the apicoposterior segment of the LUL.

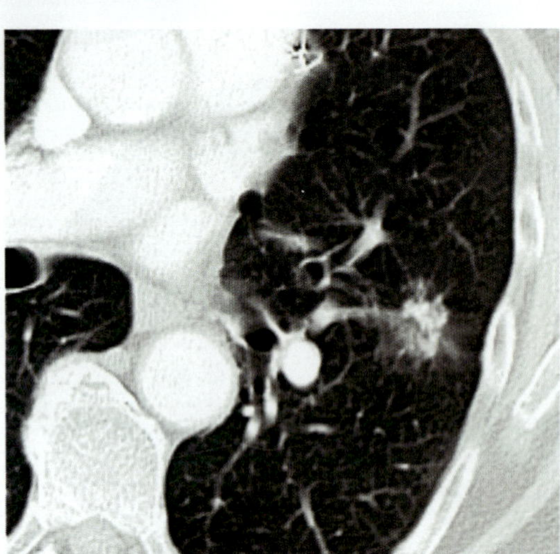

Figure 16.7 Adenocarcinoma of the lung. Part-solid and part-groundglass irregular spiculated nodule in the left lower lobe.

TABLE 16.5 Subtypes of Adenocarcinoma of the Lung

Subtypes
Adenocarcinoma *in situ*
Nonmucinous
Mucinous
Minimally invasive adenocarcinoma
Nonmucinous
Mucinous
Invasive adenocarcinoma
Lepidic predominant
Acinar predominant
Papillary predominant
Micropapillary predominant
Solid predominant
Variants of invasive adenocarcinoma
Mucinous
Colloid
Fetal
Enteric

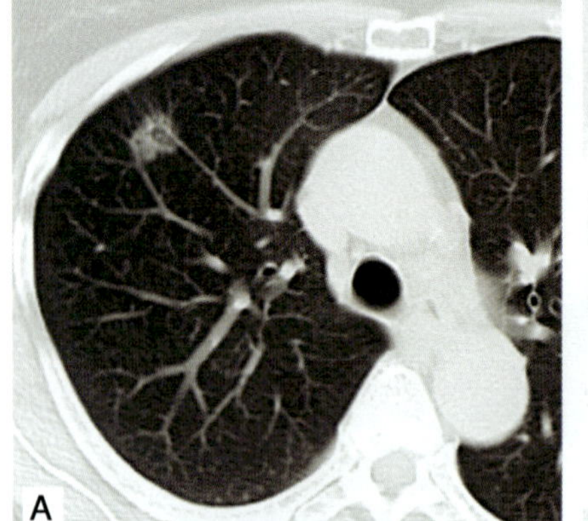

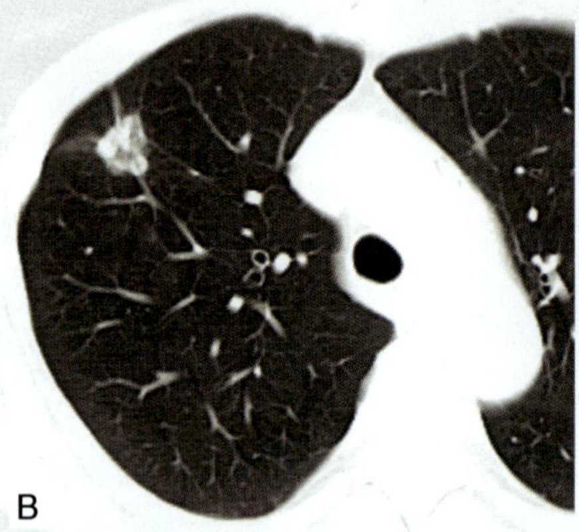

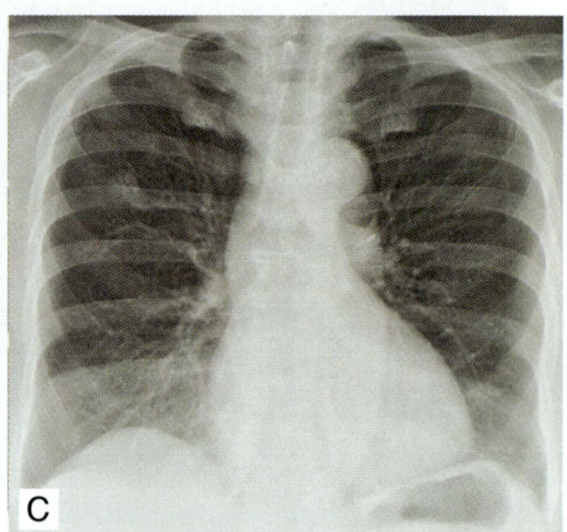

Figure 16.8 Adenocarcinoma of the lung. Initial CT image (A) and follow-up CT image (B) of the same patient demonstrate a slow-growing nodule in the RUL that initially was entirely groundglass in density. The corresponding nodule is seen in the RUL on the chest radiograph (C).

- Adenocarcinoma is typically encountered in upper lobes and peripheral location. It has surpassed squamous cell carcinoma as the commonest type of lung cancer. Although some of its subtypes are associated with very slow growth, an invasive adenocarcinoma tends to metastasize earlier in its course than squamous cells carcinoma (Figs. 16.7 and 16.8). It may be multifocal at presentation (Fig. 16.9). On histopathology, thyroid transcription factor-1 is a relatively specific marker for primary lung adenocarcinoma, and is negative for squamous cell carcinomas
- Large-cell carcinoma accounts for approximately 10% of lung cancers and typically is located in the periphery of the lung. It has poor prognosis and relatively aggressive behavior, manifested by rapid growth, large size at presentation, and early metastasis

Multiple subtypes of adenocarcinoma exist. These were classified in 2011 by International Association for the Study of Lung Cancer/American Thoracic Society/European Respiratory Society based on pathological/histological architecture, degree of invasion and mucin production (Fig. 16.10 and Table 16.5) [14].

Recently, several key driving genetic mutations were identified in NSCLC, particularly adenocarcinomas [15,16] (Fig. 16.11). Identification of such mutations allows for better prognostication and, particularly, specific targeted therapies. *Current mutations for which approved targeted therapies exist with improved outcomes are*

- EGFR mutation;
- ALK rearrangement;
- ROS1 rearrangement;
- BRAF mutation;
- NTRK gene fusions.

Additional therapies are under investigation for several other mutations.

Atypical adenomatous hyperplasia (AAH) is considered a precursor for adenocarcinoma of the lung. It represents a proliferation of atypical bronchoalveolar cells along the alveolar walls and sometimes respiratory bronchioles. It typically presents as pure groundglass nodule of less than 1 cm in size (often less than

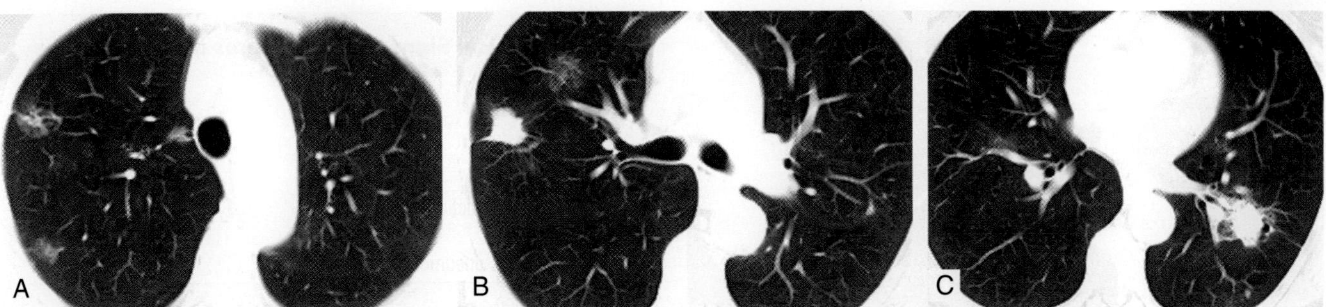

Figure 16.9 Multifocal adenocarcinoma of the lung. Three CT images (A, B, and C) of the same patient demonstrate multiple irregular nodules that are groundglass, part-solid, or solid in density.

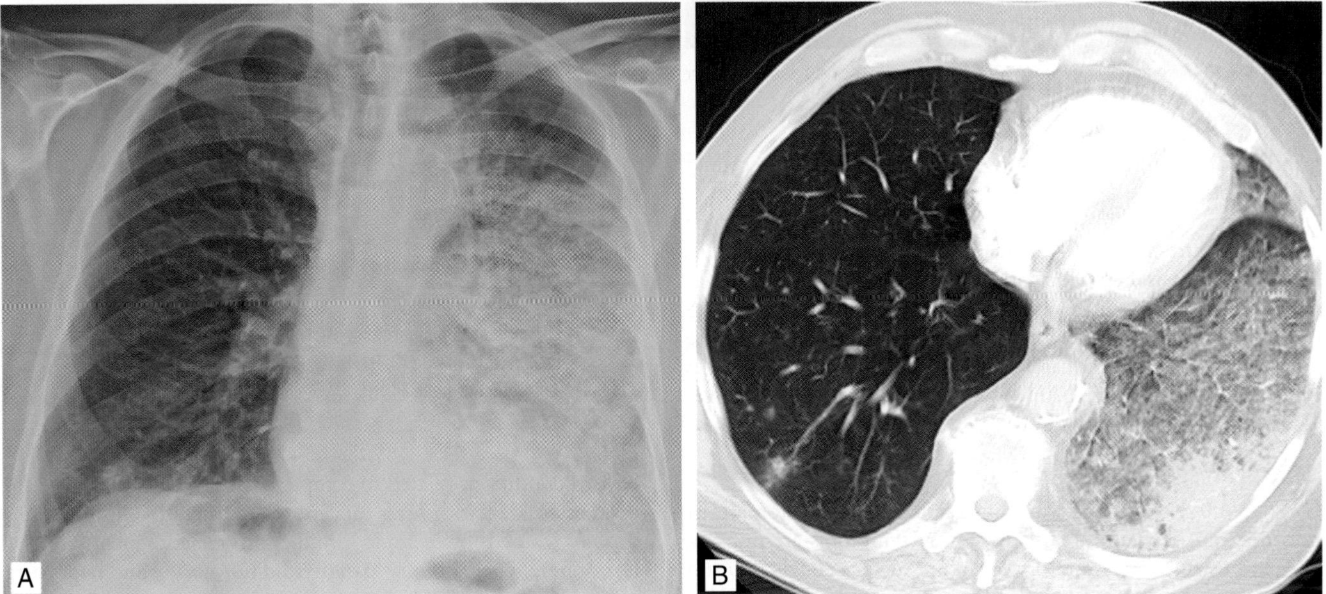

Figure 16.10 Invasive mucinous adenocarcinoma. Chest radiograph (A) and CT image (B) of the same patient demonstrate a diffuse groundglass and dense consolidation in the LLL and lingula. Additional small focus in the posterior segment of RLL.

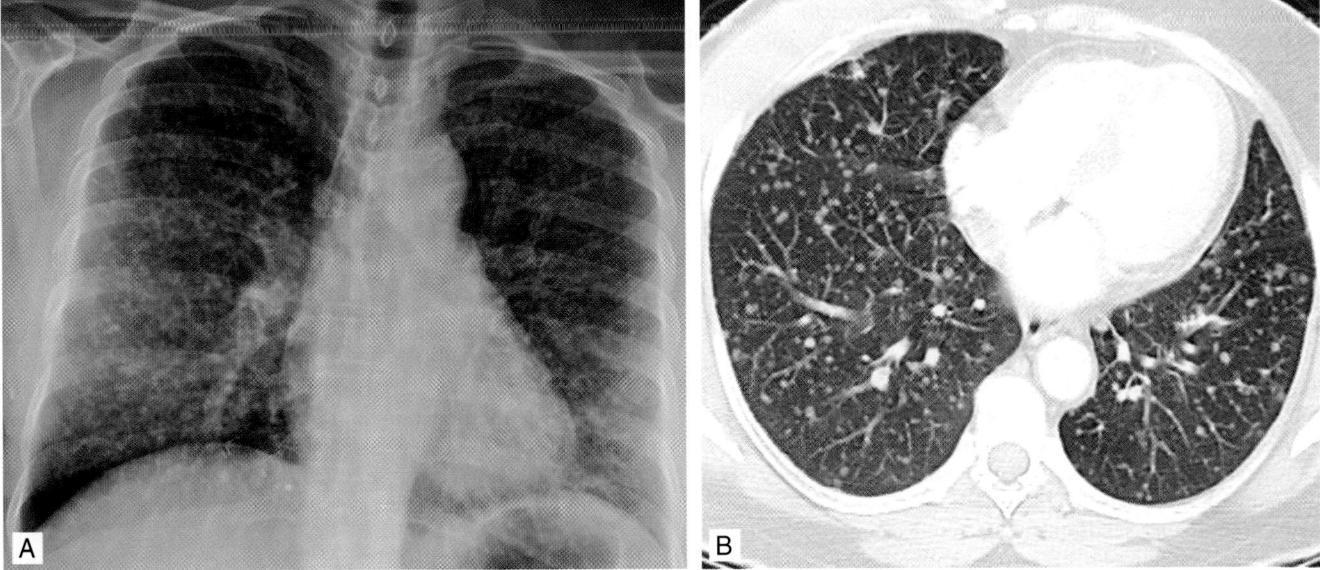

Figure 16.11 EGFR-positive adenocarcinoma of the lung. Chest radiograph (A) and CT image (B) of the same patient show innumerable scattered bilateral pulmonary nodules without dominant mass.

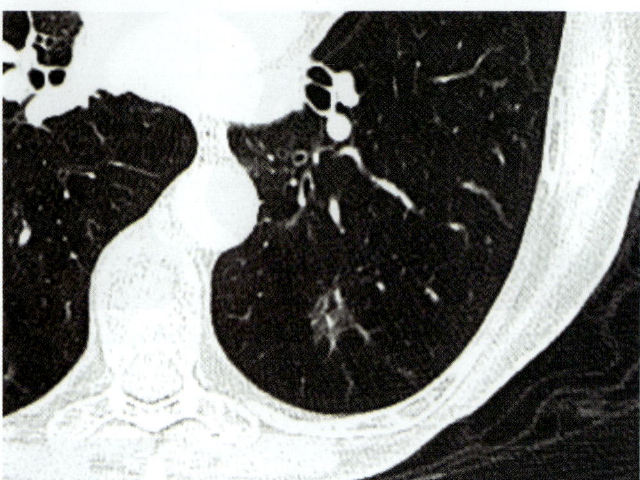

Figure 16.12 Adenocarcinoma in situ. Purely groundglass irregular 1.2-cm nodule in the posterior segment of the LLL.

5 mm). When multiple, AAH has higher frequency of preceding malignancies [17].

Adenocarcinoma in situ (AIS) is recognized as a second type of precursor lesion for lung adenocarcinoma. In contrary to AAH, AIS consists of neoplastic cells that grow along alveolar wall without destroying it or invading it (lepidic growth). AIS was part of conditions that previously were grouped under the label of bronchoalveolar carcinoma [14]. Radiographically, it is undistinguishable from AAH, except that it is commonly over 1 cm in size (Fig. 16.12).

Clinical Presentation

Only 10–20% of patients with lung cancer are asymptomatic at presentation. The commonest presenting symptoms are nonspecific and usually are respiratory in nature such as cough, sputum production, shortness of breath, hemoptysis, and chest pain/discomfort (Table 16.6). Larger central cancers may present with symptoms of major airway obstruction, particularly wheezing and postobstructive pneumonitis/pneumonia.

Locally invasive neoplasms can cause

- hoarseness (if recurrent laryngeal nerve is invaded);
- pleuritic chest pain (pleura, pericardium, or chest wall invasion);
- superior vena cava (SVC) syndrome (SVC compression/invasion);
- dyspnea from diaphragmatic paralysis (phrenic nerve invasion);
- dysphagia (esophageal invasion);
- chylothorax (thoracic duct invasion);
- local or referred neuropathic pain (brachial plexus invasion in context of superior sulcus tumors);
- Horner's syndrome (sympathetic chain invasion).

Rarely, patients may present with cerebral infarcts when cancer invades pulmonary veins and/or left atrium.

Various *paraneoplastic syndromes* are associated with lung cancer. These may rarely precede respiratory findings:

- Hypertrophic pulmonary osteoarthropathy: smooth periosteal reaction along long appendicular bones that is usually associated with bone pain
- Neuromuscular syndromes, as a result of immunologic reaction and production of various antibodies: Eaton–Lambert syndrome, visual paraneoplastic syndrome, limbic encephalitis, and peripheral neuropathy
- Migrating thrombophlebitis and clubbing

TABLE 16.6 Clinical Signs and Symptoms of Lung Cancer

Respiratory
Cough
Dyspnea
Hemoptysis
Sputum production
Wheezing
Obstructive pneumonia/pneumonitis
Local invasion
Pleuritic chest pain
Hoarseness
SVC syndrome
Dysphagia
Chylothorax
Pleural effusion
Horner's syndrome
Neuropathic pain
Paraneoplastic syndromes
Hypertrophic pulmonary osteoarthropathy
Eaton–Lambert syndrome
Limbic encephalitis
Clubbing
Migratory thrombophlebitis
Ectopic hormone production
Adrenocorticotropic hormone (ACTH)
Parathyroid hormone (PTH)
Antidiuretic hormone (ADH)

Several conditions related to ectopic hormone secretion have also been associated with lung cancers. These include Cushing's syndrome (caused by ectopic production of adrenocorticotropic hormone), hypercalcemia (parathyroid hormone), and hyponatremia (antidiuretic hormone).

Finally, lung cancer may sometimes present with signs and symptoms caused by distant metastasis. Adrenal gland is the commonest location of lung cancer metastasis (up to 60% of SCLC). *It is worth noting that in a lung cancer patient, a small adrenal mass is still statistically more likely to be an adenoma than a metastatic deposit.* Brain/central nervous system is another common place for lung cancer metastasis, shown to be involved in 3% of NCLC and 12% of SCLC asymptomatic patients.

The chest CT scans have been demonstrated to reduce mortality from lung cancer in high-risk former or current smokers. *Studies demonstrated up to 20% decrease in mortality rate with screening by annual low-dose CT scans of patients who are 55–80 years of age and have 30 or more packs per year smoking history (currently smoking or stopped smoking within the past 15 years)* [18]. Parameters of screening CTs are usually optimized to keep the dose to the patient as low as reasonably achievable. The screening CT scans is reported using the structured reporting system, Lung-RADS (Lung CT Screening Reporting and Data), whose purpose is to standardize interpretation and management recommendations [19]. Six Lung-RADS assessment categories reflect similar management guidelines to those issued by Fleischner Society for incidental pulmonary nodules.

Radiological Presentation

Nodule/Mass: Adenocarcinoma is the commonest type of lung cancer that presents with peripheral pulmonary nodule/mass, followed by large-cell carcinoma (Fig. 16.13). Several imaging

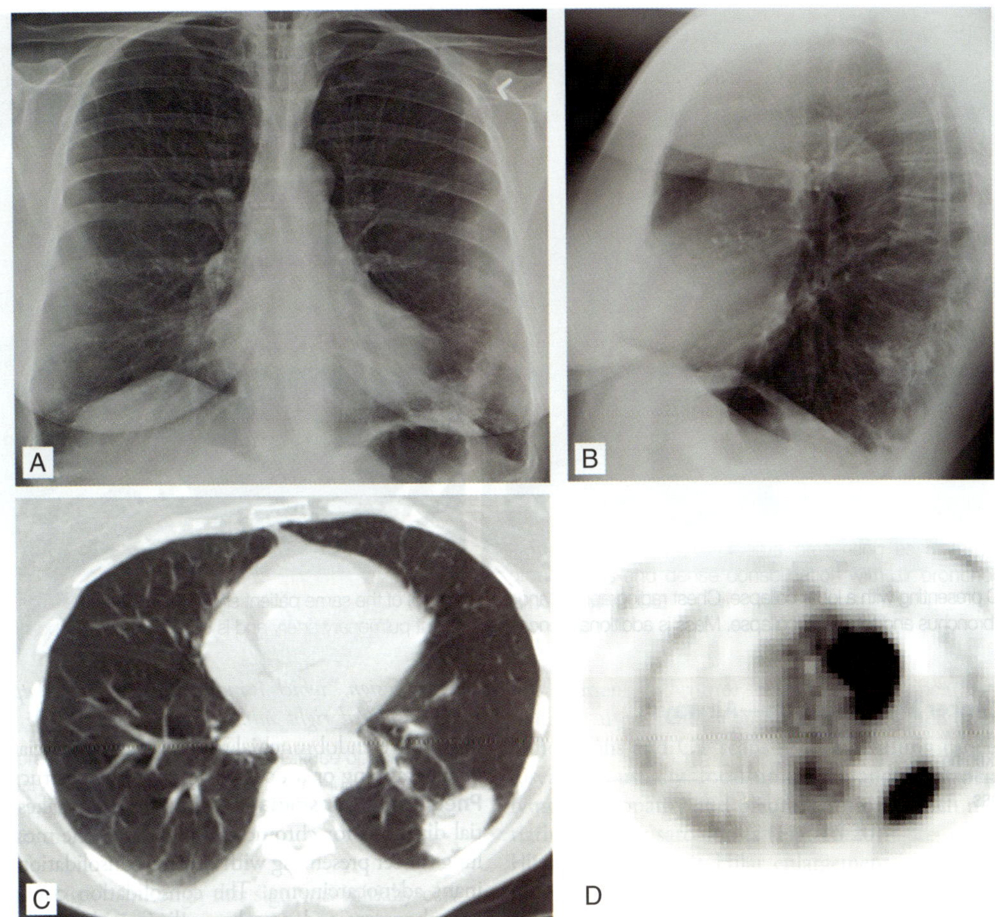

Figure 16.13 NSCLC presenting as a mass. Irregular mass in the posterior segment of the LLL on the chest radiograph (A and B) and CT scan (C), which was FDG positive on the PET scan (D).

characteristics of the nodule/mass raise a concern for malignancy [20,21], such as irregular shape, spiculated borders, large size and part-solid and part-solid density of the lesion. Cavitation with irregular thick wall is another sign of lung cancer, more commonly squamous cell carcinoma (Table 16.7). Other differentiating imaging characteristics between benign and malignant nodules were discussed in the section on solitary pulmonary nodule.

Airway: Airway involvement by lung cancer is common, particularly if cancer is central in location. By frequency, segmental bronchi are most commonly involved, followed by lobar and main bronchi. Irregular focal bronchial wall thickening, polypoid or sessile endobronchial mass, tapering of bronchial lumen, and sudden cutoff of the bronchial lumen are all radiological signs concerning for endobronchial lung cancer (Fig. 16.14 and Table 16.8).

TABLE 16.7 Lung Cancer Manifestation—Solitary Pulmonary Nodule
Irregular shape
Spiculated contours
Over 2 cm in size
Lack of satellite nodules
Eccentric calcification
Cavitation without air-fluid levels
Rapid growth (doubling in size in 1–48 months)

In addition, narrowing and occlusion of the affected airway by a growing tumor usually causes some degree of impaired aeration of distal lung parenchyma, ranging from subsegmental atelectasis to entire lung collapse depending on the level of obstruction (Figs. 16.15–16.17). *Large right central perihilar cancers associated with complete collapse of the right upper lobe characteristically cause the*

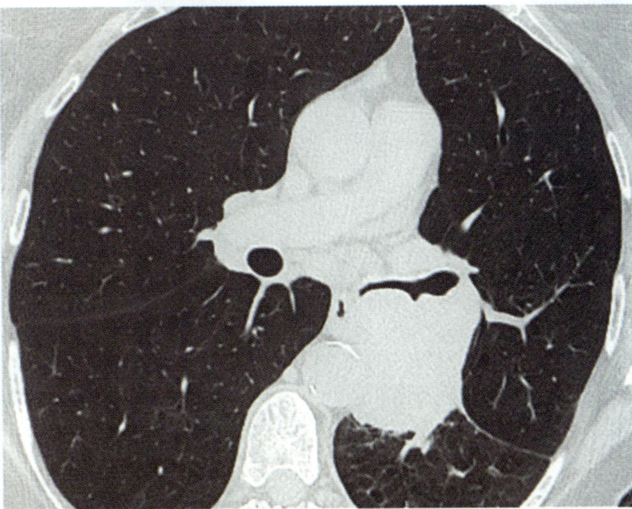

Figure 16.14 NSCLC presenting as an endobronchial mass. Large mass with endobronchial component, occluding the LLL superior segmental bronchus.

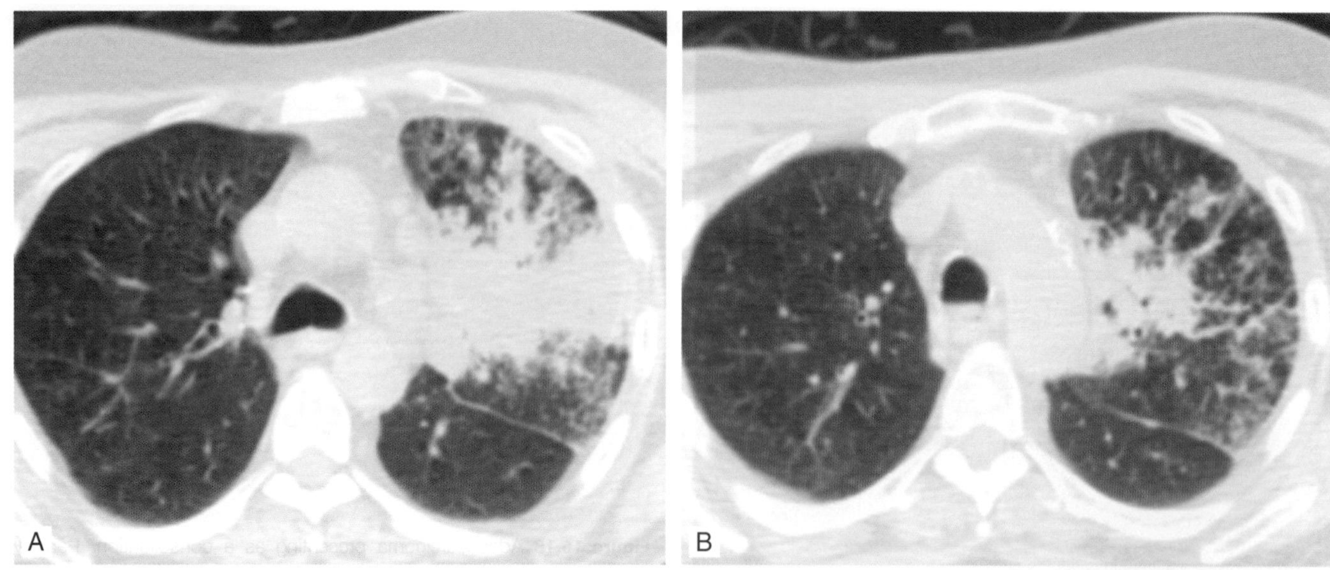

Figure 16.20 SCLC with lymphangitic carcinomatosis. Two CT images demonstrate a large left perihilar mass with LUL nodular interlobular septal thickening and peribronchovascular opacities.

- commonly invades adjacent structures at presentation, such as pleura, ribs, vertebrae, brachial plexus, cervical sympathetic chain, and axillary/subclavian vessels;
- has broad clinical presentation ranging from local pain in the upper back/lower neck to referred neurogenic pain in the upper extremity and Horner's syndrome (ptosis, myosis, and anhidrosis);
- radiographically commonly presents with obvious mass in lung apex, although not infrequently only a subtle asymmetric apical opacity may be seen.

The CT scan allows better delineation of the tumor and exact degree of local invasion [25] (Fig. 16.22). Treatment generally consists of chemotherapy and radiation; additional radical surgical resection is reserved for select cases with local invasion. Invasion of vertebrae, major vessels, and brachial plexus usually precludes surgical intervention.

Pleural Involvement: Pleural involvement by lung cancer ranges from simple benign reactive pleural effusion to direct invasion of the pleura and malignant pleural effusions (Table 16.10). Pleural effusion is seen in 2–23% of patients with lung cancer and may be caused by several different mechanisms [13,20]:

1. Sympathetic response to the tumor
2. Reactive response to postobstructive pneumonia/pneumonitis
3. Lymphatic congestion by tumor invasion of lymphatic channels or by hilar metastatic lymphadenopathy
4. Direct pleural invasion
5. Distinct pleural metastasis

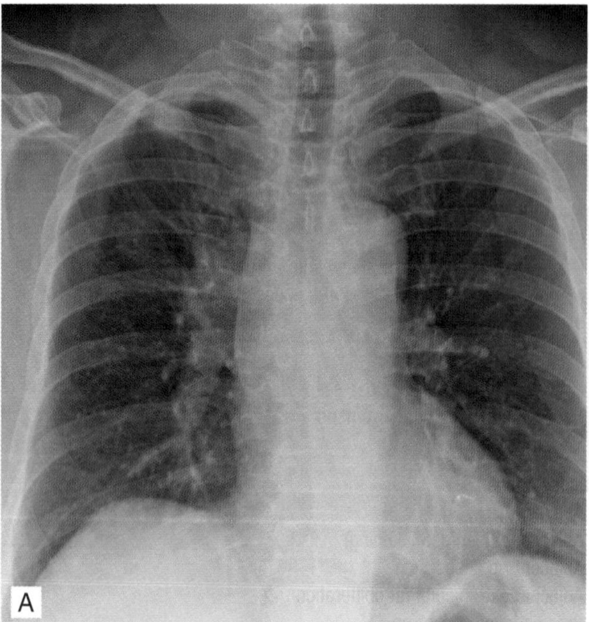

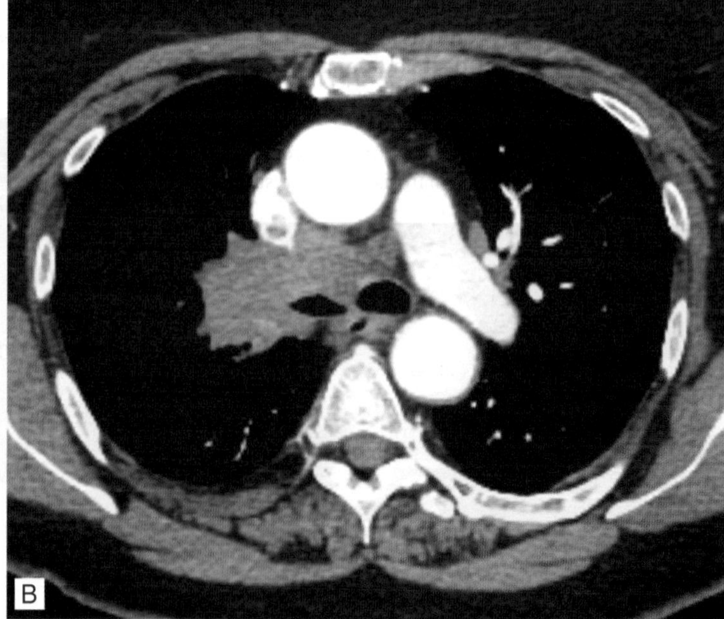

Figure 16.21 NSCLC presenting with hilar enlargement. The right hilar enlargement on a chest radiograph (A) represents hilar mass that is contiguous with the right hilar and mediastinal lymphadenopathy on the CT scan (B).

TABLE 16.10 Lung Cancer Manifestation—Pleural Involvement

Mechanism
Reactive response
Sympathetic response
Lymphatic congestion
Direct invasion
Distinct metastases
Manifestations
Linear opacities from tumor to pleura
Large contact surface between tumor and pleura
Obtuse angles between tumor and pleura
Pneumothorax
Focal pleural thickening

Although every pleural effusion is suspicious in context of lung cancer, the term "malignant effusion" should be reserved for effusions containing malignant cells. Malignant effusion is commonly accompanied by nodular pleural thickening and/or pleural masses. Infrequently, malignant pleural effusion may be a sole presenting finding of lung cancer (when measurable tumor cannot be detected on imaging). *Adenocarcinoma is the most common cancer type associated with pleural involvement* (Fig. 16.23).

- Linear opacities on CT extending from a peripherally located lung cancer to pleura suggest visceral pleural involvement, particularly if associated with pleural retraction
- Large contact surface (over 3 cm) and obtuse angle margins of a tumor with pleura are considered signs of probable parietal pleural invasion
- Infrequently, lung cancer may present with pneumothorax, which usually is seen when a cavitary/necrotic peripheral tumor invades the pleura

Chest Wall Involvement: The presence and the extent of chest wall invasion by lung cancer is important to identify because it has an impact on prognosis and management. The presence of any chest wall invasion implies higher stage while extensive chest wall invasion precludes surgical management. Chest wall invasion ranges from subtle parietal pleural thickening to frank destruction of ribs and invasion of chest wall muscles.

Radiographically, chest wall invasion is detected by osseous destruction (Fig. 16.24). CT has high sensitivity for the detection of chest wall invasion [13] (Fig. 16.25). Several CT findings have been shown to correlate with chest wall invasion with variable accuracy (Table 16.11). Thoracic magnetic resonance imaging (MRI)

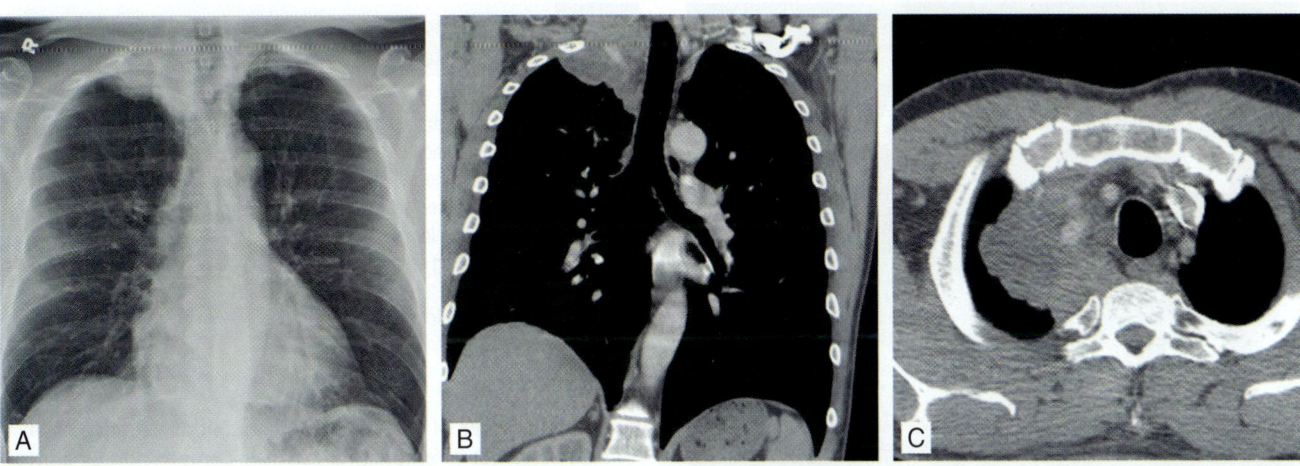

Figure 16.22 Superior sulcus tumor. Chest radiograph (A), coronal (B), and axial (C) CT images demonstrate a large mass in the right apex invading the mediastinum and superior extrapleural space, with additional encasement of the right subclavian artery.

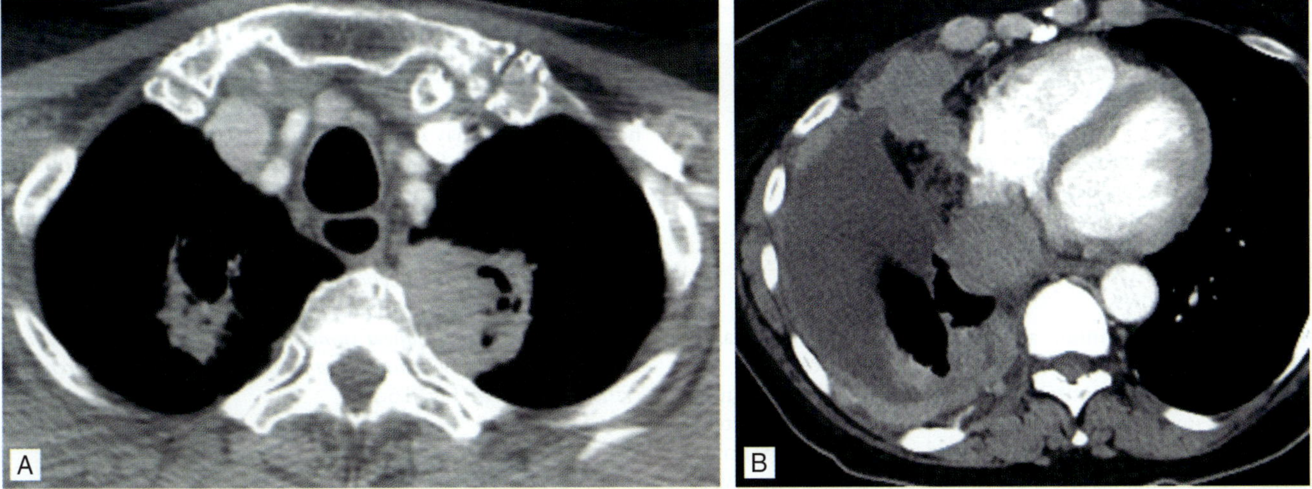

Figure 16.23 NSCLC with pleural disease in two different patients. (A) The left apical mass with large contact surface with medial pleura and obliteration of the fat plane between the pleura and thoracic vertebra. Additional synchronous lung cancer in the right apex. (B) In a different patient, right NSCLC (not seen on the image) with right pleural circumferential nodular thickening, masses, and effusion.

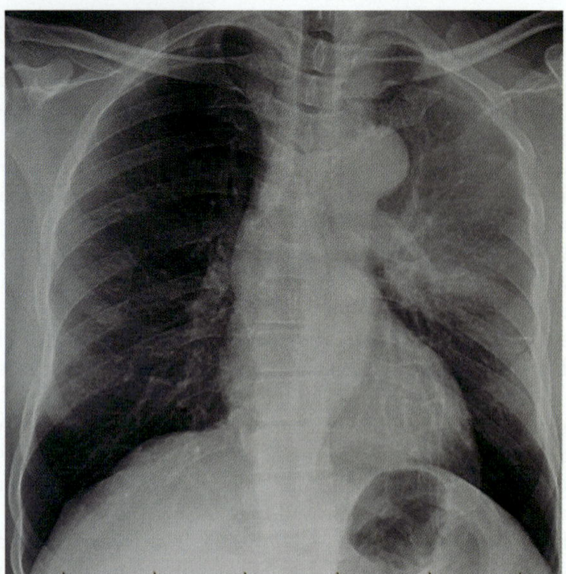

Figure 16.24 NSCLC with chest wall invasion. Large mass in the LUL, invading the posterior chest wall and destroying third to sixth left ribs.

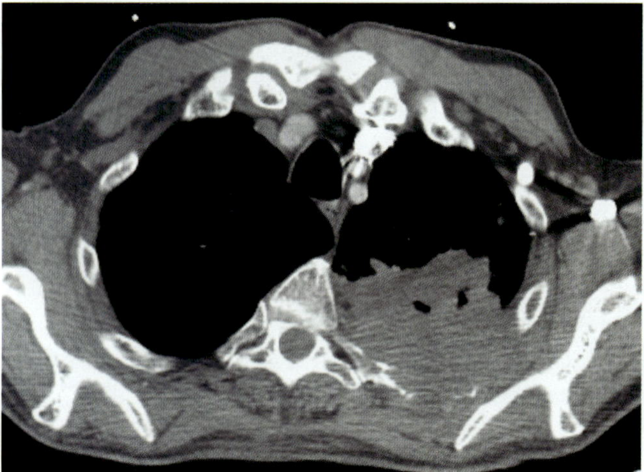

Figure 16.25 NSCLC with chest wall invasion. Large mass in the apicoposterior segment of LUL, invading the posterior chest wall and destroying the fourth left rib.

TABLE 16.11 Lung Cancer Manifestation—Chest Wall Involvement

Manifestations
Tumor contact surface with chest wall longer than 3 cm
Obliteration of extrapleural fat
Adjacent rib destruction
Adjacent muscle invasion

with or without gadolinium administration may be beneficial in select cases where subtle chest wall invasion is suspected.

Mediastinal Involvement: Similar to chest wall invasion, a mediastinal involvement by lung cancer is important to detect, because it also affects the staging and management. Clinical signs of mediastinal invasion depend on the structure involved:

- SVC invasion usually manifests with SVC syndrome (dilated neck veins, swelling and erythema of the face, neck, and upper body)

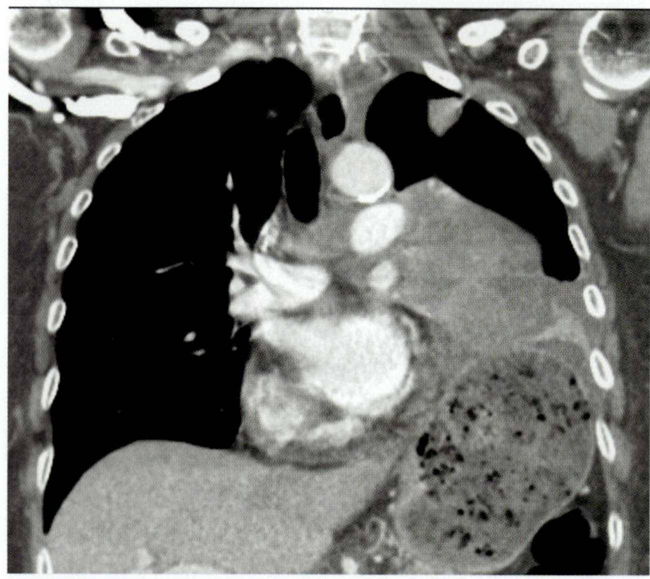

Figure 16.26 NSCLC with mediastinal invasion. Elevation and paralysis of the left hemidiaphragm caused by a large left perihilar mass invading the mediastinum and left phrenic nerve.

TABLE 16.12 Lung Cancer Manifestation—Mediastinal Involvement

Manifestations
Tumor contact surface with mediastinum longer than 3 cm
Extensive obliteration of mediastinal fat
Tumor encasing more than 90° of critical mediastinal structures
Compression of mediastinal structures
Pericardial thickening
Tumor surrounding or invading mediastinal structures
SVC syndrome
Hemidiaphragmatic elevation/paralysis

- Variable degree of dysphagia indicates either esophageal invasion by tumor or esophageal extrinsic compression by a mediastinal lymphadenopathy
- Stridor and dyspnea usually are seen with central airway and tracheal invasion
- Chest pain may be sign of a pericardial invasion, particularly if associated with pericardial effusion

Radiographically, any abnormal mediastinal contour may indicate mediastinal invasion or lymphadenopathy. Elevation of hemidiaphragm may indicate a phrenic nerve palsy (Fig. 16.26), which can be confirmed by demonstration of a paradoxical diaphragmatic motion on fluoroscopy. The CT scan is invariably better to detect and determine the extent of mediastinal invasion (Table 16.12). *CT findings with highest sensitivity for mediastinal invasion precluding surgical management include: obliteration of the mediastinal fat plane between tumor and critical structures, 3 cm or longer tumoral contact surface with mediastinum, and tumor extending more than 90° of circumference of critical structures* (Fig. 16.27).

Staging of Lung Cancer

Surgical excision is considered the lone curative treatment for NSCLC, while chemotherapy is considered the same for SCLC. As for most cancers, the TNM system (tumor, nodal

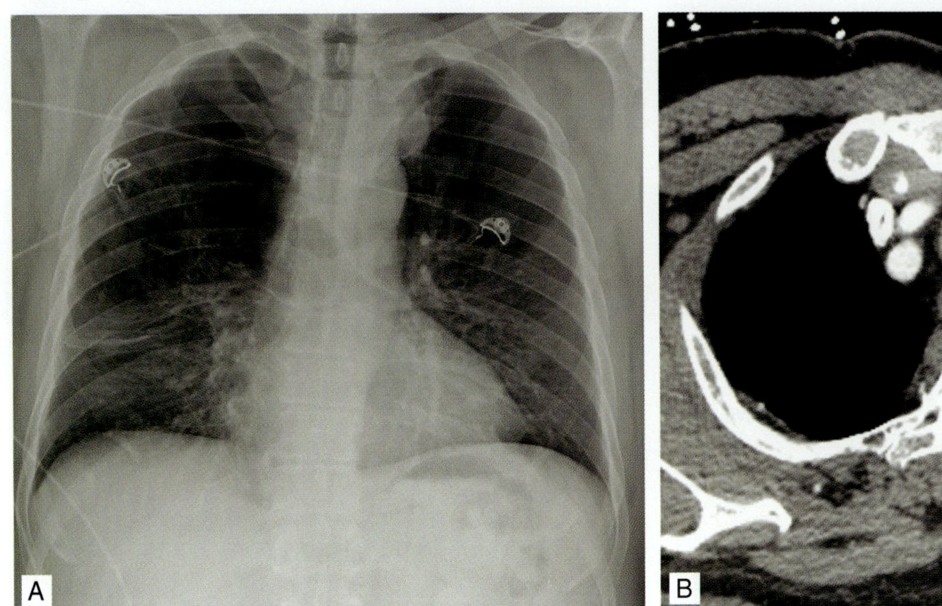

Figure 16.27 NSCLC with mediastinal invasion. Subtle left apical mass on the chest radiograph (A), which obliterates the mediastinal fat and extends into the retrotracheal space, as seen on the CT scan (B). The mass abuts/displaces the esophagus to the right and slightly erodes the anterior aspect of the thoracic vertebral body.

disease, and metastasis) is routinely used to stage lung cancers (Table 16.13).

The latest 8th edition of TNM classification for lung cancers was formulated in 2017 and contains four staging groups [26] (Table 16.14).

- Stage I includes all cancers that measure less than 4 cm in size and have no associated regional metastatic lymph nodes. Similar size cancers that invade main bronchus or visceral pleura, and those associated with atelectasis or obstructive pneumonitis are also part of the Stage I group (Fig. 16.28)

TABLE 16.13 Lung Cancer T, N, M Categories

Descriptor	Definition
Tx	Primary tumor cannot be assessed, or cytologically proved primary tumor that is not visualized by imaging or bronchoscopy
T0	No primary tumor
Tis	Carcinoma in situ
T1	Tumor <3 cm in greatest dimension
T1a	Tumor <1 cm Minimally invasive adenocarcinoma Superficially spreading tumor of any size confined to bronchial or tracheal wall
T1b	Tumor >1 cm but <2 cm
T1c	Tumor >2 cm but <3 cm
T2	Tumor >3 cm but <5 cm in greatest dimension or tumor <5 cm that is associated with: ■ invasion of main bronchus ■ Invasion of visceral pleura ■ atelectasis or obstructive pneumonitis extending to the hilum
T2a	Tumor >3 cm but <4 cm
T2b	Tumor >4 cm but <5 cm
T3	Tumor >5 cm but <7 cm in greatest dimension or tumor <7 cm that is associated with: ■ invasion of parietal pleura, pericardium, chest wall, phrenic nerve ■ separate nodules in the same lobe
T4	Tumor >7 cm in greatest dimension or tumor of any size that is associated with: ■ invasion of carina or trachea ■ invasion of mediastinum, heart, esophagus, great vessels, recurrent laryngeal nerve ■ invasion of diaphragm or spine ■ separate tumor nodules in different lobe in ipsilateral lung
Nx	Regional lymph nodes cannot be assessed
N0	No regional lymph node involvement
N1	Involvement of ipsilateral intrapulmonary, peribronchial, and/or hilar lymph nodes
N2	Involvement of ipsilateral mediastinal and/or subcarinal lymph nodes
N3	Involvement of contralateral mediastinal/hilar and/or supraclavicular lymph nodes
M0	No distant metastasis
M1	Distant metastasis
M1a	Malignant pleural effusion/nodules, or malignant pericardial effusion/nodules separate nodules in contralateral lung
M1b	Single extrathoracic metastasis
M1c	>1 extrathoracic metastases

TABLE 16.14 **Lung Cancer Stage Groups**

Category	N0	N1	N2	N3
T1a	IA1	IIB	IIIA	IIIB
T1b	IA2	IIB	IIIA	IIIB
T1c	IA3	IIB	IIIA	IIIB
T2a	IB	IIB	IIIA	IIIB
T2b	IIA	IIB	IIIA	IIIB
T3	IIB	IIIA	IIIB	IIIC
T4	IIIA	IIIA	IIIB	IIIC
M1a	IVA	IVA	IVA	IVA
M1b	IVA	IVA	IVA	IVA
M1c	IVB	IVB	IVB	IVB

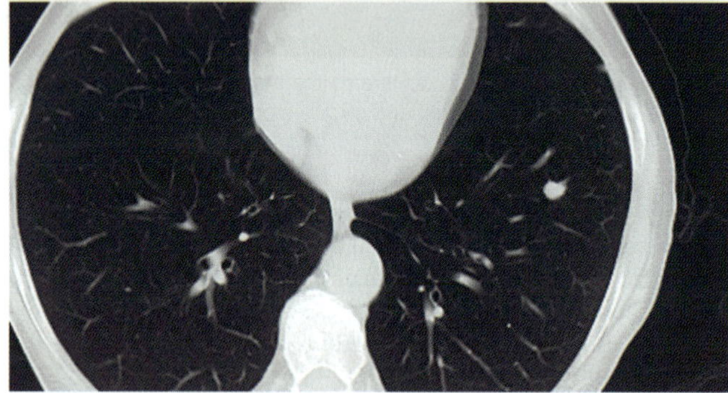

Figure 16.28 NSCLC Stage Ia. Nine-millimeter irregular nodule in the anteromedial segment of LLL, biopsy-proved NSCLC.

- In contrast, if those cancers are associated with metastatic, ipsilateral intrapulmonary, peribronchial or hilar lymph nodes, they are re-classified into Stage II group. Stage II group also includes all lung cancers that are
  1. between 4 cm and 5 cm in size with or without ipsilateral hilar lymphadenopathy;

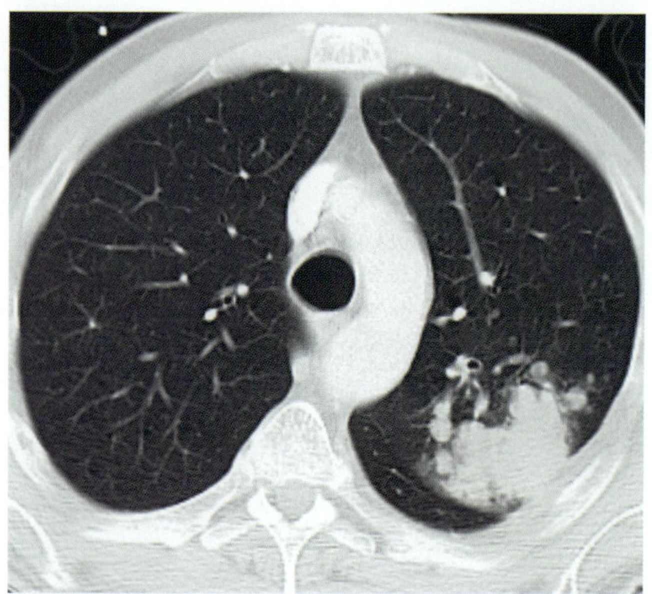

Figure 16.29 NSCLC Stage IIb. 4.5-cm mass in the apicoposterior segment of LUL abutting but-not-invading the parietal pleura. Several satellite nodules are seen in the same lobe (T3 N0).

  2. between 5 cm and 7 cm in size *without* any lymphadenopathy;
  3. less than 7 cm in size *and* invading either pericardium, chest wall and phrenic nerve; and
  4. less than 7 cm in size *with* satellite nodule(s) in the same lobe (Fig. 16.29).
- Stage III tumors are considered resectable, potentially resectable, and inoperable, depending on degree of local invasion and regional lymph node involvement (Fig. 16.30). Lung cancer greater than 7 cm and any locally invasive cancer involving carina, trachea, mediastinal structures (except pericardium), diaphragm or spine may be considered operable if regional lymph nodes are not affected or if only ipsilateral hilar lymph nodes are involved (Figs. 16.31 and 16.32). The presence of contralateral mediastinal/hilar lymphadenopathy

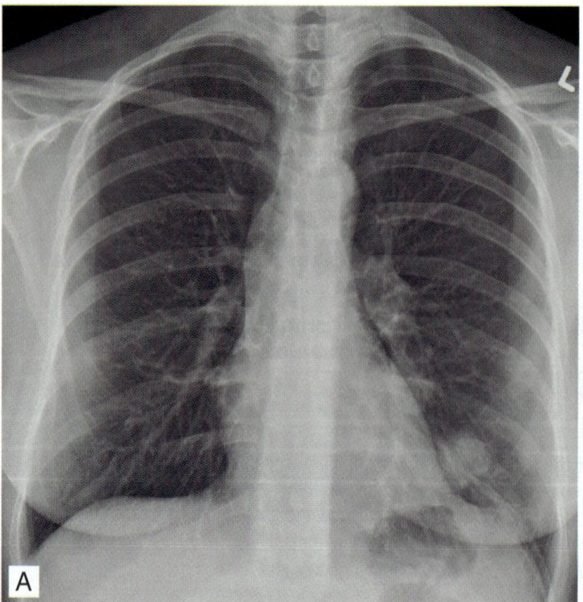

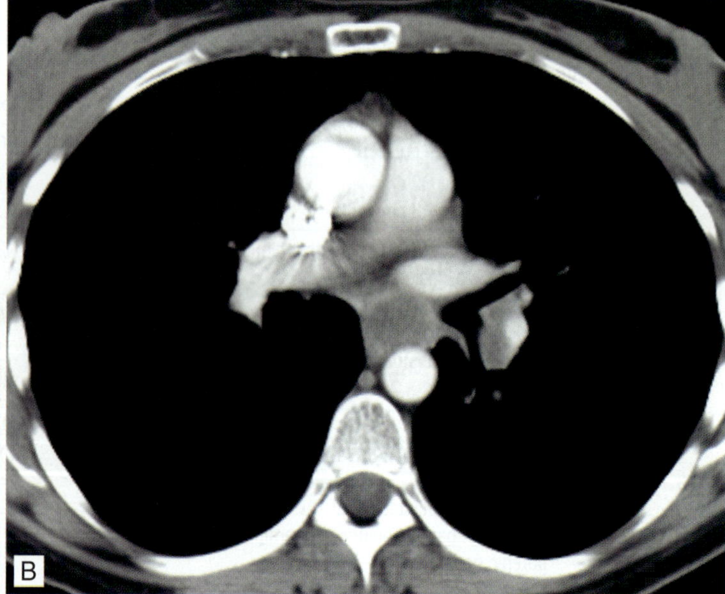

Figure 16.30 NSCLC Stage IIIa. Three-centimeter mass in the LLL seen on the chest radiograph (A). Metastatic low-density left hilar and subcarinal lymph nodes are seen on CT scan (B) (T2aN2).

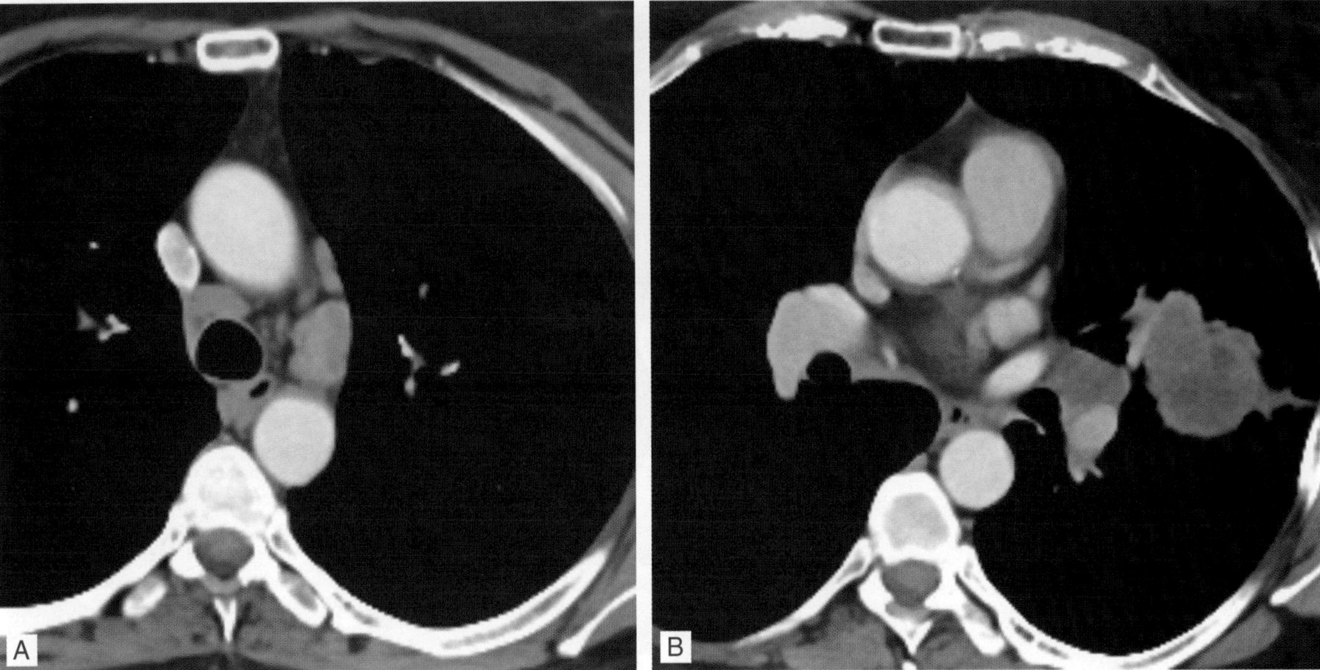

Figure 16.31 NSCLC Stage IIIb. CT images (A and B) of the same patient show a 5.1-cm mass in the LUL with metastatic left hilar and aortopulmonary window lymph nodes (T3N2).

and/or supraclavicular lymphadenopathy generally renders all cancers inoperable, unless cancers are less than 5 cm in size *and* without invasion of critical structures

- Stage IV lung cancers include tumors of any size that are associated with either
  1. malignant pleural or pericardial effusion (Fig. 16.33);
  2. malignant nodules in the contralateral lung;
  3. distant metastasis.

This staging scheme is regularly used for NSCLC. Although it can be applied to SCLC as well, the Veterans Administration Lung Study Group staging of SCLC remains widely used instead. This staging system consists of two staging groups:

- *Limited stage*, meaning any tumor with metastasis and pulmonary nodules that are not outside of single radiation field
- *Advanced* (or *extensive)* stage

Lepidic-predominant adenocarcinoma represents a special case given its propensity to be multifocal at presentation. In such situation, the tumor is classified according to the lesion with the highest TNM stage.

Investigations

Lung cancer prognosis widely varies depending on the tumor stage; notably, 5-year survival of Stage I cancers may be as high as 92%, while of some Stage III cancers as low as 13% [26] (Table 16.15).

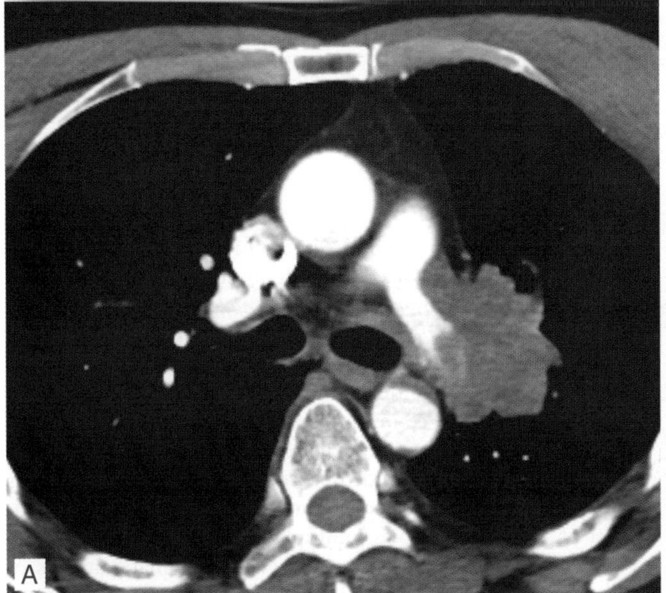

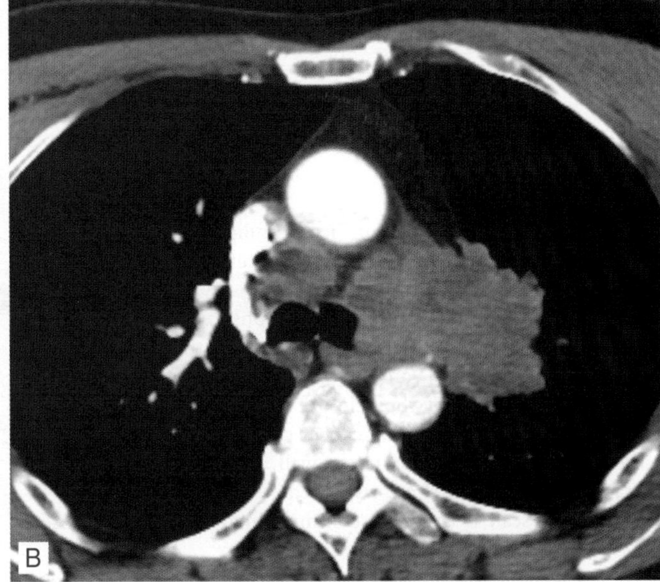

Figure 16.32 NSCLC Stage IIIc. CT scan images (A and B) show a 4.9-cm left perihilar mass invading the left upper pulmonary artery and the left recurrent laryngeal nerve in a patient who presented with hoarseness. Additional metastatic bilateral low paratracheal lymph nodes (T4 N3).

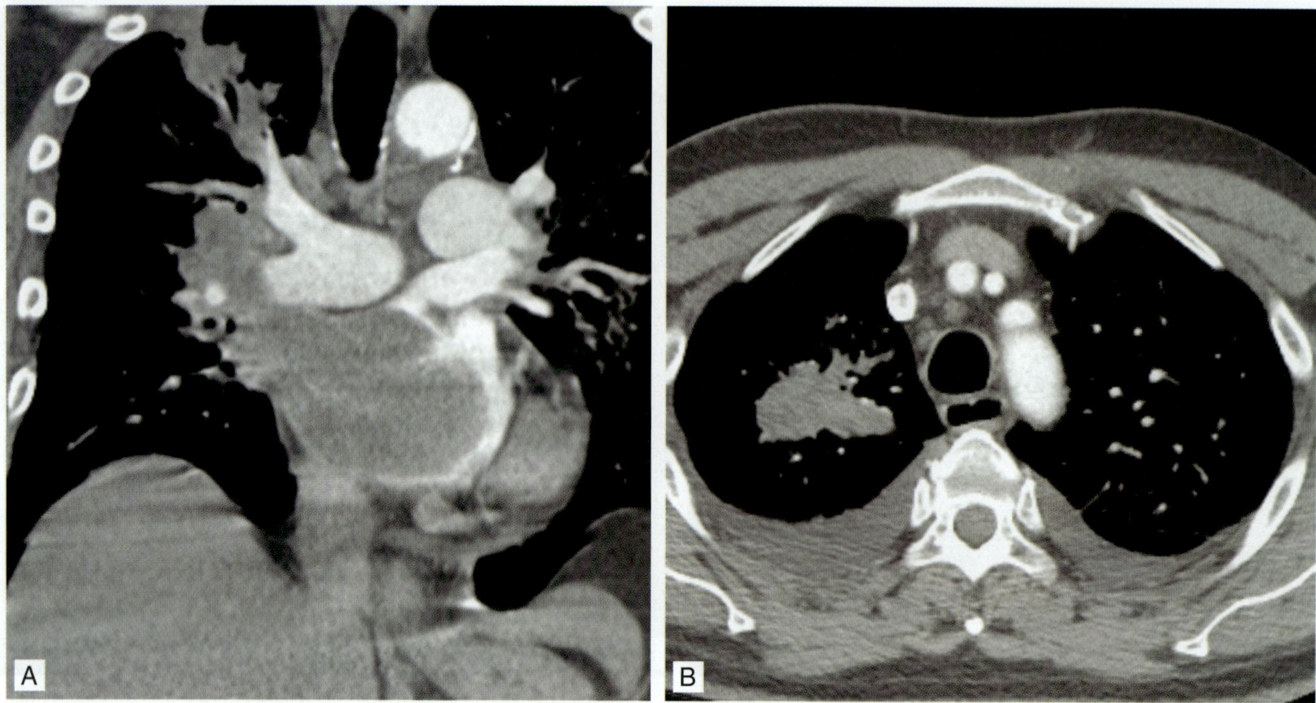

Figure 16.33 NSCLC Stage IVa. Coronal (A) and axial (B) CT images show a LUL cancer invading the right superior pulmonary vein and extending into the left atrium. Additional malignant pleural effusions (T4M1a).

TABLE 16.15 Five-Year Survival Depending on Clinical Stage

Stage	Five-Year (%)
IA1	92
IA2	83
IA3	77
IB	68
IIA	60
IIB	53
IIIA	36
IIIB	26
IIIC	13
IVA	10
IVB	0

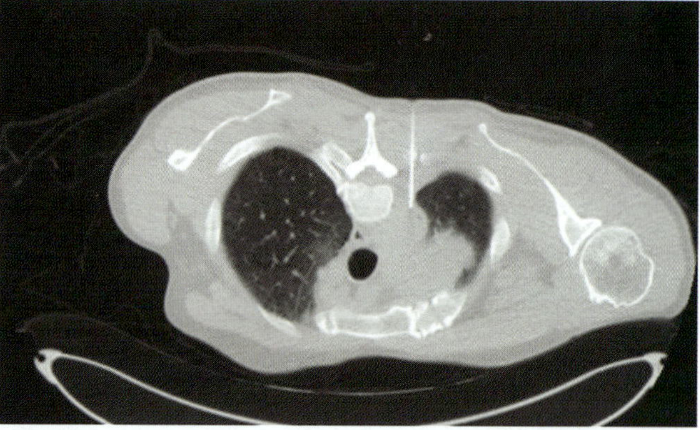

Figure 16.34 CT-guided biopsy. Image obtained during CT-guided transthoracic biopsy shows a biopsy needle inserted into the left apical cancer.

Imaging plays a primary role in determining the clinical stage of lung cancer and, therefore, has an important role in selection of appropriate treatment and prognosis.

Radiographs: Although chest radiographs commonly are the first imaging technique to detect lung cancers, these have limited role in staging process. Current practice guidelines recommend additional assessment by thoracic CT scan in all cases for staging purposes. Stage III or IV lung cancer can be diagnosed on initial radiographs when definite chest wall invasion or destructive metastatic bone lesion(s) are visualized.

CT: The CT scan is the most common imaging technique used for the diagnosis and staging of lung cancer.

- It is excellent for the evaluation of T-stage of lung cancers, particularly of T1 and T2 tumors and has variable accuracy to determine mediastinal, pleural, or chest wall invasion
- It has a major role in the detection of metastatic nodal disease in the thorax, and consequentially in determining N-stage in staging process. *Any regional lymph node larger than 1 cm in short axis is generally considered suspicious for metastasis.* The main challenges of the CT scans remain its inability to (1) detect metastatic lymph nodes that are smaller than 1 cm in short axis, and (2) confirm definite metastatic involvement of lymph nodes that are between 1 cm and 2 cm in short axis
- It is useful for image-guided procedures, such as percutaneous fine-needle aspiration and/or core biopsies (Fig. 16.34). In an era of targeted therapies, multiple core samples from image-guided biopsies are usually required for adequate analysis of the tissue for specific mutations
- It is commonly used for the detection of distant metastasis during initial investigation

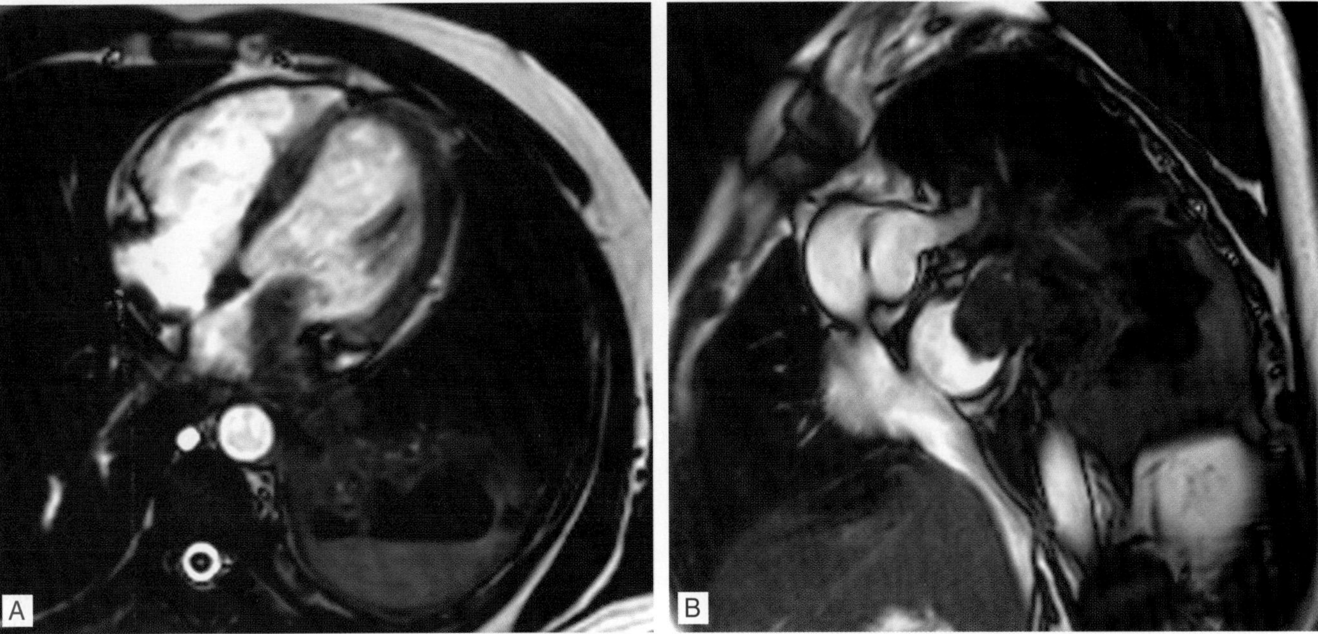

Figure 16.35 Axial (A) and two-chamber short axis (B) views of balanced coherent GRE sequence demonstrated lung mass extending across the left pulmonary vein into the left atrium. (Courtesy: Amit Choudhari, Department of Radiodiagnosis, Tata Memorial Hospital.)

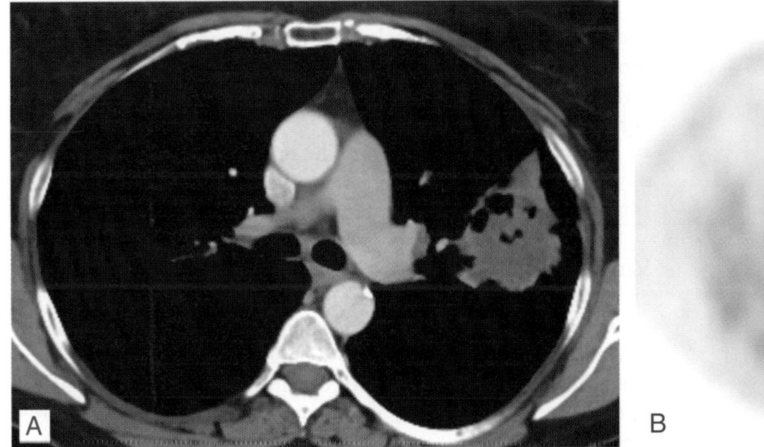

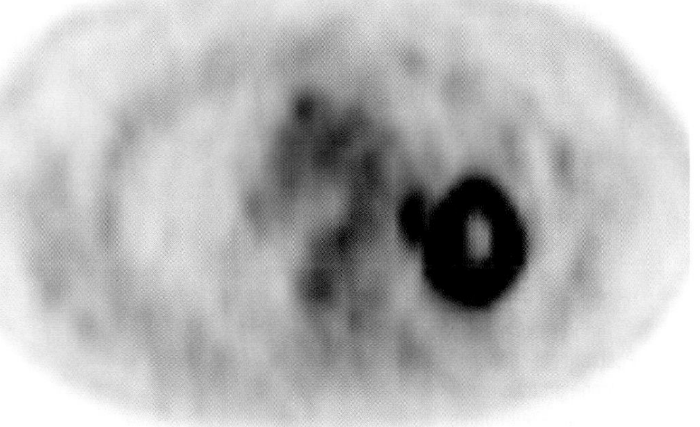

Figure 16.36 Value of PET scan. CT image (A) demonstrates a 5 mm left hilar lymph node in a patient with LUL NSCLC. The lymph node demonstrated increased uptake on ^{18}F-FDG PET scan (B) and was subsequently found to be malignant on pathology.

- It is technique of choice for follow-up imaging to assess the response to treatment (if tumor is inoperable) or cancer recurrence (if tumor was treated with surgery or curative chemo/radiotherapy)

MRI: Although MRI does not add value to CT for the assessment of thoracic nodal status, it may help in determining T-stage and tumor resectability in specific situations. In particular, MRI is better than CT in the detection of a subtle invasion of chest wall, diaphragm, and mediastinum given its higher spatial resolution (Fig. 16.35). MRI has higher accuracy in the detection of the invasion of subclavian vessels and brachial plexus by superior sulcus tumors [27]. Finally, MRI is a preferable technique for imaging of neuroaxis for the detection of metastatic disease, in

- all patients with SCLC;
- patients of clinical Stage II, III, and IV NSCLC;
- all lung cancer patients with neurological symptoms.

PET/CT and PET/MRI: Positron emission tomography (PET)/CT combination has the most value in staging of lung cancers [28,29]. It also can be used for characterization of an indeterminate lesion, assessment of response to treatment, and detection of tumor recurrence. For NSCLC staging, ^{18}F-FDG PET/CT is recommended for all patients who are considered for curative treatment. It is particularly of benefit for the evaluation of extrathoracic metastasis and of thoracic lymph nodes that are less than 1 cm in size on initial diagnostic CT scan (Figs. 16.36 and 16.37). This technique is also indicated in all patients with limited-stage SCLC [30]. Compared with CT alone, PET/CT is better in characterizing malignant pleural effusion, demonstrating bone metastasis as well as detecting distant extrathoracic metastasis.

In addition to its lack of intrinsic radiation, PET/MR integration provides better special resolution than PET/CT, particularly for neural axis, liver, bone, and breasts imaging. PET/MR further allows additional functional investigation with MR spectroscopy and MR perfusion sequences when needed [31].

Imaging with PET/CT and PET/MR has several known pitfalls, such as misregistration artifacts, and false positives and false negatives (Table 16.16) [28,32]. False-negative study may happen if a primary cancer is small (less than 8 mm in size) or in context of serum

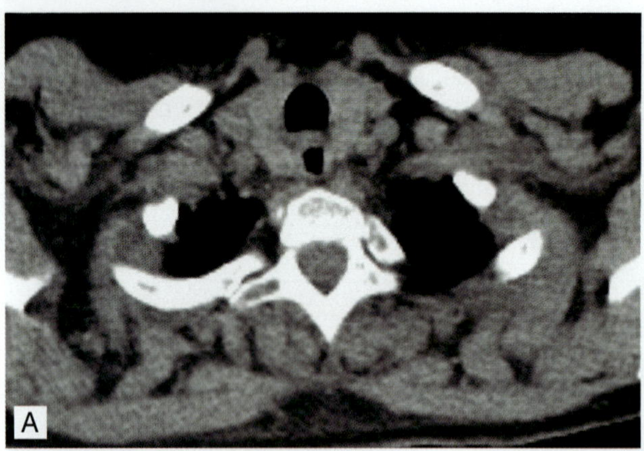

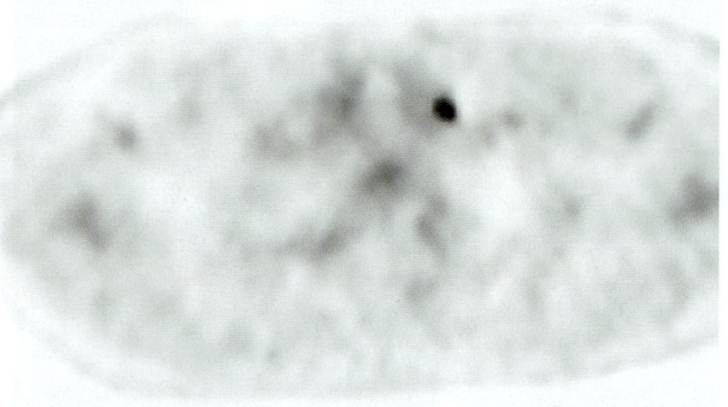

Figure 16.37 Value of PET scan. CT image shows a 4 mm left supraclavicular lymph node in a patient with LUL NSCLC (not shown). The lymph node demonstrated increased uptake on ^{18}F-FDG PET scan (B) and was subsequently found to be malignant on pathology.

TABLE 16.16 Pitfalls of Thoracic PET/CT and PET/MR Imaging

- False positive
  - Normal structures
    - Normal uptake in myocardium, brown fat, bowel
    - Misregistration artifacts
  - Benign pathological processes
    - Rheumatoid disease
    - Wegener's granulomatosis
    - Round atelectasis
    - Thymic hyperplasia
    - Reactive intrathoracic lymph nodes
    - Tuberculosis
    - Histoplasmosis
    - Bacterial pneumonia
    - Abscess
    - Pneumocystis jirovecii
    - Sarcoidosis
    - Pulmonary fibrosis
    - Progressive massive fibrosis
  - Postsurgical changes
  - Silicone granulomas
  - Radiation pneumonitis
- False negative
  - Pulmonary nodules <1 cm in size
  - Carcinoid
  - Adenocarcinoma in situ
  - Misregistration artifacts
  - Hyperglycemia
  - Normal high physiologic uptake in mediastinum preventing detection of pathologic uptake

hyperglycemia. AIS and minimally invasive adenocarcinomas are typically ^{18}F-FDG PET negative. Lepidic-predominant invasive adenocarcinoma and carcinoid tumors may not demonstrate abnormal ^{18}F-FDG uptake as well, particularly if small (Figs. 16.38–16.40). Appropriate diagnosis in such cases requires good integration with anatomic images and correlation with clinical status of a patient.

Interventional/Surgical Procedures for Staging: Bronchoscopy, endobronchial ultrasound (EBUS), endoscopic ultrasound (EUS), mediastinoscopy, anterior mediastinotomy, and video-assisted thoracoscopy (VATS) are minimally invasive techniques that can be used for diagnostic and staging purposes [33] in addition to previously mentioned CT-guided procedures (Table 16.17).

Although mediastinoscopy is still considered as "gold standard" for the evaluation of many regional nodal stations in context of lung cancer, EBUS has been shown to have similar sensitivity and specificity [34]. In addition to its good accuracy, the use of EBUS has been increasing because it can be performed in outpatient setting with conscious sedation, and has lower incidence and severity of complications than mediastinoscopy. Combination of EBUS and EUS (which additionally allows sampling of low paraesophageal and pulmonary ligament lymph nodes) can cover all regional thoracic lymph node stations. EBUS/EUS or mediastinoscopy are indicated for tissue confirmation in all patients considered for curative treatment who have

- suspicious thoracic lymph nodes on CT and/or PET/CT scan;
- normal-appearing lymph nodes on CT and PET/CT in patients with central or large (more than 3-cm size) tumors [32].

Various bronchoscopic procedures are available for the diagnosis and staging of lung cancers. Rigid and flexible (fiberoptic) bronchoscopies are used for the assessment of central and peripheral cancers, respectively. These allow endobronchial and transbronchial sampling of suspicious masses and mediastinal/hilar lymph nodes. Improved targeting and diagnostic yield of distal biopsies are achieved by navigational bronchoscopy, which benefits from integrated virtual endobronchial images obtained with preprocedure CT scan for improved guidance.

VATS is used for staging if other interventional procedures fail to adequately assess lymph nodes that appear suspicious on imaging. Furthermore, VATS may be beneficial in assessing the primary tumor, particularly to determine if invasion of critical mediastinal structures is present before curative surgical excision.

Lung Cancer Management

Stage I and II NSCLC are routinely treated by surgical excision. For selected patients who have significant comorbidities or are judged to be poor surgical candidates, focused external beam radiotherapy or stereotactic body radiotherapy can be offered. Some Stage II cancers benefit from additional neoadjuvant chemotherapy. Stage III and IV are mainly treated with some type of systemic treatment with or without additional surgery and radiotherapy:

- Chemotherapy agents most commonly used for lung cancer are platinum-based drugs (cisplatin and carboplatin)
- Targeted therapy is based on recent discoveries of specific mutation-driven oncogenes in some types of lung cancers [35]. Medications in this type of therapy target specific cancer genes

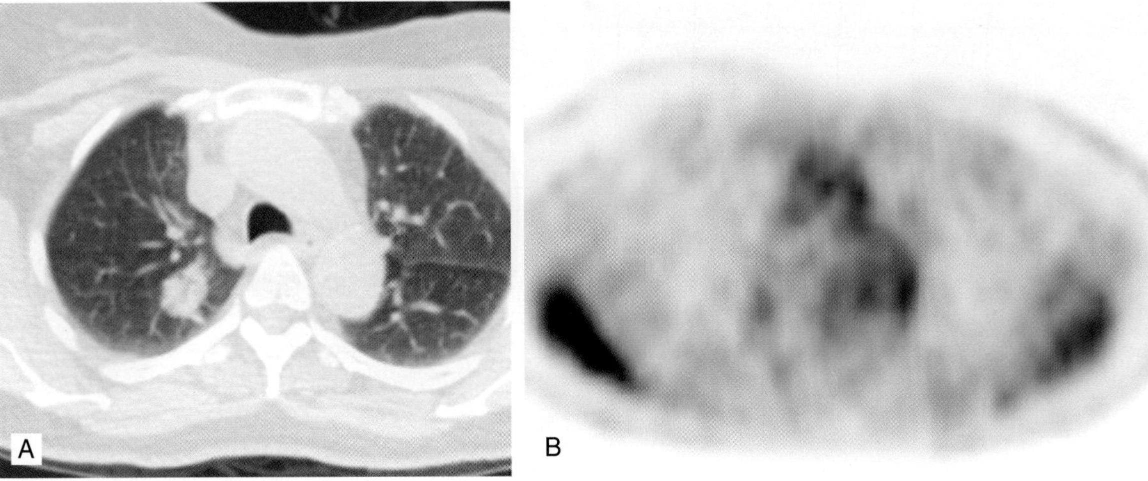

Figure 16.38 PET scan pitfalls (false negative). CT image (A) shows a 2.4-cm adenocarcinoma in the RUL, which demonstrates background uptake on ^{18}F-FDG PET scan (B) (1.7 SUV).

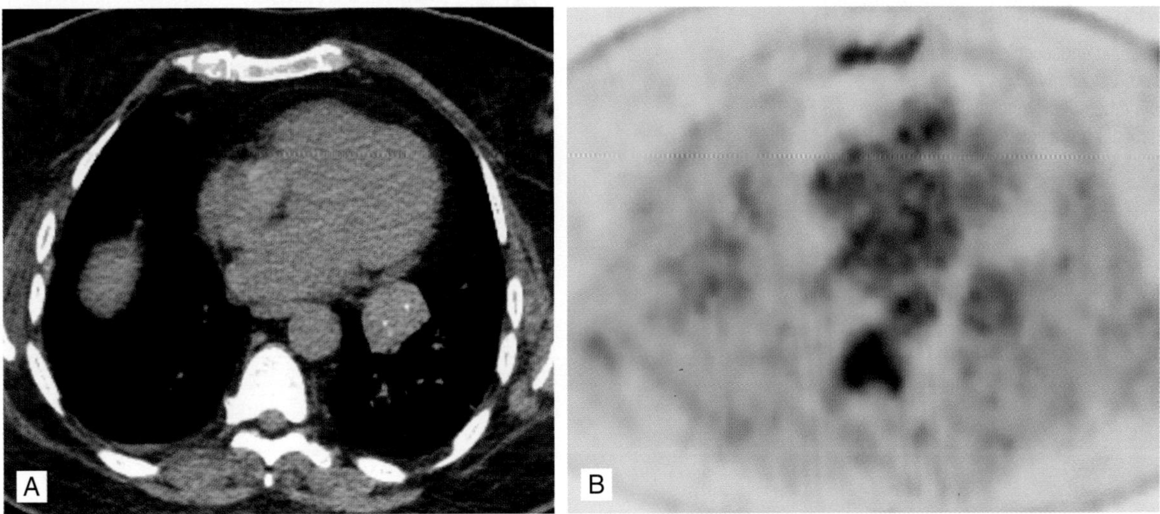

Figure 16.39 PET scan pitfalls (false negative). CT image (A) shows a 3.2-cm carcinoid in the LLL that demonstrates background uptake on ^{18}F-FDG PET scan (B) (1.8 SUV).

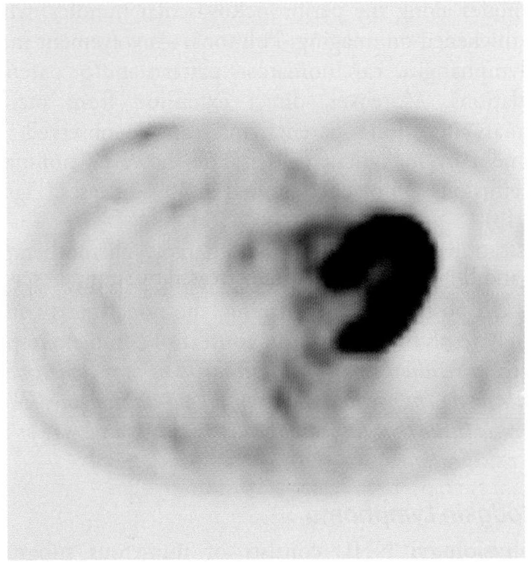

Figure 16.40 PET scan pitfalls (false positive). Normal physiological increased uptake on 18F-FDG PET scan in the left ventricular myocardium.

or proteins. The most common such drugs include EGFR inhibitors and ALK inhibitors (Fig. 16.41)

- Immunotherapy is another type of systemic treatment from which lung cancer patients may benefit. Immune therapy agents target specific checkpoint inhibitors, such as PD-1/ PD-L1 and CTLA-4 inhibitors

Lymphoproliferative Diseases/Lymphoma

Lymphoma predominantly affects mediastinal lymph nodes, but may also affect lung parenchyma, airways, pleura, and chest wall [36]. Although it is commonly seen in conjunction with systemic disease, intrathoracic lymphoma may primarily be pulmonary or mediastinal in origin. Lymphomas are generally classified into Hodgkin's disease (HD) and non-Hodgkin lymphoma (NHL) (Table 16.18).

Hodgkin's Disease

Pathophysiology: Hodgkin's lymphoma is histologically differentiated from other lymphomas by the presence of Reed–Sternberg cells. It has bimodal peak incidence, in third and eight

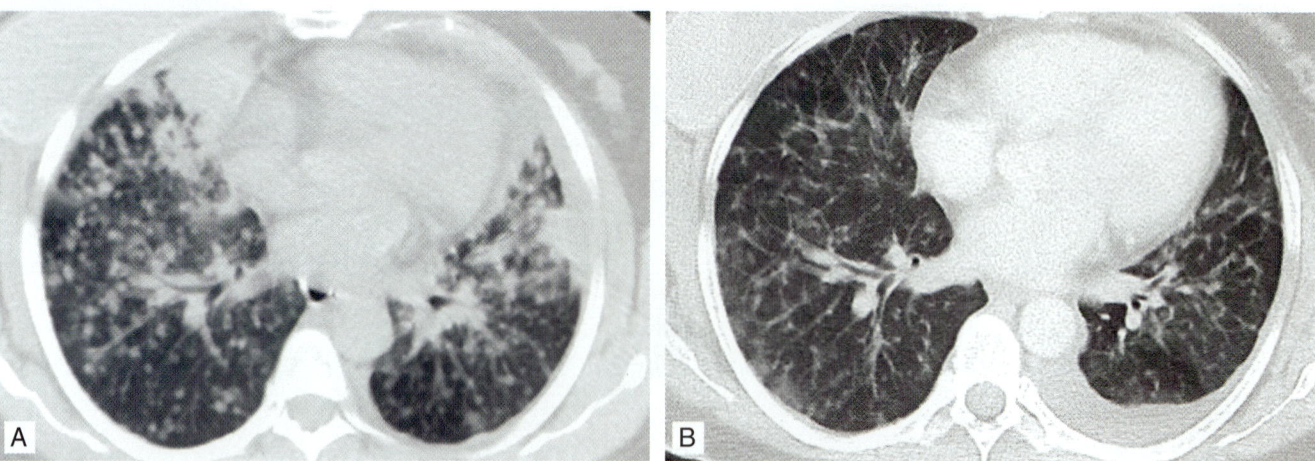

Figure 16.41 EGFR-positive adenocarcinoma of the lung. (A) Pretreatment and (B) post-targeted treatment with EGFR inhibitors.

TABLE 16.17 Lung Cancer Interventional Investigation Procedures

Bronchoscopic/endoscopic procedures
- Rigid bronchoscopy
- Flexible (fiberoptic bronchoscopy)
- Navigational bronchoscopy
- EBUS
- EUS

Surgical
- Mediastinoscopy
- Anterior mediastinotomy
- VATS

EBUS, endobronchial ultrasound; *EUS*, endoscopic ultrasound; *VATS*, video-assisted thoracoscopic surgery.

TABLE 16.19 Hodgkin's Disease

Reed–Sternberg cells on histology

Bimodal incidence (third and eighth decades)

Strong predilection for mediastinum
- Anterior and superior nodal stations
- Contiguous if multiple nodal stations
- Calcified nodes only after treatment

Pulmonary involvement
- Almost always associated with lymphadenopathy
- Direct extent from mediastinum
- Consolidations with air bronchograms
- Lymphangitic carcinomatosis

Treated by chemoradiation

decades, but may occur at all age. It has slight male predominance (Table 16.19). Prognosis of HD strongly depends on the initial staging, which is based on the anatomic extent of the disease at presentation. Although it occurs anywhere in the body, HD has strong predilection to the mediastinum. Out of all mediastinal nodal stations, anterior and superior mediastinal lymph nodes are most often affected. When multiple nodal stations are involved, the disease is usually contiguous. Hilar node involvement may be seen in 35% of cases and characteristically is bilateral and asymmetric [20].

TABLE 16.18 Thoracic Lymphoproliferative Disorders

Benign
- Focal lymphoid hyperplasia
- Lymphocytic interstitial pneumonitis
- Follicular bronchiolitis
- Lymphomatoid granulomatosis

Malignant
- Hodgkin's disease
- Non-Hodgkin's lymphoma
- Post-transplant lymphoproliferative disorder
- Leukemia

Imaging features: Radiographically, mediastinal HD typically manifests by focal abnormality in mediastinal contour, which can be smooth, lobular or irregular. *Involvement of the lung parenchyma is almost exclusively seen in conjunction with mediastinal and hilar disease.* It most often results from spread of disease from hilar lymph nodes along the peribronchovascular bundles, which are usually thickened on imaging. Pulmonary involvement may present as lymphangitic carcinomatosis pattern and/or parenchymal consolidations. Moreover, direct extension from mediastinal nodal mass into lung parenchyma can be observed. Pleural involvement by malignant cells is rare; however, nonmalignant pleural effusions can be encountered in 30% of cases (Figs. 16.42 and 16.43).

HD can be treated with radiotherapy, chemotherapy, and combined radio-chemotherapy depending on the stage of the disease. On post-treatment imaging, the nodal mass commonly completely resolves. However, in context of complete response to treatment, *a residual small mediastinal mass may sometimes persist with little or no change on long-term follow-up imaging. This represents fibrotic tissue that is metabolically inactive, and may or may not contain calcifications.*

Non-Hodgkin Lymphoma

Pathophysiology: NHL consists of numerous subgroups of malignant lymphoreticular cell proliferation. These vary in clinical presentation, histology, evolution, and prognosis [37]. NHL is

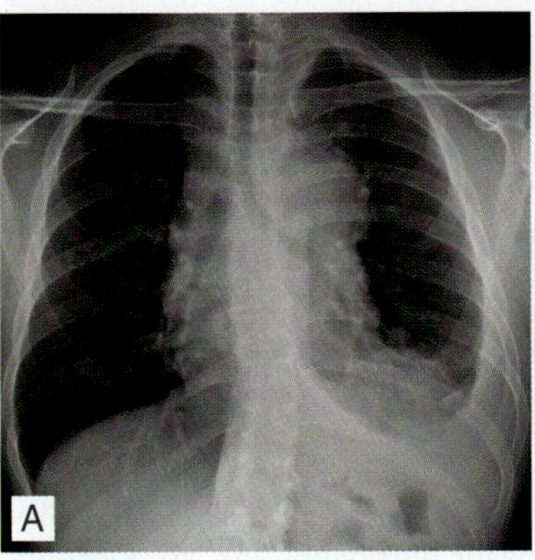

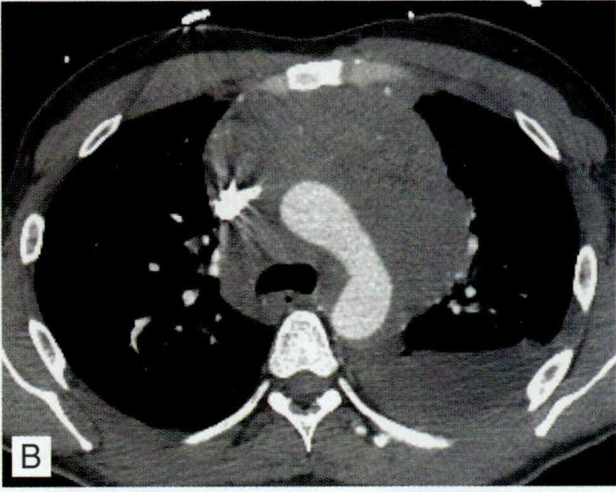

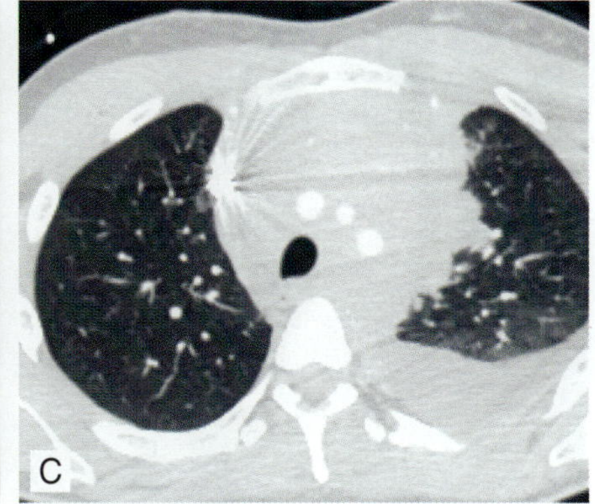

Figure 16.42 Hodgkin's disease. Chest radiograph (A) and two CT images (B and C) demonstrate a large infiltrative mediastinal mass that surrounds the aortic arch and is confluent with paratracheal lymphadenopathy. Mass extends into LUL and is associated with malignant left pleural effusion.

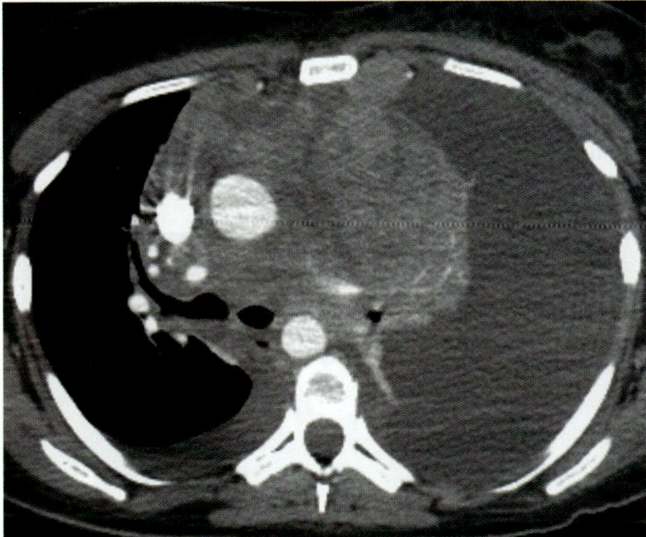

Figure 16.43 Hodgkin's disease. Large heterogeneous anterior mediastinal mass with extension into paratracheal region and left lung. Additional enlarged left internal mammary chain lymph node, large left and small right pleural effusions.

commonly graded according to aggressiveness (low grade, intermediate grade, and high grade). NHL tends to occur in older patients (40–70 years old). Predominant thoracic involvement is less common than with HD, occurring in approximately 40–50%. With respect to lung parenchyma, NHL can be divided into primary pulmonary lymphoma and secondary pulmonary involvement by lymphoma (Table 16.20).

Imaging features: As with HD, secondary involvement of the lungs by NHL is typically seen with extrapulmonary disease, particularly mediastinal and hilar lymphadenopathy and masses. Radiologically, differentiation between HD and NHL may be challenging, as both entities have similar findings in the lungs, consisting-of-but-not-limited to (1) thickening of bronchovascular bundles and interlobular septa similar to lymphangitic carcinomatosis, (2) parenchymal consolidations, and (3) direct invasion by nodal masses (Figs. 16.44 and 16.45). The main differentiating factor is the distribution of the lymphadenopathy. In contrast to HD, NHL more commonly presents with

- single intrathoracic nodal station involvement;
- discontinuous if multiple stations;
- posterior mediastinal lymphadenopathy;
- concomitant extrathoracic disease.

TABLE 16.20 Non-Hodgkin's Lymphoma

More common than HD
Older patients (fourth–seventh decades)
Thoracic involvement Usually affects multiple stations When multiple, stations can be noncontiguous
Pulmonary involvement Almost always associated with lymphadenopathy Primary or secondary pulmonary involvement Consolidations, nodules/masses, lymphangitic spread
MALT-lymphoma Groundglass or solid masses/consolidations Very good prognosis

Primary pulmonary lymphoma is rare, representing approximately 0.5% of all lung neoplasms [38]. Any type of NHL can primarily involve lungs, although B-cell lymphomas such as mucosa-associated lymphoid tissue (MALT) lymphoma and diffuse B-cell lymphoma are the most common;

- MALT lymphoma is considered low-grade lymphoma. It usually is asymptomatic at presentation and is mainly seen in patients with autoimmune disorders. Survival rate is 84–94%. Radiologically, MALT lymphoma typically presents with unifocal or multifocal ill-defined nodules and/or consolidations containing air bronchograms [34]. These may be dense or of groundglass opacity (Fig. 16.46). Often, a "CT angiogram sign" is present, representing contrast-enhanced vessel coursing and branching within the consolidation. Pleural disease is infrequent
- Primary pulmonary diffuse B-cell lymphoma is considered high-grade lymphoma and has poor prognosis. This entity predominantly affects immunocompromised patients, such as human immunodeficiency virus (HIV)-positive and post-transplant patients. It typically presents with multiple and ill-defined nodules/masses that may coalesce into consolidations (Fig. 16.47). Air bronchograms are commonly seen [38]

Post-Transplantation Lymphoproliferative Disorder

Pathophysiology: Post-transplantation lymphoproliferative disorder (PTLD) is a group of diseases that occur after solid organ or bone marrow/stem cell transplantation. PTLD includes benign conditions such as benign proliferation of lymphocytes/plasma

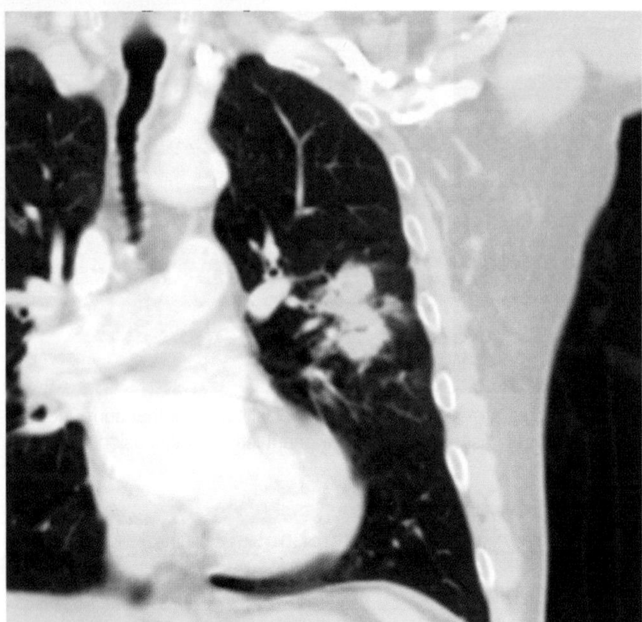

Figure 16.44 NHL. Irregular mass with air bronchograms in the LUL, in a patient with known extrapulmonary lymphoma.

cells, and malignancies such as aggressive lymphomas. Lungs are the commonest affected organ. PTLD

- is closely associated with Epstein–Barr virus;
- predominantly consists of B-cell proliferative disorders;
- commonly occurs within the first year of transplant while patient is on high immunosuppressive regimen;
- preferentially affects extranodal sites;
- may be unifocal or disseminated;
- tends to improve and/or resolve with decreasing level of immunosuppression.

Imaging features: On radiographs and CT scans, PTLD typically presents as multiple, bilateral, scattered, solid, and noncavitary large nodules or masses. Nodules/masses are well circumscribed and tend to be in perilymphatic distribution [37,38]. Occasionally, peripheral groundglass opacity ("halo-sign") and additional dense consolidations can be seen.

Lymphomatoid Granulomatosis

Pathophysiology: Considered as a neoplasm of mature B-cells, lymphomatoid granulomatosis histologically consists of an infiltrate of large atypical Epstein–Barr virus-positive B-cells, small T-cells, plasma cells, and histiocytes. These infiltrates tend to be angiocentric, potentially causing vascular occlusion, destruction, and necrosis. Despite the name, true granulomas are not present.

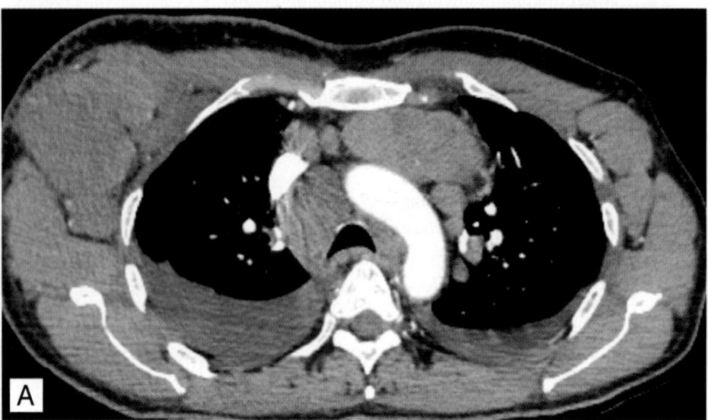

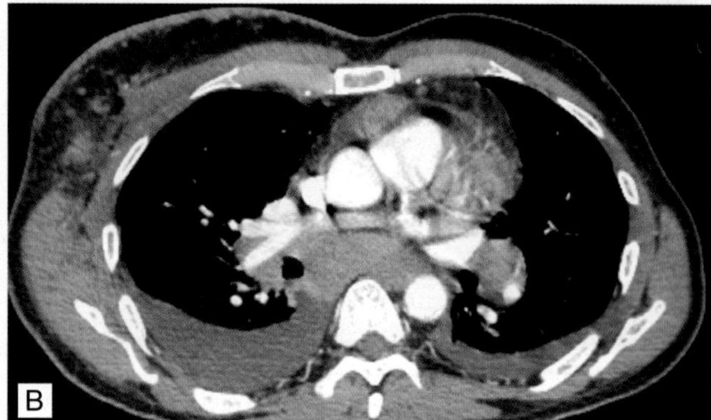

Figure 16.45 Non-Hodgkin lymphoma. Two CT images (A and B) demonstrate extensive mediastinal, hilar, and bilateral axillary nonconfluent lymphadenopathy. Additional bilateral pleural effusions.

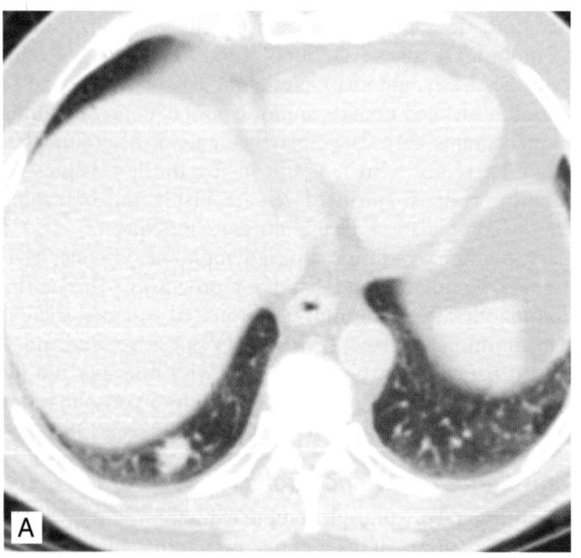

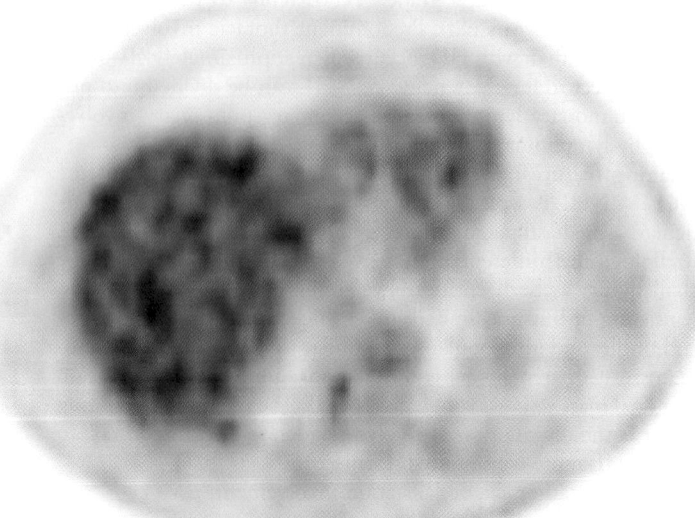

Figure 16.46 MALT lymphoma. Irregular 1.8-cm nodule in the posterior segment of RLL on a CT scan (A) with mildly increased uptake on ^{18}F-FDG PET scan (B) (2.4 SUV).

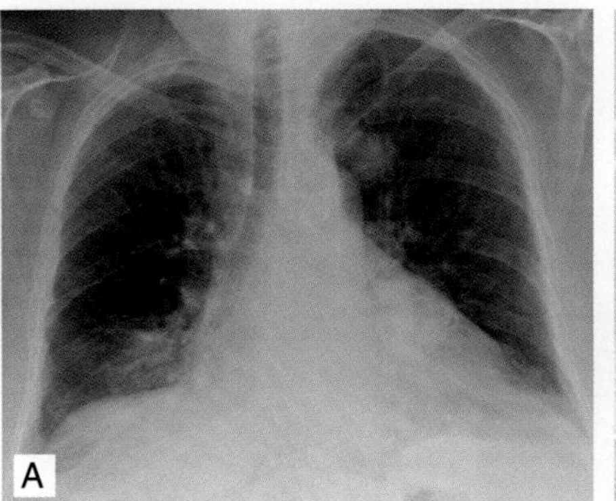

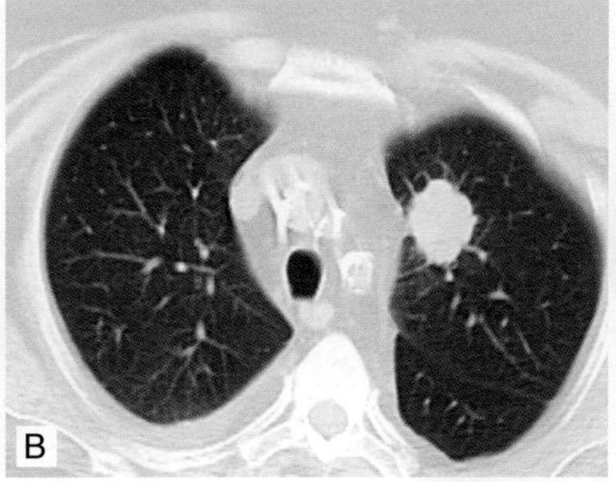

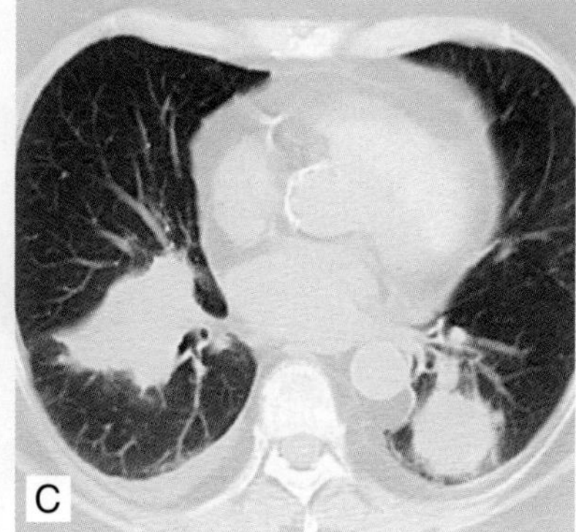

Figure 16.47 Non-Hodgkin's lymphoma, DBCL. Chest radiograph (A) and two CT images (B and C) show multiple irregular and ill-defined pulmonary masses.

This disorder may also affect other organs, such as skin and kidneys.

Imaging features: Radiologically, lymphomatoid granulomatosis manifests with lower-lobe-predominant, ill-defined and nodular opacities that predominantly are in peribronchovascular distribution [38]. These may be coalescent and form consolidations, typically with air bronchograms. The radiological appearance may resemble granulomatous polyangiitis and metastatic disease. Lesions may spontaneously resolve.

Focal Lymphoid Hyperplasia

Pathophysiology: Focal lymphoid hyperplasia, previously labeled as "pseudolymphoma," is a rare and benign entity consisting of an aggregation of mature lymphocytes, histiocytes, and plasma cells. It equally affects males and females and is associated with Sjogren's disease.

Imaging features: The most common radiological presentation is a solitary nodular or mass-like consolidation (Fig. 16.48). Focal lymphoid hyperplasia may contain air bronchogram and cavitation. It is rarely associated with lymphadenopathy, which helps differentiating this condition from MALT lymphoma. It often requires additional imaging and biopsy to differentiate from malignancy, and has benign clinical course.

Lymphocytic Interstitial Pneumonitis

Pathophysiology: Although part of lymphoproliferative disorders, lymphocytic interstitial pneumonitis (LIP) has also been classified as one of the interstitial pneumonias. LIP is histologically similar to pseudolymphoma as it consists of infiltrate of mature lymphocytes and plasma cells. In contrary to pseudolymphoma, the infiltrates in LIP are interstitial in location and diffuse in distribution. *LIP is commonly associated with connective tissue diseases (particularly Sjogren's disease) and HIV (particularly in younger patients/children).*

Imaging features: Radiologically, LIP demonstrates a combination of

1. patchy or confluent groundglass opacities;
2. small centrilobular and/or subpleural/perifissural nodules;
3. scattered thin-walled cysts (Fig. 16.49);
4. interlobular septal thickening, which together with small nodules may give appearance similar to lymphangitic carcinomatosis;
5. hilar and mediastinal lymphadenopathy [39].

Leukemia

Pathophysiology: Leukemic intrathoracic presentations are more often due to concomitant diseases or complications rather than the leukemia itself. Mediastinal and hilar lymphadenopathy is the

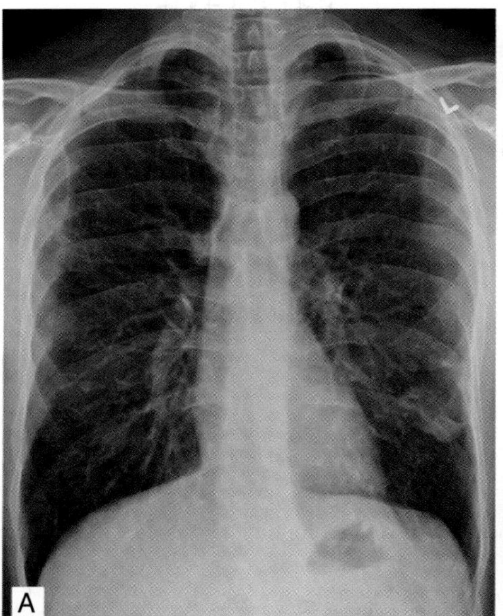

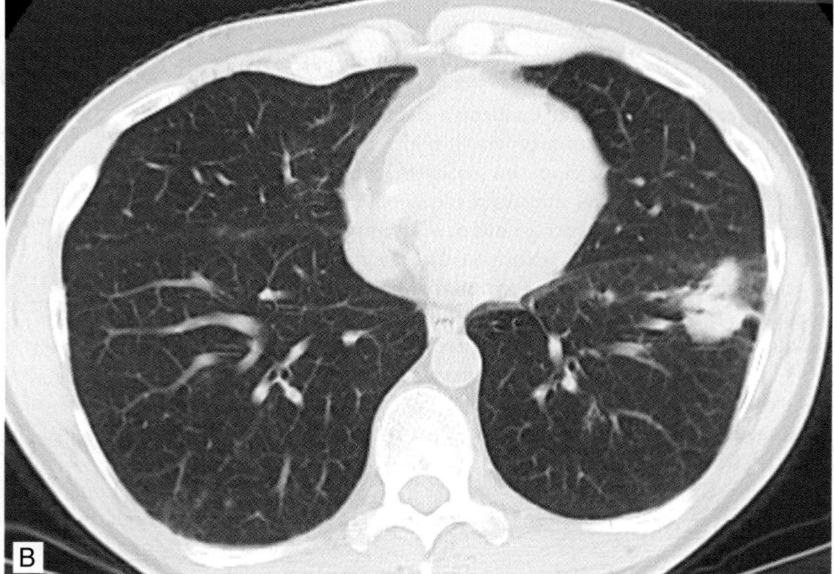

Figure 16.48 Focal lymphoid hyperplasia. Irregular mass-like consolidation with air bronchogram in the LLL on chest radiograph (A) and CT image (B).

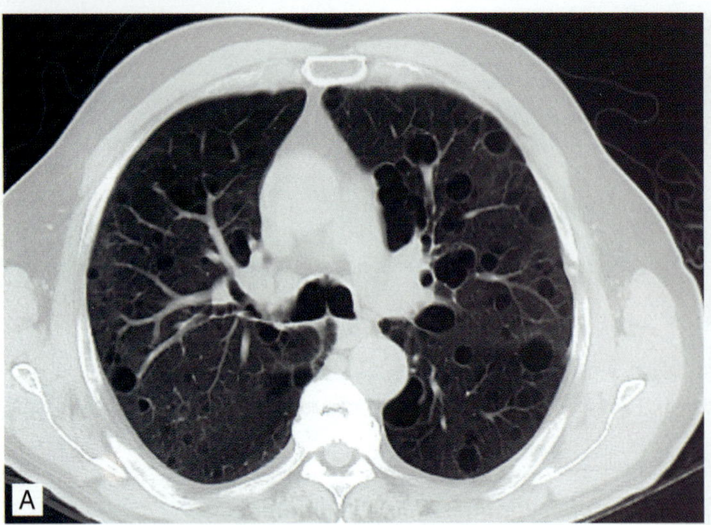
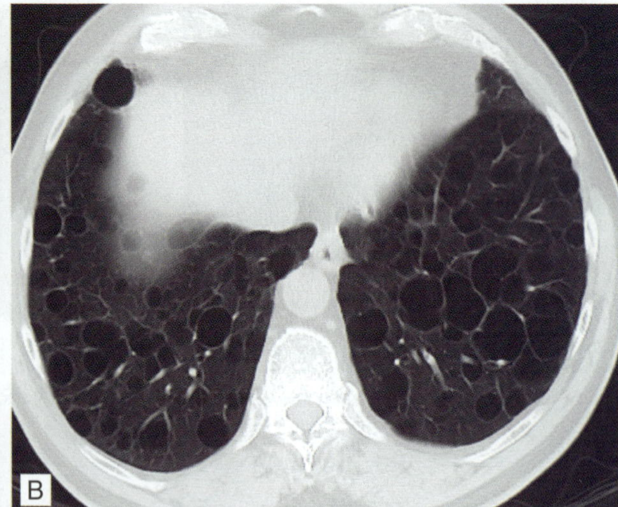

Figure 16.49 LIP. Two CT iamges (A and B) show innumerable parenchymal cysts with subtle scattered groundglass opacities in a patient with human immunodeficiency virus.

most common finding of the disease in the thorax, and commonly occurs together with extrathoracic lymphadenopathy.

Imaging features: *Predominant lung involvement usually occurs late in the disease and is characterized by peribronchovascular and septal thickening, similar in appearance to lymphangitic carcinomatosis.* Occasional patchy air-space opacities may occur. In context of acute myelogenous leukemia, these pulmonary opacities should raise a suspicion of pulmonary leukostasis, a condition characterized by occlusion of small arteries by leukemic cells. The more common causes of pulmonary findings in leukemic patients are opportunistic infections, drug reactions, pulmonary hemorrhage, and cardiogenic pulmonary edema.

Castleman Disease

Pathophysiology: Also described as angiofollicular or giant lymph node hyperplasia, Castleman disease histologically consists of hyaline vascular variant and plasma cell variant. This lymphoproliferative disorder may present as unicentric or multifocal disease. Multicentric disease is commonly associated with Kaposi-Herpes (HHV-8) and HIV viruses, and has systemic symptoms. Unicentric disease typically is found in the thorax and is asymptomatic. Castleman disease usually requires biopsy for definite diagnosis and differentiation from other lymphoproliferative disorders/lymphoma.

Imaging features: Unicentric Castleman disease presents as well-circumscribed mass or cluster of lymph nodes that are markedly hypervascular/hyperenhancing on contrast-enhanced studies (Fig. 16.50). The marked enhancement is observed in arterial phase but also persists on later venous or delayed phases. This pattern of enhancement is somewhat typical of this disease and helps in reaching the diagnosis. If a few internal components are not enhancing, this usually is due to internal necrosis. Mediastinum is the most common location of the unicentric Castleman disease [40]. In contrast, multicentric Castleman disease involves multiple parts of the body/nodal stations. Splenomegaly is often encountered. Similarly to unicentric disease, lymphadenopathy in multicentric disease is also hyperenhancing/hypervascular.

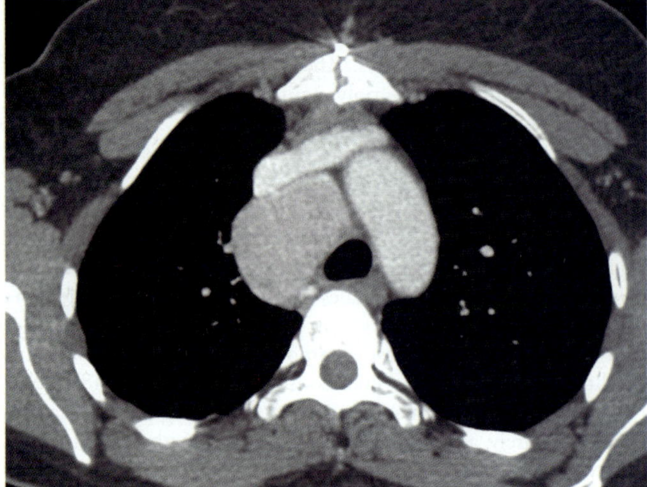

Figure 16.50 Castleman disease. Well-circumscribed hyperenhancing mass in the right paratracheal region, biopsy-proved Castleman disease.

TABLE 16.21 Thoracic Neuroendocrine Cell Spectrum of Diseases

Proliferations
Reactive neuroendocrine cell hyperplasia
Diffuse idiopathic neuroendocrine cell hyperplasia
Proliferation associated with carcinoids
Carcinoid tumor
Typical
Atypical
High-grade malignancy
Small-cell lung cancer
Large-cell neuroendocrine carcinoma

Carcinoid Tumor

Pathophysiology and clinical presentation: Carcinoid tumor is part of pulmonary neuroendocrine cell spectrum of diseases (Table 16.21). Pulmonary neuroendocrine cells are found interspersed in the mucosa of the respiratory tract. Their proliferation may be benign, most commonly in reaction to hypoxia or lung injury [41].

Diffuse idiopathic pulmonary neuroendocrine cell hyperplasia (DIPNECH) is an entity consisting of a focal proliferation of

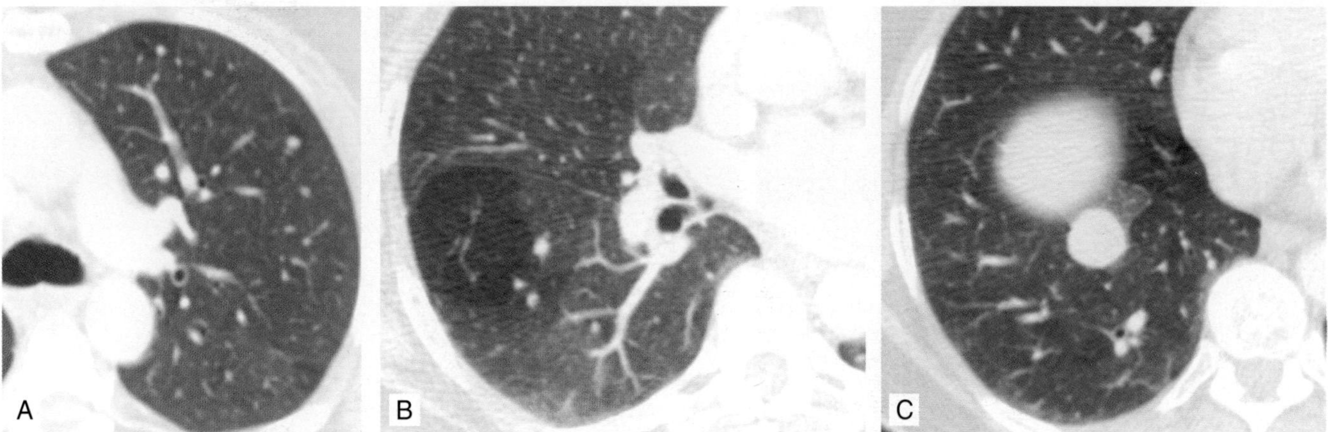

Figure 16.51 Diffuse idiopathic pulmonary neuroendocrine cell hyperplasia. Multiple small scattered pulmonary nodules associated with lobular air-trapping (A and B). Note well-defined, round, larger nodule in the basal RLL, which was confirmed carcinoid on pathology (C).

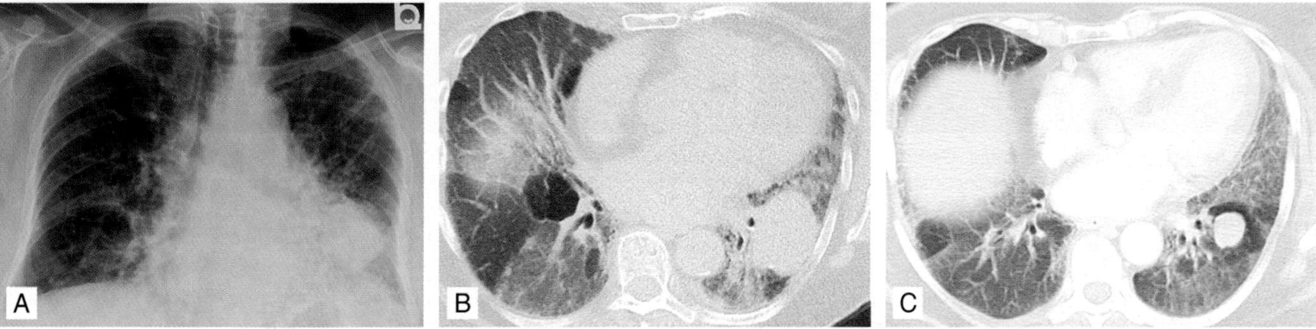

Figure 16.52 Typical carcinoid. Chest radiograph (A) and a CT image (B) show a well-defined mass in the LLL, which has grown since a prior CT scan obained 6 years ago (C).

neuroendocrine cells in distal airways. When less than 5 mm in size, these focal proliferations are called tumorlets. As they are associated with periluminal fibrosis, tumorlets are typically associated with constrictive bronchiolitis. Tumorlets are widely considered precursor for carcinoid tumor.

Carcinoid tumor is described as either typical or atypical. Approximately 90% of carcinoids are typical. These are well-differentiated tumors with low aggressiveness. They grow slowly and essentially do not metastasize. Atypical carcinoids contain higher number of mitosis and internal necrosis, tend to be more locally aggressive and metastasize in approximately 50% of cases. Almost one half of carcinoid tumors are asymptomatic at diagnosis. When endobronchial, these tumors may cause recurrent infections, cough, and hemoptysis. Carcinoids may secrete hormones, which can cause carcinoid syndrome if concomitant liver metastasis are present.

Imaging features:

- DIPNECH is usually undetectable on radiographs given small size of tumorlets. On CT scans, DIPNECH/tumorlets are characterized by 5 mm or smaller nodules that are usually seen in end-of-bronchovascular-bundle distribution and associated with distal air-trapping (Fig. 16.51)
- Typical carcinoid presents as well-circumscribed round or oval mass that is usually 2–5 cm in size and demonstrates slow growth-rate [41,42]. This tumor is sometimes difficult to differentiate from other benign pulmonary nodules such as hamartoma, particularly if the latter does not contain characteristic internal fatty components and calcifications. Given its low metabolic activity, typical carcinoid characteristically demonstrates either no or very mild FDG-uptake on PET scans (Fig. 16.52)

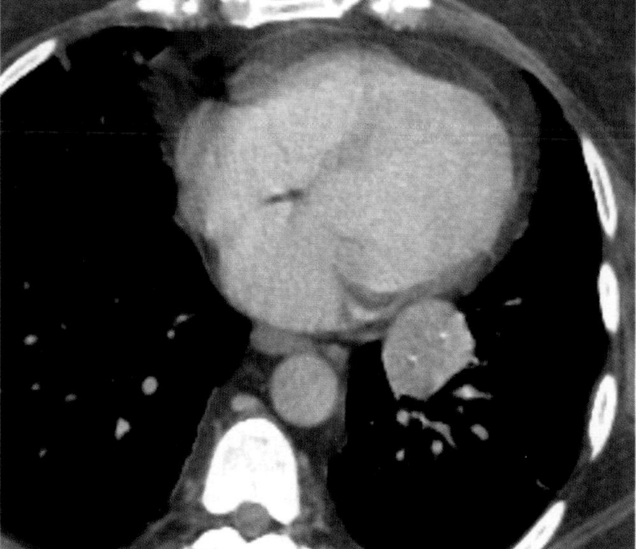

Figure 16.53 Typical carcinoid. Well-defined mass in the anteromedial segment of the LLL. The mass is hyperenhancing and contains punctate eccentric calcifications.

- Atypical carcinoid is more commonly irregular in shape and larger at the time of presentation. In contrast to typical counterpart, atypical carcinoid is peripheral in location in higher percentage of cases
- All carcinoid tumors demonstrate characteristic pronounced enhancement. Calcifications are seen in approximately 30% of cases

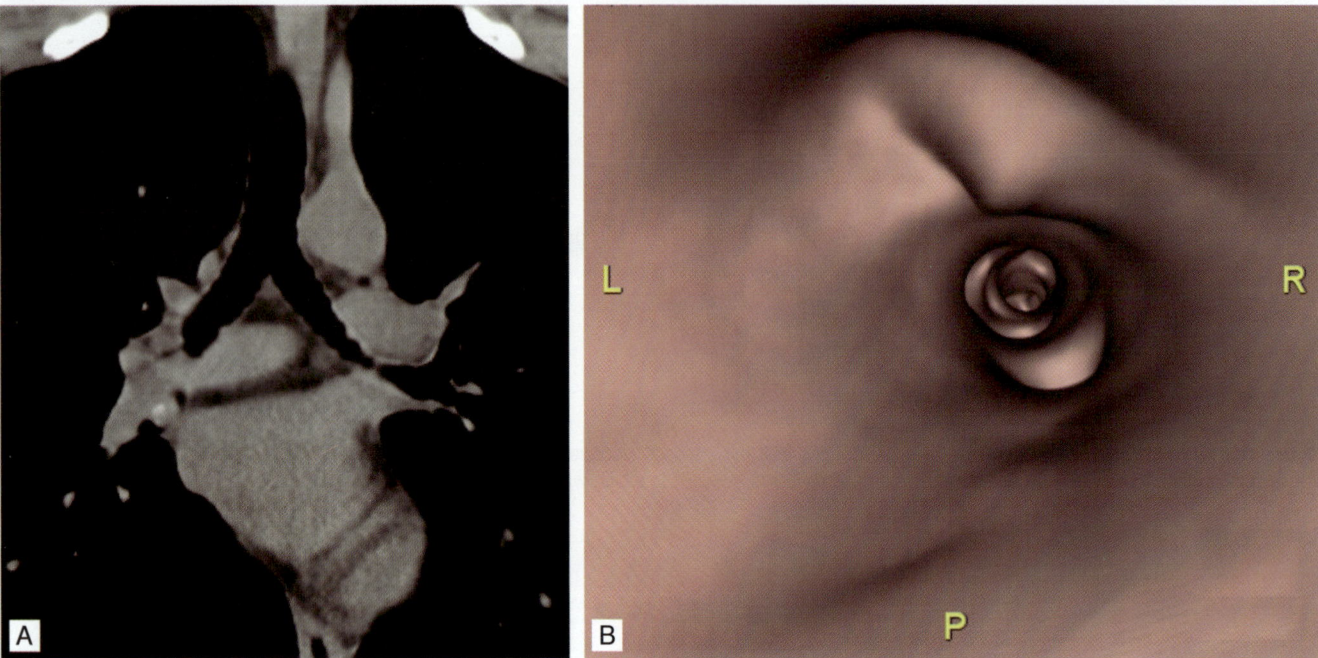

Figure 16.54 Endobronchial carcinoid. Coronal CT image (A) demonstrates partially calcified small endobronchial lesion in the right lower lobar bronchus. 3D image from virtual bronchoscopy (B) demonstrates corresponding lesion along the anterior wall protruding into lumen of the bronchus.

and are often eccentric and irregular (Fig. 16.53). *Carcinoids can be completely endobronchial, or have "tip of iceberg" appearance (small endobronchial and larger extrabronchial components).* When endobronchial, the majority of carcinoids involve lobar or segmental bronchi (Fig. 16.54). Bone metastases are typically of blastic nature when present

Minor Salivary Gland Tumors

Pathophysiology and clinical presentation: These bronchial wall tumors originate from mucus glands and have histological similarities to tumors arising in salivary glands [43] (Table 16.22). These tumors

- are not associated with smoking;
- have better prognosis than of other primary lung malignancies despite their tendency to be locally invasive;
- are most commonly found in trachea, followed by mainstem bronchi and segmental bronchi;
- Adenoid cystic carcinoma and mucoepidermoid carcinoma are the most common types.

Imaging features: Radiologically, minor salivary gland tumors present as focal, eccentric, and mass-like thickening of the tracheal/bronchial wall. They have variable endobronchial component, which, when large enough, may cause atelectasis or collapse (Fig. 16.55).

TABLE 16.22 Thoracic Salivary Gland Tumors
Adenoma
Pleomorphic adenoma
Adenoid cystic carcinoma
Mucoepidermoid carcinoma
Epithelial–myoepithelial carcinomas

Metastatic Disease

Lung is the most common organ affected by metastatic disease. Metastases can reach lung parenchyma by vessels (most common), lymphatics, airways, or direct invasion (Table 16.23). The direct invasion is reserved to intrathoracic tumors, most commonly thymic neoplasms, lymphoma, esophageal cancer, and thyroid tumors. Endobronchial spread of a tumor is very rare and is almost uniquely seen with NSCLC. Lymphatic spread of metastasis can occur from either concomitant hematogenous pulmonary metastases, hilar lymphadenopathy, or intrathoracic lymphatics/thoracic duct. This pattern of metastatic disease is usually seen with breast, prostate, cervix, and upper abdominal (pancreas, stomach) malignancies. Finally, hematogenous metastases can be seen with any primary malignancy. There are several different radiological manifestations of intrathoracic metastatic disease [44–46] (Table 16.24). Pleural metastases are discussed in a different chapter.

Multiple Lung Nodules

Multiple pulmonary nodules are typical presentation of hematogenous metastases (Fig. 16.56). Nodules are

- usually variable in size, ranging from a few millimeters to several centimeters;
- in predominant basilar distribution;
- typically round and well circumscribed, although irregular shape and angular margins may be seen;
- occasionally at the end of a vessel location;
- surrounded by groundglass halo if hemorrhagic.

Almost all primary tumors may present with this pattern of metastatic disease (Table 16.24). Thyroid cancer characteristically

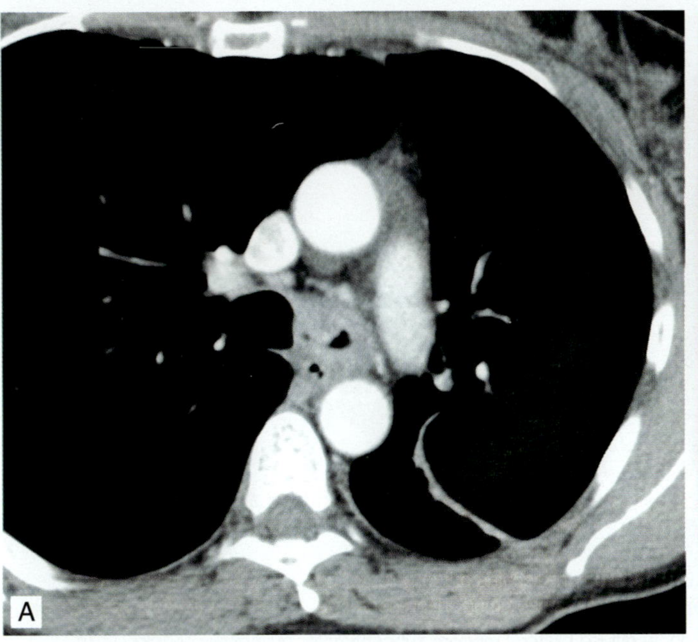

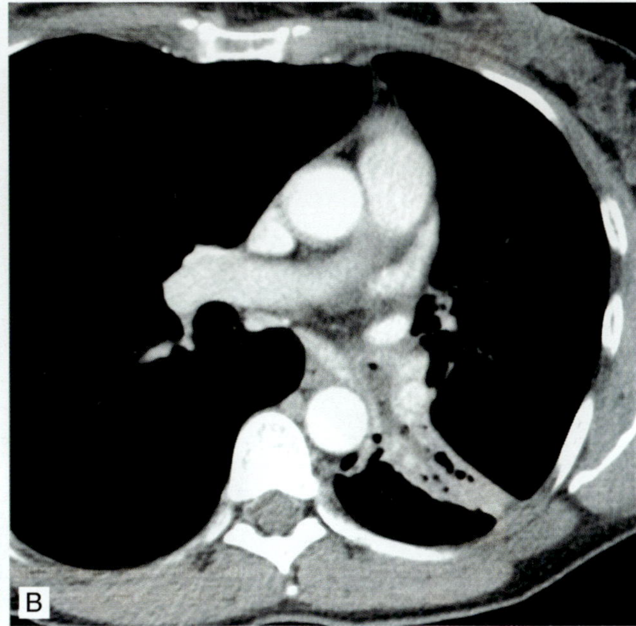

Figure 16.55 Adenoid cystic carcinoma. CT images show an irregular and nodular wall thickening of the left mainstem bronchus (A), with associated mucus plugging and partial LLL collapse (B).

TABLE 16.23 Thoracic Metastatic Disease—Mechanisms

Hematogenous spread
Lymphatic spread
Endobronchial spread
Direct invasion

TABLE 16.24 Thoracic Metastatic Disease—Manifestations

Multiple lung nodules
Large well defined (colon, stomach, sarcoma)
Miliary-type (thyroid)
Cavitary (head and neck, cervix, colon)
Hemorrhagic (melanoma, RCC)
Calcified (thyroid, osteosarcoma, colon, ovary)
Solitary nodule
Melanoma
Sarcoma
Colon
Breast
Endobronchial
Melanoma
Renal cell carcinoma (RCC)
Colon
Thyroid
Breast
Lymphangitic carcinomatosis
Lung
Breast
Pancreas
Stomach
Cervix

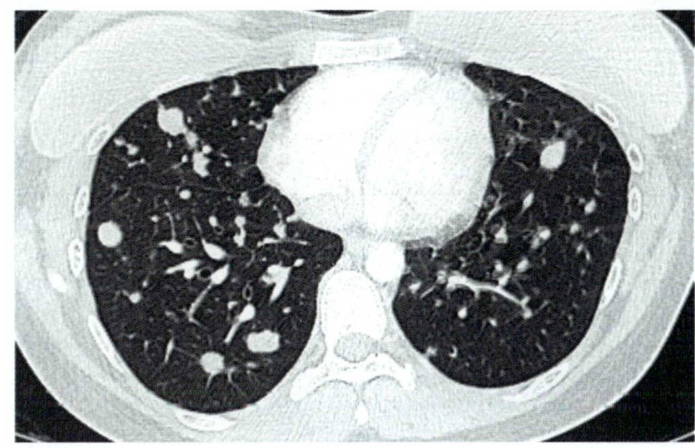

Figure 16.56 Metastases from breast cancer. Multiple scattered bilateral well-defined nodules of variable size.

produces metastases that are 2–3 mm in size and in random distribution, similar to military pattern seen with tuberculosis (Fig. 16.57). In contrast, "Cannonball" metastases, or large well-defined masses, are typically seen with colon and other gastrointestinal tract primaries. Cavitary metastases typically suggest squamous cell carcinomas (head and neck, cervix) or adenocarcinoma of the GI tract (Fig. 16.58). Finally, calcified metastases are usually seen in context of osteosarcoma, mucinous adenocarcinoma, and thyroid cancer.

Solitary Pulmonary Nodule

Melanoma, sarcoma, colon, breast, kidney, and testicular cancers are the most common primary tumors associated with solitary pulmonary metastasis. If a single pulmonary nodule is found in context of *melanoma, sarcoma, or testicular cancer*, metastatic nature of the nodule is more likely than benign process or a primary lung neoplasm. For all other primary cancers, the likelihood of single pulmonary nodule to be metastasis is either equal to or less than being benign or primary lung cancer. Solitary metastasis is typically spherical, well defined, and in

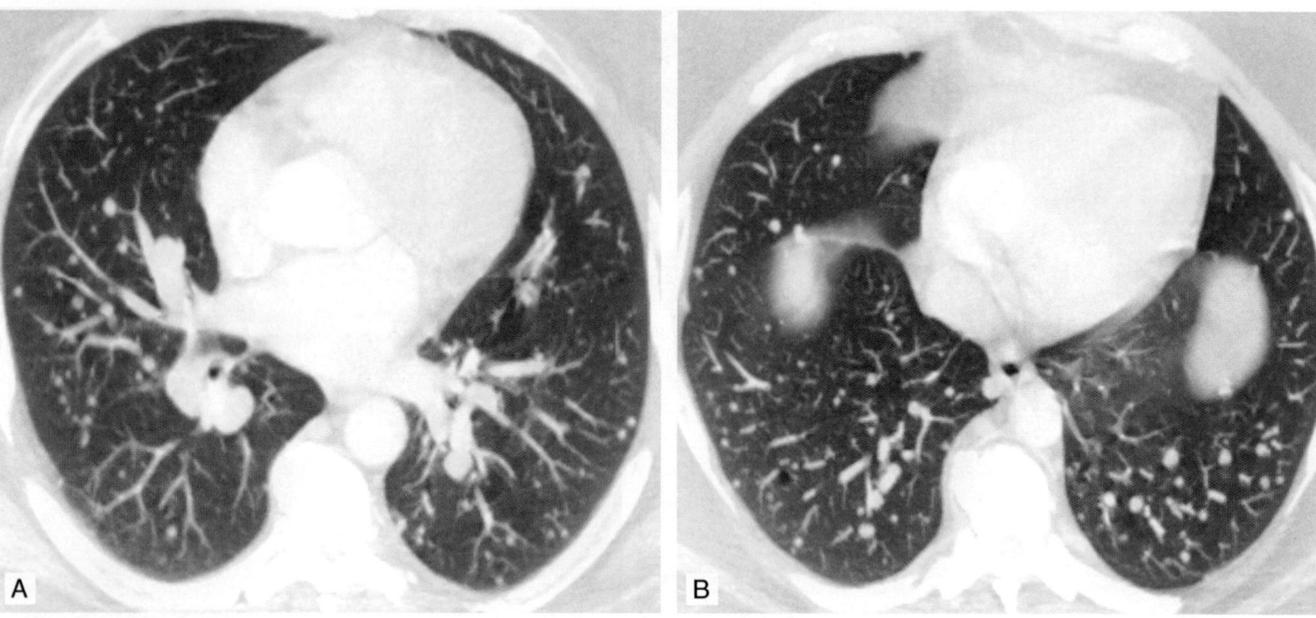

Figure 16.57 Metastases from thyroid cancer. Two CT images (A and B) show diffuse bilateral random subcentimeter pulmonary nodules.

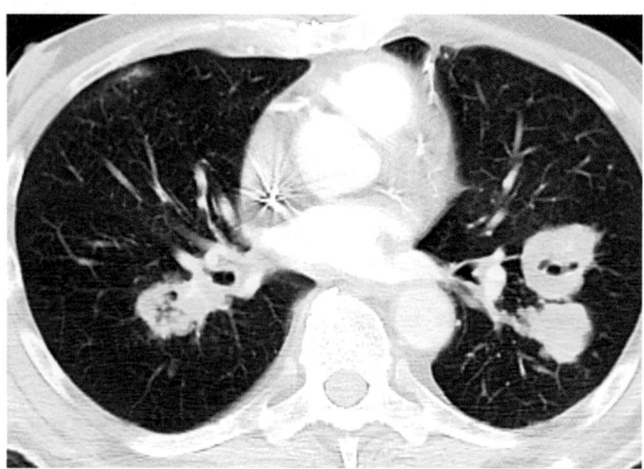

Figure 16.58 Cavitary metastases from colon cancer. Multiple pulmonary nodules and masses containing internal cavitation.

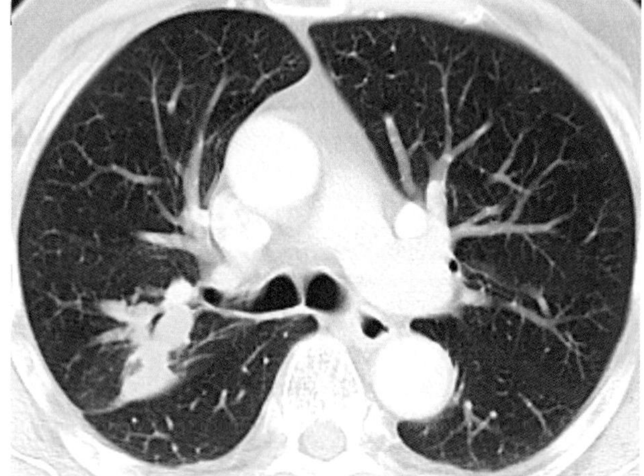

Figure 16.59 Endobronchial metastasis from melanoma. Endobronchial mass in the posterior segmental bronchus of the RUL, with associated distal subsegmental atelectasis.

lower lobes, which may help differentiating it from primary lung cancer. Approach to solitary lung nodule is discussed in detail earlier in the chapter.

Endobronchial Metastases

Similar to primary endobronchial lesions, endobronchial metastases can cause airway obstruction (Fig. 16.59). These usually are multiple, which may help differentiating them from primary endobronchial neoplasm. The commonest primary tumors that give endobronchial metastasis are *melanoma, renal cell carcinoma, colon, breast, and thyroid cancers*. Overall, endobronchial metastases are rare.

Lymphangitic Carcinomatosis

Lymphangitic carcinomatosis represents lymphatic invasion by neoplastic cells, either through direct invasion, or through hematogenous or lymphatic spread. *Primary lung, breast, GI, pancreatic and cervical cancers are usual primary neoplasms that are associated with this type of metastatic disease.* The process is usually symmetric and bilateral, although asymmetric and unilateral distribution may be seen with lung and breast cancers.

Lymphangitic carcinomatosis can be detected on radiographs by the presence of coarse linear/interstitial opacities, with or without pleural effusions. However, the high-resolution CT scan is usually required for the diagnosis (Fig. 16.60). On CT scans, carcinomatosis is suspected with the presence of

- nodular or beaded interlobular septal thickening;
- irregular nodularities along bronchovascular bundles;
- pleural effusions;
- lymphadenopathy.

Intrathoracic Lymphadenopathy

Although metastatic lymphadenopathy is associated with concomitant pulmonary metastases in majority of cases, some extrathoracic primary neoplasms metastasize to mediastinal or hilar

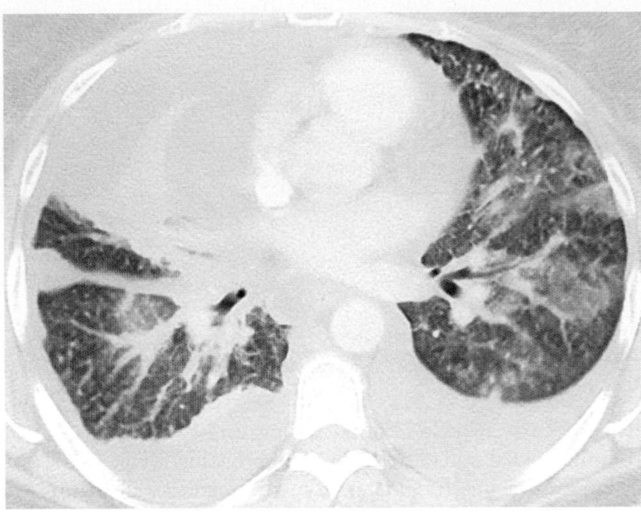

Figure 16.60 Lymphangitic carcinomatosis from gastric cancer. Diffuse nodular interlobular septal thickening with bronchovascular opacities and bilateral pleural effusions.

lymph nodes alone. Distribution of lymphadenopathy may help identifying the primary cancer:

- *Superior mediastinal* adenopathy in primary head and neck cancer
- *Internal mammary chain* adenopathy in ipsilateral breast cancer
- *Pericardial and anterior diaphragmatic adenopathy* in intra-abdominal malignancies, particularly pancreatic, gastrointestinal, and ovarian neoplasms
- *Posterior mediastinal, paravertebral, lower paraesophageal, and retrocrural adenopathy* suggests a GI and testicular cancers

The appearance of enlarged lymph nodes is usually not useful in differentiating the underlying disease or identifying the primary neoplasm. However, some characteristics may be helpful:

- Calcified adenopathy in osteogenic tumors, mucinous adenocarcinomas, and thyroid cancers
- Hyperenhancing or hypervascular lymph nodes in renal cell carcinomas, melanoma and papillary thyroid cancers
- Necrotic hypoenhancing lymph nodes in breast, lung, and testicular cancers

Suggested Readings

- J Bueno, L Landeras, J Chung, Updated Fleischner Society Guidelines for managing incidental pulmonary nodules: common questions and challenging scenarios, Radiographics 38 (5) (2018) 1337–1350.
- N Purandare, V Rangarajan, Imaging of lung cancer: implications on staging and management, Indian J Radiol Imaging 25 (2015) 109–120.
- SJ Hong, TJ Kim, KB Nam, IS Lee, HC Yang, S Cho, New TNM staging system for esophageal cancer: what chest radiologists need to know, Radiographics 34 (2014) 1722–1740.
- A Sirajuddin, VA Lewis, TJ Franks, S Dhand, JR Galvin, CS White, Primary pulmonary lymphoid lesions: radiologic and pathologic findings, Radiographics 36 (2016) 53–70.

17 Diseases of Airways

SARV PRIYA, SACHIN S. SABOO, PRASHANT NAGPAL

Tracheal Diseases

Congenital Abnormalities

Tracheal agenesis is an extremely uncommon congenital anomaly with an estimated prevalence of 1 in 50,000. Floyd et al. have described three subtypes [1,2]:

- Type 1 is seen with agenesis of the proximal trachea with a short segment of normal distal trachea and presence of a distal tracheoesophageal fistula (TEF)
- Type 2 is characterized by a complete absence of the trachea with normal bifurcating bronchi (TEF may or may not be present)
- Type 3 shows atresia of the entire trachea and carina with two main bronchi arising separately from the esophagus (Fig. 17.1)

There are several branching aberrations of the trachea and major bronchi that are commonly encountered incidentally on imaging. Tracheal bronchus [3] is the most common subtype. It usually arises as an accessory bronchus from the right side of the distal trachea within 2–6 cm of the carina and supplies the right upper lobe. Normal anatomical right upper lobe bronchus may or may not be present with this accessory tracheal bronchus. The term pig bronchus is used when the entire right upper lobe is supplied by the tracheal bronchus with the absence of normal anatomical right upper lobe bronchus. The tracheal bronchus is seen along with a separate anatomical right upper lobe bronchus in the majority of cases (Fig. 17.2). Other rare branching abnormalities that can be seen include blind-ending cardiac bronchus (arises from the medial wall of the right main bronchus) (Fig. 17.3), and bridging bronchus (originates from the medial wall of the left main bronchus and supplies the right lower or upper lobe and rarely may supply the entire right lung [4–6].

Three-dimensional (3D) computed tomography (CT) with or without virtual bronchoscopy is sometimes useful to depict these tracheal branching abnormalities and understand the relationship with surrounding structures. Tracheal bronchus should be distinguished from the tracheal diverticulum or paratracheal cyst, which is seen as a focal outpouching from the right posterolateral

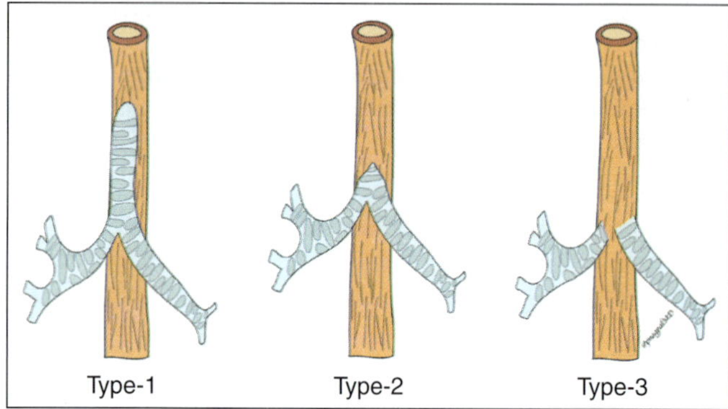

Figure 17.1 An illustrative diagram showing the types of tracheal agenesis and the morphology.

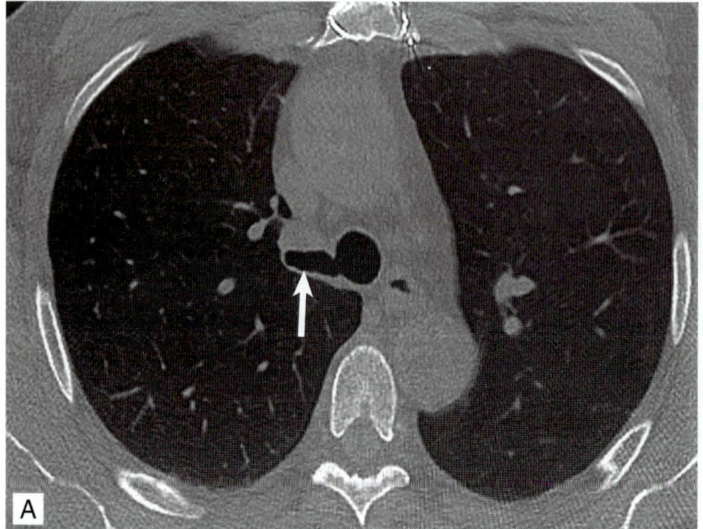

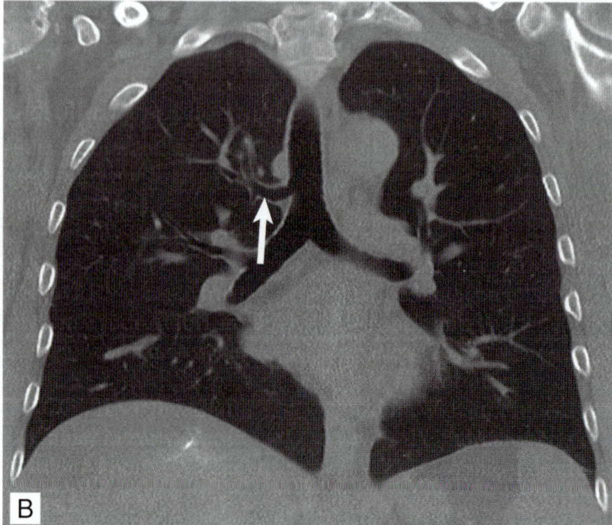

Figure 17.2 A 48-year-old female patient with tracheal bronchus. Axial (A) and coronal (B) lung window images show incidental tracheal bronchus (*arrows*) arising from distal trachea, just above bifurcation and supplying the right upper lobe.

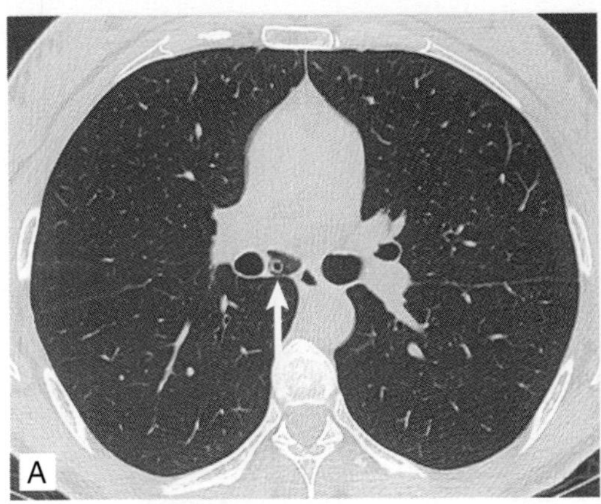

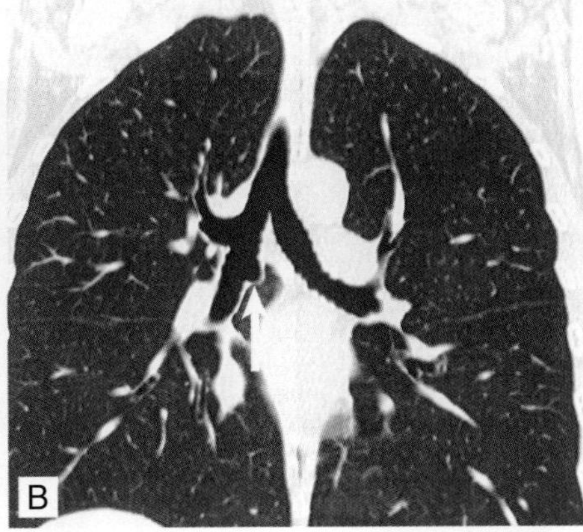

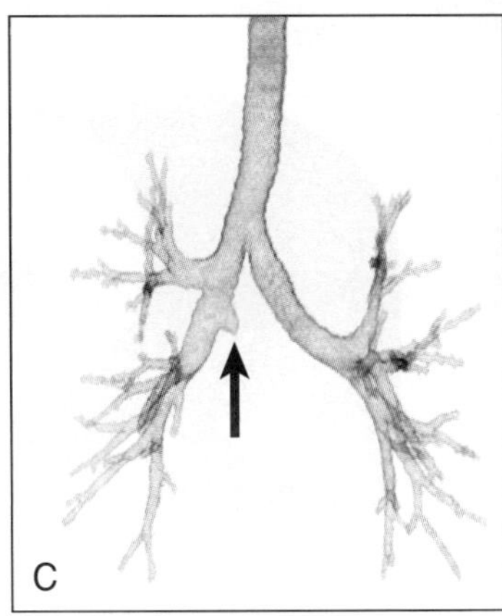

Figure 17.3 A 41-year-old male patient with cardiac bronchus. Axial (A) and coronal (B) lung window CT images and volume-rendered (C) airway images show a blind-ending accessory bronchus (*arrows*) arising from the medial wall of the right bronchus intermedius consistent with cardiac bronchus.

wall of the trachea approximately 4–5 cm below the level of vocal cords near the thoracic inlet (Fig. 17.4) [7].

Bronchial atresia is congenital obliteration of the segment of the airway [8,9]. There is a normal development of airway proximal and distal to the obstructed segment. The bronchus immediately distal to the occluded segment is dilated, and mucus-filled forming a bronchocele. Since usually there is collateral ventilation, the distal lung shows mosaic attenuation with air trapping and hypoperfusion (Fig. 17.5), which is most pronounced on expiratory images. If collateral ventilation is not adequate, atelectasis of the lung segment ventilated by the bronchial segment may be seen. The entity most frequently involves the left upper lobe followed by the right lower lobe.

TEF can be a congenital anomaly or an acquired disease [10]. Congenital TEF usually occurs in association with the esophageal atresia, but it may also occur as an isolated anomaly. TEF may be associated with other congenital anomalies such as the VACTERL complex (i.e., vertebral, anal, cardiovascular, tracheoesophageal, renal, radial, and limb anomalies). There are five types, with type C being the most common subtype. Tracheoesophageal fistula without the esophageal atresia is also referred to as H-type (Fig. 17.6A) [11].

Plain radiographs may reveal an air-filled blind pouch of the proximal esophagus, raising suspicion of the esophageal atresia. *If the radiograph shows intestinal air, it may suggest the presence of tracheoesophageal fistula.* However, the diagnosis and type of fistula are confirmed by a contrast study of the esophagus. Low or iso-osmolar nonionic contrast medium must be used due to the risk of aspiration. If a simple swallow does not show the fistula, the contrast medium should be injected into a nasogastric tube with the patient prone. As the tube is withdrawn, contrast is slowly injected to show the fistula.

Multidetector CT can also be used to detect tracheoesophageal fistula in complex cases due to its excellent multiplanar volumetric and virtual bronchoscopic reconstructions and may help in surgical planning. It can be performed with oral contrast to increase the sensitivity of the test. However, there are concerns about radiation exposure with the use of CT in pediatric patients. Recently, high-resolution structural magnetic resonance imaging (MRI) has also been employed for preoperative surgical planning that avoids the need for radiation. 3D printed or virtual reality models built from CT or MRI images can also help in presurgical planning in addition to improving patient and family education about these complex anomalies.

The acquired causes of TEF include esophageal or lung cancer in the majority of cases (Fig. 17.6B); other causes include mediastinal radiation, prolonged endotracheal intubation, surgical or endoscopic interventions, and mediastinal granuloma.

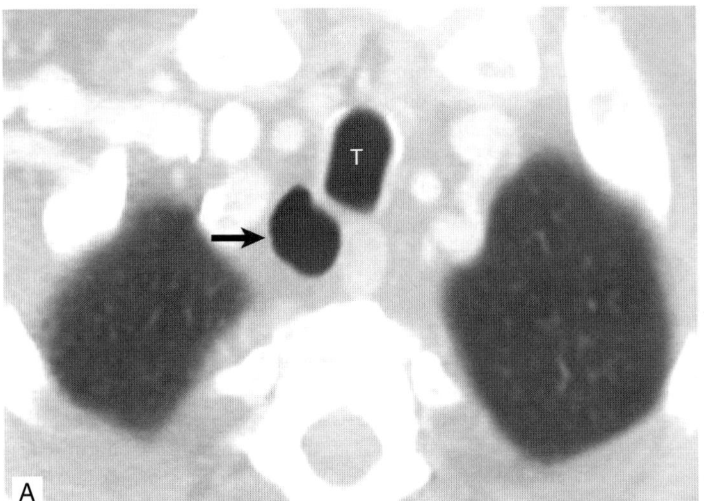

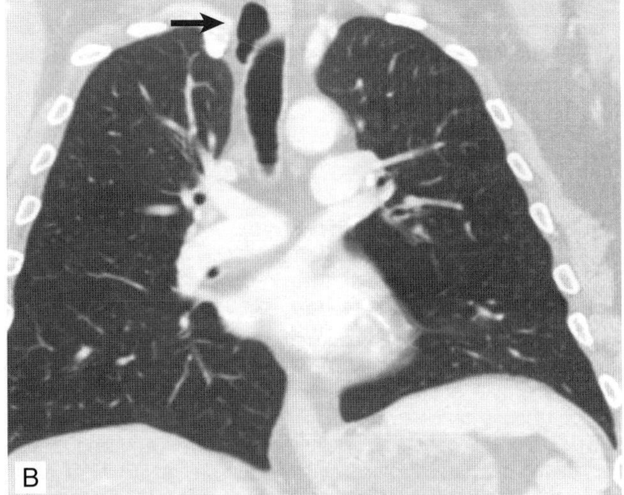

Figure 17.4 A 54-year-old female patient with tracheal diverticulum. CT chest axial (A) and coronal (B) lung window images show air-filled outpouching near right posterolateral wall of trachea at the level of thoracic inlet suggestive of right paratracheal diverticulum (*arrows*). *T:* trachea.

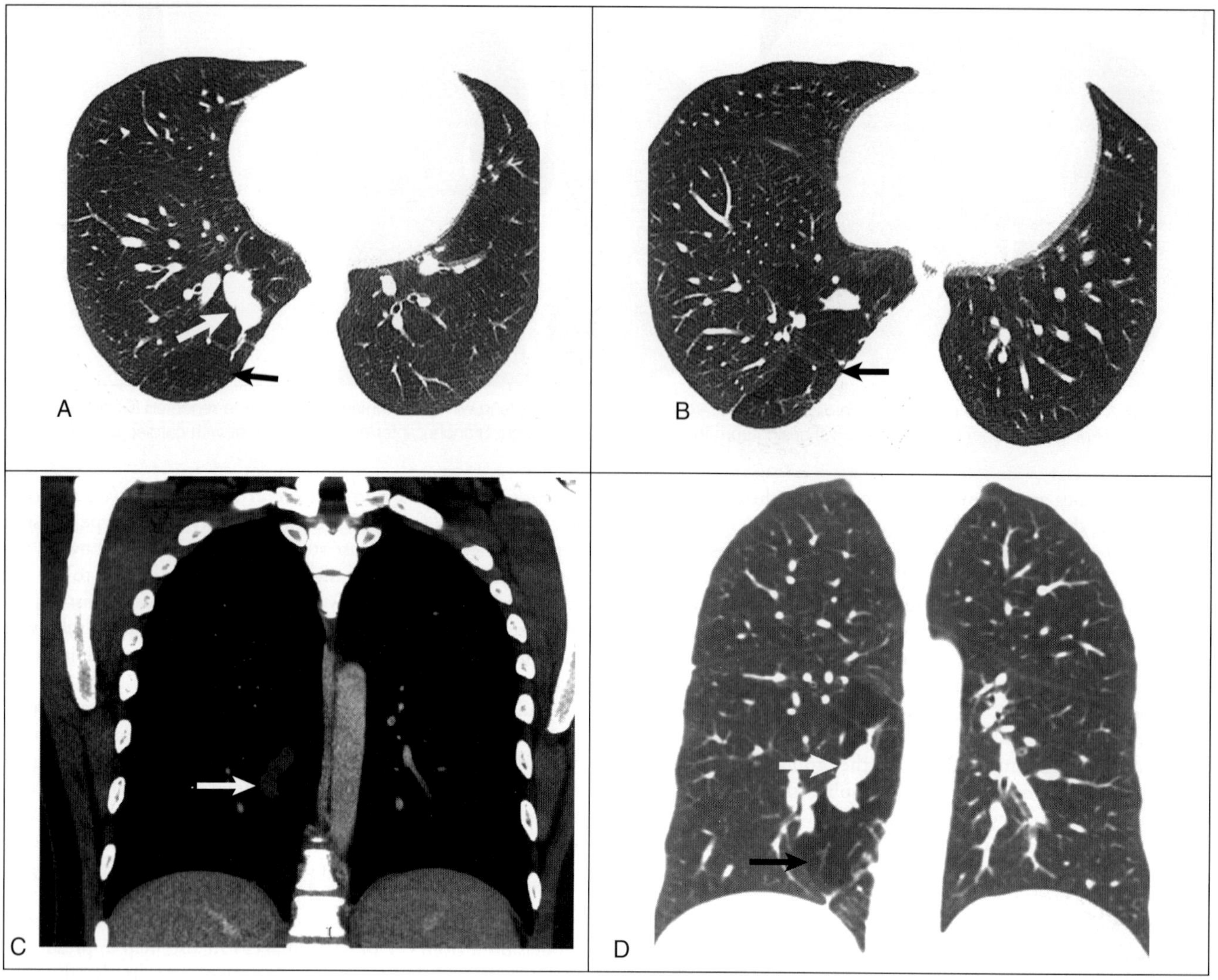

Figure 17.5 A 54-year-old female patient with bronchial atresia found incidentally on chest CT. CT chest lung window (A, B, and D) and soft-tissue window (C) images show a curvilinear mucus-filled tubular opacity in right lower lobe (*white arrow*) with adjacent air trapping (*black arrow*), suggesting bronchial atresia.

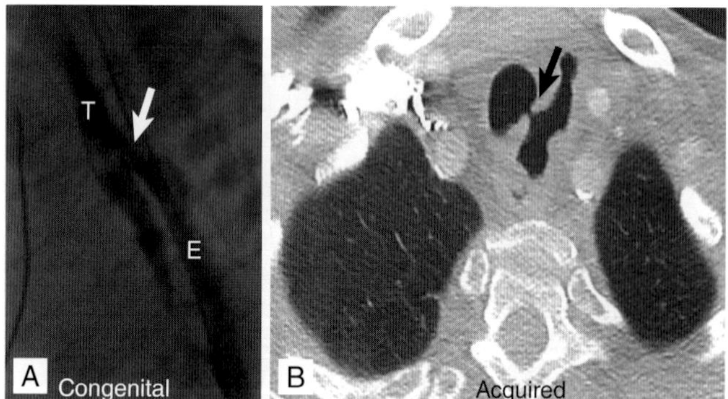

Figure 17.6 Congenital and acquired tracheoesophageal fistula. Congenital tracheoesophageal fistula: 9-month-old female with recurrent pneumonia. Lateral spot film (A) from an esophagram study shows a fistulous connection between trachea and esophagus suggesting a H-type tracheoesophageal fistula (*white arrow*). Acquired tracheoesophageal fistula: CT chest lung window image (B) from another 61-year-old male patient with a history of esophageal carcinoma shows presence of tracheoesophageal fistula at suprasternal location (*black arrow*).

Tracheal Narrowing

Tracheal stenosis can be congenital or acquired. Congenital tracheal stenosis is a rare but life-threatening condition characterized by the presence of complete cartilaginous rings of the tracheal with the absence of the membranous portion [12]. CT shows focal, diffuse, or funnel-like narrowing of the tracheal lumen without wall thickening. Some congenital vascular diseases like a double aortic arch (Fig. 17.7A), pulmonary sling (Fig. 17.7B), or anterior pretracheal course of the innominate artery (Fig. 17.7C) may cause extrinsic tracheal compression [13,14]. Innominate artery compression syndrome, if present, usually cause mild to moderate anterior narrowing of the mid-portion of the trachea while left pulmonary artery sling may cause long diffuse segment severe tracheal stenosis.

Acquired tracheal stenosis is most commonly seen secondary to iatrogenic causes, including tracheostomy and endotracheal intubation [15]. Stricture development following prolonged intubation is thought to be secondary to ischemia of the tracheal mucosa due to overinflation of the cuff of the endotracheal tube. Low-pressure cuffs have now become widespread to prevent this

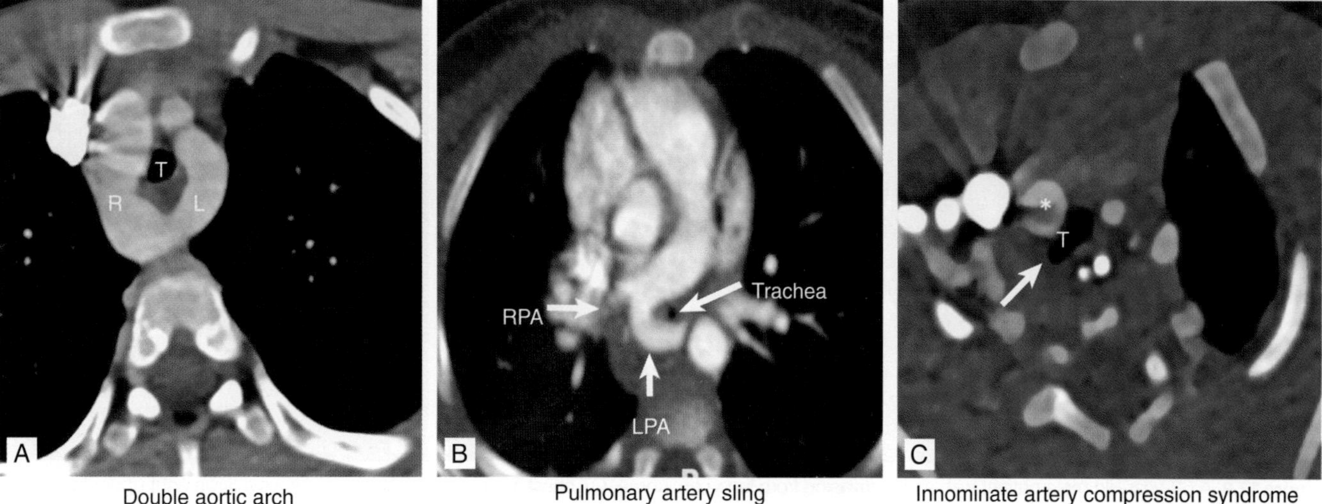

Figure 17.7 Vascular causes of tracheal narrowing. (A) A 7-year-old male child with occasional stridor. CTA axial (A) image shows well-formed double aortic arches on either side of trachea forming a complete vascular ring with mild tracheal narrowing. R: right aortic arch; L: left aortic arch. (B) A 3-year-old female child with pulmonary artery sling and tracheal stenosis. CTA axial image shows aberrant origin of the left pulmonary artery (LPA) from right pulmonary artery (RPA) with retrotracheal course of LPA causes severe tracheal narrowing. (C) A 5-year-old male child with innominate artery compression syndrome. CTA chest axial images show extrinsic narrowing of the tracheal lumen (*arrow*) secondary to the anterior course of the right innominate artery (*). *T:* trachea.

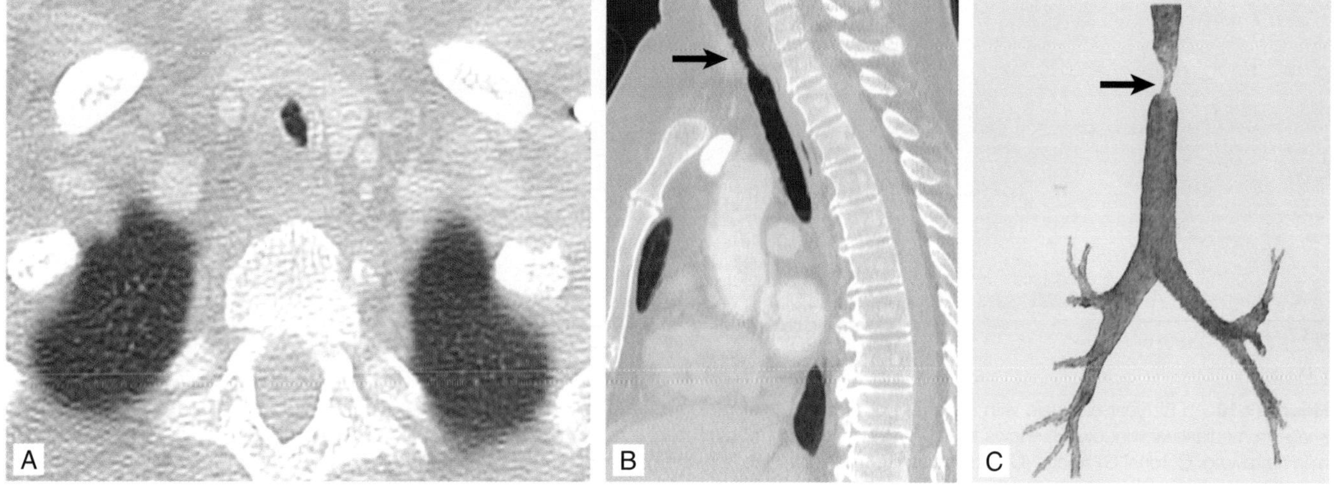

Figure 17.8 Acquired tracheal stenosis. CT chest axial (A), sagittal (B), and volume-rendered airway (C) images show typical appearance of circumferential hourglass tracheal narrowing (*arrow*) at the level of thoracic inlet, in a patient with history of endotracheal intubation for 24 days due to traumatic brain injury.

complication. *CT shows characteristic circumferential hourglass stenosis best seen on 3D volume-rendered images* (Fig. 17.8). Tracheal narrowing may also be due to an extrinsic mass or mediastinal fibrosis.

The common anatomic structures from which masses may originate that lead to tracheal narrowing include lung (Fig. 17.9), thyroid (Fig. 17.10), thymus, lymph nodal, and vessels.

Fibrosing mediastinitis [15], which may be due to tuberculosis or histoplasmosis, can cause both tracheal and bronchial stenosis and presents as infiltrative soft tissue on CT with compression of airways and adjacent vasculature. Calcifications may also be seen (Fig. 17.11). Multiple inflammatory or infiltrative diseases can also involve the trachea and the central airway. The diseases that can involve trachea are rare and include *amyloidosis* (Figs. 17.12 and 17.13), tracheobronchopathia osteochondroplastica (TBO) (Fig. 17.14), chronic relapsing polychondritis (Fig. 17.15), sarcoidosis, granulomatosis with polyangiitis, and rhinoscleroma [15]. An important diagnostic feature that can help narrow the differential diagnosis is that primary cartilaginous diseases that can involve trachea like relapsing polychondritis and tracheobronchopathia osteochondroplastica, affects the anterior and lateral cartilaginous portion of the trachea and spares the posterior wall [16]. On the other hand, infiltrative diseases like amyloidosis, sarcoidosis, and granulomatosis with polyangiitis can involve any wall of the trachea, including the membranous noncartilaginous posterior wall [16]. The features that are typical of these diseases involving the large central airway are summarized in Fig. 17.16.

Tracheobronchomalacia refers to the structural weakness of the tracheal cartilages, which leads to excessive airway collapse in expiration [17]. The tracheobronchomalacia can be congenital or acquired, and the narrowing can be focal or diffuse. The congenital form may be self-limiting that typically resolves by second year. Acquired causes are more common, and the causes include recurrent infection, prior radiation, intubation, tumors, or chronic obstructive airway disease.

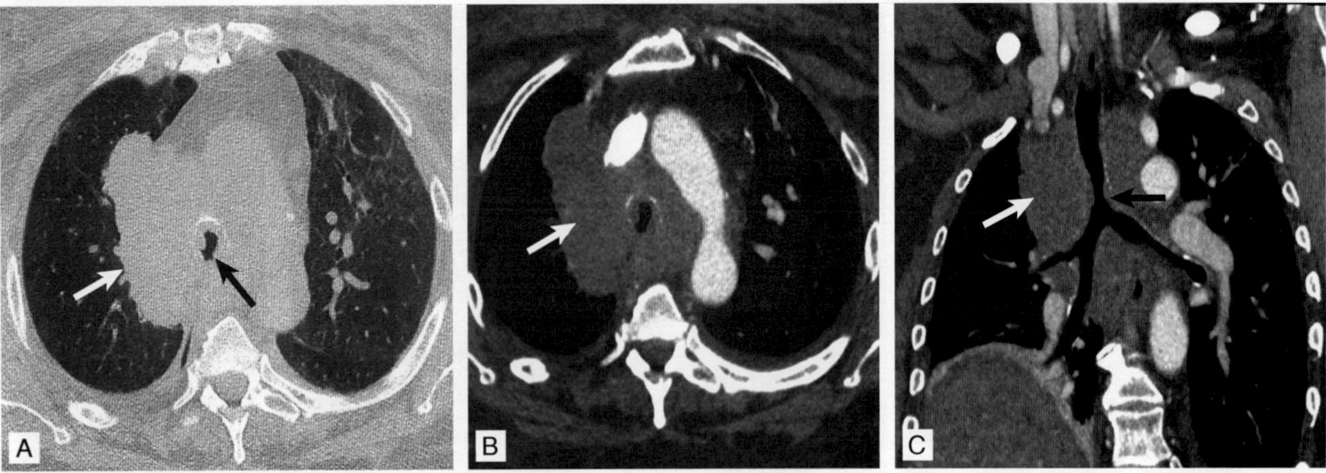

Figure 17.9 A 63-year-old male patient with airway invasion from lung carcinoma. CT chest lung window (A) image shows a large right upper lobe mass (*white arrow*) (biopsy-proven lung carcinoma) invading the mediastinum. CT axial (B) and coronal (C) mediastinal window images show circumferential invasion of the central airways (*black arrow*) with moderate luminal narrowing.

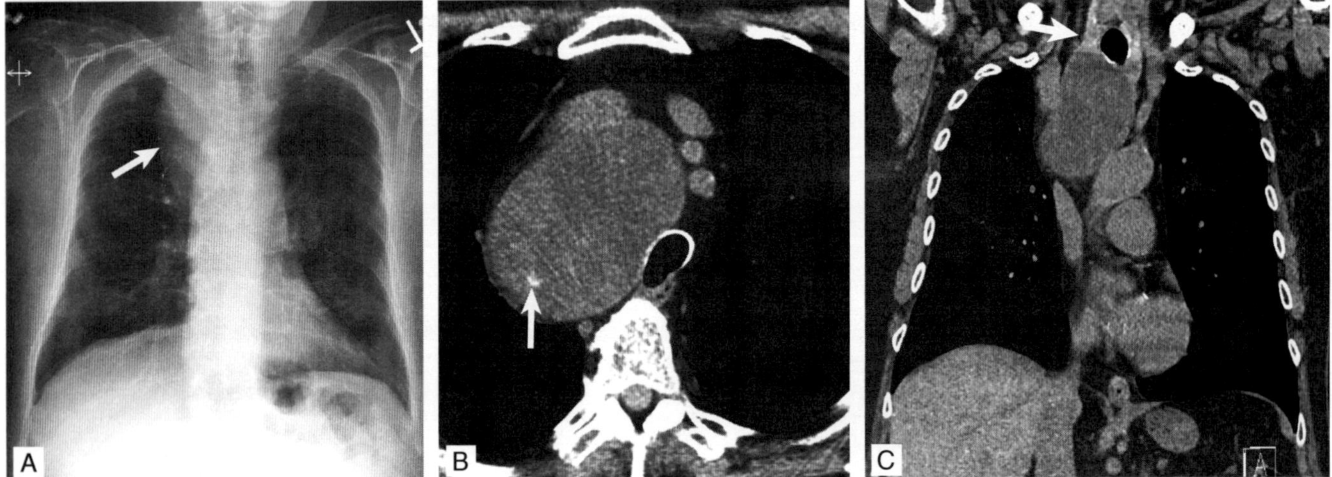

Figure 17.10 An 82-year-old male with shortness of breath. Chest radiograph (A) shows soft-tissue density right paratracheal mass (*arrow*). Axial CT image in mediastinal window (B) shows a large well-defined right paratracheal mass with foci of calcification (*arrow*) causing tracheal displacement and mild narrowing. Coronal CT image (C) shows that the mass is arising from the inferior portion of the right thyroid gland (*arrow*) with retrosternal mediastinal extension.

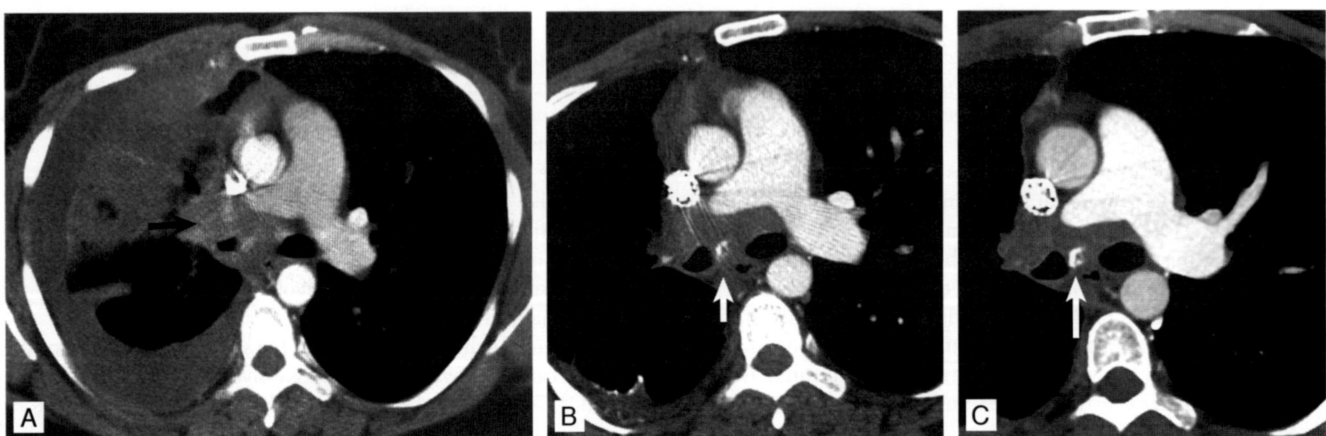

Figure 17.11 Fibrosing mediastinitis from histoplasmosis. CT chest axial (A) image in a 47-year-old female patient with acute histoplasmosis infection presenting with right lung consolidation, pleural effusion, and mediastinal soft tissue causing superior vena cava (SVC) narrowing and right pulmonary artery encasement (*black arrow*). Follow-up chest radiograph a year later (B) shows stent in SVC with developing calcification (*white arrow*) and occlusion of distal right pulmonary artery (RPA). Repeat follow-up evaluation a year later (C) shows stable RPA occlusion with increasing calcification (*arrow*) and mild narrowing of right main stem bronchus.

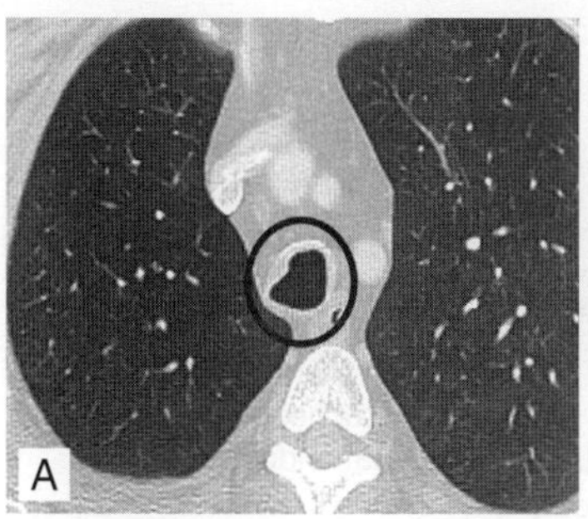

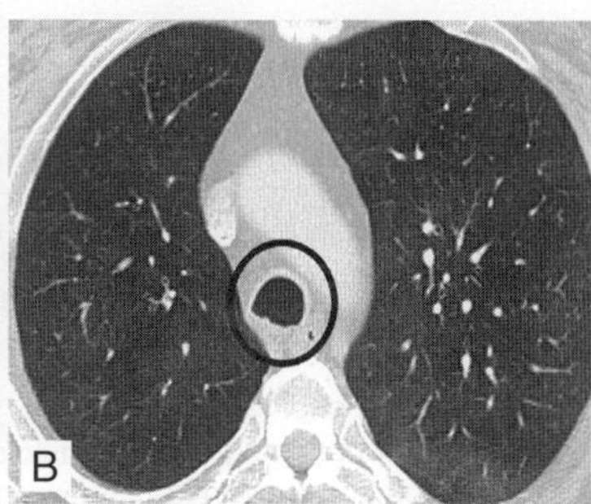

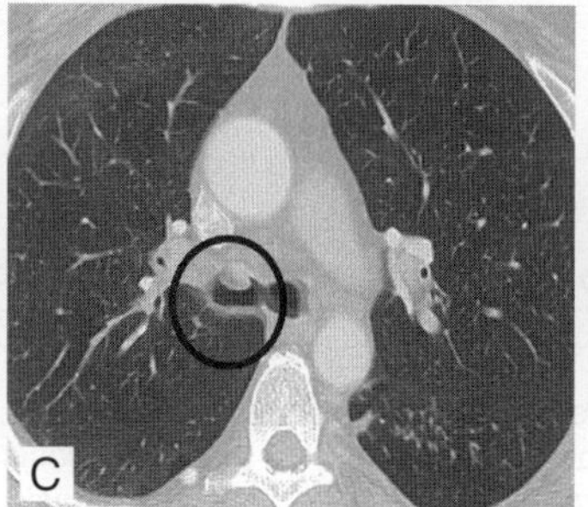

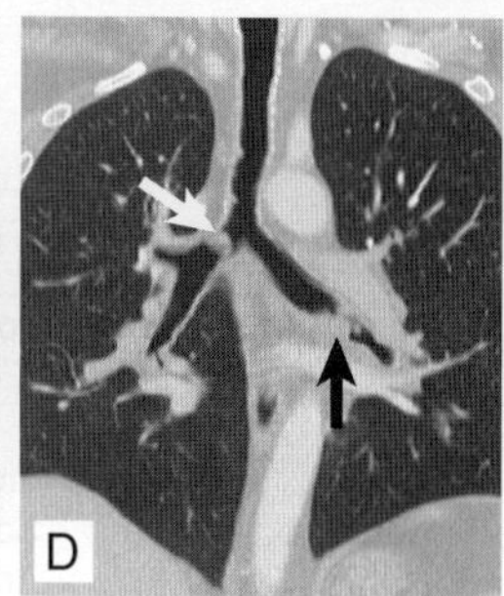

Figure 17.12 A 65-year-old female patient with biopsy-proven amyloid—focal type. CT chest lung window images (A, B, and C) images show anterior and posterior tracheal wall thickening (circle) (A, B), right main stem bronchus thickening (C) and nodularity. Coronal lung window image (D) shows multifocal tracheal and bilateral bronchial involvement (*arrows*).

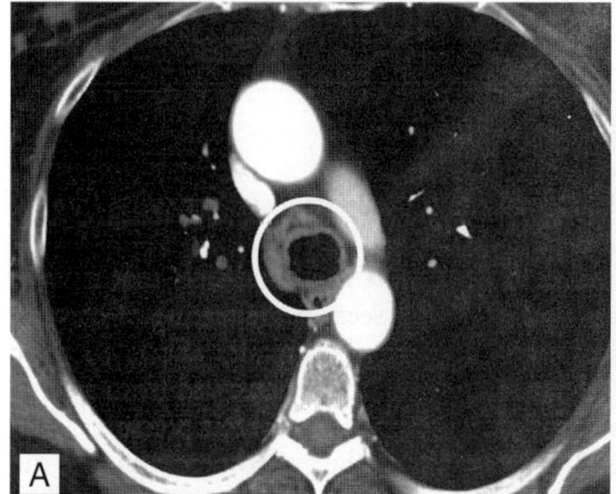

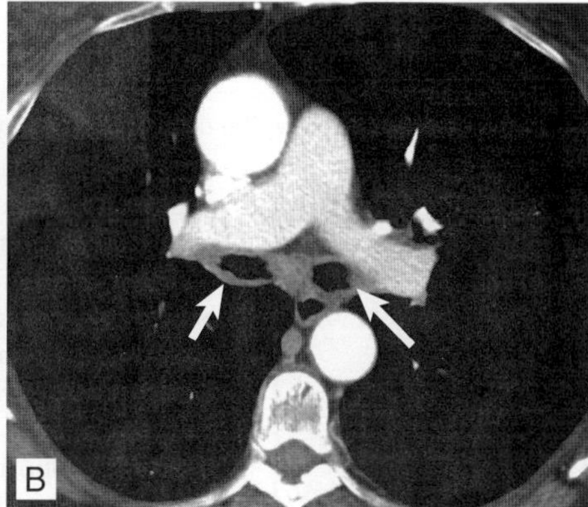

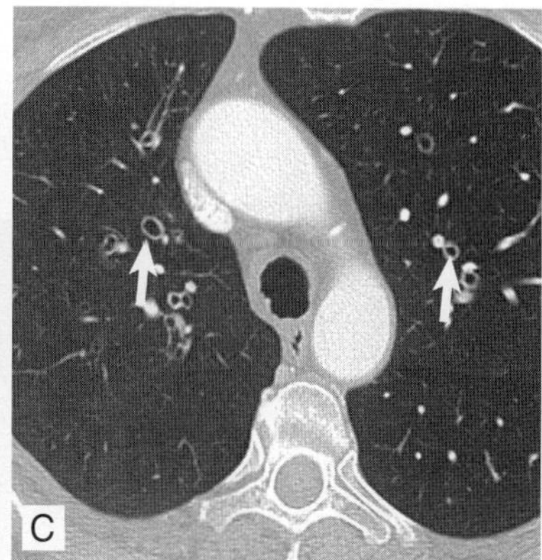

Figure 17.13 A 59-year-old male patient with biopsy-proven amyloid—diffuse type. CT chest mediastinal window axial (A, B) and lung window (C) images show diffuse tracheal thickening (A) involving the posterior wall (circle) with bilateral main stem bronchial thickening (*arrows* in B) extending into the segmental airways (*arrows* in C).

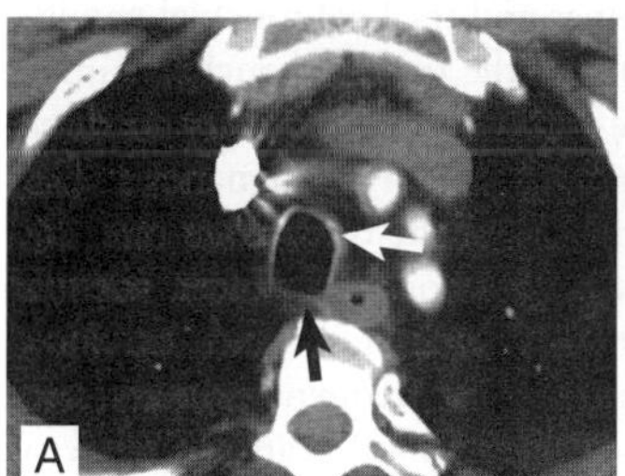

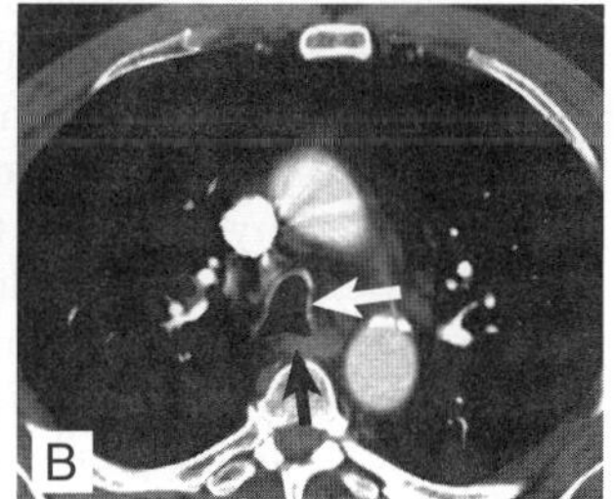

Figure 17.14 A 56-year-old male patient with tracheobronchopathia osteochondroplastica. CT chest axial mediastinal window images (A, B) show nodular thickening (*white arrows*) of airway with calcifications. Posterior membrane is spared (*black arrows*).

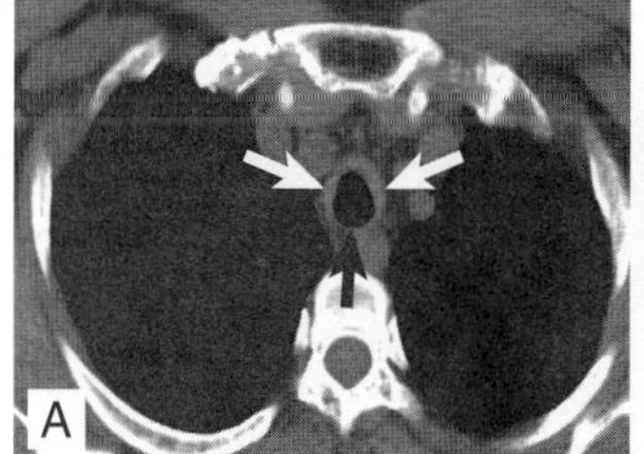

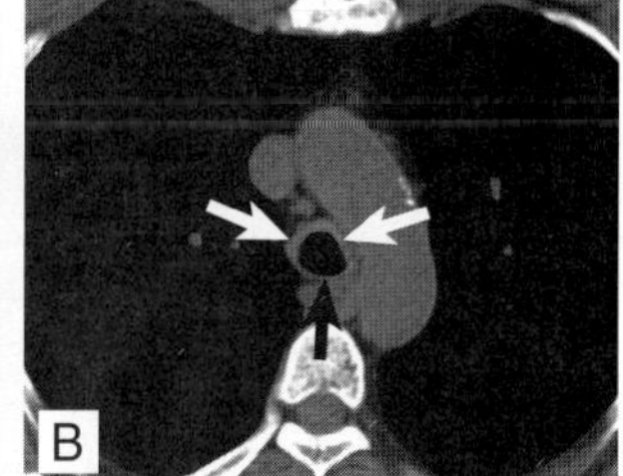

Figure 17.15 A 66-year-old female with rheumatoid arthritis and relapsing polychondritis. Axial CT chest mediastinal window images (A, B) show smooth, slightly hyperdense thickening of the anterior and lateral wall of the trachea (*long white arrows*) with sparing of the posterior wall (*black arrows*).

Multidetector CT with dynamic airway or expiratory imaging can provide quick, noninvasive assessment of airway collapse during expiration (Fig. 17.17). The degree of narrowing that defines tracheobronchomalacia is a matter of debate. Initially, the airway collapse by more than 50% on dynamic expiratory imaging was proposed. However, it was shown that some healthy individuals could have such a collapse during forced expiration. Currently, the collapse of the airway by greater than 50% in end expiration or by greater than 70% on dynamic expiratory imaging is considered more acceptable [18]. *Excessive dynamic airway collapse is a condition that is frequently confused with tracheobronchomalacia* [19]. Excessive dynamic airway collapse is not associated with cartilage weakness and is defined as excessive (>50%) collapse of the airway wall due to the laxity of the posterior wall membrane with intact airway cartilage.

Laryngotracheobronchitis or croup is the commonest cause of tracheal narrowing in children [20]. It is usually viral and affects the upper trachea, most often in young children. It is diagnosed clinically with chest radiograph only performed in uncertain cases.

Croup has a typical appearance on the frontal chest radiograph presenting as "steeple sign" (inverted V-like narrowing) of the upper trachea (Fig. 17.18). Pyogenic bacteria and tuberculosis are usually more severe infections and may cause a more generalized acute tracheitis with severe narrowing. On imaging, there is a narrowing of the upper trachea similar to croup; however, the wall

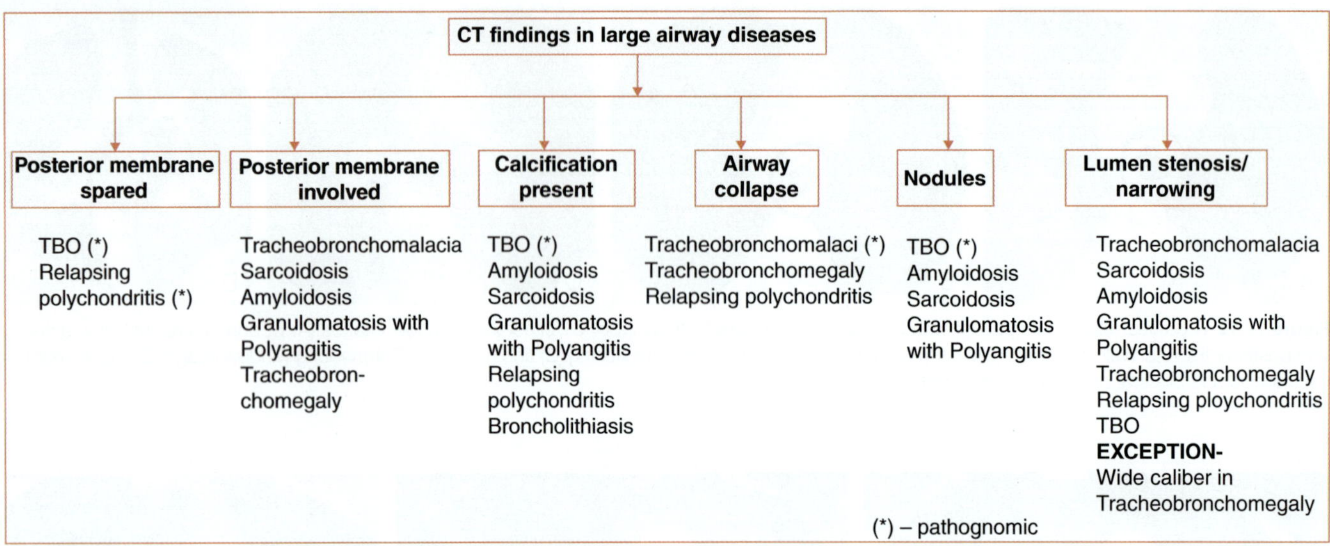

Figure 17.16 Summary of the important features of the diseases involving the central large airways.

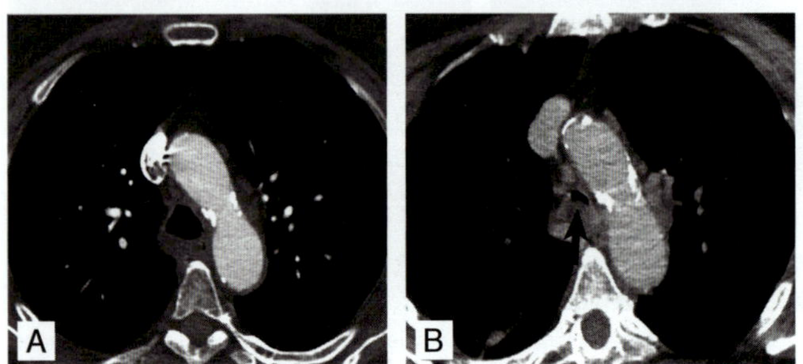

Figure 17.17 A 47-year-old female patient with tracheomalacia. CT chest axial inspiratory (A) and end expiratory (B) images show >50% collapse of the tracheal lumen (*black arrow*) on end expiration image suggesting tracheomalacia.

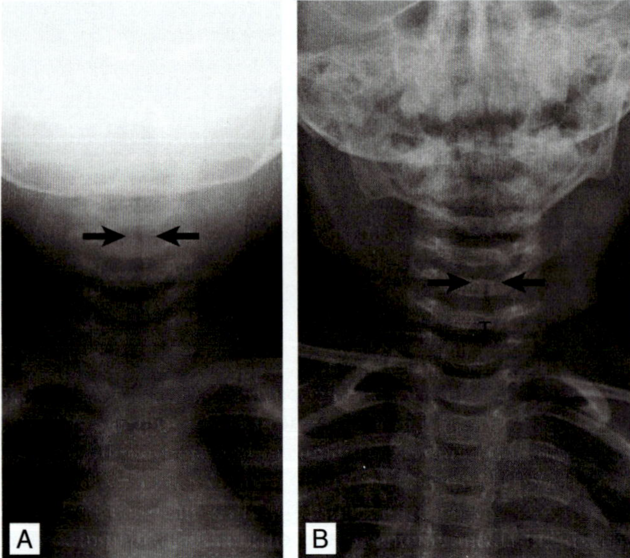

Figure 17.18 Croup on frontal soft-tissue neck radiograph. Frontal neck radiograph (A) in a 20-month old showing severe narrowing of the sub glottic airway with tapering of the upper trachea (*black arrows*) resembling steeple of the church, consistent with laryngotracheobronchitis or croup. Similar appearance of croup in another 2-year-old female child (B) associated with mild tracheal shift to the right. *T*: trachea.

appears irregular. In chronic stages, tuberculosis may cause fibrosis with tracheal stenosis.

Saber-sheath trachea (Fig. 17.19) is a condition that usually occurs in older men and is usually seen in the setting of chronic obstructive airway disease [21]. The abnormality affects only the intrathoracic part of the trachea, which is narrowed from side to side, probably as a result of abnormal intrathoracic pressures. This theory is supported by the caliber of the extrathoracic part of the trachea being normal. The best diagnostic clue on imaging is a marked decrease in coronal diameter with an increased sagittal diameter (tracheal index = coronal diameter/sagittal diameter; abnormal <0.6).

Primary tumors of the trachea are rare. Benign primary tumors present as small, well-defined intraluminal nodules. The most common benign tumors are hamartomas and tracheobronchial papillomas [22] (Fig. 17.20). About 90% of the tracheobronchial tumors in adults are malignant, and the majority are secondary to direct invasion by thyroid, lung, or esophageal malignancies [23] (Fig. 17.9). Primary malignant tumors of the trachea are rare, and common histological types include squamous cell cancer, adenoid cystic carcinoma, mucoepidermoid carcinoma, and carcinoid tumor. Squamous cell cancer is the most frequent primary neoplasm of the trachea, typically occurs in 50–60 years age range, is male predominant, and has a strong association with smoking [24] (Fig. 17.21).

Cross-sectional imaging is nonspecific for these tumor types, and imaging findings include a localized mass, polypoid or sessile lesion, eccentric narrowing, or a long stricture. CT is particularly important in the evaluation of the local spread of the disease. Carcinoid tumor is the most frequent bronchial tumor of childhood and usually presents as a smooth rounded intrabronchial mass that may contain calcifications (Fig. 17.22) [25]. The symptoms from airway obstruction are more common than symptoms from hormone secretion. Newer radioactive agents like Ga68—somatostatin receptor positron emission tomography (PET) are specific for well-differentiated carcinoid tumor localization [26] (Fig. 17.23). Of note, well-differentiated carcinoid is somatostatin receptor radiotracer avid, and poorly differentiated carcinoid tumor is not avid on somatostatin receptor PET imaging but is avid on conventional F18-deoxyglucose PET. Rarely, the trachea can be the site of metastases from a distant primary tumor. The most common

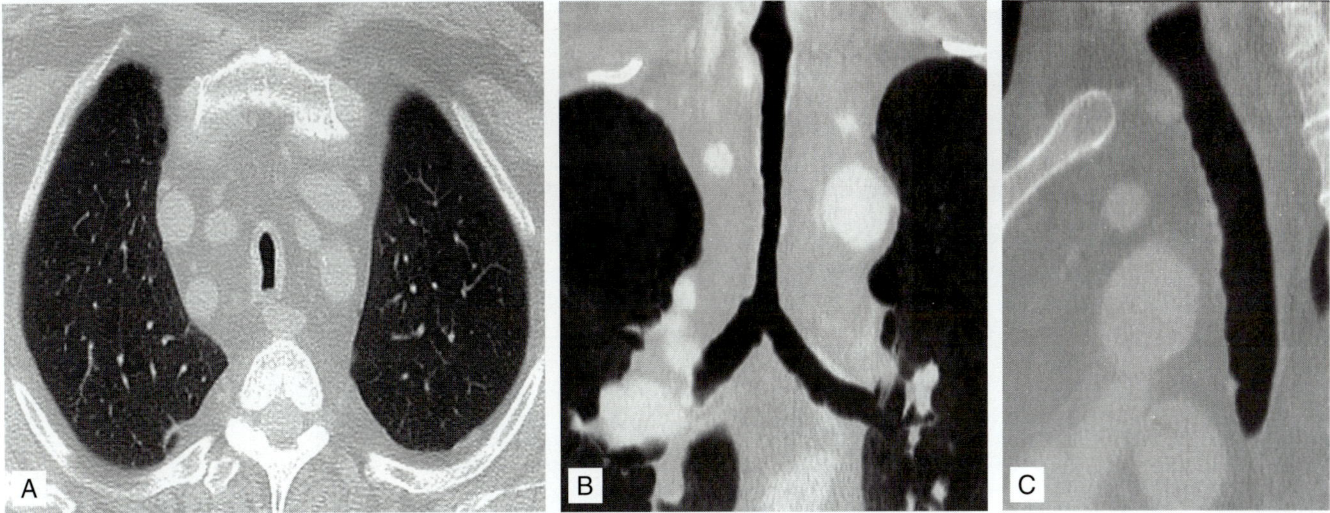

Figure 17.19 A 64-year-old man, with 40 pack-year smoking history. CT image axial (A) showing centrilobular emphysema with decreased transverse diameter and increased anteroposterior diameter. Tracheal deformity is better seen on minimum intensity projection coronal (B) and sagittal (C) view.

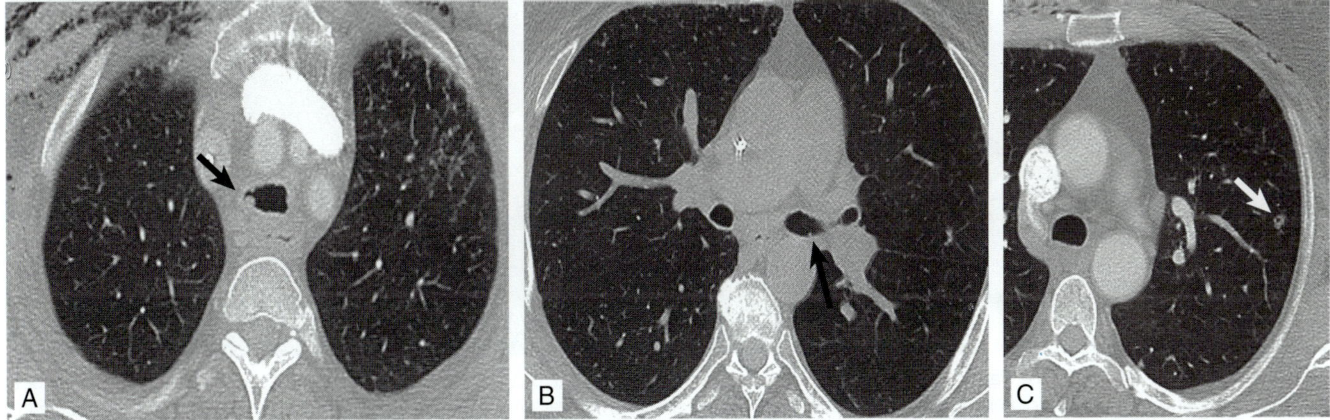

Figure 17.20 A 32-year-old female patient with tracheobronchial papillomatosis. CT chest axial lung window images (A–C) show tracheal (A) and left main bronchus (B) nodules (*black arrows*) with a cavitary nodule in left upper lobe (*white arrow*) suggesting airway papillomatosis. Also seen is incidental right chest wall subcutaneous emphysema from attempted traumatic neck central line insertion.

primary tumor that can cause tracheal metastasis is melanoma [27] (Fig. 17.24).

Tracheal Widening

The normal dimensions of the trachea have been assessed using a variety of techniques, including radiography, fluoroscopy, and computed tomography. The tracheal diameter increases with increasing age. Pathological dilatation of the trachea is rare and may result from a defect of connective tissue. This may be an isolated abnormality as in *tracheobronchomegaly* (Mounier–Kuhn syndrome) or associated with Ehlers–Danlos syndrome or cutis laxa [28].

Mounier–Kuhn syndrome is usually seen in males in their fourth to fifth decade [29]. CT imaging in Mounier–Kuhn syndrome shows the maximum coronal and sagittal diameter of the trachea exceeding 21 mm and 23 mm in females and 25 mm and 27 mm in males, respectively (Fig. 17.25). There may be associated findings of tracheal caliber corrugation, multiple diverticula, or bronchiectasis. The hypothesis that it results from a defect of connective tissue receives some support from its occasional association with Ehlers–Danlos syndrome, a generalized connective tissue disorder. The patients with tracheobronchomegaly are at increased risk of infections due to impaired mucociliary clearance.

Bronchial Diseases

Bronchiectasis

Bronchiectasis refers to permanent, irreversible dilatation of one or more bronchi and is usually the result of severe, recurrent, or chronic inflammation or infection [30]. Childhood pneumonia, especially pertussis, measles, and tuberculosis, as well as smoking, are important causes. Other predisposing factors include chronic sinusitis, bronchial obstruction, and abnormalities of the cilia, mucus, and immune system (e.g., Kartagener syndrome—(Fig. 17.26), cystic fibrosis, and agammaglobulinemia). Noninfective causes include bronchopulmonary aspergillosis and inhalation of noxious fluids or gases. In addition, bronchiectasis is seen in association with intrinsic connective tissue abnormalities such as Ehlers–Danlos syndrome, Marfan syndrome, and tracheobronchomegaly, and rarely in association with more common conditions such as rheumatoid disease and Sjögren syndrome. In patients with interstitial pulmonary fibrosis, distortion and

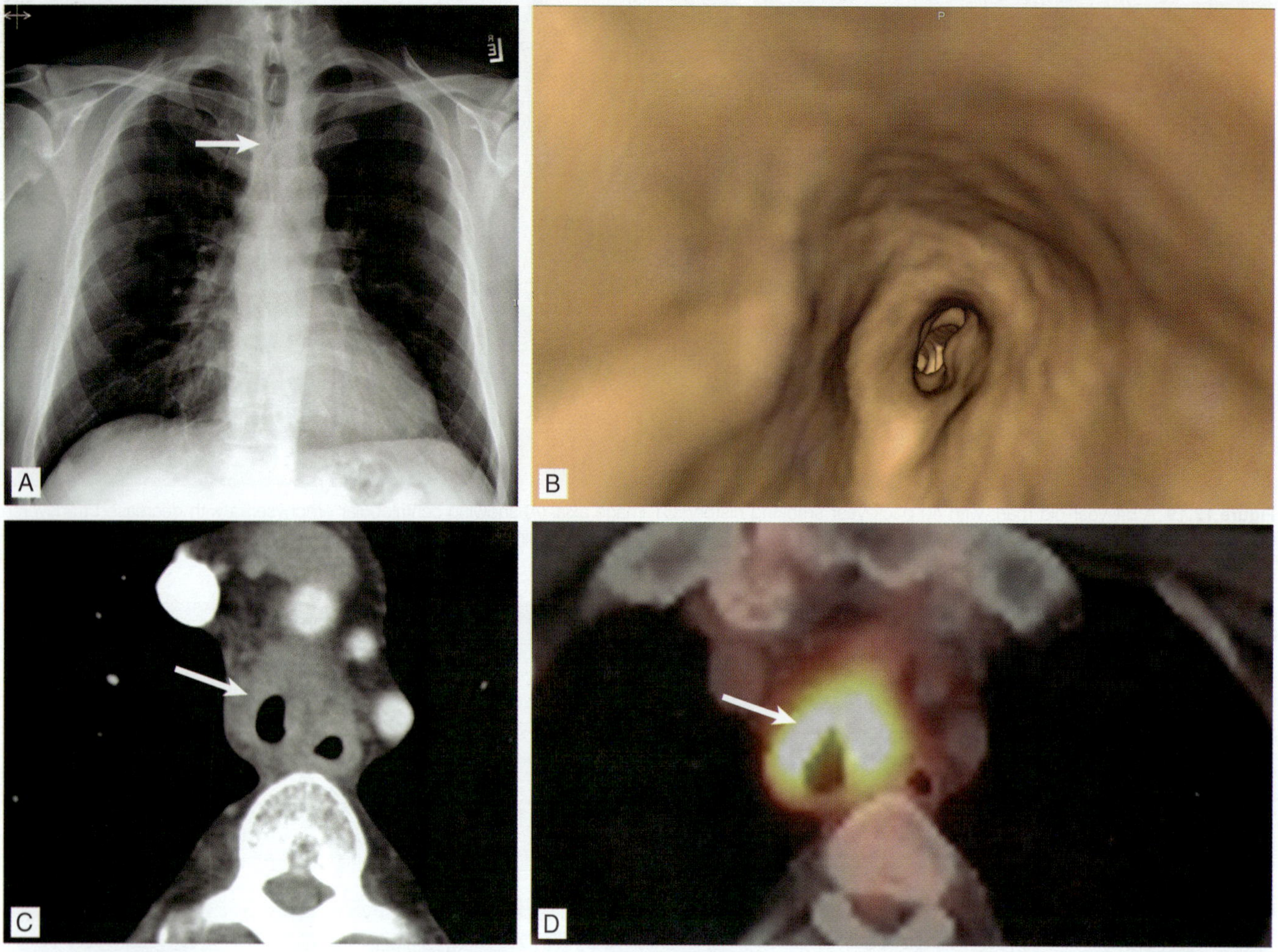

Figure 17.21 A 67-year-old male patient with biopsy-proven squamous cell cancer of trachea. Frontal chest radiograph (A) shows mild focal tracheal narrowing (*arrow*). Endoluminal virtual bronchoscopy (B) and axial CT chest (C) images show eccentric tracheal soft-tissue thickening (*arrow*) and narrowing. Fluoro-deoxy-glucose Positron Emission Tomography (FDG-PET) CT (D) axial image shows intense uptake at the site of tracheal thickening consistent in this squamous cell cancer.

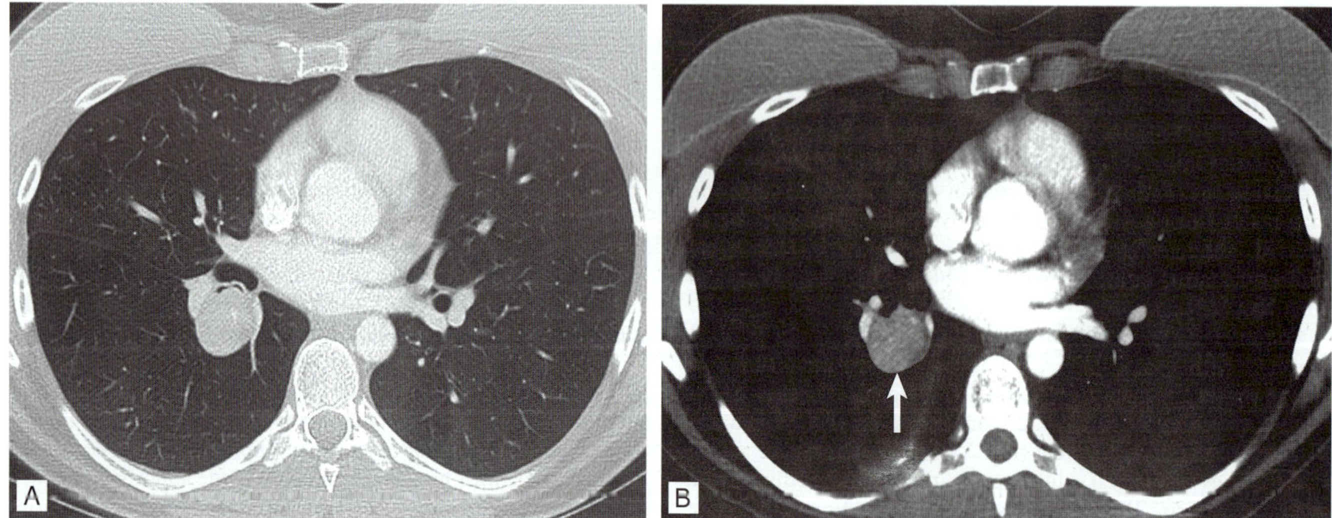

Figure 17.22 A 48-year-old female patient with bronchial carcinoid tumor. CT chest lung window (A) and mediastinal window (B) images show an enhancing intrabronchial mass along the posterior wall of the right lower lobe bronchus (*arrow*), proven to be carcinoid tumor on bronchoscopic biopsy.

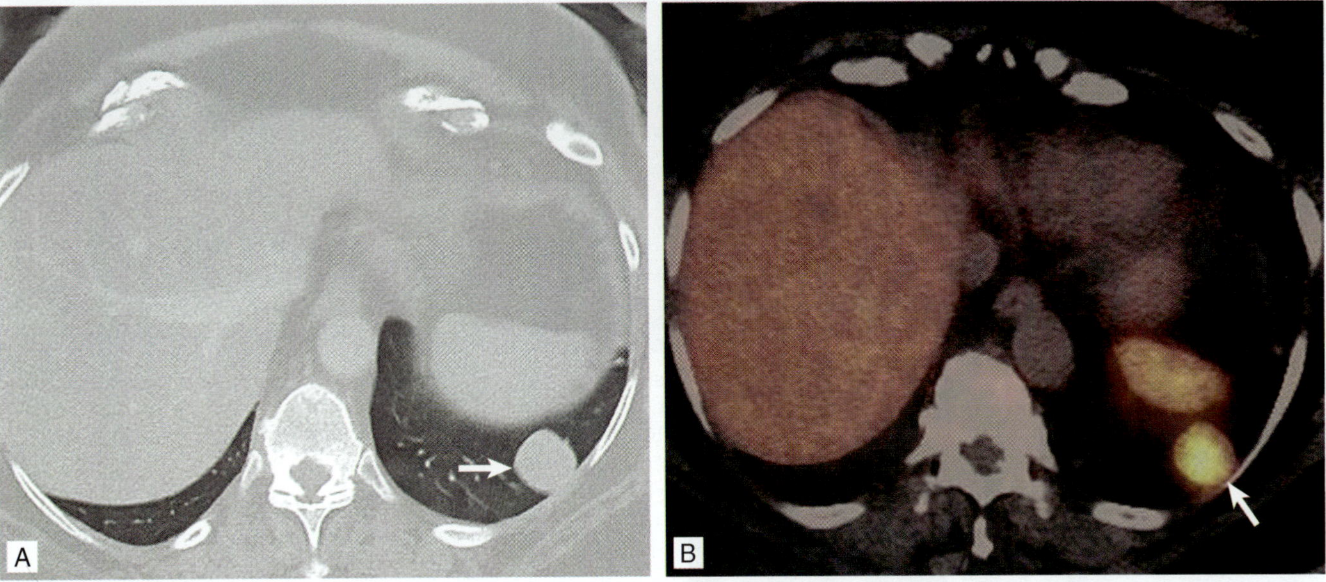

Figure 17.23 A 65-year-old male patient with pulmonary carcinoid tumor. CT chest (A) axial image shows a smooth round pulmonary 2.5 cm nodule in the left lower lobe (*white arrow*). Ga68-Dotatate PET-CT (B) shows intense uptake in the nodule (*white arrow*) (SUVmax 23). Biopsy showed a well-differentiated carcinoid tumor.

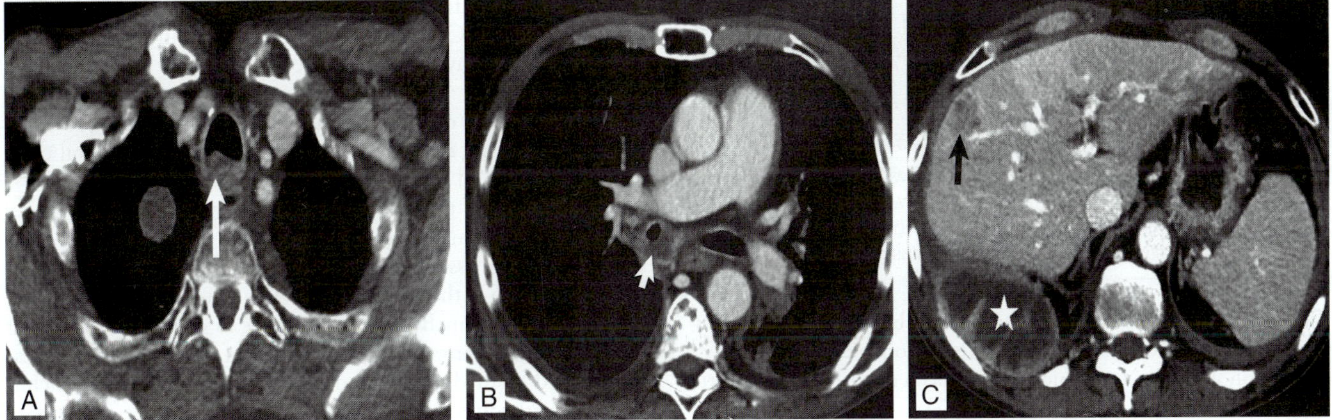

Figure 17.24 A 57-year-old male with metastasis to the airway. CT chest mediastinal window images (A–C) in a patient with malignant melanoma of the back (not shown) presents with multiple metastatic lesions including metastasis to the trachea (*long white arrow*), bronchus intermedius (*short white arrow*, B), pleura (*star*), and liver (*black arrow*, C).

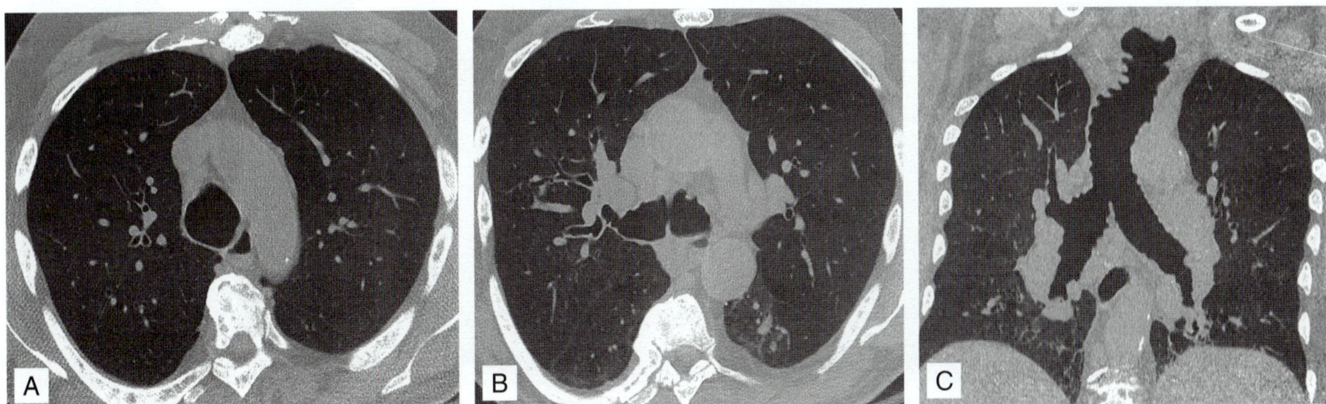

Figure 17.25 A 43-year-old male patient with Mounier–Kuhn syndrome. CT chest axial images (A–C) show diffuse tracheobronchomegaly with increased tracheal corrugation (trachea measured 4 cm in transverse dimension).

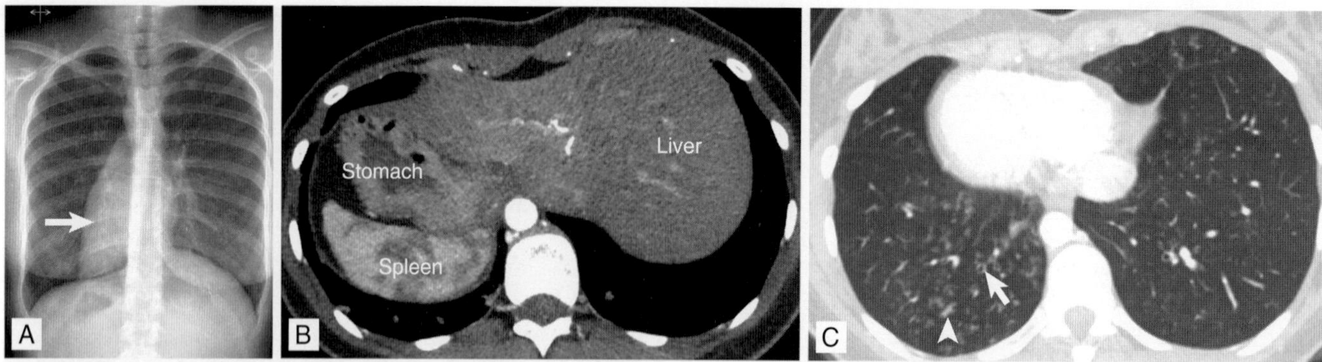

Figure 17.26 A 42-year-old female patient with Kartagener syndrome. Chest radiograph (A) in a 47-year-old female patient shows dextrocardia (*white arrow*). CT chest soft-tissue window image (B) shows situs inversus with liver on the left side and spleen and stomach on the right side. CT lung window (C) image shows mild bronchiectasis and bronchial wall thickening (*white arrow*) with multiple tree-in-bud nodules (*arrowhead*) suggesting infectious or inflammatory bronchiolitis.

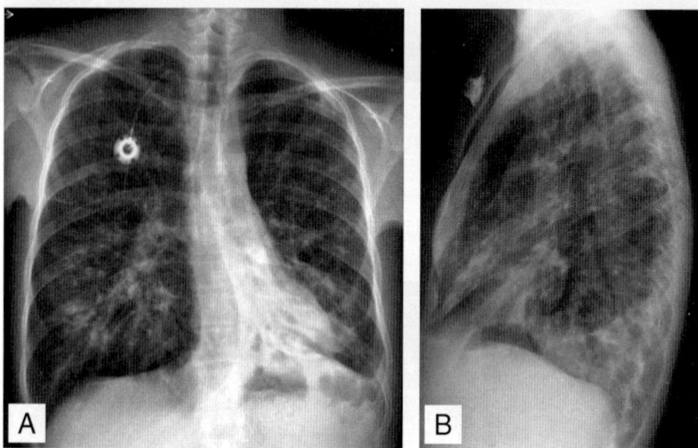

Figure 17.27 Cystic fibrosis in a 43-year-old man with florid bronchiectasis. Frontal (A) and lateral (B) chest radiograph shows diffuse parallel linear (tram-track) and "ring-like" shadows in bilateral lungs due to diffuse bilateral bronchiectasis. Additionally, a small left pleural effusion is also present.

dilatation of segmental and subsegmental bronchi is a frequent occurrence producing so-called "traction bronchiectasis."

Morphologically, bronchiectasis has been described as cylindrical, varicose, or saccular [30] (Fig. 17.27).

- Cylindrical (or tubular) bronchiectasis produces a dilated bronchus with parallel walls;
- Varicose bronchiectasis, the walls are irregular; and
- Saccular (or cystic) bronchiectasis, the airways terminate as round cysts.

In an individual patient, it is common to see more than one pattern (Fig. 17.28).

The diagnosis of bronchiectasis is primarily based on imaging and is characterized by airway enlargement. Imaging may help to narrow down the differential diagnosis and ascertain the etiology of bronchiectasis. CT imaging is the mainstay in diagnosis. Several CT criteria have been proposed to diagnose bronchiectasis. These include [31]

- bronchoarterial ratio >1.1 in adults (>0.8 in children);
- lack of tapering of bronchi extending into the peripheral third of the lung; and
- visualization of the airways within a centimeter of the costal pleura (except mediastinal pleura).

Usually, there is associated peribronchial thickening. The bronchoarterial ratio is the most reproducible criteria.

Normally, a bronchus is the same size as or fractionally larger than the adjacent artery, although attention to the arterial bifurcation should be made to avoid overdiagnosis. When the bronchus is more markedly dilated compared to the adjacent pulmonary

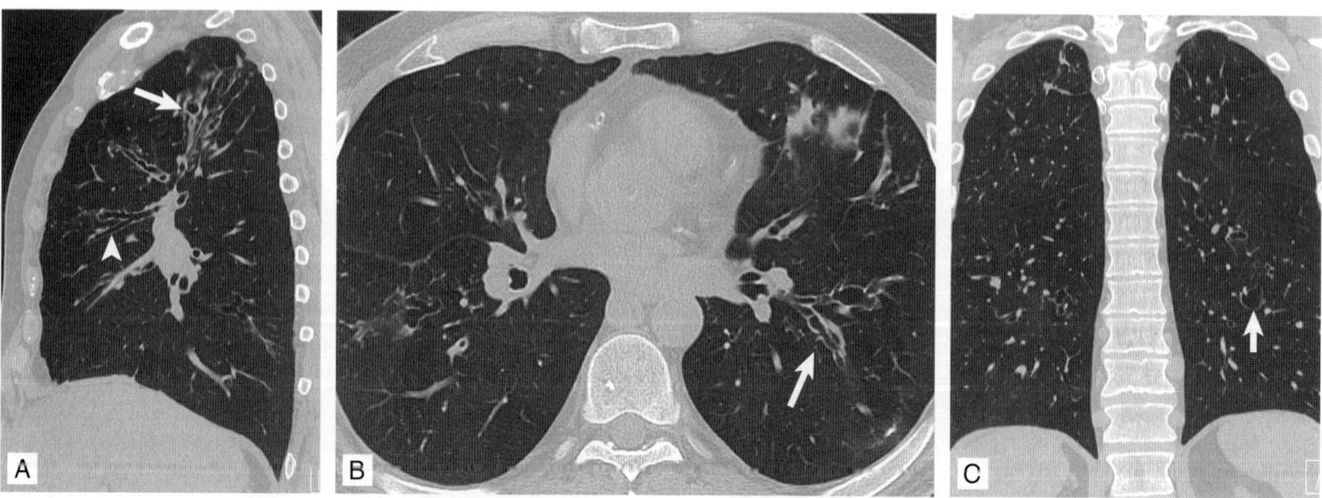

Figure 17.28 A 24-year-old male with severe asthma and recently treated allergic bronchopulmonary aspergillosis. CT chest lung window images (A–C) showing different types of bronchiectasis in the same patient: cylindrical (*arrowhead* in A), varicoid (*long arrows* A, B), and cystic bronchiectasis (*block arrow* in C).

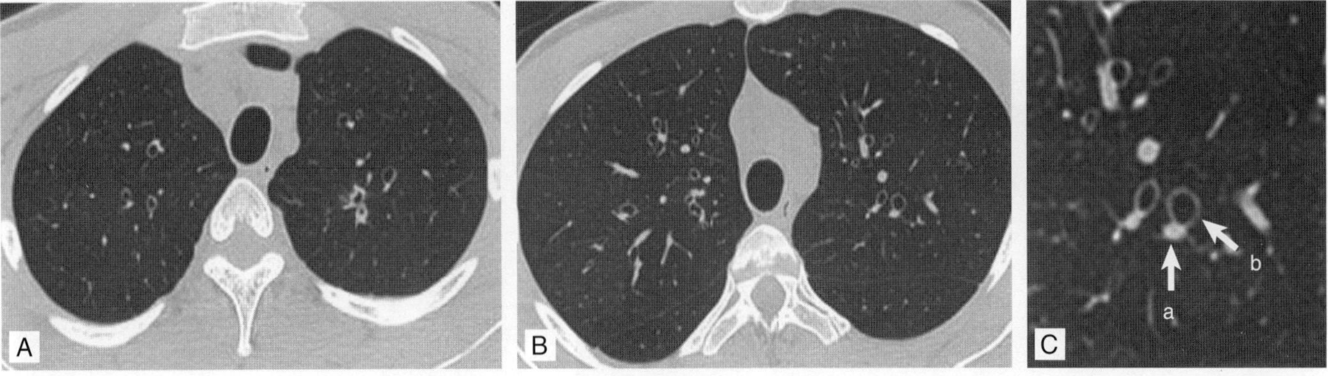

Figure 17.29 A 22-year-old woman with asthma. CT chest axial images (A, B) show bilateral dilated bronchi with bronchial diameter exceeding the pulmonary artery diameter in cross section (best seen in magnified axial CT chest image C), also known as signet ring sign. *a*: artery; *b*: bronchus.

artery, as seen in the cross section, a typical signet ring sign is seen (primary finding of bronchiectasis) (Fig. 17.29). On expiratory scans, there is frequent evidence of air trapping. Peripheral airways may become plugged, producing small subpleural branching opacities.

Bronchiectasis may be localized or generalized.

Localized bronchiectasis may be due to the mural, intramural, or extramural causes. In children, a foreign body is the most common intraluminal cause of focal bronchiectasis. Broncholithiasis may also result in a localized form of bronchiectasis or lead to lobar collapse if the occlusion is complete (Fig. 17.30). Endobronchial carcinoids may be seen on CT as an enhancing intrabronchial nodule, which can lead to bronchiectasis or obstruction distally. Extraluminal causes include bronchial narrowing secondary to mediastinal lymphadenopathy or masses.

Diffuse bronchiectasis may show a lobar predominant pattern [32,33].

- Upper lobe predominance is seen in cystic fibrosis, allergic bronchopulmonary aspergillosis (ABPA), sarcoidosis, or tuberculosis
- Nontuberculous mycobacterial infections show the right middle lobe or lingular predominance (Fig. 17.31). Lady Windermere syndrome is a pattern of atypical mycobacterial infection, which presents in middle-age women (typically white women) as bronchiectasis, centrilobular nodules, and eventual scarring and volume loss mostly affecting the middle lobe and lingula. The syndrome is typically seen in white, elderly females
- Lower lobe predominance is commonly seen due to primary ciliary dyskinesia (Kartagener syndrome) (Fig. 17.26), chronic aspiration, interstitial fibrosis, α-1 antitrypsin deficiency, or in immunodeficiency state
- A central predominant pattern is seen in ABPA and Mounier–Kuhn syndrome. Williams–Campbell syndrome is a rare cause of peripheral predominant pattern

Cystic Fibrosis

Cystic fibrosis was formerly a condition seen only in children. However, with improved management, many patients now reach adulthood and may be treated with lung transplantation. Cystic fibrosis is caused due to a genetic defect involving cystic fibrosis transmembrane regulator protein located on chromosome 7. The increased viscosity of the bronchial secretions in cystic fibrosis causes bronchial obstruction. This leads to air trapping and also predisposes to bronchiectasis [34].

Imaging findings comprise air trapping, upper lobe predominant bronchiectasis, mucous plugging, or consolidation (Fig. 17.32). Peribronchial thickening, peripheral nodular opacities, and ring shadows may be visible. Areas of emphysema may also develop.

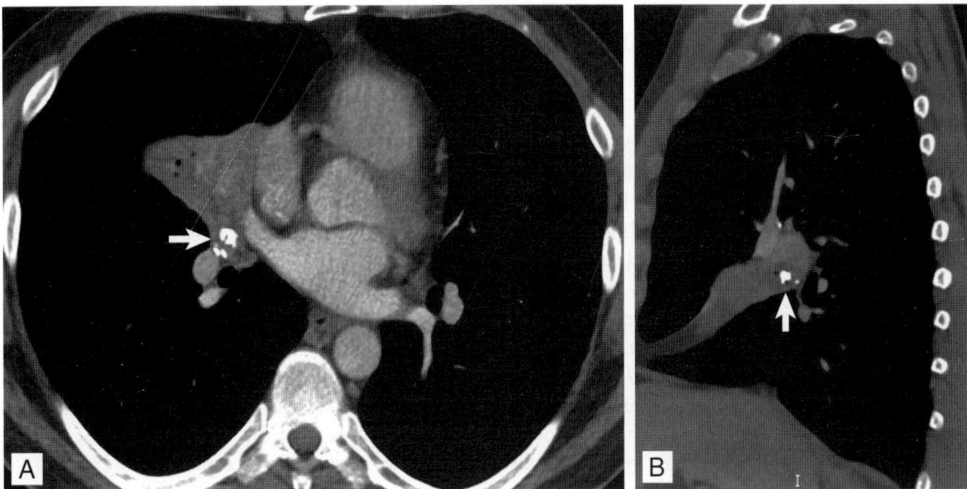

Figure 17.30 A 37-year-old man with chronic cough. Axial (A) and sagittal (B) soft-tissue window images showing complete collapse of the right middle lobe with an obstructing broncholith (*arrow*). The airways are dilated and mucus-filled due to central obstruction.

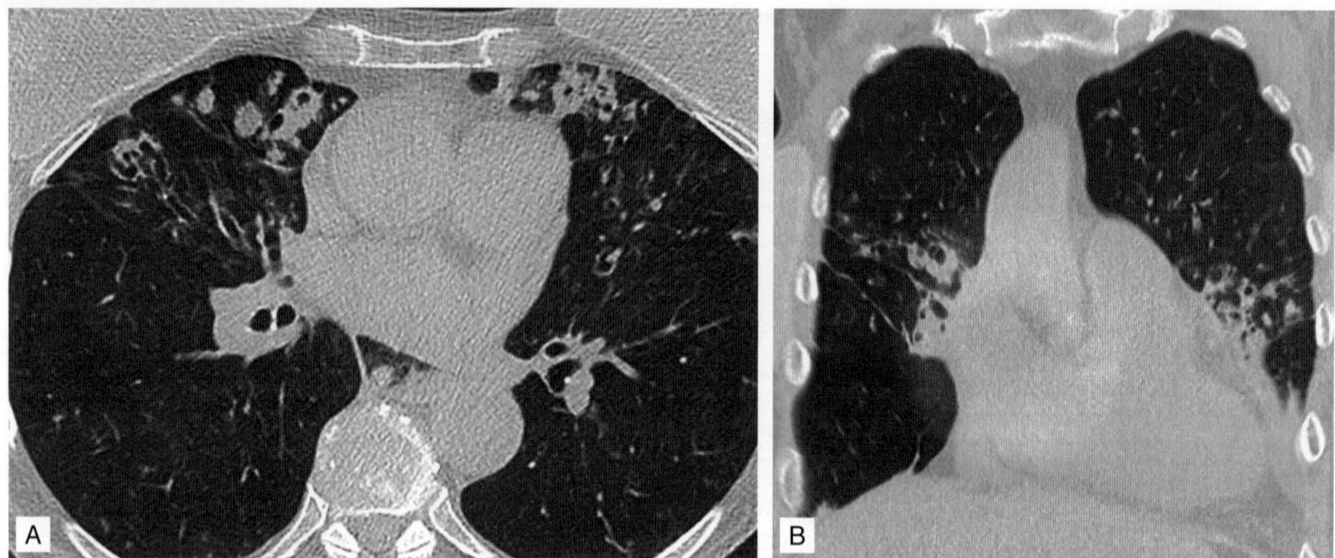

Figure 17.31 A 58-year-old female with chronic cough and shortness of breath. Axial (A) and coronal (B) lung window CT images showing middle lobe and lingular predominant bronchiectasis, bronchial wall thickening, and nodularity favoring nontubercular atypical mycobacterial infection. The constellation of findings in the middle-age female age group is also referred to as "Lady Windermere syndrome."

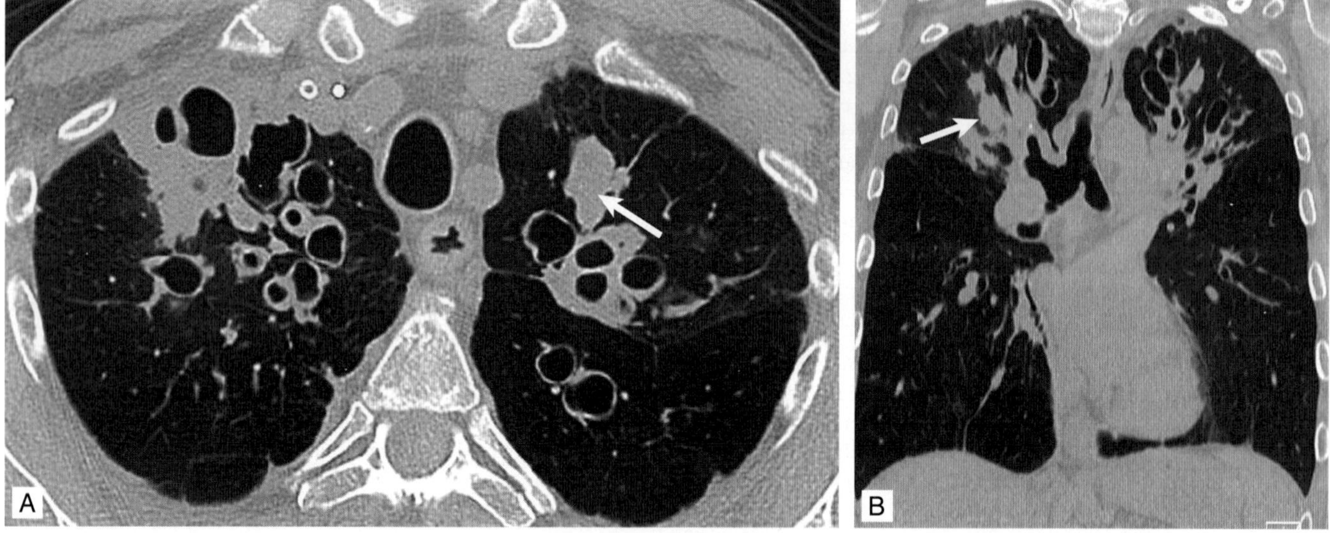

Figure 17.32 A 33-year-old female patient with cystic fibrosis. CT chest axial (A) and coronal (B) images show upper lobe predominant disease with bronchiectasis, bronchial wall thickening with mucus plugging (*arrows*). Associated scarring and small volumes of the upper lobes due to repeated infections are also appreciated on the coronal view.

CT is more sensitive and superior to radiography for the assessment of cystic fibrosis and associated complications. CT severity scores (Bhalla and Brody systems) [35] have been shown to perform better than bronchoscopy or chest radiography in predicting disease severity. Both semiautomated and automated scoring systems are available that can quantify airway thickening, bronchiectasis, bronchial diameter, air trapping, emphysema, mosaic perfusion, abscess, collapse, or consolidation. Secondary chest infections are common, staphylococci, and *Pseudomonas* being important pathogens, so areas of consolidation or centrilobular nodules or tree-in-bud opacities may be seen. In response to chronic pulmonary infection, reactive hilar lymph node enlargement is common. The central pulmonary arteries may also enlarge due to pulmonary arterial hypertension. In later stages of the disease, spontaneous pneumothorax may occur. As a response to chronic pulmonary ischemia and decreased pulmonary blood flow, bronchial artery hypertrophy may occur, which predisposes these patients to hemoptysis.

Although CT is currently the gold standard for the assessment of anatomical changes in the lungs in patients with cystic fibrosis, as the disease is predominantly seen in young patients, there is a concern for radiation exposure due to repeated scans required for disease monitoring. Hence, a low-dose chest CT protocol is preferred [36]. Recently, intravenous contrast-enhanced MRI has been used for evaluating the early lung abnormalities and in monitoring the lung function without radiation risk. This is especially significant for children where spirometry may be challenging to perform and may also remain normal in the early stages. Studies have shown a strong correlation between CT and MRI in assessing the structural and perfusion defects in the lungs. Hyperpolarized gas MRI (helium-3 or xenon-129) and multiple breath washout MRI have also been shown to provide a qualitative and quantitative assessment of the ventilatory and oxygen exchange defects [37,38]. These gas-based MRI imaging techniques have shown good correlation with spirometry, and are useful for monitoring the disease progression. Though contrast-enhanced MRI is commonly used, several nonenhanced MRI techniques like arterial spin labeling have also been used to assess for lung perfusion.

Airway Diseases

Asthma

Asthma is a chronic disorder of the airways and is characterized by recurring symptoms, reversible airflow obstruction, bronchial hyperresponsiveness, and underlying inflammation. Asthma can be seen from infancy through childhood, and patients may have variable symptoms, including wheezing, dyspnea, cough, and chest tightness [39]. According to the Global Initiative for Chronic Obstructive Lung Disease (GOLD) report 2020 [40], asthma and chronic obstructive pulmonary disease (COPD) are distinct disorders, and the term asthma and COPD overlap should not be used.

Extrinsic or atopic asthma is usually associated with a history of allergy and raised plasma IgE. An important cause of extrinsic asthma is aspergillosis. Intrinsic or nonatopic asthma may be precipitated by a variety of factors such as exercise, emotion, and infection.

The role of radiology in asthma is not to diagnose but to evaluate for potential complications like bronchiectasis (Figs. 17.28 and 17.29) or pneumothorax and to rule out conditions that can mimic asthma [41–43]. Chest radiographs show nonspecific findings in asthmatics. Most asthmatics show a normal chest x-ray during remissions. During an asthmatic attack, the chest x-ray may show signs of peribronchial wall thickening, hyperinflation, depression of the diaphragm, and expansion of the retrosternal air space (Fig. 17.33). Bronchial wall thickening, when viewed in profile, appears as ring shadows and as tram track lines on enface view (Fig. 17.27). CT chest is currently not recommended for the routine evaluation and may help in patients with atypical presentations. CT findings include air trapping on an expiratory scan, bronchial wall thickening, or tubular bronchiectasis. The most important role of imaging is to identify complications, including pneumothorax, pneumomediastinum, mucus plugging leading to atelectasis, subcutaneous emphysema, and pneumonia [44]. Asthma is seen in increasing association with disorders like ABPA, Churg–Strauss syndrome, or eosinophilic pneumonia.

Allergic Bronchopulmonary Aspergillosis

ABPA is not a primary fungal infection, but a hypersensitivity reaction to antigens released by the colonization of the tracheobronchial tree by *Aspergillus fumigatus* in patients with asthma (2–32%) or cystic fibrosis (2–15%). ABPA is diagnosed with combined clinical, laboratory, and radiographic criteria.

On imaging, the upper lobe predominant disease is a frequent feature. Chest radiograph or CT may show linear or branching opacities, parenchymal opacities (usually involving the upper lobes), and atelectasis due to mucoid impaction [45,46] (Fig. 17.34). The branching opacities, representing mucus-filled dilated airway, are also referred to as "finger-in-glove" appearance. Various clinical, laboratory, and radiographic features that support the diagnosis of ABPA include a history of asthma or cystic fibrosis, peripheral eosinophilia, elevated total IgE levels, elevated IgE against *Aspergillus*, serum precipitins against *Aspergillus*,

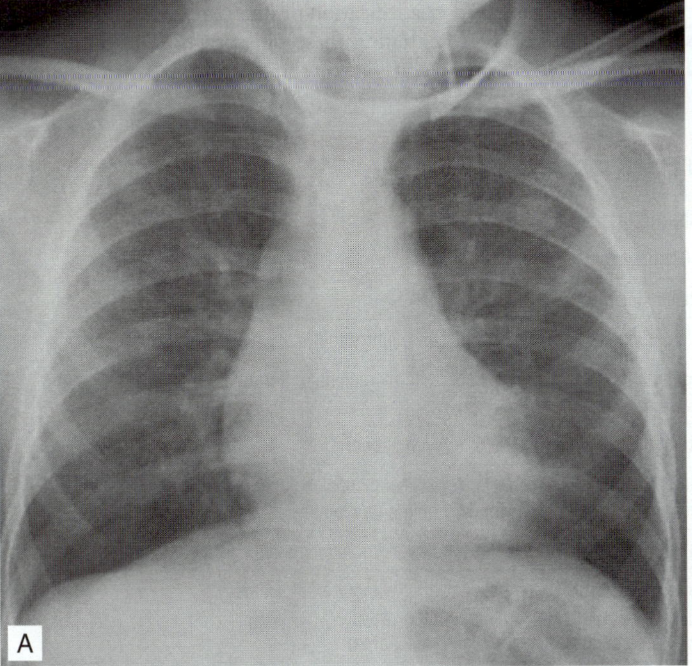

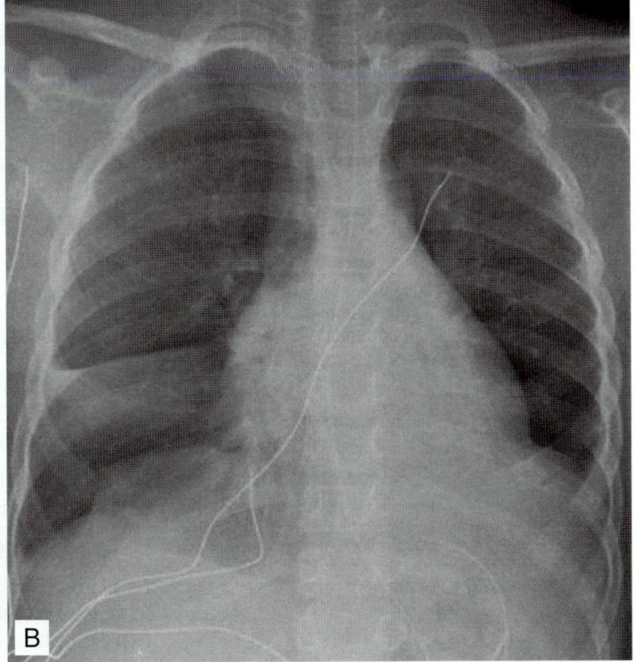

Figure 17.33 A 3-year-old female child with acute onset shortness of breath and wheezing. Frontal chest radiograph (A) shows hyperaeration of the lungs with increased bronchovascular markings and segmental atelectasis involving the lingula (obscuring the left heart border) consistent with clinical diagnosis of asthma. Follow-up radiograph (B) 2 days later show normalization of the bronchovascular markings with persistent hyperinflation and new lateral segment right middle lobe atelectasis (bordered superiorly by right minor fissure). (Courtesy: Dr. Simon Kao, MD, Pediatric Radiology, University of Iowa Hospitals & Clinics.)

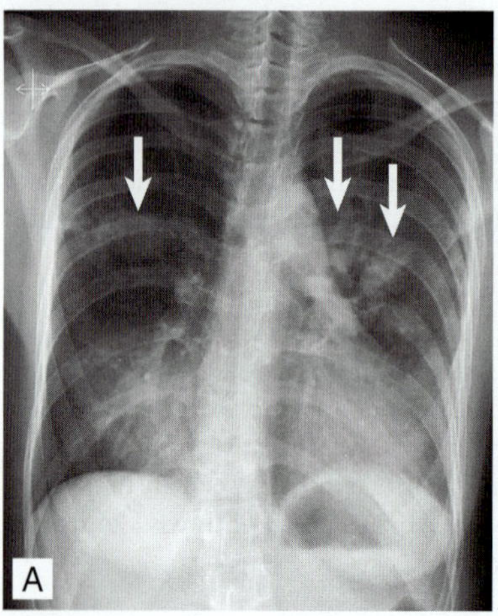

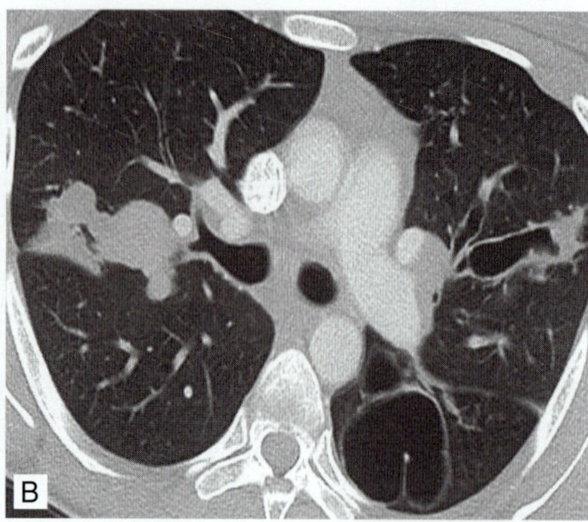

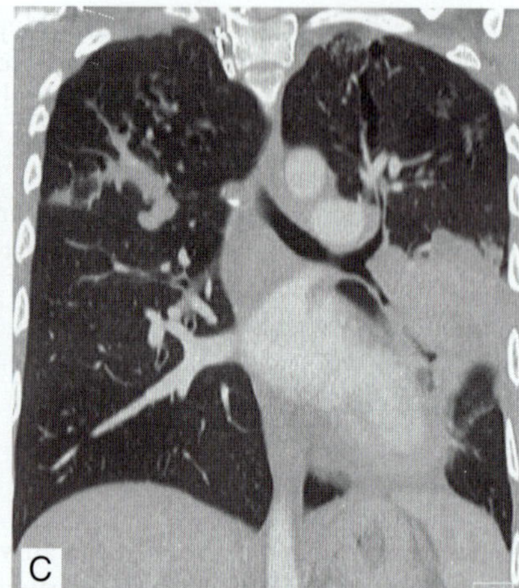

Figure 17.34 A 47-year-old man with severe asthma and allergic bronchopulmonary aspergillosis. Chest radiograph (A) showing linear or oval branching opacities resulting from mucoid impaction of bronchocele, the finger-in-glove sign (*white arrows*). Also, bilateral lung areas of homogeneous opacification is seen. CT chest axial (B) and coronal (C) images show bronchiectasis in central distribution with mucus plugging in bilateral upper lobes and centrilobular nodules in the left upper lobe.

fleeting pulmonary parenchymal opacities, central bronchiectasis, and positive skin test to *A. fumigatus*.

Chronic Obstructive Pulmonary Disease (COPD)

According to the GOLD 2020 report [40], a project initiated by the National Heart, Lung, and Blood Institute and the World Health Organization, COPD is defined as "a common, preventable, and treatable disease that is characterized by persistent respiratory symptoms and airflow limitation that is due to airway and/or alveolar abnormalities usually caused by significant exposure to noxious particles or gases and influenced by host factors including abnormal lung development." Emphysema is one of the many structural abnormalities seen in patients with COPD [40].

COPD is a heterogeneous entity with multiple phenotypes and endotypes, with imaging manifestations being large airway disease (bronchitis), small airway disease (small airways that are not seen on CT but can be assessed by inspiratory–expiratory CT), and destructive alveolar disease (emphysema) [47,48]. Both emphysema and airway disease can overlap and coexist in the same patient. GOLD staging is widely used to classify the severity of COPD and is based on pulmonary function testing. However, pulmonary function testing lacks anatomic specificity to refine COPD phenotyping, and forced expiratory volume 1 (FEV1) alone is insensitive to detect early changes of COPD. Pulmonary function tests can also not quantify changes in COPD or classify small airway disease. In addition, many patients with identical GOLD stage may have different morphology on lung CT imaging. Imaging plays a key role in the assessment of COPD and for the assessment and quantification of different COPD phenotypes (Table 17.1). Differentiating these phenotypes is important due to their pathophysiology, genetic status, and treatment strategies.

TABLE 17.1 Pathological Phenotypes and CT Assessment of COPD [52,53]

Imaging Phenotype	CT Quantification and Characterization
1. Emphysema	Voxels below –950 HU (>6% of voxel)
Pleural-based or paraseptal emphysema	Characterized by pleural-based lucencies
Trace centrilobular emphysema (CLE)	Characterized by minimal centrilobular lucencies (<0.5% of a lung zone)
Mild CLE	Characterized by scattered centrilobular lucencies, separated by regions of normal lung (0.5–5% of a lung zone)
Moderate CLE	Multiple well-defined centrilobular lucencies (>5% of any lung zone)
Confluent CLE	Coalescent centrilobular lucencies, including multiple regions of lucencies spanning several secondary pulmonary lobules without hyperexpansion of secondary pulmonary lobules or architectural distortion
Advanced destructive emphysema	Panlobularlucencies along with hyperexpansion of secondary pulmonary lobules and architectural distortion
2. Large airway disease (bronchitis)	▪ Less than 6% of voxels below –950 HU. Can occur with or without emphysema ▪ Wall thickening of central, segmental, and subsegmental airways ▪ Calculation of total airway area occupied by the wall (%wall area)
3. Small airway disease	▪ Air trapping (FEV1/FVC ratio <0.7; FEV1 <80% predicted) ▪ Quantified as voxels <856 HU on expiratory CT ▪ Parametric response maps with measurement of disease probability maps ▪ Inflammatory SAD identified by the presence of peripheral centrilobular micronodular opacities

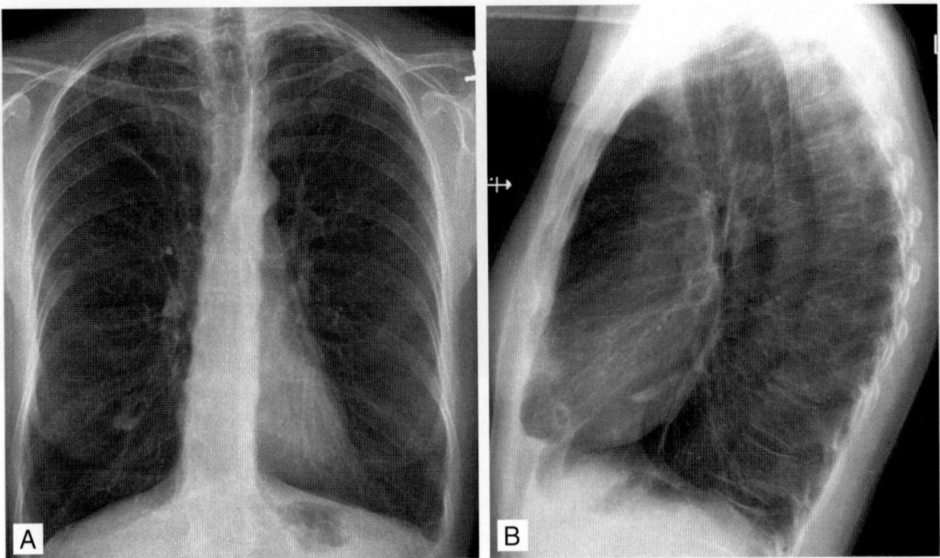

Figure 17.35 A 53-year-old female with chronic obstructive pulmonary disease (COPD). Frontal (A) and lateral (B) chest radiographs show hyperexpanded lungs with coarse bronchovascular markings, increase in anteroposterior diameter, increased retrosternal airspace with diaphragmatic flattening.

A chest radiograph is the initial technique to evaluate COPD (Fig. 17.35). Typical radiographic signs include hyperinflation of the lungs, diaphragmatic flattening, increased retrosternal airspace, intercostal space widening, pruning of peripheral pulmonary vascularity, and vertical configuration of the cardiac silhouette. However, plain radiographs are limited in COPD characterization and assessment of airway-predominant COPD. Currently, CT and, less commonly, MRI are the two primary techniques used for classification and phenotyping of COPD [49]. CT shows hyperinflation and low attenuation of lung parenchyma. Emphysema on CT appears as a focal area of abnormally decreased lung parenchymal attenuation without visible walls. The absence of a discernible wall is important to distinguish emphysema from a cyst. Sometimes, emphysema is associated with the formation of bullae. CT-based visual assessment and quantitative imaging have been used to identify patterns of lung destruction and improve the classification of different phenotypes [50]. CT can provide structural and anatomical information while MRI provides functional information regarding ventilation and perfusion. The advantage of quantitative imaging is to stratify patients into emphysema or airway-predominant disease. The stratification is important since both have a different clinical profile, and an accurate diagnosis can help to tailor the treatment.

CT-Based Visual Classification of COPD (Fleischner Criteria)

Broadly, the Fleischner's society [51] classified COPD into two types: emphysema-predominant and airway-predominant disease. The airway disease is further divided into large airway and small airway disease.

Emphysema is defined as "an increase beyond the normal in the size of the air spaces distal to the terminal bronchioles, with dilatation and destruction of their walls." Based on the disease distribution, emphysema can be further subdivided into centrilobular emphysema, paraseptal emphysema, and panlobular emphysema.

- Centrilobular emphysema is characterized by the central destruction of the secondary pulmonary lobules (Fig. 17.36).

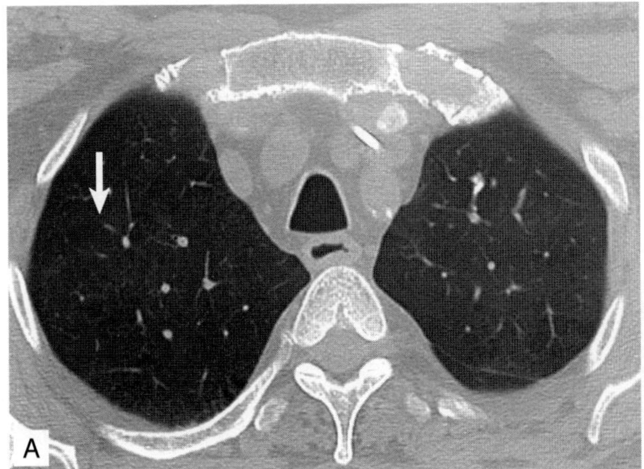

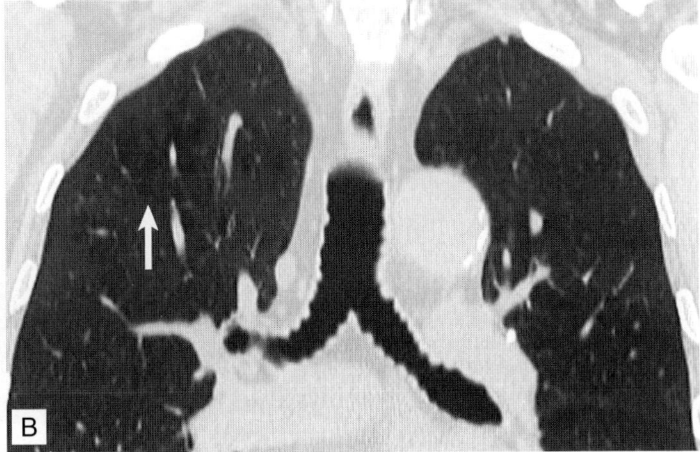

Figure 17.36 A 49-year-old male smoker with centrilobular emphysema. CT chest axial (A) and coronal (B) images show focal areas of decreased lung attenuation (*arrows*) in the location of the central region of the acinus, in upper lobe distribution—centrilobular pattern of emphysematous changes.

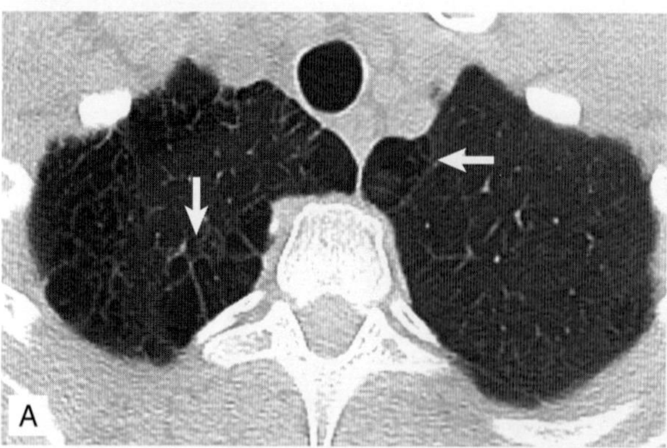

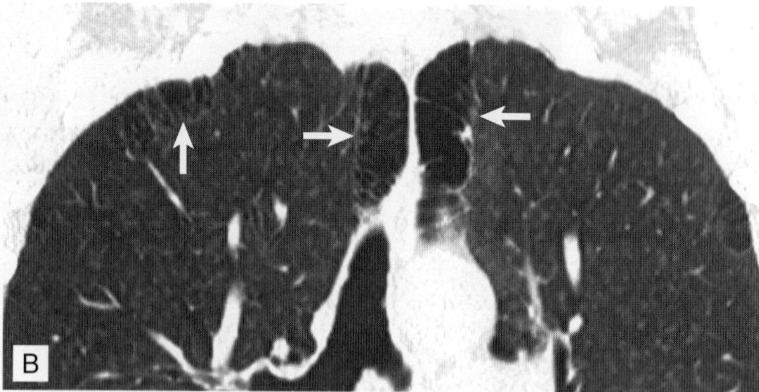

Figure 17.37 A 52-year-old man, active smoker with CT chest axial (A) and coronal (B) images showing typical appearance of paraseptal emphysema. The lucent areas larger than 1 cm suggest subpleural apical bullae (*arrows*).

The upper zones tend to be more severely involved than the lung bases. It is usually found in smokers

- Paraseptal emphysema involves the periphery of the secondary lobules, usually in the lung periphery (adjacent to visceral pleura), and is upper lobe predominant (Fig. 17.37)
- Panlobular emphysema shows uniform destruction of the secondary pulmonary lobule. It is classically associated with α1-antitrypsin deficiency, which is a lower lobe predominant pattern of emphysema (Fig. 17.38)

Paracicatricial emphysema refers to distension and destruction of terminal air spaces adjacent to fibrotic lesions and is most frequently seen as a result of tuberculosis.

Bullae may be seen in association with some form of emphysema, commonly occurring in paraseptal and panlobular emphysema. A bulla is defined as a sharply demarcated area of emphysema, 1 cm or more in diameter with less than 1 mm thick walls. They may be single or multiple and are usually peripheral. In asymptomatic patients and in those with pulmonary scarring, bullae tend to be apical, but in chronic obstructive airways, disease bullae are found throughout the lungs. Their walls may be visible as a smooth, curved, hairline shadow. If the walls are not visible, the displacement of vessels around a radiolucent area may indicate a bullous area. Bullae are usually air-filled but may become infected and filled with fluid. A large bulla may be difficult to differentiate from a loculated pneumothorax on a radiograph, and CT may be necessary to demonstrate the wall of the bulla or thin strands of lung tissue crossing it (Fig. 17.39).

Airway-predominant disease is characterized by bronchial airway disease (airway thickening) and small airway disease (disease of peripheral small airways that are beyond resolution of CT, but seen as air trapping on expiratory CT). Inspiratory and expiratory CT are needed to evaluate small airway disease which appears as relatively normal lung on inspiratory exam with geographical areas of low attenuation on expiratory CT. Small airway disease shows significant air trapping (which correlates with FEV1/FVC ratio <0.7 and FEV1 <80% predicted on spirometry) [52]. Airway disease can occur with or without emphysema. Several additional changes can also be observed, including dilated main pulmonary artery, bronchiectasis, interstitial lung disease (ILD), and large airway disease (saber-sheath trachea, tracheobronchomegaly, etc.).

Quantitative Lung CT Imaging

Quantitative features can be applied to lung CT images based on lung density (Hounsfield units), texture, and airway or vascular mapping. These tools have been developed using a consistent imaging protocol that has been validated and applied in various multicenter studies. For emphysema quantification, a cut off of −950 HU is frequently used on an inspiratory scan. Of note, the voxel is quantified as emphysema if >6% of the voxel has an attenuation of less than −950 HU (Fig. 17.37). These low attenuation areas (LAA%) are a commonly used index to show the percentage of lung voxels below −950 HU, and quantification of

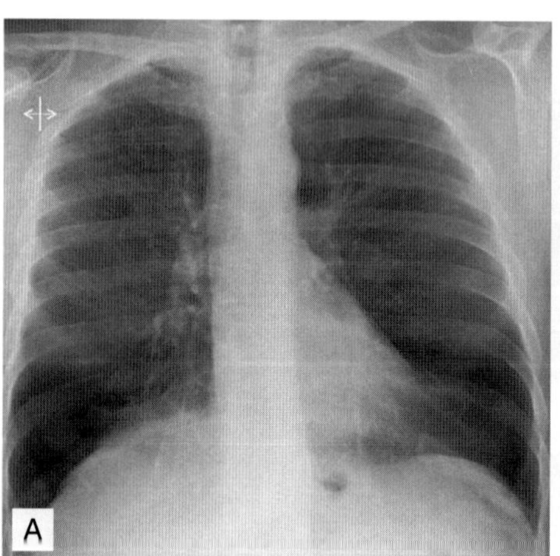

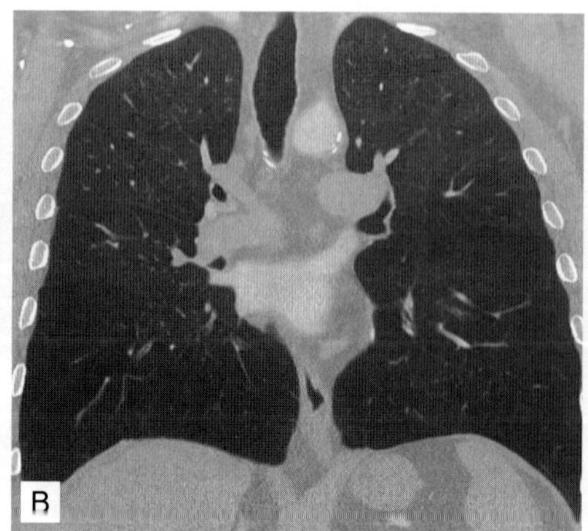

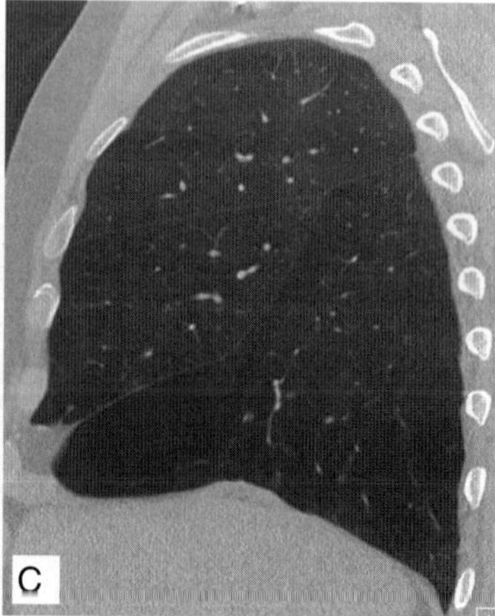

Figure 17.38 A 47-year-old male patient with panlobular emphysema. Plain chest radiograph (A) in a patient with α-1 antitrypsin deficiency shows hyperexpanded lungs with diffusely increased lower lobe lucency. CT chest coronal (B) and reconstructed sagittal (C) images show decreased lung attenuation in bilateral lower lobes suggesting panlobular type of emphysema.

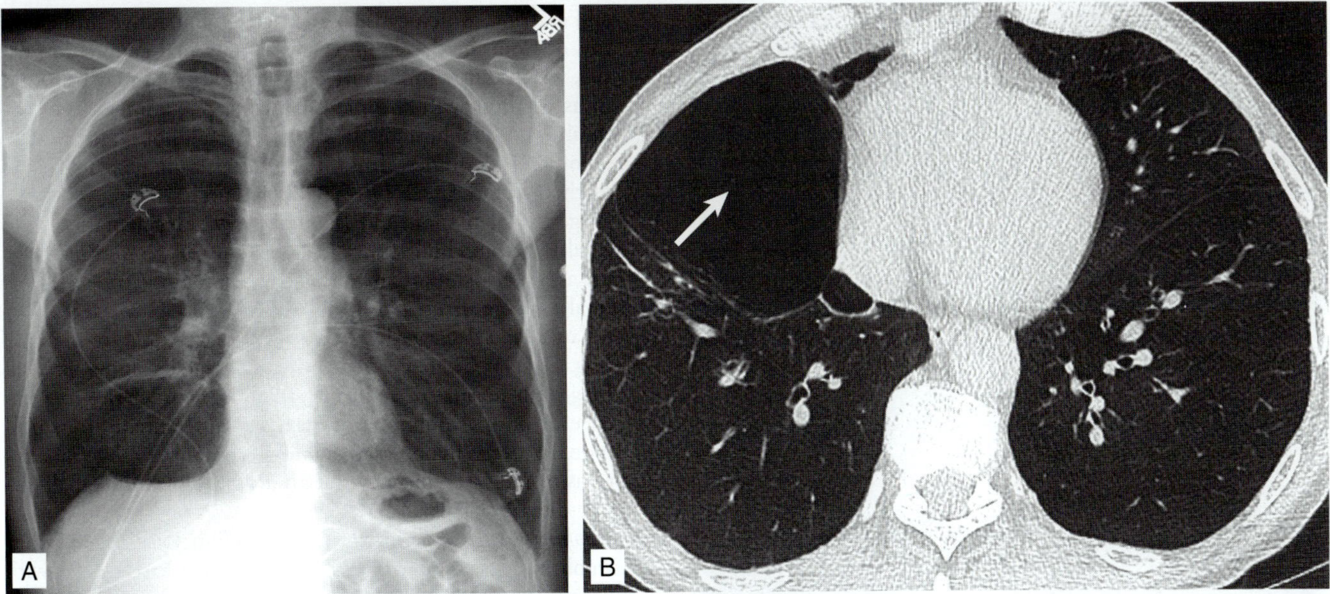

Figure 17.39 A 46-year-old male patient with large bulla in medial right lung. Frontal chest radiograph (A) shows large lung volumes with an area of lucency in the right lung adjacent to the right heart border. CT chest (B) axial image shows a large bulla in right middle lobe with a small strand traversing through the bulla (*arrow*).

these areas has been shown to correlate with FEV1, exercise capacity, and correlate with patient morbidity and mortality [53,54]. If spirometry suggests obstructive pattern disease with density characteristics showing attenuation of −950 HU in less than 6% of a voxel, the disease is characterized as an airway-predominant pattern. For functional small airway disease, CT attenuation of less than −856 HU on an expiratory scan is a marker of air trapping. Similar to low attenuation area, the quantified degree of air trapping is demonstrated to correlate with spirometric abnormalities and patient outcomes. Machine learning-based texture analysis is another novel technique for quantifying diffuse lung diseases like emphysema (Fig. 17.40), lymphangioleiomyomatosis, ILD, including recently COVID-19 lung disease [55,56]. Texture features have also been used for lung nodules to distinguish benign and malignant diseases [57].

Bronchiolitis

The term bronchiolitis encompasses a range of conditions and is characterized by inflammation/fibrosis of small bronchioles (<2 mm in diameter) [58]. Direct signs of bronchiolitis include centrilobular or ground-glass nodules and small centrilobular nodules with central lucency secondary to bronchiolectasis. Indirect signs involve the presence of air trapping as seen on expiratory CT scans and decreased attenuation and reduced vascularity (mosaic attenuation) on inspiratory CT [59–61].

1. *Infectious bronchiolitis*: This is one of the common types of bronchiolitis. This can occur in children, usually in the first year of life, and is *most commonly the result of respiratory syncytial virus infection*. The condition is usually self-limiting. In adults, this may be seen with distal airway infections like early atypical mycobacterial infections. Radiologically, the appearances are most frequently hyperinflation of the lungs and perihilar prominence and indistinctness. CT shows branching tree-in-bud opacities with bronchial wall thickening. Air trapping is more common in chronic infectious bronchiolitis
2. *Obliterative or constrictive bronchiolitis (OB)*: Bronchiolar obliteration may result from peribronchiolar inflammation

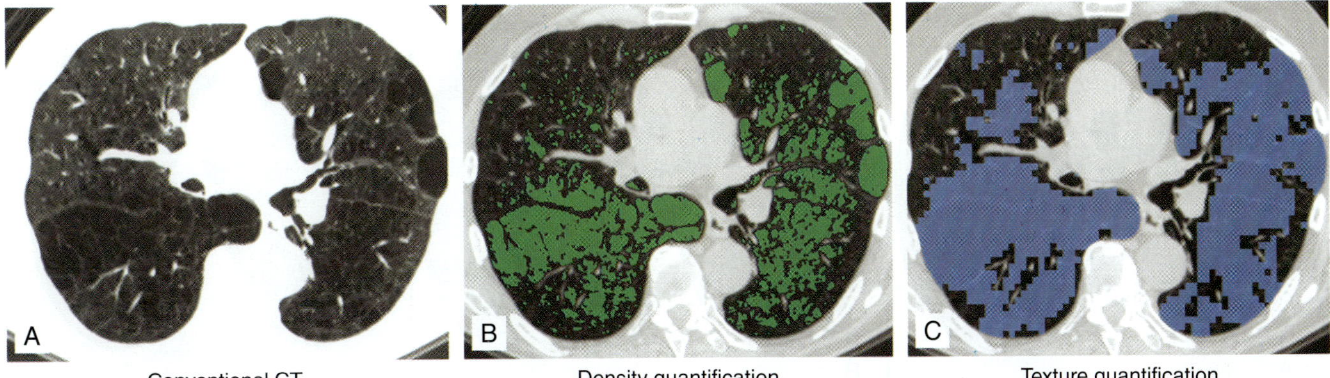

Figure 17.40 Quantitative techniques for emphysema measurement. Conventional CT image (A) showing centrilobular, and paraseptal emphysema with subpleural bullae. Density-based quantification (using −950 HU cut off) highlighting the emphysematous areas (B, green, overall quantified as 78% lung volume). Similarly, disease can be quantified using 3D texture technique (C, emphysema: blue). (Courtesy: Eric Hoffman, PhD, University of Iowa, Iowa City, USA.)

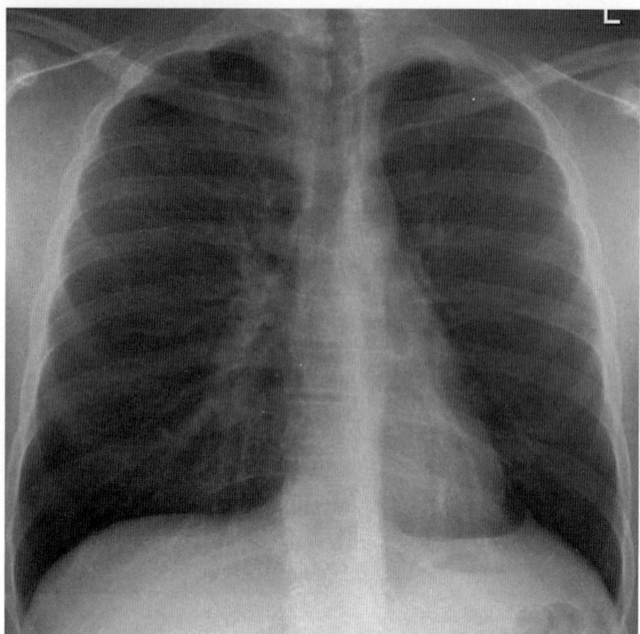

Figure 17.41 A 46-year-old man with history of recurrent respiratory infections during childhood. Chest radiograph shows lung asymmetry with hyperlucent left lung showing decreased bronchovascular markings and small hilar shadow. Asymmetry with hyperlucent small volume lung with decreased vascularity is suggestive of Swyer–James syndrome.

and scarring, which causes constrictive obliterative bronchiolitis, or from the development of intraluminal granulation tissue, which causes proliferative bronchiolitis and may be found in association with chronic organizing pneumonia. OB may result from viral bronchiolitis (often in childhood), from inhalation of toxic fumes, drug therapy (classically penicillamine), or rheumatoid disease. It may also complicate lung or heart–lung transplantation and bone marrow transplantation. OB resulting from childhood viral infection may present in adult life as Swyer–James syndrome. The chest radiograph may show small volume affected lung with evidence of pulmonary hyperinflation and decreased vascularity in the mid and lower zones (Fig. 17.41). Changes on CT include small volume affected lung with normal or reduced pulmonary vascularity in presence of normal pulmonary artery (to differentiate from pulmonary artery hypoplasia), with or without patchy (mosaic) areas of increased lucency due to air trapping from small airway disease (Fig. 17.42)

3. *Smoking-related inflammatory bronchiolitis*: Respiratory bronchiolitis (RB) is inflammation of the small bronchioles with deposition of pigment laden macrophages due to smoking. Patients with RB are usually asymptomatic with normal pulmonary function. If progressive, patients become symptomatic with abnormal pulmonary function with the development of RB-ILD. CT shows upper and mid lung predominant ground-glass opacities (Fig. 17.43). Emphysema may or may not be present. RB is usually reversible with smoking cessation

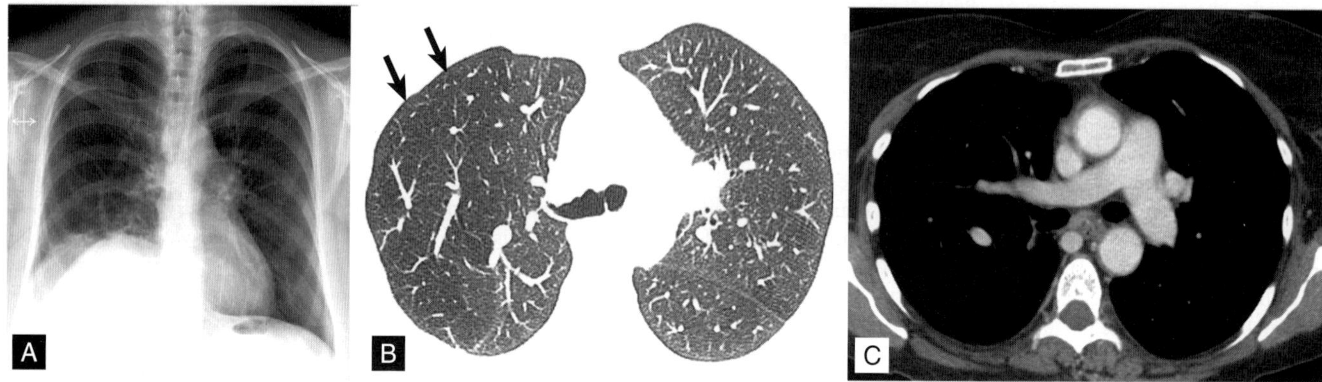

Figure 17.42 A 34-year-old woman with history of recurrent childhood pneumonia. Chest radiograph shows hyperlucent and small volume right lung. CT chest lung window (B) image shows large area of air trapping (*black arrows*) in the small volume right lung. Mediastinal window (C) image showed normal size pulmonary artery ruling out pulmonary artery hypoplasia as the etiology of these imaging findings.

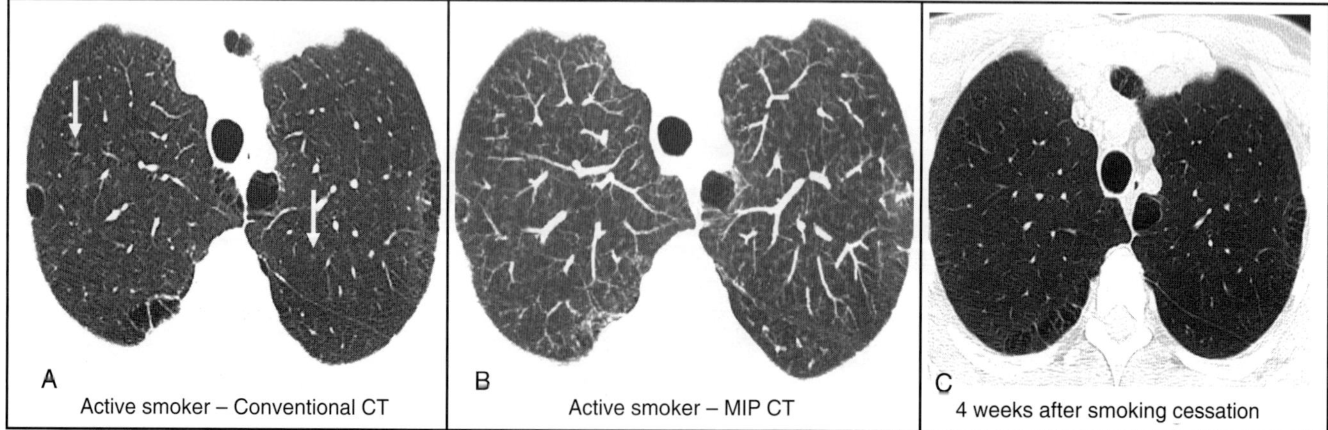

Figure 17.43 A 52-year-old man, active smoker with emphysema and chronic cough. Axial CT (A) and maximum intensity projection (MIP) CT image (B) showing ill-defined ground-glass nodules in the upper lobes (*white arrow in A*), consistent with respiratory bronchiolitis. Axial CT image 4 weeks after smoking cessation (C) showing resolution of respiratory bronchiolitis.

Collapse or Atelectasis

Atelectasis is derived from the Greek words "ateles" and "ektasis," which mean incomplete expansion. It is defined as a diminished volume affecting all or part of a lung. This contrasts with consolidation, in which a diminished volume of air in the lung is associated with normal lung volume [62]. The term "atelectasis" is typically used when there is partial collapse, whereas the term "collapsed lung" is typically reserved for when the entire lung is totally collapsed. Pulmonary atelectasis is one of the most commonly encountered abnormalities on chest radiographs. Whenever atelectasis is found, it should prompt a vigorous search for a cause as it is a sign of an underlying disease process. There are several different mechanisms that may cause pulmonary collapse (Fig. 17.44). The types of atelectasis based on the mechanisms are detailed below [63].

Obstructive/Resorptive Collapse

This is the most common type and results from the resorption of gas from the alveoli when communication between the alveoli and the trachea is obstructed (Figs. 17.45 and 17.46). The degree of collapse may be modified by collateral air drift if the obstruction is distal to the main bronchus, and also by infection and accumulation of secretions. If the obstruction becomes chronic, subsequent resorption of intra-alveolar secretions and exudate may result in complete collapse. This is the usual mechanism of collapse seen in mucous plugging, foreign body, broncholith, or carcinoma of the bronchus (Fig. 17.46).

Relaxation or Passive Collapse

This is the mechanism whereby the lung tends to retract toward its hilum when air or increased fluid collects in the pleural space (Fig. 17.47). The presence of air or fluid in the pleural space causes equalization of the intrapleural and intra-alveolar pressure resulting in lung collapse.

Cicatrization Collapse

Normal lung expansion depends upon a balance between outward forces in the chest wall and opposite elastic forces in the lung. When the lung is abnormally stiff, this balance is disturbed, lung compliance is decreased, and the volume of the affected lung is reduced. This occurs with diffuse or localized pulmonary fibrosis and may be associated with variable degrees of bronchiectasis (Fig. 17.48).

Adhesive Collapse

The surface tension of the alveoli is decreased by surfactant if this mechanism is disturbed, as in the respiratory distress syndrome, the collapse of alveoli occurs, although the central airways remain patent.

Gravity Dependent Atelectasis

This is seen secondary to decreased alveolar expansion in the dependent lung segments and is often described on CT as bibasilar/plate-like, band, discoid, or subsegmental atelectasis. It is predominantly seen in hospitalized patients with shallow breathing or patients with rib fracture or pleuritic chest pain (Fig. 17.49).

Middle Lobe Syndrome

It is a disorder of recurrent or fixed atelectasis involving the right middle lobe and/or lingula (Fig. 17.50). There is no clear definition of right middle lobe syndrome, and the etiology can be: obstructive or nonobstructive. Obstructive causes can be extraluminal (bronchial compression by surrounding lymph nodes) or by an intraluminal bronchial obstruction (Fig. 17.30). It may also

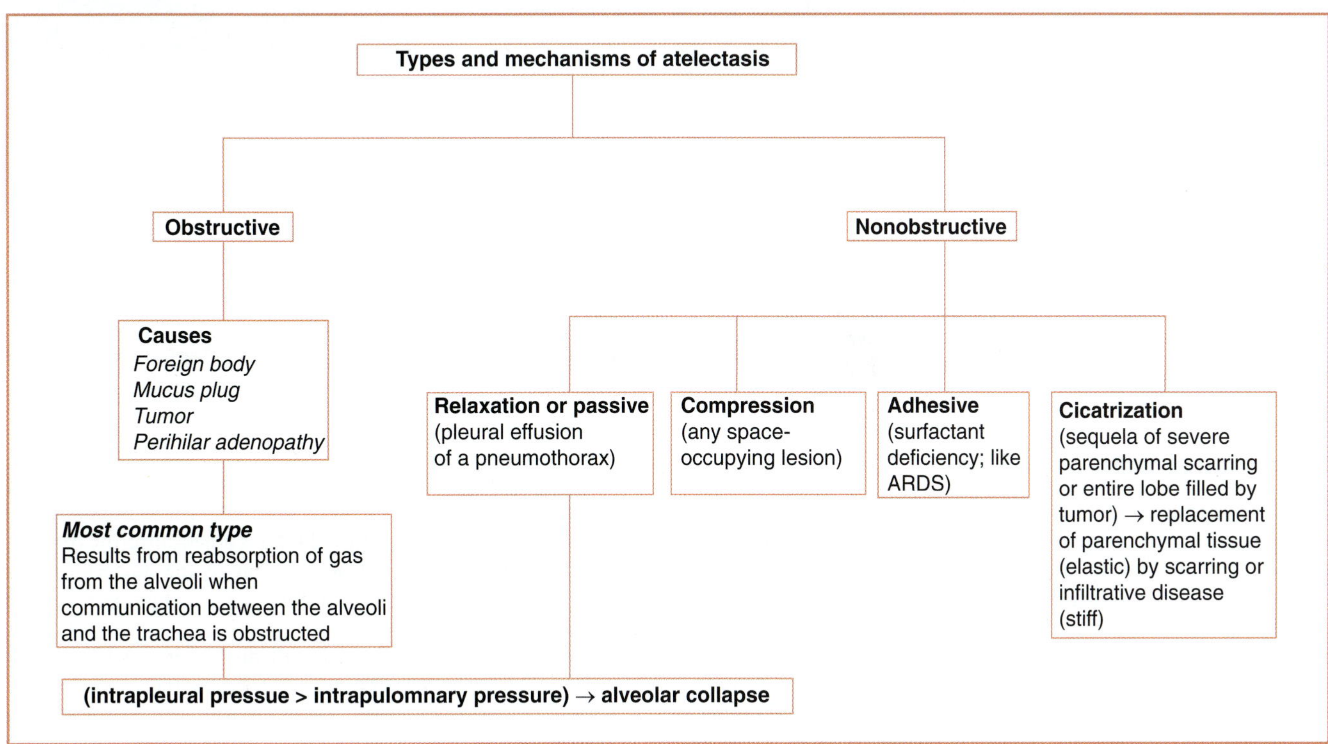

Figure 17.44 Types of atelectasis based on the mechanism of the disease.

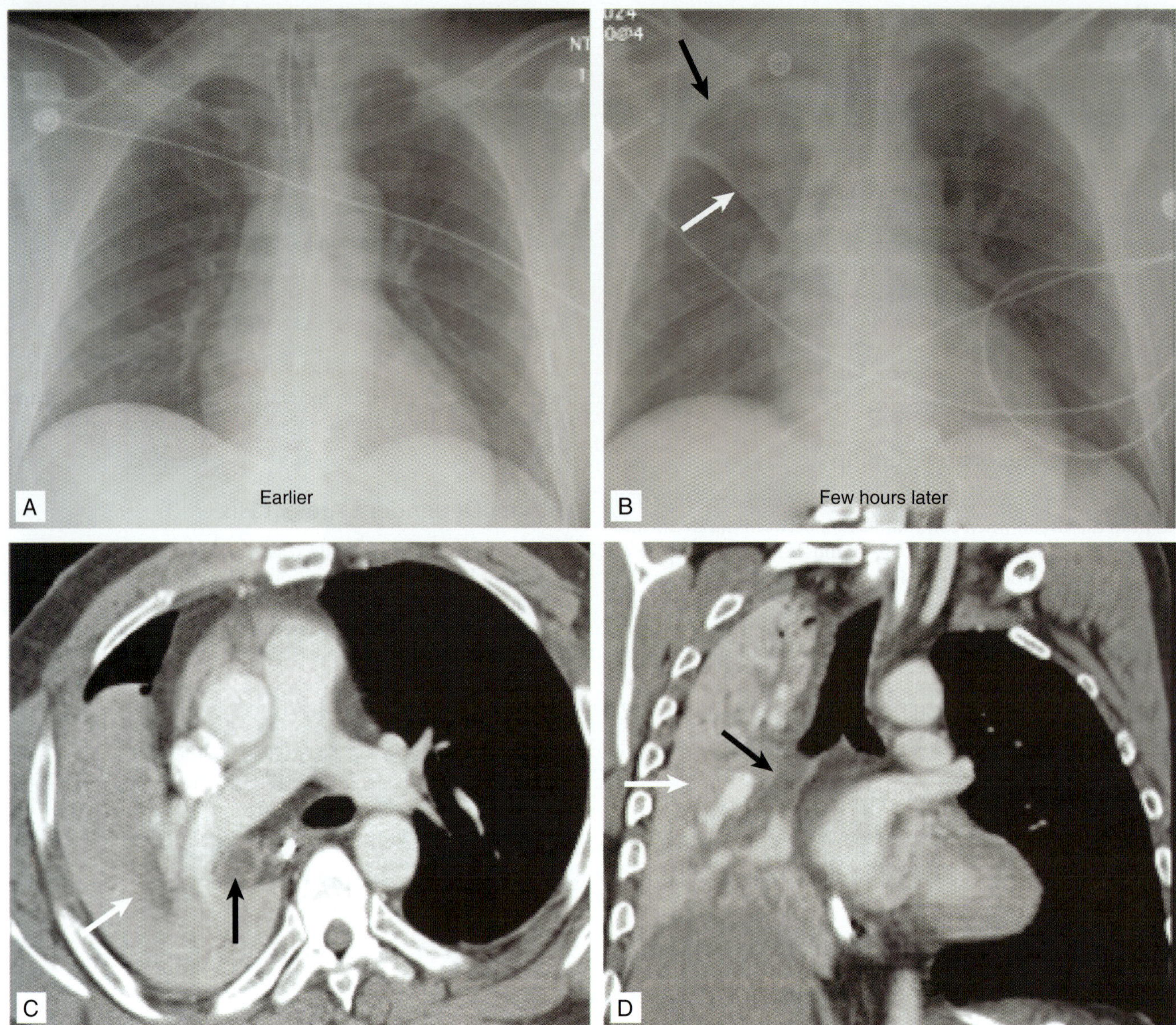

Figure 17.45 A 43-year-old man with obstructive collapse. Frontal chest radiographs (A, B) few hours apart from a patient in ICU demonstrate slightly diminished right lung volume with moderate collapse of the right upper lobe (*black arrow in B*). Notice the elevation of the horizontal fissure (*white arrow*). Axial (C) and coronal (D) CT images performed few hours after the second chest (B) radiograph showing mucus plugging (*black arrow*) of the right main bronchus few centimeters distal to the carina with enhancing collapsed right lung (*white arrow*).

develop in the presence of a patent lobar bronchus without identifiable obstruction (Fig. 17.50). Middle lobe syndrome has also been reported as a pulmonary manifestation of primary Sjögren syndrome.

Radiological Signs of Collapse

The radiographic appearance in pulmonary collapse depends upon the mechanism of collapse, the degree of collapse, the presence or absence of consolidation, and the pre-existing state of the pleura. Signs of collapse may be considered as direct or indirect (Fig. 17.51). Indirect signs are the results of compensatory changes that occur in response to the volume loss [64–66]. The chest radiograph is an excellent diagnostic tool for showing segmental or lobar atelectasis. CT is an excellent means of visualizing the lobar bronchi and proximal portions of the segmental bronchi in normal subjects.

Direct Signs of Collapse

- Displacement of interlobar fissures
  This is the most reliable sign, and the degree of displacement will depend on the extent of the collapse.
- Loss of aeration
  Increased density of a collapsed area of the lung is nonspecific and may not become apparent until collapse is almost complete. However, if the collapsed lung is adjacent to the mediastinum or diaphragm, the obscuration of the adjacent structures may indicate loss of aeration.
- Vascular and bronchial signs
  If a lobe is partially collapsed, crowding of its vessels may be visible; if an air bronchogram is visible, the bronchi may appear crowded. However, these are hard to visualize on a chest radiograph.

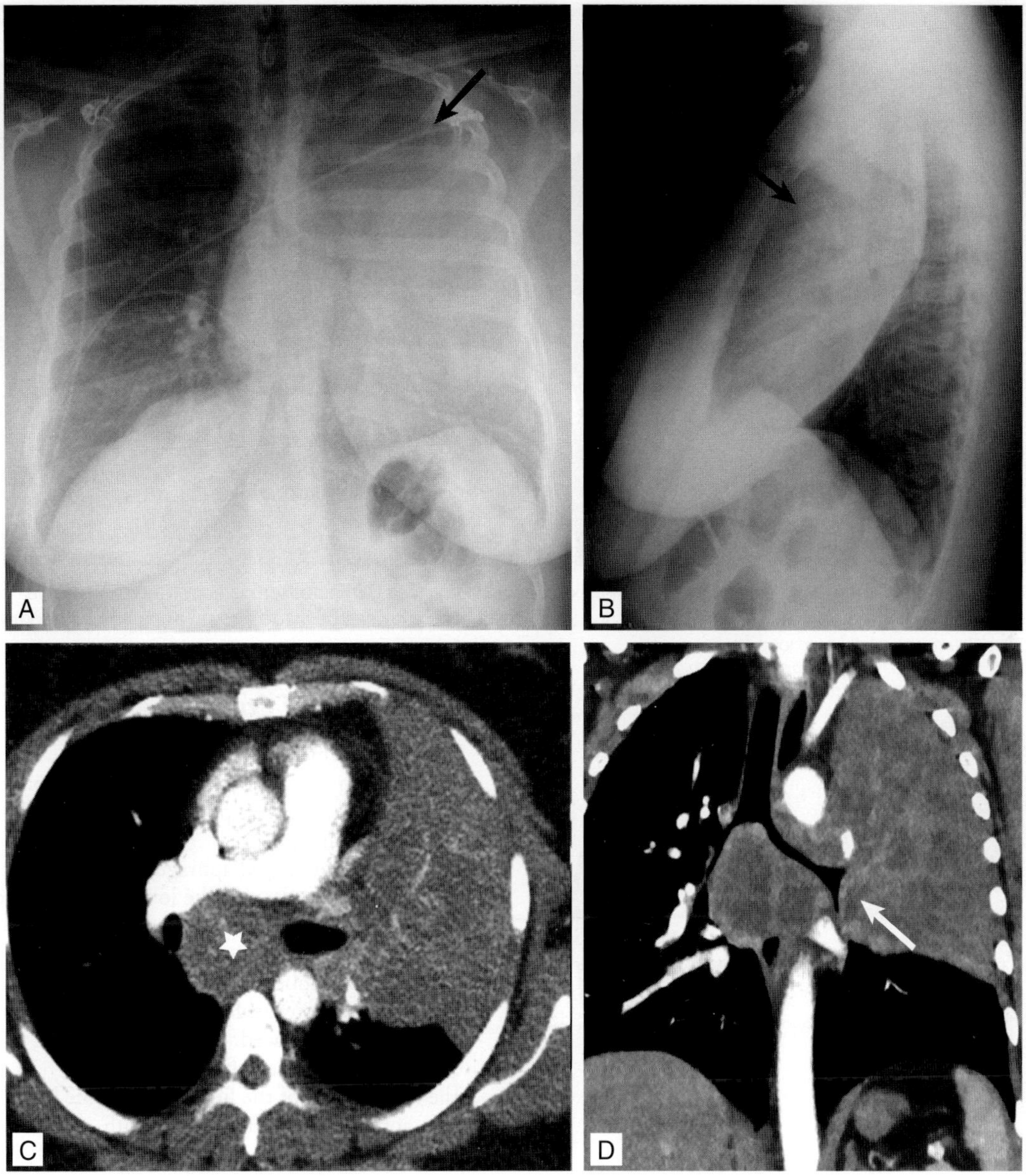

Figure 17.46 A 67-year-old female patient with obstructive atelectasis. Frontal (A) and lateral (B) chest radiographs in a patient presenting with difficulty in breathing demonstrate diffuse opacification of the left upper lobe including lingula (*black arrows*), concerning for collapse/consolidation of the left upper lobe with central obstructing hilar mass. Axial (C) and coronal (D) CT images demonstrate abrupt cut off of the left upper lobe bronchus (*arrow* in D) and associated bulky left hilar and mediastinal lymphadenopathy (*star*). Patient was diagnosed as bronchogenic carcinoma with associated metastatic lymphadenopathy with postobstruction left upper lobe collapse and pneumonia given the heterogeneous postcontrast enhancement.

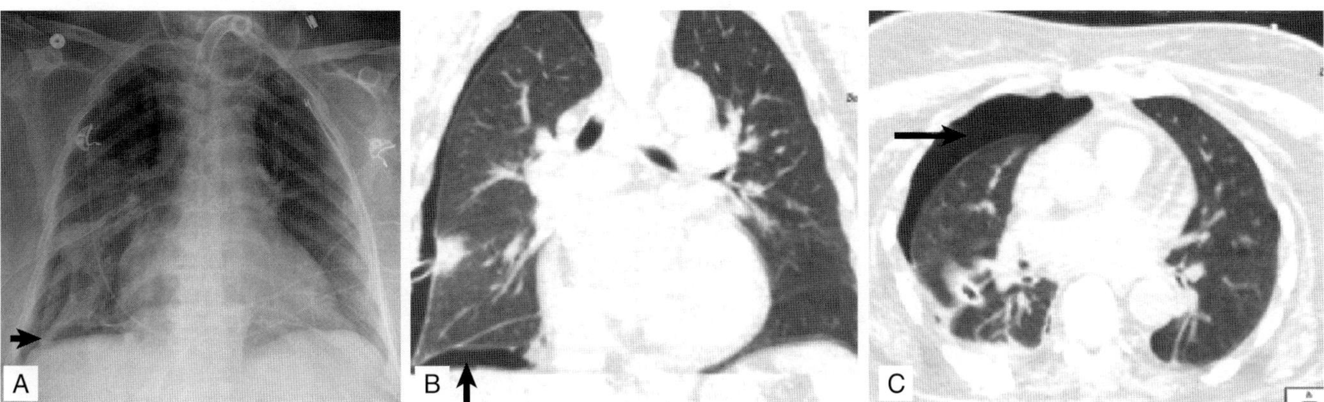

Figure 17.47 A 38-year-old woman with right pneumothorax and passive atelectasis. Frontal chest radiograph (A) demonstrating right pneumothorax (*black arrow*) with partial right lower lobe collapse confirmed on the coronal (B) and axial (C) CT images.

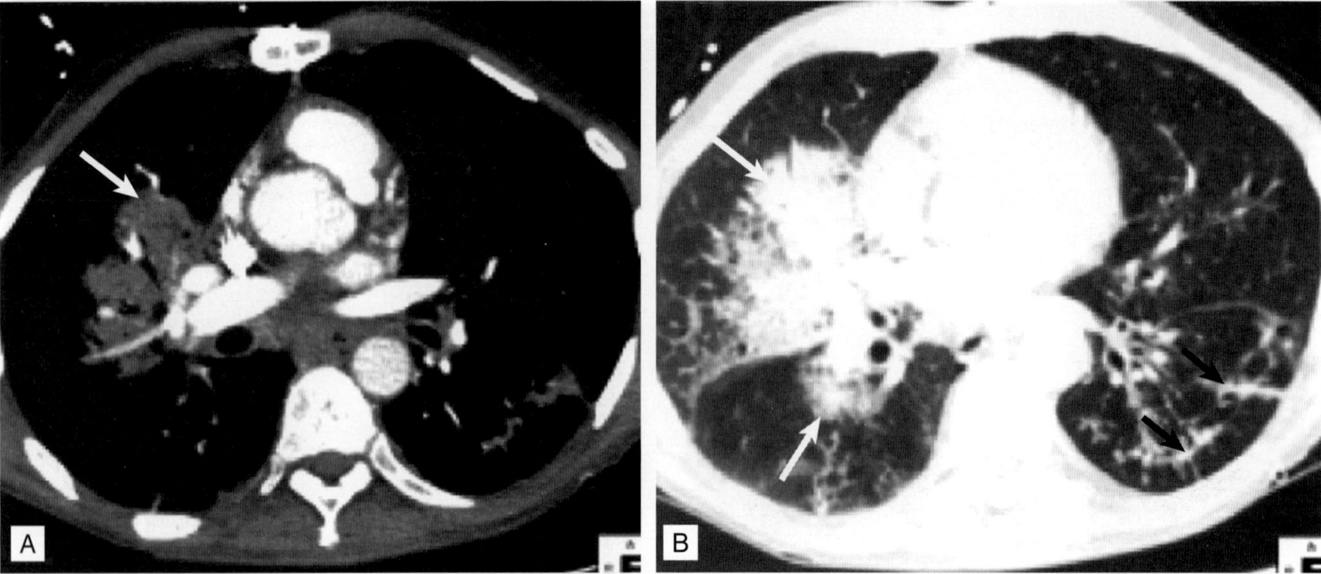

Figure 17.48 A 67-year-old man with recurrent pulmonary infections. Axial Contrast Enhanced Computed tomography (CECT) images demonstrate peribronchial pneumonic consolidative changes in right middle lobe and superior segment of right lower lobe (*white arrows*) along with subsegmental cicatrization-related atelectasis (*black arrows*) in left lower lobe.

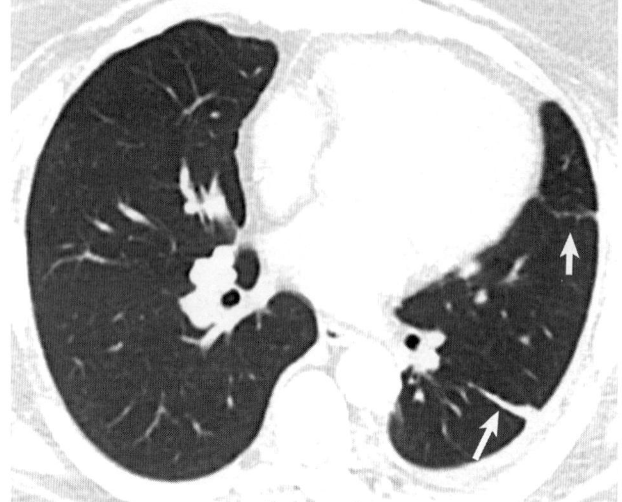

Figure 17.49 A 47-year-old hospitalized male patient with linear plate like subsegmental atelectasis (*arrows*) in the left lung.

Indirect Signs of Collapse

- Hilar displacement
  This is the most reliable indirect sign of collapse. The hilum may be elevated in the upper lobe collapse and depressed in the lower lobe collapse.
- Elevation of the hemidiaphragm
  This sign may be seen in the lower lobe collapse but is rare in the collapse of the other lobes.
- Mediastinal displacement
  In the upper lobe collapse, the trachea is often displaced toward the affected side, and in the lower lobe collapse, the heart may be displaced.
- Compensatory hyperinflation
  The normal part of the lung may become hyperinflated, and it may appear hypertransradiant, with its vessels more widely spaced than in the corresponding area of the contralateral lung. If there is a considerable collapse of a lung, compensatory hyperinflation of the contralateral lung may occur, with herniation across the midline.

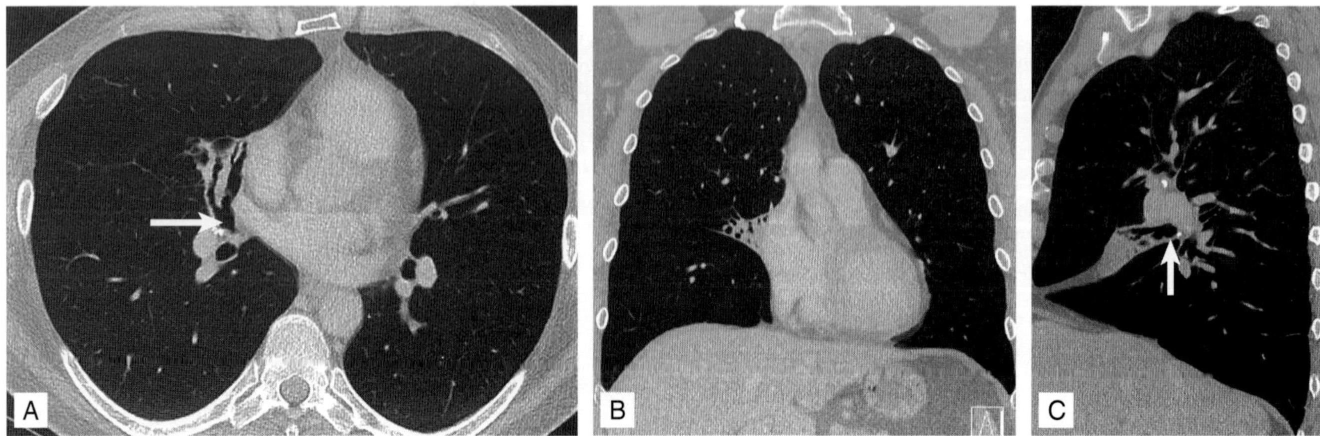

Figure 17.50 A 54-year-old man with chronic cough. Axial (A), coronal (B), and sagittal (C) lung window CT images showing near complete right middle lobe collapse and bronchiectasis without any central obstructive lesion (*arrow*).

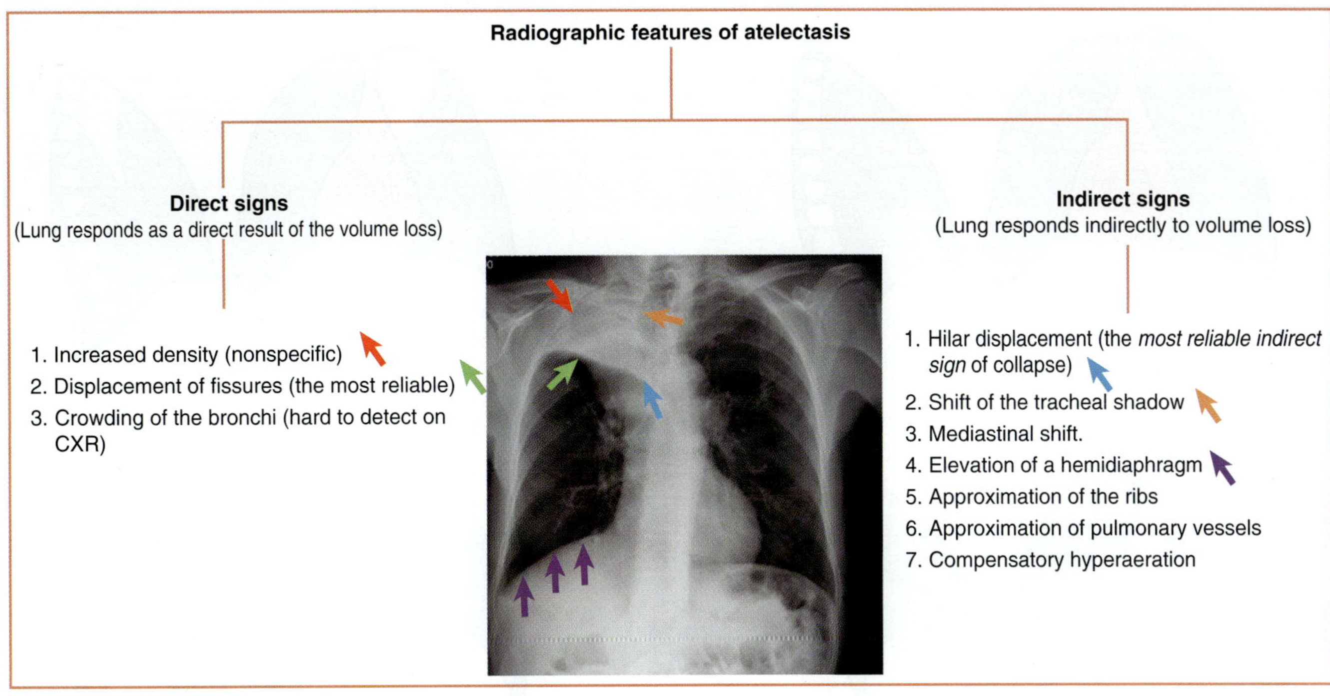

Figure 17.51 An image-based illustration of the direct and indirect signs of atelectasis.

Patterns of Collapse

An air bronchogram is almost never seen in resorption/obstructive collapse, but is usually seen in passive and adhesive collapse, and may be seen in cicatrization collapse if fibrosis is particularly dense. Pre-existing lung disease such as fibrosis and pleural adhesions may alter the expected displacement of anatomic landmarks in lung collapse. There also tends to be a reciprocal relationship between the compensatory signs: for example, in lower lobe collapse, if diaphragmatic elevation is marked, hilar depression will be diminished.

Complete Collapse of a Lung

Complete collapse of a lung, in the absence of pneumothorax or large pleural effusion or extensive consolidation, causes opacification of the hemithorax, displacement of the mediastinum to the affected side, and elevation of the diaphragm. Obstruction of the mainstem bronchus can lead to atelectasis of the entire lung. Compensatory hyperinflation of the contralateral lung occurs, often with herniation across the midline. Herniation most often occurs in the retrosternal space, anterior to the ascending aorta, but may occur posterior to the heart or under the aortic arch.

Lobar Collapse

The following descriptions apply to the collapse of individual lobes, uncomplicated by pre-existing pulmonary or pleural disease. The illustration drawings (Figs. 17.52 and 17.53) represent the alteration in the position of the fissures, as seen in the frontal and lateral projections, resulting from lobar collapse.

Right upper lobe collapse (Figs. 17.52, 17.54, and 17.55): The normal horizontal fissure is usually at the level of the right fourth rib anteriorly. As the right upper lobe collapses, the horizontal fissure pivots about the hilum, its lateral end moving upward and medially toward the superior mediastinum, and its anterior end moving upward toward the apex. The upper half of the oblique fissure moves anteriorly. The two fissures become concave superiorly. In severe collapse, the lobe may be flattened against the superior mediastinum and may obscure the upper pole of the hilum. The hilum is elevated, and its lower pole may be prominent. Deviation of the trachea to the right is usual, and compensatory hyperinflation of the right middle and lower lobes may be apparent. A juxtaphrenic peak (diaphragmatic tenting) may also be seen. Golden S-sing or reverse S-sign of golden is typically seen with right upper lobe collapse (typically in bronchogenic carcinoma) and may also be seen in the collapse of the other lobes. The upper concavity is formed by the edge of the collapsed lobe, while the more medial convexity is due to the obstructing tumor or enlarged hilar lymph node (Figs. 17.54 and 17.55).

Right middle lobe collapse (Figs. 17.52 and 17.56): In right middle lobe collapse the horizontal fissure and lower half of the oblique fissure move toward one another. This can best be seen in the lateral projection as a triangular opacity with its apex pointing toward hilum. The horizontal fissure tends to be more mobile, and therefore usually shows the greater displacement. Signs of right middle lobe collapse are often subtle on the frontal projection, since the horizontal fissure may not be visible, and increased opacity does not become apparent until collapse is almost complete. However, obscuration of the right heart border is often present and maybe the only clue in this projection. The lordotic AP projection brings the displaced fissure into the line of the x-ray beam and may elegantly demonstrate the right middle lobe collapse. Since the volume of this lobe is relatively small, indirect signs of volume loss are rarely present.

Lower lobe collapse: The normal oblique fissures extend from the level of the fourth thoracic vertebra posteriorly to the diaphragm, close to the sternum, anteriorly. The position of these fissures on the lateral projection is the best index of lower lobe

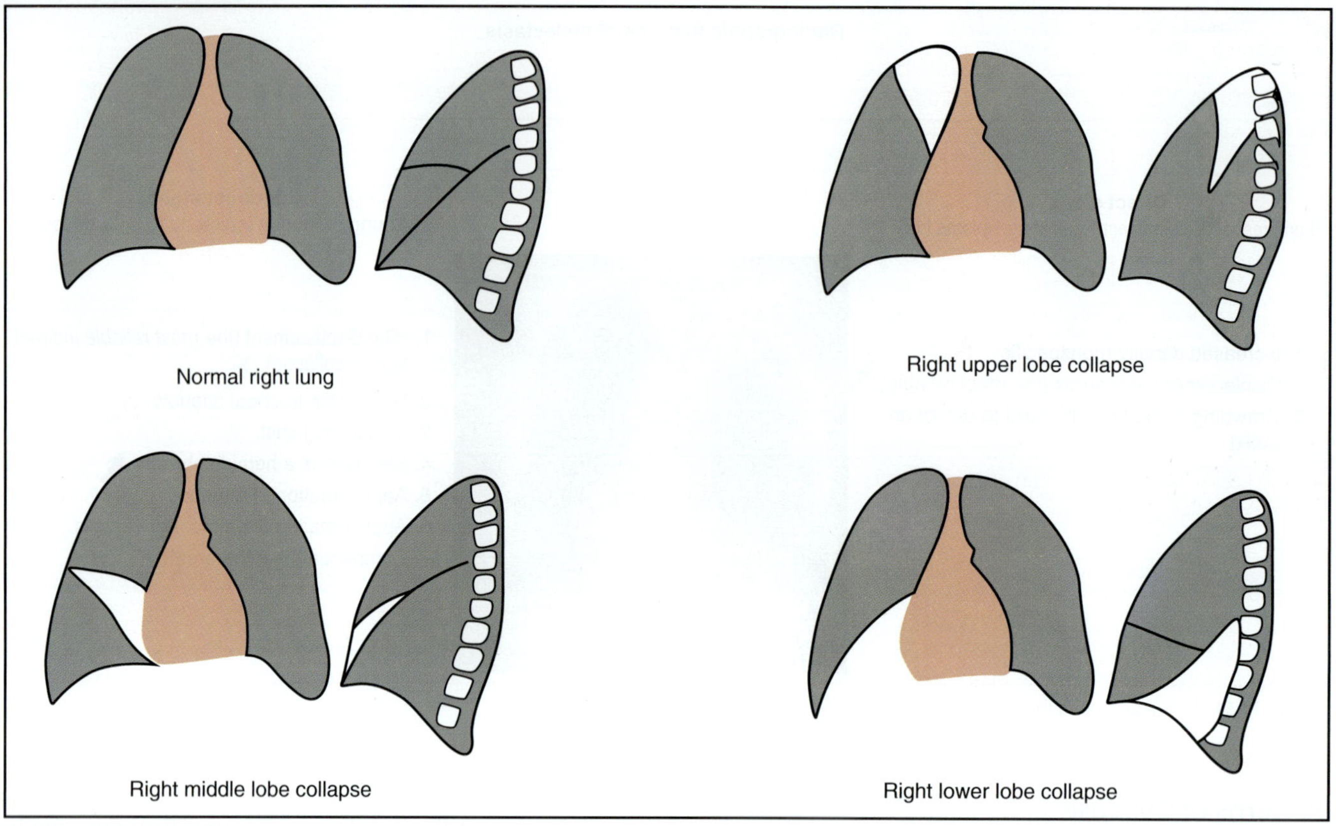

Normal right lung

Right upper lobe collapse

Right middle lobe collapse

Right lower lobe collapse

Figure 17.52 An illustrative image showing normal right lung fissures and their morphology with right-sided lobar collapse.

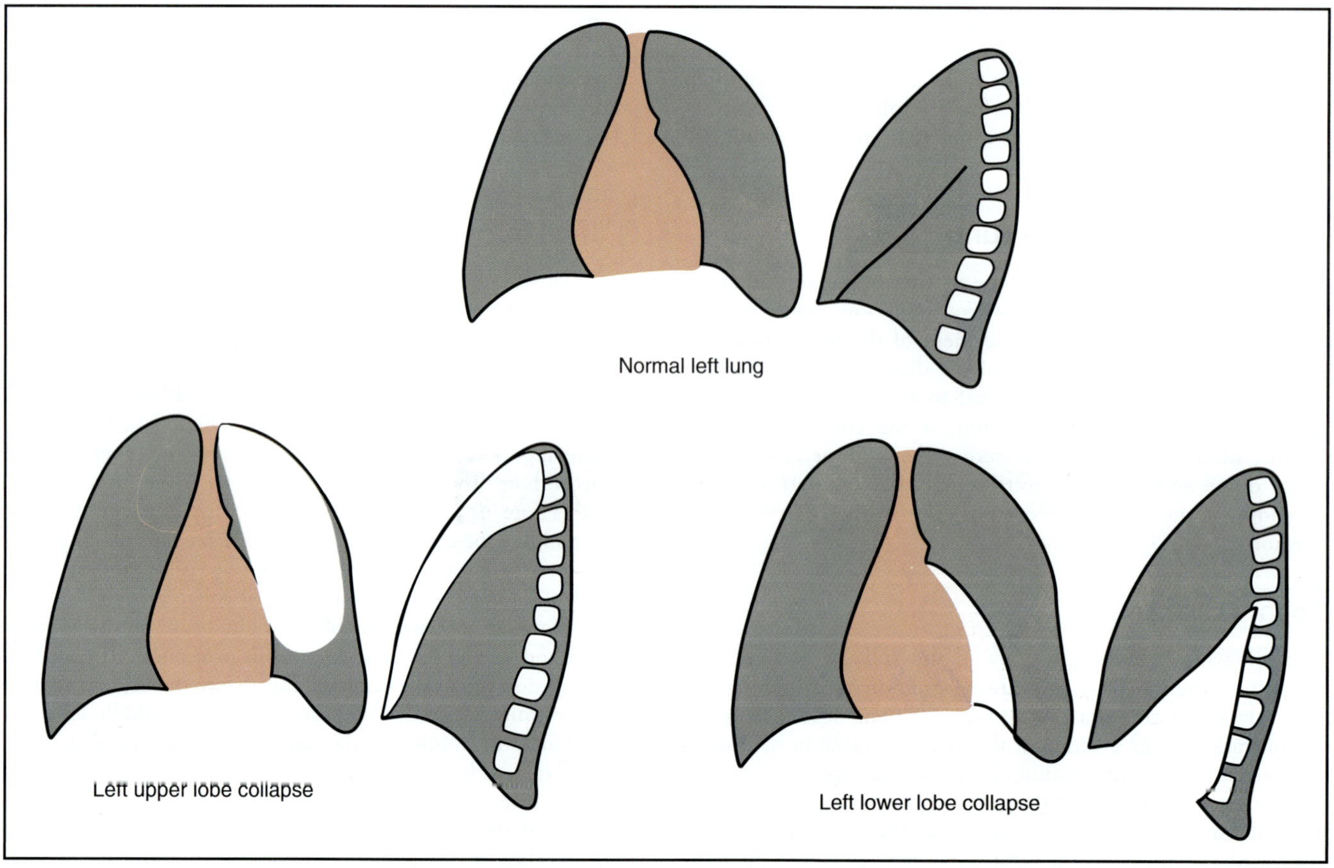

Normal left lung

Left upper lobe collapse

Left lower lobe collapse

Figure 17.53 An illustrative image showing normal left lung fissures and their morphology with left-sided lobar collapse.

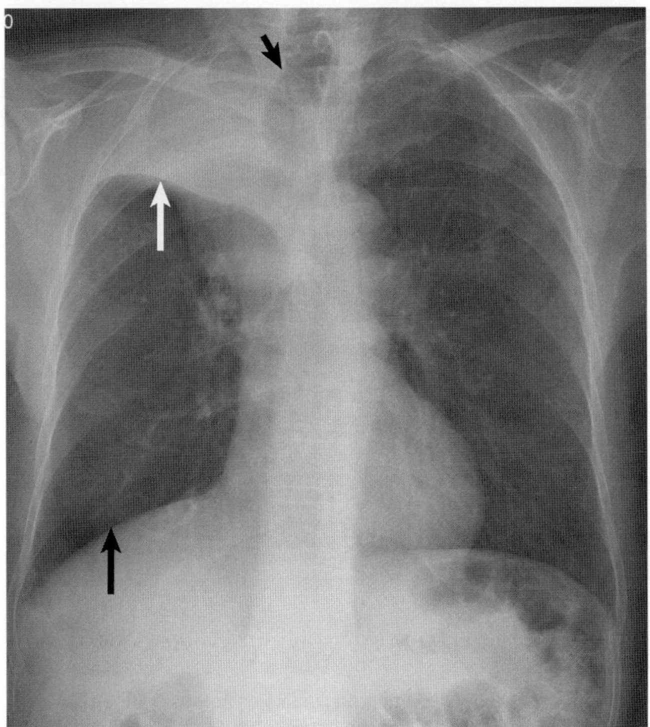

Figure 17.54 A 63-year-old smoker with cough, shortness of breath, and weight loss. Frontal chest radiograph showing right upper lobe atelectasis with elevation of the horizontal fissure (*white arrow*), elevation of the right hemidiaphragm (*long black arrow*), and right-sided deviation of the trachea (*short black arrow*).

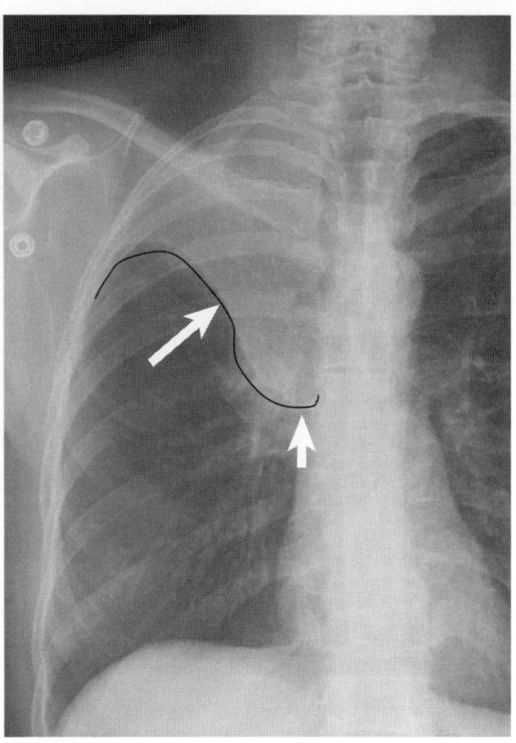

Figure 17.55 A 59-year-old smoker with right upper lobe lung cancer. Frontal chest radiograph showing golden S-sign. The upper concavity is formed by the edge of the collapsed lobe (*long white arrow*) while the more medial convexity is due to the obstructing tumor (*short white arrow*).

volumes. When a lower lobe collapses, its oblique fissure moves posteriorly but maintains its normal slope. In addition to the posterior movement, the collapsing lower lobe causes medial displacement of the oblique fissure, which may then become visible in places on the frontal projection.

Right lower lobe collapse (Figs. 17.57 and 17.58): This causes depression of the horizontal fissure, which may be apparent on the frontal projection. Increased opacity of a collapsed lower lobe is usually visible on the frontal projection as a paraspinal mass (Fig. 17.52). A completely collapsed lower lobe may be so small

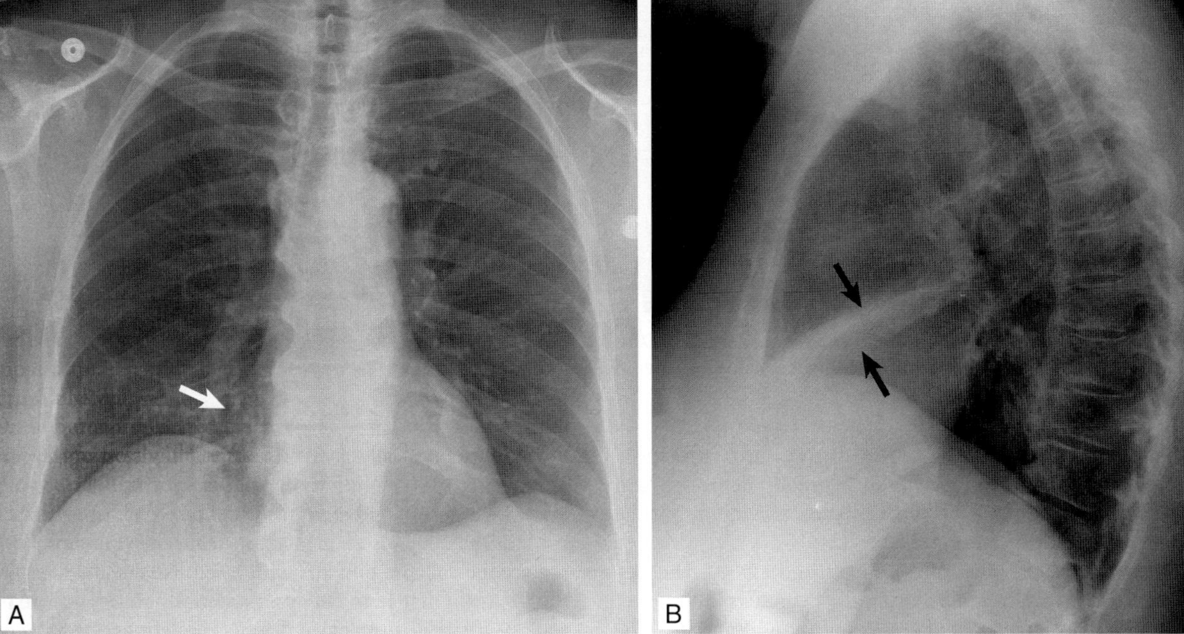

Figure 17.56 A 43-year-old male patient with right middle lobe collapse. Frontal (A) and lateral (B) chest radiographs demonstrate right middle lobe collapse with blurring of the right cardiac border on the PA view (*white arrow*) and approximation of the horizontal and oblique fissures on the lateral view (*black arrows*).

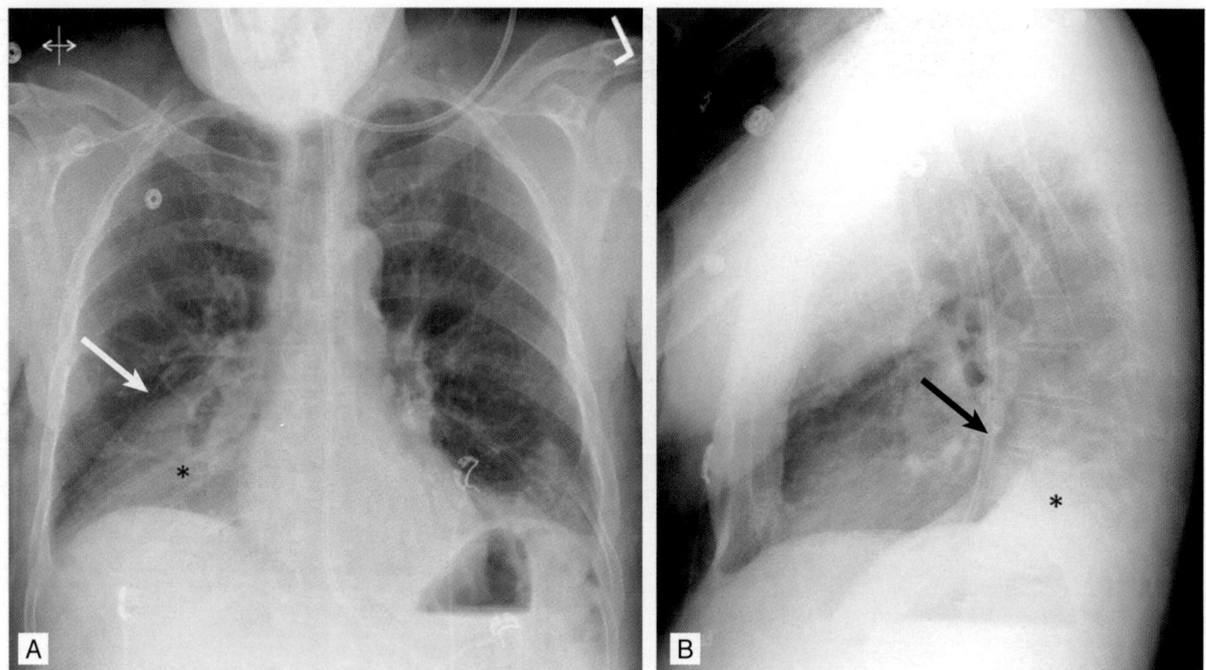

Figure 17.57 A 49-year-old man with right lower lobe collapse due to aspiration. Frontal (A) chest radiograph demonstrates collapse of the right lower lobe (*) with inferior displacement of horizontal fissure on the frontal view (*white arrow*) and posterior displacement of major fissure (*black arrow*) with obliteration of the silhouette of the right hemidiaphragmas seen on lateral view (B).

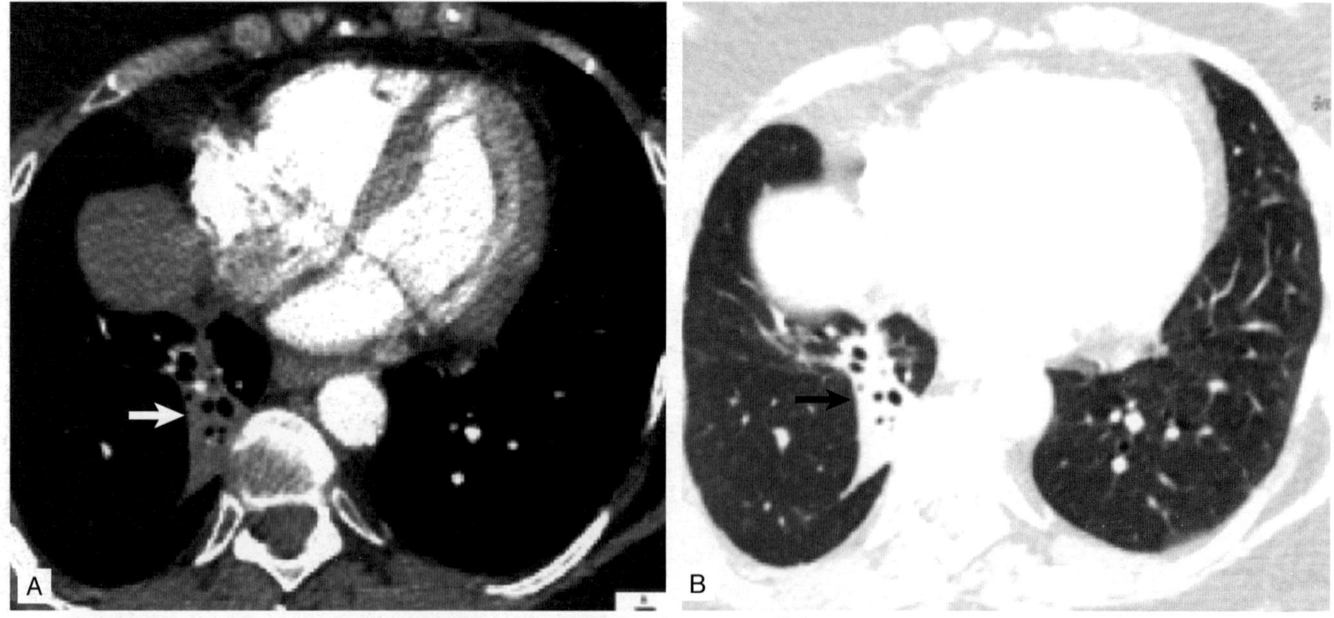

Figure 17.58 A 63-year-old female with right lower lobe atelectasis. Axial CECT chest mediastinal (A) and lung (B) window images with a lung cancer demonstrate collapse of the posterior basal segment of the right lower lobe with bronchial crowding (*arrows*).

that it flattens and merges with the mediastinum, producing a thin, wedge-shaped shadow. The hilum is usually depressed and rotated medially, and upper lobe hyperinflation is evident, but the diaphragmatic elevation is not usual.

Left upper lobe collapse (Figs. 17.53, 17.59, and 17.60): The pattern of upper lobe collapse is different in the two lungs. Left upper lobe collapse is apparent on the lateral projection as anterior displacement of the entire oblique fissure, which becomes oriented almost parallel to the anterior chest wall (Fig. 17.59). Left upper lobe collapse typically gives rise to the Luftsichel sign (Fig. 17.60). Compensatory hyperinflation of the superior segment of the left lower lobe insinuates between the collapsed left upper lobe and the mediastinum and is shaped like a crescent (Luftsichel). The left upper lobe collapse presents with a veil-like opacity over the hemithorax as the left lung collapses anteriorly to lie against the chest wall. With the complete collapse, the left upper lobe may lose contact with the chest wall and diaphragm and retract medially against the mediastinum. On a lateral film, therefore, left upper

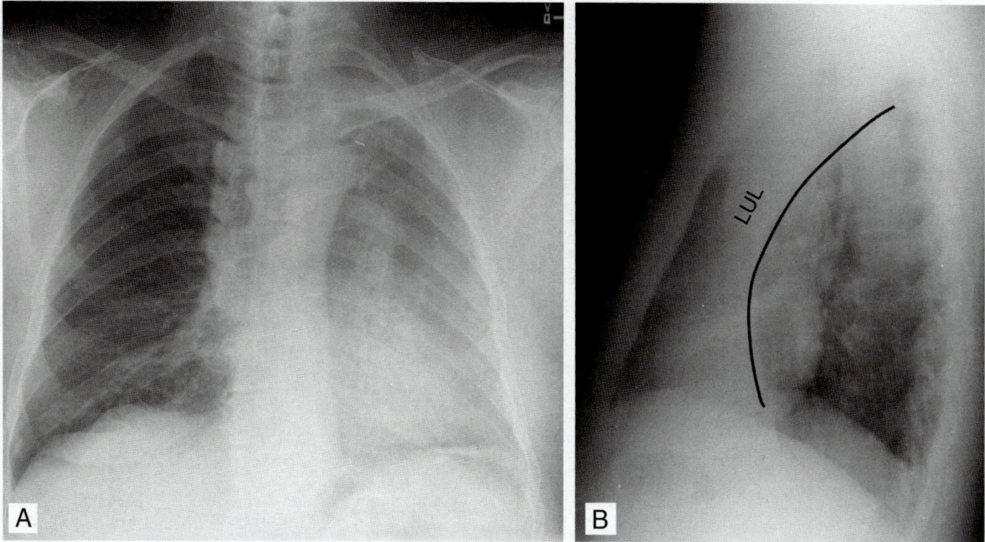

Figure 17.59 Frontal chest radiograph in a 60-year-old female patient demonstrates diffuse haziness of the left lung with volume loss and related crowding of the ribs while the lateral chest radiograph demonstrates LUL collapse with related posterior concavity of the oblique fissure (black line) and complete opacification of the left upper lobe (LUL).

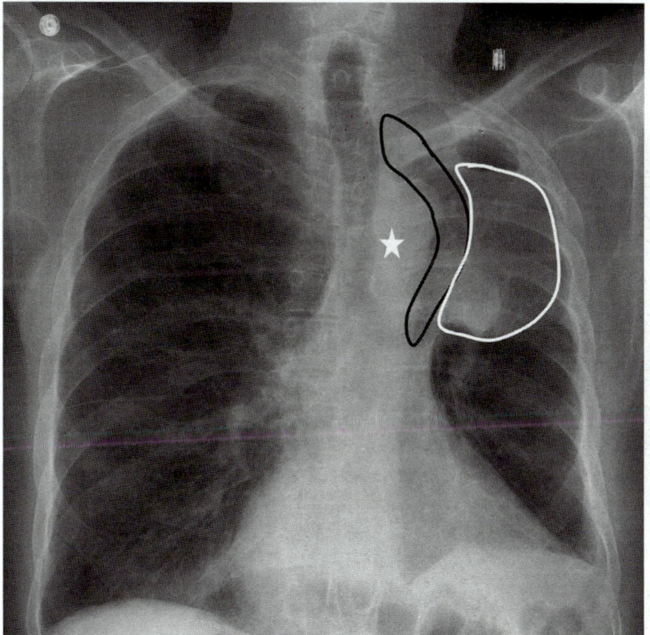

Figure 17.60 A 61-year-old male with left upper lobe collapse. Frontal chest radiograph showing compensatory hyperinflation of the superior segment of the left lower lobe (*shaped like sickle*) (*black line*), which insinuates between the collapsed left upper lobe (*white line*) and the mediastinum (*white star*).

lobe collapse appears as an elongated opacity extending from the apex and reaching, or almost reaching, the diaphragm; it is anterior to the hilum and is bounded by displaced oblique fissure posteriorly, and by hyperinflated lower lobe anteriorly.

A collapsed left upper lobe does not produce a sharp outline on the frontal view. An ill-defined hazy opacity is present in the upper, mid, and sometimes lower zones, the opacity being densest near the hilum. Pulmonary vessels in the hyperinflated lower lobe are usually visible through the haze. The aortic knuckle is usually obscured unless the upper lobe has collapsed anterior to it, allowing it to be outlined by the lower lobe. If the lingula is involved, the left heart border is obscured. The hilum is often elevated, and the trachea often deviates to the left.

Lingular collapse: The lingula is most often involved in the collapse of the left upper lobe, but it may collapse individually when the radiological features are similar to the right middle lobe collapse. However, the absence of a horizontal fissure on the left makes anterior displacement of the lower half of the oblique fissure and increased opacity anterior to its important signs. On the frontal projection, the left heart border becomes obscured.

Left lower lobe collapse (Figs. 17.53 and 17.61): The collapsed segment retracts inferiorly and posteromedially. On a frontal radiograph, there is increased retrocardiac density, inferior displacement of the left hilum, obscuration of the aortic arch knob, left hemidiaphragm, and lower lobe vessels, and parallel orientation of major fissure with the left heart border. Flat waist sign [67] (Fig. 17.61), seen in the left lower lobe collapse, refers to the straightening of the left heart border secondary to the leftward shift of the heart.

Rounded atelectasis: This is an unusual form of pulmonary collapse which may be misdiagnosed as a pulmonary mass. It appears on the plain film as a homogenous mass, usually 2–5 cm in diameter, with ill-defined edges. It is always pleural-based and associated with pleural thickening. On CT, rounded atelectasis appears as a soft-tissue density mass with or without air bronchogram, having acute angles with pleura and not completely surrounded by the lung parenchyma (Fig. 17.62). There is compression of the bronchovascular bundles giving rise to the comet tail sign [68]. It is often related to asbestos exposure but may occur secondary to any exudative pleural effusion. It is commonly seen in the lower lobe. It is not of any other pathological significance. The CT appearance is usually diagnostic and enables differentiation from other pulmonary masses.

Mimickers of Lobar Collapse

Various pathologies and artifactual summation shadows can mimic lobar collapse on a radiograph. On a lateral chest radiograph, the presence of fluid or fat in the inferior portion of the oblique fissure can mimic a partial (anterior-inferior) lower lobe

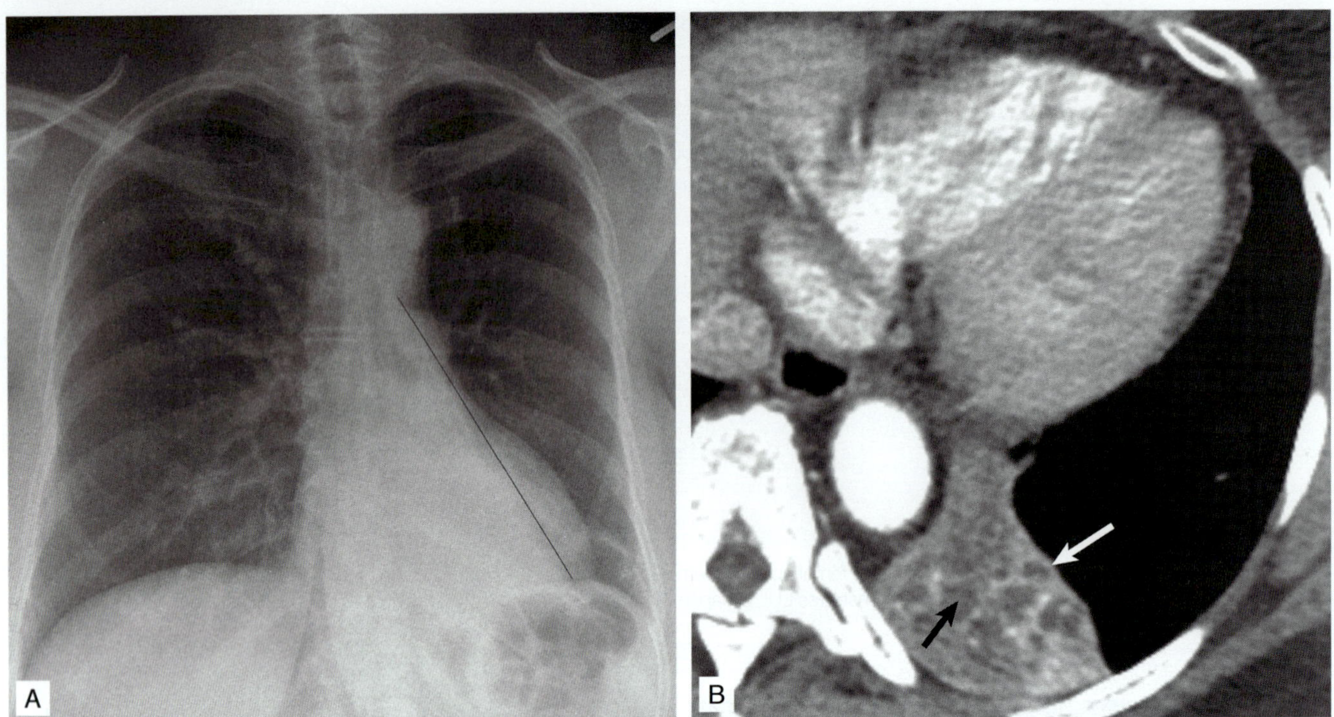

Figure 17.61 A 45-year-man with left lower lobe collapse from bronchial carcinoid. Frontal chest radiograph (A) showing retrocardiac opacification giving flat waist sign (*black line*). Axial CT (B) chest demonstrates collapsed left lower lobe (*white arrow*) with dilated mucus-filled bronchi (*black arrow*).

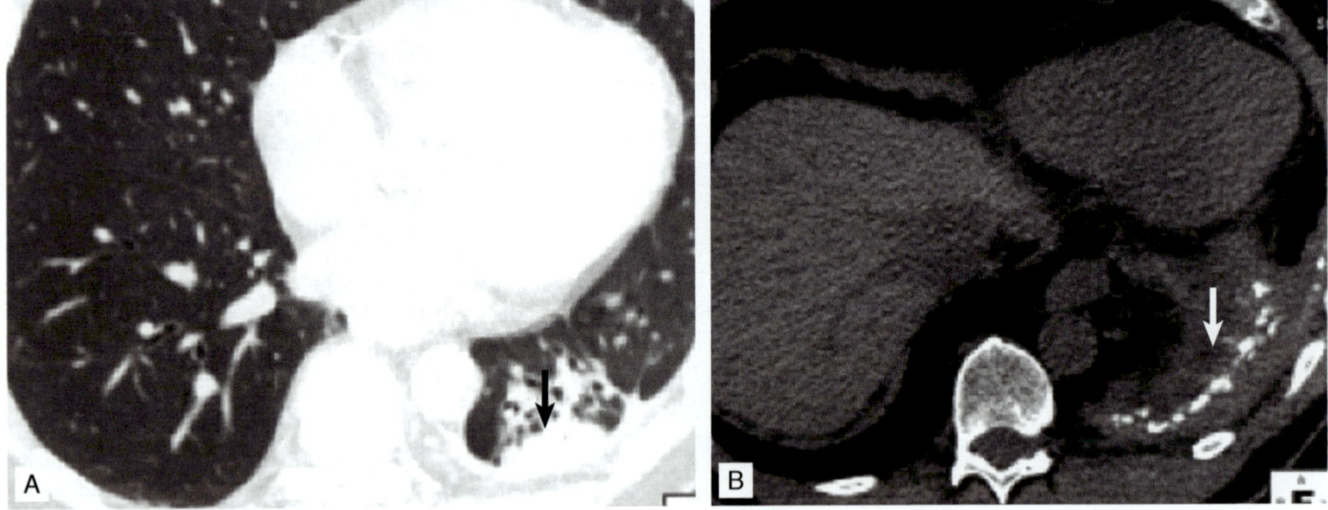

Figure 17.62 A 47-year-old male with history of prior chest trauma. Axial CT lung window image (A) showing a peripheral mass-like opacity in the left lower lobe (*black arrow*). Note decreased left lower lobe volume and crowing to the adjacent airway and vasculature. Below this lung finding, soft-tissue window CT image (B) showing thick and calcified pleura from prior hemothorax (*white arrow*). Collectively, the findings suggest round atelectasis from prior trauma.

collapse (Fig. 17.63). CT or comparison with prior exams (especially for fissural fat) can help make the correct diagnosis. On a frontal chest radiograph, pectus excavatum leads to obscuration of the right heart border, which mimics right middle lobe disease (collapse or pneumonia). However, the lateral radiograph typically shows inward bowing of the sternum (Fig. 17.64), which should suggest that the appearance on the frontal view is likely a mimic. Sometimes, lobar pneumonia can also be mistaken for lobar collapse. The identification of the fissure curvature is critical to distinguish as the collapse is associated with volume loss. Hence, the fissure is displaced toward the part of the lung that shows increased density (Fig. 17.65A). In pneumonia, the fissure can be in the normal anatomical location or can have a bulge opposite to the portion of the lung with increased density (Fig. 17.65B). Sometimes on a frontal radiograph, the medial portion of the breast shadow can mimic a lower lobe collapse. This artifactual appearance from the summation shadow can be confirmed by careful attention and identifying that the medial density is continuing with the rest of the breast shadow (Fig. 17.66).

Consolidation

Consolidation refers to the replacement of air within the alveoli from airspace or an interstitial process. It is seen as an area of

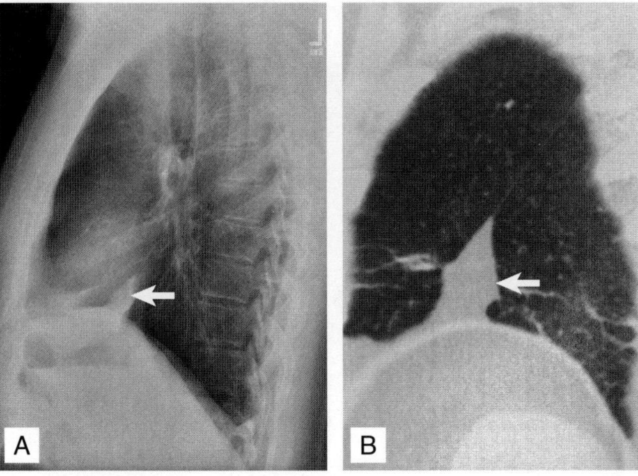

Figure 17.63 Fat in fissure mimicking partial lower lobe collapse. Lateral chest radiograph (A) demonstrates triangular opacity related to the left oblique fissure mimicking partial lower lobe collapse (*white arrow*). However, sagittal CT chest image of the lung (B) demonstrates density within the left oblique fissure with density similar to upper abdominal fat suggesting intrafissure fat (*white arrow*). Note that few linear bands of atelectasis within inferior lingula and anterior left lower lobe are seen.

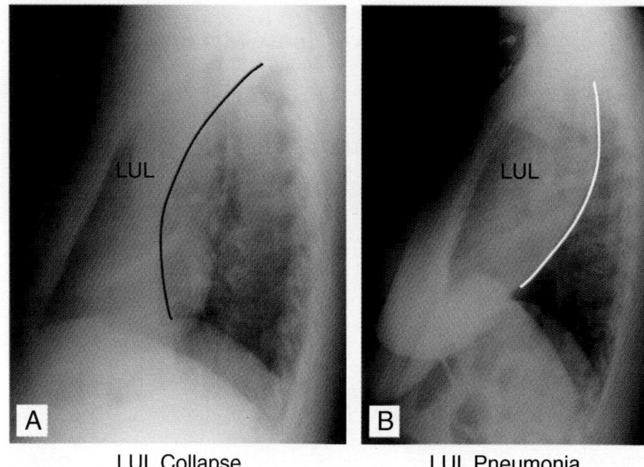

Figure 17.65 Collapse versus pneumonia. Lateral chest radiograph (A) in a patient with left upper lobe (LUL) collapse showing the increased density in the anterior lung from collapse and the curvature of the oblique fissure (black line) toward the area of increased lung density. Comparison in left upper lobe pneumonia (B) showing increased density of the LUL with oblique fissure (white line) bulging away from the region of increased lung density.

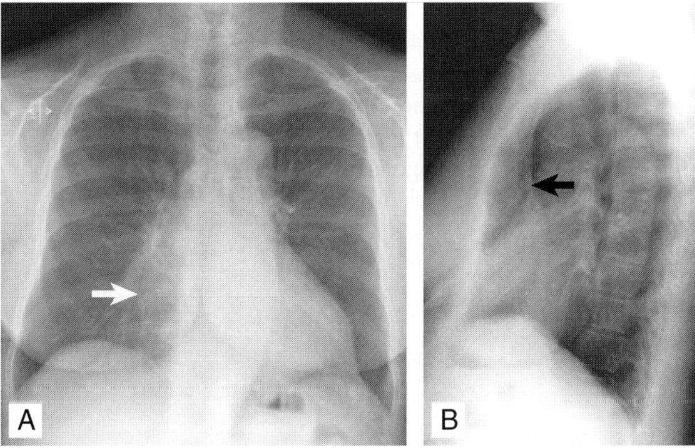

Figure 17.64 Pectus excavatum mimicking right middle lobe collapse. Frontal chest radiograph in a 43-year-old female with cough shows obscuration of right heart border (*white arrow*) suspicious for right middle lobe disease. Lateral radiograph (B) shows that the findings seen on frontal radiograph were due to inward bowing of the sternum (*black arrow*).

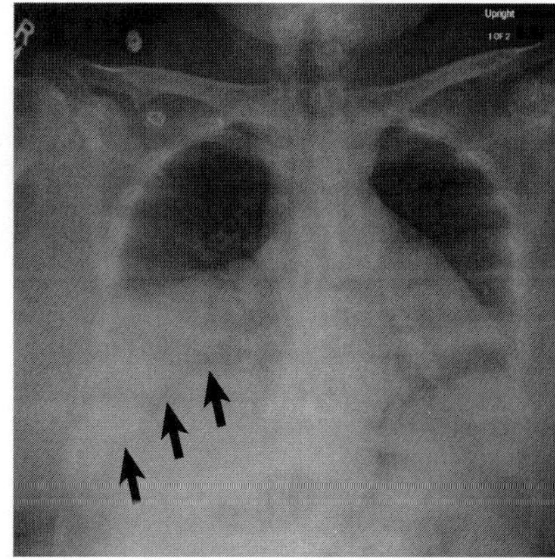

Figure 17.66 Mimic of lower lobe collapse. Frontal chest radiograph demonstrating dense large right breast mimicking right lower lobe collapse. The linear density (*black arrows*) is seen continuing with the rest of breast contour. There is only mild atelectasis in the right middle lobe which obscures the right heart border.

increased lung density, causing obscuration of the margins of walls of the lung vasculature and the airway [69]. Functionally, the pulmonary airways can be divided into two groups. The proximal airways function purely as a conducting network; the airways distal to the terminal bronchioles are also conducting structures, but, more importantly, are the site of gaseous exchange. These terminal airways are termed acini, an acinus comprising respiratory bronchioles, alveolar ducts, alveolar sacs, and alveoli arising from a terminal bronchiole. Consolidation implies the replacement of air in one or more acini by fluid, pus, blood, cells, or solid material, but does not imply a particular pathology or etiology. The smallest unit of the consolidated lung is a single acinus, which casts a shadow approximately 7 mm in diameter. Communications between the terminal airways allow fluid to spread between adjacent acini, so that larger confluent areas of consolidation are generally visible and are frequently not confined to a single segment.

The most common cause of consolidation is acute inflammatory exudate associated with pneumonia. Other causes include cardiogenic pulmonary edema, noncardiogenic pulmonary edema, hemorrhage, and aspiration. Neoplasms such as adenocarcinoma and lymphoma can produce consolidation, and alveolar proteinosis is a rare cause. In an individual patient, consolidation may be due to more than one basic etiology. For example, a patient with major head trauma may be particularly susceptible to infection, aspiration, and noncardiogenic pulmonary edema. The features of consolidation on chest radiograph and CT chest are summarized in Table 17.2. When consolidation is associated with a patent conducting airway, an air bronchogram (Figs. 17.67 and 17.68) is often visible. This sign is produced by the radiographic contrast between the column of air in the airway and the surrounding opaque acini. If consolidation is secondary to bronchial obstruction, however, the air in the conducting airway is

TABLE 17.2 Radiologic Signs of Consolidation

- Airspace opacity
- Air bronchogram
- Alveolar (ill-defined/fluffy) opacities
- Patchy parenchymal opacities
- Preserved lung volume
- CT angiogram sign
- Tree-in-bud nodules

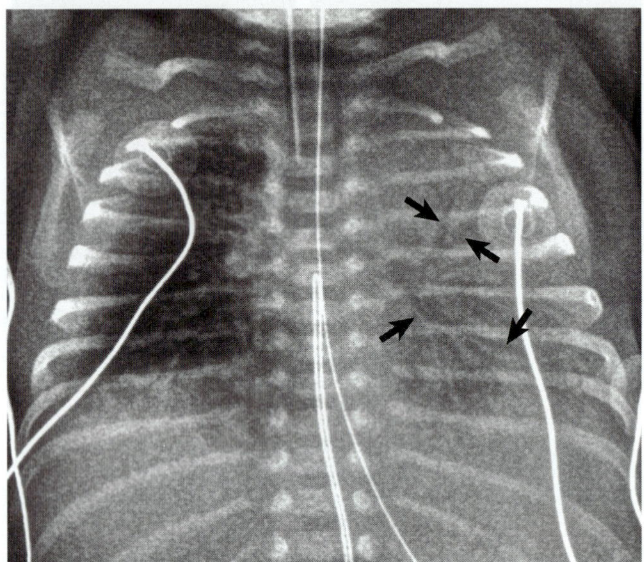

Figure 17.67 A 2-day-old, 32-week-gestational age newborn with surfactant deficiency (hyaline membrane disease). Frontal chest radiograph shows bilateral low lung volumes with diffuse left opacification showing multiple air bronchograms (*black arrows*) suggesting combined collapse and consolidation.

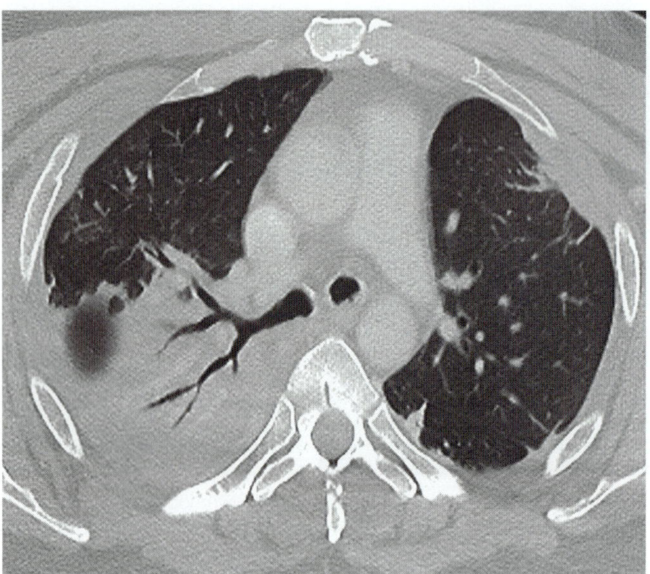

Figure 17.68 A 55-year-old male with fever. CT image showing consolidation in the right lung with air bronchogram.

resorbed and replaced by fluid, and the affected area is of uniform density.

Rarely, the appearance of the consolidation can help in the identification of the cause. Consolidation from lipoid pneumonia leads to decreased attenuation and consolidation from Amiodarone toxicity may have increased attenuation on noncontrast CT, helping narrow the differential diagnosis. Aspiration pneumonia typically occurs in the presence of risk factors like altered mental status, drug overdose, or gastroesophageal diseases. It tends to occur in lower lobes with the right lower lobe as the most common location. The presence of risk factors, typical location, and presence of contents within the central airway or within the airway of the consolidated lung may help in the diagnosis (Fig. 17.69).

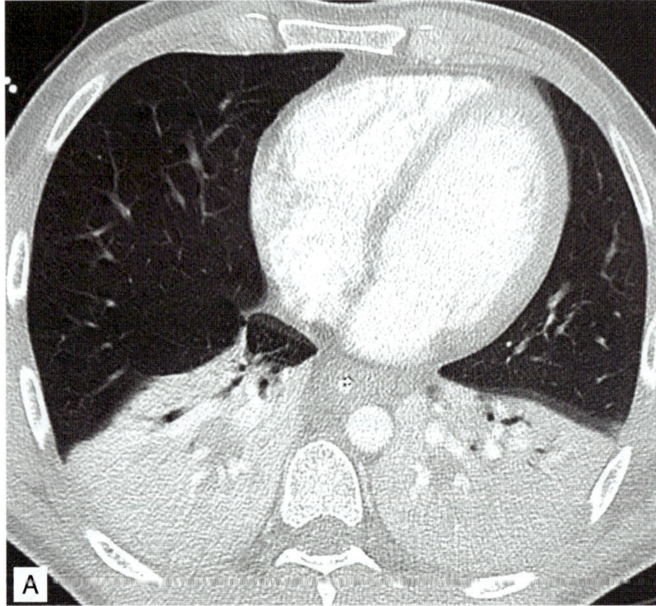

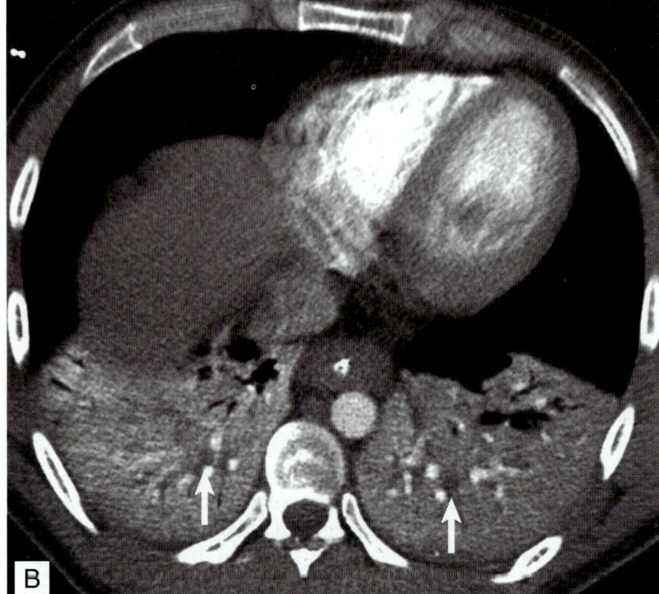

Figure 17.69 A 41-year-old male with drug overdose. Axial contrast-enhanced CT chest lung window (A) and soft-tissue window (B) images showing bilateral lower lobe consolidation. The airway within the consolidated lung shows hypodense contents (*white arrow,* B). The clinical context and the morphology suggest aspiration pneumonia.

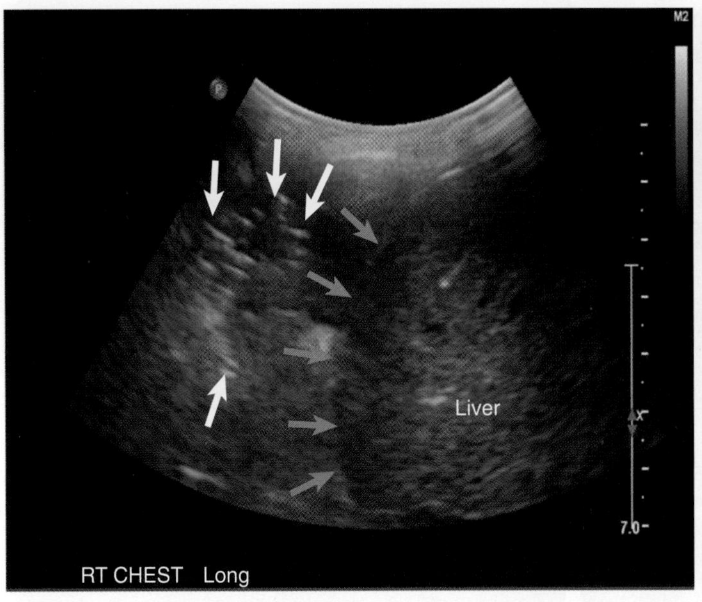

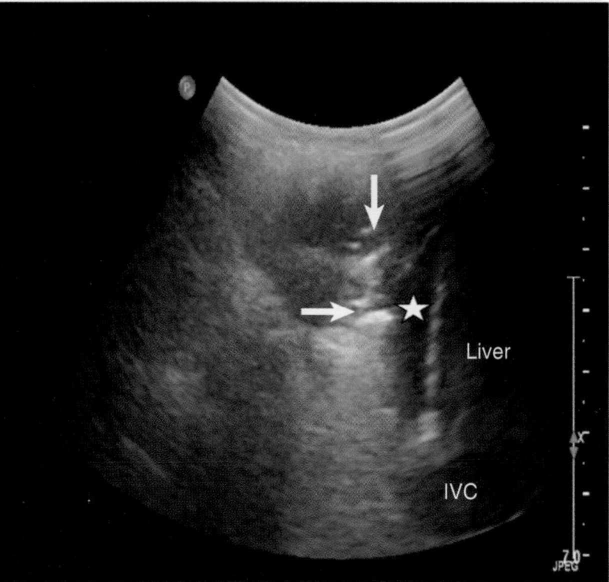

Figure 17.70 A 16-year-old patient with fever and right-sided chest and upper abdominal pain. Ultrasound abdomen showing right lower lobe lung consolidation with linear echogenic areas representing air bronchogram (*white arrows*) consistent with pneumonia in the clinical setting. Small parapneumonic right pleural effusion is also seen (*star*). Liver and inferior vena cava (IVC) are labeled and the diaphragm is highlighted by *gray arrows* in the figure.

The volume of a purely consolidated lung is similar to that of the normal lung since air is replaced by a similar volume of fluid or solid. However, collapse and consolidation are often associated with one another. Sometimes, infectious causes of consolidation can increase the lung volume leading to bulging of the fissures, also known as "bulging fissure" sign. When consolidation is due to fluid overload, its distribution is influenced by gravity. In acute pneumonitis, the consolidation is often denser and more clearly demarcated inferiorly by a pleural surface, and is less dense and more indistinct superiorly.

Ultrasound may rarely be used in an emergency setting to demonstrate consolidation in the peripheral lung. When air bronchograms are evident on the chest radiograph, these may be manifest as echogenic linear structures (Fig. 17.70). When the bronchi become fluid filled, they are more clearly demonstrated as echo-free branching structures.

Lobar Consolidation

Consolidation of an entire lobe produces a homogenous opacity, possibly containing an air bronchogram, delineated by the chest wall, mediastinum or diaphragm, and the appropriate interlobar fissure or fissures. Parts of the diaphragm and mediastinum adjacent to the nonaerated lung are obscured (Silhouette sign) and help to localize the site of consolidation [70,71].

Right upper lobe consolidation: This is confined by the horizontal fissure inferiorly and the upper half of the oblique fissure posteriorly, and may obscure the right upper mediastinum/paratracheal stripe. The fissure is usually in the usual anatomical location (Fig. 17.71).

Right middle lobe consolidation: This is limited by the horizontal fissure above, and the lower half of the oblique fissure posteriorly, and may obscure the right heart border (Fig. 17.72). The

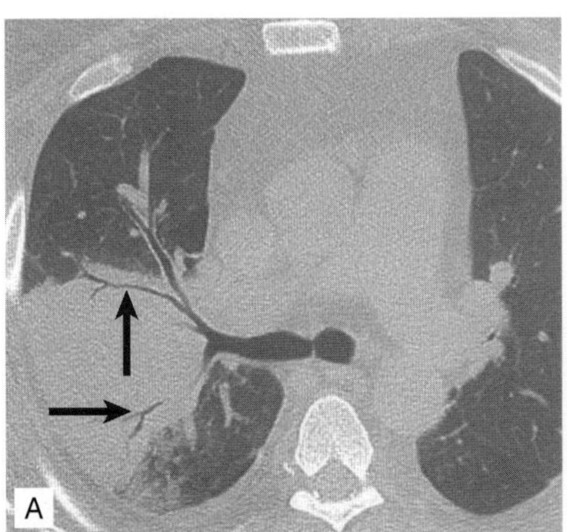

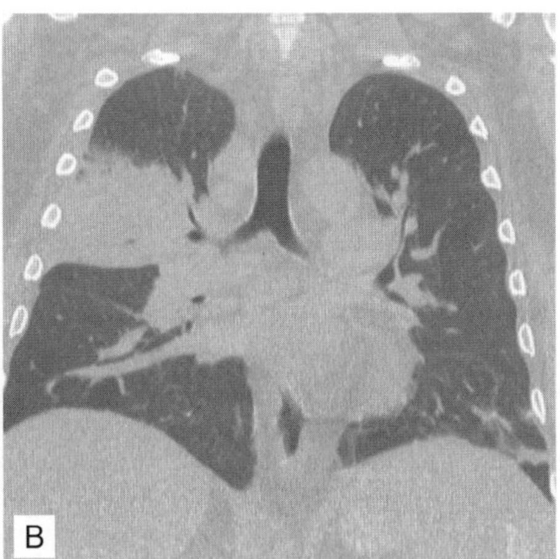

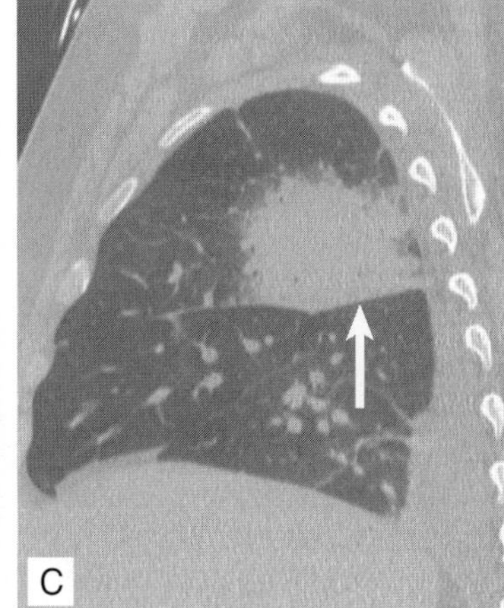

Figure 17.71 A 49-year-old male patient with right upper lobe consolidation due to pneumonia. CT chest axial (A), coronal (B), and sagittal (C) lung window images show consolidation in the right upper lobe with air bronchogram (*black arrow*). The fissure is located in the expected anatomical location (*white arrow*).

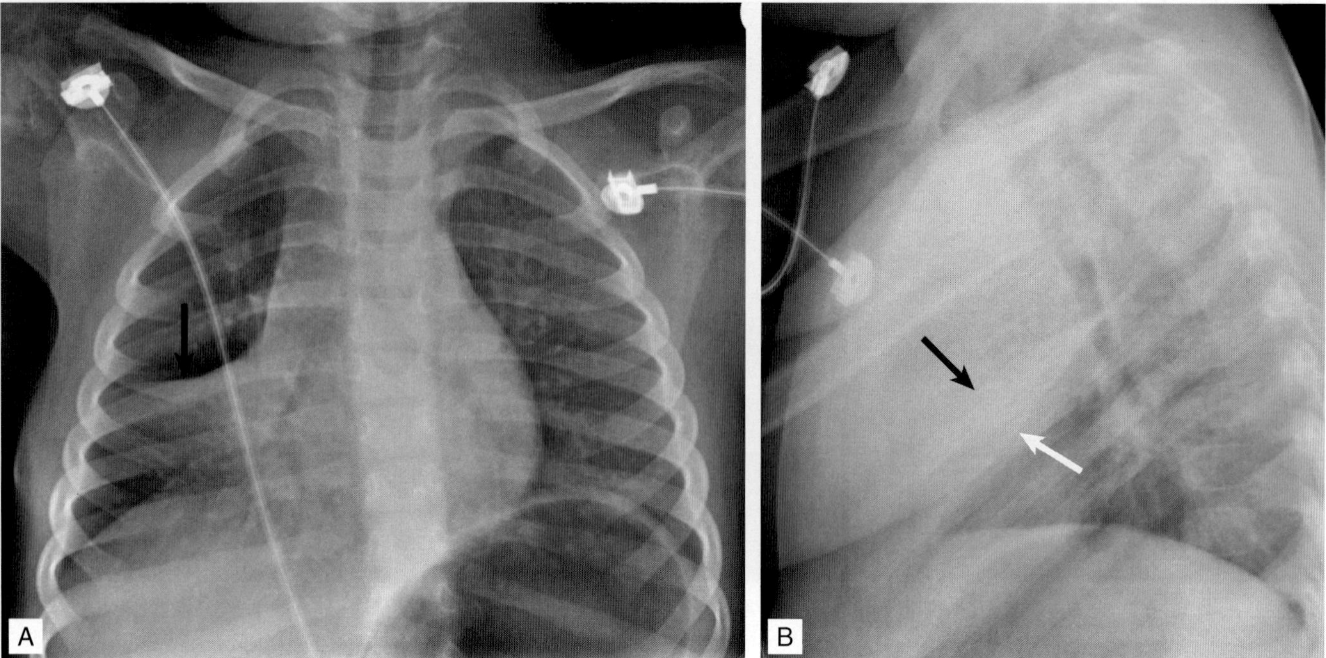

Figure 17.72 A 4-year-old boy with high-grade fever and chills. Frontal chest radiograph (A) showing increased attenuated marginated by horizontal fissure superiorly (*black arrow*) and causing obscuration of the right heart border (*arrow*) (silhouette sign). Lateral chest radiograph (B) also shows typical anterior triangular opacity between horizontal fissure (*black arrow*) and oblique fissure (*white arrow*).

right heart border is obscured only if the consolidation involves the medial segment of the right middle lobe. If consolidation spares the medial segment of the right middle lobe, the right heart border is not obscured.

Right lower lobe consolidation: This is limited by the oblique fissure anteriorly and may obscure the right hemidiaphragm. Normally, on a lateral chest radiograph, there is a decreasing density of the lower thoracic spine as compared to the upper thoracic spine. In patients with lower lobe pneumonia, there is an increased density of the lower thoracic spine as compared to the upper thoracic spine on the lateral radiograph (Spine sign).

Left upper lobe consolidation: Left upper lobe consolidation may obscure the left paratracheal stripe and aortic knuckle. If the consolidation primarily involves the lingula, the left heart border is obscured (Fig. 17.73).

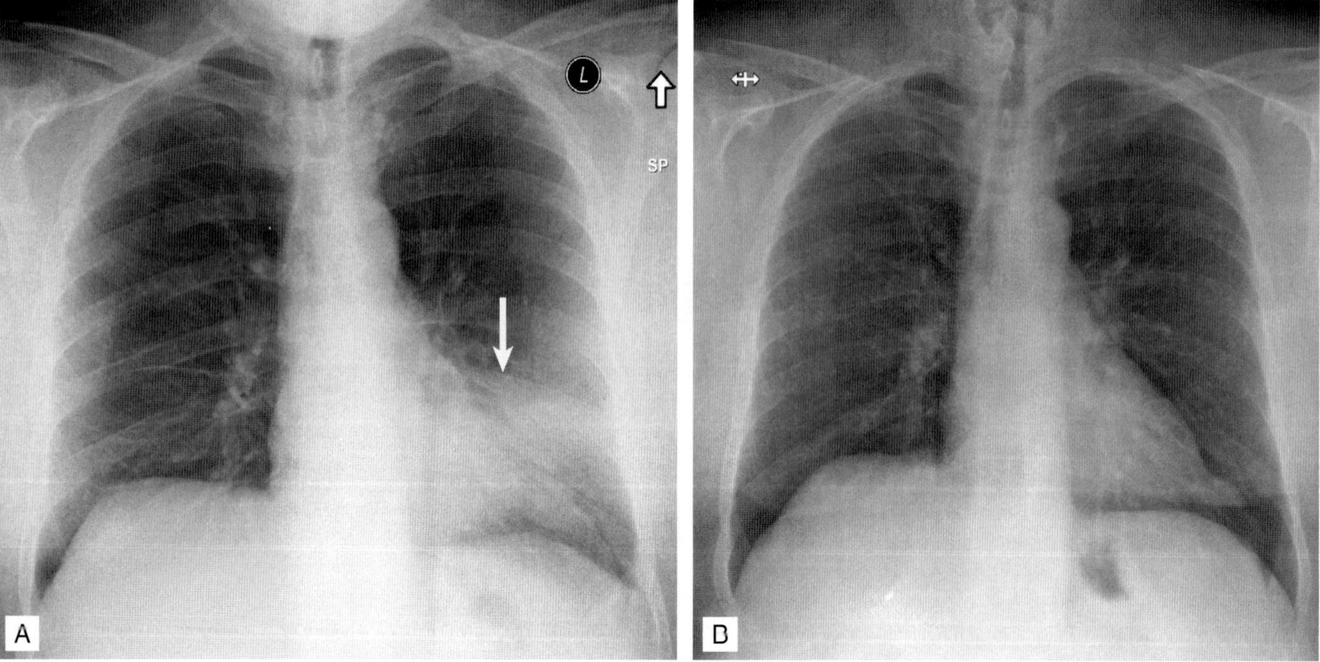

Figure 17.73 A 52-year-old female with fever and cough. Frontal chest radiograph (A) showing consolidation in the left lung (*arrow*) obscuring the left heart border. The left heart border silhouette localizes this pneumonia to the lingula of the left upper lobe. Frontal radiograph (B) obtained 3 months after treatment shows resolution of the pneumonia with clear demarcation of the left heart border.

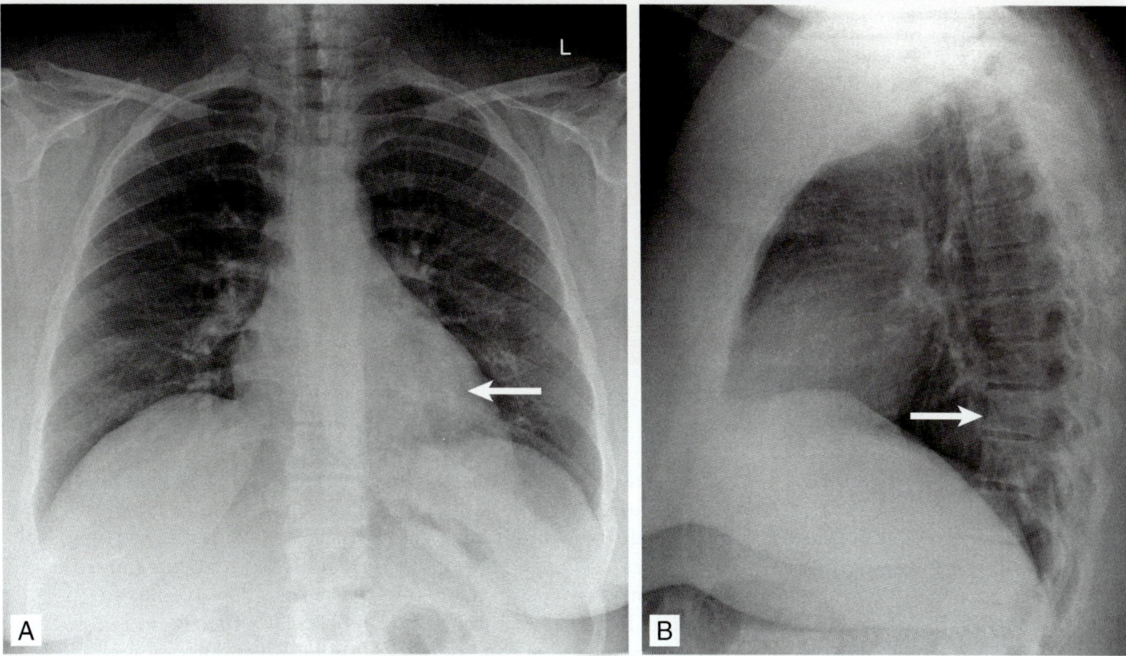

Figure 17.74 A 49-year-old female with fever. Frontal chest radiograph (A) shows increased left retrocardiac density (*arrow*) with partial silhouette of the left hemidiaphragm. Lateral chest radiograph (B) shows increased density of the lower thoracic spine as compared to upper thoracic spine (*arrow, spine sign*) confirming the posterior location of the left lower lobe pneumonia.

Left lower lobe consolidation: This may obscure the left hemidiaphragm and the descending aorta with increased density overlying the lower thoracic spine on lateral radiographs. The increased density of the lower thoracic spine as compared to the upper thoracic spine on the lateral radiograph (Spine sign) helps diagnose the lower lobe consolidation (Fig. 17.74).

Suggested Readings

- O Algin, G Gokalp, U Topal, Signs in chest imaging, Diagn Interv Radiol 17 (2011) 18–29.
- AV Ngo, CM Walker, JH Chung, et al., Tumors and tumorlike conditions of the large airways, AJR Am J Roentgenol 201 (2013) 301–313.
- CM Walker, GF Abbott, RE Greene, JA Shepard, D Vummidi, SR Digumarthy, Imaging pulmonary infection: classic signs and patterns. AJR Am J Roentgenol 202 (2014) 479–492.
- K Nowers, JD Rasband, G Berges, M Gosselin, Approach to ground-glass opacification of the lung, Semin Ultrasound CT MR 23 (2002) 302–323.
- DK Sundarakumar, AS Bhalla, R Sharma, AK Gupta, SK Kabra, P Jagia, Multidetector computed tomography imaging of congenital anomalies of major airways: A pictorial essay, World J Radiol 3 (2011) 289–297.
- S Bodduluri, JM Reinhardt, EA Hoffman, JD Newell Jr, SP Bhatt, Recent advances in computed tomography imaging in chronic obstructive pulmonary disease, Ann Am Thorac Soc 15 (2018) 281–289.

18

Diffuse Lung Disease

DEXTER P. MENDOZA, SUBBA R. DIGUMARTHY

Introduction

Diffuse lung diseases are often first identified on chest radiographs (CXR). CXR allows for the general assessment of lung volumes and disease distribution, and can help detect ancillary findings such as lymphadenopathy, pleural effusions or pleural plaques, or pulmonary arterial enlargement, providing clues as to the underlying etiology and complications related to the diffuse lung disease. CXR, however, is neither sensitive nor specific in the assessment of diffuse lung disease, often requiring further assessment with high-resolution computed tomography (HRCT).

HRCT relies on the acquisition of thin transverse sections (typically 1.5 mm thickness or less) with a high spatial resolution to visualize the lung parenchyma and interstitium. In addition, prone images are obtained to eliminate gravity-dependent atelectasis in the dependent portions of the lungs, which can obscure or be mistaken for abnormalities. Static (end-expiratory) or dynamic expiratory imaging is also routinely performed to help detect and confirm the presence of air trapping. During expiration, there is an expected increased attenuation of the lung parenchyma from incomplete expansion. Areas of air trapping would appear as areas of persistent or increased lucency.

HRCT is highly sensitive in the detection of diffuse lung disease and can characterize morphologic abnormalities that can point to a specific diagnosis, supplanting biopsy. Several terminologies are commonly used to describe these HRCT findings and patterns (Table 18.1). HRCT can also help direct the site of biopsy when necessary. It is valuable in monitoring of disease, including response to therapy, its evolution over time, and any complications. There are innumerable causes of diffuse lung disease, with the more common pathologies discussed in this chapter. Acute pathologies that can result in diffuse lung abnormalities such as acute infections, pulmonary edema, acute respiratory distress syndrome (ARDS), and diffuse alveolar hemorrhage are discussed separately.

Idiopathic Interstitial Pneumonias

Idiopathic interstitial pneumonias (IIPs) are a heterogeneous group of diffuse lung diseases without established cause and resulting in varying degrees of interstitial lung inflammation and fibrosis. They can be further subcategorized as chronic fibrosing interstitial pneumonias (idiopathic pulmonary fibrosis [IPF] and idiopathic nonspecific interstitial pneumonia [NSIP]), acute and subacute interstitial pneumonias (cryptogenic organizing pneumonia and acute interstitial pneumonia [AIP]), smoking-related interstitial pneumonias (respiratory–bronchiolitis–interstitial lung disease (ILD) and desquamative interstitial pneumonia [DIP]), and rare interstitial pneumonias (lymphoid interstitial pneumonia and pleuroparenchymal fibroelastosis [PPFE]) [1].

Usual Interstitial Pneumonia and Idiopathic Pulmonary Fibrosis

IPF is the most common IIP and is the most common type of pulmonary fibrosis. It is characterized by usual interstitial pneumonia (UIP) pattern on imaging and/or histology. Histopathologic findings of UIP are characterized by spatial and temporal heterogeneity of fibrosis, and predilection for the periphery of the lobule and subpleural regions. It is important to note that while all cases of IPF are UIP and most cases of UIP are IPF, a small subset of UIP have known causes, including connective tissue disorders, chronic hypersensitivity pneumonitis (HP), and drug or occupational exposures. The diagnosis of IPF requires the absence of alternative etiology for ILD and the presence of UIP pattern on either HRCT or histopathology [2].

IPF typically affects older patients with approximately 80% of those affected 65 years or older and is more common in men (approximately 1.5:1 ratio). It is also more commonly seen in smokers [3]. The symptoms of IPF are nonspecific and may include progressive shortness of breath, nonproductive cough, and weight loss. The disease is typically progressive with increasing severity and extent of fibrosis and worsening of symptoms. Some patients, however, may have extended periods of stability and acute episodes of exacerbation or acceleration, typically secondary to acute processes such as infections or pulmonary edema.

On CXR, IPF, and UIP typically present as reduced lung volumes and symmetric, basilar-predominant reticular opacities (Fig. 18.1). In the early stages, a fine reticular pattern may be seen in the posterior costophrenic angles on the lateral radiograph. In advanced cases, bronchiectasis and honeycombing may be discernible on CXR. A normal CXR does not exclude UIP, and UIP findings are better characterized by HRCT.

Computed tomography (CT) plays an essential role in the evaluation of suspected IPF. A UIP pattern on CT is highly correlated with a UIP pattern on pathology and is diagnostic of IPF once other causes of ILD have been excluded, supplanting the need for lung biopsy [2]. Recently, updated guidelines propose the use of four CT patterns when considering an IPF diagnosis: typical UIP, probable UIP, indeterminate for UIP, and most consistent with a non-IPF diagnosis (Table 18.2) [2,4].

"Typical UIP" pattern on CT is characterized by varying degrees of basal- and peripheral-predominant reticular pattern often accompanied by traction bronchiectasis and bronchiolectasis and associated with subpleural honeycombing and the absence of atypical features (Fig. 18.1). If these criteria are met except for the presence of honeycombing, the pattern is considered that of "probable UIP." *Honeycombing is the most specific CT finding of*

TABLE 18.1 Common Descriptive Terminologies in the HRCT Evaluation of Diffuse Lung Diseases

Terminology	Description	Examples of Pathologies
Nodule Distribution		
Perilymphatic	Distribution along the lymphatics, which are located along the peribronchovascular, interlobular, and subpleural interstitium (including along fissures)	Sarcoidosis, lymphangitic carcinomatosis, berylliosis
Centrilobular	Occur in the center of the secondary pulmonary lobule	RB, HP, pulmonary hemorrhage
Tree-in-bud	Subset of centrilobular nodules that are branching	Infection (bacterial, mycobacterial, viral, fungal), aspiration
Random	Can involve all areas of the lung	Metastasis, infection (including miliary spread)
Lung Attenuation		
Consolidation	Increased parenchymal attenuation obscuring vessels and airway walls; may have air-bronchograms	Acute: Infections, aspiration, severe pulmonary edema/ hemorrhage Chronic: malignancy (adenocarcinoma, lymphoma), OP
Ground-glass opacity	Hazy increased parenchyma attenuation with preservation of vascular and airway margins	Acute: Atypical infections, pulmonary edema/ hemorrhage Chronic: NSIP, RB, DIP, HP
Mosaic attenuation	Combination of areas of decreased and increased attenuation, typically from either small airway's disease (air trapping) or small vessel disease (decreased perfusion)	Airways: HP, asthma, obliterative bronchiolitis Vascular: CTEPH, vasculitis
Others		
Honeycombing	Clustered or stacked small cystic airspaces with thickened walls; manifestation of advanced fibrosis	UIP, DIP, chronic HP
Bronchiectasis	Irreversible bronchial dilation; bronchial lumen greater than the adjacent vessel	Chronic infections, UIP, NSIP, HP, sarcoid
Bronchiolectasis	Irreversible bronchiolar dilation	
Traction bronchiectasis and bronchiolectasis	bronchial and bronchiolar dilation resulting from retraction by adjacent parenchymal fibrosis	

CTEPH, chronic thromboembolic pulmonary hypertension; *DIP*, desquamative interstitial pneumonia; *HP*, hypersensitivity pneumonitis; *NSIP*, nonspecific interstitial pneumonitis; *OP*, organizing pneumonia; *RB*, respiratory bronchiolitis; *UIP*, usual interstitial pneumonia.

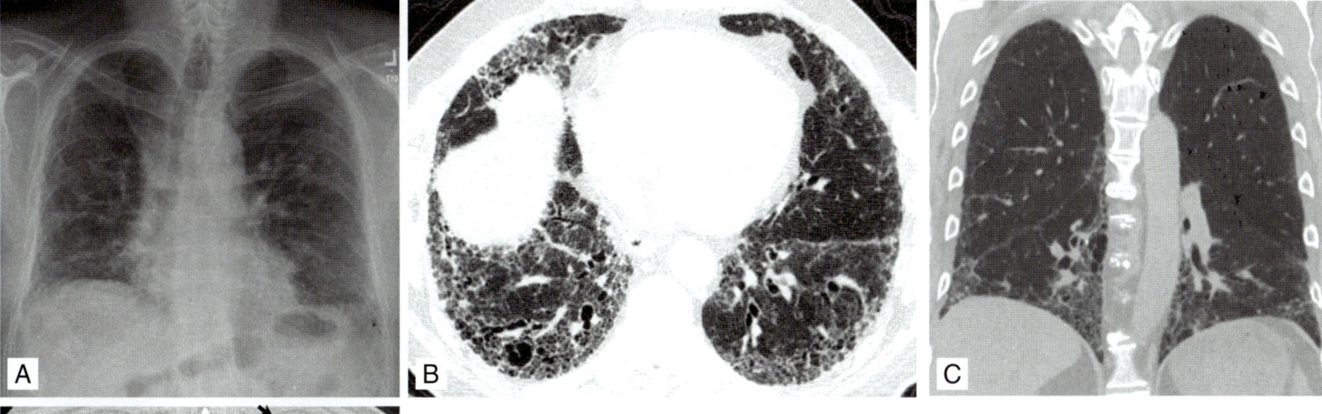

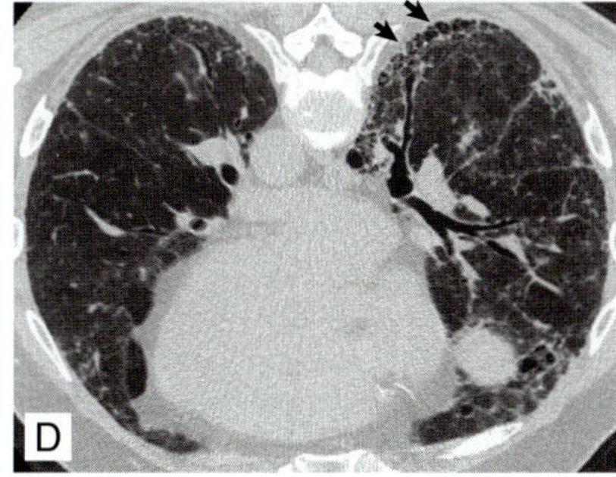

Figure 18.1 Usual interstitial pneumonia in a patient with idiopathic pulmonary fibrosis. (A) Frontal chest radiograph demonstrates decreased lung volumes with basal-predominant reticular opacities. (B) Axial CT image demonstrates extensive subpleural reticulation and interstitial thickening with traction bronchiectasis and bronchiolectasis and architectural distortion. (C) Coronal CT image confirms basal predominance of the findings. (D) Prone CT image demonstrates stacked, clustered subpleural cysts in the posterior basal right lower lobe (*arrows*) consistent with honeycombing.

TABLE 18.2 **HRCT Diagnostics Criteria for Usual Interstitial Pneumonia***

Typical UIP CT Pattern	Probably UIP CT Pattern	CT Pattern Indeterminate for UI	CT Features Most Consistent With Non-IPF Diagnosis
Basal predominant	Basal predominant	Variable or diffuse	Upper or mid-lung predominance
Subpleural predominant	Subpleural predominant		Peribronchovascular predominance; subpleural sparing
Subpleural reticulation with peripheral traction bronchiectasis and bronchiolectasis	Subpleural reticulation with peripheral traction bronchiectasis and bronchiolectasis	Fibrosis with inconspicuous features suggestive of a non-UIP pattern	Predominance of consolidations or ground-glass opacities Extensive mosaic attenuation Multiple nodules or cysts
Honeycombing present	Absent honeycombing		
Absence of features suggesting an alternative diagnosis	Absence of features suggesting an alternative diagnosis		

*Adapted from Fleischner Society Guidelines [4].

UIP and is characterized by subpleural cystic airspaces with discrete, thickened walls that are stacked or lined up in a row (Fig. 18.1). It is a finding of end-stage fibrosis and is associated with worse outcomes. When IPF is suspected and the CT pattern is determined to be either typical UIP or probable UIP, histologic sampling is generally not required.

If the pattern, however, is determined to be "indeterminate for UIP" or "most consistent with an alternative diagnosis," histologic sampling may be performed if a definitive diagnosis is necessary to direct treatment. The pattern is considered "indeterminate for UIP" if features do not meet the criteria for either typical or probable UIP patterns, but findings that suggest an alternative diagnosis are not present.

Findings that suggest an alternative diagnosis include [4]:

1. Upper or mid lung predominance;
2. Peribronchovascular or perilymphatic distribution;
3. Marked mosaic attenuation;
4. Preponderance of ground-glass opacification or consolidation;
5. Presence of profuse micronodules, centrilobular nodules, or cysts; and
6. Pleural effusion, pleural thickening, or pleural plaques.

These alternative diagnoses are discussed in the remainder of the chapter.

Nonspecific Interstitial Pneumonia

NSIP is the second most common chronic interstitial pneumonia. Unlike UIP, the interstitial abnormalities of NSIP are typically uniform and homogeneous on histology, which may be predominantly inflammatory (i.e., cellular type NSIP) or fibrotic (i.e., fibrotic NSIP).

NSIP can be idiopathic but is more commonly seen with connective tissue disorders, HP, and drug-induced pneumonitis [3,5–7]. The symptoms of NSIP are similar to those of UIP, but unlike UIP, NSIP has a much better prognosis and typically responds well to steroid therapy.

On CXR, NSIP can present as either patchy or confluent hazy (ground-glass) opacities predominantly involving the mid and lower lungs. Typical HRCT findings of NSIP include symmetric bilateral, basilar-predominant ground-glass opacities with reticulation, and traction bronchiectasis, which may be exuberant and disproportionate to the degree of parenchymal disease, particularly in fibrotic-type NSIP (Fig. 18.2). While the abnormalities in NSIP are also typically peripheral, up to half of those affected have relative sparing of the subpleural spaces, which essentially excludes UIP (Fig. 18.2) [3]. Honeycombing can be seen with NSIP but is much less common (up to 30%) and is much less extensive (typically affecting less than 5% of the lungs) compared to UIP.

Organizing Pneumonia

Cryptogenic organizing pneumonia is the idiopathic form of organizing pneumonia (OP) and was previously known as bronchiolitis obliterans with organizing pneumonia, a term that has largely fallen out of favor. Slightly more than half of OP is idiopathic, while the remainder are secondary to a variety of pathologies and exposures such as connective tissue disorders, radiation therapy, medications, and infections [8]. Common presenting symptoms of OP include shortness of breath and cough and can be associated with fever, chills, and weight loss. OP responds well to steroid therapy but can recur.

The imaging findings of OP are heterogeneous on both CXR and HRCT. Findings may be symmetric or asymmetric, may be unilateral or bilateral, may be consolidative or ground-glass, and may be nodular or mass-like (Fig. 18.3). Distribution is typically subpleural or peribronchovascular. A perilobular pattern, which appears as linear or band-like opacities in an arcade-like or polygonal morphology, is a typical appearance (Fig. 18.3). Another typical finding in OP is the "atoll" or "reversed halo sign," which is characterized by central ground-glass with surrounding consolidative edge (Fig. 18.3). This finding, however, can also be seen in other pathologies such as pulmonary infarctions, infections, and vasculitis [9].

Acute Interstitial Pneumonia

AIP is characterized by diffuse alveolar damage (DAD) on histology and is indistinguishable from ARDS. In essence, AIP is ARDS without known etiology and is a diagnosis of exclusion.

The imaging features of AIP parallel those of ARDS and occur in a stagewise progression with an exudative, an organizing, and a fibrotic phase [10]. In the exudative phase, typical findings are diffuse or dependent consolidations and ground-glass opacities (Fig. 18.4), which may improve during the organizing phase. In those who develop fibrosis, the antidependent regions of the lungs are typically more severely affected.

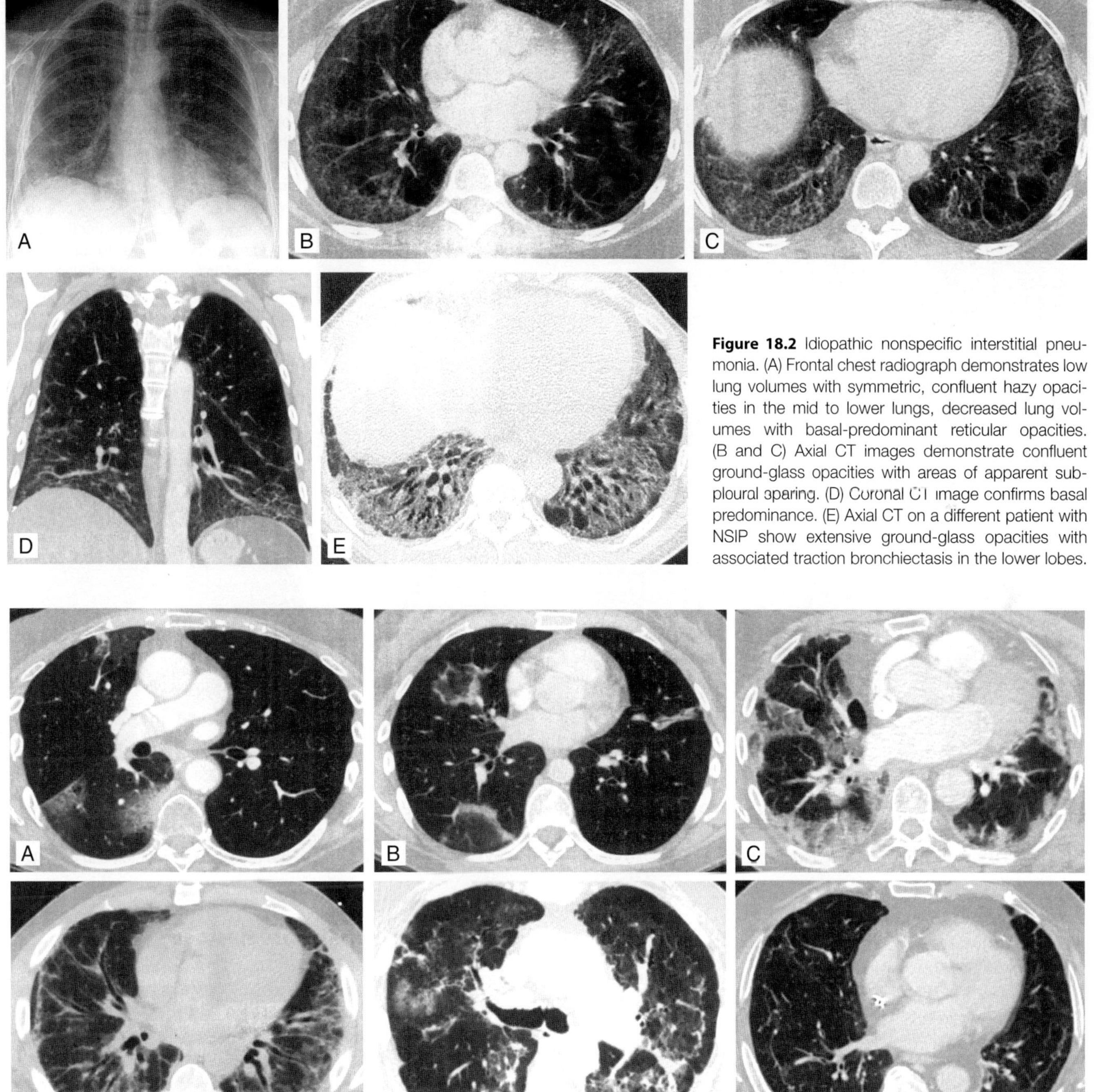

Figure 18.2 Idiopathic nonspecific interstitial pneumonia. (A) Frontal chest radiograph demonstrates low lung volumes with symmetric, confluent hazy opacities in the mid to lower lungs, decreased lung volumes with basal-predominant reticular opacities. (B and C) Axial CT images demonstrate confluent ground-glass opacities with areas of apparent subpleural sparing. (D) Coronal CT image confirms basal predominance. (E) Axial CT on a different patient with NSIP show extensive ground-glass opacities with associated traction bronchiectasis in the lower lobes.

Figure 18.3 Various imaging presentation of organizing pneumonia. Axial CT images in different patients demonstrate (A) Multifocal, subpleural mixed ground-glass, and consolidative opacities in the right lung. (B) Rounded opacities with peripheral consolidation and central ground-glass consistent with "reversed halo" sign (also known as "atoll" sign). (C) Peripheral and peribronchovascular consolidations and ground-glass opacities. (D) Peripheral and peribronchovascular consolidations and ground-glass opacities with associated traction bronchiectasis. (E) Patchy central, peribronchovascular ground-glass opacities with perilobular areas of consolidation peripherally. (F) Arcade-like perilobular thickening.

Smoking-Related Interstitial Pneumonias

Smoking-related interstitial pneumonias are a spectrum of pathologies of increasing severity, which include respiratory bronchiolitis (RB), RB-ILD, and DIP [11,12].

RB is a common finding both on imaging and pathology in individuals with significant smoking history. RB and RB-ILD are essentially identical on both imaging and histology and are only differentiated by the presence of symptoms in those with RB-ILD. Typical CT findings are upper lobe predominant or diffuse centrilobular ground-glass nodules (Fig. 18.5).

DIP is much less common than RB and RB-ILD. It is highly associated with smoking, but up to 40% of those with DIP have no significant smoking history. On CT, DIP appears as basal and

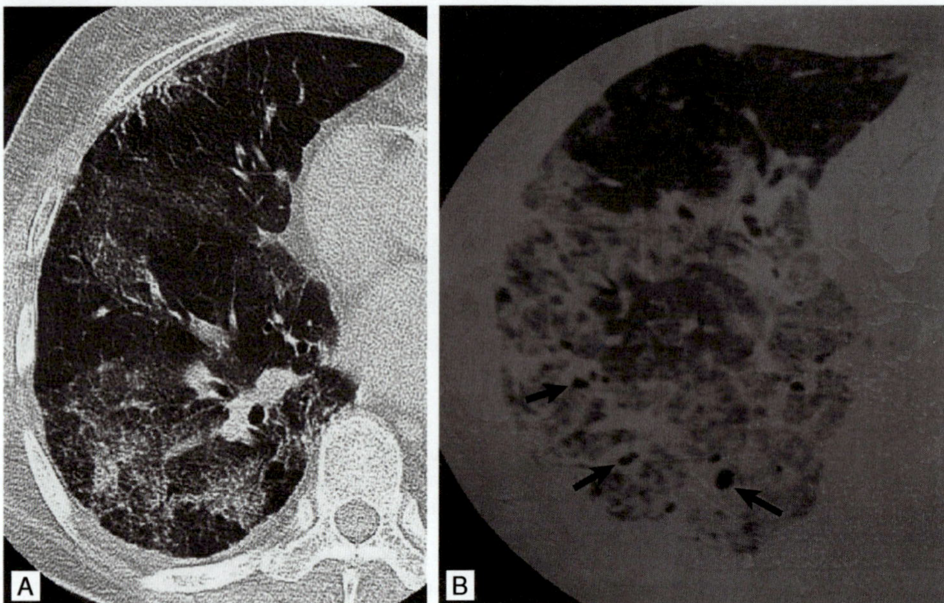

Figure 18.4 High-resolution CT findings of acute interstitial pneumonia. (A) HRCT scan at the level of right lower lobe shows multilobular ground-glass attenuation without traction bronchiectasis. The patient was a 64-year-old woman with AIP. (B) HRCT scan at the level of right lower lobe shows extensive inhomogeneous attenuation with traction bronchiectasis (*arrows*) and nondependent area of sparing. Note that inhomogeneous area with traction bronchiectasis corresponds to proliferative phase of diffuse alveolar damage, and nondependent area of sparing corresponds to exudative phase of diffuse alveolar damage. Regional differences of pathologic phase of diffuse alveolar damage are seen. The patient was a 68-year-old man with AIP. (Source: K Ichikado, Seminars in ultrasound, CT and MRI, Hematobil Imaging 35 (1) (2014) 39–46.)

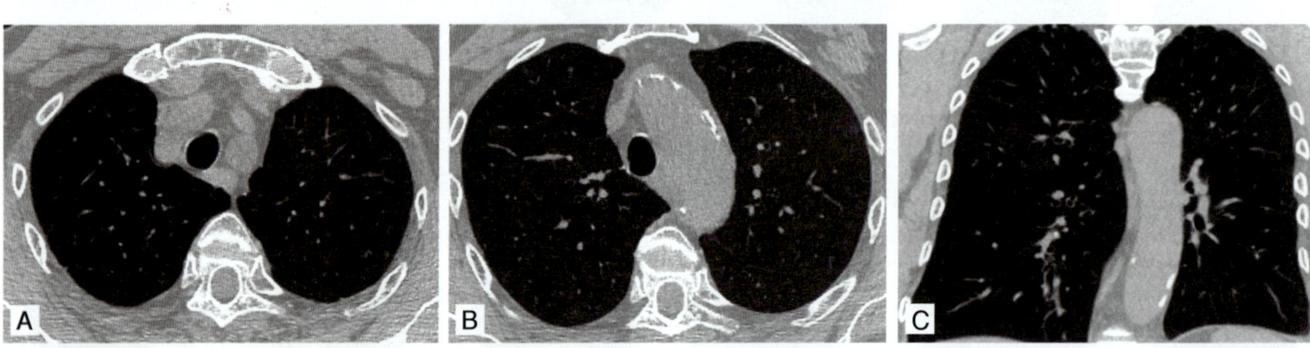

Figure 18.5 Respiratory bronchiolitis and respiratory bronchiolitis-interstitial lung disease. (A and B) Axial CT images demonstrate diffuse ill-defined centrilobular ground-glass nodules bilaterally. (C) Coronal CT image demonstrates upper lobe predominance of the findings. There is also evidence of paraseptal emphysema concordant with smoking history. RB and RB-ILD are identical on imaging and differentiated only by the presence of symptoms in RB-ILD.

peripheral confluent ground-glass opacities with superimposed clustered cystic lesions (Fig. 18.6). A subset of DIP may progress and result in fibrosis. Smoking cessation may result in clinical and radiographic improvement in some patients with smoking-related interstitial pneumonias [12].

Lymphocytic Interstitial Pneumonia

Lymphocytic interstitial pneumonia (LIP) is a rare benign lymphoproliferative disorder characterized by dense lymphoid infiltration of the alveolar septa. It is rarely idiopathic and is often associated with an underlying collagen vascular disorder (particularly Sjögren's syndrome, rheumatoid arthritis [RA], and systemic lupus erythematosus [SLE]), autoimmune disorders, infections and immunodeficiency (particularly HIV/AIDS in children), and drug toxicity [13].

HRCT findings reflect lymphoid infiltration and include patchy or confluent ground-glass opacities or consolidation, ill-defined centrilobular nodules, septal thickening with small perilymphatic nodules, and perivascular cystic airspaces, particularly in the setting of Sjögren's syndrome (Fig. 18.7) [14]. These cystic airspaces are thought to reflect follicular bronchiolitis resulting in airway obstruction. Up to a third of cases can progress to pulmonary fibrosis [15].

Pleuroparenchymal Fibroelastosis

Pleuroparenchymal fibroelastosis (PPFE) is another rare interstitial pneumonia that results in exuberant bilateral apical pleural and subpleural lung fibrosis. Approximately half of the cases of PPFE are idiopathic, and the rest have associated conditions such as lung transplantation, hematopoietic stem cell transplantation, and chemotherapy [16]. Typical HRCT findings include dense, progressive biapical pleural, and lung parenchymal thickening (Fig. 18.8). Pneumothoraces and bronchopleural fistulas have been reported as possible complications. Progressive cases may require lung transplantation.

Connective Tissue Diseases

Lung involvement is common in connective tissue disease (CTD) and may manifest as a chronic interstitial pneumonia (CTD-related ILD) that may be indistinguishable from the IIP patterns described. As CTD is more common in women, the concomitant interstitial pneumonias are also more commonly seen in women [7]. The lung abnormality can be the initial manifestation of CTD and depends on the underlying CTD.

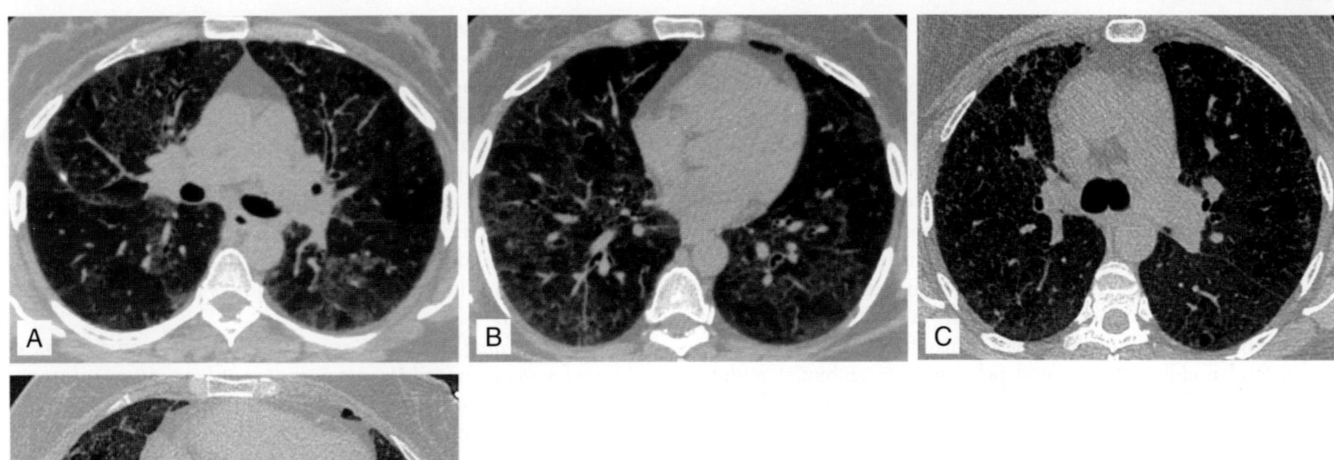

Figure 18.6 Desquamative interstitial pneumonia. (A and B) Axial CT images demonstrate patchy, multifocal ground-glass opacities with tiny clustered cysts within the areas of ground-glass. (C and D) Axial CT images on a different patient demonstrate faint diffuse ground-glass with scattered and clustered cysts bilaterally. Background of emphysema and diffuse bronchial wall thickening is also present.

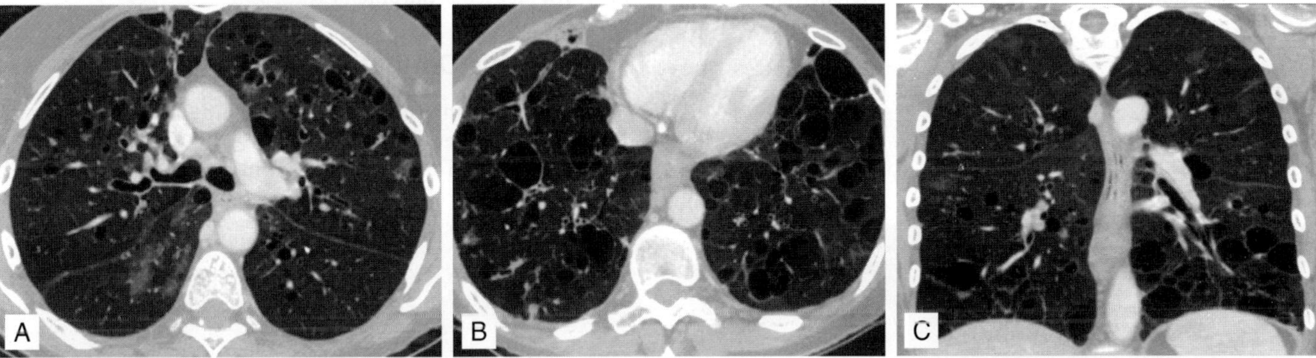

Figure 18.7 Lymphocytic interstitial pneumonia in a patient with Sjögren's syndrome. (A and B) Axial CT images demonstrate multiple peribronchovascular thin-walled cysts with scattered small solid and ground-glass nodules bilaterally. There are also geographic areas of interstitial septal thickening. (C) Coronal CT image demonstrates basal predominance of the cysts with additional patchy ground-glass opacities bilaterally.

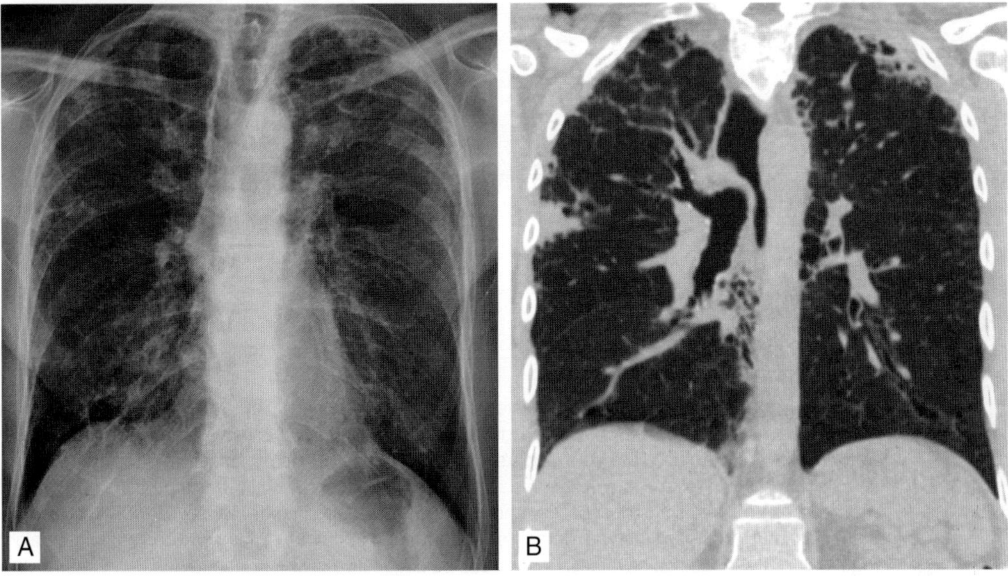

Figure 18.8 Pleuroparenchymal fibroelastosis (PPFE). (A) Frontal chest radiograph demonstrates biapical pleural-parenchymal thickening and upper lobe predominant reticular opacities. (B) Coronal CT image demonstrates biapical pleural and subpleural parenchymal thickening and upper lobe predominant fibrotic changes consistent with PPFE.

Rheumatoid Arthritis

The most common pattern of ILD to affect patients with RA is UIP, which may be indistinguishable from IPF. Certain CT findings have been reported to help distinguish UIP related to RA and other CTD from IPF such as significant anterior upper lobe fibrosis, "exuberant honeycombing," and the so-called "straight edge sign" wherein the fibrosis is isolated in the lung bases with an abrupt transition between fibrotic and relatively normal lung parenchyma (Fig. 18.9) [17].

Other pulmonary manifestations in RA include NSIP, OP, bronchiectasis, obliterative bronchiolitis resulting in significant air trapping, and rarely follicular bronchitis, which manifests as centrilobular of tree-in-bud nodules. Rheumatoid pulmonary (necrobiotic) nodules are also a rare manifestation. They are typically peripheral, may be large (up to 7 cm), may cavitate, and may regress spontaneously. Pleural involvement manifests as pleural effusions or pleural thickening [18].

Progressive Systemic Sclerosis (Scleroderma)

A majority of patients with scleroderma (up to 80%) eventually develop ILD. The most commonly seen pattern is NSIP, followed by UIP [19]. Esophageal dysmotility is commonly seen with scleroderma and can manifest as a patulous (dilated), fluid-filled esophagus (Fig. 18.10). Reflux and aspiration may exacerbate the underlying ILD. Pulmonary hypertension, either as a primary vasculopathy, or secondary to underlying pulmonary disease or cardiac dysfunction, is also commonly seen (~40%) with scleroderma and can manifest as pulmonary arterial dilation [20].

Systemic Lupus Erythematosus

SLE is a multisystem autoimmune disorder. Common presenting symptoms are arthritis, malar rash, photosensitivity, and neuropsychiatric symptoms such as seizures, psychosis, and delirium. Pneumonia is the most common form of lung involvement. Other forms of lung involvement include pulmonary hemorrhage and a variety of ILD (including OP, NSIP, UIP, and LIP), which may progress to pulmonary fibrosis [21].

Lupus pneumonitis can occur in up to 5% of patients with SLE and presents with fever, dyspnea, and cough. Imaging features are nonspecific and are typically a combination of ground-glass and consolidative opacities, which can be unilateral or bilateral and multifocal. Diagnosis requires exclusion of underlying infection.

"Shrinking lung" syndrome is another common manifestation of SLE and is characterized by progressive loss of lung volumes, particularly in the lower lobes, without apparent parenchymal abnormalities. It is thought to be due to chronic diaphragmatic dysfunction or pleuritis restricting full lung expansion. Serositis in the form of pleuritis and pericarditis are also common.

Sjögren's Syndrome

Sjögren's syndrome is a rare disease characterized by corneal and conjunctival dryness (keratoconjunctivitis sicca), mouth dryness (xerostomia), and recurrent parotitis. Most patients have a coexisting connective tissue disorder, most commonly RA. LIP is the most common ILD associated with Sjögren syndrome (Fig. 18.7). Follicular bronchitis, NSIP, UIP, and OP have also been associated with Sjögren syndrome [14].

Polymyositis/Dermatomyositis

Polymyositis/dermatomyositis are a group of connective tissue disorders characterized by proximal limb weakness. ILD is seen in more than half of the cases in the form of NSIP and/

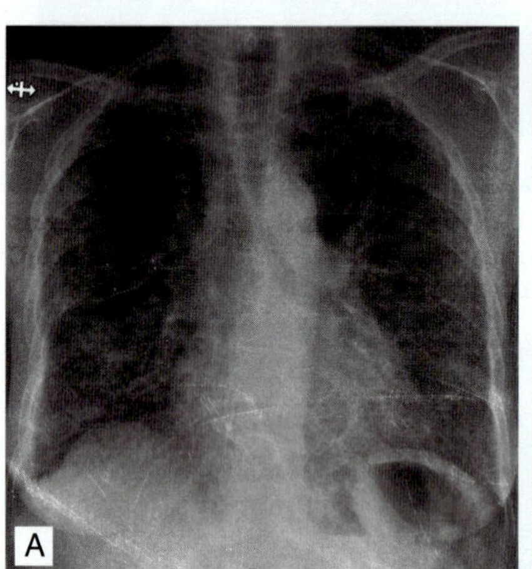

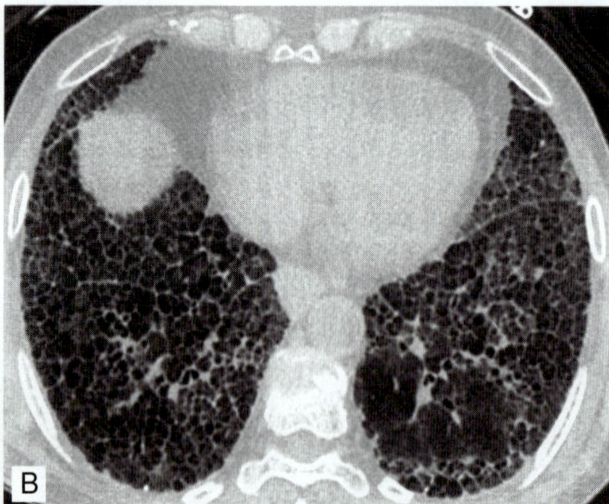

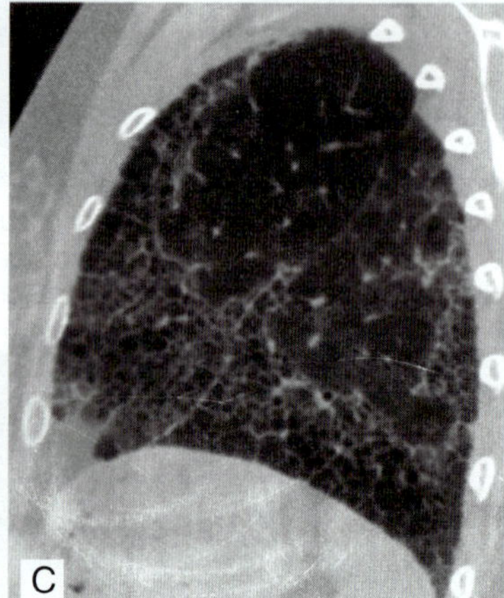

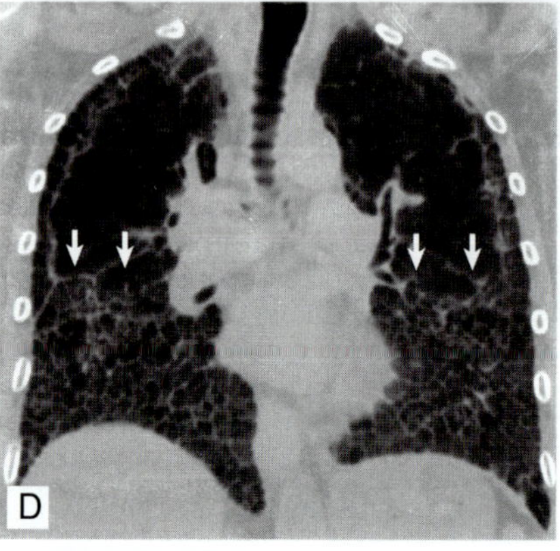

Figure 18.9 Rheumatoid arthritis-related interstitial lung disease (ILD) with usual interstitial pneumonia (UIP) pattern. (A) Frontal chest radiograph demonstrates low lung volumes with peripheral and basal-predominant reticular opacities and apparent small cystic lucencies suggestive of honeycombing. (B) Axial CT image demonstrates extensive, "exuberant" honeycombing in the lung bases. (C) Sagittal CT image demonstrates significant involvement of the anterior upper lobe. (D) Coronal CT image demonstrates abrupt transition between areas of fibrosis and normal lung parenchyma (*arrows*, "straight edge" sign). These findings have been reported to be suggestive of UIP related to underlying connective tissue disorder rather than idiopathic pulmonary fibrosis.

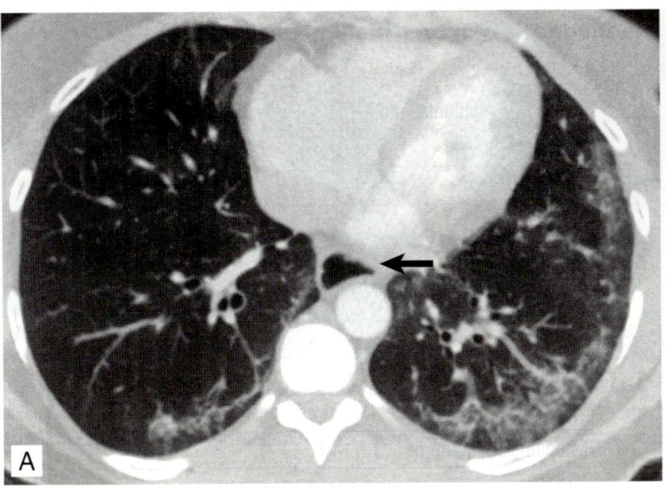

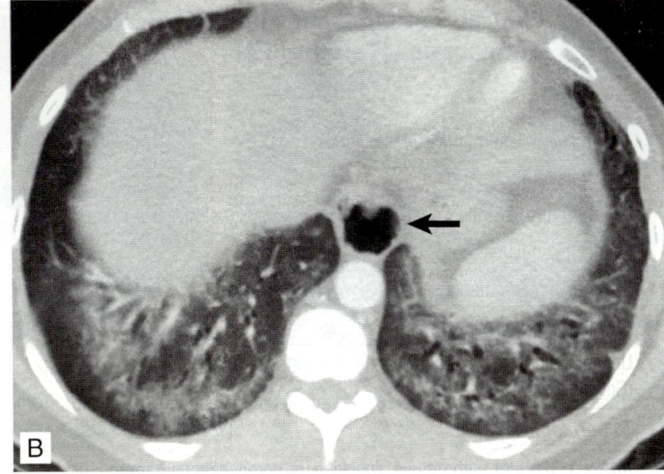

Figure 18.10 Systemic sclerosis (scleroderma) with associated nonspecific interstitial pneumonia (NSIP). (A and B) Axial CT images demonstrate confluent basal-predominant ground-glass opacities with subpleural sparing and associated traction bronchiectasis. Note the patulous esophagus (*arrows*) suggestive of esophageal dysmotility, a common finding in systemic sclerosis.

or OP. In patients with polymyositis/dermatomyositis, the presence of Jo-1 antibody is predictive of the eventual development of ILD, which is typically responsive to corticosteroid therapy.

Ankylosing Spondylitis

Upper lobe predominant fibrosis can be seen in less than 1% of patients with ankylosing spondylitis, typically presenting more than 10 years following the onset of disease. Imaging reflects apical fibrosis, typically with associated bronchiectasis, paraseptal emphysema, and pleural thickening. Cysts may also be present.

Interstitial Pneumonia With Autoimmune Features

Interstitial pneumonia with autoimmune features refer to the presence of an ILD with associated autoimmunity and clinical features suggestive of, but not diagnostic for, a connective tissue disorder. It is considered to be an intermediary within the spectrum with idiopathic ILD on one end and CTD-ILD on the other. Diagnosis is based on meeting the following criteria [22]:

1. The presence of ILD identified either on CT or lung biopsy
2. Exclusion of other causes of ILD
3. Failure to meet criteria for a classical CTD
4. The presence of at least one feature from at least two of the three domains—clinical, serologic, and morphologic (Table 18.3).

The CT patterns identified in interstitial pneumonia with autoimmune features are most commonly UIP, NSIP, HP, and OP. When a UIP pattern is present, three features have been reported to be associated with a higher likelihood of an underlying CTD [17]:

1. Significant anterior upper lobe fibrosis
2. Exuberant honeycombing
3. "Straight edge" sign

Hypersensitivity Pneumonitis

Hypersensitivity Pneumonitis (HP), also referred to as extrinsic allergic alveolitis, is an immune-mediated lung disease resulting from intense and often prolonged exposure to a variety of antigens from inhaled organic dusts. Classical HP syndromes include *farmer's lung* resulting from exposure to thermophilic actinomycetes, *bird fancier's lung* from avian proteins, and *hot tub lung* from mycobacterium avium complex, among others. Up to 40% of cases, however, do not have an identifiable exposure despite careful assessment [23].

HP most commonly affects middle-aged adults and may be more commonly seen in nonsmokers than smokers. This is thought to be due to the immunosuppressive effects of tobacco smoking. Regardless of the type of allergen exposure, the clinical, pathologic, and radiologic manifestations of HP are similar and can be classified into acute, subacute, and chronic, all of which can occur concurrently.

Acute Hypersensitivity Pneumonitis

Acute HP occurs following exposure to large amounts of antigen in susceptible individuals. It is characterized by alveolar infiltration with neutrophilic exudate with severe cases resulting in DAD with pulmonary edema or hemorrhage. Depending on the severity, imaging may be normal or may demonstrate as diffuse ground-glass opacities, multifocal ill-defined consolidations, and centrilobular nodules.

Subacute Hypersensitivity Pneumonitis

Continued exposure to offending agents can result in progressive symptoms over several weeks to months. Histologically, subacute HP is characterized by alveolitis, small, ill-defined granulomas, and cellular bronchiolitis. These findings are reflected on CT as patchy ground-glass opacity and small ill-defined centrilobular nodules, and focal areas of mosaic attenuation and air-trapping as confirmed on expiratory phase imaging (Fig. 18.11). The combination of focal areas of increased attenuation (ground-glass), decreased attenuation (mosaic attenuation), and normal lung parenchyma results in the "headcheese" sign, which is nearly pathognomonic of HP (Fig. 18.11). These findings may be reversible with treatment and removal of the offending agent.

Chronic Hypersensitivity Pneumonitis

Long-standing exposure to the antigen can result in progression of symptoms and ultimately result in pulmonary fibrosis, which can develop over months and years. Imaging findings include reticulation, architectural distortion, volume loss, traction bronchiectasis and bronchiolectasis, and honeycombing with areas of air trapping (Fig. 18.12) [24]. The distribution of the fibrotic

Other manifestations include pulmonary masses and/or nodules, pulmonary edema, and pulmonary hemorrhage. Unlike granulomatosis with polyangiitis, the masses and nodules seen in eGPA do not typically cavitate [27].

Drug-Related Lung Diseases

Certain drugs have been associated with lung toxicity, which can manifest in a variety of ways depending on the agent (Table 18.4). Common lung manifestations related to drugs include pulmonary edema, DAD, pulmonary hemorrhage, OP, hypersensitivity reactions, and chronic interstitial pneumonitis with fibrosis [28].

Amiodarone

Amiodarone is an iodinated drug used in the treatment of refractory ventricular arrhythmias. It can accumulate in the liver and the lungs, with pulmonary toxicity seen in up to 5% of patients. Lung involvement may occur in the form of DAD, OP, or chronic interstitial pneumonitis resulting in fibrosis.

Classical CT findings include consolidations, which are hyperattenuating due to the accumulation of iodine (Fig. 18.14). Hyperattenuating liver is often seen in the setting of amiodarone lung toxicity.

Bleomycin

Bleomycin is a cytotoxic drug used in the treatment of lymphoma and certain carcinomas, particularly testicular, ovarian, and cervical cancers. Pulmonary toxicity can be seen in less than 5% of patients. A wide variety of lung manifestations have been reported with bleomycin toxicity including pulmonary edema, DAD, OP, hypersensitivity reactions, and chronic pneumonitis with fibrosis.

Chronic pneumonitis with fibrosis typically presents with progressive shortness of breath and cough 1–2 months following initiation of bleomycin therapy. Imaging shows lower lobe predominant reticulations and ground-glass opacities, with or without consolidations. Bleomycin can also characteristically result in development of pulmonary nodules representing foci of OP, which can mimic metastases.

Cyclophosphamide

Cyclophosphamide is an alkylating, immunosuppressive chemotherapeutic agent used in the treatment of a wide variety of malignancies and autoimmune disorders. Lung toxicity occurs in less than 1% of patients and can manifest as chronic pneumonitis with fibrosis, OP, DAD, and pulmonary edema.

TABLE 18.4 Patterns of Lung Injury Related to Drugs

Amiodarone
Chronic interstitial pneumonitis and fibrosis
Peripheral (high-attenuation) consolidations and/or nodules
Diffuse alveolar damage (ARDS)
Bleomycin
Pulmonary fibrosis (resembling UIP)
Checkpoint Inhibitors (Immunotherapy)
NSIP
OP
Diffuse alveolar damage (ARDS)
Sarcoid-like reaction
Cyclosporin
Lung masses/nodules (with or without lymphadenopathy)
Interferon
Sarcoid-like reaction
Nitrofurantoin
Pulmonary eosinophilia
Organizing pneumonia
Pulmonary fibrosis
Crack Cocaine
Diffuse alveolar damage (ARDS)
Diffuse alveolar hemorrhage
Heroin
Noncardiogenic pulmonary edema
Intravenous Crushed Pills
Excipient lung disease
Vaping
Organizing pneumonia
Diffuse alveolar damage (ARDS)
Acute eosinophilic pneumonia
Diffuse alveolar hemorrhage

ARDS, acute respiratory distress syndrome; *UIP*, usual interstitial pneumonia.

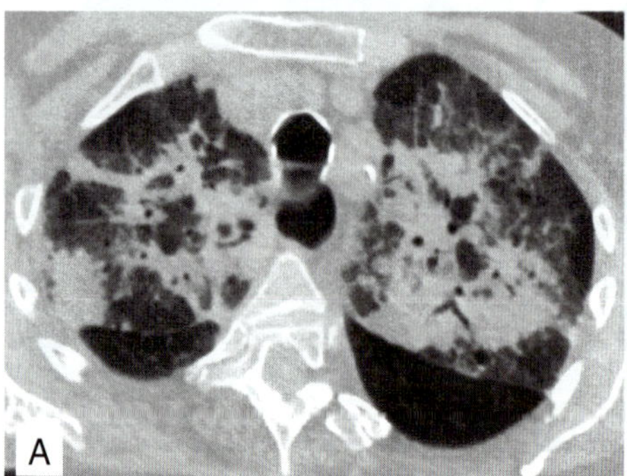

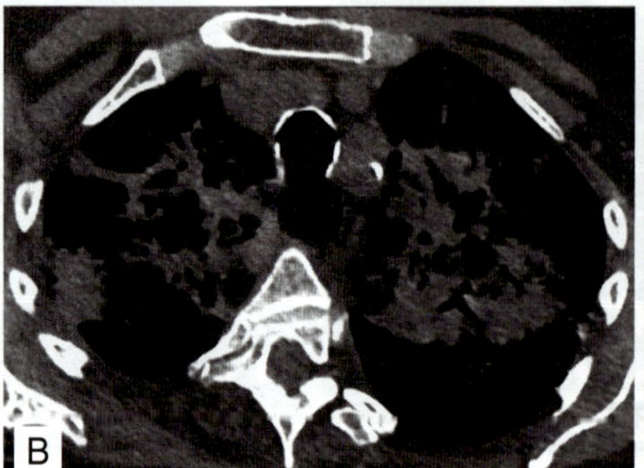

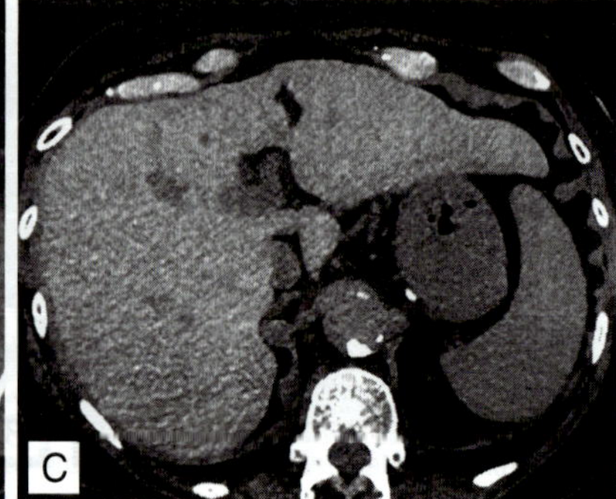

Figure 18.14 Amiodarone toxicity. (A) Axial CT image on lung window demonstrates patchy mixed consolidative and ground-glass opacities bilaterally. (B) Corresponding axial CT image on soft tissue window demonstrates relative hyperattenuation of the consolidations. (C) Axial CT images through the upper abdomen demonstrate hyperattenuation of the liver.

TABLE 18.5 Common Terminology Criteria for Adverse Events (CTACE) in the Setting of Immune Checkpoint Inhibitor-Related Pneumonitis

Grade	Definition
Grade 1	Radiographically apparent but without symptoms
Grade 2	Mild to moderate symptoms limiting instrumental ADL and requiring treatment
Grade 3	Severe symptoms limiting self-care ADL, typically requiring oxygen supplementation
Grade 4	Life-threatening respiratory compromise requiring urgent intervention
Grade 5	Respiratory failure and death

ADL, activities of daily living.

Methotrexate

Methotrexate is a commonly used antifolate agent for the treatment of a variety of malignancies and inflammatory disorders. It can cause lung toxicity in as much as 10% of patients receiving treatment, typically as a hypersensitivity reaction. Eosinophilia can be seen in up to half of patients with lung toxicity. Common imaging features include basal-predominant consolidations and ground-glass opacities, which typically resolve following cessation of treatment. Pulmonary fibrosis can occur but is rare.

Nitrofurantoin

Nitrofurantoin is an antibiotic most commonly used in the treatment of urinary tract infections. Nitrofurantoin-related lung toxicity can be acute or chronic. Acute toxicity can present as eosinophilic lung disease similar to idiopathic simple or acute eosinophilic pneumonia, which resolves following discontinuation of the medication. Long-standing nitrofurantoin use can result in chronic toxicity in the form of basal-predominant fibrosis.

Immune Checkpoint Inhibitors

Immune checkpoint inhibitors (ICIs) are a type of immunotherapy used in the treatment of a variety of cancers, including melanoma, lung cancer, urothelial cancers, head and neck cancers, and lymphoma. Commonly used ICIs include atezolizumab, durvalumab, ipilimumab, nivolumab, and pembrolizumab. They work by preventing the deactivation of T cells, allowing them to attack and kill cancer cells. This T cell activation, however, may also result in multisystemic adverse reactions.

ICI-related pneumonitis is estimated to affect 3–6% of patients under therapy with increased frequency in patients with lung cancer and those receiving combination ICI therapy. Most patients present with dyspnea and cough, with some patients presenting with chest pain and fever. Grading of the severity of ICI-related pneumonitis is largely based on symptoms (Table 18.5), ranging from Grade I, which is only clinically or radiographically observed but without symptoms to life-threatening respiratory failure (Grade IV) and death (Grade V) [29].

The imaging patterns of ICI-related pneumonitis are variable. Findings on radiographs are nonspecific and may have unilateral or bilateral hazy opacities and consolidations. On CT, several typical patterns have been observed, including OP pattern, NSIP pattern, HP pattern, AIP/ARDS pattern, and sarcoid-like reaction (Fig. 18.15). "Radiation recall" can also occur wherein lung abnormalities are limited to previously irradiated sites [30].

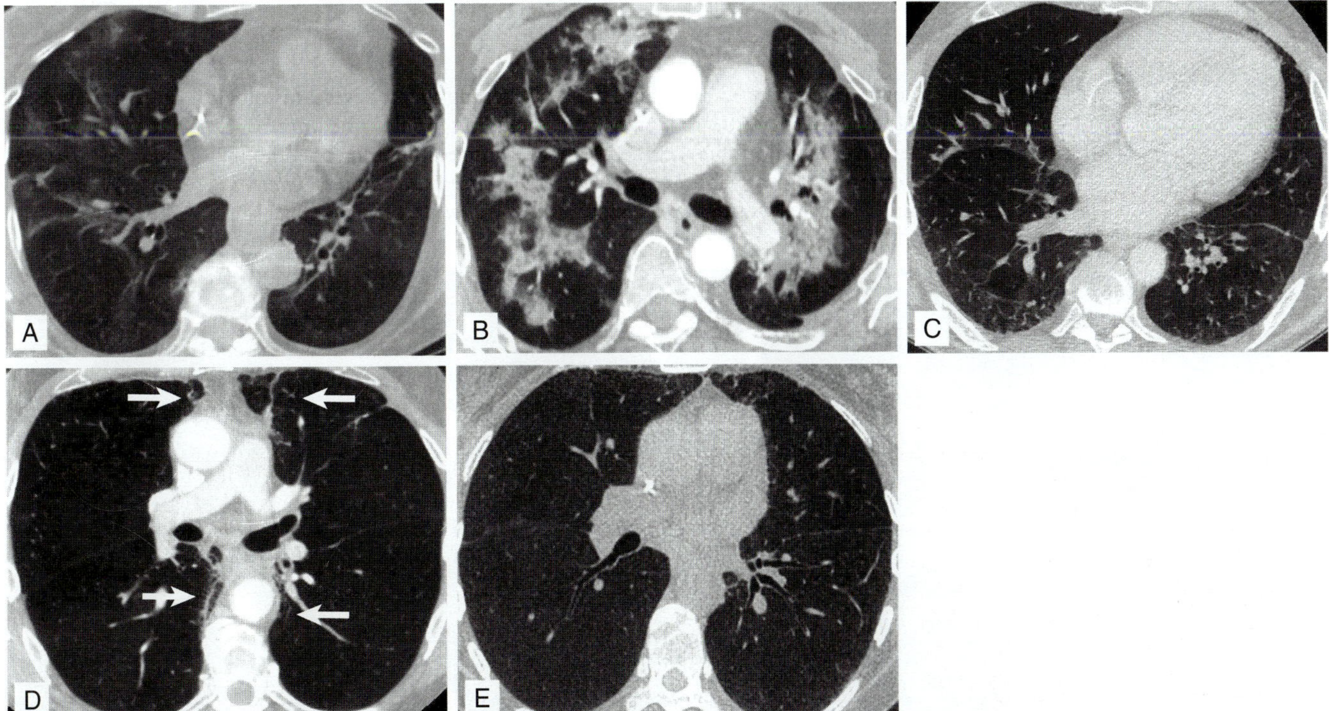

Figure 18.15 Various patterns of pneumonitis related to immune checkpoint inhibitors. Axial CT images of different patients on a variety of immune checkpoint inhibitors for the treatment of malignancy demonstrate (A) Multifocal peribronchovascular ground-glass opacities consistent with organizing pneumonia pattern. (B) Dense, confluent peribronchovascular consolidations are also consistent with organizing pneumonia pattern. (C) Basal-predominant subpleural ground-glass opacities are consistent with NSIP pattern. (D) Bilateral geographic reticular and ground-glass opacities in the paramediastinal lungs (*arrows*) in a patient with a remote history of mediastinal radiation are consistent with "radiation recall" pattern of pneumonitis. (E) Diffuse tiny 1- to 2-mm nodules with a perilymphatic distribution are consistent with a sarcoid-like reaction.

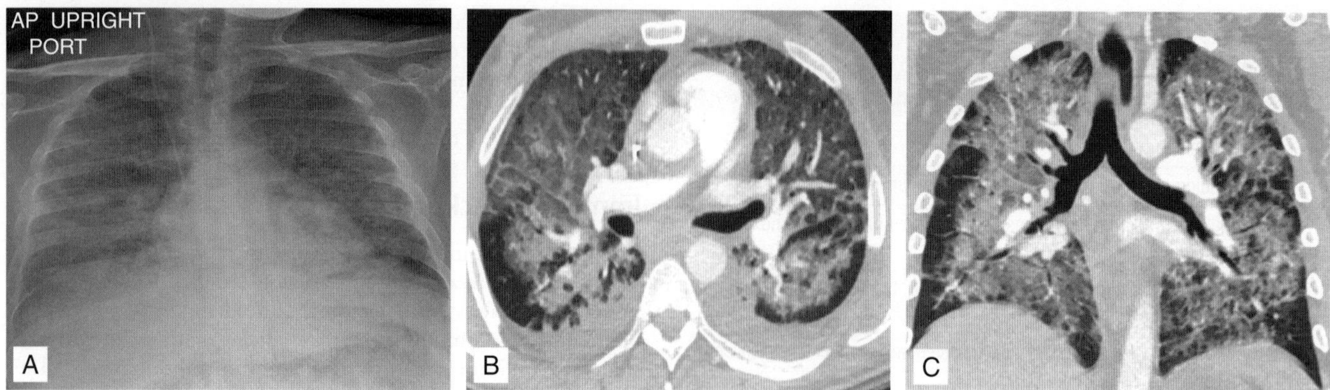

Figure 18.16 Diffuse alveolar damage related to crack cocaine use. (A) Frontal chest radiograph demonstrates diffuse, confluent hazy opacities bilaterally. (B) Axial and (C) Coronal CT images demonstrate dense ground-glass opacities with interlobular septal thickening with consolidations in the dependent lower lobes. Layering pleural effusions are also present.

Recreational Drugs

Cocaine and its derivative crack are sympathomimetic agents that can cause pulmonary edema by inducing cardiac dysfunction from ischemia or arrhythmia or cause acute lung injury with resultant noncardiogenic (high-permeability) pulmonary edema, pulmonary hemorrhage, or a combination thereof. CT commonly shows diffuse or multifocal ground-glass opacities with interlobular septal thickening or dense consolidations (Fig. 18.16).

Excipient lung disease, sometimes referred to as pulmonary talc granulomatosis, results from intravenous injection of inert fillers contained in crushed oral tablets (e.g., methadone) or other particulate matter in illicit street drugs. This results in an angiocentric granulomatous response that typically presents as centrilobular or tree-in-bud nodules on CT (Fig. 18.17). Acute pulmonary hypertension with right heart strain presenting as pulmonary arterial and right ventricular dilation may be present [31].

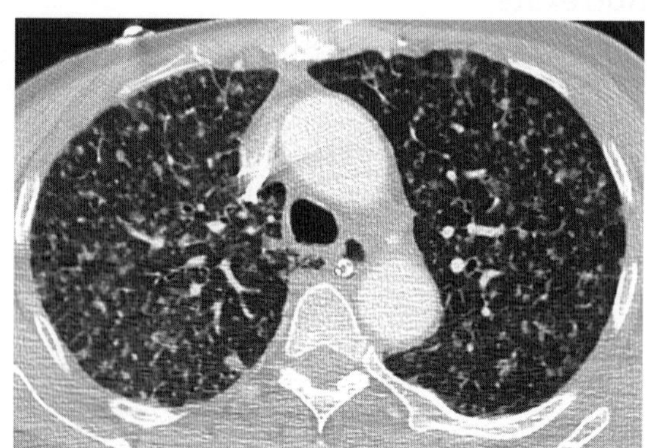

Figure 18.17 Excipient lung disease in a patient with history of intravenous injection of crushed prescription drugs. Axial CT image demonstrates diffuse centrilobular and tree-in-bud nodules bilaterally.

Vaping-associated lung disease (also known as E-cigarette or vaping-associated lung injury) is a pattern of lung injury resulting from use of electronic cigarettes and vape pens. A majority of these cases have been connected to the use of tetrahydrocannabinol-containing products containing vitamin E acetate, which is used as a thickening agent. Several histological patterns have been reported including lipoid pneumonia, DAD, diffuse alveolar hemorrhage, acute eosinophilic pneumonia, OP, and HP. *The most common CT findings are diffuse, bilateral ground-glass opacities, sometimes with subpleural sparing* (Fig. 18.18) [32].

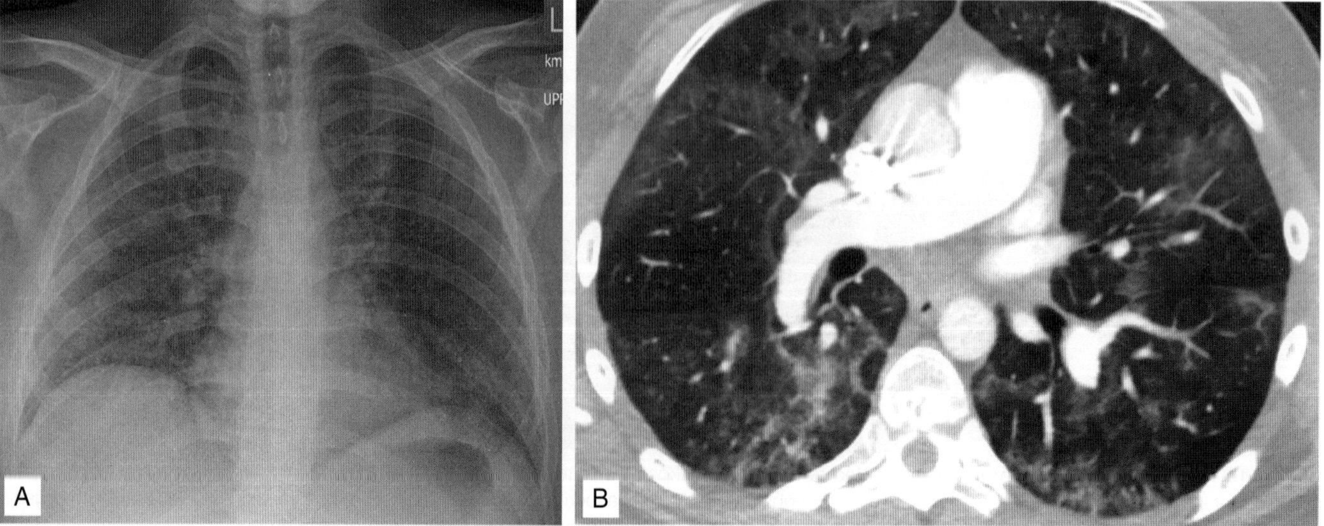

Figure 18.18 Vaping-associated lung injury. (A) Frontal chest radiograph demonstrates low lung volumes with diffuse hazy opacities bilaterally. (B) Axial CT image demonstrates diffuse ground-glass opacities with septal thickening and superimposed consolidation in the right lower lobe. Note the areas of subpleural sparing, frequently reported with vaping-associated lung injury.

Pneumoconioses

Pneumoconioses are a group of lung diseases related to inhalation of dust particles (Table 18.6) [33]. These particles may be fibrogenic and result in eventual pulmonary fibrosis and respiratory dysfunction or may be nonfibrogenic (inert) and cause minimal or no dysfunction.

Asbestos-Related Diseases and Asbestosis

Asbestos refers to a group of naturally occurring fibrous silicate minerals, which was widely used as a building material due to its great durability, tensile strength, and heat resistance. It is now a known hazardous material, prompting restrictions in its mainstream use. Intense or prolonged asbestos exposure can result in pleural and lung parenchymal diseases and is a risk factor for malignancy, which typically present decades following exposure.

TABLE 18.6 Causative Agents and Related Exposures in Pneumoconiosis

Agent	Disease	Exposure
Fibrogenic		
Aluminum	Aluminosis	Explosives manufacturing
Asbestos	Asbestosis	Construction, mining, shipbuilding, textile
Beryllium	Berylliosis	Aerospace, ceramic manufacturing
Coal	Coal-worker's pneumoconiosis	Coal mining
Silica	Silicosis	Ceramic, drilling, glass manufacturing, mining, sandblasting
Talc	Talcosis	Ceramic/paint/paper manufacturing, cosmetics
Nonfibrogenic		
Barium	Baritosis	Glass and paper manufacturing
Iron	Siderosis	Foundry work, mining, welding
Tin	Stannosis	Mining, welding

Common pleural manifestations of asbestos exposure include pleural effusions, pleural thickening, and calcified and noncalcified pleural plaques [34]. The plaques are characteristically distributed in the lower thorax and the diaphragmatic surfaces. CXR can detect most pleural effusions and pleural plaques when calcified or extensive (Fig. 18.19). Viewed en face, the pleural plaques typically have irregular, uneven borders resembling a holly leaf ("holly leaf sign"). When nodular these plaques may be mistaken for lung nodules. CT is much sensitive and can better characterize these pleural findings.

Rounded atelectasis frequently occurs with asbestos-related pleural disease and is known as Blesovsky disease. Rounded atelectasis results in characteristic imaging features on CT and presents as a rounded subpleural opacity with associated volume loss and tethering of the adjacent bronchovascular bundles resulting in the characteristic "comet tail sign." There is typically associated pleural abnormality in the form of an effusion or thickening (Fig. 18.20). Asbestos-related pleural diseases and rounded atelectasis are typically asymptomatic and are commonly found incidentally.

Asbestosis is another parenchymal manifestation of asbestos exposure resulting in a diffuse, chronic fibrosing ILD, which develops as much as 20–30 years after exposure but may be accelerated in cases of intense exposure. On CXR, findings include lower lobe predominant reticular opacities with volume loss and honeycombing in advanced cases. On CT (Fig. 18.21), asbestosis presents as subpleural, lower lobe predominant fibrosis with reticulation, subpleural curvilinear opacities often paralleling the chest wall, 2- to 5-cm parenchymal bands extending to the pleural surface, traction bronchiectasis, and honeycombing in advanced stages. It may resemble and be indistinguishable from UIP. Findings of pleural disease, which is seen in up to 80% of patients with asbestosis and a history of prior asbestos exposure, are clues to asbestosis as the underlying cause for pulmonary fibrosis.

Asbestosis is typically symptomatic with patients commonly presenting with progressive shortness of breath. While most patients have stable disease for years, some progress into end-stage pulmonary fibrosis, with eventual respiratory failure and death when left untreated. Asbestos exposure is also a known risk factor for the development of lung cancer and malignant mesothelioma. These are discussed separately.

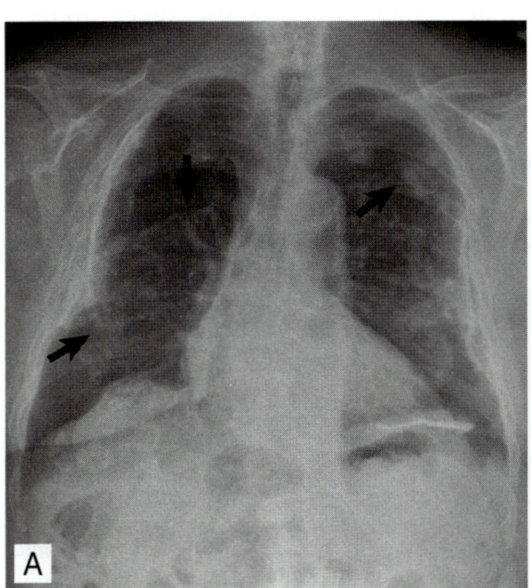

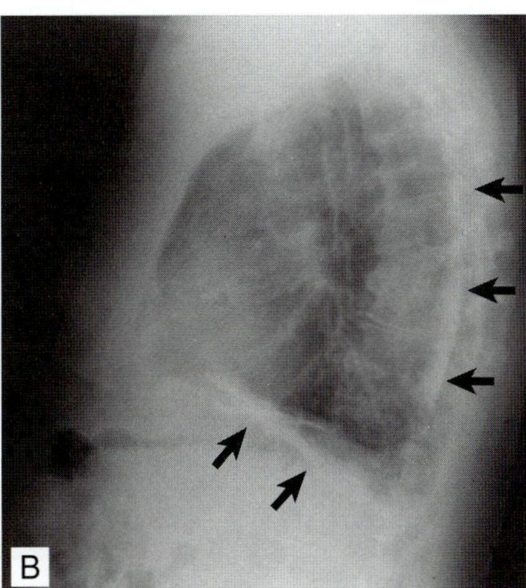

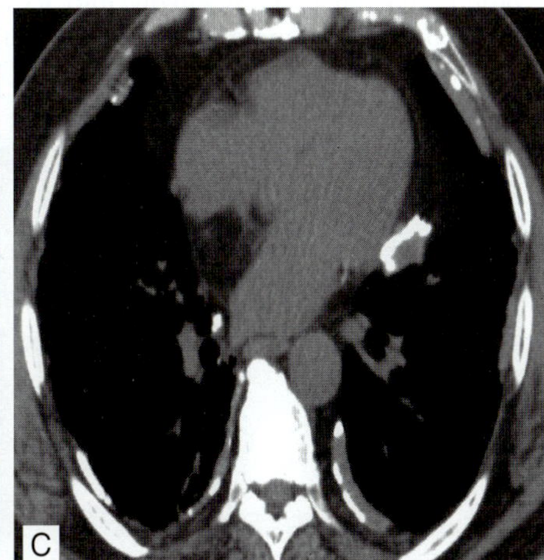

Figure 18.19 Asbestos-related pleural disease. (A) Frontal chest radiograph demonstrates bilateral pleural calcifications. Calcified plaques seen en face have irregular, uneven borders resulting in a "holly leaf" appearance (*arrows*). (B) Lateral chest radiograph shows preponderance of calcifications along the basal and posterior pleural surfaces (*arrows*). (C) Axial CT image demonstrates extensive calcified pleural plaques bilaterally.

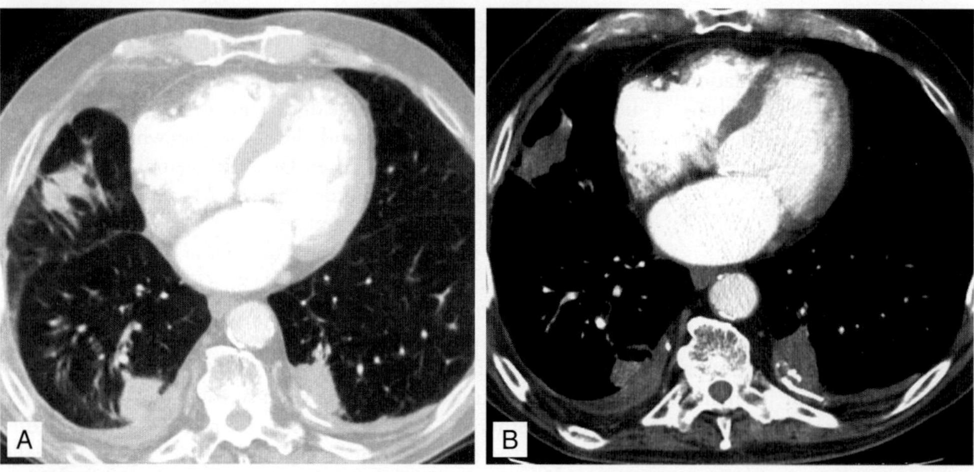

Figure 18.20 Rounded atelectasis resulting from prior asbestos exposure. (A) Axial, lung window CT image demonstrates rounded and wedge-shaped subpleural opacities in the right middle and bilateral lower lobes. Note tethering and swirling of the adjacent bronchovascular bundles resulting in a "comet-tail" appearance. (B) Axial, soft tissue window CT image demonstrates homogenous enhancement of the opacities. Note the adjacent pleural thickening, effusion, and calcification.

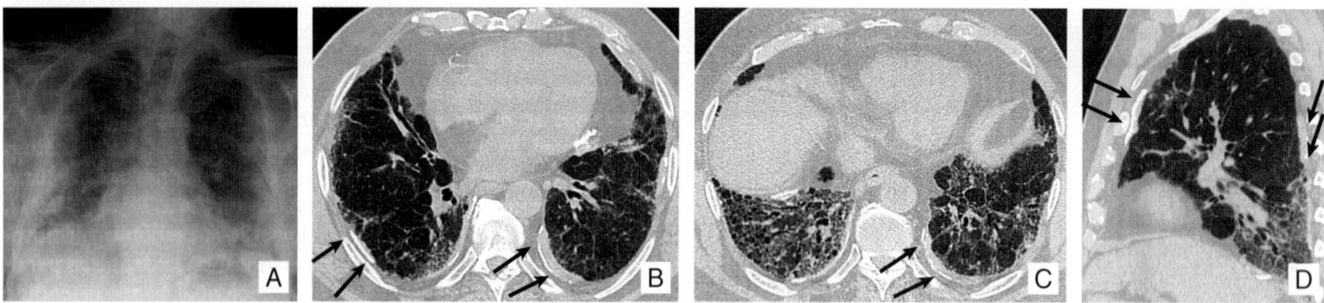

Figure 18.21 Asbestosis. (A) Frontal chest radiograph demonstrates low lung volumes with basal and peripheral-predominant reticular opacities. (B) Axial CT image demonstrates subpleural reticulation with architectural distortion with scattered parenchymal bands. (C) Axial CT image at the lung bases demonstrates extensive traction bronchiectasis and bronchiolectasis and apparent areas of honeycombing. (D) Sagittal CT image demonstrates the basal predominance of the abnormalities. Calcified pleural plaques consistent with prior asbestos exposure are also present (*arrows*).

Silicosis

Silicosis is the most common occupational lung disease and is caused by inhalation of dust containing silica. Exposure to silica is common in mining and quarrying, construction, sandblasting, and glass manufacturing. Silicosis can present as acute, classic, or accelerated.

Acute silicosis (also known as silicoproteinosis) is primarily seen in sandblasters and results from exposure to large amounts of silica over a relatively short time period. It presents shortly after exposure and can progress rapidly into respiratory failure. CT features include ground-glass opacities with septal thickening ("crazy paving" pattern), central or diffuse consolidations, and diffuse centrilobular nodules.

Classic (or chronic) silicosis usually presents 10–20 years following long-standing exposure to levels of silica. Simple, uncomplicated cases are typically asymptomatic and characterized on imaging as multiple small pulmonary nodules, which may calcify. Lymphadenopathy, which may have eggshell classifications is common (Fig. 18.22) and may precede parenchymal findings.

Classic silicosis can be complicated and may result in progressive massive fibrosis (Fig. 18.23) wherein the small nodules coalesce into larger opacities, eventually resulting in upper lobe

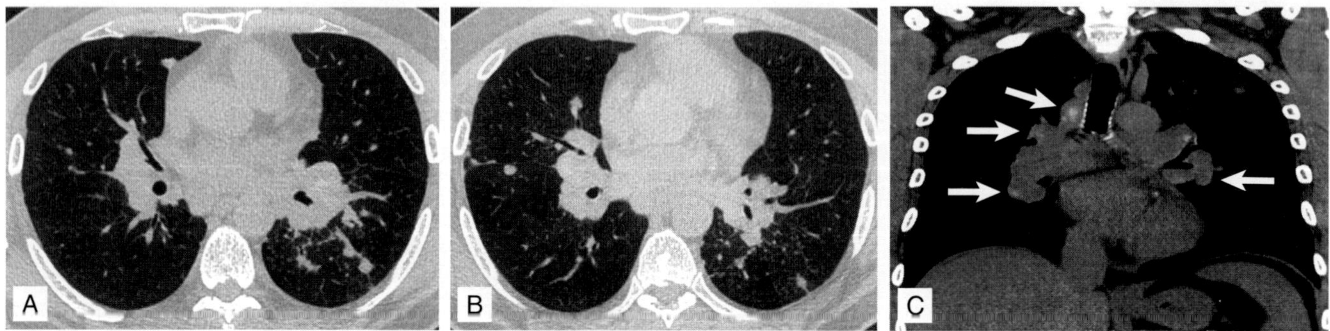

Figure 18.22 Simple, uncomplicated silicosis in a patient who previously worked as a sandblaster. (A and B) Axial CT images demonstrate multiple clustered small pulmonary nodules predominantly with a peribronchovascular distribution. (C) Coronal CT image high attenuation lymph nodes (C, *arrows*) suggestive of developing calcifications.

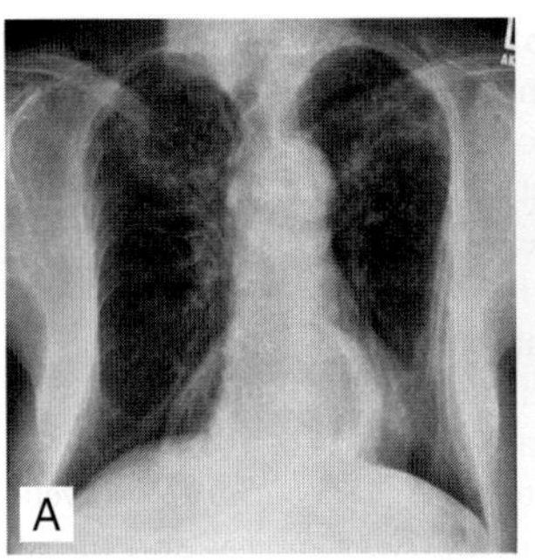

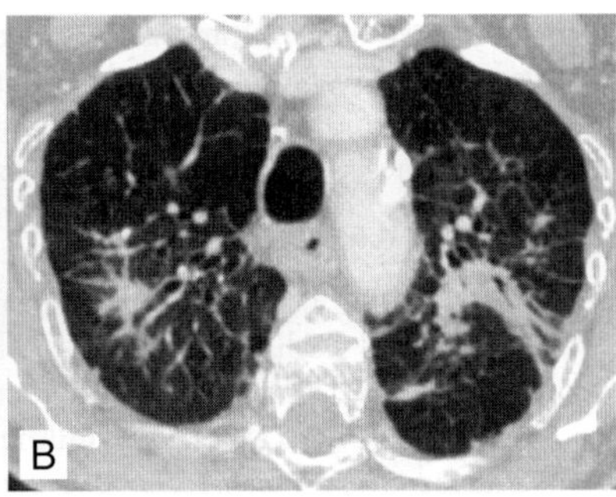

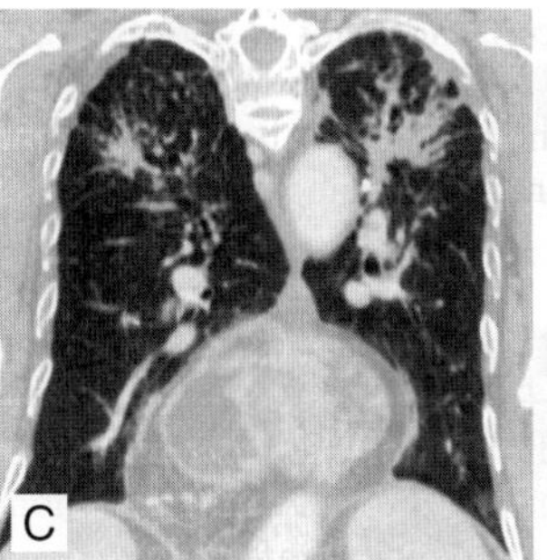

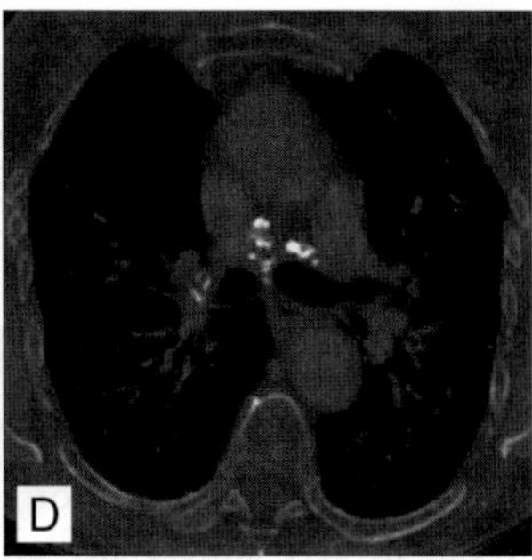

Figure 18.23 Progressive massive fibrosis due to silicosis in a former foundry worker. (A) Frontal chest radiograph demonstrates confluent opacities in the upper lobes with associated superior retraction of the bilateral hila. An incidental hiatus hernia is also seen as a retrocardiac opacity with air–fluid level. (B) Axial and (C) Coronal CT images demonstrate confluent areas of fibrosis in the upper lobes with resultant mass-like opacities. Note the associated volume loss and adjacent architectural distortion and traction bronchiectasis.

predominant fibrosis, with volume loss and architectural distortion. Larger masses may have central necrosis and cavitation. Complicated silicosis can result in significant respiratory dysfunction and failure in some patients. Accelerated silicosis has similar imaging findings as classic silicosis but presents and progresses more rapidly, usually in 4–8 years.

Coal-Workers Pneumoconiosis

Coal-workers pneumoconiosis (CWP) results from inhalation of coal dust. The clinical presentation and imaging findings of CWP overlap considerably with and may be indistinguishable from those of silicosis and can only be differentiated by exposure history.

Caplan syndrome (also known as rheumatoid pneumoconiosis) is the co-occurrence of RA and a pneumoconiosis, more commonly CWP but also with silicosis. On imaging, it is characterized by superimposition of larger necrobiotic (rheumatoid) nodules on the smaller nodules seen with the pneumoconiosis (Fig. 18.24).

Talcosis

Lung disease related to talc may result from either inhalation of dust particles or intravenous injection of crushed oral drugs. Commercially available talc is usually contaminated with other minerals, such as asbestos or silica, and may resemble asbestosis or silicosis, respectively. Findings are typically less severe compared to the other pneumoconioses.

Injection of crushed oral medications can result in talc granulomatosis, a type of excipient lung disease as discussed earlier.

Berylliosis

Beryllium exposure has historically been seen in fluorescent lamp workers but is now more commonly seen in those working in aeronautic, computer, and electronics manufacturing.

Acute, high-dose exposure can result in chemical pneumonitis that presents as pulmonary edema. Chronic berylliosis from longstanding exposures results in a multisystemic granulomatous disease with imaging features indistinguishable from those of sarcoid, including mediastinal and hilar lymphadenopathy, small perilymphatic nodules, and upper lobe predominant confluent opacities and fibrosis in advanced cases.

Nonfibrogenic Pneumoconioses

Siderosis results from dust containing iron, often associated with welding. Inhaled iron particles may accumulate and result in

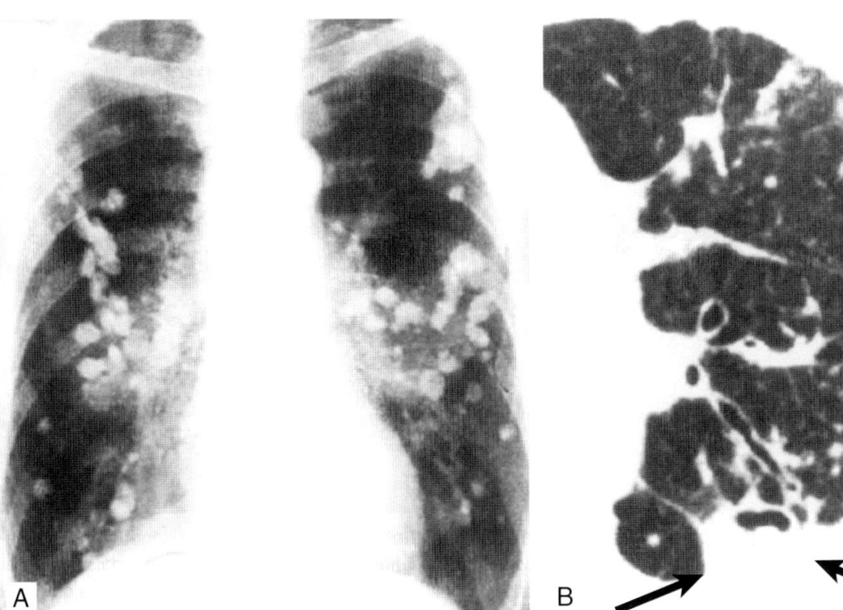

Figure 18.24 Caplan syndrome. (A) Frontal chest radiograph demonstrates multiple rounded opacities are present (some partly calcified). (B) Axial CT image shows a left lower lobe cavitary mass corresponding to a necrobiotic (rheumatoid) nodule (*arrows*) superimposed on multiple additional smaller nodules corresponding to underlying pneumoconiosis.

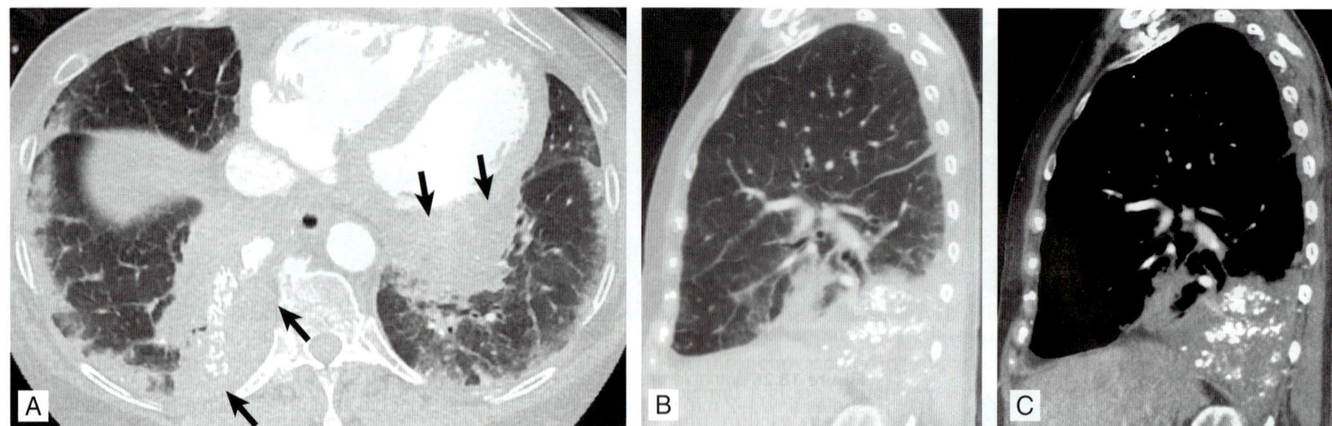

Figure 18.28 Diffuse pulmonary amyloidosis. (A) Axial CT image demonstrates subpleural consolidations predominantly in the lower lobes with larger mass-like consolidations in the right paravertebral and left paramediastinal lower lobes (A, *arrows*). There are associated diffuse ground-glass opacities with interlobular septal thickening. (B) Sagittal CT image through the right lung demonstrates extensive septal thickening and ground-glass opacities with a large consolidative opacity in the posterior basal right lower lobe. (C) Corresponding sagittal CT image in soft-tissue window shows dense calcifications within the consolidation.

sclerosis complex (TSC). Patients typically present with progressive shortness of breath or may present acutely with a pneumothorax or a chylous pleural effusion.

On radiographs, the thin-walled cysts may appear as diffuse linear opacities. CT shows multiple, uniformly distributed, thin-walled spherical cysts (Fig. 18.29) [40]. *The intervening lung parenchyma is typically normal.* In the setting of TSC, multiple nodules representing multifocal micronodular pneumocyte hyperplasia may be present. Myocardial fatty foci may also be seen in TSC. Fatty renal lesions representing renal angiomyolipoma can be seen in both sporadic LAM and TSC-LAM.

Pulmonary Langerhans Cell Histiocytosis

Langerhans cell histiocytosis (LCH) refers to a group of diseases of unclear etiology, characterized by accumulation of Langerhans cells in one or more organ systems. Lung involvement is seen in up to 40% of patients. Most cases of pulmonary LCH typically affect young or middle-aged adults, with an overwhelming proportion (90%) having a history of smoking [41].

The findings of pulmonary LCH evolve over time. In the early stages, pulmonary LCH is characterized by peribronchiolar granulomas consisting predominantly of Langerhans cells and eosinophils. These granulomas are later replaced by fibrosis and cysts, which may coalesce. Pathologic findings are reflected on imaging, with a preponderance of nodules in early stages that later turn into cysts. The cysts may coalesce giving them a "bizarre" appearance (Fig. 18.30). About a third of cases regress spontaneously, a third remain stable, and the remainder progress into diffuse cystic destruction, which can lead to respiratory failure and death in some cases.

Other Cystic Lung Diseases

Birt–Hogg–Dube syndrome is an autosomal dominant disorder classically presenting with the triad of fibrofolliculomas, trichiodiscomas, and skin tags. Other associations are renal tumors (including renal cell carcinoma and oncocytomas) and diffuse cystic lung disease. The cysts in Birt–Hogg–Dube syndrome can be round, oval, or lentiform and may septated. They are also typically subpleural and paramediastinal in distribution (Fig. 18.31).

Light chain deposition disorder is a multisystem process associated with plasma cell dyscrasias such as multiple myeloma and Waldenström macroglobulinemia. Renal involvement is almost always present and involvement of the heart and liver is also common. Lung manifestations are uncommon and usually asymptomatic. When present, it is characterized by variable-sized nodules and basal-predominant cysts. Amyloid may have similar findings of cysts and nodules and is discussed separately earlier in the chapter.

Tracheobronchial papillomatosis results from human papillomavirus infection and is characterized by the formation of

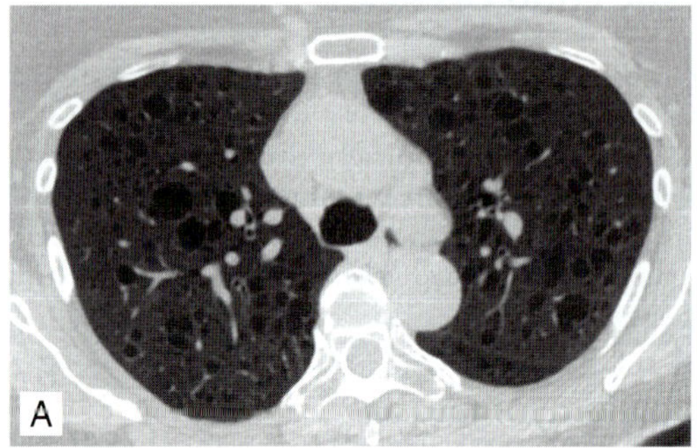

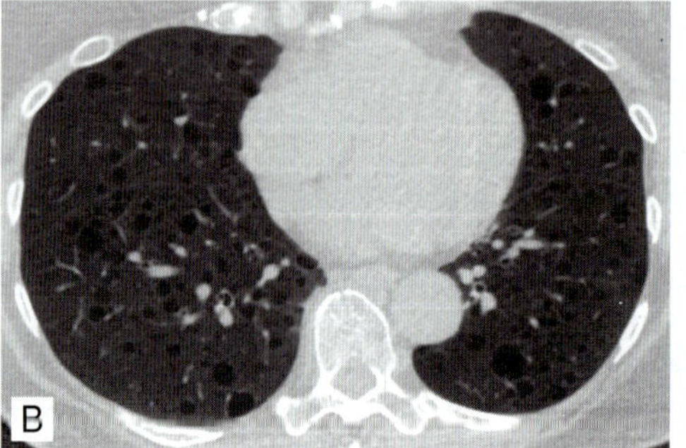

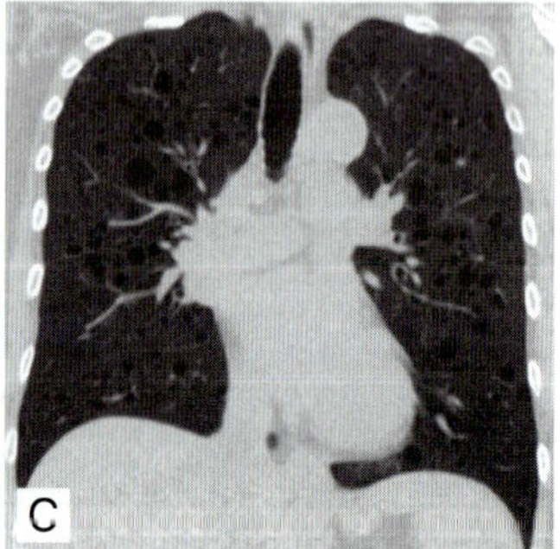

Figure 18.29 Lymphangioleiomyomatosis. (A and B) Axial CT images demonstrate uniformly distributed thin-walled round cysts seen in all lobes. The intervening lung parenchyma is otherwise normal. (C) Coronal CT image demonstrates uniform craniocaudal distribution of the cysts, including cysts in the costophrenic angles.

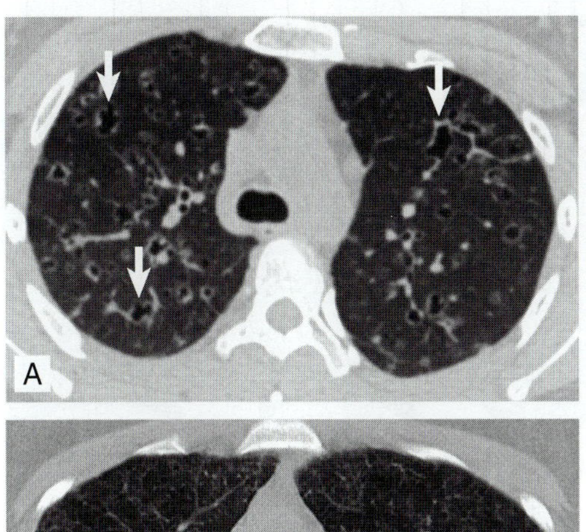
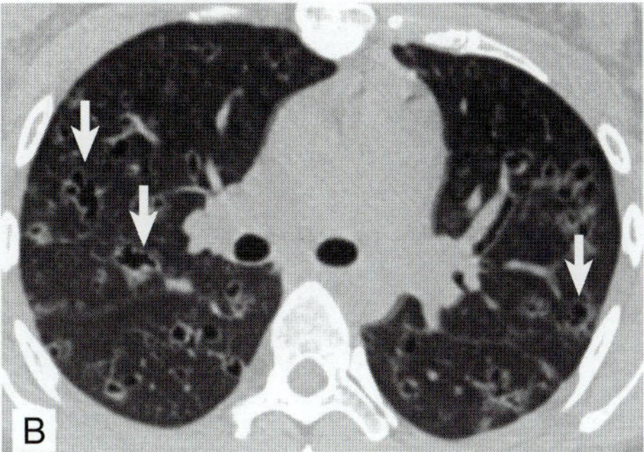
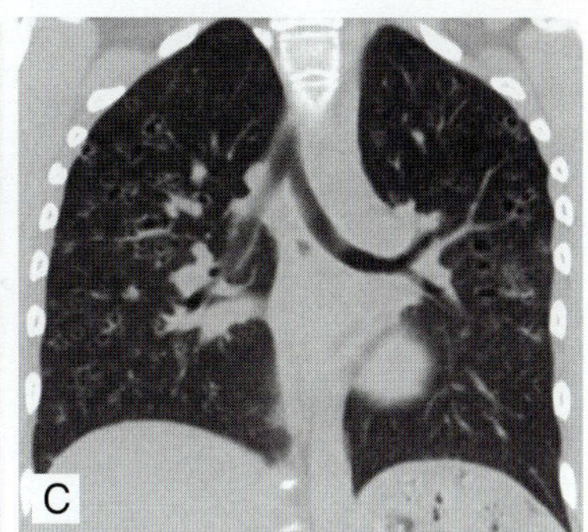
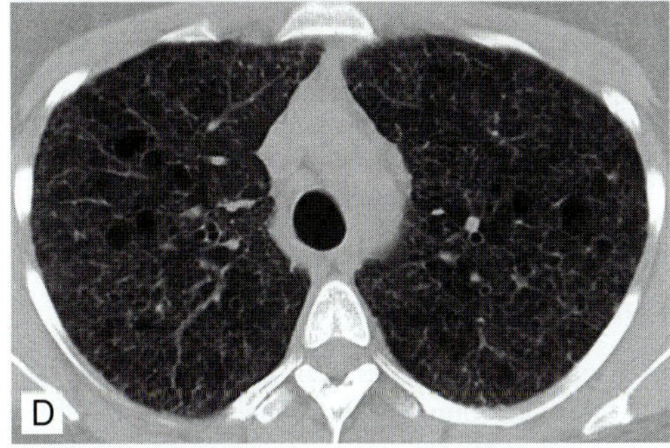

Figure 18.30 Pulmonary Langerhans cell histiocytosis. (A and B) Axial CT images demonstrate combination of nodules and cysts with varying wall thicknesses. Several of the cysts have also coalesced resulting in a "bizarre" appearance (*arrows*). (C) Coronal CT image demonstrates upper lung predominance of the cysts with sparing of the costophrenic angles. (D) Axial CT image of the same patient 5 years later show marked progression of the cystic lung disease with diffuse cysts throughout the emphysematous lungs. In advanced cases, the cysts may be indistinguishable from airspaces resulting from emphysema.

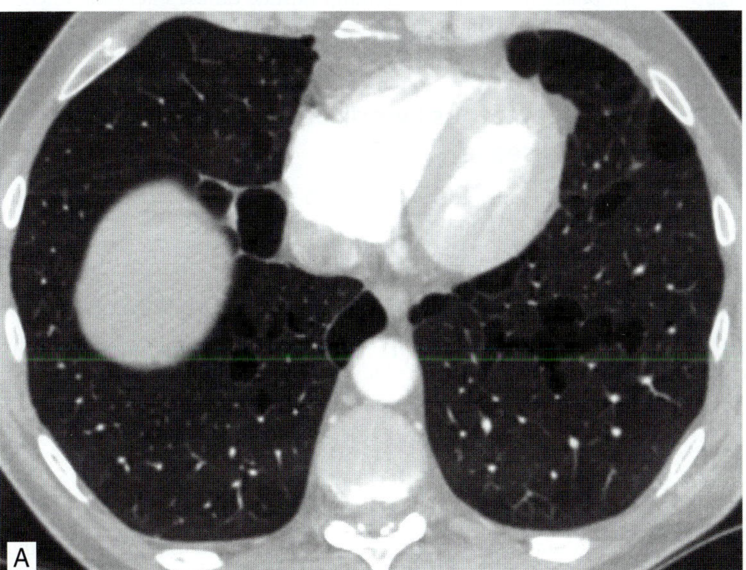
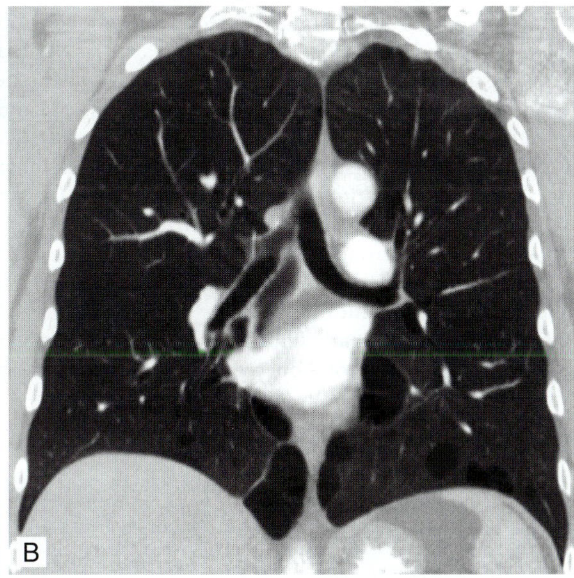

Figure 18.31 Cystic lung disease in the setting of Birt–Hogg–Dube (BHD) syndrome. (A) Axial, and (B) Coronal CT images demonstrate multiple ovoid and lentiform cysts with a predominantly paramediastinal distribution.

multiple papillomas throughout the airway. It can affect the lungs and is characterized by nodules that may cavitate and evolve into cysts, typically within the dependent portions of the lungs. In rare cases, malignant transformation into squamous cell carcinoma can occur.

Up to 20% of adults with neurofibromatosis have lung manifestations characterized by bullae formation in the upper lobes and interstitial fibrosis of the lung bases.

Several pathologies discussed earlier in the chapter may also have multiple cysts on imaging, including LIP, DIP, ankylosing spondylitis, and amyloidosis. Other causes of diffuse cysts such as malignancies (cystic metastases) and infections (e.g., *Pneumocystis jirovecii*) are discussed separately.

Other Diffuse Lung Diseases

Pulmonary Alveolar Proteinosis

Pulmonary alveolar proteinosis is characterized by accumulation of lipid-rich proteinaceous periodic acid-Schiff-positive material. Most cases (90%) are idiopathic, while the remainder are ether congenital or secondary to an underlying condition such as infections and malignancies [42]. In idiopathic pulmonary alveolar proteinosis, the presence of anti-GM-CSF IgG antibodies interfere with the degradation of surfactant resulting in its accumulation.

Typical CT findings are patchy or geographic ground-glass opacities with smooth interlobular thickening ("crazy paving"

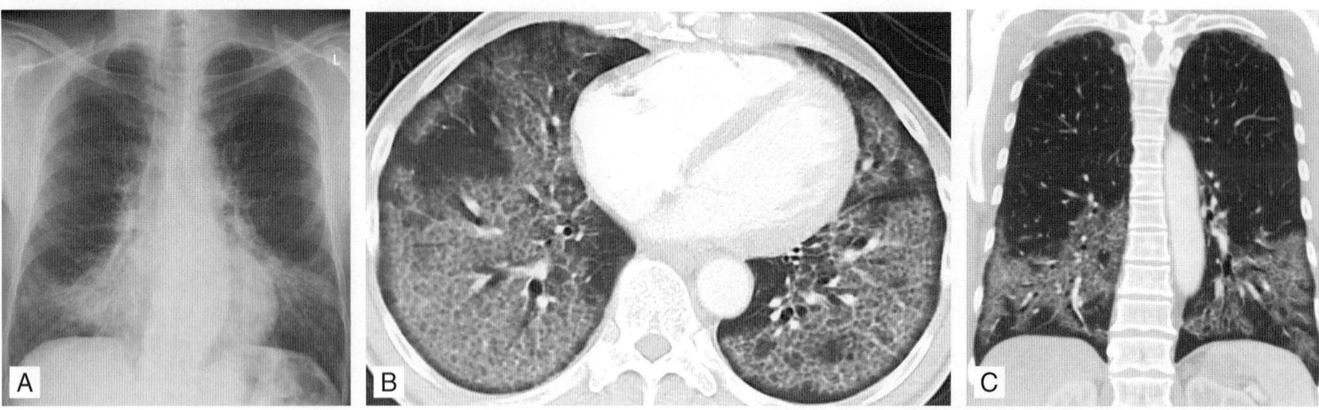

Figure 18.32 Pulmonary alveolar proteinosis. (A) Frontal chest radiograph demonstrates dense, confluent opacities in the mid and lower lungs, predominantly affecting the right middle lobe and lingula. (B) Axial CT image demonstrates diffuse ground-glass opacities with intralobular septal thickening consistent with "crazy paving" pattern. (C) Coronal CT image demonstrates mid- and lower-lung predominance of the abnormalities. There is also notable subpleural sparing and a sharp interface between affected and nonaffected lung parenchyma.

pattern). These opacities are typically well-demarcated by normal lung parenchyma and subpleural sparing is common (Fig. 18.32). Consolidations are uncommon but may also be present.

Pulmonary Hemosiderosis

Pulmonary hemosiderosis refers to diffuse pulmonary iron deposition thought to be secondary to recurrent episodes of pulmonary hemorrhage. It can be idiopathic, be associated with Goodpasture syndrome, or rarely be secondary to an underlying condition including connective tissue disorders, coagulopathy, and congestive heart failure, particularly in the setting of mitral stenosis. Lane–Hamilton syndrome refers to idiopathic pulmonary hemosiderosis with concurrent celiac disease. On imaging, pulmonary hemosiderosis is characterized by diffuse ground-glass opacities with interlobular septal thickening, small ill-defined nodules, mid to lower lung zone coarse reticulations, and pulmonary ossification, which can be confluent. Small peribronchovascular and subpleural cystic changes, thought to represent focal areas of honeycombing, may also be present (Fig. 18.33).

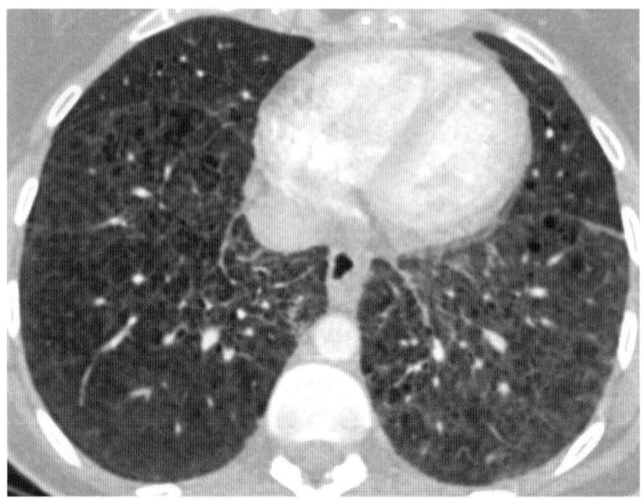

Figure 18.33 Idiopathic pulmonary hemosiderosis in the setting of celiac disease (Lane–Hamilton syndrome). Axial CT image demonstrates diffuse ground-glass opacities with areas of interlobular septal thickening thought to be due to iron deposition. Small cluster cystic changes (focal areas of honeycombing) are also present.

Diffuse Pulmonary Lymphangiomatosis

Diffuse pulmonary lymphangiomatosis is a rare condition more commonly seen in children and young adults characterized by diffuse proliferation of lymphangiomas. The lymphangiomas can proliferate in the lungs, pleura, and mediastinum resulting in dysfunction in lymphatic flow. The CT findings include diffuse interstitial thickening, patchy ground-glass opacities, pleural thickening and effusion, and infiltrative mediastinal soft tissue masses (Fig. 18.34) [43].

Granulomatous Lymphocytic Interstitial Lung Disease

Granulomatous lymphocytic ILD is a rare noninfectious complication of common variable immunodeficiency [44]. It is characterized on histology with the combination of lymphoid hyperplasia and granulomatous infiltration. CT typically shows a combination of ground-glass opacities and consolidation with nodular septal thickening with a lower lung and peribronchovascular distribution (Fig. 18.35). The findings of granulomatous lymphocytic ILD may wax and wane over time and can progress to fibrosis in some patients. *Splenomegaly is commonly seen.*

Granulomatosis With Polyangiitis

Granulomatosis with Polyangiitis (also called as Wegener's granulomatosis) is a vasculitis of small and medium-sized arteries. It is angiogenic and multi system necrotizing disease commonly involving the upper and lower respiratory tract and kidneys. Any age group can be affected, with the mean age at diagnosis being 50 year, and there is no gender predilection.

CT is the mainstay in imaging. The spectrum of CT findings in chest includes: (Fig. 18.36)

- Lung nodules (most common manifestation) are usually multiple and bilateral and occur without a zonal predilection. The size of nodules varies, most commonly measuring between 2 to 4 cm but ranging from a few millimeters to 10 cm.
- Cavitation may occur in larger nodules. The cavities may get secondarily infected and air-fluid level can be seen.
- Lung consolidation may be seen in a third of patients with Polyangiitis granulomatosis.
- Ground-glass opacity may result from alveolar hemorrhage or mosaic perfusion secondary to small-vessel vasculitis. Areas of diffuse hemorrhage may coalesce to form hemorrhagic consolidation.

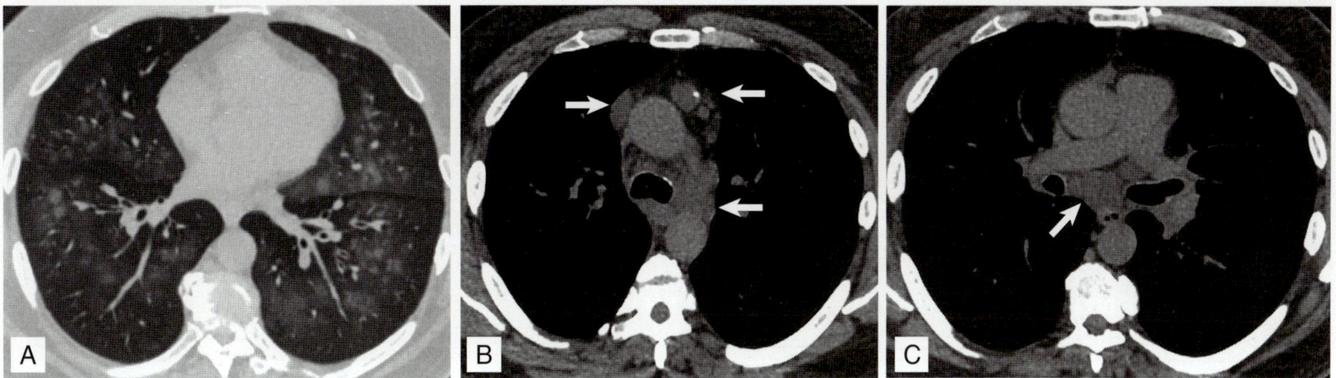

Figure 18.34 Diffuse pulmonary lymphangiomatosis. (A) Axial CT image demonstrates multifocal, patchy ground-glass opacities bilaterally with a centrilobular distribution resulting from lymphatic obstruction. (B and C) Axial CT images in soft-tissue window demonstrate multiple nodular and infiltrative soft-tissue masses (*arrows*) in the mediastinum corresponding to lymphangiomas.

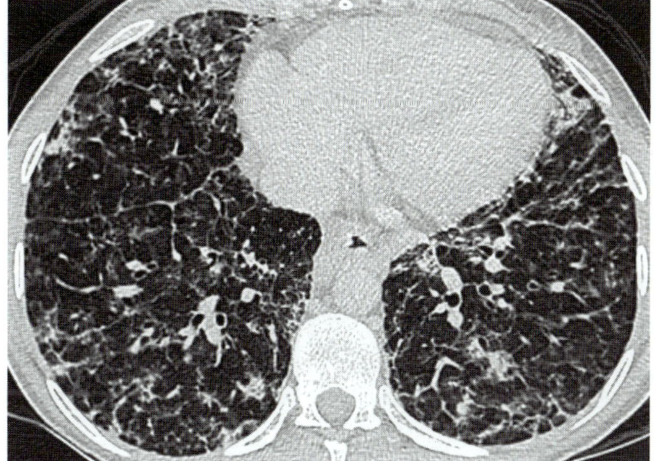

Figure 18.35 Granulomatous lymphocytic interstitial lung disease in the setting of combined variable immunodeficiency. Axial CT image demonstrates diffuse basal-predominant, peribronchovascular nodules, ground-glass opacities, and diffuse interstitial thickening.

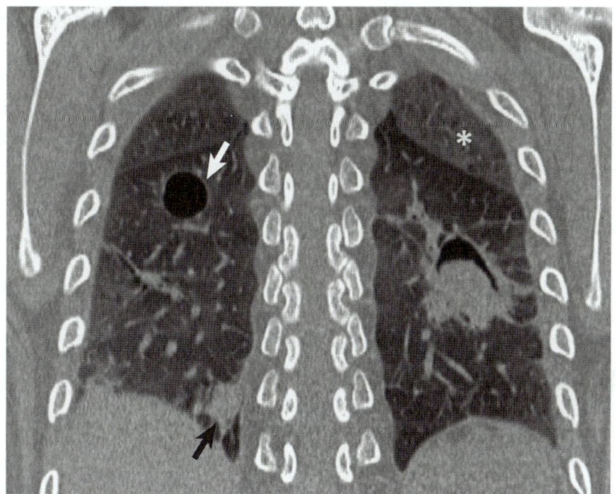

Figure 18.36 Polyangiitis granulomatosis. HRCT coronal image shows cavitation (*white arrow*), nodule (*black arrow*) and ground glass areas (*asterisk*). The large cavity in left lung shows soft tissue attenuation due to secondary fungal infection.

- Airway involvement is late. Subglottic trachea is most commonly involved which can show stenosis and or mucosal ulceration.

Suggested Readings

- JH Chung, CW Cox, SM Montner, et al., CT features of the usual interstitial pneumonia pattern: differentiating connective tissue disease-associated interstitial lung disease from idiopathic pulmonary fibrosis, AJR Am J Roentgenol 210 (2) (2018) 307–313. doi:10.2214/AJR.17.18384.
- CW Cox, CS Rose, DA Lynch, State of the art: Imaging of occupational lung disease, Radiology 270 (3) (2014) 681–696. doi:10.2214/AJR.17.18384.
- E Criado, M Sánchez, J Ramírez, et al., Pulmonary sarcoidosis: typical and atypical manifestations at high-resolution CT with pathologic correlation, Radiographics 30 (6) (2010) 1567–1586. doi:10.2214/AJR.17.18384.
- DM Hansell, AA Bankier, H MacMahon, TC McLoud, NL Müller, J Remy, Fleischner society: glossary of terms for thoracic imaging, Radiology 246 (3) (2008) 697–722. doi:10.1148/radiol.2462070712.
- JL Myers, AH Limper, SJ Swensen, Drug-induced lung disease: a pragmatic classification incorporating HRCT appearances, Semin Respir Crit Care Med 24 (4) (2003) 445–454. doi:10.1055/s-2003-42379.
- S Raoof, P Bondalapati, R Vydyula, et al., Cystic lung diseases: algorithmic approach, Chest 150 (4) (2016) 945–965. doi:10.1016/j.chest.2016.04.026.

19

Miscellaneous Conditions of Chest

DEXTER P. MENDOZA, SUBBA R. DIGUMARTHY

Thoracic Trauma

Thoracic injuries account for up to 25% of trauma-related deaths [1]. They are typically secondary to either penetrating trauma such as gunshot or knife wounds, or due to blunt trauma associated with motor vehicle collisions and falls.

Portable chest radiographs (CXRs) are the first line imaging evaluation for thoracic trauma patients as they are easily accessible and provide a general overview of injuries that may require immediate intervention. Cross-sectional imaging with computed tomography (CT) provides a more detailed evaluation of injuries, including the mediastinum, airway, lungs, and thoracic skeleton. Administration of intravenous contrast is vital to the evaluation of cardiovascular structures, allowing the detection of vascular injuries and active hemorrhage.

Thoracic Cage Injuries

Injuries involving the thoracic skeleton are common. The injuries may be isolated to the osseous structures or indicative of a more serious internal injury. CXRs are highly sensitive to fractures when they are displaced. CT may be necessary when evaluating other associated injuries and complications.

Fractures of the first and second ribs are indicative of high-impact injury and are strongly associated with injuries to the mediastinal vasculature [2]. Fractures of the lower ribs, on the other hand, may be associated with injury to the diaphragm and upper abdomen [3]. Rib fractures are also frequently associated with pneumothoraces and hemothoraces. A flail chest is a potential complication in the presence of multiple (three or more), contiguous, segmental rib fractures (Fig. 19.1). This can result in disruption of the normal chest wall mechanics and diminished ventilation and may require surgical fixation [4].

Clavicular fractures and sternoclavicular dislocations, particularly posterior dislocations, can cause life-threatening injuries to the subjacent vessels, trachea, and esophagus [5]. Sternal fractures are typically due to direct impact and can have associated cardiac and aortic injuries [6]. Monitoring for cardiac injuries with telemetry and serial cardiac enzymes is generally indicated.

Thoracic spinal injuries are most commonly due to hyperflexion mechanisms resulting in anterior wedge vertebral body compression deformities and burst fractures in severe cases. Burst fractures are vertebral body compression deformities with associated disruption of the anterior and middle columns and are strongly associated with spinal cord injury due to retropulsion of fracture fragments [7]. Thoracic spine fracture-dislocations can also result in partial or complete transection of the spinal cord (Fig. 19.2). MRI may be necessary to assess for ligamentous and spinal cord injuries when neurologic symptoms are present [8].

Pleural Injuries

Pneumothoraces can develop from chest wall injuries and rib fractures resulting in disruption of the pleural layer(s), allowing air to enter the pleural space. While pneumothoraces are most apparent as the air rises, the air may collect within the inferolateral spaces in supine CXR resulting in the characteristic deep sulcus sign (Fig. 19.3). Sharp mediastinal borders may also indicate a medial pneumothorax. Tension pneumothorax is a life-threatening condition wherein increased intrapleural pressure leads to cardiomediastinal compression and

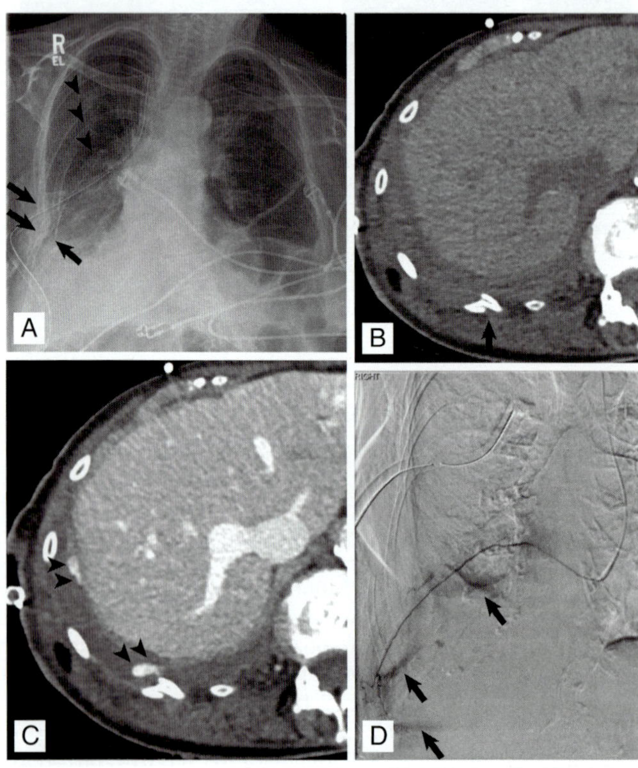

Figure 19.1 Segmental right rib fractures with a hemothorax. (A) Frontal chest radiograph demonstrates multiple right rib segmental fractures with posterior (*arrowheads*) and lateral (*arrows*) components. A right apical chest tube is in place for evacuation of pneumothorax. Contiguous segmental fractures can result in a flail chest. (B) Axial CT image without contrast shows fracture of the right posterior rib (*arrow*). There is high-density pleural fluid consistent with hemothorax. (C) Contrast-enhanced axial CT image show small foci of contrast extravasation into the collection consistent with active bleeding. (D) Targeted angiography of the right 11th intercostal artery confirmed vascular injury.

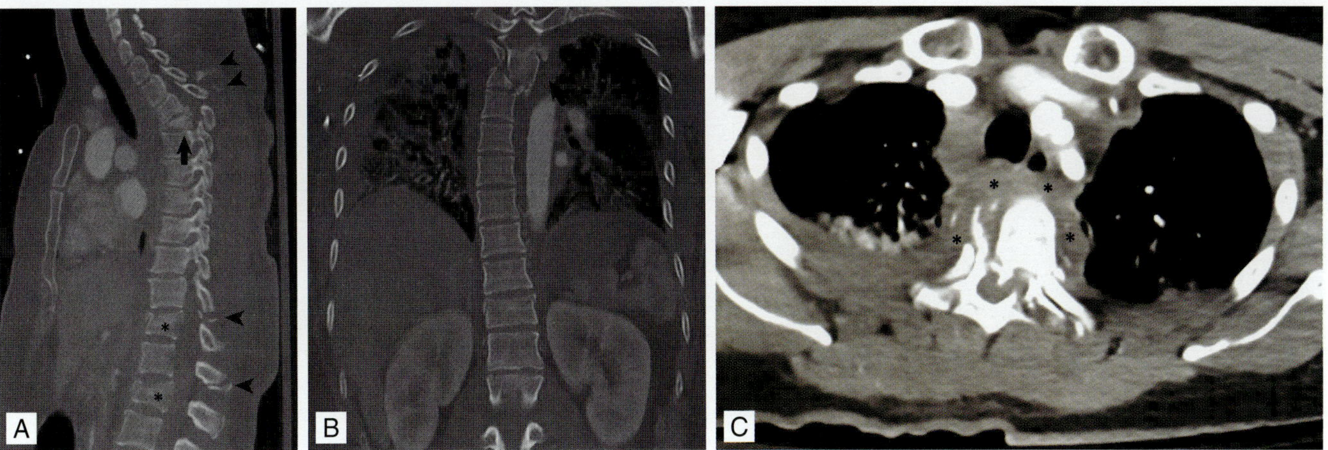

Figure 19.2 Fracture-dislocation of the thoracic spine. (A) Sagittal CT image shows severe anterior wedge compression deformity of the T4 vertebral body and associated retropulsion (*arrow*). There are also mild compression deformities of the T11 and L1 vertebral bodies (*asterisks*) as well as fractures of several spinous processes (*arrowheads*). (B) Coronal CT image shows left lateral listhesis of T3 (*arrow*) with respect to T4. (C) Axial CT image shows T4 burst fracture with surrounding paraspinal hematoma (*asterisks*).

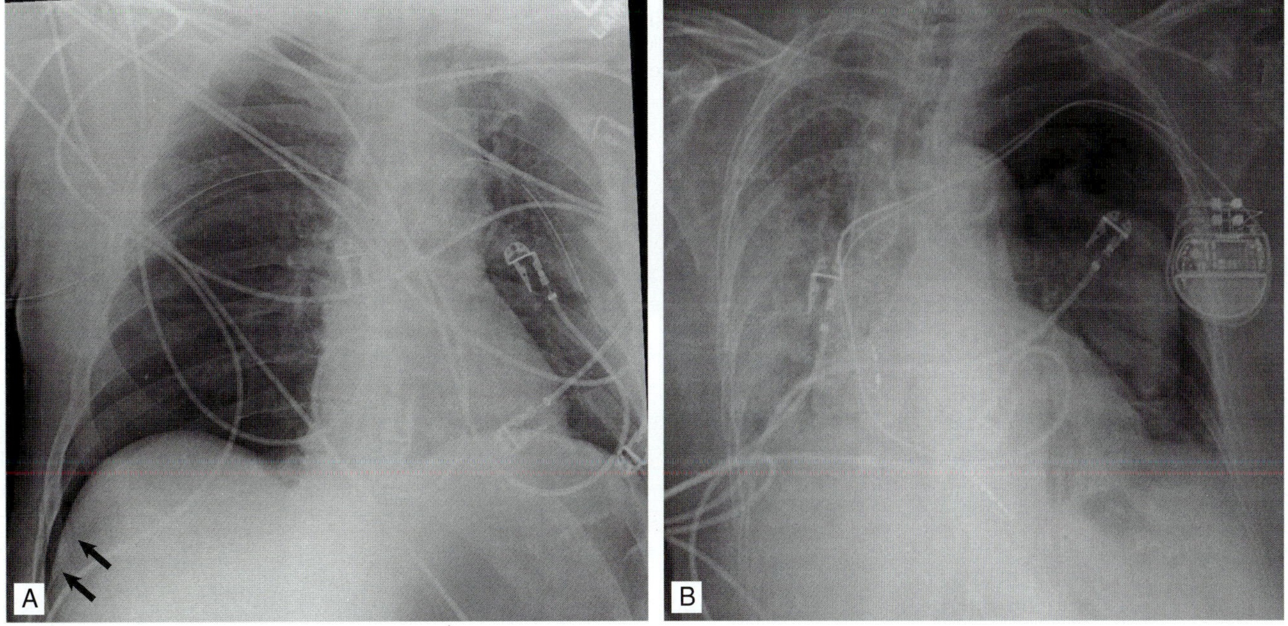

Figure 19.3 Pneumothoraces. (A) Supine chest radiograph shows a deep sulcus sign (*arrows*) consistent with a basilar pneumothorax. There is leftward mediastinal shift and splaying of the left intercostal spaces suggestive of increased thoracic pressure, which can predispose to tension physiology. (B) Semierect portable chest radiograph of a different patient shows a large left pneumothorax with complete atelectasis of the left lung.

displacement and reduction in venous return resulting in hemodynamic instability. Typical findings (Fig. 19.3) suggestive of tension physiology include a large pneumothorax, contralateral mediastinal shift, splaying or widening of the ipsilateral intercostal spaces, and depression of the ipsilateral diaphragm.

A hemothorax usually results from traumatic injury to an intercostal vessel, with blood collecting within the pleural space [2]. CXR cannot reliably differentiate between a hemothorax and pleural effusion. On CT, hyperdense blood products may pool within the dependent pleural space with varying attenuations depending on the acuity of the bleed. Administration of intravenous contrast could potentially identify active contrast extravasation (Fig. 19.1).

Lung Parenchymal Injuries

Impact to the chest wall can be transmitted to the lungs causing local disruption of the alveolar capillary network and resulting in pulmonary contusions. They present as local, geographic areas of ground-glass opacities or consolidations (Fig. 19.4). Development can be delayed by up to 12 hours and resolution or partial improvement is to be expected within 48 hours [9].

Pulmonary lacerations are tears of the lung parenchyma. Due to the elastic recoil of the lungs, lacerations typically present as spherical spaces (Fig. 19.4), which can be filled with air (pneumatocele), blood (hematocele), or both. They can take weeks or months to resolve and can leave behind a scar. Care should be

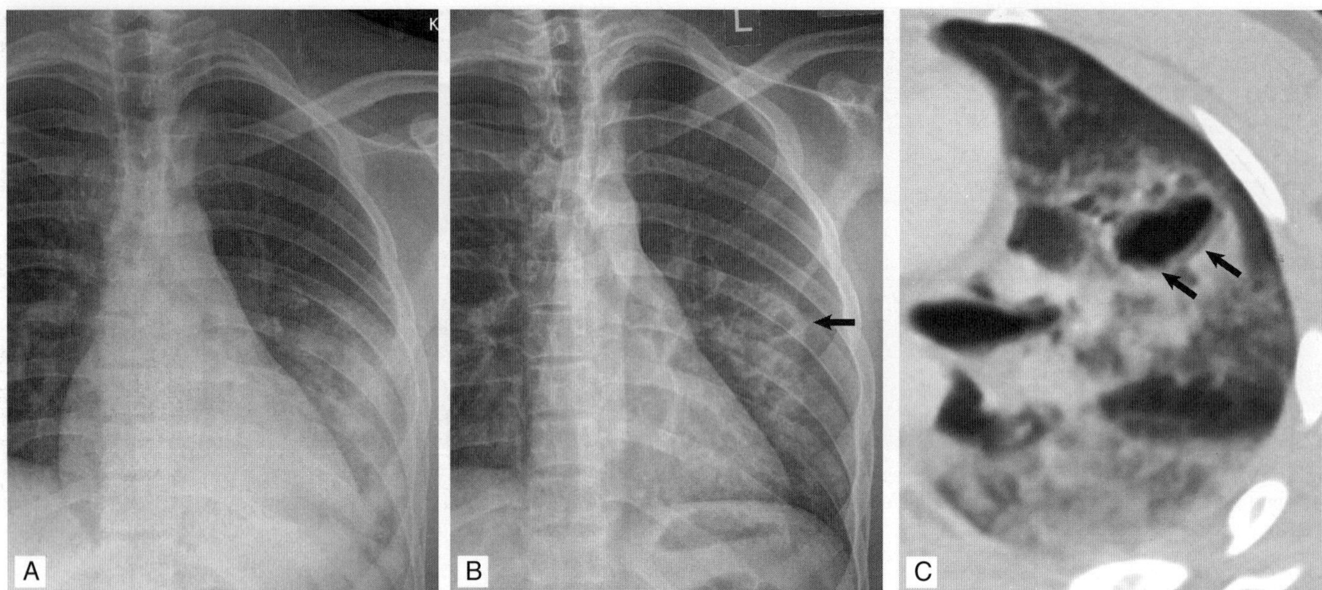

Figure 19.4 Post-traumatic pulmonary contusion and laceration. (A) Chest radiograph shows confluent dense opacities in the mid-to-lower left lung. (B) Follow-up chest radiograph 24 hours later demonstrate partial clearing of the opacities. There is a rounded lucency within the opacity suggestive of a cavitation. (C) Axial CT image of the same patient demonstrates confluent, geographic ground-glass, and consolidative opacities consistent with pulmonary contusions. A laceration (post-traumatic pneumatocele) is noted in the lingula (*arrow*).

taken to prevent mistaking a slowly resolving hematoma for a neoplastic lesion.

Airway Injuries

Traumatic injuries to the tracheobronchial tree are rare. When present, they occur within 2 cm of the carina with equal frequencies between the left and right mainstem bronchi. Delays in detection are common due to lack of recognition on imaging, necessitating careful assessment, and a high index of suspicion.

The most common findings are pneumomediastinum, pneumothorax, and subcutaneous emphysema. On CT, additional signs include sharp bronchial angulation, airway narrowing, periluminal air, and focal discontinuity of the airway. Without treatment, airway injuries can result in stenosis. In cases of complete transection, the affected lung may fall into the dependent portion of the thoracic cavity ("fallen lung" sign) [10].

Mediastinal Injuries

Cardiac and pericardial injuries result from penetrating trauma but can also result from high-impact blunt trauma, usually in association with a sternal fracture. Potential injuries include cardiac contusion, myocardial rupture, and hemopericardium that can result in tamponade physiology. These injuries are generally accompanied by electrocardiogram and cardiac enzyme abnormalities.

Traumatic aortic injuries are associated with high mortality rates [11]. Common sites of injury are those wherein the aorta is relatively fixed:

(1) The aortic root
(2) The aortic isthmus, at the level of the ligamentum arteriosum just past the origin of the left subclavian artery
(3) The diaphragmatic hiatus

They can be associated with coronary arterial injury and hemopericardium particularly when they occur at the aortic root. They can occur as a result of blunt or penetrating trauma or as a result of shear injury from rapid deceleration. On CXR, findings indicative of traumatic aortic injury include mediastinal widening (Fig. 19.5), loss of the normal contour of the aorta, and a left apical cap indicating blood in the apical pleural or extrapleural space. CT angiography is the most appropriate imaging in their evaluation. CT angiography findings include aortic dissections or transections, pseudoaneurysms (Fig. 19.5), mediastinal hematoma, hemopericardium, and active contrast extravasation [11].

Most esophageal injuries result from penetrating trauma, but they can also occur from blunt trauma as a result of increased intraluminal pressure with a closed glottis or injury against the thoracic spine [12]. CXR findings include mediastinal widening, pneumomediastinum, and pleural effusion. On CT, findings may include pneumomediastinum, mediastinal fluid and mediastinitis, extraluminal contrast, and pleural effusion. Direct esophageal findings such as focal wall thickening or esophageal wall defect may also be present. Water-soluble contrast esophagography may help confirm the diagnosis and determine the site of injury.

Diaphragmatic Injuries

Diaphragmatic injuries result from increased abdominal pressure combined with shear injury to the diaphragm [13]. Direct penetrating traumas such as gunshot wounds can also occur. Diaphragmatic injures can be associated with significant morbidities including impaired lung ventilation and abdominal visceral herniation and ischemia.

Left-sided injuries are more common than right-sided injuries due to the protective effect of the liver under the right hemidiaphragm. CXR may demonstrate only apparent elevation of the injured hemidiaphragm or intrathoracic herniation of abdominal organs. On CT, a "collar sign" can be seen as intra-abdominal organs "squeeze" through a focal defect (Fig. 19.6). A "dependent viscera sign" may also be seen as the herniated viscera fall dependently in the thoracic cavity (Fig. 19.6) with the loss of diaphragmatic support.

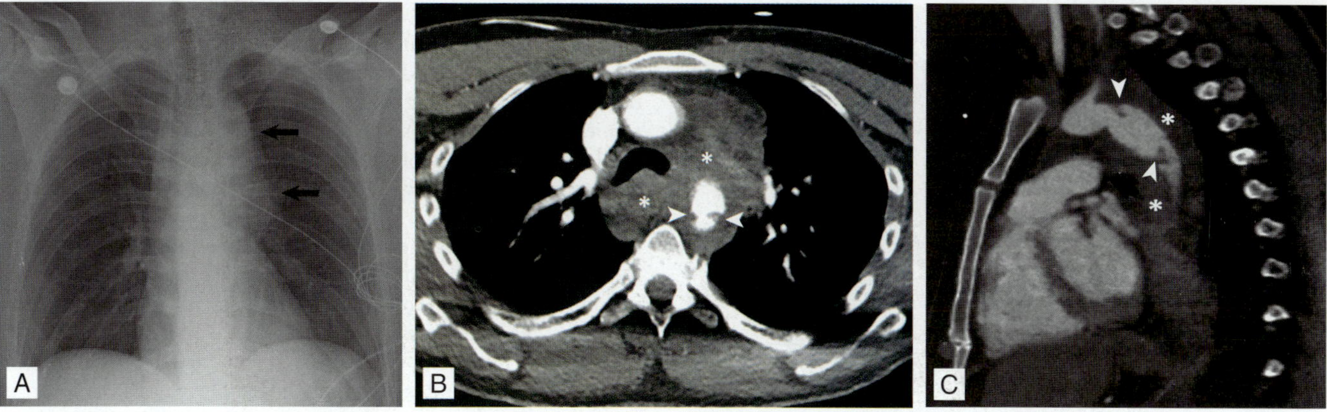

Figure 19.5 Traumatic aortic injury. (A) Chest radiograph lobulated widening of the superior mediastinum at the level of the aortic arch and descending aorta (*arrows*). (B) Axial, and (C) sagittal CTA images demonstrated irregularity of the proximal descending aorta just past the origin of the left subclavian artery with intraluminal linear filling defects (*arrowheads*) consistent with traumatic aortic dissection. There is high-density fluid surrounding the aorta (*asterisks*) consistent with mediastinal hematoma.

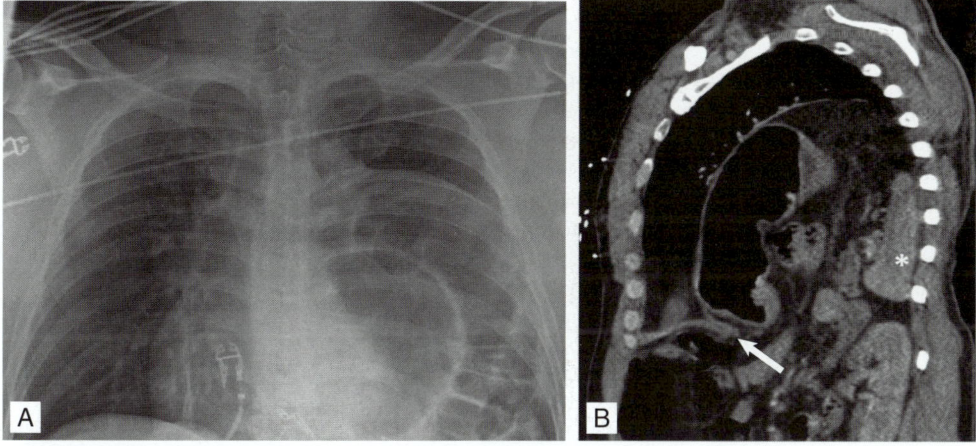

Figure 19.6 Traumatic diaphragmatic hernia. (A) Chest radiograph demonstrates excursion of the stomach and colon into the left hemithorax. (B) Sagittal chest CT image demonstrates a large diaphragmatic hernia with extension of the abdominal organs into the thoracic cavity. Note the diaphragmatic defect (*arrow*) through which the abdominal contents are "squeezed" through ("collar sign") and the posterior location of the spleen (*asterisk*) consistent with the "dependent viscera sign."

Postoperative Chest

Familiarity with the expected postoperative changes on imaging following various thoracic surgeries is necessary to prevent misinterpretation of expected pathological changes. Also, chest radiography and CT play central roles in the evaluation of potential complications following surgery.

Thoracic Access

In general, lung resections can be achieved either with an open approach or a minimally invasive approach with video assistance (VATS). An open approach involved either a sternotomy or thoracotomy, depending on the access required. The sternotomy can be partial or complete, and midline or transverse. With a thoracotomy, the hemithorax is accessed through an intercostal space which involves division of one of the muscle groups of the chest wall. It may also require partial rib resection or may result in rib fractures as the intercostal space is spread out. VATS, on the other hand, requires three to four entrance ports through which the videoscope and trocars are introduced. In general, VATS is better tolerated by patients, is associated with reduced postoperative pain, and results in a shorter length of hospital stay.

Lung Resection and Pneumonectomy

Lung resections can be classified as either nonanatomic or anatomic.

Nonanatomic resections involve resection of a nonanatomic portion of the lung such as wedge resections, bullectomies and blebectomies, and most volume reduction surgeries. Wedge resections are typically employed in surgical lung biopsies (such as in indeterminate interstitial lung disease), in excisional biopsies of indeterminate lung lesions that may be malignant, or in resections of solitary or isolated pulmonary metastases (metastasectomy). It may also be indicated in the resection of small, peripheral minimally invasive, or noninvasive primary lung cancers [14]. On imaging, wedge resections result in a dense linear opacity representing the surgical staple line with adjacent atelectasis and architectural distortion (Fig. 19.7). Surrounding hematoma may be seen early in the postoperative period.

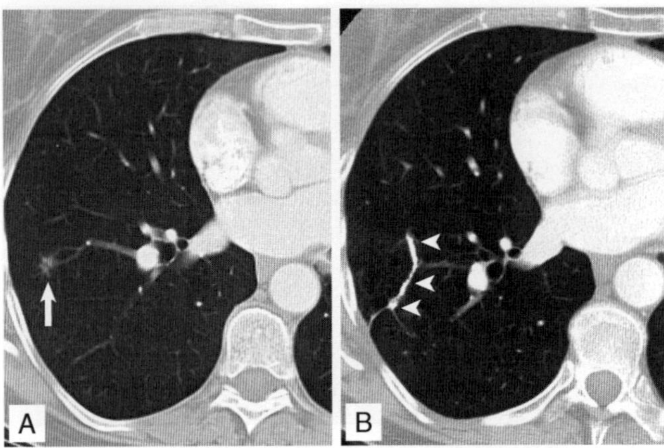

Figure 19.7 Wedge resection of a metastatic lesion. (A) Axial chest CT chows a spiculated nodule in the right lower lobe (*arrow*), which was presumed to be metastatic in the setting of known renal cell carcinoma. (B) Axial chest CT 2 months following wedge resection shows expected changes with linear hyperdensity corresponding to suture material with surrounding architectural distortion.

Anatomic resections, on the other hand, are those that follow the segmental anatomy of the lungs. These include segmentectomies, lobectomies, and pneumonectomies. A segmentectomy involves resection of one or more segments of the lungs. It is most commonly employed in the resection of lung cancers if the patient cannot tolerate a complete lobectomy due to poor lung function. It may also be employed in metastasectomies.

Lobectomy is the definitive surgical treatment for primary lung cancers. Other indications include congenital anomalies such as congenital pulmonary airway malformations and other benign pathologies such as chronic infections and bronchiectasis. A sleeve lobectomy is a modified lobectomy in which a lobe is resected en bloc with a segment of the mainstem bronchus and the remainder of the nondiseased lobes is anastomosed with the residual mainstem bronchus in an end-to-end fashion [15]. It is an alternative to pneumonectomy in patients with central tumors affecting the central airways. Occasionally, the bronchial stump may be reinforced using vascularized tissue such as muscle flaps (e.g., intercostal, latissimus dorsi, and pectoralis) or fat flaps (e.g., omentum or pericardial fat pads). This can be seen as either soft tissue of fat density, respectively, in the region of the bronchial stump (Fig. 19.8). Care should be taken not to mistake them for recurrent disease on imaging. On CXR, the findings following lobectomies may mimic those of complete lobar atelectasis [16] with resulting volume loss of the affected lung, mediastinal and hilar displacement, and elevation of the ipsilateral hemidiaphragm (Fig. 19.8).

Pneumonectomy is the surgical removal of an entire lung and is indicated for locally advanced lung cancers that invade central structures such as the mainstem bronchus and main pulmonary artery or those that cross interlobar fissure. Compared to the other types of lung resections, it is associated with higher rates of mortality and morbidity and is therefore only employed as a last resort in carefully selected patients. A pneumonectomy may require resection and ligation of affected intrapericardial structures such as portions of the pulmonary veins or arteries (intrapericardial pneumonectomy). Extrapleural pneumonectomy involves resection of the parietal pleura and portions of the pericardium and ipsilateral hemidiaphragm. It may be indicated in select cases of mesothelioma although there has been a shift away from this type of surgery given high rates of mortality and morbidity [17].

Following a pneumonectomy, the earliest postoperative imaging demonstrates predominantly air-filled pneumonectomy space that eventually filled with fluid following removal of chest tubes, typically reported as two intercostal spaces per day (Fig. 19.9). Complete resorption of the air in the pneumonectomy space may take up to weeks resulting in complete opacification of the pneumonectomy space from the accumulated fluid and mediastinal shift. The fluid may also be resorbed over time but in most cases, a small amount of fluid persists (Fig. 19.9).

Potential Complications of Lung Resection and Pneumonectomy

Small pneumothoraces are expected following lung resections. Air leaks, however, should be suspected if the pneumothorax persists beyond 10 days after surgery. A bronchopleural fistula (BPF), an abnormal connection between the pleural space and an airway, can occur as a result of dehiscence of sutures or staples, from necrosis of the bronchial stump, or as a result of infections [18,19].

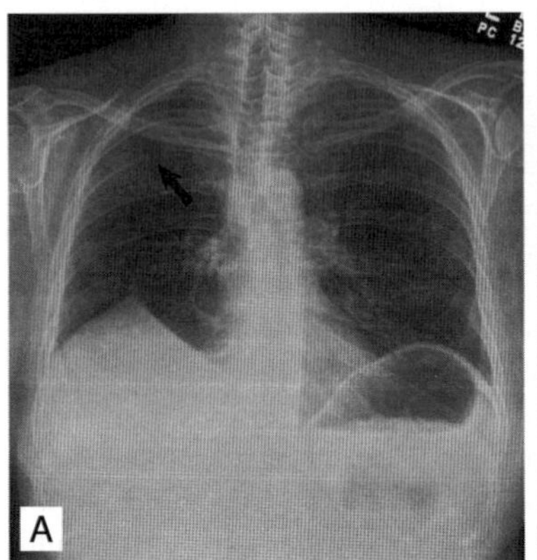

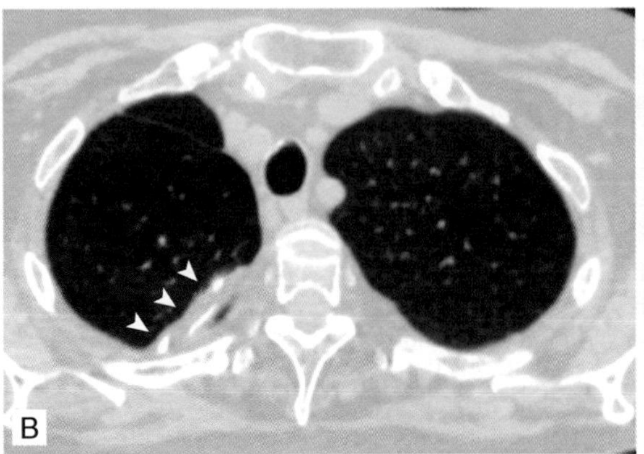

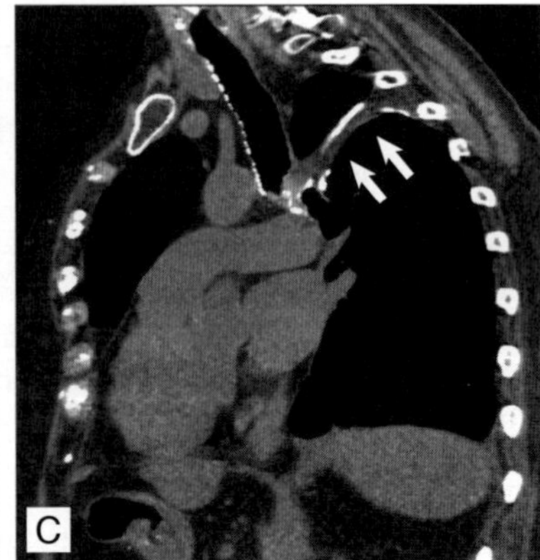

Figure 19.8 Expected postoperative changes of right upper lobectomy. (A) There is expected decreased right lung volume with elevation of the right hemidiaphragm and associated juxtaphrenic peak. There is also discontinuity of the right posterior fifth rib (*arrow*) consistent with thoracotomy. (B) Axial CT image shows a bandlike opacity in the right lung extending from the posterior chest wall to the mediastinum with associated linear hyperdense suture material (*arrowheads*). (C) Oblique sagittal CT image shows soft tissue and fat attenuating structure extending from the posterior chest wall to the hilum (*arrows*). These are consistent with an intercostal muscle flap.

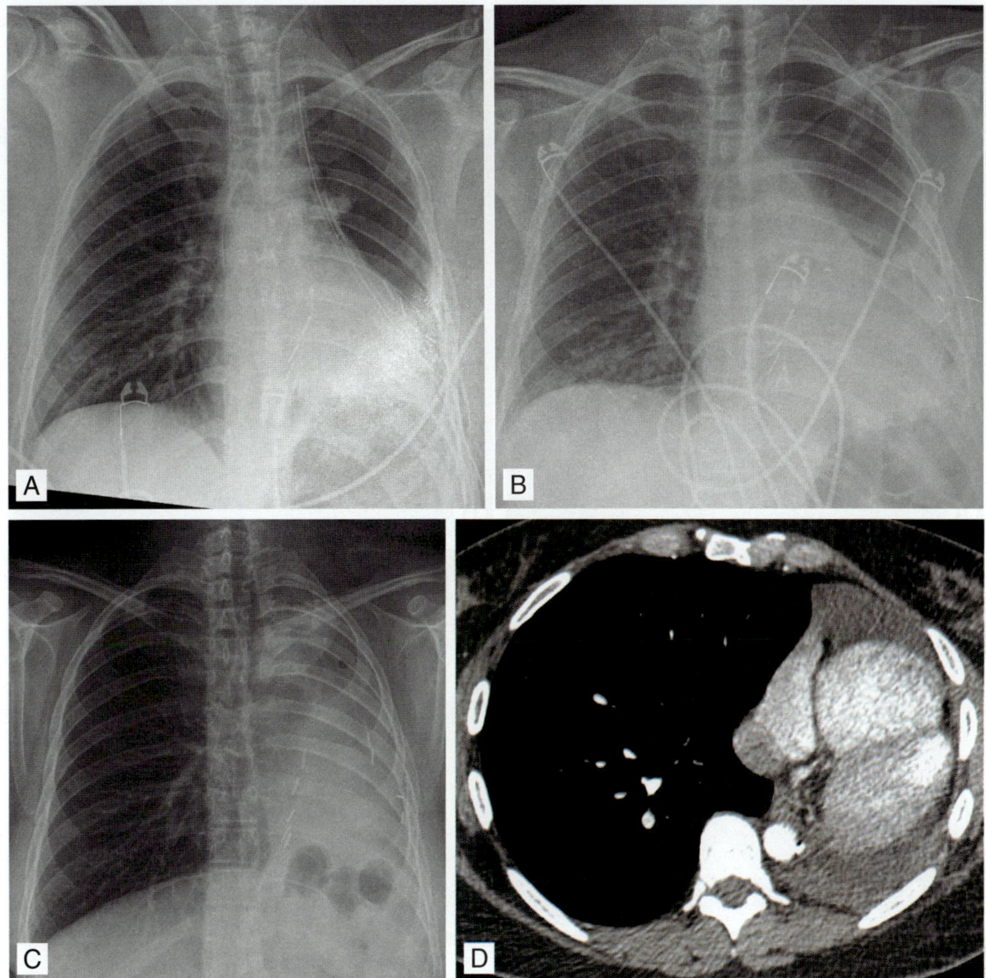

Figure 19.9 Expected postpneumonectomy changes. Sequential chest radiographs (A) immediately following left pneumonectomy; (B) 5 days following surgery; and (C) 1 month following surgery. Note the gradual filling of the pneumonectomy space with fluid and shift of the mediastinum toward the pneumonectomy space. (D) Axial chest CT image shows leftward shift of the heart with small residual fluid in the pneumonectomy space.

Treatment may involve surgical reclosure, which may require fortification with a vascularized flap. BPF may present as a new or increasing amount of air in the ipsilateral pleural space or pneumonectomy space [20]. CT may be able to directly identify a connection between the pleural space and airway.

Postoperative lobar torsion is a rare complication following partial lung resections, typically following a lobectomy but can also occur following sublobar resections. It most commonly affects the right middle lobe following a right upper lobectomy [21]. Treatment involves urgent surgical reduction to prevent infarction and necrosis of the torsed lobe. Findings of lobar torsion on CXR may be subtle and are nonspecific, including consolidation of the affected lobe and displacement into an atypical location (Fig. 19.10). On CT, the appearance of the torsed lobe varies depending on the duration and severity of the torsion. Earlier in the process, localized pulmonary edema with ground-glass opacities and interstitial thickening may be seen. As the torsion persists and progresses, consolidations, nonenhancement, and evidence of necrosis may be seen. At the hilum, an abrupt cutoff of the airway and pulmonary vessels can be seen (Fig. 19.10).

In addition to lobar torsions, pulmonary infarctions may result from venous insufficiency, which can occur in the setting of pulmonary venous thrombosis, compression, or inadvertent ligation. On CXR, venous infarctions are seen as nonspecific opacities with varying densities depending on the stage and severity of infarction. Similarly, CT findings can vary, ranging from ground-glass opacities to dense consolidations. Over time, localized fibrosis may develop.

Postpneumonectomy syndrome is characterized by excessive displacement of the heart and other mediastinal structures toward the pneumonectomy space resulting in compression of the contralateral (residual) mainstem bronchus by the pulmonary artery against the thoracic spine [22]. It usually occurs within the first 2 years of pneumonectomy and can present with shortness of breath, stridor, and recurrent pneumonia. CT best demonstrates the compression and narrowing of the mainstem bronchus (Fig. 19.11). Treatment requires surgical centralization of the mediastinum, which can involve the placement of fillers such as breast implants within the pneumonectomy space (Fig. 19.11).

Lung Transplantation

Lung transplantation involves orthotopic transplantation of both lungs, of a single lung, or of the bilateral lower lobes. The most

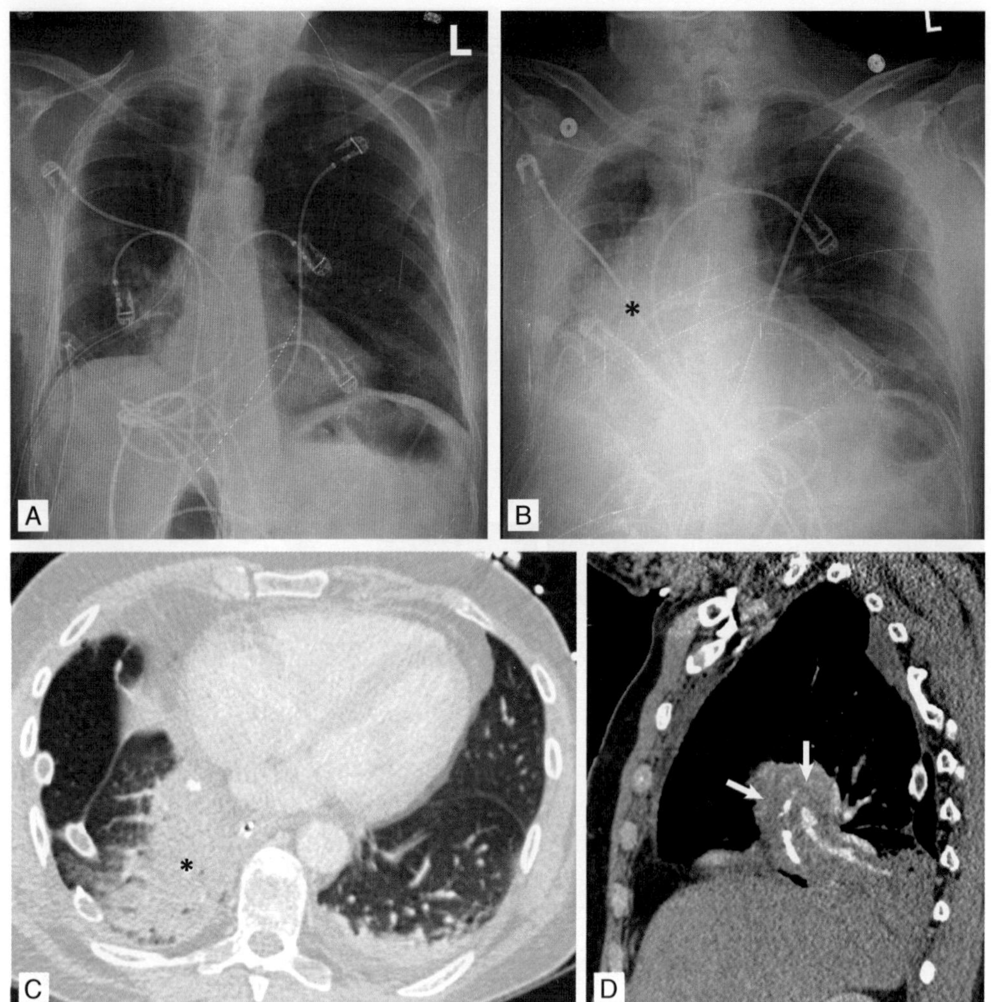

Figure 19.10 Right middle lobe torsion after right upper lobectomy. (A) Immediate postoperative radiograph demonstrates expected changes of right upper lobectomy with decreased right lung volume and chest tube in place. (B) Chest radiograph the following day showed interval development of dense paramediastinal opacity at the right lung base (*asterisk*). (C) Axial chest CT image demonstrates dense consolidation of the right middle lobe (*asterisk*), which is displaced inferiorly and posteriorly. (D) Sagittal CT image shows "swirled" appearance of the right middle lobe vasculature (*arrows*), confirming right middle lobe torsion.

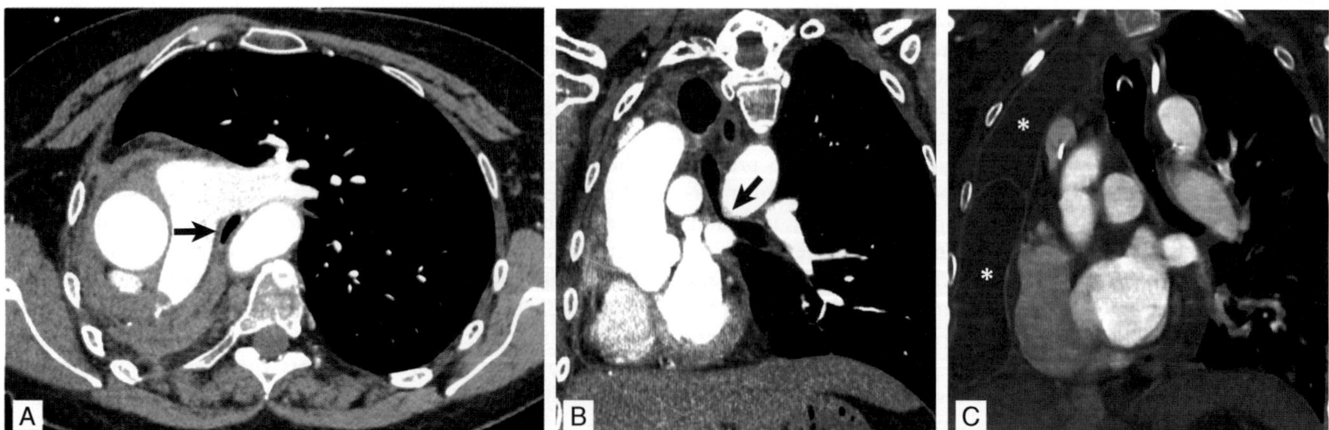

Figure 19.11 Postpneumonectomy syndrome. (A) Axial and (B) coronal CT images show changes of right pneumonectomy with rightward shift of the mediastinal structures. There is marked narrowing of the left main bronchus (*arrows*) due to mass effect from the left pulmonary artery against the descending aorta. (C) Coronal CT image following placement of breast implants (*asterisks*) into the pneumonectomy space with centralization of the heart and improvement of the left main bronchus narrowing.

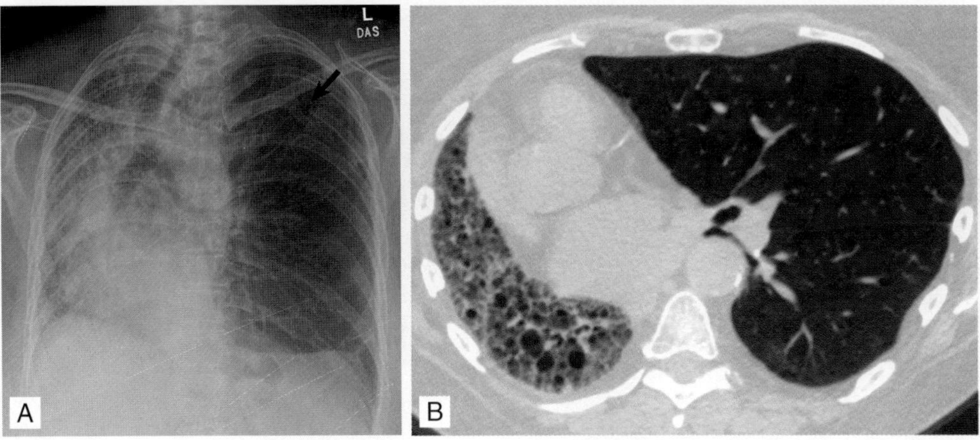

Figure 19.12 Single lung transplantation. (A) Frontal chest radiograph shows expected changes of left lung transplantation, including a left thoracotomy (*arrow*). The transplanted left lung is well-expanded and clear. There are advanced fibrotic changes to the native right lung with marked volume loss. (B) Axial chest CT shows a normal transplanted left lung and a fibrotic native right lung. There is rightward mediastinal deviation due to volume loss.

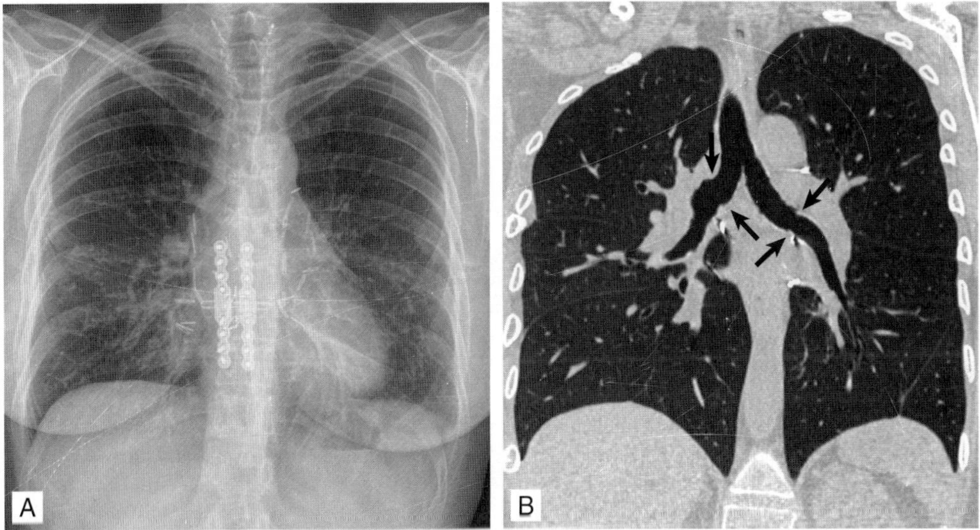

Figure 19.13 Double lung transplantation. (A) Frontal chest radiograph shows expected changes of bilateral lung transplantation with plate fixation of the clamshell sternotomy and multiple surgical clips in the mediastinum and hila. (B) Coronal CT image shows normal transplanted lungs. Note the expected focal irregularity at the level of the bronchial anastomoses bilaterally (*arrows*).

common indications for lung transplantation include advanced chronic obstructive pulmonary disease, interstitial lung diseases such as idiopathic pulmonary fibrosis and sarcoidosis, cystic fibrosis, and idiopathic pulmonary hypertension.

The airways of the transplanted lung are attached to the native airways in an end-to-end fashion. If there is a discrepancy in size between the donor and recipient bronchi, the smaller bronchi are inserted and "telescoped" into the larger bronchi. Typical postoperative appearance of *single lung transplantation* is an ipsilateral posterior thoracotomy and size discrepancy between the native and transplanted lung (Fig. 19.12). In *double lung transplantation*, a transverse (clamshell) sternotomy is seen. Multiple surgical clips are also seen in the hilar region. Vascular and airway anastomosis are readily evaluated by CT (Fig. 19.13).

Potential Complications of Lung Transplantation

Reperfusion pulmonary edema, a type of noncardiogenic edema, can occur within the first 24 hours of lung transplantation. It may progress and peak around postoperative day 5 but mostly improves by the end of the first week following surgery [23]. On CXR, reperfusion pulmonary edema presents as peribronchial cuffing, peripheral septal lines, and indistinctness of the pulmonary vascular. Unlike in cardiogenic pulmonary edema, the cardiac silhouette is usually normal in size. Other potential complications in the acute setting include acute rejection and infection.

Anastomotic dehiscence is a serious complication following lung transplantation and results from ischemia and necrosis of either the native or donor bronchus. Risk factors include a long donor bronchial stump and prolonged peribronchial dissection during harvesting. Postoperative pulmonary infections, prolonged mechanical ventilation, and acute rejection are additional risk factors. Partial dehiscence may be managed conservatively with close follow-up and antibiotics, but complete dehiscence or persistent BPF may require surgery. CXR may demonstrate new or increasing pneumothorax and/or pneumomediastinum. CT may be able to show the bronchial wall defect representing the dehiscence [24].

Anastomotic stenoses are more common than dehiscence and are usually seen 3 months or more postsurgery. Causes for late stenosis include the formation of granulation tissue secondary to bronchial

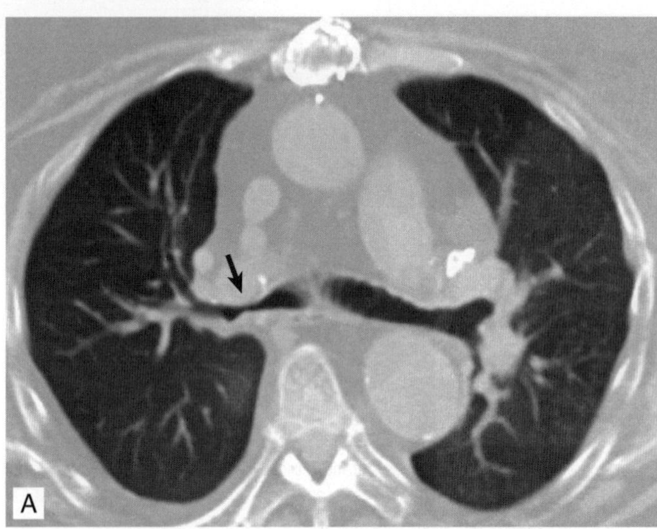

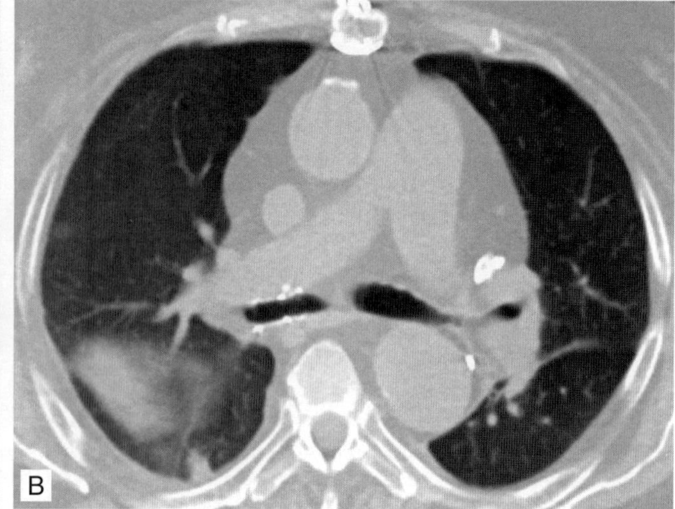

Figure 19.14 Bronchial anastomotic stricture. (A) Axial chest CT image demonstrates luminal narrowing at the right bronchial anastomosis (*arrow*). (B) Axial chest CT shows interval bronchial stent placement with improvement of the stenosis.

ischemia, healing of prior dehiscence, and infections. CXR is normal in most cases, but CT can reliably show airway narrowing (Fig. 19.14). Flexible bronchoscopy remains the gold standard for diagnosis. Several treatment options are available including balloon bronchoplasty, stenting, and surgical reconstruction.

Transplant rejection can be categorized into hyperacute, acute, and chronic [23].

- *Hyperacute rejection* occurs immediately following surgery and is due to preformed antibodies against donor-specific antigens. It is rapid and fulminant and results in homogeneous opacification of the transplanted lungs as reflected on both CXR and CT
- *Acute rejection* is a cell-mediated immune response that occurs within the first few months following the transplant, with the risk decreasing over time. Presentation is variable with some patients remaining asymptomatic while others presenting with dyspnea, worsening pulmonary function, or fevers. CT typically shows basal predominant consolidative and ground-glass opacities with interlobular septal thickening
- *Chronic rejection* sometimes referred to as chronic lung allograft dysfunction is seen in up to 50% of lung transplant patients. Patients present with progressive shortness of breath and worsening respiratory function. Chronic rejection can manifest in two ways: bronchiolitis obliterans and restrictive allograft syndrome
  - Bronchiolitis obliterans is more common and is characterized on CT as mosaic attenuation and air trapping, which are best identified on expiratory phase images (Fig. 19.15). Pulmonary function testing shows a progressive obstructive pattern
  - Restrictive allograft syndrome is characterized on CT as upper lobe predominant fibrosis (Fig. 19.16) with restrictive physiology on pulmonary function testing

Pleural Procedures

Pleurodesis involves the promotion of adhesive pleuritis with the goal of obliterating the potential space within the pleural cavity. It is performed in the setting of recurrent or persistent pneumothoraces or pleural effusions (particularly when malignant). Adhesive pleuritis can be achieved with either mechanical (pleural abrasion) or chemical (e.g., talc, bleomycin, tetracycline, cisplatin) means. Talc particles are hyperdense on CT and typically collect in the pleural space and may appear nodular (Fig. 19.17). *They can be associated with increased FDG uptake on PET and should not be mistaken for malignancy* (Fig. 19.17). Pleural thickening and residual loculated pleural fluid are common after pleurodesis.

Pleurectomy refers to the resection of either only the parietal pleura (partial) or both the parietal and visceral pleura (complete).

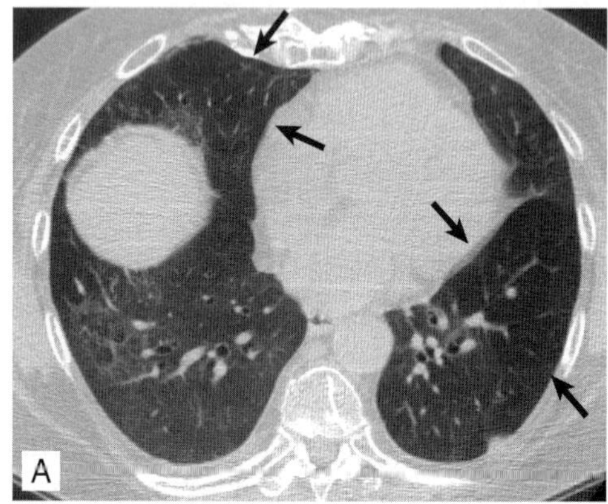

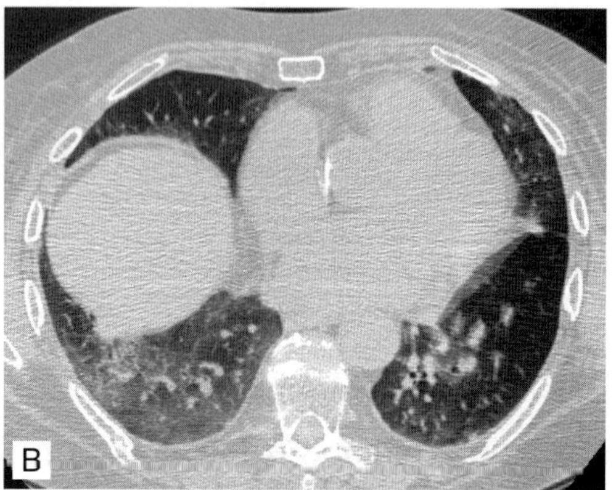

Figure 19.15 Lung transplantation complicated by bronchiolitis obliterans. (A) Axial chest CT shows mosaic attenuation of the lung parenchyma with geographic lucent areas, particularly in the left lower and right middle lobes (*arrows*). There is also bronchiectasis in the lower lobes. (B) Expiratory phase CT image shows accentuation of the lucent areas consistent with air trapping seen with bronchiolitis obliterans.

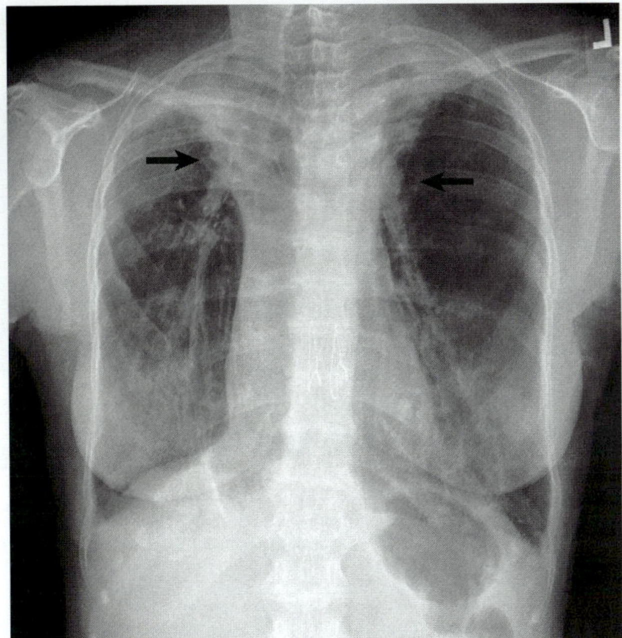

Figure 19.16 Chronic lung allograft dysfunction manifesting as restrictive allograft syndrome (RAS). Chest radiograph shows clamshell sternotomy wires and bilateral lung transplantation with fibrotic changes to the upper lobes with significant volume loss rand superior retraction of the bilateral hila (*arrows*). Patient had worsening pulmonary function consistent with RAS.

It is performed in select patients with mesothelioma or in the setting of fibrothorax or empyema. Decortication involves surgical removal of fibrous material along the pleura and pleural space. It may be indicated in the setting of failed percutaneous drainage of empyema or organized hemothorax.

Open pleural drainage is the surgical creation of a fistulous connection between the pleural space and the skin, mostly indicated in patients with chronic empyema, traditionally tuberculous in nature [25]. The most common type is an Eloesser flap, which consists of a U-shaped incision through the skin and chest wall muscles, resection of a section on the subjacent ribs, and inward folding of the musculocutaneous flap into the pleural space and fixation to the parietal pleura. CXR and CT show the chest wall defect from the flap creation and CT can readily show the direct connection between the pleural space and skin surface (Fig. 19.18).

Esophagectomy

Esophagectomy is the resection of a part of the esophagus typically to treat benign and malignant tumors and other non-neoplastic processes such as achalasia, corrosive injuries, esophageal strictures, and esophageal perforations. The resected esophageal segment is replaced by a conduit, either the stomach or a segment of the bowel (colon or jejunum). On CXR, the mediastinal silhouette may be widened resulting from the conduit (Fig. 19.19), which may be distended with fluid, air, or a combination thereof. XR, CT, and esophagography play important roles in defining the anatomy of the conduit (if unknown) and in assessing for complications.

Potential complications following esophagectomy include [26,27]:

- Anastomotic leak
- Mediastinitis
- Esophagopleural fistula (Fig. 19.20)
- Anastomotic stricture

Anastomotic leaks usually occur within 10 days of surgery and have been reported to occur in as many as 40% of patients. Small leaks may be subclinical and asymptomatic but can be potentially fatal due to resultant infection and sepsis. Anastomotic leaks are best detected with esophagography, initially using water-soluble contrast. If large leaks are absent, barium may be used to detect more subtle leaks. CT with oral contrast can also demonstrate extraluminal contrast and helps assess for complications such as mediastinitis and abscess formation.

Esophagopleural fistulas are reported in the setting of anastomotic leaks. Initial treatment involves antibiotics and percutaneous drainage, but ultimately surgical repair is required. CXR may show increasing pleural effusion or new air-fluid levels in the pleural space. CT can readily demonstrate the extension of oral contrast into the pleural space (Fig. 19.20) and can also assess the presence of empyema.

Anastomotic strictures can also result from technical complications or from wound healing in the early postoperative setting. Delayed strictures typically result from prior anastomotic leaks, infections, or local tumor recurrence. Esophagography and CT can show esophageal dilation and a transition point at the level of the anastomosis.

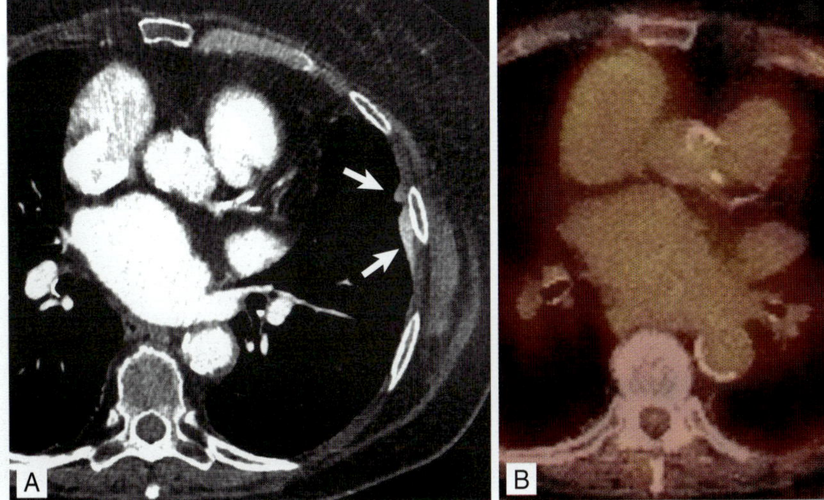

Figure 19.17 Talc pleurodesis. (A) Axial chest CT shows hyperdense material in the left lateral pleural space (*arrows*) in a patient with history of malignant pleural effusion treated with talc pleurodesis. (B) Corresponding PET/CT image shows uptake in the same location, which is expected in the setting of pleurodesis.

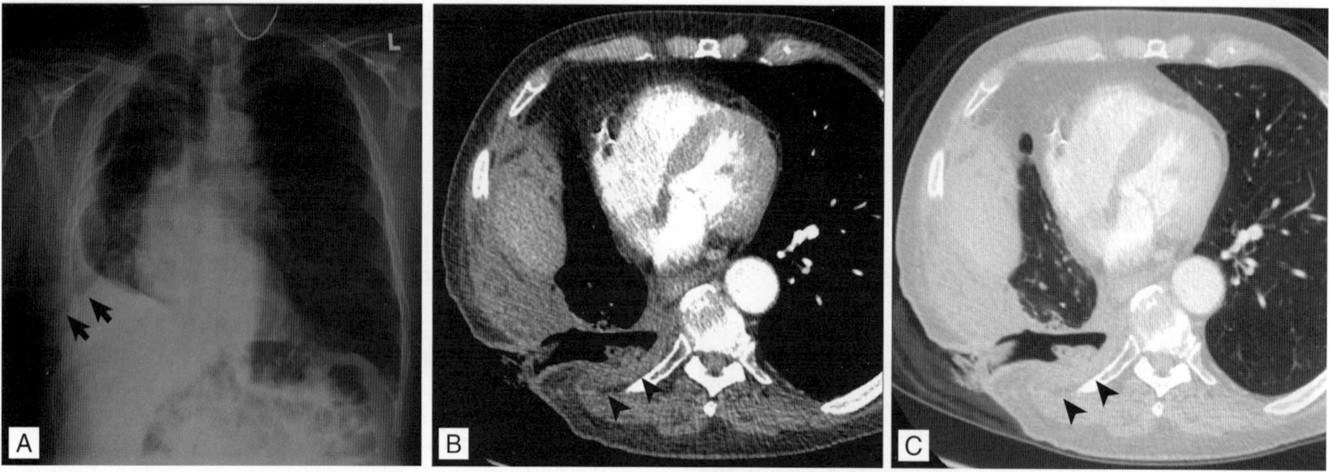

Figure 19.18 Eloesser flap. (A) Chest radiograph shows typical finding of an Eloesser flap, including chest wall soft tissue defect (which appears as a linear lucency, *arrows*) and partial resection of subjacent ribs. Axial chest CT images (B) soft tissue and (C) lung windows show typical soft tissue defect with invagination of the chest wall soft tissue (flap, *arrowheads*) into the pleural space which is now contiguous with surface.

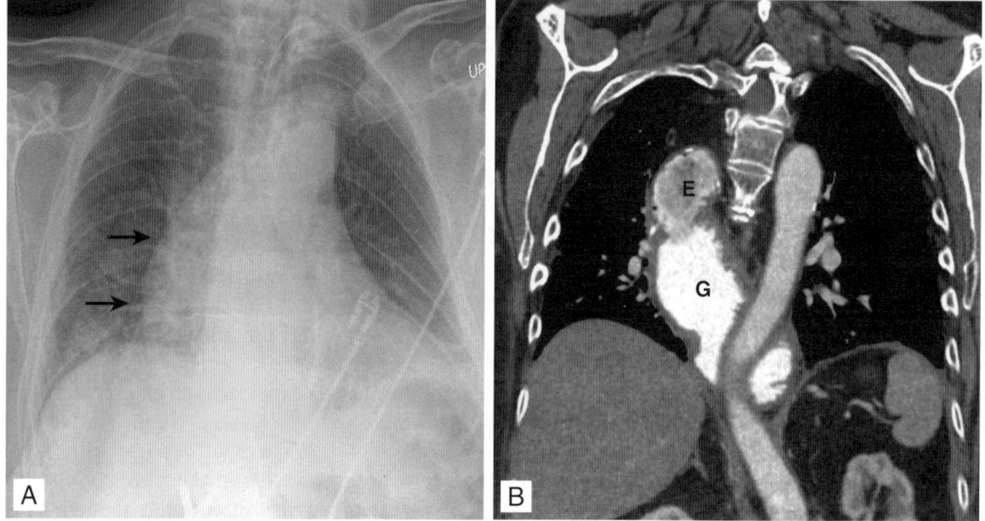

Figure 19.19 Esophageal with gastric pull-through. (A) Chest radiograph shows apparent widening of the cardiomediastinal silhouette with a large tubular structure along the right aspect of the mediastinum corresponding to the gastric conduit (*arrows*). (B) Coronal CT image shows an intrathoracic stomach which is anastomosed with the remaining proximal esophagus. There is free flow of contrast and other ingested material between the esophagus (E) and gastric conduit (G).

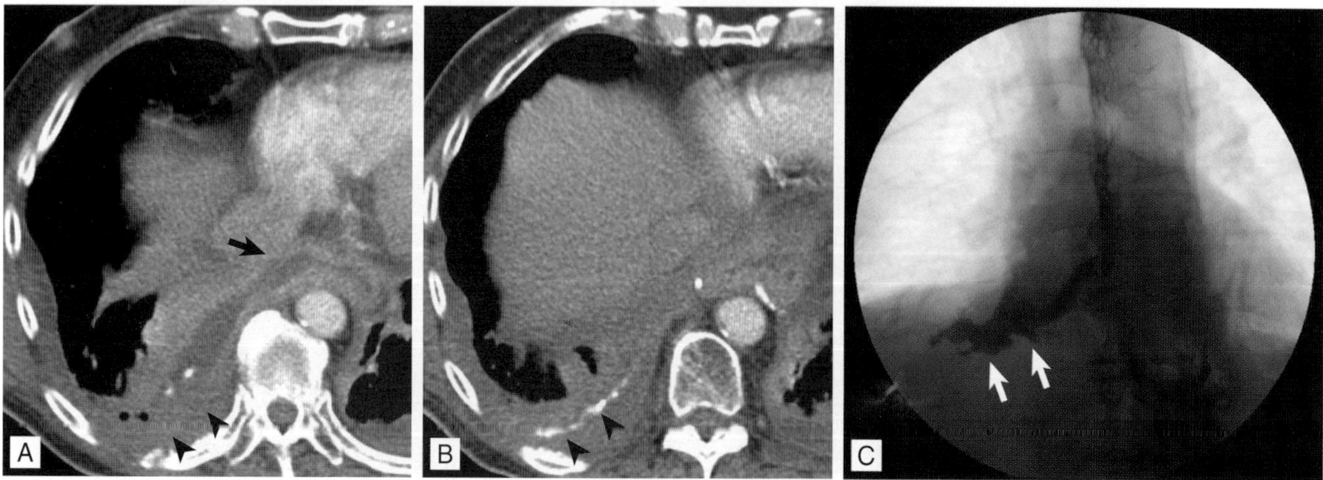

Figure 19.20 Esophagopleural fistula following esophagectomy and gastric pull through. (A) Axial CT image shows apparent focal defect along the right lateral aspect of the gastric conduit (*arrows*), which is contiguous with the pleural space (*arrowheads*). (B) Axial CT image more inferiorly shows oral contrast (*arrowheads*) layering in the pleural space. (C) Contrast esophagogram shows free flow of ingested oral contrast into the right pleural space.

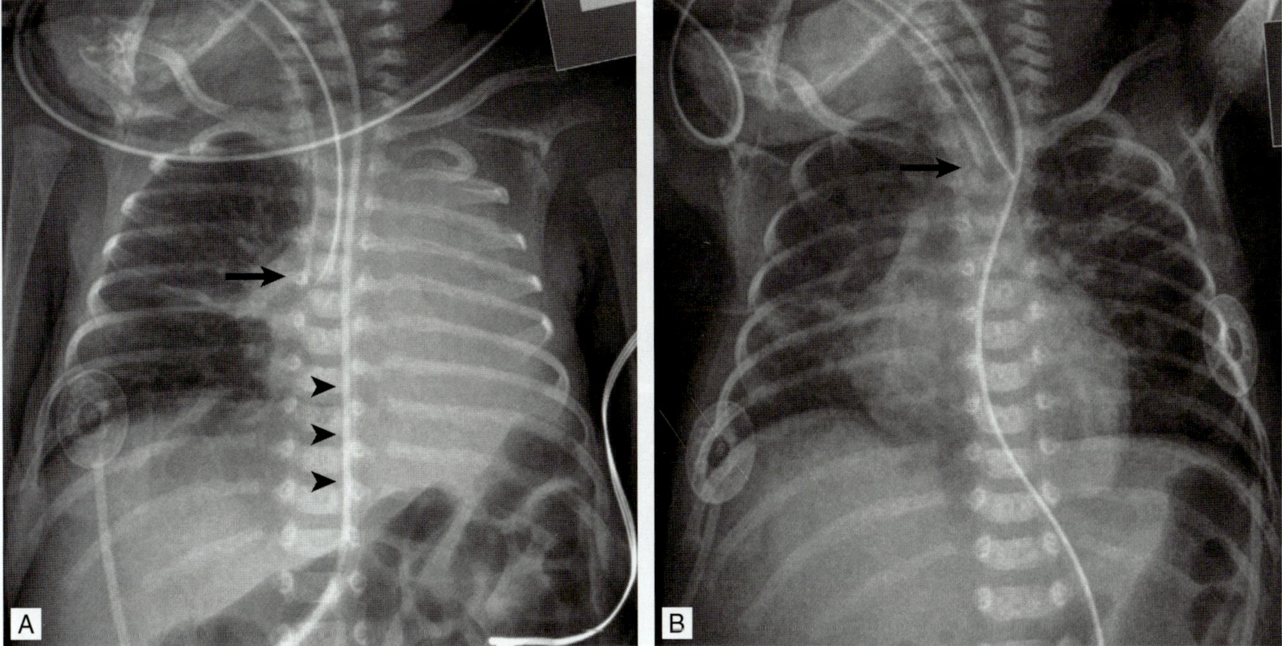

Figure 19.21 Bronchial placement of endotracheal tube. (A) Frontal chest radiograph shows the endotracheal tube terminating in the right mainstem bronchus (*arrow*) resulting in complete opacification of the left hemithorax due to left lung atelectasis. There is also an enteric tube (*arrowheads*) extending into the stomach. (B) Subsequent chest radiograph shows interval retraction of the endotracheal tube, which is now in the trachea, with improved ventilation of the left lung.

Thoracic Lines, Tubes, and Devices

CXRs play an essential role in the assessment of lines, tubes, and other thoracic devices to ensure their proper positioning and function and to assess any complications related to their placement or malpositioning [28,29]. Common devices assessed with CXR include those related to

- mechanical ventilation,
- central venous access,
- hemodynamic monitoring and support,
- pleural drainage, and
- nutrition, among others.

Airway Tubes

Endotracheal (ET) intubation is commonly employed in patients who require mechanical ventilation either due to respiratory failure or due to the inability to protect the airway adequately. Ideally, the tip of the ET tube should be 3–7 cm from the carina with the neck in the neutral position. Notably, the ET tube can be displaced up to 2 cm cephalad or caudal with neck extension or flexion, respectively. High placement of the ET tube places the patient at risk of accidental extubation or injury to the vocal cords by the inflated cuff, while low placement can lead to bronchial intubation. Bronchial intubation can lead to lobar or complete lung atelectasis of the nonintubated lung (Fig. 19.21).

Occasionally, a double-lumen ET tube may be used in cases requiring anatomic lung isolation. For example, this may be employed during surgery when controlled ventilation of one lung is necessary, in the setting of unilateral lung lavage, or in the setting of severe unilateral pulmonary hemorrhage or infection to protect the unaffected lung.

Tracheostomy tubes are placed in patients who require long-term mechanical ventilation. An appropriately placed tracheostomy tube has its tip approximately a third or halfway between the stoma and the carina. Unlike an ET tube, a properly secured tracheostomy tube typically does not change in position with head motion.

Long-term intubation or tracheostomy tube placement can be complicated by the erosion of the tracheal wall and in some instances the development of tracheoesophageal fistulas [30]. These can also result from overinflation of the ET tube or tracheostomy tube cuff resulting in distention of the tracheal wall and ischemia.

Central Venous Catheters

Central venous catheters (CVCs) are commonly used for the administration of fluids, medications, and nutrition, for hemodialysis, and for central venous pressure monitoring. Broadly, CVCs can be categorized as peripherally inserted central catheters, nontunneled CVC, tunneled CVC, and implantable ports.

The desired positioning of the distal tip of the CVC is typically the lower superior vena cava (SVC) or at the junction of the SVC and right atrium (i.e., superior cavoatrial junction). The tip may also be positioned in the high right atrium to improve blood flow, as in the case of dialysis catheters. There is an increased risk for arrhythmias and cardiac injuries when the catheter is placed too low into the right atrium.

CXR is routinely obtained following placement of CVC to ensure proper positioning and exclude complications. Detailed knowledge of the thoracic vascular anatomy as well as variants is critical to the detection of a malpositioned line [31]. Radiographic landmarks may help identify the location of the catheter tip. In most patients, the first intercoastal space approximates the cranial aspect of the SVC, although some patients may have a relatively short SVC with a lower confluence of the brachiocephalic veins. The superior cavoatrial junction is approximately where the lower border of the bronchus intermedius crosses the right heart border.

The use of radiographic landmarks, however, can be limited by reduced visibility, differences in patient positioning and rotation, and low lung volume technique. Also, it can be challenging to ascertain the precise location of the catheter on CXR as the catheter tip is not fixed and can move several centimeters based on positioning, phase of respiration, and radiographic technique.

Placement of CVC into the small thoracic veins (e.g., azygos internal mammary and superior intercostal veins; Fig. 19.22) can lead to catheter malfunction and carries the risk for venous thrombosis and venous perforation. Arterial placement of a CVC

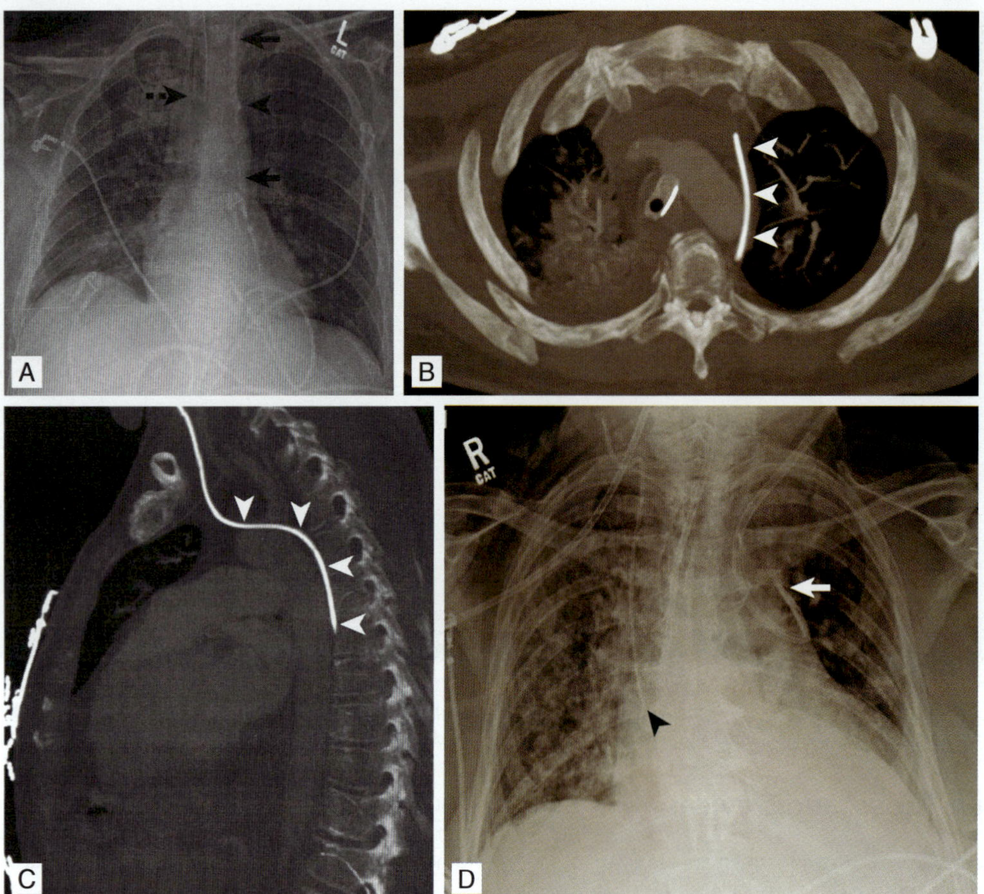

Figure 19.22 Malpositioned central lines. (A) Chest radiograph shows a left internal jugular vein approach central venous catheter coursing along the left mediastinum (*straight, solid arrows*) adjacent to the descending thoracic aorta. Note the apparent kinking of the catheter at the level of the aortic aortic arch (*arrowhead*). (B) Axial and (C) sagittal maximum intensity projection images demonstrate the course of the central venous catheter to the left of the aortic arch and posterior to the descending aorta (*arrowheads*), corresponding to the course of the left superior intercostal vein. (D) Chest radiograph of a different patient shows a right internal jugular (IJ) vein approach central venous catheter with its tip appropriately near the expected superior cavoatrial junction (*arrowhead*). A left IJ approach dialysis catheter has an abnormal course and is pointed cephalad and determined to be extravascular in location (*arrow*).

carries the risk of bleeding, air or thrombotic embolization resulting in a stroke, and inappropriate arterial infusion of medications (e.g., pressors) and other substances (e.g., parenteral nutrition). Extravascular placement can also occur (Fig. 19.22).

Other complications of CVC placement include pneumothorax, mediastinal hematoma, mediastinitis particularly with extravascular placement, catheter-associated thrombosis, and catheter-related bloodstream infections with potential for sepsis, endocarditis, and septic emboli. CVC may also fracture and migrate. Fragmentation from compression between the first rib and clavicle is termed as "pinch-off syndrome."

Pulmonary Artery Catheter

A pulmonary artery catheter (PAC) is a balloon-tipped catheter that allows for the measurement of pulmonary arterial, central venous, and pulmonary capillary wedge pressures (an indirect measurement of the left atrial pressure). This is employed in the monitoring of critically ill patients, providing information regarding volume status and may elucidate etiology of hypotension. With the balloon uninflated, the ideal location of the distal tip of the PAC is past the pulmonic valve and within the right or left pulmonary artery but no further than the proximal right interlobar of the proximal left descending pulmonary artery. The PAC tip migrates to its "wedge" position once the balloon is inflated.

Catheters that are placed too distally can result in pulmonary arterial occlusion and infarction. Pulmonary arterial injury in the form of a pseudoaneurysm or perforation can also occur (Fig. 19.23).

Pleural Drains

Pleural drains are frequently used to evacuate pleural effusion, pneumothorax, hemothorax, or empyema. Proper positioning is dependent on the type and location of pleural collection being drained. In general, apical and anterior positioning is preferred for the treatment of pneumothoraces, while basal and posterior positioning is preferred for layering pleural fluid. The desired positioning may vary in cases of loculated collections. For surgical chest tubes, the proximal-most side hole (identified on CXR as a focal discontinuity) should be within the pleural space (Fig. 19.24). A side hole outside the pleural space can lead to an air leak and ineffective drainage.

Enteric Tubes

Enteric tubes, most commonly nasogastric tubes and orogastric tubes, are frequently placed for administration of medications, nutritional support, and gastric decompression. Proper placement of orogastric tubes and nasogastric tubes is within the stomach with the distal tip and side hole past the esophagogastric junction.

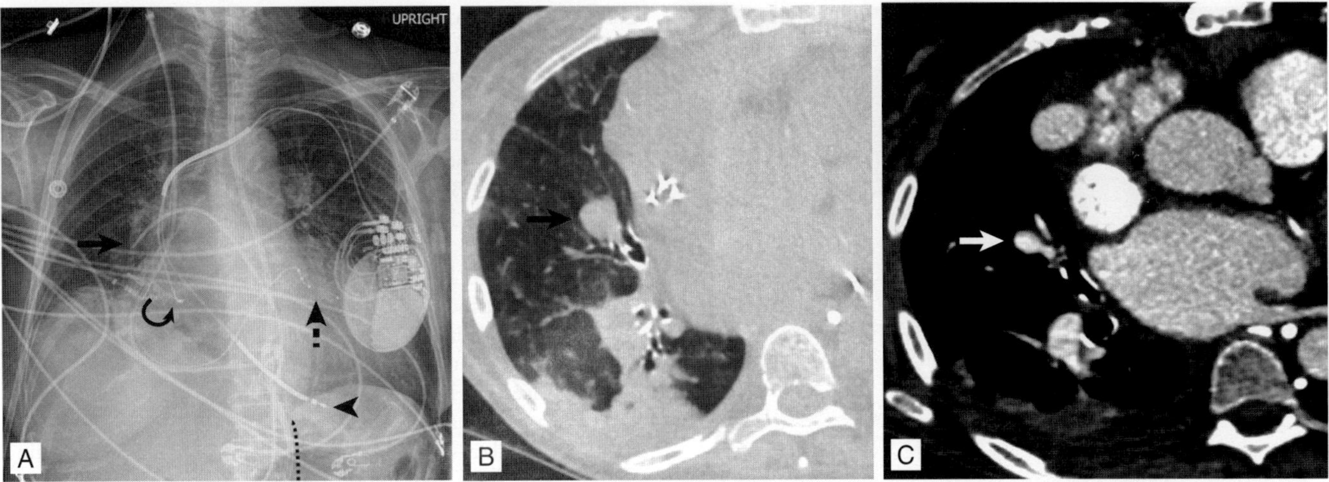

Figure 19.23 Pulmonary artery pseudoaneurysm secondary to pulmonary artery catheter placement. (A) Frontal chest radiograph shows a right internal jugular vein approach pulmonary artery catheter with tip deep in the right hilum (*straight, solid arrow*). A cardiac resynchronization therapy-defibrillator (CRT-D) device has its leads in the expected right atrium (*curved arrow*), right ventricle (*arrowhead*), and coronary sinus tributary (*dashed arrow*). An enteric tube (*dashed line*) is seen coursing below the diaphragm into the stomach. (B) Axial chest CT without contrast shows a right perihilar nodular opacity in the right middle lobe (*arrow*). (C) Subsequent contrast-enhanced chest CT confirmed a pseudoaneurysm (*arrow*) of the right middle lobe lateral segmental pulmonary artery.

Tubes used solely for feeding (not for suction) are smaller, more flexible, and commonly have a weighted tip. These are ideally placed in the postpyloric region in the second portion of the duodenum to minimize the buildup of tube feeds in the stomach, which can lead to aspiration. Gastric or duodenal placement, however, may be acceptable in some patients. Placement into the proximal jejunum, past the ligament of Treitz, may be appropriate in patients in whom the duodenum needs to be bypassed (e.g., in the setting of pancreatitis).

Enteric tubes may be inadvertently placed in the tracheobronchial tree (Fig. 19.25). In which case, immediate removal and CXR follow-up are indicated as it can result in a pneumothorax. Tubes may also be coiled within the oropharynx and esophagus requiring repositioning. Rarely, insertion may result in injury to the esophagus or stomach. In these cases, CXR may show pneumomediastinum, pneumoperitoneum, or pleural effusions.

Circulatory Assist Devices

Intra-aortic balloon pump (IABP) is a temporary assist device that provides circulatory support in the setting of cardiogenic shock. It works by inflating during diastole, increasing diastolic pressure, and improving coronary perfusion leading to improved cardiac output, and

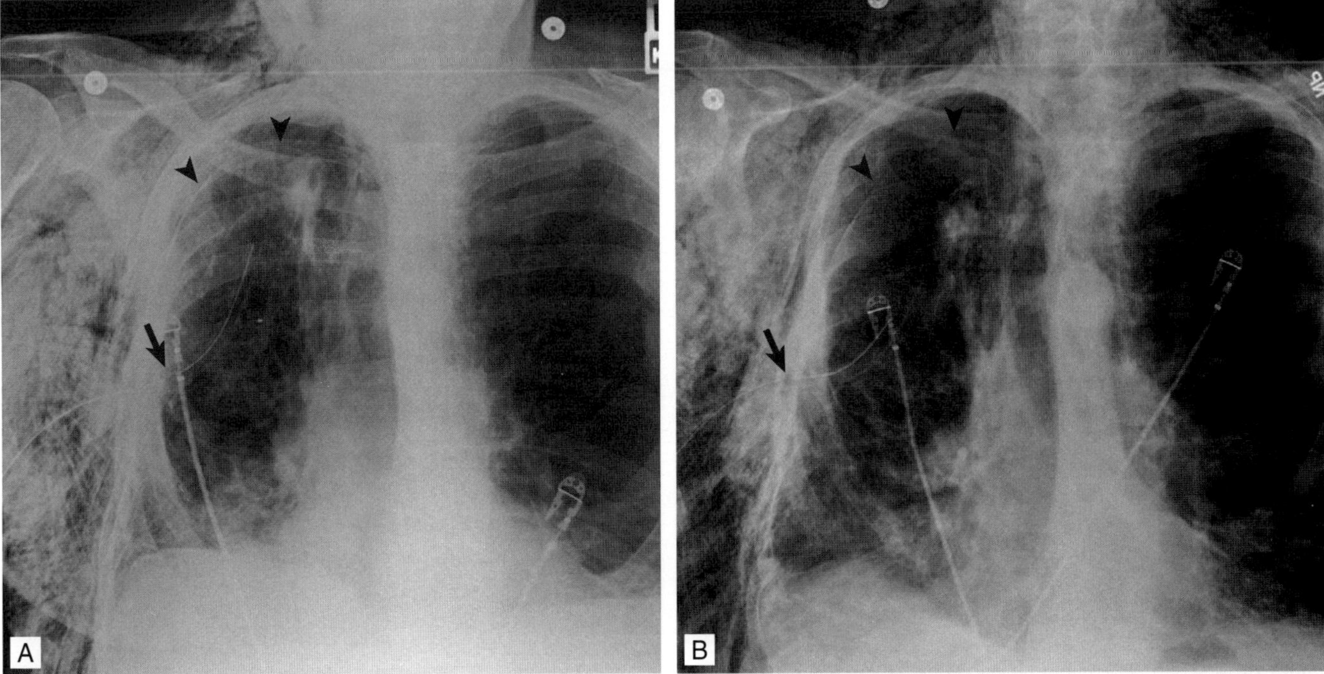

Figure 19.24 Chest tube placement for pneumothorax. (A) Frontal chest radiograph shows a chest tube in the right pleural space extending toward the apex. Note the thin radiopaque line marking the chest tube and the discontinuity of the marker (*arrow*) indicating the proximal-most chest tube hole. There is a small right apical pneumothorax (*arrowheads*) and subcutaneous emphysema along the right chest wall and supraclavicular fossa. (B) Follow-up chest radiograph the next day shows the proximal-most chest tube hole in the chest wall (*arrow*) outside the pleural space. There is an increase in size of the pneumothorax (*arrowheads*) and increased extent of extensive subcutaneous emphysema.

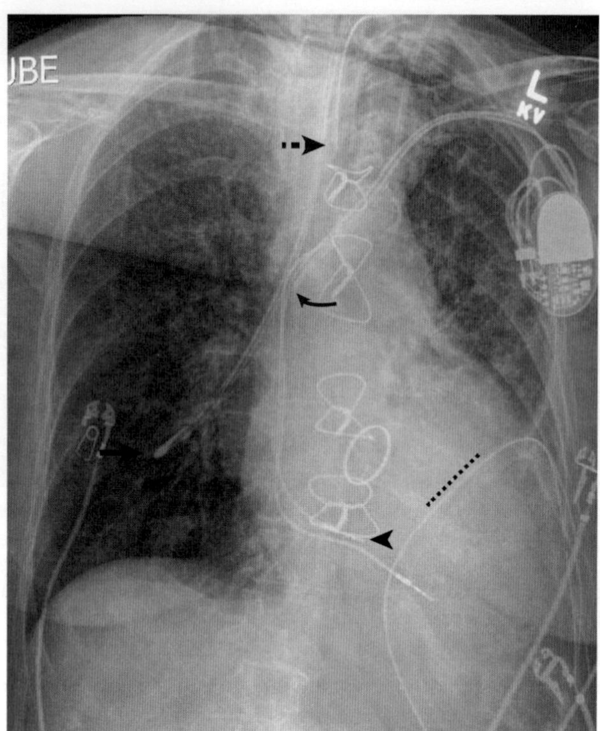

Figure 19.25 Endobronchial placement of an enteric tube. Chest radiograph shows an enteric tube inadvertently placed in the trachea, extending into the right lower lobe (*straight, solid arrow*). Also present are: tracheostomy tube in the mid thoracic trachea (*dashed arrow*), a left internal jugular vein approach central venous catheter with tip overlying the left brachiocephalic vein (*curved arrow*), and a left basilar chest tube (*dashed line*). The patient has a dual chamber pacemaker with the atrial lead dislodged inferiorly, extending toward the level of the tricuspid valve (*arrowhead*).

by deflating during systole, decreasing afterload, and decreasing left ventricular work. The IABP is usually placed through the femoral artery and advanced retrograde into the descending thoracic aorta distal to the origin of the left subclavian artery, approximately 2 cm below the superior aspect of the aortic arch. High IABP placement (Fig. 19.26) risks injury to the aortic arch and injury to or occlusion of the arch vessels. Low placement may result in ineffective counterpulsion and risks injury or intermittent occlusion of major abdominal aortic branches such as the superior mesenteric artery or renal arteries.

Left ventricular assist device (LVAD) is a mechanical pump used to augment or replace the left ventricular function in the setting of late cardiac failure [32]. It is used as a bridge to cardiac transplant or as a last resort for those ineligible for transplantation ("destination therapy"). There are a variety of LVAD models available. In general, in surgically placed LVAD, blood from the left ventricle is diverted into the LVAD (either through an inflow cannula placed into the left ventricle or directly into the LVAD placed at the left ventricular apex) and is pumped into the aorta via an outflow cannula (Fig. 19.27). An Impella device (Fig. 19.28) is a percutaneously inserted, transcatheter LVAD advanced in a retrograde fashion into the left ventricle, typically via the axillary or femoral artery. The device works by diverting and pumping blood from the left ventricle into the aorta. Complications of LVAD include bleeding, thrombus formations, obstruction of either the inflow or outflow cannula and infection.

Right ventricular assist devices are less commonly used and are indicated in right heart failure. Acute right heart failure can be seen in the setting of myocardial infarction, acute pulmonary embolism, decompensated heart failure, and decompensated pulmonary hypertension. It can also occur in up to 40% of patients following LVAD placement. The mechanics of right ventricular assist devices are similar to that of LVAD, except that blood is diverted from the right ventricle into the main pulmonary artery rather than the left ventricle into the aorta. Potential complications are similar to those of LVAD.

Extracorporeal Life Support

Extracorporeal life support is an overarching term that encompasses both extracorporeal membrane oxygenation (ECMO) and extracorporeal carbon dioxide removal. Extracorporeal life support is increasingly being used in the setting of respiratory and cardiac failure [33].

ECMO, which is more commonly employed, allows for either respiratory gas exchange support (venovenous ECMO; VV-ECMO) or both gas exchange and circulatory support (venoarterial ECMO;

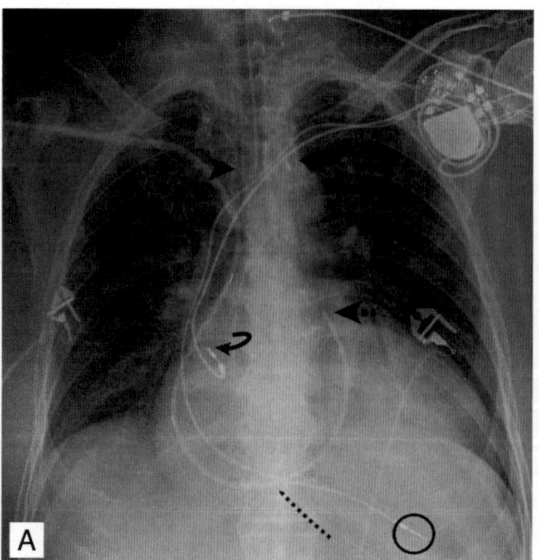

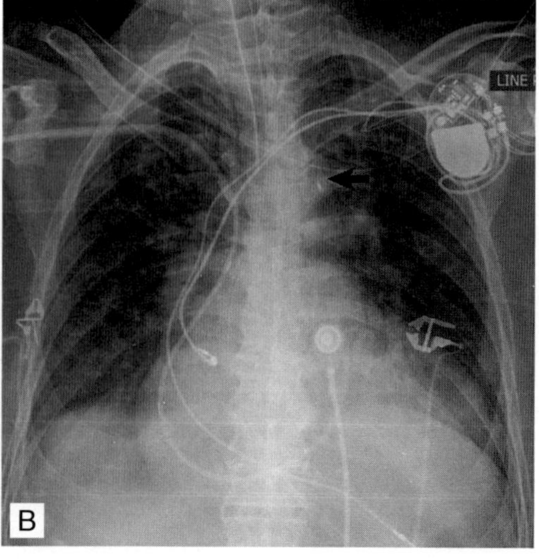

Figure 19.26 High placement of an intra-aortic balloon pump (IABP). (A) Chest radiograph shows an IABP in the descending thoracic aorta with its metallic tip (*solid straight arrow*) extending superior to the aortic arch, likely within the left subclavian artery origin. Other support apparatus includes: an endotracheal tube (*arrowhead*) in the midthoracic trachea; a right subclavian vein approach pulmonary artery catheter with tip overlying the distal main pulmonary artery trunk (*dashed arrow*); an enteric tube is seen coursing below the diaphragm into the stomach (*dashed line*); and a dual chamber pacemaker with right atrial (*curved arrow*) and right ventricular (*circle*) leads. (B) Follow-up chest radiograph shows interval retraction of the IABP, now with the tip a few centimeters below the superior aspect of the aortic arch (*arrow*).

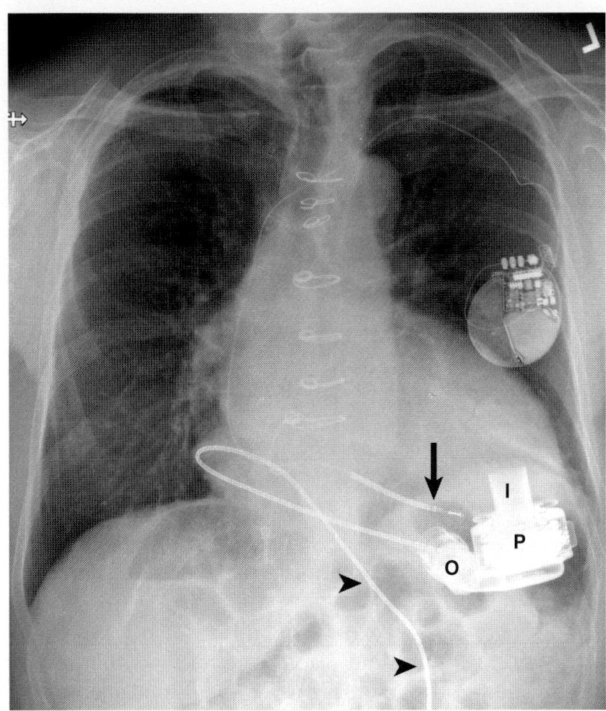

Figure 19.27 Implanted left ventricular assist device (LVAD). An LVAD is seen in the left lower thorax. The inflow conduit (I) is surgically placed into the left ventricular aspect directing blood into the pump (P), which pushes blood through the outflow conduit (O) which is connected to the ascending aorta by a nonradio-opaque graft. The driveline (*arrowheads*) is tracked subcutaneously in the anterior chest and upper abdominal wall and connects to a battery pack and control external to the patient. A left chest AICD is also seen with its lead in the right ventricle (*arrow*).

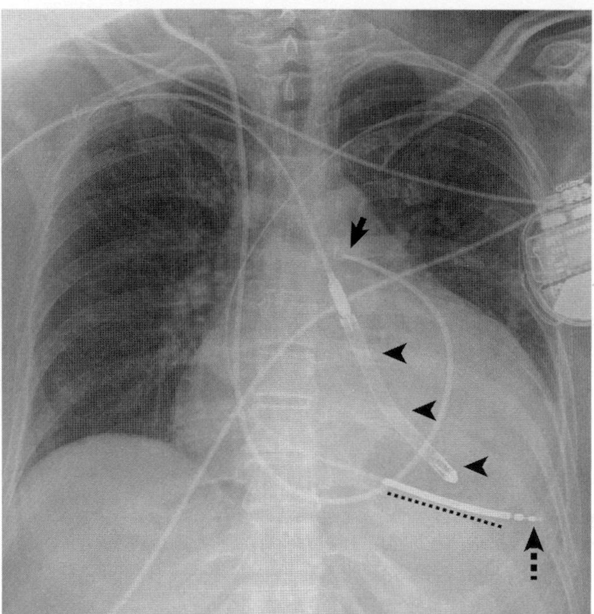

Figure 19.28 Appropriate placement of transcatheter left ventricular assist (Impella) device. The Impella device is placed via a catheter through the right axillary artery and advanced retrograde through the aorta and aortic valve into the left ventricle (*arrowheads*). A right IJ approach pulmonary artery catheter has the tip at the expected level of the distal main pulmonary artery trunk (*solid arrow*). A single chamber automatic implantable cardioverter defibrillators (AICD) has its lead in the expected right ventricle (*dashed arrow*). Note the thick defibrillator coil (*dashed line*) typical of AICD compared to pacemakers.

VA-ECMO). VV-ECMO is used in the setting of respiratory failure as can be seen with acute respiratory distress syndrome, advanced interstitial lung disease, or severe graft dysfunction following lung transplantation and as a bridge to lung transplantation. Depending on the cannula employed, VV-ECMO works by withdrawing deoxygenated blood from a central vein or the right atrium, oxygenating it within the oxygenator, and returning oxygenated blood into a central vein or right atrium (Fig. 19.29).

While VV-ECMO is entirely right-sided and only provides gas exchange support, VA-ECMO can provide both circulatory and respiratory support. It is indicated in the setting of both cardiac and respiratory failure as can be seen with acute massive pulmonary embolism and acute decompensated pulmonary hypertension. In central VA-ECMO, the drainage cannula is placed directly into the right atrium and the return cannula into the ascending aorta. In peripheral VA-ECMO, the drainage cannula is typically placed through the femoral vein and advanced to the level of the inferior cavoatrial junction and the return cannula is placed through the femoral artery to the level of the common iliac artery or the lower abdominal aorta.

Proper placement of the cannula(s) is necessary to ensure proper function. Potential complications of ECMO include pneumothorax, hemorrhage (either related to the cannulation site or due to required anticoagulation therapy), and vascular or cardiac injury.

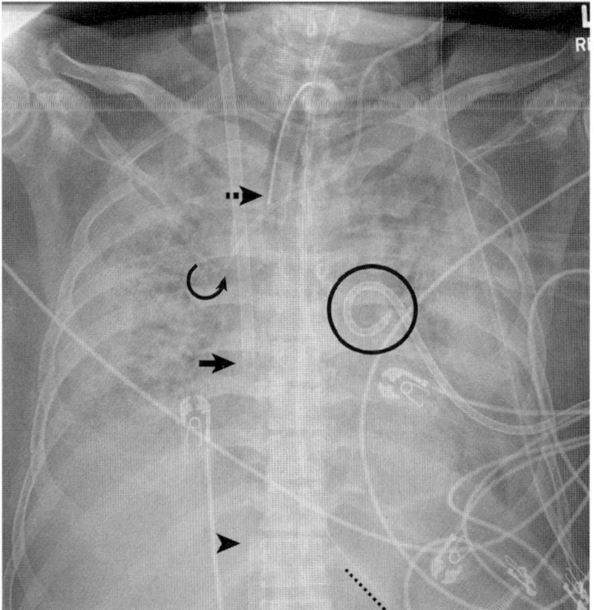

Figure 19.29 Extracorporeal membrane oxygenation (ECMO). Frontal chest radiograph shows a large bore cannula inserted through the right internal jugular (IJ) vein and terminating in the right atrium (*solid straight arrow*). An additional inferior-approach cannula (typically inserted through the femoral vein) is seen terminating in the inferior vena cava (*arrowhead*). These cannulae are typically used for veno-venous ECMO. Additional support apparatus include a tracheostomy tube in the trachea (*dashed arrow*), left IJ central venous catheter terminating in the superior vena cava (*curved arrow*), and a pigtail drainage catheter in the left pleural space (*circle*).

Cardiac Conduction Devices

Cardiac pacemakers are used to treat a variety of cardiac conduction abnormalities such as heart blocks, symptomatic bradycardias, and tachyarrhythmias. A temporary pacing lead may be

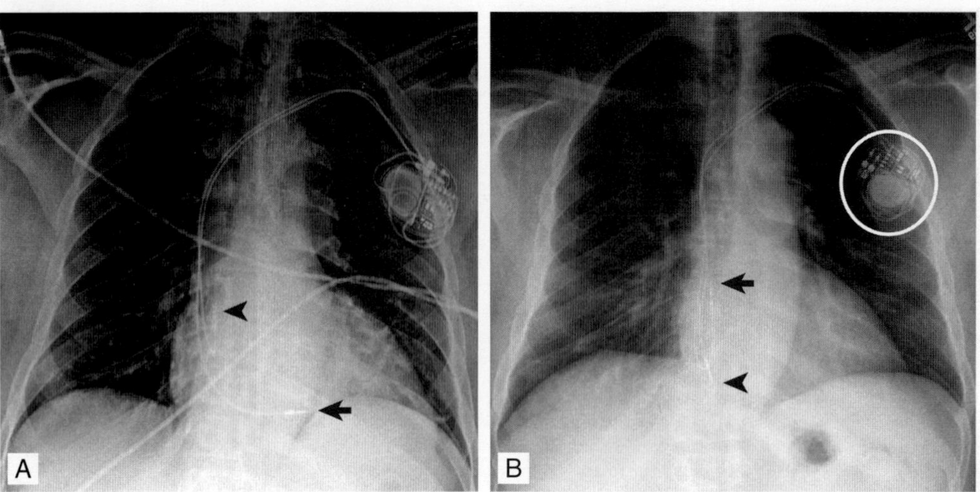

Figure 19.30 Dual chamber pacemaker and Twiddler's syndrome. (A) Chest radiograph shows appropriate positioning of the right atrial (*arrowhead*) and right ventricular (*arrow*) leads. (B) Chest radiograph obtained a month later showed interval retraction of the right atrial (*arrowhead*) and ventricular (*arrow*) leads. Note interval change in orientation of the pacemaker generator and increased coiling of wires around it (*circle*), consistent with "Twiddler's syndrome."

placed percutaneously, into the internal jugular or subclavian vein with the tip placed within the region of the right ventricular apex. This is used as a bridge in urgent or emergent cases until a permanent pacemaker can be placed.

There are several types of permanent pacemakers, which are selected based on the pathology being treated and can be placed via a transvenous, epicardial, or subxiphoid approach. A single chamber pacemaker usually has the lead in the right ventricle with the tip projecting into the apex. Dual chamber pacemakers typically have a second lead in the right atrium that is often turned cephalad into the right atrial appendage (Fig. 19.30). A similar placement is expected in single lead permanent pacemakers. A biventricular pacemaker is used for chronic resynchronization therapy to improve the synchronized contraction of the ventricles. This device has a third lead placed epicardially within the coronary sinus into a tributary (Fig. 19.23). An implantable cardioverter defibrillator can be combined with pacemakers with a similar placement of the leads. Characteristically, thick shock coils are seen along the right ventricular lead at the levels of the SVC or brachiocephalic vein and in the right ventricle (Fig. 19.23).

Potential complications of a pacemaker or implantable cardioverter defibrillator placement include pneumothorax, hemothorax, vascular or cardiac injury and hemopericardium, and lead malpositioning. The leads may also be dislodged, which usually happens shortly after placement before the development of fibrosis, which can hold the lead in place. Leads may also become displaced with the placement of other central lines or PACs (Fig. 19.31). Other potential complications include lead fracture,

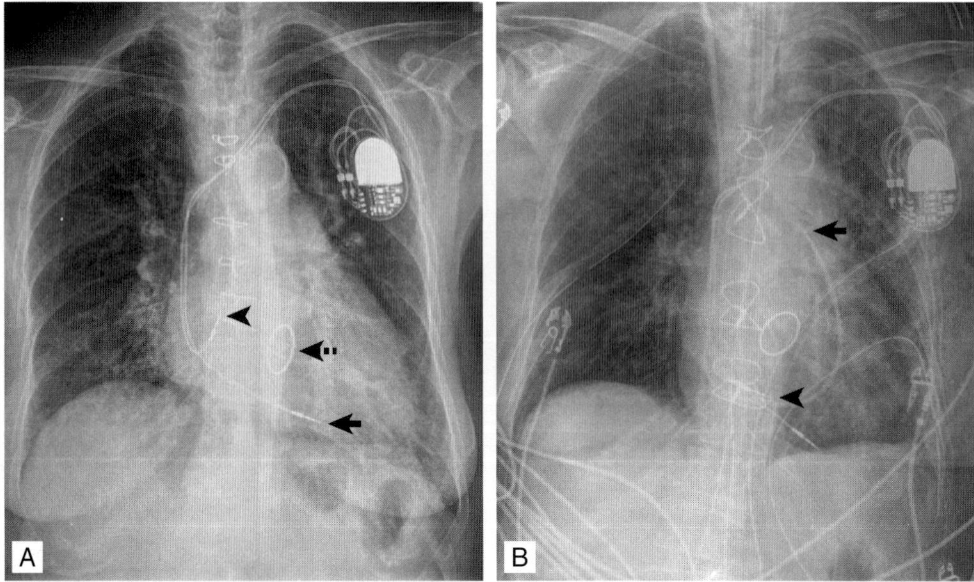

Figure 19.31 Dual chamber pacemaker lead displacement. (A) Preoperative chest radiograph shows a left chest dual chamber pacemaker with leads in the right atrium (*arrowhead*) and right ventricle (*arrow*). The patient has had prior median sternotomy and aortic valve replacement (*dashed arrow*). (B) Postoperative chest radiograph following coronary artery bypass grafting shows interval displacement of the right atrial lead (*arrowhead*), now projecting to the level of the tricuspid valve. This is likely secondary to placement of the pulmonary artery catheter (*arrow*). Endotracheal tube, enteric tube, and bilateral and midline chest tubes are in their expected location.

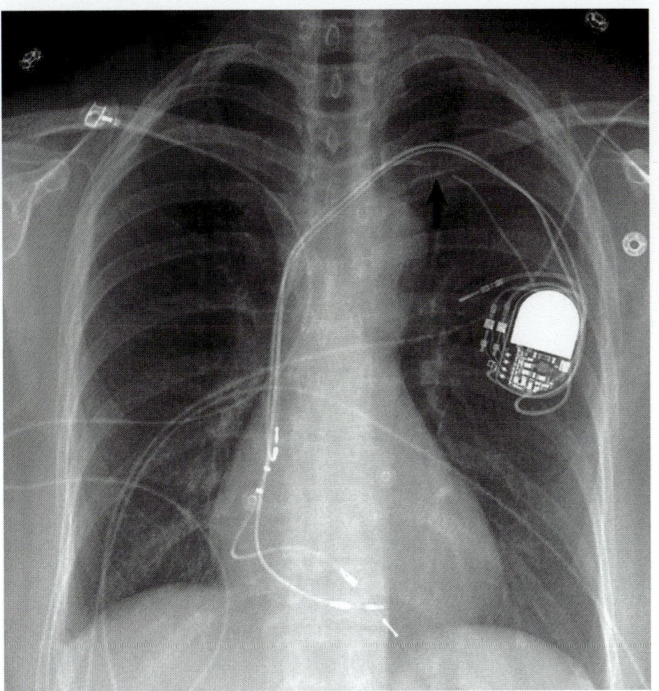

Figure 19.32 Pacemaker lead fracture. A dual chamber pacemaker has leads in the right atrium and right ventricle. One of the ventricular leads is fractured at the level of the clavicle and first rib (*arrow*), a common site of lead fracture due to compression between the two bones.

classically at the level of the brachiocephalic vein as it courses between the clavicle and first rib (Fig. 19.32). "Twiddler syndrome" results in dislodgement and coiling of the leads in the chest wall (Fig. 19.30) in patients who constantly manipulate the pulse generator.

Suggested Readings

- SR Digumarthy, PK Shukla, DP Mendoza, L Guo, YR Chretien, J-AO Shepard, et al., Postoperative imaging after lobectomy: predicting the displacement and change in orientation of nonresected lung nodules, J Comput Assist Tomogr 43 (4) (2019 Aug) 592–598.
- MCB Godoy, BS Leitman, PM de Groot, I Vlahos, DP Naidich, Chest radiography in the ICU: part 1, evaluation of airway, enteric, and pleural tubes, AJR Am J Roentgenol 198 (3) (2012 Mar) 563–571.
- MCB Godoy, BS Leitman, PM de Groot, I Vlahos, DP Naidich, Chest radiography in the ICU: part 2, evaluation of cardiovascular lines and other devices, AJR Am J Roentgenol 198 (3) (2012 Mar) 572–581.
- YL Ng, N Paul, D Patsios, A Walsham, T-B Chung, S Keshavjee, et al., Imaging of lung transplantation: review, AJR Am J Roentgenol 192 (3 Suppl) (2009 Mar) S1-S13, quiz S14–S19.
- SE Zinck, SL Primack, Radiographic and CT findings in blunt chest trauma, J Thorac Imaging 15 (2) (2000 Apr) 87–96.

20 Normal Heart

AMNA ZAFAR, SUMIT GUPTA

Introduction

The heart lies in the anterior mediastinum immediately posterior to the sternum and is closely related to the central portion of the diaphragm. The apex of the heart is normally orientated downward and leftward but there is considerable variation in the orientation according to the build of an individual patient. In tall slim individuals, particularly those with hyperinflated lungs, there is a very vertical orientation to the heart, whereas in patients with a short, wide build, and poor air entry there will be a much more horizontal orientation of the ventricular mass. The orientation of the heart is governed very much by surrounding structures as well as the intrinsic anatomy and differential chamber enlargement will often change the alignment of the heart. The normal position of the heart, with the apex pointed to the left, is classified as levocardia. When the majority of the heart mass is in the right hemithorax, and the base to apex axis is directed to the right, the patient is said to have dextrocardia [1]. There are two main types of dextrocardia: (i) dextrocardia of embryonic arrest (or isolated dextrocardia): the heart is placed further right in the thorax than is normal, and (ii) dextrocardia with situs inversus: the heart is a mirror image of the normal position on the left [1]. Caution is advised not to confuse dextrocardia with dextroversion where the majority of the heart mass is in the right hemithorax with the apex pointed toward the left. When the heart resides in the midline, with no apparent apex on a frontal chest radiograph, then the patient is said to have mesocardia [2].

The conventional terms of anterior, posterior, superior, and inferior are not used in exactly the same way with anatomical descriptions of the heart due to the oblique orientation of the heart within the thorax. For instance, the right ventricle (RV) is not situated entirely on the right, but more anterior and the left ventricle (LV) is situated more posterior. Cardiac axes (imaging planes) are used for accurate and consistent description of cardiac anatomy using all imaging techniques including nuclear imaging, coronary computed tomography angiography, magnetic resonance imaging (MRI), and echocardiography. The most commonly employed cardiac imaging planes are (i) *Vertical long-axis (two-chamber) view*: para-sagittal plane oriented along the long axis of the left ventricular lumen depicting left atrium and LV; (ii) *Horizontal long-axis (four-chamber) view*: plane bisecting all four chambers of the heart depicting both atria and both ventricles; (iii) *Three-chamber view*: oblique long axis view depicting left atrium, LV, and aortic root; (iv) *Short-axis view*: oblique coronal plane that is perpendicular to the vertical long axis view.

Pericardium

The pericardium is a thin membrane surrounding the heart and the origin of the great vessels. It is composed of two layers, outer fibrous layer and inner serous layer. The inner serous layer is further divided into two more layers, an outer parietal layer and inner visceral layer. The parietal pericardium is a thin layer lining the fibrous pericardial sac and the visceral pericardium is a thin layer over the surface of the heart itself. Normal pericardium measures 2 mm or less in thickness based on measurements made on computed tomography (CT) and MRI (Figs. 20.1 and 20.2) [3,4]. Pericardial anatomy is discussed in greater detail in a separate chapter.

Cardiac Chambers

The heart has four chambers, two atria and two ventricles. The atria and ventricles are separated by atrioventricular valves. Fibrous interatrial septum separates the two atria and the muscular interventricular septum separates the two ventricles. The right and left atrioventricular grooves (coronary grooves) demarcate the underlying atria from the ventricles. Anterior and posterior interventricular

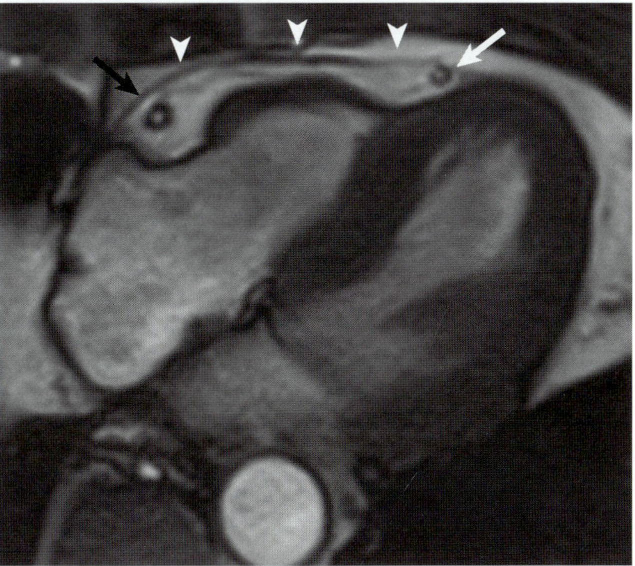

Figure 20.1 Axial steady state free precession (SSFP) cardiac magnetic resonance image showing normal thin pericardium (*arrowheads*) along the free wall of the right ventricle. Right (*black arrow*) and left anterior descending (*white arrow*) coronary arteries are also seen.

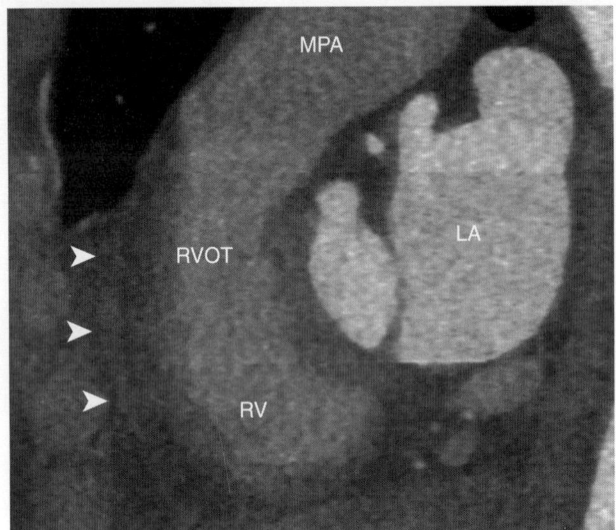

Figure 20.2 Sagittal coronary computed tomography angiography image showing normal thin pericardium (*arrowheads*) anterior to the right ventricular (RV) free wall and right ventricular outflow tract (RVOT). *LA*, Left atrium; *MPA*, main pulmonary artery.

groove demarcate the underlying right and left ventricle. At the posterior aspect of the heart, the junction of the posterior interventricular groove with the right and left atrioventricular groove is called the crux of the heart (crux cordis). The right atrioventricular groove is inferior compared to the left due to inferior position of the septal leaflet of the tricuspid valve. In the anatomical position, the LV forms the apex of the heart.

Atria

Right Atrium

The atria are divided into several components: venous component, vestibule of the atrioventricular valve, septal component, and appendage. Embryologically venous component is derived from the sinus venosus, while appendage comes from the primitive auricle. Crista terminalis (Fig. 20.3A and B) which is a remnant of the embryologic vein of the sinus venosus separates the anterior trabeculated appendage from the posterior smooth-walled portion of the right atrium. The right atrial appendage (RAA) is a triangular and broad-based structure seen extending into the free wall of the atrial chamber. Pectinate muscles (Fig. 20.4) which branch at a right angle to the crista terminalis are seen as linear filling defects in the RAA on contrast-enhanced cross-sectional studies. The superior vena cava drains into the right atrium immediately posterior to the RAA and the inferior vena cava drains into the floor of the right atrium, passing for a short distance through the pericardium before entering the atrium.

The smooth-walled vestibule incorporates the attachments for the tricuspid valve. Just below the interatrial septum and close to the tricuspid valve lies the opening of the coronary sinus that drains into the right atrium. There is frequently a fibrous fold lying between the inflow of the inferior vena cava and the tricuspid valve; this is known as the eustachian valve (Fig. 20.5). Frequently this valve extends into the right atrial chamber as a collection of mobile fronds known as the Chiari network. This is a normal variant of no clinical significance. The coronary sinus also drains into the right atrium and its opening is guarded by the Thebesian valve (Fig. 20.6).

Left Atrium

Embryological derivation and components of the left atrium are same as the right. The left atrium is about the same size as the right atrium and lies posterior, superior, and toward the left of the right atrium (Fig. 20.5). The left atrium forms the upper posterior border of the heart and lies just below the carina and anterior to the esophagus. The relationship to esophagus facilitates imaging of the left atrium and remainder of the heart by transesophageal echocardiography. The smooth-walled venous component of the left atrium lies posteriorly and typically

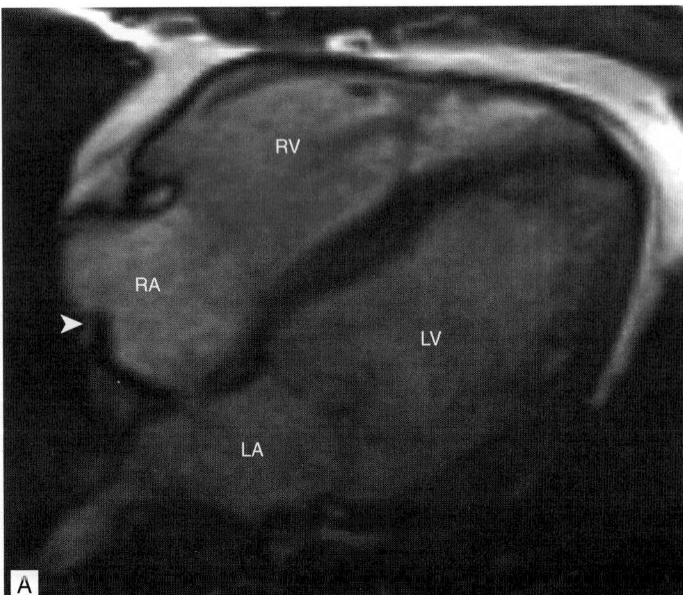

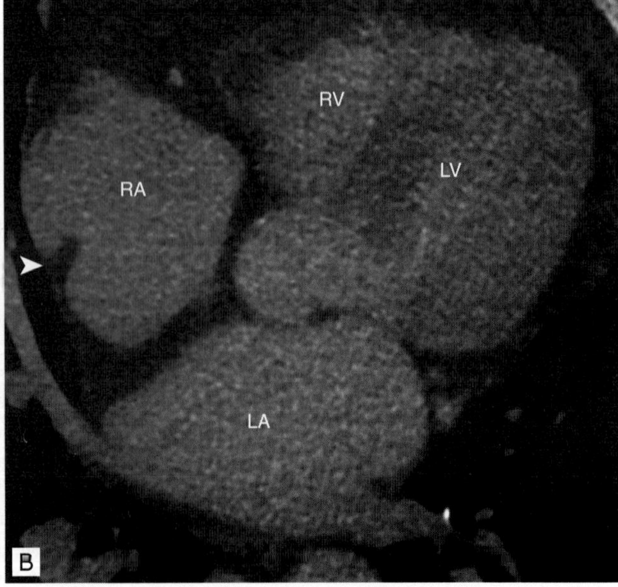

Figure 20.3 Four-chamber cardiac magnetic resonance image (A) and axial computed tomography angiography image (B) showing crista terminalis (*arrowhead*) which separates trabeculated appendage from the posterior smooth-walled portion of the right atrium (RA). *LA*, left atrium; *RA*, right atrium; *RV*, right ventricle.

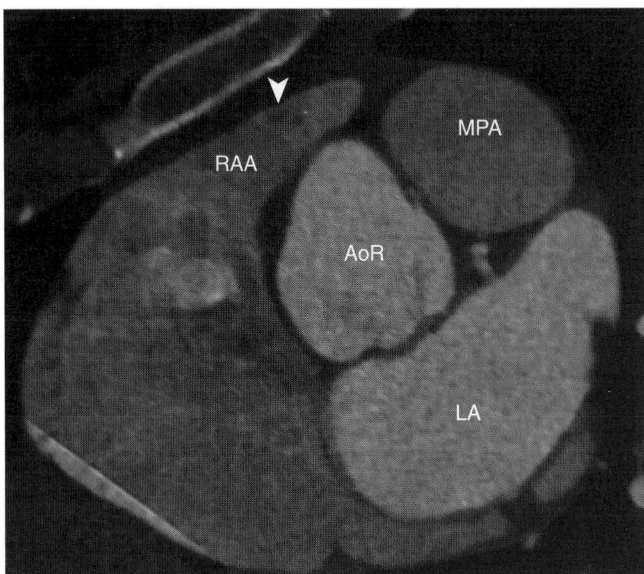

Figure 20.4 Reformatted computed tomography angiography images showing triangular broad-based right atrial appendage (RAA) with small pectinate muscles (*arrowhead*). *AoR*, aortic root; *LA*, left atrium; *MPA*, main pulmonary artery.

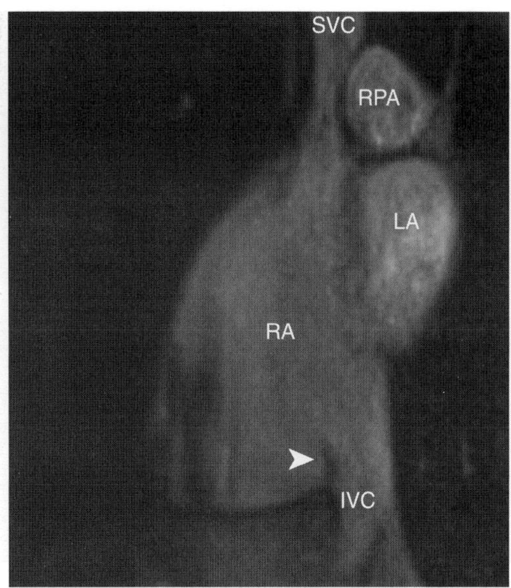

Figure 20.5 Oblique sagittal cardiac magnetic resonance image showing Eustachian valve (*arrowhead*) at the junction of inferior vena cava (IVC) and right atrium (RA). *LA*, left atrium; *RPA*, right pulmonary artery; *SVC*, superior vena cava.

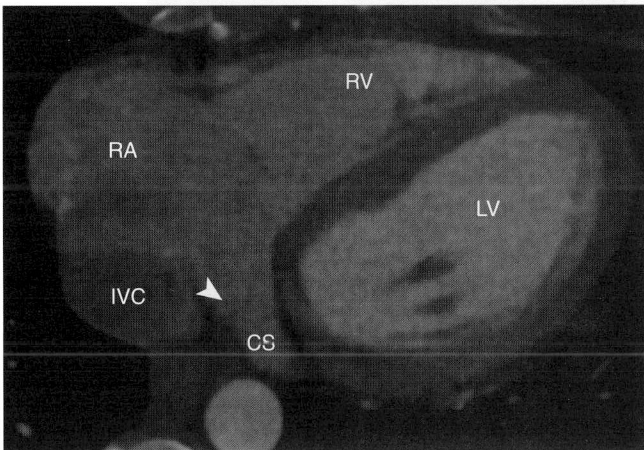

Figure 20.6 Axial coronary computed tomography angiography image showing opening of the coronary sinus (CS) into the right atrium (RA) being guarded by the Thebesian valve (*white arrowhead*). *IVC*, inferior vena cava; *LV*, left ventricle; *RV*, right ventricle.

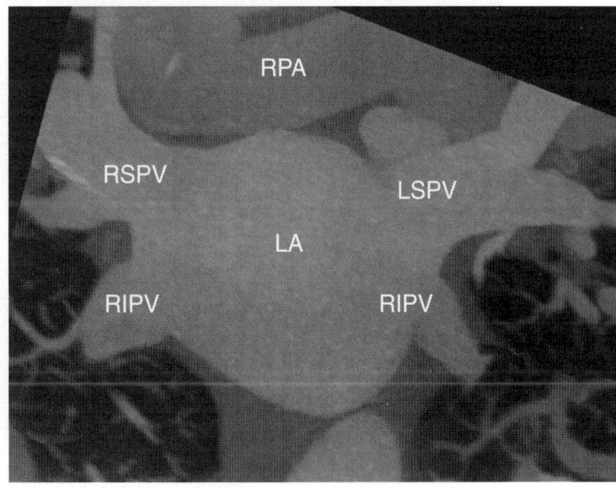

Figure 20.7 Maximum intensity projection (MIP) oblique coronal coronary computed tomography angiography image showing four pulmonary veins draining in to the left atrium (LA). *LIPV*, left inferior pulmonary vein; *LSPV*, left superior pulmonary vein; *RIPV*, right inferior pulmonary vein; *RPA*, right pulmonary artery; *RSPV*, right superior pulmonary vein.

receives four pulmonary veins (Fig. 20.7). The vestibule of the left atrium is also smooth-walled and incorporates leaflets of the mitral valve. The left atrial appendage (LAA) is a pouch like projection which runs from caudal to cranial at the left lateral aspect of the heart (Fig. 20.8). LAA shows considerable variations in morphology, size, and relationship with cardiac and extra cardiac structures. Four different morphological types of LAA were described in a recent study: (i) "chicken wing" being the most common (48%), (ii) "cactus" (30%), (iii) "windsock" (19%), and (iv) "cauliflower" (3%) (Fig. 20.9) [5]. The morphological features of LAA may become significant in the presence of atrial fibrillation. In the above study, the "cauliflower" morphology was found to be most often associated with cardioembolic events. The LAA contains pectinate muscles which are less prominent compared to the RAA and are also seen as filing defects on contrast-enhanced cross-sectional studies (Fig. 20.8). There is a prominent band-like ridge at the confluence of the LAA and left upper pulmonary vein which used to be mistaken for a thrombus, hence its name; Coumadin ridge (also known as left lateral ridge or warfarin ridge; Fig. 20.8).

The superior pulmonary veins lie anterior to their respective pulmonary arteries. The left superior pulmonary vein courses inferiorly, and anteriorly to the left pulmonary artery and enters the left atrium immediately posterior to the opening of the LAA. The right superior pulmonary vein passes in an anterior to posterior direction as it traverses inferiorly lying anterior to the right pulmonary artery. The right superior pulmonary vein opens in the left atrium immediately posterior to the confluence of the superior vena cava with right atrium. The left inferior pulmonary vein courses anterior to the descending

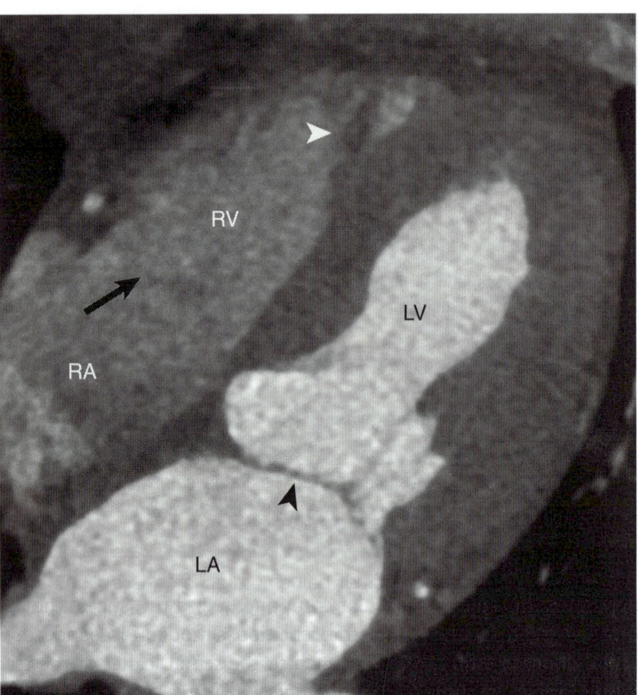

Figure 20.11 Four-chamber coronary computed tomography angiography image showing moderator band (*white arrowhead*), a distinguishing feature of morphological right ventricle. Note that the tricuspid valve (*black arrow*) is apically displaced compared to the mitral valve (*black arrowhead*). *LA*, left atrium; *LV*, left ventricle; *RA*, right atrium; *RV*, right ventricle.

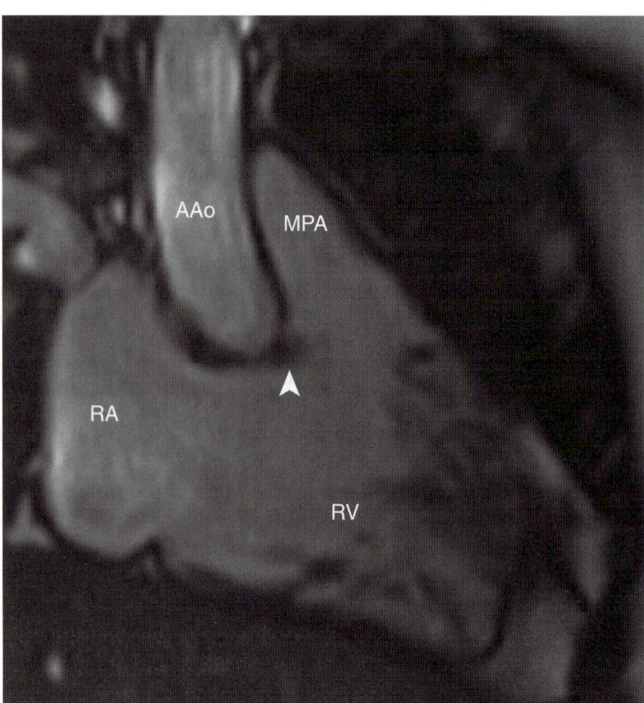

Figure 20.12 Cardiac magnetic resonance right ventricle inflow and outflow view showing supraventricular crest (*white arrowhead*), a muscular ridge separating the pulmonic and tricuspid valves. Coarse apical trabeculations of the right ventricle are also seen. *AAo*, ascending aorta; *MPA*, main pulmonary artery; *RA*, right atrium; *RV*, right ventricle.

is a continuation of the right bundle branch extending from the interventricular septum to the free wall of the RV and joins the anterior papillary muscle. The papillary muscles of RV are more in number and less prominent compared to the LV and are seen along both the septal and free wall. Unlike the LV there is no fibrous continuity between the atrioventricular and semilunar valve on the right side. The pulmonic and tricuspid valves are separated by a muscular ridge called the supraventricular crest (crista supraventricularis or ventriculoinfundibular fold; Fig. 20.12) which forms the posterior (paraseptal) wall of the infundibulum. The smooth muscular infundibulum (conus) forms the right ventricular outflow tract (Fig. 20.12) that curves around the septal and anterior surface of the LV to reach the pulmonary valve. The RV is thin walled, with free wall thickness measuring up to 3 mm.

RV enlargement occurs anteriorly resulting in obliteration of the retrosternal clear space and laterally resulting in leftward and cranial displacement of the cardiac apex. RV measurement on cross-sectional imaging at the level of tricuspid valve is normally less than the corresponding LV measurement at the level of mitral valve. The normal RV/LV ratio is less than 1. RV/LV ratio of greater than 1 is a sign of right heart strain in acute pulmonary embolism associated with poor prognosis [11].

Left Ventricle

The LV pumps oxygenated blood into the systemic circulation via the aorta and its branches. It is the most muscular chamber in the heart with thick walls and is characterized by a symmetrical conical shape, smooth interventricular septum and two large papillary muscles. The LV lies posterior and to the left of the RV (Fig. 20.13). The LV components are similar to the RV and include (i) inlet with valvular apparatus, (ii) apical–trabecular component, and (iii) subaortic outflow tract. The inlet of the LV extends from the atrioventricular junction to the attachments of the papillary muscles and includes the mitral valve. The mitral valve with anterior and posterior leaflets has no septal attachments. There is fibrous continuity between mitral and aortic valves which is distinct from the RV. Two papillary muscles seen within the LV are (i) anterolateral papillary muscle which originate between the anterolateral and inferolateral walls, and (ii) posteromedial papillary muscle which originates near the junction of inferior wall with the septum (Fig. 20.13). Fine trabeculations are seen at the left ventricular apex. Smooth septal wall is a distinguishing feature of the morphologic LV compared to morphological RV. The left ventricular outlet is short and lacks the conal muscles, in contrast to the right side. The left ventricular wall shows gradual thinning in the longitudinal direction from base to apex. The circumferential LV wall thickness is more uniform and can measure up to 1 cm at end diastole with gradual thinning in the longitudinal direction from base to apex. The apical wall can be as thin as 1–2 mm in diastole.

The 17-segment heart model developed by the American Heart Association divides the left ventricular myocardium into three slices along the long axis of the LV; basal, mid, and apical slices (Fig. 20.14) [12]. The slices are further segmented into anterior, lateral, inferior, and septal segments. The 17th segment is referred to as the true apex or the apical cap. This model allows for use of standardized nomenclature to refer to different segments of the LV, which is particularly useful for reporting wall motion abnormalities and defects in myocardial perfusion noted on noninvasive imaging.

Interventricular Septum

The interventricular septum consists of muscular as well as fibrous components. It predominantly consists of a thick-walled muscular layer that separates the RV and LV. The membranous septum is the posterior and superior aspect of the interventricular septum

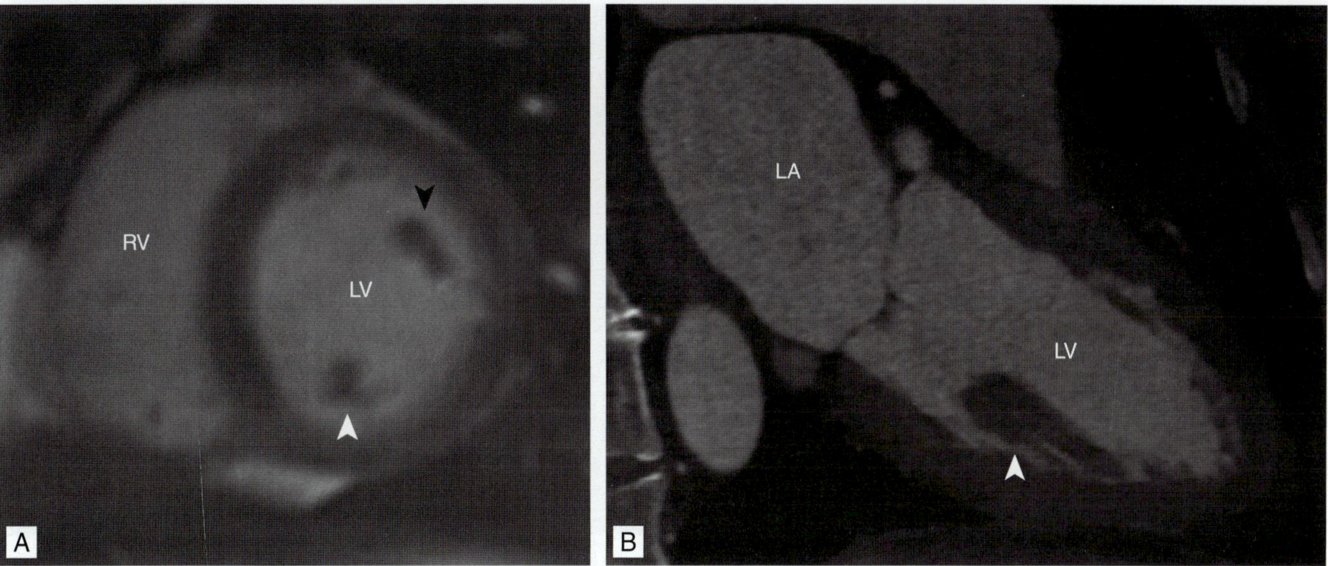

Figure 20.13 Short axis steady state free precession (SSFP) cardiac magnetic resonance image (A) and two-chamber computed tomography angiography image (B) showing anterolateral (*black arrowhead*) and posteromedial (*white arrowhead*) papillary muscles. *LA*, left atrium; *LV*, left ventricle; *RV*, right ventricle.

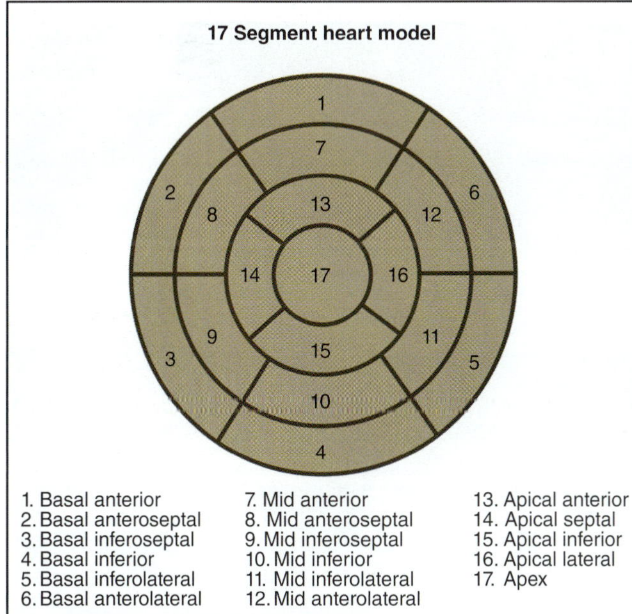

Figure 20.14 The 17-segment model of the left ventricle developed by the American Heart Association allows for use of standardized nomenclature to refer to different segments of the left ventricle.

and is much thinner compared to the muscular septum. The membranous septum forms the fibrous skeleton of the heart [13]. The interventricular septum is normally bowed toward the RV throughout the cardiac cycle due to higher pressure on the left side (Fig. 20.13A). Physiological flattening of the septum during early diastole is called ventricular coupling.

Valves

Left-Sided Valves: Mitral and Aortic

The cardiac valves are part of the fibrous skeleton of the heart [14]. There are two atrioventricular valves that guard the inlet of the ventricles; mitral (left side) and tricuspid (right side), and two semilunar valves at the outlet; aortic (left side) and pulmonic (right side). The mitral valve is located at the inlet of the LV and has an anterior and posterior leaflet (Fig. 20.15A). The anterior leaflet is deeper than the posterior leaflet but has a slightly smaller circumference. Both leaflets are anchored to two large papillary muscles (anterolateral and posteromedial) via chordae tendineae [13,14]. Chordae are thin fibrous chords that extend from the free end of the leaflets to the apices of the papillary muscles (Fig. 20.15B). The base of the anterior mitral valve leaflet is in fibrous continuity with the posterior part of the aortic valve annulus (Fig. 20.15B). Similarly, the anterior portion of the aortic valve annulus is in continuity with the interventricular septum. The aortic valve is comprised of three cusps; right, left, and posterior/noncoronary (Fig. 20.16). The right cusp is always anterior, the left cusp lies posterior and to the left, while the noncoronary/posterior cusp is just anterior to the interatrial septum. The basal hinge points of the three coronary cusps give rise to a virtual plane that defines the aortic annular plane [14]. The cusps attach to each other and the annular ring (part of the fibrous skeleton) at the commissures. There is a normal thickening in the middle of the free edge of the cusps known as the nodule [15]. Just superior to the aortic annulus are the sinuses of Valsalva, which is the space between the valve cusps and the dilated part of the aortic root [14]. The right and left coronary cusps give rise to the corresponding coronary arteries, while the noncoronary cusps aptly named, does not give rise to a coronary vessel. The angulated orientation of the ascending aorta means that all sinuses are not at the same level, the noncoronary sinus usually being the lowest and the left coronary sinus being the highest.

Right-Sided Valves: Tricuspid and Pulmonic

The tricuspid valve lies at the inlet of the RV. Unlike the atrioventricular valve on the left, the tricuspid valve has three leaflets; anterior, septal, and inferior. The anterior leaflet has chordal attachments from the anterior and septal papillary muscle, the septal leaflet from the septal and posterior papillary muscles, while the posterior leaflet from the posterior and anterior papillary muscles [14]. The anterior papillary muscle contains the moderator band that extends from the inventricular septum and contains

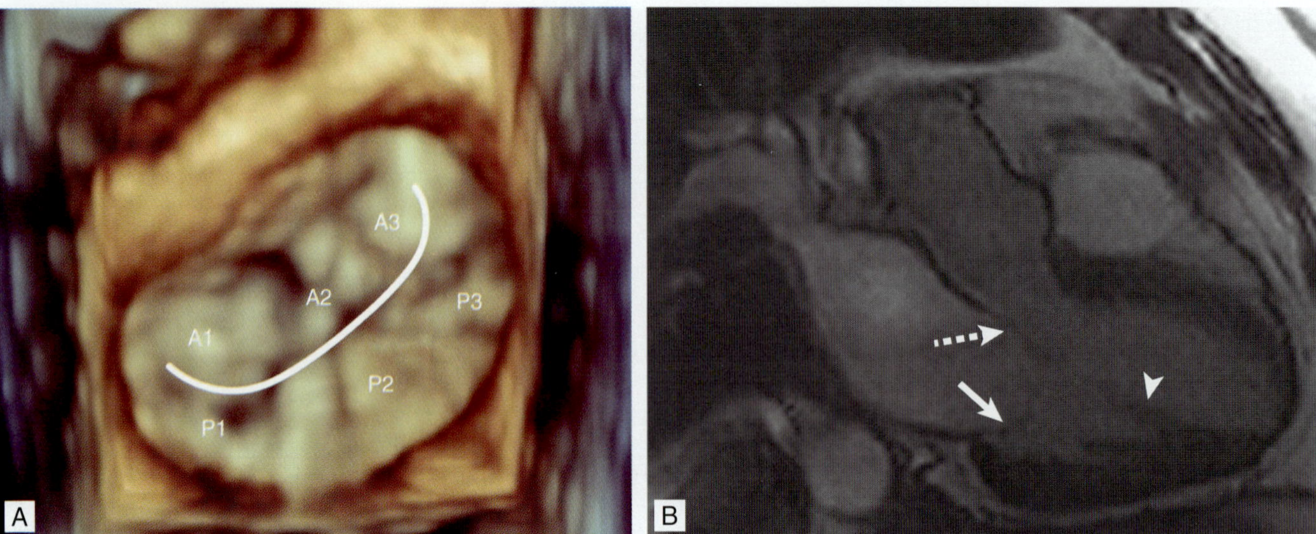

Figure 20.15 (A) Three-dimensional echocardiographic view of the mitral valve from the left atrium. A1–3 represent scallops of the anterior leaflet from the lateral to medial side, P1–3 represent scallops of the posterior leaflet. (B) Three-chamber steady state free precession (SSFP) cardiac magnetic resonance image showing the left ventricle. The posteromedial papillary muscle (*arrowhead*) is in view with chordae tendinea extending to the anterior (*dashed arrow*) and posterior (*solid arrow*) leaflet of the mitral valve. The base of the anterior mitral valve leaflet is in fibrous continuity with the posterior part of the aortic annulus.

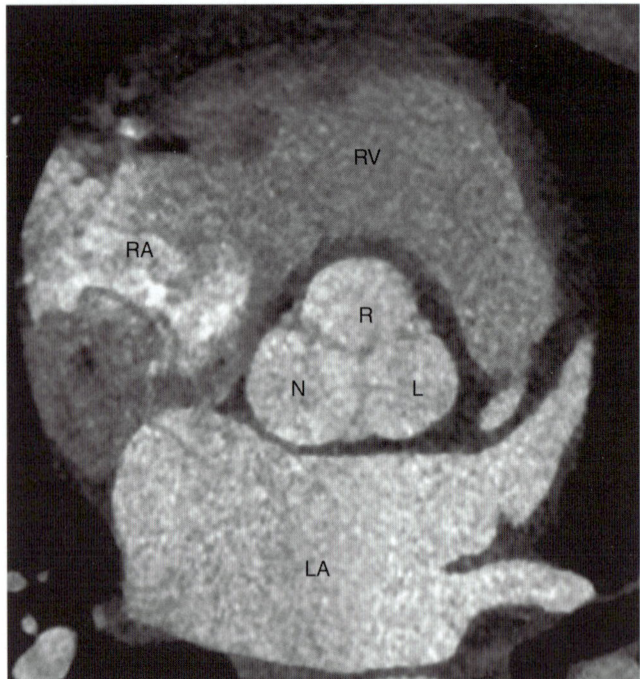

Figure 20.16 Reformatted computed tomography angiography image showing cross-sectional view of the aortic valve. Aortic valve cusps correspond to the sinuses of Valsalva. *L*, left sinus of Valsalva; *LA*, left atrium; *N*, noncoronary sinus of Valsalva; *R*, right sinus of Valsalva; *RA*, right atrium; *RV*, right ventricle.

Figure 20.17 Reformatted cardiac computed tomography angiography image showing the right ventricular outflow tract. Note that the pulmonary valve (*white arrow*) is superior and to the left of the aortic valve. *RV*, right ventricle; *MPA*, main pulmonary artery; *AV*, aortic valve.

the right bundle branch. The tricuspid valve is apically displaced compared to the mitral valve; this is an important identifier of normal atrioventricular valve anatomy (Fig. 20.11) [15].

The outflow portion of the RV forms a muscular tube that curves around the septal and anterior surface of the LV to reach the pulmonary valve. The pulmonary valve is superior and to the left of the aortic valve (Fig. 20.17). The structure of the pulmonary valve bears resemblance to the aortic valve, with three cusps; anterior, left, and right. The base of the cusps forms the pulmonary annulus, and the cusps attach to each other and the annulus at the commissures [14,15].

Coronary Anatomy

Left Coronary Artery

The left coronary artery arises as a left main stem from the left sinus of Valsalva. It is initially directed leftward and posteriorly

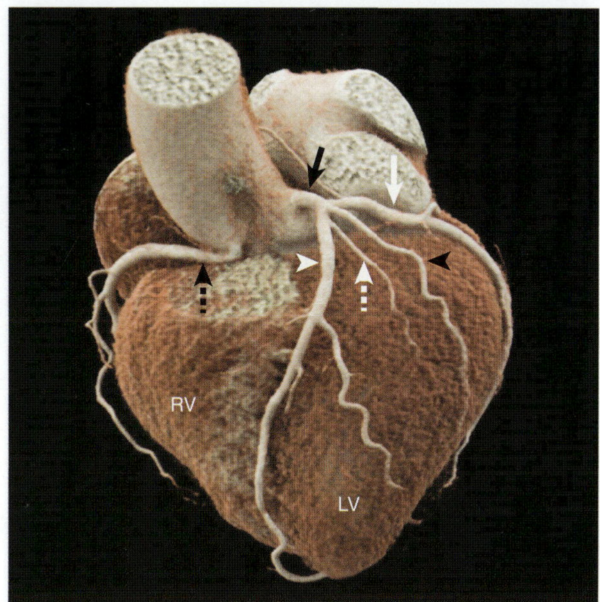

Figure 20.18 Three-dimensional volume-rendered coronary computed tomography angiography image showing trifurcation of the left main stem (LMS; *black arrow*) into left anterior descending (LAD; *white arrowhead*), ramus intermedius (RI; *black arrowhead*), and left circumflex (LCx; *white arrow*) arteries. The first diagonal branch is seen coming off the LAD (*white dashed arrow*). The right coronary artery (RCA; *black dashed arrow*) courses in the right atrioventricular groove. *LV*, left ventricle; *RV*, right ventricle.

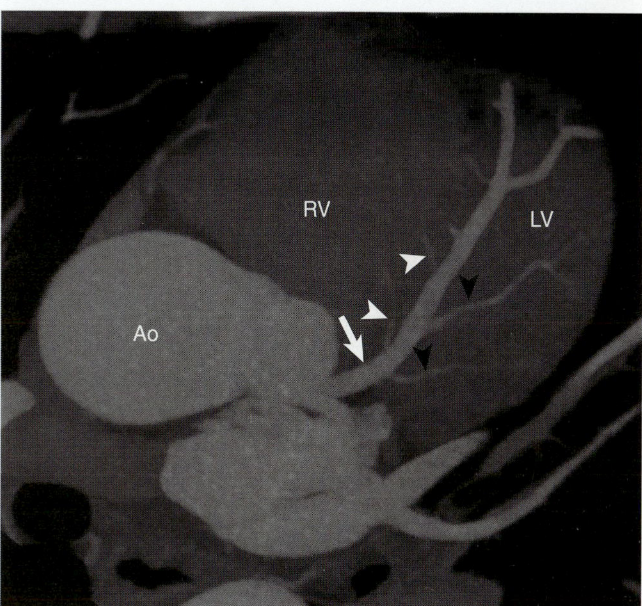

Figure 20.19 Maximum intensity projection (MIP) reformatted coronary computed tomography angiography image showing the course of the left anterior descending artery (*white arrow*) in the anterior interventricular groove and its main branches. The diagonal branches (*black arrowheads*) supply the anterior left ventricle, and the septal perforators (*white arrowheads*) supply the anterior two thirds of the interventricular septum. *Ao*, aorta; *LV*, left ventricle; *RV*, right ventricle.

but it curves immediately around to an anterior orientation where it bifurcates to the left anterior descending (LAD) artery and the left circumflex (LCx) artery.

Occasionally the LAD artery and the left circumflex artery can have separate origins from the left coronary cusp [2]. In ~20% of cases, the left main coronary artery trifurcates into three branches; LAD artery, left circumflex artery, and the ramus intermedius lying between the two branches (Fig. 20.18) [15,16]. The ramus intermedius supplies free wall muscle between the diagonal and obtuse marginal territories. The LAD artery runs along the superior aspect of the interventricular septum emerging into the anterior interventricular groove as a superficial vessel which runs right down to the apex of the heart. The LAD artery supplies the anterior two thirds of the interventricular groove through its septal perforating branches (Fig. 20.19). Along its course, the LAD artery gives off diagonal branches that supply the anterior segments of the LV (Fig. 20.19). The circumflex artery courses in the left atrioventricular groove, and gives off free wall branches, known as marginal or obtuse marginal branches, that supply the anterolateral segments of the LV. The circumflex artery also supplies LA branches [2,15]. Coronary perfusion of the LV and RV is described in terms of the nomenclature established by the AHA 17 segment heart model (Fig. 20.14). Typical coronary distribution is shown in Fig. 20.20.

Right Coronary Artery

The right coronary artery (RCA) arises from the right sinus of Valsalva and immediately turns rightward and inferiorly to follow the right atrioventricular groove (Fig. 20.21). The conus branch is one of the earliest branches of the RCA and can sometimes have a separate origin adjacent to the right coronary stem. It passes over the surface of the right ventricular outflow tract, and supplies the conus portion of the pulmonary trunk. In 55% of cases, the next branch of the RCA is the sinoatrial nodal artery [16]. In the remaining 45%, the sinoatrial nodal artery is a branch of the left circumflex artery [16]. However, it always courses toward the superior vena cava inflow, near the cephalad aspect of the interatrial septum. Along its course in the anterior AV groove, the RCA gives off several right ventricular free wall branches, called RV marginals or acute marginals that supply the right ventricular myocardium (Fig. 20.21). When the RCA reaches the crux of the heart near the posterior ventricular groove, it turns anteriorly and runs in the interventricular groove as the posterior descending artery (PDA; Fig. 20.21) [2,15].

Coronary artery dominance is determined by which artery supplies the inferior portion of the posterior interventricular septum and gives rise to the PDA; right dominant if PDA and posterior lateral ventricular branch is supplied by the RCA (~80% of the population), left dominant if PDA is supplied by the left circumflex artery [2]. If the right coronary and left circumflex arteries supply the PDA and posterior lateral ventricular, respectively, the circulation is said to be codominant (Fig. 20.22). The PDA supplies penetrating branches into the septum, and the inferior segments of the LV. Occasionally, left circumflex artery may also give rise to a second PDA. The atrioventricular nodal branch usually arises from the dominant coronary artery and may have a dual supply [17].

Segmental Anatomy of Coronary Arteries

Standardized nomenclature of the coronary arteries has been developed for proper communication of results of coronary angiography, where coronary arteries and their major branches are divided into various segments [18,19]. This nomenclature has also been adopted by several centers for reporting of coronary CT angiography. For practical purposes the coronary arteries are divided into segments as follows: The left main stem coronary

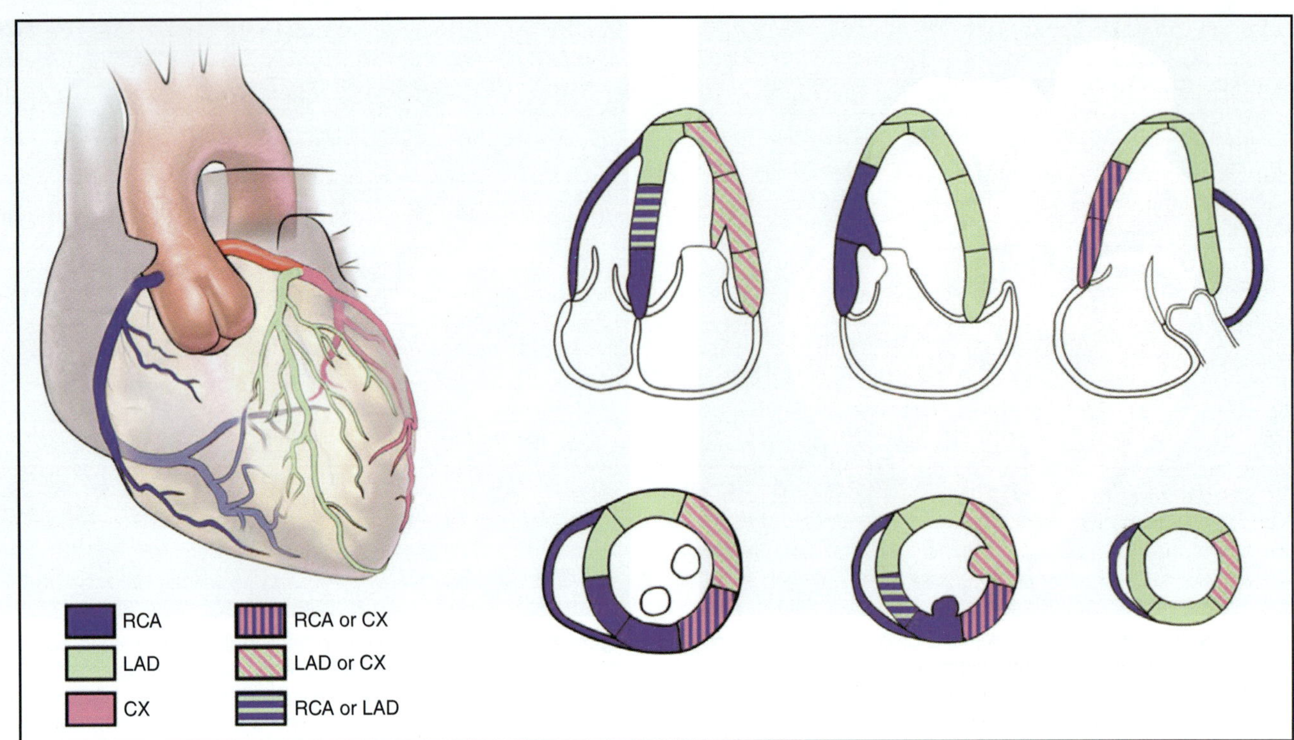

Figure 20.20 Illustration depicting the typical distribution of the right and left coronary systems. The distribution can vary among patients, and some bordering segments can have variable perfusions. Reproduced with permission from [37]. *RCA*, right coronary artery; *LAD*, left anterior descending coronary artery; *CX*, circumflex coronary artery.

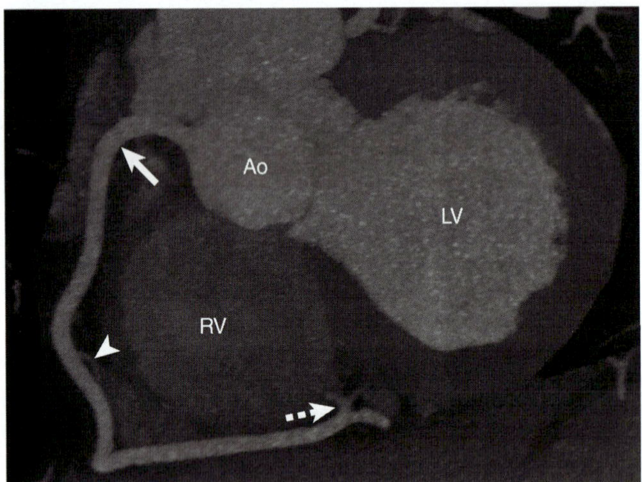

Figure 20.21 Maximum intensity projection (MIP) reformatted coronary computed tomography angiography image showing C-view of the right coronary artery (*white arrow*) with an acute marginal branch (*white arrowhead*). When the RCA reaches the crux of the heart, it turns anteriorly, and runs in the posterior interventricular groove as the posterior descending artery (PDA; dashed *white arrow*). *Ao*, aorta; *LV*, left ventricle; *RV*, right ventricle.

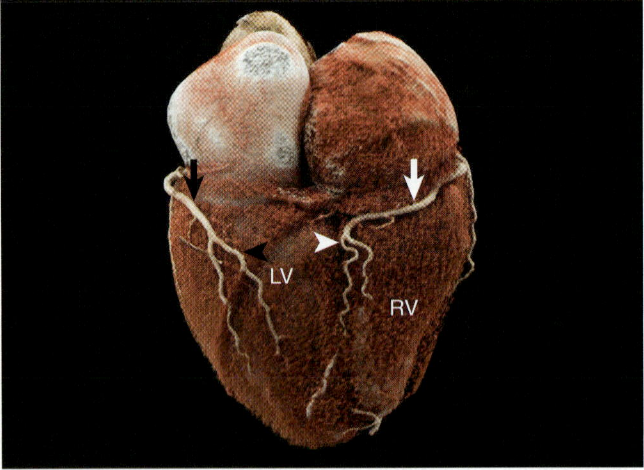

Figure 20.22 Three-dimensional volume-rendered coronary computed tomography angiography image showing codominance; posterior descending artery (*white arrowhead*) comes off the right coronary artery (*white arrow*), while the posterior left ventricular branch (*black arrowhead*) is supplied by the left circumflex artery (*black arrow*). *LV*, left ventricle; *RV*, right ventricle.

artery extends from the ostium to its bifurcation (or trifurcation). The LAD coronary artery is divided into proximal, middle, and distal segments. The proximal LAD extends from its origin to the origin of either the first diagonal or first septal perforator, whichever is first. The mid LAD extends from this point to the origin of the second diagonal branch. The distal LAD commences from the origin of the second diagonal branch and extends distally to termination. The left circumflex coronary artery is divided into proximal and distal segments. The proximal LCx extends from its origin to the origin of the first obtuse marginal branch. The artery distal to this is the distal LCx.

The RCA is divided into proximal, mid, and distal segments. The proximal RCA extends from the ostium to the origin of acute marginal branch. The mid RCA curves around the acute margin of the heart and the distal RCA traverses along the posterior right atrioventricular groove.

Normal Variant Anatomy

Duplication of coronary arteries, although rare, can be seen with the LAD, RCA, or PDA. Dual LAD system usually consists of one short LAD terminating in the proximal anterior interventricular groove and a second longer LAD which traverses out of the anterior interventricular groove and subsequently returns back to the distal anterior interventricular groove (Fig. 20.23). Initially only four types of dual LAD systems were described [20], however subsequently new variations have been described [21] (Table 20.2). In some types of dual LAD system, the long LAD arises from the RCA and takes an anomalous course to enter the distal anterior interventricular groove, for example, Type 4 dual LAD where a long LAD arising from the RCA takes a prepulmonic course (Fig. 20.24). Recognition of variation in LAD anatomy is important for accurate identification at time of surgical intervention or revascularization.

Presence of intramyocardial or intracavitary course of the coronary arteries are also considered anatomical variants. Normally epicardial coronary arteries plunge into the myocardium only at their distal end. When a portion of an epicardial coronary artery takes an intramyocardial course and then emerges back out into the epicardial space this is referred to as myocardial bridging. This is most commonly seen involving the mid LAD (Fig. 20.25) [22]. This arrangement of tunneled coronary artery passing under the "bridge" of overlying myocardium may cause systolic compression of the vessel. Recognition of myocardial bridging is important as this has been described to occasionally cause symptoms [23], and cause complications during coronary artery bypass surgery including inadvertent perforation of the RV [24]. Rarely intracavitary course of an epicardial coronary artery may be seen and two variants have been described in the literature. An intracavitary course of the proximal LAD through the RV, estimated to be present in 0.3% of population [25], and an intracavitary course of the RCA through the right atrium present in less than 0.1% of the population (Fig. 20.26) [26]. Detection of intracavitary course is of particular importance to the as the cardiac surgeon as artery may be difficult to localize at the time of bypass grafting and to the interventional cardiologist and electrophysiologists due to risk of inadvertent injury at the time of pacemaker implantation, right heart catheterization, and electrophysiology procedure.

Anatomic variant of left-sided sinoatrial node artery has been described, S-shaped sinoatrial node artery [27], which arises from the LCx and courses posteriorly between the LAA and the ostium of the left superior pulmonary vein and then courses anteriorly adjacent to the anterior wall of the left atrium (Fig. 20.27). The course of this artery predisposes it to injury during surgery or catheter-based ablation and therefore important to recognize.

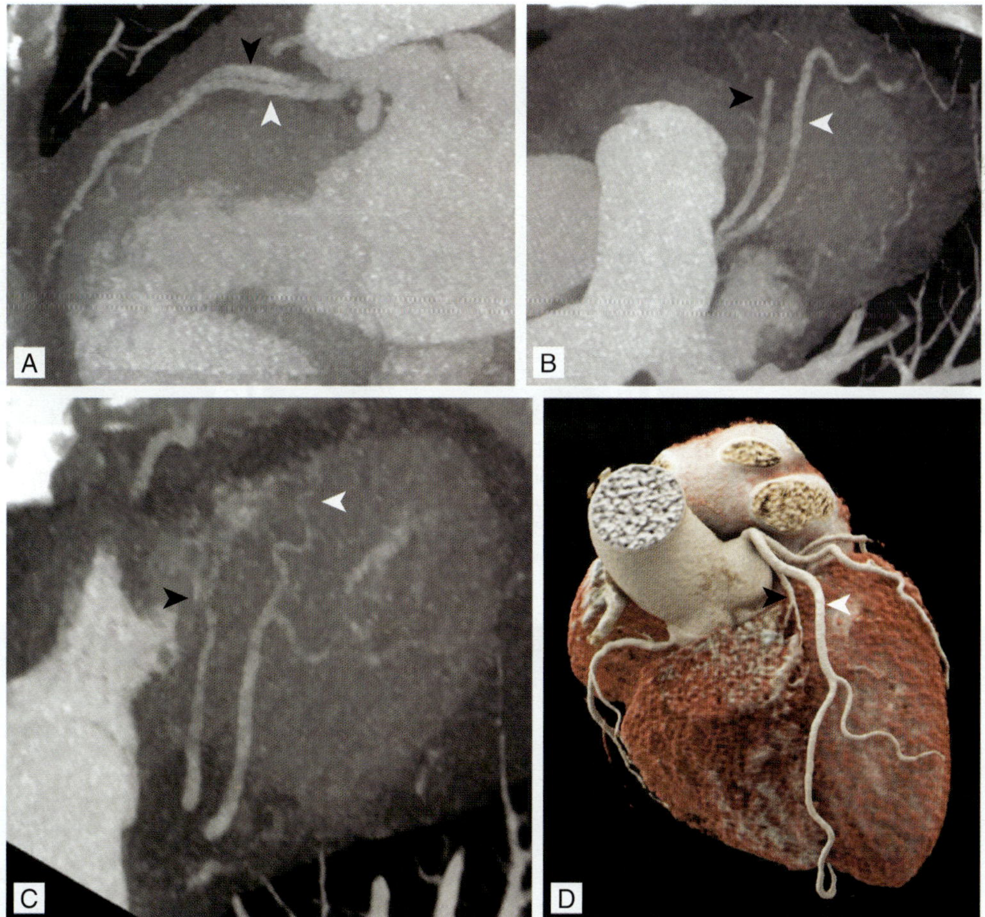

Figure 20.23 Maximum intensity projection (MIP) reformatted (A, B, and C) and three-dimensional volume-rendered (D) coronary computed tomography angiography images showing dual left anterior descending (LAD) coronary artery system with short LAD (*black arrowhead*) being rightward (B) and terminating in the proximal anterior interventricular groove (A, B, and C) and a second longer LAD (*white arrowhead*) which traverses out of the anterior interventricular groove (B) and subsequently returns back to the distal anterior interventricular groove (C). This is known as Type 1 dual LAD.

TABLE 20.2 Types of Dual Left Anterior Descending Coronary Arteries

Type	Origin		Course	
	Short LAD	Long LAD	Short LAD	Long LAD
I	Proximal LAD	Proximal LAD	Proximal AIG	LV side of the proximal AIG, re-enters the distal AIG
II	Proximal LAD	Proximal LAD	Proximal AIG	RV side of the proximal AIG, re-enters the distal AIG
III	Proximal LAD	Proximal LAD	Proximal AIG	Intramyocardial course in the proximal septum, either emerges as epicardial vessel in distal AIG or terminates as septal branches
IV	LMS	Proximal RCA	Proximal AIG	(i) Epicardial prepulmonic course anterior to RVOT, enters distal AIG (ii) Intramyocardial course within the septal crest emerging as epicardial vessel in distal AIG
V	Left SOV	Right SOV	Proximal AIG	Intramyocardial course within the septal crest emerging as epicardial vessel in distal AIG
VI	LMS	Proximal RCA	Proximal AIG	Between the RVOT and aortic root, enters mid/distal AIG
VII	Proximal LAD	Proximal LAD	Proximal AIG	LV side of the proximal AIG, re-enters the distal AIG (LMS originates form right SOV and shows interarterial course)
VIII	LMS	Mid-RCA	Proximal AIG	Inferior wall of RV, turns around the apex and reaches distal AIG (LMS originates from the right SOV with retroaortic course)
IX	Proximal LAD	Proximal LAD	Mid AIG	LV side of the mid AIG, re-enters the distal AIG, terminates before reaching the apex (PDA artery extends to distal AIG)
X	LMS	Right SOV	Proximal AIG	Epicardial prepulmonic course anterior to RVOT, enters distal AIG

AIG, anterior interventricular groove; *LAD*, left anterior descending; *LMS*, left main stem; *LV*, left ventricle; *PDA*, posterior descending artery; *RV*, right ventricle; *RVOT*, right ventricle outflow tract; *SOV*, sinus of Valsalva.

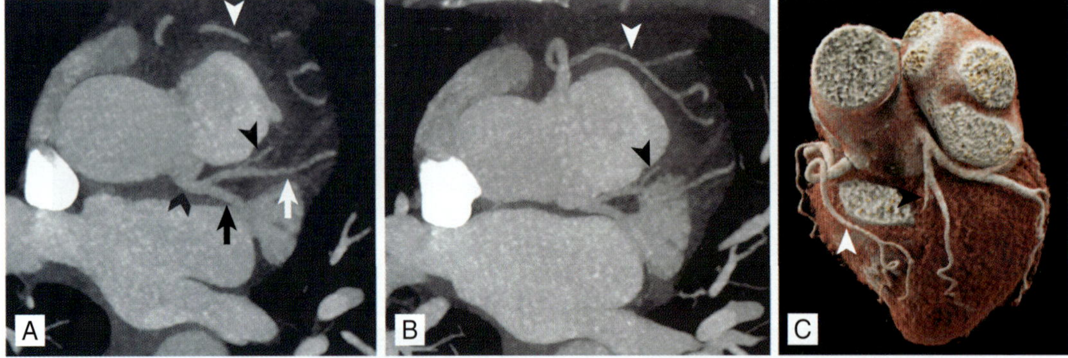

Figure 20.24 Maximum intensity projection (MIP) reformatted (A and B) and three-dimensional volume-rendered (C) coronary computed tomography angiography images showing dual left anterior descending (LAD) coronary artery system with short LAD (*black arrowhead*) terminating in the proximal anterior interventricular groove (A, B, and C) and a second longer LAD (*white arrowhead*) which arises from the right coronary artery and takes a prepulmonic course to reach the anterior interventricular groove (A, B, and C). This is known as Type 4 dual LAD. The left main (*black chevron*), left circumflex (*black arrow*), and first diagonal branch of LAD (*white arrow*) are also shown (A).

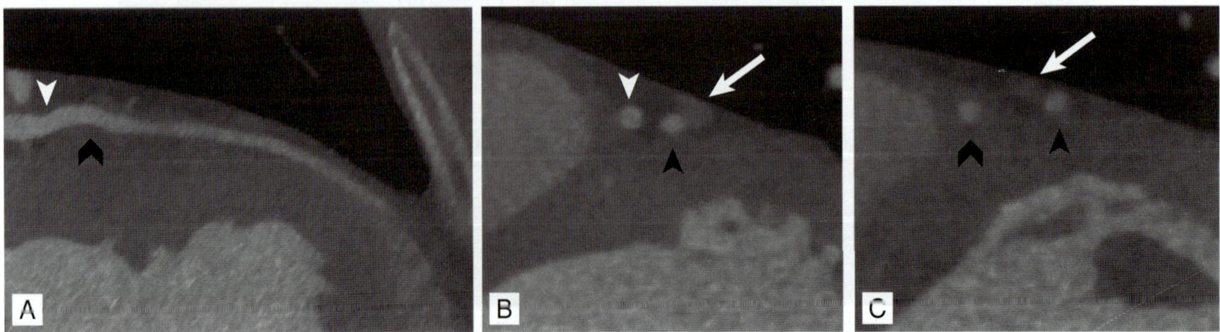

Figure 20.25 Reformatted coronary computed tomography angiography images showing proximal left anterior descending (LAD) coronary artery (*white arrowhead*) within the epicardial space (A and B) with an intramyocardial course (*black chevron*) of the mid LAD (A and C). The first diagonal branch of LAD (*black arrowhead*) and anterior interventricular vein (*whitearrow*) are also shown.

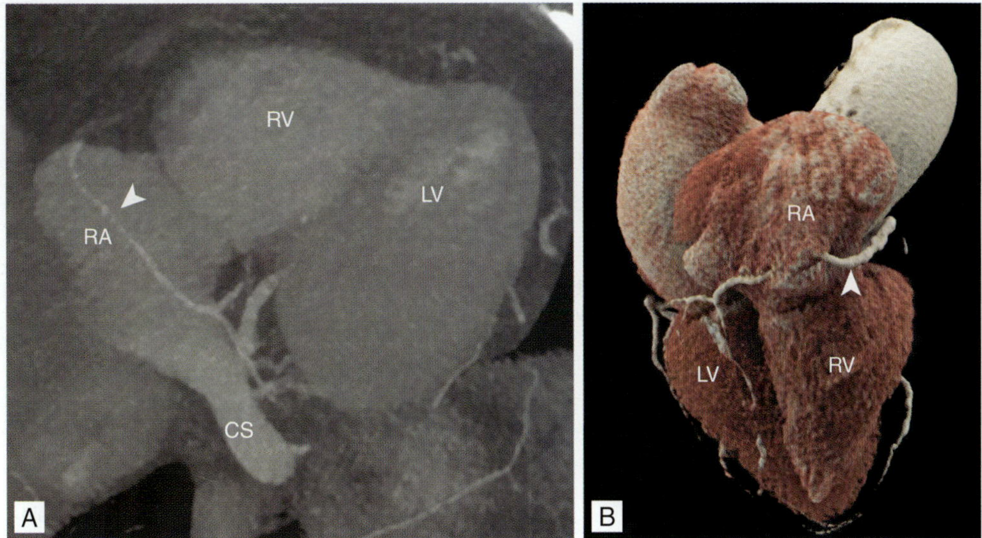

Figure 20.26 Maximum intensity projection (MIP) axial (A) and three-dimensional volume-rendered (B) coronary computed tomography angiography images showing intracavitary course of the right coronary artery (*arrowhead*) through the right atrium (RA). *CS*, coronary sinus; *LV*, left ventricle; *RV*, right ventricle.

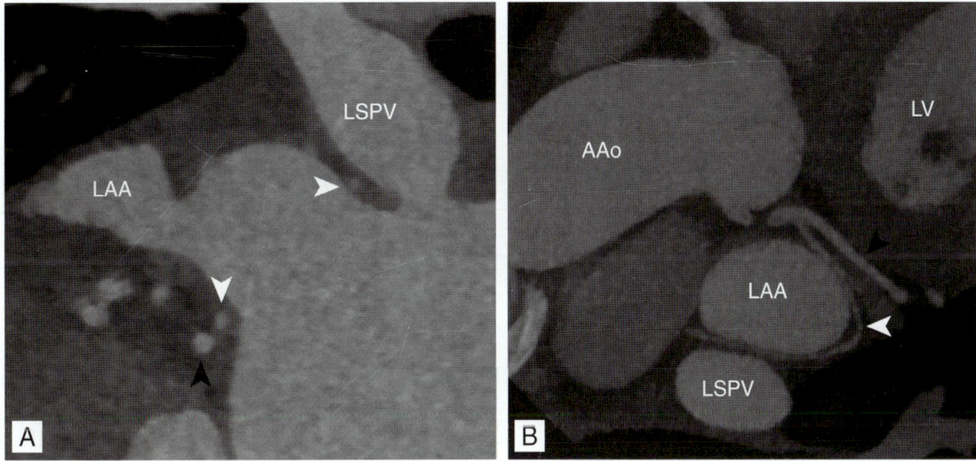

Figure 20.27 Reformatted coronary computed tomography angiography image (A) and maximum intensity projection (MIP) image showing sinoatrial node artery (*white arrowhead*) which arises from the left circumflex coronary artery (*black arrowhead*) and courses posteriorly between the left atrial appendage (LAA) and the ostium of the left superior pulmonary vein (LSPV). *AAo*, ascending aorta; *LV*, left ventricle.

Cardiac Venous Anatomy

Cardiac venous systems can be grouped based on the region of the heart being drained: (i) the coronary sinus and its tributaries which drain major portion of the heart, (ii) the anterior cardiac veins, which drain the anterior part of the RV and the right border of the heart, and (iii) the Thebesian veins which open directly into any of the four cardiac chambers. Cardiac venous anatomy is illustrated in Fig. 20.28.

The coronary sinus is a wide venous channel approximately 2 cm in length which lies in the posterior left atrioventricular groove and drains into the right atrium posteromedially. The opening of the coronary sinus into the right atrium is guarded by a semilunar valve, the Thebesian valve (Fig. 20.6). The coronary sinus is larger in men compared to women. At the crux of the heart the RCA is seen inferior to the coronary sinus. The main tributaries of the coronary sinus are as follows: (i) the great cardiac vein (GCV), (ii) small cardiac vein, (iii) middle cardiac (posterior interventricular) vein, (iv) posterior vein of the LV, and (v) oblique vein of the left atrium.

The anterior interventricular vein originates in the distal or middle third of the interventricular groove and ascends toward the base of the heart parallel to the LAD coronary artery (Fig. 20.29). The diagonal veins draining the lateral and anterolateral aspect of the LV and anterior two thirds of the interventricular septum connect with the anterior interventricular vein. The anterior interventricular vein becomes the GCV or left coronary vein in the anterior interventricular groove toward the base of the heart. It then turns laterally along the left atrioventricular groove, lies parallel to the left circumflex coronary artery. At the bifurcation of the left main coronary artery, the GCV crosses over the LAD and LCx forming the base of the triangle of Brocq and Mouchet (Fig. 20.29). The GCV then wraps around the left side of the heart in the posterior left atrioventricular groove to merge with the coronary sinus. The junction of the GCV with coronary sinus is defined by the presence of the LA oblique vein of Marshall. At the transition of the GCV to coronary sinus an intravenous valve is usually seen, the valve of Vieussens. The two main branches

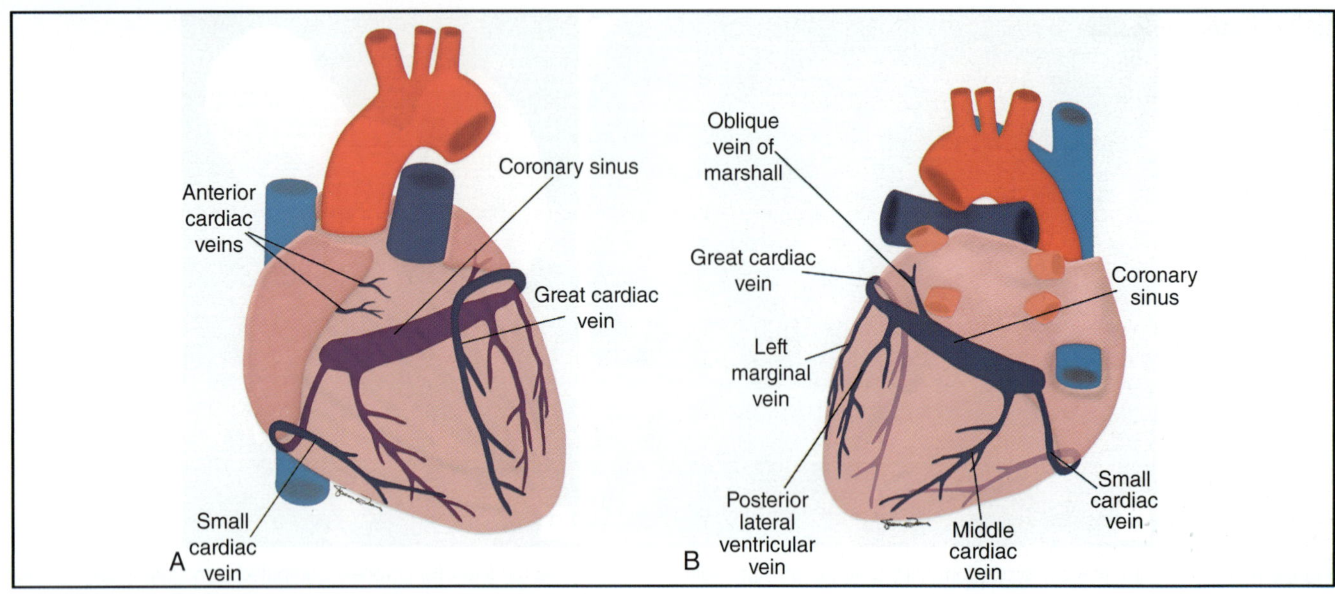

Figure 20.28 Cartoon illustration of the anterior (A) and posterior (B) views of the heart outlining cardiac venous anatomy. (Courtesy: Sussane Loomis, MS, Medical and Scientific Communications, Department of Radiology, Massachusetts General Hospital, Boston, MA, USA.)

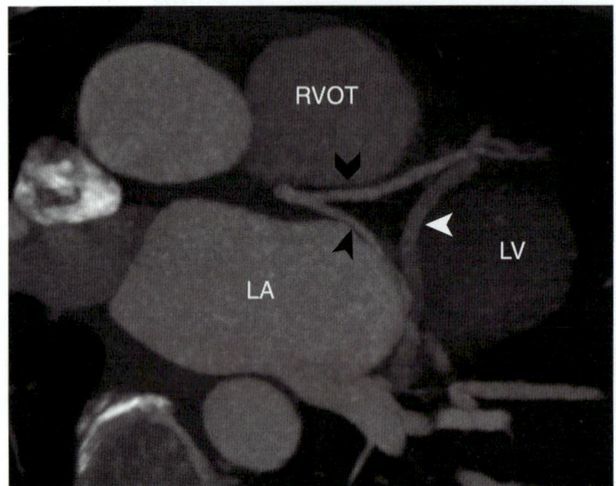

Figure 20.29 Maximum intensity projection (MIP) axial coronary computed tomography angiography image showing great cardiac vein (*white arrowhead*) crossing over the left anterior descending (*black chevron*) and left circumflex (*black arrowhead*) coronary arteries and forming the base of the triangle of Brocq and Mouchet. *LA*, left atrium; *LV*, left ventricle; *RVOT*, right ventricle outflow tract.

that drain blood in the GCV are the left marginal vein along the lateral border of the heart and the posterior lateral ventricular vein (Fig. 20.30).

The middle cardiac vein originates near the cardiac apex and ascends within the posterior interventricular groove toward the base of the heart to the left and parallel to the posterior descending coronary artery. The middle cardiac vein drains into the right atrium directly or into the coronary sinus just before it drains into the right atrium (Fig. 20.31). Blood from the posterior third of the interventricular septum is drained by the middle cardiac vein. The small cardiac vein (right coronary vein) is seen in the right atrioventricular groove and may drain into the right side of the coronary sinus, middle cardiac vein, or directly into the right atrium. The small cardiac vein receives blood from the posterior aspect of the right atrium and ventricle. The right cardiac vein may not be seen in nearly two thirds of the population.

The oblique LA vein of Marshall is seen coursing obliquely at the posterior aspect of the left atrium and draining into the left side of the coronary sinus. The anterior cardiac veins are small veins draining blood from anterior aspect of the RV into the right atrium via sinus coronaries atrii dextri. The Thebesian

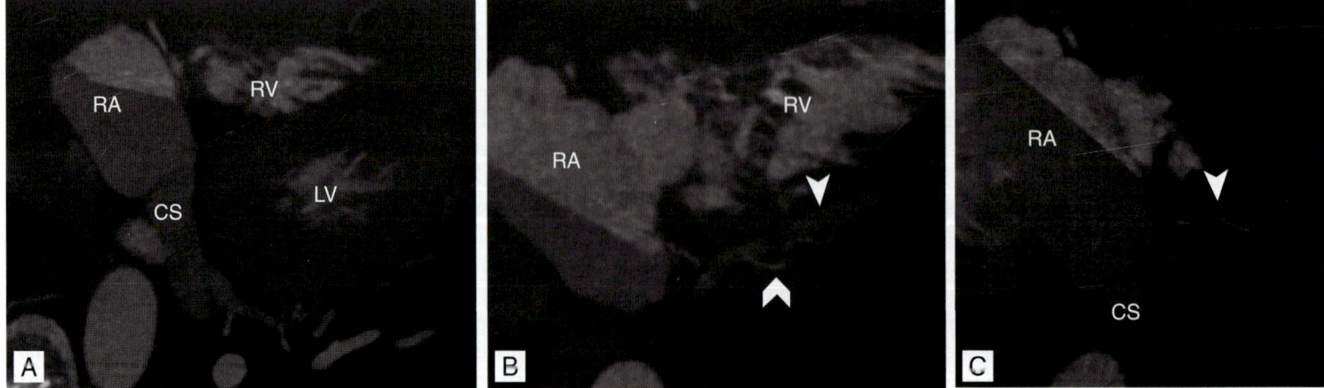

Figure 20.30 Maximum intensity projection (MIP) reformatted coronary computed tomography angiography images showing posterior lateral ventricular vein (*black arrowhead*) draining into the great cardiac vein (A); the middle cardiac vein (*white arrowhead*) running within the posterior interventricular groove (B); parallel to the posterior descending coronary artery (*white chevron*) and draining into the coronary sinus (C). *CS*, coronary sinus; *LV*, left ventricle; *RA*, right atrium; *RV*, right ventricle.

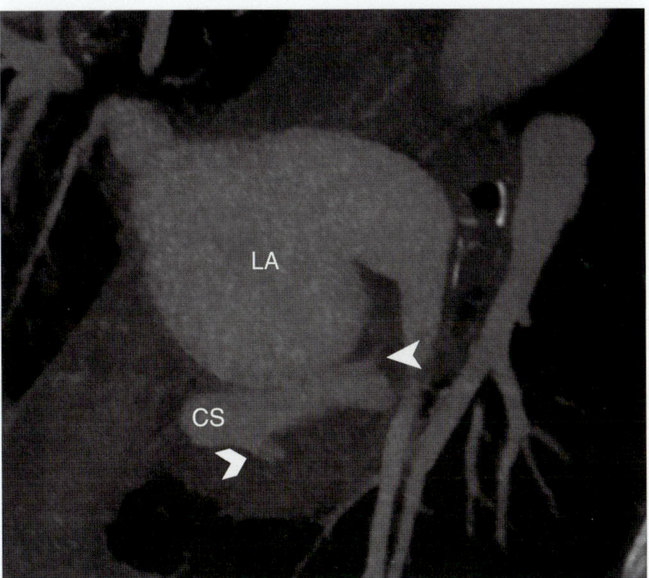

Figure 20.31 Maximum intensity projection (MIP) reformatted coronary computed tomography angiography images showing middle cardiac vein (*white chevron*) draining into the coronary sinus and left atrial oblique vein of Marshall (*white arrowhead*) draining and marking the junction of the GCV with coronary sinus. *CS*, coronary sinus; *LA*, left atrium.

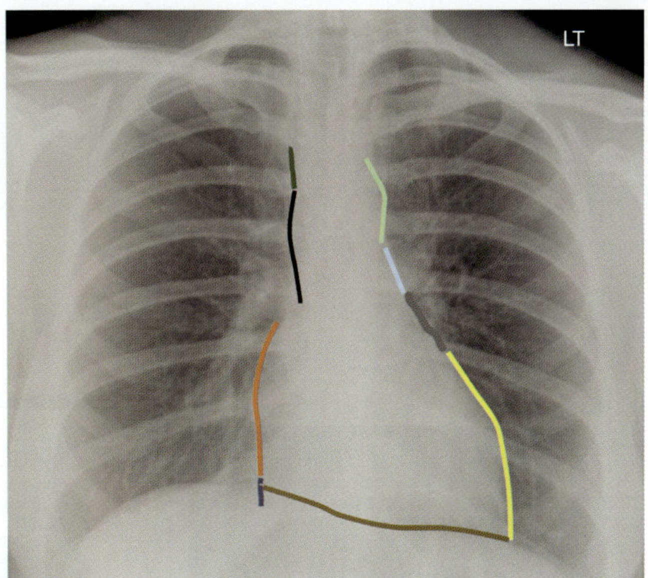

Figure 20.32 Frontal (posteroanterior) chest radiograph with structures forming the left, right, and inferior borders depicted: (i) the aortic knuckle (*light green*), (ii) the main pulmonary artery (*light blue*), (iii) the left atrial appendage (*gray*), and (iv) the left ventricular contour (*yellow*); (v) superior vena cava (*dark green*), (vi) ascending aorta (*black*), (vii) right atrium (*orange*), (viii) inferior vena cava (*dark blue*), and (ix) right ventricle (*brown*).

veins are the smallest cardiac veins which arise from the muscular walls of the cardiac chambers and drain into the respective chamber cavity.

The knowledge of the coronary venous anatomy has become increasingly important in view of diagnostic and therapeutic electrophysiological procedures including cardiac resynchronization therapy, mapping maneuvers for determination of type of arrhythmias, and delivery of ablative energy. Veins draining the lateral wall of LV may be used for LV epicardial lead placement for cardiac resynchronization. The LA oblique vein of Marshall is often cannulated for ablation procedures for atrial fibrillation [28].

Multimodality Imaging

A multimodality approach for the assessment of cardiac structure and function is most useful when different techniques complement each other. The consensus statement by the Task Force on Multimodality Imaging established by the European Association of Cardiovascular Imaging, clearly states that "All imaging specialists with expertise in one modality should be encouraged and facilitated to achieve a basic capability to perform and report in one or more additional modalities" [29]. Thus, it is imperative that cardiac imagers have a basic understanding of all the different imaging techniques, including echocardiography, cardiac CT, cardiac MRI, and invasive coronary angiogram.

Chest Radiograph

The chest radiograph is the commonest type of imaging examination of the heart, although frequently the examination is used for other aspects of examination of the thorax and the heart is examined as part of this overall investigation. The chest radiograph can be extremely valuable in cardiac assessment in three ways. First, cardiac size and contour can be clearly demonstrated and the silhouette of the heart produced in this way will give many important clues as to chamber enlargement. The second and most crucial aspect of the chest radiograph is the evaluation of the lungs. Careful analysis of the pulmonary appearances will give vital clues to the cardiac function. Third, the chest radiograph will demonstrate additional features related to cardiac disease which may include metallic or other implants, calcifications or bony anomalies which are related to the underlying heart abnormality.

The normal chest radiograph should show clear definition of the cardiac contour. The left heart border on a frontal chest radiograph is formed by (i) the aortic knuckle, (ii) the main pulmonary artery, (iii) the LAA, and (iv) the left ventricular contour. The right heart border is formed by (i) superior vena cava, (ii) ascending aorta, (iii) right atrium, and (iv) inferior vena cava (Fig. 20.32). On lateral chest radiograph, the anterior border of the heart is formed by the RV and the posterior border of the heart is formed by the left atrium (above the hilum) and LV (below the hilum). On a conventional posteroanterior chest radiograph the cardiothoracic ratio can be measured. This expresses the proportion of heart size to internal thoracic diameter. Cardiothoracic ratio is normally well below 50% but in anteroposterior radiographs (usually mobile or portable radiographs) normal value can be accepted as 55%. In infants, the normal value can also be 55%.

Echocardiography

Imaging Techniques

Transthoracic echocardiogram is a critical and usually first line tool for structural and functional assessment of the heart. Two-dimensional echocardiography provides images of cardiac structures, analogous to getting a thin "slice" through the heart (Fig. 20.33A) [30]. M-mode imaging is a one-dimensional evaluation using a single line of ultrasound interrogation down a specific orientation through cardiac structures (Fig. 20.33B). While

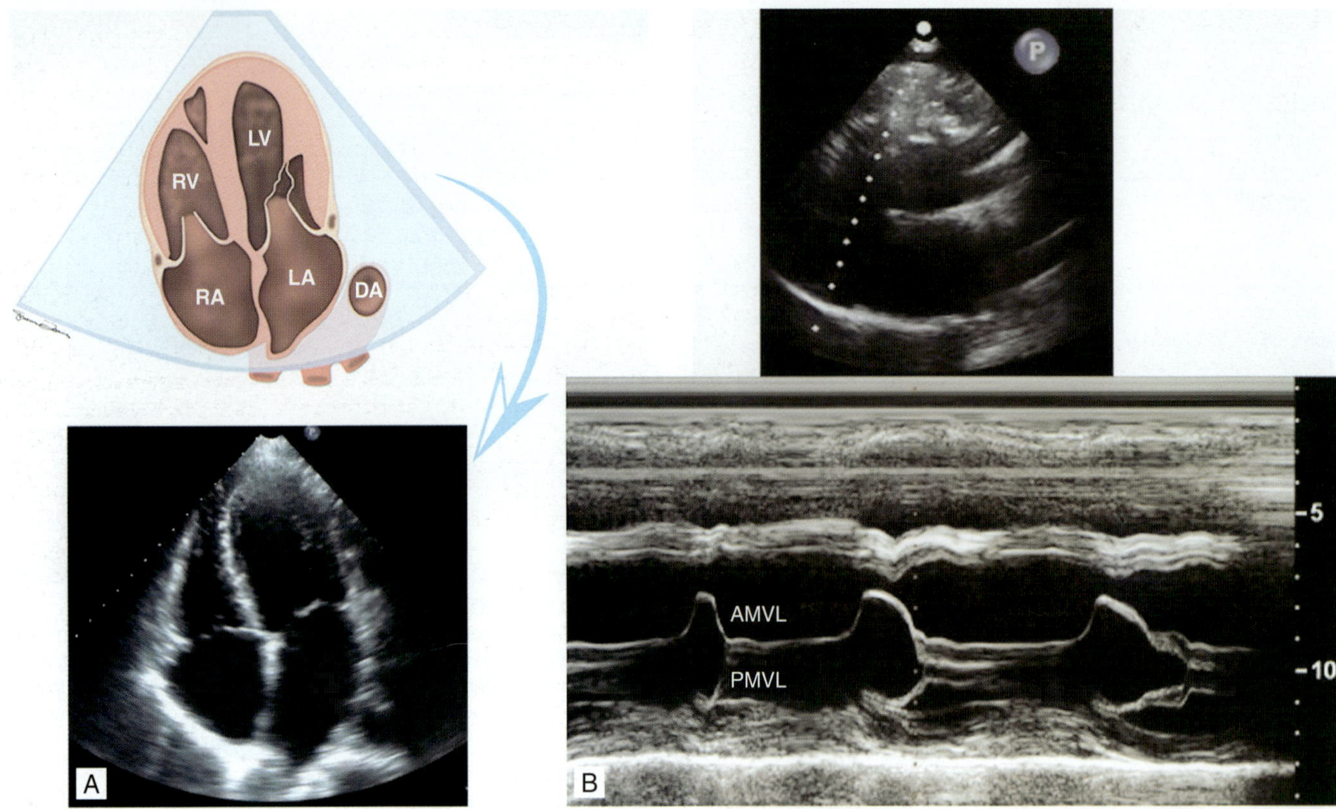

Figure 20.33 (A) Transthoracic echocardiogram image along with the illustration shows the relationships of the right atrium (RA), right ventricle (RV), left atrium (LA), left ventricle (LV), and descending aorta (DA). (Courtesy: Sussane Loomis, MS, Medical and Scientific Communications, Department of Radiology, Massachusetts General Hospital, Boston, MA, USA.) (B) M-mode of the mitral valve, the anterior mitral valve leaflet (AMVL) and posterior mitral valve leaflet (PMVL) are in view. The 2D echocardiogram image at the top shows the direction of the M-mode beam through the left ventricle.

M-mode imaging has limited spatial resolution, the temporal resolution is very high due to the high sampling rate, allowing precise timing evaluation of cardiac events (valve opening or closure) [30].

Doppler echocardiography allows evaluation of blood flow through the heart and is carried out using continuous-wave, pulsed-wave, and color flow Doppler techniques. Continuous-wave Doppler technique employs a continuously emitting transducer adjacent to a continuously receiving transducer. This allows a continuous interrogation down the length of the ultrasound beam but the technique does not allow differentiation of structures at any particular depth along the beam. This allows quantification of high-velocity flows, such as assessment of peak velocity in aortic stenosis. The velocity–pressure relationship across an orifice (e.g., valve) is defined by the modified Bernoulli equation; pressure gradient, $\Delta P = 4 \times \text{velocity}^2$ [30]. For example, velocity of the tricuspid regurgitation jet can be used to estimate the pressure gradient/difference between right atrium and RV.

Pulse-wave Doppler examination uses time delays to interrogate at specific depths along the beam. This means that measurements can be made at precise sites within the heart. For example, pulsed-Doppler evaluation is an integral component of diastolic assessment of the LV, and measurement of left ventricular outflow and inflow velocities. Color flow Doppler examination is based on the principle of pulsed-Doppler technique and as such it is limited by high-velocity flows. Color flow Doppler superimposed on two-dimensional imaging is extremely helpful in identifying abnormal blood flow within the heart, for example, color flow jet through the interventricular septum to define a ventricular septal defect, or regurgitant flow through a valve (Fig. 20.34). Furthermore, the characteristics of the color flow jet in valvular heart disease can provide quantitative and qualitative assessment of regurgitant lesions.

The cardiac cycle consists of ventricular systole and diastole. Systole is the period from mitral valve closure to aortic valve closure. It begins with ventricular depolarization, and subsequent

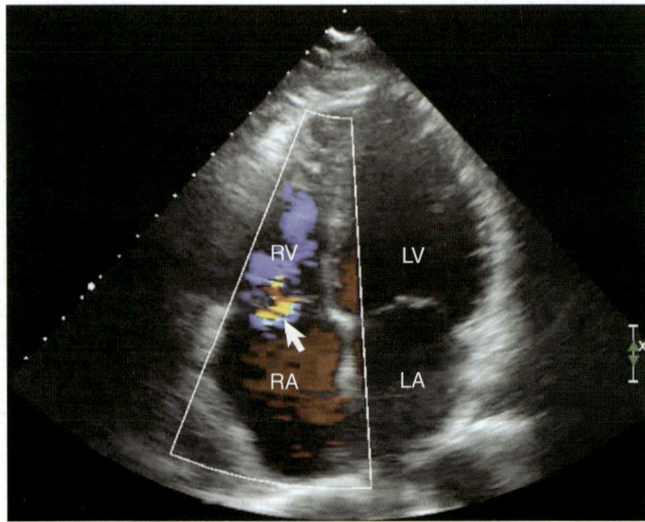

Figure 20.34 Color flow Doppler image on transthoracic echocardiography showing flow through the tricuspid valve. A trace amount of regurgitant flow is noted going back into the right atrium (*white arrow*).

left ventricular contraction, which leads to LV pressure exceeding LA pressure resulting in closure of the mitral valve. This is followed by isovolumic contraction, where ventricular pressure increases rapidly while the ventricular volume remains constant. When LV pressure exceeds aortic pressure, the aortic valve opens and blood is ejected into the aorta [30]. Diastole is initiated by closure of the aortic valve, which is followed by isovolumic relaxation, where both valves are closed and LV volume remains constant but pressure drops rapidly as LV myocardium relaxes. When LV pressure is less than LA pressure, mitral valve opens, and blood starts to come into the LV. Ventricular volume ranges from a minimum at end-systole (LVESV) to a maximum at end-diastole (LVEDV). Stroke volume (SV) is the difference between end-diastolic volume and end-systolic volume. LV ejection fraction is a measure of overall ventricular function and is defined as [30]:

$$\text{Ejection fraction (EF\%)} = \frac{\text{LVEDV} - \text{LVESV}}{\text{LVEDV}} \times 100\%$$
$$= \frac{\text{SV}}{\text{LVEDV}} \times 100\%$$

Doppler echocardiography can also be used to estimate intracardiac pressures. Normal values for intracardiac and pulmonary pressures are provided in Table 20.3 [31]. Furthermore, quantification of systemic (Qs) and pulmonary (Qp) blood through Doppler echocardiography is important in identifying the degree of shunting in cases of intra or extracardiac shunts. For example, a Qp/Qs ratio <1.5 indicates a small left to right shunt, while a ratio >2.0 signifies a large left to right shunt [31].

Standard Transthoracic Echocardiogram Views

Transthoracic echocardiography is usually performed with the patient laying in a left lateral decubitus or supine position [30]. A complete transthoracic exam includes assessment from four standard windows; parasternal, apical, suprasternal, and subcostal. Window refers to the physical location of the transducer or probe on the chest wall (Fig. 20.35). Each cardiac window can provide two-dimensional views of different cardiac planes based on the rotation and angulation of the probe at each window. For example, parasternal long axis displays the LV along its long axis, with the anteroseptal wall and the inferolateral walls in view (Fig. 20.36A), however, the parasternal short axis view is obtained by rotating the transducer in the same location to obtain a transaxial view of the LV (Fig. 20.36B).

TABLE 20.3 Normal Ranges for Intracardiac and Pulmonary Pressures

Chamber	Pressure (Systolic/Diastolic)
Right atrium/central venous pressure	Mean: 1–5 mm Hg
Right ventricle	15–30/1–7 mm Hg
Pulmonary artery	15–30/4–12 mm Hg Mean: 9–19 mm Hg
Left atrium	Mean: 2–12 mm Hg
Left ventricle	90–140/5–12 mm Hg
Aorta	90–140/60–90 mm Hg Mean: 70–105 mm Hg

Adapted from [31].

Transesophageal Echocardiography

This technique involves insertion of an echocardiography probe in the esophagus of a sedated patient. This allows images to be obtained from close proximity to the heart and without acoustic interference from lung or bone tissue. Image quality is especially improved for the posterior most structures such as left atrium, mitral valve, pulmonary veins, and interatrial septum (Fig. 20.37) [30]. Positioning of the probe at different locations within the esophagus (upper esophagus to deep gastric), and the ability to rotate the imaging plane from within the transducer, allows visualization of multiple different cardiac planes. Indications for use of transesophageal echocardiography can be divided into general and procedural settings, and are outlined in Table 20.4 [32]. It is important to note that unlike transthoracic echocardiography, transesophageal echocardiography is an invasive procedure, and while the complication rate is extremely low (death <0.01–0.02%, esophageal perforation/major bleeding <0.01%), there are absolute and relative contraindications to the procedure [30]. These are clearly outlined in the American society of Echocardiography Consensus Document on the use of transesophageal echocardiography [32].

Contrast-Enhanced Echocardiography

This study uses agitated saline containing microbubbles, injected through a peripheral IV, to allow opacification of right-sided structures. It is most useful in identifying right to left extracardiac (e.g., pulmonary) or intracardiac shunts (patent foramen ovale, atrial septal defects; Fig. 20.38), however, other uses can include detection of persistent left superior vena cava, delineating right heart borders and masses, and echo-guidance during pericardiocentesis.

Agitated saline bubbles are mostly absorbed during their transit through the lungs, and cannot be used to adequately opacify left-sided structures. Commercially available contrast agents consist of a thin and relatively permeable shell (consisting of phospholipids or human albumin), which is typically filled with an inert gas slowing diffusion and dissolution of microbubbles within the blood [33]. Availability of these agents and commercial names vary based on geographic areas [34,35]. These agents along with contrast-specific imaging techniques are used to enhance LV opacification and endocardial border definition in patients with suboptimal echocardiogram images [33]. Most importantly, the clinical use of these agents is not limited by hepatic or renal dysfunction, since the microbubbles eventually dissolve in the bloodstream.

Cross-Sectional Imaging

Multidetector row computed tomography and MRI have enabled detailed assessment of static and dynamic cardiac anatomy. Contrast-enhanced CT images allow accurate delineation of cardiac chambers, myocardium, pericardium, coronary arteries, and cardiac veins, as well as the inflow and outflow vessels. CT enables acquisition of volume of data which can then be manipulated to obtain different reconstructions including multiplanar reformats, maximum intensity projection, minimum intensity projections, curved planar reformats, and volume-rendered three-dimensional images. This enables more detailed analysis of cardiac anatomy with innumerable projections which is not possible with other imaging techniques, particularly projectional imaging techniques. The four-dimensional aspect of CT allows a very comprehensive

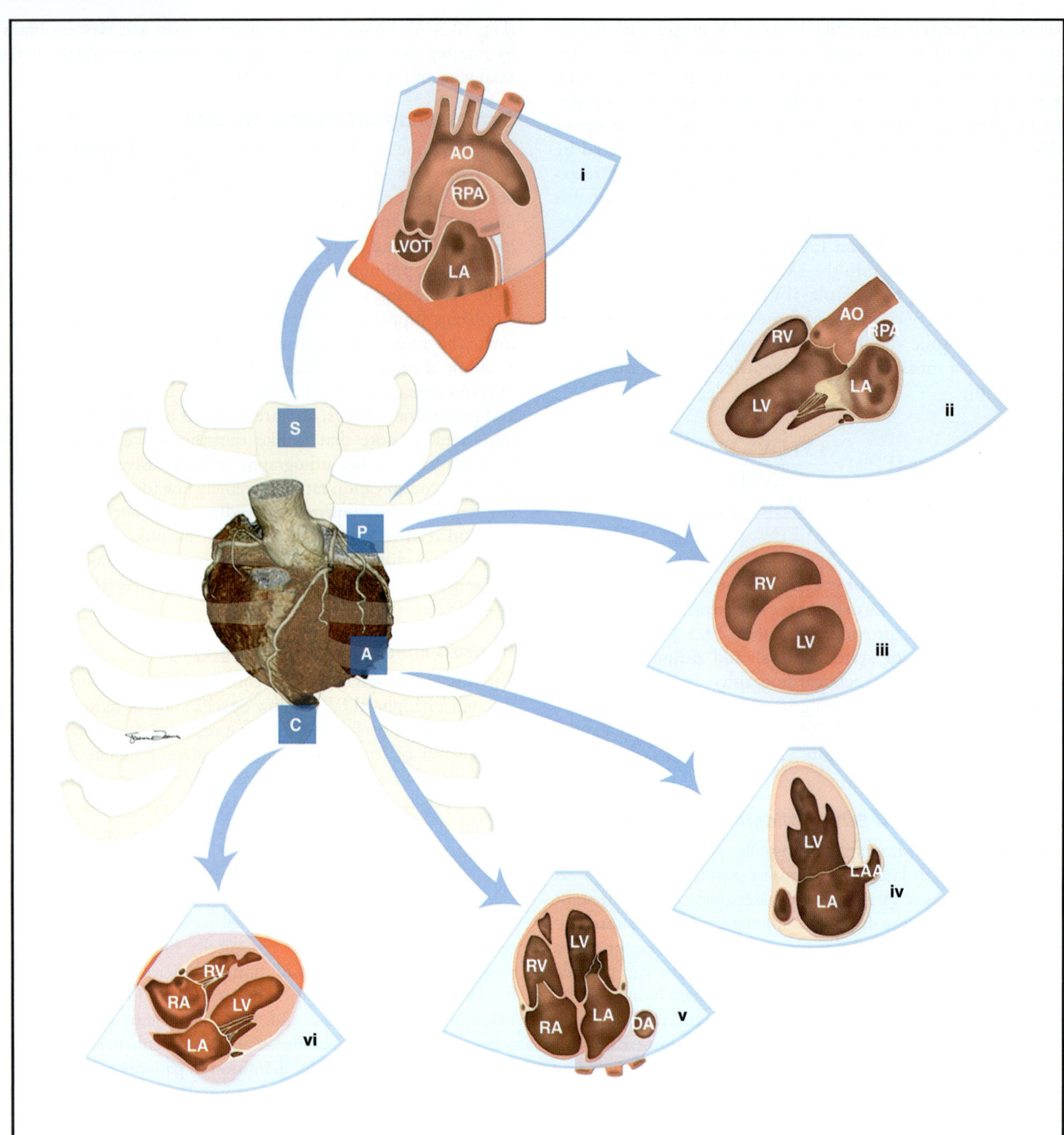

Figure 20.35 Illustration showing the physical location of the ultrasound transducer on the chest wall for various transthoracic imaging windows: (S) suprasternal, (P) parasternal, (A) apical, and (C) subcostal. The cut-outs illustrate the standard transthoracic views; (i) suprasternal notch view, (ii) parasternal long axis view, (iii) parasternal short axis view, (iv) apical two-chamber view, (v) apical four-chamber view, and (vi) subcostal view. *AO*, aorta; *LA*, left atrium; *LV*, left ventricle; *LVOT*, left ventricular outflow tract; *RA*, right atrium; *RPA*, right pulmonary artery; *RV*, right ventricle. (Courtesy: Sussane Loomis, MS, Medical and Scientific Communications, Department of Radiology, Massachusetts General Hospital, Boston, MA, USA.)

evaluation of cardiac structure and function, and is especially useful in identifying normal variants of cardiac structure from true pathology.

Optimal spatial resolution combined with higher soft tissue characterization capabilities of cardiac MRI also make it an ideal technique for distinguishing between normal anatomy and cardiac pathology. CMR can allow detailed assessment of cardiac structures even without contrast administration, however, gadolinium-based MRI contrasts do not pose a significant risk of allergic reactions or contrast mediated nephropathy like their iodine-based CT counterparts. Precise quantitative assessments of flow through regurgitant valves or intracardiac shunts are some of the important utilities of flow-based CMR techniques that make cardiac CMR superior to other imaging techniques. CMR sequences and their utility in assessment of normal cardiac anatomy and pathological processes are summarized in Table 20.5. While CT and MRI techniques and their applications are discussed in detail in their separate chapters, major indications of cardiac CT and MRI are outlined in Table 20.6.

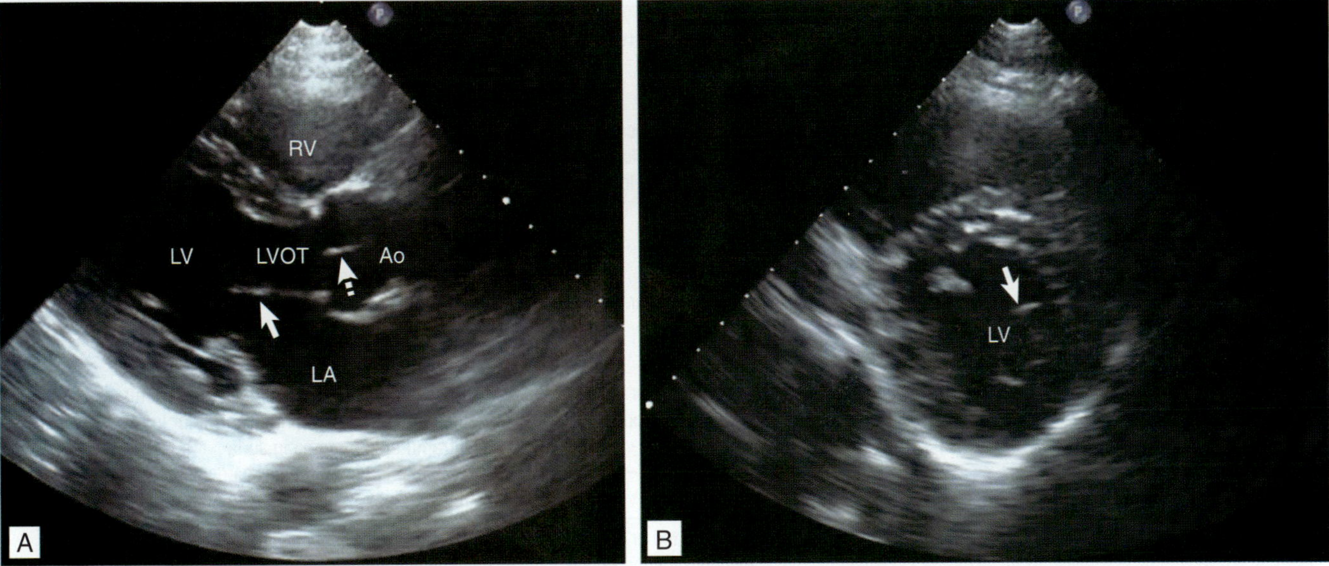

Figure 20.36 Transthoracic echocardiogram image showing parasternal long axis (A) and parasternal short axis (B) views of the heart, which are obtained from the same parasternal window on the chest wall. *Ao*, ascending aorta; *LA*, left atrium; *LV*, left ventricle; *LVOT*, left ventricular outflow tract; *RV*, right ventricle. The solid *white arrow* points to the anterior leaflet of the mitral valve, while the *dashed arrow* points to the aortic valve closure line.

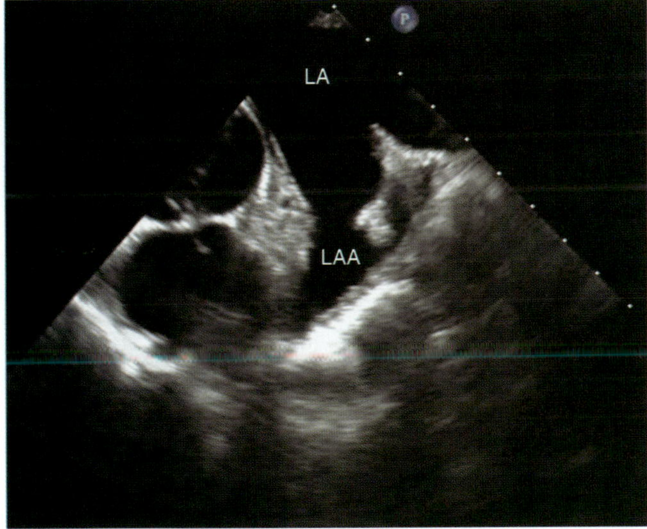

Figure 20.37 Transesophageal echocardiogram (TEE) image of the mid-esophageal view of the left atrial appendage (LAA).

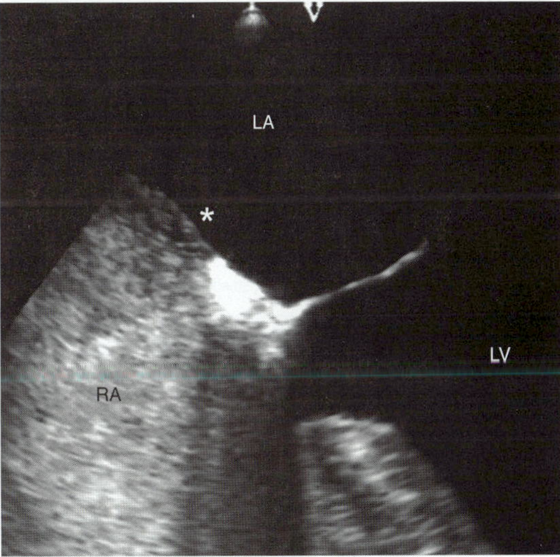

Figure 20.38 Transesophageal echocardiogram image showing agitated saline contrast in the right atrium (RA). There is no evidence of bubble contrast in the left atrium (LA), indicating an intact atrial septum. *LV*, left ventricle.

TABLE 20.4 Indications for Use of Transesophageal Echocardiography (TEE) in the Clinical Setting

General	▪ In-depth evaluation of structures that are in the far field on TTE imaging ▪ Left atrial appendage to rule out the presence of left atrial thrombi in patients with suspected cardioembolic stroke ▪ Interatrial septum in patients with suspected atrial septal defects ▪ Evaluation of prosthetic valves ▪ Evaluation of paravalvular abscess (native and prosthetic valves)
Procedural	▪ Guiding catheter placement in catheter-based intracardiac procedures, e.g., left atrial appendage closure device placement, mitral clip placement, and transcatheter valve procedure ▪ Open heart valvular and thoracic aorta procedures, e.g., assessing valvular gradients immediately after valvular repair or replacement

Adapted from [32].

TABLE 20.5 Key Cardiac Magnetic Resonance Imaging Sequences and Their Utility

Category	Sequence	Description	Utility
Localizer	Balanced SSFP	Three-plane localizer Two-chamber localizer Four-chamber localizer	Broad overview of cardiac/chest anatomy
Structure and function	Balanced SSFP	Short axis Four-chamber Two-chamber Three-chamber LVOT Axial	Global and regional myocardial function High SNR and image contrast provides good endocardial border definition
Tissue characterization	Double inversion recovery multiecho spin echo	T1-weighted or T2-weighted without fat suppression	T1-weighted imaging: (i) Anatomic structures such as pericardium and lymph nodes, (ii) fat in RV free wall or intramural hematoma in aorta T2-weighted imaging: myocardial edema in acute myocardial infarction or acute myocarditis
	Triple inversion recovery multiecho spin echo	T1-weighted or T2-weighted without fat suppression	To confirm the presence of fat
	Modified Look-Locker inversion recovery (MOLLI) Shortened modified Look-Locker inversion recovery (ShMOLLI)	T1 parametric mapping	Diffuse infiltration or scarring not detected by LGE
	Multiple TE spin echo or T2-weighted balanced SSFP	T2 parametric mapping	Diffuse myocardial edema
	Multiple TE spoiled gradient-recalled echo	T2* parametric mapping	Myocardial iron deposition and myocardial hemorrhage
Perfusion	Spoiled gradient echo	Ultrashort TE and TR T1-weighted gradient echo	Myocardial perfusion
Viability	Inversion recovery spoiled gradient echo (or balanced SSFP)	Late gadolinium enhancement	Extent and location of myocardial fibrosis
Vascular and flow	3D spoiled gradient echo (or balanced SSFP)	Magnetic resonance angiography	Vessel anatomy
	Phase-contrast gradient echo	Flow quantification	Flow velocities, profile, and volume

RV, right ventricle; *SNR*, signal-to-noise ratio; *SSFP*, steady state free precision; *TE*, echo time; *TR*, repetition time.

TABLE 20.6 Major Indications for Cardiac Computed Tomography and Cardiac Magnetic Resonance Imaging

Cardiac CT	Coronary calcium scoring Plaque burden and degree of luminal narrowing in coronary artery disease Patency of coronary artery stents and coronary artery bypass grafts Preprocedural planning, e.g., transcatheter aortic/mitral valve replacement, pulmonary vein ablation, and left atrial appendage closure Cardiac anatomy and function Cardiac masses Pericardial disease Congenital heart disease
Cardiac MRI	Cardiac anatomy and function Myocardial perfusion Myocardial viability Cardiomyopathy Cardiac masses Valvular heart disease Cardiac shunts Pericardial disease Congenital heart disease

Invasive Coronary Angiogram

Despite the wide range of noninvasive options available for coronary imaging, coronary angiography remains the gold standard for the diagnosis of coronary artery disease [36]. Coronary angiography may be combined with right and left heart catherization for the evaluation of intracardiac pressures, and/or left ventriculography for evaluation of left ventricular systolic function and wall motion abnormalities (Fig. 20.39). Lastly, the ultimate advantage of invasive coronary angiography is the ability to intervene therapeutically during the procedure, if clinically indicated. Coronary angiographic equipment has very high x-ray specifications because diagnostic demands are extremely high. Image resolution must be capable of demonstrating coronary anatomical detail down to structures of 0.3 mm or less and exposure times must be no more than 5 ms. This must be achievable with frame rates of 12.5 frames/s (digital) or 25 frames/s (cine).

The traditional standard access for coronary angiograms had been the common femoral artery, however, radial artery access has become popular in recent years. For femoral access, the aim of the proceduralist is to gain access below the take-off of the inferior epigastric artery and above the bifurcation of the common femoral artery. Access above this point increases the risk of retroperitoneal hematoma, and below this increases the risk for pseudoaneurysm formation, AV fistula formation, and

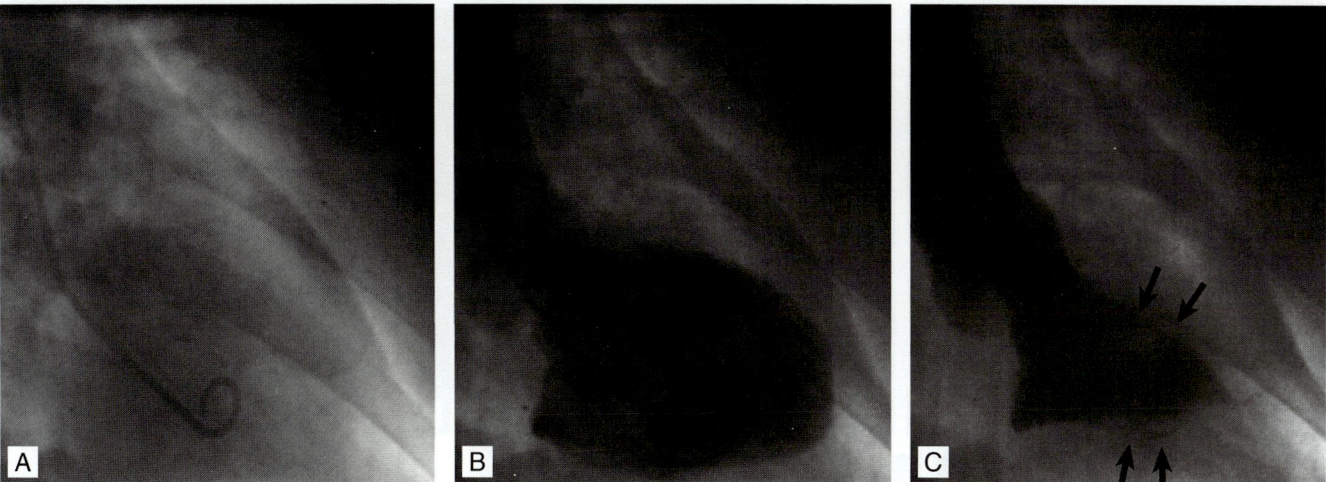

Figure 20.39 Left ventricular angiogram in the right anterior oblique projection using a pigtail catheter. (A) Plain frame. (B) Diastolic frame. (C) Systolic frame. The papillary muscles are *arrowed*.

cannulation of the superficial femoral artery which cannot accommodate vascular closure devices and large sheaths [36]. Commonly used catheter shapes such as Judkins or Amplatz allow selective cannulation of the left and right coronary ostia. Iodine as the contrast medium at 320–370 mg/mL is generally employed. This can be injected manually by hand using a multivalve manifold at flow rates of 2–4 mL/s, or using power injectors [36]. The latter technique is more commonly employed for large volume injections such as during left ventriculography or aortography.

Standard coronary angiography views allow visualization of the origin and course of the three main coronary arteries and their branches in at least two different planes. For all views, the x-ray source is under the table, and the image intensifier (II) is directly above the patient. The x-ray source and the II move in an arc around the patient, and the patient body surface facing the II determines the view, for example, for the left anterior oblique view, the II is facing the left anterior chest of the patient. In addition, the II can tilt toward the head or feet of the patient, to provide cranial or caudal projections, respectively (Fig. 20.40). The standard angiography views are depicted in Fig. 20.41.

Percutaneous revascularization is generally recommended for coronary lesions with greater than 70–80% diameter stenosis [31]. In recent years, numerous additional techniques have been developed to assess the severity and physiologic significance of borderline coronary lesions. Fractional flow reserve and instantaneous wave-free ratio depend on pressure measurements proximal and distal to the stenosis to assess the hemodynamic significance of a lesion. Both have been validated in multiple trials to predict ischemic outcomes [31].

Pulmonary angiography can be performed for the assessment of possible pulmonary embolism. The technique is relatively straightforward but it does require sufficient experience to pass a venous catheter through the right atrium, RV and main pulmonary artery. In performing such an examination the patient should be fully monitored for pressure and ECG evaluation to be aware of any cardiac irregularity caused by passage of the catheter. Pharmacomechanical catheter-directed therapy via a right heart

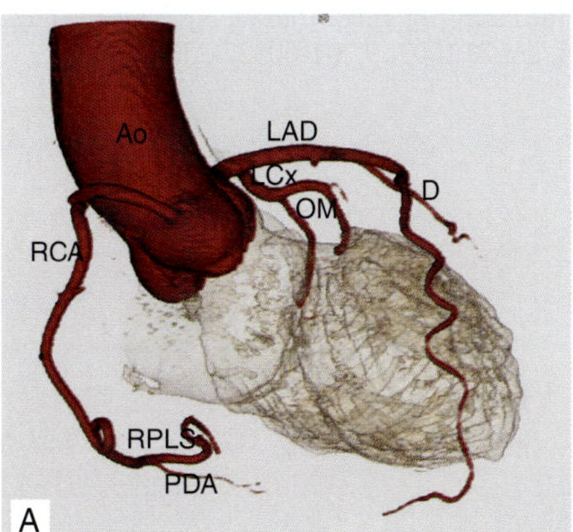

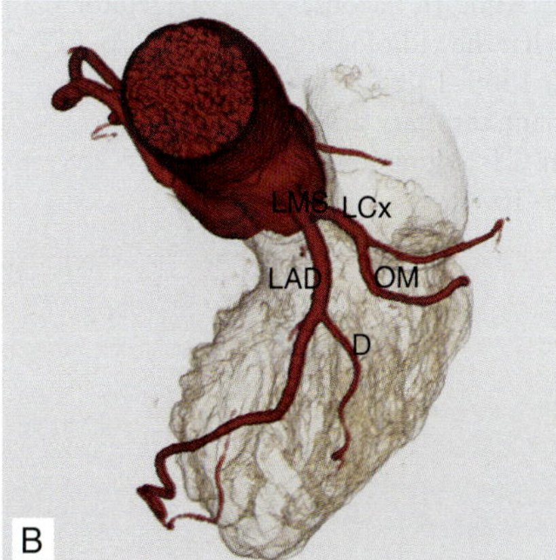

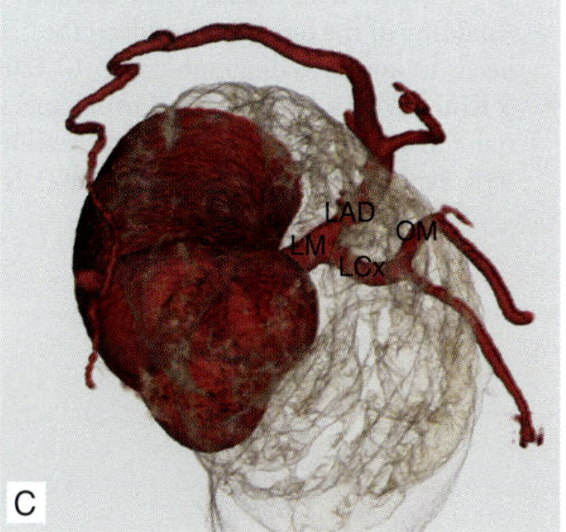

Figure 20.40 Three-dimensional volume-rendered coronary computed tomography angiography images showing the basic angiography views. (A) Right anterior oblique cranial angulation is used to display the entire length of the left anterior descending artery (LAD), and the proximal and distal segments of the right coronary artery (RCA). The LAD is seen wrapping around the left ventricular apex. (B) Left anterior oblique cranial angulation shows the LAD straight down, and the left circumflex artery (LCx) traversing the atrioventricular groove. (C) Left anterior oblique caudal angulation is an important view for the left main stem (LMS) and proximal segments of the LAD and LCx. *Ao*, aorta; *D*, diagonal branch; LAD, left anterior descending artery; *LCx*, left circumflex artery; *LMS*, left main stem; *OM*, obtuse marginal branch; *PDA*, posterior descending artery; *RPLS*, posterolateral branch.

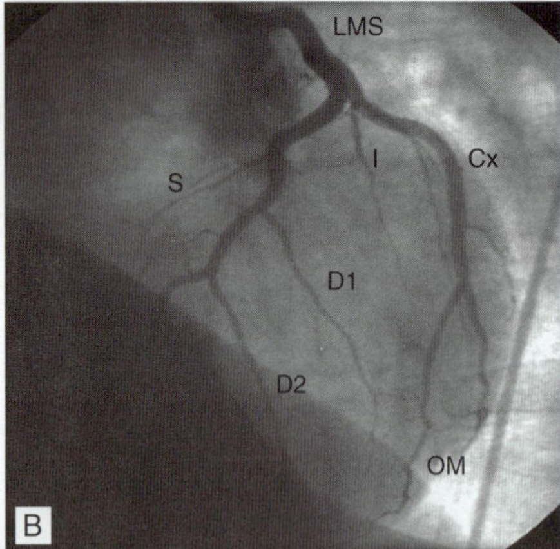

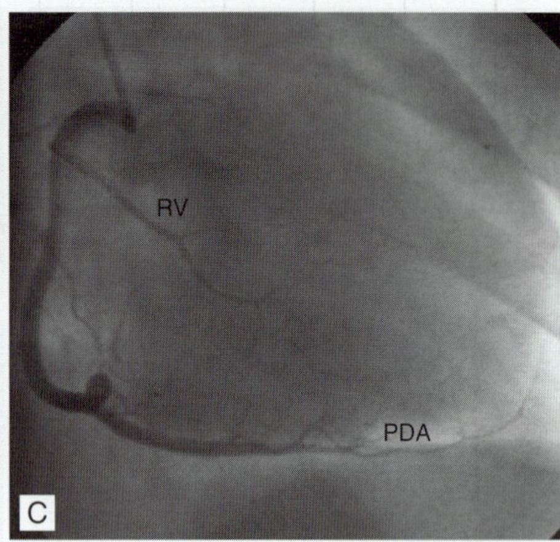

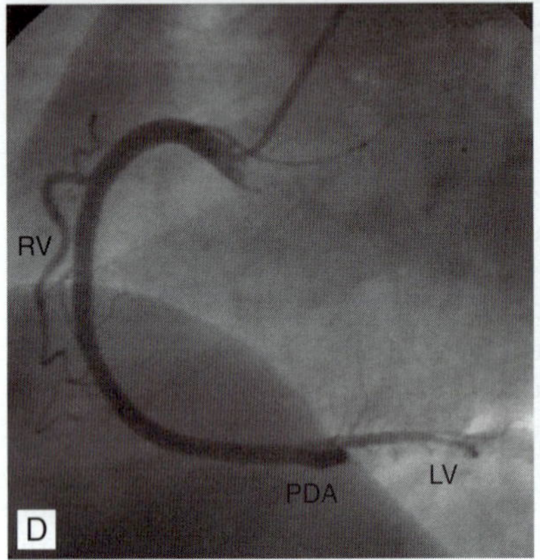

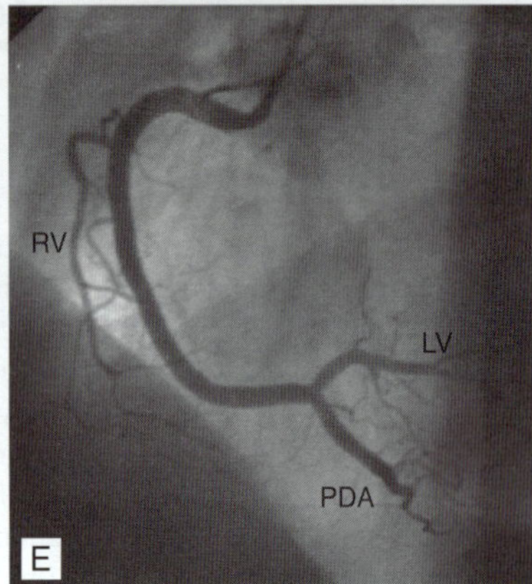

Figure 20.41 Series of normal coronary artery angiograms. *Cx*, left circumflex artery; *D*, diagonal branch; *I*, ramus intermedius branch; *LAD*, left anterior descending artery; *LMS*, left main stem; *LV*, posterolateral branch; *OM*, obtuse marginal branch; *PDA*, posterior descending artery; *RV*, right ventricular/acute marginal branch; *S*, septal branch. (A) Right anterior oblique view of the left coronary artery. (B) Cranially angulated view of the left coronary artery. (C) Right anterior oblique view of the right coronary artery. (D) Left anterior oblique view of the right coronary artery. The posterior descending artery is foreshortened. (E) Cranially angulated left anterior oblique view of the right coronary artery. The posterior descending artery is now well profiled.

catheterization approach is frequently used today for treatment of massive pulmonary embolism or high risk submassive pulmonary embolism [31]. This allows targeted delivery of a lower dose of thrombolytics to significantly decrease the accompanying risk of major bleeding [31].

Suggested Readings

- JP O'Brien, MB Srichai, EM Hecht, DC Kim, JE Jacobs, Anatomy of the heart at multidetector CT: what the radiologist needs to know, Radiographics 27 (6) (2007) 1569–1582.
- S Kini, KG Bis, L Weaver, Normal and variant coronary arterial and venous anatomy on high-resolution CT angiography, AJR Am J Roentgenol 188 (6) (2007) 1665–1674.
- PA Iaizzo, The Visible Heart® project and free-access website "Atlas of Human Cardiac Anatomy", EP Eur 18 (Suppl_4) (2016) 163–172, iv.
- F Saremi, D Sánchez-Quintana, S Mori, H Muresian, DE Spicer, C Hassani, et al., Fibrous skeleton of the heart: anatomic overview and evaluation of pathologic conditions with CT and MR imaging, Radiogr Rev Publ Radiol Soc N Am Inc 37 (5) (2017) 1330–1351.
- MA Kadoch, H-CRF Becker, CT cardiac anatomy, in: Schoepf UJ, editor. CT of the Heart [Internet]. Totowa, NJ: Humana Press; 2019. p. 227–234. doi:10.1007/ 978-1-60327-237-7_20.

21

Chest Radiograph in Acquired Heart Disease

SACHIN S. SABOO, DHIRAJ BARUAH, CARLOS S. RESTREPO

Introduction

The chest radiograph with its ready availability, low radiation dose, and relatively low expense is an easily repeatable examination. This, together with its ability to show the heart size and pulmonary vascularity, makes it an ideal monitoring examination to follow the progress of a disease or its treatment [1].

Heart Size and Shape

A posteroanterior (PA) chest radiograph is an important indicator of cardiac size. Not only can global cardiac enlargement be detected but individual chamber enlargement can also be identified, particularly when both PA and lateral radiographs are available [1].

The most common method of describing the heart size is by using the cardiothoracic ratio (CTR) (Fig. 21.1). This is derived by measuring:

1. the internal diameter of the thoracic cavity from the medial border of the ribs at the level of the right hemidiaphragm, and
2. the transverse cardiac measurement as the horizontal distance the most lateral aspects of the left and right margins of the heart.

The CTR is expressed as a percentage of the heart size with respect to the internal thoracic diameter. It is sometimes useful to record the actual measurements from the radiograph. While the most common figure used as a normal CTR is a maximum of 50% [2], some important caveats such as prominent pericardial fat pad are also needed to be observed.

The CTR is often increased in neonates and can also be increased in the elderly, often being associated with an unfolding of the aorta or thoracic scoliosis. An increased CTR can be fallacious if the radiograph is obtained during expiration or in the supine position [3].

Moderate to severe cardiomegaly can be suggested in an adult if the CTR is >0.55 [1]. On an AP chest radiograph, a CTR of 60% has higher specificity when evaluating for cardiac enlargement [3]. Differential diagnosis for moderate to severely enlarged cardiac silhouette is listed in Table 21.1.

The common causes of a small cardiac silhouette are extracardiac conditions, in particular the presence of emphysema or air trapping. Additional causes include cachexia and adrenal insufficiency.

Enlargement of the heart is often associated with the enlargement of a specific chamber and the dynamic changes can be assessed through plain film, for example, stenosis or regurgitation of a valve. Isolated enlargement of individual cardiac chambers is less common than multichamber enlargement, the latter being the consequence of sequential effects of one lesion upon several parts of the cardiovascular circulation. A dilated and failing left ventricle (LV) can lead to left atrial enlargement and this, in turn, can raise pulmonary pressure and increase the size of the right-sided chambers as well. Single chamber enlargement will be discussed in detail later in the chapter, to provide an insight into the assessment of multichamber enlargement as well as highlight several other conditions.

The vascular pedicle width (VPW) on the chest radiograph is used to estimate the intravascular volume status and can be

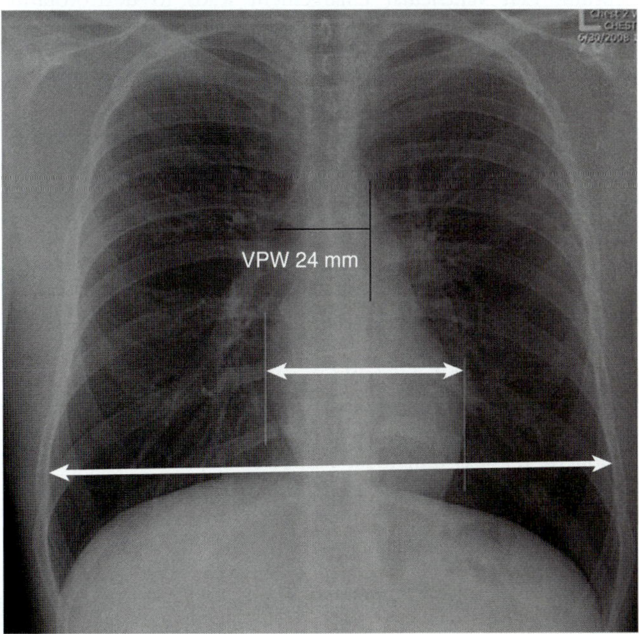

Figure 21.1 The assessment of cardiac enlargement. The cardiac diameter should be the maximum cardiac diameter (*double arrowed shorter line*). The transverse thoracic diameter is measured in various ways; here it is measured as the maximum internal diameter of the thorax (*double arrowed wider line*). Vascular pedicle width (VPW) is the distance on a horizontal line obtained from first dropping a perpendicular line at the takeoff point of the left subclavian artery from the aortic arch to the point at which the superior vena cava crosses the right main bronchus as shown by black lines. VPW is normal as shown in this radiograph and is below 49.3 mm.

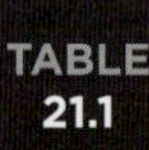

TABLE 21.1 Acquired Causes for Moderate to Severely Enlarged Cardiac Silhouette Based on Cardiothoracic Ratio (CTR)

Moderate to severely enlarged cardiac silhouette (CTR >0.55)
Volume overload: LA enlargement due to mitral valve regurgitation Aortic valve regurgitation related to enlarged ascending aorta Tricuspid valve regurgitation-related enlarged right atrium
Dilated cardiomyopathy
Ischemic cardiomyopathy
Pericardial effusion and pericardial mass

measured in either supine or erect positions (Fig. 21.1). Studies have reported the VPW to be significantly larger in patients with volume overload. Different cut-off VPW values exist based on radiographic projections with mean VPW values on supine being significantly larger than in erect radiographs, with 71 mm on supine (95% confidence interval 64.9–77.3 mm) and 62 mm (95% confidence interval 49.3–75.1 mm) on erect, respectively. VPW values can be altered by respiratory effects.

Azygos vein diameter of more than 1 cm on an erect chest radiograph is considered to be dilated and is indicative of systemic venous hypertension or right ventricular failure [4].

Cardiac rotation occurs due to enlargement of individual cardiac chambers (Table 21.2). The axis of cardiac rotation is nearly vertical and extends from the top of the aortic arch through the anterior wall of the left atrium and the proximal interventricular septum. Left ventricular enlargement leads to dextrorotation while the right ventricular enlargement leads to levorotation. Levorotation suggests leftward rotation while dextrorotation reflects rightward rotation of cardiac silhouette [5].

Approach to Acquired Heart Disease on Chest Radiograph

It is important to have a systematic checklist when evaluating chest radiographs and is particularly critical for the assessment of acquired heart diseases to not miss subtle but important abnormalities and to narrow down the differential diagnosis. This includes evaluating radiographs in patients with suspected cardiac abnormality for thoracic arteries including the thoracic aorta and central pulmonary arteries, overall pulmonary vascularity, cardiac silhouette for size, individual cardiac chamber enlargement, and thoracic osseous abnormalities [1,6–8].

The abnormal left cardiovascular silhouette on the frontal radiograph occurs from superior to inferior aspect due to enlargement of the aortic arch, main pulmonary artery, left atrial appendage, and left or right ventricles (RV) [1,6–8].

- The main pulmonary artery appears as a smooth convexity above the upper portion of the right ventricular contour just below the aortopulmonary region and in parallel just above the level of the left main bronchus. Causes of the enlargement of the main pulmonary artery are described in the pulmonary hypertension section [6–8]
- Left atrial appendage region is located inferior and adjacent to the left bronchus. The enlargement of the left atrial appendage is seen as a bulge along the left cardiac border just beneath the main pulmonary artery. Causes for enlargement in this region include enlarged left atrial appendage, enlarged right ventricular outflow tract, left pericardium partial defect, and cardiac, pericardial, or mediastinal tumors [6–8]
- Causes for enlargement along the lower left cardiac border on the frontal radiograph are described in the section for causes of left ventricular and right ventricular enlargement

The abnormal bulge of the right cardiac silhouette on the frontal radiograph occurs predominantly due to right atrial (RA) enlargement [6–8]. Other causes for bulging and enlargement of the right cardiac silhouette include

- prominent right paracardiac fat pad;
- pericardial cyst or pericardial tumor;
- right diaphragmatic eventration or hernia; and
- tumors of the heart, diaphragm, or mediastinum.

Individual Cardiac Chamber Enlargement

Left Atrial Enlargement

The left atrium is a roughly spherical posteriormost cardiac chamber and if it is enlarged, the increased density of the enlarged chamber itself is often evident, particularly on a penetrated PA; (Fig. 21.2) or a lateral view. The double density/extra shadow along the right heart border on the PA film due to the enlarged left atrium is formed by the projection of the distended rightward margin of the left atrium lying close to the usual RA margin [6–8]. *A "double" right heart border, elevation of the left main bronchus, horizontal orientation of the distal portion of the left bronchus, splaying of the carina, and enlargement of the left atrial appendage are features of left atrial enlargement* [6–9]. Posterior displacement of the left upper lobe bronchus due to left atrial enlargement is seen on the lateral radiograph. The displaced left upper lobe bronchus is seen posterior and beyond the plane of the trachea [6–9]. While these features are usually well recognized, exact measurements have been suggested as shown in Fig. 21.3. A distance

TABLE 21.2 Types of Cardiac Rotation and Their Appearance

Levorotation of Heart	Dextrorotation of Heart
Etiology: atrial septal defect, ventricular septal defect, pulmonic valvular stenosis, mitral valve disease, cor pulmonale with right ventricular dilatation, absence of the pericardium, deformity of the thoracic skeleton and left lower lobe atelectasis	*Etiology:* dilatation of the left ventricle due to heart failure as a sequelae of coronary heart disease, hypertension, cardiomyopathy, aortic regurgitation, severe aortic stenosis, severe coarctation, and patent ductus arteriosus
Radiograph appearance: convex main pulmonary artery segment, narrow mediastinal vascular pedicle elevation of the cardiac apex, rarely, filling in of the retrocardiac space on a lateral view	*Radiograph appearance:* concave pulmonary artery segment, widening of the aortic arch loop, caudal displacement of the cardiac apex, and, rarely, filling in of the retrosternal space

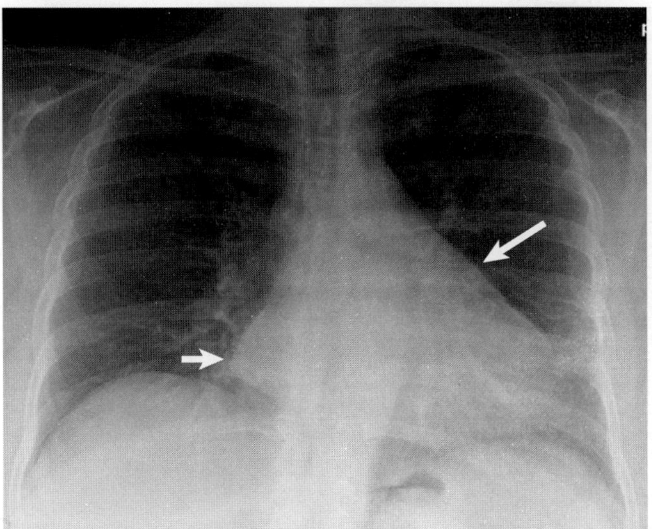

Figure 21.2 Rheumatic mitral stenosis. This frontal film shows enlargement of the left atrial appendage (*long arrow*) in addition to the increased density of the right heart border (*short arrow*).

between the middle of the double density (formed by the lateral border of the left atrium) and the middle of the left main bronchus of greater than 7 cm has been shown to indicate left atrial enlargement in over 90% of cases [6–9].

Typically acquired causes of left atrial enlargement include mitral insufficiency, mitral stenosis, decreased LV compliance due to hypertrophic cardiomyopathy, and restrictive cardiomyopathy [6–9].

Right Atrial Enlargement

The features of RA enlargement can be subtle and difficult to determine in mild and moderate cases. The right atrium enlarges in the rightward and posterior direction. *The most common finding on the frontal radiograph is a lateral prominence of the right cardiac border, often associated with an increased convexity particularly at the superior border at its junction with the SVC* [6–8]. In severe chronic cases, the right heart border can become massively distended toward the right side (Fig. 21.4). RA enlargement on PA view can result in elongation of the right heart border (Fig. 21.4). On the lateral radiograph, RA enlargement results in the sharp horizontal interface with the lung above the RV and displacement of cardiac silhouette posterior to inferior vena cava (IVC), like LV enlargement.

Typically acquired causes of RA enlargement include tricuspid stenosis and tricuspid regurgitation, dilated cardiomyopathy, and atrial fibrillation [6–8].

Left Ventricular Enlargement

As the LV enlarges there is usually an increase in the CTR and the curvature of the lower left heart border takes on a larger radius. The LV enlarges posteriorly and laterally toward the left lateral wall of the thorax and in a downward direction, displacing the apex laterally and inferiorly. Additional findings of depression of the left hemidiaphragm may present LV enlargement on a PA radiograph (Fig. 21.5A). LV enlargement on a lateral film in adults is assessed by increased posterior displacement and convexity of the posterior border of the cardiac silhouette (Fig. 21.5B).

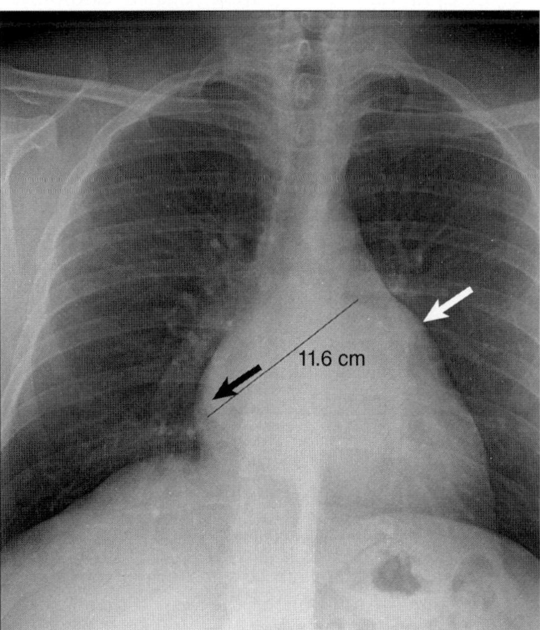

Figure 21.3 Left atrial enlargement. PA chest film demonstrates the double right heart border (*black arrow*) and splaying of the carina, due to enlargement of this posterior chamber. Left atrial appendage enlargement is also identified (*white arrow*). A distance between the middle of the double density (formed by the lateral border of the left atrium) and the middle of the left main bronchus as shown by a black line on this PA chest film of greater than 7 cm has been shown to indicate left atrial enlargement in over 90% of cases and less than 7 cm in greater than 90% of normal subjects. This measurement is 11.6 cm in the current case of left atrial enlargement.

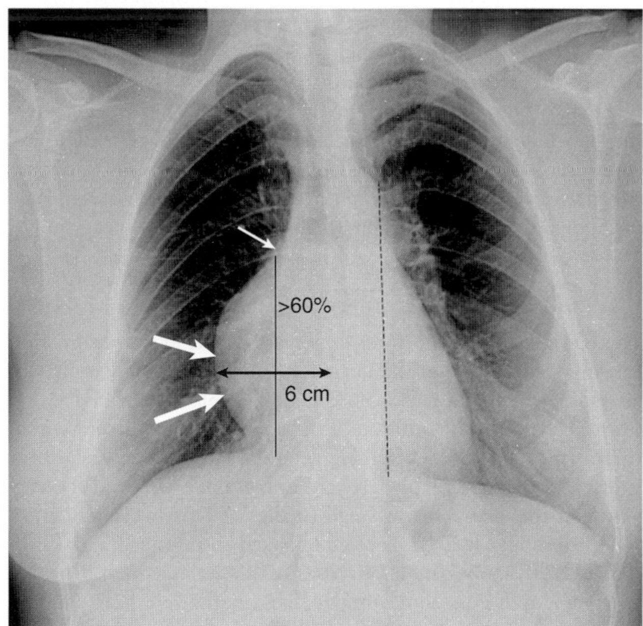

Figure 21.4 Right atrial enlargement. Right atrial enlargement (*bold arrows*) is often difficult to detect with only subtle enlargement of the right heart border present on the PA view with the *thin arrow* denotes the junction of SVC with RA. RA enlargement on PA view results in elongation of the right heart border with general consideration about the size of substantial right atrial enlargement suggested if RA border exceeding 60% in height (*bold line*) as compared to the mediastinal cardiovascular silhouette measured from the top of the aortic arch to the base of the heart (*dotted line*). Besides measurement of >5.5 cm from the midline to most lateral RA margin also suggest RA enlargement (*double arrow black line*).

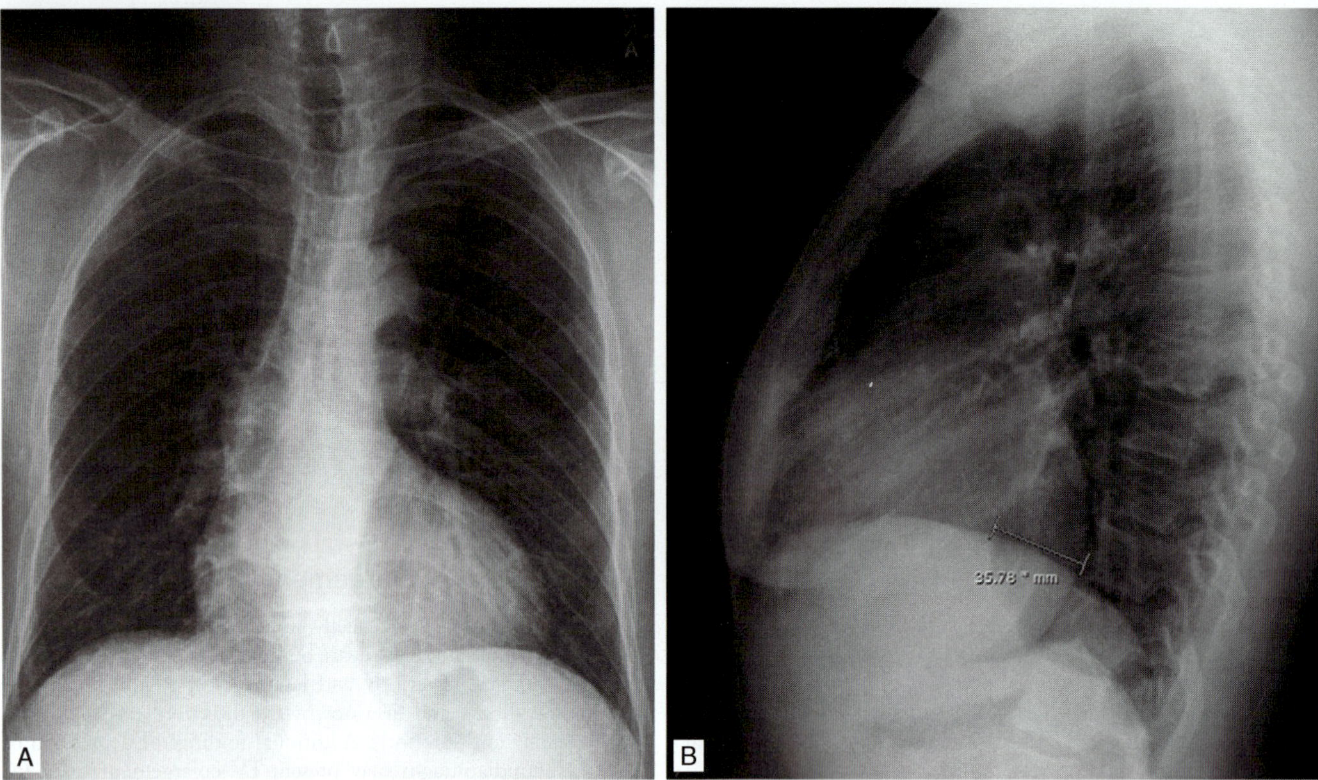

Figure 21.5 Selective left ventricular enlargement in aortic incompetence. (A) The frontal view shows that the left ventricle has enlarged along its long axis, taking the apex of the heart to the left and downward. (B) The lateral view shows the left ventricle extending behind the IVC (*line*).

This is the Hoffman–Rigler sign and is indicated by the presence of the posterior border of the LV extending horizontally and posteriorly to the posterior border of the IVC, in excess of 1.8 cm at a level 2 cm cephalad to their crossing [2,6–8,10]. Individual anatomical variation can cause discrepancies.

Some of the common acquired causes of left ventricular enlargement include pressure overload in patients with hypertension and aortic stenosis, volume overload from aortic valve regurgitation or mitral valve regurgitation and ventricular septal defect (VSD), dilated cardiomyopathy or LV wall abnormalities related to LV aneurysm [2].

Right Ventricular Enlargement

The RV enlarges in the anterior, superior, and leftward direction causing levorotation of the heart [6–8,11]. While right ventricular enlargement may also cause lateral displacement of the left heart border, it is the position of the apex and the different curvature of the heart border that suggests RV enlargement. The apex is often displaced laterally leftward but ***not inferiorly*** and the curvature at the apex remains small (if the LV remains small). Also, the cardiac apex may be directed leftward and upward with boot-shaped cardiac apex in severe cases of RV enlargement. The RV enlargement occurs somewhat higher on the left heart border, between the LV contour and the pulmonary outflow tract (Fig. 21.6A). Only a severe degree of RV dilation can be recognized on the frontal radiograph while the lateral view is more sensitive for its assessment. Associated enlargement of the main pulmonary artery segment may be noted. The lateral view will frequently show an enlarged RV extending anteriorly, causing obliteration of the retrosternal area, prominent convexity of the anterior border instead of the usual straight interface; and contact of the right heart border for greater than one third the length of the sternum (Fig. 21.6B) [6–8,11].

Acquired causes of RV enlargement typically includes cor pulmonale, tricuspid valve regurgitation, dilated cardiomyopathy, and secondary to LV failure [6–8,11,12].

Pulmonary Vascular Pattern

The pulmonary vascular pattern composed of a combination of arteries and veins can provide a great deal of information about the cardiovascular system on plain film. Visualization of the pulmonary vessels and their abnormalities can only be achieved reliably with a technically good erect PA chest radiograph. Supine radiograph or AP radiograph will often be misleading [1]. The visualization of any vessels in the lungs will depend on the silhouette sign, namely the outlining of the vascular structures by intrapulmonary air. If for any reason, such as infiltration, pulmonary edema or consolidation there is no air adjacent to the vessels, they will not be visible in their own right and conclusions about vascularity will be hard to draw. The degree of exposure of the film must not detract the radiologist from examination of the vessels and their size. A light (underexposed) film may make vessels appear more prominent but this will not alter their size, and it is the size and distribution of the vessels that are of major importance [13].

Normal Pulmonary Vascular Pattern

The main pulmonary artery divides after a variable distance into the left and right pulmonary arteries. The left upper lobe artery arises as the left pulmonary artery passes over the left main bronchus. This portion of the circulation can be identified on the plain PA radiograph as the upper part of the left hilum. The descending branch of the right pulmonary artery is the first

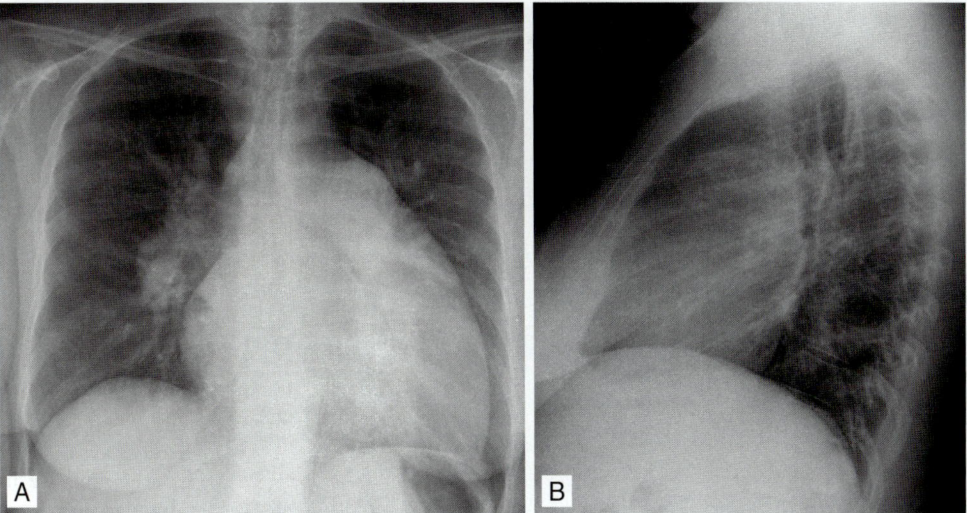

Figure 21.6 Gross right ventricular enlargement due to isolated right ventricular cardiomyopathy. The right ventricular enlargement occurs on the left heart border between the left ventricular contour and the pulmonary outflow tract (A) and is well seen on the lateral film (B).

vessel to be identified and forms, on the PA radiograph, the lower border of the right hilum. Within the lung the arteries can be identified as they divide continually, with smoothly tapered branches, and can usually be identified as far as the outer third of the lung [1,13]. The difficulty in clearly distinguishing pulmonary arteries and veins in most circumstances means that the term "pulmonary vessels" or "pulmonary vascularity" are more practical than potentially inaccurate attempts to distinguish the two types of vessels.

On a normal erect PA radiograph, the upper lobe vessels tend to be small or not visible. In the normal adult in the erect position, there is adequate pulmonary perfusion through the lower parts of the lungs with only a minimal flow in the apices [1] (Fig. 21.7). The normal diameter of the upper lobe vessels in the first interspace is rarely more than 3 mm [13]. The normal transverse diameter values have been calculated for the descending branch of the right pulmonary artery corresponding to the right interlobar artery on CT. This usually does not exceed 16 mm in men and 15 mm in women. Any size above this suggests pulmonary hypertension. The left pulmonary artery measurement on a lateral radiograph, from the orifice of the left upper lobe bronchus to the posterior aspect of the vessel, if greater than 18 mm, is suggestive of pulmonary hypertension [1,13].

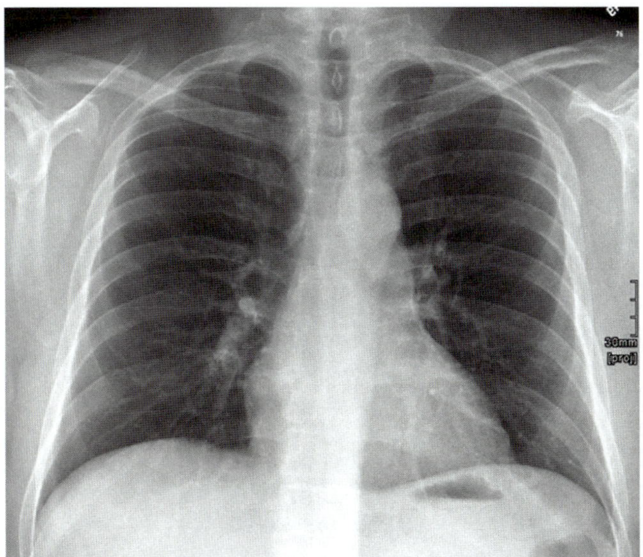

Figure 21.7 Normal chest radiograph. In the normal subject, there is a marked difference between the size of the upper and lower zone vasculature, the lower zone vessels being much more prominent.

Abnormal Pulmonary Vascular Pattern

The pressure in the pulmonary arteries may be increased (pulmonary arterial hypertension) or the pressure in the pulmonary veins may be increased (pulmonary venous hypertension [PVH]), or both of these may be present. Overall pulmonary flow may increase above normal (pulmonary plethora) or it may fall below normal (pulmonary oligemia). There may also be patchy changes in the pulmonary vascular pattern. Hence it is important to determine the type of pulmonary vascular abnormality, the severity of the pulmonary vascular abnormality, and assessing symmetry, asymmetry, or even focal distribution of the pattern [1,13].

Pulmonary Hypertension

Pulmonary hypertension is defined as a mean pulmonary artery pressure greater than 25 mm Hg at rest and is divided into precapillary and postcapillary. There are five diagnostic categories for pulmonary arterial hypertension based on the 2013 Nice Classification [14].

Pulmonary hypertension manifests on a frontal chest radiograph with a large, triangular heart with large main and central pulmonary arteries. The enlargement can often be extremely large with complete infilling of the pulmonary artery/ventricular concavity on the left heart border. There is rapid tapering of the pulmonary arteries as they run toward the periphery (Fig. 21.8) called pulmonary artery pruning [1]. In some cases, the central vessels are near normal in size but peripherally the arteries are still disproportionately small. Calcification of the main and central pulmonary arteries, although uncommon, can develop and can be identified on a radiograph (Fig. 21.9) and is typically associated with irreversible pulmonary vascular

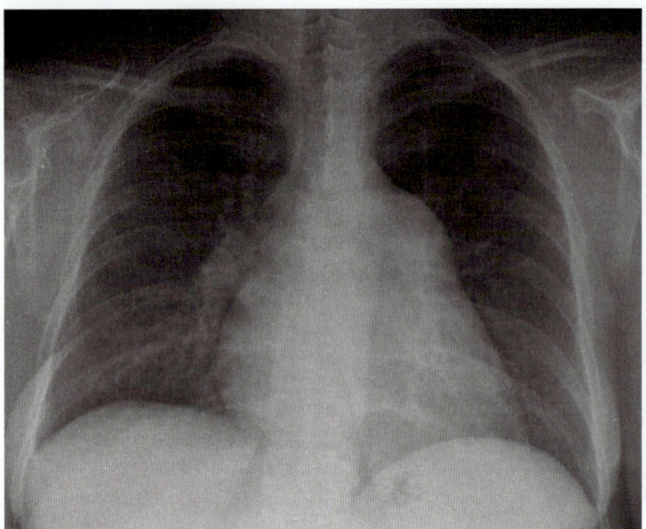

Figure 21.8 Pulmonary arterial hypertension. The heart has a large triangular shape with large main and central pulmonary arteries. There is complete infilling of the pulmonary artery/ventricular concavity on the left heart border. The pulmonary arteries within the lungs are enlarged but there is rapid tapering of the vessels as they run toward the periphery.

disease due to severe precapillary arterial pulmonary hypertension. Calcification of the pulmonary artery in combination with aortic arch calcification in young females may suggest a patent ductus arteriosus. Pulmonary artery calcification is often curvilinear in appearance and can be easily mistaken for egg-shaped calcification of enlarged hilar lymph nodes, although in the latter condition there is an absence of peripheral pruning. Pulmonary hypertension often results in RA and right ventricular enlargement (Fig. 21.6A).

Eisenmenger's syndrome develops in patients with large untreated left to right shunts, usually at the ventricular or arterial levels and results in a pulmonary-to-systemic shunt [1]. The pulmonary vascular bed is thus subjected to both high flow and high pressure. The features of Eisenmenger's syndrome on the radiograph are initially pronounced tapering of the pulmonary arteries, usually associated with cardiomegaly caused by the volume overload of the shunt. As the syndrome progresses less blood flows through the pulmonary vascular bed and the pulmonary vessels become less prominent. This change is associated with the reduction in left to right shunt and the cardiomegaly may diminish. A late radiograph in Eisenmenger's syndrome may be difficult to distinguish from normal until the old radiograph is reviewed [1].

Pulmonary Venous Hypertension

In patients with acquired heart disease, the type of pulmonary vascular abnormality is usually PVH. If impairment to the forward flow of blood through the left side of the heart develops, then left atrial pressure rises. This increase in atrial pressure is directly transmitted to the pulmonary veins, producing PVH. The changes in PVH are well defined on the radiograph and increases as the left atrial pressure increases, with the first radiological feature being enlargement of the upper zone vessels [1,13]. The physiological reasons surrounding upper lobe blood diversion are not always well understood [1].

As there is always higher pressure in the lower zones than in the upper zones due to the hydrostatic pressure across the lungs, this extravasation of fluid into the extracellular space will first occur at the lung bases. The consequence of this is redistribution of flow to the mid and upper zones of the lungs. These changes are related to lung zones, not anatomical lobes. This phenomenon is the earliest manifestation/Grade 1 phase of pulmonary edema, even though the fluid has not extended to pulmonary lymphatics or air spaces [1,15,16]. Three grades of PVH are based on mean left atrial wedge pressure/left ventricular end-diastolic pressure (Table 21.3) and are measured using Swan–Ganz catheter.

Increased production of excess extravascular lung water due to increased hydrostatic pressure gradient across the capillary wall, and/or diminished osmotic pressure gradient across the wall, results in progressive accumulation of fluid within the interstitial space thereby leading to interstitial pulmonary edema [15]

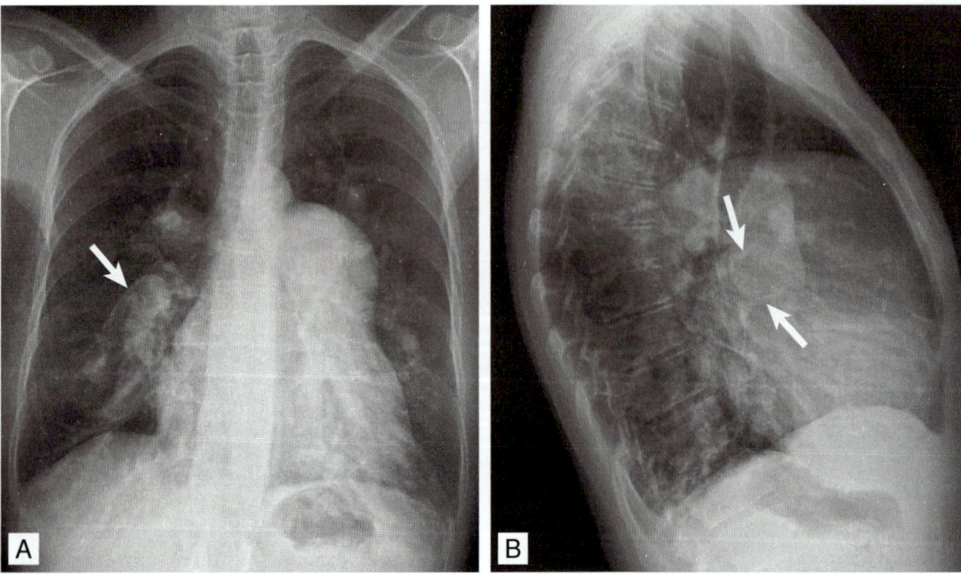

Figure 21.9 (A–B) Pulmonary arterial hypertension. If the pulmonary artery hypertension is severe and chronic, the pulmonary arteries may become very large and calcified (*arrows*).

TABLE 21.3 Grades of Pulmonary Venous Hypertension Based on Pulmonary Venous Pressure/Mean Left Atrial Wedge Pressure

Grade 1 (Upper lobe pulmonary blood diversion)	Pulmonary venous pressure between 12–19 mm Hg and 15–25 mm Hg, respectively, in acute and chronic disease
Grade 2 (Interstitial pulmonary edema)	Pulmonary venous pressure between 20–25 mm Hg and 25–30 mm Hg, respectively, in acute and chronic disease
Grade 3 (Alveolar pulmonary edema)	Pulmonary venous pressure >25 mm Hg and 30 mm Hg, respectively, in acute and chronic disease

(Fig. 21.10). This must be constantly drained back to the central circulation and this occurs via the intrapulmonary lymphatics. These intrapulmonary lymphatic channels become visible, producing the development of Kerley B lines—horizontal subpleural lines, 1–3 mm in thickness and up to 1 cm in length most frequently identified at the costophrenic angles (Fig. 21.11) [1].

Alveolar pulmonary edema can develop as the pulmonary pressure rises. It appears when the pulmonary pressure is >25 mm Hg in the acute phase or between 30 and 35 mm Hg or more in the chronic phase [1,13]. The leakage of fluid into the interstitium exceeds the drainage capacity of pulmonary lymphatics. This can occur at relatively low pressures in the acute situation but higher pressures in patients with chronic pulmonary hypertension and well-developed lymphatic channels [15,16].

- The chest radiograph appearances of PVH in the interstitial edema phase/grade II are characterized by a mild haziness in the lower zones with attenuation of the lower zone vessels and prominence of the upper zone vessels (Fig. 21.10). There may be slight loss of definition of the cardiac and mediastinal silhouette. Additional features include prominent interstitial markings, peribronchial cuffing, loss of hilar angle, enlarged and indistinct appearance of the hila and subpleural edema resulting in increased thickness of the pleura. The edema may cause thickening of the interlobar fissures, seen in the horizontal fissure in the PA radiograph and both horizontal and oblique fissures in the lateral radiograph [1,15,16]
- Radiographic features in grade III/alveolar type of pulmonary edema include confluent airspace opacities, perihilar alveolar opacities, and lower lobe or generalized alveolar opacities. Pleural effusions may also develop and can be bilateral and large [1,15,16]

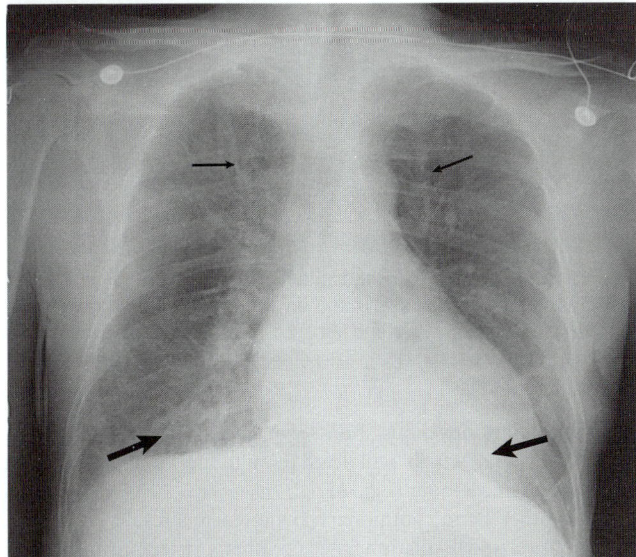

Figure 21.10 Pulmonary venous hypertension. There are peribronchial patchy ground glass opacities (*bold arrows*) in the lower zone > upper zones due to alveolar type of pulmonary edema with prominence of the upper zone vessels (*thin arrows*) which is most notable when viewing the branches of the right pulmonary artery. Note the mild left ventricular type of cardiomegaly and subpleural edema and trace pleural effusion as seen with minimal obscuration of costophrenic angles.

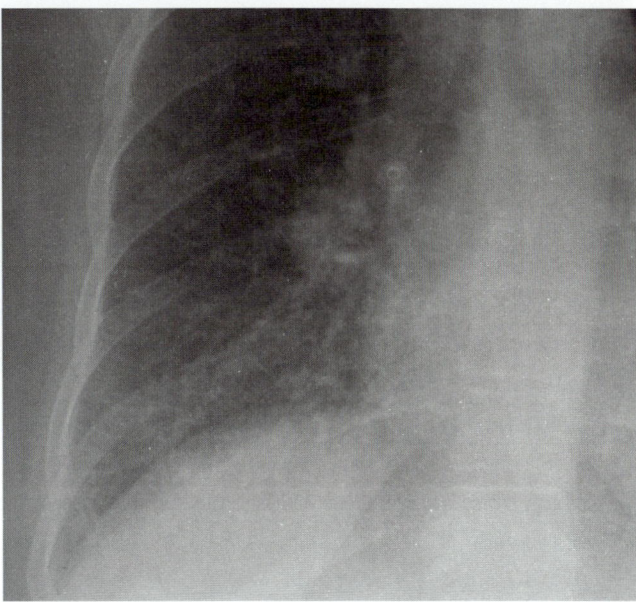

Figure 21.11 Kerley B lines are caused by interstitial fluid and are defined as subpleural perpendicular lines 1–3 cm in length in costophrenic angle.

Longstanding PVH can occasionally be associated with the development of hemosiderosis and pulmonary ossific nodules [17] (see Mitral stenosis section).

Various radiographic features can be used to differentiate cardiogenic cause from renal and capillary permeability-related pulmonary edema and are summarized in Table 21.4. Cardiogenic edema typically occurs due to myocardial or valvular heart disease while overhydration is typically caused by intravenous saline infusion or renal failure while capillary permeability edema is due to injury to lung microvasculature due to various pathological, traumatic, and infective conditions [1,13,15,16]. Capillary permeability edema causes leak of fluid into the lung at normal or near-normal pulmonary venous pressure and capillary oncotic pressure thus signifying its occurrence in the absence of underlying heart disease.

An asymmetric pattern of distribution of PVH/pulmonary edema can occur due to various etiologies with gravity being the most common etiology [1,15,16].

- Individuals with cardiac problems frequently prefer the right side while lying down due to the perception of prominent left-sided pulsation in the left lateral decubitus position
- If there is an underlying chronic obstructive pulmonary disease the edema appears in the normal or less severely abnormal portions of the lungs

TABLE 21.4 **Differentiating Typical Causes of Pulmonary Edema on Radiograph**

Factor	Cardiac	Renal/Overhydration	Capillary Permeability Edema/ Pulmonary Microvasculature Injury-Related Edema/Adult Respiratory Distress Syndrome
Cardiac size	Enlarged	Enlarged	Normal
Vascular pedicle width	Normal or increased	Increased	Normal or decreased
Pulmonary blood flow distribution	Typically, upper lobe diversion	Balanced	Normal or balanced
Pulmonary blood volume	Normal or increased	Increased	Normal
Septal lines	Common	Variable, not common	Absent
Peribronchial cuffing	Typically, present	Typically, present	Typically, absent
Air bronchogram	Uncommon	Uncommon	Very common
Pulmonary edema distribution along horizontal lung axis	Homogenous through lung	Typically, central	Typically, peripheral and patchy
Pleural effusions	Typically, present	Typically, present	Uncommon

- Asymmetric contralateral pulmonary edema may occur due to severe pulmonary artery stenosis or occlusion of the pulmonary artery in conditions such as pulmonary embolism (PE), congenital pulmonary artery stenosis or due to acquired pulmonary artery stenosis from bronchogenic carcinoma, vasculitis, fibrosing mediastinitis, and mediastinal tumors
- Unilateral obstruction of pulmonary veins due to tumors of the mediastinum, lung, heart and pericardium, and mediastinal fibrosis can also result in unilateral pulmonary edema
- Re-expansion pulmonary edema can occur due to re-expansion of the previously collapsed lung or following thoracentesis [15,16]

Pulmonary Plethora

This appearance is most commonly due to above-normal volume of blood flow through the pulmonary arteries. It is usually associated with intracardiac shunting from left to right such as atrial septal defect, VSD, patent ductus arteriosus, anomalous pulmonary venous drainage, and common arterial trunk [1,13]. The increased pulmonary blood flow results in the increased caliber of the main and both left and right pulmonary arteries and their branches. Besides, the parenchymal arterial branches are identified as extending to the lung periphery and remain sharply outlined by air-filled lungs since the shunt does not necessarily increase left atrial pressure thus distinguishing them from PVH. The increased flow may also be associated with heart failure and pulmonary edema, particularly in large high-pressure shunts in infancy, but is commonly seen without evidence of interstitial edema.

An early sign in mild cases of pulmonary plethora is the size equalization of upper and lower zone vessels.

In large longstanding shunts, the pulmonary vessels will be considerably enlarged and tortuous. Additionally, the central pulmonary arteries will also be enlarged due to pulmonary arterial hypertension, particularly if the shunt is large and between ventricles or great arteries [1].

Other less common causes of increased pulmonary flow can also cause plethora.

- Hyperdynamic circulation due to increased metabolic states can produce plethora

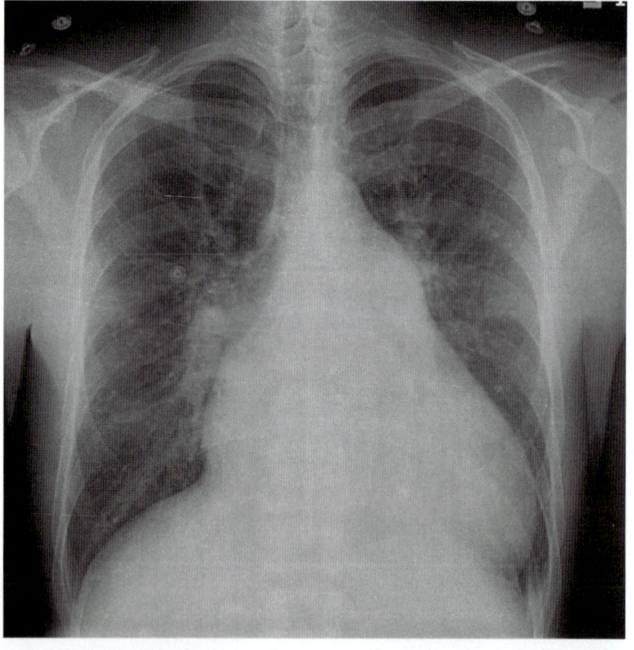

Figure 21.12 Pulmonary plethora due to high-output cardiac failure. This PA chest radiograph demonstrates pulmonary plethora (A). The pulmonary vessels are considerably enlarged and also more tortuous than usual. The central pulmonary arteries are also large. This patient had a large intracardiac shunt.

- Systemic arteriovenous shunts can give rise to a high output cardiac state, which will lead to high pulmonary flow and consequent plethora (Fig. 21.12)

On the other hand, pulmonary hypertension results in central pulmonary arterial dilation and peripheral artery pruning and sharp pulmonary vascular margins. Isolated PVH results in obscured pulmonary vascular margins although pulmonary venous caliber may be increased in the upper zone.

Pulmonary Oligemia

Pulmonary oligemia is a state of below-normal flow through the pulmonary vasculature. It is usually due to congenital heart disease with right to left shunting [1,13], taking flow away from the lungs. It is generally associated with some degree of cyanosis. In some cases of reduced overall cardiac output, there may be pulmonary oligemia but this is not commonly detected as normal circulatory compensation mechanisms act to preserve normal cardiac output wherever possible.

The appearance on the chest radiograph is of generalized decrease in size of the pulmonary vessels in all zones [1,13]. The differential between upper and lower zones is usually maintained although it is less obvious. The under perfusion of the lung parenchyma is often associated with hyperlucent lung fields but caution must be exercised in interpreting any over penetrated film as being due to oligemia. The size of the pulmonary vessels must be assessed.

Right Ventricular Failure/Right Ventricular Dysfunction

RV failure occurs most often due to left heart failure or pulmonary hypertension and can be a systolic failure or diastolic impairment. This can result in abnormal right ventricular enlargement. Systolic RV failure can result in impaired right ventricular function while diastolic RV impairment can result in central venous engorgement, pleural effusion, peripheral edema, ascites, and passive hepatic congestion.

Radiographic manifestations include

- widening of the vascular pedicle with azgous vein prominence;
- obscuration of the retrosternal lucency on the lateral radiograph due to RV enlargement; and
- findings of pulmonary hypertension related to dilation of the main pulmonary artery and at the hilar region [1,6–8]. The associated findings of left heart failure can also be present.

Thoracic Osseous Radiographic Features Associated with Cardiovascular Disease

The shape of the bony structures is important; pectus excavatum (Fig. 21.13A and B) is important to identify, as this appearance is associated with both Marfan's disease and prolapse of the mitral valve. The definition of pectus excavatum is a narrowed AP thoracic diameter, less than 8 cm, between the anterior border of the vertebral bodies and the posterior margin of the sternum as assessed on the lateral radiograph. The other cause for a narrowed AP thoracic diameter includes straight thoracic spine/straight back syndrome [1].

Another subtle abnormality is the presence of rib notching in the presence of coarctation of the thoracic aorta which usually occurs in ribs 3–8 (Fig. 21.13C) [1].

Other thoracic osseous abnormalities such as postoperative sternotomy sutures and thoracotomy changes related to rib deformities can be assessed with radiographs. Osseous erosions or destruction can happen with osteomyelitis in cases from septic endocarditis, also observable on the radiographs [1].

Thoracic Cardiovascular Calcifications in Acquired Heart Disease

Thoracic cardiovascular structures calcification is not uncommon and can be a marker of significant and specific finding of a disease entity. The coronary arteries and cardiac valves are typical structures to calcify [18]. It is important to remember that valvular calcifications could be indicative of valve stenosis and would require further evaluation with an echocardiogram for grading of stenosis.

Following is the radiographic approach for assessment of thoracic cardiovascular calcifications

- Aortic valve calcification is best seen on the lateral chest radiograph and can be obscured on the frontal radiograph. This can be located on the lateral radiograph as a calcification superior and anterior to the line connecting carina and anterior costophrenic angle [6–8,18]. Significant aortic valve calcification on radiograph could represent significant valve stenosis with a pressure gradient of more than 50 mm Hg [18]. The most common causes for aortic valve calcification include bicuspid aortic valve, which is typically seen in young adults followed by atherosclerotic valve degeneration which is typically seen in elderly patients

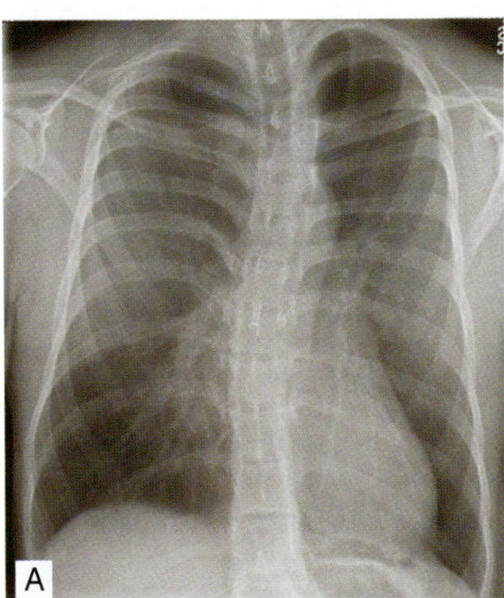

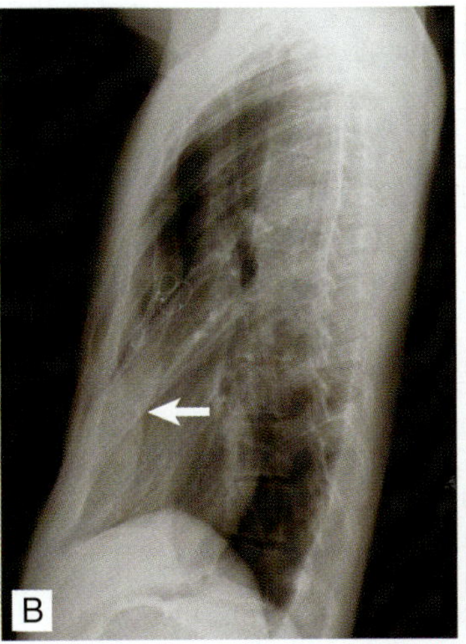

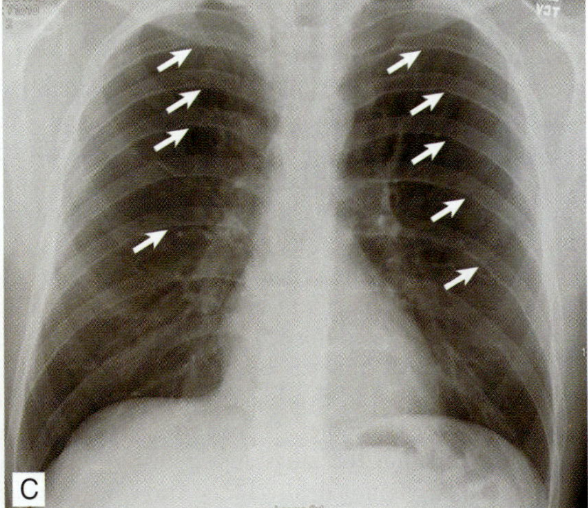

Figure 21.13 Depressed sternum. (A) Frontal view. The heart is displaced to the left. Its left border is straight and there is a prominence in the position of the main pulmonary artery. There is an ill-defined shadow to the right of the vertebral column. The clue to those appearances is given by the visualization of the intervertebral disks at the level of the lower thoracic spine where normally they would disappear. Sternotomy sutures are related to remote cardiac surgery. (B) Lateral view. This demonstrates the enormous sternal depression (*arrow*). This patient was thought to have a normal heart. (C) Coarctation of aorta. This PA film demonstrates inferior rib notching of multiple bilateral ribs (*arrows*) from third to seventh ribs due to prominent intercostal collateral arterial circulation. It can rarely be unilateral on the left side only in the presence of an anomalous right subclavian artery. It is unusual to identify this appearance in the asymptomatic adult as most cases are now identified in childhood, but it is important to assess the ribs in the young hypertensive patient.

above 65 years of age. Aortic valve stenosis is typically associated with poststenotic dilatation of the ascending aorta [6–8,18]

- Aortic annular calcification appear as circular calcification just below the aortic valve region and is typically associated with degenerative aortic valve calcification [18]
- Ascending aortic calcification is commonly atherosclerotic and is noted along the right anterolateral margin of the ascending aorta in an elderly person. Other causes include syphilitic vasculitis and aortic valve disease [18]
- Mitral annular calcification are typically degenerative in etiology or physiologic in the elderly, appear as a dense band-like "C-" or "O-" or "U-shaped" calcification in the mitral valve location and is better seen on lateral radiograph than the frontal view. Mitral valve calcification is less common than mitral annular calcification [6–8,18]
- Coronary arterial calcification is less commonly noticed on radiographs. The presence of coronary arterial calcification on a radiograph is suggestive of severe coronary artery disease. On the lateral chest radiograph, they are seen as parallel calcified linear density [18]. Most coronary artery stents are composed of stainless steel and appear as sharply defined parallel linear density that is denser than calcification
- LV myocardial calcifications are typically suggestive of prior transmural MI or LV aneurysm and typically located in the apical or anterolateral wall of the LV. These appear as thin linear calcifications outlining the aneurysm or as irregular laminated calcification due to calcification of mural thrombus [18]
- LA wall calcification is typically diffuse, sheet-like wall calcification occurring in patients with cardiac failure concomitant with atrial fibrillation [18]
- Pericardial calcification: Please refer to the section of constrictive pericarditis (CP) [6–8,18]
- Other rare thoracic cardiovascular sites of calcifications include calcification in primary or metastatic osteosarcoma of heart, left atrial myxoma, healed myocardial tuberculoma, endocardial fibrosis, endocardial fibroelastosis, and trauma [18]

The General Postoperative Chest Radiograph

The chest radiograph obtained from the intensive care unit is often obtained in suboptimal conditions; the patient is supine or semierect, ventilated and the radiograph is portable. The daily chest radiograph is, however, an important integral part of the management of seriously ill patients. The image is used to assess the position of the lines and tubes and to identify any potential complications such as change in the cardiopulmonary status of the patients, and to assess the lungs.

As the portable film is taken in an AP projection, this will lead to an increase in the magnification of the cardiac shadow, which can be increased in size by up to 20%. The upper limit of a CTR in the AP film has been reported at 57%. Often the patients are supine and that makes the examination of lungs difficult. In this position there is poor air entry (Fig. 21.14A), and without ventilation the lungs appear to be smaller in volume. The loss of gravitational forces can also lead to redistribution through both lungs. This appearance can mimic upper lobe blood diversion. Comparison with prior PA chest radiograph is always useful (Fig. 21.14B). In addition, the supine position makes the diagnosis of a pleural fluid (Fig. 21.14C) and pneumothorax (Fig. 21.14D) extremely difficult. Due to the redistribution of fluid, the only clue available is a small veil-like opacity (Fig. 21.14C) in the apex. Pneumothorax is supine position can be suggested with the presence of deep suclus sign (Fig. 21.14D). Air in the pleural cavity also rises to the nondependent portion of the chest which can either be medial or lateral, producing an area of radiolucency.

Postcardiac Surgery

Most adult cardiac operations are performed through a central midline sternotomy with wire midline sutures being used to close the wound.

- Following cardiac surgery some widening of the mediastinum occurs, due to a combination of bleeding and edematous change. Marked mediastinal widening can represent major mediastinal hemorrhage, and the necessity to re-explore the chest
- Pneumopericardium is also common in the early postoperative period
- The increased use of the right and left internal mammary arteries for coronary grafting has led to an increase in damage to the underlining pleura during dissection of the vessels, with an increase in the pneumothorax rate. The distribution of metal clips can indicate which vessels have been used when performing the surgery (Fig. 21.15)

The standard endotracheal tube in adults should be two thirds the width of the normal trachea and the tip of the tube in neutral position should ideally be 5 cm (±2 cm) above the carina. In flexion endotracheal tube can be 3 cm (±2 cm) above the carina while in extension the ET tube can be 7 cm (±2 cm) above the carina. Endotracheal tube in neutral position should ideally be 1.5 cm above the carina in a pediatric patient [19,20].

This position allows up to 4 cm of movement that can occur when the head is moved from flexion to extension. Any deviation from this position should be interpreted in the context of the patient's head position at the time of the radiograph. The carina is often easily visualized but can be estimated at the level of T4–T7.

Complications of ventilation should also be considered and the lungs inspected for the presence of pneumothorax or pneumomediastinum.

Pulmonary artery catheters are used in patients with cardiac failure to measure capillary wedge pressure and its tip should be ideally located in the main or interlobar pulmonary artery within 2 cm of the mediastinal border on the chest radiograph [19,20].

Following most cardiac surgery, mediastinal and chest drains are placed before the closure of the sternotomy wound. Often there is a straight tube into the anterior mediastinum and an angled tube over the left diaphragm respectively, which tends to lie in a more posterior position. These tubes allow both air and fluid to escape in the immediate postoperative period.

Apically oriented thoracostomy tube is used for drainage of the pleural air, while the basilar oriented thoracostomy tube is used for drainage of the pleural effusion. On the chest radiograph, the radiologist should make sure that all the fenestrations of the thoracostomy tube are within the thorax for its appropriate functioning and avoidance of large subcutaneous emphysema [19,20].

Most central lines are placed via the subclavian or the jugular veins and the tip should be within the distal subclavian vein wherever possible. It can also be placed at the superior cavoatrial junction which is located about 4 cm below the level of the carina or two vertebral body levels below the level of the carina [21] on radiograph or at the level of the right anterior third costal cartilage or seventh thoracic vertebral body. Following percutaneous placement, a check radiograph should be obtained to assess the position of the catheter tip and to identify any complications (Fig. 21.16) [19,20].

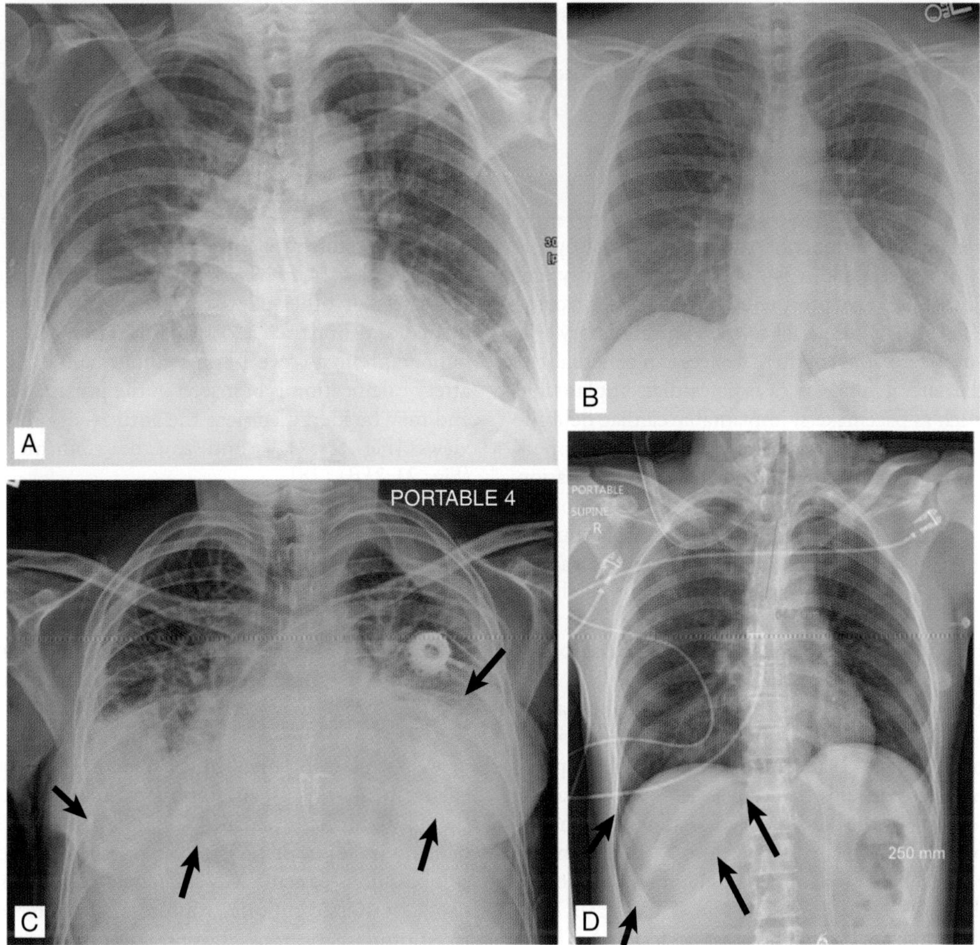

Figure 21.14 Portable AP view. (A) The supine AP view demonstrates a magnified cardiac silhouette with low lung volume, as well as even distribution of the pulmonary circulation between the upper and lower lung zones. (B) PA view in the same patient 24 hours earlier shows a very different appearance of the cardiac silhouette. (C) The supine AP view in postlung transplant patient demonstrates veil like hazy opacity in both lower hemithorax due to layering pleural effusion (*arrows*). (D) The supine AP view demonstrates increased lucency in the right lower hemithorax and projecting over right upper abdomen (deep suclus sign) due to right pneumothorax (*arrows*).

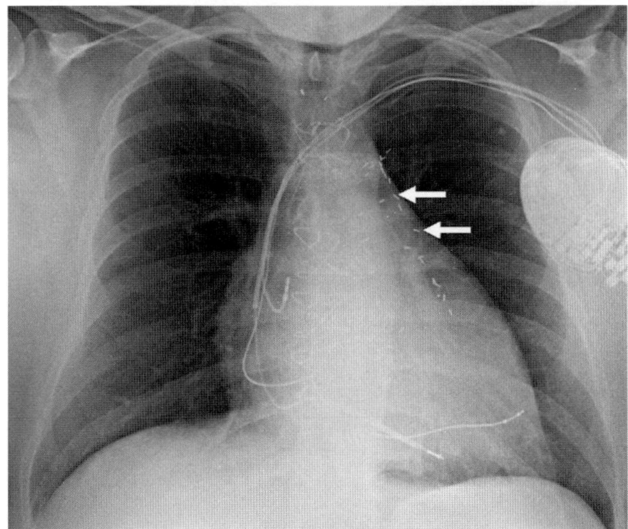

Figure 21.15 Postcardiac surgery. The midline sternotomy sutures are difficult to visualize on the PA film. There are surgical clips in the anterior mediastinum which have been used to occlude small side branches of the left internal mammary artery (*arrow*), which has been used as a graft. There is also an AICD with electrodes in the usual position.

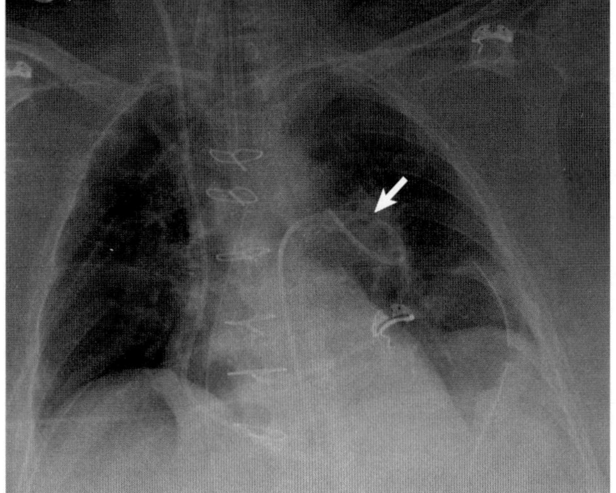

Figure 21.16 Cardiac surgery complication. Portable AP radiograph after open-heart surgery demonstrates malposition Swan–Ganz catheter from a right internal jugular approach, coiled in the left pulmonary artery (*arrow*). Ideally these are located in the main or right or left central pulmonary artery at the level of hila. Note that more proximal or distal positions are considered misplacements, typically a tip too distally inserted into a peripheral branch (more than 2 cm lateral to the Hilum).

The early postoperative chest radiograph may demonstrate basal collapse, lobar collapse (left > right), linear atelectasis, consolidation, pleural effusion, pericardial effusion, pneumothorax, and pneumomediastinum [19,20].

Implants

In recent times, an increasing number of patients have prior operative interventions to the heart and it is important to identify any sternal wires, surgical clips, valve prostheses, pacemakers, or coronary artery stents (Fig. 21.17). Referral to the clinical history will usually resolve the problem. Some of these devices can be visualized more clearly on the lateral film. In case of cardiac implantable electronic devices such as pacemakers, implantable cardiac defibrillators, and cardiac resynchronization therapy devices, it is important to exclude pneumothorax on the immediate postimplantation radiograph [22,23]. It is also important to check the course of the electrode on successive films in case of possible lead displacement.

Current pacing technology is developing rapidly and a variety of lead patterns will be seen including single lead pacing, dual lead pacing (one atrial and one ventricular lead) and biventricular pacing (one lead in the RV and the other to the LV via the coronary sinus in the epicardial coronary vein (Fig. 21.18)).

Implantable cardiac defibrillators resemble permanent pacing systems but they have a larger generator box and a more bulky intracardiac electrode (Fig. 21.19) are best distinguished from pacemakers on CXR by electrode coils that appear as more thickened radio-opaque structures on the lead. A chest radiograph should routinely be taken in PA and lateral projections after pacemaker implantation to exclude lead displacement, pneumothorax, other complications, or location in an anomalous vein (Fig. 21.20). Cardiac implantable electronic devices can be broadly classified as MR-conditional and non–MR-conditional, or legacy devices. Cardiac MR can be securely performed in patients with MR Conditional devices by following safety precautions with robust institutional guidelines and workflow utilizing a well-trained multidisciplinary team [23]. In any case of doubt it is important to check on the MRI compatibility of any devices per the manufacturers' instructions.

Coronary Heart Disease

The chest radiograph of a patient with stable angina is usually normal unless there have been previous events such as myocardial infarction or other coexisting heart disease which can result in dilated and impaired LV. Careful examination of the penetrated radiograph may reveal some abnormalities [24–28]. Coronary artery calcification is best seen in the proximal left coronary artery and may be identified near the aortic root on both PA and lateral views (Fig. 21.21A) and can be confirmed on cardiac CT (Fig. 21.21B) [28].

Acute Myocardial Infarction

The chest radiograph is usually obtained in all patients presenting with acute myocardial infarction. The common feature identified is the development of PVH or pulmonary edema [25–28].

The chest radiographic feature of acute myocardial infarction include progressive enlargement of the cardiac silhouette (Fig. 21.22). If the serial radiographs taken over the first few days or weeks following myocardial infarction show progressive cardiac enlargement, this is an important adverse prognostic sign that should be further evaluated [24–28]. The chest radiograph is particularly useful in demonstrating primary or secondary findings of complications of acute MI, such as acute mitral regurgitation from papillary muscle rupture, rupture of the interventricular septum, LV rupture; pericardial effusion and cardiac tamponade; true and false LV aneurysm; and congestive heart failure [25–28].

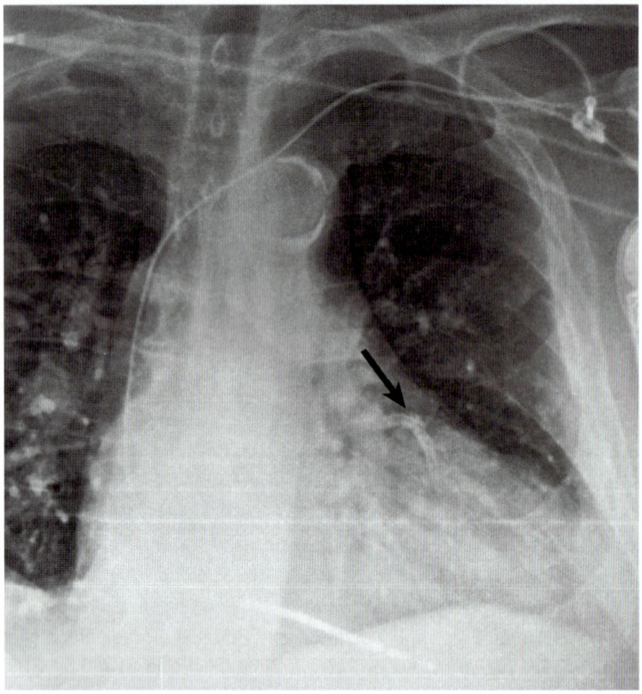

Figure 21.17 Coronary artery stent. This patient presented with chest pain. On the PA chest radiograph, a stent is seen in the left anterior descending coronary artery (*arrow*).

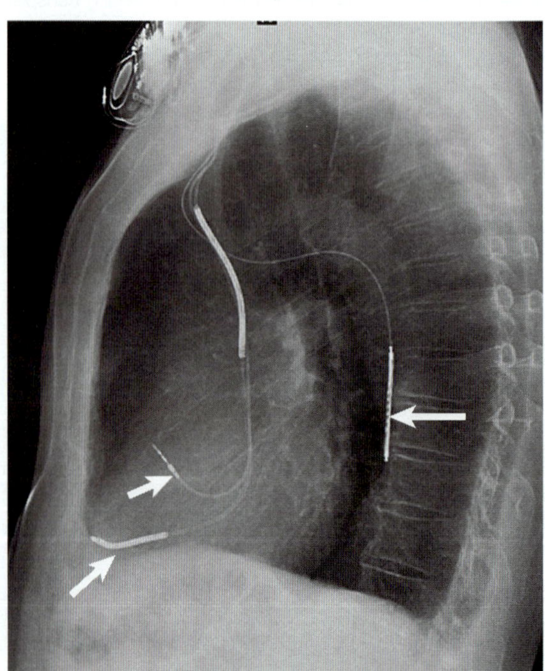

Figure 21.18 Malposition electrode after biventricular pacemaker/AICD insertion. The lateral radiograph demonstrates two anterior electrodes in the right atrium and right ventricle in appropriate position (*short arrows*), and a third electrode that went posteriorly into the azygos vein (*long, bold arrow*).

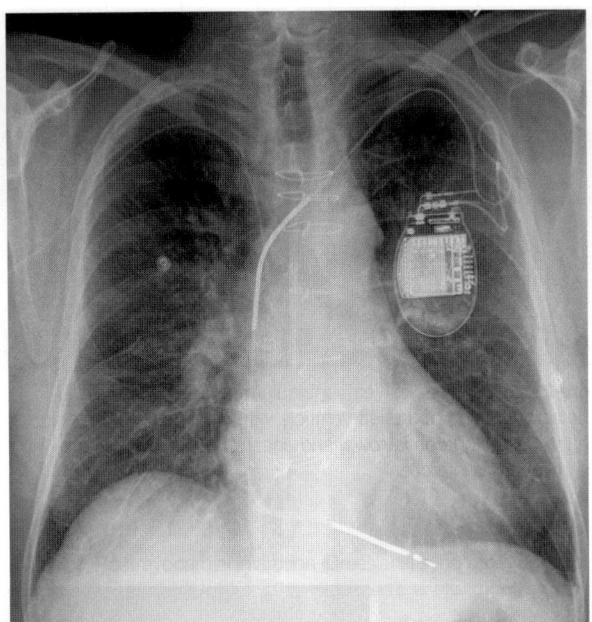

Figure 21.19 Automatic implantable defibrillator. The electrode is heavier than a normal pacing electrode with additional discharge electrodes in the SVC and the right ventricle. The generator is larger than the current generation pacemaker generators.

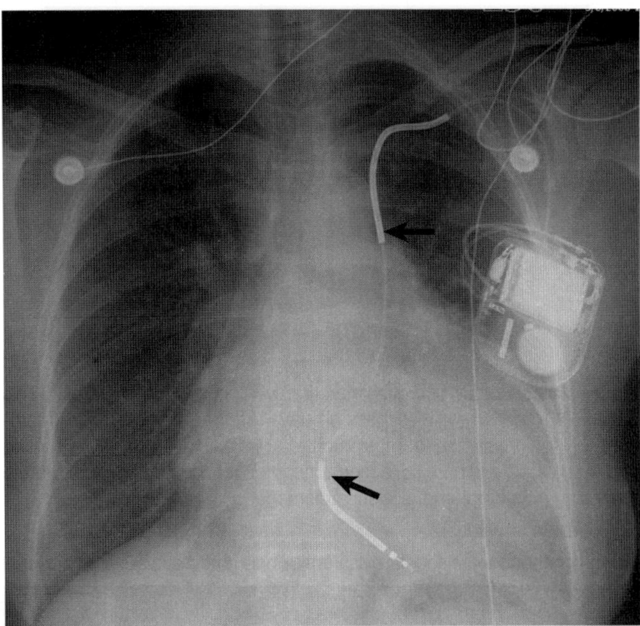

Figure 21.20 Single chamber AICD in an atypical position. The AP radiograph demonstrates the left subclavian approach electrode (*arrow*) descending to the heart to the left of the aorta, in a persistent left superior vena cava. The distal shock-coil and electrode are in the right ventricle.

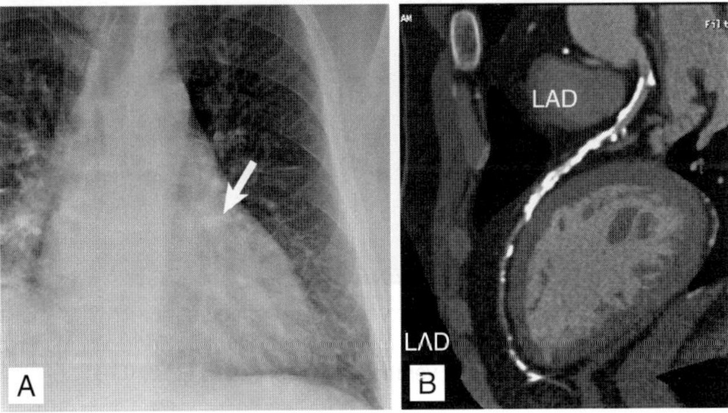

Figure 21.21 Coronary artery calcification. Calcification of the vessels is shown well on this magnified PA view (*arrow*). Calcification of the coronary arteries is often best seen on the lateral view. Corresponding Coronary CTA in the same patient confirms extensive coronary artery calcification. *LAD*: Left anterior descending.

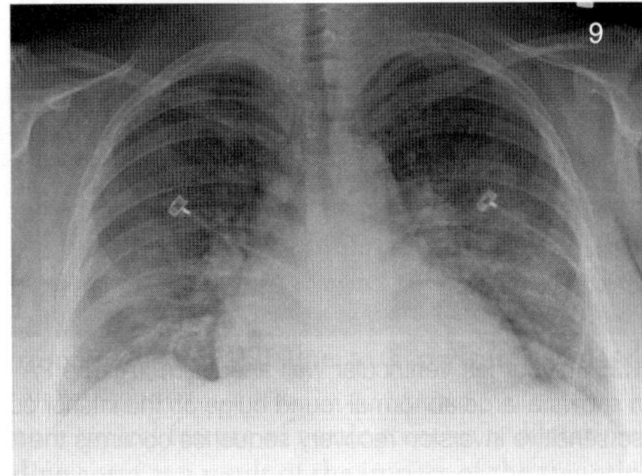

Figure 21.22 Cardiogenic pulmonary edema postacute myocardial infarction. A previous PA film obtained before the infarction (not shown) was normal. Patient returns with worsening dyspnea and chest pain with ST-elevation myocardial infarction. The AP radiograph shows an enlarged heart and vascular indistinctness from pulmonary edema.

- *Acute mitral regurgitation*

The papillary muscle rupture leads to acute mitral valve insufficiency. On the chest radiograph, pulmonary edema develops with little increase in the cardiac size or more particularly the left atrium. Asymmetric right upper lobe pulmonary edema can occur due to acute rupture of the papillary muscle. Follow-up imaging in a patient who survives the acute episode can reveal varying degrees of left atrial dilation and cardiomegaly [24–28].

- *Rupture of the interventricular septum/ventricular septal defects*

This is also a rare complication of a transmural acute MI and is most likely to rupture between 4 and 21 days postinfarction, leading to rapid-onset left to right shunting and heart failure. There is engorgement of the pulmonary arterial vasculature (pulmonary plethora) and pulmonary edema is frequently seen (Fig. 21.23) [25–28].

- *Left ventricular aneurysm*

If an infarcted segment is large and transmural, then it may develop over a few weeks into a left ventricular aneurysm. This is most commonly seen at the cardiac apex or anterolateral wall typically due to a true aneurysm in association with an anterior infarct (Fig. 21.24A and B), but it can also occur in the posterior/inferior wall of LV near the diaphragmatic surface. In this case it typically signifies a false aneurysm in the left circumflex or right coronary artery territory (Figs. 21.25A–C). Identification of a contour bulge or double density to the left cardiac silhouette should raise concern for a LV aneurysm. The wall of a longstanding aneurysm (or a nonaneurysmal infarct) may also show calcification (Figs. 21.26A and B) [25–28].

- *Pericardial effusion*

Acute pericardial effusion is a poor prognostic marker as it is also commonly associated with partial ventricular rupture and Dressler's syndrome. Postcardiac injury syndrome/*Dressler's syndrome* is a global pericardial inflammatory reaction to the infarct (Fig. 21.27), occurs 2 weeks to several months after myocardial infarction and may present with mild cardiomegaly [25–28]. Pericardial effusions with or without tamponade can

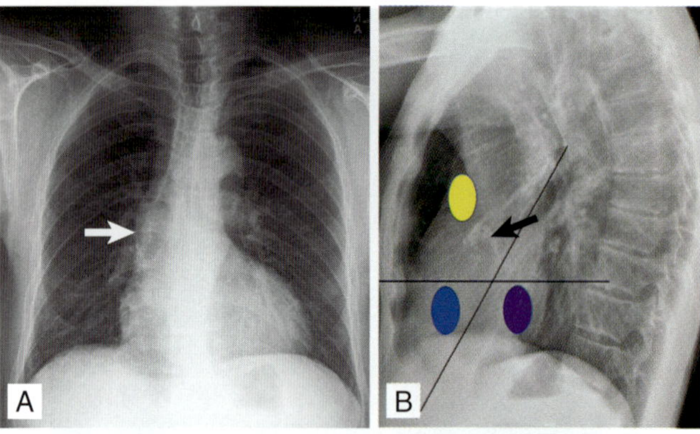

Figure 21.30 Calcified aortic stenosis. The heart has a slightly prominent left ventricular contour on the PA chest radiograph and there is dilatation of the ascending aorta (*white arrow*) caused by the poststenotic dilatation (A). Calcification of the aortic valve (*black arrow*) is more apparent on the lateral film (B). Note that the native cardiac valve position and valve devices can be grossly localized on frontal and lateral chest radiographs through bisecting the cardiac silhouette with an imaginary line drawn perpendicular to the long axis of the heart on the frontal view and parallel to the long axis of the heart on the lateral view from the carina to the cardiac apex. The aortic valve (*black arrow*) typically projects cranially while the mitral valve (*purple*) projects below these lines in the posterior quadrant. The pulmonic valve (*yellow*) is typically is the most cranially located cardiac valve on both the views while the tricuspid valve (*blue*) is positioned most inferiorly and in the anterior quadrant.

The intrinsic aortic valve pathology category includes bicuspid aortic valve (most common cause in the developed countries) damage to the valvular cusps as a result of rheumatic fever (most common cause in the developing countries), endocarditis, and atherosclerosis-related degeneration [6–8]. The condition can occur in combination with aortic stenosis. Occasionally AR can develop as a complication of primary disease of the aortic wall, such as aortitis. A dissection of the aorta can produce valvular regurgitation if the false lumen dissects toward the aortic valve ring.

The appearances described are those that develop in association with chronic AR.

- The chest radiograph demonstrates a large cardiac silhouette due to LV enlargement with normal pulmonary vascularity in the initial phase [6–8]. The heart size reflects the severity of the disease
- The ascending aorta and often the aortic arch are enlarged especially in systemic diseases and may have aortic wall calcification [18]. The dilated aorta can sometimes be visualized as a bulge on the right of the mediastinum
- In many patients with pure AR, there is excellent compensation for the increased flow in the LV and there is normal pulmonary vasculature
- The combination of a large LV, no other chamber enlargement and normal pulmonary vessels is suggestive of severe chronic AR [6–8]

Mitral Valve Disease

Mitral Stenosis

The most common cause of mitral stenosis is rheumatic fever. The reduction of flow occurs as a result of a fusion of the leaflet commissures resulting in a pressure overload condition. Also, thickening of the valve leaflets occurs with shortening and thickening of the chordae tendinae which further restricts valve movement. The symptoms of flow restriction (dyspnea and heart failure) may be minimal until the valve becomes critically narrowed. The condition does however predispose to thrombus formation in the left atrium and consequent systemic embolus. The condition may present with a systemic embolism [6–8].

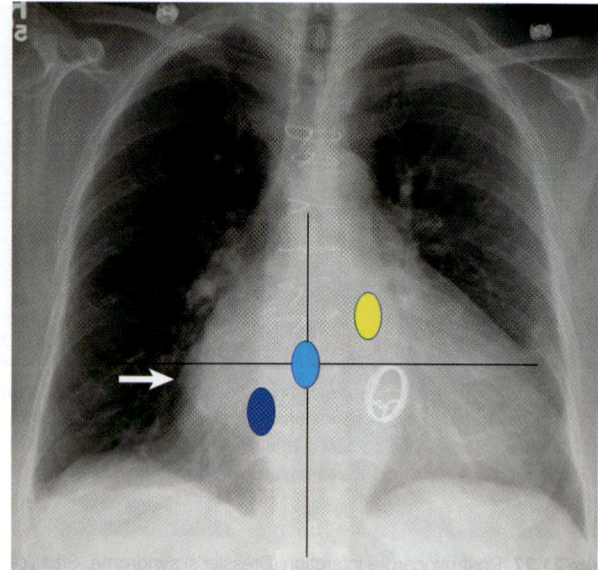

Figure 21.31 Left atrial dilatation in mitral stenosis in a patient with malfunctioning prosthetic mitral valve. The grossly enlarged left atrium (*arrow*) extends beyond the right heart border on the frontal view. Note prosthetic mitral valve projects below the lines drawn on the frontal CXR as explained in this image and as shown on lateral CXR in Fig 21.30B. *Light blue*: aortic valve, *dark blue*: tricuspid valve, *yellow*: pulmonic valve. It should be noted that cardiac valve localization based solely on a radiograph is relatively unreliable and correlation with clinical history should be considered as physiological variations in cardiac size, axis, and position, along with variations in radiographic techniques can affect them.

- The chest radiograph demonstrates selective left atrial enlargement, which can vary from trivial to gross (Fig. 21.31). If the mitral stenosis is a result of rheumatic fever there is often marked enlargement of the left atrial appendage, which forms a bulge on the left heart border just below the main pulmonary artery (Fig. 21.32). This enlargement can again range from the trivial to the marked with a large protrusion
- In chronic disease, there is often a normal heart size with only subtle signs of left atrial enlargement being evident (Fig. 21.32)

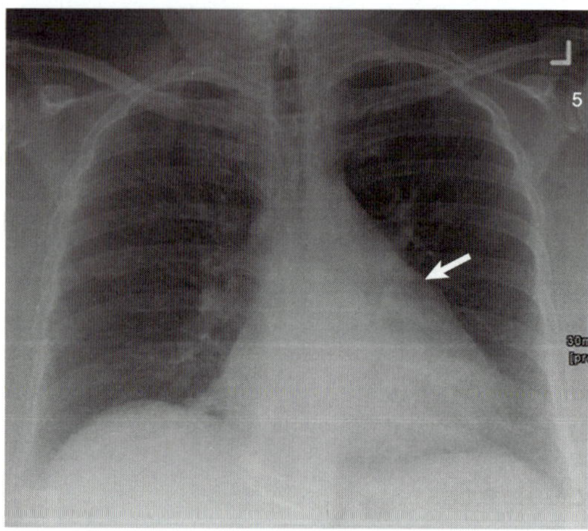

Figure 21.32 Mitral stenosis with a normal size heart. In the early years of this chronic disease, there is often a normal heart size with only subtle signs of left atrial enlargement being evident. The left atrial appendage is prominent and there is pulmonary venous hypertension.

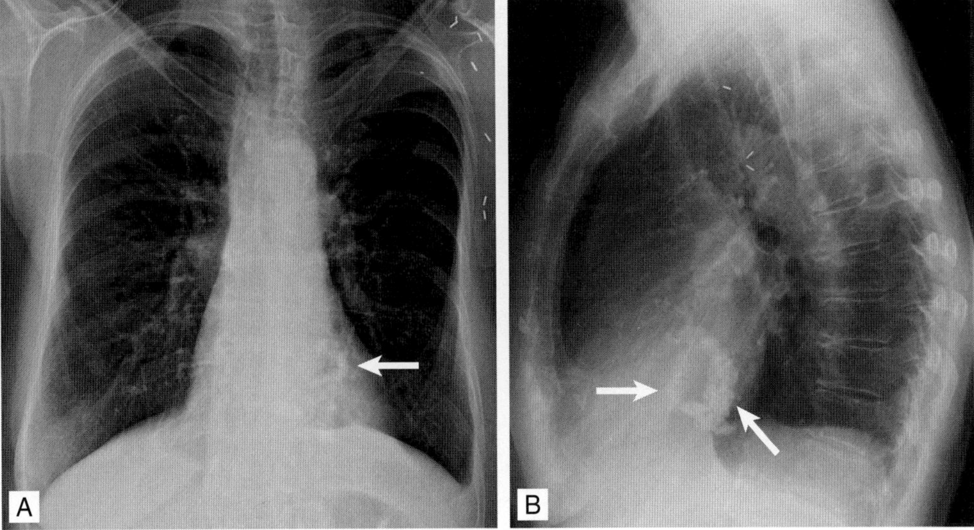

Figure 21.33 (A, B) Calcified mitral valve in rheumatic mitral stenosis. The calcification is best seen in the lateral view (*arrow*).

[6,8]. In cases of unexplained heart failure with a normal heart size, it is important not to overlook mitral stenosis. Even in the late stages of the condition, the atria may be large but the left ventricular contour is still small, indicating the small size of the ventricular chamber [7]

- If the mitral stenosis is both severe and longstanding then calcification of the valve can develop. This feature can sometimes be visualized in the PA projection if the film is penetrated (Fig. 21.33A) however it *is best visualized in the lateral projection* (Fig. 21.33B) [6–8]. This calcification needs to be differentiated from the far more common C- or J-shaped calcification that occurs in the valve annulus (Fig. 21.34)
- In severe mitral valve disease with associated atrial fibrillation, calcification of the left atrium, or thrombus within the left atrium, can occur [6,8]

Mitral stenosis-related chronically raised left atrial pressure results in left atrial dilation, upper lobe blood diversion, PVH, or pulmonary edema, with enlargement of the main and central pulmonary arteries indicating pulmonary arterial hypertension [7].

The right-sided cardiac chambers including the RV and right atrium may be considerably enlarged which could be related to pulmonary hypertension or associated tricuspid regurgitation. Subsequently, right heart failure could also occur. A very large left atrium, aneurysmal if it reaches within 2.5 cm of the thoracic wall, may be associated with segmental or even lobar collapse. This is more common on the right side. In general, the ascending aorta and aortic arch are not enlarged in isolated mitral stenosis and their enlargement should raise concern for associated aortic valve disease [6–8].

Mitral stenosis-related hemosiderosis and pulmonary ossific nodules may occasionally be seen [6–8]. Pulmonary hemosiderosis manifests on radiograph and CT as 1–3 mm ill-defined punctate nodules along with reticular opacities predominantly in the mid and lower lungs (Fig. 21.35) representing fibrotic nodules in patients with multiple episodes of edema and pulmonary hemorrhage. Pulmonary

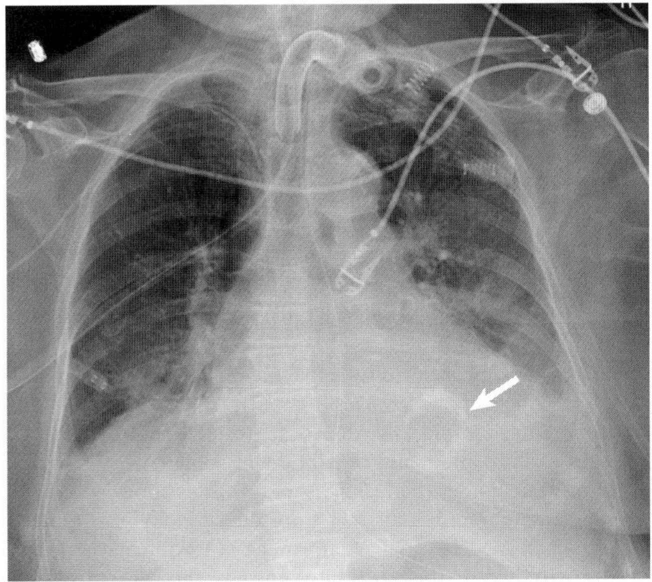

Figure 21.34 Calcification in the mitral ring. In this AP view the calcified mitral valve ring (*arrow*) appears as a characteristic C-shape; it may take a J-shape.

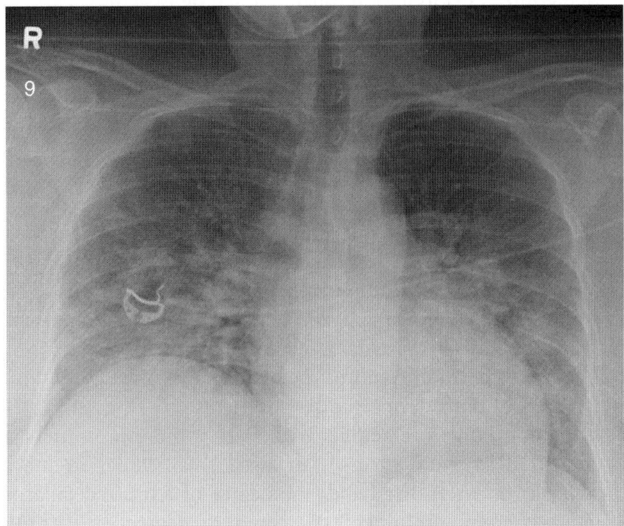

Figure 21.35 Pulmonary hemosiderosis in a patient with longstanding mitral valve disease. The fine granular and ground-glass background pattern in the lung is typical of hemosiderosis. Also, note changes suggestive of mitral valve disease: cardiomegaly, straightening of the left heart border and some upper lobe blood diversion.

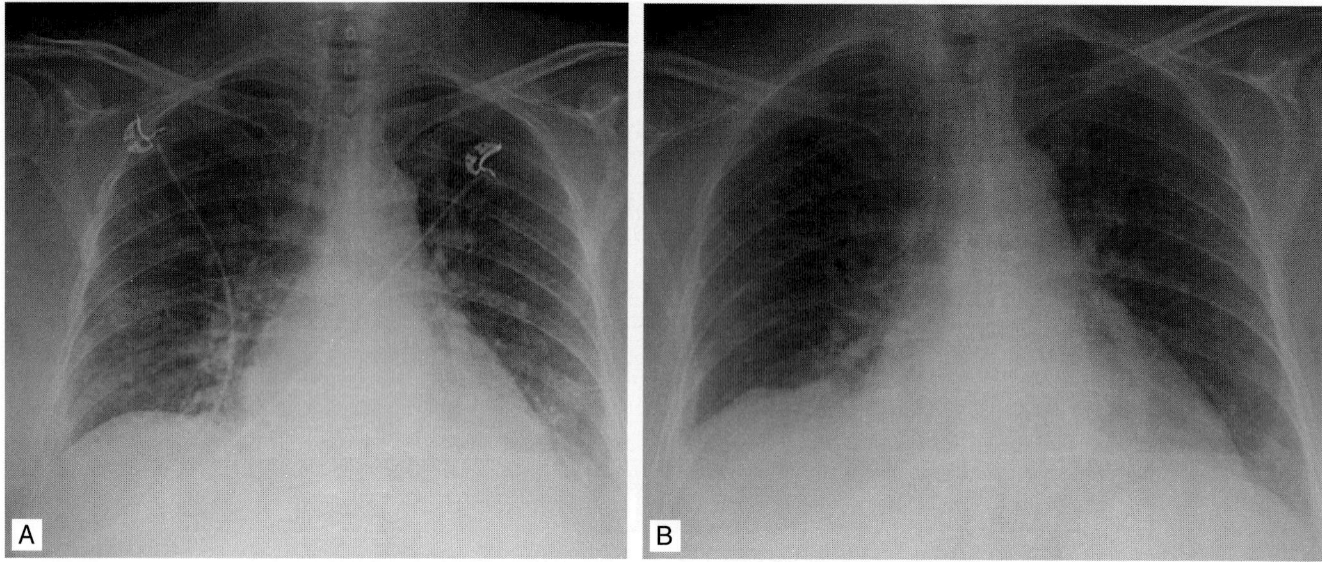

Figure 21.36 Acute nonrheumatic mitral regurgitation. (A) Frontal view in the acute phase. The heart size is virtually normal, even in the presence of high left atrial pressure as evidenced by the preferential dilatation of the upper lobe vessels and interstitial edema. (B) Frontal film 2 weeks later shows clearing of the pulmonary edema.

ossific nodules on radiograph and CT are densely calcified/ossified 1–5 mm nodules and reticular opacities mainly in the mid and lower lungs and occur due to severe longstanding PVH [17]. Left atrial appendage dilation and left atrial wall calcification is considered to pathognomonic sign of rheumatic heart disease [6–8].

Mitral Regurgitation

Mitral regurgitation occurs due to dysfunction of any component of the mitral valve—dysfunction of the valve leaflet, annulus, chordae tendineae, or papillary muscle [6–8].

Mitral regurgitation can be acute or chronic and the most common cause of mitral regurgitation in western countries is degeneration of the valve. Infective endocarditis will also cause damage of the valve with consequent regurgitation but this will usually be on an already abnormal valve. In the case of an impaired LV, mitral regurgitation can occur due to annular dilatation or papillary muscle dysfunction.

- Acute mitral regurgitation usually caused by ischemic heart disease is associated with marked elevated left atrial pressure causing PVH and acute pulmonary edema (Fig. 21.36A). However *heart size remains normal with a resolution of pulmonary edema after acute episodes resolve* (Fig. 21.36B) [6–8]. In most cases, the chest radiograph appearances are very different from those of mitral regurgitation associated with rheumatic disease
- In the chronic mitral regurgitation, the heart tends to enlarge with a left ventricular and left atrial enlargement (Fig. 21.37) with very marked left atrial enlargement in longstanding cases. Mitral annular calcification is frequently noted [6–8]
- If the mitral valve prolapse is associated with Marfan's disease there may also be an enlargement of the aortic root
- The most common result of rheumatic valve disease is a combination of both stenosis and regurgitation [6–8]
- It is important to remember that PVH is more prominent as compared to the degree of left atrial enlargement in mitral stenosis; on the other hand, the degree of left atrial enlargement is more prominent compared to degree of PVH in patients with mitral regurgitation [6,8]
- The presence of left ventricular dilatation in mitral regurgitation (seen as enlargement of the left ventricular contour with a larger radius curve) will indicate left ventricular volume overload or end-stage left ventricular dilatation/left heart failure [6–8]

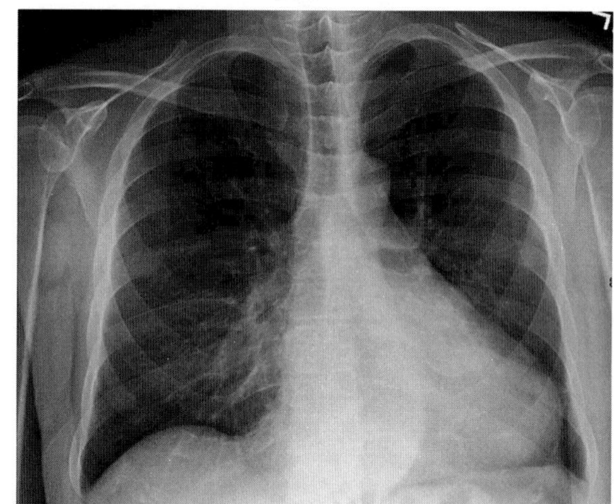

Figure 21.37 Longstanding severe mitral regurgitation due to mitral valve prolapse in a patient with Marfan syndrome and pectus excavatum. There is prominence of the left ventricular contour without obvious signs of left atrial enlargement. There is also pulmonary venous hypertension.

Tricuspid Valve Disease

The tricuspid valve is very commonly regurgitant as a consequence of left-sided heart disease but it is unusual for the secondary effects to cause diagnostic changes on the chest radiograph. Several congenital conditions will affect tricuspid valve function. Metastatic carcinoid disease will also affect the right-sided heart valves, producing deformity and some regurgitation of both tricuspid and pulmonary valves [6–8].

- Important tricuspid valve disease will cause enlargement of the right atrium, producing a prominent, bulging or elongated right heart border (Fig. 21.38A and B). This appearance has a single margin and is distinct from the "double heart border" produced by left atrial enlargement. The difference can be distinguished by the position of entry of the IVC, this structure limiting the expansion of the right atrium
- Significant cardiomegaly can be caused by RA enlargement [6–8]

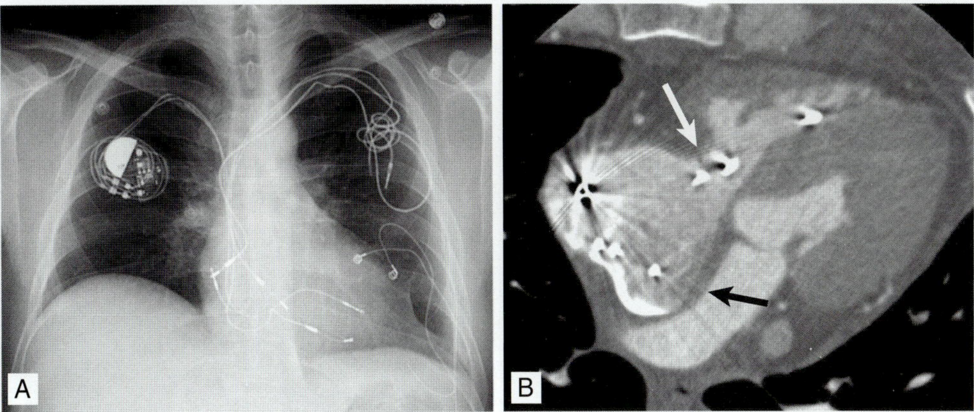

Figure 21.38 Tricuspid stenosis. Mild atrial enlargement can be difficult to identify on chest radiography. (A) Patient with severe tricuspid stenosis with no obvious enlargement of the right atrium on AP radiograph. (B) Contrast-enhanced CT demonstrates the severe tricuspid stenosis (*white arrow*) with right atrial dilation with leftward bowing of the interatrial septum (*black arrow*).

Pulmonary Valve Disease

It is very rare to see acquired disease of the pulmonary valve. Carcinoid disease and endocarditis can occasionally affect the valve [6–8,30].

Pericardium

On a chest radiograph, the pericardium has the same radiographic density as the heart. However, sometimes a substantial amount of epicardial fat is present and this leads to the identification of the pericardium and the radiolucent fat line lying within the cardiac silhouette. Pericardial fat pads, which develop in the cardiophrenic angles, are often visualized as low-density triangles and can occasionally be large and alter the cardiac silhouette. In the assessment of cardiac size on the chest radiograph the fat pads should be ignored.

Pericardial Effusion

Physiologically, the normal pericardial cavity contains 15–50 mL of fluid. Generally, more than 200 mL of pericardial fluid accumulation is required for radiographic visualization of cardiac silhouette enlargement. A moderately large pericardial effusion greater than 250 mL can cause massive symmetric enlargement of the cardiac silhouette with rounded, globular appearance (water bottle configuration) on PA radiograph with absence of any particular chamber enlargement and the presence of normal superior mediastinum. Pulmonary edema may be absent.

The cardiac contour is very clearly demarcated in pericardial effusion due to the static outer margin of the distended pericardial sac.

The other feature often demonstrated is a rapidly increasing cardiac silhouette on serial chest radiographs (Figs. 21.39A, 21.40A and B) as the effusion accumulates.

On the lateral radiograph, loss of retrosternal lucency and presence of a fat pad sign (Oreo cookie sign, sandwich sign, or bun sign), comprised of radio-opaque pericardial fluid stripe outlined by lower attenuation retrosternal mediastinal and epicardial fat, can help with the diagnosis (Fig. 21.39B).

Constrictive pericarditis: This condition is a result of inflammation of the pericardial sac leading to its thickening, fibrosis, adhesions, and/or calcification.

Radiographically, the cardiac silhouette is often normal but can be nonspecifically enlarged. Straightening of the right heart border and roughening of the cardiac outline as a result of pleuropericardial adhesions have been described. Biatrial dilation has also been described in CP. Calcification has been described in approximately half of the cases of CP; it often has a characteristic distribution involving the anterior and lateral aspects of the heart,

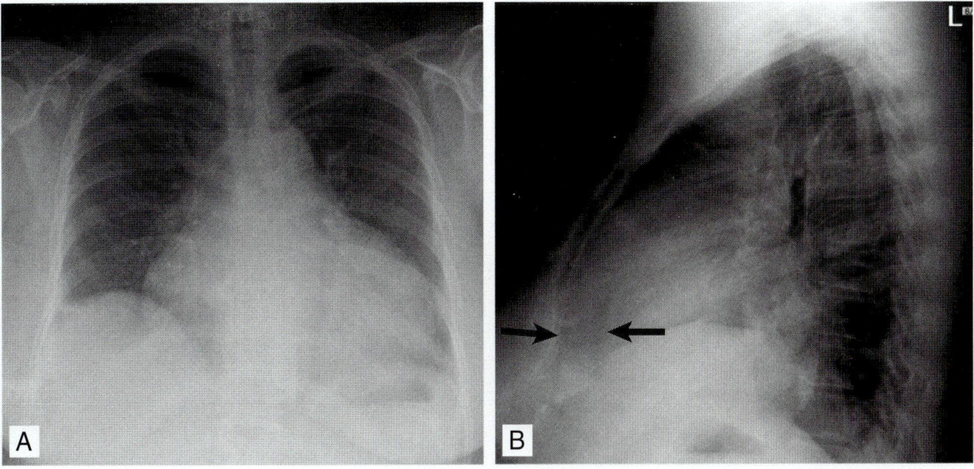

Figure 21.39 Pericardial effusion. (A) Frontal chest film. The heart silhouette has dramatically increased in size. The lungs show no features of cardiac failure, which might be expected if this were a dilated heart. (B) Lateral chest film. Epicardial fat is identified (*arrows*), displaced away from the edge of the cardiac silhouette and indicating the presence of a pericardial effusion.

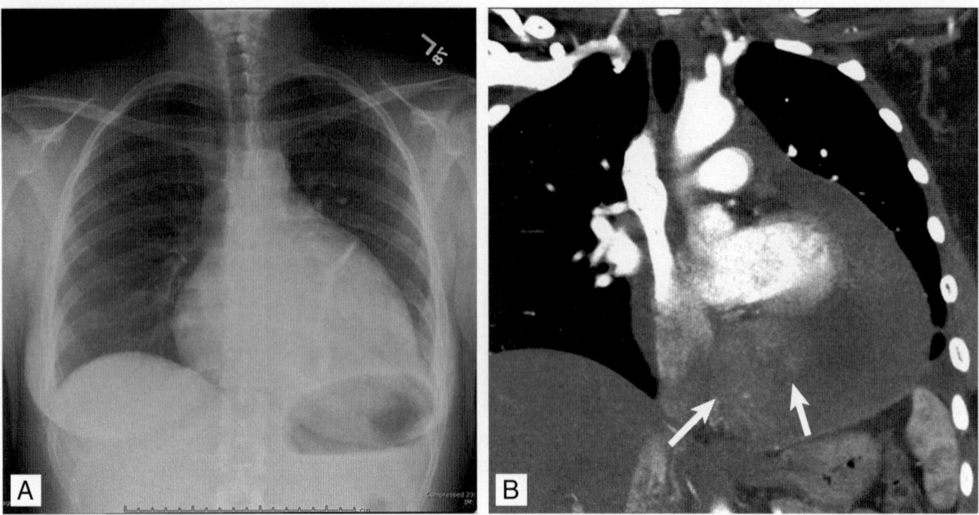

Figure 21.40 Pericardial effusion. (A) The AP view demonstrates an enlarged cardiac silhouette due to malignant pericardial effusion in a patient with a primary pericardial sarcoma. (B) Contrast-enhanced CT demonstrated the pericardial effusion with intrapericardial soft tissue mass (*arrows*).

along the diaphragmatic surface, atrioventricular groove, and pulmonary trunk (Fig. 21.41) [18,31].

Pericardial Mass and Mimics

- The most common "masses" associated with the heart are the pericardial fat pads. These arise from the cardiophrenic angle but can mimic disease as well. The triangular nature of the lesion with the characteristic position suggests the diagnosis (Fig. 21.42). The thickness of these fat pads increases in obesity and is typically asymmetric, with significantly more presence along the RV as compared to the LV [31]
- A benign *pericardial cyst* is usually an incidental finding, asymptomatic, unilocular, fluid-filled, and is intimately related to the pericardium. The cyst is thin-walled, occurring in the lower half of the mediastinum, and is more common in the right anterior cardiophrenic angle (Figs. 21.43A and B) [31]

Pericardial defect/absent pericardium typically manifests radiographically as the interposition of the lung between the pulmonary trunk and aortic arch, and also as lung interposition between the left hemidiaphragm and base of the heart. The partial defect can result in a bulge of the left upper heart border or prominent pulmonary artery due to herniation of the left atrial appendage through the defect beyond the normal left heart contour (Fig. 21.44) [31].

Other uncommon masses adjacent to or in continuity with the heart border include aneurysmal dilated coronary artery fistulas, multiple infective pericardial cysts, tuberculous (Figs. 21.45A and B), and hydatid cysts (Figs. 21.46A and B). Radiographically appearance of hydatid cysts is variable with enlarged cardiac silhouette or well-defined paracardiac opacity [31].

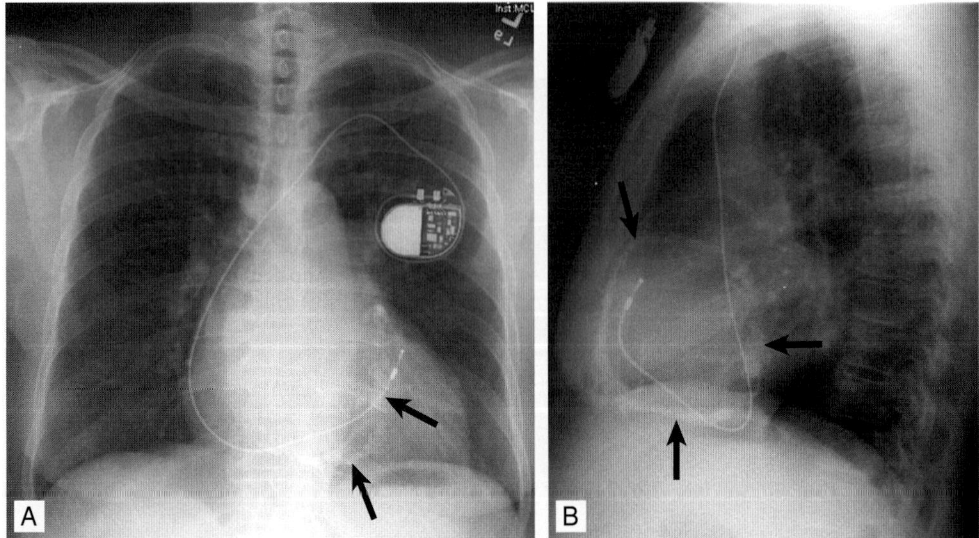

Figure 21.41 Constrictive pericarditis with calcification of the pericardium. Often with constrictive pericarditis there is straightening of the right heart border and roughening of the cardiac outline as a result of pericardial thickening. Calcification often has a characteristic distribution involving the anterior and inferior aspects of the heart as shown on the PA (A) and lateral films (B) (*arrows*).

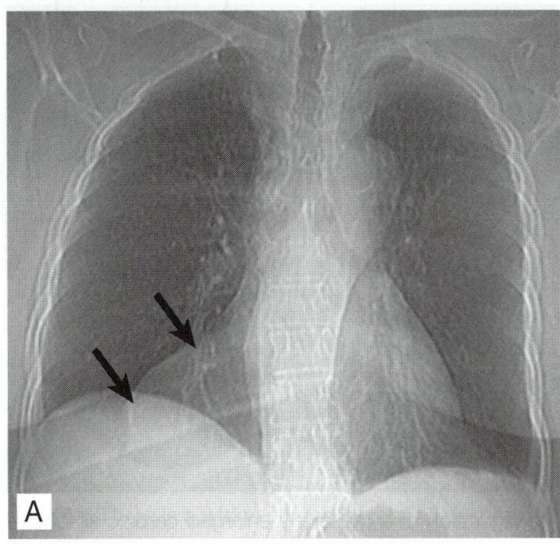

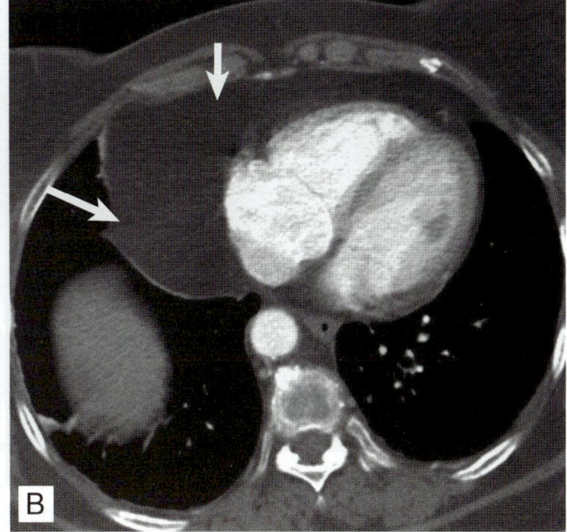

Figure 21.42 Cardiac fat pad. Frontal radiograph (A) and axial contrast CT (B). There is a low-density soft-tissue opacity adjacent to the right heart border (*arrows*). The triangular nature of the lesion with the characteristic position suggests the diagnosis of a pericardial fat pad.

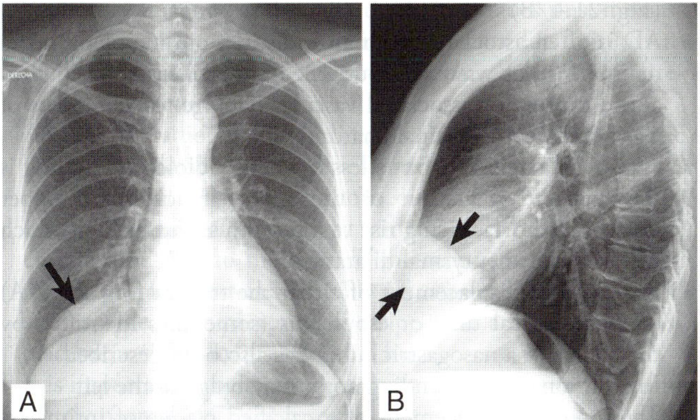

Figure 21.43 Pericardial cyst. (A) Frontal chest radiograph shows a sharply defined abnormal opacity in the right pericardiophrenic angle (*arrow*). (B) Lateral view. This is seen to lie anteriorly and is one of the characteristic sites for a pericardial cyst (*arrows*).

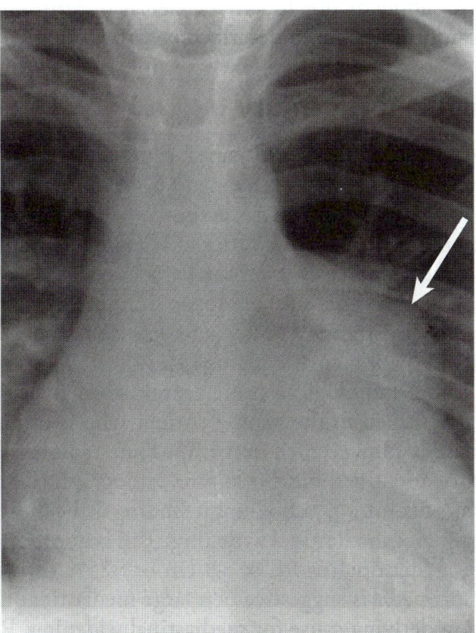

Figure 21.44 Congenital pericardial defect. An isolated pericardial defect is usually left-sided (*arrow*) and can allow prolapse of the left atrium or left atrial appendage beyond the normal left heart contour.

Thoracic Aorta

Enlargement of Thoracic Aorta on CXR

The aorta is considered to be enlarged if the diameter of the aorta is more than 50% above the higher end of the normal range for the individual depending on the age, sex, body size, and segment of the aorta [32–34].

The aortic arch is considered to be enlarged on the frontal chest radiograph if it measures more than 4 cm from the location of the indented trachea to the most lateral margin of the aorta. Features of enlargement of ascending aorta include convex right contour above RA margin/mid-right heart margin and lateral displacement of the superior vena cava on the frontal radiograph with a forward bulge of the anterior border of the aorta on the lateral view.

Role of Chest Radiographs in Acquired Aortic Pathologies

The frontal projection is the most used radiographic projection for the exclusion of acute aortic disease in an unstable patient or patients who cannot be moved due to a normal chest radiograph with a 98% negative predictive value in the setting of blunt trauma. However, the detailed workup of thoracic aortic diseases is limited using chest radiographs due to lack of anatomic details and suboptimal contrast resolution. Acute aortic abnormalities such as dissection, penetrating aortic ulcer, and intramural hematoma are usually not directly visualized on radiographs [32–34]. Posterior–anterior and lateral chest radiograph projections obtained in an upright position help in better assessment of the mediastinal and aortic contours as compared to portable radiographs. These have a role in the detection of calcification of the thoracic aorta, cardiac valve leaflets, and annulus [18]. Besides cardiovascular support devices and prostheses such as prosthetic cardiac valves, aortic endograft, stents, and pacemaker leads can be localized using radiographs.

Aortic Dissection

Aortic dissection (AD) is a devastating disease that typically occurs as a result of degeneration of the thoracic aorta. In many cases, there is associated aneurysmal dilatation of the aorta.

There are two major types of classifications, the De Bakey and the Stanford [32–34].

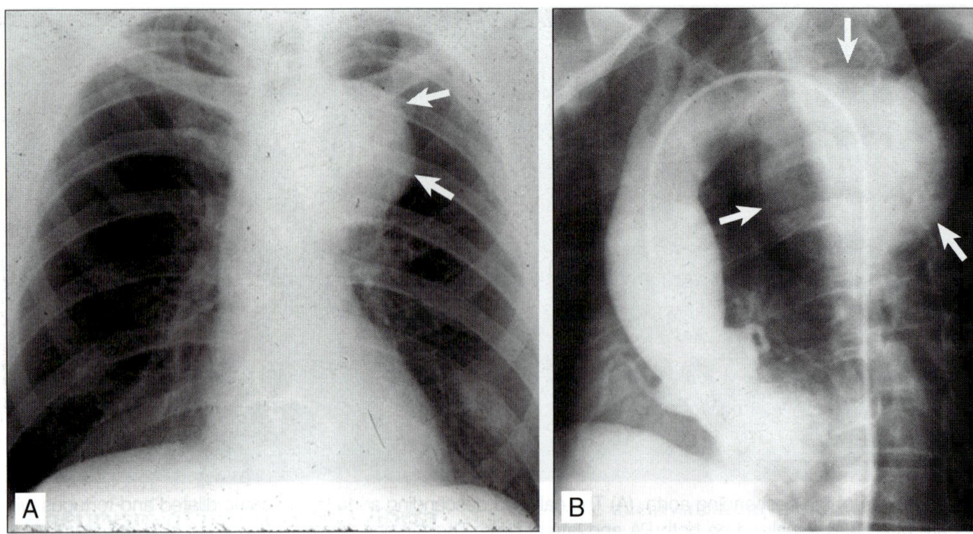

Figure 21.54 Syphilitic aortic aneurysm. (A) frontal view shows abnormal aneurysmal dilation of the aorta (*arrows*). (B) Catheter angiography demonstrates the fusiform aneurysm of the distal aortic arch and proximal descending aorta (*arrows*).

outpouching or as a mass on a radiograph. Patients can present with abnormal widened cardiomediastinal silhouette and minimal to moderate increased pulmonary vascularity. However, patient with right ventricular outflow tract obstruction from SOV aneurysms can manifest with decreased pulmonary vascularity [36].

Pulmonary Embolism

This condition represents a spectrum of clinical outcomes, from the devastating acute massive central PE to pulmonary arterial hypertension as a result of multiple or chronic pulmonary embolic disease.

Chest radiography is the initial examination of choice in patients suspected of having a PE, especially in the outpatient setting. Prospective Investigation of Pulmonary Embolism Diagnosis I study showed chest radiographs were abnormal in 84% of patients with proven PE and 66% of those without PE [39,40]. Radiographs show nonspecific and transient findings and usually do not allow a specific diagnosis of PE. The radiographic diagnosis of pulmonary artery embolism is very difficult particularly in cases without infarction. The current role of chest radiography is limited to excluding entities mimicking symptoms of PEs, such as pneumonia, pulmonary edema, pneumothorax, and pleural effusion. A recent PA and lateral chest radiograph are also required for the interpretation of abnormal ventilation perfusion (V/Q) scan since perfusion defects substantially larger than corresponding chest radiographic abnormalities are suggestive of PE, whereas perfusion defects substantially smaller than corresponding chest radiographic abnormalities are not commonly associated with PE [1,39].

Acute Massive Pulmonary Embolism

It is frequently stated that the presenting film is normal but often the plain film is not normal, with signs that can be difficult to visualize and interpret.

- There is often slight enlargement of the heart
- Westermark described (a) a wedge-shaped shadow in patients with pulmonary infarcts and (b) pulmonary oligemia (Fig. 21.55A) in cases without infarction (the Westermark sign)

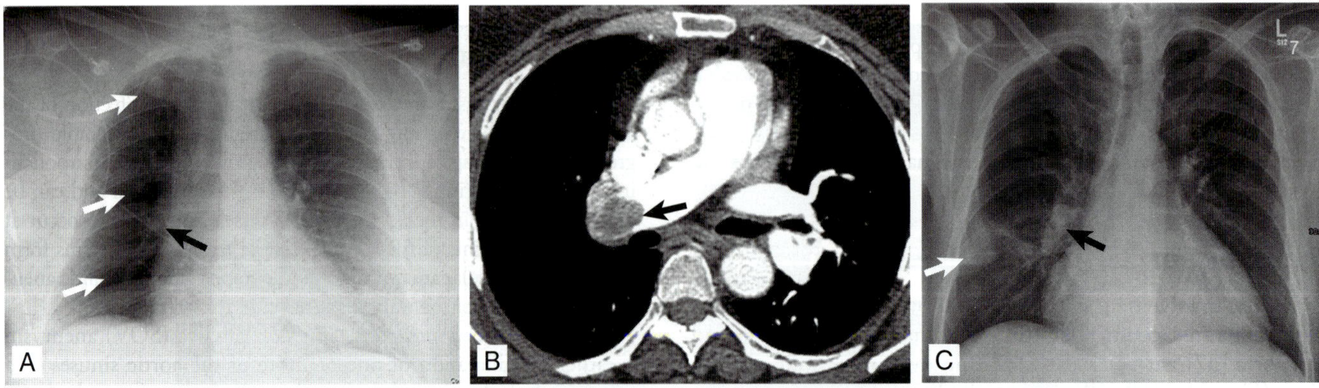

Figure 21.55 Acute massive pulmonary embolism. (A) Frontal chest film (portable). The right lung is hypertransradiant (*white arrows*) due to oligemia (Westermark sign), and there is over perfusion of the left mid and lower zones and prominent right main pulmonary artery (Fleischner sign, *black arrow*). (B) CT angiogram in the same patient demonstrates a large embolus impacted in the right pulmonary artery (*arrow*), producing virtually complete obstruction. (C) Frontal chest film (portable) in different patient shows subpleural peripheral nodular opacity in the right mid zone (*white arrow*) due to pulmonary infarct (Hampton hump), and mildly dilated right main pulmonary artery (Fleischner sign, *black arrow*) at the right hilum due to acute pulmonary embolus. Note mild cardiomegaly.

caused by embolic obstruction of the pulmonary artery (Fig. 21.55B) or hypoxic vasoconstriction secondary to the ventilation of poorly perfused lung, although this can be extremely difficult to detect and can be mimicked by emphysematous lucency. Although the Westermark sign of oligemia is more specific, the low prevalence of this finding in patients with PE limits its utility [1]. Any previous films are of considerable use as they allow direct comparison, highlighting changes

- Fleischner described a prominent central pulmonary artery (Fig. 21.55A) as another sign of PE, a finding caused by either pulmonary hypertension from acutely increased pressure from PE in peripheral arteries or distention of the pulmonary artery by a large thromboembolus [1,39]

Non-massive Pulmonary Embolic Disease

Pulmonary infarction can occur due to these smaller emboli but this is relatively uncommon as the bronchial circulation usually protects the lungs. Often nonspecific but often reversible ancillary findings develop such as:

- Plate-like atelectasis, which can be seen secondary to inhibited respiratory excursion, mucous plugging, or distal airway closure or focal depletion of surfactant. Persistence of this linear atelectasis may represent small areas of scarring as a sequelae of prior infarction. The plate-like atelectasis appears as a linear shadow when projected on end and is commonly termed a *Fleischner line.*
- The classic peripheral subpleural triangular or wedge-shaped area of infarct with a sharply convex medial margin appearing as focal consolidation can sometimes be detected but remains rare, this being termed “Hampton’s hump” representing hemorrhage without necrosis that resolves within a few days. A true infarct with ischemic necrosis of the lung can also occur and takes few weeks to months to resolve or can persist as a focal scar. Hampton’s hump is neither sensitive nor specific of a pulmonary infarct.
- Studies report atelectasis and/or pulmonary parenchymal abnormalities and pleural effusion as the most common radiographic findings in patients with angiographically proven PE [1].
- Pleural effusion usually is unilateral and small.
- Cavitation within a bland infarct is rare and occurs more commonly in larger infarcts >4 cm and <2 weeks of occurrence [1,39].

However, these findings and the above-described signs described by Hampton and Fleischner do not occur any more frequently in patients with PE than in patients without PE. Although the Westermark sign of oligemia is more specific, the low prevalence of this finding in patients with PE limits its utility [41].

Radiographics Features of Subtypes of Pulmonary Embolisms

- *Chronic pulmonary thromboembolic disease*
  If the patients suffer from continued small pulmonary emboli over a long period, irreversible pulmonary hypertension will eventually become established, leading to right heart failure/cor pulmonale. The chest radiograph will show the changes of pulmonary arterial hypertension in the form of enlarged main, right, and left pulmonary arteries, along with enlargement of the RV and right atrium [1,42].
- *Septic pulmonary emboli* are thrombi-containing microorganisms that become lodged in the peripheral pulmonary arteries. On a radiograph, these manifests as variably 1–3 cm sized ill-defined peripheral pulmonary nodules which may cavitate [43].
- *Cement embolism* occurs as a rare complication of percutaneous vertebroplasty. These appear as bilateral, branching, linear radiopaque structures in the expected course of pulmonary arteries in a postvertebroplasty setting, corresponding to the embolized cement on the chest radiograph [44].
- *Fat embolism* refers to the embolization of fat into the systemic or pulmonary circulation and is typical of bone marrow origin. These appear as bilateral patchy or diffuse air space opacities with a predilection for the lower peripheral lungs, resembling the findings in acute respiratory distress syndrome on chest radiographs [1,45].
- *Amniotic fluid embolism* occurs due to passage of amniotic fluid into the maternal venous blood due to tearing of uterine veins during labor. These appear as diffuse bilateral air space opacities resembling severe pulmonary edema and acute respiratory distress syndrome on chest radiographs [46].

Pulmonary Artery Aneurysm

Generalized dilatation of the pulmonary artery occurs in many situations where there are altered pulmonary hemodynamics. This can result from the presence of a left to right shunt, an increase in pulmonary artery pressures or even longstanding mitral valve disease. These dilatations do not constitute aneurysms. Localized aneurysm of the pulmonary artery is very rare and appears as focal dilatation of pulmonary artery. Central pulmonary artery aneurysm appears as a lobulated contour of the central pulmonary artery or as round perihilar opacity or hilar enlargement on the radiograph. On the other hand, segmental and subsegmental pulmonary aneurysms appear as nonspecific pulmonary nodules or as hemorrhagic consolidation which can evolve into nodules or masses [47].

Pulmonary Arteriovenous Malformation

This is a rare abnormal direct connection between the pulmonary artery and pulmonary vein resulting in a right-to-left shunt. This occurs between small pulmonary arteries and veins in the vast majority of cases (95). These are typically located in the peripheral lower lobes (50–70%) and vary in size from 1 to 5 cm in diameter along the course of the pulmonary vasculature.

Radiographs have low to moderate sensitivity in the range of 50–70% for their detection. PAVM appear as round, oval, or lobulated well-defined nodules with feeding artery(ies) and draining vein(s) or as consolidative lesions in diffuse types of PAVM (Figs. 21.56A and B) [1]. Multiple PAVM appear as multiple small nodular opacities that can enlarge rapidly in the case of the Osler–Weber–Rendu syndrome or hereditary hemorrhagic telangiectasia [48].

Scimitar syndrome: One relatively common form of partial anomalous pulmonary venous drainage that can often present in adult life is the Scimitar syndrome/hypogenetic lung/pulmonary veno-lobar syndrome which results in a left-to-right shunt. The syndrome describes an anomalous pulmonary vein draining the right lower lobe, inserting below the diaphragm (Fig. 21.57), usually into the IVC while sometimes can insert into right atrium, SVC, portal vein, and hepatic vein [49].

Heart Transplantation

Cardiac transplantation is now widely accepted as a form of treatment for end-stage heart disease. Over 5000 cardiac transplants are performed worldwide annually and 2000–3000 in the United

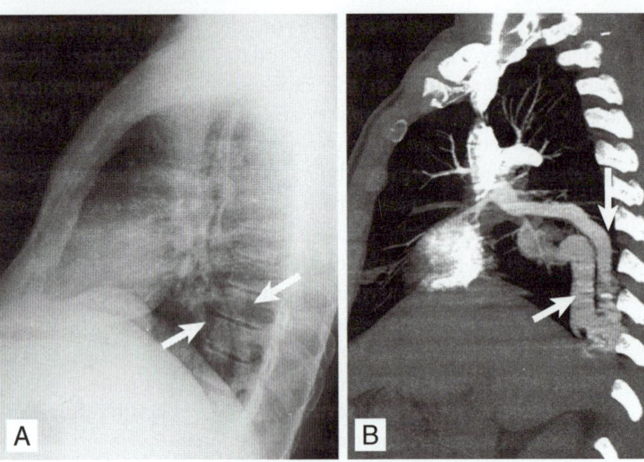

Figure 21.56 Pulmonary arteriovenous malformations. (A) Lateral chest film. Abnormal pulmonary elongated shadows can be identified in the posterior lower zone, overlying the lower thoracic spine (*arrow*). (B) Pulmonary CT angiogram, the sagittal view shows the pulmonary arteriovenous malformations in the posterior right lower lobe (*arrows*).

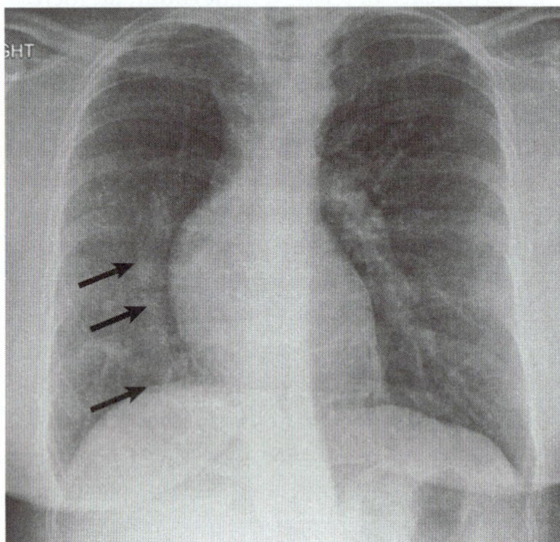

Figure 21.57 Scimitar syndrome. This PA film demonstrates a characteristic appearance of a soft-tissue curved opacity with increased caliber in its lower portion shaped like an inverted Scimitar sword/Turkish sword (*arrows*) within the right lower zone near right medial costophrenic angle representing partial anomalous right lower lobe pulmonary vein, terminating below the diaphragm into IVC. Note associated with a hypoplastic right lower lobe, with associated shift of the heart toward the right side (dextroversion).

States each year [50]. Two methods of transplantation exist; the first is heterotopic heart transplant where the donor heart is "piggy-backed" into the recipient's heart with the native right atrium being preserved (Fig. 21.58). The second method is for the native heart to be completely or near completely removed as in orthotopic heart transplants [50].

The complications may be categorized into early (<1 month), intermediate (1–12 months), and late (>12 months).

The common complications of heart transplantation are pulmonary infection, pulmonary edema, and allograft rejection, of which the infection is the most common post-transplant complication in all the stages. The chest radiograph can reveal the expected early postoperative cardiac surgery findings including minimal pneumothoraces, pleural effusions, pneumomediastinum, pneumopericardium, atelectasis, enlarged cardiac silhouette, sternal dehiscence, and infections [50,51]. In addition the chest radiograph can

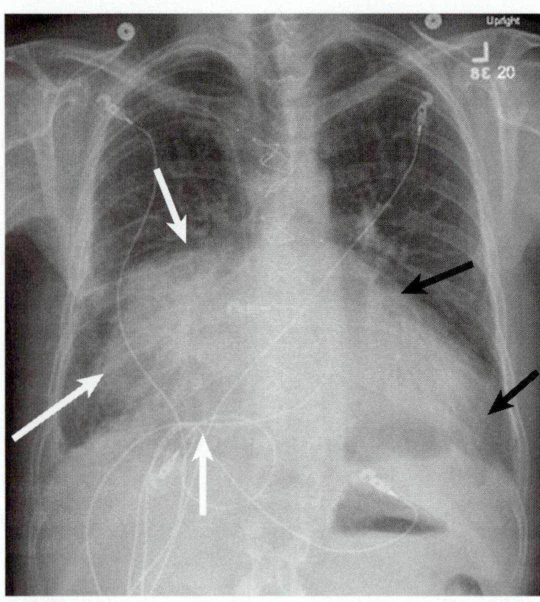

Figure 21.58 Heterotopic heart transplant in-patient with ischemic cardiomyopathy. Frontal chest film shows donor transplanted heart (*white arrows*) to the right of the native heart connected to the native heart (*black arrows*) in a parallel fashion with connections between the donor and native aortas, pulmonary arteries, left atria, and right atria. Note sternotomy sutures due to heart transplant. Cardiac transplantation is the treatment for patients with end-stage myocardial failure. Note that this procedure is technically more demanding than orthotopic heart transplantation.

demonstrate an altered configuration of the cardiac contour with a double heart border where there is a double RA contour produced by the overlap of donor and recipient right atria in heterotopic transplant with lateral position of the native right atrium. The enlarged cardiac silhouette in the immediate postoperative period could be related to a discrepancy between the native pericardium and the donor heart or a small pericardial effusion however beyond this period this increase in size can suggest cardiac rejection [50,51]. If there is a discrepancy in the size of the donor and native aorta, there can be an abrupt change in diameter at the site of anastomosis. Additionally, one may notice residual cardiac pacer wire fragments in the thoracic veins [50].

Cardiac Devices on Chest X-Ray

- A left ventricular assist device is used to augment cardiac output in the setting of LV dysfunction
  - On radiograph, HeartMate II VAD is identified by its location below the diaphragm in the preperitoneal pocket while HeartMate 3 and HeartWare VAD System are located above the diaphragm in the pericardial space
  - HeartMate II VAD has a typical radiopaque bell-shaped impeller housing unit/pump, partly radiopaque inflow and outflow cannulas and uniformly radiopaque driveline. A normal radiographic angle between the inflow cannula and the pump should be greater than 55° while a more acute angle representing device malposition
  - On the contrary, the Heartmate 3 and HeartWare HVAD systems reveal a radiopaque circular impeller/pump unit with a centrally located inflow cannula. The radiopaque part of the outflow cannula is angled in the case of the HeartMate 3 and is straighter in the HeartWare HVAD System [52]

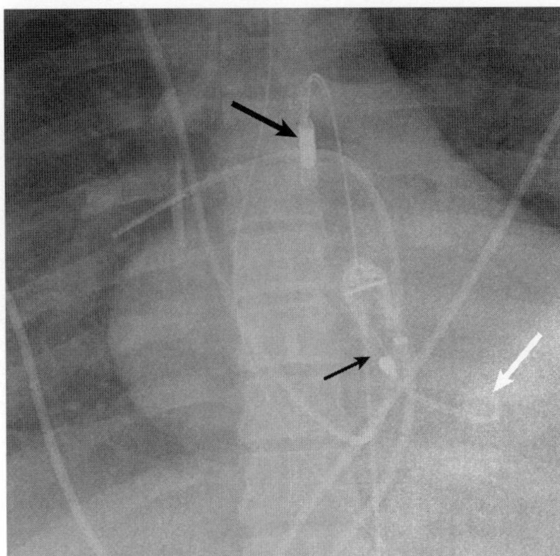

Figure 21.59 Magnified PA chest film demonstrates a typical location of the percutaneously placed left-sided Impella system with its radiopaque coiled appearance of the distal tip located centrally within the left ventricle (*white arrow*). For this left-sided Impella system, note that the inlet area is in the left ventricle (*small black arrow*), the outlet area is situated above the aortic valve (*large black arrow*), and the impeller is in between these two areas along the length of the catheter. The ideal location of the distal tip is 3–4 cm across the aortic valve. Note that for the right heart failure or biventricular failure, the Impella may be placed with the inflow area in the inferior vena cava, and the outflow tip may be positioned within the main pulmonary artery.

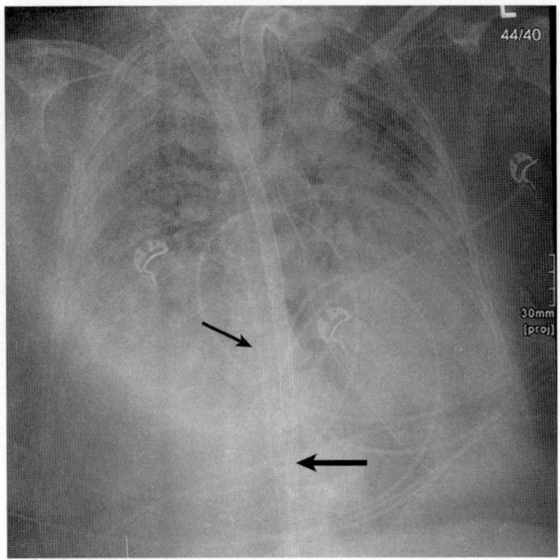

Figure 21.60 Venovenous ECMO on a portable radiograph in severe COVID-19 pneumonia-related acute lung injury/ARDS in a middle-aged woman shows the location of the tip of the femoral venous approach ECMO cannula being located at IVC to right atrium junction (ideal location), while the tip of the internal jugular venous approach cannula is in the lower right atrium (ideally located near SVC to right atrium junction). Diffuse multifocal consolidative and ground glass airspace opacities in both lungs due to acute lung injury from COVID-19. ECMO allows reduction of barotrauma to the lung parenchyma since it results in bypass of venous blood. Note the normal location of the tracheostomy tube and esophagogastric tube.

  - Impella ventricular support systems is temporary, percutaneously implanted VAD which can be left ventricular assist device (Fig. 21.59) or RVAD [52]
- *Extracorporeal membrane oxygenation (ECMO)* support venous bypass system is used for patients with acute respiratory and/or cardiac failure. Venoarterial and venovenous (Fig. 21.60) are the two types of vascular access used for ECMO therapy. For venoarterial ECMO, cannulation sites vary, with femoral vein-femoral artery access being the most common [52]
- The Watchman device is a percutaneous LAA occlusion device with a jellyfish-like appearance and consisting of a self-expanding nitinol frame and polyethylene terephthalate fabric. On a radiograph, the device appears radio-opaque due to the nitinol frame over the LAA location [23]
- On radiographs, the MitraClip appears as two adjacent metallic clips made from cobalt–chromium in the anatomical mitral valve position (Fig. 21.61A) [23]
- The AtriClip on a radiograph is seen as a metallic hair clip-appearing structure due to two parallel titanium tubes, projecting over the expected location of the LAA [23] (Fig. 21.61B)
- The Amplatzer Septal Occluder appears as a circular double nitinol disk on radiographs over the expected location of the interatrial septum for ASD closure (Fig. 21.62) or over the interventricular septum in cases of VSD closure [23]

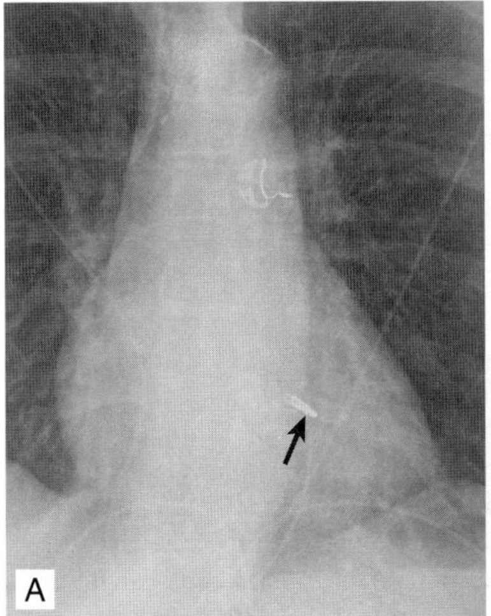

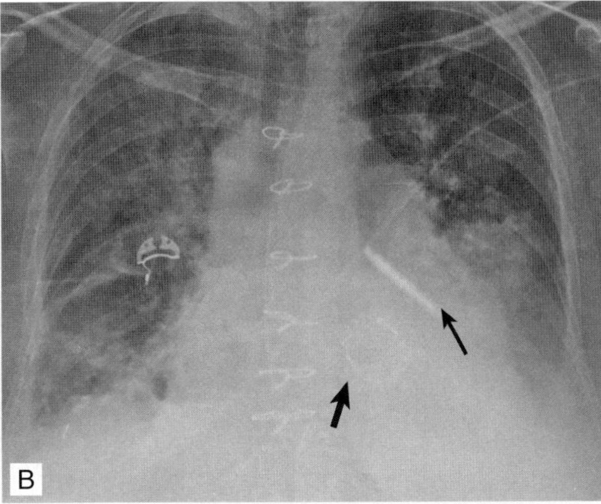

Figure 21.61 Mitraclip device (A) and Atriclip (B) on the magnified frontal views of the central cardiac silhouette. Image A demonstrates a small tubular metallic device projecting in the typical location of mitral valve due to Mitraclip (*arrow*). Image B demonstrates a metallic linear construct corresponding to an Atriclip device projecting over the left heart in the expected location of the left atrial appendage ostium (*thin arrow*). Note the TAVI placement (*thick arrow*).

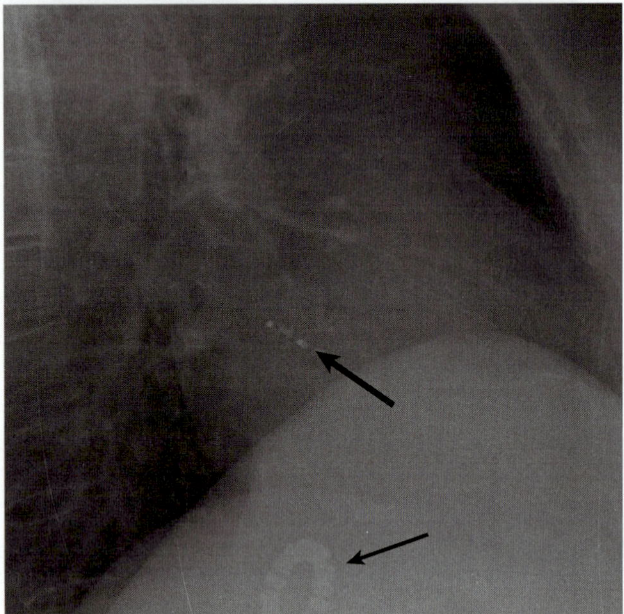

Figure 21.62 Lateral zoomed radiograph of an atrial septal occluder of a patient following percutaneous closure of an ASD demonstrates a double disk, atrial septal occlusion device (*bold black arrow*) projecting over the expected position of the interatrial septum. The primary treatment option for atrial septal defects (ASD) is percutaneous, transcatheter closure. Note ring-like radiopaque density projecting over the upper abdomen midline at the gastroesophageal junction (*thin black arrow*) used for the treatment of reflux.

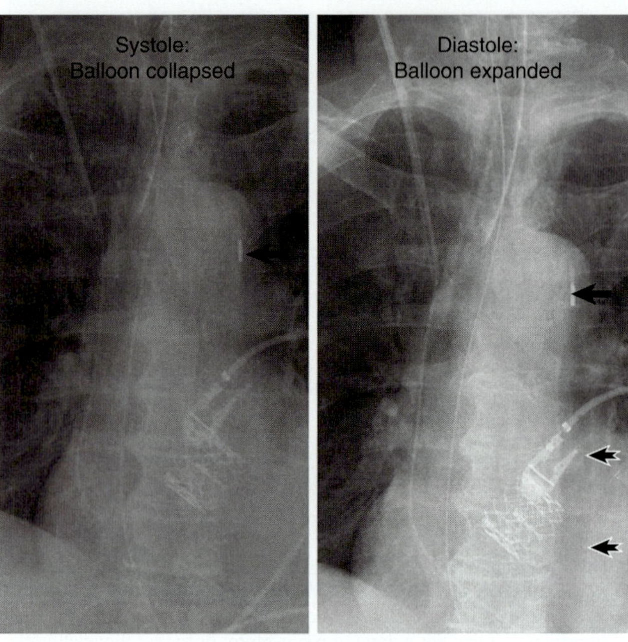

Figure 21.64 Intra-aortic balloon pump (IABP). The composite PA film in systole demonstrates the distal end of IABP consisting of a radiopaque marker tip positioned in the proximal descending aorta, 2–3 cm distal to the origin of the left subclavian artery and the radiopaque tip is in the center of the aortic knob (*black arrow*) as ideally expected. The PA film in diastole also shows lucency due to the intra-aortic balloon expansion during diastole (*notched arrows*) as compared to systole to maintain cardiac perfusion. Note that additional and better radiographic reference point being tip position of IABP being approximately 2 cm above the carina (*thick black arrow*).

- Transcatheter pulmonary and aortic valve devices can be anatomically localized over the pulmonic valve and aortic valve positions respectively on chest radiographs due to the metallic stent portion of these percutaneously placed valves [23]
- On a radiograph, multiple radiopaque markers of the EndoWave catheter denoting the treatment segment of pulmonary arteries can be identified to overlap the embolus-containing pulmonary artery region [53]

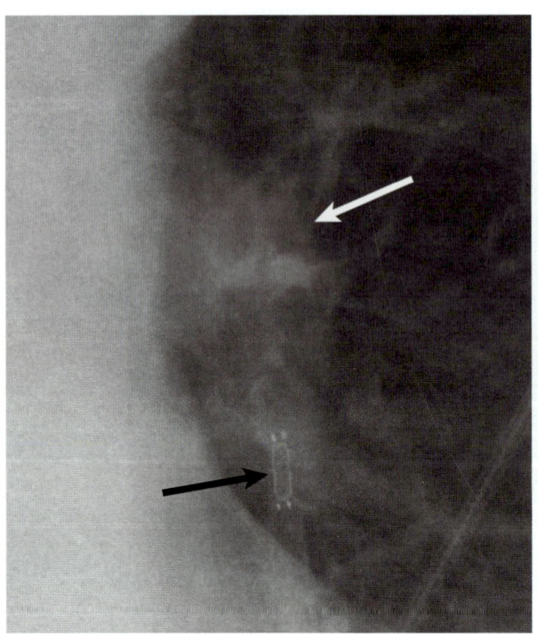

Figure 21.63 Frontal zoomed radiograph of the CardioMEMS device appearing as a linear radiopaque density seen in the left lower proximal segmental pulmonary artery (*black arrow*) just below the left hilum (*white arrow*) in a middle-aged man with dilated ischemic cardiomyopathy.

- On the radiograph, CardioMEMS Heart Failure System device appears as a small radiopaque line due to sensor with an adjacent radiopaque dot due to nitinol on either end within the expected location of the branch pulmonary artery (Fig. 21.63) [23,54]
- An intra-aortic balloon pump is a counter pulsation circulatory assist device used to improve coronary and cerebral blood flow consists of an electrocardiographically synchronized helium inflated balloon mounted on a flexible catheter (Fig. 21.64). Typically, it is inserted through the common femoral artery [52]

Suggested Readings

- C Chiles, CE Putman, Pulmonary and cardiac imaging. New York: Marcel Dekker; 1997.
- CB Higgins, Essentials of cardiac radiology and imaging. New York: J. B. Lippincott; 1992.
- WF Dahnert, Radiology review manual. LWW; Wolters Kluwer N.V.; 2017.
- S Digumarthy, S Abbara, J Chung, Problem solving in chest imaging. Elsevier; 2019.
- WR Webb, CB Higgins, Thoracic imaging: pulmonary and cardiovascular radiology. Wolters Kluwer N.V.; 2016.
- D Hansell, D Lynch, HP McAdams, A Bankier, Imaging of diseases of the chest. Mosby Elsevier; 2009.
- W Manning, D Pennell, Cardiovascular magnetic resonance a companion to Braunwald's heart disease. Elsevier; 2018.
- MS Norell, J Perrins, Essential interventional cardiology. Philadelphia: W. B. Saunders; 2001.
- S Abbara, S Achenbach, P Rajiah, CT and MR in cardiology. Elsevier; 2019.

22

Coronary Artery Disease

ANDERSON H. KUO, SANDEEP S. HEDGIRE, BRIAN B. GHOSHHAJRA

Introduction

Ischemic heart disease represents the leading cause of mortality worldwide [1]. Coronary artery disease, the underpinning substrate of ischemic heart disease, denotes the culmination of several metabolic, hemodynamic, genetic, and inflammatory factors [2]. While the exact pathogenesis of coronary artery atherosclerosis continues to be deciphered, a nonlinear series of events starting with intimal thickening and xanthoma formation is now thought to play a central role [3], Fig. 22.1. The resultant narrowing of the arterial lumen may be sufficient in causing myocardial injury in the case of supply and demand mismatch, but is less frequently fatal until the advanced stage due to compensatory mechanisms afforded by its gradual evolution. Importantly, plaque rupture and thrombosis can lead to acute arterial occlusion, accounting for majority of acute coronary syndrome [4]. This complication can occur even in the absence of significant baseline narrowing.

Clinically, the presentation of coronary artery atherosclerosis is diverse, hinging on complex interactions between the myocardium, coronary circulation, and timing. The reduced coronary reserve may cause episodic self-limited chest pain (stable angina pectoris), shortness of breath that is aggravated by increased myocardial demand, or may manifest as diminished exercise capacity. Plaque rupture or erosion may lead to acute chest pain at rest (unstable angina), arrhythmia, or various complications of myocardial infarction. Alternatively, some patients exhibit only nonspecific symptoms such as sweating, weakness, nausea, and dizziness or even remain asymptomatic. On imaging, coronary artery disease may have a similarly multifaceted appearance.

In this chapter, the role of computed tomography (CT) imaging in detection, quantification, and risk stratification of coronary artery disease, its various manifestations, and post-treatment surveillance of coronary blood flow are discussed. Myocardial sequelae of coronary artery disease and their significance on reperfusion are introduced.

Coronary Artery Calcification

Introduction

As coronary artery atherosclerosis can be clinically silent, many tools have been developed in identifying patients who have atherosclerosis and might benefit from therapy before symptom onset. One of the most commonly used risk stratification methods, the atherosclerotic cardiovascular disease (ASCVD) score [5], estimates the patient's 10-year risk for fatal or nonfatal myocardial infarction or stroke using several demographic, clinical, and laboratory parameters. While experts generally agree that patients with high risk (>20%) for cardiovascular event will likely benefit from therapy and those with low risk (<5%) will likely benefit little, management for the intermediate-risk group is less clear. Side effects of therapy, patient adherence/effort, and cost add to the complexity of the issue. In this situation, coronary calcium scoring has emerged as a potent supplementary stratifying factor for cardiovascular event.

Methods and Technique

Calcium scoring leverages identification of coronary artery calcification in estimating the overall atherosclerotic disease burden. Using an ECG-gated, breath-held, noncontrast CT scan obtained from the level of the hilum to the diaphragm, the amount of calcification in each coronary artery territory is quantified (Fig. 22.2). Technical aspects of calcium scoring to consider include:

- Electron beam CT (originally developed but no longer manufactured) or multidetector CT
- Calcification detection using a threshold of 130 Hounsfield units
- Scan acquisition at 120 kVp due to energy-level dependent measurement of Hounsfield unit
- Contiguous count of at least 3 pixels (1 mm^2) of calcification to minimize inclusion of noise
- Slice thickness of 3 mm (some software allows conversion of other slice thickness images)
- Low (<75 beats per minute) heart rate [6] to avoid excessive motion artifacts (may be relaxed with high speed scanner)
- A scan time of a few seconds and radiation exposure of approximately 1 mSv or less is now typical

Interpretation

The Agatston method [7] is the most widely used scoring strategy. In this measurement, each positive area (in mm^2) is assigned a weighting factor depending on its density (1 for 130–199 HU, 2 for 200–299 HU, 3 for 300–399 HU, and 4 for 400+ HU). The individual artery score is derived as the summed products of the calcified area and weighting factor. An overall calcium score is given as the summation of individual artery scores and the value of interest. A nonzero score is considered positive. *While the divisions are somewhat arbitrary and not uniform across literature, a nonzero total score is sometimes categorized as minimal (less than 10), mild (10–99), moderate (100–399), severe (400–999), and extensive (1000 or above).* It should be noted that alternatives to the Agatston method for better depiction of the calcified disease burden are available, such as the volume method [8] and mass method [9]. However, these alternatives are rarely used clinically since the vast majority of the available clinical literature is based on Agatston measurements. Regardless of the method used, it is prudent to assess the myocardium for signs of prior infarction, such as subendocardial fatty metaplasia (Fig. 22.3), as they may be occasionally seen [10].

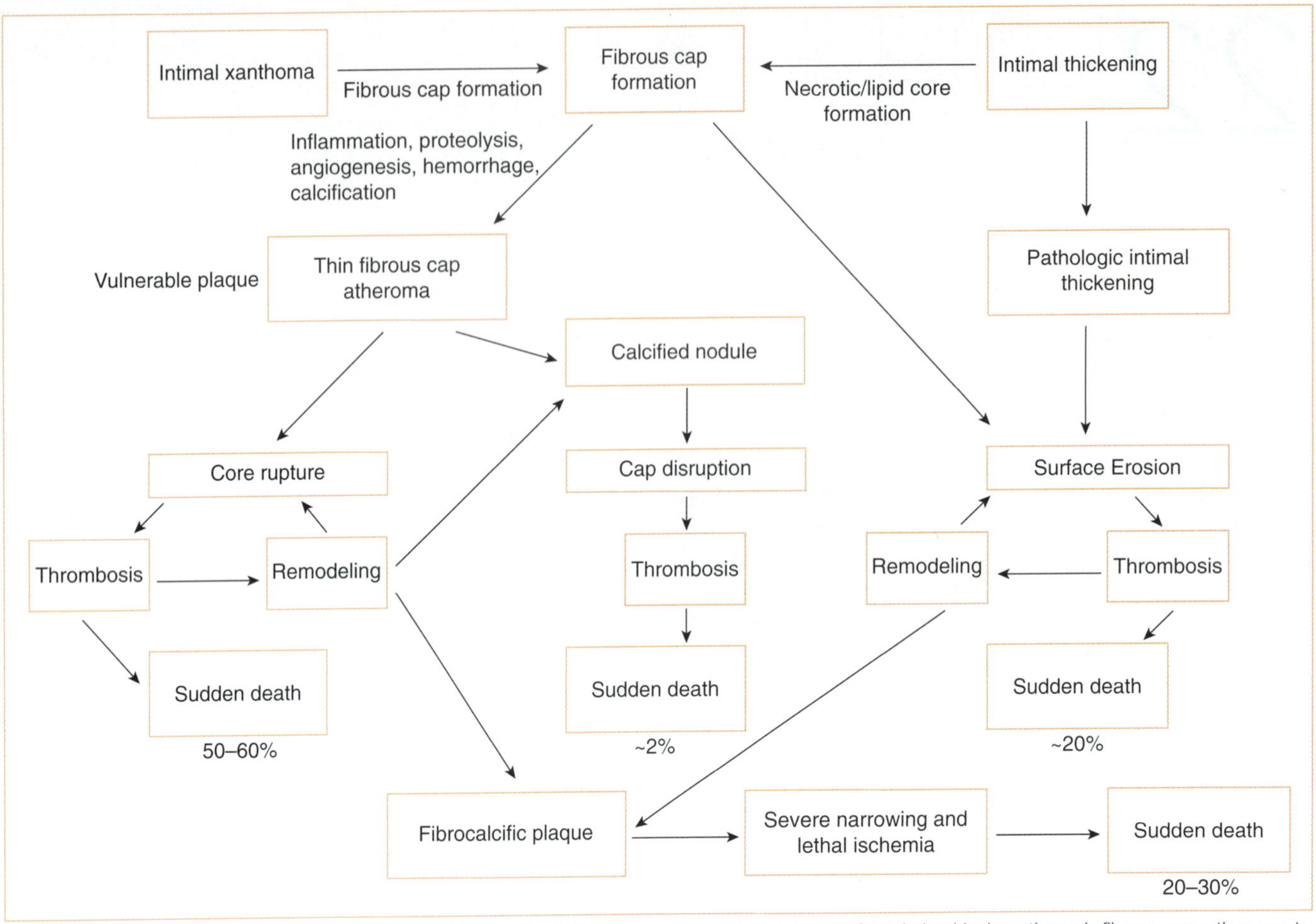

Intimal xanthoma → Fibrous cap formation → Fibrous cap formation

Intimal thickening → Necrotic/lipid core formation → Fibrous cap formation

Fibrous cap formation → Inflammation, proteolysis, angiogenesis, hemorrhage, calcification → Thin fibrous cap atheroma

Vulnerable plaque: Thin fibrous cap atheroma

Thin fibrous cap atheroma → Core rupture; Thin fibrous cap atheroma → Calcified nodule

Core rupture → Thrombosis → Remodeling → Core rupture

Thrombosis → Sudden death (50–60%)

Remodeling → Calcified nodule; Remodeling → Fibrocalcific plaque

Calcified nodule → Cap disruption → Thrombosis → Sudden death (~2%)

Intimal thickening → Pathologic intimal thickening → Surface Erosion

Fibrous cap formation → Surface Erosion

Surface Erosion → Thrombosis → Remodeling → Surface Erosion

Thrombosis → Sudden death (~20%)

Remodeling → Fibrocalcific plaque

Fibrocalcific plaque → Severe narrowing and lethal ischemia → Sudden death (20–30%)

Figure 22.1 Progression of atherosclerotic lesions. Atherosclerotic lesions are thought to progress from intimal lesions through fibrous cap atheroma to thin fibrous cap atheroma (TFCA), which can then undergo episodes of rupture, thrombosis, and healing/remodeling. Early intimal lesions may erode, leading to thrombosis and acute coronary syndrome (accounting for ~20% of deaths). Rupture and thrombosis of TFCAs account for 50–60% of the deaths, making identification of these lesions critical. Some imaging features help identify these lesions on CT. On repeated plaque erosion, rupture, and remodeling, fibrocalcific plaques ensue, which may lead to severe narrowing and lethal ischemia, accounting for 20–30% of deaths. Very rarely, cap disruption of protruding calcified nodule can lead to thrombosis and acute coronary syndrome.

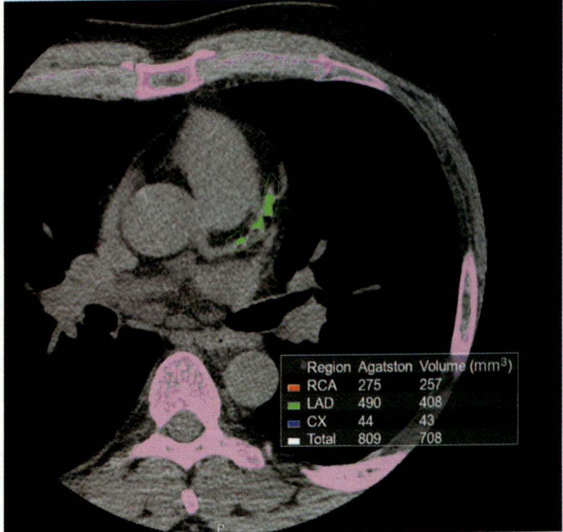

Figure 22.2 Coronary calcium scoring. Upon completion of the ECG-gated noncontrast scan, the calcifications are discerned from the underlying tissue using hounsfield unit thresholding. The coronary artery calcifications are then manually isolated into separate coronary artery territories, giving the calcium score (here quantified using both the Agatston and volume methods). Note that the left main coronary artery is also analyzed but not shown in table due to a value of zero.

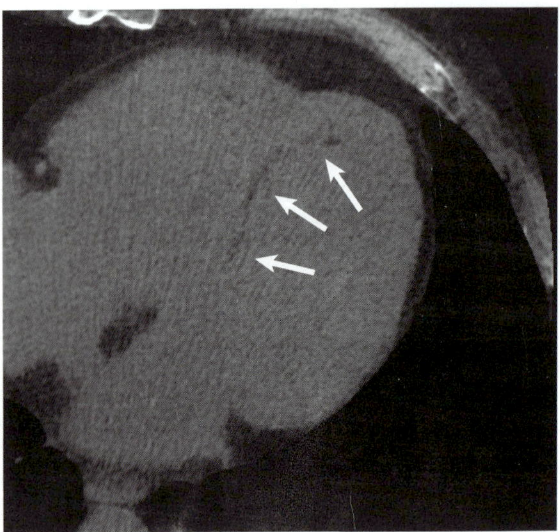

Figure 22.3 Subendocardial fatty metaplasia on calcium score CT. Linear low attenuation foci in a subendocardial distribution (*arrows*) are suggestive of fatty metaplasia, a result of prior myocardial infarction. Myocardial wall thinning and contour irregularity/aneurysm formation (not seen in this case) are additional clues to prior infarction but may be difficult to detect on noncontrast scans.

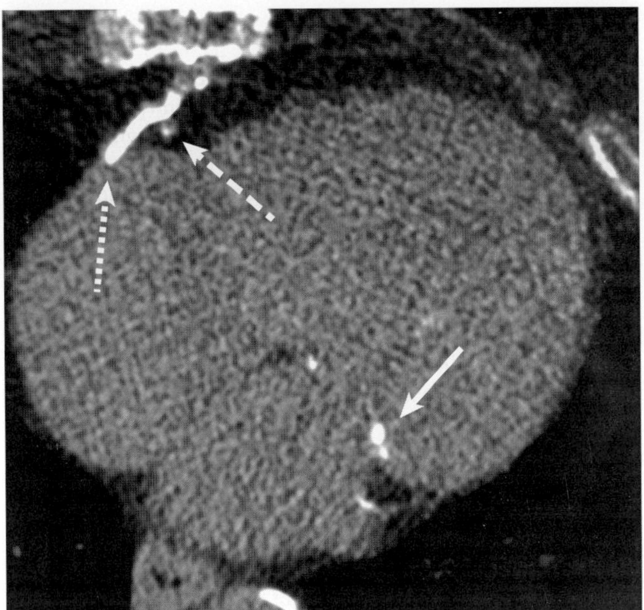

Figure 22.4 Mimics of coronary artery calcification. Mitral annular calcification (*solid arrow*) and pericardial calcification (*dotted arrow*) should not be mistaken for coronary artery calcifications. Notice the partially calcified right coronary artery (*dashed arrow*) underlying the pericardial calcification.

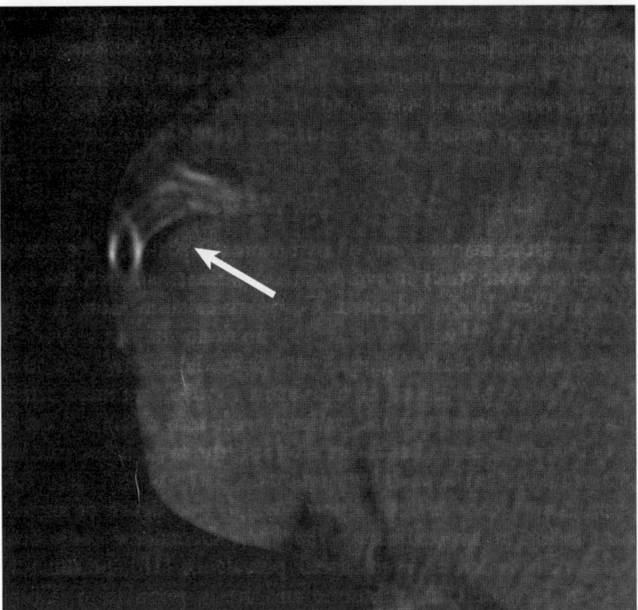

Figure 22.5 Calcium scan with excessive motion. With motion degradation, the coronary calcifications exhibit a swirling appearance (*arrow*). If quantification is attempted in this setting, the result may be over- or underestimated.

Some centers elect to provide age, sex, and ethnicity matched percentile scores to provide context of the measurement and facilitate patient communication. However, absolute calcium scores have been shown to be more predictive than percentile scores [11]. Despite routine noncontrast chest CTs not being acquired under the same setting, the Society of Cardiovascular Computed Tomography and Society of Thoracic Radiology jointly recommend evaluating and reporting coronary calcification estimates as none, mild, moderate, or severe [12]. This recommendation is based on studies that show decent agreement between nonstandard estimates and Agatston scores. Certainly, if the only clinical question is whether there is coronary artery calcification as per risk stratification and the exact score is not needed, identification of calcification on routine noncontrast chest CT is sufficient.

Three common pitfalls should be given attention:

1. Careful examination of the artery course is needed to prevent inclusion of noncoronary calcifications, such as that of the mitral annulus, aortic root, pericardium, or rarely adjacent bronchi (Fig. 22.4). This determination may be particularly difficult in the presence of anomalous coronary artery course, which warrants a dedicated contrast-enhanced scan
2. Care must be given when excessive motion is present as motion degradation may cause severe over- or underestimation of the calcium score. Cardiac motion may be evidenced as swirling of the calcifications (Fig. 22.5). Respiratory motion artifacts may manifest on coronal or sagittal views as stair-stepping or mismatch in the cardiac contour
3. It is essential that indwelling devices, especially coronary stents, are not mistaken for calcification (Fig. 22.6). In the absence of sufficient clinical history, examination of the area on multiplanar views may help distinguish the sharply demarcated, geometric, and circumferential coronary stents from dense calcifications

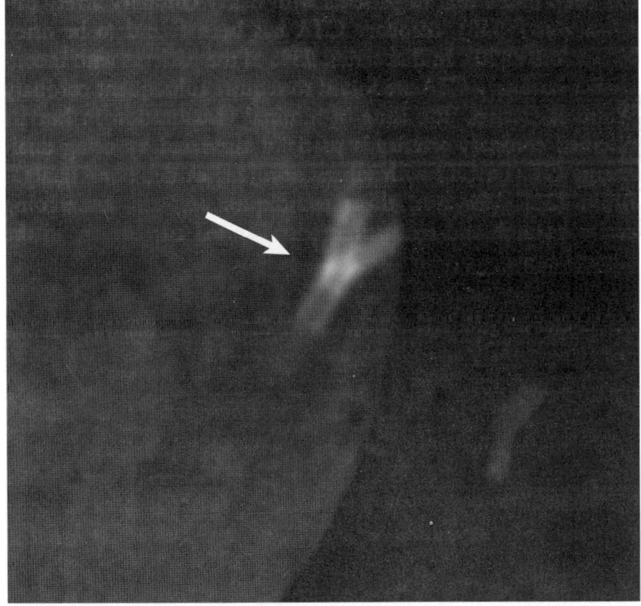

Figure 22.6 Stent on calcium scoring scan. Coronary artery stents (*arrow*, bifurcation stent) can appear very similar to atherosclerotic calcifications. In general, presence of hardware precludes accurate assessment of coronary calcium score.

Calcium Scoring in Asymptomatic Patients

In asymptomatic patients, the calcium score has been shown to be an independent predictor of mortality controlling for patient demographic and other risk factors. Compared to patients without calcification, adjusted relative risk ratios of all-cause mortality are 2.2, 4.5, 6.4, 10.4, and 12.5 fold for patients with minimal, mild, moderate, severe, and extensive calcifications [13]. A negative calcium score is a particularly important marker. The Multi-Ethnic Study of Atherosclerosis shows that in participants with ASCVD risk between 5% and 7.5% and nonzero calcium score, an actual event rate of 7.4% is indeed seen, compared to an actual event rate of only 1.5% in those with zero calcium score [14]. An event rate of 1.5% is well below the recognized threshold for statin therapy and effectively reclassifies these patients. Similarly, in subjects with ASCVD risk between 7.5% and 20%, zero and nonzero calcium scores are associated with actual event rates of 4.6% and 10.4%, respectively, suggesting statin therapy would only be indicated in the latter.

Calcium Scoring in Symptomatic Patients

In contrast to management of asymptomatic patients, the role of a calcium score study in symptomatic patients is much less certain and less likely indicated. Coronary calcium score is only weakly correlated with stenosis [15], no doubt in part secondary to possible noncalcified plaques and potential positive remodeling. Whereas prevalence of significant (>50%) coronary artery narrowing in asymptomatic patients with zero calcium score is very low, documented at about 1% [16], the same is not true for symptomatic patients. In symptomatic patients with zero calcium score, meta-analysis reports overall prevalence of significant lesion at approximately 7% [17]. Occasional individual studies document an even higher prevalence [18], presumably due to variations in technique and study population. Commonly, calcium score images are acquired as a component of the stenosis evaluation during coronary CT angiography (CTA). Calcium score images in this setting serve primarily as a noncontrast reference, given calcified plaque can sometimes blend in with the opacified vessel lumen [19] (Fig. 22.7). Nonetheless, it has been noted that in patients with heavy coronary artery calcifications (>540), coronary CTA has been found to be often inconclusive [20]. In that series, 93% of the patients with inconclusive coronary CTA are found to require subsequent coronary revascularization. The issue of luminal visualization in heavily calcified coronary arteries is partially alleviated by using dual-energy CT (DECT) with subtraction [21] or deblooming algorithm [22]. However, these techniques are still undergoing active research and refinement with limited current use in the clinical arena.

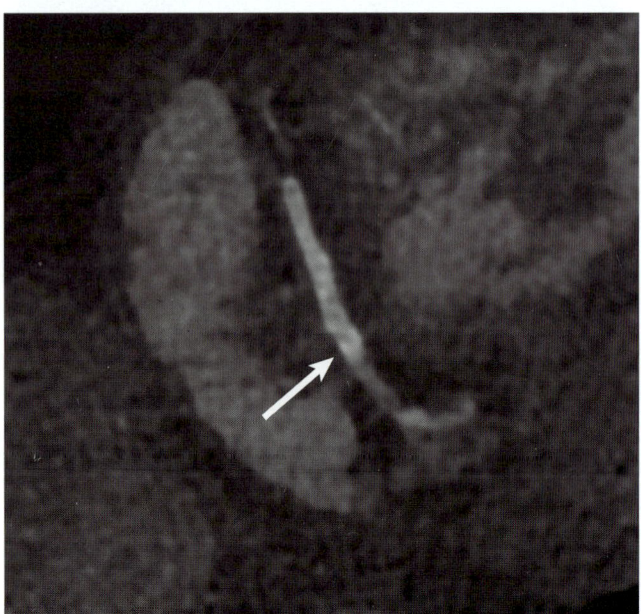

Figure 22.7 Poor delineation of calcification from opacified vessel lumen. When the arterial contrast opacification is robust, calcified plaques (*arrow*) may be difficult to detect. This issue is circumvented by comparison with the noncontrast or calcium scoring scan.

Repeat Calcium Scoring

The utility of repeat calcium score testing is equally poorly established. Literature documents that development/progression of coronary calcifications between scans is associated with increased hazard for cardiovascular events [23]. However, studies also suggest that the progression/development of coronary calcium score may be reasonably predicted using the baseline score and available clinical parameters [24]. Further, analysis shows inclusion of calcium score progression in large cohort studies adds little to risk prediction [25]. Adding to the issue is rescan reproducibility, which varies by about 20 points for the Agatston method [26]. Combined, these findings indicate routinely repeat calcium scoring is of very questionable clinical benefit at this time.

Summary—Calcium Scoring

In summary, calcium scoring is performed in asymptomatic patients with intermediate risk for coronary artery disease since the risk/benefit of preventive treatment may be further stratified. Because the result is viewed in light of existing literature with specified acquisition parameters, care is needed to ensure the scanning protocol allows for valid interpretation. A numeric result is given, with higher values corresponding to higher all-cause mortality. Currently, there is no clear benefit of calcium scoring in symptomatic patients or repeat testing.

Stenosis and Plaque Evaluation

Advancement in imaging techniques has led to improving capability of CTA in noninvasive evaluation of the coronary arteries. In contrast to calcium scoring, where only calcified plaques are assessed, coronary CTA allows direct assessment of both calcified and noncalcified plaques, luminal narrowing, and plaque characteristics as well as more subtle aspects of anatomy.

Technical Considerations in Coronary CT Angiography

Coronary CTA represents the pinnacle of CT imaging in terms of technical demands. In contrast to most body parts, spatial resolution, temporal resolution, and contrast resolution all need to be addressed.

Spatial Resolution

With the importance of luminal narrowing quantification in mind, the constraint imposed by spatial limitation is first considered. With 0.5 mm isovolumetric CT acquisition, a 3 mm coronary artery is represented by 6 voxels in profile and 28 voxels in cross section. In contrast, a 1.5 mm coronary artery is represented by 3 voxels in profile and 7 voxels in cross section. With increasing voxel size, this insufficient voxel representation worsens. Consequently, Society of Cardiovascular Computed Tomography guideline recommends a slice width of at most 1.0 mm and slice increment of 50%, although thinner slice width is preferred [27]. Also because of this limitation, it should be kept in mind that a vessel under 1.5 mm in size may be visible if patent but rarely adequately displayed for narrowing assessment on CT. In aiding with the issue of spatial resolution, coronary CTA may be performed following administration of nitroglycerin, which results in significant coronary artery vasodilation, increases the number of evaluable artery segments, and improves the diagnostic accuracy

TABLE 22.1 Contraindications to Nitroglycerin

Contraindications of Nitroglycerin
Hypotension (SBP <90 mm Hg)
Recent type five phosphodiesterase inhibitor use
■ Sidenafil
■ Tadalafil
■ Vardenafil
■ Avanafil
■ Udenafil
Severe left ventricular outlet obstruction
■ Aortic stenosis
■ Obstructive hypertrophic cardiomyopathy
■ Subaortic membrane or ring
■ Supravalvular stenosis
Severe anemia
Elevated intracranial pressure
Allergic reaction

of the exam [28]. Sublingual tablet, sublingual spray, and dermal patch have all been used with success, albeit with differences in timing and duration [29]. Side effects of nitroglycerin are generally mild and transient, which may include headache, dizziness, flushing, and hypotension. Contraindications should be kept in mind (Table 22.1). To avoid inadequate display of the voxels due to image matrix size limitation, a small field-of-view reconstruction (200–250 mm) is recommended as is a larger (512 × 512) default image matrix size [27].

Temporal Resolution

Temporal resolution is the second hurdle in successfully imaging the coronary arteries. Similar to other cardiac CT exams, the acquisition of coronary CTA is performed with ECG-gating and breath-holding. Either prospective triggering or retrospective gating can be used, each with its own advantages and disadvantages (Table 22.2). In contrast to the remaining portions of the heart, even a small amount of motion can prove problematic in the coronary arteries due to their small size. For this reason, coronary CTA is best acquired over one of the two critical windows to generate motion-free images: the end-systolic quiescent period (corresponding to isovolumetric relaxation) or end-diastolic quiescent period (corresponding to ventricular diastasis). In patients with a heart rate less than 70 beats per minute, the diastolic quiescent period lasts more than 200 milliseconds [30], sufficient for most modern scanners capability. However, this period progressively shortens with increasing heart rate, such that the duration is less than 65 milliseconds at a heartbeat of more than 100 beats per minute. In contrast, the end-systolic quiescent period is less dependent on heart rate but brief in general, lasting 70–90 milliseconds at most heart rates. Hence, most centers aim for imaging during the end-diastolic quiescent period following heart rate control via beta-adrenergic blockage with a goal of 60 beats per minute [27]. With advancing scanner technology, especially the introduction of dual source scanning that significantly improves temporal resolution, it is now possible to perform the scan in the end-systolic window without having to control the heart rate. It should be noted that above the heart rate of 90 beats per minute, the end-systolic window is longer than end-diastolic window. Additionally, retrospective scanning mode overall achieves higher temporal resolution compared to prospective mode. On the whole, multiphase image sets of the coronary arteries are obtained, and each cardiac phase should be examined as motion artifacts may be more pronounced in certain areas of one phase but not the other [31].

Contrast Resolution

Last, the contrast-to-noise ratio needs to be appropriate for clear delineation of the coronary arteries. A mean arterial opacification of at least 250 Hounsfield units is normally sufficient, which is achieved via use of high iodine concentration contrast at a high injection rate of 5–7 cc/s [27]. Due to the need for this injection rate, an 18-gauge peripheral venous access line is often required, especially in larger patients. Bolus tracking or test bolus is preferred over fixed scan delay to ensure adequate contrast timing. Either a biphasic injection

TABLE 22.2 Prospective Versus Retrospective Gating in Coronary Artery Imaging

	Prospective Triggering	Retrospective Gating
Image acquisition	Occurs during defined segment of the cardiac cycle, typically during the end-diastolic or end-systolic quiescent period	Occurs continuously through the entire cardiac cycle
Triggering	Set time delay following QRS complex- poor peak detection leads to uninterpretable images, beat rejection, or scan halt	Continuous acquisition followed by retrospective image sorting- poor peak definition may be salvaged by manual editing
Gantry movement	"Step and shoot" movement	Continuous feed
Pitch	>1 (180° tube rotation for complete image or 90° with dual source scanners)	<1 (needs overlapping coverage to include whole heart at all phases)
Cardiac function	Generally inadequately assessed due to large portion of missing data; however, some but not all scanners do allow full or near-full cardiac cycle acquisition	Adequately assessed as images are acquired at all phases
Radiation dose	Low and heart rate independent	High but heart rate dependent
Temporal resolution	Set by scanner rotation speed	Can span multiple heartbeats at the expense of lower pitch and longer scan time, bettering temporal resolution than scanner rotation allowed (multisegment reconstruction)
When to use	When only coronary artery assessment is needed Low heart rate Compliant patient Irregular heart beat (if beat rejection available)	Adequate functional assessment is needed High heart rate Questionable patient compliance Irregular heart beat (with technical expertise for ECG editing)

TABLE 22.3 **Contrast Administration Schemes**

Technique	OPACIFICATION AIM: Coronary Artery and Left Cardiac Chambers	Pulmonary Arteries and Right Cardiac Chambers	Inlet Systemic Veins	Advantage	Disadvantage
Biphasic, short contrast bolus 1. Pure contrast component 2. Saline tracer	Dense contrast	Saline	Saline	Low contrast dose Can detect intracardiac shunt	Precise timing can be difficult Nonvisualization of right cardiac chamber structures Nonopacification of the pulmonary arteries
Biphasic, long contrast bolus 1. Pure contrast component 2. Saline tracer	Dense contrast	Dense contrast	Saline	Easier contrast timing Can evaluate right cardiac chamber structures Can evaluate for pulmonary artery embolism	High contrast dose Cannot detect intracardiac shunt
Triphasic 1. Pure contrast component 2. Mixed contrast-saline 3. Saline tracer	Dense contrast	Intermediate or faint contrast	Saline	Medium contrast dose Can evaluate right cardiac chamber structures[a] Can evaluate for pulmonary artery embolism[a] Can detect intracardiac shunt	Precise timing can be difficult Higher technical/equipment demand

[a]With triphasic contrast, the mixed contrast-saline component enables some visualization of the right cardiac chambers and pulmonary arteries, although to a lesser/limited extent.

(composed of a contrast component and a saline chaser) or triphasic injection (composed of a contrast bolus, a mixed contrast/saline component, and a saline chaser) may be used, depending on preference of right heart opacification (Table 22.3). The actual contrast volume is tailored to the duration of the scan and patient habitus. Most commonly, the tube potential (kVp) and current (mA) are both adjusted for patient size, either manually or by anatomy/weight-based algorithms. In larger patients, where radiation penetration is a major concern, the image noise may be decreased by either increasing the tube potential or current. However, it should be kept in mind that while the radiation dose increases linearly with increase in tube current, it is directly proportional to the square of the tube potential. In very large patients, the noise will likely remain an issue. Increasing the slice width to a reasonable extent may help alleviate the issue at the expense of spatial resolution.

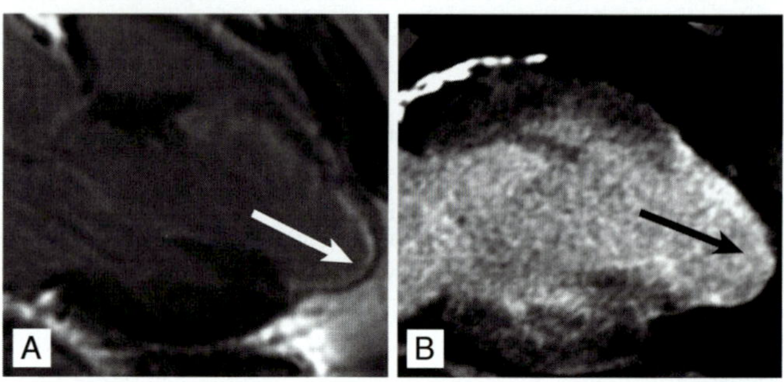

Figure 22.8 DECT. MRI late gadolinium enhancement image depicts a prior apical infarct in a patient with prior LAD territory myocardial infarction (A, *arrow*). With improved soft tissue and contrast differentiation afforded by dual-energy CT, a similar late iodinated contrast enhancement image is obtained demonstrating the similar finding of apical scarring (B, *arrow*).

Dual-Energy CT

Coronary artery imaging using DECT is an area in early adaptation and ongoing research (Fig. 22.8), briefly discussed here as it will likely have an increasing role in the clinical setting. In DECT, the scan is performed at different energy levels, once at low energy (~80 kVp) and once at high energy (120–140 kVp). Because the principle mechanism of attenuation, photoelectric effect, is dependent on both the energy level and atomic number of the substance, the change in attenuation at different energy levels is distinct to the material. Consequently, this technique enables tissue decomposition, allowing for generation of tissue specific maps (such as calcification or iodine map) and subtraction algorithms (by selectively remove all voxels of certain tissue type, such as iodine subtraction in virtual noncontrast map).

Further, the data can be used to simulate scan performed at specified energy level (kVp), termed virtual monochromatic imaging, which has additional benefits. Foremost, because the images are computationally derived, beam hardening is significantly reduced, partially alleviating blooming artifacts, decreasing metallic streak artifacts from surgical hardware, and improving estimating of lumen patency. Radiation dose may be reduced since energy level may be manipulated to maximize contrast-to-noise ratio and in some instances eliminate the need for a noncontrast scan. A lower intravenous contrast dose can be used since only a small amount of contrast is sufficient in altering the tissue characteristics to allow for identification. These benefits lend DECT as a promising tool that awaits more widespread use.

Image Display

Following scanning, the acquired images may be displayed in several ways: standard multiplanar reformat (MPR, Fig. 22.9A), curved MPR (Fig. 22.9B), vessel view (Fig. 22.9C), maximum intensity projection (MIP, Fig. 22.9D), and volumetric rendering technique (VRT, Fig. 22.9E).

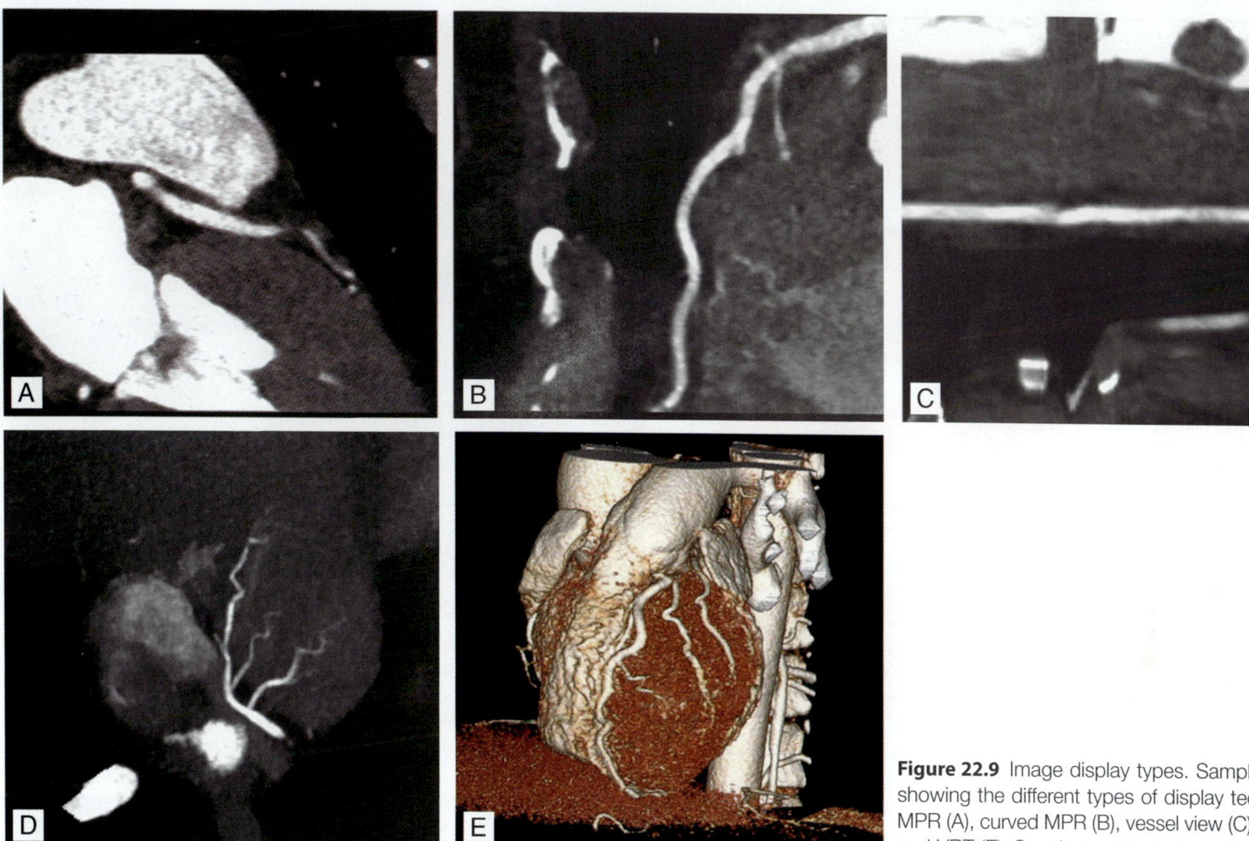

Figure 22.9 Image display types. Sample images showing the different types of display techniques: MPR (A), curved MPR (B), vessel view (C), MIP (D), and VRT (E). See the text for further details.

- Due to the tortuosity of the coronary vessels, MPR is absolutely essential for accurate interpretation. With MPR, the vessels are manually aligned and should be examined both in profile and en face, as atherosclerotic plaques are often eccentric
- Postprocessing software nearly ubiquitously allows for automatic extraction of the coronary arteries and display the entire course of the selected artery in a single image (curved MPR) to allow for easy interpretation. Care must be given when using these images, however, as it is easy to forget that the artery as laid out by either curved MPR is only one 2D representation of a 3D structures. There is thus a need to rotate the curved MPR to assess the artery from all angles as well as examine the cross-sectional view
- The curved MPR may be straightened to create dedicated "vessel view." Vessel view is advantageous in the measurement of stenosis as it eliminates the issue of vessel angulation. However, it is easy to lose track of the relationship between the coronary artery and the myocardium in this view
- While the use of MIP images in the assessment of coronary arteries may seem counterintuitive, they are helpful in two respects. One, MIPs serve to confirm high-grade narrowing or occlusion of the vessel, as residual luminal opacification by contrast and abrupt cutoff are clearly visible from the background of myocardium or pericardial fat. Two, in the distal small branches of the coronary arteries, MIPs help to confirm continuity of the vessels, which are often difficult to clearly follow on MPRs due to their small size
- VRT allows a 3D version of the coronary tree to be displayed. The value of VRT is most evident in the display of aberrant coronary artery anatomy, especially to referring physicians

Appropriate Use of Coronary CT Angiography

Appropriate use of coronary CTA is nuanced and has been evaluated per specific situation in detail in collaborative efforts [32,33]. In general, coronary CTA is deemed appropriate mainly in the work-up of symptomatic patients with intermediate risk/pretest probability for obstructive/significant coronary artery disease.

- In high-risk patients (such as those with presumed diagnosis of myocardial infarction), the lower resolution and sensitivity of CT compared to catheter angiography imply a negative CT does not exclude presence of significant narrowing with certainty, especially in the small distal arteries. If high disease burden and significant narrowing are found, catheter angiography is indicated for confirmation and possible intervention, making the CT exam redundant and cost ineffective
- In low-risk patients, where there is neither clinical suspicion nor objective (laboratory/electrocardiographic) evidence of disease, the chance of discovering significant narrowing is too low to justify its generalized use
- As such, coronary CTA is best utilized in symptomatic patients with intermediate risk/pretest probability for significant coronary artery disease, where it may serve as an arbitrator of clinical suspicion and objective evidence mismatch. Used appropriately in the acute emergency department setting, coronary CTA has been shown to reduce length of stay significantly compared to standard care while maintaining similar cumulative cost [34]

Stenosis Evaluation

Intuitively, the extent of luminal narrowing associated with atherosclerotic plaques is a major determinant of blood flow and thus clinical importance. Because the gold standard for coronary artery

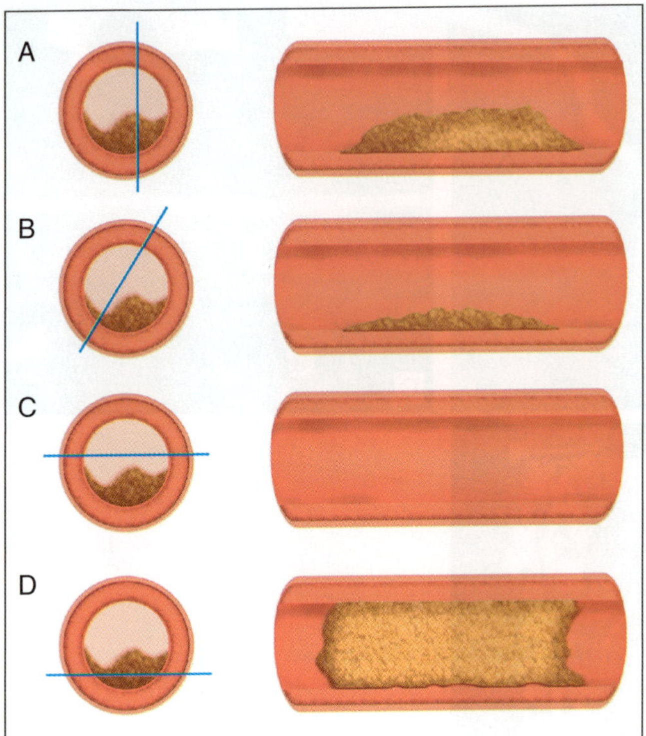

Figure 22.10 Eccentric plaque and accurate measuring. Evaluation of the coronary arteries in profile can be misleading due to the fundamentally three-dimensional nature of the plaque and two-dimensional nature of profile viewing. For a case in point, an arterial segment with moderate amount of plaque that results in close to 50% narrowing may appear properly as narrowed if assessed in the correct slicing plane (A). However, improper slicing can lead to poor visualization and overestimation or underestimation (B) of luminal narrowing. In extreme cases, the vessel may appear widely patent (C) or occluded (D).

evaluation, catheter angiography, visualizes blood flow in two dimensions, luminal narrowing is reported in diameter reduction by convention. *This custom should be kept in mind as to not underestimate the effect of narrowing: a 50% diameter reduction corresponds to 75% area narrowing, and less than 10% of the luminal area remains patent at 70% diameter reduction.* Early studies report that decreased coronary flow reserve is seen starting around 50% luminal diameter reduction and reduction of resting blood flow past 70% [35], making any narrowing past 50% potentially significant. Because the plaque is often eccentric, any suspected narrowing should be viewed in both cross section and in profile to gauge the true extent of stenosis (Fig. 22.10). Viewing the coronary arteries in multiple views will also help with detection of "flushed" occlusion, where occlusion of the artery occurs within the first 5 mm segment and may be easily dismissed as the rest of the artery is not seen. During vessel evaluation, the noncontrast portion of the exam, if obtained, should be viewed in conjunction, as dense calcified plaque may easily blend into the opacified vessel lumen.

Because of the resolution limit on CT (generally just under a millimeter), instead of an exact percentage, the extent of coronary artery narrowing is typically reported in rough quartile ranges, reflecting limit of uncertainty in measurement. This difference in method is compared to the less than 0.2 mm resolution achieved in catheter angiography and resultant estimates of exact narrowing. Discrimination of vessel occlusion (Fig. 22.11) from subtotal occlusion (severe narrowing, Fig. 22.12) is often difficult but important due to prognostic implications and

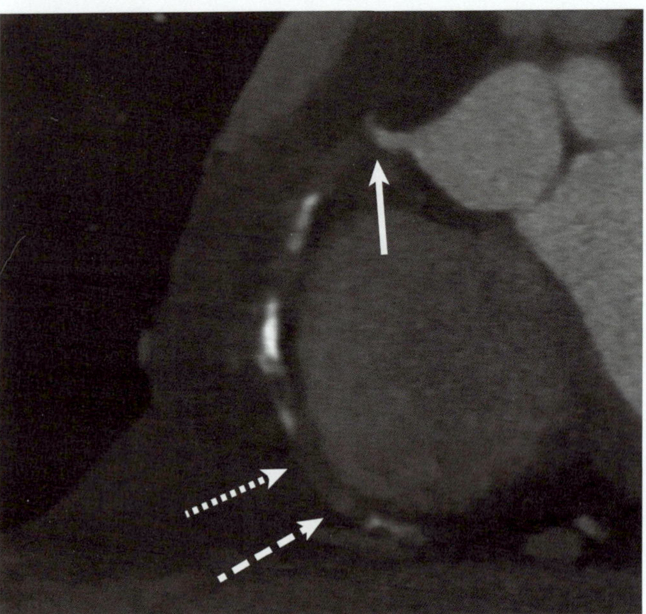

Figure 22.11 Total vessel occlusion. In an occluded artery, the segment of involvement is often long (>1.5 cm). A blunted stump (*solid arrow*) is suggestive. Distal to the occlusion, reverse contrast gradient may be seen, where the distal segment (*dashed arrow*) opacifies more strongly than the proximal segment (*dotted arrow*), a result of backward collateralization flow.

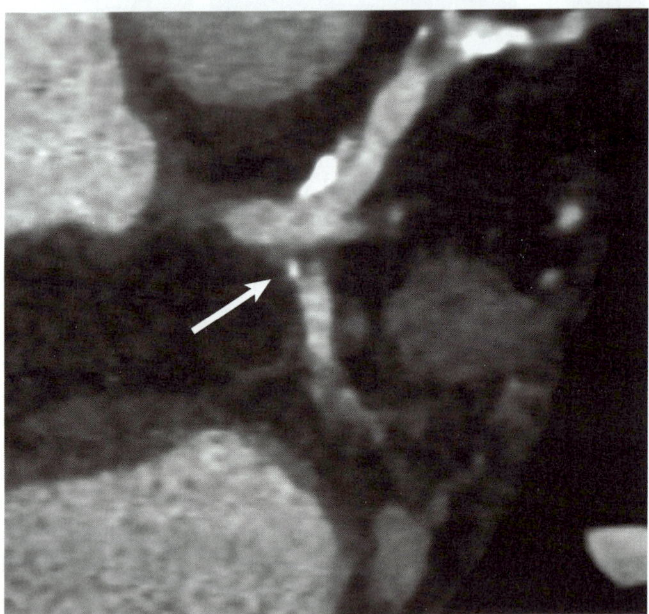

Figure 22.12 Subtotal vessel occlusion/severe narrowing. An apparent very short segment of occlusion (*arrow*) is likely to have residual contrast flow on follow-up angiography. This configuration is thus more appropriately termed subtotal occlusion/severe narrowing.

technical requirements in recanalization. Features that are suggestive of vessel occlusion [36,37] include:

- Apparent occlusion length >1.5 cm
- Higher distal attenuation gradient (denser opacification distal to the occlusion compared to proximal to the occlusion)
- Distal reverse attenuation gradient (denser opacification in the terminal portion of the vessel compared to just after the occlusion)
- Increased number of side branches
- Blunted stump

- Cross-sectional calcification >50%
- Presence of significant collateralizing vessels

Plaque Characterization

In addition to luminal narrowing, the plaque should be examined for high-risk/vulnerable features. Because acute coronary events, as mentioned, are thought to be the result of plaque rupture and thrombosis more than half of the time [38], identification of such factors prompts consideration of treatment even in the absence of significant luminal narrowing. Further, the ability to evaluate the extraluminal structures is a distinct advantage of CT over routine catheter angiography, an added value that should not be overlooked.

Our understanding of plaque vulnerability is coupled to studies examining the natural course of coronary atherosclerosis (Fig. 22.1). The advanced atherosclerotic lesion with a lipid/necrotic core and thin smooth muscle fibrous cap, the so-called thin-cap-fibroatheroma (TCFA), is found most vulnerable to rupture. In fact, by histology, TCFA is differentiated from ruptured plaque only by the integrity of the overlying cap. Unfortunately, the spatial and contrast resolution of clinical CT precludes direct identification of TCFA. Instead, a few findings that are associated with TCFA and acute coronary events [39–41] are:

- Low-density plaque, defined by <30 HU, believed to correspond to lipid/necrotic core of TCFA (Fig. 22.13)
- Small spotty calcifications (<1 mm in size), likely representing fragmented calcifications of TCFA (Fig. 22.14)
- A noncalcified ring of hyperdensity (<130 HU) surrounding low-density plaque, so-called "napkin ring sign," likely representing subtle peripheral inflammatory enhancement (Fig. 22.15)

With DECT, studies suggest potential in improving atherosclerotic plaque characterization via its ability to decompose different tissue types. For example, when compared to pathology and virtual histology intravascular ultrasound, Obaid et al. showed necrotic cores can be discriminated from fibrous plaques in postmortem arteries using DECT but not single-energy CT [42]. However, much weaker results were found with in vivo imaging on that study. Nonetheless, improved plaque characterization represents an area of active research that is expected to play an increasing role in clinical care.

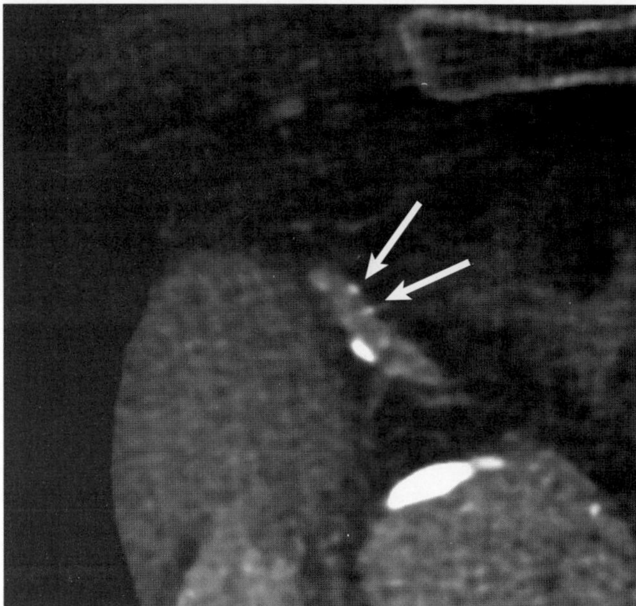

Figure 22.14 Small spotty calcification. Small spotty calcifications (*arrow*) are less than 1 mm in size. This finding is believed to represent fragmented calcification of an advanced atheroma. In contrast, larger calcifications are thought to be more stable.

Outside of the plaque, the contour of the coronary artery and surrounding pericardial/epicardial soft tissues should be examined.

- Remodeling refers to the change in the outer vessel margin in response to developing atherosclerosis. In positive remodeling, the outer border of the atherosclerotic vessel expands compared to the adjacent disease-free segments (Fig. 22.16). This expansion signifies that considerable amount of local plaque burden can develop before notable luminal area reduction. Because plaque rupture is dependent on plaque size rather

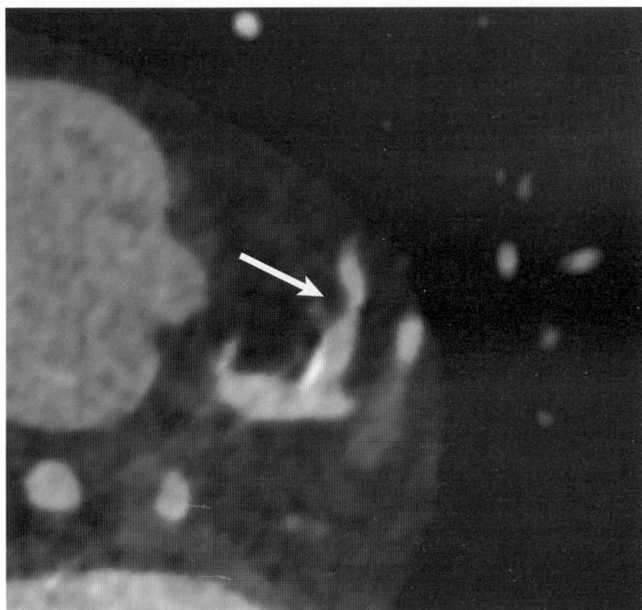

Figure 22.13 Low-density plaque. Low-density plaque (*arrow*), defined by Hounsfield units of 30 or less, is a vulnerable plaque feature. This finding is thought to represent the lipid rich/necrotic core of an advanced atheroma.

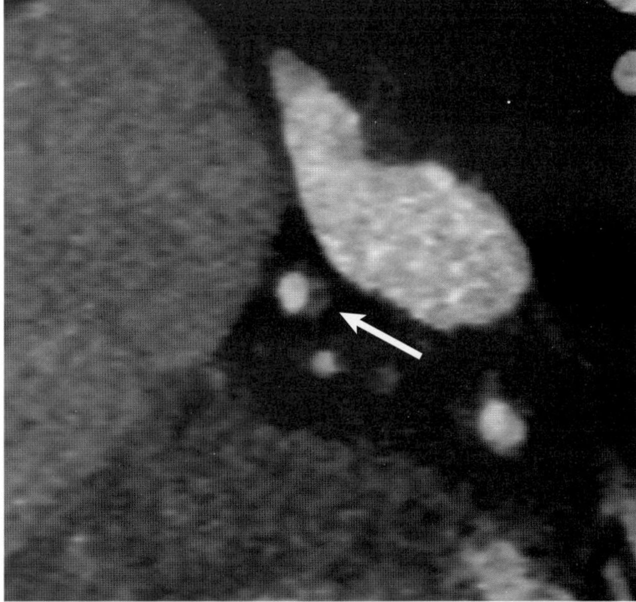

Figure 22.15 Napkin ring sign. The napkin ring sign (*arrows*) describes complex appearance of a plaque with hyperdense but noncalcified rim and lower attenuation center.

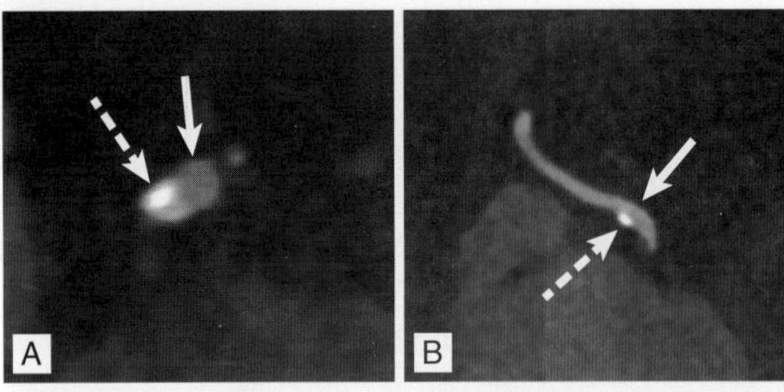

Figure 22.16 Positive remodeling. Positive remodeling refers to outward expansion of the growing atherosclerotic plaque (*dashed arrow*) that results in little luminal narrowing in the early stages (*arrow*), seen both on short axis image (A) and long axis (B) views. The lack of significant narrowing early on may result in its escape from clinical detection until the advanced stage.

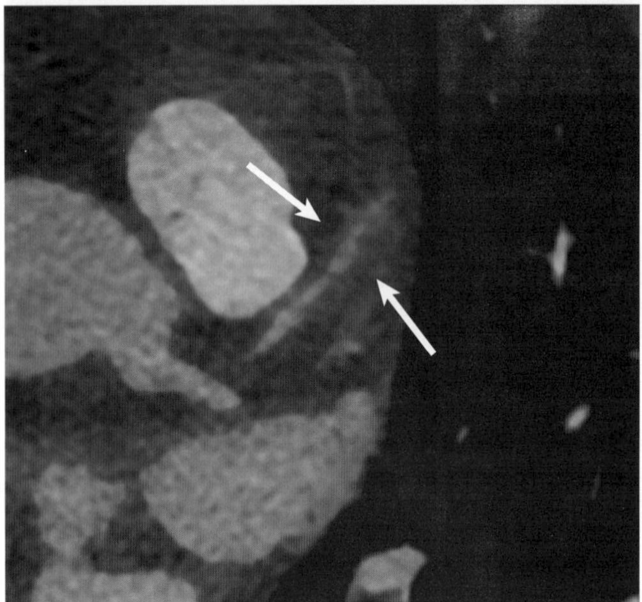

Figure 22.17 Perivascular soft tissue stranding. Perivascular fat stranding (*arrows*) describes dirty appearance of the epicardial fat surrounding the coronary lesion. This sign has been suggested to occur in culprit atherosclerotic or dissection lesions in acute coronary syndrome. Notice in this case the concurrent luminal narrowing and irregularity.

than luminal narrowing, positive remodeling is associated with more advanced, hence unstable, plaques [43]. In contrast, the outer boundary of the artery shrinks in negative remodeling, where a significant degree of narrowing can result with only modest amounts of plaque formation, leading to earlier onset of symptomatology

- Recently, perivascular epicardial fat stranding has been reported as a marker of acute plaque rupture and dissection (Fig. 22.17), a finding that may help localize the causative lesion [44]
- Last, extrinsic compression of the coronary arteries by other structures (such as enlarged pulmonary arteries) is an uncommon but easily evaluated pathology that warrants attention (Fig. 22.18)

CAD-RADS Reporting

In keeping with efforts of standardized reporting in other fields, Coronary Artery Disease Reporting and Data System (CAD-RADS) has been created to streamline CT angiographic findings of atherosclerotic disease and assist in result interpretation [45], Table 22.4. In CAD-RADS, coronary arteries and major branches greater than 1.5 mm in size are graded by stenosis severity, to include:

- No visible stenosis (0% narrowing, Fig. 22.19A)
- Minimal stenosis (1–24% narrowing, Fig. 22.19B)
- Mild stenosis (25–49% narrowing, Fig. 22.19C)
- Moderate stenosis (50–69% narrowing, Fig. 22.19D)
- Severe stenosis (70–99% narrowing, Fig. 22.19E)
- Occluded (100% narrowing, Fig. 22.19F)

The exception is made for the left main coronary artery, where 50–99% stenosis is considered severe. The overall CAD-RADS grade is determined by the highest degree of vessel stenosis, giving rise to CAD-RADS 0 through 5. To account for significant multivessel disease, CAD-RADS 4 is further divided into 4A for single or two vessel severe narrowing and 4B for three vessel disease or left main severe (>50%) disease. In patients presenting with acute or stable chest pain, the CAD-RADS grading is provided with standardized interpretation and management suggestions, which facilitate patient care.

In the case evaluation for any vessel is deemed nondiagnostic and no significant narrowing is found, a grading of N is given (CAD-RADS N). In a partially nondiagnostic exam where significant narrowing (>50%) is identified, the score is given with an additional N as a modifier (CAD-RADS #/N). The modifiers S (CAD-RADS #/S) and G (CAD-RADS #/G) are used to denote presence of stent and bypass graft, respectively. In-stent-restenosis (ISR) grading follows grading of native coronary arteries. Presence of vulnerable plaque (defined by two or more: low attenuation plaque, positive remodeling, spotty calcification, and "napkin ring sign") should be noted by the modifier V (CAD-RADS #/V). It is important to note that in the presence of a bypass graft, the bypassed proximal native artery segment no longer contributes to the CAD-RADS grading. The modifiers are used in the order of N, S, G, V, and separated by "/" symbol as dictated in the guideline. As an example,

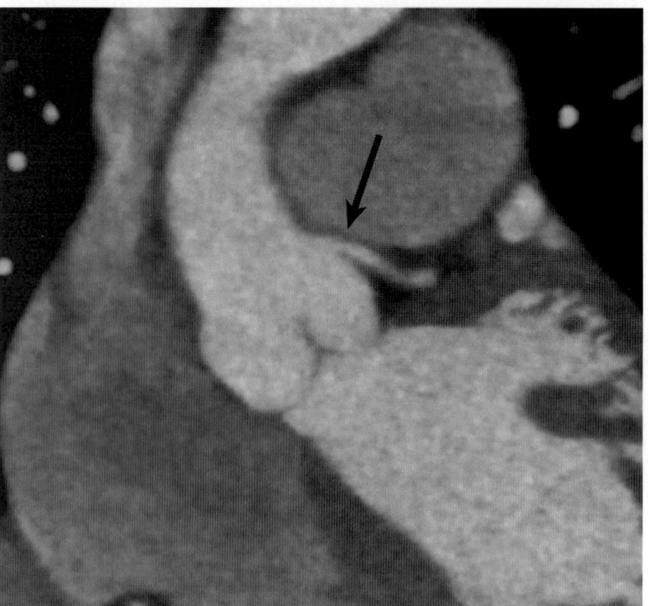

Figure 22.18 Extrinsic compression of the coronary artery. Infrequently, the coronary artery (*arrow*) may be extrinsically compressed by adjacent structures, such as the enlarged pulmonary artery in this case. Other causes of extrinsic compression may include paravalvular pseudoaneurysm, and mediastinal mass.

TABLE 22.4 CAD-RADS Grading Interpretation and Recommendations

	STABLE CHEST PAIN		ACUTE CHEST PAIN	
	Further Investigation	Management	Interpretation	Management
CAD-RADS 0 No plaque or stenosis	None	Nonatherosclerotic causes of chest pain	ACS highly unlikely	Nonatherosclerotic causes of chest pain
CAD-RADS 1 Minimal stenosis	None	Nonatherosclerotic causes of chest pain Preventative therapy	ACS highly unlikely	Nonatherosclerotic causes of chest pain Outpatient preventive therapy
CAD-RADS 2 Mild stenosis	None	Nonatherosclerotic causes of chest pain Preventative therapy	ACS unlikely	Nonatherosclerotic causes of chest pain Outpatient preventive therapy If high suspicion for ACS or high-risk plaque present, admission with cardiology consultation
CAD-RADS 3 Moderate stenosis	Functional assessment	Symptom-guided anti-ischemic and preventive pharmacotherapy	ACS possible	Admission with cardiology consultation, functional testing and/or ICA Anti-ischemic and preventive treatment
CAD-RADS 4 A: Severe stenosis B: Left main severe stenosis or 3 vessel obstructive disease	A: ICA or functional assessment B: ICA	Symptom-guided anti-ischemic and preventive pharmacotherapy	ACS likely	Admission with cardiology consultation, ICA and revascularization as appropriate Anti-ischemic and preventive treatment
CAD-RADS 5 Total occlusion	ICA and/or viability assessment	Symptom-guided anti-ischemic and preventive pharmacotherapy	ACS very likely	Expedited ICA and revascularization as appropriate Anti-ischemic and preventive treatment
CAD-RADS N Nondiagnostic	Additional or alternative evaluation	–	ACS not excluded	ICA and/or viability assessment

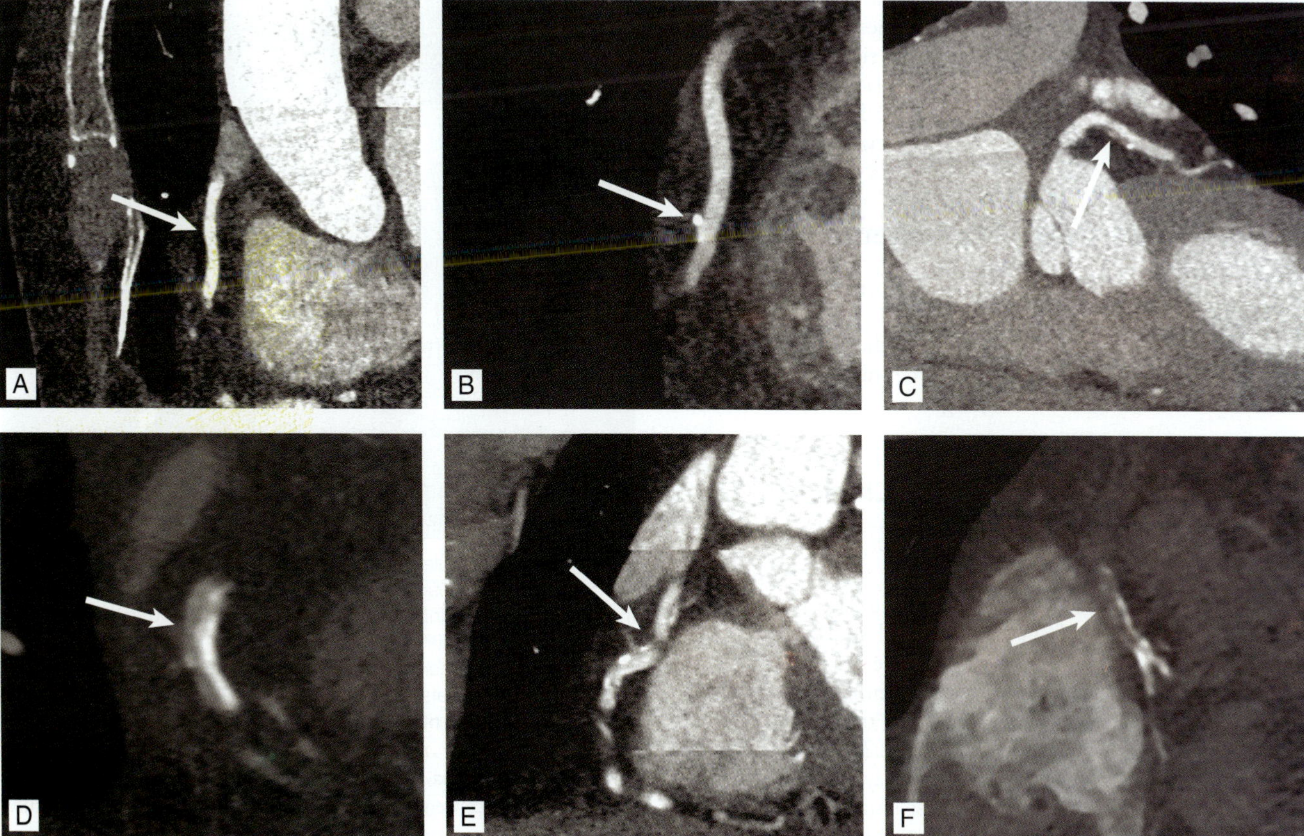

Figure 22.19 Coronary artery stenosis grading. In the CAD-RADS system, the coronary arteries are graded by extent of luminal narrowing into no significant narrowing (A), minimal/less than 25% narrowing (B), mild/25% to less than 50% narrowing (C), moderate/50% to less than 70% narrowing (D), severe/70% narrowing to subtotal occlusion (E), and total occlusion (F).

a patient with patent left internal mammary artery graft to the distal left anterior descending (LAD) artery, occluded proximal LAD artery, patent stent in the left circumflex artery, 60% narrowing in the proximal right coronary artery (RCA) with vulnerable plaque features, and nondiagnostic views of the distal RCA would be graded CAD-RADS 3/N/S/G/V. Last, it should be kept in mind that the CAD-RADS rating is developed for the assessment of coronary artery atherosclerosis and does not apply in other coronary artery pathology.

Triple Rule-Out

In a "triple rule-out" study, three potentially life-threatening conditions are assessed: acute coronary syndrome, acute aortic syndrome, and pulmonary embolism. The study is performed as an extended coronary CTA exam, starting with a noncontrast acquisition that serves as a calcium score study and helps to exclude intramural aortic hematoma. The field of view is extended to the aortic arch to include both the thoracic aorta in whole and the central pulmonary vasculature. Unlike a standard coronary CTA study, where the contrast is aimed at the systemic arterial vasculature, the contrast bolus is expanded to attain concurrent opacification of the pulmonary arterial vasculature. This goal is often achieved via adding approximately 30 cc of contrast volume. While this all-encompassing exam seems helpful in theory, these modifications have practical trade-offs that should be kept in mind. First, the extended field of view requires a longer breath hold, resulting in often motion degradation of the inferior heart with cranial-caudal scanning. With caudal-cranial scanning, the reversed scanning direction may result in inadequate opacification of the distal aorta or coronary arteries in addition to motion degradation of the aortic arch. The addition of extra contrast may preclude repeat scanning if daily allowance of contrast dose is not to be exceeded. The opacification of the right heart chambers also leads to impaired evaluation of intracardiac shunts. Therefore, in a patient with acute chest pain, ideally clinical evaluation narrows the differential to allow for a more dedicated exam.

Cardiac Manifestations of Ischemia

Equally important to evaluation of the coronary arteries is the assessment of the myocardium. Indeed, while the coronary arteries typically require dedicated study and technique to accurately examine, the myocardial changes can sometimes be seen on nondedicated studies as incidental findings.

Myocardial Perfusion and Acute Changes of Myocardial Ischemia

The regional decrease or cessation of coronary artery perfusion may be imagined with CT or MRI. Since coronary arteries penetrate and perfuse the myocardium from the epicardial surface inward, the subendocardial myocardium is most vulnerable and involved first in ischemia. On MRI, first pass perfusion identifies the perfusion defect as area of hypoenhancement involving the subendocardium with variable degree of transmurality (Fig. 22.20). On CT, similar detection of myocardial hypoenhancement may be sought in a CT perfusion study, albeit with lower contrast resolution and requirement for postprocessing for more consistent interpretation. Nonetheless, a relatively high sensitivity has been reported, documented at 90% in one series [46]. Accordingly, care should be exercised when a hypoattenuating area is seen on a contrasted CT exam, given

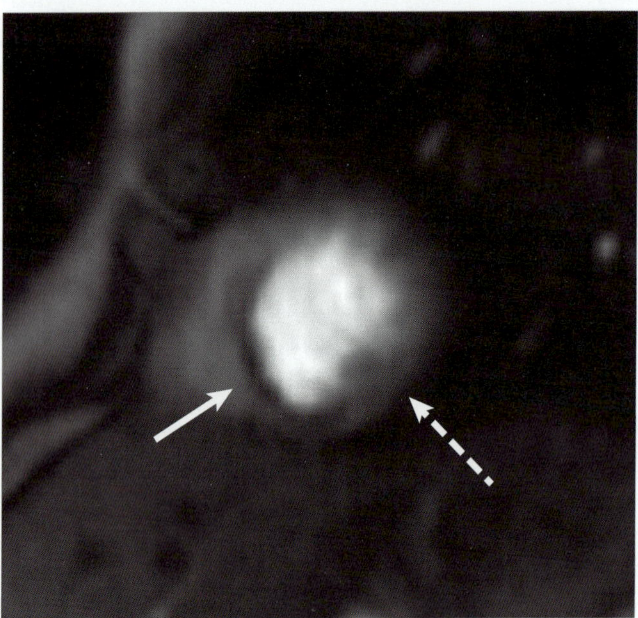

Figure 22.20 Perfusion defect on MRI. Myocardial perfusion can be assessed by examining the first pass enhancement, termed first pass perfusion. On this short axis image, there is hypoenhancement of the subendocardial inferior septal and inferior walls (*solid arrow*) compared with the normal homogeneous enhancement of the remaining walls (*dashed arrow*), consistent with a perfusion defect.

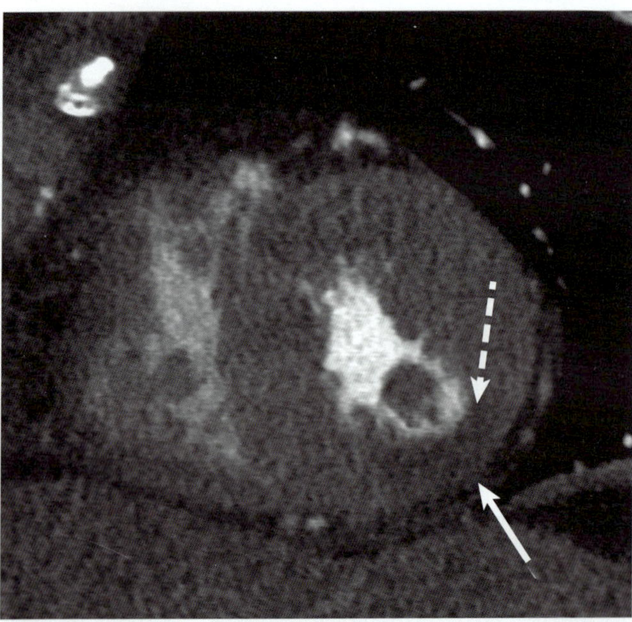

Figure 22.21 Ventricular wall thinning and hypoattenuation. On this short axis image through the mid-ventricular level, there is focal wall thinning involving the inferior and inferolateral wall (*solid arrow*), suggestive of prior myocardial infarction. Concurrent hypoattenuation of the subendocardial myocardium is seen (*dashed arrow*), which may be secondary to fatty metaplasia (intrinsic hypoattenuation) or hypoperfusion (hypoenhancement).

both fatty metaplasia from prior infarction and acute hypoperfusion/hypoenhancement can appear similar (Fig. 22.21). Thankfully, the clinical picture typically helps differentiate. When significant myocardial necrosis occurs with expansion of the extracellular volume, delayed contrast enhancement is seen in the acute setting before the onset of true scar formation. Myocardial edema as

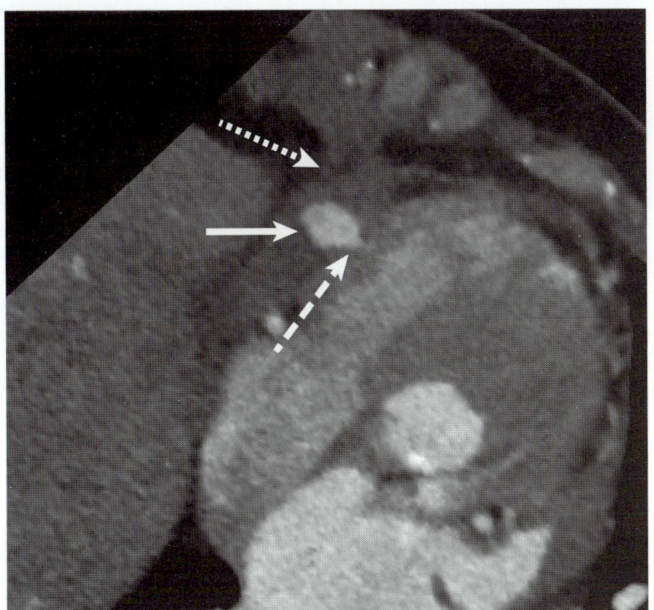

Figure 22.22 Ventricular pseudoaneurysm. On this oblique image of the right ventricle, there is focal outpouching seen arising from the free right ventricular wall (*solid arrow*). The narrow neck (*dashed arrow*, width of neck less than half of outpouching width) suggests this is a pseudoaneurysm. In the acute setting, surrounding inflammatory changes and/or hemorrhage (*dotted arrow*) is typically observed, giving evidence that a pseudoaneurysm is a contained rupture.

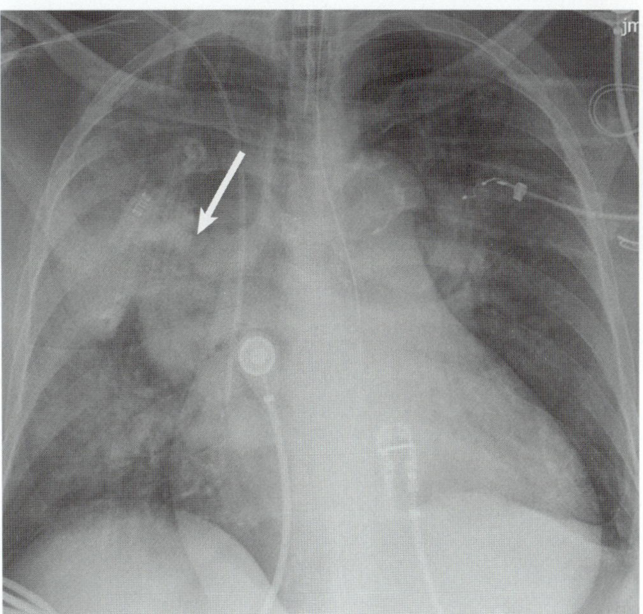

Figure 22.23 Acute mitral regurgitation. Acute mitral regurgitation is a potential complication of acute infarction that occurs when the infarction results in rupture of the papillary musculature. On radiograph, a focal opacity (*arrow*) may develop superimposed on findings of pulmonary edema due to poor cardiac function and vascular congestion.

revealed by T2 hyperintense signal alteration serves as an ancillary but nonspecific feature of acute myocardial ischemia and thus may be helpful. Lastly, focal wall motion abnormality accompanies many causes of myocardial injury, including ischemia. In cases where the other imaging findings are indeterminate or insufficiently clear, correlation with myocardial wall motion should always be considered.

Apart from acute heart failure that ensues if the infarction is sufficiently severe, a few additional complications should be kept in mind. First, the injured myocardium may rupture, typically occurring within the first 2 weeks of infarction. While frank rupture of the left ventricle is in general fatal and not imaged, contained rupture may be seen, termed a pseudoaneurysm. Held by pericardial tissue, the pseudoaneurysm is identified by disruption of the endomyocardial contour and outpouching with a narrow neck (Fig. 22.22), compared to the broader neck of a true aneurysm. Surrounding soft tissue stranding and/or hemorrhage will be present in the acute and subacute setting. Second, if the infarction involves the papillary musculature with rupture, acute valvular regurgitation may occur, typically within the first week of infarction. Acute mitral regurgitation may be seen as unifocal upper lobe pulmonary edema on radiograph (Fig. 22.23). This diagnosis should thus be considered when a focal opacity is found in a patient with clinical features of infarction and not infection. Last, in patients with recent infarction (typically within 2 months), there may be immune-mediated pericarditis with pericardial effusion (Dressler's syndrome). This possibility should be entertained when a patient with high-risk factors of myocardial infarction presents with apparent pericarditis of unclear etiology.

Chronic Findings of Myocardial Ischemia

Compared to acute changes of infarction, the chronic findings of myocardial ischemia are more often and perhaps easier seen. Following infarction of the myocardium when perfusion is not

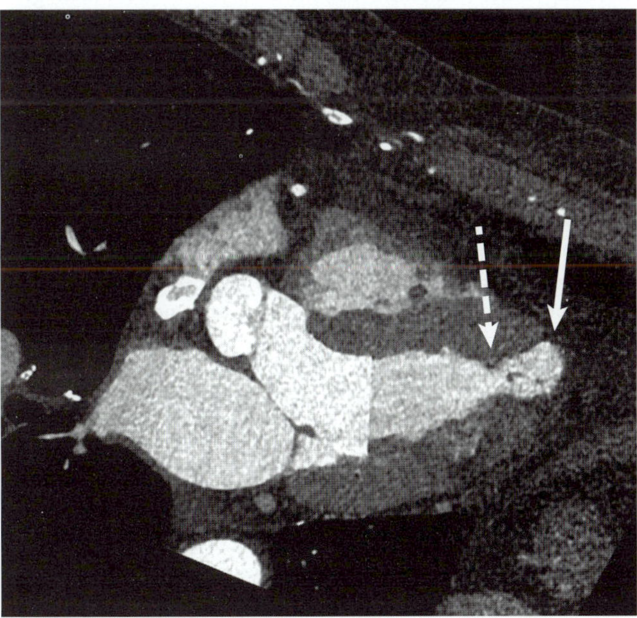

Figure 22.24 Ventricular aneurysm. On this three-chamber view, there is focal wall thinning and outpouching of the left ventricular apex (*solid arrow*). The relative broad neck of the outpouching (*dashed arrow*, width of neck greater than half of the aneurysm width) suggests this is an aneurysm.

re-established, permanent tissue loss results. This tissue loss manifests as wall thinning confined within a vascular territory on contrast CT, MRI, or echocardiography exam. This finding is most clearly evident on short axis images when there is well demarcated asymmetric thinning of the ventricular wall (Fig. 22.21). At times wall thinning may lead to stretching and outpouching, forming a ventricular aneurysm (Fig. 22.24). As aneurysms arise from

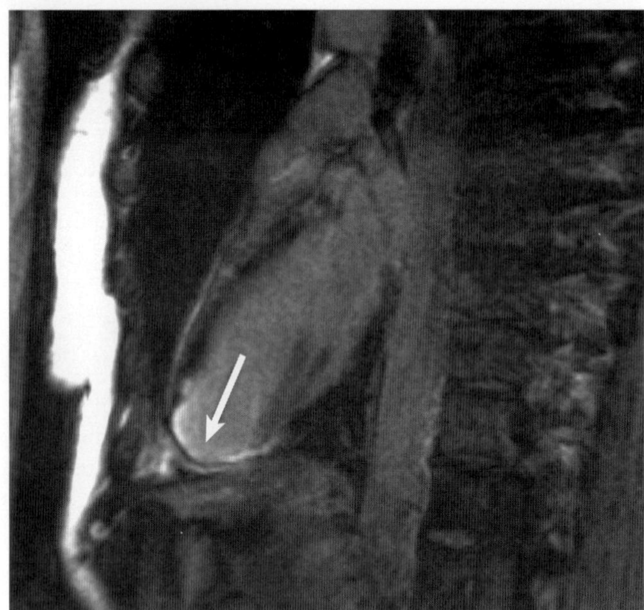

Figure 22.25 Late gadolinium enhancement and scar detection. On this two-chamber late gadolinium enhancement image, there is enhancement of the ventricular apex (*arrow*) extending to the apical anterior and apical inferior segments, consistent with scarring from prior infarction. Wall thinning and contour abnormality (aneurysm formation) are also noted.

stretching of the ventricular wall, the aneurysm neck is broad, generally measuring more than half of the sac width. On cine images, the aneurysm sac exhibits dyskinetic movement, indicating the regional wall force generation is insufficient to overcome the chamber pressure (the underlying reason for outpouching). This paradoxical movement differentiates it from anatomic variants ventricular crypt and diverticulum.

The infarcted tissue is replaced by fibrofatty scar. On MRI, myocardial scarring is best detected after contrast administration. The gadolinium contrast that diffuses into the expanded extracellular space containing the fibrotic changes is retained due to impaired resorption. Following washout of contrast from normal tissue, the area of fibrosis is prominently displayed on delayed phase images (late gadolinium enhancement, LGE, Fig. 22.25). A CT equivalent of delayed enhancement imaging has been used with some success ([47], Fig. 22.8) but is not currently in routine use. On noncontrast CT, the fibrofatty infiltration or fatty metaplasia is evidenced as curvilinear fat attenuation of the subendocardium (Fig. 22.3). This predilection for subendocardial tissue in myocardial ischemia helps distinguish it from other causes of myocardial fatty deposition. Occasionally dystrophic calcifications develop in the infarcted myocardial wall or the papillary musculature. However, myocardial calcification may occur from a host of other processes, such as hypercalcemia, senescence, or prior infection [48]. The lack of additional discriminating factors makes this finding nonspecific.

Viability Assessment by MRI

Viability, as defined by whether revascularization will improve ventricular systolic function, hinges on two conditions: the myocardium in question must be [1] alive and [2] dysfunctional due to ischemia. While the second criterion is typically established by the time revascularization is considered, MRI has emerged an excellent tool for the evaluation of the first criterion by virtue of LGE. As mentioned above, in either chronically scarred or acutely necrosed myocardium, LGE is seen and correlates with areas of infarcted cardiomyocytes that cannot be salvaged even if blood flow is re-established, previously validated in animal studies [49]. Most commonly in infarction, a small zone of myocardial necrosis is seen surrounded by a larger area of ischemic, injured, or at-risk tissue. Conceptually, the more injured but viable myocardium that is present, the higher potential for functional recovery. There is thus a need for quantification of necrosis extent. Transmurality has been in favor for use, reported as a percentage of myocardial thickness exhibiting LGE. Appropriately, studies suggest the lower extent of transmural LGE, the more favorable the functional outcome following reperfusion [50]. Nevertheless, two issues should be kept in mind. First, common with most quantitative measures, the exact threshold for determining viability is unclear. Because studies report that the proportion of patients that respond preferably drops significantly above 50% transmural involvement [50], 50% transmurality is considered as a reasonable cutoff. However, a decent number of patients over 50% transmural involvement improved still and labeling the group as "nonviable" may not be justified. Second, the transmural involvement is frequently not constant across the injured region. For example, the central region may demonstrate 75% transmural LGE while only 25% transmural LGE is seen in the more peripheral parts. Reporting a simple measure of 75% transmural LGE may thus be misleading. Instead, a description of overall ischemic involvement and estimated amount of viable myocardium is generally more helpful.

Coronary Artery Dissection

Coronary artery dissection is discussed here due to its close relationship with atherosclerosis and as an important alternate etiology of myocardial ischemia. Coronary dissection refers to separation of the coronary artery wall with or without intimal tear that may lead to narrowing of the arterial lumen. The dissection may be primary when it takes origin from within the coronary system or secondary when the dissection forms as a result of extrinsic injury (most commonly iatrogenic from catheterization) or as an extension of aortic dissection. When primary, coronary artery dissection may be a result of atherosclerosis, likely representing complications of plaque ulceration. In the remaining cases (termed spontaneous coronary artery dissection, SCAD), multiple causes are recognized, including emotional stress, vasospasm, neurohormonal dysregulation, inflammation, connective tissue abnormality/arteriopathy, genetic factors, and mechanical compression. *As such, three typically younger patient populations appear particularly vulnerable: those in the peripartum period, those who recently performed high intensity exercise, and those with fibromuscular dysplasia.*

Because findings of coronary artery dissection on imaging can be subtle, appropriate clinical history is critical to make the correct diagnosis. Two manifestations of coronary dissection may be seen on imaging:

- In some, a dissection flap analogous to the classical appearance of dissection seen in other vascular territories is identified, the intimal tear type (Fig. 22.26). This finding is more readily made but not frequently seen
- More commonly, an abrupt caliber change (Fig. 22.27) or apparent focal occlusion (Fig. 22.28) is visualized, corresponding to the intramural hematoma type, where there is no contrast opacification of the false lumen. This finding may appear identical to atherosclerosis in some cases. Lack of adjacent atherosclerotic changes, nonatherosclerotic appearance of the

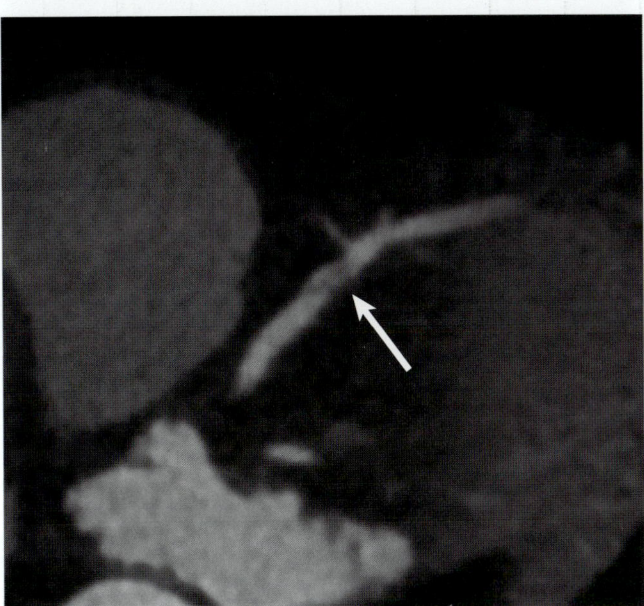

Figure 22.26 Intimal tear type of coronary artery dissection. Compared to dissection occurring elsewhere in the body, an artery dissection flap (*arrow*) is only rarely seen in the coronary arteries due to the small size of the arteries and spatial resolution of CT.

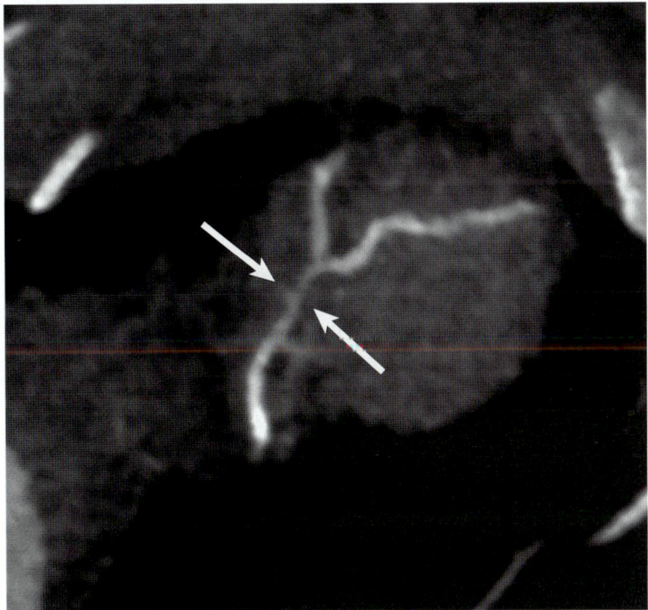

Figure 22.27 Intramural hematoma type coronary artery dissection—caliber change. Most often, coronary artery dissection appears as focal caliber change (*arrow*) or focal occlusion on CT. This appearance is often difficult to distinguish from atherosclerotic narrowing saved for appropriate clinical history/demographic and lack of identified plaque locally or disease elsewhere.

other coronary arteries, and appropriate clinical history are paramount in making the diagnosis

The LAD artery territory is thought to be most frequently involved in SCAD, seen in up to 71% of the cases [51]. However, it should be noted that coronary artery dissection is believed to be underdiagnosed [52], making true distribution difficult to report.

A few pitfalls should be kept in mind.

- Avoid misidentification of calcified portion of a mixed density plaque as contrast, as this may lead to a misdiagnosis of double

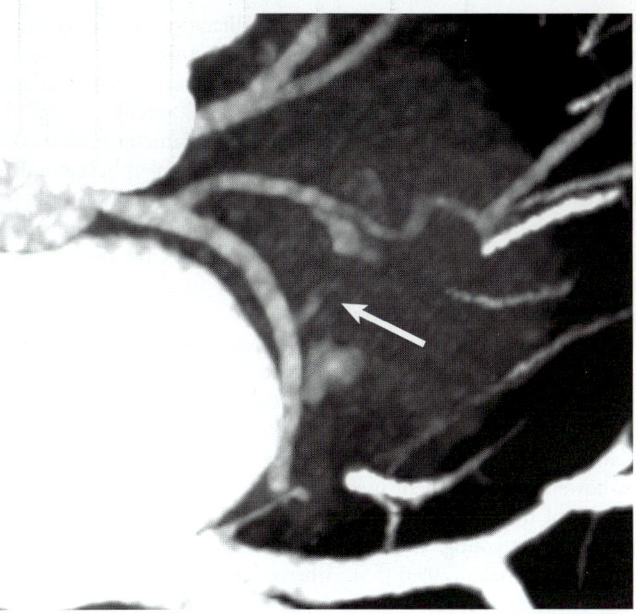

Figure 22.28 Intramural hematoma type coronary artery dissection—focal occlusion. Here focal occlusion (*arrow*) is seen as a result of coronary artery dissection. This finding may be difficult to distinguish from plaque rupture and focal thrombosis.

lumen/dissection. Apparent dissection should be examined on the noncontrast portion of the exam for calcifications
- Avoid mislabeling of artifact within the arterial lumen as a dissection flap. This pitfall may be safeguarded by ensuring the abnormality in question is seen on more than one phase of the image set
- Identification of one dissection site warrants a close inspection for a second, as up to a quarter of the patients may have multivessel SCAD [51]
- When short segment caliber change is seen, the coronary artery should be examined in relation to the myocardium to avoid misdiagnosis of myocardial bridging as dissection

It should be noted that in patients with SCAD, catheter angiography carries increased risk of dissection propagation [53]. Therefore, recommendation of catheter angiography should not be routinely made in patients with suspected coronary dissection on CT. If artifact and dissection cannot be readily differentiated initially, a tailored repeat coronary CT scan may be helpful. Because coronary artery dissection may occur in small and distal arteries and the resolution of a CT scan is limited, a negative coronary CT does not exclude its presence.

In the initial period, up to 14% of the patients with SCAD require urgent revascularization [52]. Major adverse cardiac events are reported in up to 30% within the first 3 years and estimated at 50% in 10 years. Ten-year recurrence rate for SCAD is estimated at 29% [51]. In patients where a predisposing factor is not identified, evaluation of the systemic vasculature for underlying arteriopathy should be considered.

Coronary Artery Ectasia, Aneurysm, and Pseudoaneurysm

Ectasia and aneurysm are uncommon phenomena of the coronary arteries that belong to a spectrum of the same disease. In either case, there is arterial dilatation that exceeds 50% of normal (150% baseline size). The term aneurysm is suggested when the length of the involved segment is under 50% of the total vessel length, whereas ectasia refers to diffuse dilatation involving more than 50% of the total vessel length [54]. Aneurysm is further characterized as fusiform if the transverse diameter of the dilatation is smaller than the length of involvement. Saccular morphology refers to aneurysm where the transverse diameter exceeds the length of involvement. The term "giant aneurysm" is best avoided due to lack of universally agreed definition. Seemingly simplistic in definition, description of dilatation in practice may be sometimes difficult as the baseline normal vessel size is not always clear, especially in the case of ectasia. Further, focal aneurysm may occur in an otherwise ectatic vessel.

Three etiologies of coronary artery dilatations are responsible for the majority of the coronary artery dilatations: atherosclerosis, Kawasaki disease, and vascular shunting. The classic teaching prescribes atherosclerosis as the most common cause in the Western countries and Kawasaki disease as the primary etiology in the East. This distinction is, however, of infrequent usefulness as atherosclerosis is generally a disease of mid to late adulthood whereas Kawasaki disease affects primarily the young. Overall, coronary artery dilatations are more common in males (79%) [55]. Atherosclerosis-associated dilatation may manifest as ectasia or aneurysm with aneurysm being more common distal to focal narrowing, likely in similar mechanism to poststenotic dilatation (Fig. 22.29). In a study of 978 patients with coronary dilatation, 888 patients had >70% stenosis [56]. Kawasaki disease is classically aneurysmal (Fig. 22.30) compared to other vasculitis, in which ectasia is more common. Congenital disease and shunting constitute the last major cause and must be considered when the dilatation is diffuse and smooth in morphology (Fig. 22.31). Notably, conditions included in this category include coronary-pulmonary fistula, coronary-cameral fistula, and anomalous coronary artery arising from pulmonary artery, as well as extensive collateralization that occurs as result of proximal vessel occlusion. Other rarer causes include connective tissue disorder and other inflammatory diseases.

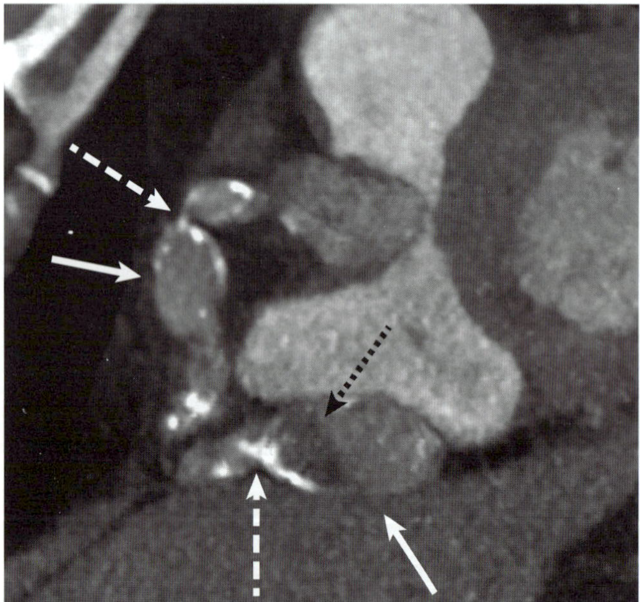

Figure 22.29 Coronary artery aneurysm in atherosclerosis. Coronary artery aneurysms may be the result of advanced atherosclerosis. In this case, fusiform aneurysms (*arrows*) are seen distal to foci of severe narrowing (*dashed arrows*). The arteries are typically diffusely diseased. Note presence of luminal thrombus (*dotted arrow*) within the inferior aneurysm, a common finding.

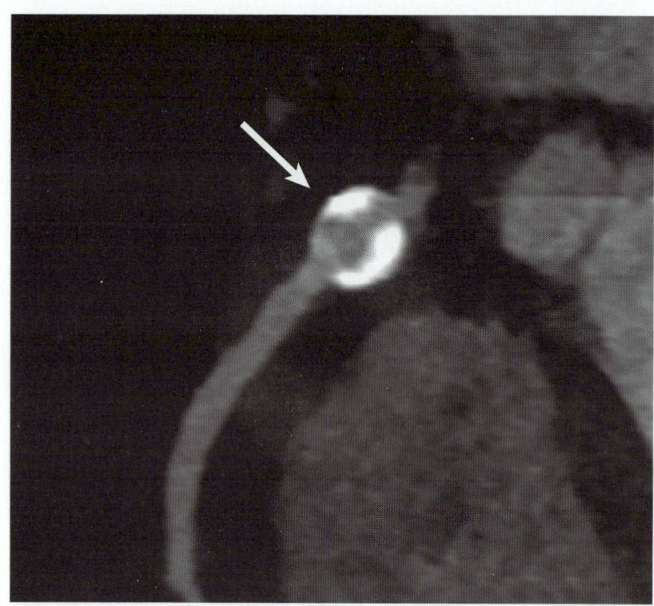

Figure 22.30 Coronary artery aneurysm in Kawasaki disease. In Kawasaki disease, the aneurysm (*arrow*) is typically seen without the background of diffuse atherosclerosis. Single or multiple aneurysms may be seen. The age of presentation is an additional important factor to consider.

The differentiation of pseudoaneurysm from aneurysm is a pathologic one. An aneurysm is contained by three-layer vessel wall, whereas the tunica intima and media of a pseudoaneurysm are ruptured or incomplete. This distinction on imaging is often difficult and more readily suggested by etiology. Coronary artery dilatations in the setting of traumatic injury, following catheter-based interventions, infection, and drug use (notably cocaine) are most commonly pseudoaneurysms (Fig. 22.32), as the intima and media are rarely intact in acute dilatation. Nonetheless, any true aneurysm that enlarges sufficiently may rupture and, when contained, become a pseudoaneurysm. Perivascular soft tissue stranding/inflammation and associated fluid collection are rarely seen with uncomplicated aneurysm and suggestive of pseudoaneurysm formation.

In addition to the dilatation, important features to identify in imaging include presence or absence of luminal thrombus (Fig. 22.29), which is reported in up to 67% of the aneurysms in

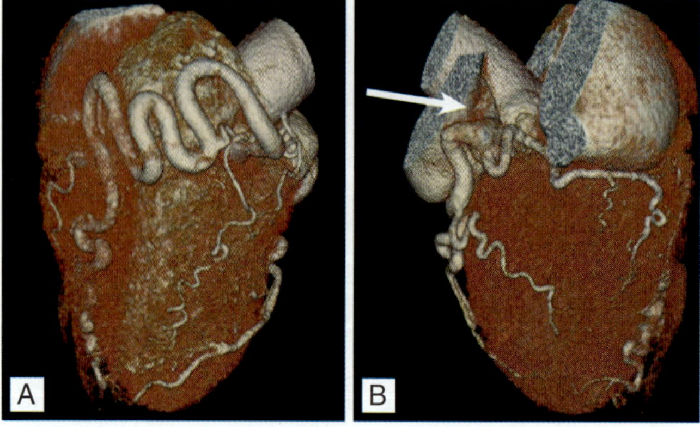

Figure 22.31 Coronary artery ectasia in congenital heart disease. If identified, coronary artery ectasia should prompt consideration of vascular shunting or anomalous vascular connection. In this case, ectasia of both the right coronary artery (A) and left coronary arteries (B) is shown in a patient with anomalous left coronary artery from the pulmonary artery (*arrow*, ALCAPA, Bland–White–Garland syndrome).

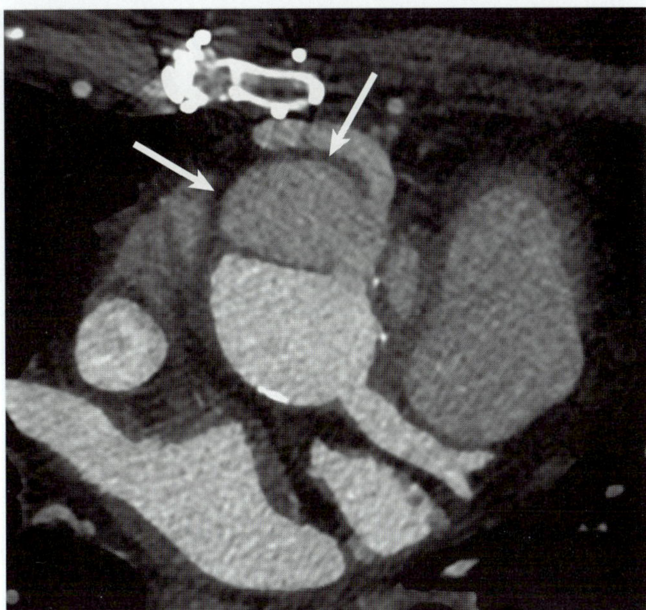

Figure 22.32 Coronary artery pseudoaneurysm. Coronary artery pseudoaneurysms may be difficult to differentiate from aneurysms. Most commonly, the etiology of the finding helps to discriminate, with pseudoaneurysms being more commonly the result of trauma (accidental or iatrogenic) or infection. The acute onset, surrounding soft tissue stranding, and wall irregularity can provide additional clue. In this case, a pseudoaneurysm (*arrows*) is seen arising from the proximal right coronary artery that is the result of recent intervention.

a small series [57]. To avoid confusing uneven contrast opacification with luminal thrombus, delayed phase images are helpful. The location of the aneurysm should be discussed in conjunction with distance of the aneurysm sac to the artery ostium or large branch vessel and presence of proximal narrowing in anticipation for possible catheter-based intervention. Attention needs to be paid to look for focal outer wall irregularity, which may hint to impending rupture/pseudoaneurysm formation. Similarly, any fat stranding around the dilated vessel should be viewed with suspicion. Comparison to prior studies is essential. It is worth noting that Kawasaki disease and dilatation secondary to shunting may regress with appropriate treatment.

The prognosis of patients with coronary artery dilatation is dependent on the etiology. In the largest international registry to date with 1565 patients and a median follow-up of 37 months, 31% of patients with coronary artery aneurysms displayed a major cardiovascular event and 15% died [55]. However, this poor prognosis may reflect the underlying atherosclerotic disease burden and not additional risk conferred by presence of aneurysm per se. In Kawasaki disease, the size and location of the aneurysm may be used for risk stratification [58]. Prognosis of patients with coronary ectasia due to vascular shunting is favorable barring underlying complex pathology [59]. The natural history in other vasculitis and connective tissue disorders is not well established due to their rarity. Mycotic and drug use-related pseudoaneurysms have a higher chance for complications and should be closely monitored, especially in the acute period.

Myocardial Bridging

Myocardial bridging is discussed here due to its effects on coronary artery atherosclerosis. Myocardial bridging refers to anomalous course of the coronary artery through the myocardium instead of the normal epicardial space, also termed intramyocardial, intramural, or intramuscular coronary artery. This congenital anomaly is common, estimated at roughly 40% in frequency by both autopsy and CT series, although a wide range of values has been reported [60]. The mid segment of the LAD artery is the most common site, followed by its distal segment. The intramyocardial segment (termed tunneled segment) may be of varying length and depth. The overlying myocardium (termed myocardial bridge) may provide a complete or partial covering.

Clinical Significance

The clinical significance of myocardial bridging is debated. Earlier reports suggest an association of myocardial bridging with various cardiac complications such as arrhythmia, angina, myocardial infarction, and sudden cardiac death. However, its high prevalence on later studies has led others to consider it as a benign anatomic variant. This view is perhaps supported by the classic teaching that coronary perfusion occurs in diastole, but compression of the tunneled artery is mainly a systolic phenomenon. Nevertheless, a recent meta-analysis inclusive of 21 prior studies finds that myocardial bridging is in fact associated with myocardial ischemia and major adverse cardiac events [61]. Together, these findings suggest that there is likely only a small subpopulation of the patients in which this common finding has pathologic consequences. The morphology and degree of narrowing are presumed influencing factors. However, there is currently no consensus on what constitutes pathologic bridging.

Pathology

The pathology of myocardial bridging is now believed to extend beyond systolic artery compression [62]. In some patients, the arterial compression persists into early diastole, shortening the perfusion window. Moreover, the early diastolic relaxation and dilatation generate transient negative pressure and a "sucking phenomenon" that disrupts normal coronary blood flow [63]. The hemodynamic alterations are likely further compounded by the angulation of the tunneling and resurfacing vessel. The locoregional endothelial function of the tunneled segment is impaired [64], predisposing to vasospasm [65]. Not surprisingly, the degree of narrowing and duration of compression are dependent on cardiac effort. In some cases, the associated flow dysregulation is evident only under exercise or pharmacologic stress.

An important consequence to the altered physiology is that myocardial bridging predisposes the coronary artery segment proximal to the bridge to atherosclerosis but spares the tunneled and more distal segments. The atherosclerotic changes may be seen earlier in life than normally expected and contribute to the association to myocardial ischemia. This accelerated atherosclerosis is typical at the junction of the proximal and mid segments of the LAD, given the mid segment is the most common location of myocardial bridging and bifurcation points are already susceptible to the development of atherosclerosis. Systolic narrowing or compression of the tunneled segment is thought to protect against lipid and infiltrate deposition and should not be mistaken for atherosclerotic narrowing. In young patients where no other etiology for myocardial ischemia is identified, myocardial bridging may warrant consideration particularly if the tunneled segment is long and deep. In patients where coronary artery bypass grafts are planned, myocardial bridging should be mentioned to reduce the possibility of intraoperative confusion.

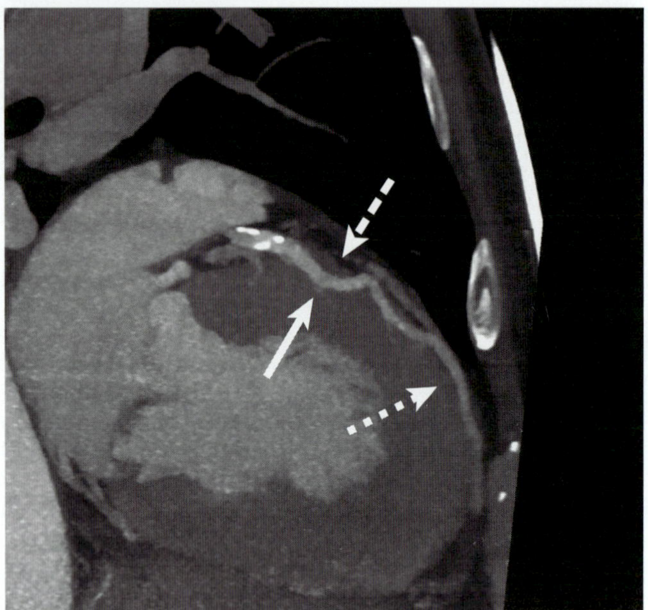

Figure 22.33 Myocardial bridging with proximal atherosclerosis. In myocardial bridging, the coronary artery dives into the myocardium for a distance before re-emergence. Note the tunneled segment (*arrow*) underlying the outer myocardial wall (*dashed arrow*) and the normal epicardial position of the artery (*dotted arrow*). While the tunneled segment is thought to be protected against atherosclerosis, the segment proximal to the myocardial bridge is at an increased risk, as in this case.

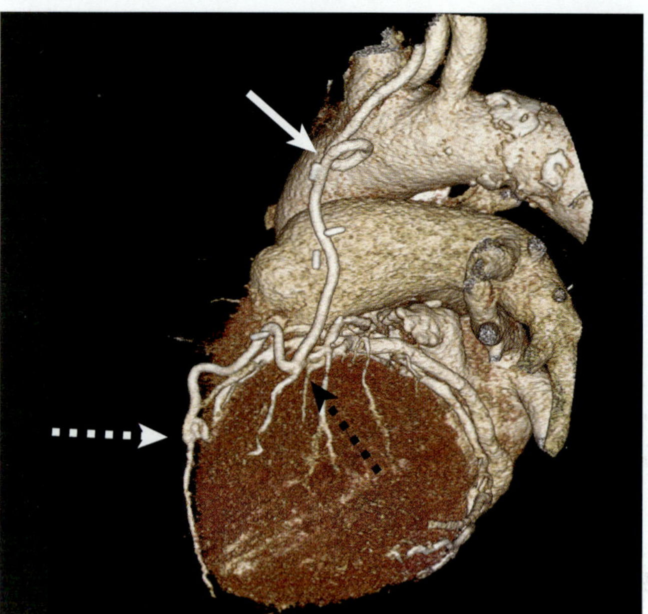

Figure 22.34 Sequential coronary artery bypass graft. In a sequential or "jumped" graft, a single bypass artery is used to provide blood flow to two diseased arteries. Here, a left internal mammary artery bypass graft (*solid arrow*) is seen anastomosing to both the first diagonal artery (*dashed arrow*) and the mid-distal left anterior descending artery (*dotted arrow*).

Imaging

Contrast-enhanced coronary CTA has high sensitivity in detection of myocardial bridging. On CT, myocardial bridging is best shown on MPRs and MIP images, where the traversing artery can be clearly viewed in relation to the myocardium and epicardial fat (Fig. 22.33). As mentioned, close attention should be paid to the artery segment proximal to the bridge for atherosclerotic narrowing. The inability to assess physiology is a weakness of CT, and suspected cases of pathologic bridging typically undergo physiologic testing. It should also be noted that measurement of artery compression/narrowing extent is best avoided on CT due to spatial resolution limitation, image noise (especially when ECG dose modulation/pulsing is used), and common use of beta-adrenergic blockade in heart rate control that may lessen the compression. The inability to visualize extraluminal structures makes catheter angiography less sensitive in the detection of myocardial bridging. Instead, the dynamic change in caliber of the vessel ("milking effect") and in course/angulation of the tunneling and resurfacing segments ("step down–step up phenomenon") are examined.

Coronary Artery Intervention

Upon identification of coronary artery atherosclerosis, therapeutic options consist of (a) medical therapy that aim at symptomatic control and halting or even reversing plaque progression and (b) revascularization via percutaneous coronary intervention (PCI) or coronary artery bypass grafting (CABG). Here, we describe the postprocedural appearance of the coronary system that may be encountered.

Coronary Artery Bypass Grafts

Types of Bypass Grafts: In CABG, revascularization is achieved by creation of collateral supply using either a venous or an arterial conduit. In venous bypass, a segment of the saphenous vein is harvested from the lower extremity. This venous segment is then reversed in direction or valvectomized and used to connect the ascending aorta to the obstructed coronary artery. Radio-opaque graft anastomosis markers are sometimes placed to help identify the bypass graft ostia on follow-up. In arterial bypass, the arterial segment may be either used as an in situ graft or a free graft. In an in situ graft, a noncoronary artery near the heart is mobilized without disruption of its origin and anastomosed to the diseased artery. Most commonly, the left internal mammary artery (internal thoracic artery) is used due to its normal course in close proximity to the anterior cardiac wall. The right internal mammary artery may be used in the same fashion, although more often anastomosing to the RCA or inferior aspect of the heart. Very rarely, the right gastroepiploic artery or the inferior epigastric artery are utilized. In a free graft, the arterial segment (most commonly the radial artery, although internal mammary arteries are also used in decent frequency) is transplanted to create the aortocoronary connection. Occasionally, a single graft is used for reperfusion of two native arteries in a "jumped" or sequential graft by a mid-graft side-to-side anastomosis and an end-graft end-to-side anastomosis (Fig. 22.34).

Imaging: On radiographs, radio-opaque markers provide easy clue to prior CABG if present (Fig. 22.35). Surgical clips from internal mammary artery harvest are sometimes visible. However, changes of sternotomy may be the only provided sign. On CT, internal mammary grafts can be identified by examining the expected course of the arteries, where the mobilized artery is seen displaced posteriorly (Fig. 22.36). Venous grafts and free arterial grafts are seen as anomalous vessels arising from the ascending aorta if patent (Fig. 22.37). If occluded, focal outpouching/irregularity of the ascending aorta is suggestive of the remnant anastomotic ostium (Fig. 22.38). Care needs to be paid to safeguard against mistaking the cannulation site used for cardiopulmonary bypass for an occluded graft by searching for the

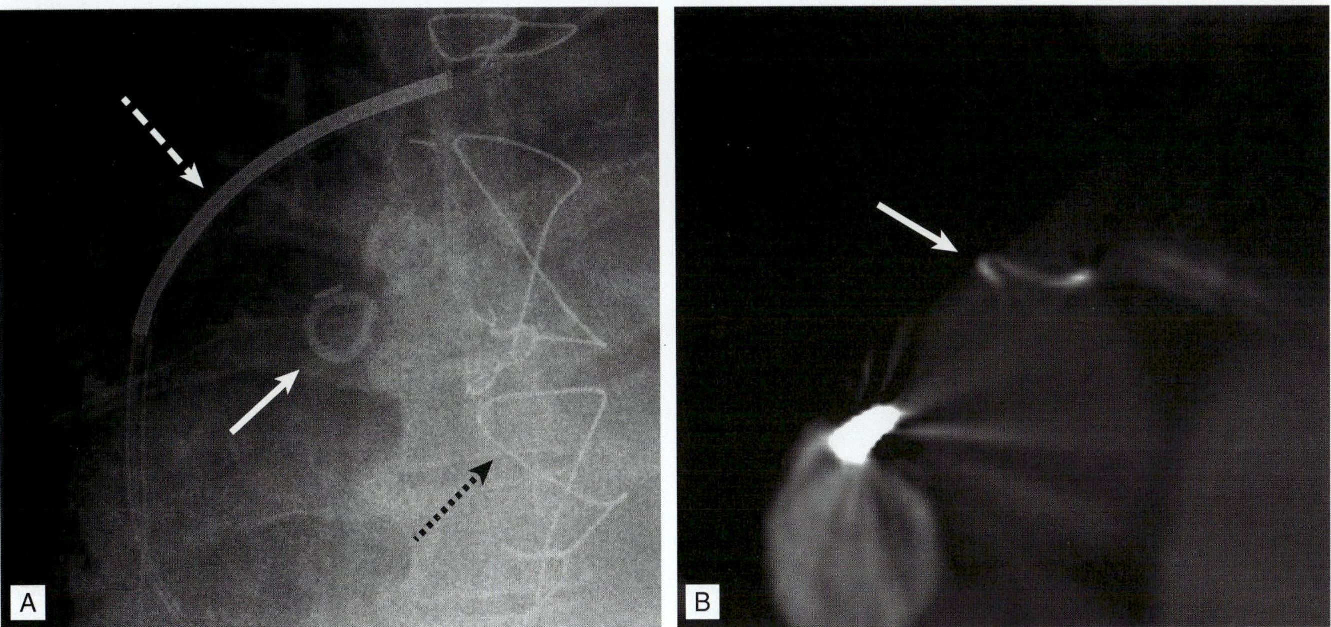

Figure 22.35 Coronary bypass graft anastomosis markers. On radiograph (A), changes of prior coronary artery bypass grafting may be identified by the presence of radio-opaque anastomosis markers (*arrow*). Sternotomy wires (*dotted arrow*) and pacer/ICD leads (*dashed arrow*) are partially seen. On CT (B), the radio-opaque marker is identified on the anterior aspect of the ascending aorta (*arrow*). Note that several markers are in use with variable appearance. Occasionally, the ostia may be marked impromptu using surgical wires.

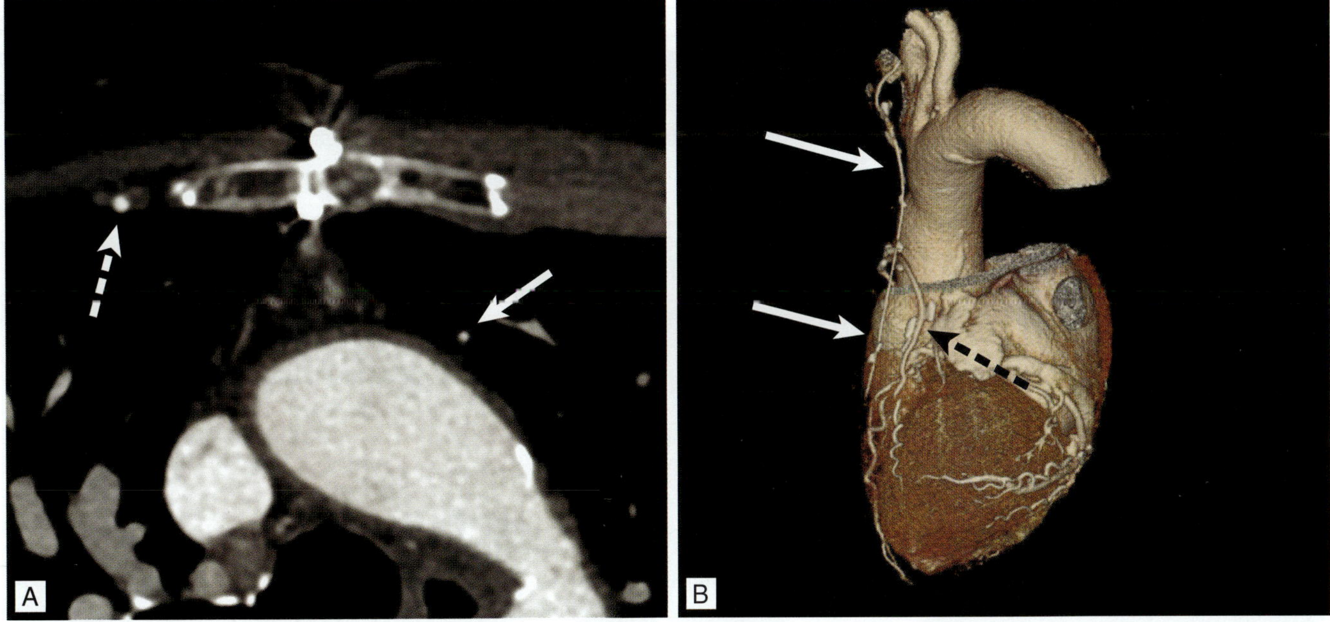

Figure 22.36 Arterial in situ coronary bypass graft. On CT (A), in situ arterial coronary bypass grafts are easily identified by the abnormal positioning of the redirected internal mammary artery (*arrow*), which can be followed to the coronary anastomosis. Note the normal positioning of the internal mammary artery on the contralateral side (*dashed arrow*). Corresponding volumetric rendering (B) shows the typical course of the left internal mammary graft (*arrow*). Also note a partially seen venous bypass graft (*dashed arrow*).

hyperdense felt pledget on noncontrast images (Fig. 22.39). In addition to luminal narrowing and occlusion, the grafts should be evaluated for malpositioning and kinking (Fig. 22.40).

Similar to the native coronary arteries, the bypass grafts are examined for narrowing and occlusion in their entirety. In the case of in situ internal mammary artery grafts, the field of view is extended to the clavicular heads to ensure adequate coverage of the artery origin (Fig. 22.41). *Three etiologies of graft stenosis and occlusion include graft thrombosis, neointimal hyperplasia, and atherosclerosis.* Similar in appearance, these complications are best distinguished by differences in time course of their occurrence. Graft thrombosis is an acute complication of bypass surgery that occurs predominantly within the first month postsurgery. Neointimal hyperplasia is a result of smooth muscle proliferation and extracellular matrix deposition that occurs within the first year. Atherosclerosis,

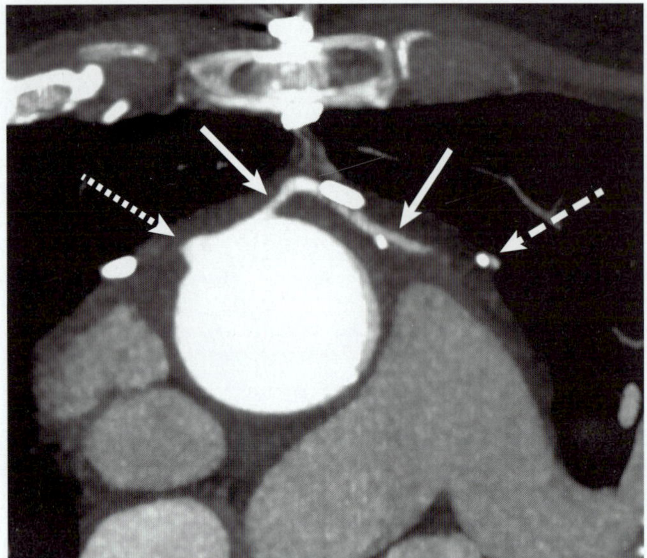

Figure 22.37 Patent venous coronary bypass graft. In a venous coronary bypass grafts (and free arterial bypass grafts, which have a very similar appearance), the aortic anastomosis is typically identified in the anterior aspect of the ascending aorta instead of the sinuses of Valsalva. Inevitably, the graft displays a course in the prevascular space (*arrows*), where it can be identified. Note a concurrent in situ left internal mammary bypass graft (*dashed arrow*) as well as focal irregularity of the right anterolateral ascending aorta (*dotted arrow*), representing a partially visualized ostium of an additional bypass graft.

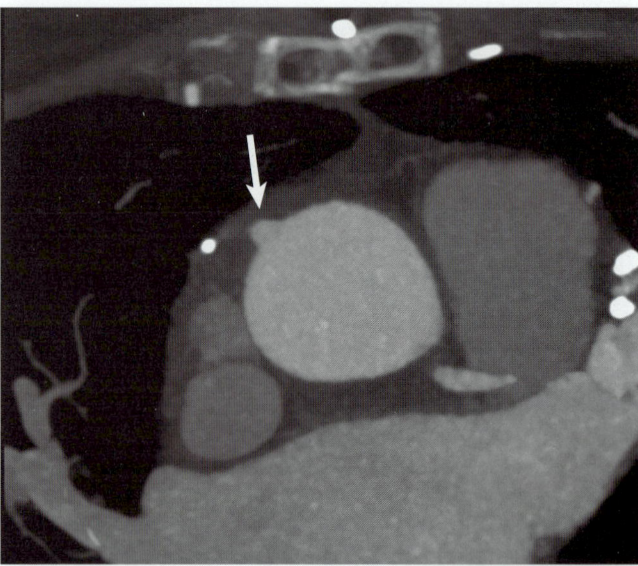

Figure 22.38 Occluded venous coronary bypass graft. When occluded, venous and free arterial bypass grafts can be difficult to identify. In some cases, the graft occludes just distal to the ostium, facilitating its detection (*arrow*). Surgical clips around the course of the bypass graft may also provide a clue. The area should be evaluated on noncontrast images as to not misidentify prior aortic cannulation site as patent ostium of an occluded graft.

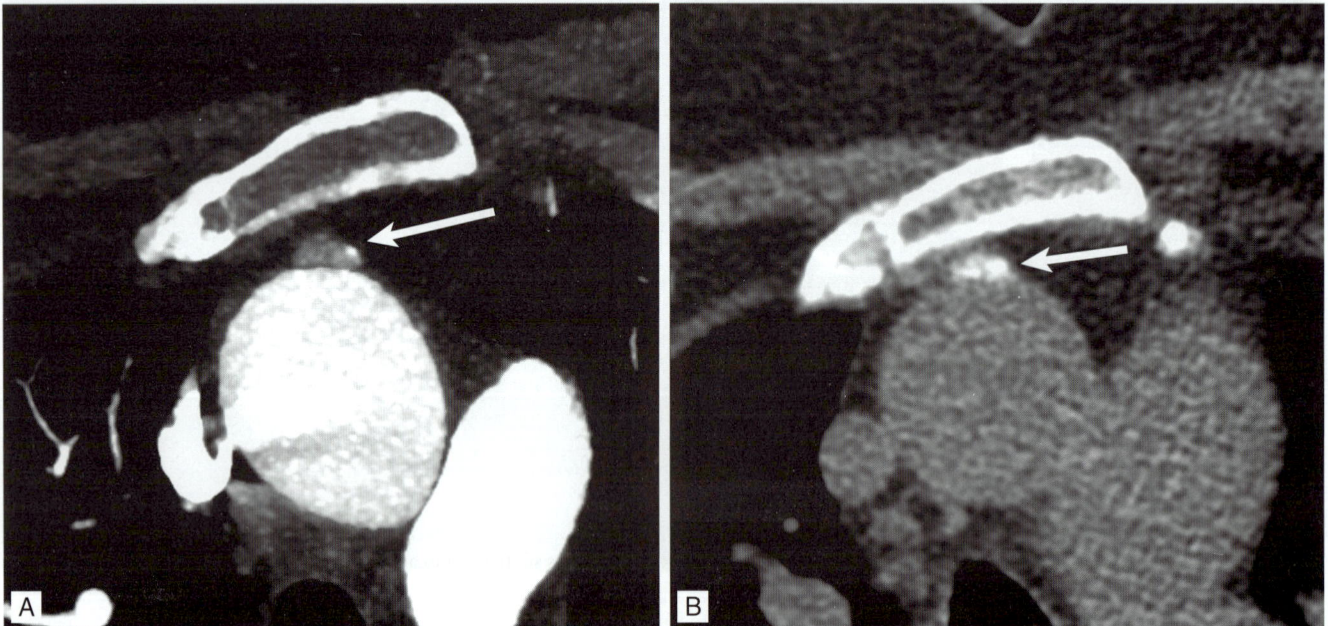

Figure 22.39 Cardiopulmonary bypass cannulation site. In patients who underwent prior cardiopulmonary bypass, the aortic cannulation site is most often closed and reinforced with hyperdense felt pledgets (*arrow*), which may be mistaken for pseudoaneurysm or ostium of an occluded graft on contrast-enhanced images (A). Examining area on noncontrast images (B) helps correctly identify as neither pseudoaneurysm nor ostium should appear hyperdense before contrast administration.

although may initiate early, is typically not sufficiently visualized or obstructive until after the first year. Also similar to native coronary arteries, the bypass grafts may develop aneurysm and pseudoaneurysm. Pseudoaneurysm is generally considered a surgical complication that is seen in the acute period. Akin to that of native coronary artery, a graft aneurysm is a result of atherosclerosis, a late complication.

Percutaneous Coronary Intervention

In PCI, the diseased arterial segment is accessed via a transcatheter approach. The stenosis or occlusion is crossed and balloon angioplasty performed to re-establish blood flow. Because prior clinical trials have demonstrated improved clinical and angiographic outcome by the addition of stents [66], coronary stents are now deployed as standard of care.

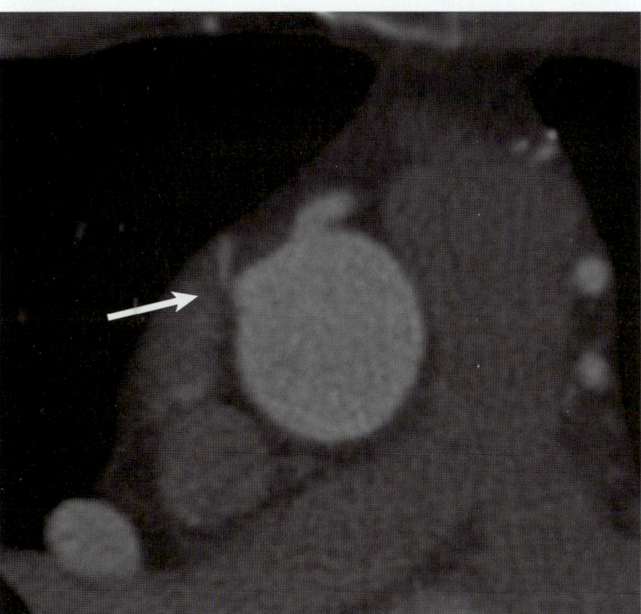

Figure 22.40 Focal coronary artery bypass graft kinking. Occasionally, focal kinking of the arterial bypass graft results in hemodynamically significant narrowing. Here, there is subtotal occlusion of a venous bypass graft (*arrow*) as a result of focal kinking.

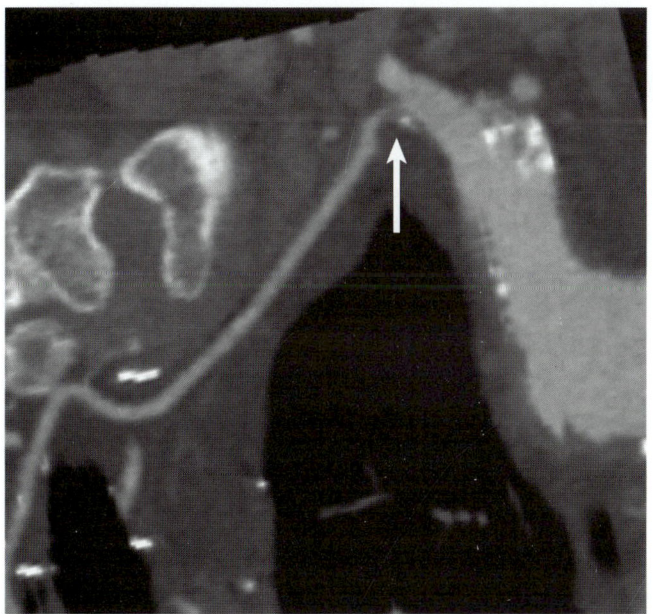

Figure 22.41 Origin of the internal mammary artery graft. In the evaluation of coronary bypass grafts, the field of view should be extended to the level of the clavicular heads in the case of an in situ internal mammary graft. Here, focal severe narrowing of the left internal mammary artery origin is seen (*arrow*) secondary to atherosclerotic changes.

In-Stent-Restenosis

On imaging, coronary artery stents appear as hyperdense geometric structures, which may be easily mistaken for coronary artery calcifications (Fig. 22.6). Appropriate clinical history is key to its identification. ISR represents a feared complication that results from either thrombus organization or neointimal proliferation and subsequent narrowing or occlusion of the stent lumen

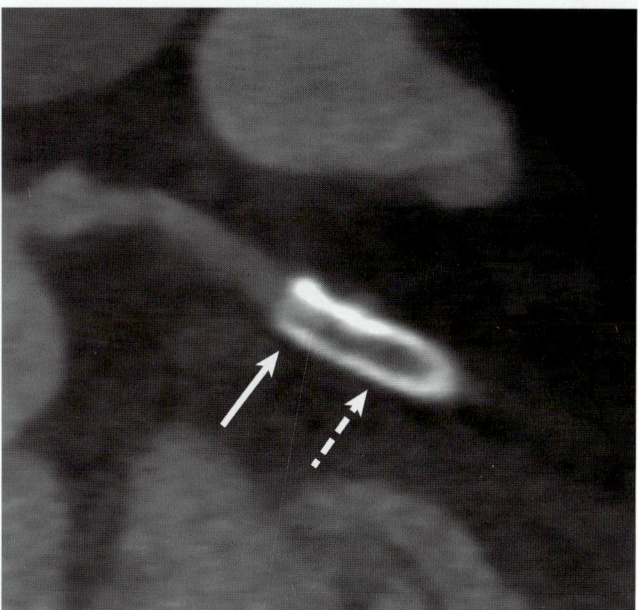

Figure 22.42 Coronary artery stent occlusion. Because metallic artifacts may obscure the in-stent lumen, lack of contrast opacification is alone not a sufficient sign of in-stent-restenosis unless both an opacified segment (*solid arrow*) and a nonopacified segment (*dashed arrow*) are seen. In occluded cases, lack of contrast flow distal to the stent is helpful in making the diagnosis.

(Fig. 22.42). Unfortunately, the high density of the stent material and adjacent bulky calcification often result in obscuration of the stent lumen, which limits evaluation. There is general consensus based on studies that stents of 2.5–3 mm or more are evaluable, more so than stents of smaller sizes [67]. Using 64-slice CT, 93% of the stents ≥2.5 mm are deemed evaluable with ISR sensitivity of 95% [68]. In practice, the evaluability of the stent should be judged on a case by case basis and clearly conveyed.

Stent Fracture and Protrusion

Rarely, a coronary artery stent may be fractured (Fig. 22.43), requiring targeted revascularization in the case of flow compromise. In the absence of obstruction, the clinical significance of this abnormality is not clear nor studied in detail due to its rarity. This finding should not be confused with overlapping or serial stents. The distinction between the two is best made by clinical history and comparison to prior exam. Last, extracoronary positioning of a stent should be described. Most commonly, the coronary artery stent protrudes slightly into the aortic lumen, which may be purposefully positioned in treating ostial stenosis (Fig. 22.44). However, this placement may interfere with future procedures such as transcatheter replacement of the aortic valve and is thus worth noting. Rarely, extraluminal stent migration occurs, which is potentially devastating. Thankfully, this finding is rarely a diagnostic challenge.

Coronary CT Fractional Flow Reserve

Computed tomography derived fractional flow reserve (FFR) is a promising technique with growing interest that has not yet reached widespread clinical use. This topic is briefly mentioned here for completeness as it addresses a major weakness of CT imaging in coronary atherosclerosis. As discussed above, CT provides anatomic description of the arteries. While powerful, it has been noted that not all cases of significant narrowing on CT is associated with functional myocardial ischemia even when confirmed on catheter

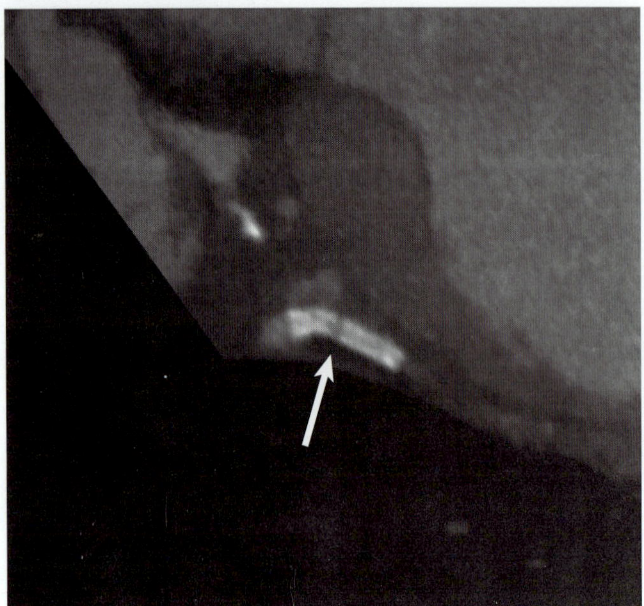

Figure 22.43 Fracture coronary artery stent. Stent fracture (*arrow*) is an uncommon complication that may be suggested on CT images by discontinuity of the stent wall or separation of the components. Clinical history should be examined as to not mistaken serial stents as a fracture. Also note the mild kinking of the proximal stent component.

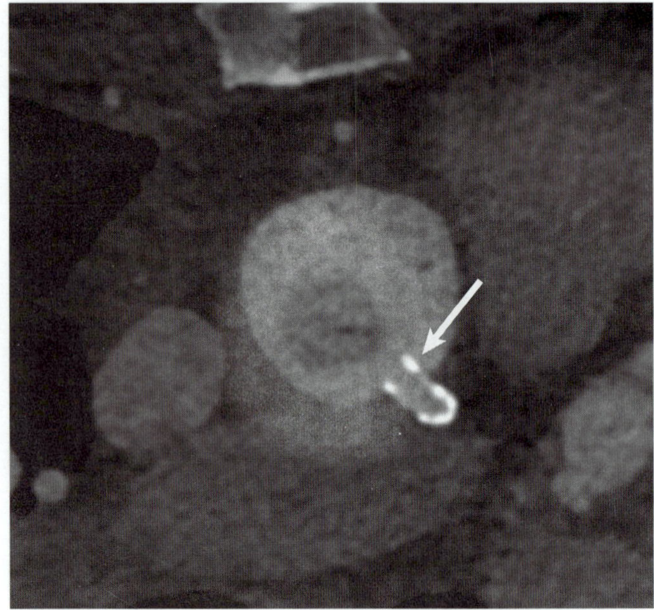

Figure 22.44 Protruding coronary artery stent. In ostial disease and narrowing, the coronary stent may be placed such that the proximal component protrudes partially into the aorta. This configuration may cause confusion or complication with future procedure if not identified.

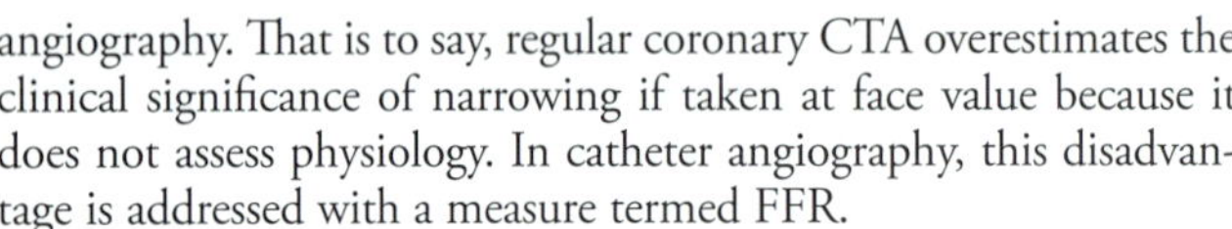

angiography. That is to say, regular coronary CTA overestimates the clinical significance of narrowing if taken at face value because it does not assess physiology. In catheter angiography, this disadvantage is addressed with a measure termed FFR.

In FFR, a catheter with an attached pressure transducer is maneuvered across a stenotic lesion to obtain proximal and distal pressure readings after pharmacologic (adenosine) induction of hyperemia to serve as a suitable surrogate for the blood flow reduction. Calculated as the ratio of distal coronary pressure to proximal pressure, FFR is reduced in the presence of a pressure gradient. Studies show that FFR reliably discriminates functionally significant lesions: a lesion with FFR >0.80 is rarely clinically important whereas FFR <0.75 is nearly always associated with inducible ischemia [69]. When FFR >0.75 is used to defer versus perform PCI in patients with intermediate lesions, long-term (15 year) follow-up indicates this deferral is safe and associated with lower rate of myocardial infarction compared to the stented group [70]. Studies like this have cemented the use of FFR in angiography, which is now considered standard of care. A relatively newly established measurement using similar principle, instant wave-free ratio, may be obtained without use of hyperemic agent [71].

The advent of computational modeling in the last decades has led to the possibility of a similar measurement to be obtained using CT imaging. In essence, a simplified closed-loop model of the cardiovascular system is constructed to enable estimation of the hemodynamic properties including FFR at each location, giving rise to computational fluid dynamics models [72]. The result of the process is a 3D, personalized, dynamic model that may be interpreted alongside the structural images (Fig. 22.45). The noninvasive acquisition is a major advantage, which may be performed using the coronary CTA dataset if certain requirements are achieved. The technical complexity and lack of widespread availability represent its major weaknesses. Currently, HeartFlow FFR$_{CT}$ (processing algorithm by commercial company HeartFlow, Redwood City, CA) is the only clinical CT FFR tool approved for use in the United States.

Overall Approach

1. Calcium scoring is used for risk stratification in asymptomatic patients with intermediate to high risk for coronary artery atherosclerosis.
2. Coronary CTA is mainly used to evaluate symptomatic patients with intermediate risk/pretest probability for significant/obstructive coronary artery obstruction.
3. In performing coronary CTA, spatial, temporal, and contrast resolutions all need to be considered. Nitroglycerin may be given to induce coronary artery dilatation and increase the number of evaluable segments. Beta adrenergic blockade helps with heart rate control but is becoming less critical with improving scanner temporal resolution. Adequate contrast opacification is achieved with injection of high concentration contrast at a high rate, necessitating a relatively large bore access line.
4. In interpreting coronary CTA, both extent of atherosclerotic narrowing and plaque features should be assessed (keeping in mind that acute coronary events are more frequently the result of plaque rupture than narrowing).
5. CAD-RADS allows for standardized reporting that provides the referring physician with interpretation and management suggestions.
6. Coronary artery dissection is a major differential for atherosclerotic disease that is distinguished by patient demographic, risk factors, and global atherosclerotic disease burden. Visualization of a dissection flap, although possible, is a rare finding.
7. Coronary artery aneurysm and ectasia are predominantly the result of atherosclerosis, Kawasaki disease, and vascular shunting. Coronary artery pseudoaneurysms are more frequently the result of trauma and infection.
8. Myocardial bridging is a very common anomaly that is pathologic in only a very small proportion of the patients. The arterial segment proximal to the bridge is prone to develop

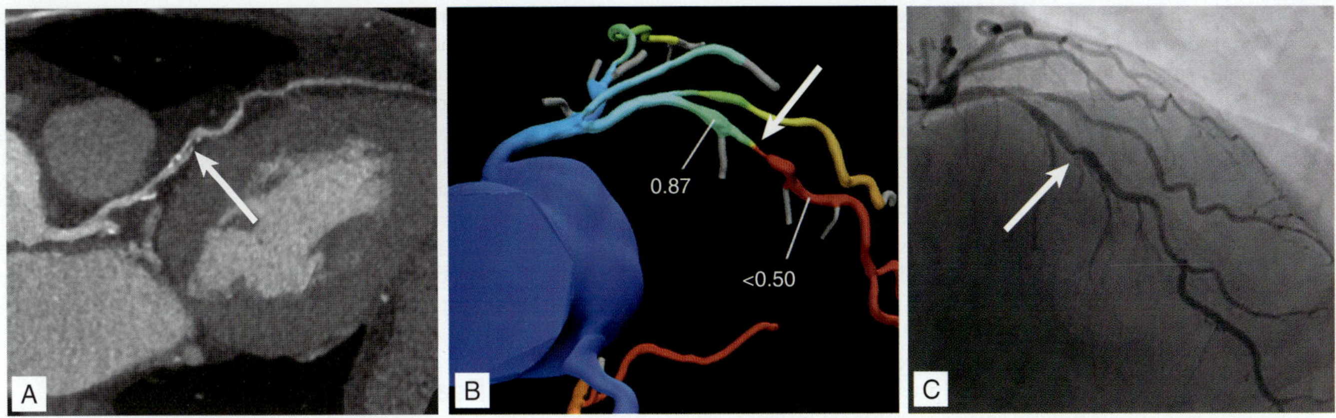

Figure 22.45 CT fractional flow reserve. In the mid LAD, a focus of moderate narrowing by partially calcified plaque is seen (A, *arrow*), which may or may not be functionally significant. Using HeartFlow FFR_{CT} (HeartFlow, Redwood City, CA), CT FFR is computed throughout the entire coronary tree (B). The associated concurrent drop in CT FFR to less 0.75 indicates the lesion is likely hemodynamically significant (*arrow*). On catheter angiography (C), the moderate stenosis is redemonstrated (*arrow*) and iFR recapitulated a similar drop across the lesion (not shown). (Courtesy: Dr. Praveen G. Ranganath, Massachusetts General Hospital Boston, MA, USA.)

atherosclerosis, whereas the tunneled segment is protected against atherosclerosis.

9. Interpreting coronary CTA in patients with prior bypass without proper clinical history is ill-fated as occluded grafts may be very difficult to detect. Similarly, clinical history is key to avoid misidentification of coronary artery stent as dense calcific plaque.
10. CT FFR is a promising technique that assesses physiology using structural data that is not yet widely used.

Sample Report Templates

Coronary Calcium Score

EXAM: CORONARY CALCIUM SCORE CT
CLINICAL HISTORY: [ ]
COMPARISON: [ ]
TECHNIQUE: Scout images of the chest were obtained. Noncontrast CT of the heart was then performed with parameters specified by the Agatston method. The scan was acquired using prospective ECG-triggering and under breath-holding using a [scanner type]. Calcium scoring was completed by manual segmentation and according to the Agatston method.
HEART RATE AND RHYTHM: The patient was in [sinus rhythm] with heart rate of approximately [ ] beats per minute at the time of acquisition.
QUALITY: [Excellent, with no artifacts; Good, with minor artifact of no consequences; Fair, with moderate artifacts but diagnostic quality; Poor, with severe artifacts that limit evaluation].
FINDINGS:
Coronary arteries:
The Agatston calcium score is [ ], corresponding to [ ] percentile for subjects of the same age, sex, and ethnicity who are free of clinical cardiovascular disease and treated diabetes. The calcium score distribution is as follows: left main coronary artery: [ ]; left anterior descending artery: [ ]; left circumflex artery: [ ]; right coronary artery: [ ].
The coronary arteries are [normal in origin and course]. There is [right; left; co-] coronary artery dominance.
Cardiac morphology: The atria and ventricles are [normal in morphology and size], allowing for limitations of a noncontrast study.
Cardiac valves: There is [no significant calcifications] of the aortic and mitral valves.
Pericardium: There is [no significant pericardial effusion or calcifications].
Extracardiac findings: [There are no significant extracardiac findings in the limited views of the great vessels, lungs, mediastinum, and upper abdomen.]
IMPRESSION:

1. [No evidence of coronary atherosclerosis, coronary calcium score 0; Coronary atherosclerosis, calcium score __].
2. [Other important findings.]

Coronary CT Angiography

EXAM: CORONARY CT ANGIOGRAPHY
CLINICAL HISTORY: [ ]
COMPARISON: [ ]
TECHNIQUE: Scout images of the chest were obtained followed by noncontrast CT of the heart. Following administration of intravenous contrast, [0.6] mm collimated images were obtained through the coronary arteries. Delayed images [were; were not] obtained. The scan was acquired using [prospective; retrospective] ECG-triggering and under breath-holding using a [scanner type]. 3D reconstructions including curved MPRs were performed.
MEDICATIONS IF APPLICABLE: Dose and route of administration such as beta blocker and nitroglycerine The patient experienced [no significant side effects or complications].
HEART RATE AND RHYTHM: The patient was in [sinus rhythm] with heart rate of approximately [ ] beats per minute at the time of acquisition.
QUALITY: [Excellent, with no artifacts; Good, with minor artifact of no consequences; Fair, with moderate artifacts but diagnostic quality; Poor, with severe artifacts that limit evaluation].
FINDINGS:
Coronary arteries (description can be altered to document presence, characteristics of plague and degree of luminal narrowing

when present) For example the following description refers to reporting template for CAD-RADS 0:

The coronary arteries are [normal in origin and course]. There is [right; left; co-] coronary artery dominance.

Left main coronary artery: The left main coronary artery is a [small; medium; large] sized vessel with [bifurcation; trifurcation]. It is [patent without evidence of plaque or stenosis]. [The ramus intermedius is patent without evidence of plaque or stenosis.]

Left anterior descending artery: The LAD is [patent with no evidence of plaque or stenosis]. Its evaluable major branches are [patent without evidence of plaque or stenosis]. [A __ mm segment of myocardial bridging is seen in the mid; distal LAD.] The distal LAD terminates [before; at; around] the apex.

Left circumflex artery (LCx): The LCx is [patent with no evidence of plaque or stenosis]. Its evaluable major branches are [patent without evidence of plaque or stenosis]. [It gives off a patent posterior descending artery and a patent posterior left ventricular branch.]

Right coronary artery: The RCA is [patent with no evidence of plaque or stenosis]. Its evaluable major branches are [patent without evidence of plaque or stenosis]. [It gives off a patent posterior descending artery and a patent posterior left ventricular branch.]

[No vulnerable plaques were identified.] [There were no evidence of dissection or abnormal dilatation.] [No bypass grafts or stents were seen.]

[The Agatston calcium score is __, corresponding to __ percentile for subjects of the same age, sex, and ethnicity who are free of clinical cardiovascular disease and treated diabetes. The calcium score distribution is as follows: Left main coronary artery: __; LAD: __; LCx: __; RCA: __.]

Cardiac morphology and function: The atria and ventricles are [normal in morphology and size]. The cardiac function is [normal without evidence of focal wall motion deficit].

Cardiac valves: There is [no significant thickening or calcifications] in the aortic and mitral valves.

Pericardium: The pericardial contour is [preserved]. There is [no significant pericardial effusion, thickening, or calcifications].

Extracardiac findings: [There are no significant extracardiac findings in the limited views of the great vessels, lungs, mediastinum, and upper abdomen.]

IMPRESSION:

1. CAD-RADS [0- no plaque or stenosis by coronary CT angiography]. [Consider nonatherosclerotic causes of chest pain.]
2. [Other important findings.]

Suggested Readings

- P Greenland, MJ Blaha, MJ Budoff, R Erbel, KE Watson, Coronary calcium score and cardiovascular risk, J Am Coll Cardiol 72 (2018) 434–447.
- RC Cury, S Abbara, S Achenbach, A Agatston, DS Berman, MJ Budoff, et al., Coronary Artery Disease – Reporting and Data System (CAD-RADS): an expert consensus document of SCCT, ACR and NASCI: endorsed by the ACC, JACC, Cardiovasc Imaging 9 (2016) 1099–1113.
- F Saremi, S Achenbach, Coronary plaque characterization using CT, Am J Roentgenol 204 (2015) W249–W260.
- SN Hayes, CESH Kim, J Saw, D Adlam, C Arslanian-Engoren, KE Economy, et al., Spontaneous coronary artery dissection: Current state of the science: a scientific statement from the American Heart Association, Circulation 137 (19) (2018) e523–e557.
- S Abou Sherif, O Ozden Tok, Ö Taşköylü, O Goktekin, ID Kilic, Coronary artery aneurysms: a review of the epidemiology, pathophysiology, diagnosis, and treatment, Front Cardiovasc Med 4 (2017).
- G Murtaza, D Mukherjee, SM Gharacholou, A Nanjundappa, CJ Lavie, AA Khan, et al., An updated review on myocardial bridging, Cardiovasc Revascul Med 21 (9) (2020) 1169–1179.

23

Noncoronary Artery Heart Disease

MUHAMMAD USMAN AZIZ, PRABHAKAR RAJIAH, SATINDER SINGH

Introduction

Nonischemic heart disease accounts for nearly half of the cardiac deaths and includes heterogenous diseases, including valvular heart disease, cardiomyopathies, cardiac masses, and pericardial diseases. Noninvasive imaging techniques have increased the diagnostic accuracy for all these diseases and consequent decrease in invasive procedures. In this section, we will review valvular heart disease, cardiomyopathy, and cardiac tumors emphasizing the current and evolving role of noninvasive imaging techniques.

Valvular Heart Disease

Valvular heart disease is common and is one of the leading causes of hospitalization and mortality worldwide [1]. With prevalence of 2.5%, it accounts for up to 20% of all cardiac surgeries performed in the United States [2,3]. Most common cause of valvular heart disease now is degenerative in the western world (rheumatic heart disease remains the most common cause in developing countries). Often these are diagnosed in early stages with echocardiography; hence chest radiographic findings are minimal to nil.

Echocardiography remains the initial technique of choice for diagnosis due to its noninvasive nature, accessibility, well-established strong evidence-based data, no radiation exposure, and high temporal resolution enabling excellent visualization of cardiac valves. It is, however, limited by limited field of view due to obesity, chest deformity, or scarring from prior surgery, artifacts, and operator skill.

Cardiac magnetic resonance imaging (MRI) and computed tomography (CT) are used if echo is suboptimal and in select patients requiring additional risk assessment [4]. Cardiac MRI offers excellent contrast and temporal resolution and is often the second choice after echocardiography. It can, however, be time-consuming, is susceptible to hardware artifacts and cannot be performed in patients with claustrophobia. Newer CT scanners have excellent spatial resolution and much improved temporal resolution for evaluation of heart structures. It is also fast, widely available, not restricted by hardware and is less limited by claustrophobia. Nonetheless, it does require intravenous iodinated contrast administration, and there is exposure to radiation. The latter, however, has decreased in the latest generation of scanners due to low kVp imaging, iterative and model-based reconstructions, EKG dose modulation and newer techniques like high pitch scanning available on dual source CT machines.

The purpose of this section is to review the major cardiac valvular abnormalities, their pathophysiology, and appearance on different imaging techniques.

Echocardiography

Echocardiography is widely used in the diagnosis of valve disease, assessment of valve morphology, and assessing the morphology and function of both ventricles. In patients scheduled for surgery, echo is used preoperatively, intraoperative transesophageal echo (TEE), perioperative, and for postoperative surveillance.

MRI of Cardiac Valves

Valves can be difficult to visualize on MRI due to their low proton density, especially on the traditional "black blood" spin-echo sequences. The balanced steady state free precession (b-SSFP) sequence has replaced the previously commonly utilized spoiled gradient echo imaging as the mainstay of MRI assessment of the valves [5]. In stenosis and regurgitation, dephasing from turbulent flow appears as dark or black jets in the forward (stenosis) and backward (regurgitation) directions [6,7] (Table 23.1).

MR can also readily identify ventricular response to valve disease: chamber hypertrophy in valve stenosis, and dilatation from increased volumes in regurgitation. Ventricular contour tracing on dedicated software allows calculation of ventricular volume and mass, which can be indexed to the patient's body surface area and compared to reference values to assess severity of the valve disease affecting management, including surgical intervention.

The severity of stenosis and regurgitation can be subjectively assessed from signal loss on cine images. Regurgitant fraction can also be indirectly calculated by comparing the ventricular volumes and stroke volumes but this method can be limited by presence of shunting. Direct flow assessment with acquisition of velocity encoded cine (VENC) magnitude and phase contrast sequences is the most accurate MR method in assessing the severity of the stenosis or regurgitation. Voxel grayscale encoding can display flow velocity and direction on the phase contrast images and in cases of stenosis, can help calculate pressures across the valve plane. The resultant values can then be compared to the reference tables for grading. Similarly, in cases of regurgitation, flow velocities from each phase of the cardiac cycle are multiplied by the region of interest area, and the resultant flow is divided by forward flow to get regurgitant fraction.

CT of the Cardiac Valves

CT is often considered when additional information is needed or when echocardiography and MRI cannot be performed or are suboptimal due to reasons listed earlier. CT is also used preoperatively to evaluate coronary arteries in patients with valvular endocarditis to avoid dislodging vegetation with catheter. CT is the technique of choice to evaluate suspected obstruction from thrombosis or

TABLE 23.1 Sample MR Cardiac Protocol for Valvular Assessment

Plane	Sequence
Axial	Black blood-gated HASTE/SSFSE through chest
Axial	White blood SSFP through chest
2 Chamber	Vertical long axis—cine SSFP
4 Chamber	Horizontal long axis—cine SSFP
3 Chamber	LVOT view—cine SSFP
Short axis	Stack of cine SSFP cine through entire heart
Aorta/PA flow	Mid ascending aorta phase contrast flow
Optional/Selective Postcontrast Sequences	
Short axis	Look locker sequence for assessment of inversion recovery time
Short axis/2 chamber/3 chamber/4 chamber	10 minutes postcontrast magnitude or phase sensitive inversion recovery (late gadolinium enhanced)

pannus in post-transcatheter aortic valve replacement (TAVR) and even postsurgical valve replacement (SVR) population where echo cannot evaluate the valve apparatus optimally (Box 23.1).

Aortic valve calcification scoring obtained from a noncontrast EKG-gated cardiac CT is known to correlate directly with severity of aortic valve stenosis and is now routinely done in all patients who are being evaluated for TAVR [8].

BOX 23.1 Sample Cardiac CT Technique for Valvular Assessment

Noncontrast CTA for Aortic Calcium Score

Slice thickness (mm)	2.5–3
Field of view (mm)	From carina to cardiac apex
EKG gating	Prospective
Dedicated 3D postprocessing for evaluation of aortic valvular calcium	

Contrast CTA for Valve Assessment

Slice thickness (mm)	1.5–2
Field of view (mm)	From carina to cardiac apex (may be extended up to the aortic arch if required; for assessment of associated findings)
EKG gating	Retrospective or prospective
IV access	Optimally 18-gauge caliber
Contrast injection and flow rate	Dual or triphasic injection—contrast, contrast + saline, saline
	Flow rate of 4–5 cc/s
Acquisition parameters	Slice thickness of 0.5–0.9 mm (vendor dependent)
Postprocessing	Phase reconstruction from the entire R-R cycle (0–90%); typically at 10% intervals
Dedicated 3D postprocessing for valvular evaluation	

Aortic Stenosis

Degenerative aortic stenosis (AS) with valve leaflet thickening and calcification is the most common cause of AS especially in elderly in the developed world with prevalence of 2–5%. Rheumatic fever is a less common cause in developed countries. Bicuspid aortic valve is the most common cause of AS in younger patients. Aortic valvular calcification is thought to be present in up to 25% of individuals at 65 years of age [9].

AS can occur at the supra-, sub-, or at the valvular levels. Valvular stenosis is the most common type (Boxes 23.2–23.4).

AS is a slowly progressive disease and therefore remains asymptomatic for a long duration before clinical presentation. However, once it becomes symptomatic, there is rapid decline associated with high mortality if not treated. Most common symptoms include chest pain, dyspnea, and syncope. Heart failure develops in later stages with an elevated risk of sudden death. On physical examination, a systolic murmur may be heard in the right second intercostal space on auscultation.

Aortic valve calcification can be seen on lateral radiograph as faint speckled calcification (Fig. 23.1). Dilatation of ascending aorta may be present in long-standing AS (Fig. 23.2), but it correlates poorly with severity of AS. There is also cardiomegaly with

BOX 23.2 Causes of Aortic Stenosis

Valvular

- Congenital; bicuspid, unicuspid, or tricuspid partially fused valves
- Acquired; degenerative calcific, rheumatic, infective endocarditis

Subvalvular

- Subaortic stenosis from muscular or membranous diaphragm
- Hypertrophic cardiomyopathy with LVOT obstruction

Supravalvular

- Diffuse aortic hypoplasia or interrupted aortic arch
- Membrane above the aortic root
- Williams' (Beuren) syndrome

BOX 23.3 Bicuspid Aortic Valve

- Most common congenital cardiac malformation (0.5–2.0% of population)
- Most common cause of aortic stenosis in younger patients
- Associations: coarctation of aorta (Turner syndrome)
- Can be treated surgically or by TAVR

BOX 23.4 Williams Syndrome

- Hypercalcemia in infancy
- Elfin faces with low nose bridge
- Supravalvular aortic stenosis; produces hour glass narrowing
- Stenosis in peripheral pulmonary arteries, hypoplasia of thoracic and abdominal aorta, isolated stenosis in arch vessels, renal or celiac or superior mesenteric artery
- Dilated and tortuous coronary arteries due to subjection to elevated left ventricular systolic pressure

rounding of the LV apex due to hypertrophy (Fig. 23.2). In congenital AS presenting in infancy, chest radiograph shows pulmonary edema with cardiomegaly.

Echocardiography can determine aortic valve area, its restricted opening, leaflet thickening, and calcification as well as elevated velocity and pressure gradient across the stenotic valve (Figs. 23.3A–C). Severity of AS has been described on echocardiography (Box 23.5) [10]. It also provides ventricular systolic and diastolic function and morphology. In select patients with asymptomatic severe AS, exercise or dobutamine stress echocardiography has a role in selection for surgery; (1) if patient develops symptoms, (2) fall in blood pressure from baseline, or (3) increased mean gradient of >20 mm Hg.

MRI also shows valve thickening, susceptibility from valve calcification, limited mobility, and reduced aortic valve orifice area. Geometric aortic valve area measured by planimetry on MR tends to underestimate in comparison with TEE [11]. Systolic flow void is seen extending into the aorta in systole representing dephasing from flow jet (Figs. 23.3D–E). On phase contrast flow sequences, peak velocity and flow can be quantified. Adjustment

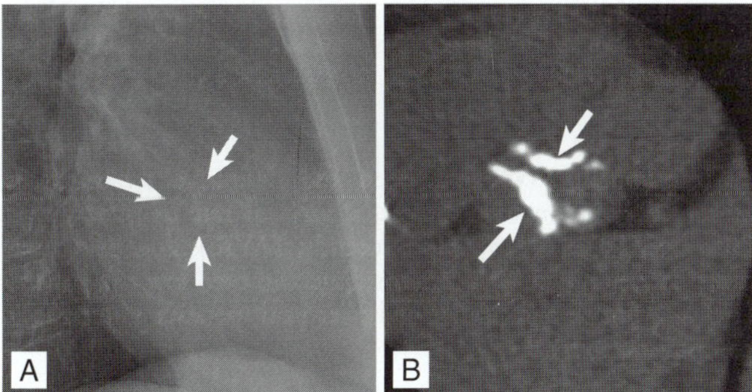

Figure 23.1 Aortic valve calcification. (A) Lateral chest radiograph shows speckled calcification of the aortic valve (*arrows*) and confirmed on noncontrast chest CT (B).

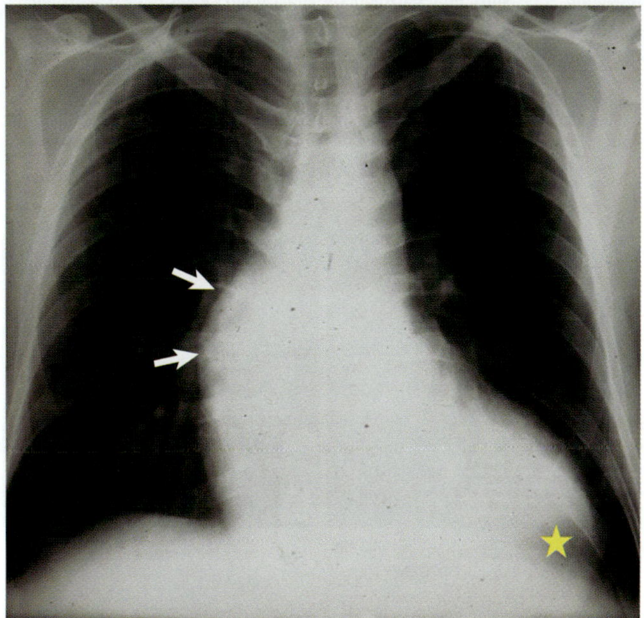

Figure 23.2 Chronic aortic stenosis frontal chest radiograph. The left ventricle is dilated with apex shifted downward and to the left (*star*). There is also dilatation of the ascending aorta (*arrows*).

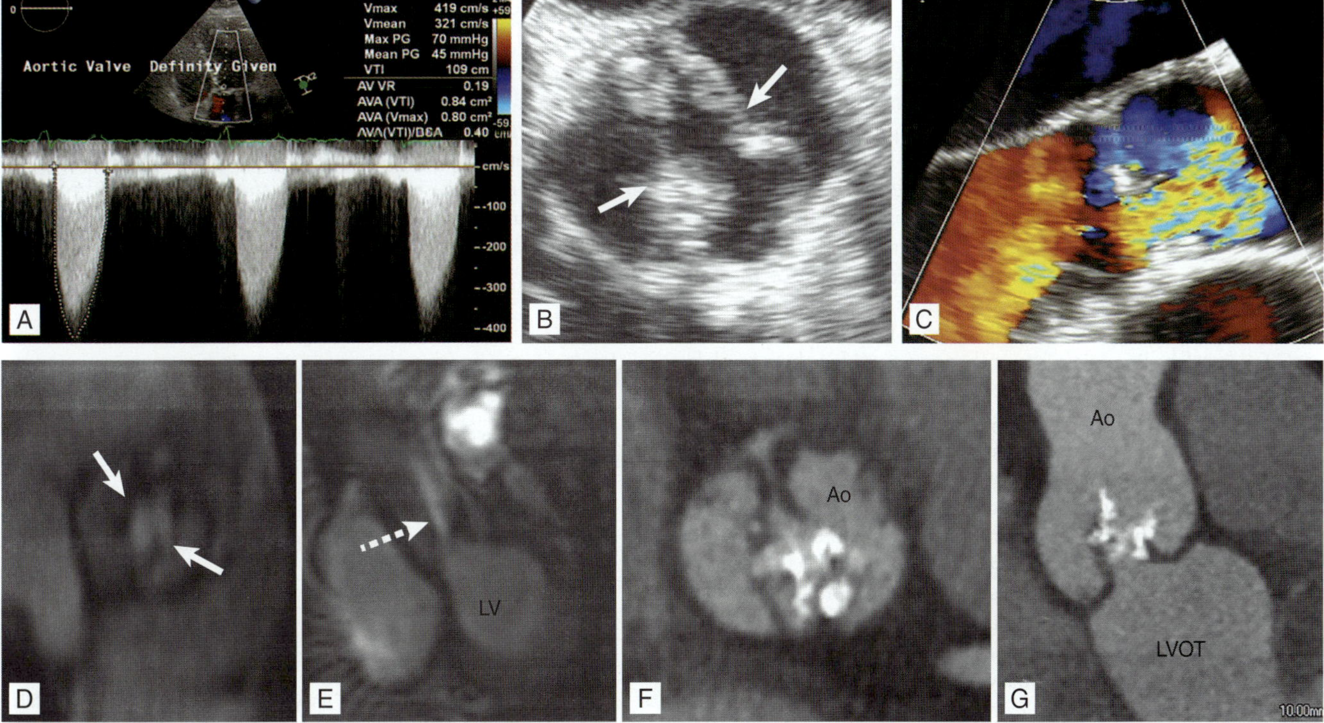

Figure 23.3 Bicuspid aortic stenosis. (A) TTE showing aortic valve area of 0.84 cm^2 and Vmax 419 cm/s. (B, C) TEE. Bicuspid aortic valve leaflets are thickened and calcified with severe aortic stenosis, AVA of 0.8 cm^2 and a mean pressure gradient of 43 mm Hg. (D, E) Aortic valve and coronal SSFP cine images through the aortic valve and ascending aorta show thickened stenotic aortic valve with fusion of the right and noncoronary cusps (D). Systolic dephasing in the ascending aorta (*dotted arrow*) from stenotic flow into the aorta. (F, G) Axial and coronal CT in a different patient with severely calcified bicuspid aortic stenosis. *Ao*, aorta; *LV*, left ventricle; *LVOT*, left ventricular outflow tract.

BOX 23.5 Severity of Aortic Stenosis on Echocardiography

Mild	Valve area of 1.5 cm^2 or greater, peak velocity of less than 3 m/s, pressure gradient of less than 25 mm Hg
Moderate	Valve area between 1.0 and 1.5 cm^2, peak velocity between 3 and 4 m/s, pressure gradient between 25 and 40 mm Hg
Severe	Valve area less than 1.0 cm^2, peak velocity greater than 4 m/s, pressure gradient of greater than 40 mm Hg

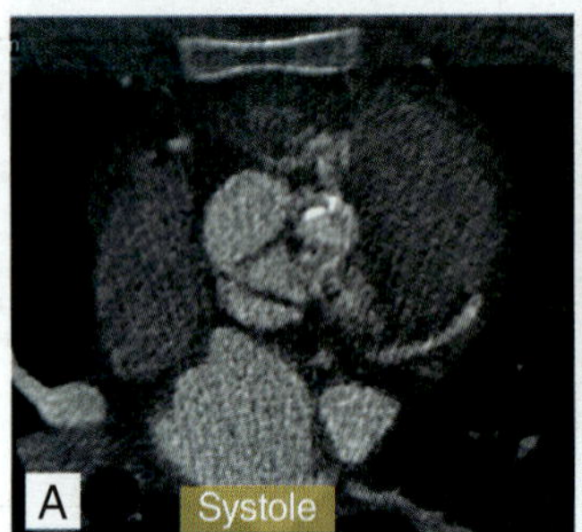

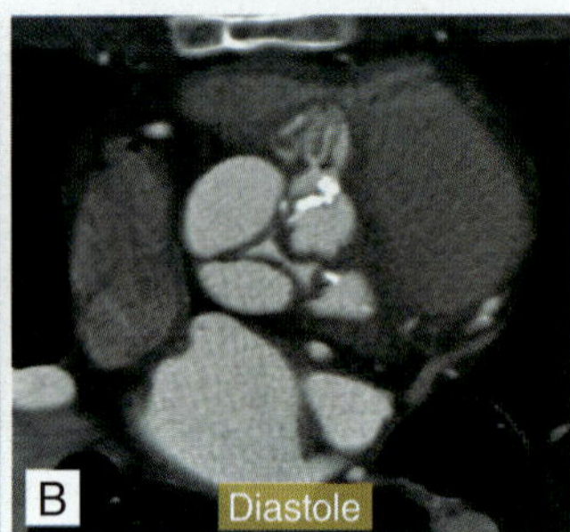

Figure 23.4 Tricuspid aortic calcific stenosis. Thickened calcified aortic leaflets show restricted systolic opening suggesting aortic stenosis (A) and incomplete cooptation in diastole suggesting concomitant presence of aortic regurgitation (B). Systolic images are noisier due to EKG modulation where the radiation exposure is maximum in diastole and reduced in systole. Ideally for TAVR CT where annulus measurements are done in systole, the EKG modulation if used should be reversed, that is, regular radiation in systole and decreased radiation in diastole.

of the VENC may be required in cases of aliasing secondary to very high velocities. From an optimal aortic root plane, the peak transaortic velocity can be obtained and using Bernoulli equation ($4V^2$), peak gradient can be estimated. On postcontrast imaging, patchy and subendocardial late gadolinium enhancement (LGE) can be seen in up to one-third of patients indicating presence of fibrosis and carries poor prognosis [12]. On T1 mapping there are higher native T1 values in severe AS. Myocardial tagging assessing myocardial contraction has shown increased twisting of the left ventricle leading to increased torsion in cases of AS, with improvement noted 1 year after valve replacement [13,14].

CT is not first line investigation but can provide valve area, left ventricular (LV) volume and function, ascending aortic measurements, and quantification of aortic calcification (Figs. 23.3F–G, 23.4). On postcontrast cardiac CT, valve leaflet thickening of greater than 2 mm, fixation, limited mobility, and calcification are noted. Decreased aortic valvular orifice area, LV wall thickening of more than 12 mm indicating hypertrophy, and poststenotic ascending aortic dilation in long-standing AS can be seen (Fig. 23.5).

CT is the technique of choice and essential for pre-TAVR planning as well as post-TAVR evaluation for thrombosis or pannus. Aortic valve calcification has association with subclinical atherosclerosis without known coronary artery disease and has a high correlation with stroke and cardiovascular events. Severe CT aortic calcium score of 1274–1377 Agatston units (AU) in women, and 2062–2065 AU in men have shown a high reproducibility and predict severe disease [8]. This is of particular value in cases with discordant echocardiography pressure gradients—low-flow, low-gradient AS.

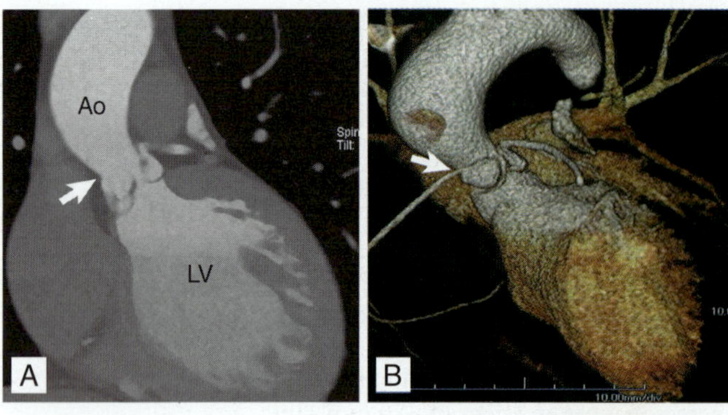

Figure 23.5 Isolated supravalvular aortic stenosis. (A, B) Coronal and 3D volume rendered reconstruction images from a gated cardiac CTA. An 11-year-old male with supraaortic stenosis (*white arrows*) due to elastin gene mutation and abnormal array CGH analysis result consistent with a 5p14.1 duplication. Similar imaging findings are seen in patients' with Williams syndrome. In this patient, the aortic valve was tricuspid but was deformed and thickened. *Ao*, aorta; *LV*, left ventricle.

Traditionally, SVR has been the definitive treatment in advanced symptomatic AS with a survival rate of greater than 80% after 10 years [15]. More recently, TAVR is now being used more commonly in high, intermediate and even low risk patients [16] and has shown similar or better postoperative outcomes in comparison to SVR.

Aortic Regurgitation

Aortic regurgitation is commonly seen in males with prevalence increasing with age (Box 23.6). Presentation includes gradually worsening signs and symptoms of heart failure. There is high mortality (25%) in patients with advanced heart failure. Patients with type A aortic dissection or infective endocarditis (IE) can present acutely (Box 23.7).

Chest radiograph may be normal in acute cases. In chronic cases, there is often significant LV dilatation.

Incomplete coaptation of the valve leaflets, delayed opening, and premature closure are readily visualized on echocardiography. LV dilation can be seen in chronic cases. Color Doppler evaluation shows regurgitant jet which can be central or eccentric (Fig. 23.6).

BOX 23.6 Causes of Aortic Regurgitation

A. Leaflet abnormality
- Rheumatic valvular disease
- Bicuspid aortic valve with thickening and calcification
- Valvular endocarditis
- Aortic valve leaflet prolapse in Marfan's syndrome or patients with perimembranous VSD

B. Ascending aortic dilatation
- Systemic hypertension
- Annuloaortic aneurysm in Marfan's syndrome
- Ehlers–Danlos syndrome
- Aortitis in rheumatoid arthritis, ankylosing spondylitis, giant cell aortitis

C. Aortic root abnormality
- Type A dissection
- Sinus of Valsalva aneurysm
- Trauma (rare)

BOX 23.7 Consequences of Aortic Valve Infective Endocarditis

- Aortic regurgitation
- Left ventricular failure from aortic regurgitation or coronary emboli
- Aortic root/periaortic root abscesses
- Systemic embolization
- Mycotic aneurysms, splenomegaly and infarction, and renal failure

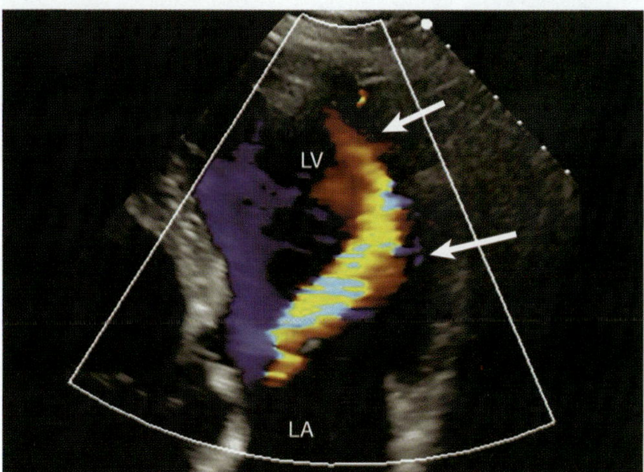

Figure 23.6 Doppler transthoracic echocardiographic images showing severe aortic regurgitation with the regurgitant jet (*white arrows*) reaching up to the left ventricular apex. *LA*, left atrium; *LV*, left ventricle.

AR is identified as backward diastolic flow into the LV outflow track on SSFP cine MR imaging, especially in left ventricular outflow tract (LVOT) or three-chamber view (Fig. 23.7A). Phase contrast velocity encoding is the most accurate way of regurgitation quantification, preferably in double oblique planes to ensure complete visualization of the flow void (jet) (Fig. 23.7B–C). VENC may need to be adjusted depending on the concomitant presence of AS. Grading of regurgitation on MRI have been proposed [17] based on regurgitating fraction; 30% for mild, 30–49% for moderate, and greater than 50% for severe AR. It has also been proposed that regurgitant fraction on MR may be a more accurate prognostic parameter than left ventricular volumes.

BOX 23.8 Causes of Mitral Stenosis

Acquired
- Rheumatic heart disease (most common)
- Prolapse of left atrial tumor or rarely thrombus through the mitral valve
- Leaflet carcinoid, valve vegetation

Congenital (rare)
- Part of hypoplastic left heart syndrome
- Obstructing large papillary muscles
- Parachute mitral valve deformity

Role of CT is limited, but if performed for other reasons such as coronary artery evaluation, a retrospective-gated CT can provide information about aortic valve morphology and malcoaptation of the valve leaflet (Fig. 23.4B), which has high sensitivity and specificity for detecting moderate to severe aortic regurgitation compared to transthoracic echocardiography [18].

Conservative management of AR includes control of arrhythmias and vasodilators. Antibiotic prophylaxis may be required to prevent superimposed infections and endocarditis. In acute cases, conservative measures are employed as a bridge to surgical management. Surgical intervention has a better outcome before advanced left heart failure develops with a 5-year survival rate of 85% in patients with a higher than 45% LV ejection fraction.

Mitral Stenosis

Rheumatic heart disease is the most common cause. Other causes include degeneration, endocarditis, tumors, and rarely congenital (Box 23.8). Thickening and calcification of the valve leaflets result in restricted opening leading to a decrease in the normal cross-sectional valve area of 4–6 cm^2. Obstruction at the level of the inflow tract of the left ventricle results in inadequate diastolic LV filling. Left atrial dilation, pulmonary hypertension, and arrhythmias may occur, with atrial fibrillation being most common.

Symptoms typically develop 5–10 years after the initial acute rheumatic fever in younger age. Patients, usually present with dyspnea. Shortness of breath and cough may also develop due to pulmonary edema. Thrombi may form due to atrial fibrillation, with added risk of stroke. Ten-year survival rates vary from about 60% to less than 15%, in asymptomatic patients at diagnosis or patients with severe symptoms at presentation, respectively [19].

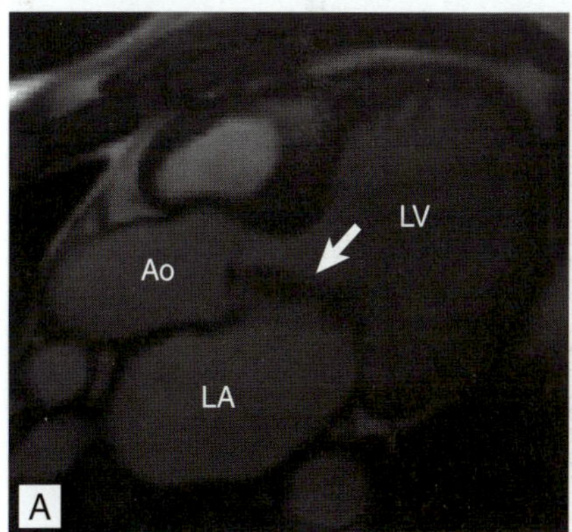

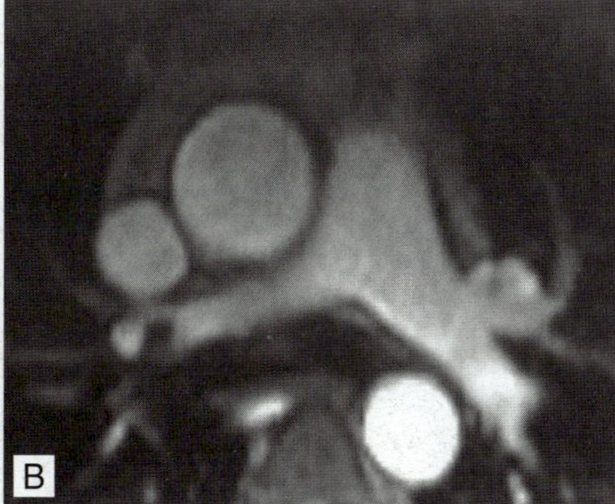

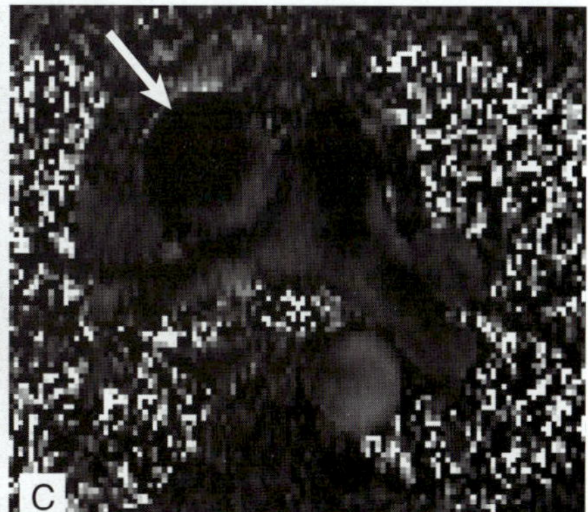

Figure 23.7 Aortic regurgitation. (A) Cine SSFP sequence LVOT view shows severe aortic regurgitation with a large eccentric dephasing jet extending into the left ventricular cavity and originating from the aortic valvular plane (*white arrow*). (B, C) Through plane phase contrast images acquired just above the level of the aortic valve show dephasing on the phase contrast image (C) in the ascending aorta (*white arrow*) due to significant regurgitation. Calculated regurgitant fraction was of 48% consistent with severe aortic regurgitation. *Ao*, aorta; *LA*, left atrium; *LV*, left ventricle.

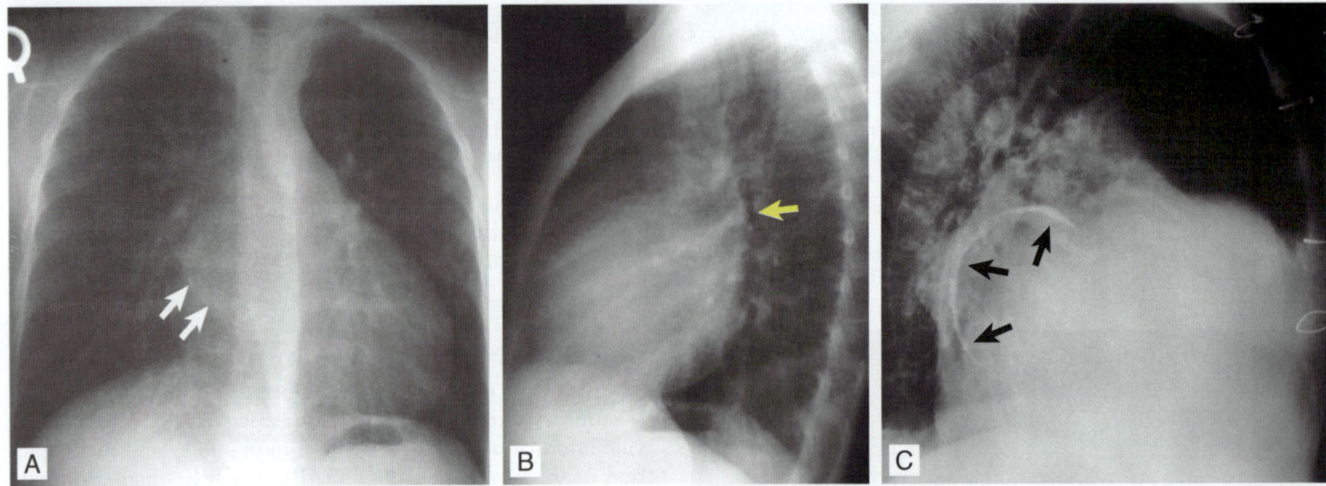

Figure 23.8 Mitral stenosis. (A, B) Left atrial enlargement seen as double density along right cardiac margin (*white arrows*) on frontal view and as bulge along upper heart border on lateral view displacing the left upper lobe bronchus posteriorly (*yellow arrow*). There is also upper lobe vascular redistribution due to pulmonary venous hypertension (PVH). (C) In chronic mitral stenosis, there can be calcification in left atrial wall or in the mural thrombus seen as curvilinear arrows on lateral view (*black arrows*).

Left atrial enlargement seen as retrocardiac increased density with double right cardiac border, splaying of the carina, and upward displacement of left main bronchus on frontal view and posterior bulge of upper cardiac margin on lateral view (Figs. 23.8A–B). Features of pulmonary venous hypertension such as upper lobe redistribution of blood flow, peribronchial, and septal thickening (Kerley B lines) may be present. In later stages, features of pulmonary artery hypertension may be seen as dilated pulmonary arteries with right ventricle (RV) enlargement. Rarely nodular calcifications of the mitral valve may be seen. In long-standing chronic cases with atrial fibrillation eccentric thrombus with calcification may be seen in the dilated left atrium (Fig. 23.8C) and rarely hemosiderosis may be seen as dense tiny nodular densities in the lungs.

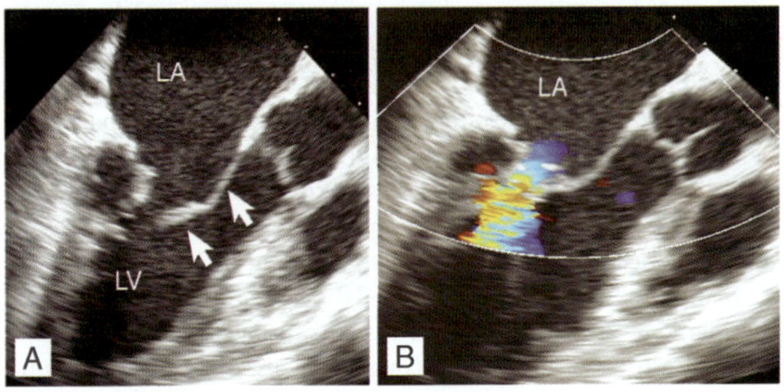

Figure 23.9 Mitral stenosis. (A, B) TEE shows thickened mitral leaflets, restricted opening, stenotic turbulence and increased velocities across mitral valve and hockey stick appearance (*arrows*). There is dilatation of the left atrium. *LA*, left atrium; *LV*, left ventricle.

Rheumatic mitral stenosis on echocardiography has typical appearance with thickened leaflets and commissural fusion resulting in bowing deformity of leaflets mimicking hockey stick (Figs. 23.9 and 23.10A–B). Valve planimetry is done in mid diastolic phase and Doppler across the valve provides the mean transmittal gradient. Patients with severe symptoms but only moderate mitral stenosis on echo may also benefit from exercise echocardiography.

Due to the presence of atrial fibrillation and problem with EKG gating, cardiac MR is not routinely used. Signal loss occurs due to the presence of calcification. Restriction motion of the leaflets, fish mouth appearance due to fused commissures, bowing of the anterior leaflet, dephasing from increased velocity flow across the narrow orifice can be seen with measurements of the velocities with phase contrast imaging (Fig. 23.11). Secondary findings may include chamber dilatation and back pressure changes from pulmonary hypertension.

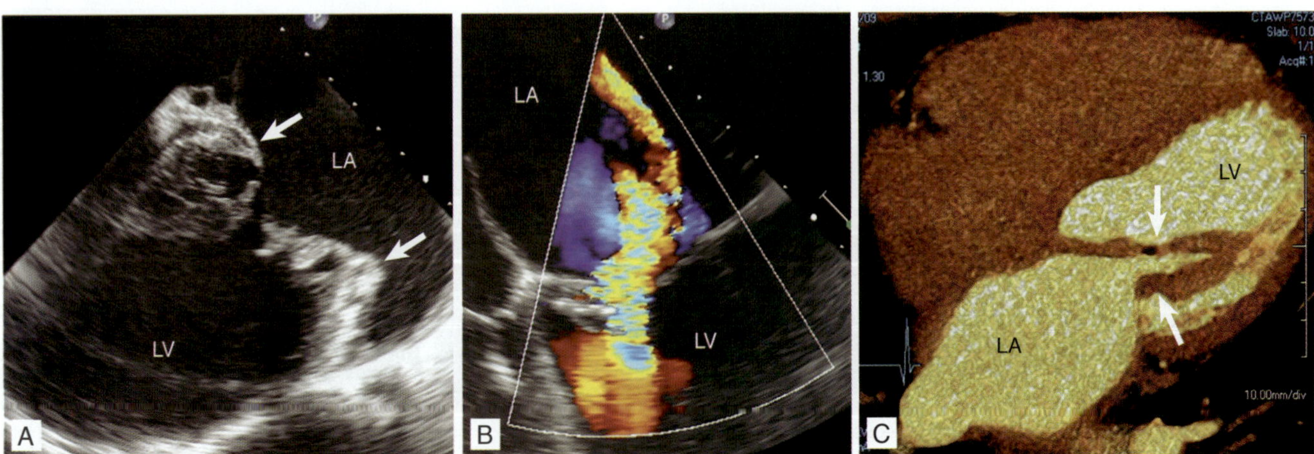

Figure 23.10 Rheumatic mitral stenosis and regurgitation. (A, B) TEE shows irregularly thickened and calcified mitral valve leaflets (*arrows*) with turbulent flow across the stenotic valve along with backward flow. (C) Chordae tendineae thickening and fusion (*arrows*) is also common in as seen in the axial color rendered CT image. *LA*, left atrium; *LV*, left ventricle.

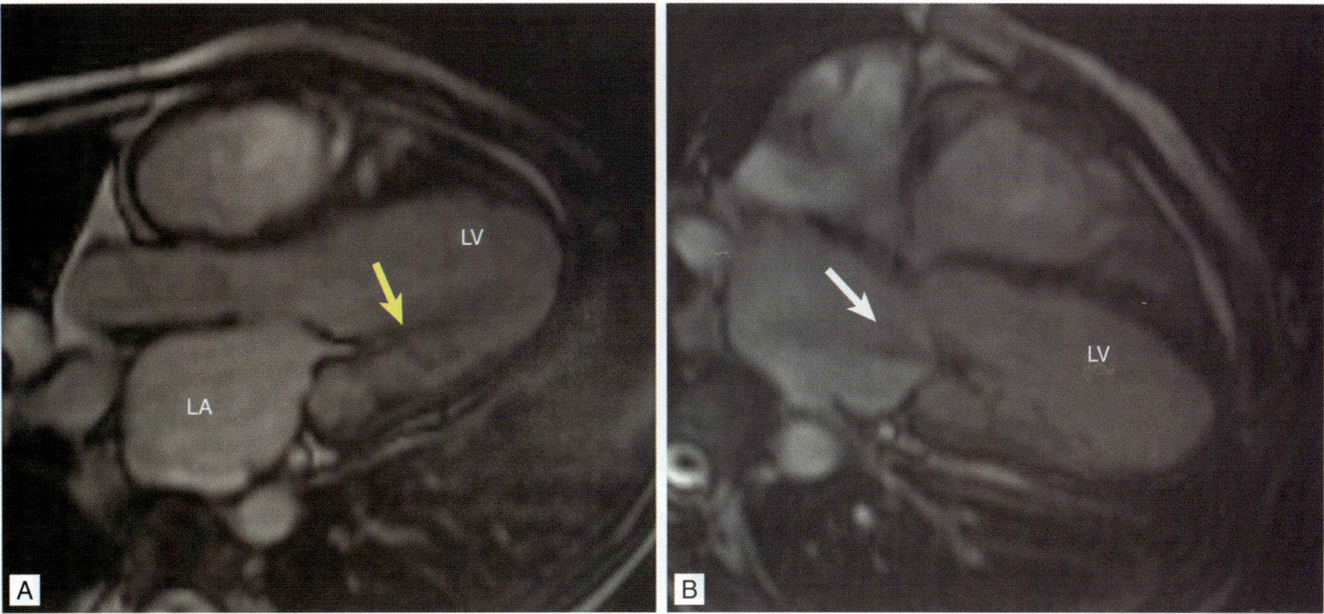

Figure 23.11 (A) LVOT view cardiac MR shows the dephasing jet (*yellow arrow*) in the left ventricle from mitral valvular stenosis. (B) Mitral insufficiency was also present as shown in four-chamber view (*white arrow*). *LA*, left atrium; *LV*, left ventricle.

Due to its high spatial resolution, CT is particularly useful in detecting calcification in the mitral apparatus. CT can also provide orifice area in addition to left atrial size, detect left atrial appendage thrombus, pulmonary edema, pulmonary hypertension, and right ventricular hypertrophy. Chordae tendineae may also be thickened and matted together (Fig. 23.10C).

Medical therapy includes anticoagulation for arrhythmias and reducing cardiac effort. More invasive treatment options include balloon valvuloplasty with excellent survival rate, and surgical replacement. Lately, robotic replacement of mitral valve has gained grounds with decreased postoperative morbidity and fast recovery leading to increased patient acceptance.

Mitral Regurgitation

Mitral valve regurgitation represents backward flow into the left atrium from the left ventricle during systole and is the most common valvular abnormality in the United States. Multiple etiologies can result in valve degeneration, leaflet retraction, and incomplete coaptation resulting in regurgitation (Box 23.9). Myxomatous degeneration of the mitral leaflets results in prolapse (Barlow's disease)—which is a billowing of the leaflet into the left atrium of more than 2 mm. "Flail" leaflet can occur secondary to chordal thinning and rupture in advanced disease. Chronic regurgitation can result in chamber dilation. In patients with inferior wall myocardial infarction (MI) acute papillary muscle rupture often present as acute atypical pulmonary edema.

BOX 23.9 Causes of Mitral Regurgitation

Primary

A. Leaflet

Rheumatic endocarditis, mitral Valve Prolapse, left atrial myxoma or thrombus, tumor deposit

B. Chordae tendineae

Rupture from endocarditis, cystic medial necrosis or trauma

C. Papillary muscle

Infarction

Secondary (Functional)

Mitral annulus dilatation due to LV dysfunction (ischemic heart disease, dilated cardiomyopathy, hypertension)

Mitral valve prolapse affects 1–3% of general population and usually presents in the second to fourth decades of life [20]. The variable clinical outcome depends on patient age, degree of mitral regurgitation, LV ejection fraction, atrial diameter, and ventricular arrhythmia. Although MVP may remain asymptomatic, it can lead to significant MR and heart failure, increases risk for IE and ventricular arrhythmia including sudden cardiac death (SCD). The ventricular arrhythmia related to MVP tend to occur more often in young females who also tend to have bileaflet prolapse and more valve thickening. Characteristic T-wave abnormality (biphasic or inverted T-waves in inferior leads II, III, and aVF) are seen in majority of patients with MVP-related SCD and its presence should prompt further investigation. Due to mechanical traction exerted by the prolapsing leaflet a localized area of myocardial fibrosis seen as delayed enhancement on MRI can be seen in inferolateral wall of LV or the papillary muscles.

In acute presentation, heart size is often normal with pulmonary edema present. In acute posteromedial papillary muscle rupture due to acute inferior wall MI, there can be focal right upper lobe edema due to direction of acute MR jet and this can mimic pneumonia on chest radiograph. In chronic cases, enlarged cardiac silhouette is present with or without pulmonary hypertension (Fig. 23.12).

Due to excellent evaluation of mitral valve apparatus, echocardiography can detect underlying cause for mitral regurgitation. Color Doppler can detect and quantify severity of MR from the width of vena contracta (the high velocity central color Doppler jet from the regurgitating flow occurring at or just below the level of the valve orifice) or effective regurgitant orifice area. MR is considered severe if the vena contracta width is >7 mm with peak transmitral velocity >1.5 m/s and mitral velocity time integral: aortic velocity time integral ratio >1.34 [21]. TEE provides better

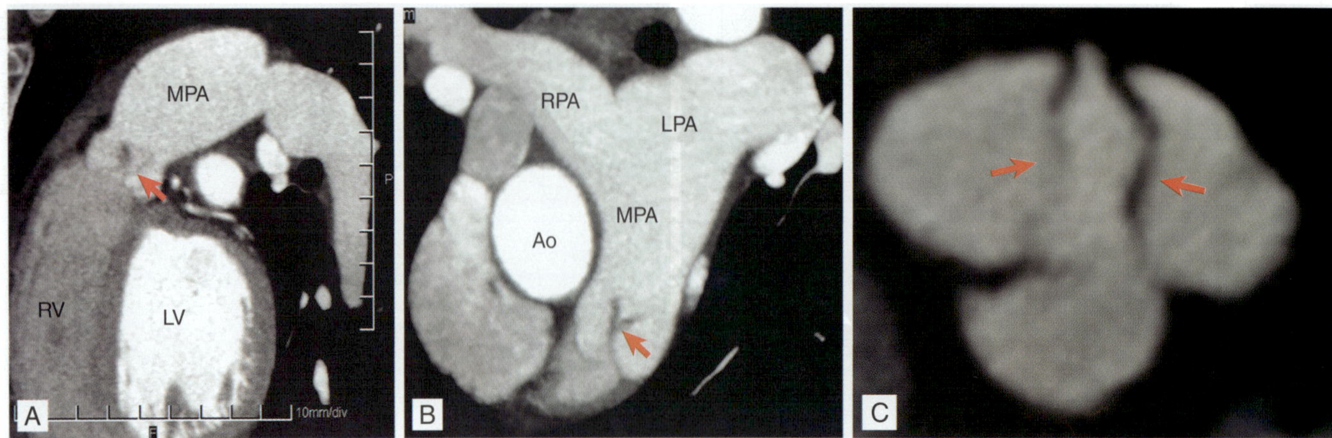

Figure 23.15 Valvular pulmonary stenosis. Multiplanar MPR (A, B) and cross-section images (C) show thickened stenotic pulmonary valves (*red arrows*) with dilatation of main (MPA) and left pulmonary artery (LPA). *Ao*, aorta; *LPA*, left pulmonary artery; *LV*, left ventricle; *MPA*, main pulmonary artery; *RPA*, right pulmonary artery; *RV*, right ventricle.

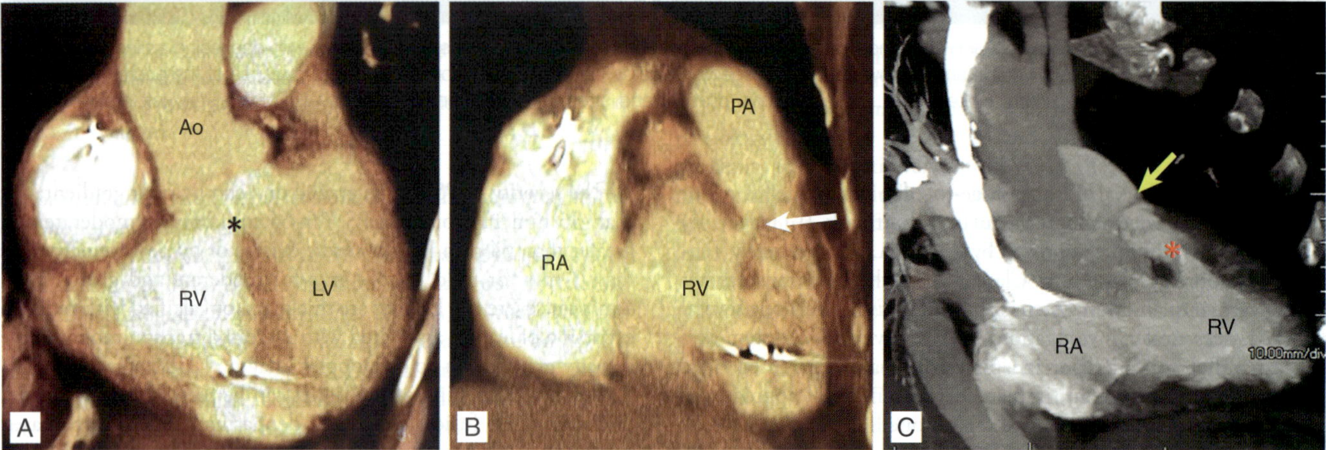

Figure 23.16 A 64-year-old female with prior Blalock–Taussig palliation for tetralogy of Fallot. (A) Oblique coronal 3D volume rendered CT reconstruction demonstrating right ventricular (RV) hypertrophy, overriding aorta (Ao), and subaortic VSD (*asterisk*). (B) 3D volume rendered reconstruction illustrating the right ventricular outflow tract obstruction (*white arrow*). (C) Another patient with infundibular narrowing (*red star*) as well as hypoplasia of pulmonary annulus (*yellow arrow*). *Ao*, aorta; *LV*, left ventricle; *PA*, pulmonary artery; *RA*, right atrium; *RV*, right ventricle.

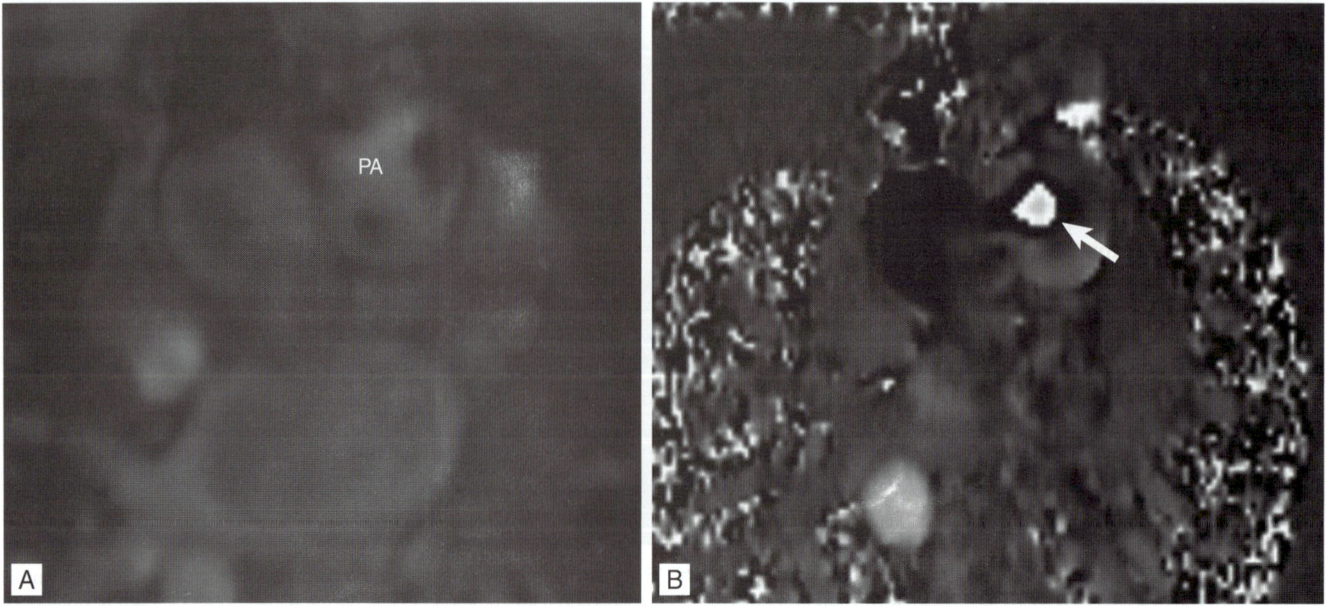

Figure 23.17 (A, B) Phase contrast sequence image through the pulmonary valve showing restricted opening of the pulmonary valve leaflets. Aliasing is seen due to increased velocity flow through the narrow orifice (*white arrow*). *PA*, pulmonary artery.

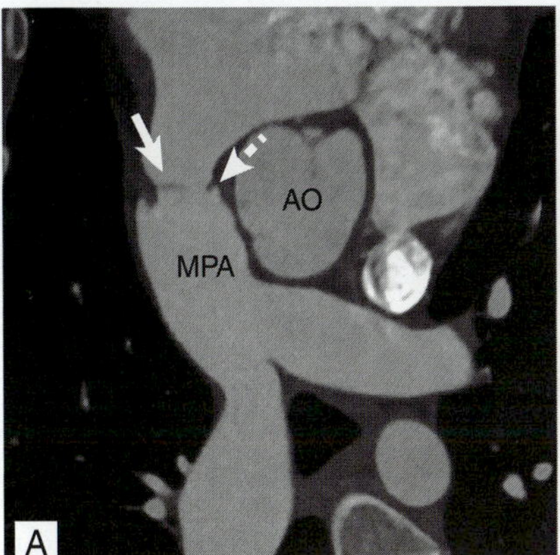

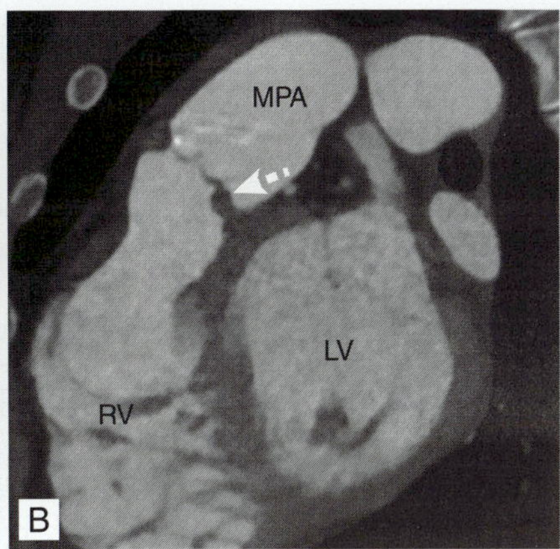

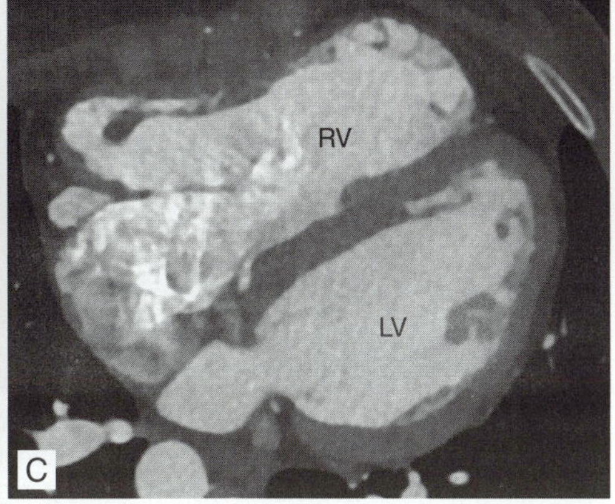

Figure 23.18 (A–C) Follow-up TOF patient with bioprosthetic valve replacement. Multiplanar reconstruction (MPR) images (A, B) showing narrowing at the level of the pulmonic valve (*dashed arrows*) with restricted leaflet opening (*white arrow*) suggesting pulmonary valve stenosis. (C) Right atrial and ventricular dilation and flattening of interventricular septum due to pressure overload are seen on the four-chamber cardiac CTA. Optimal contrast opacification of both ventricles as in this patient is critical in evaluation of biventricular function. *Ao*, aorta; *LV*, left ventricle; *MPA*, main pulmonary artery; *RV*, right ventricle.

function and any associated complex congenital heart defects can also be evaluated.

CT can show valvular leaflet thickening, reduced valvular annular opening area, right ventricular hypertrophy, and dilation. Flattening or bulge of the interventricular septum toward the left ventricle due to increased right cardiac pressures. Main and left pulmonary artery are usually more dilated due to post-stenotic flow directed more into the left branch due to more acute angulation of the right branch of the pulmonary artery (Fig. 23.15). Various congenital cardiac anomalies associated with pulmonary stenosis can be well assessed on a gated cardiac CT performed with optimal contrast opacification of both systemic and pulmonic cardiac chambers (Fig. 23.18).

In symptomatic congenital valvular PS, balloon angioplasty shows good results.

However, patients with dysplastic pulmonary valve with thick and stiff leaflets usually do not respond to percutaneous balloon valvuloplasty and often require surgical valvotomy.

Pulmonic Regurgitation

Trivial or mild pulmonic regurgitation (PR) is common in patients with normal heart and usually is of no clinical significance. More commonly PR results from surgical repair of TOF (Box 23.11). Transannular patching with pericardium, Dacron or polytetrafluoroethylene provide excellent relief of right ventricle outflow tract (RVOT) obstruction but invariably lead to PR, hypokinesis, aneurysm of the RVOT (Fig. 23.19), and fibrosis.

Echocardiogram is used for surveillance follow-up after corrective surgery of TOF. Color Doppler can show a jet directed into the RV during ventricular systole, can calculate pressure half time to determine the severity of PR.

Cardiac MR is the technique of choice to evaluate PR especially in post-treated TOF patients to determine the degree of PR, severity of RV dilatation and dysfunction which help in determining the optimal timing for intervention. Artifacts from the reversed flow into the RV are readily visualized using cine MRI sequences (Fig. 23.20). Phase contrast MR sequence using VENC can quantify the regurgitant fraction; up to 25% is mild, 25–35% moderate, and greater than 35% is considered severe. Right ventricular function and volume assessment using MRI is of utmost importance in determining time to intervene. A cut

BOX 23.11 Causes of Pulmonary Regurgitation

A. *Acquired (more common)*
- After repair of TOF
- PV endocarditis
- Pulmonary HTN causing annulus dilatation

B. *Congenital*
- Absent pulmonary valve in TOF

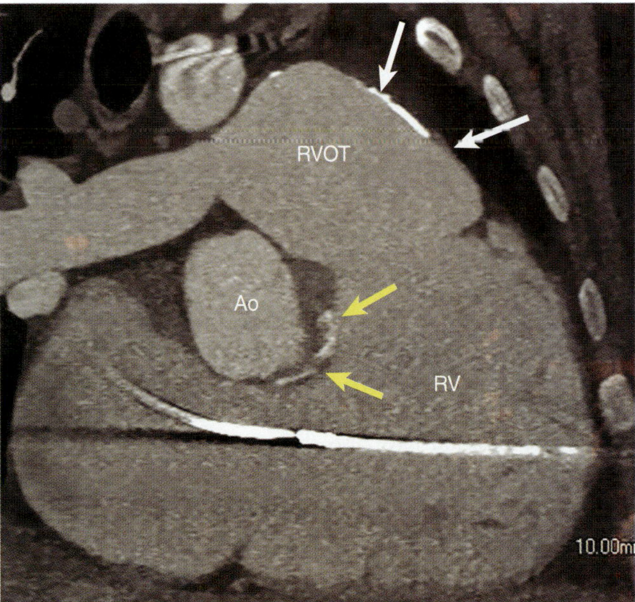

Figure 23.19 Surgically corrected TOF now with significant biventricular dysfunction by echo. Cardiac MR could not be performed due to the presence of non-MR compatible AICD. A gated cardiac CTA was done and the coronal oblique reformat bone window image shows aneurysmal dilatation of the RVOT patch repair (*white arrows*). Surgical sutures are also seen at the site of VSD closure (*yellow arrow*). The indexed RV end diastolic volume was 230 mL/m^2 and RVEF was 25%, both suggesting need for pulmonary valve replacement. *Ao*, aorta; *RV*, right ventricle; *RVOT*, right ventricular outflow tract.

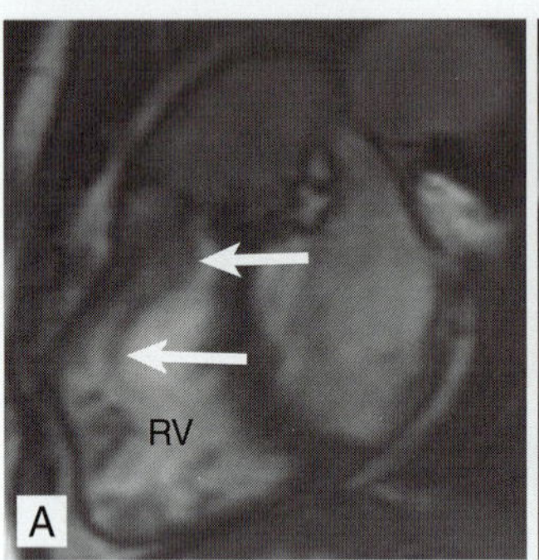

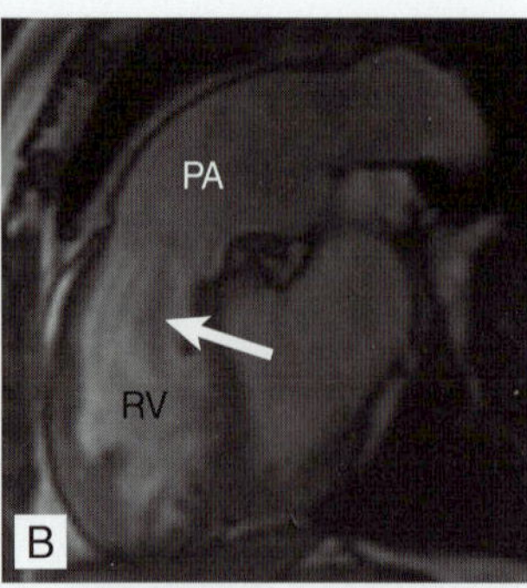

Figure 23.20 Pulmonary regurgitation. Right ventricular outflow tract (RVOT) view from cine SSFP sequence from two different cardiac MRIs (A, B) showing dephasing artifacts from pulmonary regurgitation (*white arrows*). *PA*, pulmonary artery; *RV*, right ventricle.

BOX 23.12 MR Criteria for Pulmonary Intervention [24,25]

- Indexed RVED volume >150 mL/m^2
- Indexed RVES volume >80 mL/m^2
- RV function <47%

off ranging from a right ventricular end diastolic volume of 150–170 mL/m^2 is usually considered optimal for pulmonary valve replacement (Box 23.12) [26,27].

CT is of limited value in direct assessment of PR but can provide information regarding the RVOT morphology, degree of RVOT dilatation or calcification (Fig. 23.19), branch pulmonary artery stenosis, and biventricular function in patients where MR or echo could not be done or are suboptimal.

Surgical replacement is usually indicated in severe advanced patients with significant RV dilatation and reduced systolic function. Treatment options include repair, replacement, or transcatheter valve replacement.

Transcatheter Pulmonary Valve Replacement

Transcatheter pulmonary valve replacement is now the treatment of choice in most congenital heart patients with degeneration of previous RVOT repair. Transcatheter pulmonary valve replacement with the Melody valve is safe and effective in relieving the RVOT/conduit obstruction, restoring the valve function, improving the functional status of the patient, and delaying the next surgical intervention. Edwards's pulmonic balloon expandable valve as well as the Edward TAVR technology in pulmonary position have also shown good hemodynamic and functional results with high success rate and low mortality [28]. It is important to know the coronary artery anatomy and its proximity to the RVOT/pulmonary valve to avoid extrinsic compression by the stent. This information is usually derived from simultaneous coronary angiography and large balloon inflation in the RVOT. Similar information can also be derived from a gated cardiac CTA.

Tricuspid Stenosis

Rheumatic disease is the most common cause of obstruction at the level of the tricuspid valve resulting in thickening and fusion of the valve leaflets. Carcinoid syndrome can also result in tumor deposition on the right heart valves, especially the tricuspid

BOX 23.13 Causes of Tricuspid Stenosis

- Rheumatic heart disease
- Carcinoid
- Endocarditis
- RA myxoma prolapsing across TV

valve which can result in plaque formation and fibrosis (Box 23.13). Normal tricuspid valve leaflet area is between 3 and 5 cm^2. Doppler gradient of greater than 5 mm HG is considered significant.

Symptoms secondary to long-standing tricuspid stenosis include edema, syncope, fatigue, and other signs of reduced heart output. *Distention of SVC, IVC, and presence of ascites suggest congestive heart failure.*

Thickened and fused leaflets, doming of the leaflets, turbulent, high velocity flow across the tricuspid valve with an elevated pressure gradient can be easily seen on echocardiogram.

Tricuspid valve leaflet orifice narrowing and dephasing jet into the RV through the narrowed tricuspid orifice can be seen on double oblique, short-axis, vertical, or horizontal long axis MR images. Right atrial dilation and systemic vein enlargement may be present.

Cardiac CT has limited value in evaluating tricuspid valve disease. It can detect secondary findings of right-sided chamber dilatation, and contrast reflux into distended IVC and HV's. An optimized cardiac CTA with three-phase contrast injection can identify valve vegetation, thrombus, or right atrial tumor. CT can also identify lung causes for pulmonary HTN including pulmonary fibrosis, chronic pulmonary embolic disease, and COPD.

Conservative management is initially employed to improve cardiac functioning. Invasive treatment includes balloon valvuloplasty, valve repair, or replacement.

Tricuspid Regurgitation

Trace tricuspid regurgitation (TR) may be seen in up to 90% of asymptomatic individuals, of no clinical significance. TR can be due to rheumatic disease or IE, carcinoid, or prolapse. Secondary (functional) TR is often due to RV abnormality such as infarction, volume, or pressure overload.

Color Doppler imaging is the primary technique to quantify severe TR shown by a vena contracta width >7 mm, peak velocity >1 m/s, and prominent flow reversal in hepatic veins. RV may be normal in size but hyperdynamic in patients with compensated severe TR but it gradually dilates and becomes hypokinetic with time.

Symptoms from TR vary from being asymptomatic in mild cases, to symptoms of right heart failure.

Significant TR or tricuspid insufficiency can be identified as turbulent flow across the tricuspid valve into dilated right atrium (Fig. 23.21A). Quantification of the regurgitant fraction is possible by assessment of the pulmonary artery flow, and subtraction of the right ventricular stroke volume. Direct measurement is possible by 4D flow technique.

Annuloplasy is the most common surgical intervention for TR, however, it is associated with significant residual regurgitation. Surgical tricuspid valve replacement carries 70% 5-year survival.

Transcatheter Tricuspid Valve Replacement

Transcatheter tricuspid valve replacement is in its early stages of development due to complex tricuspid valve apparatus. The

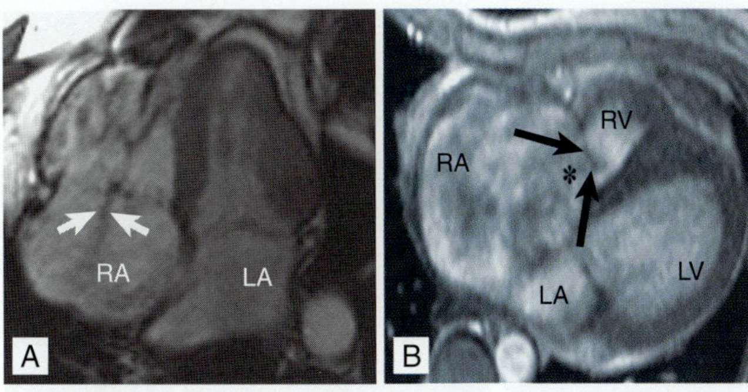

Figure 23.21 Tricuspid insufficiency. (A) Functional TR due to tricuspid annulus dilatation from RV dilatation. (B) Ebstein's anomaly with apically displaced septal tricuspid leaflet along with valve dysplasia (*black arrows*) leading to TR. The portion of RV up to displaced leaflet is atrialized (*star*). *LA*, left atrium; *LV*, left ventricle; *RA*, right atrium; *RV*, right ventricle.

tricuspid annulus is less fibrous compared to the mitral valve, the right coronary artery is in close proximity to the parietal attachment of the valve, the conduction system is in close proximity to the valve and the valve is a nonplanar dynamic structure which changes its size and shape throughout the cardiac cycle making it very challenging to evaluate with noninvasive imaging. The large size of the tricuspid valve requires a large caliber venous access system either via jugular or femoral approach.

Ebstein's anomaly is a developmental anomaly of tricuspid valve in which the septal hypoplastic leaflet is displaced toward the RV apex while the anterior larger leaflets maintain its normal attachment site but are often dysplastic. The RV is divided into two portions, a proximal dilated atrialized part and smaller more distal RV with limited pumping capacity. The right cardiac chambers are enlarged but pulmonary artery is of normal size or small. Increased volume in right chamber lead to septal bowing of interventricular septum which can cause decreased diastolic LV volume (Fig. 23.21B). Depending on the severity of RV dysfunction and TR, patients can remain asymptomatic into adulthood. Symptoms often develop from conduction abnormalities, most common of which is Wolf–Parkinson–White syndrome and right bundle branch block. This anomaly can be easily identified on Echo, cardiac CT or cardiac MR (Fig. 23.21B). Currently, MR is the technique of choice and is especially useful in determining leaflet size and location, annulus and atrial size along with RV function, findings which help in deciding type of surgical repair.

Prosthetic Valves

Prosthetic valves can be mechanical or bioprosthetic (Box 23.14). Patients with prosthetic heart valve require follow up with clinical assessment and imaging to detect rare but life threatening complications.

Prosthetic valve localization on a radiograph can be done by drawing an imaginary line from the left atrial appendage to the right cardio phrenic angle on a frontal projection, and from carina to the cardiac apex on a lateral view. Aortic and pulmonic valves typically lie above these lines, and mitral and tricuspid below, with the tricuspid being more anterior on the lateral view (Figs. 23.22 and 23.23). Cine fluoroscopy is commonly used for assessment of leaflet motion, but is limited in evaluating leaflet thickening or determining the cause of dysfunction.

Transthoracic echocardiography is often the first imaging technique used but can be limited by artifacts from metallic valve components. Latest generation of multidetector CT (MDCT) can evaluate prosthetic valve with minimal beam hardening artifacts. Retrospective-gated contrast cardiac CT scanning can readily access the dynamic motion of the leaflets and their opening and closing angles, presence of thrombus or pannus, and valve dehiscence (Figs. 23.24A–C).

BOX 23.14 Types of Prosthetic Valves

A. Mechanical valves—made of carbon, plastic, or metal. Ball in cage, tilting disk, bileaflet

More durable, requires lifelong anticoagulation. Bileaflet most common mechanical valve used. Indicated in younger patients (less than 50 years of age); in repeat replacements or with concomitant aortic root placement

B. Bioprosthetic valves—made of pericardium, bovine, or porcine tissue

Less durable, do not require lifelong anticoagulation—better safety profile. Preferred treatment choice in elderly patients and in patients planning pregnancy [25]

C. Transcatheter valve replacement

Less invasive, lower complications

Aortic (TAVR)

Edward-SAPIEN—balloon expandable valve, a stainless steel frame and leaflets from bovine pericardium

Medtronic core valve—self-expanding, contain leaflets from porcine pericardium attached to an alloy stent made from nitinol

Mitral and Tricuspid (TMVR, TTVR) (experimental at few centers)

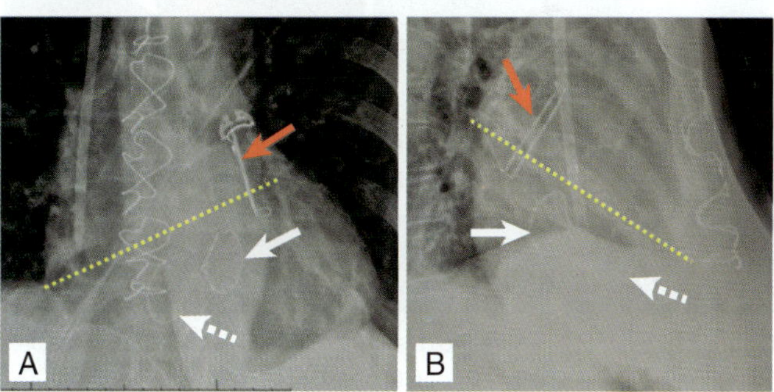

Figure 23.22 (A, B). An example of valve localization using the imaginary lines on frontal and lateral views. Mitral (*white arrow*) and tricuspid (*dashed arrow*) repaired valves are seen. Note more anterior position of tricuspid valve on lateral view. A left atrial appendage clip is also seen (*red arrows*).

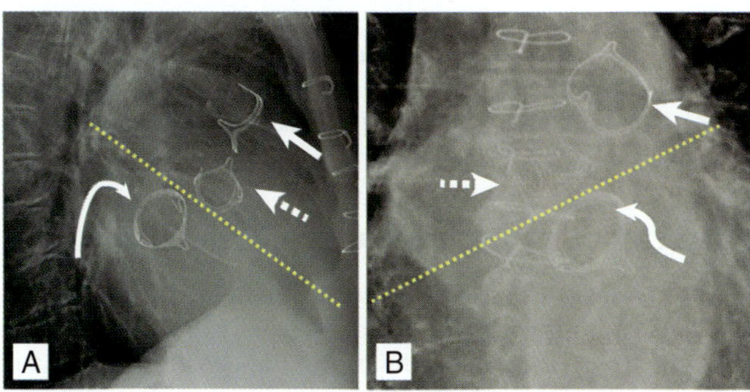

Figure 23.23 Chest radiographs, lateral (A) and frontal (B) views demonstrating multiple bioprosthetic valves in pulmonic (*white arrow*), aortic (*dashed arrow*), and mitral (*curved arrow*) locations. Note the respective locations of the valves in relation to the imaginary localization planes on frontal and lateral views.

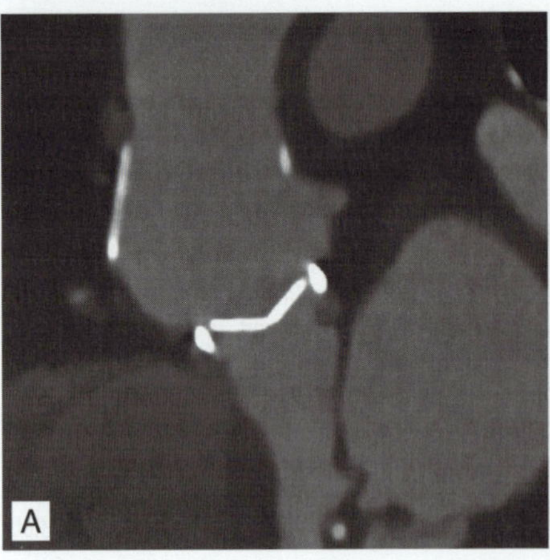

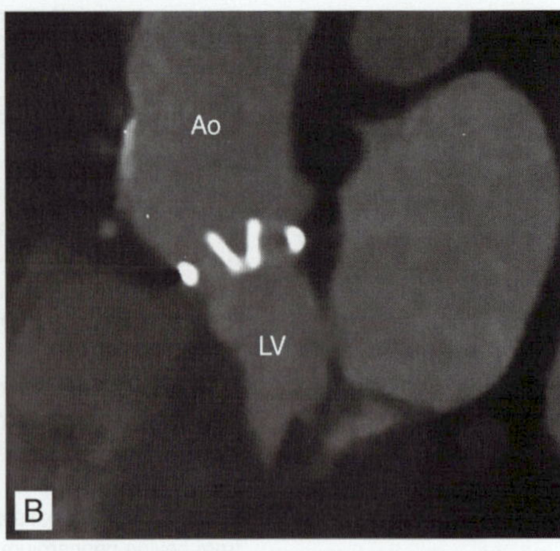

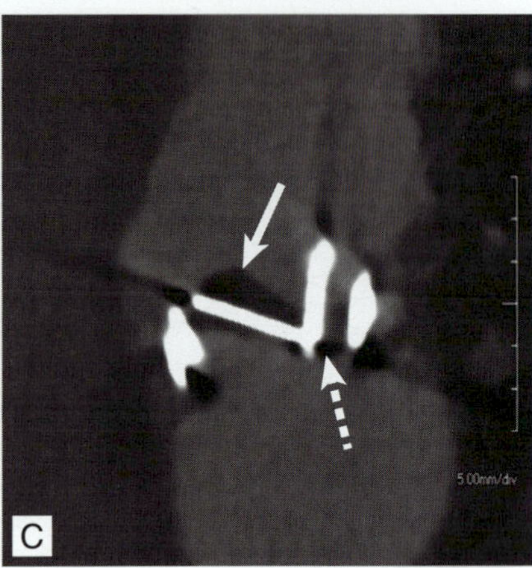

Figure 23.24 (A, B) Coronal oblique images from a retrospectively gated cardiac CTA demonstrating normal opening and closing of the metallic aortic valve. (C) MPR reconstruction from a retrospective cardiac CTA demonstrating immobile aortic metallic valve leaflet (*dotted arrow*). Note presence of thrombus along the aortic surface of the leaflet (*white arrow*). *Ao*, aorta; *LV*, left ventricle.

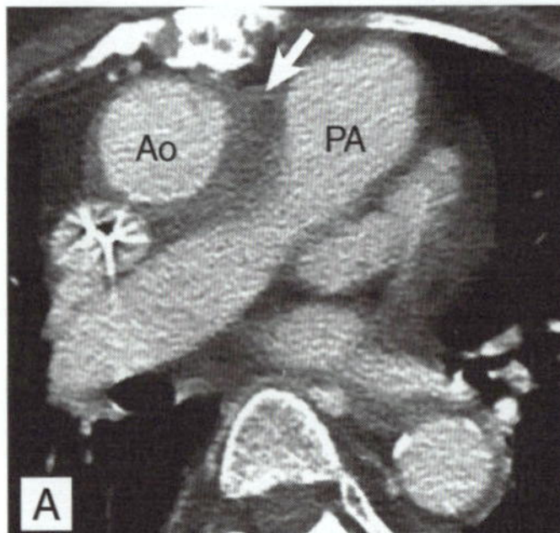

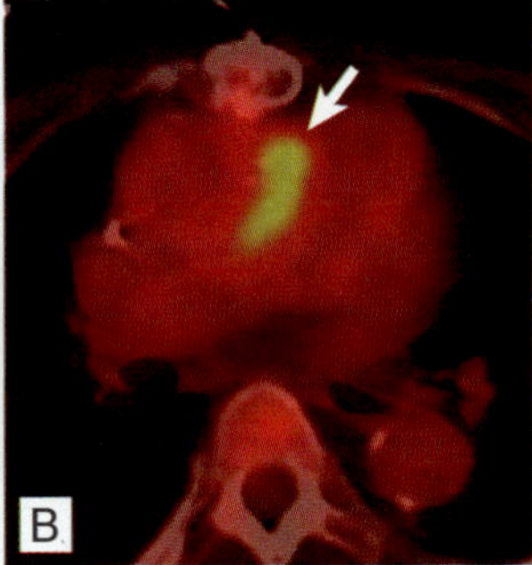

Figure 23.25 (A, B) A 71-year-old female s/p TAVR with CORE valve presented with fever and blood culture positive for coagulase positive staphylococcus bacteremia (MRSA) despite IV antibiotics. CTA chest showed a heterogenous attenuating fluid collection around the ascending aorta just above the core valve (*white arrow*). A subsequent FDG PET showed intense uptake in the corresponding area suggesting this to be the infective nidus. *Ao*, aorta; *PA*, pulmonary artery.

In patients with suspected infected valve prosthesis, SPECT/CT with indium 111 oxime, or technetium 99m hexamethyl propylene amine oxime and F-18 FDG PET/CT may show increased activity with infection (Fig. 23.25A–B).

Transcatheter Aortic Valve Replacement

With careful patient selection, increasing operative experience, advances in imaging evaluation and technical refinements, the outcome from TAVR has significantly improved. Symptomatic patients with AS are first evaluated with transthoracic echo (TTE) to determine if they meet the criteria for severe AS. A pre-TAVR CTA of the heart and chest, abdomen, pelvis is done for annulus measurements and to determine appropriate access site (Boxes 23.15 and 23.16, Table 23.2) [29]. In patients with renal insufficiency, oral or intravenous hydration along with lower amount of intravenous contrast is used to limit renal damage. Post-TAVR follow-up usually involves clinical assessment and TTE to determine any change in transaortic gradient. In patients with increasing gradient further evaluation with a retrospective-gated cardiac CTA and/or TEE is indicated to determine presence of valve thrombosis and leaflet motion restriction (Box 23.17) (Fig. 23.26). Pannus is defined as a linear hypodensity on the ventricular side of the valve and appears contiguous with the adjacent LVOT walls. In contrast, thrombus is usually located on the aortic side of the prosthetic valve and can result in pressure gradients on echocardiography (Box 23.18). This may also be nodular in appearance. Hypoattenuating leaflet thickening (HALT) is a manifestation of subclinical thrombosis appearing as thin centrifugal hypodensities without a pressure gradient or increased velocities on echocardiography. HALT with restricted motion is termed hypoattenuation affecting motion.

BOX 23.15 MDCT TAVR Protocol

- Noncontrast CT for aortic valve calcification
- Systolic prospective or retrospective-gated CTA for heart, nongated for chest, abdomen & pelvis
- Contrast: single injection, usual 60–100 (based on BMI), renal insufficiency 30–40 cc
- If no contrast could be given: noncontrast CT or noncontrast MR; supplemented with TEE or IVUS
- Single breath hold imaging: 4–8 seconds
- *Postprocessing of images (systolic phase): dedicated workstation*

BOX 23.16 MDCT TAVR CT Annulus Evaluation

- Done in systolic phase using phase with maximal valve opening
- Use double oblique method
- To define basal ring and accurate measurements the plane must be balanced so that all three leaflets come to view when scrolling cephalad at the same time
- When the inferior aspect of all three aortic cusps are identified in the same plane a true double oblique transverse image of the root is achieved
- Measure annulus diameter and area/perimeter
- Annulus to LM and RCA distance
- Mitral annular calcification especially anterior near the anterior mitral leaflet
- LVOT size and status of outlet septal thickness
- Optimal deployment angle
- Other findings:
  Lung nodule/mass, PTE, mediastinal adenopathy, interstitial lung disease or COPD, degree of thoracic aortic atherosclerotic disease, radiation fibrosis in patients with known lung cancer

TABLE 23.2 TAVR Valve Sizes and Normal Measurement Ranges

Edwards LifeSciences Sapien Valve Sizes	20 mm	23 mm	26 mm	29 mm
Native annulus area (mm^2)	273–345	338–430	430–546	540–683
Area-derived diameter (mm)	18.6–21.0	20.7–23.4	23.4–26.4	26.2–29.5
Valve height (mm)	15.5	18	20	22.5
Ilio-femoral vessel diameter	≥5.5 mm			≥6.0 mm
Edwards eSheath introducer set	14F or equivalent			16F or equivalent

BOX 23.17 Role of CT in TAVR-Related Complications

- Vascular access related (arterial injury at access, problems with closure, LV apex injury)
- Aortic injury during procedure
- Coronary artery obstruction
- Myocardial injury in transapical approach leading to pseudoaneurysm formation
- Valve thrombosis during postprocedure follow-up

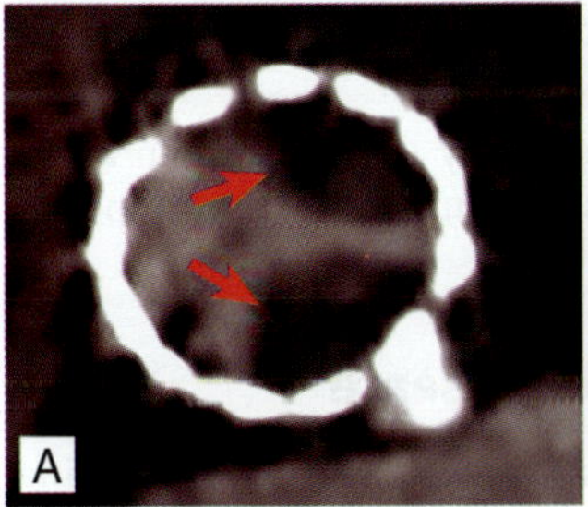

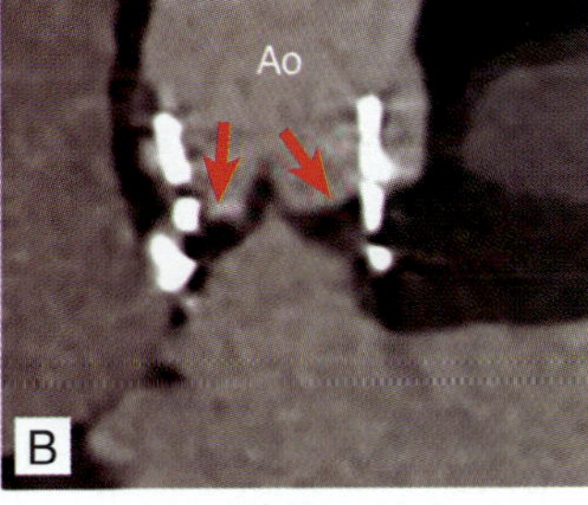

Figure 23.26 Post-TAVR thrombosis. A 52-year-old male with severe aortic stenosis underwent TAVR and at 6-month F/U echo transaortic gradient increased from 13 to 26 mm Hg. (A, B) A retrospective-gated CTA done showed hypodense thrombus (*red arrows*) in the right and left coronary cusps. *Ao*, aorta.

BOX 23.18 Post-TAVR Valve Thrombosis

- Post-TAVR thrombosis is underdiagnosed in asymptomatic patients
- Increase in valve hemodynamic deterioration (VHD) should raise concern
- Gated CTA can detect thrombus as hypoattenuation along valves (HALT)
- Reversible with anticoagulation

Infective Endocarditis

IE is a complex, deadly disease which involves heart and associated multiorgan complications. Its prognosis depends on prompt detection leading to aggressive treatment with appropriate antibiotics and early SVR when indicated. Up to 40% of patients with endocarditis have prosthetic valves (Box 23.19). In patients with prosthetic heart valve, IE is most common in first 5 years after surgery. *Staphylococcus epidermidis* and *S. aureus* infection from devices, surgery, and skin wound are the causative organisms within 2 months of surgery. After 2 months, *Streptococcus* is the most common organism spread via hematogenous route.

BOX 23.19 Predisposing Factors to Infective Endocarditis

- Presence of prosthetic valves
- H/O prior endocarditis
- Cyanotic congenital heart disease
- Degenerative valve disease
- H/O intravenous drug abuse
- Nosocomial bacteremia
- Indwelling leads or pacemakers

Patients present with fever, shortness of breath, and other signs of heart failure. Fluctuating cardiac murmurs may be present. Right-sided IE may present with septic emboli in lungs while left-sided IE from systemic spread to brain, abdominal viscera, mesenteric ischemia, joint infection, spondylodiscitis, and mycotic aneurysms (Figs. 23.27 and 23.28).

Echocardiography remains the first imaging technique for diagnosis, assessing severity, risk for embolization (size and mobility), and follow-up serial evaluations. Echo features suggesting IE include presence of vegetation on valve, valve perforation, perivalvular abscess or pseudoaneurysm, or presence of intracardiac fistula. TEE is more sensitive in detecting small vegetations, perivalvular abscess, and evaluating prosthetic valves (Fig. 23.29C). Retrospectively, EKG-gated cardiac CTA can assess both native and prosthetic valve along with any perivalvular lesion. The sensitivity and specificity of CT to detect perivalvular abscess and pseudoaneurysm compared to surgical findings is very high (>95%) especially in the aortic valve [30] (Figs. 23.29A and 23.30). Cardiac CT also allows noninvasive evaluation of coronary arteries preoperatively in patients undergoing valve surgery as catheter angiography is often contraindicated. CT can also detect extra cardiac IE-related lesions in both right and left-sided endocarditis. MR is of limited value (Fig. 23.29B) in some cases.

FDG-PET/CT or radiolabeled leukocyte SPECT/CT may show abnormal increased activity/uptake especially around the prosthetic valves [31,32] (Fig. 23.25).

Carcinoid Syndrome

Approximately half of all patients with carcinoid syndrome develop cardiac involvement. Thickening of the right-sided heart valves with retraction and fibrosis of the valve leaflets and papillary muscles result in dysfunction including incomplete coaptation and restricted opening. In a minority of cases, involvement of the left-sided cardiac valves is possible when a right to left shunts or left-sided bronchial carcinoids are present.

Secretion of the vasoactive substances results in clinical symptoms with flushing being the most common symptom. Signs of heart failure can be seen in advanced stages. Diagnosis is based on urinary and plasma 5-hydroxy indoleacetic acid levels.

Both MR and CT can show leaflet thickening, restricted leaflet motion, incomplete coaptation, carcinoid deposit, and secondary chamber dilation (Fig. 23.31). SPECT imaging using

Figure 23.27 A 69-year-old male with a PMH of CAD, CVA, HTN, hyperlipidemia, s/p CABGx1, Asc Ao and transverse arch replacement, and AVR (tissue) in 2017. He presented for increasing confusion and difficulty ambulating. TTE revealed a large thrombus on the aortic valve. A subsequent Cardiac CT was done for further evaluation of coronary arteries before surgery which showed aortic valve endocarditis. There was also acute septic embolism of SMA branch. Blood culture grew *Staph. epidermidis*. (A) TTE: There is an echogenic mass in the aortic valve orifice (*yellow arrow*). (B) CTA LVOT view shows an irregular soft tissue-filling defect across the prosthetic aortic valve. In addition there was a small extra luminal contrast along the right cusp (*red arrow*) suggesting small perivalvular abscess. (C) Acute thrombus in the distal portion of the right lower quadrant SMA with surrounding stranding due to septic emboli (*green arrow*). (D) Diffusion restriction of pre- and postcentral gyri (*arrow*) compatible with acute infarction, in a distribution concerning for embolic etiology. *Ao*, aorta; *LA*, left atrium; *LV*, left ventricle.

radiolabeled octreotide and specific tracer somatostatin agents including DOTATE PET/CT have excellent sensitivity (Fig. 23.32).

Somatostatin agents and serotonin inhibitors are the main treatment options along with symptomatic treatment for right heart failure. More invasive options may include balloon angioplasty in advanced cases of stenosis, or surgical treatment in cases of severe regurgitation.

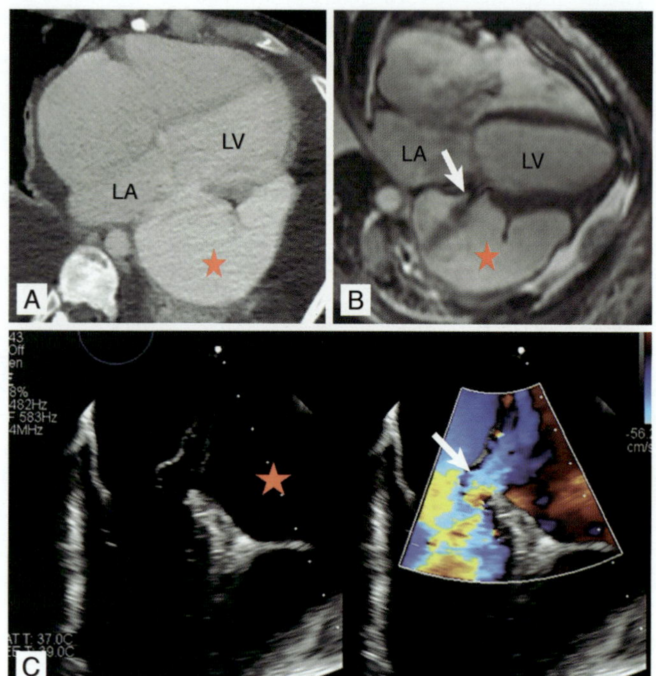

Figure 23.29 Pseudoaneurysm due to infective mitral valve endocarditis. Gated CTA (A) and four-chamber SSFP image from cardiac MRI (B) showing a large contrast filled cavity (pseudoaneurysm— *red star*) communicating with the left ventricle cavity (*white arrow*) with dephasing artifact from the flow through the narrow neck. (C) TEE confirmed the large patent PSA (*red star*) near the left AV valve with a large defect along the mitral annulus (*white arrow*) communicating with LV. *LA*, left atrium; *LV*, left ventricle.

Radiation-Induced Valvular Disease

Rare, usually develops decades after significant mediastinal radiation treatment usually >30 Gy [24]. In one autopsy survey, up to 81% of valves were involved by radiation-induced damage [33]. Vast majority of patients are asymptomatic and valve disease is incidentally detected, often with development of coronary artery disease-related symptoms. Cardiac CT can show valve leaflet fibrosis and calcification, along with aortic or pulmonary artery calcifications (Fig. 23.33).

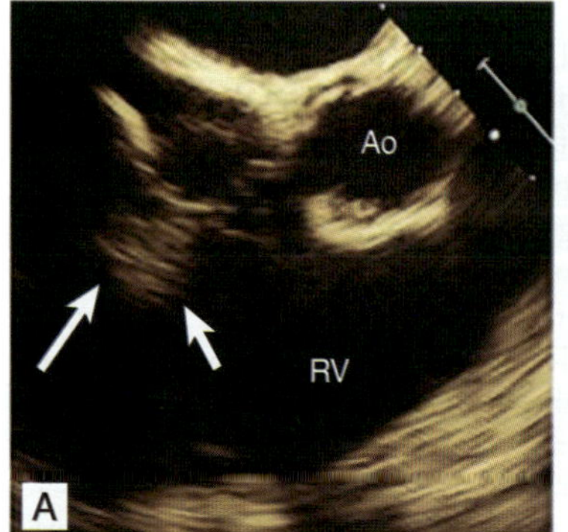

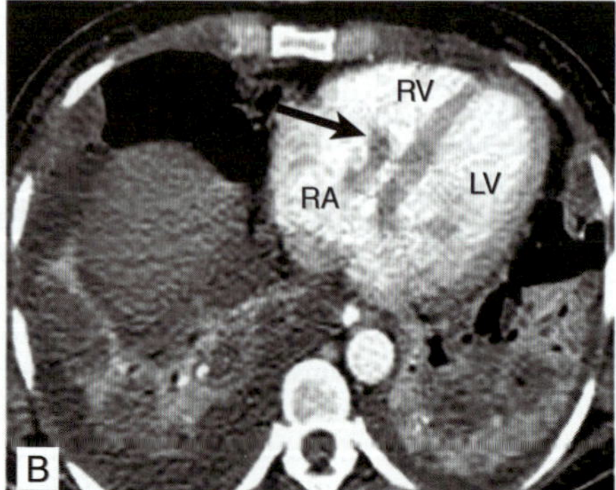

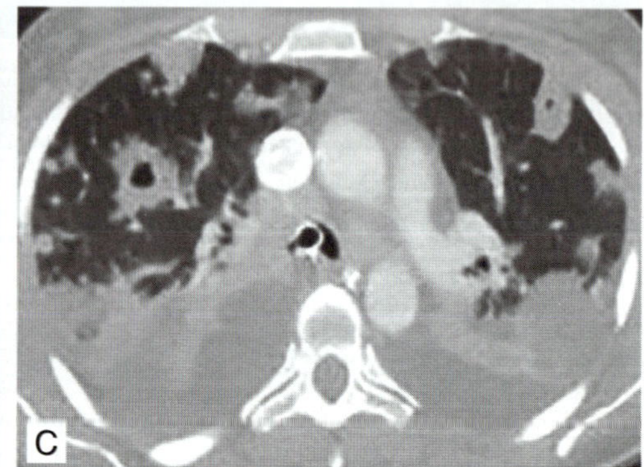

Figure 23.28 Tricuspid valve endocarditis with septic embolism. (A) TTE image showing vegetation along the tricuspid annulus (*white arrows*). (B) Mediastinal and (C) lung window images from nongated CT examination showing large vegetation at the tricuspid valve (*black arrow*). Note multiple cavitary lesions in both lungs—septic emboli. *Ao*, aorta; *LV*, left ventricle; *RA*, right atrium; *RV*, right ventricle.

Imaging of Cardiomyopathies

Cardiomyopathies refer to a diverse group of diseases of the myocardium that result in mechanical and/or electrical dysfunction. Inappropriate myocardial hypertrophy or dilation is seen, without associated hypertension, coronary artery disease, congenital heart disease, or valvular heart disease. Approximately 6.5 million people are affected with heart failure in the United States, with almost 25,000 deaths annually [1,34]. Cardiomyopathy can be either primary or secondary to other systemic diseases. Morphologically, it can be classified as hypertrophic, restrictive, dilated, arrhythmogenic, and inflammatory types, all of which can be either primary or secondary [34]. Recently a MOGE(s) classification has been proposed, which describes the morphofunctional phenotype (M), organ (O), genetics (G), etiology (E), and functional status (S) [35].

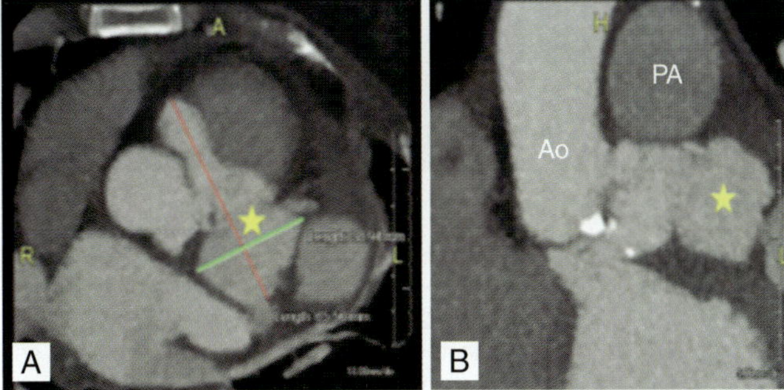

Figure 23.30 Preoperative-gated cardiac CTA in patient with aortic valve endocarditis. Axial (A) and coronal (B) images show a large irregular extraluminal contrast collection (*yellow star*) along the left cusp abutting the LM and LAD consistent with aortic root abscess and pseudoaneurysm. Patient underwent successful surgical aortic root homograft and aortic valve replacement. *Ao*, aorta; *LV*, left ventricle; *PA*, pulmonary artery.

Cardiomyopathies can clinically present in several ways, typically with heart failure, arrhythmia, SCD, or chest pain. Symptoms include dyspnea, fatigue, edema, ascites, chest pain, palpitations, and syncope. Cardiomyopathy is the underlying etiology for cardiac failure in 2–15% of patients. Imaging plays an important role in the evaluation of cardiomyopathies [36]. The specific imaging approach depends on the initial presentation. For those patients who present with heart failure, imaging is necessary to establish the diagnosis of heart failure, quantify the function (i.e., ejection fraction) and to distinguish patients who present with reduced EF from those with preserved EF [37]. The next important step is to establish the etiology of the cardiomyopathy, since the treatment strategies can vary significantly depending on the etiology [38]. Broadly, cardiomyopathies are classified as ischemic and nonischemic.

Imaging Techniques

Several imaging techniques are used in the evaluation of cardiomyopathies (Table 23.3). Chest radiograph has a limited use as an

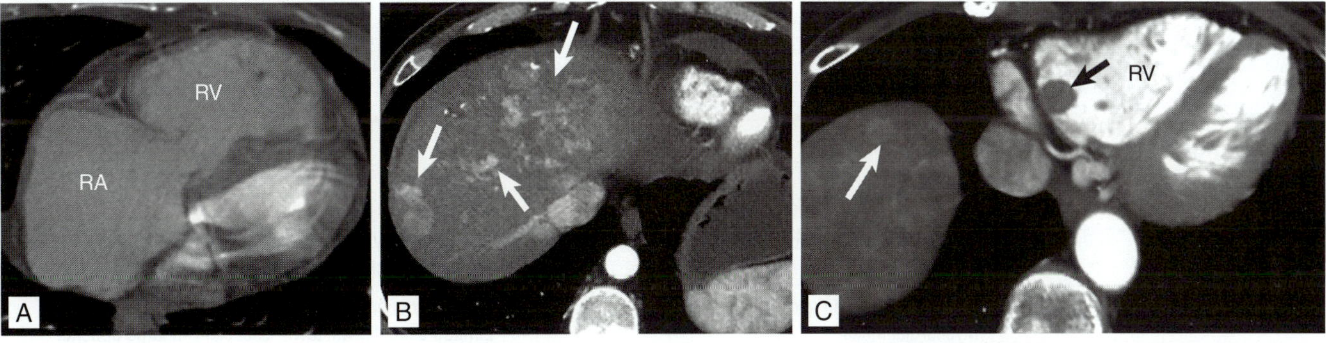

Figure 23.31 (A, B) Cardiac CTA in a patient with history of metastatic carcinoid disease to the liver demonstrating dilated right atrium and ventricle consistent with carcinoid heart disease. (C) Different patient with metastatic carcinoid disease shows enhancing nodule (118 HU) along the tricuspid valve within the right ventricle in early arterial enhanced phase imaging (*black arrow*) consistent with a metastatic deposit. There are multiple enhancing liver metastasis (*white arrow*). *RA*, right atrium; *RV*, right ventricle.

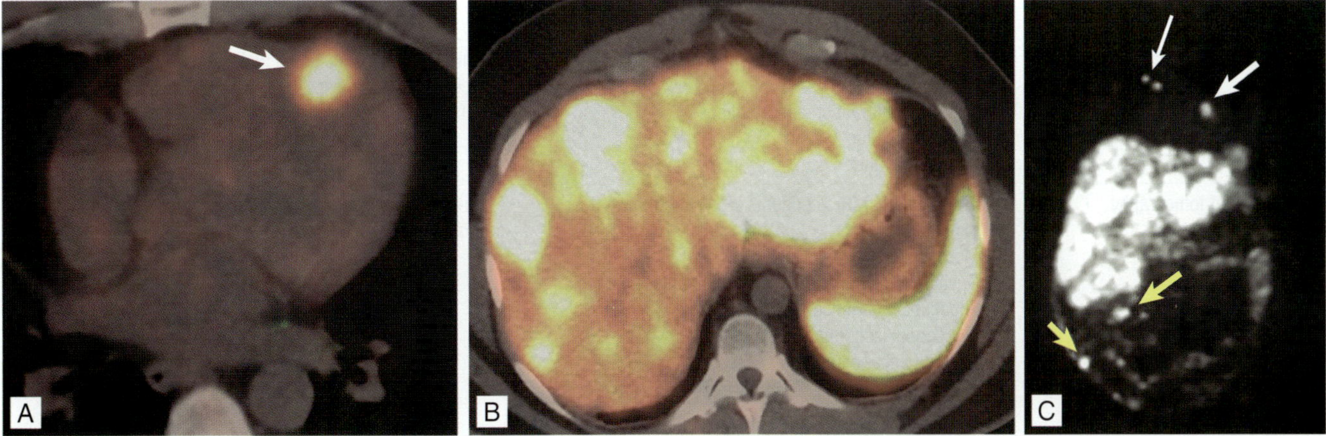

Figure 23.32 (A–C) A 43-year-old male with metastatic neuroendocrine tumor presents for initial staging and subsequent treatment planning. PET CT DOTATATE performed shows increased tracer activity in interventricular septum thick (*thick white arrow* in A,C), several nodes in the mediastinum (*thin white arrow* C), liver metastases (B,C) and peritoneal nodules (*yellow arrows* C).

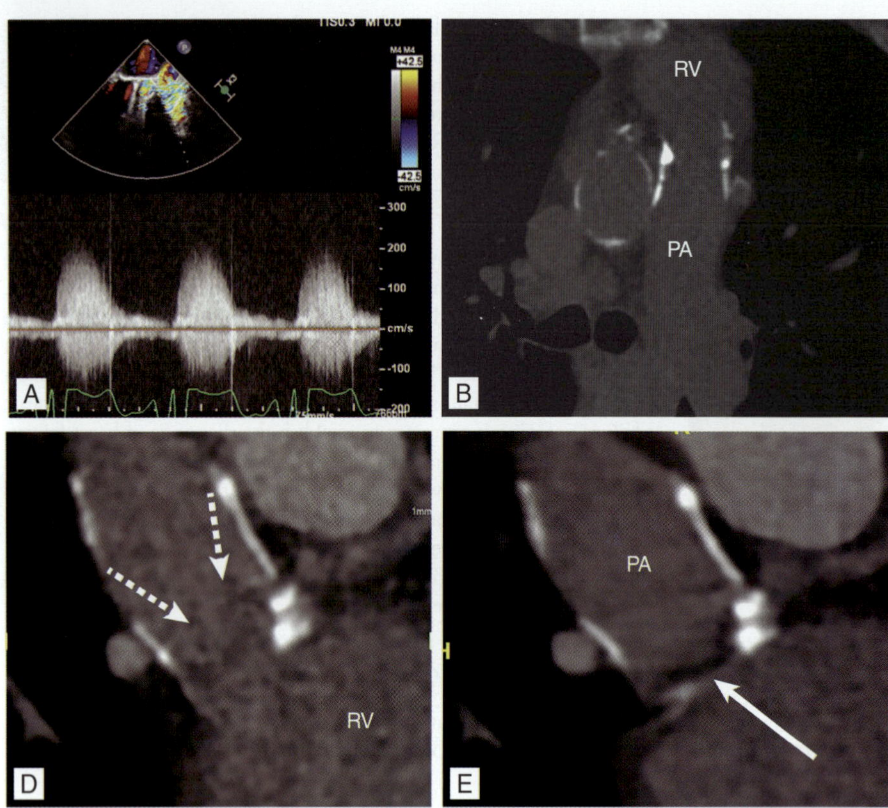

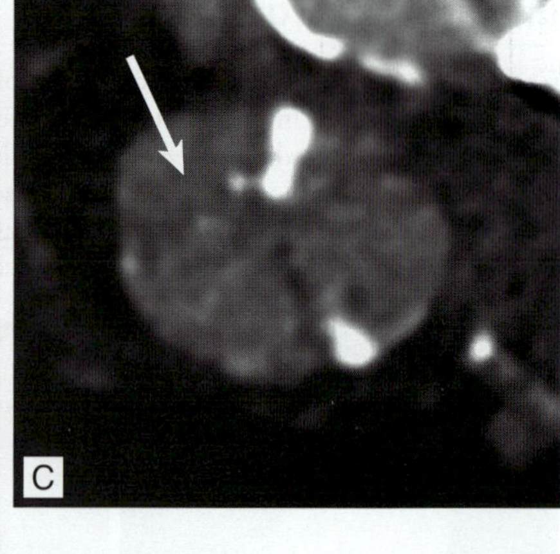

Figure 23.33 (A) TTE image in a 57-year-old patient with history of Hodgkin's disease and radiation to mediastinum at 6 years of age, showing severe pulmonic stenosis with mean gradient of 15–17 mm Hg. (B) Noncontrast cardiac CT image showing severe calcifications along the RVOT and pulmonic valve annulus. (C, D, E) Retrospective-gated cardiac CT images showing leaflet thickening and calcifications (*white arrows*) and restricted opening (*dashed arrows*). *PA*, pulmonary artery; *RV*, right ventricle.

TABLE 23.3 Role of Imaging in Cardiomyopathies

Technique	Utilities	Limitations
Radiography	Evaluation of heart failure	Low sensitivity and specificity Cannot characterize abnormality
Echocardiography	Ventricular function (global, regional) and volumes Myocardial mass Regional wall motion abnormalities Diastolic function Valvular function	Operator dependence Limited acoustic windows- especially in large patients and COPD; particularly for RV and apical regions Cannot characterize cardiomyopathies
Nuclear medicine	Quantification of ventricular function Myocardial ischemia Sarcoidosis Amyloidosis	
Magnetic resonance imaging	Ventricular function (global, regional) and volumes Myocardial mass Regional wall motion abnormalities Valvular function Characterization	Contraindications including metallic devices and claustrophobia Artifacts in patients with metallic devices
Computed tomography	Alternative to MRI in patients who cannot have it or expected artifacts Morphological evaluation Qualitative global and regional ventricular function Functional quantification Myocardial ischemia Delayed enhancement	Potentially nephrotoxic iodinated contrast media Ionizing radiation
Cardiac catheterization	Hemodynamics Constrictive pericarditis Coronary arterial morphology and function	

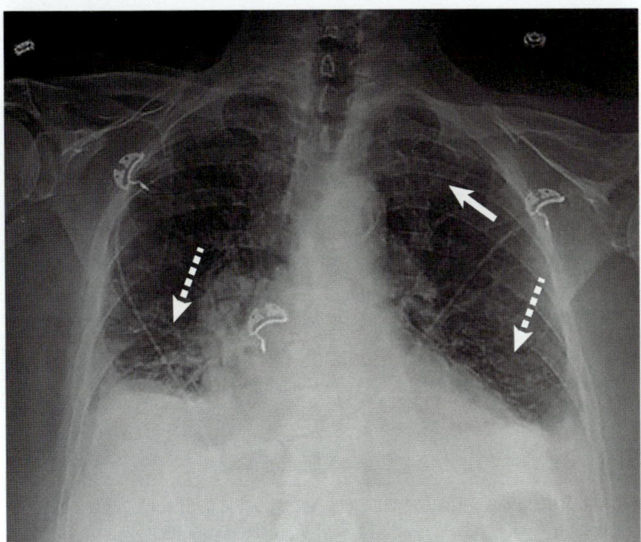

Figure 23.34 Chest radiograph of cardiomyopathy. PA chest radiograph shows enlargement of the cardiac silhouette with perihilar congestion (*dashed arrows*) and dilated veins (*white arrow*), consistent with cardiac failure.

initial imaging technique to evaluate heart failure and associated vascular abnormalities [37]. Enlargement of the cardiac silhouette may be seen in some cardiomyopathies. Heart failure manifests as pulmonary congestion, blurred margins of vessels, dilated of pulmonary veins, septal lines, pleural effusions, and alveolar opacities (Fig. 23.34). Dilated pulmonary arteries can be seen with pulmonary hypertension. Echocardiography is often the initial cross-sectional imaging technique that is used to evaluate cardiac failure and cardiomyopathy. Echocardiography provides information on ventricular function and volumes, myocardial mass, wall motion abnormalities, and valvular function. Echocardiography can also evaluate diastolic dysfunction, which is seen in the early stages of cardiac abnormalities. Using contrast improves the quantification of ventricular volumes and function. Echocardiography is widely available, portable and noninvasive, but limitations include operator dependence and limited acoustic windows which limit its ability to visualize the RV and apical regions. Echocardiography is also limited in tissue characterization [37,38].

MRI is a valuable imaging technique in the evaluation of cardiomyopathies (Tables 23.4). It can provide morphological information that is superior to echocardiography due to its ability to visualize the entire heart, including RV and LV apical and lateral regions as well as surrounding structures. MRI is considered the gold standard in the quantification of cardiac volumes and function, with high accuracy and reproducibility. In addition, MRI also has the ability to characterize tissues which helps in narrowing the specific etiology of cardiomyopathy. Using different sequences, several specific features can be extracted. Cine SSFP sequence is used to evaluate morphology and qualitative assessment of ventricular and valvular function. This sequence is also used for accurate and reproducible quantification of ventricular volumes. Cine sequence in real-time mode is used to evaluate the respiratory changes of the ventricular septum, which is useful in evaluation of constrictive pericarditis which can be clinically confused with restrictive cardiomyopathy. Strain imaging provides an evaluation of regional myocardial function, which is often deranged earlier than ejection fraction in several cardiac diseases. Parametric mapping techniques provide quantitative assessment of intrinsic myocardial properties such as T1, T2, and T2*, with the pixels color-coded based on these values. Native T1-mapping

TABLE 23.4 MRI Sequences and Utility in the Evaluation of Cardiomyopathies

Sequence	Utility
Cine steady state free precession	Morphological evaluation Global and regional function Quantification of function Qualitative valvular function
Real-time cine imaging	Pericardial function
Strain imaging	Regional myocardial function
First-pass perfusion imaging	Ischemia
Early gadolinium enhancement	Capillary hyperemia in myocarditis Microvascular obstruction in myocardial infarction
T2-weighted fat suppressed images	Myocardial edema
Late gadolinium enhancement	Characterization of cardiomyopathies based on pattern of enhancement Prognosis and risk stratification
T1 mapping	Edema, fibrosis, infiltration
T2 mapping	Edema
Extracellular volume mapping	Fibrosis, scarring
T2* images and mapping	Myocardial iron
Phase contrast	Quantification of flow and stenosis

is used for evaluation of myocardial fibrosis, edema, infiltration, and iron. T2 mapping is used for evaluation of myocardial edema, seen in acute myocarditis and MI. Extracellular volume (ECV) maps are obtained from pre- and postcontrast T1 values of the myocardium and blood pool along with hematocrit. T2* is used for evaluation of myocardial iron deposition. T2-weighted images with fat suppression are used for evaluation of myocardial edema. Following contrast, first-pass perfusion images, both at stress and rest can be used for identification of myocardial ischemia. Early gadolinium enhancement is obtained in the first few minutes after contrast administration. Abnormal enhancement in these images can be seen due to capillary hyperemia in acute myocarditis as well as in acute MI. LGE is an important sequence which allows characterization of cardiomyopathies based on the pattern of enhancement. This sequence is obtained 7–10 minutes following administration of intravenous gadolinium-based contrast media with an inversion recovery pulse. Contrast washes away from normal myocardium by this time, whereas it is retained in scar/fibrotic tissue. LGE also is a predictor of future adverse events, including the development of ventricular arrhythmia and SCD [39,40]. The salient imaging features of key cardiomyopathies and differential diagnosis for LGE of myocardium are listed in Tables 23.5A and 23.5B.

CT scan has a limited role in the evaluation of cardiomyopathies. Its main utility is in the exclusion of coronary artery disease in a patient who presents with heart failure and/or dilated cardiomyopathy. CT has high accuracy and negative predictive value in the exclusion of coronary artery disease. CT is also valuable in patients who cannot get an MRI due to contraindications including claustrophobia and metallic devices or due to expected artifacts from such devices. Using retrospective ECG-gating, that is, acquisition of data throughout the cardiac cycle, ventricular function, and volumes can be obtained with

TABLE 23.5A Salient Imaging Findings of Key Cardiomyopathies

Cardiomyopath	Key Findings
Ischemic	Regional wall motion abnormalities in vascular distribution Subendocardial or transmural perfusion defect in vascular distribution Subendocardial or transmural LGE in vascular distribution Ventricle may be dilated Global systolic dysfunction may be seen
Dilated nonischemic	Dilated ventricle Global systolic dysfunction Linear mid-myocardial LGE in the septum may be seen
Amyloidosis	Concentric ventricular thickening Biatrial enlargement Diffuse subendocardial to transmural LGE High native T1, extracellular volume
Sarcoidosis	Ventricle—May be dilated or thickened Global/regional hypokinesis Mid-myocardial/subepicardial LGE Mid-myocardial/subepicardial edema in acute phase
Hypertrophic cardiomyopathy	Classic type—Asymmetric hypertrophy of the basal ventricular septum Systolic anterior motion of the mitral valve may be seen Mitral regurgitation may be seen Left ventricular outflow tract obstruction may be present Patchy mid-myocardial, RV insertion, or diffuse LGE Elevated native T1 and ECV
Myocarditis	Global/regional hypokinesis Mid-myocardial/subepicardial LGE Mid-myocardial/subepicardial edema in acute phase Elevated T1, T2, and ECV may be seen Ventricle dilation or global systolic dysfunction may be seen Pericardial effusion may be associated
Iron deposition	Concentric thickening Dark signal of myocardium in gradient echo images Low myocardial T2* (<20 ms)
LV noncompaction	Prominent trabeculations—Trabeculated/nontrabeculated myocardial ratio at end diastole >2.3 Ventricle dilation or global systolic dysfunction may be seen
Arrhythmogenic right ventricular cardiomyopathy	Major wall motion abnormalities of the RV—Aneurysm, akinesia, dyssynchrony along with either RV dilation or RV dysfunction Fat or LGE may be seen in the RV myocardium
Stress-induced cardiomyopathy	Classic type—Apical ballooning (akinesis) with hyperkinesis of basal segments Edema may be seen in the apical segments No abnormal LGE

TABLE 23.5B Patterns of Late Gadolinium Enhancement

Pattern	Etiology
Subendocardial in vascular distribution	Myocardial infarction
Subendocardial—Diffuse	Cardiac amyloidosis Hypereosinophilic syndrome Systemic sclerosis Cardiac transplant
Mid-myocardial—Linear	Idiopathic dilated cardiomyopathy Myocarditis
Mid-myocardial—Patchy	Myocarditis Sarcoidosis Chagas disease Fabry's disease
Mid-myocardial—RV insertion points	Hypertrophic cardiomyopathy RV pressure overload
Subepicardial	Myocarditis Sarcoidosis Chagas disease Fabry's disease
Transmural	Myocardial infarction (vascular distribution) Cardiac amyloidosis Chronic/severe myocarditis Chronic/severe sarcoidosis

accuracy comparable with MRI. Regional wall motion abnormalities can also be calculated. CT can provide morphological evaluation of valves, but cannot provide quantification of valvular function. CT perfusion, both at rest and stress can be used to evaluate myocardial ischemia. CT can also be used to evaluate delayed enhancement, but this is limited by the low contrast-to-noise ratio of this technique [41].

Several scintigraphic techniques are also used in the evaluation of cardiomyopathies. Myocardial ischemia following stress and rest are evaluated either using SPECT (thallium-201, Tc-99m-sestamibi/tetrofosmin) or PET (Rb-82) techniques. Gallium-67, thallium-201, and 18F-FDG PET are useful in the evaluation of cardiac sarcoidosis. Several isotopes such as Tc-pyrophosphate, tc-DPD (3,3,0 diphosphon-1,2 propanodicarboxylic acid), I-123 serum amyloid P component, Pittsburgh compound B, and 18F-florbeapir are useful in diagnosing cardiac amyloidosis. Cardiac function can also be quantified using Tc- labeled human albumin serum or red blood radionuclide ventriculography or using SPECT with Tc-sestamibi/tetrofosmin or thallium-201 [38,42].

Cardiac catheterization is an invasive technique that provides hemodynamic information and prognostic value, particularly for the evaluation of pulmonary hypertension and constrictive pericarditis. Coronary angiography is also the gold standard in the evaluation of coronary arteries with invasive fractional flow reserve used for lesion-specific ischemia. Endomyocardial biopsy can also be performed to obtain confirmatory diagnosis [38].

Ischemic Cardiomyopathy

Most of the classification systems of cardiomyopathies exclude ischemia as a type of cardiomyopathy. However, this remains the most common cause of dilated cardiomyopathy and cardiac failure. Ischemic cardiomyopathy is secondary to coronary artery disease, which decreases blood flow to the myocardium. This can eventually culminate as MI that progress as a wavefront from subendocardium to the subepicardium. Diagnosing ischemic etiology is important, since this can be treated using medicines and

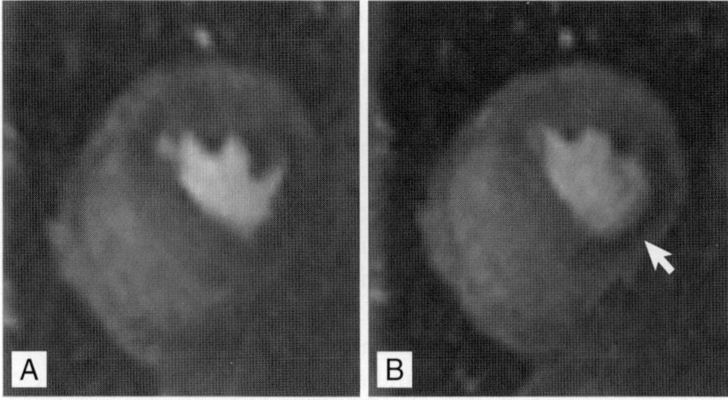

Figure 23.35 Myocardial ischemia. (A) First-pass perfusion MRI at rest shows normal perfusion of the myocardium. (B) First-pass perfusion MRI obtained after injection of IV regadenoson shows a subendocardial perfusion defect in the basal inferior wall (*arrow*), consistent with inducible ischemia.

revascularization procedures. Patients can present with symptoms of cardiac failure. Echocardiography may show ventricular dilation and global systolic dysfunction. Regional wall motion abnormalities are seen in a vascular distribution. In patients with suspected ischemic cardiomyopathy, a coronary CTA can be performed to evaluate for coronary artery disease as an etiology for cardiomyopathy. This obviates the need for an invasive angiographic procedure. On MRI, the ventricle is dilated and there may be global systolic dysfunction. Regional motion abnormalities, such as hypokinesis, akinesis, or dyskinesis are seen in a vascular distribution. For example, left anterior descending artery supplies the basal and mid anterior, anteroseptum, and most of the apical segments; the left circumflex artery supplies the lateral wall; and the right coronary artery supplies the basal and mid inferoseptum, inferior segments, and apical inferior segment. On first-pass perfusion images, myocardial ischemia is seen as a subendocardial or transmural perfusion defect on stress, but not on rest images (Figs. 23.35A–B), whereas MI is seen as perfusion defect in both stress and rest images [37]. Subendocardial to transmural LGE can be seen in patients with MI (Figs. 23.36). *If the LGE involves <50% of the myocardium thickness, the myocardium is more likely to recover function after revascularization procedure. LGE > 75% indicates that the myocardium is not viable and unlikely to recover function. LGE 50–75% is indeterminate* [43]. In acute MI, myocardial edema is seen as high signal in STIR images with elevated T2 values (>50 milliseconds) and T1 values. The edema is usually more extensive than the LGE, and the difference between the two represents the myocardium that can be salvaged with revascularization. Acute microvascular obstruction is seen as a dark filling defect within a bright scar tissue. Complications of MI can also be evaluated with MRI, including thrombus, aneurysm, pseudoaneurysm, rupture (free wall or septum), pericarditis, and mitral regurgitation. Ischemia can also be evaluated by scintigraphic techniques, including SPECT and PET-CT [44]. In ischemic cardiomyopathies, AICD is placed for prevention of SCD in New York Heart Association (NYHA) class II or III heart failure despite medical therapy and LV EF ≤ 35% of NYHA class I heart failure and LV EF ≤ 30%, at least 40 days post-MI and 90 days postrevascularization, if meaningful survival of >1 year is expected [45].

Dilated Nonischemic Cardiomyopathy

Dilated cardiomyopathy can also be idiopathic or due to toxins, familial, infections, infiltrative disorders, autoimmune diseases, metabolic abnormalities, and arrhythmias. This is characterized by dilation of the left ventricle with global systolic dysfunction (Fig. 23.37A). Typically, no regional wall motion abnormalities are seen. Note that dilation of the heart can been in other causes of cardiac failure and also with valvular regurgitation and shunts. This is usually a diagnosis of exclusion, after coronary artery disease has been excluded. In the absence of any specific etiology, it is considered to be idiopathic. Most of these cases do not have any LGE. A linear mid-myocardial enhancement can be seen, particularly in the ventricular septum (Fig. 23.37B). This is due to replacement fibrosis and associated with poor prognosis. Nevertheless, the main role of imaging, particularly MRI is to exclude coronary artery disease as a cause of dilated cardiomyopathy [36,38]. In nonischemic cardiomyopathies, AICD is placed for primary of SCD in NYHA class II or III heart failure and LV EF ≤ 35%, if meaningful survival of >1 year is expected [45]. In patients with SCD due to VT/VF or hemodynamically unstable VT or stable sustained VT, it is placed for secondary prevention [45].

Hypertrophic Cardiomyopathy

Hypertrophic cardiomyopathy is generally an inherited disease characterized by inappropriate myocardial hypertrophy. Clinical manifestations include dyspnea, syncope, arrhythmias, and

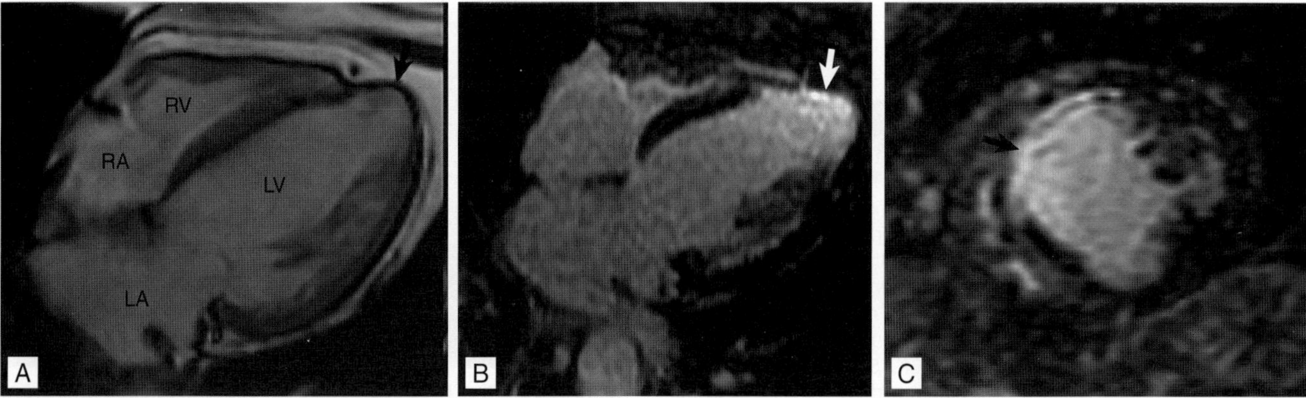

Figure 23.36 Myocardial infarction. (A) Four-chamber cine balanced steady-state free precession (b-SSFP) image shows dilation of the left ventricle with apical thinning and aneurysm (*arrow*). (B) Four-chamber postcontrast inversion recovery image shows full-thickness late gadolinium enhancement (LGE) of the LV apical region (*arrow*), consistent with an established infarction in the left anterior descending (LAD) artery territory. (C) Short-axis postcontrast inversion recovery image in the same patient shows the myocardial infarction as a full thickness late gadolinium enhancement (*arrow*). The involvement of full thickness of the myocardium makes this nonviable and will not benefit from a revascularization procedure.

SCD. *Myocardium is considered to be thickened when the end-diastolic diameter is >15 mm.* MRI is accurate in measurement of myocardial thickness and evaluation of morphology. The most common morphological type is the asymmetric basal type, in which the basal septum is hypertrophied (Fig. 23.38A). This may produce obstruction of the LVOT, which is seen as a dark jet in the LVOT (Fig. 23.38B). This obstruction provides a Venturi effect and systolic anterior motion of the mitral valve, which results in mitral regurgitation. LGE may be seen in a mid-myocardial pattern, especially in hypertrophied segments and at the insertion points of the right into left ventricle (Fig. 23.38A). MRI also shows abnormalities of the papillary muscles, which may contribute to LVOT obstruction. In the apical variant HCM, the hypertrophy involves the apical segments and there is ace-of-spade appearance of the LV cavity (Fig. 23.39A–B). This may be complicated by apical aneurysm and thrombosis. Other variants include mid-ventricle type, mass-like type, concentric and spiral types. Concentric type of HCM may be challenging to distinguish from other etiologies such as hypertension, AS, and athlete's heart. In systemic hypertension, the thickening is milder, EF can be lower, ventricle can be dilated, LGE is absent or minimal. There is increased LV wall stress and lower anteroseptal systolic strain. In AS, restricted opening of the aortic valve in systole and flow acceleration can be seen in MRI. In athlete's heart, there is mild concentric hypertrophy, with mild LV dilation (end-diastolic diameter <6.5 cm), normal EF, and no LGE. Athlete's heart also improves with 3 months of deconditioning. For suspected HCM, CT is performed if MRI is contraindicated and can provide similar morphological information. Echocardiography is often the first imaging technique used, and it provides morphological and hemodynamic information [38,46]. Risk factors for SCD in HCM include: cardiac arrest or sustained ventricular arrhythmias, family history of SCD, cardiac arrest, or sustained ventricular arrhythmia attributable to HCM and syncope caused by arrhythmias or LVOT obstruction. MRI also provides evaluation of indicators of SCD including—massive LV hypertrophy ≥30 mm in any segment, LV systolic dysfunction (EF < 50%), apical aneurysm, and extensive LGE, involving multiple segments or ≥15% of total myocardial mass [47]. These features typically warrant the placement of an ICD.

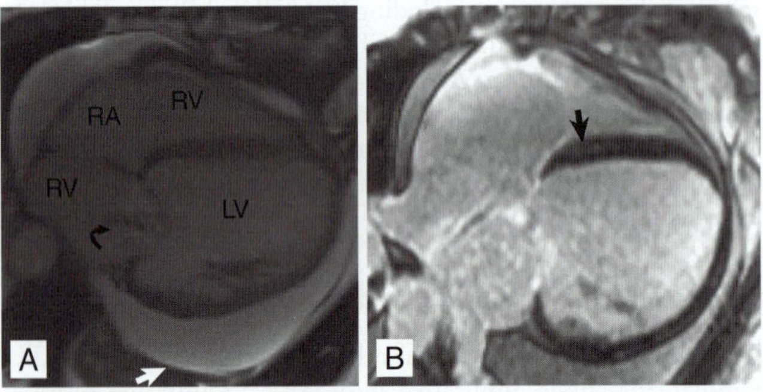

Figure 23.37 Dilated nonischemic cardiomyopathy. (A) Four-chamber cine SSFP image shows severe dilation of the left ventricle (LV). There was also severe global systolic dysfunction with ejection fraction of 21%. There is also moderate central mitral regurgitation (*curved arrow*) secondary to mitral annular dilation from LV enlargement. Note also the large circumferential pericardial effusion (*straight arrow*). (B) Four-chamber postcontrast inversion recovery image shows a linear mid-myocardial LGE in the ventricular septum (*arrow*), which is frequently seen in nonischemic dilated cardiomyopathy.

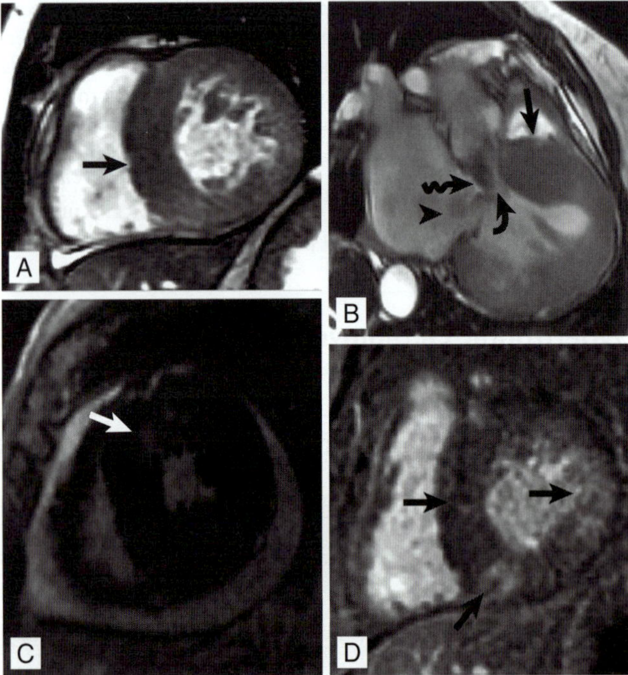

Figure 23.38 Hypertrophic cardiomyopathy. (A) Short-axis cine SSFP MRI shows asymmetric thickening of the ventricular septum (*arrow*). (B) Three-chamber SFFP image in the same patient shows the asymmetric thickening of the basal septum (*arrow*). There is also flow acceleration in the left ventricular outflow tract (*curved arrow*), indicative of obstruction. There is systolic anterior motion of the mitral valve (*serpiginous arrow*) and posteriorly directed mitral regurgitation (*arrowhead*). (C) Short-axis postcontrast inversion recovery image shows a focal, patchy mid-myocardial LGE in the basal anteroseptum at the site of RV insertion (*arrow*), consistent with hypertrophic cardiomyopathy. (D) Short-axis postcontrast inversion recovery image in another patient shows extensive patchy mid-myocardial LGE throughout the myocardium (*arrows*).

Myocarditis

Myocarditis is inflammation of the myocardium, usually secondary to infection, but can also be due to toxins, drugs, or idiopathic etiologies. This can manifest either in acute, subacute, or chronic fashion. Acute myocarditis presents similar to acute MI, with chest pain, ECG abnormalities, and elevated cardiac enzymes.

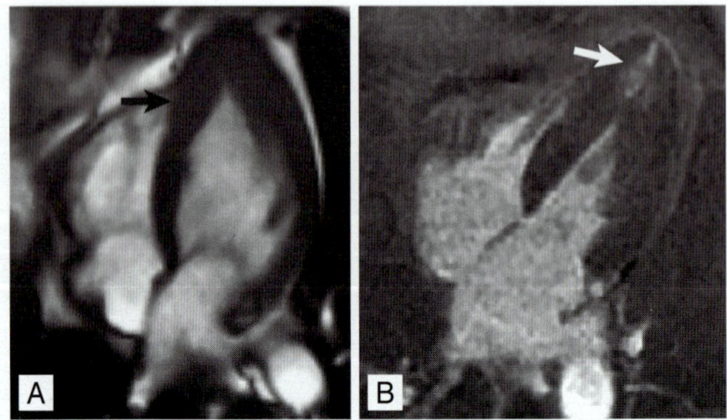

Figure 23.39 Apical hypertrophic cardiomyopathy. (A) Four-chamber cine SSFP shows hypertrophy of the apical myocardial segments (*arrow*), consistent with apical hypertrophic cardiomyopathy. (B) Four-chamber postcontrast inversion recovery image shows a patchy area of LGE in the apical myocardium (*arrow*).

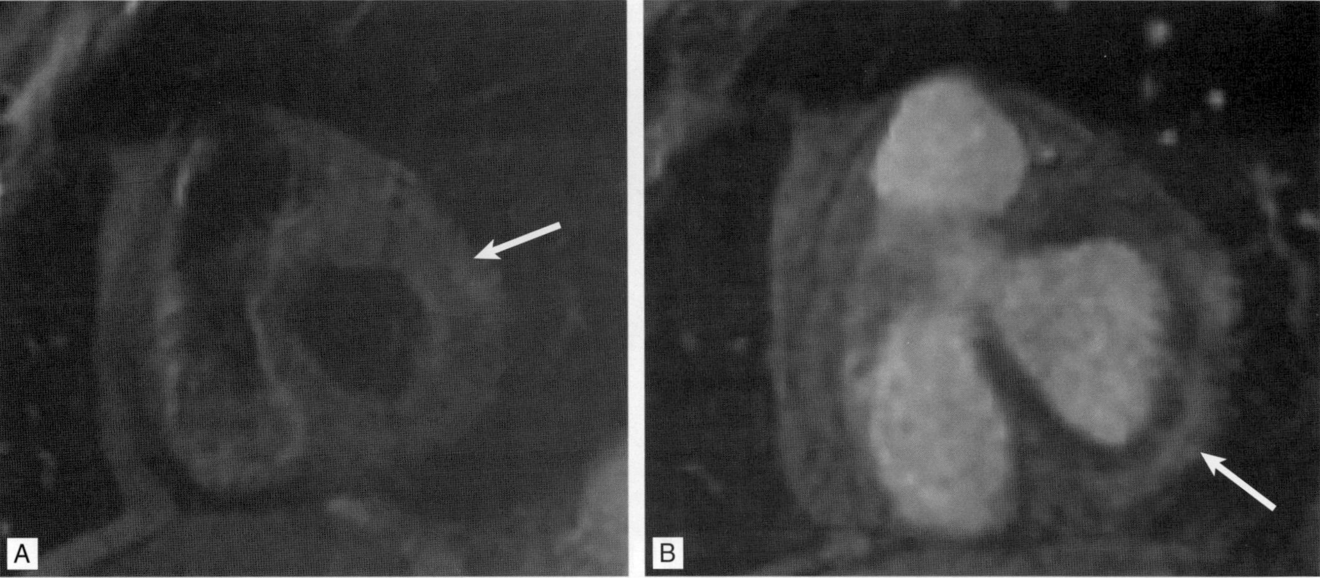

Figure 23.40 Acute myocarditis. (A) Short-axis triple inversion recovery black blood image shows a focus of high signal in the basal anterolateral wall (*arrow*), consistent with myocardial edema. (B) Short-axis postcontrast image in the same patient shows subepicardial late gadolinium enhancement in the basal lateral wall (*arrow*), consistent with acute myocarditis.

Myocarditis can also present with heart failure, cardiac arrhythmia, and SCD. On MRI, global systolic dysfunction or regional wall motion abnormalities can be seen. In acute myocarditis, edema is seen as high signal on T2-weighted images (Fig. 23.40A) and high native T1 and T2 values. Subepicardial or mid-myocardial LGE can be seen (Fig. 23.40B). Pericardial effusion and inflammation can be associated. The diagnosis of acute myocarditis is based on 2018 Lake Louise criteria based on presence of at least one T1-based criterion (high T1 values, ECV, or LGE) and one T2-based criterion (high T2 signal, high T2 values) [48]. Chronic myocarditis does not have myocardial edema, but LGE may be present.

Sarcoidosis

Cardiac sarcoidosis is characterized by the presence of noncaseating granulomas, seen in 5–50% of patients with systemic sarcoidosis. This can either manifest acutely similar to acute myocarditis or in the chronic stage with conduction abnormalities such as heart block. In the acute phase, the imaging features are similar to that of myocarditis, with wall thickening, myocardial edema (high T2 signal, high T2 values) and occasionally granulomas. Global systolic dysfunction and regional wall motion abnormalities may be seen. LGE is seen in a mid-myocardial or subepicardial distribution (Fig. 23.41B). In the chronic stages,

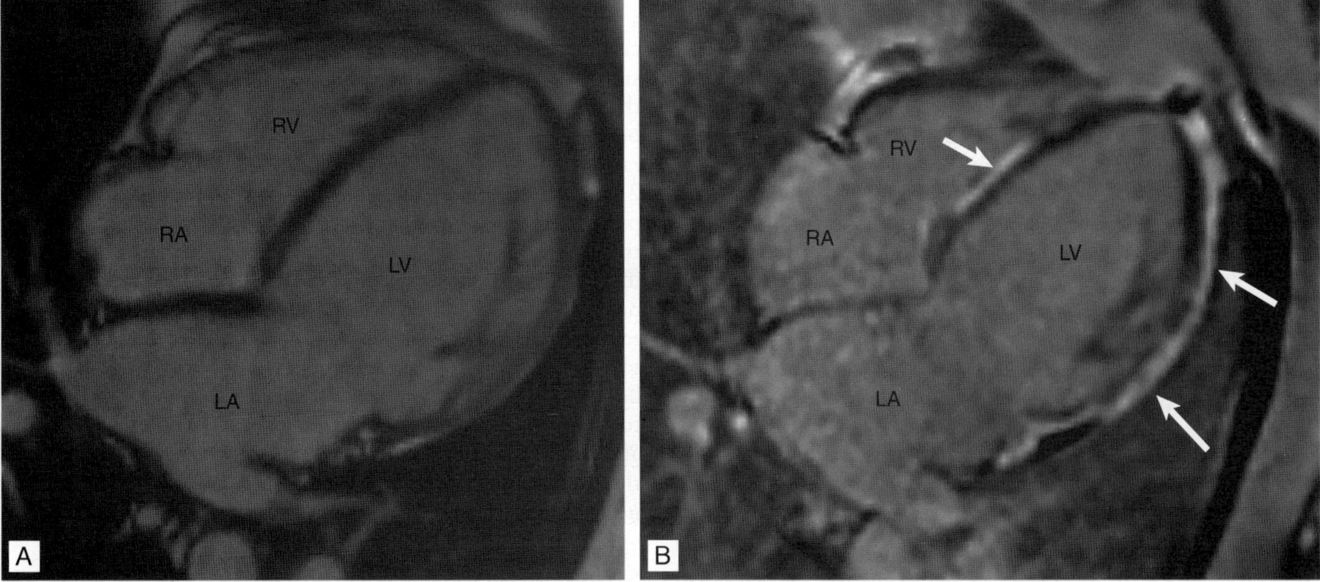

Figure 23.41 Sarcoidosis. (A) Four-chamber cine SSFP image shows severely dilated left ventricle (LV). (B) Four-chamber-contrast inversion recovery image demonstrate extensive subepicardial late gadolinium enhancement (*arrows*), indicative of cardiac sarcoidosis in this patient with systemic sarcoidosis.

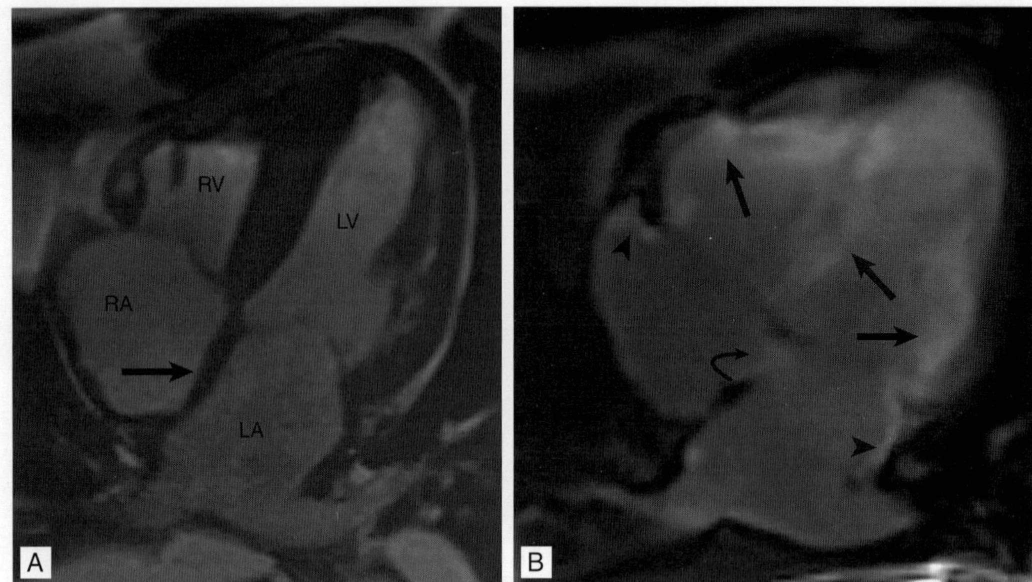

Figure 23.42 Cardiac amyloidosis. (A) Four-chamber cine SSFP image shows mild concentric thickening of the ventricles. There is also mild thickening of the atrial wall and interatrial septum (*arrow*). Bilateral pleural effusions are also partially visualized. (B) Four-chamber postcontrast inversion recovery image shows extensive late gadolinium enhancement of the myocardium of the ventricles (*straight arrows*). In addition, there is also enhancement of the atrial walls (*arrowheads*) and interatrial septum (*curved arrow*). These imaging findings are classic for cardiac amyloidosis.

the myocardium can be thinned with associated wall motion abnormalities (Fig. 23.41A). LGE may be subepicardial or mid-myocardial, but occasionally in burnt out stage, can be transmural. Sarcoidosis features can be seen in other systems, particularly in the lungs and mediastinum [39,49].

Amyloidosis

Cardiac amyloidosis is characterized by deposition of β-pleated proteins in the myocardium. It is typically of the light chain, AL type, or transthyretin type. It can clinically present with heart failure or arrhythmia. On echocardiography, concentric thickening and a speckled pattern can be seen. Abnormal longitudinal strain is seen in the apical region. On MRI, concentric thickening of the ventricles as well as the atria and interatrial septum is seen (Fig. 23.42A). Biatrial enlargement can be seen (Fig. 23.42A). Diffuse subendocardial LGE progressing to transmural enhancement is seen in the ventricles as well as the atria and interatrial septum (Fig. 23.42B). The blood pool appears dark due to rapid washout of contrast resulting from excessive ECV throughout the body. High native T1 values and ECV are seen due to the infiltration. Global systolic function can be normal or reduced. Scintigraphic techniques such as Tc-99m pyrophosphate and methylene diphosphonate can be used to diagnose transthyretin type of amyloidosis [38,39,50].

Siderotic Cardiomyopathy

Siderotic cardiomyopathy is characterized by excess deposition of iron in the myocardium, seen in hemochromatosis, sickle cell disease, and thalassemia. It is important to diagnose this entity early, since chelation therapy can prevent the development of heart failure and improve the overall outcome. Multiecho gradient echo images, that is, gradient echo images with different echo times (TE) are necessary to make this diagnosis. In these images, the myocardium with iron deposition appears darker than normal myocardium (Fig. 23.43). This can be quantified by drawing a region of interest in the ventricular septum and plotting the signal intensity against TE values. Curve fit for T2* decay provides the myocardial T2* value, which is usually around 33 milliseconds. Myocardial T2* <20 milliseconds is considered to be iron deposition, whereas T2* <10 milliseconds is considered severe iron deposition. Native T1 values are low in these patients. In advanced cases, LV dilation, global systolic dysfunction, and mid-myocardial LGE may be seen [38,51].

Left Ventricular Noncompaction

LV noncompaction is an uncommon cardiomyopathy caused by persistence of embryonic ventricular sinusoids, resulting in a spongy, noncompacted myocardium. Clinical presentation can be with heart failure, thromboembolism, arrhythmia, or sudden death. On MRI, there are prominent trabeculations in the LV cavity, usually involving the apical region. These trabeculations are considered abnormal when the end-diastolic ratio of noncompacted to compacted myocardium is >2.3 (Fig. 23.44). Occasionally diagnosis can be challenging, especially in patients with dilated cardiomyopathy who have prominent trabeculations. In addition, prominent trabeculations are seen in a large number of normal people. In challenging cases diagnosis can be suggested when the trabecular mass >15 g/m^2, ratio of trabecular to myocardial mass >20–25%, involvement of basal segments and one segment with ratio >3.0. LGE can be seen in the trabeculations, although this may be challenging to evaluate. Complications include heart failure, arrhythmia, and thrombus. The RV may be involved and is diagnosed when the thickness of the noncompacted RV is >75% of total thickness [52].

Stress-Induced Cardiomyopathy

Stress-induced cardiomyopathy, also called Takostubo cardiomyopathy or apical ballooning syndrome, is more common in

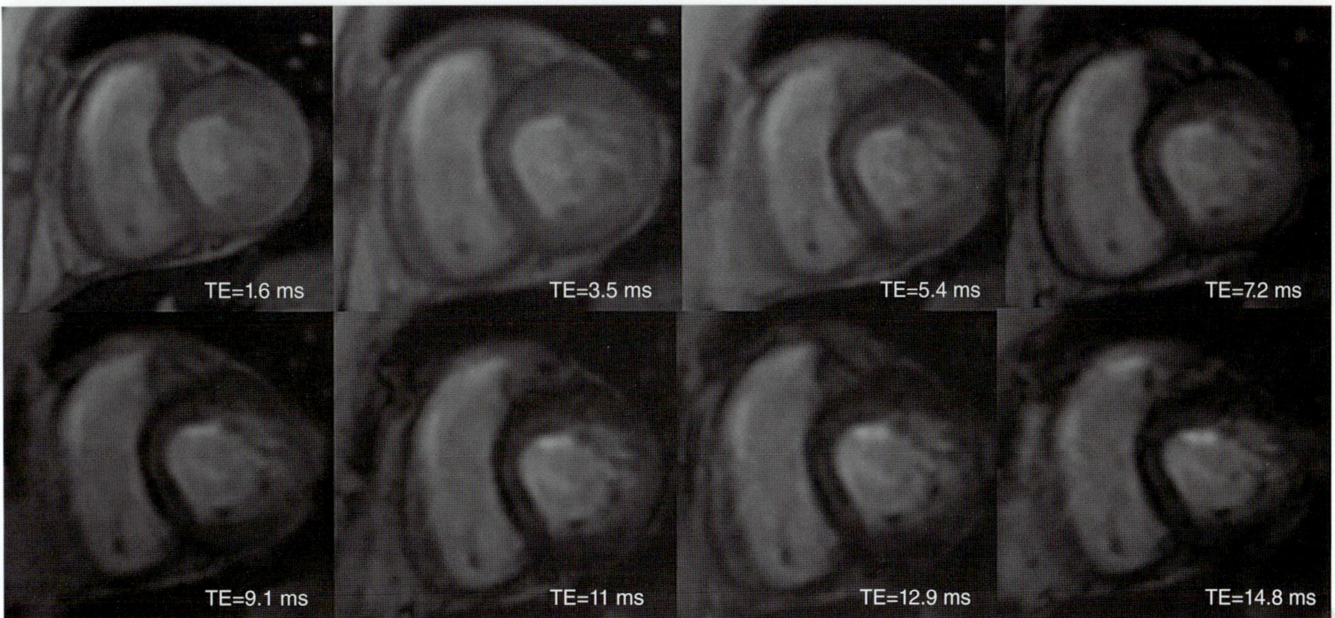

Figure 23.43 Siderotic cardiomyopathy. Short-axis gradient-echo images obtained at progressively increasing echo times (TE) shows that the myocardial signal progressively decreases and appears dark at longer TE, consistent with myocardial iron deposition. The myocardial T2* value was 12 milliseconds (Normal >20 milliseconds).

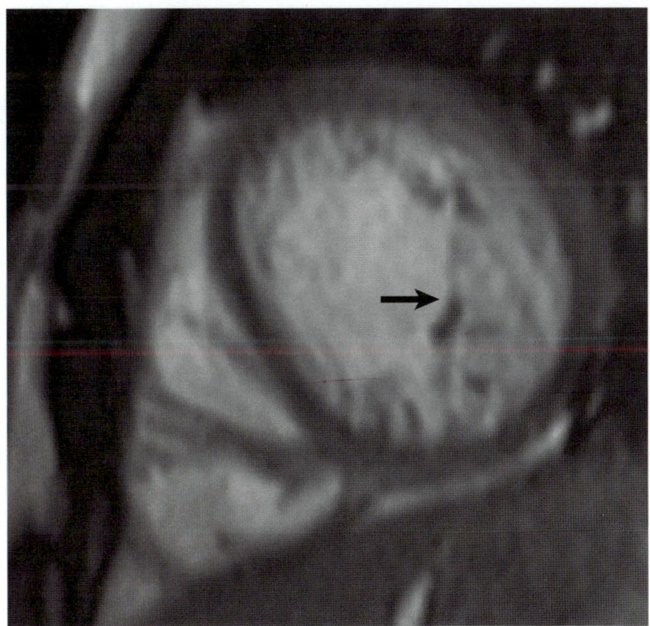

Figure 23.44 Left ventricular noncompaction. Short-axis cine SSFP image shows prominent trabeculations in the left ventricular apex (*arrow*), consistent with LV noncompaction. The ratio of noncompacted to compacted myocardium in end-diastole was 4.1.

postmenopausal women. It classically presents with a transient and reversible cardiac failure following a major stressful event. Clinical presentation is often similar to acute MI, with chest pain, ECG abnormalities, and elevated enzymes, but there is no coronary artery disease. Echocardiography and MRI show the classical wall motion abnormalities of akinesis or ballooning of the mid and apical segments and hyperkinesis of the basal segments in a nonvascular distribution (Fig. 23.45A–B). Myocardial edema may be seen, but there is typically no LGE. Follow-up imaging usually reveals resolution of the cardiac failure. In the reverse type, akinesis is seen in the basal segments with hyperkinesis of the apical segments [53].

Arrhythmogenic Right Ventricular Cardiomyopathy

Arrhythmogenic right ventricular cardiomyopathy (ARVD) is an inherited, autosomal dominant disorder characterized by fibrofatty replacement of the RV myocardium. Clinically this presents with arrhythmia, SCD, or heart failure. The diagnosis is made using 2010 ARVD Task Force criteria, which has family history, pathology, ECG depolarization, ECG repolarization, and RV wall motion abnormalities. On MRI, major RV motion abnormalities such as aneurysm, akinesis, dyskinesis, and dysynchronous contraction can be seen with either low RVEF (<40%) or dilated RV (end-diastolic volume index ≥110 mL/m^2 in men; ≥100 mL/m^2 in women) is a major criterion for ARVD (Figs. 23.46A–B). RV EF in the 40–45% range and mildly dilated RV (end-diastolic volume index 100–110 mL/m^2 in men, 90–100 mL/m^2 in women) is a minor criterion for ARVD. Fat and LGE may be seen in the RV myocardium (Figs. 23.46B–C), but are not necessary for diagnosis. LV changes are seen in 76% of ARVD patients, with some having a dominant LV disease. In the LV-dominant form, LGE is seen often in the septum, whereas it is seen in the inferior and lateral LV walls in the RV-dominant form [36,54].

Storage Disorders

Cardiomyopathies are seen in storage disorders, including glycogen storage, lysosomal storage, and mitochondrial diseases. Anderson–Fabry disease is caused by α-galactosidase deficiency, which results in accumulation of glycosphingolipid. Concentric LV thickening and regional wall motion abnormalities can be

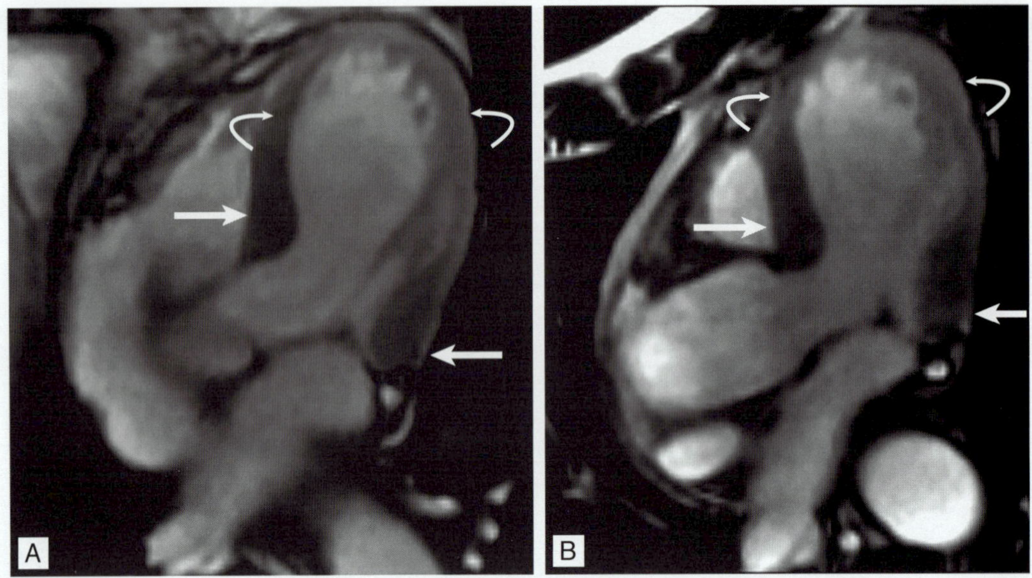

Figure 23.45 Stress-induced cardiomyopathy. (A) Four-chamber and (B) three-chamber cine SSFP images show ballooning and thinning of the apical segments (*curved arrows*) with normal thickness of the basal segments (*straight arrows*). Note also the presence of high signal edema in the apical segments (*curved arrows*).

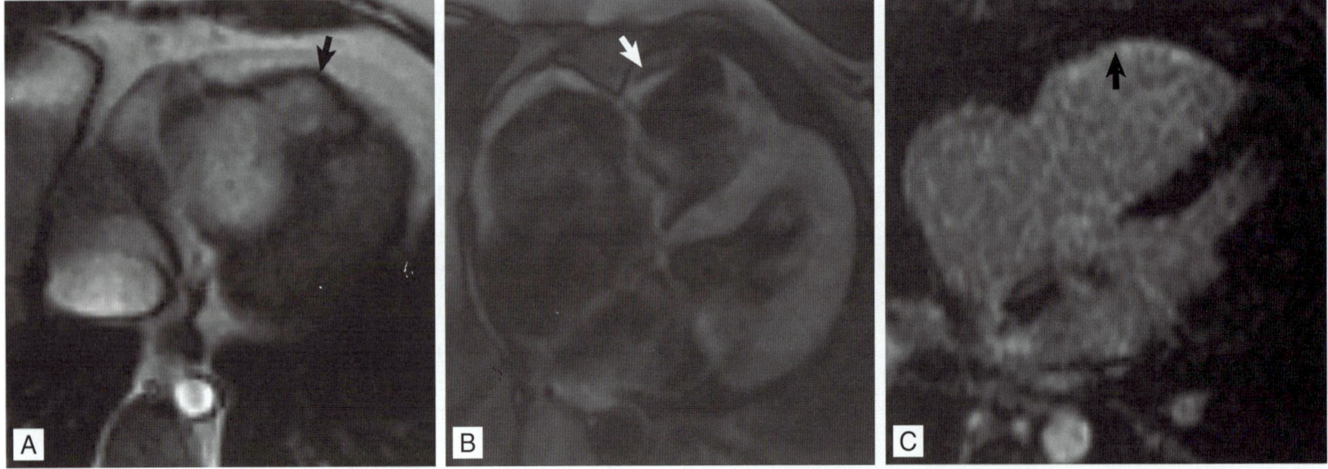

Figure 23.46 Arrhythmogenic right ventricular cardiomyopathy. (A) Axial cine-SSFP image shows a focal outpouching of the RV apical region (*arrow*). This patient also had mild RV systolic dysfunction (EF, 39%), which fulfills the criteria for ARVD. (B) Axial fat saturated black-blood double inversion recovery image shows the presence of fat within the RV myocardium (*arrow*). (C) Axial postcontrast inversion recovery image shows mild subendocardial late gadolinium enhancement (*arrow*) of the RV myocardium.

seen. Native T1 values are low due to the presence of sphingolipid. High T1 and ECV can be seen with fibrosis. LGE is typically seen in the basal inferolateral wall in a mid-myocardial or subepicardial distribution (Figs. 23.47A–B) [55]. Danon disease is a lysosomal storage disorder due to mutation of lysosomal associated protein-2, which also manifests with concentric LV thickening, cardiac failure, and arrhythmia. LGE is usually seen in a mid-myocardial distribution, typically sparing the ventricular septum.

Cardiac involvement is also seen in muscular dystrophies including Duchenne's, Becker, Emery Dreifuss, and myotonic dystrophy. MRI is used to diagnose cardiac involvement. Dilated ventricles, global or regional systolic dysfunction, mid-myocardial to subepicardial LGE and noncompacted myocardium may be seen. Abnormal strain and elevated T1 and ECV may be seen [56].

Other Cardiomyopathies

Chemotherapy cardiotoxicity is seen with agents such as anthracyclines, tyrosine kinase inhibitors, interferon, and trastuzumab. It is diagnosed when there is a reduction of EF >10% or a reduction of EF >5% in symptomatic individuals in patients who are on chemotherapy. Early diagnosis of this entity can be made with abnormal myocardial strain, increased LV mass, high signal in T2-w images, high T1, T2, and ECV values. LGE in mid-myocardial to subepicardial distribution can be seen [57].

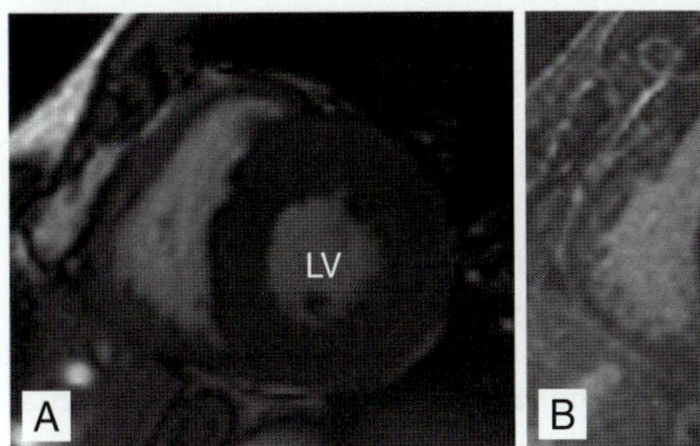

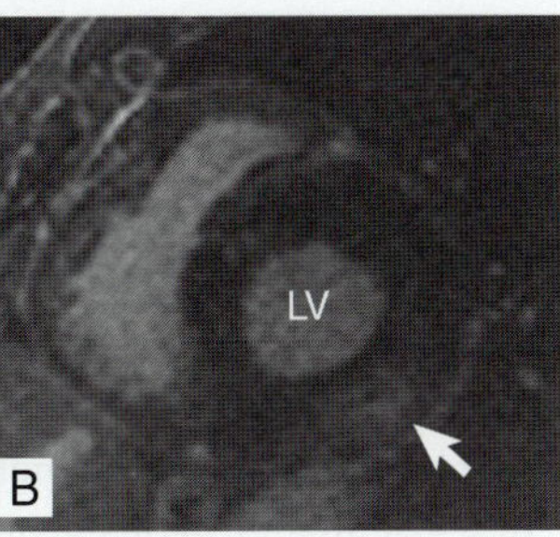

Figure 23.47 Fabry Anderson disease. (A) Short-axis SSFP image shows concentric left ventricle hypertrophy. (B) Short-axis postcontrast image shows late mid-myocardial Gd enhancement in the mid inferolateral wall, a typical site of enhancement seen in these patients. It has been hypothesized that cardiac involvement might predispose to subclinical myocarditis leading to tissue injury, or it could impair myocardial resistance to physical stress that is most prominent in the inferolateral wall of the LV.

Peripartum cardiomyopathy is seen in late stages of pregnancy or in the first 5 months after pregnancy. LGE can be seen in subepicardial to mid-myocardial distribution.

Chagas disease is caused by the parasite, *Trypanosoma cruzi*, which is endemic in South and Central America. Cardiac involvement may present with heart failure, arrhythmia, sudden death, and thromboembolism. Global systolic dysfunction, regional wall motion abnormalities, LV dilation, aneurysm, and thrombus may be seen. LGE is commonly seen, typically in apical and basal inferolateral segments, either in a subendocardial, transmural, mid-myocardial, or subepicardial pattern [58].

Endomyocardial fibrosis is the most common cause of restrictive cardiomyopathy worldwide, which is a spectrum of hypereosinophilic syndrome. This has necrotic, thrombotic, and fibrotic phases. Apical thickening may be seen. A three-layered pattern of LGE may be seen, with an inner layer of dark thrombus, middle layer of subendocardial enhancement from fibrosis, and outer dark layer of normal myocardium.

Scleroderma may show linear mid-myocardial LGE, either in the septum or LV free wall [38].

Cardiac Tumors

Cardiac masses are rare and can be divided as neoplastic versus nonneoplastic. The neoplastic lesions can be primary or secondary tumors (Table 23.6). The primary tumors of the heart are rare with necropsy incidence of only 0.05% while the secondary tumors are much more common, seen in 1% of postmortem examinations [59].

Up to 90% of primary cardiac tumors are benign and can arise from the myocardium or the pericardium [60]. The secondary cardiac tumors are much more common and are mostly malignant [61]. In an autopsy series, metastatic involvement of heart is seen in up to one in five patients dying from cancer [59–63].

Clinical Presentations

Cardiac tumors may be asymptomatic and found incidentally during evaluation of an unrelated problem or can be symptomatic. Symptoms include dyspnea, chest discomfort, syncope or presyncope and can be due to mass effect on the myocardial function or blood flow, arrhythmias, interference with heart valves causing stenosis or regurgitation or due to pericardial involvement leading to effusion or even tamponade. Tumors may also present due to embolic events either due to pulmonary thromboembolism from right chamber masses or systemic thromboembolism from left-sided chamber masses [62,64]. Lastly, there can be systemic manifestation in the form of constitutional symptoms such as fever, fatigue, arthralgia, weight loss, and paraneoplastic syndromes.

TABLE 23.6 Cardiac Masses

Benign	Malignant	Tumor-Like Masses
Myxoma	Metastasis	Thrombus, vegetation
Lipoma	Sarcoma (angiosarcoma, liomyosarcoma, rhabdomyosarcoma, undifferentiated sarcoma, osteosarcoma, malignant fibrous histiocytoma)	Prominent crista terminalis
Papillary fibroelastoma	Primary cardiac lymphoma	Lipomatous hypertrophy of IAS
Fibroma	Mesothelioma	Caseous necrosis of mitral annular calcification
Rhabdomyoma		
Hemangioma		
Paraganglioma		
Teratoma		

Goals of imaging in patients with suspected cardiac mass are

1. to establish if a cardiac tumor is present or not,
2. determine location of the mass in the heart,
3. characterization of the mass to determine if it is benign or malignant, and
4. evaluate effect of the mass on the adjacent structures.

Echocardiography is often the first technique as it is widely available, noninvasive and can be done bedside. It can easily identify and locate the mass in a cardiac chamber, determine its mobility and obstructive effect on adjacent valve. Echo can also determine if the myocardium or pericardium is involved. When TTE evaluation is limited due to poor acoustic window, TEE though invasive usually provides excellent evaluation of a cardiac mass.

Cardiac MRI is often the second technique of choice to evaluate cardiac mass. In addition to determining its location, mobility, and obstructive effects on valves, MR can also characterize a mass using T1-, T2-weighted, and postcontrast imaging (Table 23.7) [65]. CMRI is limited by its less wide availability, long exam time, claustrophobia, and inability to scan due to an incompatible cardiac hardware. Cardiac CT is an excellent technique with high spatial and temporal resolution, widely available and fast which can be performed in patients with cardiac hardware. In clinical practice, due to their complementary nature often more than one technique is used to evaluate a suspected cardiac mass.

TABLE 23.7 MR Tissue Characteristics of Common Cardiac Tumors

Cardiac Tumor	T1	T2	Postcontrast (Delayed Enhancement)
Myxoma	Isointense	High	Heterogenous
Lipoma	High	High	None
Fibroma	Isointense	Low	Yes
Angiosarcoma	Heterogenous	Heterogenous	Heterogenous
Lymphoma	Isointense	Isointense	Minimal to none
Metastasis	Low (melanoma: high)	High	Heterogenous

Cardiac Myxoma

The most common benign primary cardiac tumor derived from mesenchymal cell precursors. Most commonly found in the left atrium though can also occur in the right atrium and rarely in the ventricles and great vessels (Figs. 23.48 and 23.49) [66]. In the left atrium, they are most commonly attached by a stalk to the interatrial septum near the fossa ovalis. The right atrial myxoma is more common in children. The majority of these tumors occur in women and mean-age at diagnosis is 50s. Tumors vary in size from 1 to 15 cm in diameter [66].

Morphologically, two types of myxomas are described: polypoid and papillary. The polypoid myxomas when large enough can prolapse into the mitral valve thereby causing mitral stenosis symptoms. The papillary variety is more often associated with embolic phenomena [67,68]. Rarely, constitutional symptoms including fever, fatigue, and weight loss have been described. In approximately 7% of patients, cardiac myxomas can occur in association with multiple endocrine neoplasia and hyperpigmentation of skin (lentiginosis syndrome); also known as Carney complex [66,69], not to be confused with *Carney's triad* (gastrointestinal stromal tumors, pulmonary chondroma, and extra adrenal paraganglioma) or *Carney Statakis syndrome* (GISTs and paragangliomas; Box 23.20).

On echocardiography, seen as variable echogenicity mobile mass in the left atrium attached by a stalk along the interatrial septum near the fossa ovalis (Fig. 23.48A–B). On CT they are often low attenuating masses attached to the interatrial septum with smooth or slightly irregular surface (Fig. 23.49). In up to 15% of patients, these masses are calcified and calcification is more commonly seen in the right atrial myxomas [65,66,68]. These tumors often demonstrate heterogeneous enhancement only recognized on delayed CT images [70]. On cardiac MR, the tumors demonstrate heterogeneous signal intensity on T1- and T2-weighted images due to the presence of grading amount of hemorrhagic, myxoid, necrotic, and ossific tissue. There is often patchy delayed enhancement after gadolinium administration (Figs. 23.48C–F) [65,68,71]. Depending on their location, these tumors can prolapse into the left or RV in diastole. Myxoma can be confused with thrombus (Figs. 23.50 and 23.51) and the common distinguishing features are listed in Table 23.8.

Complete surgical resection has best long-term outcome with very low operative mortality [72]. After resection, annual

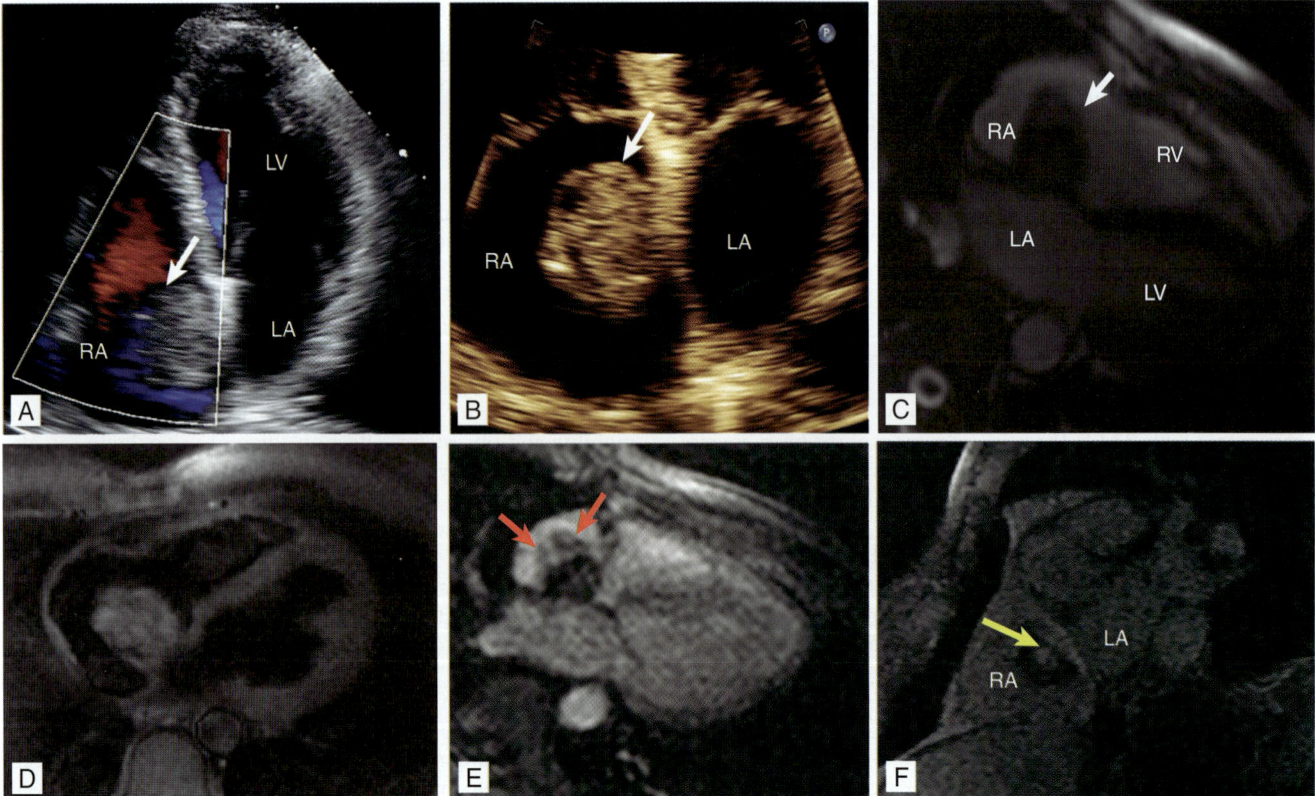

Figure 23.48 RA myxoma. (A, B) Echocardiogram four-chamber view shows a large slightly heterogeneous mass in the right atrium attached to the interatrial septum. (C–F) Four-chamber bright blood gradient echo, triple inversion, postcontrast first pass and delayed images of cardiac MR confirm the echo findings and also shows vascularity in the tumor in first pass images (*red arrow*) and enhancement on delayed images (*yellow arrow*). *LA*, left atrium; *LV*, left ventricle; *RA*, right atrium; *RV*, right ventricle.

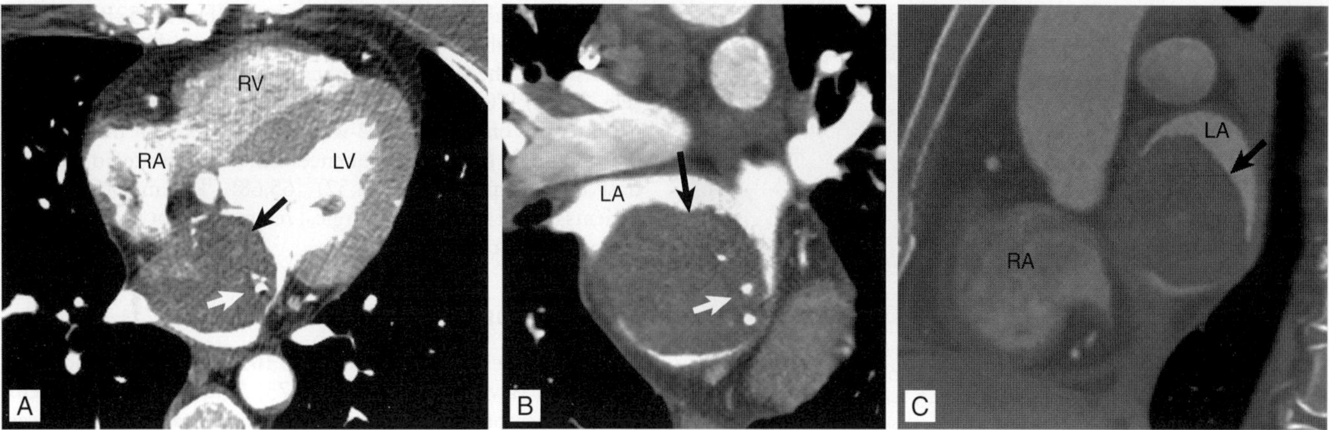

Figure 23.49 LA myxoma. (A–C) Axial, coronal, and sagittal contrast-enhanced CT images show a large well-circumscribed homogenous mass (*black arrows*) seen in the left atrium attached to the interatrial septum with calcification (*white arrows*). *LA*, left atrium; *LV*, left ventricle; *RA*, right atrium; *RV*, right ventricle.

BOX 23.20 Carney Complex

- Autosomal dominant
- Multiple myxomas; often diagnosed at earlier age, increased tendency to recur
- Schwannomas
- Endocrine tumors
- Pigmented lentigines and blue nevi on face, trunk, and neck

follow-up with TTE is often recommended for at least 4 years since these tumors can reoccur, often at the site of original primary tumor.

Lipoma

Second most common primary benign tumor of the heart, occurs commonly in middle aged and older patients [61]. Fifty percent of lipomas originate from the subendocardial layer and the rest

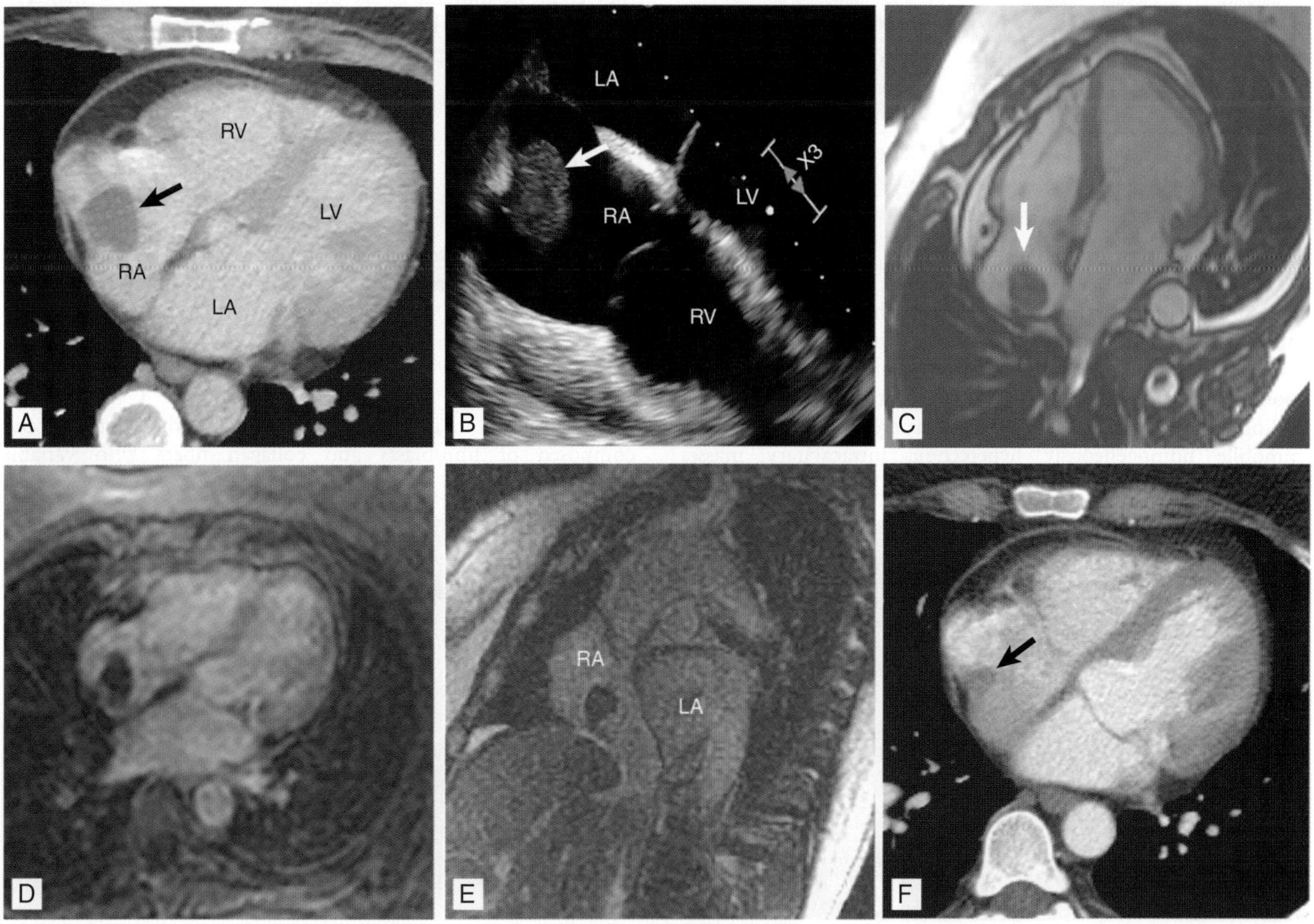

Figure 23.50 RA thrombus. A well-defined filling defect is seen in the right atrium (*arrows*) on contrast enhanced CT (A) and four-chamber view of echocardiogram (B). The mass was isointense to myocardium on T1-weighted images (C) and there was no vascularity seen during postcontrast first pass images (D) and no delayed enhancement seen on short-axis atrial view of CMR (E). Patient was anticoagulated and the mass decreased significantly in 2 months on follow-up CT (F). *LA*, left atrium; *LV*, left ventricle; *RA*, right atrium; *RV*, right ventricle.

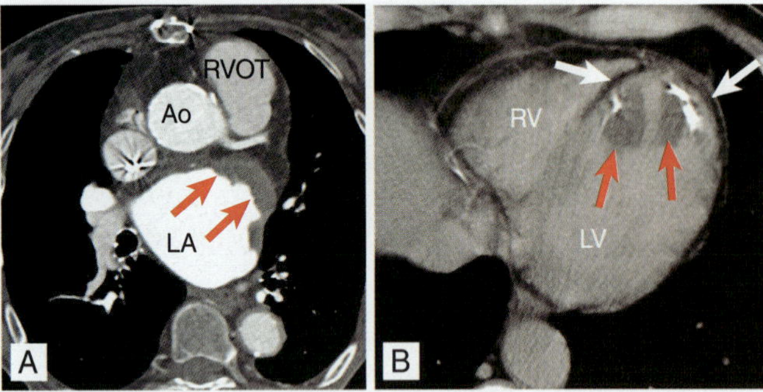

Figure 23.51 (A) Left atrial eccentric filling defect (*arrows*) due to thrombus in this patient after Maze procedure. (B) LV apical thrombus with calcification (*red arrows*) in patient with prior LAD territory MI as shown by thinned and hypodense distal interventricular septum and apical walls (*white arrows*). *Ao*, aorta; *LA*, left atrium; *LV*, left ventricle; *RA*, right atrium; *RVOT*, right ventricle outflow tract.

TABLE 23.8 Differentiating Features of Myxoma and Thrombus

Feature	Myoma	Thrombus
Location	LA>RA>Ventricles, along IAS in LA	LA, LAA>LV Apex>RA>RV
Clinical information	Asymptomatic or SOB, mitral stenosis features in LA myxoma	H/O atrial fibrillation, prior MI, indwelling central line
Mobility	Often mobile, can be sessile	Often immobile, can be mobile
Calcification	May be present, more common in RA myxoma	Rare, can be seen in chromic organized thrombus
Postcontrast enhancement (MR, CT)	Variable; slight to moderate	None except in chronic vascularized thrombi

from subepicardial or myocardial tissue. The majority of these patients are asymptomatic but can present with arrhythmia or less commonly valvular dysfunction. Very rarely the subepicardial lipomas can cause extrinsic mass effect on the coronary arteries leading to myocardial ischemia. Lipomas are well-circumscribed immobile homogeneously hyperechoic intracavitary masses without any calcification as seen on echo (Fig. 23.52B). On CT they are nonenhancing homogeneous masses with fat CT attenuation within the cardiac chamber, myocardium, or pericardium (Fig. 23.52) [70]. On MR, lipomas have homogeneous high signal intensity on T1- and T2-weighted images with marked suppression on fat saturation sequences and demonstrate no postcontrast enhancement (Fig. 23.52) [65,68]. The majority of the patients do not require any surgical removal except in rare severely symptomatic scenarios.

Fibroelastoma

Papillary fibroelastomas account for 10% of cardiac tumors and 75% of all valvular neoplasms [68,73]. Their appearance resembles sea anemones with fronds around a central core. These cardiac tumors are often found on the valvular endocardium of the aortic and mitral valve, followed by tricuspid valve. They often are found on the downstream side of the valve, for example, LV side of the mitral valve or aortic side of the aortic valve. Patients often are middle age and present with embolic cerebral complications leading to imaging evaluation.

Fibroelastoma is composed of collagen and elastic fibers with endothelial covering and a short connective tissue pedicle. Thrombus may form on their surface and can embolize. On echo they are small in size, echogenic tumors attached on the endothelial surface with slightly stippled margins due to finger-like projections causing vibration at the tumor blood interface. Due to its small size, TEE is more sensitive than TTE (Fig. 23.53B–C). On cardiac CT, they could be difficult to see due to their small size. When seen they appear as focal low attenuating nodules attached to the valve and often better appreciated on a retrospective-gated study (Fig. 23.53A, D). These tumors are isointense on T1-weighted and hypointense on T2-weighted images due to high fibrous content, although rarely they can have hyperintense signal (Fig. 23.54) [65,68].

Surgical excision is often reserved for large mobile left-sided fibroelastomas. The right-sided papillary fibroelastomas are usually managed medically unless there is risk of paradoxical embolism due to intracardiac shunts or significant hemodynamically obstructing lesions.

Fibroma

More common in infants, often located in the ventricles and composed of fibroblasts and collagen fibers with variable

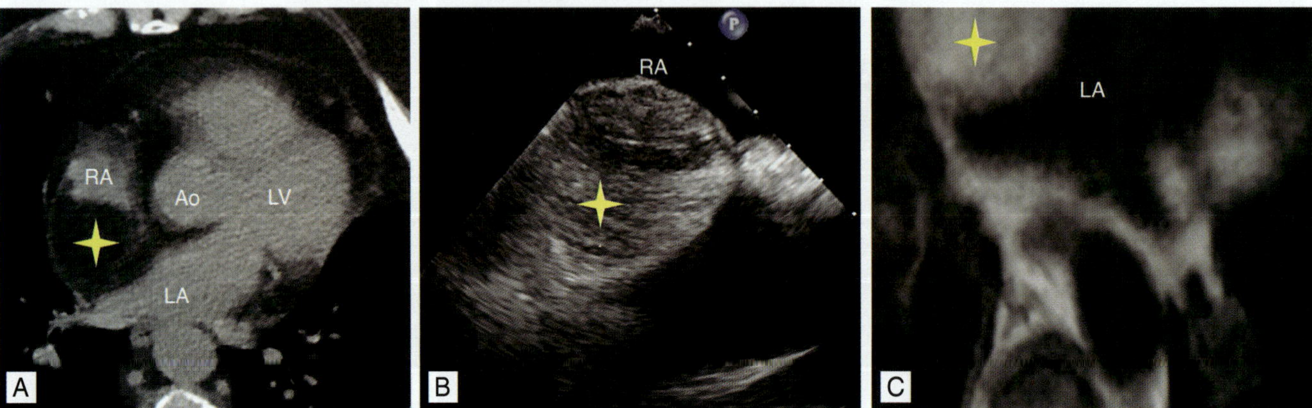

Figure 23.52 Right atrial lipoma. (A–C) Contrast-enhanced CT axial images (A) show a well-circumscribed noncalcified low-density mass in the right atrium (*star*) with CT attenuation values of fat. (B) Lipomas are hyperechoic heterogenous masses on echo. (C) They are hyperintense on T1 MR images (*star*). These can be associated with interatrial septal fatty hypertrophy. The majority of these lesions are benign and do not need resection. *Ao*, aorta; *LA*, left atrium; *LV*, left ventricle; *RA*, right atrium.

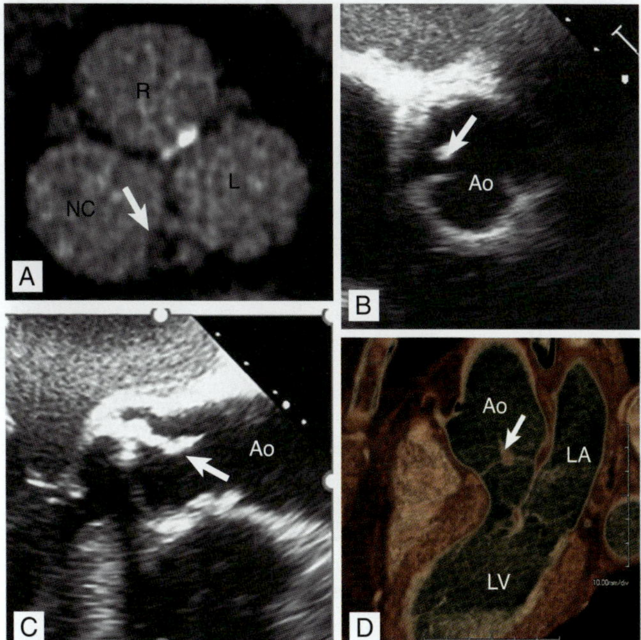

Figure 23.53 Fibroelastoma. (A–D) A small nodular lesion is seen attached to the noncoronary aortic valve cusp (*white arrow*, A, D) in aortic valve short-axis and LVOT 3D images. It is seen as echogenic nodule attached to aortic leaflet on echo (B, C *white arrow*). Fibroelastomas are attached along the aortic side of the valve and have tendency to form thrombus and embolize; therefore, they are resected as surgical cure. *Ao*, Aorta; *L*, left; *LA*, left atrium; *LV*, left ventricle; *NC*, noncoronary; *R*, right.

calcification. They are most commonly located in the left ventricle myocardium or interventricular septum and can mimic hypertrophic cardiomyopathy. These patients can present with ventricular arrhythmia and sudden death due to conduction disturbances. Larger tumor can also produce shortness of breath from obstruction to blood flow [74,75]. These tumors can be associated with familial adenomatous polyposis and Gorlin syndrome and in these scenarios, the fibromas are often located in the atria.

On echo they are well demarcated solid echogenic masses within the myocardium ranging in size from 1 to 10 cm with central calcifications. Cardiac CT clearly shows their intramyocardial location with homogeneously low attenuation and often with central calcification (Fig. 23.55) [70]. There is often minimal or no contrast enhancement. Fibromas are isointense compared to the myocardium on T1-weighted images and are also homogeneous and hypo intense on T2-weighted images with minimal to no postcontrast enhancement [65,68,71,75]. Since these tumors do not regress spontaneously and there is increased risk of arrhythmia and sudden death, surgical resection is recommended regardless of the symptoms.

Rhabdomyoma

Most common primary cardiac tumor in first year of life [75]. Often they are multiple and involve apical ventricles. They can cause arrhythmias and rarely flow obstruction leading to heart failure symptoms. Their association is well known in patients with tuberous sclerosis [68,76–78]. On echo they are small well

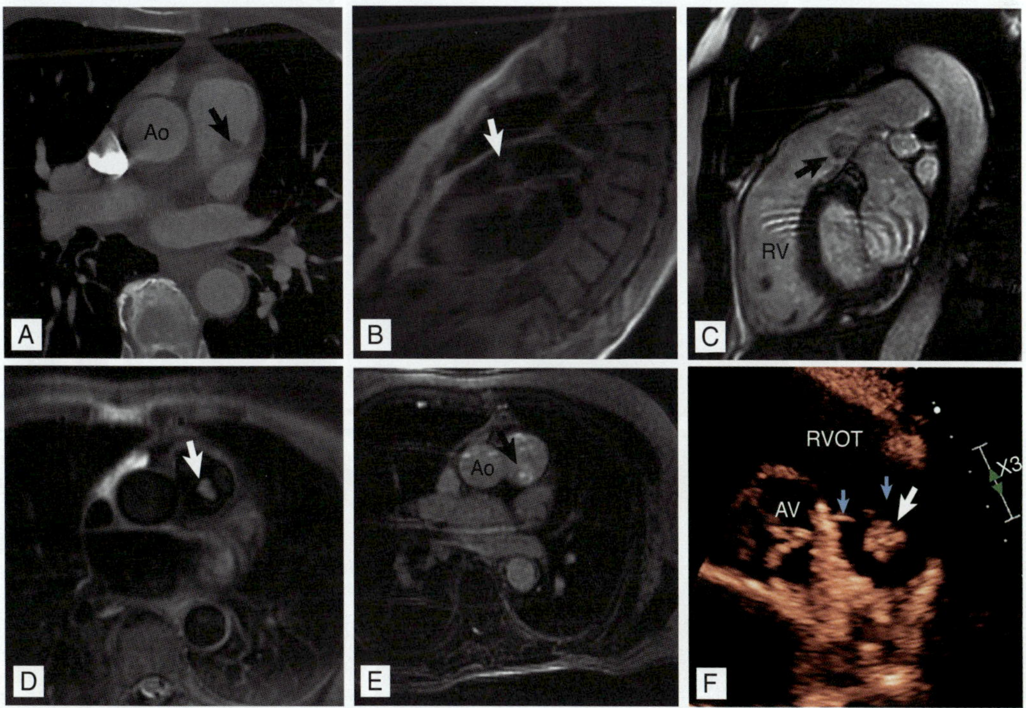

Figure 23.54 Pulmonary valve fibroelastomas are rare as seen in this patient. (A) On axial contrast-enhanced CT, there is a small slightly irregular filling defect in the main pulmonary artery near the pulmonary valve (*arrow*). (B) On oblique sagittal T1-weighted image, the nodule is isointense to the myocardium and is slightly hyperintense on balanced turbo field echo (bTFE) sequence (C) and hyperintense on triple inversion fat suppressed sequence (D). The lesion was very mobile on cine images. There is contrast enhancement seen on delayed postcontrast images (E, *arrow*). Better seen in transesophageal echocardiogram (F) as pedunculated mobile nodule (*white arrow*) attached to the pulmonary valves (*small blue arrows*). *Ao*, aorta; *AV*, aortic valve; *RV*, right ventricle; *RVOT*, right ventricular outflow tract.

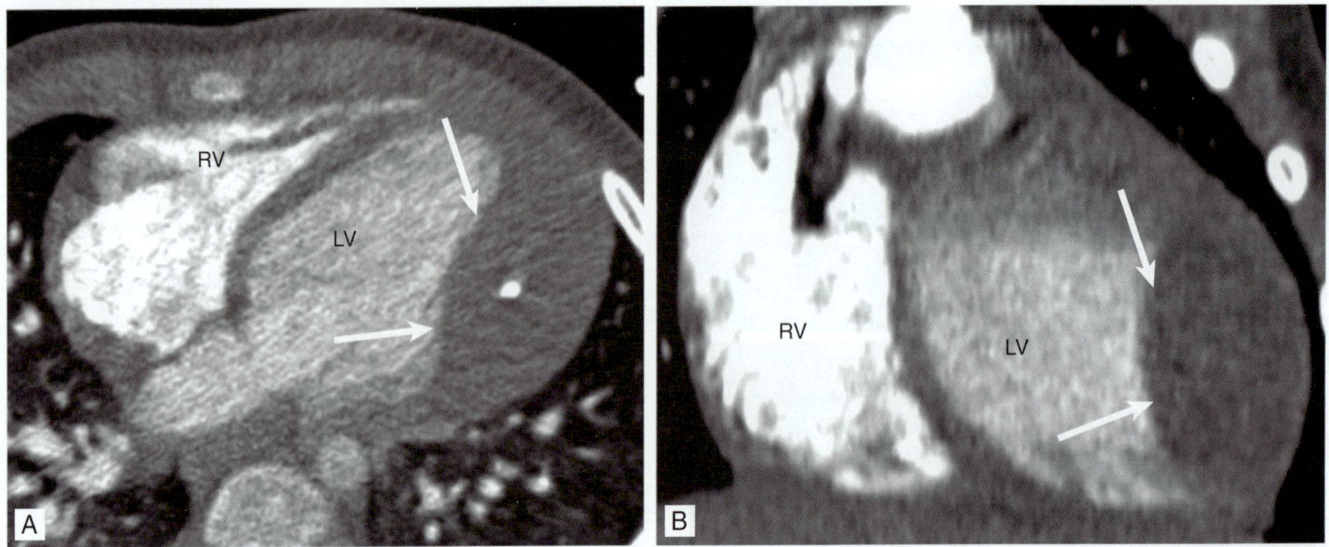

Figure 23.55 LV fibroma. (A–B) In contrast-enhanced axial and coronal reformat CT, a well-defined homogenous hypodense mass is seen in the left ventricle lateral wall myocardium (*arrows*) with focal calcification. Most commonly seen in infants or young children and resection is recommended as these tumors do not spontaneously regress unlike rhabdomyomas. *LV*, left ventricle; *RV*, right ventricle.

circumscribed multiple nodules or one large pedunculated mass in the cardiac cavity. Occasionally, they appear as lobulated homogeneous and hyperechogenic masses within the myocardium due to myocardial embedding. Cardiac CT shows intramural location with homogeneous low attenuation and variable intracavitary extension. Presence of multiple masses and association with tuberous sclerosis distinguish rhabdomyomas from myomas. These tumors are isointense on T1-weighted images and hyperintense compared to the myocardium on T2-weighted images without any postcontrast delayed enhancement (Figs. 23.56A, B) [65,76–78]. Tuberous sclerosis has high association with renal angiomyolipomas, fat containing hepatic

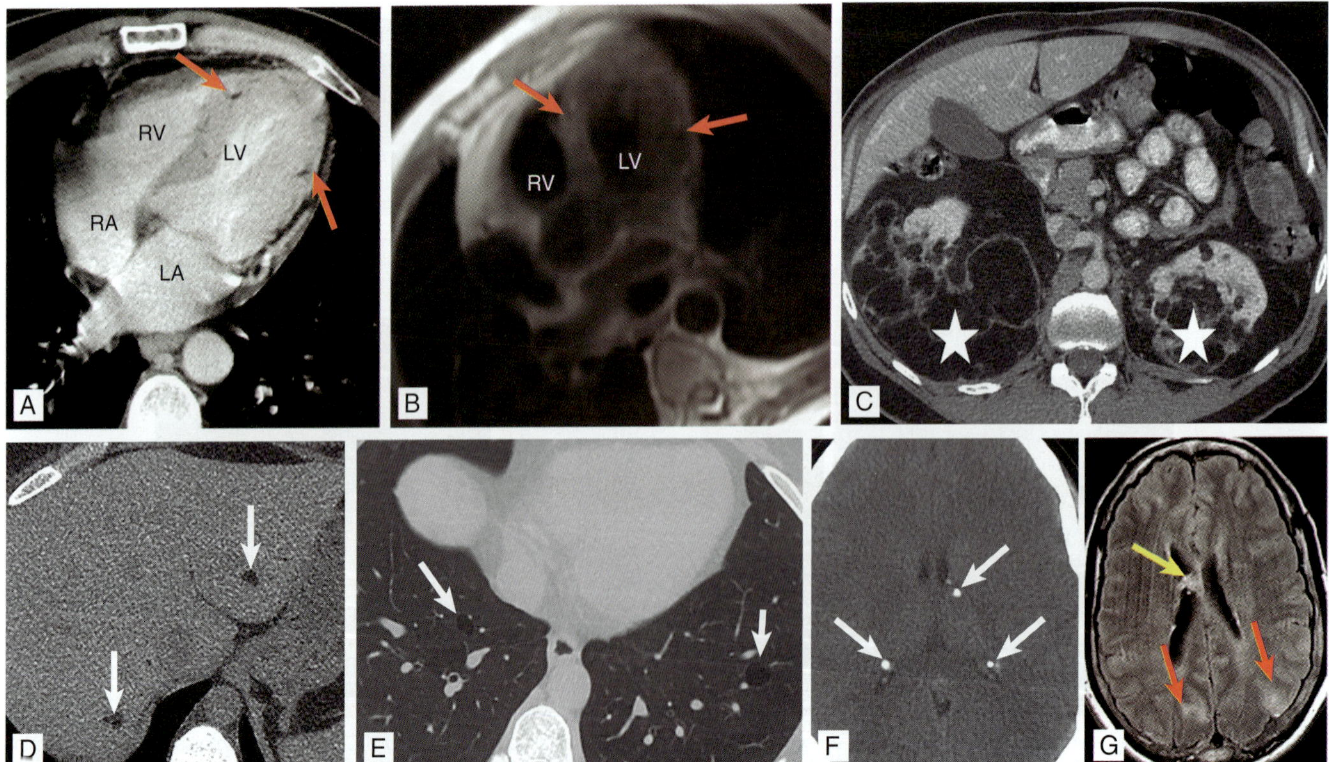

Figure 23.56 Tuberous sclerosis. (A) On CT, the hamartomatous lesions are low or fat density intramyocardial areas lesions of variable sizes in LV myocardium (*red arrows*). (B) On T2-weighted MR, these lesions are hyperintense (*red arrows*). There is high association of renal angiomyolipomas (C, *stars*), liver fat containing angiomyolipomas (D), lung cysts (E), subependymal calcified tubers on brain CT (F), subcortical hyperintense signal (*red arrows*) and subependymal giant cell astrocytoma (*yellow arrow*) on FLAIR brain MR (G). *LA*, left atrium; *LV*, left ventricle; *RV*, right ventricle.

angiomyolipomas, cystic lesions in lungs, subependymal calcified tubers seen on head CT, subcortical hyperintensities and subependymal giant cell astrocytoma as seen on brain MRI (Figs. 23.56C–G). In comparison to fibromas, rhabdomyomas are known for undergoing spontaneous regression. Therefore, usually patients are followed with serial echocardiography and surgery is only reserved for patients with arrhythmia or heart failure.

Cardiac Paraganglioma

Rare neuroendocrine tumor originates from the paragangliomic cells located in relation to the atria, great arteries, as well as coronary arteries. They most often arise in the visceral paraganglia of the left atrium in its posterior wall or roof and less commonly in the interatrial septum, coronary arteries, or aortic root [68,79]. Secretory paragangliomas lead to excessive sympathetic discharge causing Cushing-like symptoms such as palpitations, flushing, and tremors. A large size of the tumor can cause dyspnea and angina due to compression of the cardiac chamber or coronary artery. On echo, paragangliomas are usually broad-based hyperechoic masses. On cardiac CT, they are heterogeneous masses with low attenuation and often marked enhancement on contrast-enhanced imaging due to high vascularity [70,79]. On MR, these tumors show high signal intensity on T2-weighted images and often demonstrate FDG uptake on PET imaging (Fig. 23.57) [65,71,79]. Surgical resection is difficult but is recommended if possible with preoperative medical optimization to prevent catecholamine surges. Preoperative transcatheter embolization can also be helpful in highly vascular tumors.

Malignant

Secondary Cardiac Tumors

Cardiac metastases are 20–40 times more common than primary cardiac tumors [59–61,63]. Pericardial involvement is more common than myocardial metastasis (Fig. 23.61). Melanoma has the greatest propensity for cardiac involvement; however, cancer of the lung, breast, kidney, and esophagus are the most common carcinomas that metastasize to the heart. Cardiac metastases can occur either hematogeneously, via lymphatics, transvenous spread via IVC, or direct invasion (Figs. 23.58–23.61).

Clinically, myocardial metastases can present with conduction disturbances or rarely from coronary artery obstruction leading to ischemia. Other presentations include heart failure, valvular dysfunction, or symptoms from pericardial effusion and tamponade (Fig. 23.61).

Echocardiography is often the initial technique. On MR most cardiac metastasis are low signal intensity on T1 weighted and high signal intensity on T2 weighted except for metastatic melanoma, which is hyperintense on T1 imaging due to the paramagnetic T1 shortening effects of melanin. Heterogeneous

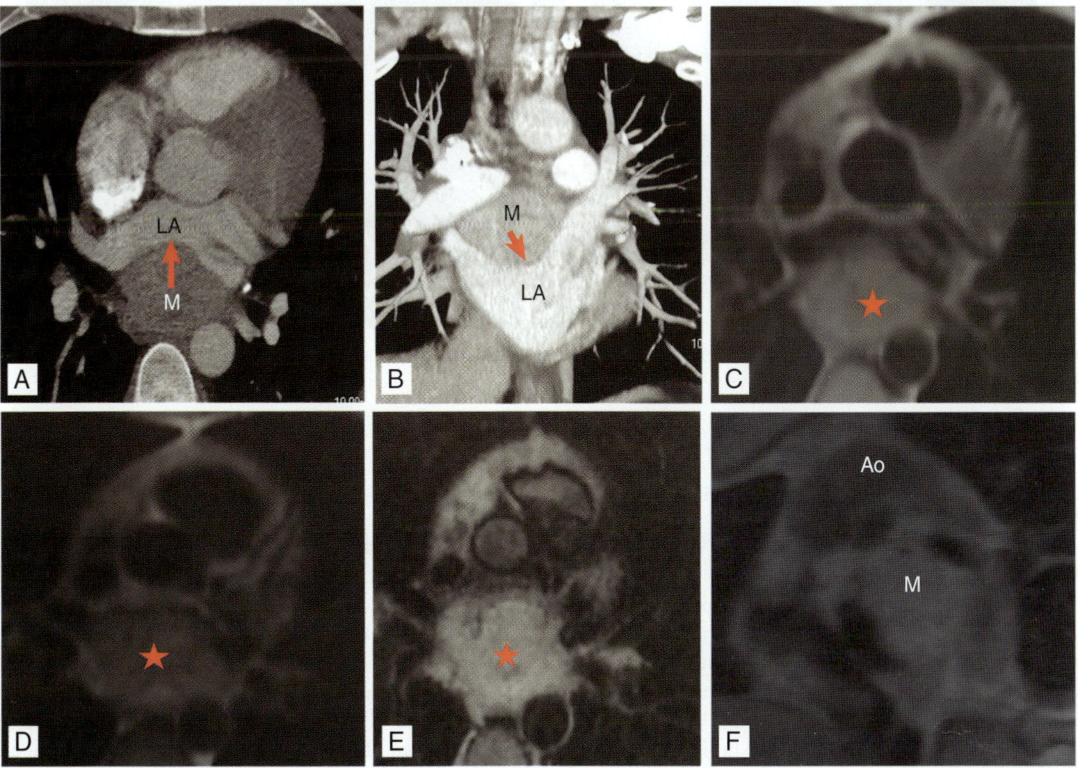

Figure 23.57 Cardiac pheochromocytoma. Axial (A) and coronal (B) CT images demonstrate heterogeneously enhancing noncalcified soft tissue middle mediastinal mass (M) located posterosuperior to the left atrium (LA). The mass is displacing and indenting the posterior wall and roof of the left atrium (*red arrow*). These tumors often are hypervascular and therefore are difficult to resect surgically. T1 (C), T2 (D) and triple inversion recovery (E) axial MR images demonstrate a slightly hyperintense middle mediastinal mass (*stars*) in comparison to myocardium. The mass shows intense contrast uptake as seen on postcontrast T1 sagittal oblique images (F). *Ao*, aorta; *LA*, left atrium; *M*, mass.

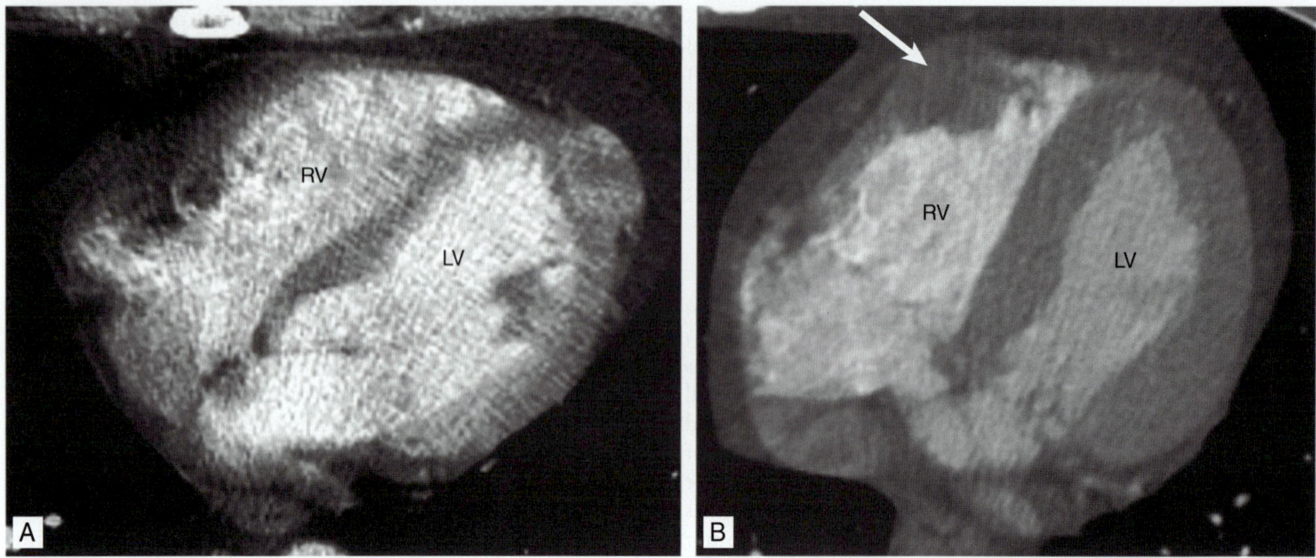

Figure 23.58 Cardiac metastasis. Two different patients (A) with renal cell cancer metastatic to LV myocardium and (B) with colon cancer and RV myocardium metastasis. In a patient with known malignancy, any focal nodular myocardial abnormality should be suspected for metastasis. *LV*, left ventricle; *RV*, right ventricle.

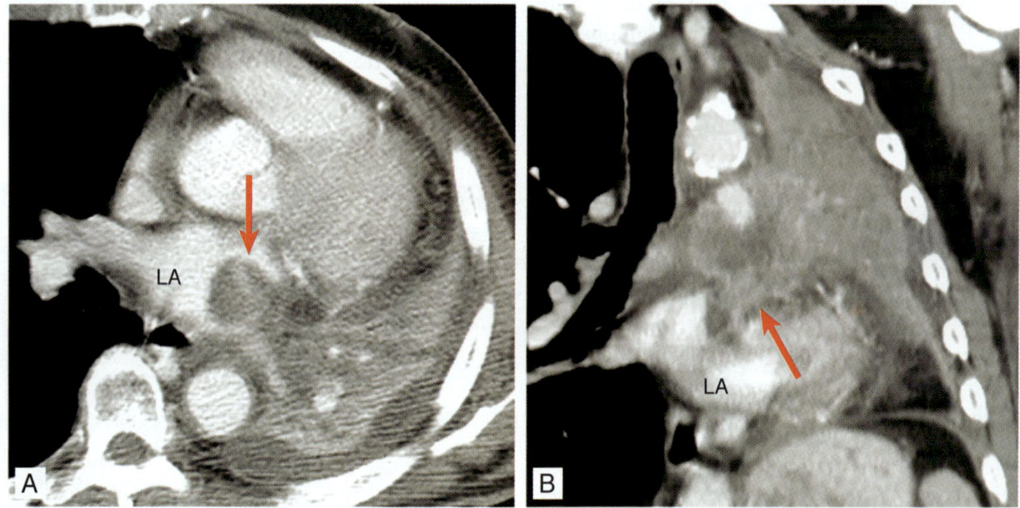

Figure 23.59 Direct invasion from left upper lobe bronchogenic carcinoma. (A–B) There is lobular soft tissue mass (*red arrows*) seen in the left atrium (LA) which extended via left upper lobe pulmonary vein. *LA*, left atrium.

enhancement distinguishes tumoral thrombus from bland thrombus (Figs. 23.60A–C) [68,71,80].

Primary Cardiac Malignant Tumors

Extremely rare, represent only 5–6% of all primary cardiac tumors [59–61,80,81]. Most common tumors are sarcomas, followed by primary cardiac lymphoma, and mesothelioma. Their clinical presentations can be variable but typically are according to the location of the tumor.

Features suggestive of malignancy include rapid growth, local invasion, hemorrhage, or necrosis within the mass, involvement of more than one cardiac chamber, extension into the pericardium with pericardial effusion (Box 23.21).

Primary Cardiac Sarcoma: Primary cardiac sarcomas represent two third of all malignant primary cardiac tumors [59,60,81]. Often seen in younger patients in their 40s and carry worst prognosis in comparison to extracardiac soft tissue sarcomas. Histologically, sarcomas include angiosarcoma, leiomyosarcoma, liposarcoma, rhabdomyosarcoma, synovial sarcoma, myofibrosarcoma, and undifferentiated pleomorphic sarcoma [82].

Angiosarcoma: The most common type of cardiac sarcomas, composed of malignant cells that form vascular channels, usually very aggressive, often originate in the right atrium and extend into RV, right AV groove often encasing the RCA and pericardium (Fig. 23.62). There is often evidence of metastasis to lungs at the time of presentation. Men in their 40s are affected more than females [81,82]. Presenting symptoms are due to right heart failure, arrhythmia, or shortness of breath due to pericardial involvement. On echo these tumors are echogenic lobular or nodular masses in the right atrium often with

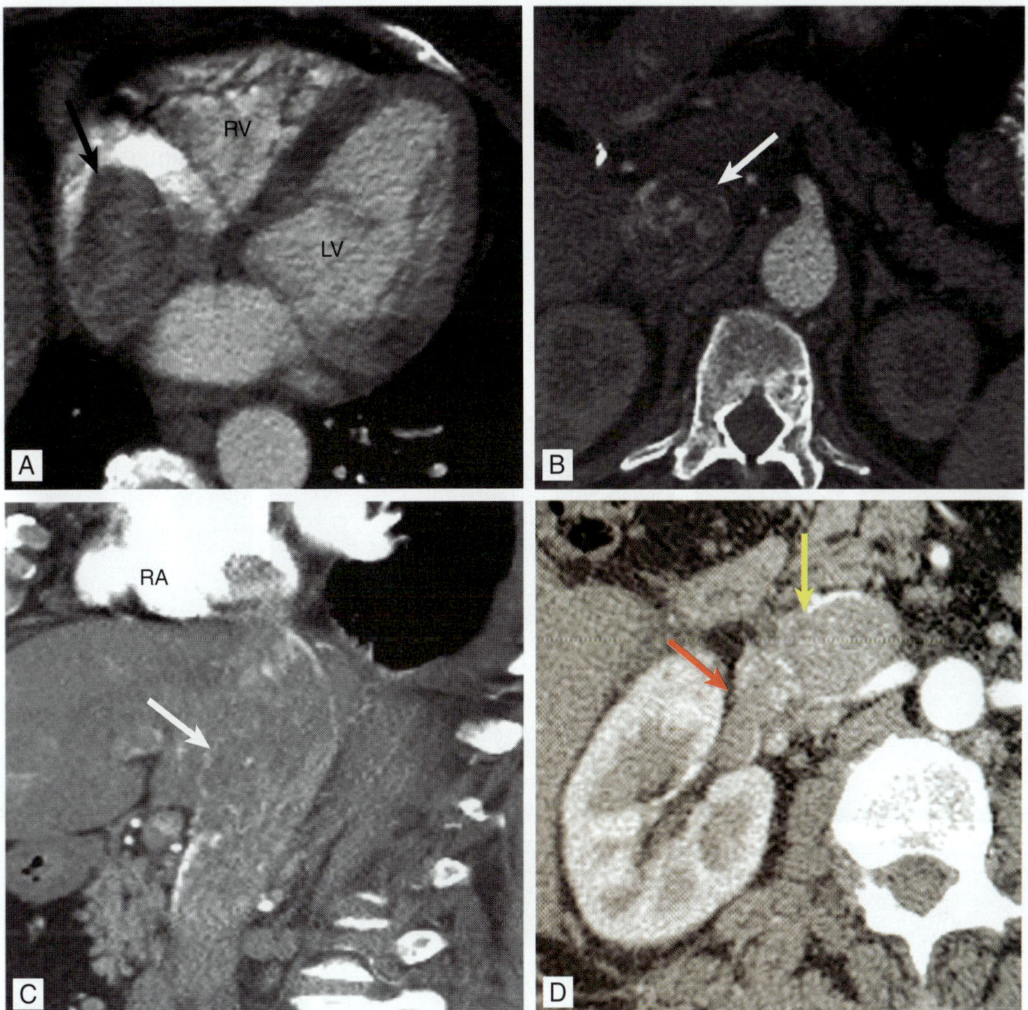

Figure 23.60 A 59-year-old female with right renal cell carcinoma. (A–D) Nongated chest and abdomen CT. A large mass is present in the right atrium (*black arrow*) which is contiguous with mass in the IVC (*white arrow* and *yellow arrow*) and right renal vein (*red arrow*) (B–D). There is increased vascularity with the IVC thrombus best seen in arterial phase axial and coronal CT images (B, C) suggesting it to be tumor thrombus. Patient underwent open right radical nephrectomy, caval thrombectomy, and right atrial thrombectomy. *LV*, left ventricle; *RA*, right atrium; *RV*, right ventricle.

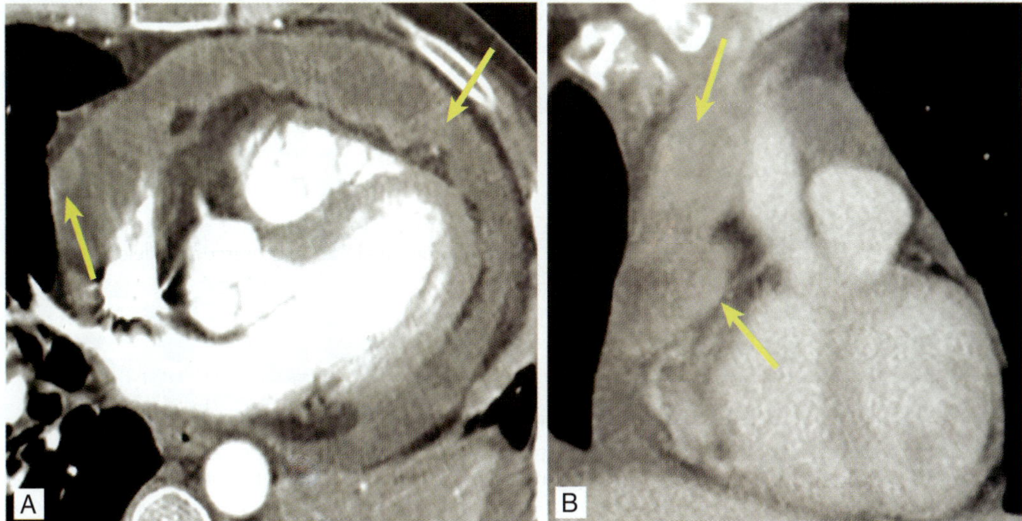

Figure 23.61 Pericardial metastasis. Much more common than myocardial metastasis. (A) There is nodular enhancing thickening of the pericardium (*yellow arrows*) with moderate complex pericardial effusion in this patient with known lung cancer. (B) There are much larger solid enhancing masses (*arrows*) in the pericardium associated with pericardial effusion in this patient with metastatic synovial sarcoma. Rarely such patients present with large pericardial effusion or tamponade.

BOX 23.21 Features Suggesting Malignant Nature of Tumor

- Rapid growth
- Large size with necrosis and hemorrhage
- Involvement of multiple cardiac chambers
- Evidence of local invasion
- Presence of pericardial effusion

pericardial effusion due to direct pericardial extension (Fig. 23.62A). On CT these tumors are highly vascular and demonstrate gross hemorrhagic and heterogeneous appearance with evidence of invasion into adjacent structure commonly present (Figs. 23.62B, C and 23.63) [82]. Pericardial effusion and thickening is common. On T1-weighted images on MR, these tumors are often isointense to hyperintense multiple nodules on which demonstrate LGE surrounding a large central necrosis (Figs. 23.62D–F) [71,80]. Cardiac angiosarcomas carry a poor prognosis without surgical resection. Neoadjuvant chemotherapy in conjunction with surgical debulking offers the best survival.

Leiomyosarcoma: Highly aggressive and second most common sarcomas following angiosarcomas. These tumors are usually present in the posterior left atrium though can also involve other cardiac chambers. Clinical presentation depends on the size and

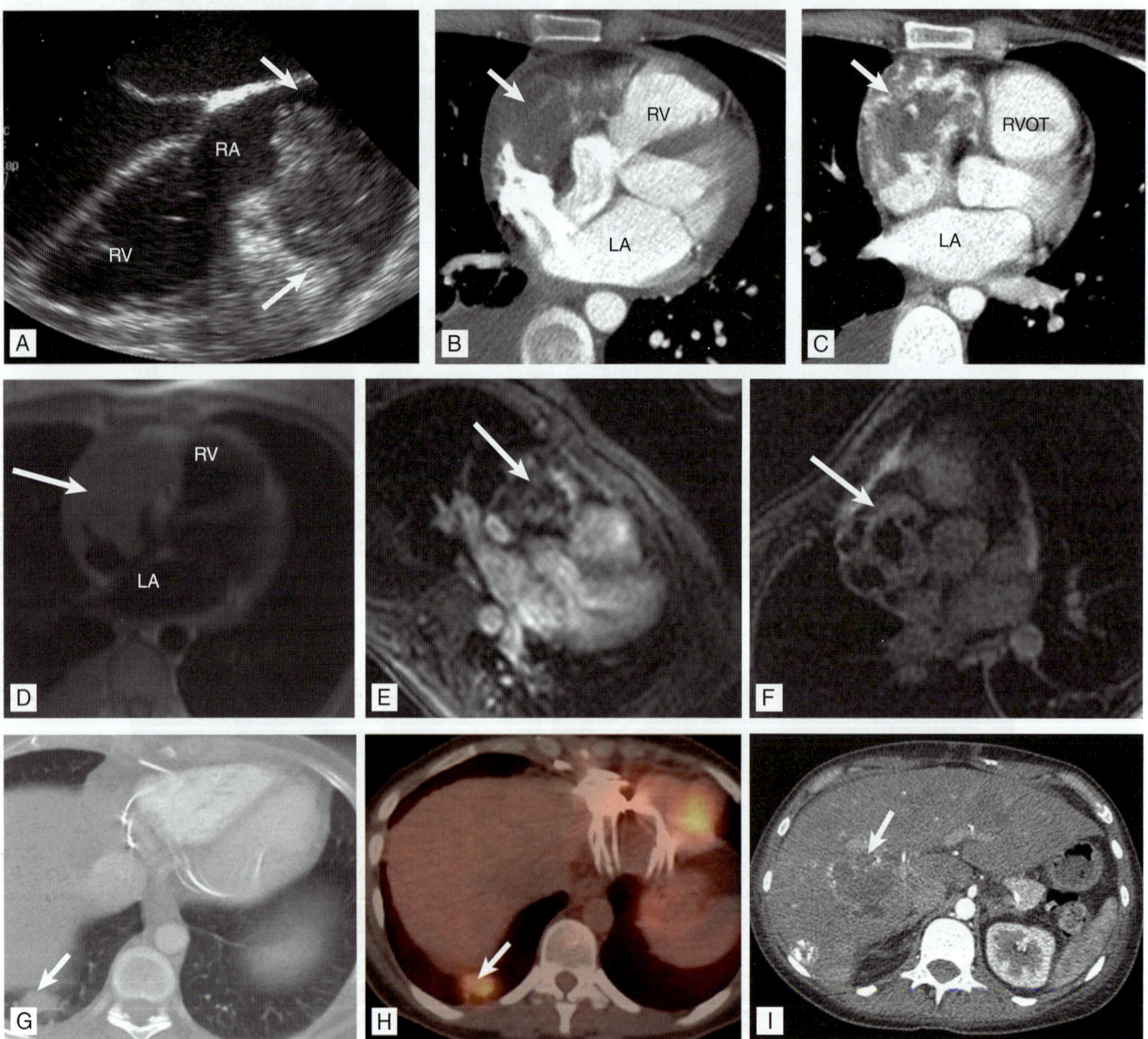

Figure 23.62 Metastatic right atrial angiosarcoma. A 35-year-old female presented with SOB and transthoracic echo (A) showed large pericardial effusion causing tamponade along with large right atrial mass (*arrows*). Pericardial effusion was tapped and was bloody but negative cytology. Contrast-enhanced chest CT (B, C) showed a large heterogenous vascular right atrial mass (*white arrows*) extending into the right atrioventricular groove with suspected pericardial extension. The mass was isointense to slightly hyperintense on T1 imaging and showed increased peripheral vascularity on postcontrast first pass images along with delayed enhancement (*white arrows*) on MR (D, E). The mass was resected and proved to be high-grade angiosarcoma. At 4-month follow-up, patient developed a right lower lobe nodule (*white arrows*) which showed FDG uptake (G, H). She was given chemotherapy, but unfortunately she developed hepatic (*white arrow* on I) and bone metastasis along with local recurrence. *LA*, left atrium; *LV*, left ventricle; *RA*, right atrium; *RV*, right ventricle; *RVOT*, right ventricle outflow tract.

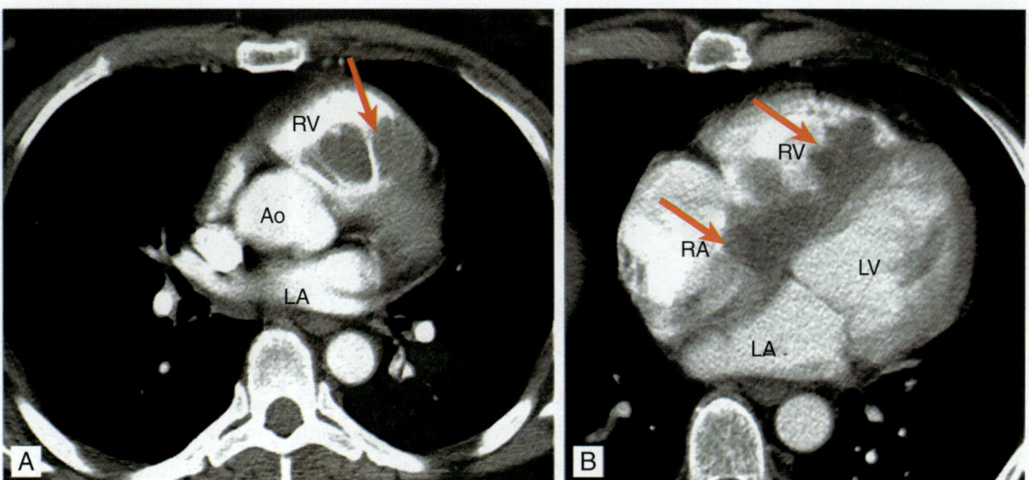

Figure 23.63 Primary cardiac sarcoma. (A–B) A lobulated soft tissue mass (*red arrows*) is seen in the right ventricle along the interventricular septum and extends into the right atrium. Multiple chamber involvement is one of the features for malignant mass. *Ao*, aorta; *LA*, left atrium; *LV*, left ventricle; *RA*, right atrium; *RV*, right ventricle.

location of the tumor. Tumors infiltrating the myocardium are frequently associated with arrhythmias with less common presentation include venous and intra-arterial thrombosis. On CT leiomyosarcomas are lobulated with irregular low attenuating masses usually associated with pericardial effusion. Rarely dystrophic calcification can be seen. When pulmonary veins are invaded, they are often seen as filling defects in the pulmonary veins. These tumors also have poor prognosis with high incidence of distant metastasis. Surgical resection offers palliation with the relief of obstructive symptoms.

Rhabdomyosarcoma: Most common pediatric malignant primary cardiac tumors and involve striated muscle. These tumors arise from the myocardium and have a tendency toward valvular involvement with no chamber predilection. Often these are large bulky and invasive tumors, more than 10 cm in size, presenting typically with symptoms relating to cardiac invasion or obstruction. On CT they are seen as irregular or smooth low attenuating mass within the cardiac chamber. They are isointense on T1-weighted and hypointense on T2-weighted images with moderate homogeneous postcontrast enhancement. Both CT and MR can detect extra cardiac extension including pulmonary artery metastasis [68,70,71,80,82]. Combination of surgery, chemotherapy, and radiation therapy are often the standard treatment for rhabdomyosarcoma. Despite treatment, prognosis is dismal with survival less than 1 year in most cases.

Primary Cardiac Lymphoma: Primary cardiac lymphoma is much less common than secondary cardiac involvement (approximately 30% of patients with lymphoma have cardiac involvement) [83]. Majority are aggressive B-cell lymphomas, most commonly seen in immunocompromised patients with increasing incidence due to lymphoproliferative disorder from Epstein–Barr virus in patients with AIDS and those who received transplant. They most commonly involve the right side of the heart, particularly the right atrium although any chamber can be involved. Often there are multiple lesions and the mean age of diagnosis is often 60 years of age. Primary cardiac lymphoma symptoms may include arrhythmias including heart block, syncope, or even restrictive cardiomyopathy. Patients can have fever, chills, sweats, and weight loss along with chest pain and dyspnea and rarely acute heart failure could be the presentation (Box 23.22).

On echo they are homogeneous infiltrative masses causing wall thickening or nodular masses protruding into the cardiac chamber (Fig. 23.64D). The coronary artery can be encased due to involvement of the adjacent atrial ventricular groove (Fig. 23.64B). Similarly, pericardium involvement leads to effusion or rarely tamponade. On cardiac CT, they appear as focal or diffuse soft tissue masses or infiltrating multiple nodules demonstrating heterogeneous postcontrast enhancement (Figs. 23.64A–B) [68,70]. Often there is associated mediastinal adenopathy. On T1-weighted images, tumors are isointense and usually show mild hyperintensity due to edema on T2-weighted images [71,83]. FDG PET can show uptake, degree of which is directly proportional to degree of the malignancy of the lesion (Fig. 23.64). Diagnosis often involves evaluation of pericardial fluid and/or endomyocardial biopsy. These tumors do respond to chemotherapy although recurrence rate is very high. Recurrence often develops at extra cardiac extra nodal sites.

BOX 23.22 Primary Cardiac Lymphomas: Poor Outcome Predictors

- Immune status
- Left ventricular involvement
- Presence of dyspnea
- Presence of extracardiac disease

Mesothelioma: These tumors are derived from the pericardial mesothelial cell layer. By definition, these tumors must be localized within pericardial space without any pleural involvement. Association with asbestos exposure as cause relationship is unclear. These tumors often present with pericardial effusions with or without tamponade and have male sex predominance with most patients in their fifth or sixth decades. Echo often shows pericardial effusion and echogenic tumor mass encasing the heart. Both cardiac MR and CT can show multiple enhancing pericardial nodular masses with associated effusion [68,70,71,80,83]. These tumors demonstrate FDG uptake, therefore PET CT is very useful in staging and monitoring the disease during treatment. Primary pericardial mesotheliomas are highly aggressive tumors with extremely poor prognosis and median after diagnosis survival of only 6 months. Poor prognosis is due to late presentation, diagnostic difficulties, difficult for complete resection, and poor response to therapies.

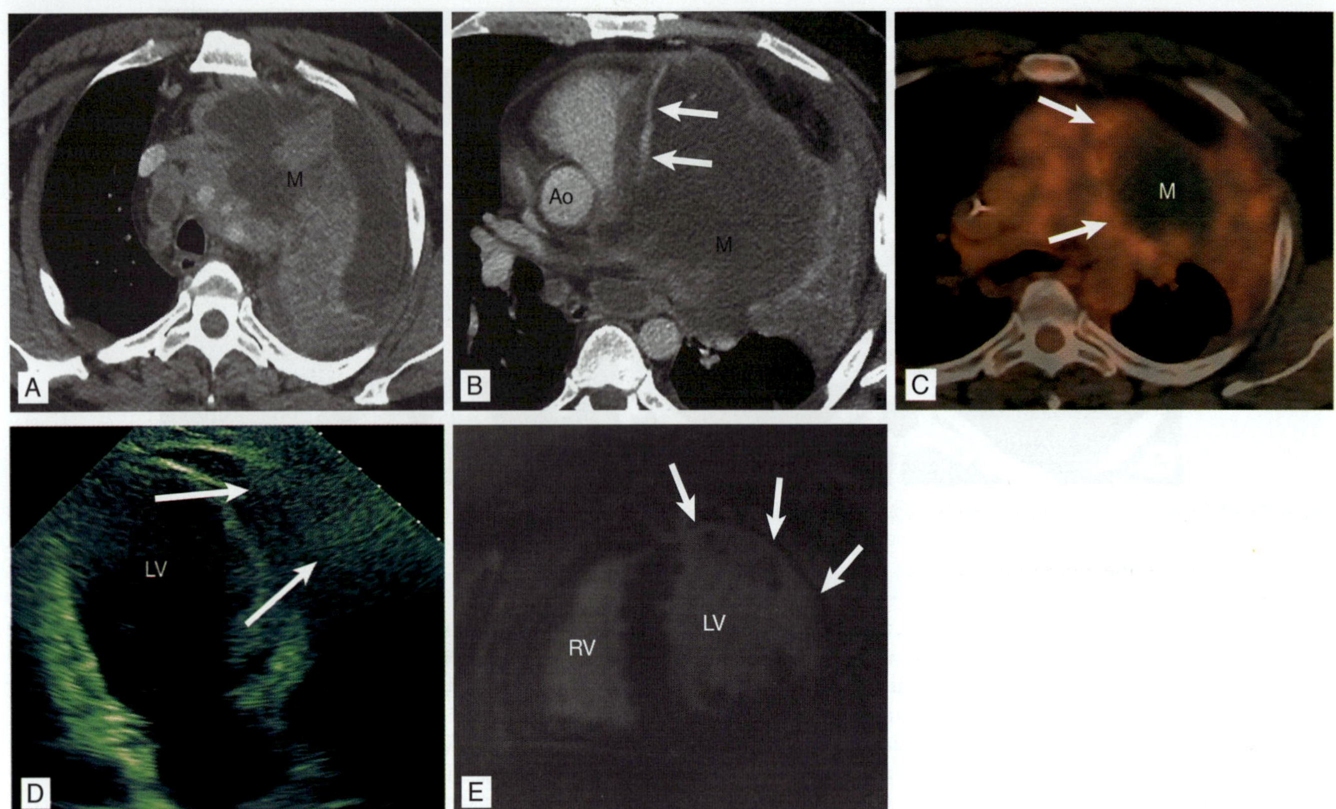

Figure 23.64 B-cell lymphoma involves pericardium and coronary arteries. (A, B) Contrast-enhanced CT shows a large heterogeneous necrotic soft tissue mass in the anterior and middle mediastinum (M) inseparable from the LV anterolateral myocardium and encases the left anterior descending (*white arrows*) and circumflex (not shown) coronary artery as well as all three neck vessels. There is complex pericardial effusion and thickening. (C) The mass shows peripheral nodular uptake (*white arrows*) on PET scan. (D) Transthoracic echo also shows mass infiltrating the LV myocardium and pericardium (*white arrows*). (E) On postcontrast MR, there was transmural delayed enhancement of the anterior and anterolateral LV wall in the LAD and Cx territory (*white arrows*). *Ao*, aorta; *LV*, left ventricle; *M*, mass; *RV*, right ventricle.

Suggested Readings

- J Vogel-Claussen, H Pannu, PJ Spevak, EK Fishman, DA Bluemke, Cardiac valve assessment with MR imaging and 64-section multi-detector row CT, Radiographics 26 (6) (2006) 1769–1784.
- SG Myerson, Heart valve disease: investigation by cardiovascular magnetic resonance, J Cardiovasc Magn Reson 14 (7) (2012), doi:10.1186/1532-429X-14-7.
- JK Lempel, MA Bolen, RD Renapurkar, et al., Radiographic evaluation of valvular heart disease with CT & MR correlation, J Thorac Imaging 31 (2016) 273–284.
- P Blanke, UJ Schoepf, JA Leipsic, CT in transcatheter aortic valve replacement, Radiology 269 (3) (2013) 650–669.
- H Aung, EE Williamson, SP Singh, Transcatheter aortic valve replacement: preprocedure and postprocedure imaging, Adv Clin Radiol 1 (2019) 119–134.
- PA Erba, MN Pizzi, A Roque, et al., Multimodality imaging in infective endocarditis: an imaging team within the endocarditis team, Circulation 140 (2019) 1753–1765.
- P Rajiah, S Raza, SS Saboo, B Ghoshhajra, S Abbara, Update on the role of cardiac magnetic resonance in acquired non ischemic cardiomyopathies, J Thorac Imaging 31 (6) (2016) 348–366.
- AJ Baxi, CS Restrepo, D Vargas, A Marmol-Velez, D Ocazionez, H Murillo, Hypertrophic cardiomyopathy from A to Z: genetics, pathophysiology, imaging and management, Radiographics 36 (2) (2016) 335–354.
- DH O'Donnell, S Abbara, V Chaithiraphan, K Yared, RP Killeen, R Martos, et al., Cardiac MR imaging of non ischemic cardiomyopathies: imaging protocols and spectra of appearances, Radiology 262 (2) (2012) 403–423.
- CM Kramer, Role of cardiac MR imaging in cardiomyopathies, J Nucl Med 56 (2015) 39S–45S.
- K Kalisz, P Rajah, Computed tomography of cardiomyopathies, Cardiovasc Diagn Ther 7 (5) (2017) 539–556.
- ET Hoey, M Shahid, A Ganeshan, S Baijal, H Simpson, RW Watkin, MRI assessment of cardiac tumours: part 1 & 2, multiparametric imaging protocols and spectrum of appearances of histologically benign lesions, Quant Imaging Med Surg 4 (6) (2014) 478–497.
- ML Grebenc, ML Rosado-de-Christenson, CE Green, AP Burke, JR Galvin, Cardiac myxoma: imaging features in 83 patients, Radiographics 22 (3) (2002) 673–689.
- PA Araoz, SL Mulvagh, HD Tazelaar, PR Julsrud, JF Breen, CT and MR imaging of benign primary cardiac neoplasms with echocardiographic correlation, Radiographics 20 (5) (2000) 1303–1319.
- P Rajiah, JP Kanne, V Kalahasti, P Schoenhagen, Computed tomography of cardiac and pericardiac masses, JCCT 5 (1) (2011) 16–29.
- PJ Sparrow, JB Kurian, TR Jones, MU Sivananthan, MR imaging of cardiac tumors, Radiographics 25 (5) (2005) 1255–1276.
- TY Tao, N Yahyavi-Firouz-Abadi, GK Singh, S Bhalla, Pediatric cardiac tumors: clinical and imaging features, Radiographics 34 (4) (2014) 1031–46.
- J Jeudy, J Kirsch, F Tavora, AP Burke, TJ Franks, TL Mohammed, et al., From the radiologic pathology archives: cardiac lymphoma: radiologic-pathologic correlation, Radiographics 32 (5) (2012) 1369–1380.

24 Pericardium

JENA N. DEPETRIS, UDO HOFFMANN, SANDEEP HEDGIRE

Introduction

The pericardium is a fibrous structure that surrounds both the cardiac chambers and the origins of the great vessels. Composed of two layers, visceral and parietal, normally separated by a small amount of fluid [1], the pericardium plays several important roles in normal physiology, including decreasing the friction between the beating heart and surrounding structures, preventing excessive dilatation of the cardiac chambers, and limiting the spread of infection or inflammation from the adjacent mediastinum or lungs [2,3].

Numerous pathologies can affect the pericardium, including infectious, inflammatory, traumatic, acquired, congenital, and neoplastic processes. This chapter will discuss the characteristic imaging features of both the normal and diseased pericardium with an emphasis on cross-sectional imaging techniques such as computed tomography (CT) and magnetic resonance imaging (MRI), and review the advantages and limitations of various imaging techniques for assessment of the pericardium.

Imaging Techniques

Transthoracic Echocardiography

Transthoracic echocardiography is the standard initial noninvasive imaging technique used for the evaluation of pericardial disease [4]. Although this technique has the advantages of easy accessibility and real-time imaging without the use of ionizing radiation, pericardial assessment is frequently limited by the available acoustic window and image quality can be easily degraded, particularly in the setting of a hemorrhagic pericardial effusion or gas within the intervening soft tissues. Although transesophageal echocardiography can be an alternative approach, it is a more invasive imaging technique with many of the same limitations, which may still preclude full evaluation of the pericardium. In settings where echocardiography is nondiagnostic or challenging to interpret, cross-sectional imaging with either CT or MRI can be advantageous for further characterization of the pericardium. In fact, the American College of Radiology 2020 appropriateness criteria considers both cardiac CT and cardiac MRI more appropriate diagnostic tests in the evaluation of dyspnea due to suspected pericardial disease compared with transesophageal echocardiography and invasive angiography with ventriculography [5].

Advanced Cross-Sectional Imaging

By comparison, cross-sectional imaging techniques, including CT and MRI, are valuable adjuncts to echocardiography and offer unique advantages in assessing the pericardium, including a larger field of view with superior soft tissue contrast for anatomic assessment. These techniques are particularly useful to characterize loculated or complex pericardial effusions, constrictive pericarditis, and pericardial masses. In addition, given that both CT and MRI are performed in standard imaging planes, these techniques are less operator dependent compared with echocardiography. Given the numerous potential applications of these techniques in the workup of pericardial disease, familiarity with these imaging techniques is important for all radiologists.

Computed Tomography

Cardiac CT, with the implementation of cardiac gating and increase in both spatial coverage and temporal resolution, now allows for motion-free imaging of the pericardium. These features, combined with multiphase, multiplanar reformatting capabilities allow for precise anatomic visualization of the normal pericardium and detailed assessment of anatomic variations or other pericardial abnormalities [3]. Additionally, CT allows for reasonable tissue characterization including the detection of pericardial calcifications, differentiation of simple and complex pericardial fluids, and characterization of certain pericardial masses. The obvious disadvantages of CT include the use of intravenous iodinated contrast and ionizing radiation, especially in patients with impaired renal function and young patients, respectively.

Magnetic Resonance Imaging

By comparison, cardiac MRI can provide a comprehensive assessment of the pericardium utilizing a variety of sequences tailored for morphologic and functional assessment without the use of iodinated contrast media or ionizing radiation. Similar to CT, MRI has a wider field of view and multiplanar reformatting capabilities with excellent spatiotemporal resolution [3]. Evaluation of the pericardium by MRI involves the use of numerous cardiac- and respiratory-gated sequences (summarized in Table 24.1), including steady-state free precession or gradient-recalled echo cine sequences, real-time cine imaging of the interventricular septum during respiration, double and triple inversion recovery black-blood sequences, myocardial tagging, phase contrast or velocity encoded sequences, and late gadolinium-enhanced sequences, among others. T1- and T2-weighted sequences allow for superior fluid and soft tissue characterization compared with echocardiography or CT, while cine sequences and myocardial tagging sequences enable dynamic assessment of the pericardium during cardiac motion, enhancing sensitivity for pericardial adhesions, and constrictive physiology. Despite its unique strengths, there are several disadvantages of MRI including far more limited availability, the use of intravenous gadolinium, and long image acquisition times requiring a great deal of patient focus and cooperation. Furthermore, cardiac rhythm abnormalities,

TABLE 24.1 MRI Techniques Commonly Used for Assessment of the Pericardium

MR Technique	Clinical Utility for Pericardium
Steady-state free precession (SSFP)	Assess myocardial (septal) wall motion Assess for the presence of pericardial effusion
Double/triple inversion recovery fast spin echo (FSE) black-blood	Assess pericardial thickness Assess for the presence of pericardial effusion
T1-weighted gradient echo myocardial tagged cine	Assess for pericardial adhesions
Real-time GRE cine during dynamic respiration	Assess for ventricular interdependence
T2-weighted fast spin echo (FSE)	
T1 and T2 fat saturation	Assess tissue characteristics (e.g., pericarditis or pericardial neoplasm)
Postcontrast (gadolinium)	

Adapted from Czum et al. [2].

which are frequently associated with pericardial pathologies, can make cardiac gating difficult to achieve and produce profound artifacts that significantly degrade image quality. Table 24.2 provides a summary of the strengths and weaknesses of the imaging techniques discussed in this section.

Normal Pericardial Anatomy

The normal pericardium is a uniformly thin fibrous structure, typically measuring less than 2 mm in thickness, with any measurement of 4 mm or greater being considered abnormally thickened [2,3,6]. Although the pericardium is typically indistinguishable from the adjacent myocardium by chest radiography, cross-sectional imaging with CT or MRI provides excellent delineation of the pericardium in a majority of patients. Clear discrimination of the pericardium from the adjacent myocardium by cross-sectional imaging requires the presence of at least a thin layer of epicardial fat or pericardial fluid, and the pericardium is often most clearly seen over the right-sided cardiac chambers (Fig. 24.1).

Cranially the pericardium attaches to the main pulmonary artery (proximal to the bifurcation), the proximal ascending thoracic aorta (approximately halfway between the aortic valve and the brachiocephalic artery), and the superior vena cava [7,8]. Posteriorly the pericardium incompletely covers the left atrium, attaching to the proximal pulmonary veins. The pericardium is additionally stabilized within the mediastinum by several so-called pericardial ligaments, namely, the pericardiophrenic and sternopericardial ligaments, which are often difficult to appreciate by imaging.

Due to the relatively closer apposition of the inner visceral pericardium to the heart contours compared with the outer parietal pericardium, a small volume of normal physiologic pericardial fluid can accumulate in pockets near the pericardial attachment sites, known as pericardial sinuses or recesses (Fig. 24.2) [2,7]. These recesses can best be understood by

TABLE 24.2 Summary of the Strengths and Limitations of Various Imaging Techniques in the Evaluation of Pericardial Disorders

Technique	Strengths	Weaknesses
Transthoracic echocardiography (TTE)	▪ First-line technique in suspected pericardial disease ▪ Widely available at low cost ▪ Portable/available at bedside ▪ Functional hemodynamic assessment ▪ Respirometry available for respirophasic assessment ▪ TEE as adjunct ▪ Can be performed in the acute setting and in hemodynamically unstable patients	▪ Operator-dependent image quality ▪ Diagnostic utility limited by available acoustic window ▪ Narrow field of view ▪ Low signal-to-noise ratio (SNR) of pericardium ▪ Limited capacity for tissue characterization
Cardiac CT	▪ Excellent assessment of pericardial calcifications ▪ Detailed anatomic assessment of pericardium and extracardiac structures ▪ Simultaneous preoperative planning/clearance ▪ Functional assessment available	▪ Ionizing radiation ▪ Iodinated contrast relatively contraindicated in patients with poor renal function ▪ Functional assessment available at relatively higher radiation doses ▪ Image quality susceptible to arrhythmias ▪ Requirement for breath hold ▪ Patients must be hemodynamically stable ▪ Modality not portable
Cardiac MRI	▪ Second-choice technique for pericardial assessment (excluding calcifications) ▪ Detailed adjunctive anatomic assessment of pericardium ▪ Superior tissue characterization ▪ Ability to assess for pericardial inflammation (edema and late gadolinium enhancement) ▪ Functional assessment available	▪ Limited availability at high cost ▪ Limited assessment of pericardial calcifications ▪ Gadolinium relatively contraindicated in patients with poor renal function ▪ Image quality susceptible to arrhythmias ▪ Requirement for breath hold ▪ Patients must be hemodynamically stable ▪ Modality not portable

Adapted from Xu et al. [4].

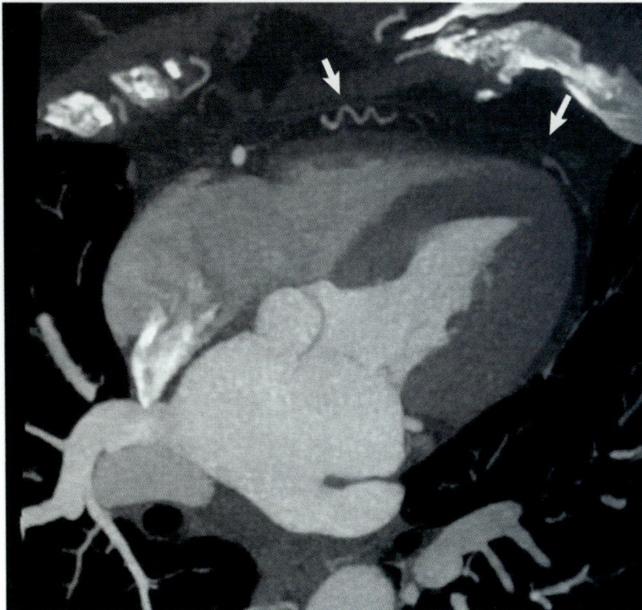

Figure 24.1 Axial contrast-enhanced EKG-gated cardiac CT demonstrating the normal (<2 mm thick) pericardium (*arrows*) best visualized over the right ventricle anteriorly.

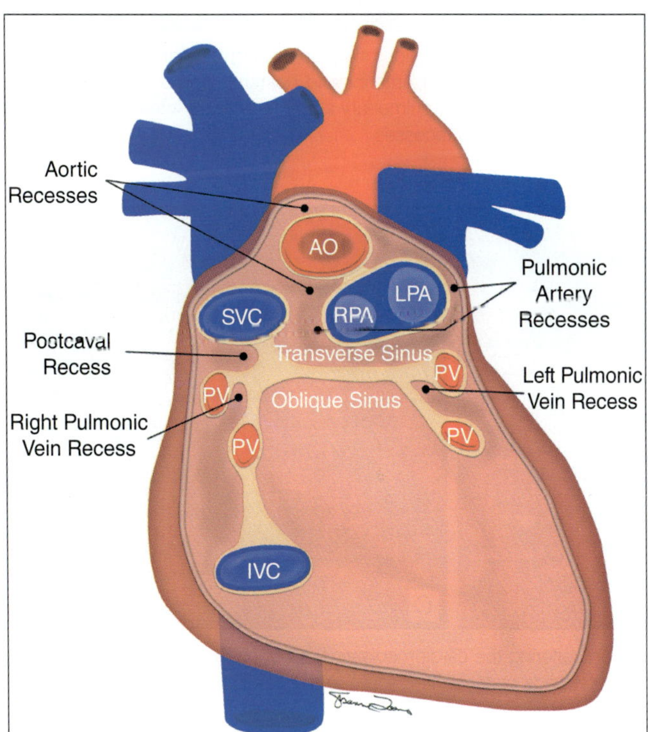

Figure 24.2 The posterior aspect of the pericardial space. The transverse sinus lies between the aorta/pulmonary artery and the great veins, giving rise to the aortic and pulmonary (*artery*) recesses. The oblique sinus lies posterior to the left atrium between the right and left pulmonary venous confluences. The pulmonary vein recesses and postcaval recess arise from invaginations of the pericardium. *AO*, aorta; *IVC*, inferior vena cava; *PV*, pulmonary vein; *RPA/LPA*, right/left pulmonary artery; *SVC*, superior vena cava.

TABLE 24.3 Origin and Location of the Various Anatomic Pericardial Recesses

Site of Origin	Pericardial Recesses	Location
Pericardial cavity	Pulmonary vein recesses	Along lateral borders of heart between the superior and inferior pulmonary veins
	Postcaval recesses	Posterior and to the right of the SVC
Transverse sinus	Aortic recesses	*Superior aortic recess* extends superiorly from the transverse sinus surrounding the ascending aorta *Inferior aortic recess* extends inferiorly from the transverse sinus posterior to the aortic root and anterior to the left atrium
	Pulmonary (artery) recesses	Inferior to the right and left pulmonary arteries
Oblique sinus	Posterior pericardial recess	Posterior to the right pulmonary artery, medial to the bronchus intermedius, and anterior/adjacent to the esophagus

categorizing them according to their different sites of origin, which include the pericardial cavity proper, the transverse sinus, and the oblique sinus (Table 24.3) [3,7–9]. Knowledge of the anatomic location and imaging appearance of these pericardial recesses is extremely important to avoid misdiagnosis and unnecessary imaging follow-up, as they can be mistaken for lymphadenopathy, masses, esophageal lesions, bronchogenic cysts, or even aortic dissection (Fig. 24.3).

Adjacent to the pericardium in the cardiophrenic angles, triangular-shaped low-density pericardial fat pads can often be seen both on plain film and cross-sectional imaging (Fig. 24.4). These benign structures can be quite large in some patients and can alter the appearance of the cardiomediastinal silhouette, although they should not be included in an overall assessment of cardiac size, particularly when interpreting radiographs.

Pericardial Disorders

Congenital Absence of the Pericardium

Embryology and Epidemiology

Pericardial defects, both congenital and acquired, are rare. The most common among them is congenital absence of the pericardium (also referred to as *pericardial agenesis*), which results from premature atrophy of a cardinal vein leading to underdevelopment of the pleuropericardial membrane and thus failure of pericardial formation [1,3,6].

Congenital absence of the pericardium is more common in men and may be partial or complete, with partial absence of the left pericardium

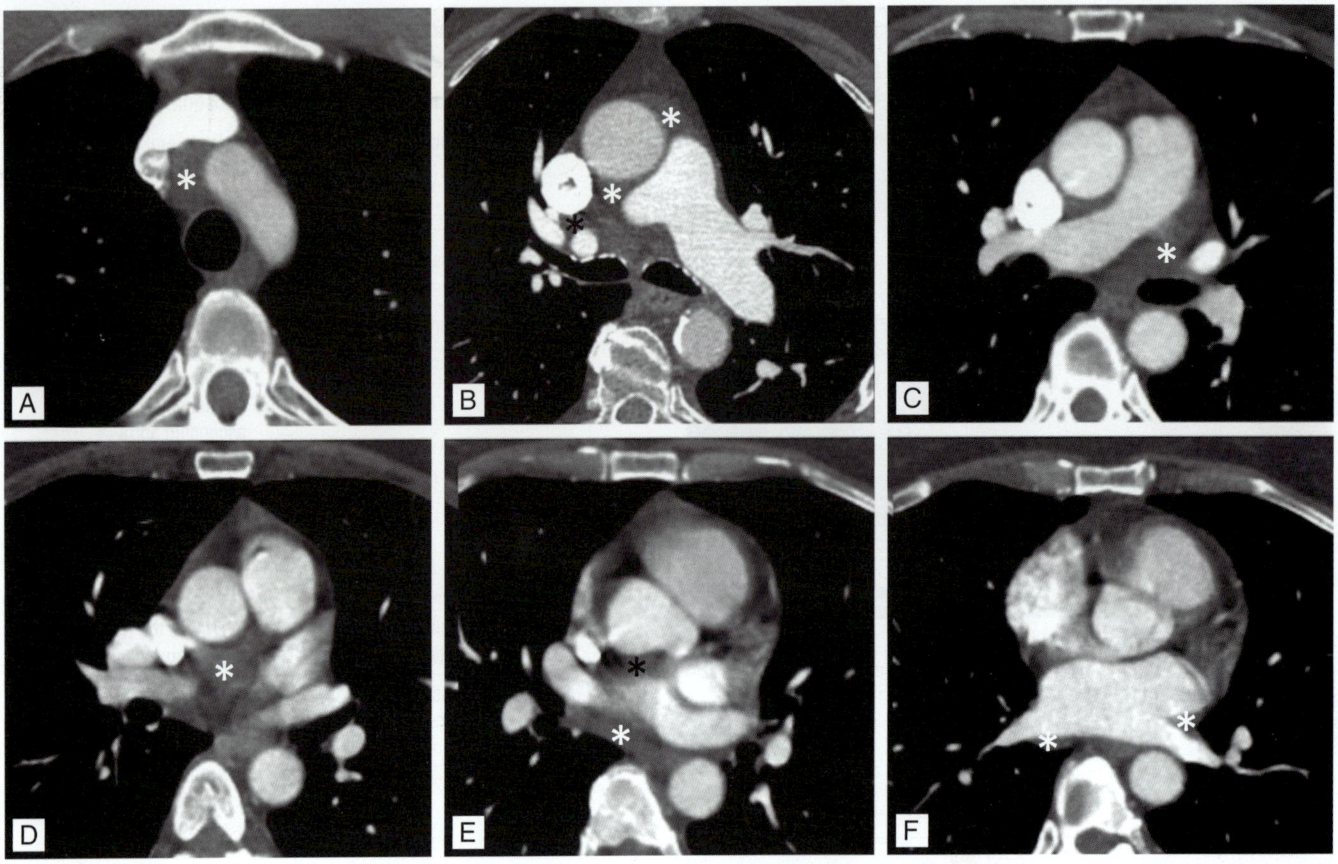

Figure 24.3 Multiple axial contrast-enhanced CT images demonstrating the normal appearance of various fluid-containing pericardial recesses and sinuses (*asterisks*). (A) Superior extension of the superior aortic recess—a normal anatomic variant. (B) Anterior and posterior portions of the superior aortic recess (*white*) as well as the postcaval recess (*black*). (C) Left pulmonary artery recess. (D) Right pulmonary artery recess. (E) Inferior aortic recess (*black*) and oblique sinus (or posterior pericardial recess; *white*). (F) Right and left pulmonary venous recesses.

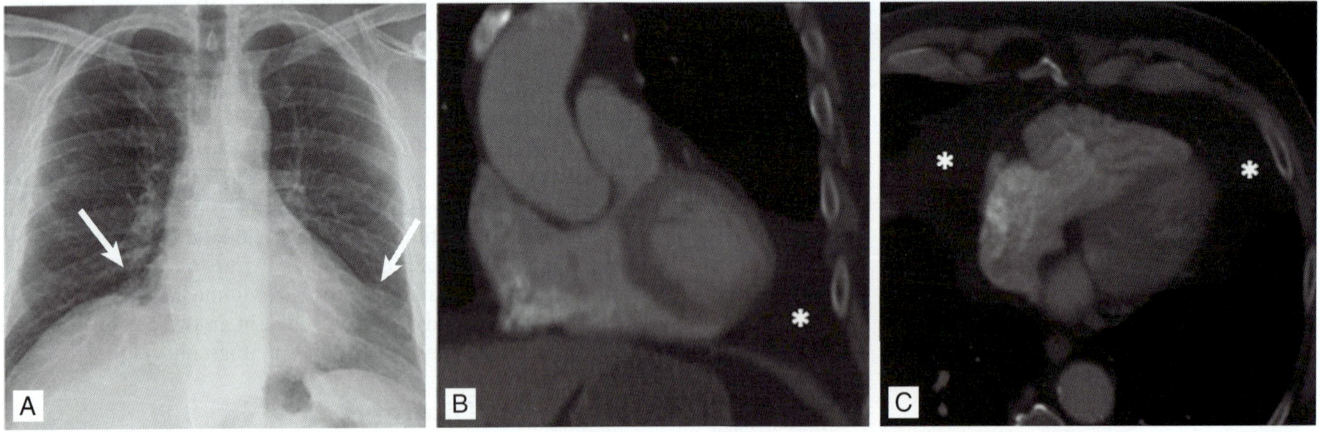

Figure 24.4 Frontal chest radiograph (A) demonstrates prominent pericardial fat pads altering the cardiomediastinal silhouette (*arrows*). Corresponding coronal (B) and axial (C) contrast-enhanced chest CT demonstrates large triangular fat pads (*asterisks*) adjacent to the cardiac borders, which explains the appearance noted on the radiograph.

being the most common variant. Acquired pericardial defects, from trauma or previous surgery (e.g., pericardiectomy for constrictive pericarditis or CABG), typically do not share imaging findings seen in congenital absence of the pericardium, and should only be considered in the appropriate clinical context (Fig. 24.5).

Clinical Features

Congenital pericardial defects are frequently asymptomatic, but have been found to be associated with other congenital abnormalities of the heart (e.g., atrial and ventricular septal defects, patent ductus arteriosus, tetralogy of Fallot, etc.), lungs (e.g., pulmonary sequestration, bronchogenic cyst), chest wall, and diaphragm (diaphragmatic hernia) in approximately one third of cases [1,3,6,9]. Depending on the degree of pericardial agenesis/size of the pericardial defect, imaging findings may be subtle.

In rare instances, herniation of the cardiac chambers through the pericardial defect can occur, including left atrial appendage

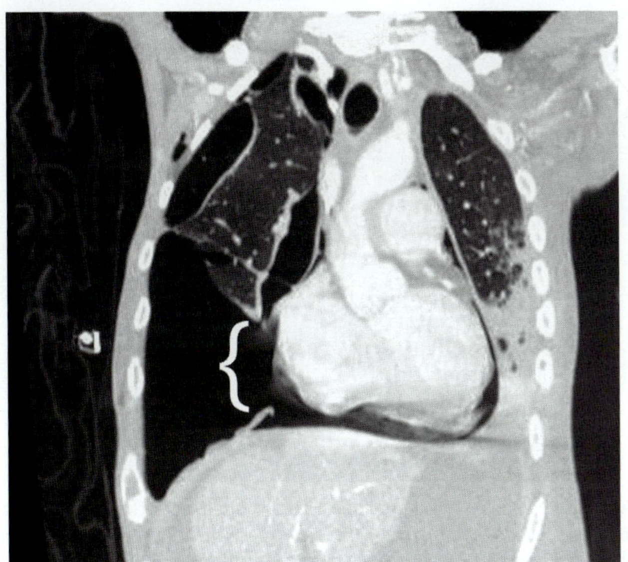

Figure 24.5 Coronal chest CT in lung windows demonstrating air within the right pleural space and pericardium with an open (acquired) pericardial defect (bracket) along the right heart border.

herniation, which in severe cases may result in entrapment, ischemia/necrosis due to coronary artery compression, and even death [3,6]. In addition, patients who develop a pneumothorax may concurrently develop pneumopericardium or even pneumomediastinum, due to open communication between these anatomic spaces through the existing pericardial defect.

In the setting of cardiac herniation, entrapment, or ischemia, urgent surgical repair is required to relieve compression of the herniated structures and surgically close the pericardial defect. Asymptomatic cases, in contrast, often require no treatment.

Imaging Features

On chest radiograph, the classic appearance of congenital absence of the pericardium is the *snoopy sign* (Fig. 24.6) [10], which refers to a combination of leftward shift or levorotation of the heart, flattening and elongation of the left heart border, and a lucency representing lung interposition between the aorta and main pulmonary in the absence of normal pericardial coverage [6,11]. There may alternatively be apparent elevation of the cardiac apex with lung interposed between the left hemidiaphragm.

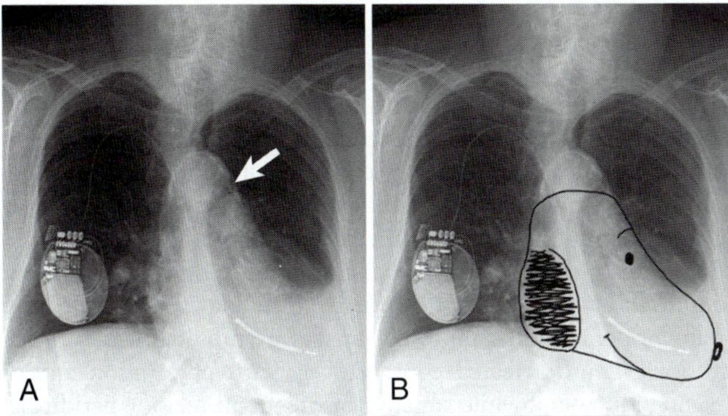

Figure 24.6 Frontal chest radiograph (A) demonstrating the classic *snoopy sign* (B) of congenital (partial) absence of the pericardium, which refers to the straightening of the left heart border causing the heart to take on this characteristic appearance. This radiograph also demonstrates a lucency in the aortopulmonary window (*arrow*) suggestive of lung interposition in this area due to the lack of pericardial coverage.

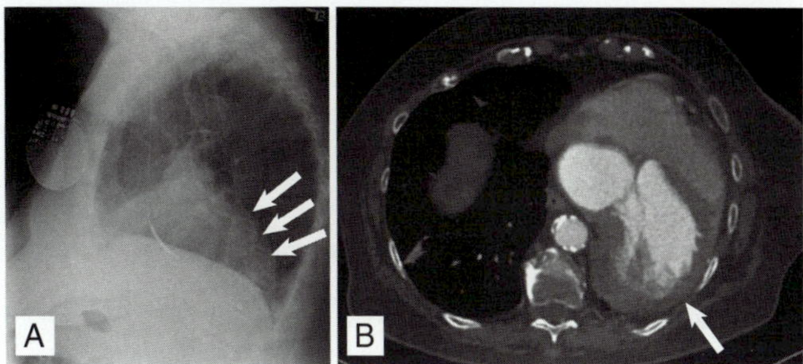

Figure 24.7 A lateral chest radiograph (A) and an axial contrast-enhanced chest CT (B) both demonstrating the pronounced levorotation and posterior deviation of the heart (*arrows*) in a patient with congenital absence of the pericardium.

Complete or partial absence of the pericardium can be detected by both CT and MRI, with MRI being the method of choice due to its excellent capacity for direct visualization of the pericardium and thus identification of pericardial defects. In addition, these cross-sectional techniques can confirm and provide greater evaluation of the findings identified on chest radiograph (Fig. 24.7). Functional assessment by CT or MRI may also show increased cardiac mobility (particularly excessive apical motion) in the absence of the restrictive forces of the fibrous pericardium. Imaging findings are summarized in Table 24.4.

Pericardial Calcification

Epidemiology

Calcification of the pericardium is a relatively uncommon finding and is most often thought to be a consequence of previous pericardial inflammation (pericarditis). The specific underlying etiology is frequently unknown, particularly if discovered as an incidental finding. Table 24.5 lists etiologies of pericardial calcification.

Clinical Features

At least half the patients with pericardial calcifications will have associated constrictive physiology [2] with features such as jugular venous distention and Kussmaul's sign on physical examination. Constrictive pericarditis will be discussed in the subsequent section, but it is important to note that pericardial calcifications,

TABLE 24.4 Direct and Indirect Imaging Features of Pericardial Agenesis

	CXR	CT/MRI
Direct	■ None	■ Pericardial defect/absence
Indirect	■ Snoopy sign ■ Posterior displacement of the cardiac shadow on lateral radiograph ■ Elevation of the cardiac apex ■ Lucency between aorta and main pulmonary artery ■ Lucency between the cardiac apex and left hemidiaphragm	■ Leftward shift or levorotation of the heart ■ Lung interposition between aorta and main pulmonary artery ■ Lung interposition between the cardiac apex and left hemidiaphragm ■ Increased cardiac motion (excessive apical motion)

TABLE 24.5 Etiologies for Pericardial Calcification

Infectious pericarditis (TB, histoplasmosis, coxsackievirus, influenza)
Uremic pericarditis
Connective tissue diseases (SLE)
Rheumatic heart disease
Chronic/previous hemopericardium (trauma, surgery)
Mediastinal radiation
Pericardial neoplasm

although suggestive, are not diagnostic of constrictive physiology in isolation.

If discovered as an incidental finding, treatment is rarely necessary. In situations of pericardial calcification with constrictive physiology, surgical pericardiectomy (or pericardial stripping) may be considered, as will be discussed in a later section.

Imaging Features

On a chest radiography, pericardial calcifications are most commonly seen along the anterior and diaphragmatic aspects of the heart, which can best be appreciated on a lateral projection (Fig. 24.8). *Pericardial calcifications commonly involve the atrioventricular groove and right atrium but frequently spare the left atrium and left ventricular apex* [1] (Fig. 24.9), a feature which may further help in making the correct diagnosis. Differential diagnosis for pericardial calcifications includes myocardial calcifications from previous infarct, mitral annular calcifications, or a mediastinal teratoma.

Given its high sensitivity for detection of calcifications, CT is a particularly useful technique in this disease, allowing for detailed assessment of the extent of pericardial involvement. Although MRI is more limited in assessing for pericardial calcifications, you may see a circumscribed signal void on multiple sequences in the region of pericardial calcification, commonly surrounded by T1 hyperintense epicardial fat.

Both CT and MRI may also allow for assessment of extracardiac structures, which can provide additional information about

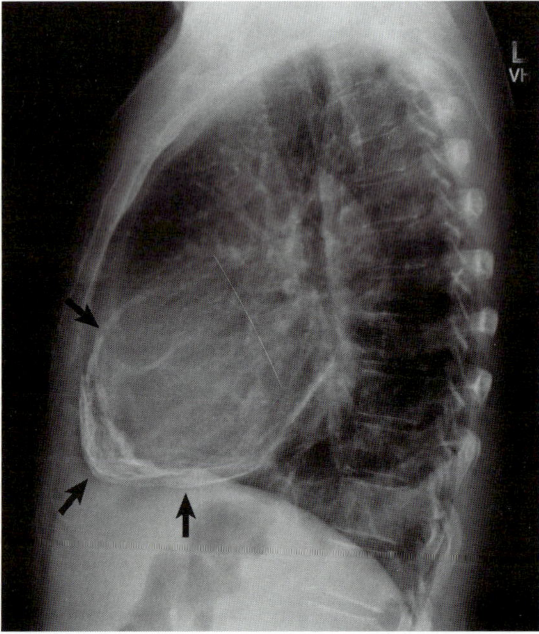

Figure 24.8 Lateral projection chest radiograph demonstrates calcification of the heart border (*arrows*), characteristic of pericardial calcifications.

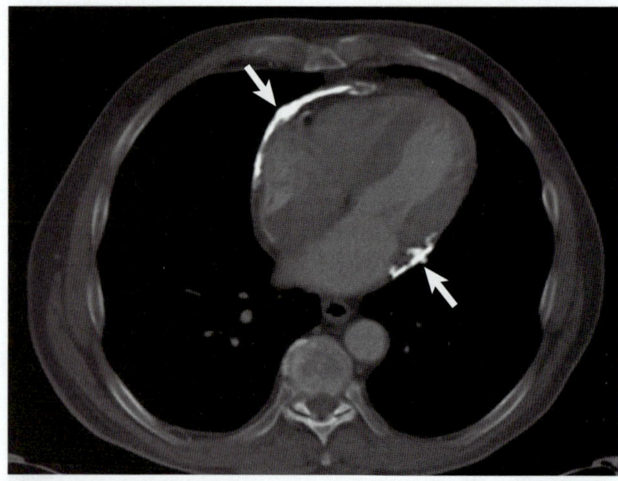

Figure 24.9 Chest CT is highly sensitive and specific for detecting pericardial calcifications, which are shown in a typical distribution here involving the atrioventricular grooves (*arrows*) while sparing the left ventricular apex.

the underlying etiology of pericardial calcifications. For example, if pericardial calcifications are seen in conjunction with fibrotic changes in the adjacent lung, previous mediastinal radiation as the likely etiology can be suspected. Similarly, a tubercular etiology may be considered in the setting of coexisting calcified and/or necrotic lymph nodes or fibrocalcific, fibronodular pulmonary opacities in the upper lobes or apical segments of the lower lobes.

Pericardial Effusion/Fluid

Epidemiology

Pericardial effusion, the most common abnormality of the pericardium encountered in clinical practice, is defined as an accumulation of excess *fluid in the potential space between the parietal and visceral pericardial layers exceeding 50 mL* [1,3,6,11]. Although pericardial effusion most frequently occurs as a result of obstruction of venous or lymphatic drainage from the heart, several types of fluid may collect in the pericardial space, including transudates, exudates, purulent fluid, and blood. There are many potential causes of pericardial effusion, including congestive heart failure, renal insufficiency, infection, myocardial infarction, malignancy, and iatrogenic or traumatic injury (Table 24.6), but can often be narrowed based on the clinical presentation.

Clinical Features

Depending on the volume and acuity of fluid accumulation within the pericardial space, the clinical presentation of pericardial effusion can range from asymptomatic to cardiac tamponade, which will be discussed later on in this chapter. It is important to remember that a rapid accumulation of even a small volume of pericardial fluid may be more dangerous and clinically significant than a slow accumulation of potentially large pericardial effusions.

The treatment of a pericardial effusion depends heavily on the volume and type of fluid, the underlying etiology, and the presence or absence of clinical symptoms. Smaller, asymptomatic pericardial effusions may be treated conservatively with observation and/or imaging follow-up, while larger or rapidly accumulating pericardial effusions can often require intervention with pericardiocentesis, pericardial drainage catheters, or a pericardial window.

Imaging Features

The amount of fluid in the pericardial space determines the appearance on plain chest radiograph, with a large pericardial

TABLE 24.6 Etiologies of Pericardial Fluid/Effusion

Infectious	Viral Bacterial (suppurative) Tuberculous Fungal/parasitic
Inflammatory/autoimmune	Rheumatoid arthritis Systemic lupus erythematosus (SLE) Sarcoidosis Sepsis (sympathetic effusion) Other connective tissue disorder
Metabolic	Hypoalbuminemia Malnutrition Chronic hypothyroidism (myxedema) Uremia
Systemic/hemodynamic	Cirrhosis Congestive heart failure Dressler syndrome (post-MI)
Traumatic/iatrogenic	Traumatic hemorrhage/hematoma Postpericardiotomy syndrome Radiation pericarditis Postcardiac surgery Postcatheter intervention/perforation
Neoplastic	Pericardial metastasis Primary pericardial neoplasm lymphoma
Other	Drug reaction Chylopericardium Bleeding disorders/anticoagulation Idiopathic

Adapted from Czum et al. [2].

effusion causing massive enlargement of the cardiomediastinal silhouette (Fig. 24.10). Rapid enlargement of the cardiac silhouette over serial radiographs is also suggestive of acutely enlarging pericardial effusion. Consequently, drainage of a large effusion will lead to an abrupt decrease in the cardiac silhouette on imaging. The classic sign of a pericardial effusion on a lateral chest radiograph is the *Oreo cookie sign*, which refers to the parallel lucencies of the epicardial and pericardial fat separated in the middle by the relatively opaque pericardial effusion (Fig. 24.11).

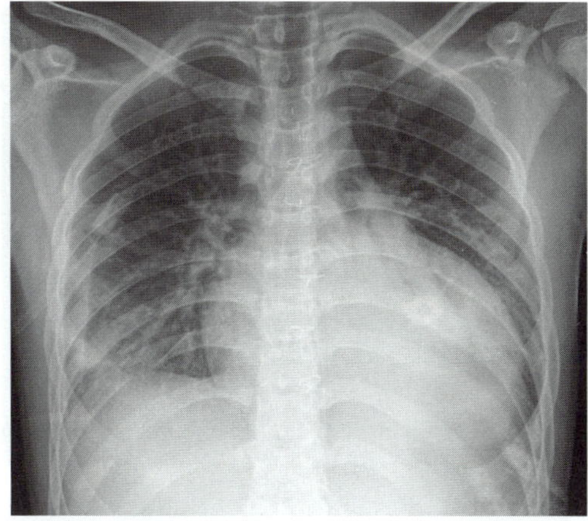

Figure 24.10 Frontal chest radiograph demonstrating enlargement of the cardiomediastinal silhouette due to a large pericardial effusion.

Echocardiography is considered the first-line imaging technique, given its availability, low cost, lack of ionizing radiation, and high sensitivity and specificity for the detection of pericardial effusion [1]. A simple pericardial effusion will appear sonographically as a largely anechoic collection surrounding the cardiac chambers, and this characteristic echo-free space around the heart is well demonstrated using both two-dimensional and M-mode imaging.

When there is a clinical suspicion for a complex pericardial effusion or if the results of echocardiography are inconclusive, CT and MRI are excellent tools for further assessment. Loculated pericardial effusions (Fig. 24.12) in an anterior position, for example, can be particularly difficult to assess by echocardiography due to their retrosternal location, meanwhile CT and MRI can assess this area without difficulty. Since the majority of thoracic imaging by CT and MRI occur with patients in a supine position, any excess fluid will tend to accumulate in a dependent portion of the pericardium. If an effusion becomes large, it tends to surround the heart and motion artifact from the fluid may sometimes be detected.

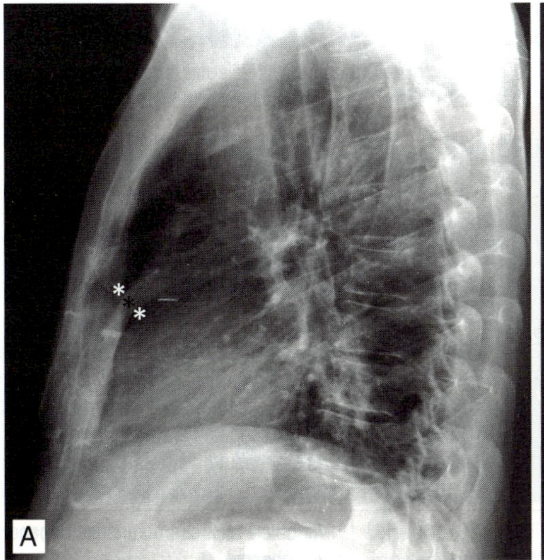

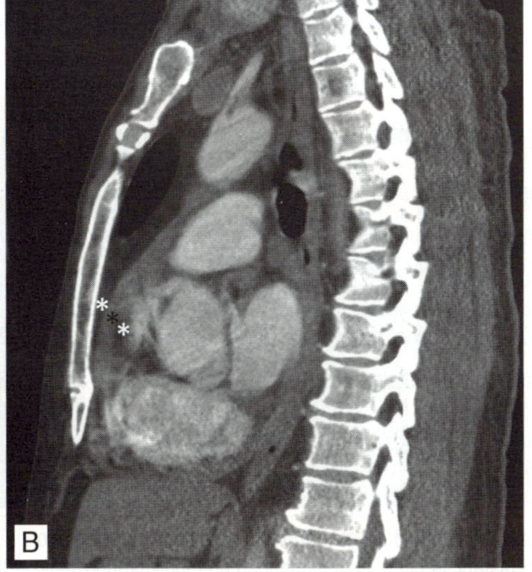

Figure 24.11 Lateral chest radiograph (A) demonstrating the classic *Oreo cookie sign*, which refers to a vertical radiopaque line of pericardial fluid (*black asterisk*) between two vertically oriented lucent lines (*white asterisks*) of retrosternal fat (anteriorly) and epicardial fat (posteriorly), as demonstrated on the corresponding sagittal contrast-enhanced chest CT (B).

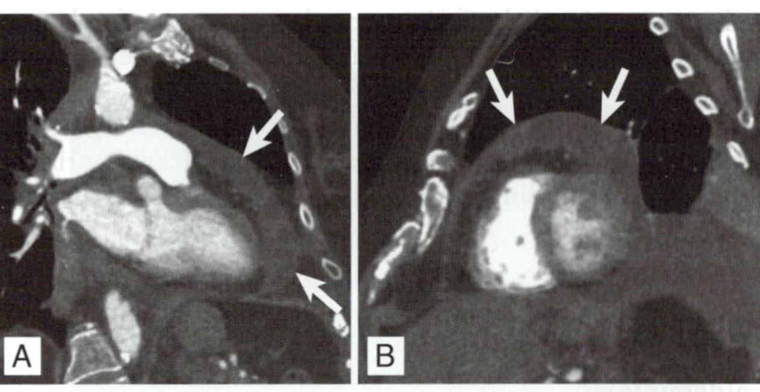

Figure 24.17 Oblique coronal (A) and short-axis (B) contrast-enhanced chest CT demonstrate a malignant pericardial effusion with high density, complex pericardial fluid, and associated nodularity of the pericardium (*arrows*), in a patient with known primary lung malignancy.

TABLE 24.8 Etiologies of Pneumopericardium

Accidental (penetrating or blunt) trauma
Iatrogenic trauma (thoracic surgery/pericardial drainage)
Positive pressure ventilation (barotrauma)
Infectious pericarditis (gas-producing organisms)
Fistulous connection with adjacent air-containing organ (airways/GI tract)

Imaging Features

Unlike other pericardial disorders, pneumopericardium is often visible on plain radiograph as a lucency outlining the heart borders. Although pneumopericardium can commonly co-occur with pneumomediastinum, it is important to differentiate air tracking up into the superior mediastinum (as seen in pneumomediastinum) from air confined within the pericardial cavity, which should stop at the pericardial attachment site at level of the great vessel origins (Fig. 24.18). The *continuous diaphragm sign* can be seen on a frontal projection chest radiograph; however, this is not a specific sign and can be seen in either pneumopericardium or pneumomediastinum.

Cross-sectional imaging with cardiac CT can be particularly useful in assessing the extent of pericardial air accumulation (Fig. 24.19), detecting imaging features of tamponade physiology (discussed later), and evaluating extracardiac structures to determine the underlying etiology. Cardiac MRI remains impractical as a diagnostic technique in pneumopericardium due to the artifact that air can produce and long imaging times, as patients with pneumopericardium frequently require urgent or emergent care.

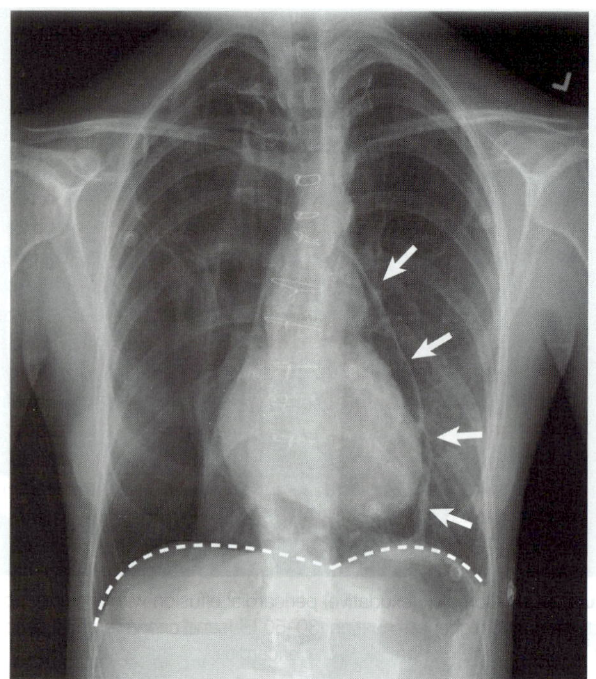

Figure 24.18 Frontal chest radiograph demonstrating a large right pneumothorax and a concurrent large pneumopericardium with the *continuous diaphragm sign* (dotted line) and a sharply defined pericardial line (*arrows*). Pnuemopericardium can be differentiated from pneumomediastinum in this case, given that you can see the air surrounding the heart stops at the level of the pericardial attachment to the great vessels.

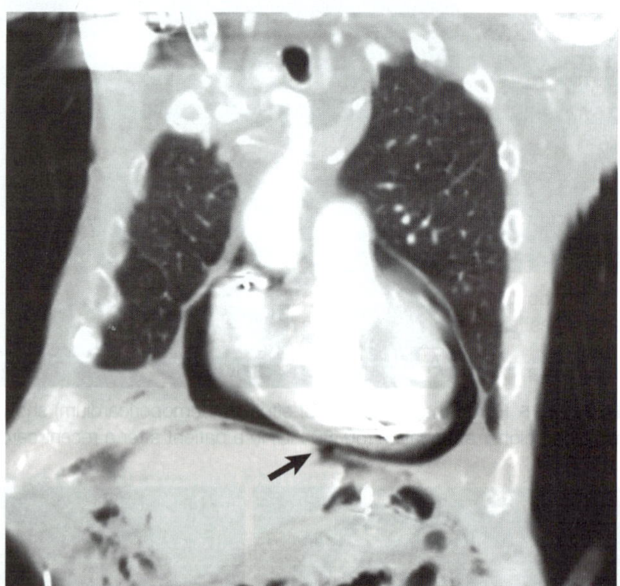

Figure 24.19 Coronal chest CT in lung windows demonstrates another case of pneumopericardium. In this case, there is coexisting free intraperitoneal air that is communicating with the pericardial space inferiorly through a diaphragmatic defect (*arrow*) at the site of a previous pericardial drain.

Pericarditis Without Constriction

Epidemiology

Pericarditis is a fibrotic inflammatory reaction affecting part or all of the pericardium with many potential underlying etiologies similar to the causes of pericardial effusion, including infectious, inflammatory, metabolic, traumatic, and toxic processes [9].

Clinical Features

Pericarditis can present clinically as an acute, chronic, or recurrent process, and may ultimately lead to constriction (discussed in a subsequent section). Common presenting symptoms include abrupt pleuritic positional chest pain, worse when lying supine, and a pericardial friction rub on auscultation.

Therapy of pericarditis, particularly acute pericarditis, should be targeted to the underlying etiology as much as possible. Although mild cases of pericarditis without constriction may resolve without any treatment, colchicine and nonsteroidal anti-inflammatory drugs or steroids are commonly used to reduce inflammation and control pain. Adjunctive interventional

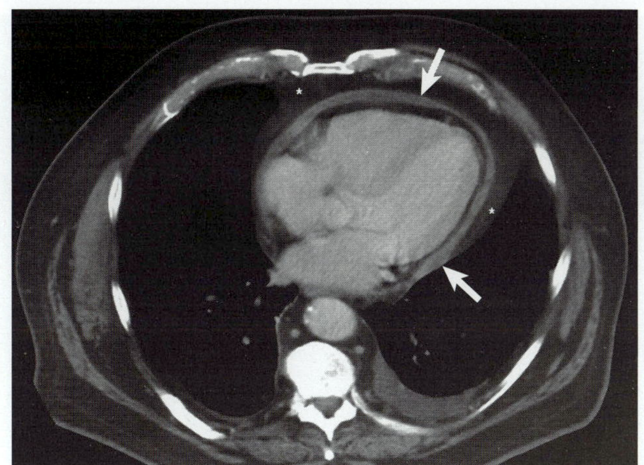

Figure 24.20 Axial contrast-enhanced chest CT demonstrates marked pericardial thickening and enhancement (*arrows*) with subtle stranding of the adjacent fat (*asterisks*), compatible with pericarditis.

TABLE 24.9 Differentiating the Imaging Features of Constrictive Pericarditis versus Restrictive Cardiomyopathy

	Constrictive Pericarditis	Restrictive Cardiomyopathy
Physical exam	Elevated JVP Kussmaul sign Pericardial knock	Elevated JVP ± Kussmaul sign
Pericardial thickness	Thickened	Normal
Pericardial calcification	Commonly present	Not present
Atrial enlargement	Mild–moderate	Moderate–severe
Septal motion	Septal bounce (respirophasic variation)	Normal

therapies such as pericardial drainage or pericardiotomy/pericardiectomy are rarely considered in complicated or refractory cases.

Imaging Features

Pericardial inflammation in isolation is a pathologic diagnosis and can be difficult to detect by imaging unless other key features are present, including pericardial thickening, pericardial enhancement, increased attenuation or stranding of the adjacent fat, and/or a concurrent pericardial effusion (Fig. 24.20). It is important to note that subtle regional pericardial thickening can sometimes be difficult to differentiate from small volume physiologic pericardial fluid, and care must be taken to ensure correct diagnosis.

Although echocardiography may be used to detect associated pericardial effusions, pericarditis is much better assessed with cross-sectional imaging techniques when suspected clinically. Thickening and enhancement of the pericardium can be identified by both CT and MRI, with MRI having greater sensitivity as well as the ability to detect pericardial edema on T2 weighted sequences [7]. MRI has the additional advantage of being able to differentiate pericardial enhancement in pericarditis from myocardial enhancement seen in myocarditis, which can present similarly, with the use of gadolinium.

Constrictive Pericarditis

Epidemiology

Constrictive pericarditis is both a clinical and imaging diagnosis caused by thickened/fibrotic pericardium or pericardial adhesions, defined as an abnormal fusion of the parietal and visceral pericardium, which can be seen as the long-term sequelae of chronic/recurrent pericardial inflammation (pericarditis). The most common cause of constrictive pericarditis worldwide is tuberculosis, with less common etiologies including viral/bacterial infections, hemopericardium, radiation, and cardiac surgery [11].

Pathophysiology

Inflammation and/or thickening of the pericardium reduce pericardial compliance, which in turn leads to a reduction in left ventricular diastolic filling and ultimately diastolic failure [6]. The thickened, rigid pericardium also prevents transmission of intrathoracic pressures to the cardiac chambers. These changes taken together result in a physiologic phenomenon known as *ventricular interdependence (ventricular coupling)*, wherein the filling of one ventricle is dependent upon the filling of the other ventricle [2,6]. This ventricular interdependence manifests on imaging as a *septal bounce*, which will be discussed later.

Clinical Features

Clinically, patients with constrictive pericarditis will present with features of congestive heart failure, including progressive dyspnea, fatigue, and lower extremity edema. By symptomatology alone, constrictive pericarditis can be difficult to distinguish from restrictive cardiomyopathy, and care must be taken to differentiate these two pathologies by imaging. Table 24.9 summarizes the key differences between constrictive pericarditis and restrictive cardiomyopathy. The definitive treatment for constrictive pericarditis is complete pericardiectomy.

Imaging Features

On plain chest radiograph the heart is often normal, but can be nonspecifically enlarged. Straightening of the right heart border and roughening of the cardiac outline as a result of pleuropericardial adhesions have been described. The lungs are usually clear due to constriction most commonly involving the right heart, although a pleural effusion is not uncommon.

One of the most common and important imaging features of constrictive pericarditis is pericardial calcification, often present in a characteristic distribution involving the front and lateral aspects of the heart (Figs. 24.8 and 24.9). Approximately 50% of patients with pericardial calcification will have constrictive physiology and up to 90% of patients with constrictive physiology will have pericardial calcifications [2]. Pericardial calcifications, when extensive, can be identified on plain film, however, as previously discussed, CT is particularly sensitive for the detection of pericardial calcifications.

Echocardiography can be used to assess diastolic septal motion for the presence of a *septal bounce*, wherein the interventricular septum moves toward the left ventricle in early diastole as the right ventricular pressures increase and subsequently moves back toward the right ventricle in late diastole as the ventricular pressures equalize and systemic pressures increase [2]. The presence of a *septal bounce* is suggestive *ventricular interdependence (ventricular coupling)*, which occurs when the filling of one ventricle is dependent upon the filling of the other ventricle.

In constrictive physiology, there is classically variation of the abnormal septal motion during respiration, with the diastolic flattening becoming more pronounced during inspiration. This

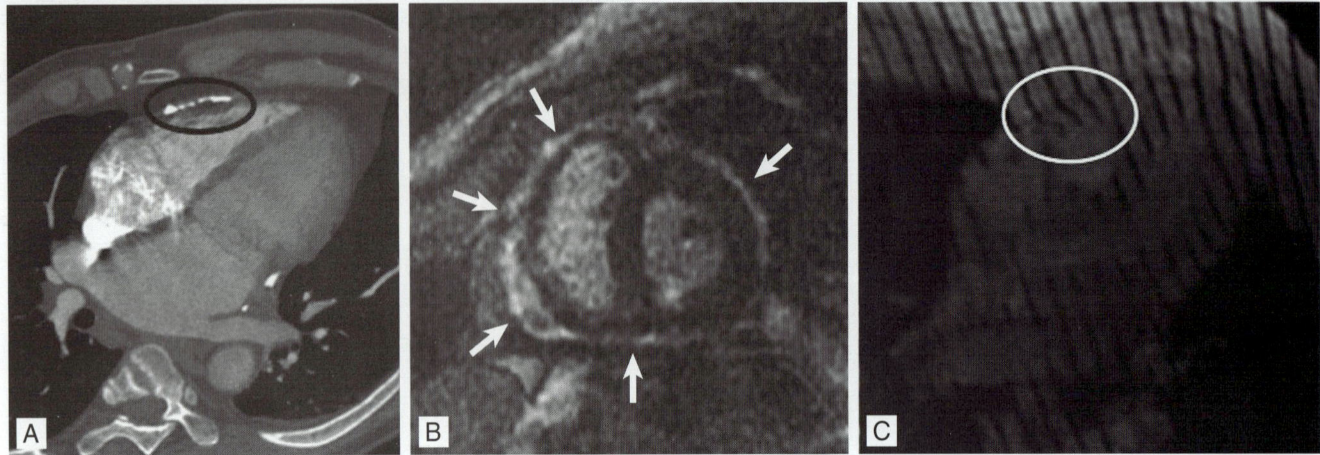

Figure 24.21 (A) Four-chamber contrast-enhanced cardiac CT demonstrates pericardial calcifications, particularly along the right ventricular free wall with a tubular ventricular configuration and biatrial enlargement. (B) A corresponding short-axis late gadolinium enhancement sequence of the same patient demonstrates marked circumferential pericardial thickening and enhancement (*arrows*), particularly adjacent to the right ventricle in the region of calcification. (C) A tagged cine sequence demonstrates bending of the tag lines along the right ventricular free wall during systole (*circled*), a finding that is compatible with pericardial adhesions in the setting of constrictive pericarditis.

respirophasic variation in septal motion is considered to be a pathognomonic sign for constriction. It is important to remember that a septal bounce and ventricular interdependence can be seen both in constrictive pericarditis and tamponade.

Cross-sectional imaging techniques, CT and MRI, are valuable adjunctive techniques in the diagnosis of constrictive pericarditis and effectively demonstrate additional features suggestive of constrictive pericarditis including a tubular ventricular morphology with disproportionate biatrial dilatation, interventricular septal flattening, and pericardial thickening (>4 mm) with or without a concurrent effusion (Fig. 24.21) [6,11]. Contrast-enhanced CT may additionally demonstrate dilatation and contrast reflux into the inferior vena cava, hepatic veins, and azygos vein, suggesting elevated right heart pressures due to constriction.

MRI techniques in particular have evolved significantly and now have greater diagnostic capacities than both echocardiography and CT in detecting constriction, most notably with the use of tagged cine sequences aimed at assessing for regions of pericardial adhesion. The absence of normal pericardial slippage manifests as tag lines which bend but do not break as expected with ventricular contraction (Fig. 24.21). MRI is also especially useful in assessing for the characteristic respirophasic variation of abnormal septal motion with respiratory-gated steady-state free precession cine sequences (Fig. 24.22). The combination of pericardial adhesions with an exaggerated inspiratory septal bounce is suggestive of constrictive physiology.

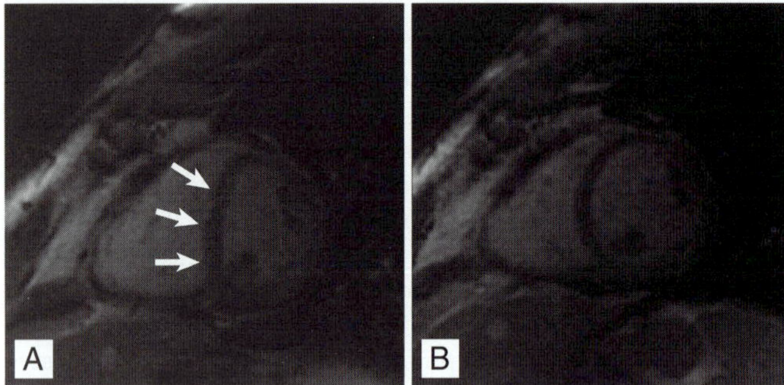

Figure 24.22 Respirophasic dynamic SSFP cine imaging during (A) inspiration and (B) expiration demonstrates early diastolic septal flattening during inspiration (*arrows*) compatible a *septal bounce*. This finding confirms *ventricular interdependence* with respirophasic variation and is considered to be pathognomonic of constrictive physiology.

Cardiac Tamponade

Pathophysiology

Cardiac tamponade describes the physiologic result of large or rapid accumulations of fluid/air/material in the pericardial space wherein diastolic function becomes impaired to the point of failure. As mentioned in an earlier section, the absolute volume of material within the pericardial cavity is somewhat less important than the rate of accumulation, because over short periods of time the pericardium is unable to remodel and adjust to the rising intrapericardial pressure. The result is progressive extrinsic compression of the ventricular chambers resulting in an emergent impairment of cardiac output [2].

Clinical Features

Presenting symptoms of cardiac tamponade often include the so-called *Beck triad* of muffled heart sounds, hypotension, and jugular venous distension, along with pulsus paradoxus. Tamponade is frequently considered a life-threatening emergency and typically warrants immediate intervention in the form of ultrasound-guided pericardiocentesis.

Imaging Features

The imaging features of cardiac tamponade are uncommonly encountered in clinical practice, but it is crucial for radiologists to recognize them when present and make a timely diagnosis and prompt appropriate therapy.

Echocardiography is a quick and affordable first-line technique that can be utilized at the bedside when suspicion of cardiac tamponade is raised. Echocardiography may demonstrate abnormal motion of the interventricular septum in the form of a *septal bounce* suggestive of *ventricular interdependence* (also seen in constrictive pericarditis) with concurrent visualization of a large collection of fluid, blood, or other material within the pericardial space. Doppler evaluation of the tricuspid and mitral valve inflow can also assist in the diagnosis of tamponade, which will demonstrate exaggeration of the normal inspiratory increase

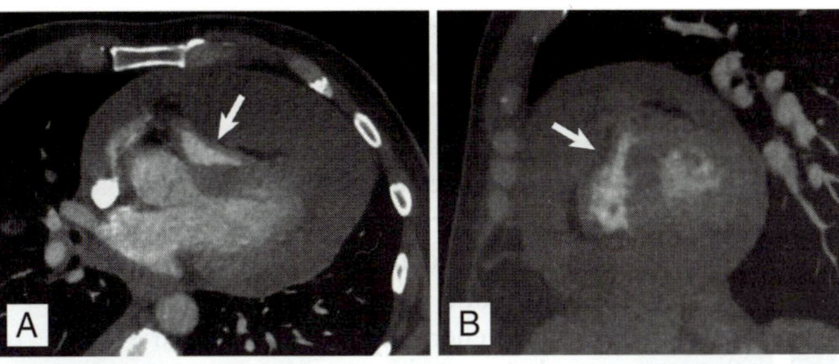

Figure 24.23 Axial (A) and short-axis (B) contrast-enhanced cardiac CT demonstrate a large pericardial effusion resulting in inversion of the right ventricular free wall (*arrows*), consistent with cardiac tamponade physiology.

in tricuspid inflow as well as the normal inspiratory decrease in mitral flow velocity.

Cross-sectional imaging with CT can provide additional diagnostic information on a relatively quick time course, and should be considered in the case of equivocal echocardiography findings. Pericardial collections of fluid, blood, or even air can be easily identified by CT, especially if loculated or in locations not well visualized by ultrasound, and contrast may be seen refluxing into dilated inferior vena cava, hepatic veins, or azygos vein due to impaired diastolic right ventricular filling. The most specific sign for tamponade physiology by CT is deformation or inversion of a ventricular free wall in diastole (Fig. 24.23). Unsurprisingly, due to the acute and emergent nature of cardiac tamponade, MRI remains impractical as a diagnostic technique.

Pericardial Cyst

Epidemiology

Pericardial cyst is the most common benign pericardial mass and represents a congenital abnormality typically resulting from an excluded portion of a pericardial recess [1,3]. These masses are frequently asymptomatic and often are discovered incidentally by imaging, although larger cysts can rarely exert mass effect on the heart and adjacent structures. The most common location for a pericardial cyst is the right anterior cardiophrenic angle [1–3,11], although they can be seen in any location attached to the pericardium, directly or through a short pedicle, and they may grow slowly over time, sometimes measuring up to 8 cm or larger.

Clinical Features

The majority of pericardial cysts are asymptomatic and require no therapeutic intervention. Complications including cardiac compression, superimposed infection, and cyst rupture are exceedingly rare. In the unusual setting of large, symptomatic, or infected cysts, percutaneous aspiration or surgical resection may be considered.

Imaging Features

Small pericardial cysts are likely to be radiographically occult on plain film, although larger cysts may distort or enlarge the cardiomediastinal silhouette. CT often demonstrates a well-circumscribed hypodense rounded or ovoid lesion adjacent to the heart with a smooth, nonenhancing wall and no internal septations. Although the majority of pericardial cysts will measure water attenuation (between 10 and 30 HU), they may rarely contain internal debris, which may cause them to appear more hyperdense on CT. Occasionally pericardial cysts contain calcification and differentiation from other mediastinal masses can be difficult.

MRI can be a valuable diagnostic tool in differentiating pericardial cysts from other more concerning lesions. MR features of simple pericardial cysts include T1 hypointensity, homogeneous T2 hyperintensity, lack of enhancement with intravenous gadolinium administration, and lack of restricted diffusion on DWI sequences (Fig. 24.24). Pericardial cysts containing internal debris may demonstrate altered T1 and T2 characteristics; however, the lack of enhancement and lack of restricted diffusion should help clarify the diagnosis in this rare situation. The differential diagnosis for a pericardial cyst is summarized in Table 24.10.

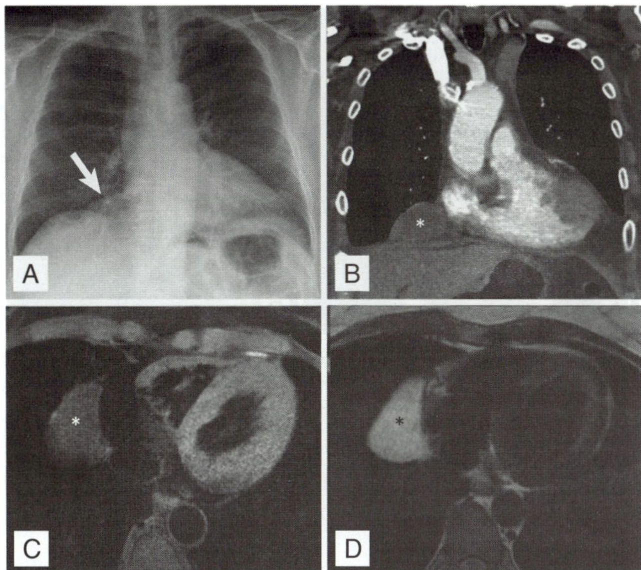

Figure 24.24 Frontal chest radiograph (A) demonstrates an abnormal contour at the right cardiophrenic angle (*arrow*) partially obscuring the right heart border, which corresponds with coronal chest CT; (B) findings of a well-circumscribed, low-density ovoid lesion near the right anterior costophrenic angle (*asterisk*). Axial T1 with fat saturation (C) and T2 (B) sequences demonstrate T1 hypointensity and T2 hyperintensity, of the same lesion which are characteristics of a simple pericardial cyst (*asterisks*).

Pericardial Neoplasms

Epidemiology

Pericardial neoplasms, both benign and malignant, are rare entities. Metastatic disease is far more common than primary pericardial neoplasms, with pericardial metastases most often originating from lung cancer, breast cancer, melanoma, or lymphoma primaries [1,6]. Metastatic involvement of the pericardium may occur as a result of direct extension/invasion from adjacent structures, lymphatic spread, or hematogenous spread, and autopsy studies have suggested that pericardial metastatic disease can be detected in up to ~20% of patients with known

TABLE 24.10 Differential Diagnosis of a Pericardial Cyst [2]
Pericardial cyst
Foregut duplication cysts (bronchogenic, neurenteric, etc.)
Pericardial diverticulum
Thymic cyst
Pericardial hydatid disease
Diaphragmatic eventration or Morgagni hernia
Thoracic pancreatic pseudocyst
Cystic neoplasm

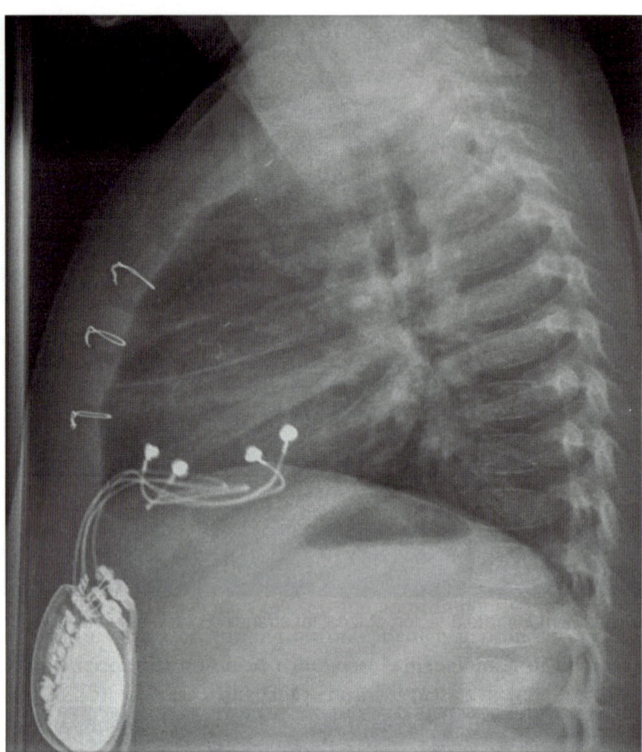

Figure 24.30 Lateral chest radiograph demonstrates an epicardial pacemaker device in the soft tissues of the upper abdomen with multiple leads terminating in the inferior pericardial space.

discussed in the preceding sections, pericardial fluid collections are commonly treated with the use of percutaneous pericardial drainage catheters, which will appear on radiographs and CT as linear radiodense/hyperdense catheters entering and terminating within the pericardium, often surrounding a portion of the heart (Fig. 24.29).

Another occasionally encountered device is the epicardial pacemaker. Although much less commonly used compared with the traditional transvenous or transcutaneous pacemakers, epicardial pacemakers are an alternative device treatment of arrhythmias in certain patients. Their appearance on lateral chest radiograph is distinct from a transvenous pacemaker device because the leads will follow the epicardial contour, rather than entering the cardiac chambers as in transvenous leads (Fig. 24.30). Similarly epicardial pacing wires can be encountered on imaging postcardiac surgery.

Finally, it is important to be aware of the appearance of surgical material that may be used for repair or reconstruction of the pericardium in cases of trauma or extensive pericardial surgery. Various patches and meshes may be used for pericardial reconstruction, mostly to prevent the dreaded and potentially fatal complication of cardiac herniation. On noncontrast-enhanced chest CT, pericardial patch material is likely to appear hyperdense in a contour surrounding the heart (Fig. 24.31).

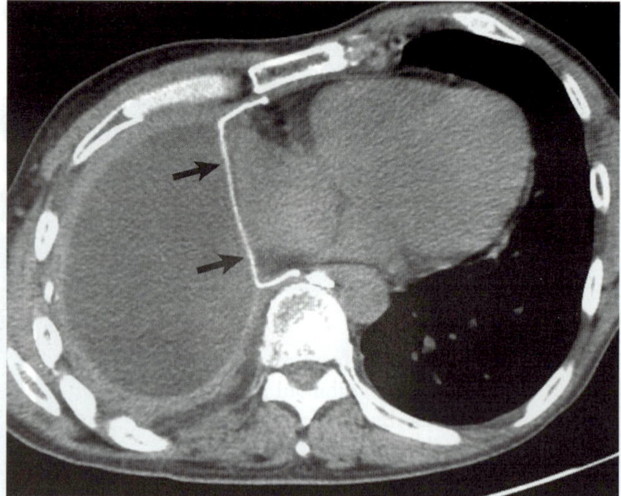

Figure 24.31 Axial noncontrast chest CT demonstrates postoperative changes of a right extrapleural pneumonectomy with right pericardial reconstruction using hyperdense surgical mesh material (*arrows*).

Overall Approach to the Pericardium/ Take Home Points

- Echocardiography is considered the first-line imaging tool for assessment of suspected pericardial pathology
- CT and MRI are useful adjuncts in evaluating pericardial disease, particularly in the characterization of loculated or complex pericardial effusions, constrictive pericarditis, and pericardial masses
- Detailed functional/physiologic assessment can be performed using CT or MRI and is extremely important for diagnosing many pericardial diseases, including pericardial adhesions, constrictive pericarditis, cardiac tamponade in the appropriate clinical settings

Suggested Readings

- E Ünal, M Karcaaltincaba, E Akpinar, OM Ariyurek, The imaging appearances of various pericardial disorders, Insights Imaging 10 (1) (2019) 42.
- J Bogaert, M Francone, Pericardial disease: value of CT and MR imaging, Radiology 267 (2) (2013) 340–356.
- SM O'Leary, PL Williams, MP Williams, AJ Edwards, CA Roobottom, GJ Morgan-Hughes, et al., Imaging the pericardium: appearances on ECG-gated 64-detector row cardiac computed tomography, Br J Radiol 83 (987) (2010) 194–205.
- N Oyama, N Oyama, K Komuro, T Nambu, WJ Manning, K. Miyasaka, Computed tomography and magnetic resonance imaging of the pericardium: anatomy and pathology, Magn Reson Med Sci 3 (3) (2004) 145–152.
- LS Broderick, GN Brooks, JE Kuhlman, Anatomic pitfalls of the heart and pericardium, Radiographics 25 (2) (2005) 441–453.

25
Diseases of Arteries

VIKY S. LOESCHER, MICHAEL STEIGNER

General Concepts

The introduction of helical computed tomography with its capability of single breath-hold rapid acquisitions has led to the development of computed tomography angiography (CTA). This produces even higher quality images with better contrast enhancement than conventional CT and has the added advantage of being able to reformat oblique and curved multiplanar reconstructed (MPR) images, maximum intensity projection images, as well as three-dimensional (3D) images. Automated tube current modulation, a technique that now is widely available in all new scanners, should be used in conjunction with automatic tube potential selection. Vascular imaging uses a threshold-based test bolus or bolus-tracking algorithm using a region of interest typically placed in the ascending, proximal descending thoracic aorta or proximal abdominal aorta [1–3].

CTA is a noninvasive method of imaging used to assess any vasculature. When used to assess the aorta and arteries, it is generally performed before and after intravenous injection of iodinated contrast medium. Unenhanced images show calcification in the wall of arterial vessels, depict features of an intramural hematoma (IMH), helps differentiating high density surgical material such as pledgets from pseudoaneurysms, or identifies postoperative hematomas; whereas contrast-enhanced images show flowing blood, degree of stenosis, thrombus, or atheroma within the vessel lumen. Delayed phase images can be obtained to assess for endoleaks, iodine contrast extravasation such as in gastrointestinal bleeding or in post-traumatic or postprocedural settings, or to fully assess for mesenteric ischemia with venous etiology. The use of ECG-gated CTA significantly decreases the effect of cardiac motion in the evaluation of the aortic root and allows for accurate measurements and assessment of the thoracic aorta. The design of vascular imaging protocols is particularly challenging due to the nonuniform velocity of blood, differences in cardiac outputs, and different effects of underlying conditions on blood flow that many times cannot be predicted before the scan [3].

CTA is commonly used in vascular imaging for the assessment of thoracic and abdominal aortic aneurysms (AAAs) to see if they are suitable for endovascular repair, and in the diagnosis of acute aortic syndrome [3]. CTA is also used-in the investigation of carotid and renal vascular disease.

MR angiography (MRA) is also a noninvasive method of imaging the aorta and arteries which can be performed with or without the intravenous injection of a paramagnetic intravascular gadolinium-based contrast agent (GBCA). GBCA shortens blood longitudinal relaxation (T1). 3D spoiled gradient echo (GRE) pulse sequences with a short repetition time and a short echo time are ideal for MRA. 3D GRE T1 pulse sequence provides images with high signal-to-noise ratio and good spatial resolution. Time-resolved MRA is an acquisition mode of postcontrast images over successive time points and has specific vendor acronyms such as TWIST (Siemens, Germany), TRICKS (General Electric, USA), 4-D TRACK (Phillips, Netherlands), or TRAQ (Hitachi, Japan). This sequence is particularly helpful in small arteries such as run offs of feet and hands, as well as the arteries below the knee, or in cases of arteriovenous shunts. The core of this time-resolved sequence is also a 3D-spoiled GRE [3]. A typical MRA protocol includes localizers, coronal, and axial T2-weighted single-shot fast spin echo sequences, which allow a general assessment and planning of the 3D-MRA. The 3D-MRA noncontrast (mask) is acquired followed by two successive arterial phase acquisitions, as well as a delayed T1-weighted 3D spoiled GRE sequence with fat saturation. GBCA is administered to all patients with GFR >30 mL/min, followed by saline chaser. The decision to administer GBCA in patients with a lower GFR should be made on a case-by-case basis. For patients who cannot receive GBCA, a balanced steady-state free precession (SSFP) sequence is used because it provides bright blood imaging without gadolinium. It has been shown that MRA without contrast can detect aortic dissection with high accuracy when compared to MRA with contrast [4]. The associated off-resonance artifact seen on SSFP sequences can be decreased using lower strength magnetic fields (1.5 T).

Doppler imaging is one of the principal diagnostic tools for the assessment of arterial diseases. The term Doppler is an eponym after Christian Johann Doppler (1803–1853), the Austrian physicist who first described the Doppler effect. Arterial ultrasound has three basic components, the first component is the standard brightness mode (B-mode) grayscale assessment. The second component uses color Doppler interrogation, allowing assessment of luminal narrowing severity. The third component uses interrogation of a small segment of an arterial vessel, producing the spectral Doppler waveform. Duplex Doppler refers to an ultrasound using the two first components, grayscale and color Doppler. Technically, the use of the three components should be denominated as "triplex," however, the inclusion of spectral analysis is also commonly referred as duplex Doppler imaging [5].

Spectral analysis interrogates usually a small 2–4 mm segment of a vessel of interest, ideally the midportion of the lumen, rather than the periphery, for optimal assessment of the laminar flow. The degree of stenosis is obtained by measuring peak systolic velocity (PSV) using spectral analysis. The Doppler angle is the angle between actual Doppler beam and the Doppler interrogation vessel sample, and it should always be less than 60° [5]. Doppler angles greater than 60° affect the accuracy of PSVs, and it could underestimate or overestimate the level of stenosis. There is an inverse relationship between stenosis and velocity, so decrease in sectional area increases velocity of flow if there are no branches. Resistive index is defined as the ratio between the difference of systolic and diastolic velocities and the systolic velocity [6].

Aorta

Normal Anatomy of the Aorta

Thoracic Aorta

The aortic root involves the annulus, sinuses of Valsalva, and the sinotubular junction. The ascending thoracic aorta extends from the sinotubular junction to the origin of the brachiocephalic trunk, and the aortic arch extends from the origin of the brachiocephalic trunk to the ligamentum arteriosum. The aortic isthmus is between the distal aortic arch and the descending thoracic aorta. The proximal descending thoracic aorta always appears more dilated and it is known as the aortic spindle [7,8] (Fig. 25.1).

The three-vessel aortic arch consists of the brachiocephalic trunk (innominate artery), the left common carotid artery, and left subclavian artery; this is the most common branching pattern of the aortic arch and is seen in about 70% of patients. The combined origin of the brachiocephalic trunk and the left common carotid artery is seen in about 20–30% of patients. This is the so-called "bovine" aortic arch, a misnomer since the bovine aortic arch shows a single trunk with common origin of the great vessels. The vertebral arteries usually arise from the subclavian arteries. When the left vertebral artery instead arises directly from the aortic arch, it is called a four-vessel aortic arch and it is seen in about 5–10% of patients [9]. The most common aortic arch anomaly is a left aortic arch with aberrant right subclavian artery arising directly from the aortic arch. The aberrant right subclavian is the last vessel arising from the arch and shows a retroesophageal course, but not forming a vascular ring (Fig. 25.2). Another variant of the aortic arch is the ductus diverticulum, a small bulging along the inner aspect of the aortic isthmus representing an embryological remnant of the ductus arteriosum and should not be mistaken with an aneurysm or pseudoaneurysm [8] (Fig. 25.3).

There are four major aortic arch types; left aortic arch, right aortic arch, double aortic arch, and cervical aortic arch [9,10]. With a right aortic arch, the most common anomalies include:

1. *Retroesophageal aberrant left subclavian artery with diverticulum of Kommerell*, which is associated with the presence of a left

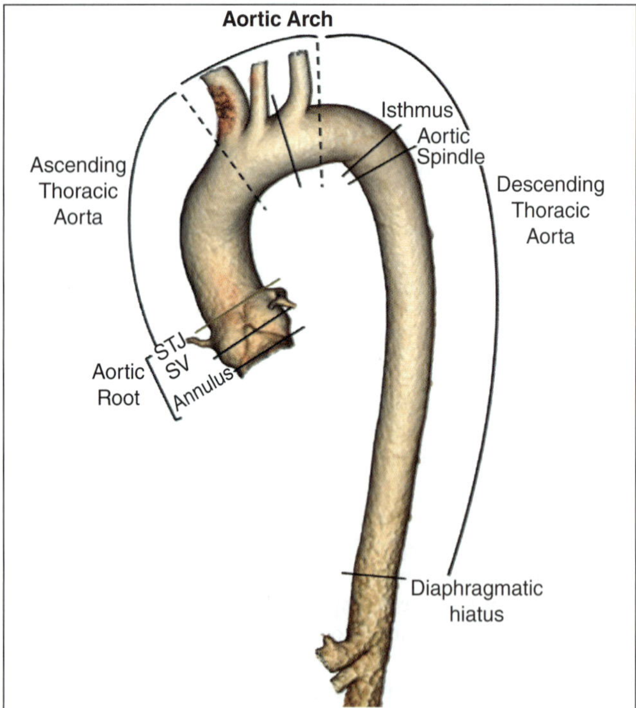

Figure 25.1 Normal anatomy of the thoracic aorta. The aortic root is composed of the annulus, sinuses of Valsalva (SV) and sinotubular junction (STJ). The ascending aorta extends from the level of the STJ to the origin of the brachiocephalic trunk. The aortic arch extends from right after the origin of the brachiocephalic trunk to the last aortic arch branch (between *dashed lines*). The descending thoracic aorta extends from right after the takeoff of the last branch of the aortic arch to the level of the diaphragmatic hiatus. The aortic spindle is a normal bulge of the proximal descending thoracic aorta.

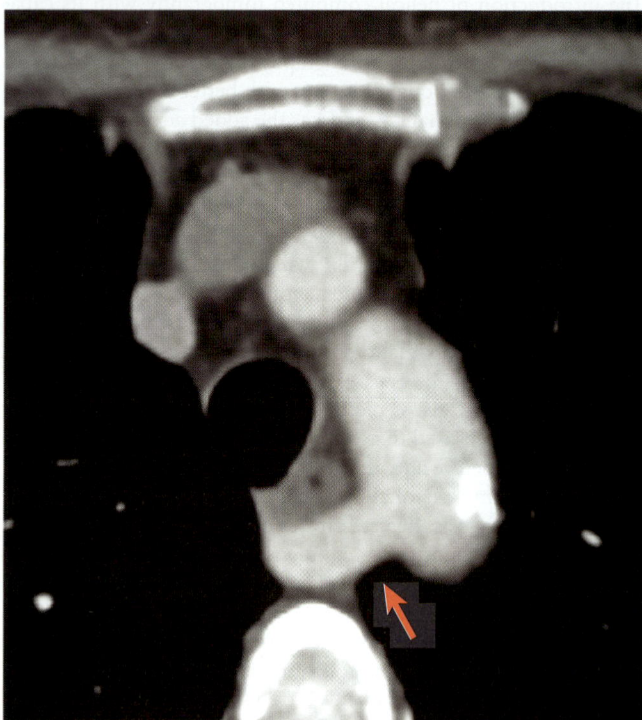

Figure 25.2 Left aortic arch and aberrant right subclavian artery. The right subclavian artery (*red arrow*) arises directly from the aortic arch and courses posteriorly to the esophagus and is associated with dysphagia lusoria.

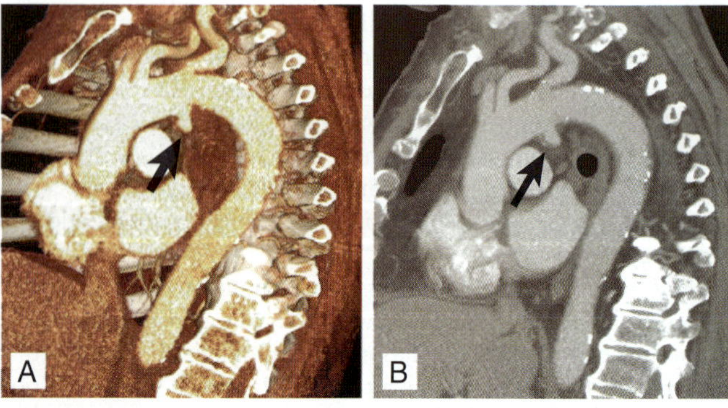

Figure 25.3 Aortic diverticulum. (A and B) CTA three-dimensional (3D) and oblique multiplanar reconstructed (MPR) images show a protrusion along the inner aspect of the isthmus with smooth contours (*black arrows*). (Courtesy: Sandeep Hedgire, MD from Massachusetts General Hospital, Boston, USA.)

ductus or ligamentum forming the second most common vascular ring [9].
2. *Mirror image right aortic arch*, which refers to the fact that the origin of the great vessels follows the opposite order of the left aortic arch. This type of aortic arch is also associated with other cardiac congenital abnormalities.
3. *Double aortic arch* refers to the persistence of both the left and right embryologic fourth arches forming the most common vascular ring. In the majority of cases, the right arch is superior and larger than the left (dominant right arch). The role of vascular imaging is to identify which arch is nondominant so it can be surgically ligated to relieve the vascular ring [9].
4. The *cervical aortic arch* is a rare anomaly characterized by a high-lying aortic arch extending above the level of the clavicles [11] (Fig. 25.4).

The Abdominal Aorta

The proximal abdominal aorta extends from the crura to the origin of the celiac artery. The renal arteries are used as a landmark to help recognize the suprarenal, juxtarenal, and infrarenal abdominal aorta. The infrarenal abdominal aorta extends to the level of the L4 vertebral body where it bifurcates into the bilateral common iliac arteries [2].

Aortic Diseases

Aortic disease presentation ranges from asymptomatic (aneurysms or penetrating atherosclerotic ulcers [PAUs] incidentally detected on MDCT) to acute chest pain (IMHs, dissections, trauma, ruptures, etc.), as well as inflammatory and traumatic disorders [7]. Currently, there are 64-detector row and newer generation CT scanners that can evaluate the entire aorta in a single short breath hold. MDCT permits the evaluation of the entire aorta with 3D reconstructions in any orientation using MPR. Moreover, when compared with regular invasive angiography, MDCT allows the evaluation of extravascular structures using less radiation, as well as decreasing the radiation exposure of the patient and the operator. The use of ECG gating should also be encouraged for the evaluation of the aortic root and ascending thoracic aorta, as cardiac motion could result in significant artifact decreasing the accuracy of aortic dimensions or mimicking dissections or pseudoaneurysms.

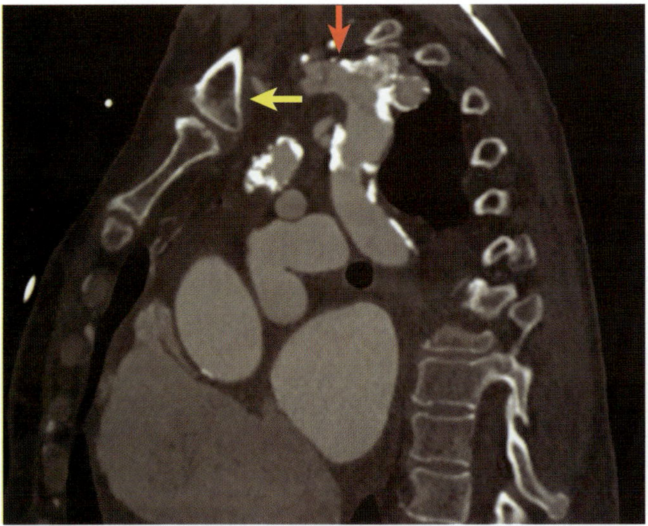

Figure 25.4 Cervical aortic arch. CTA sagittal oblique multiplanar reconstructed (MPR) image shows the aortic arch (*red arrow*) extending above the head of the clavicle (*yellow arrow*).

Aneurysms

The normal dimensions of the thoracic and abdominal aorta have been established based on large population studies [7–10]. An aneurysm is defined as a dimension exceeding the normal measurement by more than 2 SDs, or greater than the 95% confidence interval (Table 25.1).

The prevalence of thoracic aneurysms increases with age, with an incidence of approximately 450 per 100,000 and a 3:1 male predominance. In aneurysms, all three layers of the vessel wall (intima, media, and adventitia) are involved. Aneurysms can be *fusiform* involving all of the circumference of the vessel (Fig. 25.5) or *saccular* with a narrow neck. Overall, atherosclerosis is the most

TABLE 25.1 Maximum Normal Dimensions for the Aorta and Aneurysmal Size by Segments [2,8]

Maximum Normal Dimensions of the Aorta		Aneurysmal Dimensions of the Aorta
Segment	Size (mm)	Size (mm)
Sinuses of Valsalva	36.9 ± 3.8 (2 SD)	≥40
Sinotubular junction	29.7 ± 3.4 (2 SD)	≥35
Ascending thoracic aorta	32.7 ± 3.8 (2 SD)	≥40
Aortic arch		≥35
Descending thoracic aorta	17–26 (95% CI)	≥35
Proximal abdominal aorta		≥30
Infrarenal abdominal aorta		≥30

CI, confidence of interval; *SD*, standard deviation.

These are reference maximum dimensions that are used in common imaging practice. A new more individual approach is currently recommended, and maximum dimensions that trigger treatment currently vary according to the age, gender, body surface area, and other risk factors, as recently reviewed by the last American Association of Thoracic Surgery consensus guidelines [66]. These thresholds may vary across institutions.

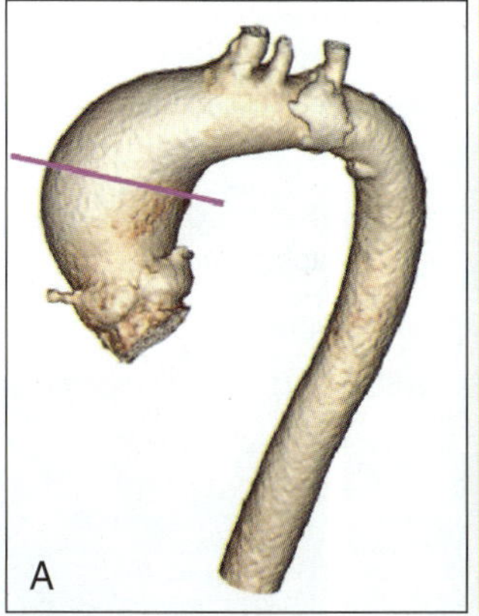

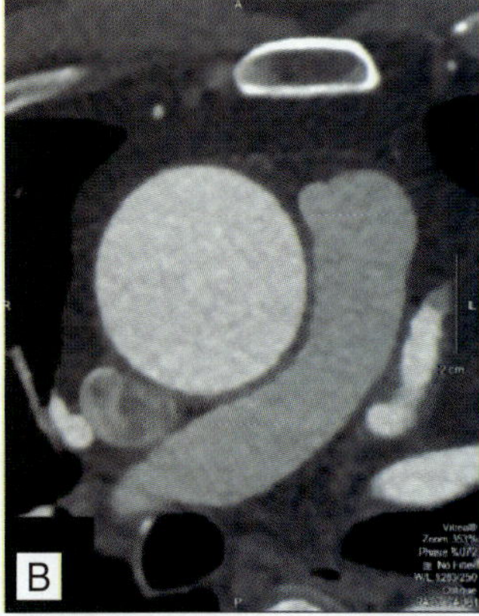

Figure 25.5 Fusiform aneurysmal dilation of the ascending thoracic aorta. (A) Three-dimensional (3D) and (B) oblique multiplanar reconstructed (MPR) images depicting fusiform aneurysmal dilation of the ascending thoracic aorta. Pink line shows level of the measurement, orthogonal to the aorta at the level of maximum dimension.

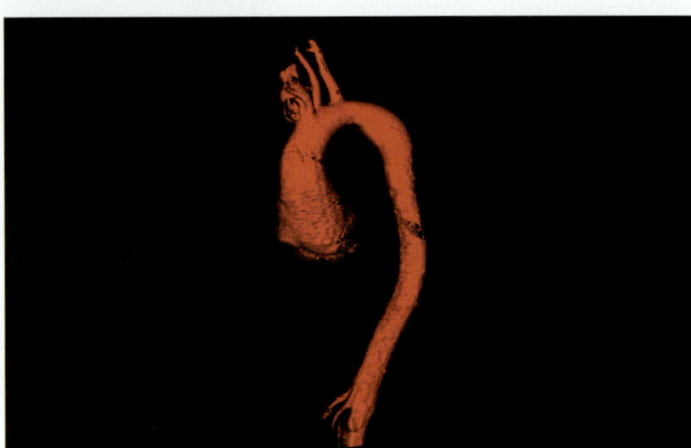

Figure 25.6 Classic tulip bulb aortic root appearance. MRA 3D of the thoracic aorta on a patient with Marfan's syndrome shows aneurysmal dilation at the level of the sinuses of Valsalva with effacement of the sinotubular junction.

common cause of aneurysms of the aorta. While cystic medial necrosis (e.g., Marfan, Ehler–Danlos, and Loeys–Dietz syndromes) is the major cause of aortic aneurysms involving the aortic root and the ascending aorta, causing effacement of the sinotubular junction and resulting in a classic tulip bulb appearance (Fig. 25.6). Aortic root aneurysms are also associated with bicuspid aortic valves and familial thoracic aortic aneurysm syndrome.

When a saccular aneurysm shows a wide neck and is present in the aortic root or ascending thoracic aorta, it is suggestive of a mycotic aneurysm due to the proximity to regions affected by endocarditis. Common associated factors are intravascular intervention, intravenous drug abuse, *Staphylococcus*, and *Salmonella* infections. Syphilitic aortitis shows a characteristic increased wall thickness thought to be related to neutrophilic infiltration of the arterial wall, which at the same time triggers enzyme pathways leading to the breakdown of the saccular dilation (Fig. 25.7). Paradoxically, this leads to very large aneurysms that typically do not rupture but can have mass effect on adjacent structures.

AAA is rare before the age of 50 years old, can be seen in about 3.5% of European men population older than 65 years old, and most commonly involves the infrarenal abdominal aorta. The current prevalence in the United States is unclear due to the low rate of AAA screening. Nevertheless, the prevalence of AAA has decreased over the last two decades and this is believed to be related to the overall decreased of associated smoking. AAA can be assessed with ultrasound (Fig. 25.8), CTA, or MRA.

The 2019 update of US Preventive Services Task Force (USPSTF) recommends:

- One time ultrasound screening for AAA in men aged 65–75 years who have ever smoked (B recommendation)
- For men aged 55–75 years who have never smoked, the USPSTF recommends selective screening in a case-by-case basis with relevant medical or family history, other risk factors, and personal values (C recommendation)
- The USPSTF also recommends against routine screening in women who have never smoked and no family history of AAA (D recommendation)
- Also concludes that the evidence is insufficient to assess the benefits of screening in women aged 65–75 years who have ever smoked or have a family history of AAA (I recommendation) [12]

Crawford and DeNatale classified thoracoabdominal aneurysm in four types:

- Type I involves from the proximal descending thoracic aorta to the hiatus
- Type II involves the descending thoracic aorta and most of the abdominal aorta
- Type III only the distal descending thoracic aorta
- Type IV the majority of the abdominal aorta from the hiatus to its bifurcation

Another definition to indicate aneurysmal arterial dilation below the abdominal aorta is greater than half of the aneurysmal dilation on the level above. For example, an aneurysmal dilation of the common iliac arteries will be greater than 15 mm, given that the level above maximum dimension is 30 mm for the infrarenal abdominal aorta.

Pseudoaneurysm

Pseudoaneurysms usually show disruption of one (intima) or two (intima and media) of the three layers of the vessel, while the blood is contained by the adventitia and periadventitial tissues. In situations of trauma such as motor vehicle accidents, the most common location for a pseudoaneurysm in the isthmus, given that it is the location with most survival after deceleration accidents. In the postoperative setting,

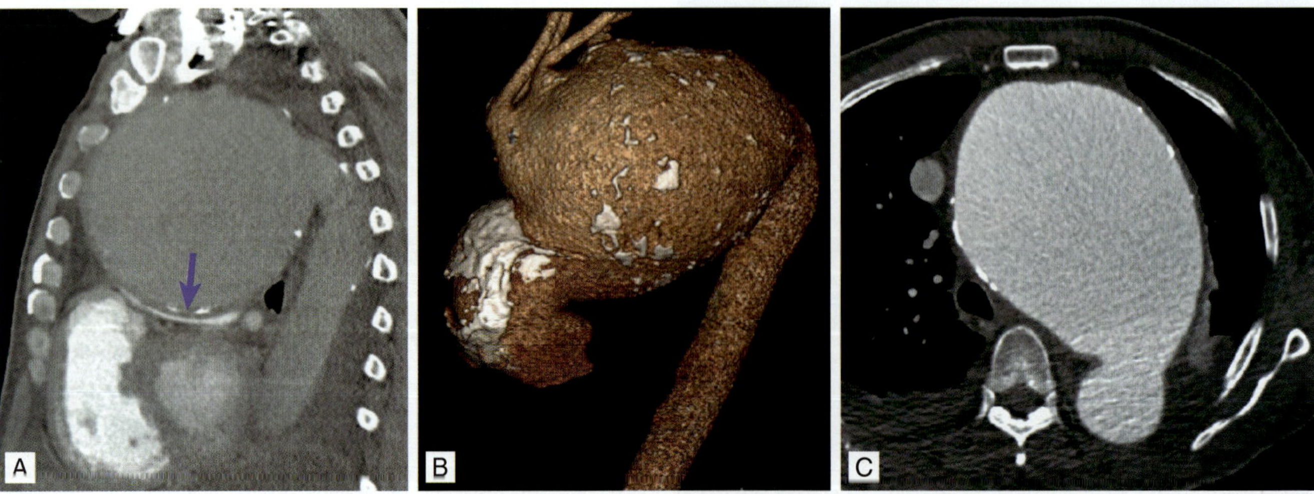

Figure 25.7 Syphilitic aortitis. (A and B) Oblique multiplanar reconstructed (MPR) and three-dimensional (3D) images show tertiary syphilis in a patient from a developing country who had never sought medical care in his entire life who presented with dyspnea on exertion. The cause is compression of the main pulmonary artery from the massive aortic aneurysm (*blue arrow*). (A and C) Oblique MPR and axial images depict the wall thickening as a hallmark of the disease (*blue arrow*).

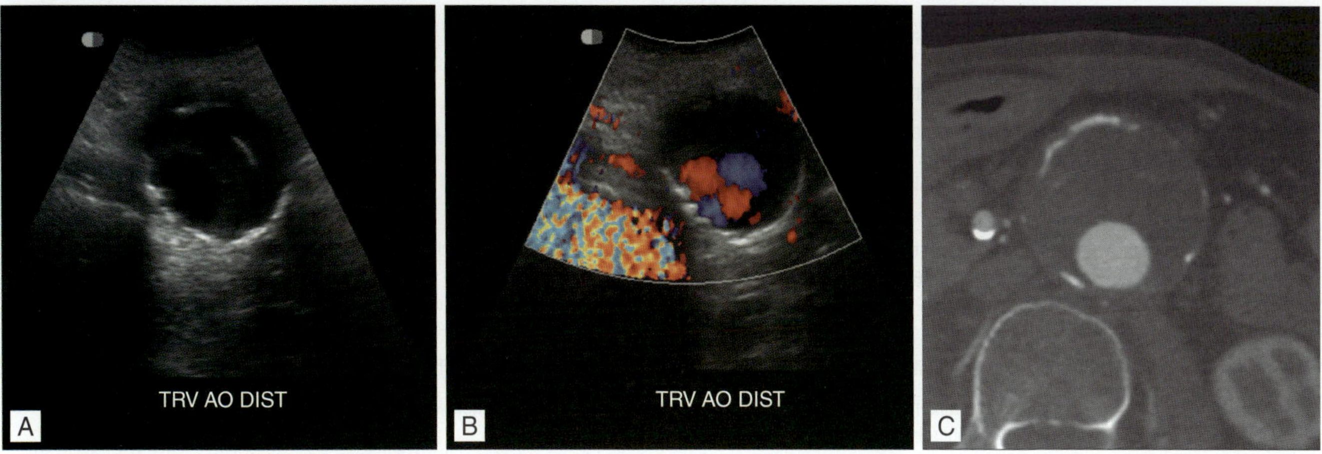

Figure 25.8 Fusiform aneurysmal dilation of an infrarenal abdominal aorta. (A) Grayscale ultrasound and (B) color Doppler imaging, and (C) axial CTA show a 5.0 × 4.8 cm infrarenal abdominal aortic aneurysm, associated with a near circumferential intraluminal thrombus.

pseudoaneurysms are seen at the level of the graft anastomosis with the native aorta (Fig. 25.9). Features that can help differentiate a pseudoaneurysm from a true aneurysm are depicted in Table 25.2.

Aortoenteric and Aortocaval Fistulas

Aortoenteric fistulas can occur in patients that present with hematemesis, melena, sepsis, and pain, but sometimes patients can also be asymptomatic. Aortoenteric fistulas maybe primary or secondary. Primary fistulas are rare and almost always occur in the setting of a pre-existing aortic disease such as a PAU or aneurysm with different etiologies including syphilis, tuberculosis, mycotic infections, or connective tissue disease. Secondary fistulas are also rare and are related to early or late postprocedural complications with or without a stent graft. About 80% of this complication occur at the third or fourth portion of the duodenum, followed by the esophagus, gastroesophageal junction. Secondary fistulas could be related to the combination of chronic low-grade infection of the aortic graft and repetitive pressure on the bowel from aortic pulsations [13]. The presence of soft tissue edema, fluid and ectopic gas adjacent to or within the aorta, is also expected findings in the immediate postoperative setting, but abnormal 3–4 weeks after. *Any ectopic gas 2 or 3 months after the procedure, should raise the suspicion of infection with or without a fistula.* CTA plays an important role identifying this entity [14], and the key finding is either extravasation of contrast from the aorta to the bowel lumen, or leakage of oral contrast from the bowel lumen to the aortic wall or para-prosthetic space [13].

TABLE 25.2 Pseudoaneurysm Versus Aneurysm [8]

	Pseudoaneurysm	Aneurysm
Vessel wall layer	One or two layers involved	Three layers are intact
Etiology	Trauma, infection	Intrinsic
Shape	Saccular	Fusiform
Margins	Lobulated	Smooth
Rupture	Higher risk of rupture than aneurysms	Risk increases with size

Aortocaval fistula is a very rare complications of AAA and it is associated with a high mortality rate. It can present with

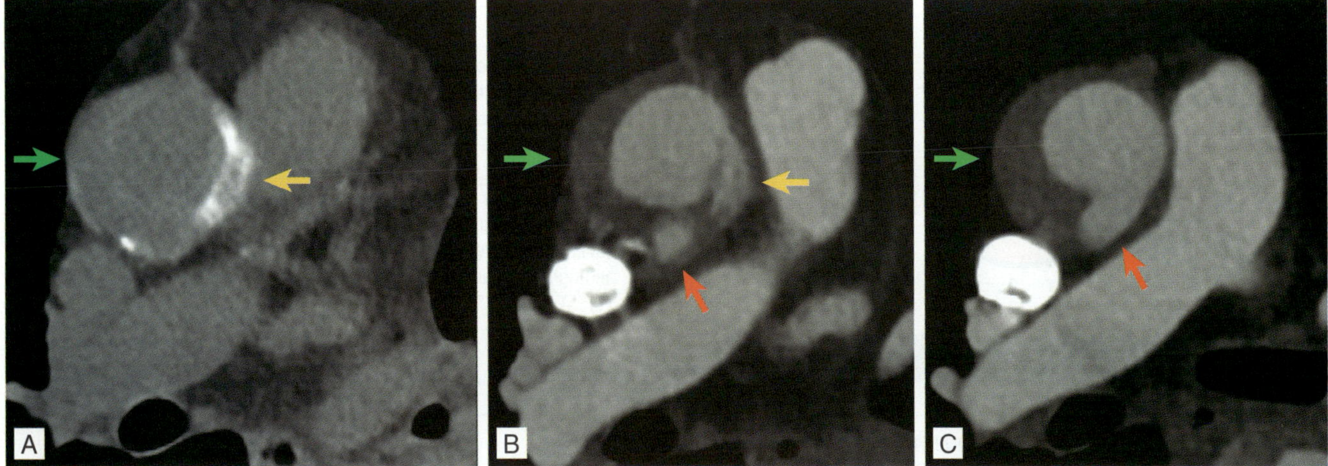

Figure 25.9 Pseudoaneurysm. A saccular pseudoaneurysm at the proximal anastomotic site between an aortic graft and the native thoracic aorta. Patient had a repair of a type A IMH 5 years before this CT. (A–C) These images depict a fluid collection (*green arrows*) surrounding the graft with hyperdense components on the noncontrast CT (left). There is an associated pseudoaneurysm (*red arrows*) adjacent to the surgical material (*yellow arrows*) of the proximal anastomosis.

TABLE 25.3 Imaging Features of Acute Aortic Disease [8,18]

Disease	Noncontrast Imaging	Postcontrast CTA
Penetrating atherosclerotic ulcer	Atheromatous plaque ulcerates the deepest layer of the intima known as the internal elastic lamina and displaces calcified plaque forming an outpouching beyond the contours of the aorta	Localized outpouching beyond the contours of the aorta with intraluminal enhancement
Intramural hematoma	Hyperdense crescent-shaped due to rupture of the vasa vasorum that feeds the media	Smooth crescentic thickening along its course without enhancement or identifiable flap Intramural blood pool (IBP) and ulcer like projections (ULP) are associated findings. ULP is a high-risk feature
Dissection	Central displacement of intimal calcification	Intimomedial flap which separates the true and false lumen
Impending rupture	Periaortic fat stranding Displaced peripheral calcifications of the aortic wall Draped aorta sign	Irregular aortic lumen with disruption of the aortic wall Draped aorta sign Displacement of mural calcifications Surrounding fat stranding
Transection	Hemopericardium, hemothorax, mediastinal hematomas in 75% of cases. Retroperitoneal hematoma	Extraluminal contrast It happens most commonly at three locations, aortic root, isthmus, and diaphragmatic hiatus
Rupture	Hemopericardium, hemothorax, mediastinal hematomas in 75% of cases. Retroperitoneal hematoma	Irregular aortic wall, active extravasation of contrast Contained ruptures will not show active extravasation

abdominal pain, bilateral pedal edema, renal insufficiency, heart failure when it is a chronic fistula, and hemodynamically instability. It consists of an abnormal communication between an aortic aneurysm and the inferior vena cava (left to right arteriovenous shunt), most commonly between the posterolateral aortic wall and the adjacent IVC. CTA shows an early filling of a dilated inferior vena cava during arterial phase imaging. Aortocaval fistulas have to be treated emergently with open surgical repair and patch angioplasty of the inferior vena cava and endovascular repair of the aorta [15,16].

Acute Aortic Syndrome

Acute aortic syndrome is a spectrum of emergencies that include PAUs, IMH, dissection, aneurysm rupture, and traumatic transection. The imaging features of aortic disease spectrum are depicted in Table 25.3 and Graph 25.1.

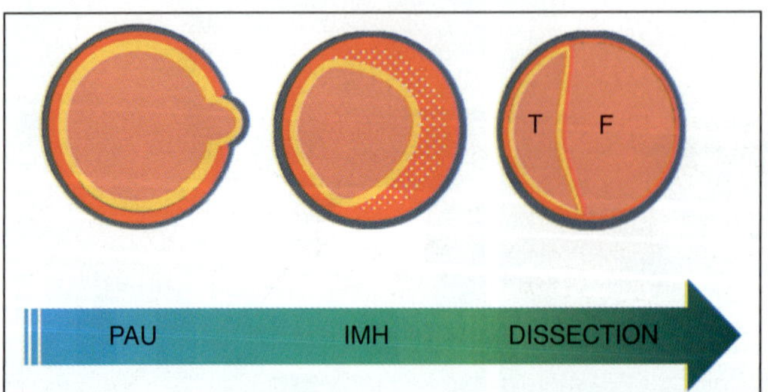

Graph 25.1 Spectrum of arterial disease. Aggressive PAU can progress to IMH or dissections. *F*, false lumen; *gray*, adventitia layer; *IMH*, intramural hematoma; *PAU*, penetrating atherosclerotic ulcer; *pink*, blood pool; *red*, medial layer; *red with white dots*, vasa vasorum; *T*, true lumen; *yellow*, intimal layer.

Aortic Dissection

The incidence of acute aortic dissection is 2.9 per 100,000 persons per year. The risk factors include pre-existing aneurysm, hypertension, bicuspid aortic valve, Marfan syndrome, and prior cardiovascular rupture. *A typical dissection will show an entrance and exit tear between the intima and the inner layer of the media*, forming the intimomedial flap which separates the true and false lumen. The blood in the false lumen is usually lateral, larger, may be free flowing or thrombosed, and usually feeds the left renal artery (Table 25.4). There are different types of complex dissection flaps; for

TABLE 25.4 Typical Features of True Versus False Lumen in Aortic Dissection [7,17]

True Lumen	False Lumen
Medial lumen	Lateral lumen
Smaller size	Larger size
Better opacified on early arterial phase with washout on delayed phases	Poor opacification on early arterial phase or thrombosed with persistent enhancement on delayed phases
It may collapse	It often dilates
Usually, supplies flow to the coronaries, celiac trunk, superior mesenteric artery, and right renal artery	Usually, supplies the left renal artery
	"Cobweb sign" is described as slender linear areas that represent strands of media that have incompletely sheared away during when the dissection occurred
	"Beak sign" is described as a wedge of hematoma and it is thought to create space for the propagation of the false lumen

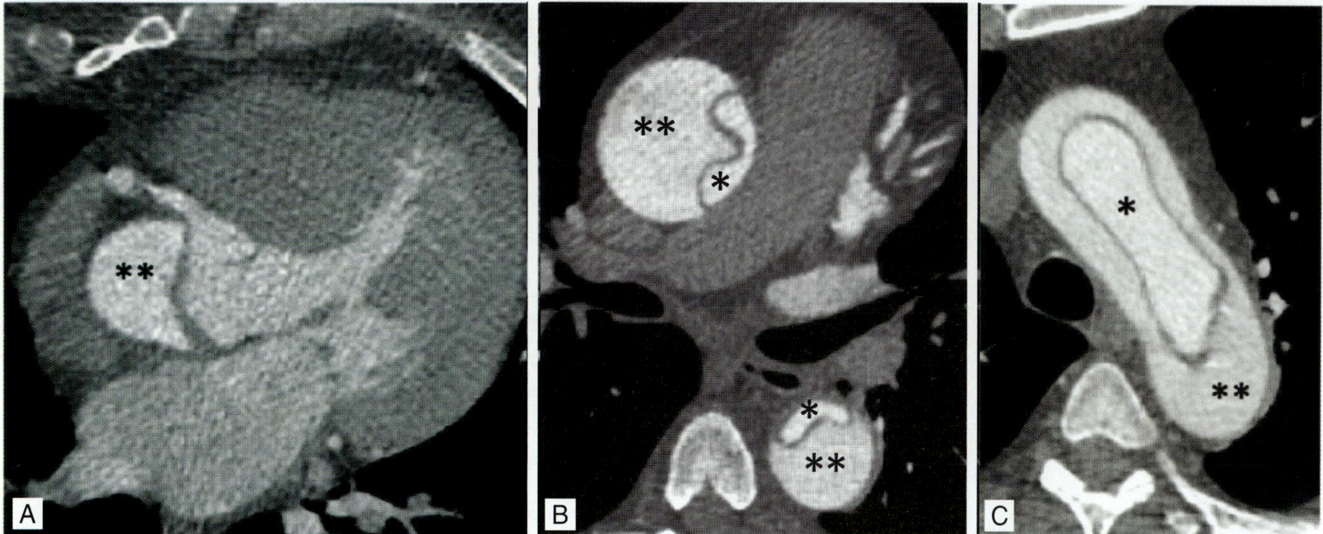

Figure 25.10 Type A Stanford aortic dissection. (A–C) CTA axial views show a dissection flap originating at the level of the sinuses of Valsalva and extending to the descending thoracic aorta (center), consistent with type A dissection. There is sparing of the origin of the coronary arteries (left main not shown but also spared). *asterisk*, true lumen; *double asterisk*, false lumen.

example, when there is diffuse involvement of the entire intima, there will be a circumferential intimal flap with a narrow and filiform circumferential true lumen that can result in intimointimal intussusception and a "windsock" appearance. There is also a three channel dissection flap that is known as the Mercedes-Benz sign, which occurs when there is a secondary dissection within one of the lumens resulting in a three channel appearance [17].

The classification of aortic dissections is based on the location of the aortic dissection, and the most common systems are DeBakey and Stanford.

- Type I DeBakey, the dissection involves the ascending and descending thoracic aorta
- Type II DeBakey, the dissection involves the ascending aorta only
- Type III DeBakey, the dissection is limited to the descending thoracic aorta

In Stanford type A, the aortic dissections involve the ascending thoracic aorta with or without extension to the descending thoracic aorta (Fig. 25.10); in Stanford type B, the dissection involves the descending thoracic aorta only (Fig. 25.11) [18].

A complicated thoracic aortic dissection can be lethal due to acute aortic regurgitation, major aortic branch obstruction, pericardial tamponade, or aortic rupture. Approximately 75% of aortic ruptures result in hemopericardium, hemothorax, and mediastinal hematomas. A case of aortic rupture also shows irregular aortic wall accompanied by active extravasation of contrast (Fig. 25.12). Contained ruptures do not show active contrast extravasation [17].

Whereas impending rupture signs include irregular aortic lumen with disruption of the aortic wall and displaced peripheral calcifications, periaortic fat stranding changes, and draped aorta sign. The draped aorta sign is the disruption of the posterior aortic wall following the contours of an adjacent vertebral body (Fig. 25.13).

Penetrating Aortic Ulcer

Penetrating atherosclerotic ulcer or penetrating aortic ulcer (PAU) are two terms that are interchangeable. In PAU, an atheromatous plaque ulcerates the deepest layer of the intima, known as the internal elastic lamina, and displaces calcified plaque forming an outpouching, or also known as a collar-button, beyond the contours of the aorta. A PAU also shows a variable extension to the media. When an atherosclerotic plaque penetrates into the media, the hemorrhage of the media will lead to either an IMH, localized aortic dissection, saccular pseudoaneurysm, or mediastinal hematoma. PAUs are often multifocal and most common in the descending thoracic aorta. It can be distinguished from an atheromatous plaque by the presence of a focal, contrast filled outpouching surrounded by an IMH, which is also consistent with aggressive behavior of a PAU. A PAU can be differentiated

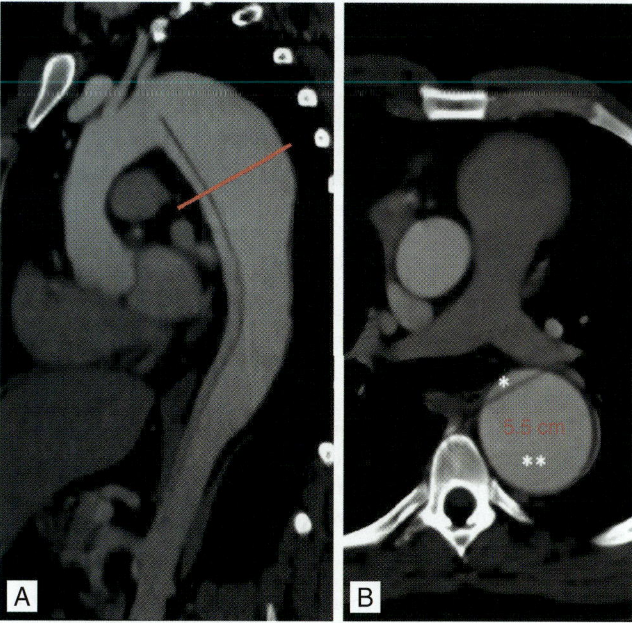

Figure 25.11 Type B Stanford aortic dissection. CTA multiplanar reconstructed (MPR) images show a dissection flap extending from the proximal descending thoracic aorta until just above the level of the origin of the celiac trunk. There is an associated aneurysmal dilation of the proximal descending thoracic aorta measuring up to 5.5 cm. Red line depicts the area of maximum dimension of the aneurysm, *asterisk* shows the true lumen and *double asterisk* shows the false lumen.

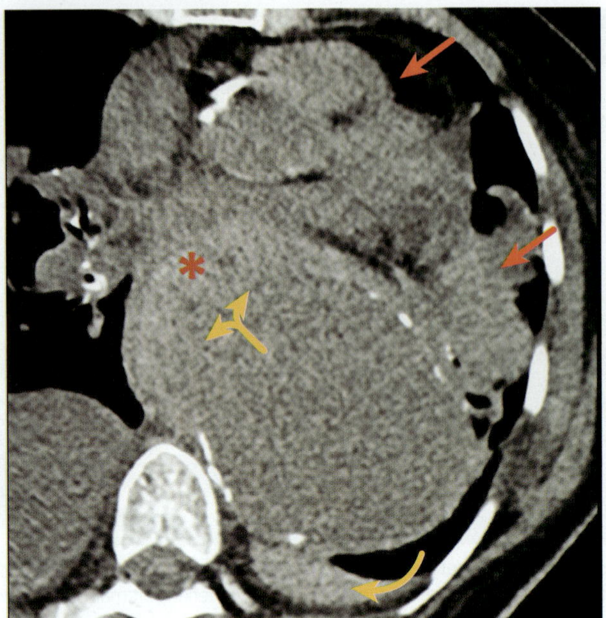

Figure 25.12 Aortic rupture. Axial CT noncontrast images show rupture of the descending thoracic aorta. There is marked aneurysmal dilation of the descending thoracic aorta with discontinuation of the peripheral calcifications (bidirectional *yellow arrow*) and periaortic hematoma (*red asterisk*). There is also associated mediastinal hematoma (*red arrows*) and hemothorax (*curved yellow arrow*).

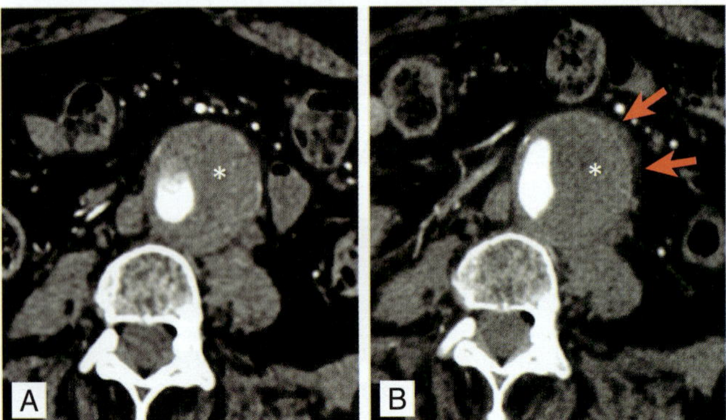

Figure 25.13 Progression of impending rupture of the aorta. CTA axial shows (A) an infrarenal abdominal aortic aneurysm (AAA) associated with near circumferential intraluminal thrombus (*asterisk*), which is known to increase the risk of aortic rupture due to wall destabilization. Short-term CTA follow-up shows (B) interval development of surrounding moderate fat stranding changes (*red arrows*) consistent with impending AAA rupture.

TABLE 25.5 Differences Between PAU and Pseudoaneurysm [7,8]

	PAU	Pseudoaneurysm
Atherosclerosis	Very common	Incidental
Location	Most common in the descending thoracic aorta	Most common in the arch, then descending, ascending, and abdominal aorta
Penetrates	Internal elastic lamina (deepest layer) of the media layer	External elastic media of the media layer
Neck	Variable	Narrow
IMH	Aggressive PAU are associated with IMH	Less common

IMH, intramural hematoma; *PAU*, penetrating atherosclerotic ulcer.

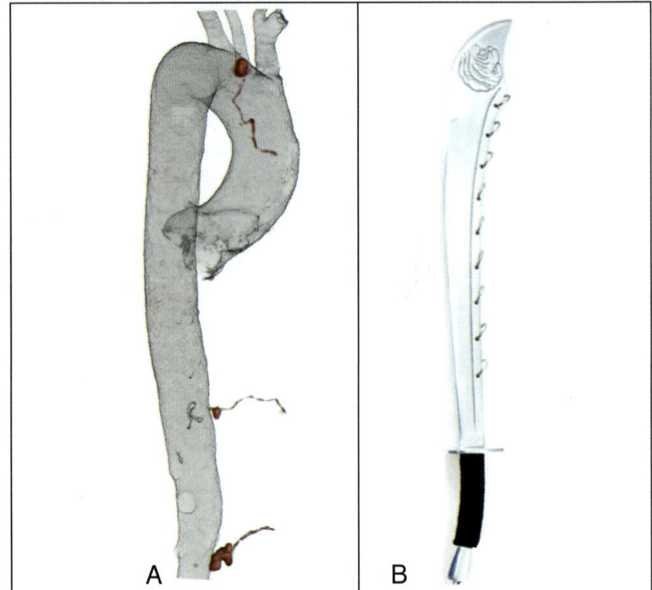

Figure 25.14 Chinese ring sword sign. (A) 3D CTA shows multilevel branch artery pseudoaneurysms of the intercostal arteries (depicted in red) in a patient with known intramural hematoma (IMH). This appearance is known as the Chinese sword sign due to the resemblance of the branch artery pseudoaneurysms with the rings of this sword. (B) The blade of the sword represents the thoracic aorta.

from a pseudoaneurysm by its more frequent association with atherosclerotic plaque, its more common location in the descending thoracic aorta, involvement of the internal elastica media and its more frequent association with IMH (Table 25.5).

Intramural Hematoma

An IMH is related to the spontaneous rupture of the aortic vasa vasorum of the medial aortic layer, and it is also understood as a hemorrhage localized to the aortic media in the absence of an intimal tear. A typical IMH is identified with a hyperdense crescentic thickening seen better in an unenhanced CT. IMH is differentiated from a thrombosed false lumen, because it does not enhance, lacks an intimal tear, as well as its constant shape along its course; whereas the false lumen of a dissection has a longitudinal spiral configuration; however, these two can be challenging to distinguish.

Intramural blood pool is described as a benign finding that can regress overtime in the setting of underlying IMH; it shows a small pool of contrast within the IMH that communicates with the aortic lumen through a tiny intimal orifice, and also connects to an intercostal or lumbar arterial branch [19]. The more appropriate term is branch artery pseudoaneurysm, which refers to the dilation of the origin of the injured branch artery. When an IMH occurs, and the origin of the branch artery is sheared off. A hole is left between the aortic lumen and the thrombosed IMH, so blood flows into the pseudoaneurysm and finally into the branch artery [20]. On some occasions, there can be progressive branch artery tears accompanied by hemodynamic instability. The appearance of multiple branch artery pseudoaneurysm has been described as the Chinese sword sign, because of the resemblance of the pooling of contrast and branch artery pseudoaneurysms with the rings of this sword [21] (Fig. 25.14).

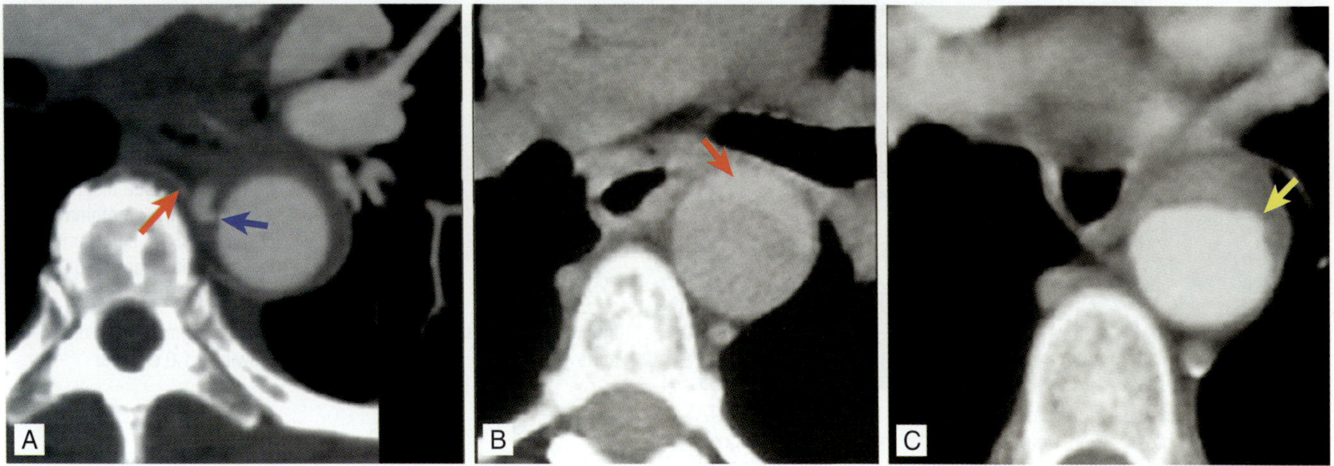

Figure 25.15 Associated findings of intramural hematomas (IMH). CTA of the aorta showing associated findings in intramural hematomas. (A) Intramural blood pool (IBP), a benign finding that communicates with the aortic lumen through a tiny intimal orifice (*blue arrow*) and is accompanied by a branch artery (intercostal artery depicted by *red arrow*). (B) Noncontrast image showing the crescentic rim of hyperdensity (*red arrow*). (C) Ulcer like projection (ULP) shows a wide intimal disruption adjacent to the aortic lumen (*yellow arrow*) and no communication with adjacent arteries. ULP indicates a high risk feature when measured more than 10 mm.

An ulcer like projection is morphologically distinct from an intramural blood pool and it has been associated with poor prognosis. An ulcer like projection is a pool of contrast protruding into the IMH and with a wider intimal disruption and no connection with any arterial branch [19] (Fig. 25.15).

Minimal aortic injury (MAI) is defined as a subcentimeter intimomedial abnormality, which could be a tear or a thrombus, and without any wall contour deformity. This usually involves the isthmus (60–72%), aortic root (3–14%), ascending aorta (8–27%), aortic arch (8–18%), distal descending thoracic aorta (11–21%), and abdominal aorta (7–22%). The most common imaging findings of MAI includes a subcentimeter rounded or triangular intraluminal filling defect, or a thin focal intimal flap. A subcentimeter IMH is also included as part of a MAI. The importance of recognizing the imaging features of MAI is based on the conservative approach of these aortic injuries, with the majority of them resolving in a period of 4–8 weeks short-term imaging follow-up [22].

On the other hand, a significant aortic injury is defined as the presence of aortic contour abnormality and includes an IMH with contour alteration, pseudoaneurysms, and aortic rupture [22]. Traumatic significant aortic injury can also occur at the aortic root, isthmus, and hiatus (Figs. 25.16–25.18).

Important pseudoaneurysm-mimics to recognize in the isthmus are the aortic diverticulum, spindle, and branch vascular infundibulum. The aortic diverticulum has smooth contours and is present in the inner contour of the isthmus and may or may not show associated calcifications, depicting the embryological remnant at the point of the ligamentum arteriosum. The aortic spindle is the normal mild "dilation" of the proximal descending thoracic aorta. The aortic infundibulum refers to the area of origin of the branches of the thoracic aorta (e.g., intercostal, bronchial, or spinal arteries), which could look more prominent and be mistaken for a small pseudoaneurysm [7,22].

Traumatic Aortic Transection

A traumatic aortic transection is a tear involving the three layers of the aortic wall, usually by rapid deceleration and osseous pinching at the aortic root (4%), the arch or isthmus (95%), and the diaphragmatic hiatus (1%). The mortality rate of aortic transections is very high and most of the time, only patients with injury at the isthmus make it to the hospital [8]. Of the 10–20% of patients who arrive to the hospital, most will survive (60–80%).

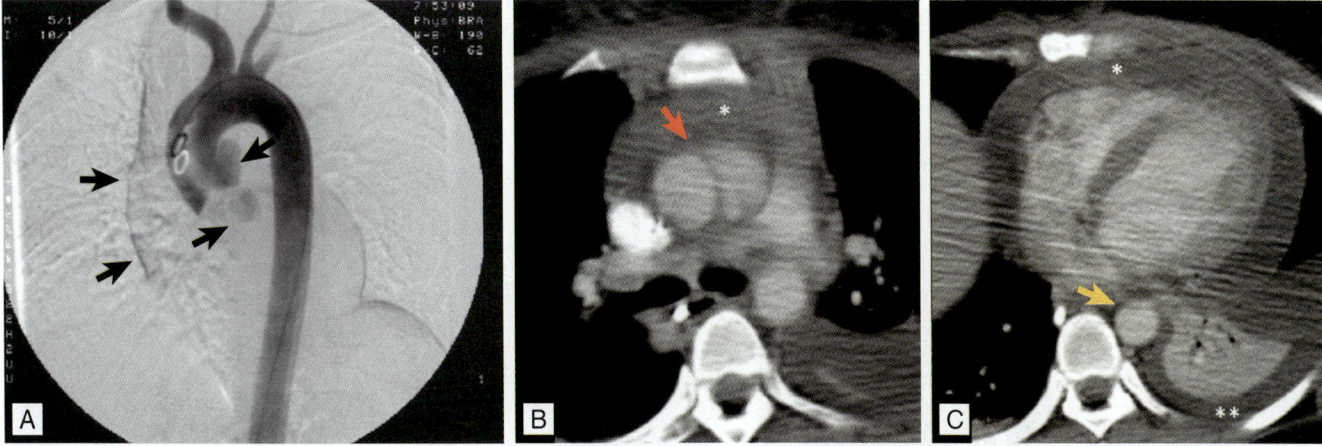

Figure 25.16 Traumatic significant aortic injury at the aortic annulus after a motor vehicle accident. (A) Digital subtraction angiogram (DSA) shows significant aortic injury (SAI) associated with extravasation of contrast (*black arrows*) consistent with rupture at the level of the aortic annulus. (B and C) CTA shows extension of SAI throughout the ascending (*red arrow*) and descending thoracic aorta (*yellow arrow*), and associated hemopericardium (*asterisk*) and hemothorax (*double asterisk*) with mixed hyperdense products.

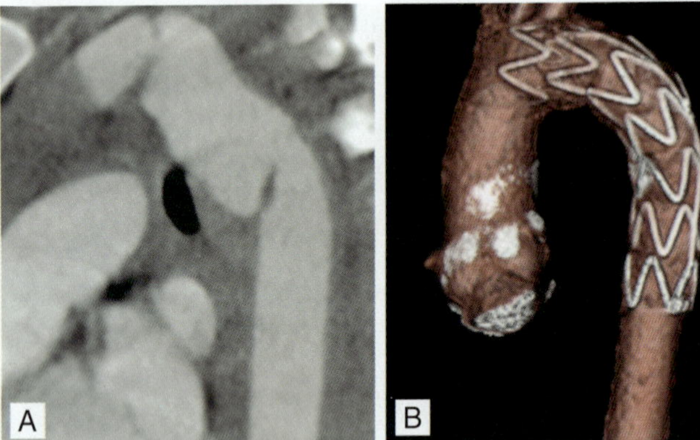

Figure 25.17 Traumatic significant aortic injury at the isthmus. (A) CTA shows intimal flap greater than 1 cm associated with contour disruption of the isthmus. (B) 3D reconstructions showing interval repair with placement of a stent graft extending from the distal aortic arch to the proximal descending thoracic aorta.

TABLE 25.6 Intervention Criteria for Aortic Aneurysms [2,7,8]

Aortic Segment	Aneurysmal Size	Intervention Criteria
Aortic root or ascending thoracic aorta	>4.0 cm	≥5.5 cm, symptomatic or growing >0.5 cm/year Connective tissue disorders: ≥4.0–5.0 cm, symptomatic or growing >0.3 cm/year Bicuspid aortic valve: ≥ 5.0 cm or growing >0.5 cm/year
Aortic arch or descending thoracic aorta	>3.5 cm	
Infrarenal abdominal aorta	>3.0 cm	≥5.5 cm, symptomatic or growing >1.0 cm/year

Management

Criteria for management of the thoracic and abdominal aorta are depicted in Table 25.6.

Management of aneurysmal dilation of the ascending thoracic aorta or acute aortic syndrome (e.g., dissection or IMH) most commonly involves open surgical repair. Intervention of the aortic aneurysm depends on its size and risk of rupture, given that an aneurysmal size of the thoracic aorta greater than 6.0 cm is associated with up to 15% per year increased risk of dissection, rupture, or death. A size of 6.0 cm for the abdomen is associated with risk of rupture of up 20% and a size equal or greater than 8.0 cm is associated with a risk of rupture of 30–50% [1,23,24]. Generally, elective surgery is performed with a diameter equal to or greater than 5.5 cm [25]. Earlier surgical repair can be performed in patients with connective tissue disorders with maximum dimension in the 4–5 cm range or bicuspid aortic valves with a maximum dimension of 5.0 cm. Aneurysms that grow in a rate of greater than 0.5 cm per year or symptomatic patients, also merit earlier intervention. Most common surgical techniques to repair the ascending thoracic aorta include placement of a supracoronary ascending aortic graft, which could be done with aortic valve replacement (Wheat procedure), or without it (David valve-sparing procedure). The ascending aortic graft could be synthetic (Bentall and Cabrol procedures) or biologic (Ross procedure which uses pulmonary valve homograft, or cadaveric grafts). The surgical intervention can also include repair of the aortic arch (elephant trunk and arch first procedures). In general, the diseased native aorta is excised, and a synthetic or biologic graft is placed. The graft is then reanastomosed with the native structures using felt pledgets, which are hyperattenuating, and in postcontrast images could be mistaken for a pseudoaneurysm. The addition of noncontrast phase images help identify the synthetic grafts and felt pledgets and becomes crucial in the assessment of postoperative changes [3,23,24] (Fig. 25.19).

Management of aneurysmal dilation of the descending thoracic aorta without complications mainly involves medical therapy with the main objective to control high blood pressure [8,26]. Endoluminal stent graft placement is preferred over

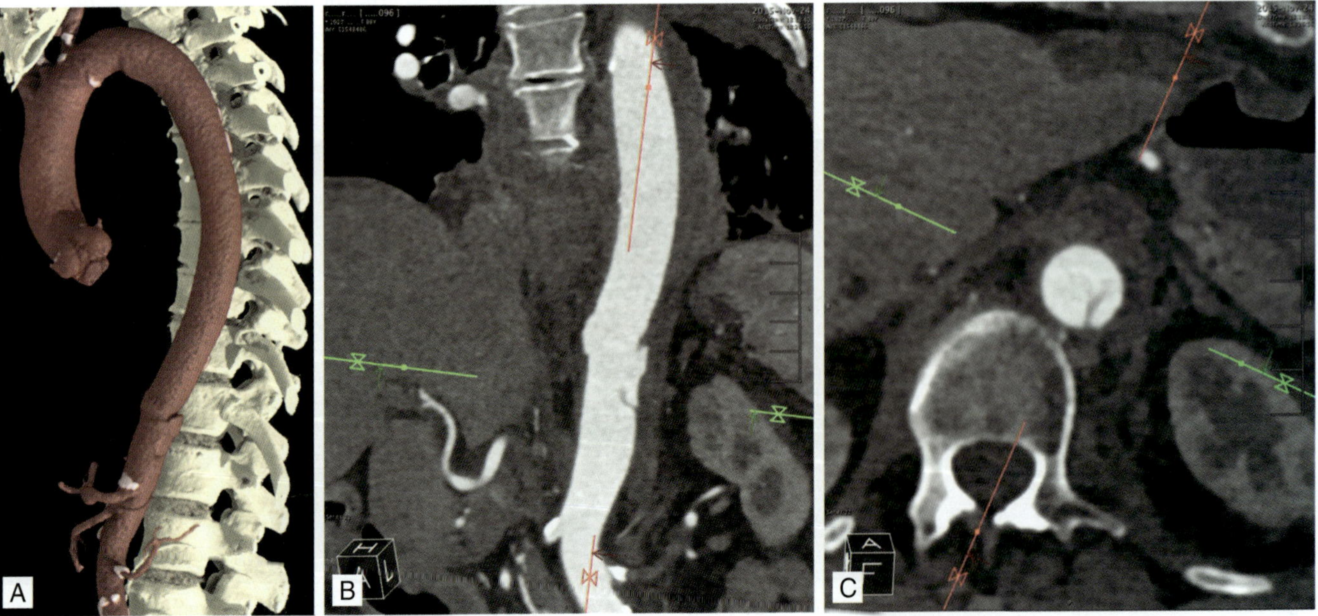

Figure 25.18 Traumatic significant aortic injury at the hiatus. (A) 3D global illumination rendering (GIR) and (B and C) CTA multiplanar reformats (MPR) show significant aortic injury with an intimal flap greater than 1 cm associated with contour abnormality.

surgical repair of the descending thoracic aorta and is generally indicated in complicated type B aortic dissection with progression of the dissection flap or associated aneurysmal dilation, intractable pain, and failure to control hypertension [8,26]. Endoluminal stent graft is also the main treatment for enlarging PAUs in the descending thoracic aorta (Fig. 25.20), and aneurysmal dilations of the abdominal aorta [27]. There are different types of abdominal aortic stent grafts; some of the approved and commonly used devices are depicted by Eliason and Upchurch [27] (Fig. 25.21).

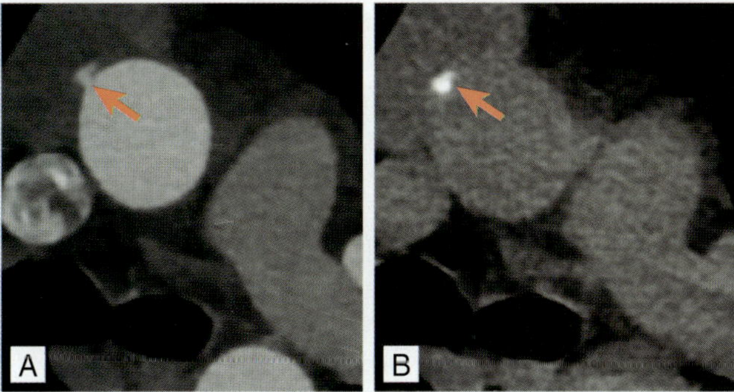

Figure 25.19 Mimic of pseudoaneurysm in the postoperative setting. (A) The felt material used for the aortic graft mimics a pseudoaneurysm (*red arrow*) in the postcontrast axial images. (B) The noncontrast axial images help identifying the felt material.

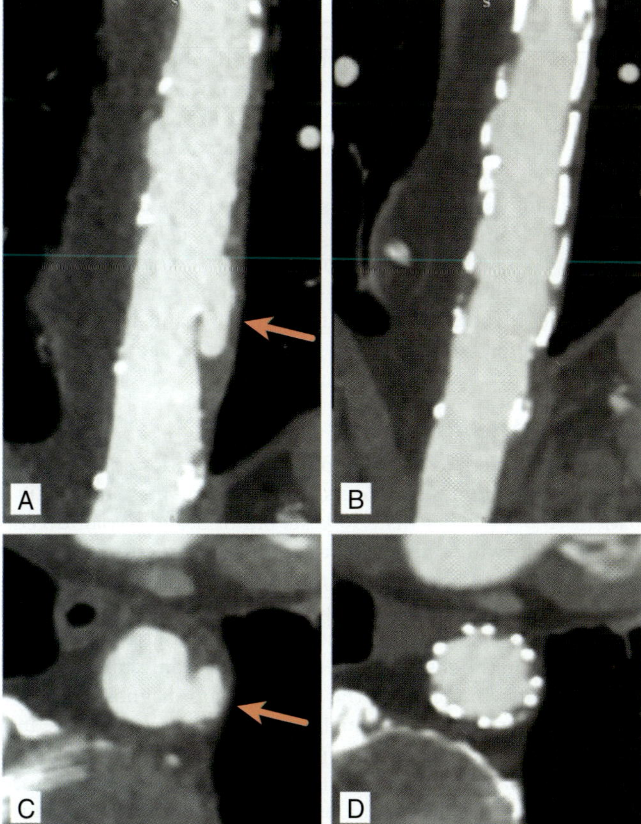

Figure 25. 20 Penetrating atherosclerotic ulcer repair. Penetrating atherosclerotic ulcer before (A & C) and after (B & D) repair. CTA oblique multiplanar reconstructed (MPR) and contrast-enhanced CTA images show a penetrating atherosclerotic ulcer (PAU) in the descending thoracic aorta (*red arrows*) measuring approximately 2.4 cm in length, and changes after endovascular repair with interval placement of a stent graft (B & D).

Endoleak is defined as persistent blood flow within the excluded aneurysm sac following endovascular aneurysm repair with placement of an endoluminal stent graft. Endoleaks are seen in 20–40% of the cases, and some of them are expected due to the presence of preexisting branch vessels such as bronchial, thoracic, lumbar branches, or inferior mesenteric artery (IMA). There are five types of endoleaks:

- Type I at the proximal (Ia) or distal (Ib) graft attachment site (Fig. 25.22)
- Type II is an enlarging aneurysmal sac associated with a collateral vessel (Fig. 25.23)

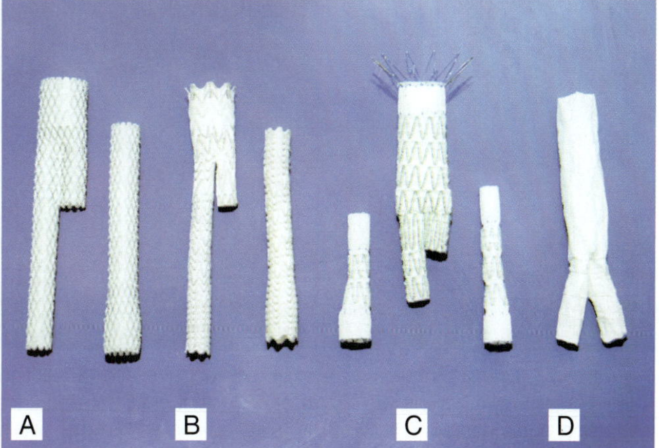

Figure 25.21 Types of abdominal aortic stent grafts. FDA-approved and currently marketed stent graft devices including (A) Medtronic, (B) Gore, (C) Cook, and (D) Endologix. An endologic stent graft has the metallic cover inside, which is important to recognize given that the normal blood flowing between the metallic and nonmetallic components can mimic an endoleak. (Reprinted with permission from: JL Eliason, GR Upchurch Jr, Endovascular abdominal aortic aneurysm repair, Circulation 117 (13) (2008) 1738–1744.)

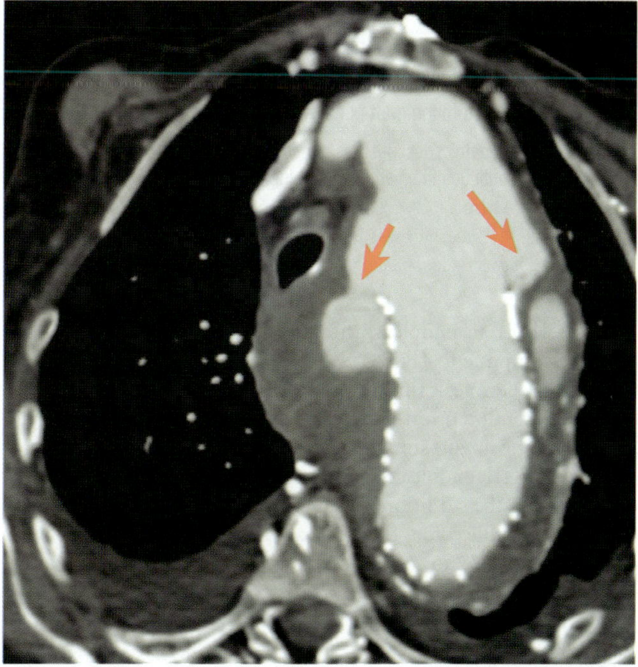

Figure 25.22 Type 1a endoleak. CTA oblique axial MPR images in this patient with history of prior stent graft placement for thoracic aortic aneurysm show a large amount of contrast within the aneurysmal sac which is not excluded by the proximal aspect of the stent-graft (*red arrows*) consistent with a type 1a endoleak.

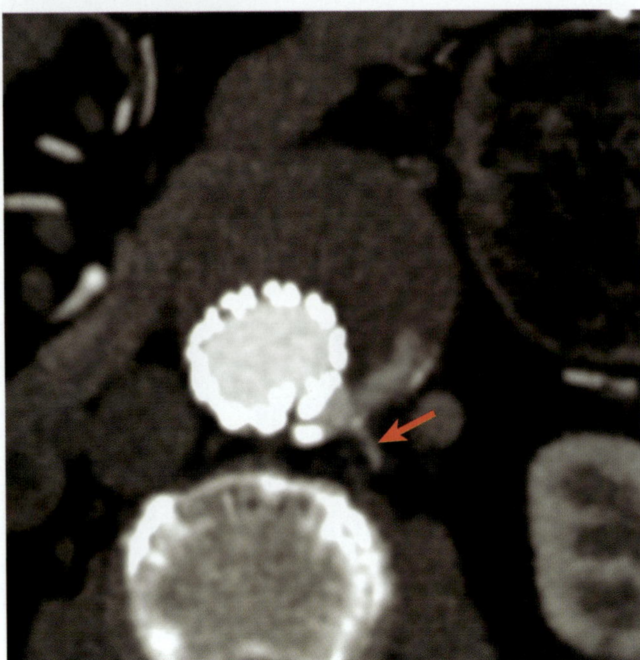

Figure 25.23 Type 2 endoleak. CTA axial maximum intensity projection (MIP) images in this patient with history of prior stent graft placement for abdominal aortic aneurysm show a moderate amount of contrast within the excluded aneurysmal sac extending from the lumbar artery (*red arrow*), consistent with a type 2 endoleak.

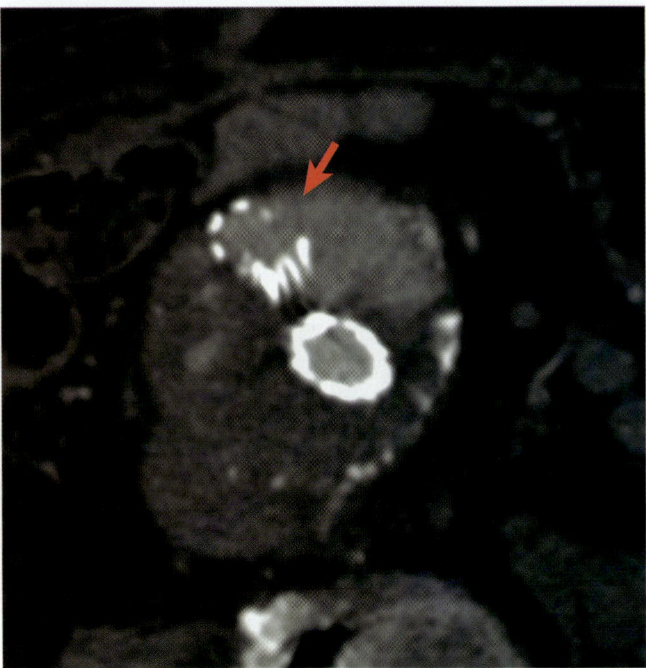

Figure 25.24 Type 3 endoleak. CTA axial images in this patient with history of prior stent graft placement for abdominal aortic aneurysm show a large amount of contrast within the excluded aneurysmal sac extending from the graft defect (*red arrow*) consistent with a type 3 endoleak.

TABLE 25.7 Endoleak Types [2,7]

Type 1*	Inadequate sealing at the proximal (type 1a) or distal (type 1b) seal of the graft
Type 2**	Associated with a collateral feeding and outflow artery, typically lumbar arteries, IMA, or bronchial arteries
Type 3*	Inadequate seal of the graft components, it is a mechanical failure of the graft
Type 4	Leak through graft porosity
Type 5	Idiopathic, described as endotension because excluded sac continues to enlarge without identifiable source for the leak

IMA, inferior mesenteric artery; *, considered emergencies and grant a call to the surgical team; **, most common Endoleak type treated conservatively and it usually resolves spontaneously.

- Type III is an endoleak through a defect in the graft or the graft components (Fig. 25.24)
- Type IV endoleak through the graft porosity
- Type V endotension endoleak refers to the continued expansion of the aneurysm without an identifiable endoleak

Type I and III endoleaks are considered emergent and usually treated with the addition of endovascular grafts or balloon re-expansion, while type II endoleaks are usually followed with imaging to ensure no continuous expansion of the excluded aneurysmal sac, but if found, then treated via percutaneously embolization techniques (Table 25.7).

Vasculitis

Vasculitides can be primary (idiopathic) or secondary. Primary vasculitis includes large-vessel vasculitis such as giant cell arteritis (GCA) or Takayasu arteritis (TA), and medium sized vessels such as Kawasaki disease (KD), polyarteritis nodosa (PAN), primary CNS angiitis, and thromboangiitis obliterans (Buerger's disease). Secondary vasculitis includes processes secondary to infections, inflammatory changes related to treatment response such as radiation, or other diseases like sarcoidosis, IgG4 vasculitis, Wegener's granulomatosis, Behcet disease, rheumatoid arthritis, ankylosing spondylitis, systemic lupus erythematosus, Cogan syndrome, or mimicking conditions such as neoplasias.

Whereas GCA and TA have similar pathology mechanisms involving T-cells, macrophages and antigen-presenting cells; other vasculitides involve autoantibodies [28]. GCA and TA have imaging similarities, and some of the differences are depicted in Table 25.8.

Giant Cell Arteritis

GCA is characterized by granulomatous infiltration in the wall of large and medium size arteries. The classical presentation is a patient (F > M) older than 50 years old of Scandinavian decent, who presents with a headache, claudication of the tongue or jaw upon swallowing, abrupt visual disturbances, and/or claudication of the upper extremities, asymmetric blood pressures, elevated inflammatory markers and abnormal temporal artery pulsation. Sometimes, in the absence of all these features, only constitutional symptoms may be present. The gold standard diagnostic test is a temporal artery biopsy, although this can be falsely negative in a third of the patients. Color Doppler ultrasound is a noninvasive technique to assess the temporal artery, and it has been proposed by some to replace invasive biopsy. GCA is most of the time associated with long, skip areas of stenosis and dilation, segmented lesions with increased wall thickness. The increased edema and inflammatory extent can be assessed using MRA and 18F-FDG PET [29] (Fig. 25.25).

The most important sequence in the MRA protocol is the postcontrast T1-weighted 3D spoiled GRE sequence with a fat

TABLE 25.8 Giant Cell Arteritis Versus Takayasu Arteritis [28,29]

	Giant Cell Arteritis	Takayasu Arteritis
Age	Elderly	Young (<50 years old) is most common
Ethnicity	Scandinavian decent	Asian decent
Gender	Women > Men	Women >>> Men
Vessels involved	Aorta (65%)	Aorta (95%)
	Branches	Branches
	Temporal arteries	Pulmonary artery (less common)

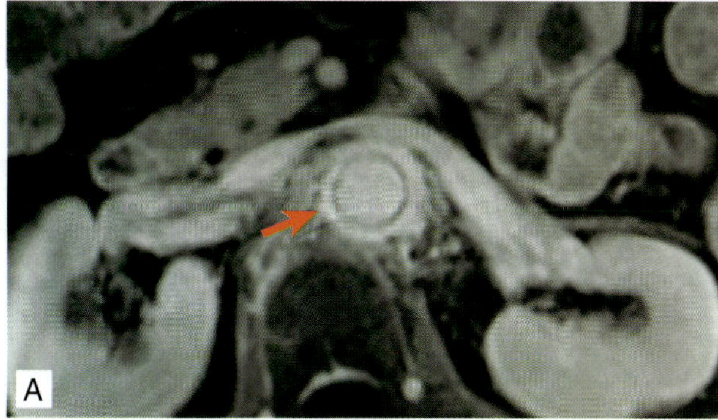

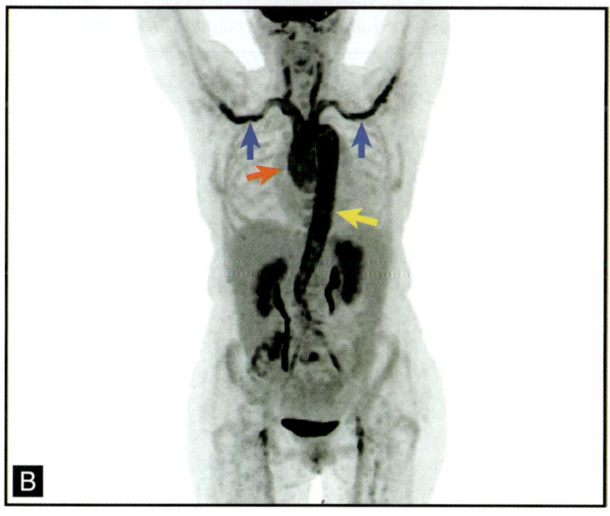

Figure 25.25 Giant cell arteritis. (A) Contrast-enhanced T1-GRE with fat saturation depicts diffuse transmural enhancement of the aortic wall. (B) Note correspondingly increased 18F-FDG uptake on three-dimensional maximum intensity projection (3D MIP) image throughout the thoracic aorta (*red arrow*), abdominal aorta (*yellow arrow*), and bilateral subclavian arteries (*blue arrows*) with a standardized uptake value (SUV) of 6.5, which confirms long-segment inflammation of the aorta.

saturation. This is acquired in a single breath hold with excellent spatial and contrast resolution. Traditionally, T1 double inversion recovery (DIR) has been used to image the aortic wall. DIR involves two successive 180 radiofrequency inversion pulses to null signal from moving blood and preserve the signal of nonmoving structures such as the aortic wall. DIR is excellent to depict aortic wall increased thickness and enhancement. Disadvantages of using DIR are incomplete nulling of the lumen, inconsistent tissue weighting, thick slices (8 mm), and excessive scan time since each slice requires a breath hold which adds considerable amount of time to the study, approximately 20–30 minutes.

Takayasu Arteritis

TA presents primarily in women between 10 and 40 years old with Asian background, low-grade fevers, fatigue, weight loss. TA progresses to a diverse variety of symptoms according to the arterial involvement, such as upper extremity claudication, decreased pulses and asymmetric blood pressures due to involvement of the subclavian arteries, secondary hypertension due to involvement of the renal arteries, gastrointestinal symptoms due to involvement of the mesenteric arteries, chest pain and dyspnea due to involvement of the pulmonary arteries, as well as neurologic symptoms due to involvement of the carotid and vertebral arteries. TA typically involves the left subclavian artery and progresses to involve the aorta in half of the patients (Fig. 25.26). The pulmonary artery can also be involved, but is less common than the aorta (Fig. 25.27).

Kawasaki Disease

KD is a predominantly medium-vessel vasculitis of unknown etiology, which affects infants and children younger than 4 years. KD can occur in any artery but has a predilection for coronary vessels. Other common arteries include axillary, subclavian, brachial, femoral, iliac, splanchnic, and mesenteric arteries, usually near or at branching points [30].

This vasculitis is known to have at least two phases, the acute and the late phase. The acute phase is defined as the first 30 days of illness with development of coronary aneurysms in about 15–25% of untreated patients and only around 5–7% for patients treated with high-dose intravenous immunoglobulin [31]. The late phase is when small aneurysms can either regress completely

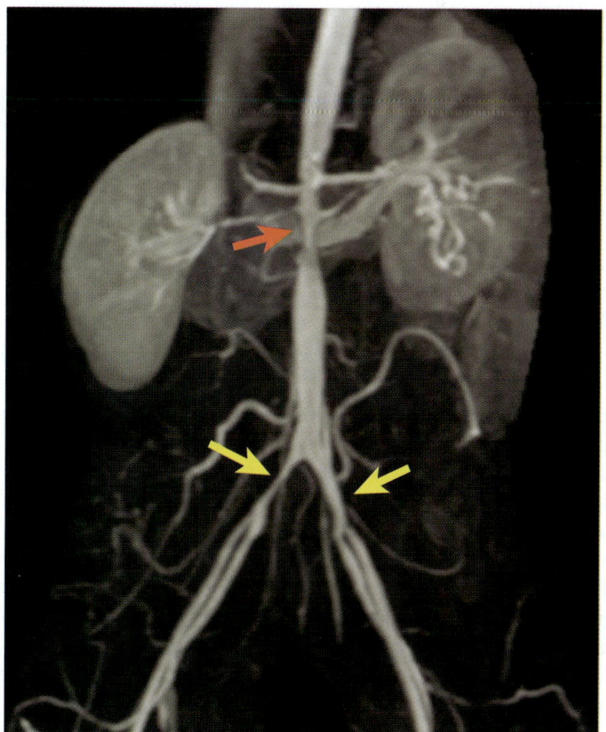

Figure 25.26 Takayasu's arteritis. Maximum intensity projection (MIP) image from an MRA showing long segment smooth stenosis of the juxtarenal abdominal aorta (*red arrow*) and both common iliac arteries (*yellow arrows*).

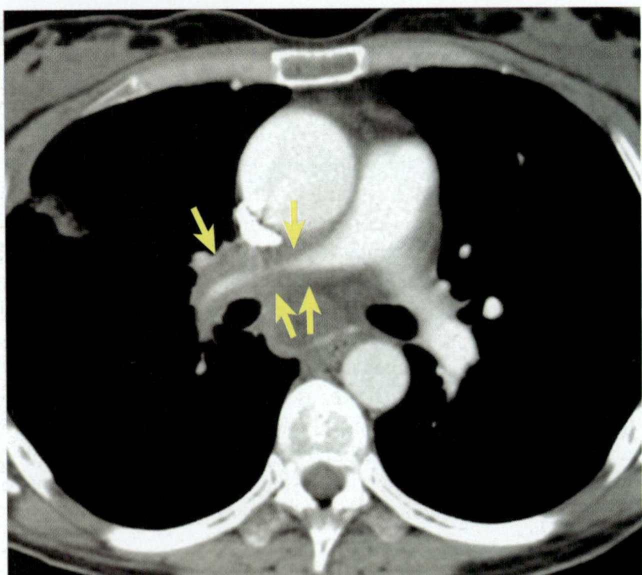

Figure 25.27 Takayasu's arteritis. Axial CTA shows smooth circumferential thickening of the right pulmonary artery (*yellow arrows*).

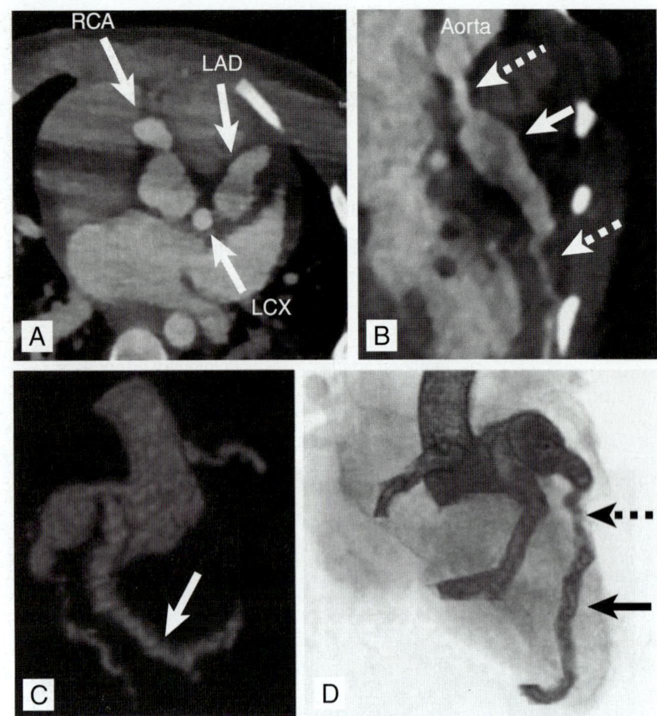

Figure 25.28 Kawasaki disease. CTA axial of the coronary arteries (A) depicting aneurysms in multivessel distribution involving the proximal left anterior descending artery (LAD), left circumflex (LCX), and right coronary artery (RCA). Multiplanar reformatted image (MPR; B) of the proximal LAD with a giant aneurysm (*solid arrow*), a normal caliber left main (LM) and distal LAD (*dotted arrows*). In addition (C and D) volume-rendered three-dimensional images show distal ectatic segments (*solid arrows*) and (D) intervening unaffected vessel segment (*dotted arrow*). (Reprinted with permission from: S Hedgire, B Pulli, M Lahoud-Rahme, RS Beroukhim, AM Rosales, B Ghoshhajra, Kawasaki disease with giant coronary artery aneurysms, Coron Artery Dis 28 (2) (2017) 177–179).

within 2 years; or progress to occlusion or localized stenosis, even 10 or 20 years after the onset of the disease. A *z*-score of >2.5 to <5 is considered a small aneurysm (<5 mm); a *z*-score ≥5 to <10 is a medium aneurysm (5 to <8 mm); and a *z*-score of ≥10 is a large or giant aneurysm (≥8 mm). The *z*-score adjusted for body surface area is also used and it has been adopted by the American Heart Association [30,31].

Imaging of the coronary arteries is critical for stratification and therapeutic management and can be done with echocardiography, invasive conventional angiography, CCTA, or MRA [32]. Conventional angiography entails risks related to anesthesia, puncture site, bleeding, and others; but it is still the gold standard for stratification. Echocardiography is also performed as primary imaging technique due to its availability and broad use, as well as it allows for assessment of the left ventricular function, aortic root, mitral, and aortic valves. However, echocardiography is many times limited in uncooperative children or due to the lack of anesthesia. CCTA and MRA (3D Navigator) are imaging techniques preferred for follow-up of these lesions (Fig. 25.28) [30,31,33,34].

Polyarteritis Nodosa

PAN is a type of necrotizing vasculitis and is characterized by inflammatory reactions in small and medium size vessels that lead to necrosis of the wall in a segmental fashion. PAN occurs more frequently in men with a male to female ratio of 2–3:1, and it affects all ages with a higher rate during the fourth and fifth decades. Approximately one third of the patients with PAN have been reported to have hepatitis B antigen. The clinical scenario includes a variety of signs and symptoms making it challenging for the clinician. These include abdominal pain, hypertension, arthralgias or arthritis, peripheral and central nervous system dysfunction, retinopathy, cardiac, respiratory, and hepatic involvement [35,36]. The American College of Rheumatology describes 10 diagnostic criteria of PAN. A conventional angiogram with characteristic PAN findings is one of the 10 diagnostic criteria, and three of the 10 criteria have to be present for PAN diagnosis [37].

PAN occurs predominately in the kidney (80–100%), heart (up to 70%), gastrointestinal tract (50–70%), liver (50–60%), spleen (45%), and pancreas (25–35%), skin (50%), skeletal muscles and mesentery (30%). Most cases of PAN have positive angiographic findings in medium and small arteries such as microaneurysms, ectasia, occlusions, hemorrhages and thrombosis, and in some occasions, lack of vascularity in a wedge shape appearance, corresponding to prior infarcts (Fig. 25.29) [38]. However, similar angiographic findings can also be seen with drug abuse. Microaneurysms are approximately 2–3 mm in diameter, which may be under the spatial resolution of MRA and CTA, even with dedicated protocols. CTA and MRA help identifying aneurysms, stenosis, occlusions, arterial wall irregularity, as well as extra-arterial findings, such as renal parenchymal changes, bowel wall thickening, perinephric hematomas, and multiple small bilateral infarcts of various ages distributed among the interlobar and arcuate arteries. Without angiography, the correct diagnosis is problematic due to sampling errors and lack of disease specificity. Therefore, a positive biopsy of a symptomatic organ site, subcutaneous nodule, or skeletal muscle can help establish the diagnosis, but if negative or nonconclusive, does not rule out the disease.

If untreated, PAN is usually fatal as a consequence of renal failure and gastrointestinal complications, and the 5-year survival is around 15%. When treated with corticosteroids and cytotoxic drugs (cyclophosphamide), the 5-year survival can increase to 80%, however, about 40% of treated patients can relapse [35,36].

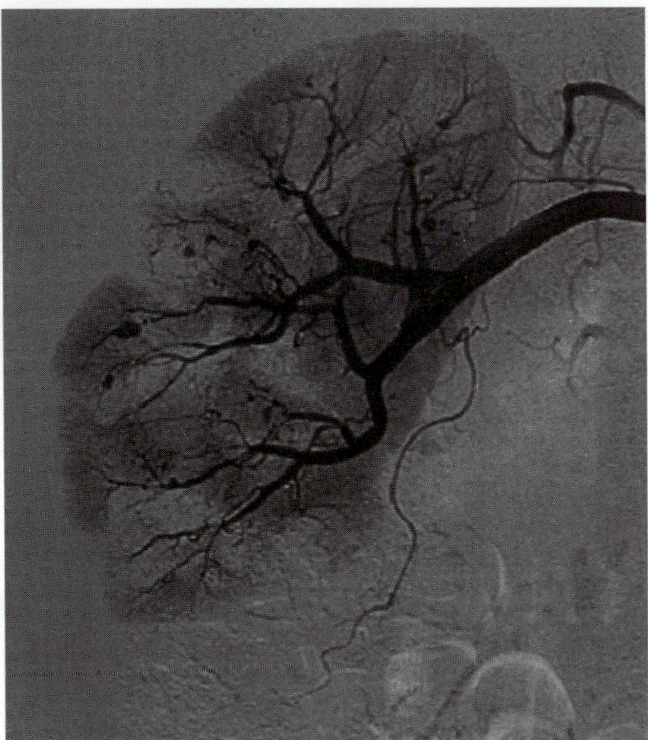

Figure 25.29 Polyarteritis nodosa involving the renal arteries. Conventional arteriogram of the right renal arteries shows multiple microaneurysms in the distal interlobar and arcuate arteries. Multifocal distal segmental renal arterial stenosis, ectasia, and occlusion of these small arteries are also seen. Multiple wedge-shaped hypoperfusion areas are also present. (Reprinted with permission from: K Ozaki, S Miyayama, Y Ushiogi, O Matsui, Renal involvement of polyarteritis nodosa: CT and MR findings, Abdom Imaging 34 (2) (2009) 265–270).

Coarctation and Pseudocoarctation

Coarctation of the aorta is the most common congenital anomaly of the aorta with an incidence of 5 per 100,000 in the general population. It refers to a hemodynamically significant narrowing of the distal aortic arch. Collateral circulation is formed by prominent internal mammary and intercostal arteries due to the blood flow demands below the level of coarctation. Their presence are considered a reliable indicator of significant coarctation [39] (Fig. 25.30). Normally, the blood flow is lower at the distal thoracic aorta than in the proximal segments. This normal relationship is reversed in hemodynamically significant aortic coarctation. The imaging technique of choice to evaluate for differences in blood flow, blood volume, and gradient is velocity-encoded cine MR with phase contrast imaging. Phase contrast imaging is helpful for both preoperative planning and postprocedural monitoring of residual or recurrent aortic coarctation [40].

Pseudocoarctation occurs when the third to seventh embryological dorsal segments fail to fuse properly, resulting in kinking of the redundant aorta without a hemodynamical significant stenosis. This lack of stenosis results in the lack of collaterals which are usually present in aortic coarctation [39] (Fig. 25.31).

Abdomen

The pathology underlying the renal arteries and rest of the arteries arising from the abdominal aorta involve different mechanisms. Therefore, we will discuss separately the different causes of renal artery stenosis, and then proceed to discuss the most common diseases involving the celiac trunk and the mesenteric arteries.

Renal Arteries

Bilateral renal arteries arise directly from the aorta (immediately below the superior mesenteric artery [SMA] at the L2 level), iliac arteries, or rarely from the IMA. Accessory renal arteries are present in approximately 30% of cases and 10% bilaterally. Accessory renal arteries enter the kidney through the hilum, while polar (aberrant) arteries enter the kidney through the capsule outside the hilum. Main renal arteries offer blood supply to the adrenal gland, ureter, perinephric tissue, and renal capsule. Early bifurcation of renal arteries (1.5 cm after the origin) should be described in possible renal donors since it may complicate the arterial anastomosis. Anomalous renal arteries are more common in cases of renal fusion or positional anomalies, including horseshoe kidney and fused renal ectopia [41].

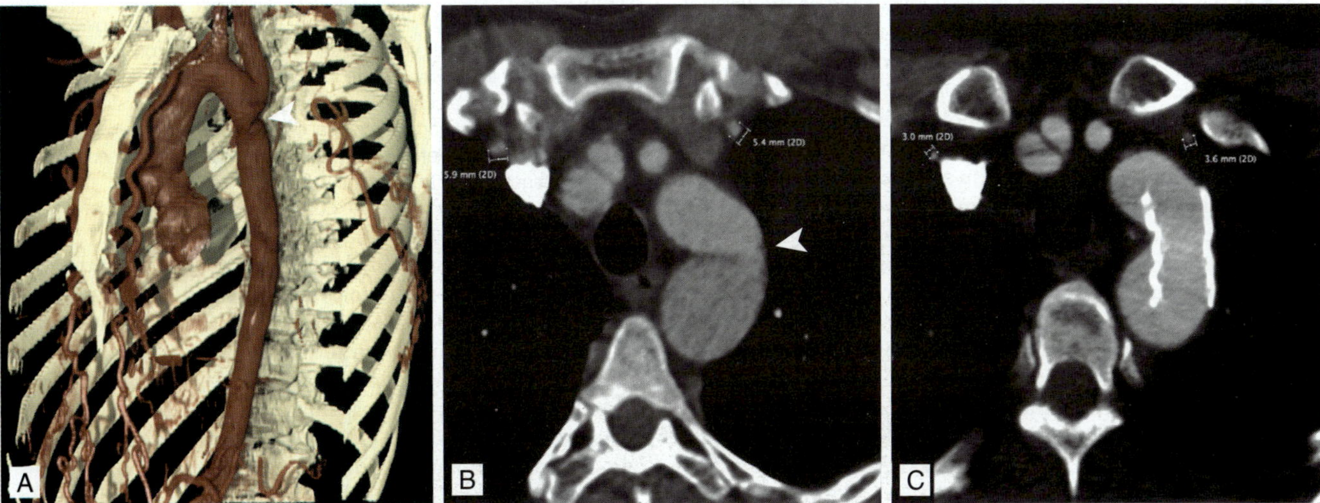

Figure 25.30 Coarctation of the aorta. (A and B) 3D global illumination rendering (GIR) and CTA axial imaging shows kinking of the aorta at the level of the isthmus associated with a hemodynamically significant stenosis, depicted by the presence of collateral flow with prominent bilateral internal mammary arteries (IMAs) measuring 5–6 mm. (C) Follow-up CTA shows interval repair with placement of a stent graft and successful decrease of collateral flow with interval significant decrease in size of the bilateral IMAs measuring 3–4 mm.

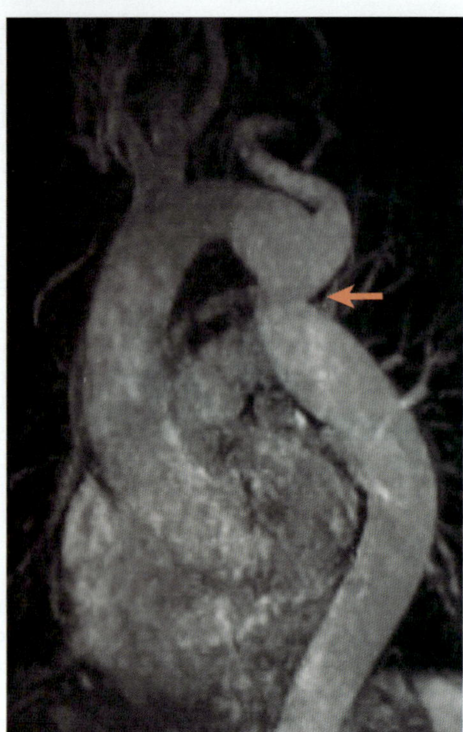

Figure 25.31 Pseudocoarctation. Pseudocoarctation of the aorta was identified incidentally on an MRA of the thoracic aorta. Maximum intensity projection (MIP) shows kinking (*red arrow*) of the aorta without collaterals.

Doppler imaging, CTA, and MRA offer diagnostic information of the renal arteries. Doppler imaging offers additional physiological real-time information, while CTA and MRA offer more accurate anatomical and diagnostic information of the renal parenchyma (cortical atrophy, decreased cortical enhancement, infarcts), poststenotic dilations, distal and accessory arteries, which can also result in secondary hypertension. In patients who cannot receive iodine or gadolinium, MRI with time of flight, and SSFP sequences provide valuable information.

Normal renal artery PSV is 60–100 cm/s, the waveform is antegrade, low resistive, monophasic, and with a normal resistive index of 0.6–0.7. The resistive index is calculated at the level of the arcuate arteries.

Renal artery stenosis (RAS) is the most common cause of secondary hypertension. About 60–70% of cases of RAS are caused by atherosclerosis, and it is more commonly seen in men older than 50 years old. RAS causes decreased perfusion to the kidneys, which activates the renin–angiotensin system and then results in hypertension. RAS due to atherosclerosis occurs at the ostium or within the proximal renal artery, and it occurs bilaterally in approximately 30% of cases (Figs. 25.32 and 25.33). Fibromuscular dysplasia (FMD) is the second most common cause of RAS and it occurs more frequently in younger female (F:M ratio 9:1) patients. RAS secondary to FMD is seen in the middle to distal renal arteries and is bilateral in about 70% of cases.

Doppler imaging criteria to detect renal stenosis greater than 60% stenosis include direct signs, such as PSV > 180 cm/s, renal artery to proximal (prerenal) aorta ratio (RAR) of PSV > 3.5:1, lack of color Doppler indicating stenosis or occlusion, and aliasing artifacts. In cases of RAS, the waveform remains antegrade, low resistive and monophasic in the absence of additional distal stenosis or intrinsic renal parenchymal disease. Additional indirect signs of RAS are obtained distal to the stenosis and are usually

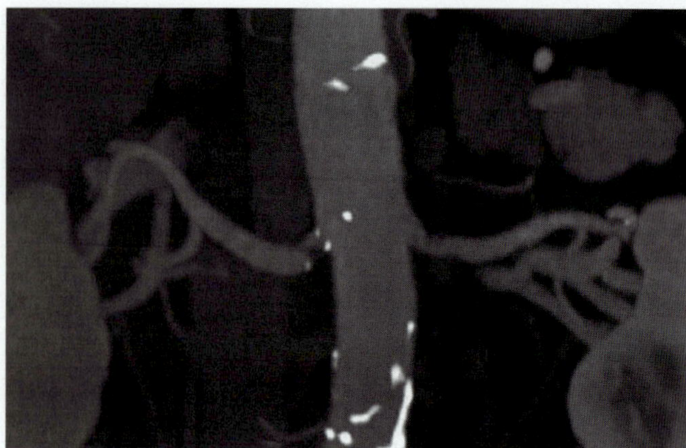

Figure 25.32 Renal artery stenosis associated with atherosclerotic disease. CTA oblique MPR shows severe stenosis of the proximal right renal artery secondary to atherosclerotic disease with calcified and noncalcified plaque.

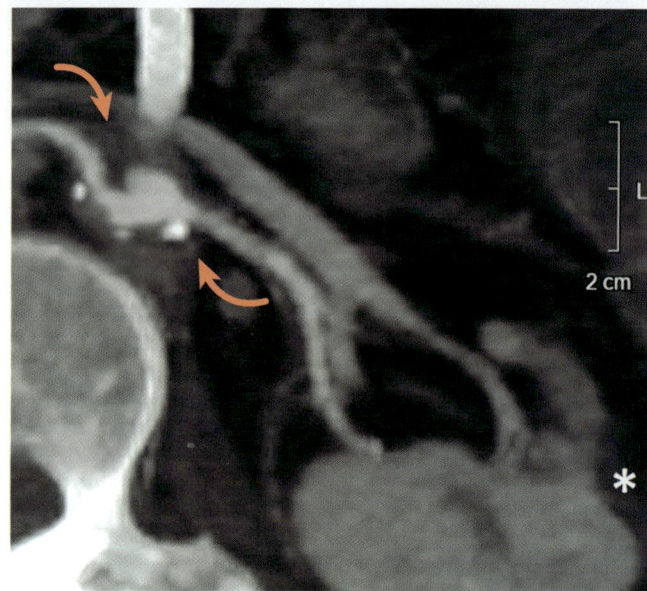

Figure 25.33 Renal artery stenosis associated with advanced atherosclerotic disease (aortoiliac disease). CTA of the abdomen shows at least moderate stenosis of the bilateral renal arteries (*red arrows*) secondary to advanced aortoiliac disease, the latter is depicted as a large amount of predominantly noncalcified plaque resulting in moderate stenosis of the juxtarenal abdominal aorta. A cortical defect in the left kidney is also present (*asterisk*), likely related to a prior infarct from RAS. There is also a partially imaged celiac trunk stent.

interrogated at the segmental renal arteries. The indirect signs of RAS are obtained by interrogating segmental or arcuate arteries distal to the area of RAS and include an acceleration time >70 milliseconds (time from the start of systole to peak systole), acceleration index <300 cm/s (slope of the systolic upstroke), turbulent flow (spectral broadening), and increase resistive index values (≥0.8; Fig. 25.34) [6,41]. An elevated resistive index can also be seen with medical renal disease or ureteric obstruction.

The American College of Cardiology and American Heart Association recommend the use of revascularization strategies to treat patients with RAS secondary to atherosclerosis [41,42]. Endoluminal stent placement is generally considered superior to balloon angioplasty, and surgical reconstruction is reserved in

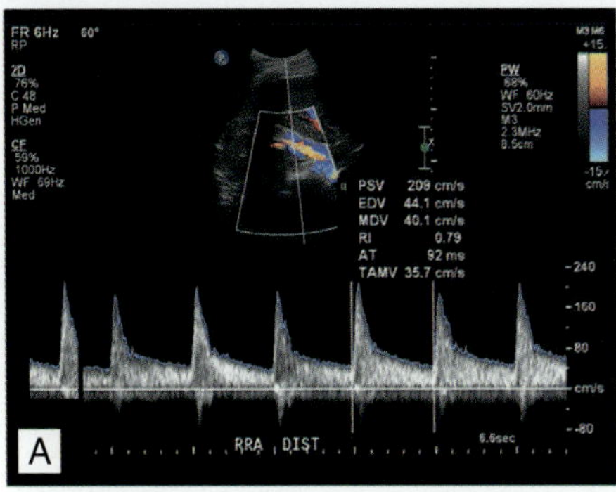

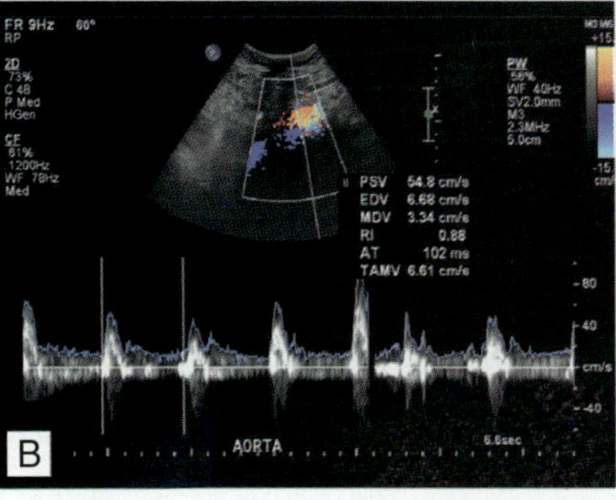

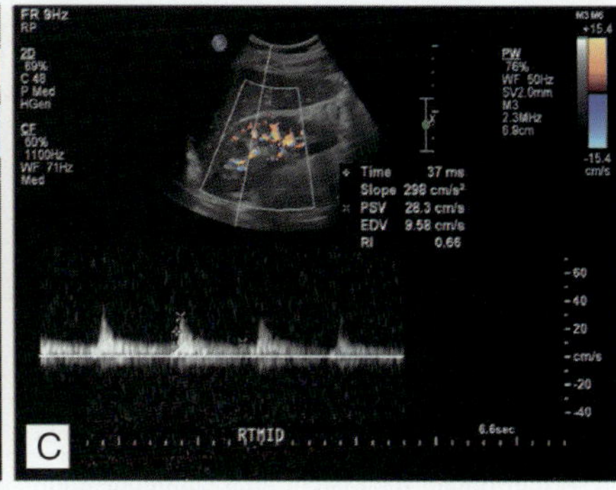

Figure 25.34 Renal artery stenosis (RAS). (A and B) Spectral Doppler analysis of the distal right renal artery and aorta shows three Doppler ultrasound direct signs of RAS; (1) Elevated peak systolic velocity of 209 cm/s (RAS criteria >200 cm/s) at the distal right renal artery, (2) increased renal aorta ratio (RAR) of 3.8 (RAR >3.5 meets RAS criteria), and (3) aliasing artifact which indicates turbulent flow. (C) Indirect signs of RAS with interrogation of the right kidney at the segmental arteries (distal to the arterial stenosis), it shows a decreased acceleration index of 298 cm/s^2 (RAS criteria <300 cm/s^2), and a tardus parvus waveform.

patients with unsuccessful endovascular therapy. An associated resistive index higher than 0.8 has been suggested as a poor indicator of revascularization response [42]. This approach changes in RAS secondary to FMD where percutaneous angioplasty is the treatment of choice [41].

Other causes of RAS include renal artery entrapment, dissection, and systemic disorders such as neurofibromatosis type 1 (NF-1), drugs, PAN, and other vasculitides. Renal artery entrapment is seen in young patients with secondary hypertension in whom there is an anomalous course of the renal artery and extrinsic compression from the diaphragm or psoas muscle. These patients usually need surgical correction of the anomalous course of the renal artery. Dissection of the renal arteries can also result in RAS, and it can be seen as an extension of an aortic dissection (Fig. 25.35), secondary to segmental arterial mediolysis, trauma or related to complicated endovascular procedures. Known predisposing factors to renal artery dissection are FMD, atherosclerosis, cystic medial necrosis, cocaine abuse, and extreme physical exertion. NF-1 is an autosomal dominant disorder with many vascular complications and hypertension secondary to RAS is seen in pediatric patients. RAS in NF-1 usually presents as a long segment of stenosis that extends to the segmental arteries, and usually needs surgical correction [43]. Drugs that can result in RAS include cocaine, methamphetamines, vinblastine, cisplatin, and bleomycin. RAS secondary to PAN and other vasculitides, such as lupus, Takayasu, and others are usually the result of chronic inflammation that can result in scarring and, consequently, stenosis and occlusion [41].

Celiac Axis and Mesenteric Arteries

The celiac axis gives rise to the left gastric artery, splenic artery, and the common hepatic artery in about 70% of the cases. The latter commonly gives origin to the gastroduodenal artery and the proper hepatic artery. The SMA arises just caudal to the celiac axis, and the IMA arises above the level of the aortic bifurcation. The common origin of the celiac axis and the SMA occurs in less than 1% of the cases. The SMA gives rise to the inferior pancreaticoduodenal, jejunal, ileal, ileocolic, and right and middle colic arteries. The IMA gives rise to the left colic, sigmoid branches, and the superior rectal artery. The most common variations are the replaced right hepatic artery arising from the SMA in about 10% of cases, and the origin of the left hepatic artery from the left gastric artery in about 7% of cases. Key collateral pathways become more robust and are recognized whenever there is a significant stenosis of one of these vessels. Pancreoticoduodenal arteries, dorsal pancreatic artery, and the Arc of Buhler (persistent fetal communication between the SMA and the celiac axis in less than 1% of the cases) are the key collateral pathways with celiac artery or SMA stenosis. The arcade of Riolan and the marginal artery of Drummond

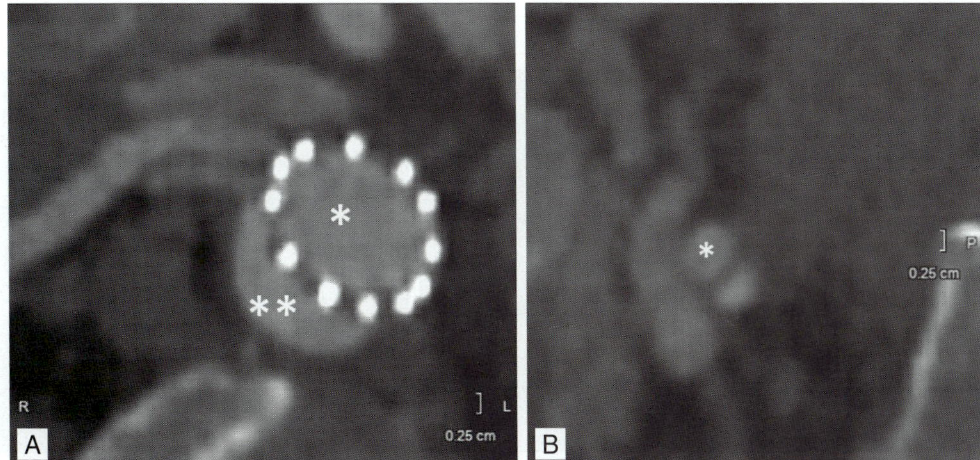

Figure 25.35 Renal artery stenosis (RAS) associated with an aortic dissection. (A and B) CTA shows axial images of a patient with prior aortic dissection with an endovascular aortic stent seen in the true aortic lumen (*asterisk*). The dissection flap extends to the proximal right main renal artery, consequently the kidney receives blood supply from both the true (*asterisk*) and the nonthrombosed false lumen (*double asterisk*), but still resulting in at least mild stenosis of the true lumen.

TABLE 25.9 Key Collateral Pathways [2,44]

Celiac Artery or SMA Stenosis	SMA or IMA Stenosis	IMA Stenosis
Pancreoticoduodenal arteries	The arcade of Riolan is constituted from the left branch of the middle colic artery (arises from the SMA) and the ascending branch of the left colic artery (arises from the IMA)	Hemorrhoidal, branch of the anterior division of the internal iliac artery
Dorsal pancreatic artery	The marginal artery of Drummond is formed by the terminal branches of the middle colic from the SMA and the left colic from the IMA	Hypogastric collateral bed
Arc of Buhler (persistent fetal communication between the SMA and the celiac axis in less than 1% of the cases)		

IMA, inferior mesenteric artery; *SMA*, superior mesenteric artery.

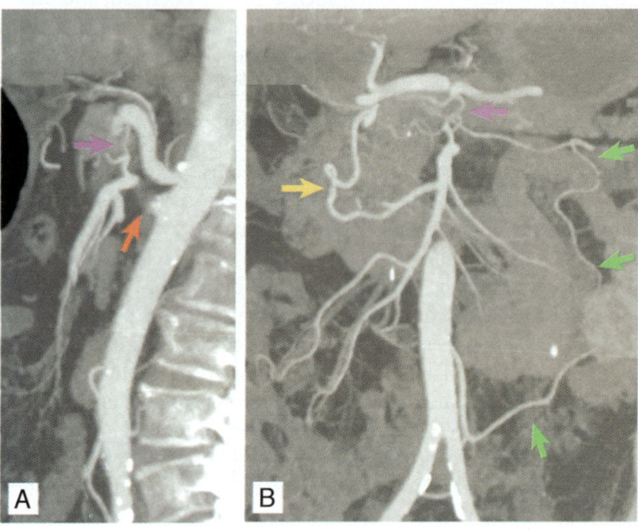

Figure 25.36 Key collateral pathways of the superior mesenteric artery (SMA). Occlusion of the SMA and distal reconstitution of flow via key collateral pathways. Maximum intensity projection (MIP) of sagittal (A) and coronal (B) shows the arc of Buhler between the SMA and the celiac trunk (*pink arrow*), pancreoticoduodenal artery (*yellow arrow*), and the arcade of Riolan (*green arrows*) between the inferior mesenteric artery and the SMA.

are the key collateral pathways with SMA or IMA stenosis. The arcade of Riolan is constituted from the left branch of the middle colic artery (arises from the SMA) and the ascending branch of the left colic artery (arises from the IMA). The marginal artery of Drummond is formed by the terminal branches of the middle colic from the SMA and the left colic from the IMA and runs along the inner margin of the transverse and left colon [2,44] (Table 25.9 and Fig. 25.36).

Spectral Doppler imaging of a normal celiac trunk shows a constant forward flow throughout systole and diastole due to the high demands of the liver and spleen. The normal celiac artery Doppler waveform is antegrade, low resistive, and monophasic. A flow-limiting stenosis of the celiac trunk with a reduction of >70% in luminal diameter shows a PSV >200 cm/s. The Doppler waveform is still antegrade, low resistive, and monophasic.

Median arcuate ligament syndrome, also known as celiac artery compression syndrome, is characterized by chronic upper abdominal pain in the setting of worsened compression during end-expiration by the diaphragmatic crurae. The typical imaging appearance is that of a hooked or "J" appearance of the celiac trunk. Imaging evaluation can be obtained during end-expiration and end-inspiration with arterial Doppler ultrasound or MRA, which show worsened stenosis during end-expiration and resulting increased mean PSV >350 cm/s during end-expiration (Figs. 25.37 and 25.38) [45]. CTA may be used but typically

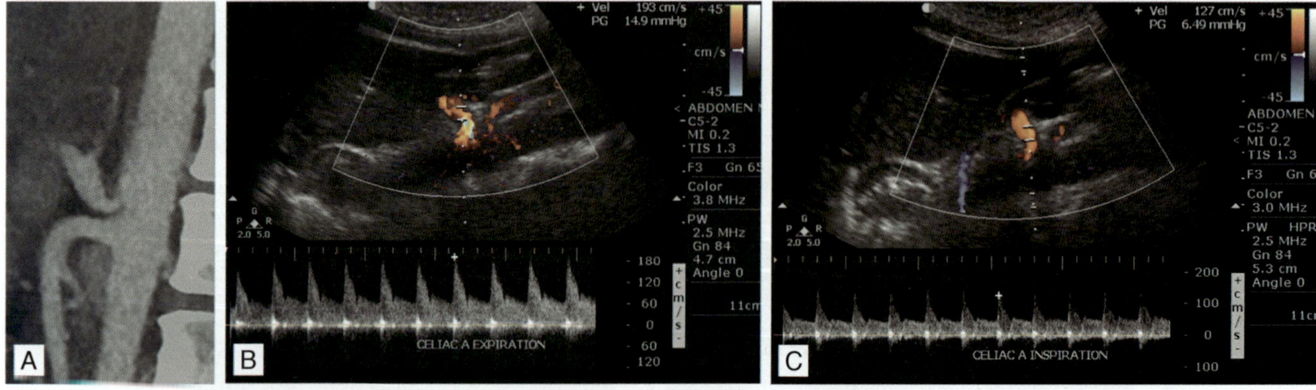

Figure 25.37 Median arcuate ligament syndrome (MALS). (A) CTA shows characteristic hooked appearance of the celiac trunk associated with median arcuate ligament compression on a patient with history of chronic abdominal pain. (B and C) Dynamic arterial Doppler images with spectral analysis at the celiac trunk, which shows a greater increased peak systolic velocity (PSV) during expiration (193 cm/s), than during inspiration (127 cm/s). Note aliasing artifact in the celiac trunk during expiration, indicating even a greater PSV during expiration.

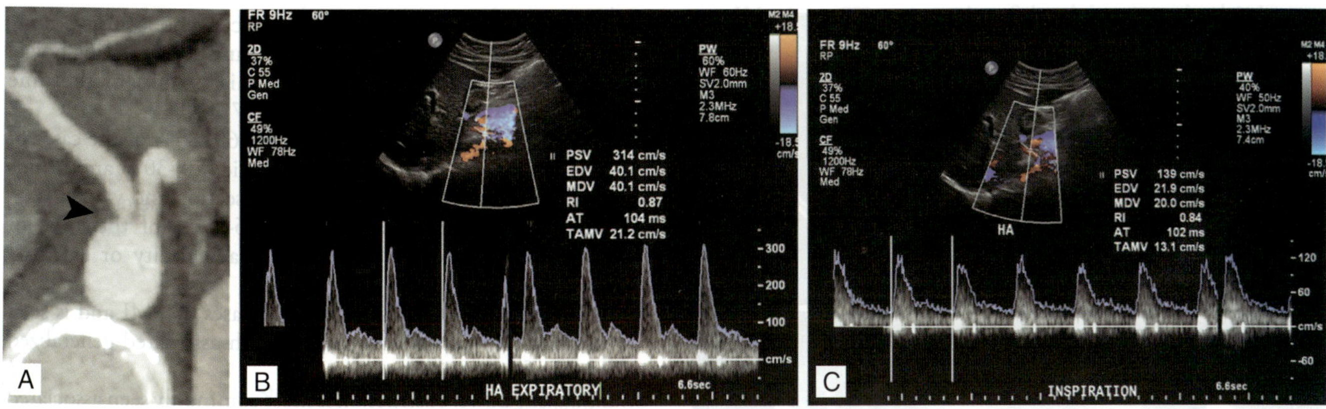

Figure 25.38 Median arcuate ligament syndrome (MALS) involving the common hepatic artery. (A) CTA axial image shows a separate origin of the common hepatic artery arising directly from the aorta. There is a typical appearance of a band like hypoattenuation (*black arrowhead*) related to median arcuate ligament compression. (B and C) Dynamic arterial Doppler ultrasound with spectral analysis at the common hepatic artery, which shows a greater increased peak systolic velocity (PSV) during expiration (314 cm/s), than during inspiration (139 cm/s).

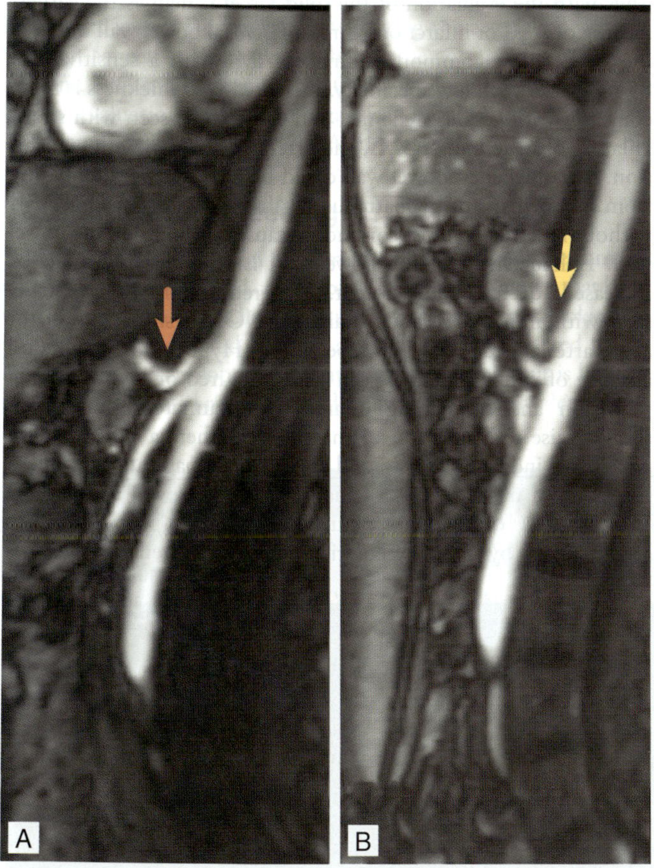

Figure 25.39 Median arcuate ligament syndrome (MALS). MRA shows (A) typical hooked appearance of the celiac trunk (*red arrow*) during inspiration due to median arcuate ligament compression, (B) and significant worsening of this morphology during expiration with resulting severe stenosis of the proximal celiac trunk (*yellow arrow*). Note the differences in positioning of the diaphragm between (A) inspiration and (B) expiration.

these patients are younger when the radiation exposure should be minimized, which is why MRA is preferred (Fig. 25.39). Symptomatic patients are treated with surgical decompression, which is usually performed laparoscopically [46].

The normal SMA Doppler waveform changes during fasting and postprandial stages. During fasting it is antegrade, high resistive, and multiphasic with early diastolic flow reversal often apparent; and during a postprandial stage is antegrade, but waveform becomes low resistive and monophasic (REF). A flow-limiting stenosis of the SMA with a reduction of >70% in luminal diameter shows a PSV >275 cm/s. The Doppler waveform is antegrade, low resistive and monophasic (REF).

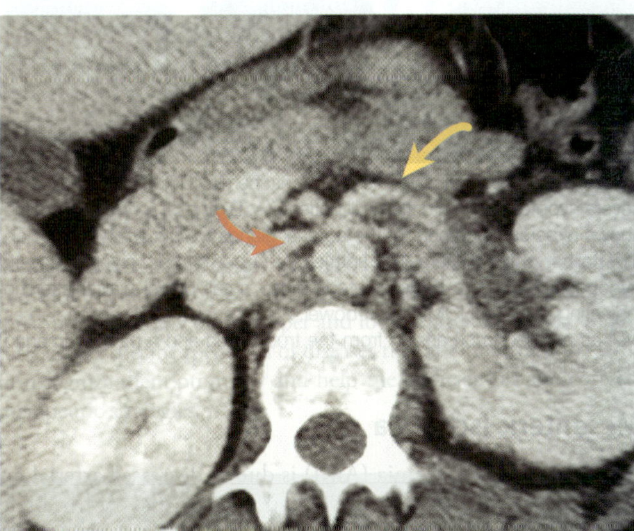

Figure 25.40 Superior mesenteric syndrome (SMA) and associated Nutcracker syndrome. Contrast-enhanced axial image shows decreased distance (<6 mm) between the aorta and the proximal SMA (*curved red arrow*) in a patient with history of chronic postprandial abdominal pain depicting SMA syndrome. These findings are present concomitantly with a nonocclusive thrombosis of the left renal artery (*curved yellow arrow*) on this patient who presented with hematuria. The hematuria and associated thrombosis of the left renal vein are components of the Nutcracker syndrome.

Superior mesenteric syndrome occurs when there is compression with or without obstruction at the level of the third portion of the duodenum between the aorta and the proximal SMA. The typical presentation is acute on chronic postprandial upper abdominal pain. There are factors that can precipitate these symptoms such as significant weight loss resulting in loss of the fat around the SMA. Imaging findings reveal decreased aortomesenteric angle to 6–22° (normal 28–65°), and decreased aortomesenteric distance to 2–8 mm (normal 10–34 mm) [2] (Fig. 25.40).

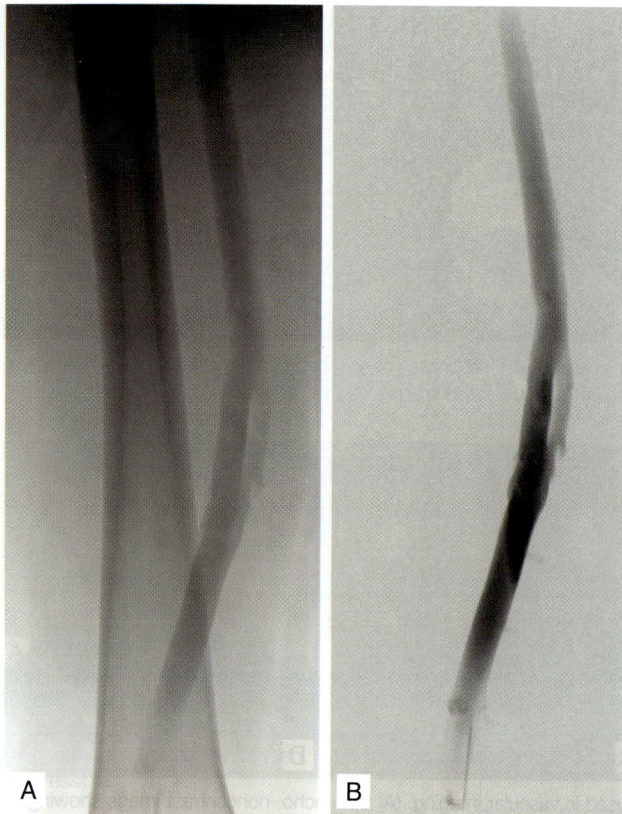

Figure 26.6 Venography of the left femoral vein. (A) Fluoroscopic image with contrast opacification of the vein lumen. (B) Same image but with digital subtraction angiography (DSA).

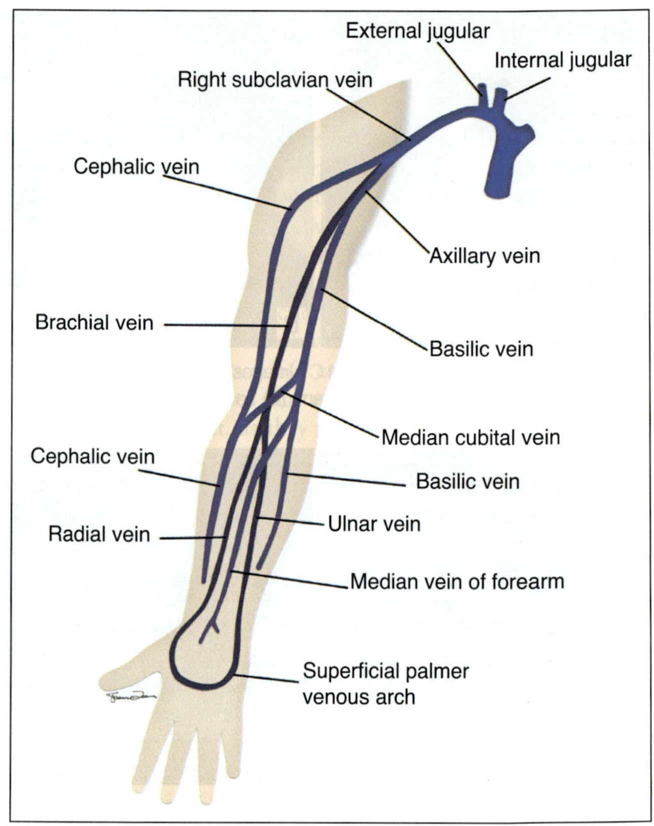

Figure 26.7 Illustration of the normal upper extremity venous anatomy. (Courtesy: Susanne Loomis).

Venography

Venography or phlebography, refers to the invasive imaging approach of directly injecting contrast material into a peripheral vein while simultaneously recording an image or video clip of serial images, in real time. Therefore, conventional venography is typically performed in a fluoroscopy suite by an interventionalist using fluoroscopy and digital subtraction angiography (DSA). As appropriate, USG guidance is often used in obtaining initial venous access. DSA is a fluoroscopic technique that generates an image or series of images, after a computer subtracts the initial precontrast image. DSA is helpful for removing or subtracting out, superimposed structures that obscure detail (Fig. 26.6). Direct venography refers to the direct injection of contrast material followed by imaging, whereas, indirect venography refers to the approach where venous anatomy is imaged a specific time after contrast material has been injected into the arterial circulation.

Upper Extremity Venous System

Anatomy and Variants

The upper extremity venous system is comprised of deep and superficial veins with numerous communicating vessels (Fig. 26.7). Bicuspid valves are present in the upper extremity veins which serve to promote unidirectional blood flow. The named upper extremity *deep veins* include:

- Radial
- Ulnar
- Interosseous
- Brachial
- Axillary
- Subclavian

The named *superficial* veins include:

- Cephalic
- Basilic
- Median cubital
- Median antebrachial

The superficial basilic and cephalic veins join the axillary vein at the shoulder; the basilic vein inferiorly and the cephalic vein superiorly. In most patients, the basilic vein joins the axillary vein inferomedial to the cephalic vein. Distal to the shoulder, upper extremity venous drainage occurs disproportionately in the superficial vessels lending them a larger diameter compared to their deeper counterparts. Once the superficial and deep veins converge at the shoulder in the axillary vein, deep venous drainage predominates [12]. Variant venous anatomy in the upper extremity is common. The most important variants relevant to dialysis access are listed in Table 26.1 [13].

TABLE 26.1 Common Upper Extremity Venous Variant Anatomy
Paired brachial veins
Paired brachial veins with low brachial–basilic junction
Single brachial vein with low basilic vein junction in the lower third of the upper arm

Superficial and Deep Venous Thrombosis

Compared to the lower extremities, venous thrombosis of the upper extremities is less common. DVT of the upper extremity has an estimated annual incidence of 0.4–1 per 10,000 [14]. Upper extremity DVT can be classified as either primary or secondary, based on the underlying cause.

Pathophysiology

Primary etiologies of upper extremity DVT, comprising approximately 20% of cases, include Paget–Schroetter (discussed in the next section) and idiopathic causes, including occult malignancy and inherited or acquired thrombophilias [14]. Secondary upper extremity DVT refers to cases caused by the presence of a central venous catheter (CVC) or pacemaker leads (Fig. 26.8). CVC-related thrombosis currently represents the most important preventable risk factor for upper extremity venous thrombosis. Upper extremity CVCs promote thrombus formation potentially through damage to the venous endothelium and by disrupting normal blood flow [15].

Clinical Presentation

Common presenting symptoms of upper extremity venous thrombosis include pain or discomfort, heaviness, paresthesia, swelling, and discoloration. Interestingly, many patients with a catheter associated thrombosis have no associated signs or symptoms [14]. In severe cases, patients may develop post-thrombotic syndrome which is characterized by chronic limb pain and swelling. D-dimer, a fibrin degradation product, is a very sensitive biomarker for venous thrombosis. A low D-dimer level is useful for ruling out venous thrombosis. However, D-dimer is not specific and increases with age, so imaging evaluation is often required in patients with a high pretest probability or an intermediate or elevated D-dimer [16].

Imaging Evaluation

The most appropriate first imaging technique for suspected upper extremity venous thrombosis is Duplex USG [17]. USG is widely available, relatively inexpensive and portable, permitting examination of critically ill patients unsafe for transport to the radiology department or dedicated imaging area. Objective findings of subacute or chronic thrombosis on venous compression USG include a non- or partially compressible vein with echogenic material filling the lumen (Fig. 26.9). Compression USG findings for acute thrombosis may only be manifest through abnormal compressibility, as acute thrombi may appear anechoic or hypoechoic. Indirect Duplex USG findings suggestive of a thrombus include abnormal flow patterns, loss of augmentation, and blunted or loss of the normal variation with respiration and the cardiac cycle. Abnormal flow patterns can include slow or absent velocity of flow and in some cases, reversal of flow distal to a chronic occlusion due to collateral flow (Fig. 26.10). For example, when a proximal thrombus is present during distal venous evaluation, the only finding may be loss of the normal respiratory variation or cardiac pulsatility on spectral Doppler. Thus, in addition to Duplex USG, chest radiography should be considered to help exclude a centrally located, obstructing lesion, as a broad differential exists for the patient presenting with unilateral upper extremity swelling and discomfort.

MRV and CTV are useful for evaluating the central venous structures: the jugular and brachiocephalic veins, and superior vena cava (SVC) (Fig. 26.11). MR with or without contrast material may be performed, with contrast-enhanced studies being preferred. Nonenhanced MRV is typically reserved for patients with a contraindication to contrast material, such as in allergic patients or patients with abnormal renal function. CTV images are typically acquired 90–120 seconds following intravenous contrast material injection. When administering contrast material through

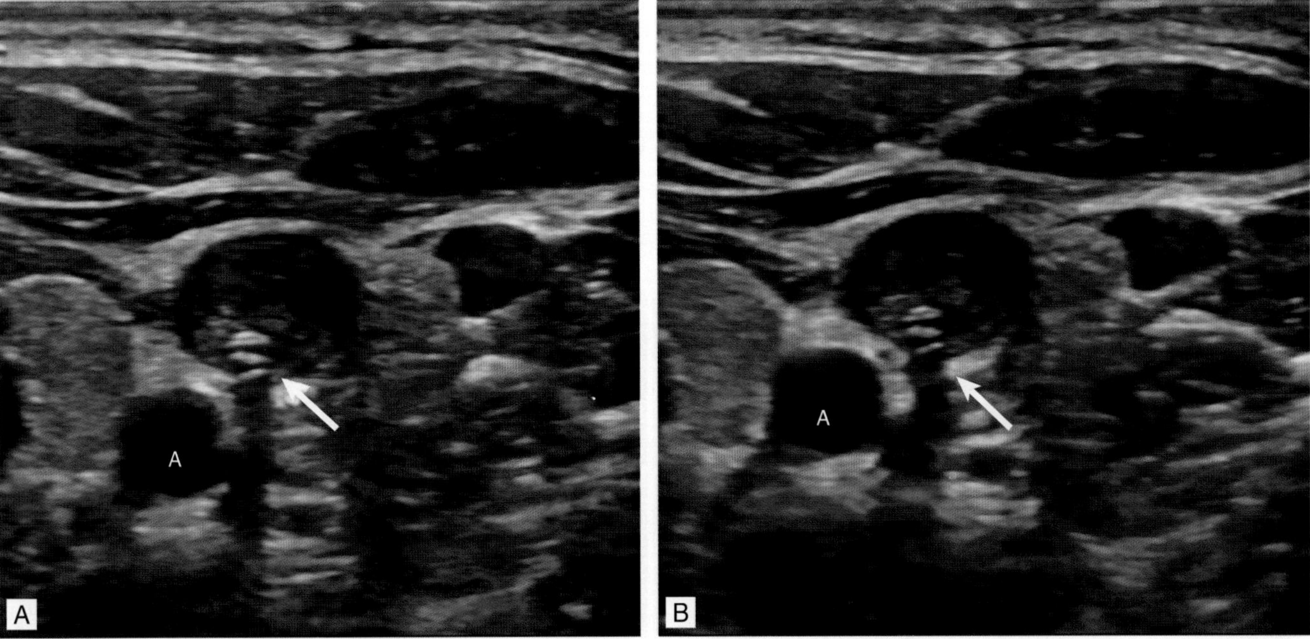

Figure 26.8 Grayscale compression ultrasound images of a patient with a catheter associated DVT involving the left internal jugular vein. (A) Left internal jugular vein and left common carotid artery ("A") with arrow showing central line (*arrow*) and surrounding echogenic material in the lumen. (B) Lack of compression.

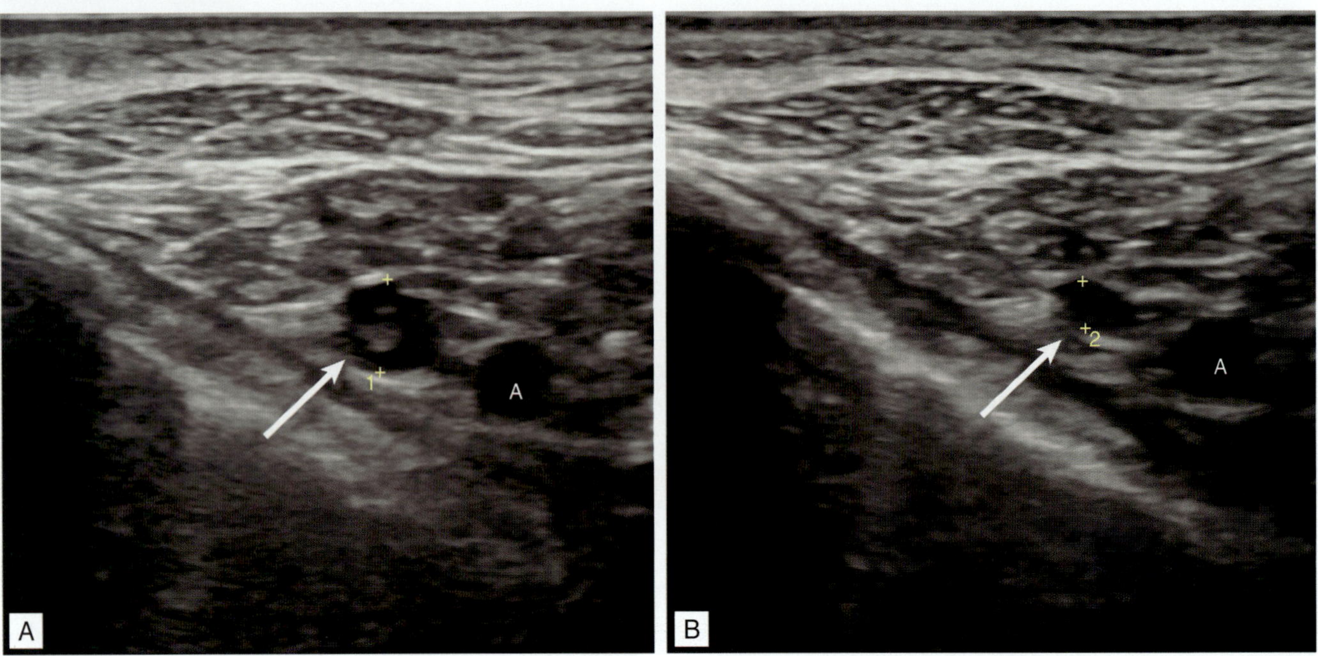

Figure 26.9 Grayscale compression ultrasound demonstrating a subacute thrombus within the left axillary vein. (A) Echogenic thrombus within the lumen (*arrow*) and nearby axillary artery (A). (B) Partially compressible.

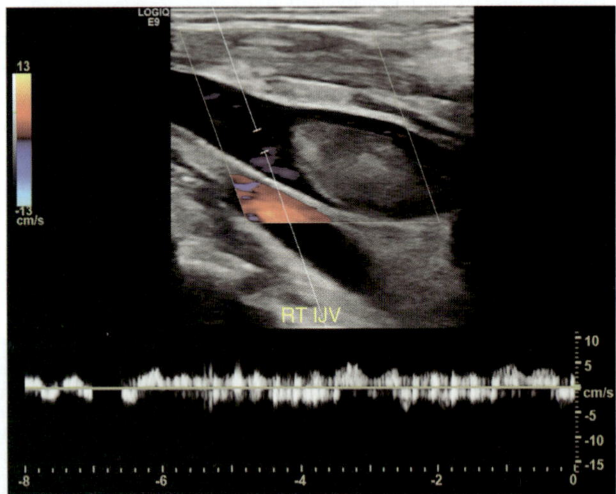

Figure 26.10 Duplex ultrasound of the right internal jugular vein with a partially occlusive thrombus. Note the blunted wave form on the spectral image at the bottom.

upper extremity peripheral venous access, injection contralateral to the suspected venous thrombosis is preferred. Since images are acquired relatively late, it is important to administer a relatively large volume of contrast material (up to 150 mL) to account for losses due to renal excretion [17]. Although it is less commonly used than USG, CT, or MR, venography remains the reference standard for evaluating venous obstruction. Venographic imaging findings in upper extremity thrombosis include a luminal filling defect or complete loss of contrast filling the lumen with an abrupt cutoff and the presence of collateral flow (Fig. 26.12).

Management

Management of upper and lower extremity venous thrombosis overlaps considerably, as much of the initial treatment recommendations were based on lower extremity disease. Treatment decisions should be made on an individual patient basis based on symptoms, disease extent, etiologies, risk of complications if untreated, and risk of hemorrhage from anticoagulation. Consensus recommendations continue to evolve as data emerge and newer anticoagulation agents are approved. The goal of

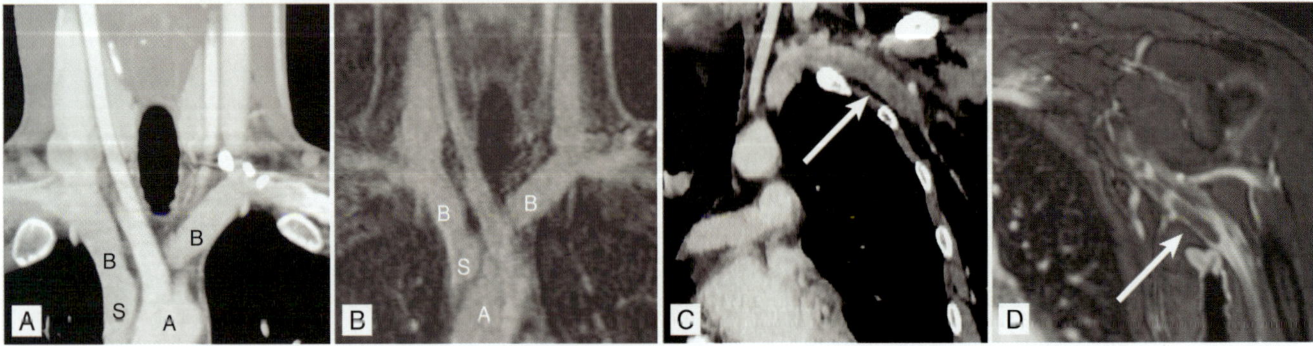

Figure 26.11 Normal appearance of contrast-enhanced CT and MR images of the central veins and in two patients with upper extremity venous thrombosis. (A) CTV image. Vessels label "A," "B," and "S" denote the aorta, brachiocephalic veins, and superior vena cava, respectively. (B) Similarly, normal contrast-enhanced MR coronal reconstructed image. (C) Contrast-enhanced CT coronal reconstructed image showing a patient with a subacute left subclavian thrombosis (*arrow*). (D) Contrast-enhanced coronal MR image showing a left axillary venous thrombosis (*arrow*).

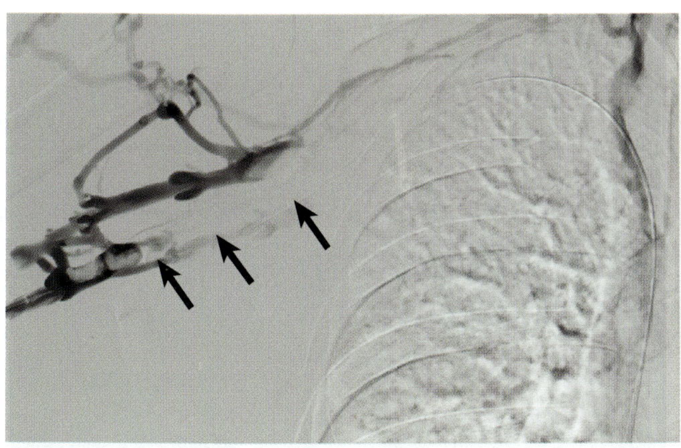

Figure 26.12 Venography in a patient with right axillary and subclavian vein thrombosis (*arrows*). Note the development of collateral flow superiorly.

treatment is to alleviate symptoms (when present), prevent progression, reduce the risk of PE, and reduce the rate of recurrence [18]. Briefly, in patients with an acute, initial proximal (axillary vein or more proximal) upper extremity DVT and no history of cancer, it is recommended that anticoagulation treatment be used for at least 3 months. In patients with a CVC associated DVT, anticoagulation may be discontinued after 3 months [18], provided the CVC is removed. In patients with an acute distal (peripheral) deep vein thrombosis (distal to axillary vein) it is reasonable to treat with surveillance or anticoagulation based on patient factors [18].

Percutaneous catheter-directed thrombolysis (CDT) and thrombectomy are minimally invasive interventional techniques reserved for patients with severe symptoms involving the proximal veins. The objective of CDT is to decrease clot burden and symptoms associated with post-thrombotic syndrome. CDT for DVT should be utilized when the benefits overweigh the risks. Table 26.2 summarizes the imaging for DVT based on chronicity across multiple imaging techniques.

Paget–Schroetter Syndrome

Thoracic outlet syndrome represents multiple disorders that occur secondary to the compression of either the brachial plexus, subclavian vein, or artery at the thoracic outlet. Paget–Schroetter syndrome (PSS) represents a form of thoracic outlet syndrome resulting from primary subclavian venous thrombosis at the costoclavicular junction. PSS is often grouped with venous compression syndromes, including May–Thurner syndrome (MTS) and Nutcracker syndrome (NS), which are discussed in later sections. The etiology of PSS is thought to be secondary to repetitive and strenuous upper extremity activity that results in subclavian vein compression at the costoclavicular triangle predisposing to thrombosis, illustrating why the condition has been referred to as *effort thrombosis*. The disorder is rare with an annual incidence of 1–2 per 100,000 and is seen most often in young, muscular men [19]. Patients often present with acute onset ipsilateral pain and swelling, frequently involving their dominant arm. Imaging evaluation is important as prompt diagnosis and treatment are necessary for good outcomes. The best first imaging study for PSS is Duplex USG, as it has an estimated sensitivity and specificity of 80–100% for diagnosis of venous thrombosis. For cases with equivocal USG findings, CT or MR venography may be considered for further imaging evaluation (Fig. 26.13). CT and MR are also helpful to identify the venous compression at the costoclavicular triangle and exclude secondary causes of venous compression, such as bone tumors or fractures of the first rib or clavicle, hypertrophy of costoclavicular ligament, or presence of cervical ribs. Dynamic imaging with the upper arm abducted and external rotated may identify the venous compression, especially in patients without a venous thrombosis. It is important to note that the subclavian vein

TABLE 26.2 Summary of Common Imaging Findings for DVT

	DURATION OF DVT		
Technique	**Acute**	**Subacute**	**Chronic**
Grayscale USG	Non- or partially compressible vein *Anechoic/hypoechoic* luminal material Venous distention	Non- or partially compressible vein *Hyperechoic* luminal material Venous distention	Non- or partially compressible vein *Hyperechoic* luminal eccentric material Smaller caliber, irregular wall
Color flow USG	Absent Doppler signal or blunted Doppler signal	Absent Doppler signal or blunted Doppler signal	Absent Doppler signal or blunted Doppler signal
Spectral Doppler	No signal or loss of flow phasicity Loss of response to augmentation or on Valsalva	No signal or loss of flow phasicity Loss of response to augmentation or on Valsalva	No signal or loss of flow phasicity Loss of response to augmentation or on Valsalva
CTV	*Hypoattenuating* filling defect Focal venous enlargement Surrounding fat stranding	*Hypoattenuating* filling defect Focal venous enlargement Surrounding fat stranding	*Hypoattenuating* filling defect Evident collateral flow Diminutive vein Fibrotic changes (e.g., web formation) Endothelial calcifications
Contrast-enhanced MR	Loss of luminal contrast enhancement Focal venous enlargement	Loss of luminal contrast enhancement Focal venous enlargement	Loss of luminal contrast enhancement Irregular wall thickening Diminutive vein Evident collateral flow
Venography	Luminal filling defect Lack of venous opacification None or limited collateral flow	Luminal filling defect Lack of venous opacification Limited collateral flow	Luminal filling defect Lack of venous opacification Evident collateral flow

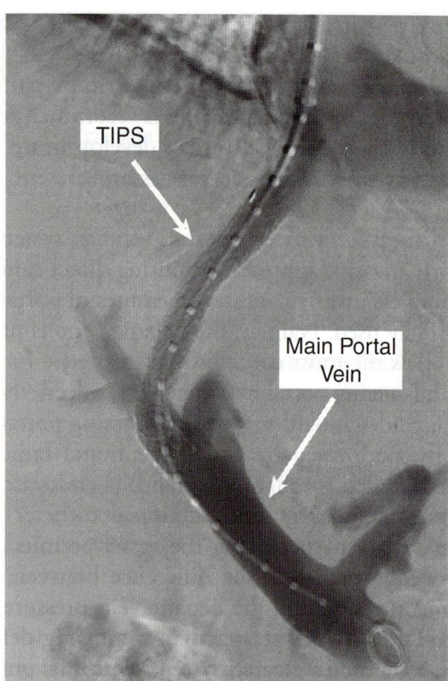

Figure 26.44 DSA image of patient following successful TIPS creation.

- Abnormally low or high peak velocities within the shunt (<90 or >190 cm/s)
- Main portal vein velocity <30 cm/s
- Reversal of left portal venous flow from hepatopetal flow (toward the liver) to hepatofugal (away from liver)
- A change in the peak systolic velocity within the shunt with either a decrease <40 cm/s or an increase >60 cm/s

Other percutaneous endovascular treatments utilized in the management of portal hypertension include direct intrahepatic portosystemic shunt, percutaneous splenic artery embolization, variceal embolization, and balloon occluded retrograde transvenous obliteration are discussed in more detail elsewhere.

Portal and Mesenteric Vein Thrombosis

Portal and mesenteric vein thrombosis are not uncommon disorders seen most commonly in patients with chronic liver disease and cirrhosis. Risk factors promoting splanchnic vein thrombosis are listed in Table 26.10.

Tumor-related PVT is most commonly seen with HCC. Patients may or may not be symptomatic, and symptoms often depend on disease extent. For acute PVT, patients may present with abdominal pain, fever, nausea, and diarrhea [77]. Left untreated, PVT may result in cavernous transformation of the portal vein, which is defined as the formation of venous collateral vessels around or within the thrombosed vein. The changes associated with cavernous transformation can increase overtime, eventually causing mass effects on adjacent structures. Mesenteric or splenic vein thrombosis demonstrates similar image features to PVT, shares similar risk factors and is similarly managed. Mesenteric vein thrombosis causing significant venous congestion can lead to mesenteric ischemia. Gallbladder varicosities are often seen in cases of extrahepatic PVT.

Duplex USG represents the best first imaging technique for evaluating PVT. USG findings consistent with PVT include [77]:

- Echogenic material within the portal vein on grayscale USG
- PV distension
- Slow or absent flow on Duplex USG

CT is very useful for evaluating for PVT, as this technique has the advantage of helping determine the underlying cause, as well as overall extent of disease (Fig. 26.45). Cavernous transformation on CT frequently manifests as numerous periportal vessels (Fig. 26.46). CT findings consistent with PVT include [77]:

- Lack of contrast enhancement within the vessel lumen
- Acute thrombus: *hyperattenuating* focus within the vessel on noncontrast-enhanced scan
- Chronic thrombus: *hypoattenuating* focus within the vessel with or without calcifications on both contrast-enhanced and noncontrast CT images
- Cavernous transformation (presence of multiple collateral veins around the porta hepatis replacing the main portal vein)
- Decreased hepatic parenchymal enhancement on portal venous CECT

Similar to CT, MR is also very useful for determining the extent of the venous thrombosis as well as the potential underlying cause. MR findings consistent with PVT include [77]:

- T1-weighted image isointensity
- Acute/subacute thrombus: T2-weighted image hyperintensity
- Cavernous transformation

Differentiating bland versus tumor PVT on imaging is important, as this often affects management. Contrast-enhanced MR with diffusion-weighted imaging is helpful in discriminating tumor versus bland thrombus in patients with HCC. In cases of HCC-related PVT, MR diffusion-weighted images demonstrate similar restricted diffusion compared to the concurrent HCC lesion(s), whereas bland PVT often demonstrates decreased restricted diffusion compared to the concurrent HCC lesion(s) [78].

For most patients, anticoagulation is the first-line treatment for patients with portal or mesenteric vein thrombosis [79]. In patients with severe symptoms refractory to anticoagulation, such as in patients with PVT with symptomatic cavernous transformation (e.g., portal biliopathy), endovascular recanalization may be beneficial. Endovascular recanalization involves catheter-directed pharmacomechanical thrombolysis/thrombectomy, venoplasty, and stenting. A TIPS is also recommended following a successful intervention to increase long-term patency.

TABLE 26.10 Risk Factors For Splanchnic Vein Thrombosis [42]

Malignancy
Oral contraceptives
Acquired or inherited thrombophilias
Congenital absence of the portal vein
Infectious/inflammatory processes (e.g., cholecystitis, pancreatitis, hepatitis, diverticulitis, or appendicitis)

Arterioportal Fistula

Abnormal vascular connections between the arterial or portal venous systems are an uncommon finding that may be sporadic or congenital. Sporadic cases may be seen in patients following hepatic interventions (e.g., biopsy or transhepatic cholecystostomy tube placement), abdominal trauma, or surgery (e.g., Whipple) and are associated with malignancy. Some are detected incidentally on imaging while others may be detected on imaging evaluation for symptomatic patients. Arterioportal fistula can lead to elevated pressures and flow within the portal system potentially leading to

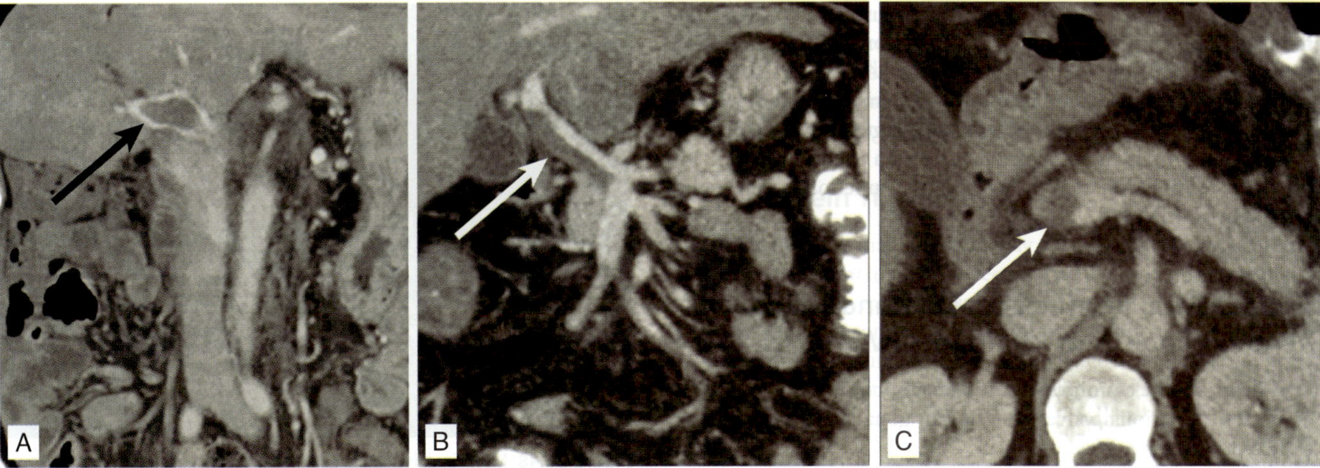

Figure 26.45 Contrast-enhanced CT images of the abdomen. (A) Coronal reconstructed image demonstrating acute portal vein thrombosis (*black arrow*). (B) Coronal reconstructed and (C) axial images demonstrating a chronic portal vein thrombosis (*white arrow*).

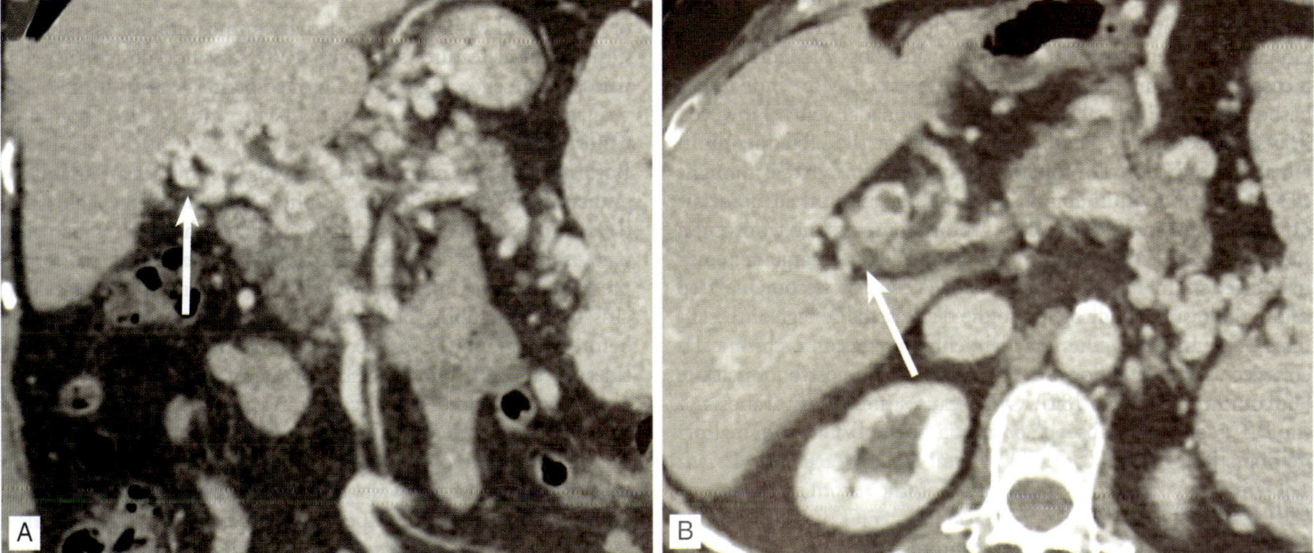

Figure 26.46 Contrast-enhanced CT (A) coronal and (B) axial reconstructed images demonstrating cavernous transformation of the portal vein with the formation of numerous small collaterals (*arrow*).

portal venous hypertension and the associated sequela. USG findings consistent with arterioportal fistulae include direct visualization of the AV connection, elevated arterialized flow velocities in the portal system and turbulent blood flow. Findings on dynamic CT or MR demonstrate early enhancement of the portal venous structures during the arterial phase. Treatment is often necessary, especially in cases with associated pseudoaneurysm formation, as spontaneous rupture may occur leading to life-threatening hemorrhage (Fig. 26.47). In many cases, endovascular treatment with embolization or covered stenting can be curative [80].

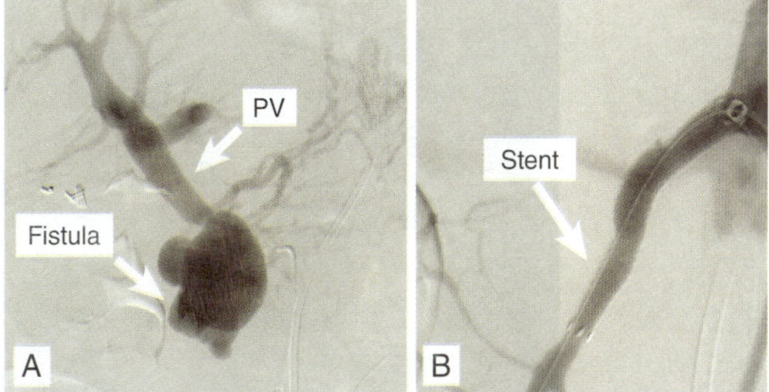

Figure 26.47 Arteriovenous fistula. (A) DSA image of a patient with a superior mesenteric artery pseudoaneurysm-to-portal vein fistula that developed over the course of a few months following a Whipple procedure for pancreatic cancer. (B) DSA image of the same patient after treatment with a superior mesenteric artery covered stent, excluding the pseudoaneurysm and fistulous connection to the portal venous system. *PV*, portal vein.

Gonadal Veins

Anatomy and Variants

Normally, there are single bilateral gonadal veins, draining each respective ovary in females and testis in males. The veins arise in the pelvis and travel cranially traveling over the ipsilateral psoas muscle. The left gonadal vein usually terminates in the mid left

Adrenal Vein Imaging and Sampling

CECT, MR, and venography are the most useful imaging techniques for evaluating the bilateral adrenal veins. Focused imaging evaluation of the adrenal veins is principally aimed at planning in preoperative adrenalectomy patients and preprocedural patients undergoing adrenal venous sampling for suspected functional adrenal adenoma(s). Preoperative knowledge of both the number and location of the adrenal vein(s) helps the surgeon perform a safe and efficient surgery. CECT appears to be the preferred technique, as it demonstrates better visualization compared to noncontrast-enhanced MR [91]. Thin slice CECT images acquired 60 seconds following injection with coronal reconstruction increase the likelihood of accurate identification [92].

Venography is reserved for cases where adrenal venous anatomy needs to be defined for accurate venous blood sampling to localize a functioning adrenal adenoma, predominately for cases of Conn syndrome (primary hyperaldosteronism) and less commonly in cases of suspected adrenal Cushing syndrome [92,93]. Patients diagnosed with hyperfunctioning adrenal adenomas are cured with surgical resection. For patients with laboratory evidence suggestive of primary hyperaldosteronism (elevated plasma aldosterone:plasma renin assay ratio), a CECT scan is routinely performed in the initial work up to look for CT evidence of one or more adrenal adenomas. Unfortunately, CT performs poorly at accurately identifying culprit hyperfunctioning adenomas. Venography with adrenal venous blood sampling is performed to determine lesion laterality and has an accuracy rate of up to 97% (Fig. 26.51) [93].

Central Thoracic Veins

Anatomy and Variants

The thoracic central venous anatomy is comprised of the bilateral subclavian, brachiocephalic, azygos, hemiazygos veins, and SVC. As each axillary vein passes under its respective clavicle, it continues medially as the subclavian vein eventually merging with the ipsilateral internal jugular vein forming the respective brachiocephalic veins. The SVC, the largest central vein in the mediastinum, is formed posterior to the manubrium within the superior mediastinum by the confluence of the brachiocephalic veins. Descending inferiorly within right aspect of the mediastinum toward the right atrium the distal SVC receives blood draining from the azygos vein. Noteworthy, congenital variant anatomy includes a double SVC (Fig. 26.52), occurring in 0.3% of individuals [12], a persistent left SVC (Fig. 26.53), occurring in less than 0.5% of patients and right upper lobe partial anomalous pulmonary venous return (PAPVR) occurring in 0.5–0.7% of the population (Fig. 26.54) [94]. A double SVC arises when

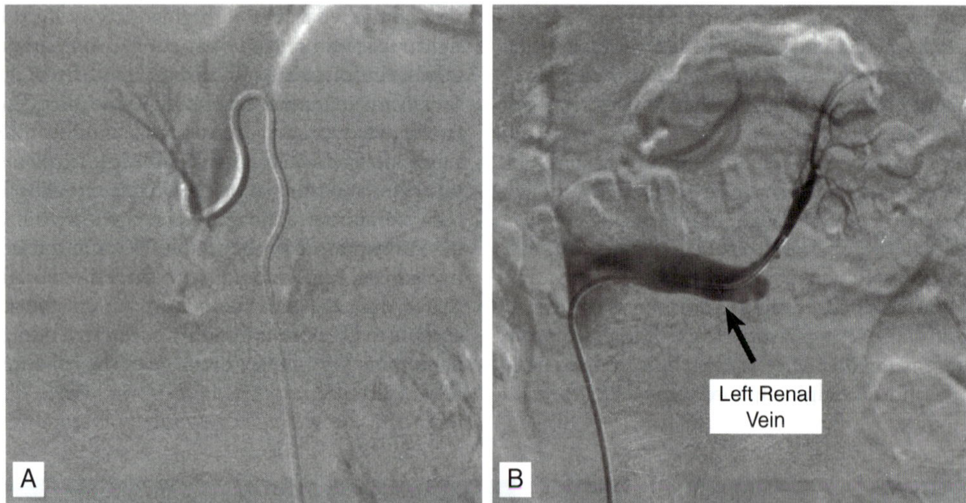

Figure 26.51 DSA images of a patient who underwent successful sampling of the (A) right adrenal and (B) left adrenal veins.

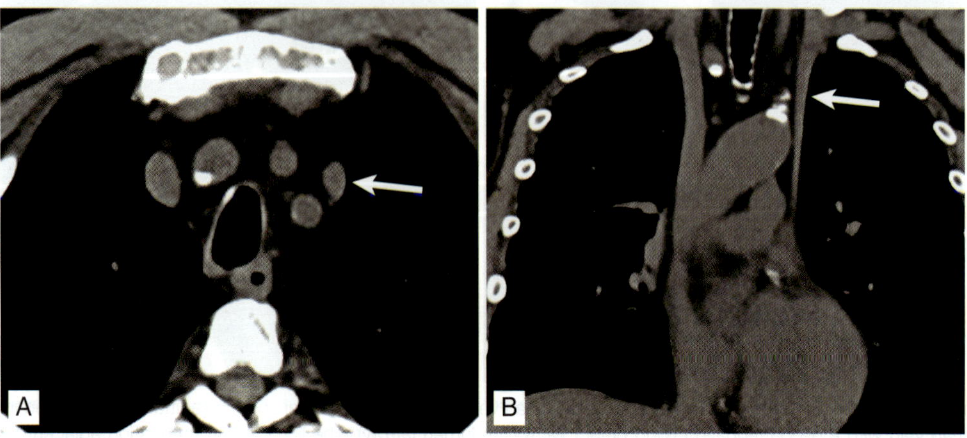

Figure 26.52 Noncontrast CT (A) axial and (B) coronal reconstructed images of a patient with a double SVC. The arrow denotes the aberrant left SVC.

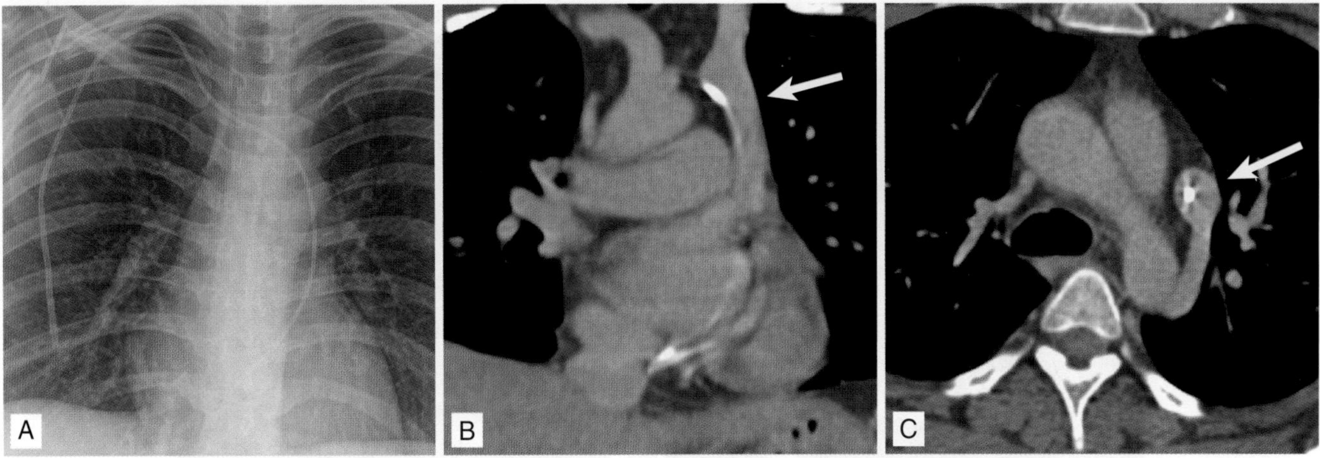

Figure 26.53 Patient with persistent left SVC. (A) Chest radiograph illustrating the course of the persistent left SVC via the course of the patient's central catheter. (B) CT coronal reconstructed and (C) axial images of a left SVC (*arrow*).

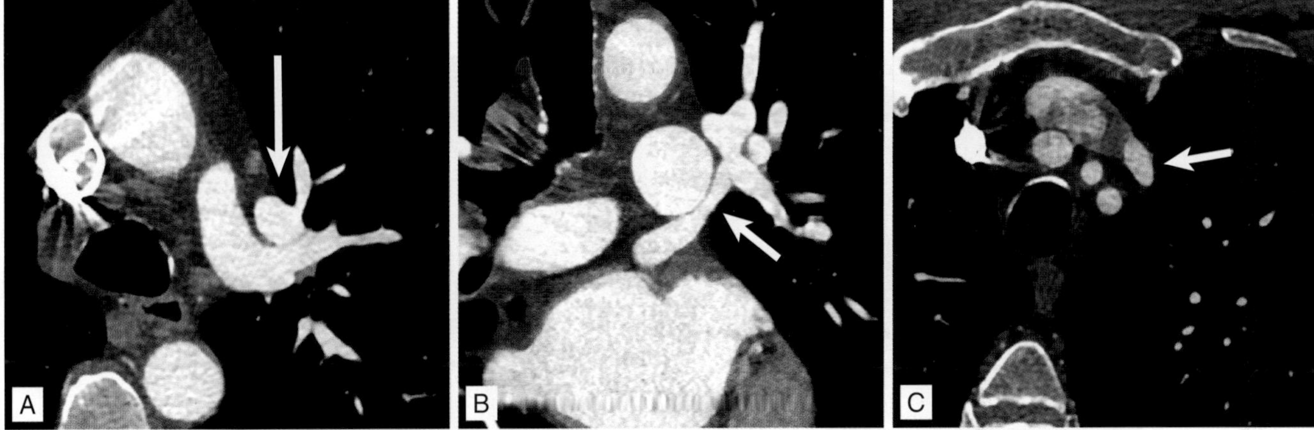

Figure 26.54 Cardiac CT (A) axial and (B) multiplanar reconstructed images demonstrating a patient with a levoatriocardinal vein (connection of the left superior upper lobe pulmonary vein, left brachiocephalic vein, and left atrium). (C) Demonstrates the connection to the left brachiocephalic vein.

the left anterior cardinal vein fails to regress, whereas a left SVC arises secondary to the abnormal regression of the right anterior cardinal vein instead of the left.

On cross-sectional imaging, a persistent left SVC is seen arising at the confluence of the left subclavian and jugular veins descending inferiorly where it drains into the right atrium via a dilated coronary sinus. It is seen lateral to the aorta and should be suspected if the coronary sinus appears dilated. This anomaly is important to recognize as the anatomy becomes important for patients requiring a left-sided CVC, pacemaker, or pulmonary artery catheter [94].

Superior Vena Cava Syndrome

SVC syndrome refers to the constellation of clinical findings seen in patients with obstruction of the SVC. In the United States, each year approximately 15,000 patients present with SVC syndrome [95]. Obstruction of the SVC is frequently classified by etiology: benign or malignant. Benign etiologies comprise approximately 35% of cases [95] with examples including infection (tuberculosis and syphilitic aortic aneurysm), fibrosing mediastinitis, prior radiation therapy and iatrogenic SVC stenosis or thrombosis secondary to CVCs, pacemakers, and defibrillators [96]. Malignant SVC syndrome arises as a result of a cancer progressively compressing the SVC with the most common cancers including small cell and nonsmall cell lung cancer, lymphoma, and metastases. The most common cancer known to cause SVC syndrome is nonsmall cell lung cancer [95]. Patients present with variable symptoms on a spectrum of severity based on the degree of venous obstruction. Symptoms frequently include swelling of the head, neck, and arms with associated cyanosis, as well as, headaches, blurry vision, cough, hoarseness, stridor, dyspnea, and dysphagia [95]. Acute SVC syndrome is a vascular emergency.

The best imaging technique for efficient evaluation of possible SVC syndrome is CECT of the chest. CT demonstrates variable loss of SVC contrast-enhancement based on the degree of venous obstruction (Figs. 26.55–26.57). In cases of complete obstruction, there will be prominent collateral vessels demonstrating contrast enhancement. CT also has the advantage of helping to define the underlying cause as benign or malignant. When performing CECT, to minimize mixing artifact from peripheral intravenous contrast material injection, image acquisition may be performed after 60–75 seconds [94].

Given lesions causing SVC syndrome are centrally located, Duplex USG is limited in evaluating SVC obstruction due to the lack of an adequate acoustic window. However, on Duplex USG of the upper extremity veins or the jugular veins, the indirect findings include a blunted or complete loss of normal waveform variability with respiration and the cardiac cycle. In patients where CECT is less desirable (such as in patients with an iodinated contrast allergy or in pediatric patients), gadolinium-enhanced

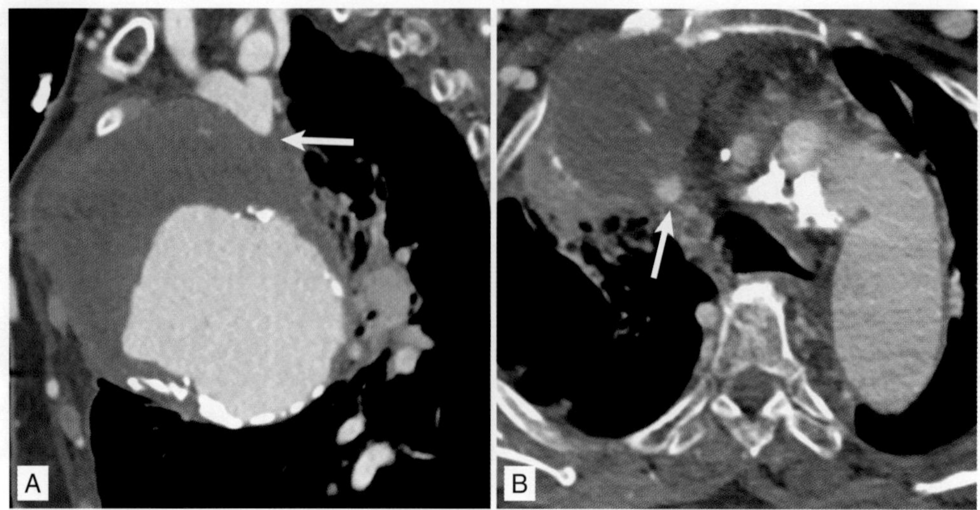

Figure 26.55 Contrast-enhanced CT showing (A) sagittal reconstructed and (B) axial images of a patient with benign SVC syndrome secondary to compression of the SVC (*arrows*) by a large partially thrombosed thoracic aortic aneurysm.

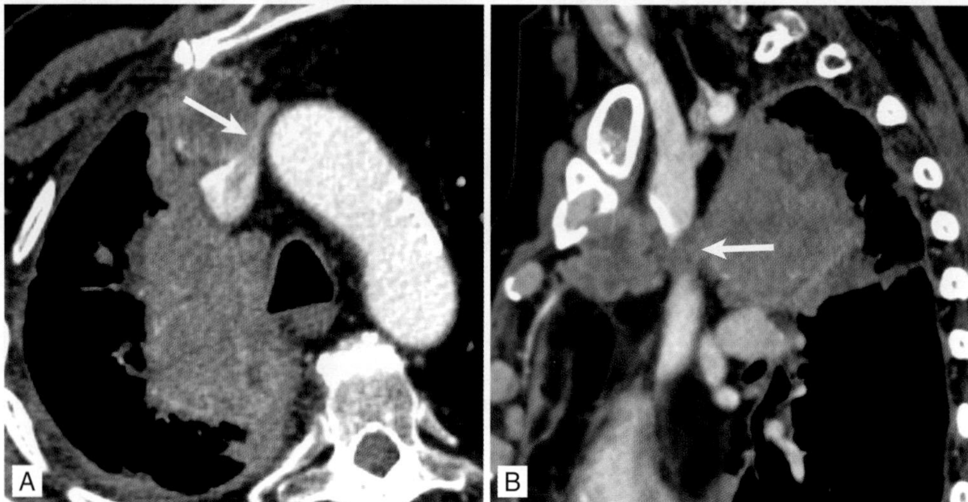

Figure 26.56 Contrast-enhanced CT showing (A) axial and (B) sagittal reconstructed images of a patient with malignant SVC syndrome secondary to compression of the SVC (*arrows*) by a large right upper lobe nonsmall cell lung cancer.

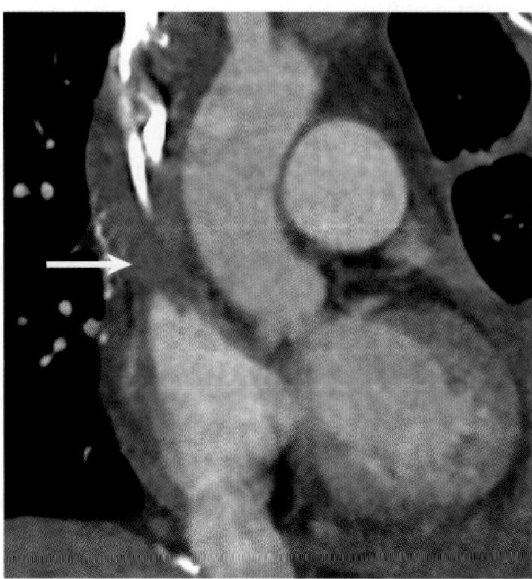

Figure 26.57 Contrast-enhanced CT coronal reconstructed imaging showing a patient with benign SVC syndrome secondary to a central line associated occlusive SVC thrombus (*arrow*).

MRV is equally sensitive and specific for evaluation of central venous obstruction. MRV will demonstrate similar findings of obstruction and development of collateral vessels. In patients with chronic renal insufficiency, noncontrast MR may be performed using SSFP sequences [94].

Venography provides the best overall imaging evaluation of the obstruction but is typically reserved for patients where endovascular treatment may be indicated, as this approach is more invasive. Depending on disease severity, venography may demonstrate a luminal filling defect within the SVC or complete SVC obstruction with development of collateral vessels. A notable collateral pathway is through the left portal vein via the internal mammary and paraumbilical veins, where focal contrast enhancement may be seen in the quadrate lobe (Fig. 26.58). Historically, this has been referred to as the *hot-quadrate sign* due to the accumulation of radiopharmaceutical at this site due to SVC obstruction.

Treatment decisions for SVC syndrome are made at the individual level largely based on the severity of disease and toward addressing the underlying cause. In cases of malignant obstruction

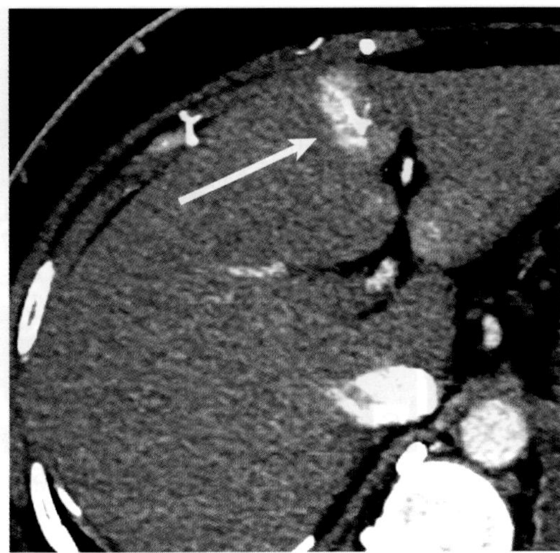

Figure 26.58 Contrast-enhanced CT showing focal contrast enhancement of the quadrate lobe (*arrow*) in a patient with benign SVC syndrome.

where disease severity is mild–moderate, chemotherapy, and radiation maybe used as first-line treatments, usually following pathologic tissue evaluation. Endovascular treatments with stenting of the SVC represent an important management strategy for cases of malignant obstruction in patients with severe symptoms, patients with persistent symptoms refractory to chemotherapy and in patients where chemoradiation are contraindicated. Endovascular angioplasty with stenting may also be used as adjuncts to anticoagulation in cases of SVC obstruction secondary to thrombosis [97].

Pulmonary Veins

Anatomy and Variants

The pulmonary veins are responsible for returning oxygen replenished blood from the lung's capillary beds to the left atrium for systemic distribution. Within the population, there is considerable anatomic variation of the pulmonary veins. In most individuals, blood returns to the left atrium via four distinct openings, or ostia, within the left atrium. Common variant anatomy consists of a single left pulmonary vein, separate right middle lobe vein and a separate right top pulmonary vein draining the apical right upper lobe. Supernumerary pulmonary veins are usually seen on the right with the most common variant being a right middle lobe vein. In up to 20% of individuals, drainage of the left lung into the left atrium arises from a common ostium [98].

Anomalous anatomy primarily consists of PAPVR and total anomalous pulmonary venous return. Both scenarios result in pulmonary venous drainage in the systemic system resulting in a left-to-right shunting. In PAPVR seen on the left, usually one or more pulmonary veins drains into the left brachiocephalic vein through a cardinal vein. When PAPVR is detected it is important to carefully define the aberrant venous course, as in some cases a perceived PAPVR may actually represent a levoatriocardinal vein, which is another anomalous pulmonary vein connection to both a systemic vein and the left atrium (Fig. 26.54). A levoatriocardinal vein represents a possible route for a paradoxical embolus to travel from the venous system to the arterial system. The *scimitar sign,* a curvilinear right lower lung zone opacity on frontal chest radiograph, represents another form of PAPVR where there is drainage of the right lower lobe pulmonary veins into the IVC. The scimitar sign is often seen in patients with scimitar syndrome [98] (Fig. 26.59).

Pulmonary Vein Imaging

Both CT and MR are useful for evaluating the pulmonary venous anatomy (Fig. 26.60). Imaging evaluation of the pulmonary veins is important in cancer imaging, congenital heart disease, perioperatively for cardiac and thoracic surgery, and preprocedurally for pulmonary vein ablation planning (commonly referred to as pulmonary vein isolation) for management of selected patients with atrial fibrillation who are refractory to medical management. For pulmonary vein isolation planning, several important components should be present in the radiology report, including [98]:

- Number, arrangement, and size of pulmonary veins
- Ostial size and arrangement (independent or shared)
- Size of fossa ovalis
- Thickness and height of the ridge between the left superior pulmonary vein and the left atrial appendage
- Relationship of left atrium and esophagus

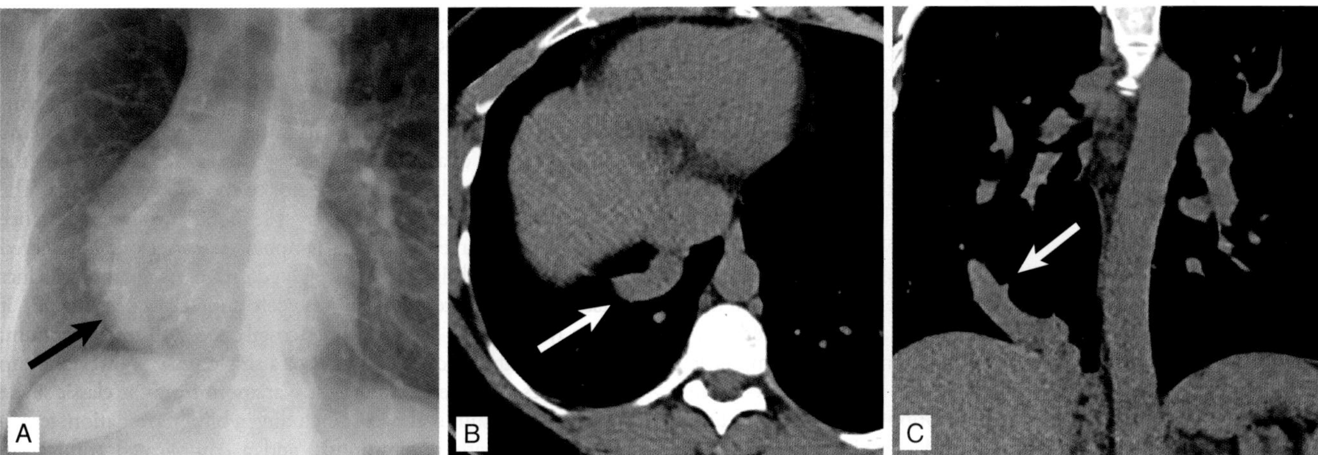

Figure 26.59 Aberrant pulmonary venous drainage. (A) Chest radiograph demonstrating the scimitar sign (*black arrow*). (B) Noncontrast-enhanced CT coronal reconstructed and (C) axial images showing the right lobe pulmonary venous drainage into the IVC.

4. Normal chest radiograph: Normal chest radiograph acts as a valuable baseline. Comparison with a previously normal film may detect subtle new changes or to detect postoperative complications, to enable early diagnosis and treatment [11].

Abdominal Radiographs

There is inherent contrast provided by soft tissues, fat, and intraluminal gas within the abdomen, and abdominal radiographs make use of this subject contrast caused by the differential attenuation of the x-ray beam in the patient. Abdominal radiographs taken in the radiology department use regular equipment with low kilovoltage exposures ranging between 60 and 75 kV (adjusted depending on the size of the patient), and short exposure times to avoid unsharpness [12,13]. The image quality in extremely ill or hospitalized patients might be slightly degraded, given their inability to adequately hold breath [14]. This degradation is compounded by the use of portable x-rays units with fixed milliampere settings, requiring higher peak voltage, which in turn causes reduced tissue contrast.

The anteroposterior view of the abdomen with the patient supine is obtained for maximum detail of the anatomy and pathology. It allows the distribution of gas showing the caliber of bowel, displacement of bowel by soft-tissue masses, and allows the visualization of obliteration of fat lines [15].

The view of abdomen with the patient standing erect is obtained to demonstrate

(i) free air under the diaphragm,
(ii) fluid levels,
(iii) more detailed double-contrast view of the intestinal wall,
(iv) possible separation of the bowel and thickness of bowel wall when one loop is layered upon the other,
(v) change in position of the bowel loops or a particular region of interest in changing from supine to erect.

If gas shadows are demonstrated which are suspected as lying outside the bowel, then horizontal-ray films are often particularly helpful by demonstrating that air–fluid levels lie within a confined space and are thus likely to represent an abscess cavity.

In patients who are unable to sit or stand for an erect film, left lateral decubitus abdominal radiograph is the projection of choice to show small pneumoperitoneum. Additionally, in this position, free air originating from a perforated duodenal or antral ulcer, or air from the lesser sac after posterior gastric ulcer perforation, enters the main abdominal cavity. With left lateral decubitus abdominal radiograph, there is better visualization of focal duodenal ileus, which is one of the commonest signs of acute pancreatitis. In some instances oblique views of the abdomen are obtained, the patient lying 30 degrees on either side and are most often performed for localizing foreign bodies or lines within the abdomen [13]. These oblique views have now become rare and obsolete.

There are numerous causes of small-bowel fluid levels and the number, distribution, and length will not usually help to distinguish between the two commonest causes, obstruction and paralytic ileus, or any of the other causes (Box 27.2). Although there is a very high interobserver variability in the interpretations of gas patterns, short air–fluid levels may be seen in the stomach, duodenal cap, and in the small bowel centrally. *Three or more small-bowel fluid levels longer than 2.5 cm are abnormal, and indicate dilated small bowel, usually with stasis.*

BOX 27.2 Causes of Abnormal Small-Bowel Fluid Levels

Small-bowel obstruction
Large-bowel obstruction
Paralytic ileus
Gastroenteritis
Mesenteric thrombosis
Diverticulosis
Uremia
Hypokalemia
Osmotic enemas
Congestive cardiac failure

Fluoroscopy

There is significant decline in the use of contrast agents and fluoroscopy techniques in the imaging of the hollow viscera given the ease of use and availability of CT scanners, MR, and endoscopy [16]. There are many causes which resulted in the progressive decline of fluoroscopy studies. However, these are still performed due to the following advantages.

- Study gastrointestinal (GI) motility and function
- Important role in evaluating postoperative patients and postoperative complications like leaks
- Esophagogram and double-contrast upper GI examinations are safe and cost effective method for evaluation of the esophagus and stomach

Contrast Agents and Techniques

Single- and double-contrast examinations continue to have a role in modern radiology. There are three techniques of imaging the GI tract.

- Mucosal relief views: Small volume of barium in collapsed or partially collapsed bowel lumen to assess the mucosa
- Single-contrast views: Large volume of low-density barium filling the bowel lumen to evaluate strictures and growths within the lumen
- Double-contrast views: Large amount of air and small volume of high-density barium coating the mucosa of the bowel lumen, to assess malignancy/ulcerations and inflammatory bowel disease

Normal Anatomy on Abdominal Radiographs

As mentioned previously, the abdominal soft tissues, and the presence of gas, fluid, or food residue within the bowel provide a natural contrast to delineate soft-tissue planes and visceral surfaces on abdominal radiographs [9]. The surfaces best visualized are the ones smoothly marginated and tangential to the x-ray beam. Localization of pathologic processes requires familiarity with the normal anatomy (Fig. 27.1). The duodenal cap is often gas-filled and frequently contains a fluid level on erect films.

Stomach

The stomach usually contains large amounts of air and fluid, seen in the left upper quadrant with its characteristic rugal folds. In the supine position, the stomach gas rises to the anterior antrum and fluid settles in the fundus. The stomach gas serves as an important landmark for identifying space-occupying lesions in the spleen laterally, liver medially, and pancreas and lesser sac posteriorly.

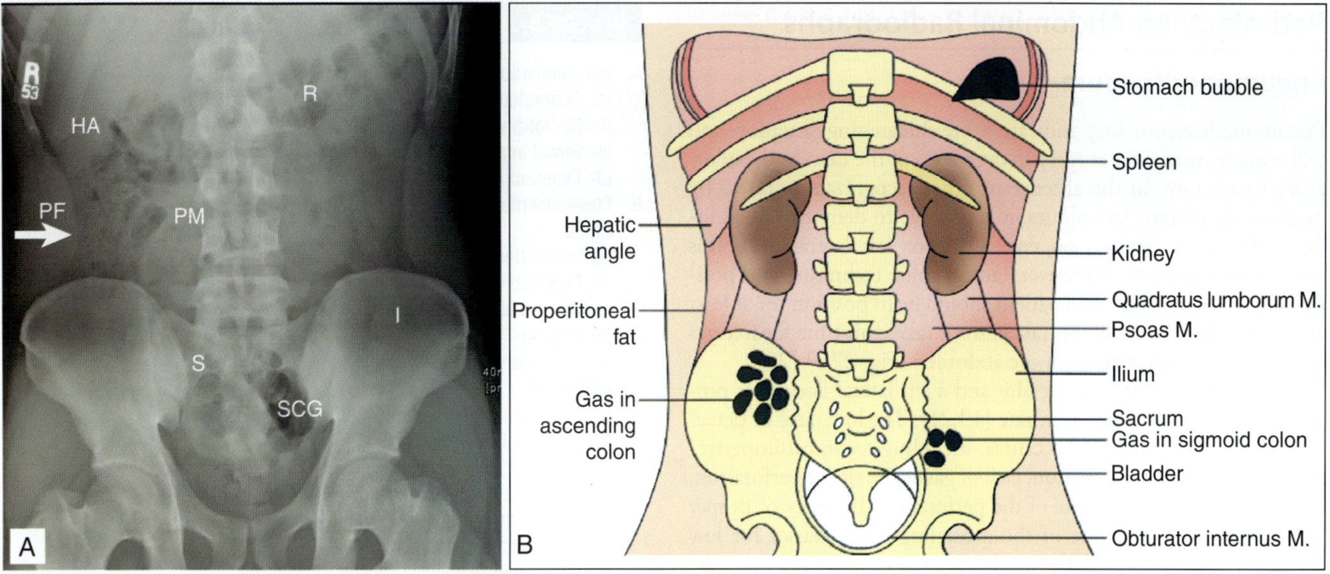

Figure 27.1 (A) Normal supine abdominal radiograph. (B) Pictorial illustration of the normal anatomy of the abdomen as seen on radiographs. *HA*, hepatic angle; *I*, Ilium; *PF*, properitoneal fat; *PM*, psoas muscle; *R*, renal shadow; *S*, sacrum; *SCG*, sigmoid colonic gas.

Small Bowel

The radiographic appearance of the small bowel is extremely variable. The small bowel along with the mesentery occupies the central portion of the abdomen. The small bowel is smaller in caliber, with typical mucosal folds called *valvulae conniventes*; these folds are usually thin and extend across the entire lumen of the bowel. *Small-bowel caliber exceeding 3.0 cm is abnormal and indicates dilatation*. Scattered gas and fluid within normally dilated bowel is seen in aerophagia and in minimally dilated bowel seen in pathological conditions such as gastroenteritis, inflammatory or infectious bowel disease, and pancreatitis (Fig. 27.2). Adynamic ileus or prolonged bowel transit caused by mechanical obstruction results in multiple air–fluid levels in a dilated bowel [17].

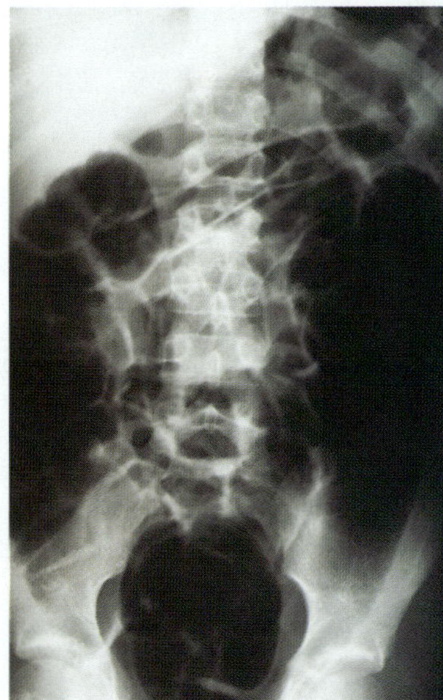

Figure 27.2 Air swallowing. There is gaseous distension of both small and large bowel, but this extends down to the rectum. A 7-year-old girl admitted to hospital with abdominal pain and distension after a single episode of vomiting. At the time of admission, she was distressed and crying. Shortly after admission her bowels were opened normally, and the abdominal distension and pain disappeared.

Large Bowel

The adult colon consists of gas and fecal material and frames the abdomen. The large bowel consists of haustrations which are more widely spaced and usually do not cross the entire lumen. *The colon caliber varies from 3 to 8 cm, with the largest diameter seen in the cecum. Persistent cecal diameter of 9–10 cm or more may indicate a risk of impending perforation from mechanical obstruction or ileus.* In inflammatory bowel disease, however, a transverse colonic diameter exceeding 5.5 cm has been suggested as the upper limit of normal, and above this megacolon should be diagnosed [18]. Colonic fluid levels are a normal finding, and some of which are several centimeters long may be seen. Eighteen percent of normal people also have a cecal fluid level. In severe pain, or when respiration is labored, as in pneumonia or asthma, increased swallowing of air often results in a dramatic plain abdominal radiograph. The gas-filled, slightly dilated loops of bowel so produced contain relatively little fluid; the term "*meteorism*" is applied to this appearance. It is sometimes difficult to distinguish meteorism produced, for example, by renal colic, from intestinal obstruction. A clinical history and examination frequently enable the radiological findings to be correctly interpreted.

Muscles, Retroperitoneum, and Pelvis

The posterior extraperitoneal fat pad, which completely surrounds the kidneys, psoas muscles, and the posterior borders of the liver and spleen, extends anteriorly and laterally to surround the parietal peritoneum and is also intimately related to intraperitoneal organs. The fat lines produced are responsible for the visualization of most of these intra-abdominal organs. These fat lines can be displaced if the organs are enlarged and may be blurred or effaced by inflammation or fluid [12]. However, the visualization of these structures by fat lines is not universal. In 19% of normal people the right psoas outline is blurred, and the lower border of the spleen can only be visualized in 58%. This is particularly important in children, where the psoas outlines are lost in 52% and the properitoneal fat line is lost in 18% of normals [9]. Delineation of the various muscles and visceral structures in the pelvis is also variable and depends on a variety of factors, including the amount of extraperitoneal pelvic fat, bowel contents, degree of bladder distention, position, and body habitus of patient.

Pathology on Abdominal Radiographs

Pneumoperitoneum

Pneumoperitoneum may indicate a life-threatening situation and will require emergency surgery in over 90% of the cases and exploratory laparotomy in the absence of other recognizable causes. By careful radiographic techniques, it is possible to demonstrate as little as 1 mL of free gas on erect chest or left lateral decubitus abdominal films [19]. However, radiographic technique and positioning are important and a patient should be in position for at least 10 minutes before the film is taken, for it takes this time for free gas to rise to the highest point in the abdomen (Fig. 27.3) [20].

A combination of an erect film and a left lateral decubitus projection increases the detection rate [19,21]. The low rates of detection are due to a number of causes, including technical imperfections, sealing of the perforation, lack of gas at the site of perforation, or adhesions around the site of the perforation. Inability of proper patient positioning is one of the most important causes for low detection rates—particularly in those patients after trauma, the elderly or the critically ill, and those who are unconscious. About 56% of patients with pneumoperitoneum may have free gas detectable on a supine radiograph [19]. The causes of pneumoperitoneum are varied (Box 27.3) and can be benign, spontaneous, iatrogenic/surgical, secondary to barotrauma or trauma, hollow visceral rupture, pneumatosis, or due to gynecological or pelvic pathology. It is essential to understand and recognize the signs and patterns of pneumoperitoneum on both supine and erect radiographs. Some radiographic signs commonly seen are as follows [22,23]:

- Collection of gas in the right upper quadrant adjacent to the liver, mainly in the subhepatic space and the hepatorenal fossa (Morison's pouch), visible as an oval or linear collection of gas—"Morison pouch" sign or "doge cap" sign (Fig. 27.4)
- The visualization of the outer as well as the inner wall of a loop of bowel—"Rigler's" sign (Fig. 27.5). This sign may be misleading if gas-distended loops of bowel are in contact, with apparent visualization of outer and inner walls, when in fact the inner walls of two loops of bowel are seen
- Small triangular collections of gas between loops of bowel on supine radiographs—"telltale triangle" sign

BOX 27.3 Causes of Pneumoperitoneum

A. Pneumoperitoneum with peritonitis
   (a) Perforated hollow viscera—traumatic and nontraumatic
   (b) Necrotizing enterocolitis
   (c) Bowel infarctions, infections, and inflammations
   (d) Penetrating abdominal injuries

B. Pneumoperitoneum without peritonitis

Chest
(a) Intermittent positive pressure ventilation
(b) Penetrating air from pneumomediastinum and pneumothorax
(c) Chronic obstructive airway disease
(d) Asthma
(e) Pulmonary peritoneal fistula

Abdomen
(a) Postoperative/laparotomy/laproscopy, endoscopy
(b) Peritoneal dialysis
(c) Perforated jejunal diverticulosis
(d) Sealed perforations of hollow viscus
(e) Pneumatosis cystoides coli/intestinalis
(f) Iatrogenic—postparacentesis

Female pelvis
(a) Iatrogenic or postinstrumentation such as hysterosalpingography
(b) Postpartum pelvic examination or exercises
(c) Vaginal douching

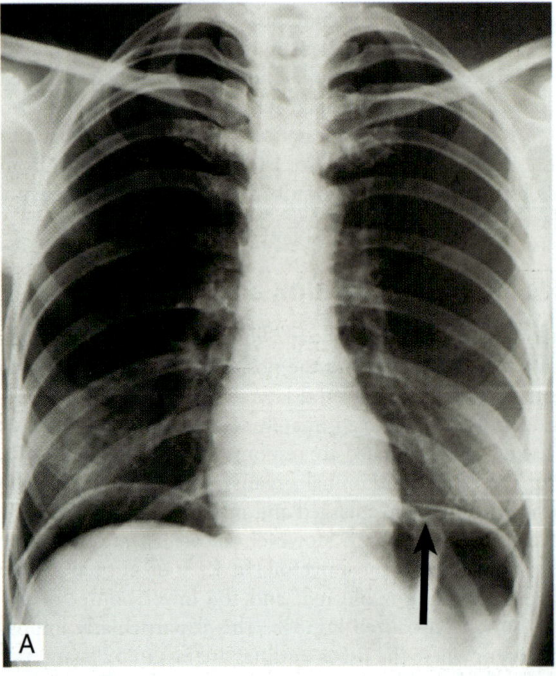

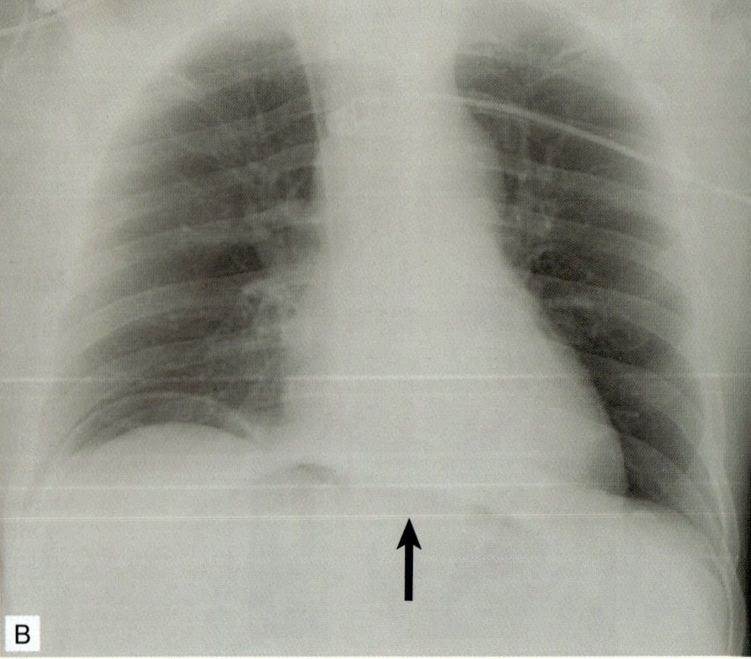

Figure 27.3 Pneumoperitoneum. (A) Erect chest film. Free intra-abdominal gas is clearly demonstrated under the right hemidiaphragm. Under the left hemidiaphragm a small triangular collection of free gas can be identified between loops of gas-filled bowel (*arrow*). (B) Portable supine chest film of an ICU patient. Free intra-abdominal gas is clearly demonstrated under the diaphragm as the "continuous diaphragm sign" (*arrow*). Large amounts of gas may accumulate underneath the central tendon of the diaphragm in the midline—the "cupola" sign.

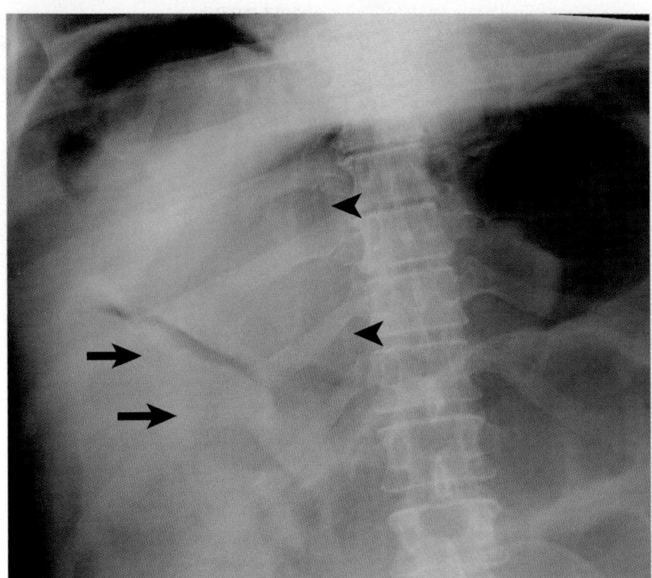

Figure 27.4 Pneumoperitoneum. Abdomen, supine. A triangular collection of free gas is demonstrated in the subhepatic region (*arrows*). The falciform ligament is also outlined (*arrowheads*).

- Reflections of the peritoneum normally present on the inner surface of the anterior abdominal wall are not usually identified, but may be visualized by large amounts of free gas when it lies on either side. Thus, the falciform ligament (Fig. 27.4), medial and lateral umbilical ligaments, and the urachus can occasionally be identified when relatively large amounts of gas are present
- Relatively large amounts of gas may accumulate underneath the central tendon of the diaphragm in the midline—the "cupola" sign or in the center of the abdomen over a fluid collection—the "football" sign
- Free gas in the fissure for the ligamentum teres

CT is the most sensitive and most accurate diagnostic technique for the detection of peritoneal free gas, with even tiny bubbles of gas being visible. CT also aids in identifying the cause of perforation without delay. The radiologist should review the images on wide window settings to appreciate small volumes of gas, as the gas adjacent to neighboring fat and bowel loops is otherwise easy to miss. Free gas tends to collect over the liver, anteriorly in the mid abdomen, and in the peritoneal recesses (Fig. 27.6). Some studies have shown the pararectal and mid-rectal recesses (Fig. 27.7) as preferential spaces for collections of free air among other more commonly known areas such as the midline/parahepatic region, pelvis, and mesenteric spaces.

Pneumoperitoneum Without Peritonitis

Occasionally, asymptomatic patients or those with very minimal signs and symptoms are found to have pneumoperitoneum. Many of these patients will subsequently be found to have a perforated ulcer which has sealed itself, or to have not yet developed the signs of peritonitis. Numerous other conditions that may produce a spontaneous pneumoperitoneum without peritonitis have been described (Box 27.3).

Postoperative Pneumoperitoneum

About 60% of all postlaparotomy patients will have evidence of pneumoperitoneum. Although, in most patients, the air will have been absorbed within a few days, a delay of up to 24 days before all the air has disappeared has been reported. Any increase in the volume of gas postoperatively indicates an anastomotic leak or further perforation [11].

Pseudopneumoperitoneum

A number of conditions have been described which simulate free air in the peritoneal cavity on the plain film (pseudopneumoperitoneum). One of the commonest of these conditions is distended bowel, usually hepatic flexure of the colon, interposed between the liver and the diaphragm—the Chilaiditi syndrome [24]. Subdiaphragmatic fat, an extension from the posterior pararenal fat, is a common normal finding and frequently can be identified as a lucent crescent under the diaphragm; this may simulate a pneumoperitoneum. Its constant position in decubitus views will enable the correct diagnosis to

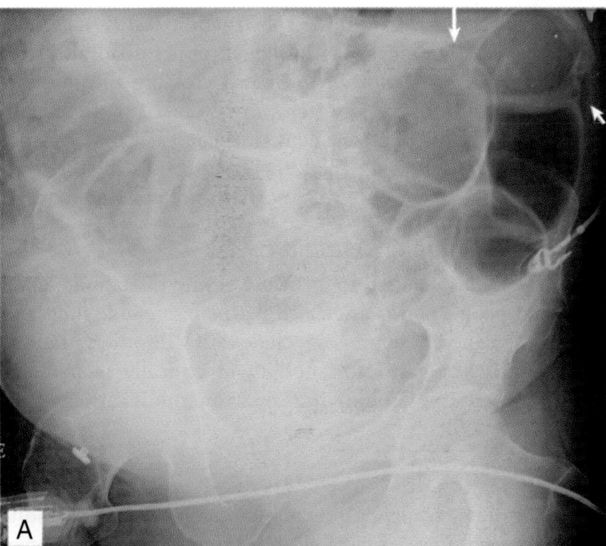

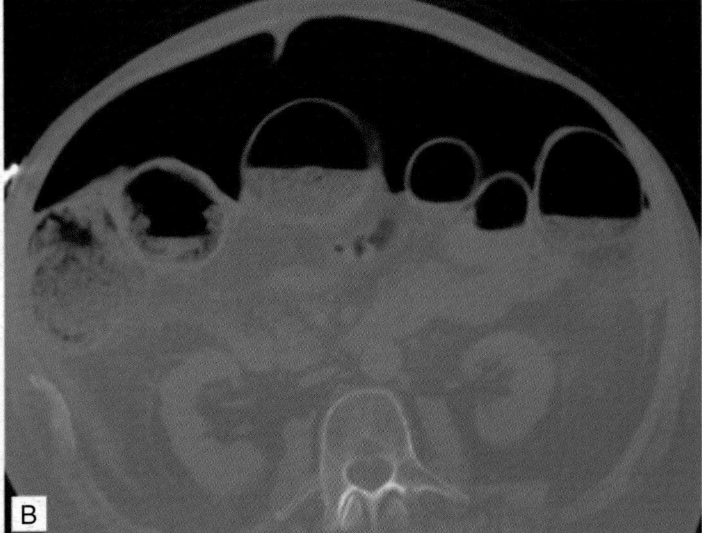

Figure 27.5 (A) Pneumoperitoneum on the abdominal supine film. The visualization of both sides of the bowel wall "Rigler's sign" (*white arrow*). Both the inside and outside wall of multiple loops of small bowel can be clearly identified. (B) Pneumoperitoneum on CT abdomen showing how the Rigler's sign is depicted on the radiograph.

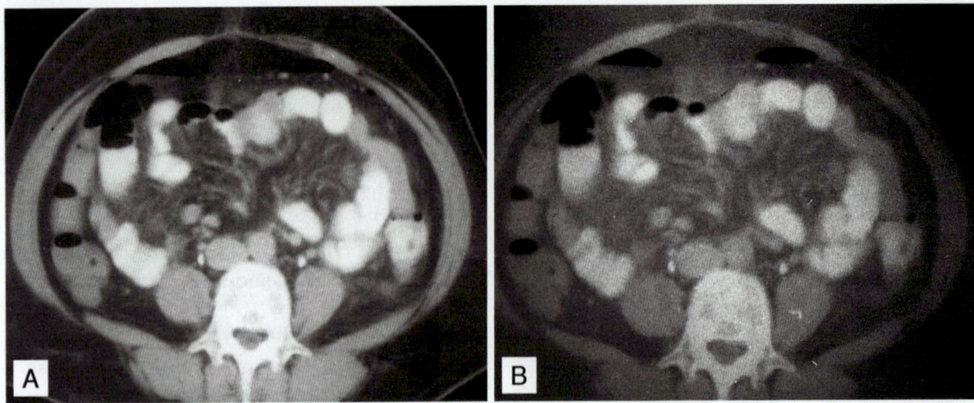

Figure 27.6 Free intraperitoneal gas. (A) On abdominal windows the free gas is not well seen anteriorly. (B) On wide window settings, the free gas is much more obvious.

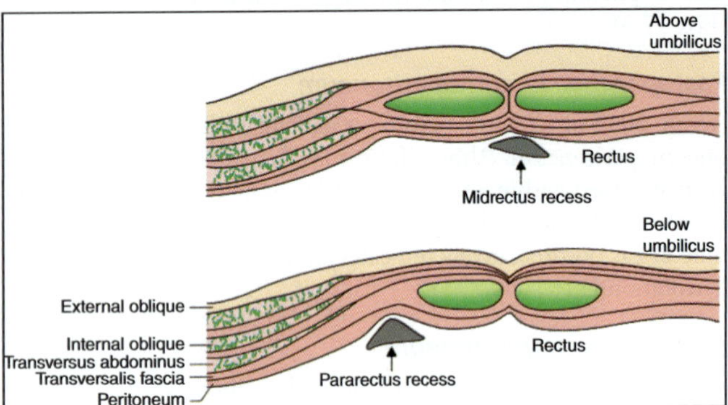

Figure 27.7 Pictorial illustrations of the mid-rectus and pararectus recesses. Preferential spaces for collections of free air within the peritoneum.

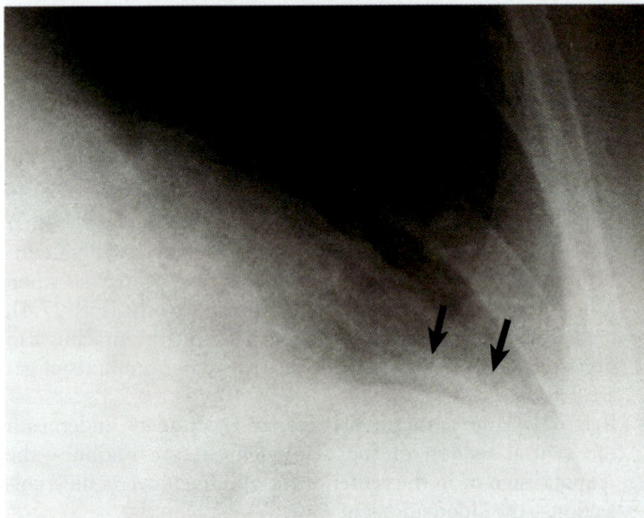

Figure 27.8 Pseudopneumoperitoneum. A band of curvilinear pulmonary collapse (*arrows*) with a crescent of normal lung beneath it simulates a pneumoperitoneum almost exactly.

be made. Sometimes curvilinear pulmonary collapse parallel to and just above the diaphragm may simulate a pneumoperitoneum (Fig. 27.8). An uneven diaphragm, omental fat between the liver and the diaphragm, subpulmonary pneumothorax may also simulate free gas on occasions [1].

Intestinal Obstruction

Conventional abdominal radiographs remain the first line of imaging for those patients presenting to the ED with clinical features of intestinal obstruction. Determination of the site of obstruction on abdominal radiograph requires adequate knowledge about normal anatomy, demonstration of dilated loops of bowel proximally and nondilated/collapsed bowel loops distally to the presumed point of obstruction, and familiarity of the distinguishing features of small and large bowel depending mainly on their size, mucosal appearance, and distribution. Dilatation of bowel occurs in mechanical intestinal obstruction, pseudo-obstruction, paralytic ileus, air swallowing, and several other conditions [25,26].

Gastric Dilatation

The "stomach bubble" on an upright abdominal radiograph is the most important anatomical radiographic landmark is formed by the gastric fundus—the part of the stomach above a line drawn tangential to the gastro-esophageal junction. It is the most superior portion of the stomach when the patient is upright, and the most dependent portion in supine position. The pylorus is the narrowest part of the stomach and the commonest portion of the stomach involved in gastric outlet obstruction (GOO) [27]. A "normal" stomach bubble is seen in the left upper quadrant, with the distal end, if filled with air, seen just crossing the midline. Abnormal dilatation of the stomach can be caused by four main groups of conditions: paralytic ileus, mechanical GOO, gastric volvulus, and air swallowing [28,29]. Other causes include postintubation, secondary to intestinal obstruction, and some drugs.

Paralytic Ileus Group of Conditions

These are frequently referred to as "acute gastric dilatation," often occurs in old people and is associated with considerable fluid and electrolyte imbalance; other causes include eating disorders, trauma, diabetes mellitus, or gastric dysmotility in critically ill patients. Delay in treatment can result in necrosis, as a result it carries a high mortality (Fig. 27.9).

Mechanical GOO

This is usually caused by peptic ulceration or carcinoma of the pyloric antrum, often leads to a massive fluid-filled stomach which occupies most of the upper abdomen and is demonstrable as a large soft-tissue mass with little or no bowel gas beyond. Fortunately, a little gas is usually present within the stomach and this can be identified on horizontal-ray films, which allow the organ to be identified [27].

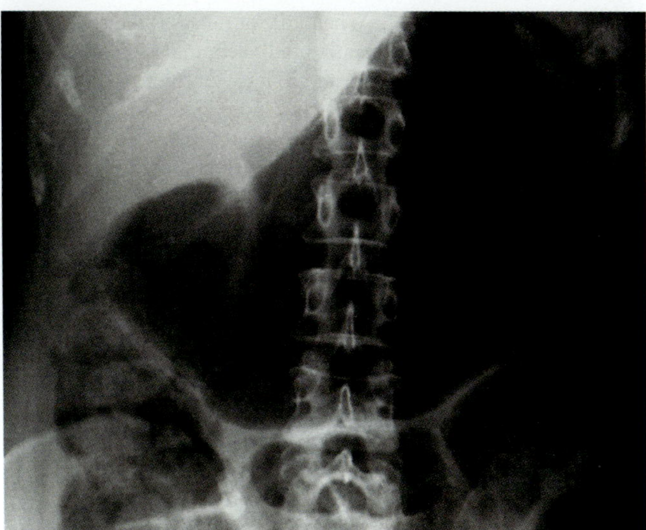

Figure 27.9 Acute gastric dilatation. Abdomen, supine. A 38-year-old woman admitted in diabetic precoma.

Gastric Volvulus

Stomach is an uncommon site for volvulus, but when it does occur the patients present to the ED with acute epigastric pain, nausea, and vomiting. It can be identified by a useful clinical triad which consists of *sudden epigastric pain, intractable retching, and inability to pass a nasogastric tube into the stomach, named the Borchardt triad.* It is of two subtypes—organoaxial and mesenteroaxial (Fig. 27.10) [29,30]. The fluid- and air-filled stomach is identified as a spherical viscus, displaced upward and to the left, and is associated with elevation of the hemidiaphragm. It is usual for the small bowel to be collapsed and it is uncommon to see any gas shadows beyond the stomach. If contrast medium is given in a case of suspected gastric volvulus, there may be complete obstruction at the lower end of the esophagus, or if contrast medium does enter the stomach it may not pass beyond the obstructed pylorus.

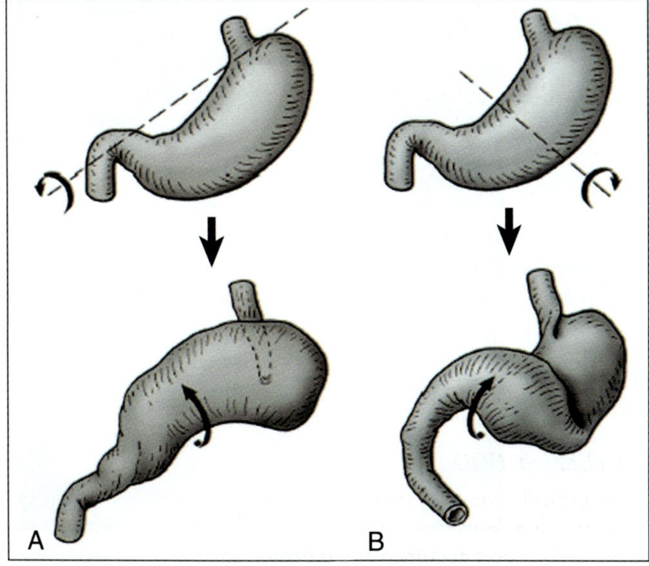

Figure 27.10 Pictorial illustrations of stomach volvulus. It is of two types: organoaxial (A) where the stomach rotates along its long axis and mesenteroaxial (B) where the stomach rotates along its short axis.

Miscellaneous

Frequently after resuscitation and intubation large amounts of gas enter the stomach and may lead to massive dilatation. This may sometimes be seen just after air swallowing, for example, in hysteria or in near-drowning.

It is very important to differentiate a distended stomach from a cecal volvulus, which may also be positioned beneath an elevated left hemidiaphragm. However, with cecal volvulus, one or two haustra can frequently be identified and the inferior part of the cecum usually points caudally, in contrast to the pyloric antrum which points cranially.

Distinction Between Small- and Large-Bowel Dilatation

Conventional abdominal radiography is the preferred initial radiologic examination for patient with obstruction and it is important to try to determine whether it is small- or large-bowel dilatation, or both. Useful differentiating features depend on the size, distribution, and marking of the loops and are summarized in Table 27.1 [31].

The valvulae conniventes usually form thin complete lines across the dilated small bowel and are prominent in the jejunum, but become less marked and widely spaced in the ileum. If the small-bowel blood supply becomes compromised and the bowel becomes edematous or gangrenous, the valvulae conniventes may become greatly thickened and may then be extremely difficult to distinguish from colonic haustra [31–33].

Haustra usually form thick, incomplete bands across the colonic gas shadow, interspaced with plicae semilunaris; however, rarely they may form complete transverse bands. Haustra may be completely absent from the descending and sigmoid colon, although they can usually still be identified in other parts of the colon even when it is massively distended [9].

The causes and management of small-bowel obstruction (SBO) are very different from those of large-bowel obstruction (LBO) and so it is essential to differentiate between them wherever possible. In most patients, this is relatively easy but some can present a major diagnostic problem, and further investigation may be needed.

Small-Bowel Obstruction

- As discussed earlier conventional abdominal radiography is the preferred initial radiologic examination despite its low diagnostic accuracy and specificity. It is usually diagnostic in up to 50–60% of cases, equivocal in about 20–30%, and normal or nonspecific in 10–20%

TABLE 27.1 Differentiating Characteristics of the Small- and Large-Bowel Loops

	Small Bowel	Stomach	Large Bowel
Number of loops	Many	Sac-like structure	Few
Position	Central abdomen	Left upper quadrant	Peripheral/frame the small bowel
Mucosal/wall pattern	Valvulae conniventes	Rugal folds	Haustral folds
Diameter	3–5 cm	Variable	5–6 cm, Caecum 9 cm
Contents	Variable, some air/fluid levels	Air and fluid	Faeces of variable consistency

BOX 27.4 Causes of Small-Bowel Obstruction

Intrinsic:
Infection, Inflammation (inflammatory bowel disease, tuberculosis)
Midgut volvulus
Enteric duplication or mesenteric cysts
Jejunal, ileal atresias
Diverticuli
Intussusception
Extrinsic:
Adhesions
Hernias (external, internal, and incisional)
Masses (benign/malignant), metastasis
Iatrogenic (radiation enteritis)
Vascular compromise causing intestinal ischemia
Intraluminal causes
Foreign body
Bezoar
Gallstones

- There are multiple causes for SBO, some of which are listed in Box 27.4. The greater the number of dilated small-bowel loops that are visible on the abdominal radiograph, the more distal the obstruction. Plain film changes in complete SBO may appear after 3–5 hours, and such changes are usually marked after 12 hours
- The commonest appearance is the presence of multiple fluid levels (Fig. 27.11). However, the presence of fluid levels alone may not be indicative of obstruction, as there are many other causes for dilatation, the most common being ileus. Ileus can be generalized (postoperative) or localized (adjacent to inflammatory conditions—pancreatitis or appendicitis) [34–37]
- In dilated small bowel which is almost completely filled with fluid, small bubbles of gas may be trapped in rows between the valvulae conniventes on horizontal-ray films; this is known as the "string of beads" sign which is traditionally considered a pathognomic radiographic finding [38]. When little or no gas is present and the dilated loops are predominantly fluid-filled, the classic obstructive bowel sounds may be absent, and so it is even more important for the radiologist to consider fluid-filled loops in SBO
- If the initial radiographs are considered normal, CT scanning is used for further diagnosis because it demonstrates the presence of bowel caliber change, fluid-filled bowel loops, and most times, the cause and the level of obstruction. The CT sensitivity for adhesions is around 73% [31]
- Plain films are generally poor at detecting bowel strangulation and ischemia
- The cause of obstruction is occasionally evident on plain film, for instance, when there is a groin hernia, volvulus, or gallstone ileus; however, obstructing lesions are better identified by CT. CT should be performed whenever there is a history of previous abdominal malignancy, as extraluminal disease in the peritoneum, nodes, and liver will be demonstrated, and may change the management of the patient

Closed loop obstruction: Closed loop obstruction (Fig. 27.12) means mechanical SBO caused when two limbs of a loop are incarcerated by a band or in a hernia, frequently compromising the blood supply due to compression of the mesenteric vessels, resulting in its "strangulation." The closed loop may fill with fluid and be palpable, or it may be visible on the radiograph as a soft-tissue mass or "pseudotumor." The strangulated loop uncommonly contains gas; the limbs of the loop, separated only by the thickened intestinal walls, may resemble a large coffee bean. If gangrene occurs, lines of gas may be seen in the wall of the small bowel. However, the appearance in strangulating obstruction, with all its lethal potential, may be indistinguishable from that of simple SBO [17]. CT is much more sensitive for bowel loop strangulation than plain films.
Volvulus of the small intestine: Volvulus of the small bowel may present as intermittent or persistent obstruction. It may occur as an isolated lesion or be combined with obstruction due to adhesive bands. In children, incomplete rotation, malrotation, or

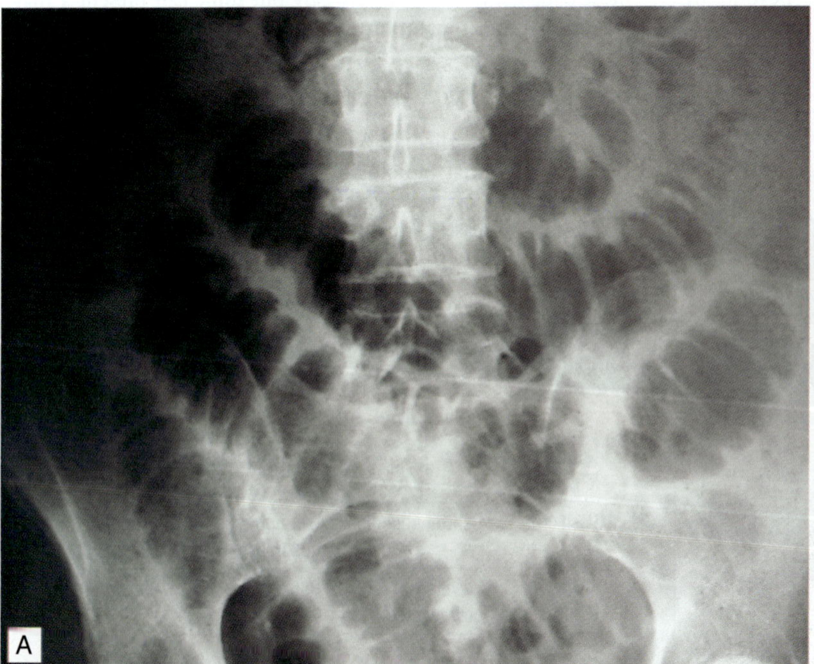

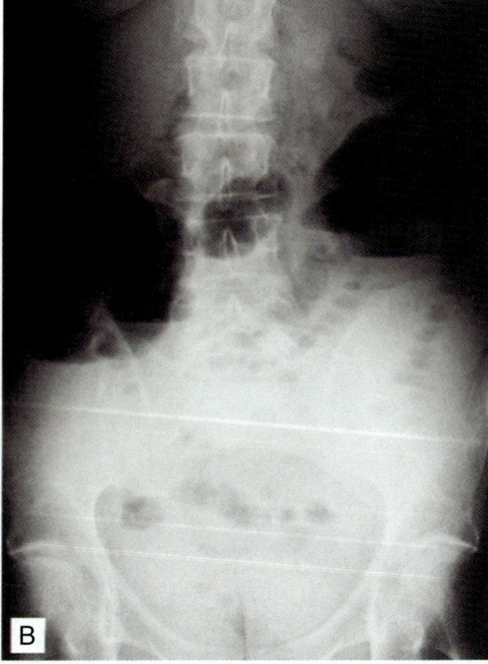

Figure 27.11 Small-bowel obstruction: (A) supine; (B) erect. Multiple dilated loops of both gas-filled and fluid-filled small bowel are readily identified. There is little or no gas in the large bowel. Multiple fluid levels are noted on erect film. Patient was a 77-year-old woman with past history of several abdominal surgeries. The small-bowel obstruction was presumed to be due to adhesions and resolved with conservative management.

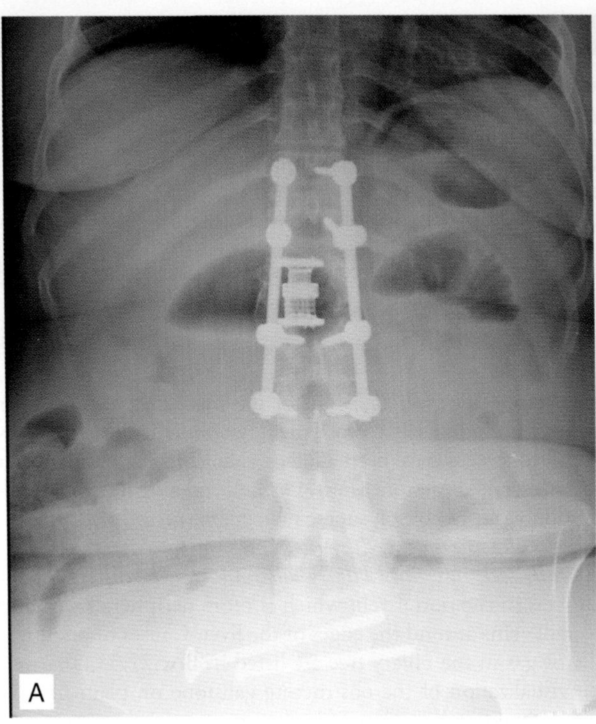

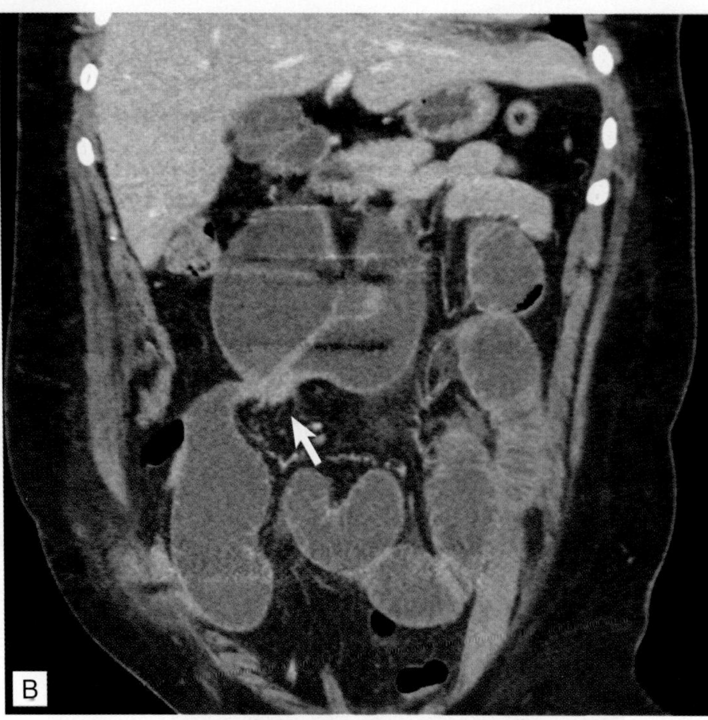

Figure 27.12 (A) abdominal plain film shows air–fluid levels within the upper abdomen indicative of bowel obstruction. (B) Coronal image of the abdomen shows high-grade closed loop small-bowel obstruction from an internal hernia involving the mid and distal small-bowel loops. It is worth noting that this patient has a history of multiple complex abdominal surgeries in the past, predisposing the formation of adhesions and increased risk of bowel obstructions.

nonrotation of the gut may be associated with a massive small-bowel volvulus which may occur in the neonatal period, or months or even years after birth [29]. There is frequently an impaired blood supply in the small bowel so that intramural gas or thumb-printing may be seen. However, it is not usually possible to distinguish simple obstruction, strangulating obstruction, or small-bowel volvulus on plain radiographs alone [29].

Strangulated external hernia: This is usually detected clinically. However, sometimes this is overlooked due to obesity, and so it is important to search the radiograph for evidence of a hernia (Fig. 27.13). Many strangulated hernias will be fluid-filled and not visible on a plain film; furthermore, the mere presence of a hernia does not mean this is the cause of obstruction. However, if dilated bowel is identified ending at a hernial orifice, then the hernia is probably the cause of obstruction.

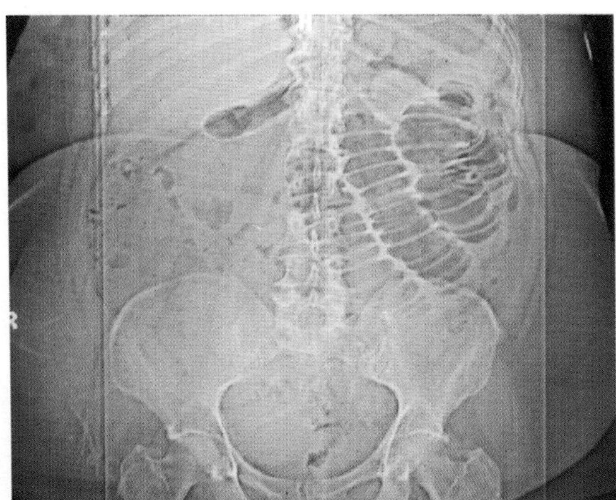

Figure 27.13 Small-bowel obstruction due to an incisional hernia in an obese patient. CT scout image showing dilated small bowel and illustrating the degree of obesity.

CT is very effective at detecting hernias, not only at the groin, but also elsewhere in the abdominal wall and within the peritoneum. It will also help establish if the hernia is the cause of the obstruction.

Appendix abscess: It may present as SBO due to small bowel becoming adherent to the wall of the abscess. The appendix abscess may be identified as a soft-tissue shadow which may contain gas and indent the cecum (Fig. 27.14) [35].

Gallstone Ileus

- Gallstone ileus or biliary ileus is a rare mechanical cause of intestinal obstruction [39]. The patient, most commonly a middle-aged or elderly woman, will often have had recurrent episodes of right hypochondrial pain characteristic of cholecystitis
- The obstruction is caused by the impaction of one or more gallstones which pass into and obstruct the distal stomach or proximal duodenum (*Bouveret's syndrome*) or the terminal ileum (classic gallstone ileus) by eroding through the inflamed gallbladder wall resulting in bilioenteric fistulas. The most common of bilioenteric fistulas is between the gallbladder and the duodenum, seen in approximately 85% cases
- The stones have to be typically 2–2.5 cm in diameter to cause obstruction. Smaller stones just pass through the lumen without causing obstruction
- The diagnosis relies heavily on imaging. Abdominal radiography is the ideal imaging technique of choice in the ED, with sensitivity for the diagnosis of gallstone between 40% and 70%. The Rigler's triad describes the typical radiological signs in plain film:
  - Air within the biliary tree (pneumobilia) (Fig. 27.15)
  - Signs of SBO
  - Ectopic radio-opaque gallstones

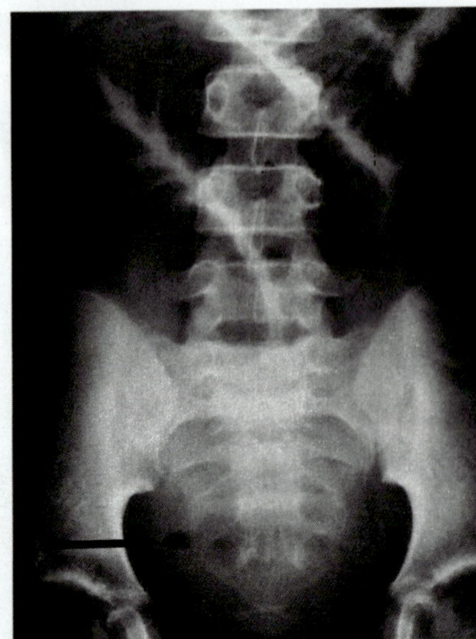

Figure 27.14 Appendicular abscess causing small-bowel obstruction. A small gas bubble which lies within the abscess (*arrow*) is seen in the right iliac fossa. Age 11 years, vomiting with diarrhea for 1 week.

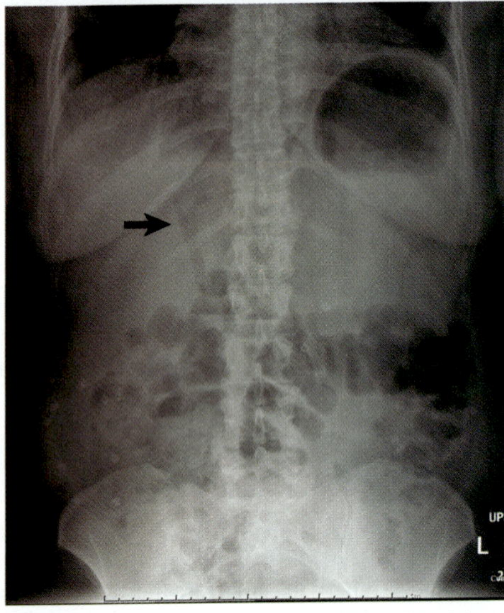

Figure 27.15 Gallstone ileus. Supine film. Multiple dilated loops of small bowel are seen. A band of gas in the right hypochondrium (*arrow*) lies within the common bile duct. The obstructing gallstone cannot be identified.

BOX 27.5 Causes of Gas in the Biliary Tree

Incompetent sphincter of Oddi—sphincterotomy
Biliary surgery or instrumentations
Biliary stent placements
Endoscopic retrograde cholangiopancreatography (ERCP)
Biliary-enteric surgical anastomosis
Fistulous communication of the biliary tree with GI tract—gallstone fistula, trauma, and perforated peptic ulcer
Infections—emphysematous cholecystitis, cholangitis, and abscesses
Malignancy causing fistula

- Often times only two signs out of the triad are present. Rigler defined his triad in 1941. Since then, two more radiological signs for gallstone ileus have been added—change in the location of a previously noted gallstone (*Rigler's tetrad*), and a right upper quadrant double air bubble on supine radiograph (*Rigler's pentad*) [40]
- *Pneumobilia is recognized by its branching pattern in that it is classically seen in central biliary ducts and can be* differentiated from gas in the portal vein which is more peripherally located in small veins around the edges of the liver. Causes of pneumobilia or gas in the biliary tree are listed in Box 27.5
- The visualization of the obstructing gallstone on plain films is frequently difficult, because it is often composed almost entirely of cholesterol, with only a thin rim of calcium within it. Sometimes gas in the biliary tree may be identified in SBO which is not due to gallstone ileus. In these cases the gas is presumed to have entered through a physiologically lax sphincter
- The small-bowel dilatation, gas within the biliary tree, and the gallstone at the point of obstruction may all be demonstrated elegantly on CT

Bezoars

In recent times there is a small increase in these cases because of the increasing numbers of gastric outlet surgeries; these surgeries prevent digestion of fibers which become impacted, causing obstruction [41]. On radiographs and CT, bezoar is seen as an ovoid intraluminal mass with a mottled gas pattern (Fig. 27.16A).

Enteroliths

Enteroliths are usually seen as ovoid high-density calcified densities usually in a patient presenting with repeated attacks of obstruction. Tubercular strictures, closed loop obstructions,

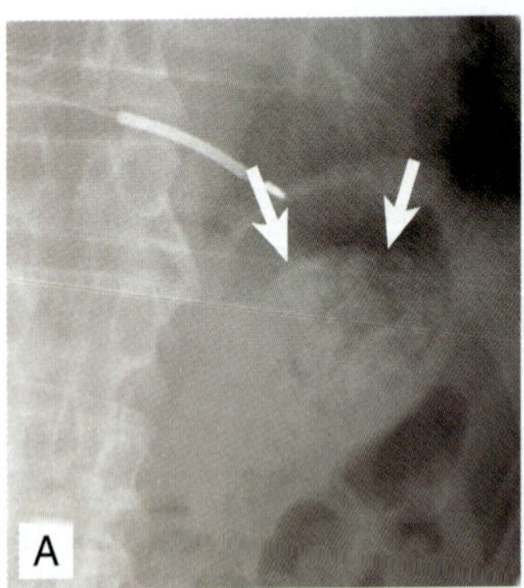

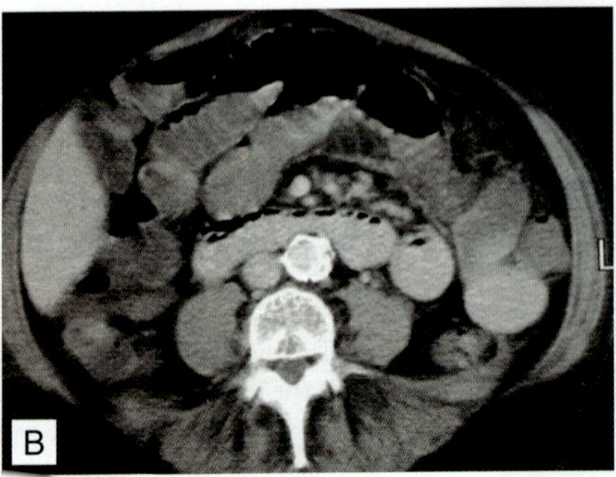

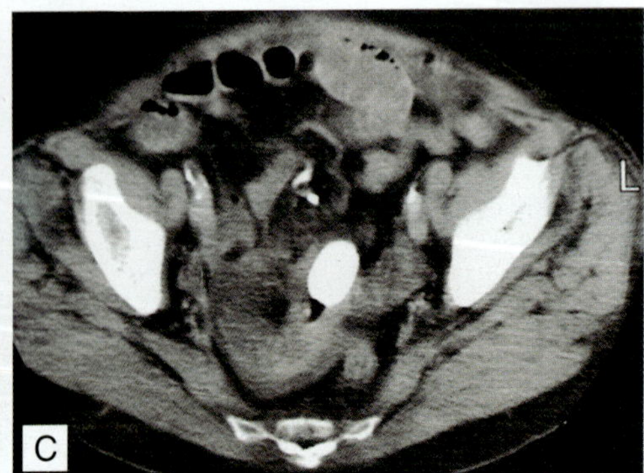

Figure 27.16 (A) Gastric bezoar: supine abdominal radiograph shows a gastric bezoar as a mottled soft-tissue mass (*arrows*) floating in the stomach at the air–fluid interface. (B-C) Small-bowel obstruction due to an ileal fecolith. (B) Dilated small-bowel loops. The gallbladder appeared normal. (C) Image through the pelvis. At the transition from dilated to collapsed bowel is a large densely calcified intraluminal fecolith.

and adhesions are common causes of detecting enetroliths in patients with recurrent attacks of subacute or acute obstruction. Associated features of obstruction depend on the timing of obtaining the radiograph or CT (Fig. 27.16B and C).

Intussusception

The incidence of intussusception varies considerably in different countries, but in general it is most frequently seen in children under 2 years of age [42,43]. In children it usually commences in the ileum as the result of inflammation of the lymphoid tissue and tends to be associated with mesenteric adenitis [44,45]. The enlarged lymphatic patches are forced into the ileum by peristaltic movement and, acting as a tumor, one part of the ileum is pulled into the other and finally pulled into the colon. Although the condition is usually recognized clinically by pain, vomiting, blood in the stool, and a palpable tumor, the diagnosis may not be apparent initially and further investigations may be needed.

Plain films may show evidence of SBO, or the intussusception itself may be identified as a soft-tissue mass sometimes surrounded by a crescent of gas and most frequently identified in the right hypochondrium (Fig. 27.17). The "*target sign*" has been described, comprising two concentric circles of fat density lying to the right of the spine—often superimposed on the kidney. It is probably due to the layers of peritoneal fat surrounding and within the intussusceptum alternating with the layers of mucosa and muscle but seen "end on" as it passes forward from the right paraspinal gutter in the transverse colon.

In adults, an intussusception is a rare condition responsible for less than 5% of SBO, with lead point intussusceptions resulting from tumors (classically lipoma of the terminal ileum, lymphoma, and metastases from melanoma), foreign bodies, and adhesions [46]. Transient intussusceptions do not cause SBO. Any part of the small bowel may be involved, although the terminal ileum is still the most common site for the underlying pathology.

USG is the technique still widely used for the diagnosis of this condition and CT readily demonstrates intussusception.

Enema therapies are still popular in treating intussusceptions. These include:

- Barium enema
- Water-soluble contrast enema
- Air enema
- Ultrasound-guided saline enema
- Ultrasound-guided air enema

Air enema has become widely popular in the western world, as it is quick, clean, uses lesser radiation than barium and has high success rates [45]. However, there is an increased risk of perforation and it is advised that the increase in pressure must be slow and progressive. Ultrasound-guided saline enema is also popular as it does not use ionizing radiation and gives high success rates [45].

Mesenteric thrombosis—Small Intestinal Infarction

Stenosis or thromboembolic occlusions of the mesenteric arteries and veins result in bowel ischemia and necrosis which leads to bowel wall thickening resulting in SBO. The clinical diagnosis is often uncertain, but the sudden onset of abdominal pain, often associated with bloody diarrhea, in an elderly person is very suggestive of this condition. CT findings are more specific and are covered in detail in the following chapters. Plain film findings are nonspecific, some of which are:

- Gas-filled or fluid-filled, slightly dilated small-bowel loops
- Thickened walls of the small bowel—secondary to submucosal hemorrhage and edema
- Linear gas streaks in the bowel wall (pneumatosis coli; Fig. 27.18), from possible infarction
- Free intraperitoneal air—from possible perforation
- Colonic distension—from generalized paralytic ileus

Large-Bowel Obstruction

LBO differs considerably from SBO in its clinical findings and pathophysiology. The marked distension of colon proximal to the level of obstruction leads to mucosal edema, bowel ischemia,

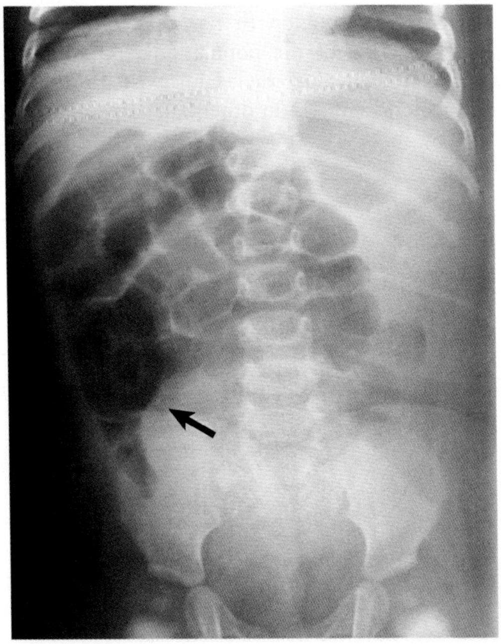

Figure 27.17 Intussusception. Supine film. There are multiple gas-filled loops of slightly dilated small bowel. In addition, there is a soft-tissue mass in the right iliac fossa (*arrow*). A 5-month-old child with mesenteric adenitis.

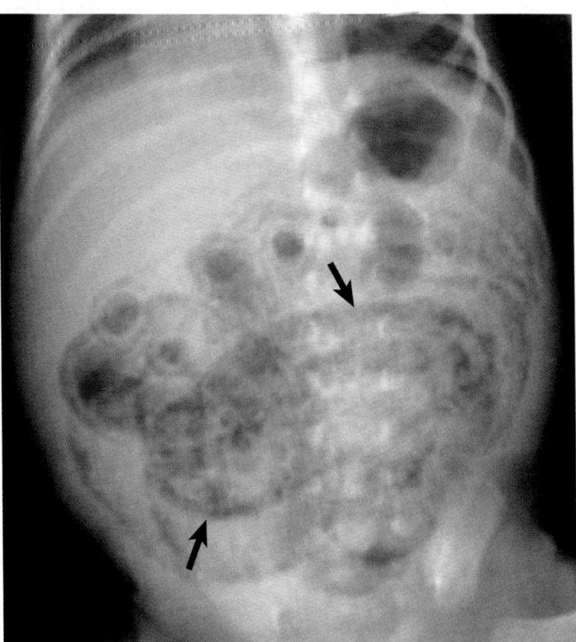

Figure 27.18 Small intestinal infarction. Supine radiograph shows dilated small-bowel loops with thickened walls and linear gas streaks in the wall (*arrows*).

BOX 27.6 Causes of Large-Bowel Obstruction

Neoplasm—adenocarcinoma of colon
Volvulus—sigmoid, cecum, and transverse colon
Intussusception
Hernias—external, internal, and incisional
Infection, inflammation—diverticulitis and inflammatory bowel disease
Intraluminal—foreign body, gallstone, and fecal impaction

and subsequently leads to bowel infarction and perforation. There are many causes for LBO, listed in Box 27.6; the commonest however is carcinoma (>60%) [32], with the two most frequent locations being the splenic flexure and sigmoid colon.

The commonest site of perforation in LBO is the cecum. Diverticular disease as a cause of obstruction has decreased in frequency since the introduction of high-fiber diets. Acute colonic volvulus comprises about 10–15% of LBO [32]. In volvulus, the colon twists upon itself and if the twist is greater than 360 degree, then surgical intervention is necessary. Sigmoid volvulus is 3–4 times more common than cecal volvulus while volvulus of transverse colon and splenic flexure are rare.

The key to the radiological appearance of LBO depends on the state of competence of the ileocecal valve. Three patterns (Fig. 27.19) of obstruction have been described.

- Type IA—Ileocecal valve is competent and the radiological appearance is one of dilated colon with a distended thin-walled cecum but no distension of small bowel (Fig. 27.20)
- Type IB—Progression of type 1A resulting in small-bowel distension, probably secondary to the tightly closed ileocecal valve opening up

Both type I obstructions can lead to massive cecal distension, which is then at risk of perforation secondary to ischemia. A transverse cecal diameter of 9 cm has been suggested as the critical point above which the danger of perforation exists.

- Type II—The ileocecal valve is incompetent, and the cecum and ascending colon are not distended, but the back pressure from the colon extends into the small bowel and there are numerous dilated loops of small bowel which may simulate SBO

The obstructed colon almost invariably contains large amounts of air and can usually be identified by its haustral margin around the periphery of the abdomen. However, on occasions the right half of the colon may be filled with fluid and massive cecal distension may be overlooked. Even more rarely, the whole colon up to the point of obstruction may be filled with fluid and so the diagnosis may be overlooked initially.

When both small- and large-bowel dilatation is present in LBO, the radiographic appearance may be identical to that of paralytic ileus. However, the clinical signs will usually help differentiate. Demonstration of air in the rectum may differentiate paralytic ileus from low LBO.

There are numerous causes of colonic distension without obstruction. These include all forms of paralytic ileus and pseudo-obstruction.

Pseudo-Obstruction

Pseudo-obstruction is a disorder of bowel which symptomatically, clinically, and radiologically may mimic intestinal obstruction. It may be acute and self-limiting and associated with pneumonia, septicemia, or certain drugs; or chronic with acute flare-ups, as seen in diabetes mellitus, collagen disorders, neurological disorders, and amyloid disease.

A large proportion of patients, however, have no associated medical condition and these cases are called "*idiopathic intestinal pseudo-obstruction*" (Fig. 27.21). A large quantity of bowel gas is usually present and there may be gastric, small- or large-bowel distension with associated fluid levels just as great as in true obstruction. CT imaging can help avoid an unnecessary surgery.

Large-Bowel Volvulus

A prerequisite for the formation of a volvulus is that a long and freely mobile mesentery must be present. This occurs normally in the sigmoid, which is the commonest organ involved. Occasionally, the cecum and ascending colon are on a mesentery, which is often associated with a degree of malrotation, and they comprise the second most common organs involved.

Cecal Volvulus (Right-Colon Volvulus)

Cecal or right-colon volvulus can only occur when the cecum and ascending colon are on a mesentery, and this is often associated with a degree of malrotation (it has been estimated that this occurs in about 11% of the population) [32]. In half of the patients with cecal volvulus, the cecum twists in the axial plane, rotating on its long axis and in other half of patients, the cecum

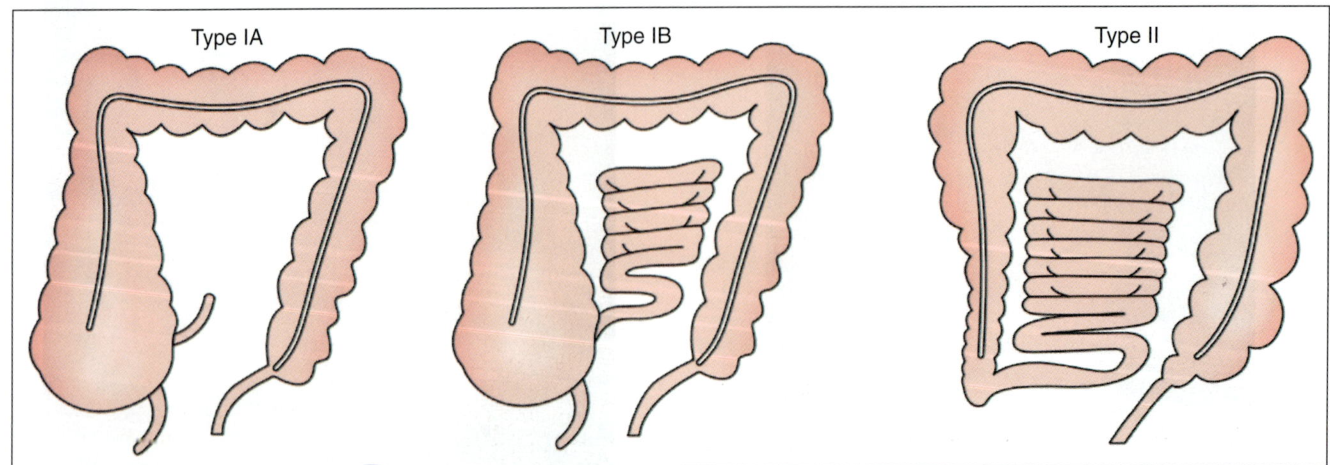

Figure 27.19 Large-bowel obstruction: Type IA: Competent ileocecal valve. Distended large bowel, particularly ascending colon and cecum. No distension of small bowel. Type IB: Competent ileocecal valve. Cecal distension and small-bowel distension. Type II: Incompetent ileocecal valve. No distension of cecum and ascending colon but distension of small bowel. Cecal perforation is much more likely to occur in type I large bowel obstruction.

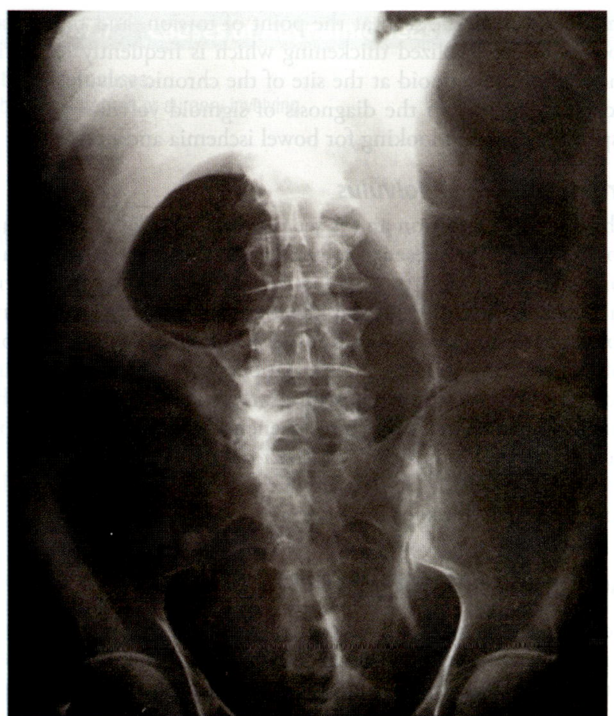

Figure 27.20 Large-bowel obstruction type IA (competent ileocecal valve). Supine film. There is gaseous distension of the large bowel from the sigmoid backward, including the ascending colon and cecum. The dilated cecum lies in the pelvis. There is no visible small-bowel distension. (Carcinoma of the sigmoid.)

twists and inverts resulting in apex of the cecal twist in the left upper quadrant. It is usually found in a relatively young age group of about 30–60 years. Gangrene may occur early in the course of the condition, and it is therefore vital that an accurate diagnosis be made promptly.

The diagnosis can be made from radiographs in about 75% cases [29]. Even though there is considerable distension of the volved cecum, one or two haustral markings can usually be identified, unlike sigmoid volvulus where haustral markings are usually absent. The distended cecum can frequently be identified as a large gas- and fluid-filled viscus situated almost anywhere in the abdomen. Identification of an attached gas-filled appendix confirms the diagnosis. Moderate or severe small-bowel distension is present in about half the cases, but the remainder only show minimal small-bowel distension. The left half of the colon is usually collapsed (Fig. 27.22).

Sigmoid Volvulus

This is the classic volvulus, occurring in old, mentally subnormal, or institutionalized population. The usual mechanism is twisting of the sigmoid loop around the mesenteric axis which leads to a closed loop obstruction. Sigmoid volvulus is usually chronic, with intermittent acute attacks; less commonly, a true acute torsion occurs.

Although plain film diagnosis is often easy with the diagnosis evident in about 57–90% of cases; up to one-third can present diagnostic difficulty with the main problem being able to differentiate the sigmoid volvulus from distended but nontwisted sigmoid, or distended transverse colon looping down into the pelvis (pseudovolvulus) [29,32].

- The essential radiological feature for diagnosis is to identify the wall of the twisted sigmoid loop separate from the remaining distended colon. When a sigmoid volvulus occurs, the inverted U-shaped loop is usually massively distended and it is commonly devoid of haustra (ahaustral). This is a most important diagnostic point. The ahaustral margin can often be identified overlapping the lower border of the liver shadow—the "liver overlap" sign. Where the ahaustral margin of the volvulus overlies the haustrated and dilated descending colon, the term "left flank overlap sign" has been used. The apex of the sigmoid volvulus usually lies high in the abdomen, under the left hemidiaphragm, with its apex at or above the level of T10

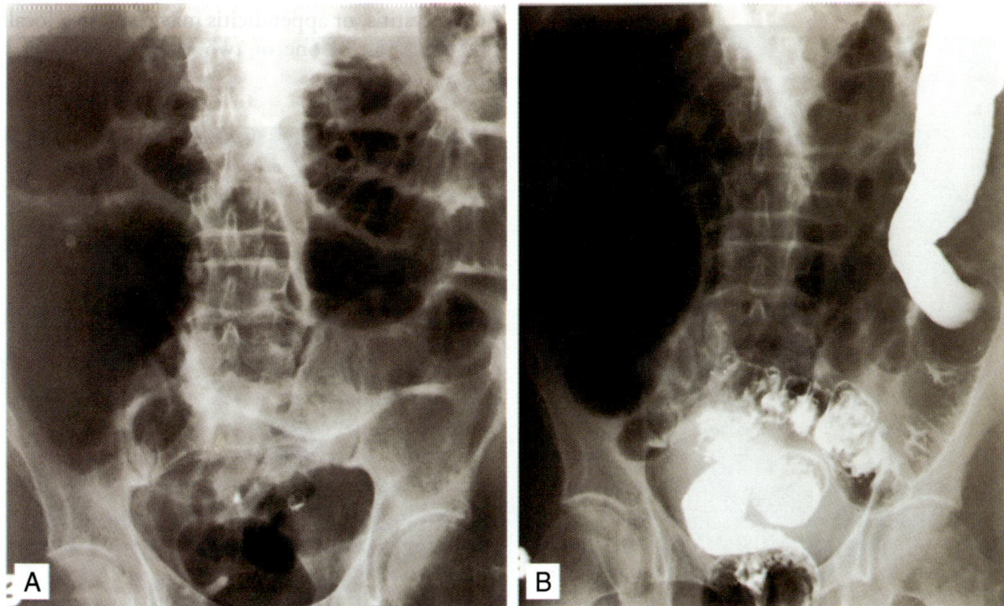

Figure 27.21 Pseudo-obstruction: (A) supine abdomen; (B) barium enema. On the plain film, gas-filled loops of both small and large bowel can be identified, with gas extending down to the rectum. The barium examination demonstrates diverticular disease in the sigmoid, but this is not obstructing, and barium flows freely into the dilated descending colon. Conservative management, using a flatus tube, failed and a laparotomy had to be undertaken. Dilated small and large bowel were found but there was no obstructing lesion. A cecostomy was performed.

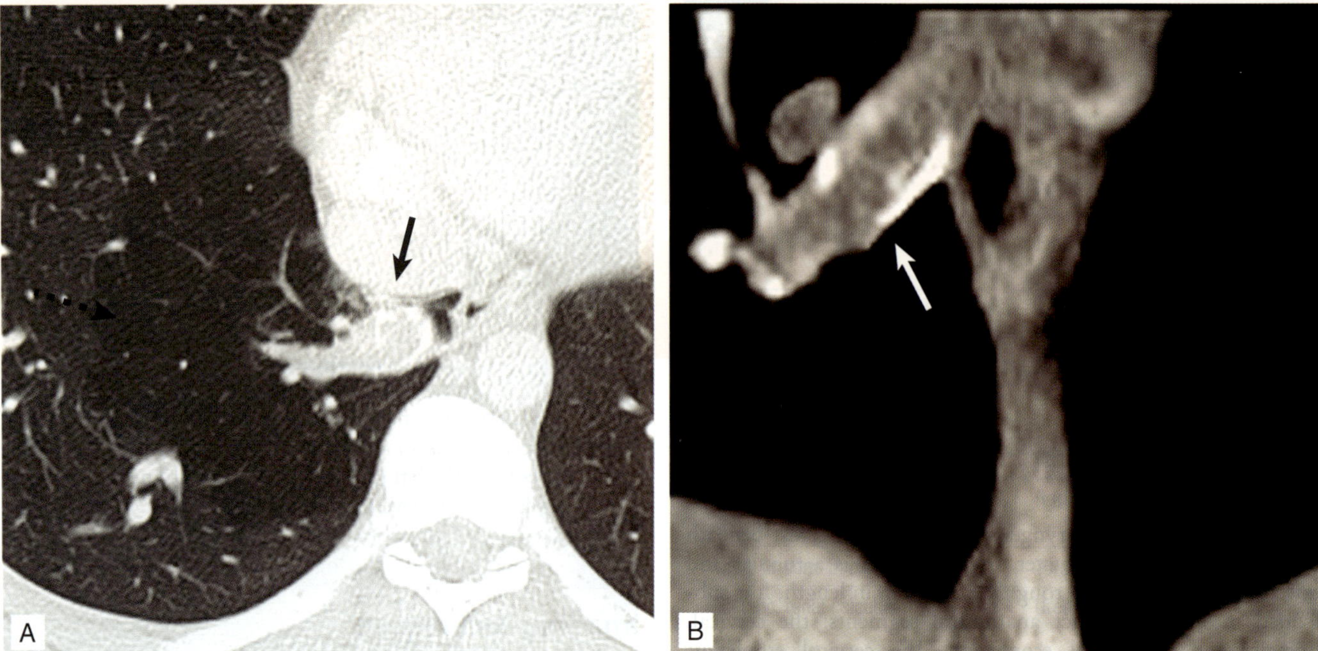

Figure 28.1 Axial CT of the chest with lung windows (A) demonstrates a tubular structure (*black arrow*) emanating from the esophagus which is filled with debris compatible with an esophageal bronchus. The supplied lung is hyperlucent secondary to air trapping (*dashed arrow*) as the bronchus does not communicate with the tracheobronchial tree. Soft tissue windows (B) demonstrate communication within the esophagus (B). This was detected in an asymptomatic individual.

condition is often termed "esophageal lung." These almost always present early in life with a clinical history of recurrent pneumonias or worsening respiratory failure. Diagnosis can be made with a combination of contrast esophagography and chest CT (Fig. 28.1) [6].

Esophageal Duplication Cyst

Pathophysiology and Clinical Presentation: While mediastinal foregut duplication cysts are rare, the esophagus is the second most common location (~20%) for a gastrointestinal duplication cyst [7]. Esophageal duplication cysts are believed to result from an aberrant diverticulum of the dorsal bud of the primitive foregut or arise from abnormal recanalization of the gut during development [8]. Usually, they are found closely applied to or within the esophageal wall, but rarely they can be sequestered from the esophagus and develop remotely within the pulmonary parenchyma.

These are most often asymptomatic and detected incidentally due to workup for another medical complaint. Symptoms include dysphagia, regurgitation, chest pain, or fevers in the setting of superinfection.

Imaging Features

- On CT, esophageal duplication cysts are single, smooth, round, or elliptical cystic masses. While there can be thin linear enhancement of the wall, there should be no solid enhancing component or nodular thickening of the wall. Attenuation of the cysts can be the same as water, while others are more hyperdense due to hemorrhagic or proteinaceous debris (Fig. 28.2)
- On MRI, lesions which are closer to water in attenuation on CT will be hyperintense on T2-weighted sequences and hypointense on T1 weight sequences. If the contents are hemorrhagic or proteinaceous, they will be hyperintense on the T1-weighted sequences [9]. With either technique pre- and postcontrast imaging can confirm there is no internally enhancing component

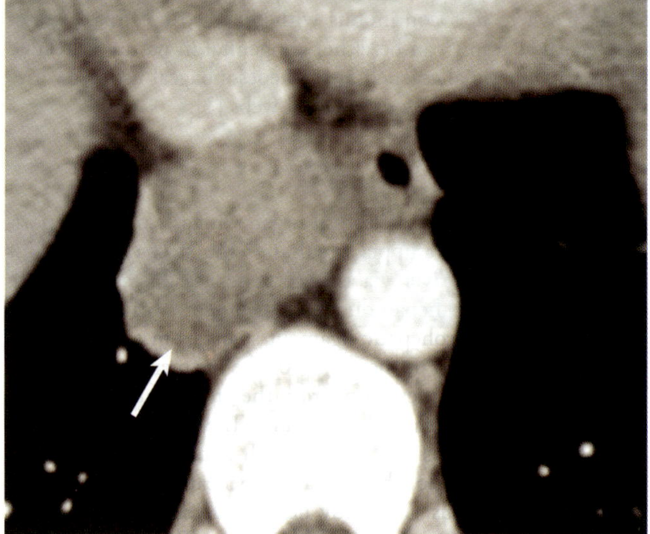

Figure 28.2 Axial CT of the chest with intravenous contrast shows a nonenhancing well-circumscribed cystic lesion in close association with the esophagus representing a foregut duplication cyst.

Stomach

Situs Inversus/Heterotaxy Syndrome

Situs anomalies arise due to failure of normal lateralization and/or duplication of the chest and abdominal viscera. In patients with situs anomalies, the stomach can be on either side; however, a right-sided stomach bubble or location of the heart and stomach on opposite sides on plain radiographs is a clue that there is an underlying heterotaxy (Fig. 28.3A). With polysplenia, the spleen and stomach are located on the same side. CT delineates additional findings such as azygos continuation of the inferior vena cava and intestinal malrotation (Fig. 28.3B) [10].

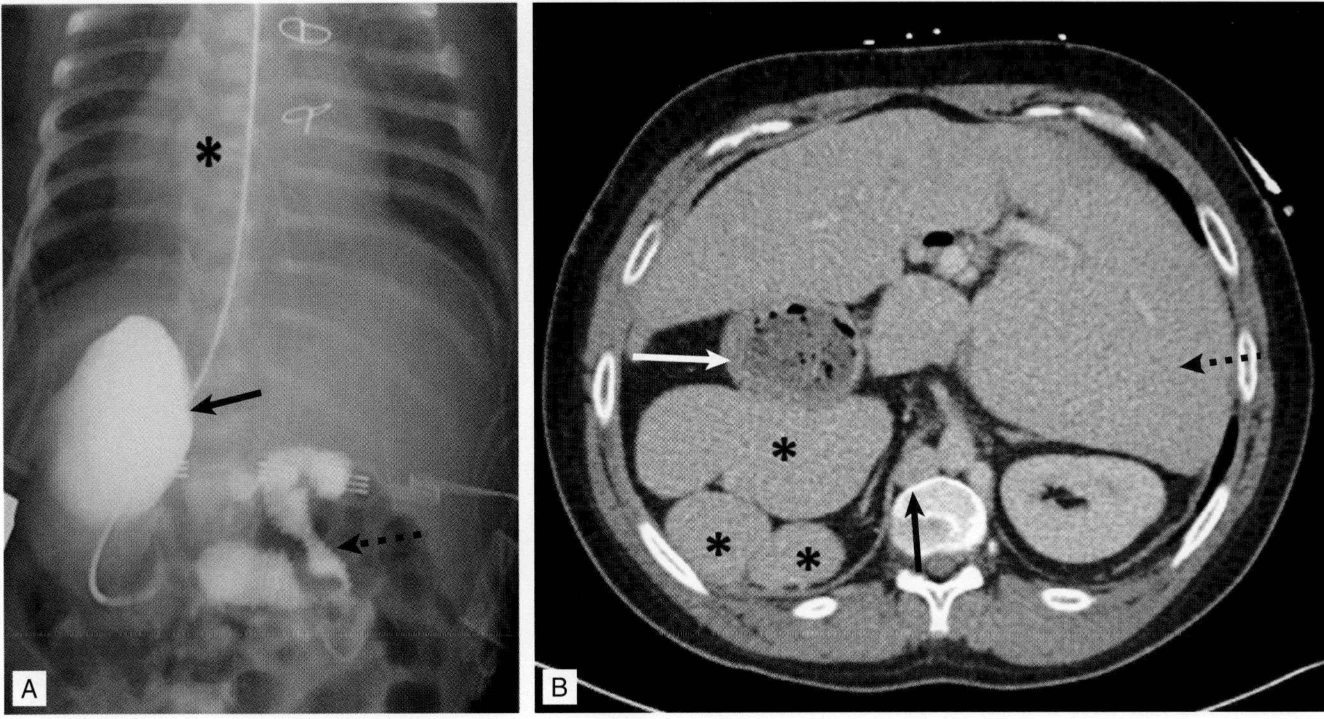

Figure 28.3 (A) Injection of contrast through a gastric tube demonstrates right-sided stomach (*arrow*), and other findings of heterotaxy including dextrocardia (*) and presence of the duodenal sweep to the left of midline (*dashed arrow*) compatible with malrotation. (B) A 23-year-old man with heterotaxy. CT of the abdomen with contrast shows stomach (*arrow*) and polysplenia (*) in the right upper quadrant. There is a left-sided liver (*dashed arrow*) and dilated azygos vein (*black arrow*) that continues as the inferior vena cava (not shown).

Gastric Duplication Cyst

Pathophysiology and Clinical Presentation: Gastric duplication cysts are rare congenital malformations thought to result from aberrant embryonic budding or ineffective recanalization of the alimentary tract in utero. They are the least common location for gastrointestinal tract duplications accounting for roughly 4% of cases [11]. Duplication cysts have epithelial lining similar to GI tract epithelium. At times, they can contain heterotopic tissue (e.g., pancreatic). They can be either cystic round or tubular depending on whether they communicate with the stomach or not. About 80% of cases are cystic in nature and usually, do not communicate with the stomach, while the remainder is tubular and show some form of communication with the stomach [12].

Majority are symptomatic within the first year of life presenting as an abdominal mass or gastric outlet obstruction (GOO). Adults can present with abdominal pain, nausea, vomiting, or abdominal distension. Rarely, these cysts can become secondarily superinfected or ulcerate leading to gastrointestinal bleeding. Cystic lesions are often resected if the patient is symptomatic. Typically, tubular duplication cysts that communicate with the stomach are asymptomatic.

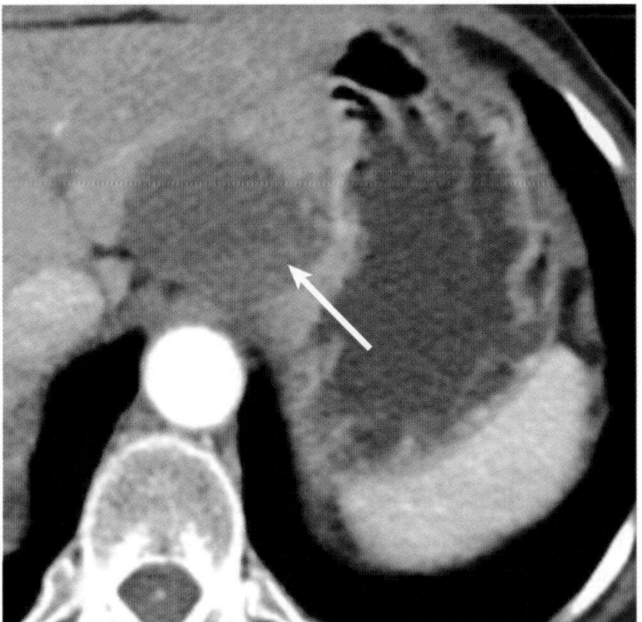

Figure 28.4 Axial CT of the abdomen with contrast shows a nonenhancing cystic round lesion in the gastrohepatic ligament, compatible with a gastric duplication cyst.

Imaging Features

- Ultrasound can be utilized as a first-line test, particularly in infants given it is noninvasive and imparts no radiation. There will be an anechoic or hypoechoic structure within the upper abdomen in close relationship to the stomach, pancreas, or liver with the wall sometimes demonstrating the gut signature sign
- Upper gastrointestinal series can aid in demonstrating a communication of the duplication cyst within the lumen of the stomach
- CT can help confirm both the cystic nature of the lesion as well as relationship of the cyst with adjacent structures for surgical planning (Fig. 28.4)

Esophagus: Inflammatory Processes

Reflux and Barrett's Esophagitis

Pathophysiology and Clinical Presentation

Gastroesophageal reflux disease (GERD) is the most common disease affecting the gastrointestinal tract with an estimated prevalence of 10–20% in western countries [13]. As such, reflux esophagitis is the most common inflammatory process in the esophagus.

Barrett's esophagus is characterized by progressive columnar metaplasia in response to chronic reflux esophagitis. It is estimated to occur in 10% of patients with reflux esophagitis [14]. Barrett's esophagitis is considered a premalignant condition that can lead to adenocarcinoma of the esophagus. Chronic inflammation predisposes to progressively worsening dysplasia followed by carcinoma in situ and eventually invasive carcinoma. Patient's with Barrett's esophagitis often undergo surveillance with periodic endoscopy with or without biopsy.

Imaging Features

- With esophagography, reflux esophagitis is seen as granularity and nodularity in the distal esophagus from edema and mucosal inflammation. Reflux ulcers can be seen in advanced disease and can have a linear or punctate pattern with radiating folds or rims of edematous mucosa. They are almost always found in the distal esophagus. Sparing of the distal esophagus should prompt consideration of another diagnosis [14]
- The classic imaging appearance of Barrett's on fluoroscopy is a mid to high esophageal stricture or ulcers associated with contrast reflux and/or gastroesophageal hernias. A reticular mucosal pattern is thought to be relatively specific for Barrett's esophagitis (Fig. 28.5), although use of this criterion alone is not sufficient [14]. Ultimately, these features are more of a screening tool before endoscopy and biopsy is required for definitive diagnosis
- On CT, low attenuation circumferential wall thickening in the distal esophagus indicates esophagitis. Although there is no absolute measurement which one can say there is unequivocally pathological wall thickening, 5 mm is often used as the cutoff [15]. If present, reflux esophagitis will have circumferential esophageal wall thickening involving at least the distal esophagus. At times, the wall thickening can appear mass-like making differentiation with early malignancy difficult that further warrants evaluation with upper endoscopy

Eosinophilic Esophagitis

Pathophysiology and Clinical Presentation

Eosinophilic esophagitis is a chronic inflammatory condition occurring predominantly in children or young men with a clinical history of long-standing dysphagia and recurrent food impactions which do not respond to antireflux medication. There is association with atopy and peripheral eosinophilia and the condition may be due to a chronic allergic reaction to food allergens. Diagnosis is achieved by identifying intraepithelial eosinophils on biopsy [16].

Imaging Features

With esophagography, the most common findings are upper and mid thoracic esophageal strictures. Alternatively, there can be small caliber of the esophagus manifested as long segment narrowing (>10 cm) of the esophagus. This typically has smooth borders with gradual tapering and dilation, as opposed to other strictures that are generally shorter (mean length <5 cm) and have more discrete margins [17]. Often, there will be closely spaced concentric rings (<2 mm in thickness) traversing the length of the strictures or esophageal narrowing, creating a characteristic "ringed" esophagus (Fig. 28.6) [18].

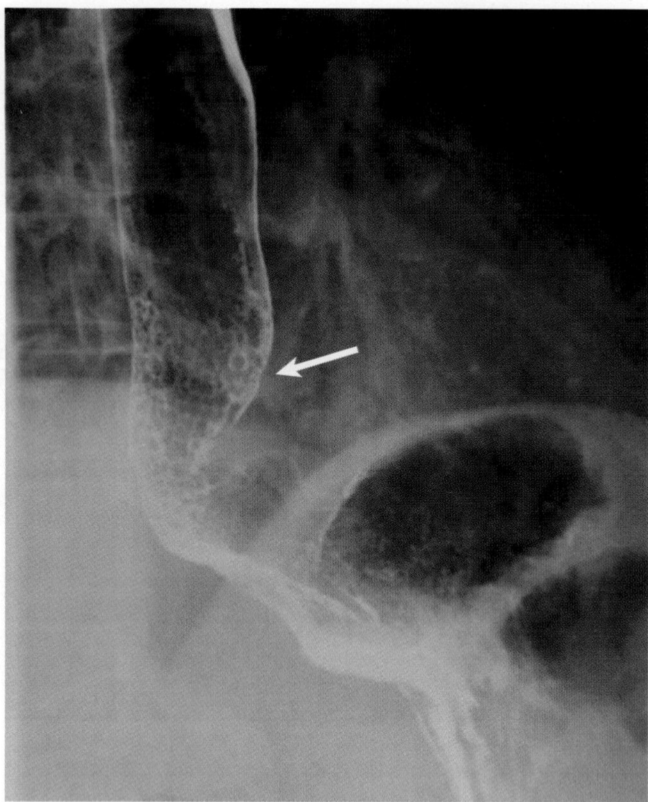

Figure 28.5 A 35-year old man with gastroesophageal reflux disease. Double contrast barium swallow examination shows fine reticular pattern (*arrow*) of the distal esophageal mucosa consistent with Barrett's esophagitis.

Infectious Esophageal Ulcers

Pathophysiology and Clinical Presentation

Infectious esophageal ulcers are secondary to infection with opportunistic pathogens, such as candida, cytomegalovirus (CMV) or herpes simplex virus (HSV). Increasing use of immunosuppressive medications, such as in transplant patients and for chronic inflammatory conditions, as well as immunocompromising illnesses, such as AIDS or diabetes mellitus, are the main risk factors [18]. Clinically these entities present with odynophagia, dysphagia, chest pain, and less commonly gastrointestinal bleeding.

Imaging Features

Endoscopy has largely supplanted esophagography in diagnosis of these conditions as it allows direct visualization and biopsy for definitive diagnosis.

- *Candida esophagitis* is the most common cause of infectious esophagitis. Candida lesions appear as plaque-like defects with intervening normal mucosa. In patients with acquired

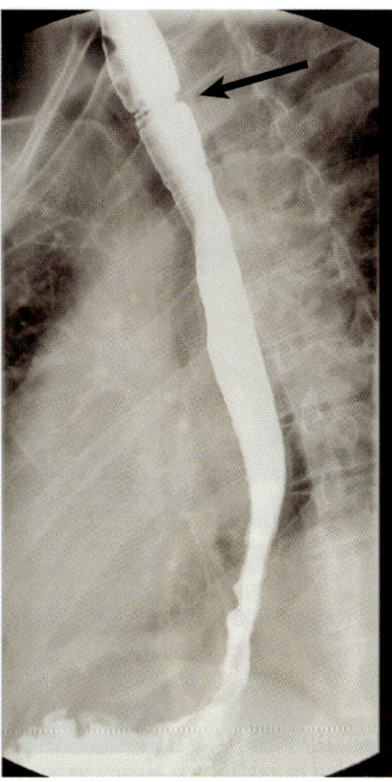

Figure 28.6 A 53-year old man with dysphagia. Double contrast barium swallow examination shows multiple concentric rings in the upper third of the esophagus (*arrow*) representing eosinophilic esophagitis.

immunodeficiency syndrome, there can be a more fulminant form in which there is a "shaggy" esophagus resulting from confluent plaques and pseudomembrane formation due to severe esophagitis (Fig. 28.7). If ulcers do form, it will be on a background of esophageal plaques that help differentiate ulcers due to HSV and CMV [18]

- Herpes esophagitis begins as mucosal blisters and vesicles, which rupture to form small (<1 cm) discrete punched out ulcers that are arranged in a linear, clustered, or punctate configuration (Fig. 28.8) [18]
- The ulcers in CMV esophagitis are often indistinguishable from those of HSV; however, CMV is also associated with formation of one or more giant ulcers (>1 cm). Definitive diagnosis is by endoscopy and biopsy [18]

Esophageal Vascular Disease

Esophageal Varices

Pathophysiology and Clinical Presentation

Abnormally dilated submucosal veins of the esophagus that can be subdivided into "uphill" and "downhill" varices. The upper two-thirds of the esophagus are drained by the esophageal veins, which empty into the azygos venous system and the superior vena cava (SVC). The lower third of the esophagus is drained by the left gastric vein, which in turn empties into the portal venous system.

When physicians refer to esophageal varices, they are most commonly referring to "uphill" varices. Uphill varices result from portal hypertension, which is most commonly due to hepatic cirrhosis. Cirrhosis leads to reversal of flow in the portal venous system resulting in reflux of blood into the left gastric vein and therefore the submucosal veins in the distal esophagus. Approximately 80–90% of cirrhotic patients develop gastric varices, of which one-third will have an episode of esophageal hemorrhage during their lifetime [19].

"Downhill" esophageal varices are less common and occur due to thrombosis of the SVC or its draining vessels. Primary lung cancer, thrombosis related to chronic or recurrent central venous catheterization, mediastinal lymphadenopathy, or mediastinal tumors can obstruct the SVC. Nonocclusive causes are rare and include large thyroid masses or pulmonary hypertension [20]. Downhill varices tend to bleed less compared to their uphill counterparts comprising only 0.1% of all variceal bleeds. This is in part due to lack of coagulopathy, which is often seen in patients with cirrhosis, as well as to their higher location away from potential erosive reflux disease [20].

Imaging Features

In the case of uphill variceal disease, there will be ancillary imaging features of cirrhosis. Additionally, there may be evidence of portal hypertension, including splenomegaly, a recanalized umbilical vein and portosystemic collateral formation in the upper abdomen. With downhill varices, there may be thrombosis or narrowing of the SVC due to in situ thrombus from a catheter or extrinsic compression from a mass or lymphadenopathy.

- On CT, the varices themselves will appear as dilated, enhancing serpiginous tubular structures within the submucosal esophagus (Fig. 28.9)

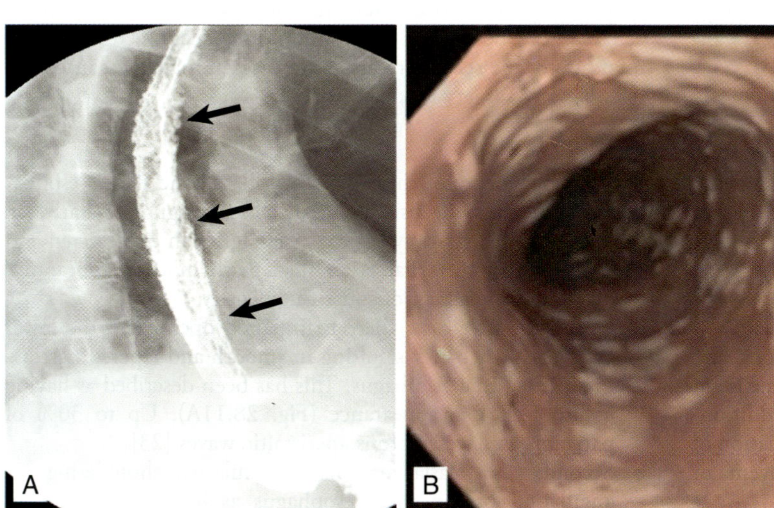

Figure 28.7 A 63-year old man with HIV and progressive dysphagia with odynophagia. Double contrast barium swallow examination (A) shows diffusely "shaggy" appearance of the esophageal mucosa with multiple plaque-like filling defects (*arrows*) and diffuse ulceration. This appearance is most consistent with *Candida esophagitis* which was confirmed on upper endoscopy (B).

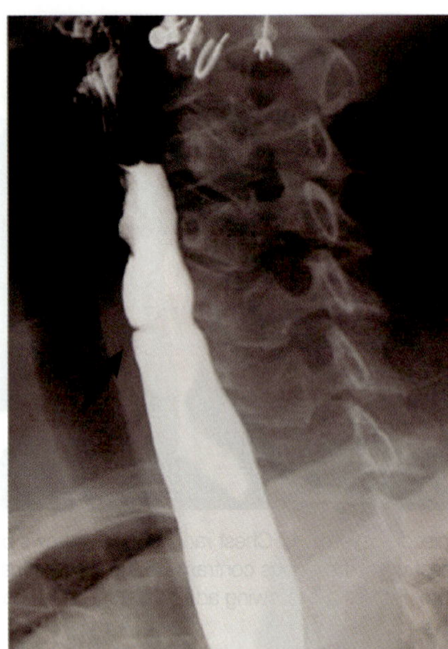

Figure 28.12 Oblique view of the cervical esophagus in a patient with globus sensation. Along the anterior aspect, there is a thin horizontal filling defect (*arrow*) that has become conspicuous with a full column barium swallow.

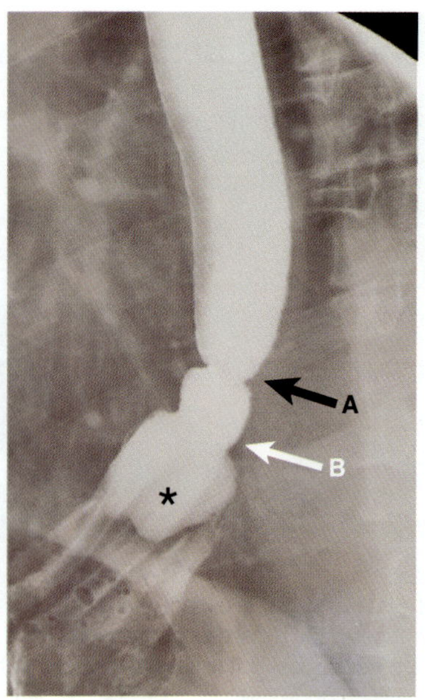

Figure 28.13 Double contrast barium esophagram shows a sliding type hiatal hernia (*) above which a concentric, fixed narrowing is present compatible with a B ring (*white arrow*). Above this, a separate concentric ring is noted (*black arrow*) compatible with an A ring.

Rings

Pathophysiology and Clinical Presentation

Esophageal rings are smooth ring-like constrictions of the distal esophagus frequently encountered on esophagography. There are two commonly described types of esophageal rings. A rings are muscular rings covered in squamous epithelium and occur due to smooth muscle hypertrophy in the distal esophageal body. Muscular rings are transient and occur from active muscle contraction and can vary in appearance during the examination. These are very rarely symptomatic and noticed incidentally on esophogram. B rings, also referred to as lower esophageal rings, are fixed and reproducible mucosal rings at the squamocolumnar junction. Rarely, they are symptomatic and referred to as Schatzki's rings [26].

Imaging Features

Distal esophageal rings are best demonstrated as circumferential narrowing on full column esophagography. These rings are best visualized when the esophagus is distended with barium during single column views with patient in the right anterior oblique position. A rings are located superior to B rings, and B rings are almost always located just superior to a hiatal hernia (Fig. 28.13). A barium tablet (~13 mm) can be administered to aid in diagnosis. Rings with maximum diameter less than 13 mm are usually associated with dysphagia [25].

Cricopharyngeal Dysfunction and Hypertrophy

Pathophysiology and Clinical Presentation

The cricopharyngeus muscle is the main contributor to the upper esophageal sphincter. It normally closes between swallows and has to effectively relax to allow for passage of a food bolus. Dysfunction of this muscle can be due to incomplete relaxation, early closure, or related to hypertrophy of the muscle itself. Cricopharyngeal dysfunction can lead to proximal trapping of ingested consents and potentially aspiration/penetration. The upstream pressure can be associated with Zenker's diverticulum, which is discussed separately in the diverticulum section in this chapter. Treatment can include endoscopic myomectomy, botulinum toxin injection, or esophageal dilation [26,27].

Imaging Features

On barium studies, prominence of the cricopharyngeus can be seen as a posterior indentation on the esophagus (Fig. 28.14). Some

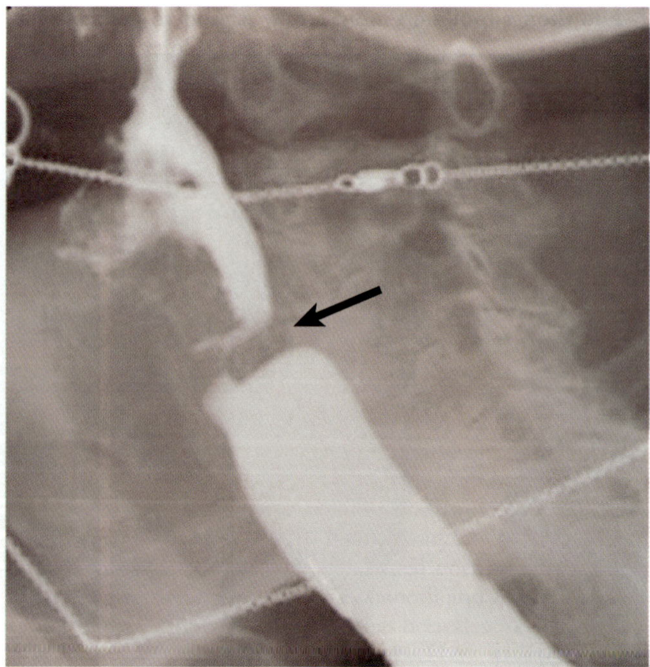

Figure 28.14 Barium swallow demonstrates a posterior indentation on the esophagus at the level of C4–C5 (*black arrow*) compatible with the cricopharyngeal impression.

argue that this can be an incidental finding, while others suggest presence of a cricopharyngeal indentation on any swallow study signifies underlying pathology. If the indentation takes up greater than 50% of the maximal esophageal luminal diameter there can be suggestion that this could be contributing to dysphagia [27].

Benign Strictures

Pathophysiology and Clinical Presentation

Strictures develop from chronic or severe episodes of esophageal inflammation leading to scarring and fibrosis. Benign esophageal strictures are one of the leading causes of dysphagia. Location, appearance, and clinical history play a part in determining the cause. Within the upper to mid-esophagus, etiologies include eosinophilic esophagitis, Barrett's esophagitis, mediastinal radiation, dermatologic conditions (such as bullous pemphigoid or epidermolysis bullosa), drug, and caustic ingestions. Within the distal esophagus, the most common cause of stricture is chronic GERD. Less common causes include prior long-term enteric tube placement or conditions that secondarily cause reflux such as scleroderma (where there is an incompetent lower esophageal sphincter) [28].

Caustic injuries to the esophagus from substances such as lye or acid can lead to some of the most extensive esophageal strictures. Caustic esophagitis leads to stricture formation 1–3 months after the initial insult. Chronic lye strictures are associated with an increased risk of developing esophageal cancer [28]. Depending on the degree of scar formation and severity, there can be segmental or diffuse strictures. Sometimes, this will be so severe as to require esophageal replacement surgery.

Imaging Features

Benign strictures demonstrate smooth margins and are concentric as opposed to eccentric narrowing (Fig. 28.15). Eccentric appearance and shouldered margins are suggestive of a malignant stricture. Retention of barium tablets (13 mm) at the level of the stricture can help to quantify the severity of narrowing. For cervical/upper esophageal strictures, rapid sequence fluoroscopy can be performed as these can be difficult to identify with routine spot images. Ancillary features and clinical history can help elucidate the etiology. For example, a mid-esophageal stricture in the presence of a hiatal hernia and/or reflux disease is suggestive of Barrett's esophagus.

Esophageal Spasm

Pathophysiology and Clinical Presentation

Diffuse esophageal spasm is a motility disorder where there are multiple spontaneous and uncoordinated esophageal contractions. This ineffective form or peristalsis can present with dysphagia or severe chest pain that can last from minutes to hours. It can occur at any age but is most commonly seen in those over the age of 50 [29]. It is often intermittent, occurs in the distal two-thirds of the esophagus and has an association with lower esophageal sphincter dysfunction. Diagnosis is often on the basis of clinical history, esophagography, and most importantly manometry studies. There are multiple treatment options with varied

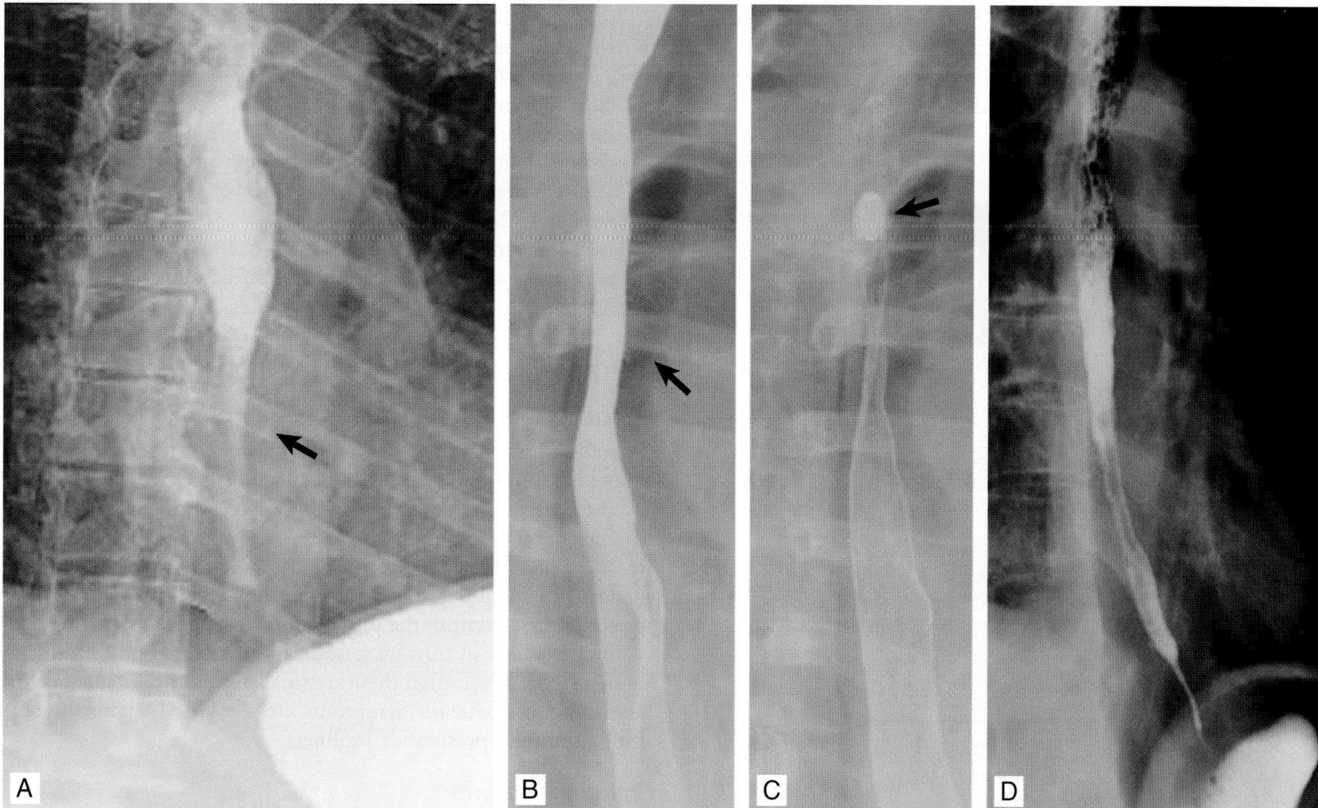

Figure 28.15 Barium swallow (A) shows long segment narrowing of the distal esophagus (*arrow*) compatible with a distal esophageal stricture in the setting of chronic reflux in a patient with Zollinger–Ellison syndrome. In a different patient, there is upper to mid-esophageal narrowing with associated pseudodiverticula (B, *arrow*) from prior radiation therapy for lymphoma. A barium tablet (C, *arrow*) is lodged within the proximal aspect of the stricture indicating the severity. In both cases there is smooth tapering with concentric narrowing suggesting a benign etiology which was confirmed via endoscopy. Long segment esophageal narrowing in patient with history of lye ingestion (D) due to a corrosive stricture.

results, including pharmacotherapy (calcium channel blockers, botulinum long-acting nitrates, anticholinergics), balloon dilation of the lower esophageal sphincter and *botulinum* toxin injection.

Imaging Features

The classic appearance of diffuse esophageal spasm on barium studies is due to repetitive, simultaneous esophageal contractions resulting in obliteration of the lumen producing a "cork screw" appearance (Fig. 28.16). This appearance is only seen in severe cases and it is important to be mindful that patient's can simultaneous contractions of varying amplitude which may not completely obliterate lumen. Additionally, as mentioned above there are associations with impaired opening of the lower esophageal sphincter.

Diverticular Disease

Pathophysiology and Clinical Presentation

Esophageal diverticula are defined by their anatomical location. Diverticula contain one or more layers of the esophageal wall. The three categories of esophageal diverticula are pharyngoesophageal, parabronchial (midthoracic), and epiphrenic. Traction diverticula can occur as a result of surrounding inflammatory process (e.g., tuberculosis, histoplasmosis, or sarcoidosis). Pulsion diverticula occur due to altered pressure gradients within the esophageal lumen. Most diverticula are asymptomatic and discovered incidentally. Overall, esophageal diverticula are rare and most commonly in the seventh to eighth decades of life [30]. Younger patients who get these are often the traction variant due to an adjacent infectious or inflammatory process (e.g., tuberculosis). Symptoms include dysphagia, regurgitation of undigested food, halitosis, and aspiration.

Esophagopharyngeal diverticula are usually pulsion diverticula. The most common type is Zenker's diverticulum, which is a posterior outpouching herniating through an area of congenital weakness proximal to the cricopharyngeus muscle (Killian dehiscence). Killian–Jamieson diverticulum occurs below the level of the cricopharyngeus muscle in the anterolateral wall of the cervical esophagus.

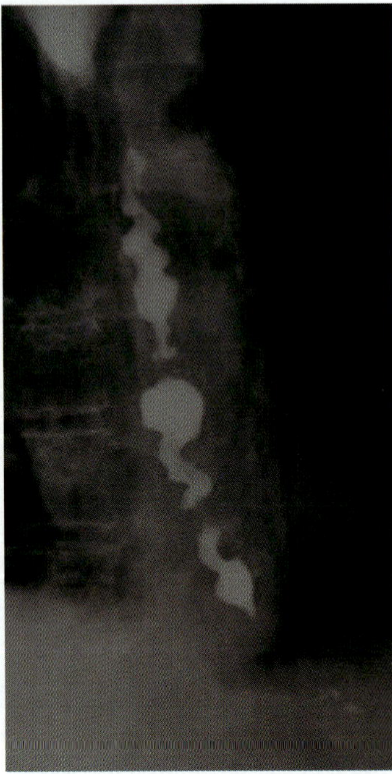

Figure 28.16 Barium swallow demonstrates near complete obliteration of the esophagus with "cork screw" like esophageal filling. In this patient with dysphagia these findings are consistent with diffuse esophageal spasm.

Mid-esophageal diverticula were previously thought to be primarily due to periesophageal adhesions due to inflammation (traction), however now thought to occur commonly from dysmotility. The pathogenesis is theorized to result from a functional distal esophageal obstruction when peristaltic waves encounter a spastic distal esophagus.

Epiphrenic diverticula are pulsion diverticula, which occur due to motility abnormalities and hypertrophy of the circular muscle of the terminal esophagus.

Pseudodiverticulosis is not true diverticula and represent an inflammatory condition where there is dilation of the ducts of submucosal glands related to chronic reflux esophagitis. Patients may require treatment with proton pump inhibitors (PPIs) [25].

Imaging Features

- Traction diverticula commonly have a triangular or tented appearance secondary to the adjacent fibrotic process and occur most commonly in the mid-esophagus (Fig. 28.17A)
- Zenker's diverticula are located posteriorly and above the cricopharyngeus muscle. There can be associated prominent cricopharyngeal impression on the posterior esophagus (cricopharyngeal bar). These diverticula can range from subcentimeter to a few centimeters in size. When these become large, contrast often pools within them on barium swallow examinations (Fig. 28.17B)
- Killian–Jamieson diverticula are smaller, typically less than 2 cm in size, and located anterolaterally and inferior to the cricopharyngeus (Fig. 28.17C) [30]
- Epiphrenic diverticula are usually single and are very large, greater than 5 cm. On plain radiographs, they often appear as a retrocardiac soft tissue opacity with or without an air fluid level (Fig. 28.17D)
- Pseudodiverticulosis appears as 1–5 mm flask-shaped outpouchings arranged longitudinally on barium swallow examinations (Fig. 28.18) [25]

Hernias

Pathophysiology and Clinical Presentation

Hiatal hernias reflect herniation of abdominal structures through the elliptically shaped esophageal hiatal orifice, which is formed by the muscular bands of the right diaphragmatic crus.

The main restraining structure is the phrenoesophageal ligament, which is made from the fascia transversalis that runs beneath the diaphragm and the endothoracic fascia. The amount of elastic tissue within the phrenoesophageal membrane increases with age, which in turn increases laxity that predisposes to hiatal hernias [31]. Most often these are small and found incidentally in asymptomatic patients. Symptoms include GERD, nausea, vomiting, and early postprandial fullness.

Imaging Features

On radiographs, hiatal hernias can present as retrocardiac soft tissue opacities with or without air fluid levels (Fig. 28.19A). Hiatal hernias are often incidentally detected on cross-sectional imaging; however, most often assessed with esophagography.

- Type I hiatal hernias are the most common (80–85%) and referred to as sliding hiatal hernias. There is widening of the

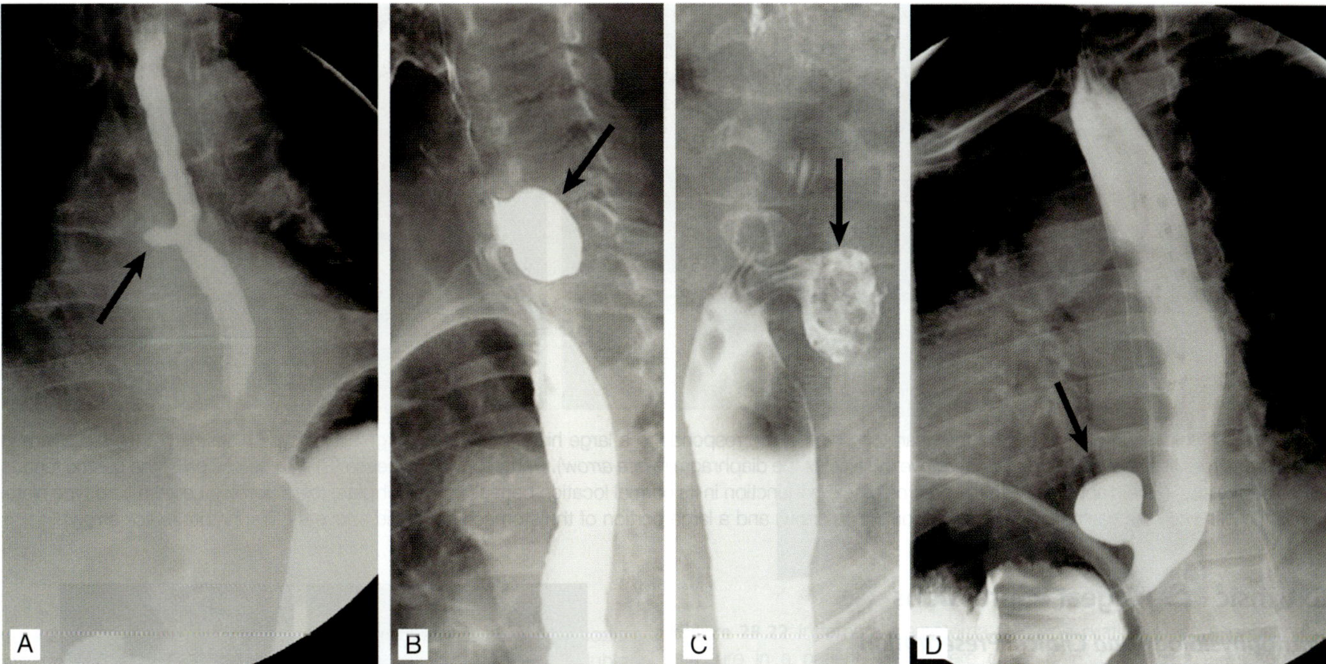

Figure 28.17 Small triangular outpouching from the mid-esophagus in a patient with radiation fibrosis (A) is compatible with a traction diverticulum (*arrow*). Barium swallow in a 75-year-old man with halitosis and regurgitation of undigested food (B) demonstrates a large outpouching filled with barium (*arrow*) arising from the posterior aspect of the cervical esophagus. Both the location and appearance are classic for a Zenker's diverticulum. In a different patient (C), an outpouching filled with barium arising from the anterior and lateral aspect of the cervical esophagus (*arrow*) is compatible with a Killian–Jamieson diverticulum. There are multiple filling defects within the diverticulum from debris. A contrast-filled outpouching arises from the distal esophagus (D) in another patient, situated above the level of the diaphragm compatible with an epiphrenic pulsion diverticulum (*arrow*).

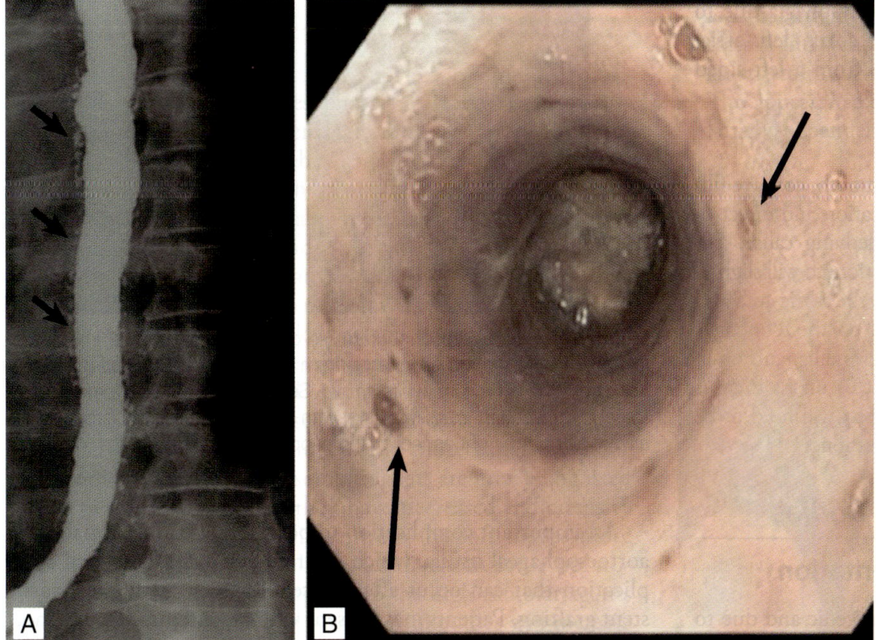

Figure 28.18 Barium swallow shows numerous approximately 1–4 mm flask-shaped outpouchings from the esophageal wall (A, *arrows*) compatible with esophageal pseudodiverticulosis. Upper endoscopy confirms the pseudodiverticula (B, *arrows*). There is also refluxed/residual food material in the distal esophagus (*).

muscular hiatus allowing the gastric cardia to herniate superiorly. For diagnosis, there should be greater than 2 cm of displacement of the gastroesophageal junction (or B ring) above the diaphragmatic hiatus (Fig. 28.19B) [31]

- Type II through IV hernias are variations of paraesophageal hernias. In Type II hernias, there is a localized defect in the phrenoesopahgeal membrane that allows the stomach to herniate above the hiatus but the gastroesophageal junction remains below the diaphragm. In Type I hernias, the gastric cardia is the leading edge of the hernia, while in Type II hernias the fundus is the leading edge (Fig. 28.19C) [31]
- Type III hernias represent a mix of both Type I and II hernias, where there is a paraesophageal hernia as well as superior displacement of the gastroesophageal junction (Fig. 28.19D)
- Type IV hernias are mixed type hernias with inclusion of the abdominal viscera

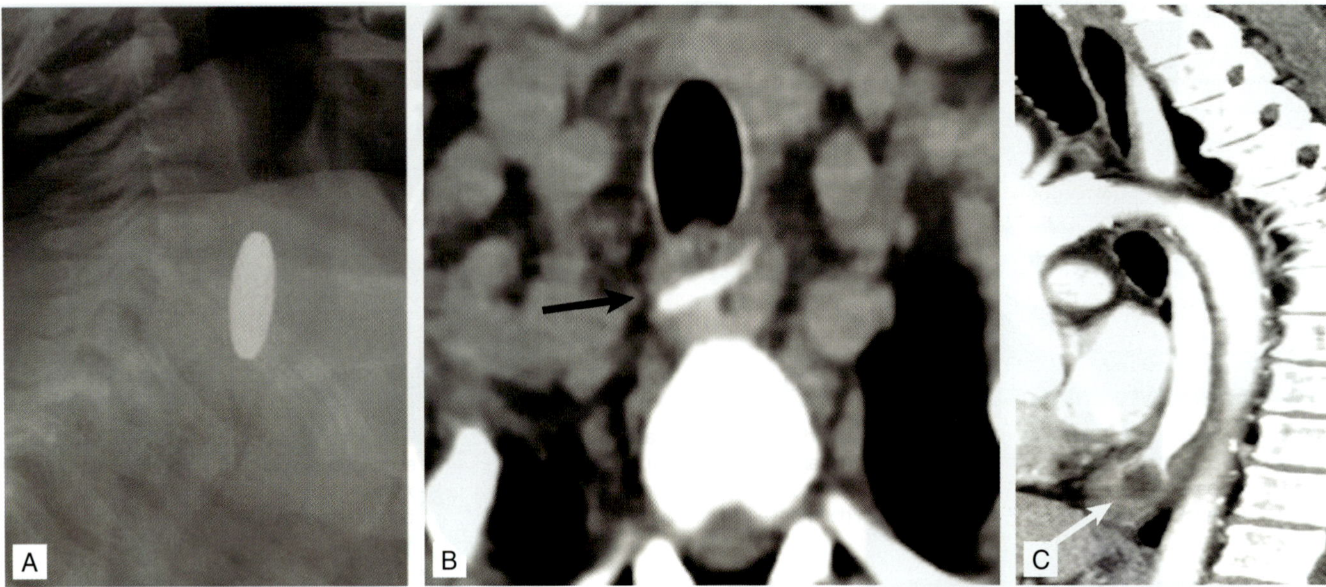

Figure 28.24 Lateral radiograph (A) demonstrates a rounded metallic density projecting anterior to the cervical corresponding to an ingested coin by an infant. Axial CT (B) demonstrates a thin linear hyperdense (*black arrow*) foreign body within the esophagus near the thoracic inlet due to an ingested fish bone. Sagittal section of a CT with oral and intravenous contrast (C) demonstrates a rounded fat attenuating object (*white arrow*) in the distal esophagus which is an impacted meat bolus, resulting in obstruction and pooled contrast within the esophagus above this level.

material (discussed in further detail under the stomach section later in this chapter). In the adult population, common foreign bodies are due to food impaction such as fish bones or meat (Fig. 28.24). In pediatrics, smaller nonedible objects can be encountered including coins

Esophageal Neoplasms

Fibrovascular Polyp

Pathophysiology and Clinical Presentation

Fibrovascular polyps are rare benign slow growing intraluminal tumors of the esophagus which rarely undergo malignant degeneration. They are composed of varying amounts of adipose cells, fibrovascular tissue, and stroma. Most commonly, they arise from the upper third of the esophagus near the level of the cricopharyngeus muscle [34].

Fibrovascular polyps can become quite large and extend to the distal third of the esophagus or prolapse into the stomach. Symptoms include dysphagia, hematemesis, weight loss, and respiratory symptoms. Polyps with long stalks can regurgitate into the pharynx and cause death from asphyxiation.

Imaging Features

- On esophogography, there will be a smooth, sausage-shaped expansile intraluminal filling defect within the upper or middle third of the esophagus. There should be free passage of barium on all sides of the lesion and absence of asymmetrical narrowing of the esophageal lumen [35]
- CT will demonstrate a long, pedunculated mass extending into the distal esophagus. Attenuation will vary with lower areas of attenuation corresponding to adipose tissue and higher areas of attenuation representing fibrovascular component (Fig. 28.25). High signal intensity on T1 weight imaging is typical and is due to the presence of adipose tissue. If this persists on fat-suppressed sequences, it may represent foci of hemorrhage [36]

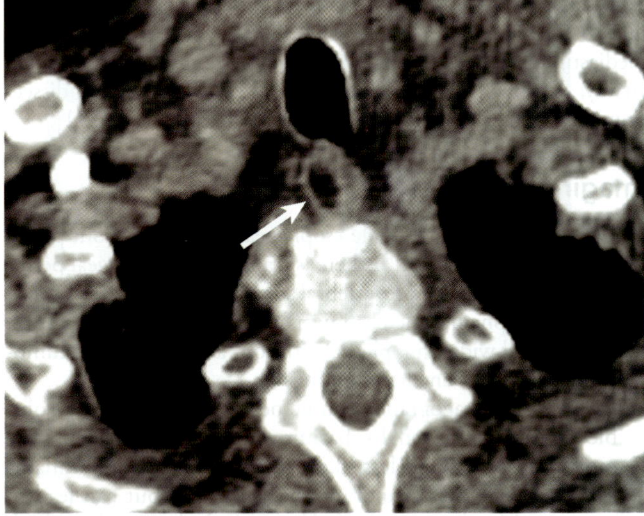

Figure 28.25 Axial CT of the chest with intravenous contrast shows a smooth oval submucosal fat attenuation mass in the cervical esophagus (*arrow*) consistent with a fibrovascular polyp.

Leiomyoma

Pathophysiology and Clinical Presentation

Leiomyomas are the most common benign esophageal tumor, although relatively rare with an incidence of 8–43 per 10,000 on autopsy and 50 times less common than esophageal carcinoma [37, 38]. Unlike malignant tumors, patients often have long-standing symptoms (>2 years) of dysphagia and odynophagia. They are usually less than 3 cm in size and located within the middle and lower thirds of the esophagus where the esophagus is lined by smooth muscle cells [38]. Arise from the muscularis mucosa or muscularis propria, with 97% being intramural [38].

Imaging Features

- With upper gastrointestinal studies, leiomyomas appear as broad based, eccentric but smooth elevations of the mucosa owing to their intramural location (Fig. 28.26)
- On CT, they are smoothly marginated, round, or ovoid homogenous hypoattenuating lesions that mirror the attenuation of the chest wall musculature. Occasionally, they may have internal calcification, but almost never have necrosis or cystic degeneration

Esophageal Carcinoma

Pathophysiology and Clinical Presentation

The two most common subtypes of esophageal carcinoma are squamous cell carcinoma (SCC) and adenocarcinoma. The esophagus is lined by squamous cells, so SCC is the predominant histologic subtype of esophageal cancer worldwide. The incidence of SCC increases with age, peaking in the seventh decade of life, and is four times more likely in African-American men. Incidence has been decreasing, most likely due to decreasing tobacco consumption [38,39]. The main independent risk factors for developing SCC include excessive alcohol consumption and long-term cigarette smoking. Other predisposing conditions include prior radiation, Plummer Vinson syndrome, achalasia, or prior caustic esophageal injuries. Adenocarcinoma typically arises in the distal esophagus almost always due to Barrett's esophagus which increases the risk of developing cancer 50–100 times compared to the general population. In the Western population, adenocarcinoma has begun to surpass SCC as the predominant histologic subtype. As opposed to SCC, adenocarcinoma is five times more prevalent in white men [38,39].

The most common symptoms of SCC or adenocarcinoma are dysphagia and unintentional weight loss. At the time of clinical presentation, metastasis has usually already occurred. The rapid spread of tumor is due to a rich lymphatic supply and lack of a serosal layer surrounding the esophagus.

Assessment of cancer location is made during endoscopy and defined by the epicenter of the lesion. For treatment planning, it is important to identify the upper border for cancers of the upper thoracic esophagus and lower borders for lower esophageal and esophagogastric cancers. The most important prognostic features of esophageal cancer are the depth of tumor penetration and lymph node involvement. This refers to high-grade dysplasia confined to the basement membrane.

- T1 is invasion of the lamina propria, muscularis mucosa, or submucosa
- T2 is invasion of the muscularis propria
- T3 is invasion of the adventitia
- T4 is invasion of adjacent structures including the pleura, pericardium, diaphragm (4a), or aorta, vertebral body, or trachea (4b)

An important point to mention is description of the degree of aortic invasion if present which will classify as T4b disease and preclude resection. A suggested marker to use is indicating the angle of contact and can be subclassified by:

- No contact
- <45°—no aortic invasion
- 45–90°—indeterminate
- Greater than 90°—aortic invasion

Nodal metastasis is classified according to number of positive regional nodes (N0: 0, N1: 1–2, N2: 3–6 regional nodes, and N3: >7). Nodal metastasis is purely classified on number of metastasis regardless of location of the primary esophageal cancer. Locoregional lymph nodes can range from lower cervical and paratracheal lymph nodes superiorly to gastrohepatic and celiac axis nodes within the abdomen. M0 refers to absent of metastases and M1 is divided into M1a (cervical lymphadenopathy in upper esophageal cancer or celiac lymphadenopathy in lower esophageal cancer) or M1b (all other distant metastases) [40].

Currently, there is no single test sufficient for the workup of esophageal cancer. There are no recommendations regarding using PET/CT over CT, or vice versa. Often the order of testing is variable depending on presentation, availability, and cost. A common strategy is to first pursue EGD with or without endoscopic ultrasound (EUS) to determine cell type and evaluate for tumor invasion/regional lymphadenopathy. CT and/or PET/CT can be performed to asses for tumor extension beyond the esophagus in higher T stages, as well as identify distant nodal or solid organ metastases [41]. Lymph nodes greater than 1 cm in short axis on CT are suspicious for metastasis, although this can under estimate the disease burden. Smaller nodes with increased FDG uptake can be detected on PET increasing sensitivity of nodal detection. PET/CT has lower spatial resolution than conventional CT and can underestimate presence of nodes adjacent to the primary lesion. Often, both techniques are used synergistically. Ultimately, nodal staging is made at the time of dissection if the patient is a surgical candidate.

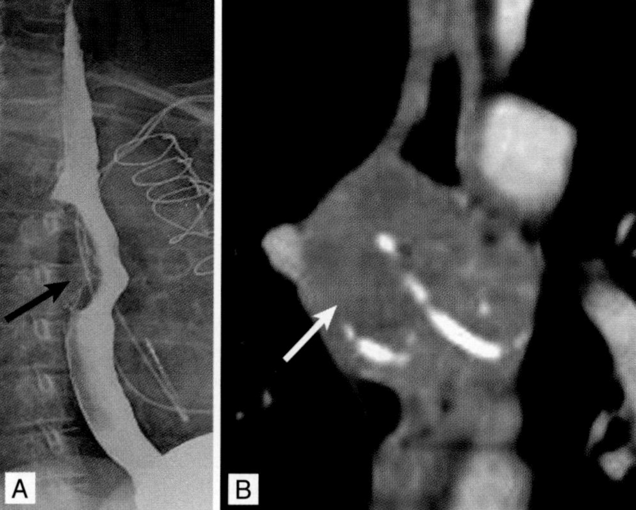

Figure 28.26 Barium swallow (A) in a patient with dysphagia shows an eccentric smooth filling defect (*arrow*) in the mid-esophagus. Coronal CT of the chest (B) with intravenous contrast shows a partially calcified enhancing mass in the wall of the esophagus (*arrow*) consistent with a leiomyoma.

Imaging Features

- Barium studies may be the first test performed in the evaluation of dysphagia. Esophageal cancers can present as polypoid, infiltrative, varicoid, or ulcerating lesions (Fig. 28.27). Nodularity of the mucosa can be seen in cancers with a superficial spreading pattern. Adenocarcinomas in the distal esophagus tend to invade the gastric cardia and fundus, which is not seen with SCC that typically occurs in the upper to mid-esophagus [42]
- When the esophagus is distended normal wall thickness should be less than 3 mm, with any thickness greater than 5 mm usually pathologic in nature. T1 and T2 esophageal tumors appear as subtle asymmetric thickening of the esophagus on CT. Thus, PET/CT and endoscopy with EUS are superior compared to conventional CT in detection of T1 and T2 lesions. Cross-sectional imaging is helpful in

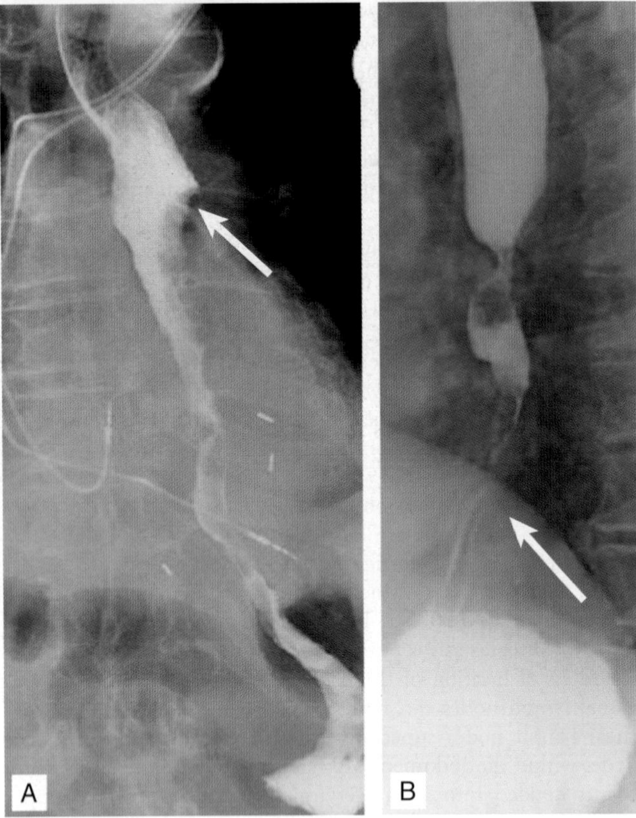

Figure 28.27 Esophogram (A) demonstrates irregular narrowing of the mid to distal esophagus with shouldered margins (*white arrow*). This lesion was proven to be a SCC by endoscopic biopsy. Esophogram in a separate patient (B) demonstrates irregular narrowing of the distal esophagus proven to be adenocarcinoma in biopsy.

identifying locoregional invasion which would upstage the patient's disease (Fig. 28.28) [43]

- PET/CT can be used for locoregional staging, evaluating for metastasis, and to evaluate response to neoadjuvant chemotherapy. With conventional CT or PET/CT, normal lymph nodes are typically less than 10 mm in short-axis diameter, have a smooth and well-defined border, and contain a fatty hilum. However, using this criterion alone, one can both over and under stage nodal disease. False positives include nodes enlarged due to inflammation and false negatives include nodes normal by size criteria containing metastases [42]
- EUS is the preferred technique to assess for determining degree of tumor invasion. On EUS, the specific layers of the esophageal wall are seen by alternating hyperechoic and hypoechoic layers. Additionally, EUS has greater accuracy rates for assessing for metastatic lymph nodes (72–80%) compared to conventional CT (46–58%) [41]. Ultrasound relies on both the size of the node (>1 cm) but also the intrinsic nodal echogenicity. Nodes with a round, sharply demarcated border, and hypoechogenicity are more likely to be metastatic in nature. EUS can also allow for FNA for cytologic confirmation

Postsurgical Esophagus

Description and Imaging Appearance: Surgery remains the standard of care in patients with early stage esophageal cancer. One of the most commonly performed approaches for esophagectomy for treatment of mid to lower esophageal carcinomas is the Ivor Lewis procedure (Fig. 28.29A). In this surgery, there is an initial laparotomy to mobilize the stomach and esophagus at the diaphragmatic hiatus, followed by celiac trunk lymph node dissection and pyloromyotomy to prevent GOO due to postvagotomy pylorospasm. Then, the patient is positioned in the left lateral decubitus position and a posterolateral thoracotomy is performed to divide the azygos and en-bloc resect the esophagus, thoracic duct, and other adjacent structures. Periesophageal, aortopulmonary, and subcarinal nodes are often dissected. Finally, the gastric conduit is pulled into the chest and anastomosed above the level of the azygos vein. Higher anastomoses are preferred to achieve adequate surgical margins and reduce gastroesophageal reflux [44].

A rarer major esophageal surgery is the esophageal bypass surgery (Fig. 28.29B and C). This provides an alternative passageway for food in the setting of esophageal obstruction, whether it be due to malignancy, strictures, or motility issues. Options for bypass conduits include the stomach, jejunum, and colon. There are multiple routes

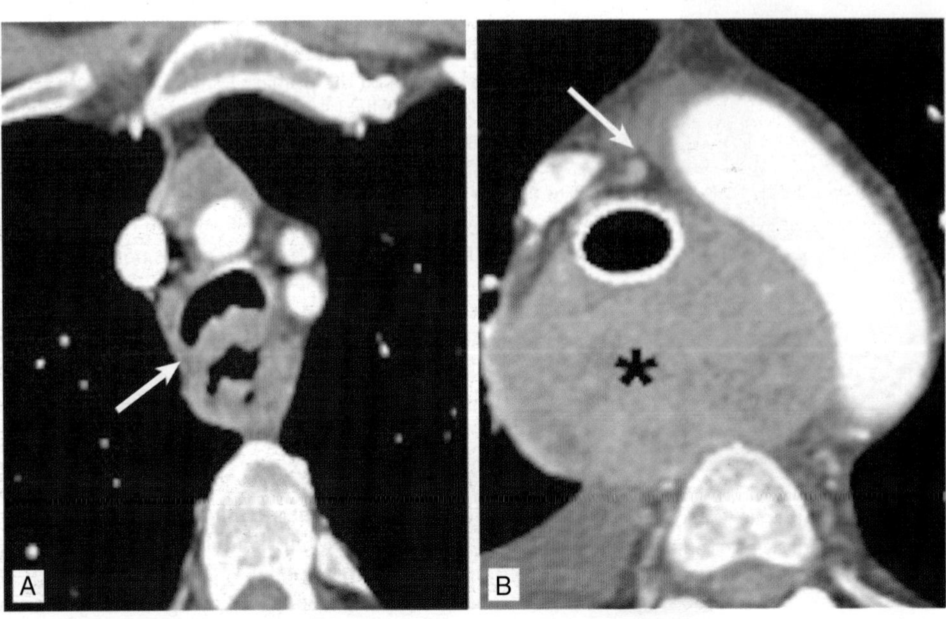

Figure 28.28 Axial CT of the chest with contrast (A) shows irregular, eccentric esophageal thickening with soft tissue invading into the posterior tracheal wall (*white arrow*). This was biopsy and proven to be esophageal SCC with local invasion. Axial CT of the chest with contrast in a separate patient (B) demonstrates a large heterogeneously enhancing esophageal mass partially encasing the trachea which contains a stent and with long segment (>90°) abutment of the aortic arch (*white arrow*).

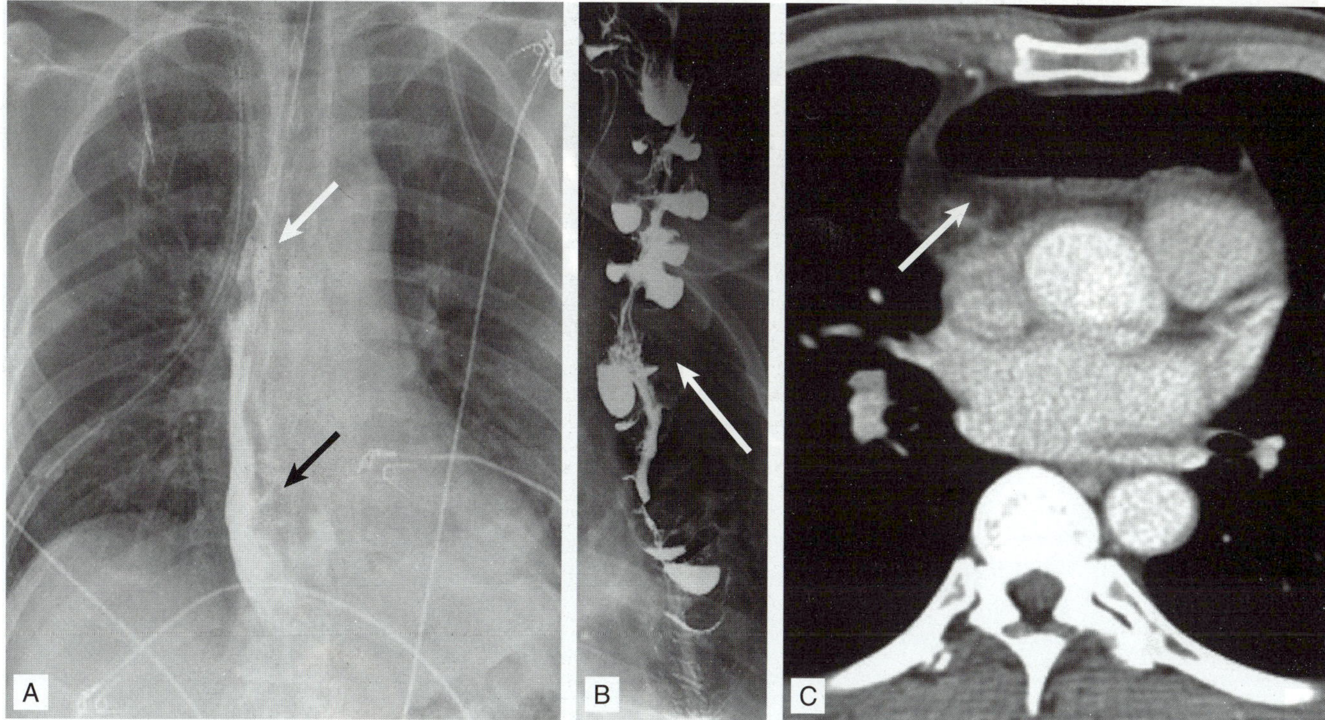

Figure 28.29 Chest radiograph (A) of a patient who has undergone Ivor-Lewis esophagectomy for adenocarcinoma showing normal appearance of contrast within the intrathoracic stomach (*black arrow*) and a nasogastric tube (*white arrow*) terminating in the thoracic stomach. Esophogram (B) in a patient who has undergone esophageal bypass for a long segment esophageal stricture due to Lysol ingestion shows interposition of the transverse colon (*arrow*) in this case. CT (C) further demonstrates transposition of the transverse colon (*arrow*) within the anterior mediastinum.

including most commonly the substernal and less commonly posterior mediastinal or subcutaneous approaches. One important benefit of the substernal approach is anatomical separation from tumor when bypass is performed in the setting of malignancy [44].

Much of the postoperative appearance for esophagectomy (Fig. 28.29) depends on both the choice of conduit (stomach, small bowel, or colon) and the location (most commonly in the posterior mediastinum for Ivor Lewis esophagectomy and substernal for bypass surgeries). It is important to interrogate the site of anastomoses if performed for malignancy to evaluate for recurrence (Fig. 28.30).

Stomach—Inflammatory Conditions

Gastritis

Pathophysiology and Clinical Presentation

Gastritis is focal, segmental, or diffuse mucosal inflammation of the stomach, which can present with loss of appetite, nausea, vomiting, and epigastric pain. The most common cause is nonsteroid anti-inflammatory drugs, *Helicobacter pylori* infection or severe systemic illnesses. The gastric mucosa is protected by mucus production, bicarbonate secretion, and ion exchange at the cell surface.

NSAIDS disrupt prostaglandin synthesis, which decreases gastric blood flow reducing bicarbonate and mucin secretion. Similarly, systemic processes, such as traumatic brain injuries, systemic shock, and burn injuries, result in mucosal ischemia and stress-induced hemorrhage.

H. pylori is a helical gram-negative bacterium that colonizes the gastric mucosa (most frequently the gastric antrum) and can penetrate into the intercellular spaces. It is found in more than 50% of adults greater than the age of 60. Chronic colonization leads to prolonged antigen exposure, which in turn can lead to the development of low-grade gastric mucosal associated lymphoid tissue lymphomas [45].

Imaging Features

- On upper gastrointestinal series, manifestations of gastritis include mucosal erosions and gastric fold thickening. Erosions are 1–5 mm punctate, linear, or stellate collections of barium due to a focal area of mucosal necrosis, which histologically does not extend through the muscularis mucosae [45]
- CT is often the first test performed in patients who present with nonspecific abdominal symptoms and can be the first study to suggest gastritis. The most common finding on CT is gastric fold thickening. Generally speaking, greater than 5 mm of thickness is suggestive of gastric pathology, however this can vary with the degree of luminal distension. The gastric antrum can measure up to 12 mm in normal patients. With severe gastritis there can be stratification of the bowel layers with hyperenhancing mucosa and muscularis with intervening hypoattenuating submucosal edema (Fig. 28.31) [46,47]

Gastric Ulcers

Pathophysiology and Clinical Presentation

Unlike erosions, gastric ulcers are mucosal defects which penetrate through the muscularis mucosa. Most commonly, these are due to *Helicobacter pylori* and NSAID usage. With the advent of H2 receptor antagonists, PPIs and *H. pylori* treatment, peptic ulcer disease incidence has decreased but still affects approximately 10% of the world's population [47]. Symptoms include dyspepsia,

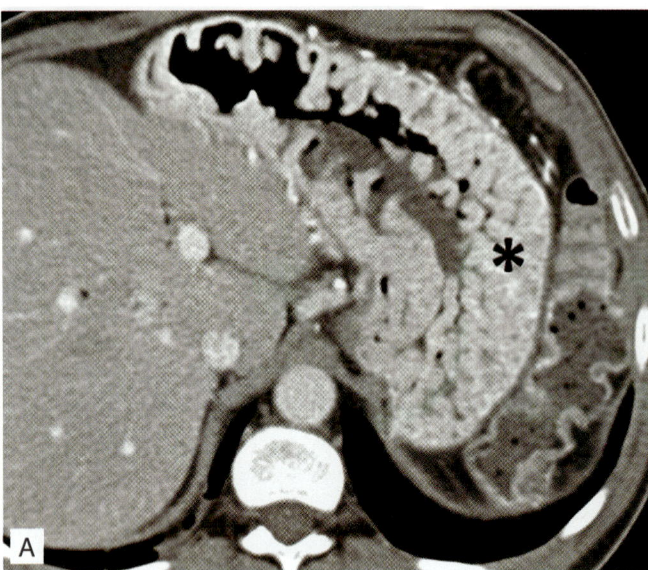

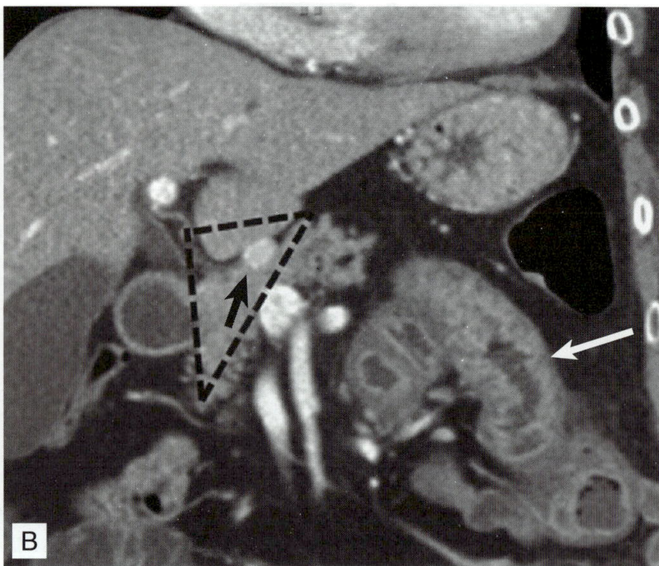

Figure 28.33 Axial CT of the abdomen with contrast (A) shows diffuse rugal fold thickening of the gastric body and antrum (*). Coronal CT of the abdomen with contrast (B) shows diffuse postbulbar enteritis (*arrow*) within the distal duodenum and proximal jejunum. There is a hyperenhancing nodule (*black arrow*) within the gastrinoma triangle (dotted black lines) representing a gastrinoma. Constellation of findings is compatible with Zollinger–Ellison syndrome.

Imaging Features

The hallmark of Menetrier's disease is massive foveolar hyperplasia with relative sparing of the antrum. On fluoroscopy, there are giant and tortuous rugal folds in a pattern described similar to the convolutions of the brain. Linear strands of barium contrast can become trapped between the enlarged folds [54,55]. Similarly, on CT, the thickened gastric rugae protrude into the gastric lumen, with relative sparing of the antrum (Fig. 28.34). The stomach is often distended due to increased gastric secretions.

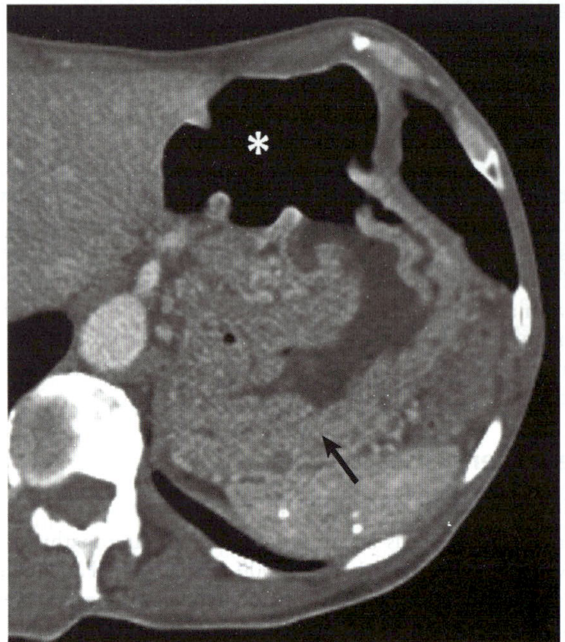

Figure 28.34 A 52-year-old man with hypoalbunemia. Axial CT of the abdomen with contrast shows marked rugal fold thickening involving fundus and body (*arrow*) with relative sparing of the antrum (*) compatible with Menetrier's disease.

Crohn's Disease

Pathophysiology and Clinical Presentation

Crohn's disease is a granulomatous process with transmural involvement. Although the small bowel and colon are the most common sites of disease, there is an estimated 0.5–4% prevalence of gastroduodenal involvement. Most patients with Crohn's disease of the stomach are asymptomatic. Symptoms include epigastric pain, anorexia, weight loss, nausea, and vomiting. Given overlap with symptoms of small and large bowel Crohn's (covered in detail in another chapter), as well as misattribution of symptoms to medication side effect, a high clinical suspicion along with radiographic and endoscopic findings is required to diagnose gastric involvement [56,57]. Complications of gastric Crohn's include GOO due to strictures and fistulization between the stomach and duodenum or colon. About 30% of patients with gastrocolic fistulas report with a triad of diarrhea, feculent vomiting, and weight loss [56].

Imaging Features

- Features of gastric Crohn's on fluoroscopy include thickening or cobblestoning of the gastric mucosa, apthoid ulcers, strictures, and fistula formation most commonly with the duodenum and transverse colon [56]
- Apthous ulcers can appear slit-like and punctate, mimicking erosive gastritis
- Chronic inflammation leads to nondistension and smooth appearance of the antrum, widened pylorus, and narrowed bulb, also known as the rams horn sign on upper GI examination [58,59]

Vascular

Gastric Varices

Pathophysiology and Clinical Presentation

Gastric varices occur due to reversal of flow in the gastric fundal venous plexus, which is most commonly due to portal hypertension in the setting of cirrhosis or splenic vein thrombosis from pancreatitis. The short gastric veins drain the fundus into the splenic vein, the gastric veins drain directly into the portal vein along the lesser curvature, while the right and left gastroepiploic veins drain into the superior mesenteric and splenic veins, respectively [60].

Gastric varices are present in 5–33% of patients with portal hypertension, the most common cause of which is hepatic cirrhosis [61]. Gastric varices bleed less commonly than esophageal varices, 25% versus 64%; however, given the large size and greater flow, gastric variceal bleeding carries higher morbidity with a mortality rate of approximately 45% [61]. Two distinct forms of gastric fundal varices are seen: submucosal and perigastric (adventitial). Almost all cases of fundal variceal bleeding are due to the submucosal variant [62].

Imaging Features

- On upper gastrointestinal series, gastric varices appear as thickened, tortuous folds, most commonly within the gastric fundus. A conglomeration of varices can produce lobulated submucosal mass-like appearance that can be mistaken for polypoid gastric malignancy [62].
- With CT, one can not only detect submucosal varices but also evaluate for the underlying cause such as changes of pancreatitis and splenic vein thrombosis or findings of cirrhosis. Additionally, CT aids in evaluating afferent and efferent venous vasculature which can be useful in the setting of any planned intervention (e.g., balloon occluded retrograde transvenous obliteration). On contrast-enhanced CT, gastric varices appear as multiple enhancing tubular vessels conforming to the contour of the stomach (Fig. 28.35) [63].

Arteriovenous Malformation

Pathophysiology and Clinical Presentation

Gastric arteriovenous malformation (AVM) is an uncommon source of upper gastrointestinal bleeding, representing 1.4% of all intestinal AVMs [64]. They are often confused with gastrointestinal ectasias which occur in elderly patients. AVMs are congenital lesions present from birth with persistent direct connections between arteries and veins. They are more commonly seen in patients with Osler–Weber–Rendu syndrome (hereditary hemorrhagic telangiectasia).

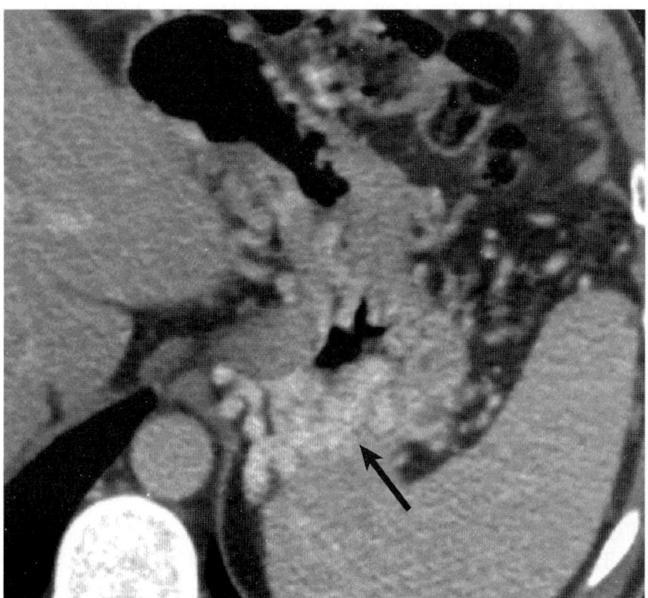

Figure 28.35 Axial CT of the abdomen with contrast in a patient with chronic pancreatitis and splenic vein thrombosis. Multiple dilated, serpiginous structures are seen along the gastric submucosa and perigastric region (*arrow*) compatible with gastric varices.

Imaging Features

AVMs result in dilated submucosal arteries and veins which can simulate variceal disease. On multiphase CTA, there will be early venous opacification with contrast seen on the arterial phase of the examination due to the direct arteriovenous connection (Fig. 28.36). CT can define extramural extent of the malformation that will not be appreciated on endoscopy and therefore very useful in surgical or pre-embolization planning [65,66].

Gastric Artery Aneurysm

Pathophysiology and Clinical Presentation

Gastric and gastroepiploic artery aneurysms are rare comprising 4% of all abdominal visceral aneurysms. Spontaneous rupture can lead to massive hemorrhage, with a mortality estimated to be greater than 70% [67]. Patients can have chronic unexplained left upper quadrant pain or be asymptomatic with incidental detection. Etiologies include atherosclerotic disease, trauma, vasculitis, infection, or adjacent to inflammatory processes such as pancreatitis or peptic ulcer disease [68].

While a true vascular aneurysm contains all three layers of the vessel wall (intima, media, and adventitia), a pseudoaneurysm contains only the adventitial layer with weak integrity and increased risk of rupture. The majority of gastric artery aneurysms are along the lesser curvature involving left or right gastric arteries, as opposed to the epiploic vessels along the greater curvature with a reported 10:1 ratio [69].

Imaging Features

- On a noncontrast CT, aneurysms will be a rounded soft tissue structure of varying attenuation depending on their degree of thrombosis. Thrombosed segments will be higher attenuation on noncontrast imaging. With injection of

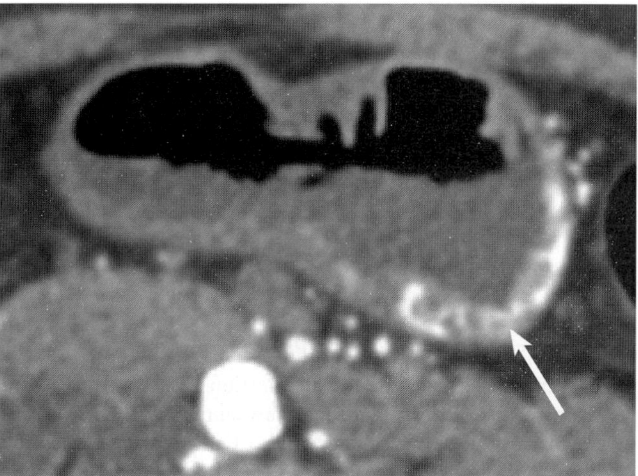

Figure 28.36 Axial CT of the abdomen with contrast shows enhancing serpiginous tangle of vessels (*arrow*) representing a gastric arteriovenous malformation in this patient with Osler–Weber–Rendu syndrome.

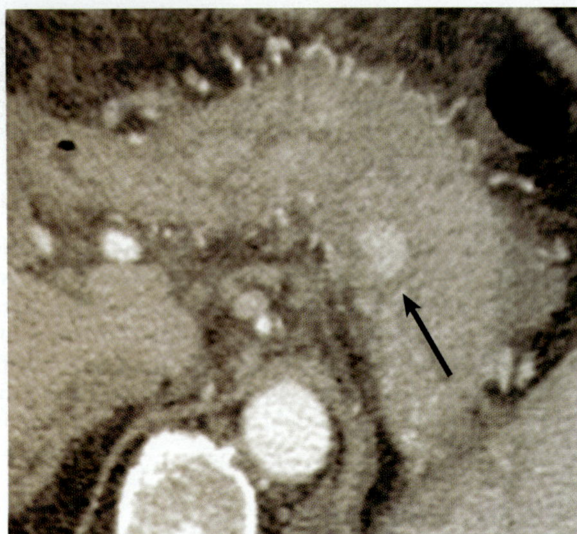

Figure 28.37 Axial CT of the abdomen with contrast in a patient with acute alcohol-induced pancreatitis and hematemesis shows an enhancing round lesion (*arrow*) along the lesser curvature of the stomach representing a left gastric artery aneurysm.

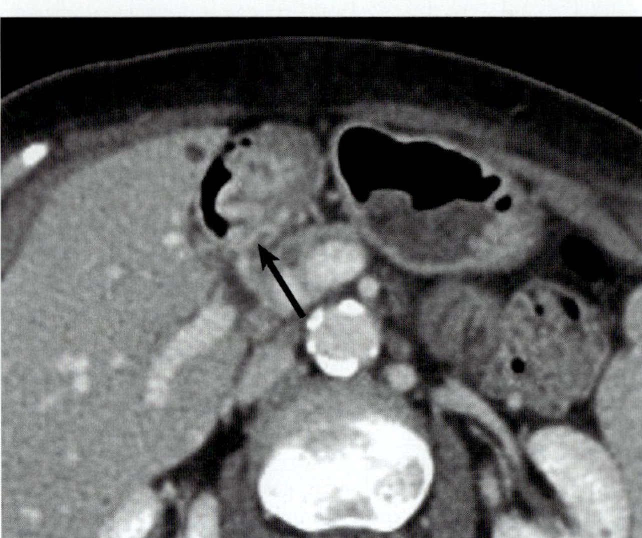

Figure 28.38 Axial CT of the abdomen with contrast of a 79-year-old woman with melena. There is antral thickening (*arrow*) with alternating bands of attenuation that was proven as gastric antral vascular ectasia on endoscopy.

contrast, the nonthrombosed aspects of the aneurysm will follow the attenuation of the aorta on multiphase examinations (Fig. 28.37)

Gastric Antral Vascular Ectasia

Pathophysiology and Clinical Presentation

Gastric antral vascular ectasia (GAVE) is a rare and often underdiagnosed vascular condition involving the gastric antrum that may lead to chronic occult bleeding or acute hemorrhage in older patients. The cause is unknown, but one proposed theory is that gastric peristalsis results in prolapse of the loose antral mucosa resulting in elongation and ectasia of vessels [70]. GAVE is most commonly seen in middle aged or older women. There is an association with CREST syndrome, atrophic gastritis, autoimmune, and connective tissue disorders. About 40% of reported cases of GAVE are associated with portal hypertension or cirrhosis [70].

Imaging Features

Tortuous, dilated submucosal vessels radiating from the pylorus lead to alternating bands of hyperemic and normal mucosa on endoscopy, akin to the stripes on the surface of a watermelon, hence referred to as "watermelon stomach." On upper gastrointestinal series and CT there are thickened, scalloped mucosal folds extending from the gastric antrum to the pylorus (Fig. 28.38) [71,72].

Emphysematous Gastritis and Gastric Emphysema

Pathophysiology and Clinical Presentation

Emphysematous gastritis (EG) is an infection of the gastric wall due to gas-forming organisms with high mortality and often requiring emergent surgical management with partial or total gastrectomy. Many organisms have been associated with EG, including gram positive, gram negative, anaerobic, and fungal. There are associations with diabetes mellitus, corrosive ingestion, vasoocclusive disease resulting in ischemia or acute gastroenteritis [73].

In benign gastric emphysema (interstitial gastric emphysema) air is introduced into the gastric wall following trauma to the gastric mucosa or due to air entering via mucosal defects in the setting of GOO. It can also be seen with patients undergoing chemo- or immunotherapy [74]. Gastric emphysema is a benign and self-limiting process that resolves with conservative management. On the other hand, EG presents with shock, severe abdominal pain, fever, and hematemesis [73].

Imaging Features

It is difficult to differentiate the two entities with imaging alone. In both conditions, there will be focal or diffuse intramural gas which outlines the contour of the stomach. This can be seen on radiographs and CT. Gastric distension is often associated with both entities, however ancillary features such as rugal fold thickening, portal venous gas, fluid collections, or surrounding perigastric fat stranding should prompt consideration of EG especially in patients with a toxic clinical picture (Fig. 28.39A). If the patient is clinically well, gastric emphysema should be the primary consideration (Fig. 28.39B). Serial radiographs can be obtained that will show a gradual decrease and eventual resolution of intramural gas.

Gastric Ischemia

Pathophysiology and Clinical Presentation

Ischemia of the stomach is uncommon given its rich collateral blood supply discussed in the anatomy section. Gastric ischemia can result from diffuse or local vascular insufficiency. Causes include systemic hypotension, vasculitis, thromboembolism or vascular stenosis, vasoconstriction, or volvulus. It can manifest with acute abdominal pain or chronic abdominal angina [75].

Imaging Features

- The most common finding is gastric wall thickening. With contrast administration, the target sign may be seen as alternating high and low attenuation layers resulting from submucosal edema. Findings seen later in the course of ischemia include diminished gastric wall enhancement, pneumatosis, portal venous gas, and gastric distension with thinning of the

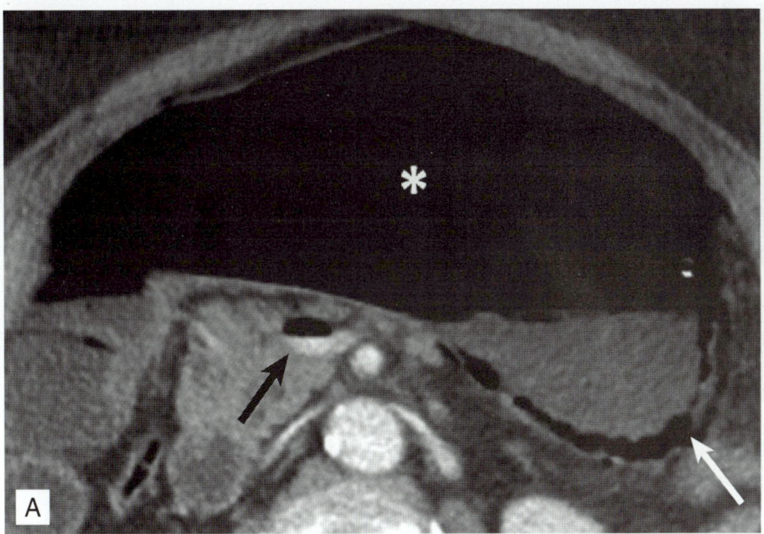

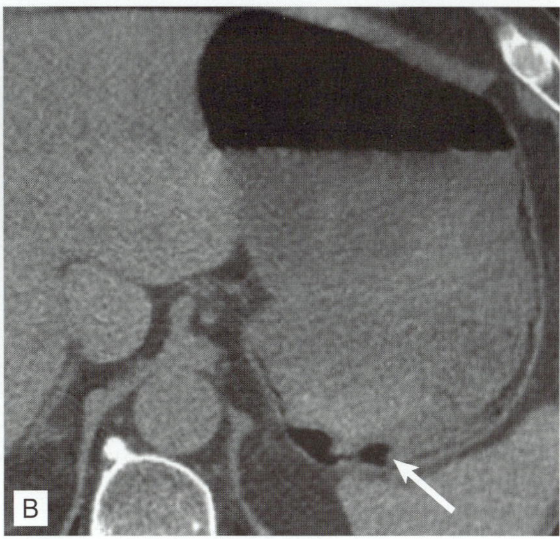

Figure 28.39 Axial CT of the abdomen with contrast in a patient with septic shock (A) shows a markedly distended stomach (*) with diffuse foci of intramural gas (*white arrow*) representing EG. Gas is also seen in the superior mesenteric vein (*black arrow*). A partial gastrectomy revealed transmural necrosis of the fundus and lesser curvature. Axial CT of the abdomen without intravenous contrast (B) in a patient with gastric outlet obstruction. There is gas within the wall of the stomach (*arrow*) without evidence of portal venous gas or pneumoperitoneum. Increased pressure due to gastric outlet obstruction resulted in benign gastric emphysema that resolved once obstruction was relieved.

gastric wall (Fig. 28.40). Free intraperitoneal air is indicative of transmural perforation [75]

- With vascular etiologies, one may see arterial occlusion in the setting of chronic atherosclerotic arterial insufficiency, thromboembolism, or dissection. Alternatively, venous thrombosis or volvulus will show significant mesenteric edema and mesenteric venous engorgement due to outflow obstruction [75]

Mechanical Gastric Disease

Foreign Bodies and Bezoars

Pathophysiology and Clinical Presentation

While uncommon, foreign bodies are an important and often challenging diagnosis to make. Populations at risk include children, psychiatric or mentally handicapped patients, adults with unusual sexual or criminal behavior, trauma patients, and those with accidental ingestions. It is important to note that sharp and elongated objects can predispose to bowel wall injury and perforation. Objects such as magnets can result in bowel wall necrosis and erosion if they are in adjacent loops of bowel. Batteries can lead to corrosive mucosal bowel injury with bowel wall necrosis and perforation [76].

Bezoars are an accumulation of ingested foreign or undigested food material within the gastrointestinal tract named by the materials that form them. The most common include: trichobezoars which are formed of hair and seen in patients with trichotillomania, and phytobezoars which are composed of poorly digested fruit and vegetable fibers in patients with gastroparesis. The most common presentation in these cases is bowel obstruction [77].

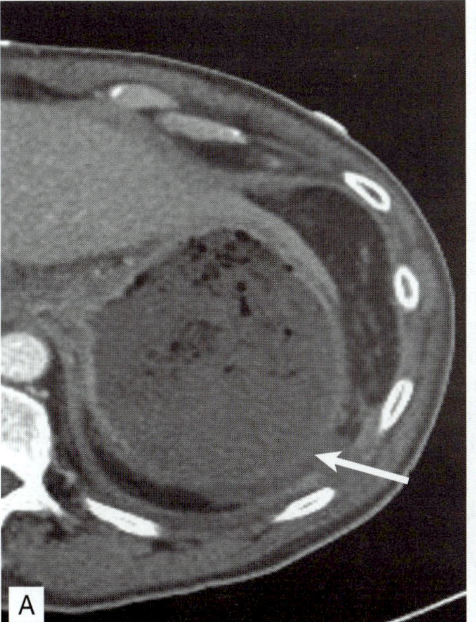

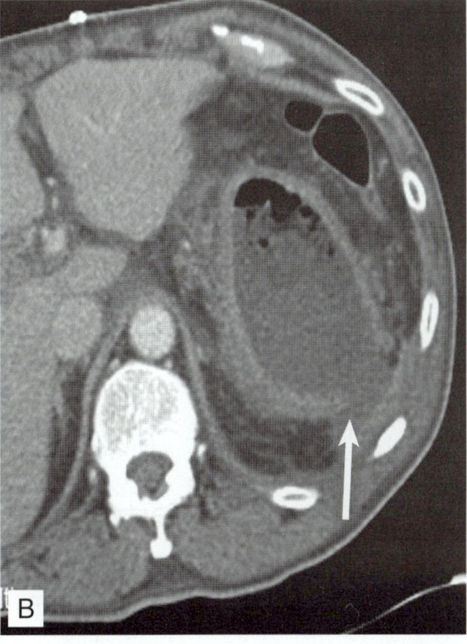

Figure 28.40 Axial CT of abdomen with contrast (A) of a 40-year-old man who is recently status post-Whipple surgery. There is loss of normal gastric rugal fold pattern and hypoenhancement of the wall at the fundus (*arrow*) with surrounding fat stranding. CT performed 3 days later (B) shows a nonenhancing transmural defect (*arrow*) with extraluminal fluid consistent with perforation form gastric ischemia.

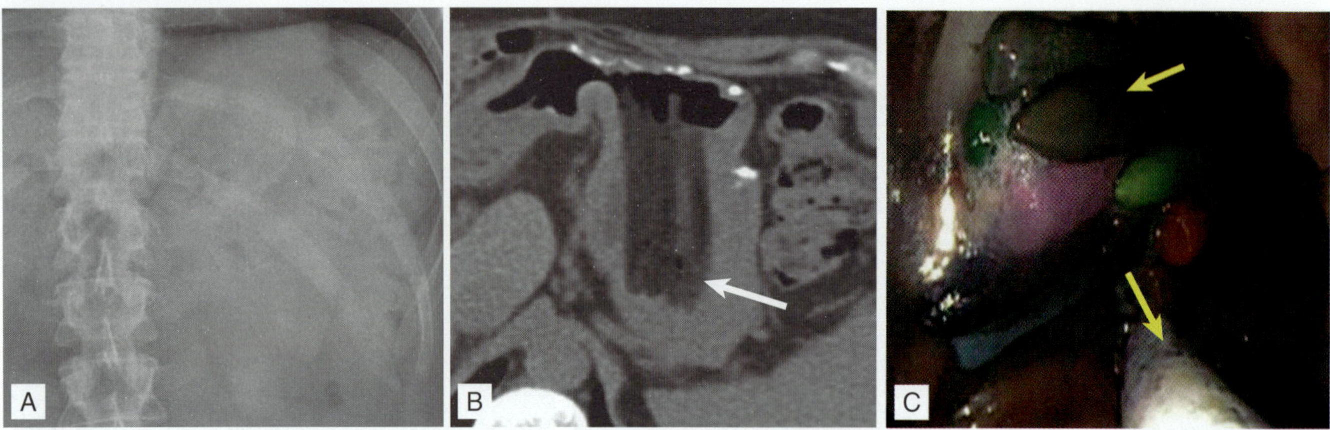

Figure 28.41 Abdominal radiograph (A) shows no radiopaque foreign bodies in a suspected case. Axial CT of the abdomen without contrast (B) confirms multiple linear foreign bodies of fat density (*arrows*), which were confirmed to be crayons on endoscopy (C).

A body packer is a drug courier who conceals packages of illicit drugs within their alimentary tract. Increased sophistication of drug traffickers and variety of packaging materials can make diagnosis difficult. In the setting of package perforation, patients can present with florid overdose of the illicit drug [78].

Imaging Features

- Radiographs are initial imaging technique to diagnose and follow-up ingested foreign bodies. Visibility on radiographs is incumbent both on the attenuation characteristics of the foreign body, surrounding structures, and the overlying soft tissues
- An object that is less radio dense will be easily visualized in an air filled and distended stomach; however, if the stomach were collapsed it would be obscured by the surrounding gastric wall and overlying soft tissue. Metal and ingested bones are the most radiodense objects. Glass can have a varying radiodensity. Wood and other organic foreign bodies are radiolucent and often radiographically occult (Fig. 28.41) [79]
- CT can be used to diagnose foreign bodies and delineate exact anatomical location with increased sensitivity to diagnose complications such as bowel perforation
- A gastric bezoar appears as a mottled, intraluminal soft tissue mass often simulating the appearance of stool (Fig. 28.42). When large, there is less diagnostic dilemma. In contrast to retained food within the stomach, small bezoars are rounded or ovoid, have a lower density than food (Hounsfield units of -150 to 50) and they tend to float on the water–air interface [77]
- With the appropriate clinical history, multiple well-defined small rounded or oval-shaped radiodense objects on abdominal radiographs should raise suspicion of drug packing. Parallelism of the small packages within the bowel or the "condom" sign in which there is a clear crescent of air surrounding an ovoid object are described findings. Often, these patients are aware that attempts to degrade image quality such as motion will decrease diagnostic accuracy [78]

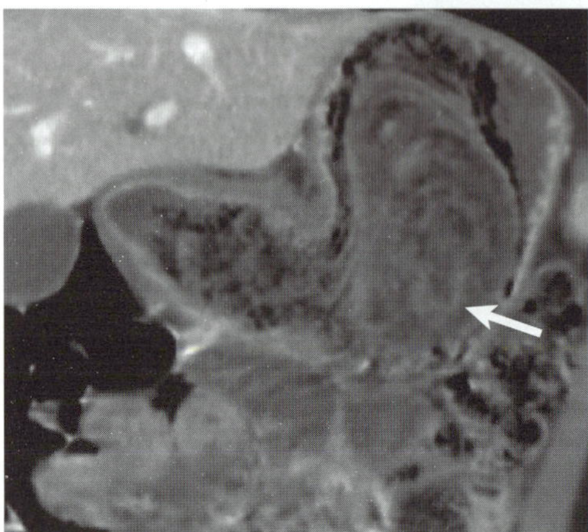
Figure 28.42 Coronal CT of the abdomen with contrast of a 17-year-old psychiatric patient shows distended stomach with mixed attenuation material in the lumen composed of soft tissue density and gas compatible with an obstructing trichobezoar (*arrow*).

Bouveret Syndrome

Pathophysiology and Clinical Presentation

Bouveret syndrome is a complication of cholelithiasis where a cholecystoduodenal fistula results in GOO due to an impacted gallstone within the distal stomach or proximal duodenum. Gallstone ileus with GOO is rare accounting for 1–3% cases. It occurs most commonly in elderly woman with a mean age of approximately 69 years [80,81]. Patients will present with nausea, vomiting, epigastric pain, and rarely hematemesis if there is gastric wall ulceration.

Imaging Features

- On radiographs, an ectopic gallstone, pneumobilia, and gastric distension is specific for gallstone ileus, but has a low sensitivity only seen in 30–35% of cases [81]
- CT is the most often used technique for diagnosis, effectively confirming the presence of GOO, pneumobilia, an impacted ectopic gallstone and a biliary-enteric fistula (Fig. 28.43). One drawback is that 15–25% of gallstones can be isoattenuating to the bile or fluid and can be difficult to identify on CT. Oral contrast will surround the stone and can help confirm diagnosis [80]
- In cases when gallstones are not visualized on radiographs or CT, MRCP can help distinguish between bile and the stone. Additionally, the site of the cholecystoduodenal fistula can be better delineated on MRCP if there is enough fluid present within the fistulous tract [81]

Gastric Volvulus

Pathophysiology and Clinical Presentation

Gastric volvulus is twisting of the stomach resulting in GOO. Patients present with the Borchardt triad of intractable vomiting,

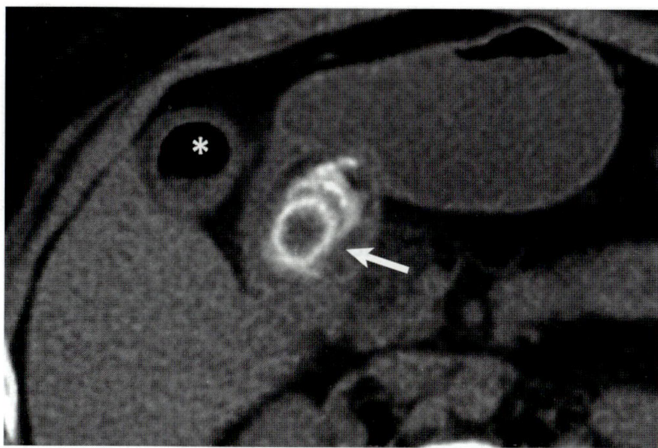

Figure 28.43 Axial CT of the abdomen without intravenous contrast shows a large impacted gallstone in the pylorus (*arrow*) with upstream gastric distension compatible with outlet obstruction in the setting of Bouveret syndrome. There is gallbladder wall thickening and intraluminal gas (*) secondary to a cholecystoduodenal fistula (not shown).

sudden epigastric abdominal pain, and inability to pass a nasogastric tube into the stomach [49,82]. Depending on the axis of rotation, gastric volvulus is divided into organoaxial and mesenteroaxial subtypes. In some cases, there will a complex mixed volvulus with both organoaxial and mesenteroaxial components.

Imaging Features

- With organoaxial volvulus, the antrum rotates anterosuperiorly and fundus rotates posteroinferiorly, resulting in the greater curvature lying superior to the lesser curvature (Fig. 28.44). Some patients will have less than 180° of rotation, with incomplete or partial volvulus in which there is not complete obstruction. Patients with paraesophageal hernias are predisposed to developing abnormal orientation of the stomach. When there is lack of clinical symptoms and outlet obstruction, it is more appropriate to use the terminology organoaxial orientation as opposed to volvulus [49,82]
- Mesenteroaxial volvulus is much less common and occurs when the stomach twists about its short axis/mesentery in which the antrum is displaced above the gastroesophageal junction (Fig. 28.44)
- Upper gastrointestinal series will delineate the anatomy and rotation of the stomach, as well as assess for passage of contrast into the duodenum that is useful in cases of partial volvulus
- The appearance of volvulus is often confusing to unexperienced viewers on CT. Coronal reformatting often aids in delineating the anatomy and demarcating the anatomic relationships. Imaging findings include GOO, gastric wall thickening. It is important to evaluate for complications of gastric ischemia or perforation [49]

Gastric Diverticulum

Pathophysiology and Clinical Presentation

Gastric diverticula are the rarest types of gastrointestinal diverticula with a reported incidence of 0.02% on autopsy studies [83]. They are true congenital diverticula containing all layers of the gastric tissue, and commonly located on the posterior wall of the gastric cardia. Most are asymptomatic and incidentally found on endoscopy, upper gastrointestinal fluoroscopy, or cross-sectional imaging. Rarely, they can present with vague symptoms of fullness or upper abdominal discomfort.

Imaging Features

- On upper gastrointestinal series, gastric diverticula can be mistaken for hiatal hernias or hypertrophic gastric folds. They can range in size from 1 to 11 cm [84]
- CT can confirm an outpouching arising from the gastric cardia. Inexperienced observers can mistake these diverticula for an adrenal mass. Presence of intraluminal fluid and gas is diagnostic (Fig. 28.45)

Gastric Trauma

Blunt and Penetrating Trauma

Pathophysiology and Clinical Presentation

Penetrating trauma is the most common cause of gastric injury, with an incidence of approximately 20% cases of gunshot wounds and 10% cases of stab wounds. A single site of gastric injury is seen in nearly 50% of stab wounds to the left thoracoabdominal region, while gunshot wounds often result in two or more foci of injury in 90% of cases [85]. High velocity blunt trauma to the

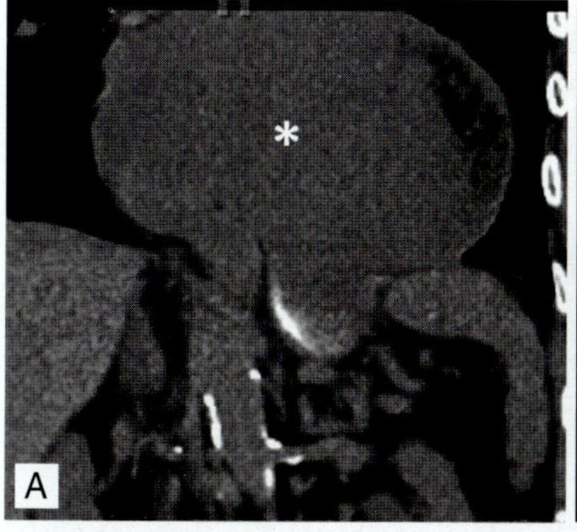

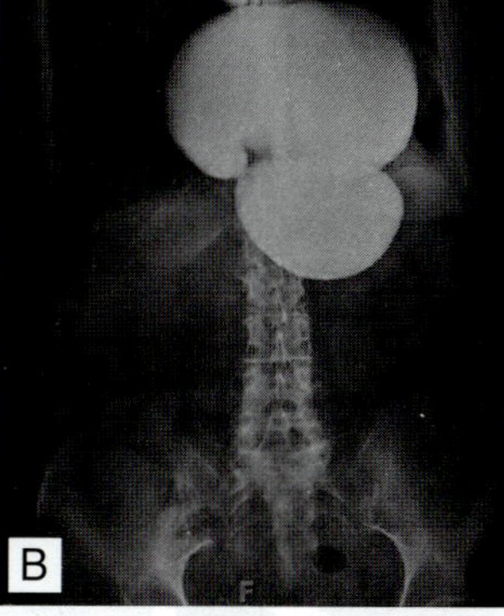

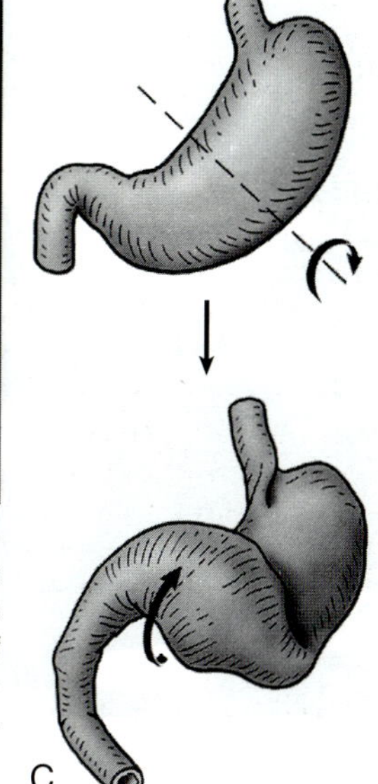

Figure 28.44 Organoaxial gastric volvulus in an 85-year-old woman with vomiting and epigastric pain. Coronal CT of the abdomen without contrast (A) shows that the stomach is almost entirely intrathoracic with an upside down orientation (*). Follow-up radiograph after drinking oral contrast (B) shows no passage of contrast into the duodenum compatible with complete obstruction. Mesenteroaxial volvulus with rotation about the short axis of the stomach along its mesentery (C).

TABLE 28.1 Differentiating Gastric Ulcers [110]

Benign	Malignant
Round or ovoid shape	Irregular shape
Projects outside of the lumen margin	Remains inside the lumen margin
Smooth ulcer mound	Irregular ulcer mound with rolled edge
Smooth, symmetric radiating folds extending to lip of ulcer	Nodular and fused radiating folds that do not extend to the lip of ulcer
Improves with conservative treatment	Fails to improve or worsens
Hampton's line—thin line radiolucent line seen at the neck of benign gastric ulcers	Carman meniscus sign—lenticular shape of barium seen on compression views with contrast trapped between the margins of a large, flat ulcer

- Metastatic sites include lymph nodes (Fig. 28.58) and peritoneal metastases. Peritoneal metastases can be subtle on CT and often, ascites may be the only indicator. Other CT findings of peritoneal disease include nodularity of the peritoneal fat, peritoneal surface nodularity of abnormal thickening of the serosal surface of intra-abdominal organs such as the small bowel (Figs. 28.55B and C)
- Cross-sectional imaging is important in the diagnosis of gastric linitis because it can provide an earlier diagnosis compared to endoscopy. There is diffuse or segmental gastric wall thickening that appears regular, concentric, and symmetric. Homogenous wall enhancement is most pronounced in delayed phases of imaging [104]

Gastric Lymphoma

Pathophysiology and Clinical Presentation

About 5–20% of extra-nodal lymphomas involve the gastrointestinal tract, with the stomach being the most common site of

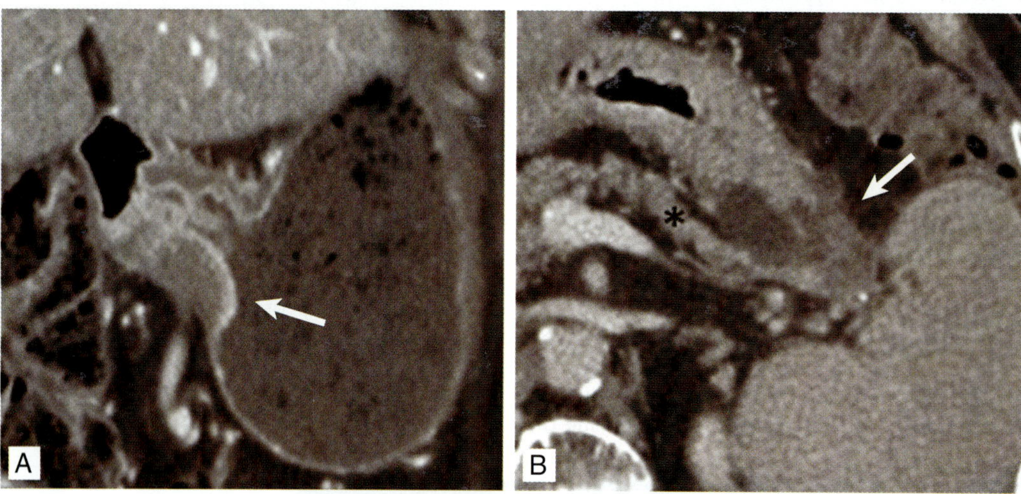

Figure 28.57 (A) Coronal CT of the abdomen with contrast shows marked asymmetric wall thickening and enhancement of the gastric antrum (*arrow*) resulting in gastric outlet obstruction proven to be secondary to gastric antral adenocarcinoma. (B) Axial contrast-enhanced CT shows a hypoenhancing mass arising from the gastric body which extends to the splenic hilum (*white arrow*) and also abuts the pancreas (*) posteriorly. This was biopsied and found to be locally invasive gastric adenocarcinoma.

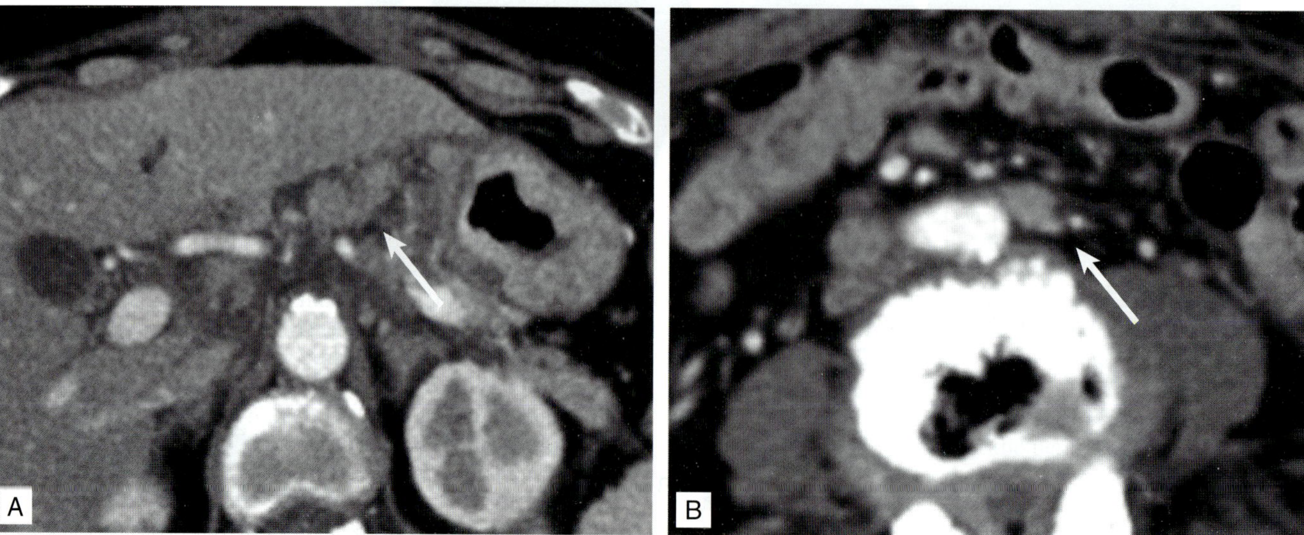

Figure 28.58 Axial contrast-enhanced CT of a patient with gastric adenocarcinoma (not shown) demonstrates locoregional metastatic lymphadenopathy involving the gastrohepatic ligament (A, *white arrow*) and left para-aortic chain (B, *white arrow*).

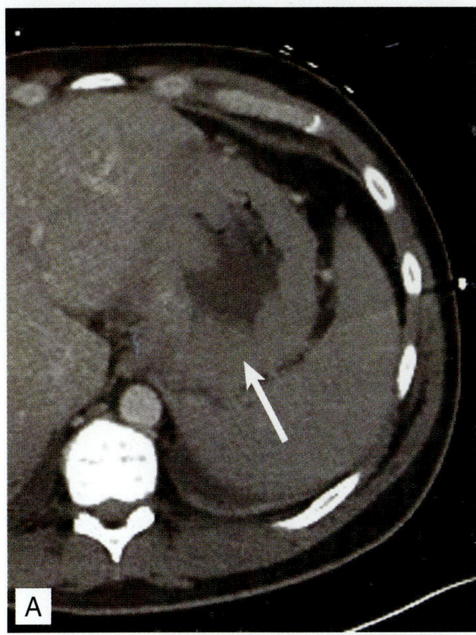

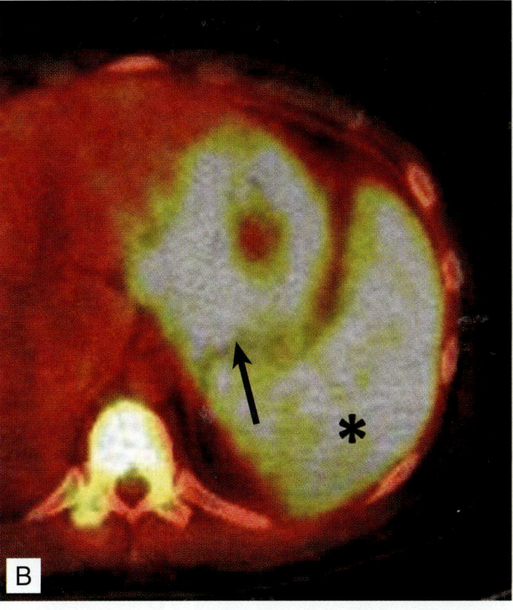

Figure 28.59 Axial CT of the abdomen with contrast (A) shows marked thickening of the gastric wall (*arrow*) without evidence of obstruction. There is extensive corresponding radiotracer uptake on the PET/CT (B) along with increased FDG avidity in the enlarged spleen (*) and bone marrow consistent with lymphoma.

involvement [111]. Lymphoma accounts for less than 5% of all gastric malignancies, with non-Hodgkin's B cell lymphoma being the most common subtype [111]. Risk factors for gastric lymphoma include HIV or *H. pylori* infection, celiac disease, inflammatory bowel disease, and immunosuppression after solid organ transplantation [111].

Most low-grade gastric lymphomas arise from mucosal associated lymphoid tissue lymphoma in the setting of chronic *H. pylori* infection. There is normally no lymphoid tissue within the gastric mucosa, however chronic infection with *H. pylori* leads to development of lymphoid tissue within the lamina propria. This type of gastric lymphoma often regresses with treatment of the infection with antibiotics [111].

Imaging Features

The most common CT finding is diffuse or segmental gastric wall thickening, often measuring 2–5 cm (Fig. 28.59) [111]. High-grade lymphoma may have greater thickening of the gastric wall and presence of extra-gastric lymphadenopathy. Lymphoma can less likely present as an ulcerative, polypoid, or infiltrative lesion, similar to that of gastric carcinoma. There is extensive gastric wall thickening without reduced distensibility of the stomach or obstruction, as opposed to linitis plastica which restricts the stomach (Table 28.2) [112]. When treated, there is increased risk of spontaneous gastric perforation.

TABLE 28.2 Differentiating Gastric Adenocarcinoma and Lymphoma

Gastric Adenocarcinoma	Gastric Lymphoma
More commonly associated with gastric outlet obstruction	Uncommon to cause gastric outlet obstruction
Nodal involvement can be present, but more commonly in the perigastric nodal stations including along the lesser and greater curvature, regional stations around the celiac artery branches or distantly to the diaphragmatic stations or para-aortic region	Nodal involvement common, often larger and beyond the normal gastric drainage pathways (above the diaphragm and below the renal veins)
Can invade through serosa and into the surrounding perigastric fat	Predominately lateral/submucosal tumor extension without serosal invasion into the perigastric fat
Focal, asymmetric gastric wall thickening, or diffuse gastric wall thickening in advanced disease	More commonly presents as marked (>2 cm) segmental or diffuse gastric wall thickening

Postsurgical Stomach

Description and Complications

Obesity is a chronic multifactorial illness affecting patients of all ages and with an increasing prevalence. Bariatric surgery is an increasingly popular form of treatment for patients with morbid obesity. The most common procedures include laparoscopic Roux-en-Y gastric bypass, laparoscopic gastric banding, and laparoscopic sleeve gastrectomy.

Roux-en-Y gastric bypass is the most popular bariatric surgery performed because it has a higher long-term success rate compared to its counterparts. It involves separating the stomach into a small fundal gastric pouch (approximately 15–30 mL in volume) and a larger excluded gastric component. The jejunum is divided 25–50 cm distal to the ligament of Treitz and the distal (Roux or efferent limb) is brought up and anastomosed in an end to end or side to side fashion with the gastric pouch (gastrojejunostomy). The distal jejunum limb can be brought up in anterior to the colon or posterior to the colon (ante- or retrocolic). The proximal jejunal limb (afferent, biliopancreatic limb) is anastomosed with the distal limb in a side-to-side fashion. Complications include leaks, marginal ulcers at the gastrojejunostomy secondary to chronic acidic exposure or obstruction. With regards to obstruction, adhesive disease is the most common cause in patients who undergo open Roux-en-Y gastric bypass. With laparoscopic technique the most common sites are usually internal hernias, either at the transverse mesocolon (for retrocolic approach), a defect in the jejunal mesentery (for creation of jejunojejunal anastomoses), or posterior to the Roux limb (Peterson's defect) [113].

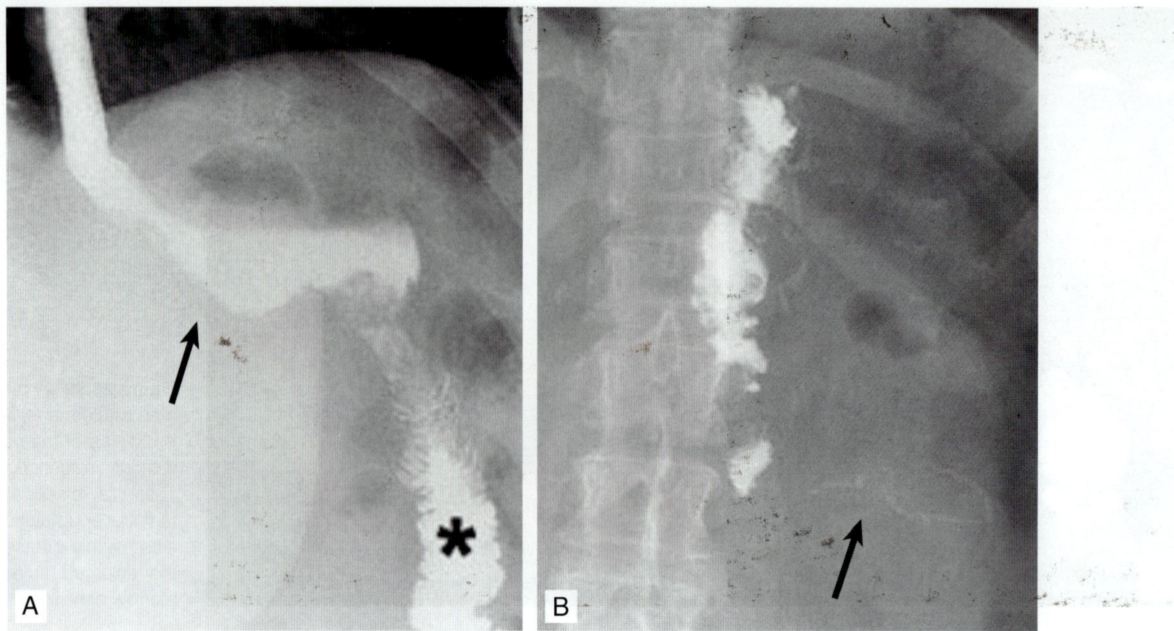

Figure 28.60 Upper gastrointestinal series (A) demonstrates normal anatomy after Roux-en-Y with a proximal gastric pouch (*black arrow*) which directly communicates to the jejunum (*) via the gastrojejunostomy. Note the staple line more distally (B, *black arrow*) which demarcates the distal anastomoses of the jejunojejunostomy.

Sleeve gastrectomy involves dividing the stomach along its long axis with resection of the greater curvature removing approximately 75% of the stomach volume [114]. This creates a narrow gastric pouch along the lesser curvature of the stomach. This reduction in stomach volume creates early satiety. Although this technique has the longest staple line given the length of resection, postoperative leaks are reported in less than 1% of cases.

Laparoscopic gastric banding is the least invasive surgical procedure performed for morbid obesity. It is a restrictive procedure in which a silicone band is placed around the proximal stomach to create a small pouch. The band is attached to a reservoir placed in the abdominal wall which can be used to inflate or deflate the cuff to adjust the stoma size. Complications include band slippage, erosion, and esophageal dilation if the band is too tight. Gastric band slippage can occur when the stomach herniates upward from below the band which can predispose to chronic stoma stenosis. Gastric band erosion results from overdistension of the band leading to ischemia and infection with a 0.3–14% prevalence [115,116]. Perforation is a rare complication occurring in 0.1–0.8% of cases [115].

Imaging Features

- Upper gastrointestinal imaging via fluoroscopy is commonly performed both in the immediate postoperative setting and afterward to evaluate for complications. All procedures can be complicated by leaks at the staple lines or anastomoses
- Evaluation of Roux-en-Y patients will demonstrate a rounded gastric pouch which empties directly into the jejunum (Fig. 28.60). Gastric sleeve appears as a long, tubular gastric pouch with preservation of the gastric antrum, and eventual filling into the duodenum (Fig. 28.61). Gastric bands are radiodense rounded structures, which form an oblique orientation to the adjacent spine when reviewed on AP radiography (Fig. 28.62)
- Roux-en-Y gastric bypass can develop marginal ulcers, which manifest as discrete ulcers at either the gastrojejunal anastomosis or proximal Roux limb (Fig. 28.63). If there is a breakdown of the gastric staple line, a gastrogastric fistula can develop in which food is able to enter the excluded stomach (Fig. 28.64). This negates the restrictive effects of forming a small gastric pouch and can lead to recurrent weight gain. Small bowel obstructions may be due to adhesions, internal hernias from the defects created during surgery or strictures at the anastomoses (Fig. 28.65)

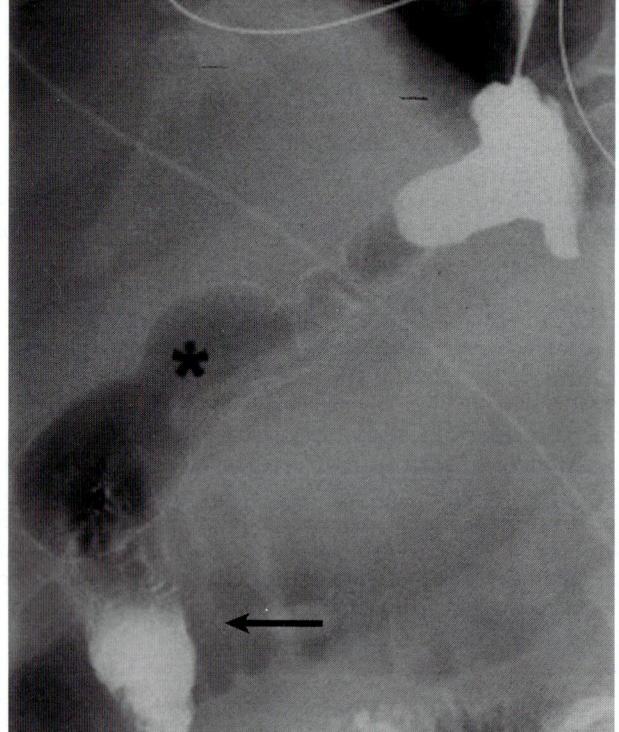

Figure 28.61 Upper gastrointestinal series (A) demonstrates normal anatomy after gastric sleeve in which there is long tubular remnant stomach (*) after resection along the greater curvature. Note the normal distal anatomy with the pylorus emptying into the duodenum (*black arrow*).

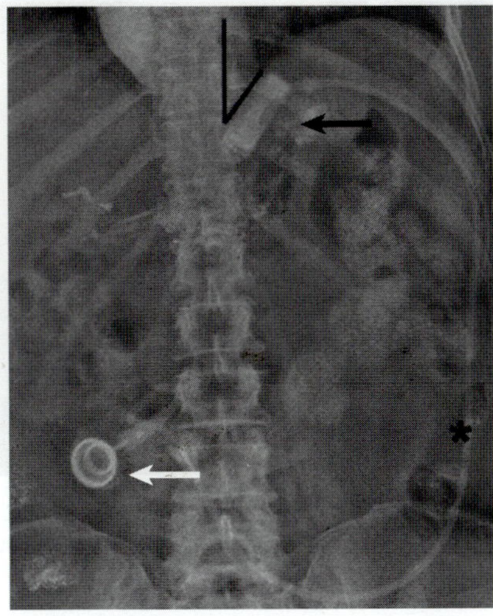

Figure 28.62 Normal gastric band anatomy with inflated band (*black arrow*) which has an acute angle (black lines) with the adjacent spine. There is long tubing (*) which connects the band to the reservoir (*white arrow*) in the abdominal wall.

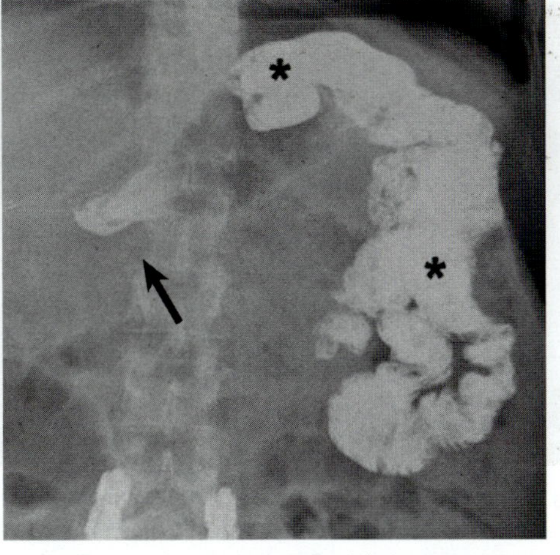

Figure 28.64 Upper gastrointestinal series (A) demonstrates contrast filling the gastric pouch and proximal jejunum (*), however note the faint opacification of the excluded stomach (*black arrow*) which was due to a gastrogastric fistula.

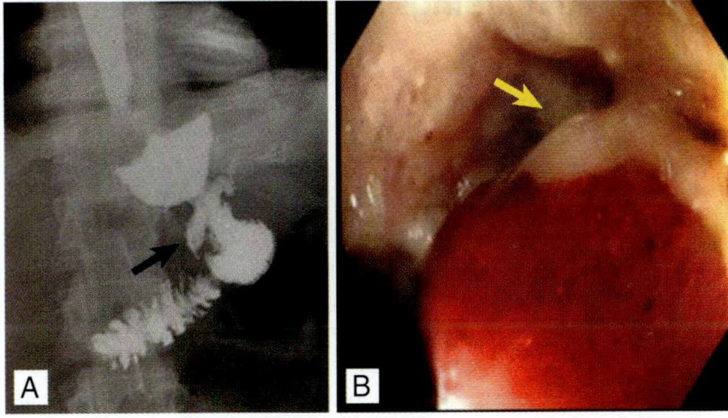

Figure 28.63 Upper gastrointestinal series (A) demonstrates a focal outpouching from the proximal aspect of the jejunum (*black arrow*) just distal to the gastrojejunostomy. Endoscopy (B) confirmed the presence of a marginal ulcer which commonly occur either at or just distal to the gastrojejunostomy.

- On AP abdominal radiographs, the angle between longitudinal axis of the gastric band and spinal column, referred to as the (phi) angle, should be between 4 and 58 [115,116]. Malposition can suggest underlying issues such as gastric band slippage or erosion. In the case of slippage, a characteristic finding is the "O" sign when the band is viewed en-face. Gastric band erosion is manifested by the band surrounded by gastric wall on CT (Fig. 28.66). Perigastric stranding and fluid is often present due to leakage of gastric contents. On fluoroscopy, the band appears as a filling defect in the gastric lumen with extra luminal contrast seen with active leak. If the band is tightened too tightly patients can experience nausea and vomiting from a functional obstruction (Fig. 28.67). The band can be deflated by withdrawing saline from the reservoir that rests in the abdominal wall

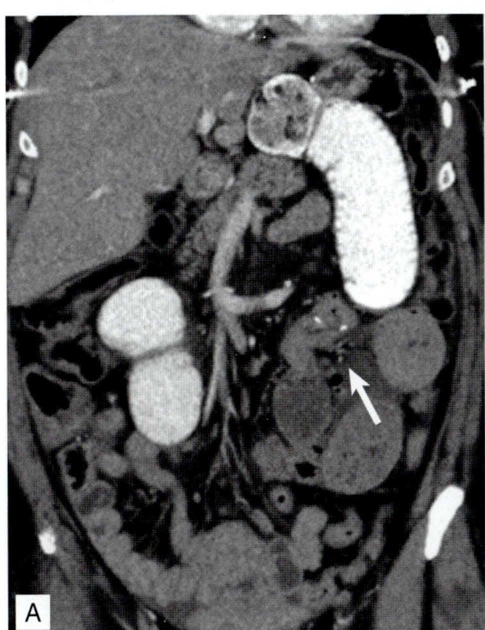

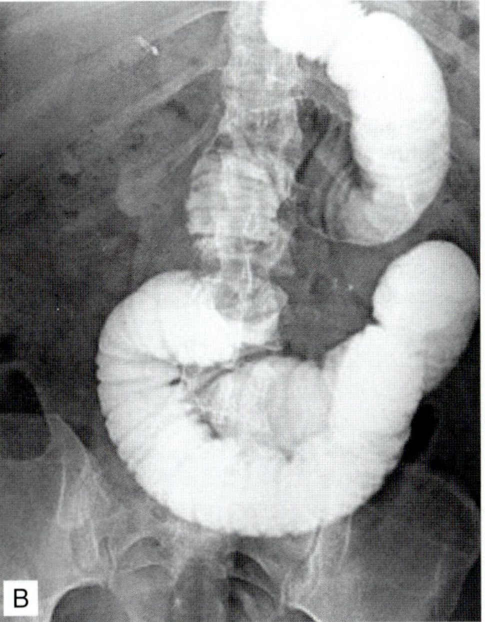

Figure 28.65 Coronal image of an abdominal CT with both oral and intravenous contrast (A) demonstrates a patient status post-Roux-en-Y gastric bypass with markedly dilated contrast-filled loops of small bowel. There is pseudofecalization and a transition point in the distal jejunal mesentery near the jejunojejunostomy staple line (*white arrow*). Upper gastrointestinal series (B) after decompression with nasogastric tube confirmed persistent high-grade obstruction. This patient was found to have an obstruction due to adhesive disease at time of operation.

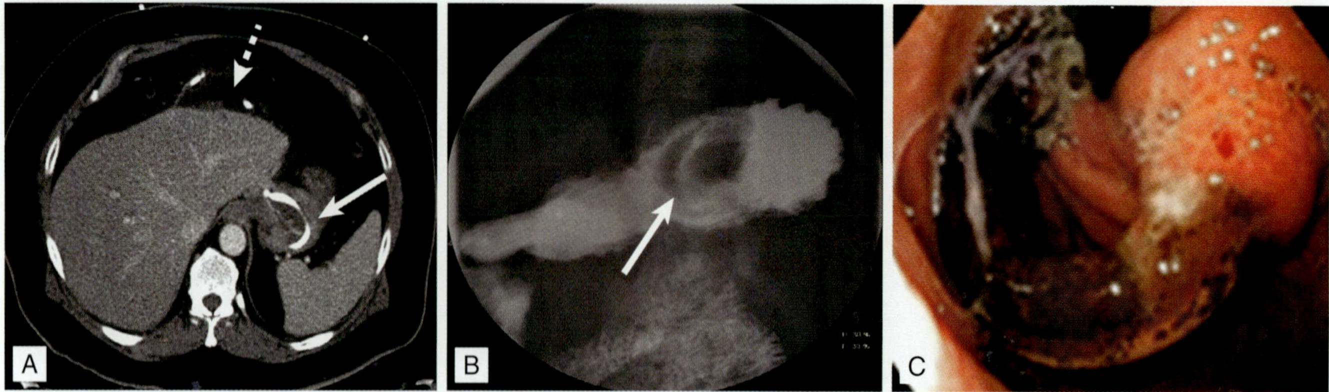

Figure 28.66 Axial CT of the abdomen with intravenous contrast (A) shows the gastric band surrounded by gastric wall (*arrow*) along with fat stranding along the connecting tube (*dashed arrow*). Follow-up upper GI study (B) shows a round doughnut-shaped filling defect (*arrow*) within the gastric lumen representing the eroded band which was confirmed on endoscopy (C).

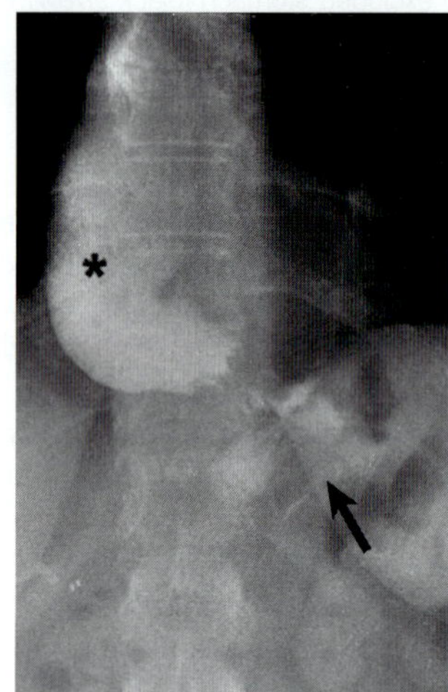

Figure 28.67 In this patient with a gastric band (*black arrow*) and significant nausea/vomiting postprocedurally, there is distension of the distal esophagus (*). This is compatible with functional obstruction due to a tight band. The band was deflated by withdrawing saline from the reservoir, at which time the patient's symptoms improved.

Summary

A wide variety of esophageal and gastric disease is encountered on imaging, the majority of which is benign. Barium swallow remains the preferred technique for initial evaluation of the esophagus while gastric disease and its complications may be better evaluated with CT especially in the emergent setting. Endoscopy remains the gold-standard for both in majority cases. A thorough knowledge regarding the imaging appearance of various entities is paramount for the radiologist to correctly diagnose the various non-neoplastic and neoplastic conditions and drive appropriate management.

Suggested Readings

- CA Young, CO Menias, S Bhalla, SR Prasad, CT features of esophageal emergencies, Radiographics 28 (6) (2008) 1541–1553.
- MS Levine, SE Rubesin, Diseases of the esophagus: diagnosis with esophagography, Radiology 237 (2) (2005) 414–427.
- RB Lewis, AK Mehrotra, P Rodriguez, MS Levine, From the radiologic pathology archives: esophageal neoplasms: radiologic-pathologic correlation, Radiographics 33 (4) (2013) 1083–1108.
- RB Iyer, PM Silverman, EP Tamm, JS Dunnington, RA DuBrow, Diagnosis, staging, and follow-up of esophageal cancer, J Am Roentgenol 181 (3) (2003) 785–793.
- P Guniganti, CH Bradenham, C Raptis, CO Menias, VM Mellnick, CT of gastric emergencies, Radiographics 35 (7) (2015) 1909–1921.
- M Zulfiqar, A Shetty, V Shetty, C Menias, Computed tomography imaging of non-neoplastic and neoplastic benign gastric disease, Curr Probl Diagn Radiol 48 (1) (2019) 75–96.
- HC Kang, CO Menias, AH Gaballah, et al., Beyond the GIST: mesenchymal tumors of the stomach, Radiographics 33 (6) (2013) 1673–1690.
- DM Richman, SH Tirumani, JL Hornick, et al., Beyond gastric adenocarcinoma: multimodality assessment of common and uncommon gastric neoplasms, Abdom Radiol 42 (1) (2017) 124–40.
- MS Levine, LR Carucci, Imaging of bariatric surgery: normal anatomy and postoperative complications, Radiology 270 (2) (2014) 327–341.

29

Imaging of Small and Large Bowel

PRIYA PATHAK, PUNEET BHARGAVA

Anatomy

The small bowel extends from the pyloric sphincter to the ileocecal valve with an average length up to 5–6 m. It consists of the duodenum, jejunum, and ileum; the duodenum measures approximately 20–25 cm in length, the jejunum 2.5 m, and the ileum approximately 3 m. The duodenum consists of four parts (first, superior; second, descending forming the C loop; third, horizontal; and fourth, ascending) and continues as jejunum at the *ligament of Treitz* in the left upper quadrant. Distinct mucosal folds of the small intestines, known as *valvule conniventes*, are well identified on imaging [1].

Small bowel layers (from outer to inner) consist of serosa encircling the jejunum and ileum and covering only the anterior portion of retroperitoneal duodenum; muscularis with outer longitudinal and inner circular layers of smooth muscles; submucosa containing blood vessels, nerves, and lymphatics; and mucosa covered with villi containing tall columnar cells. The crypts of Lieberkühn are the glands present in between the villi of the intestinal epithelium.

The large bowel consists of cecum, ascending colon (right iliac fossa to hepatic flexure), transverse colon (hepatic to splenic flexure), descending colon, sigmoid colon, and rectum, with an average total length of approximately 1.5 m. Three outer longitudinal muscle layers called taenia coli give distinct sacculations, which are interrupted by incomplete rings called haustra. The cecum is the proximal pouch of ascending colon, containing appendix along the posteromedial wall. Ascending and descending colons are retroperitoneal organs [2]. Transverse colon is the longest and most mobile part of the large intestine. It is attached to the retroperitoneum by transverse mesocolon. Descending colon continues as the S-shaped sigmoid colon of variable length. The rectum starts at approximately S3 level and runs along the sacrococcygeal curvature to continue as anal canal at the anorectal angle formed by the puborectalis sling.

To briefly review the vascular anatomy:

- The celiac artery originates from the aorta at T12 level, superior mesenteric artery (SMA) at L1 level, and inferior mesenteric artery (IMA) at L3 level. The celiac artery supply extends from the distal esophagus to the second portion of the duodenum. It trifurcates into the common hepatic artery (which further divides into gastroduodenal artery and proper hepatic artery [PHA]), splenic artery, and left gastric artery. The PHA further divides into the right and left hepatic arteries. Variant anatomy may be seen in the form of an accessory (if along with a corresponding PHA branch) or replaced (if without a corresponding PHA branch) left hepatic artery arising from the left gastric artery and an accessory or replaced right hepatic artery arising from the SMA
- The SMA supplies the third and fourth portions of the duodenum, jejunum, ileum, and colon up to the midtransverse colon. Branches of the SMA are; inferior pancreaticoduodenal artery; left-sided branches including the jejunal and ileal arteries; and right-sided branches including the ileocolic, right colic, and middle colic arteries (Fig. 29.1). Relatively common variant SMA branches include a replaced or accessory right hepatic artery (most common variant), common hepatic artery, splenic artery, celiac trunk, and gastroduodenal artery
- The IMA supplies the distal transverse colon up to the rectum and branches into the left colic artery, sigmoid arteries, and superior rectal artery

Terminal branches of SMA and IMA supplying the colon are linked together by an arterial arcade known as the *marginal artery of Drummond*, which provides collateral flow in the event of stenosis or occlusion (Fig. 29.2).

The arcade of Riolan is an additional anastomotic arterial arcade between the SMA and IMA; however, it is inconsistently present. These arterial arcades can be small or underdeveloped, leading to formation of watershed area in the splenic flexure (Griffith point). The rectum is supplied by the inferior mesenteric and internal iliac arterial branches consisting of superior, middle, and inferior rectal arteries.

The superior and inferior mesenteric veins run parallel to the respective arteries and drain into the portal vein [3–5].

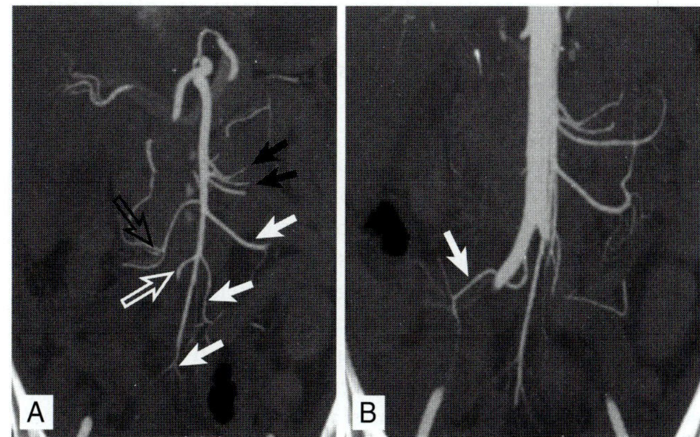

Figure 29.1 (A) Coronal three-dimensional multidetector computed tomography scan demonstrates the normal superior mesenteric artery branches: the jejunal branches (*black arrows*), ileal branches (*white arrows*), ileocolic artery (*white open arrow*), and middle colic artery (*black* open *arrow*). (B) Image delineating the ileocolic artery (*white arrow*).

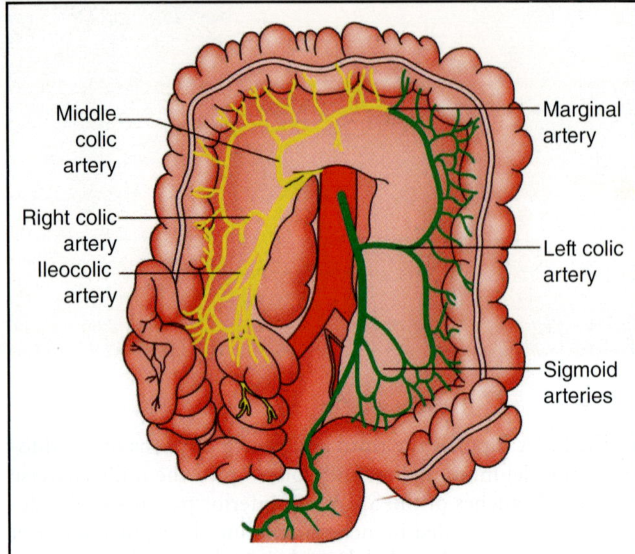

Figure 29.2 Illustration shows the marginal artery of Drummond.

Imaging Techniques

Abdominal radiographs, fluoroscopic contrast studies with barium or water-soluble agents (small bowel follow-through, enema, enteroclysis), ultrasonography (USG), computed tomography (CT), magnetic resonance imaging (MRI), enterography, and CT colonography are the available imaging techniques for evaluation of the small and large bowel. Of these, multidetector CT has emerged as the imaging technique of choice for primary evaluation and follow up of the majority of small and large bowel pathologies. The overall role of fluoroscopic contrast studies has markedly declined over the years; for example, in Crohn's disease, contrast fluoroscopy may lead to obscuration of pathology because of overlapping bowel loops and is less accurate for evaluation of active disease than other techniques. Fluoroscopy may not be tolerated in acutely ill patients and is technically challenging. In addition, colonoscopy is superior to contrast enema for detection of early inflammatory changes [5].

Computed tomography enterography includes peroral (noninvasive, more common) and enteroclysis (requires placement of nasojejunal tube) techniques for enteric contrast administration. The major advantage of enteroclysis is superior distension of the jejunum, which imparts a specific role in elective evaluation of conditions such as Crohn's disease, small bowel obstruction, and unexplained occult gastrointestinal (GI) bleed [7]. However, oral administration of contrast is more convenient and faster and demonstrates superior patient experience. Neutral oral contrast agents are more commonly used, such as Brezza (combination of sorbitol, mannitol, and xanthan gum), water, water with methylcellulose, polyethylene glycol, and low-density barium sulfate suspension (VoLumen). The major limitation of neutral oral contrast is suboptimal bowel distension because of rapid absorption [8]. Positive oral contrasts agents include dilute barium and water-soluble iodinated contrast. The predominant limitation of these agents is obscuration of mucosal enhancement pattern. Intravenous (IV) contrast with a single enteric phase at 60–70 seconds is usually adequate for small bowel imaging. Certain specific indications of CT enterography are provided in Box 29.1 [9].

BOX 29.1 Specific Indications for Computed Tomography Enterography

- Crohn's disease
- Ulcerative colitis
- Small bowel tumors
- Occult gastrointestinal bleeding
- Partial small bowel obstruction
- Celiac disease

Similar to CT enterography, MR enterography involves administration of oral contrast agents (commonly Brezza or VoLumen) for adequate bowel distension. Antiperistaltic agents are crucial to minimize motion artifacts. Standard sequences include T2-weighted imaging with and without fat suppression, fat-suppressed T1-weighted imaging with multiphase postcontrast acquisition including delayed phase, and steady-state coherent sequences to evaluate for bowel peristalsis and fixed stenosis. Scanning with the patient in a prone position decreases scan time by minimizing the scan area and elevating and separating the small bowel loops; however, a supine position is usually more comfortable for the patients.

MR and CT enterography demonstrate similar sensitivity for detecting small bowel inflammation; however, image quality is better with CT enterography. CT enterography has the advantages of superior assessment of perienteric abnormality, shorter scan time, lesser artifacts, and ability to scan uncooperative patients. Advantages of MRI enterography are elimination of ionizing radiation and the ability to image patients with impaired renal function [10].

CT colonography is a minimally invasive examination indicated for the screening of colorectal cancer, to evaluate colon after incomplete or unsuccessful colonoscopy, or to evaluate proximal to an obstructing neoplasm. The technique involves

1. Adequate bowel preparation with administration of laxatives because residual stool and fluid produce false-positive and false-negative results. Dilute barium is used for residual fecal tagging
2. Gaseous distension of colon with air or CO_2
3. Administration of antispasmodic agents such as buscopan or glucagon

Scanning is performed with patient in both supine and prone positions. Two- and three-dimensional intraluminal reconstructions are used for image interpretation along with the raw images [11] (Fig. 29.3).

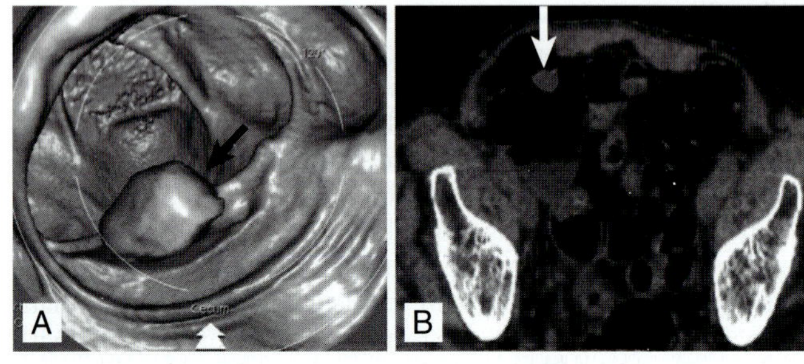

Figure 29.3 Computed tomography (CT) colonography three-dimensional endoluminal view shows a small polyp (benign on pathology) in the cecum (*black arrow*) (A), correlated as soft tissue nodule on axial CT (*white arrow*) (B).

General Causes of Non-neoplastic Bowel Wall Thickening

Inflammatory Disorders

Crohn's Disease

Pathophysiology: Crohn's disease is a chronic inflammatory disease of the GI tract characterized by a relapsing–remitting course. It can occur from the mouth to the anus, with *small bowel involvement present in 80% of cases. The terminal ileum is the most commonly affected site.* The colon is involved with the small bowel in 50% of the cases. Several proposed causative factors are immune dysfunction, infections, genetic, familial, vascular, and dietary; however, the exact cause remains unclear [12].

On pathology, *multiple discontinuous sites of bowel involvement or skip lesions are present.* Active inflammation starts with neutrophilic infiltration into the mucosa with cryptitis, lymphoid hyperplasia, and aphthoid ulceration. Progression of inflammation causes transmural involvement with deeper ulceration, fistulation, sinus tract formation, and mesenteric involvement. Chronic inflammation leads to fibrosis with progressive increased extracellular matrix deposition by mesenchymal cells, which causes luminal narrowing and strictures. Long-standing disease causes progressive mucosal atrophy and submucosal fat deposition [13].

Clinical Features: Peak involvement occurs between 15 and 25 years of age with similar gender prevalence. The second peak is in the sixth and seventh decades of life [13]. Variable clinical features depend on the disease site and activity, which includes abdominal pain, diarrhea, fever, weight loss, perianal fissures, and anemia caused by chronic GI bleed. The condition is associated with myriad of extraintestinal manifestations such as dermatologic (erythema nodosum, aphthous ulcer, and pyoderma gangrenosum), musculoskeletal (ankylosing spondylitis, polymyositis), primary sclerosing cholangitis, and calcium oxalate stones [14]. *Patients are at increased risk of colorectal cancer and lymphoma; increased risk of lymphoma is linked to immunomodulator therapies used in Crohn's disease treatment* [13].

Imaging Features: Features can be categorized into following subtypes:

1. Active inflammatory disease
2. Penetrating disease
3. Fibrostenotic disease
4. Reparative and regenerative disease

Of note, there is extensive overlap between these subtypes without a stepwise progression [15].

Fluoroscopy: Mucosal abnormalities on barium studies are thickened, nodular folds and a cobblestone pattern produced by a combination of longitudinal and transverse ulcers. Aphthous ulcers present as areas of barium collection within the mounds of mucosal edema (Fig. 29.4). Penetrating disease shows deep ulcers, fistula (enteroenteric, enterocolonic), and sinus tracts (Fig. 29.5). Strictures, stenosis, and wall sacculations are features of chronic stage (Fig. 29.6). The *string sign of Kantor* refers to a beaded string-like appearance of the bowel caused by multifocal narrowing or strictures [16].

Ultrasonography: Inflamed bowel segments show concentric mural thickening (Fig. 29.7), stratification, and hyperemia. Interbowel fluid and increased echogenicity of perienteric fat are seen.

CT and MRI enterography: Imaging features can be divided according to the subtypes; however, patients usually present with varying combinations of active, fibrostenotic or chronic, penetrating, and reparative disease.

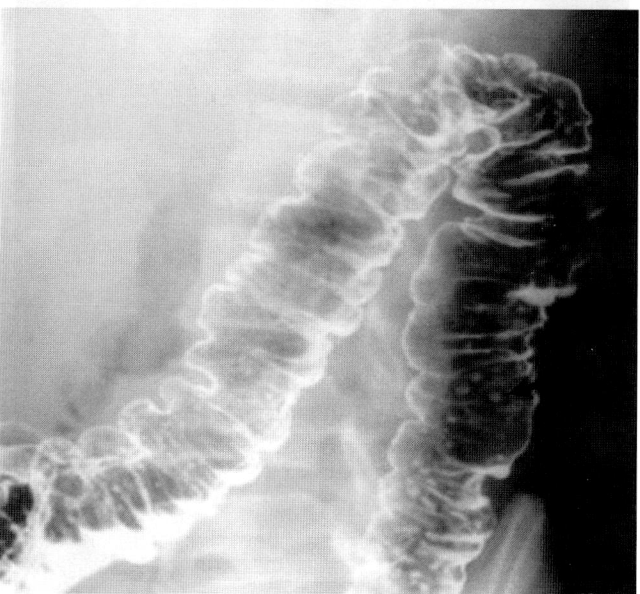

Figure 29.4 Double-contrast barium enema from a 34-year-old man with Crohn's disease demonstrates numerous aphthous ulcers in the transverse and descending colon as tiny barium collection within mounds of mucosal edema (*black arrow*).

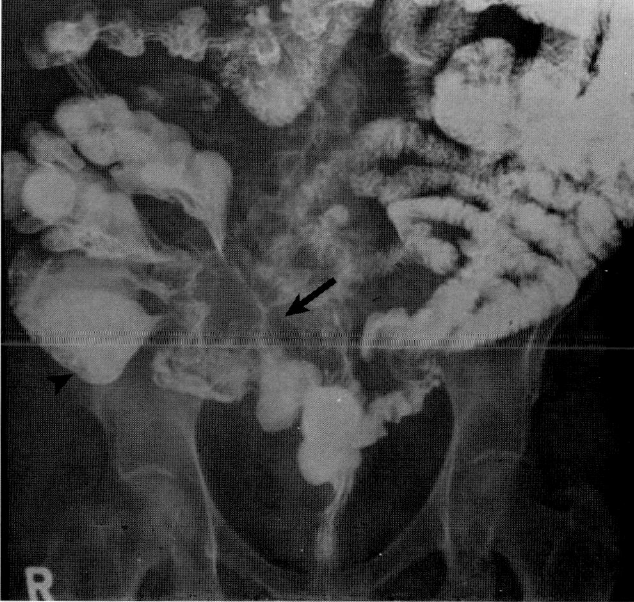

Figure 29.5 Small bowel follow-through in a 39-year-old man with penetrating Crohn's disease demonstrates distortion of the mid sigmoid colon (*arrow*) and complex fistulation with the ileal loops (*arrowhead*).

On contrast-enhanced CT, **active inflammatory disease** presents with the following features:

- Mural thickening (commonly asymmetric), stratification, edema, and segmental mural hyperenhancement (the term *mucosal hyperenhancement* is not preferred because bowel involved by Crohn's disease may lack a mucosal layer secondary to inflammatory damage) (Fig. 29.8). Mural thickening is measured in a bowel segment adequately distended by enteric contrast and is graded into mild, 3–5 mm; moderate, 5–9 mm; and severe, 10 mm or greater
- Ulcerations are indicated by extension of air or contrast into the bowel wall

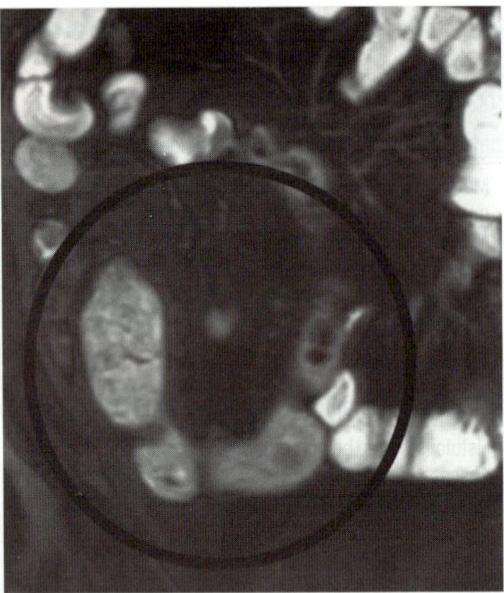

Figure 29.11 Coronal fat-saturated T2-weighted magnetic resonance imaging of the abdomen shows distal ileal sacculations in chronic Crohn's disease.

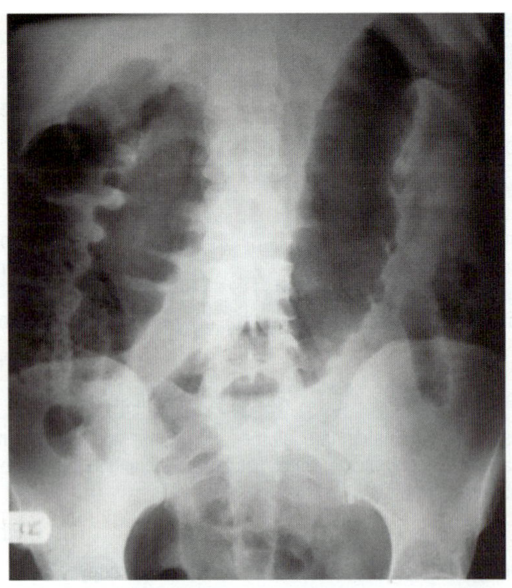

Figure 29.13 Toxic megacolon.

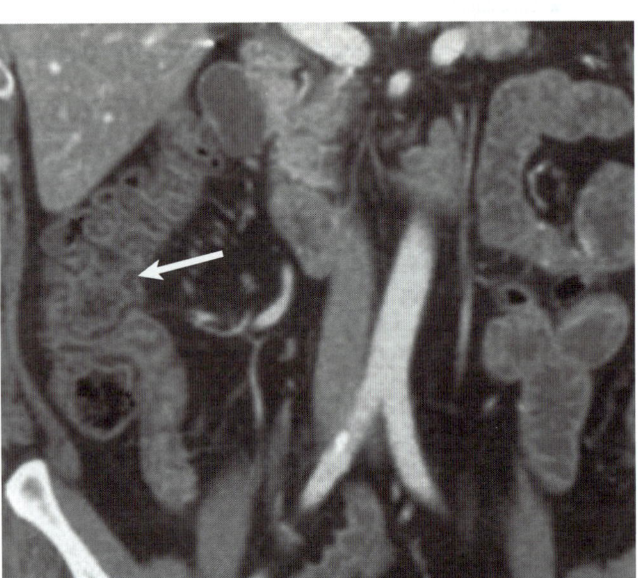

Figure 29.12 Coronal contrast-enhanced computed tomography of the abdomen and pelvis from a 64-year-old woman shows submucosal fat deposition in the terminal ileum and ascending colon as a sequela of Crohn's disease (*white arrow*).

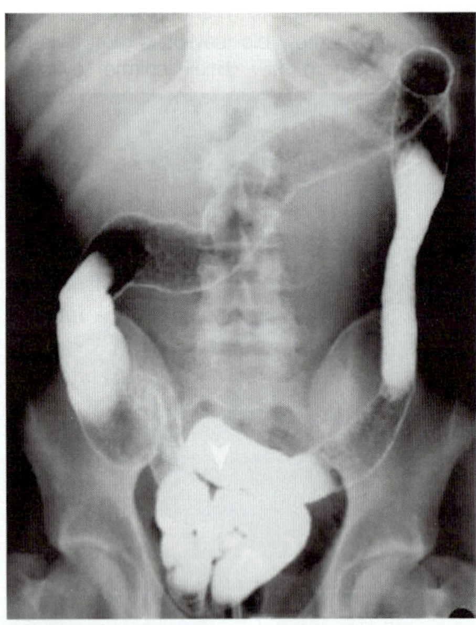

Figure 29.14 Double-contrast barium enema in a 58-year-old man with chronic ulcerative colitis demonstrates diffusely irregular colonic mucosal pattern with a grainy appearance. There are narrowing and foreshortening of the descending colon with loss of haustration (*lead pipe colon*).

on supine radiographs (Fig. 29.13). Other findings include air-fluid levels, loss of colonic haustrations, mucosal islands, and absence of formed stool [20].

Fluoroscopy: Single- or double-contrast barium enema delineates mucosal abnormalities as granular and stippled mucosa, superficial erosions, and ulcers. *Deeper ulcers or collar button ulcers are formed because of undermining submucosal extension limited by the muscle layer.* Pseudopolyps are seen as nodular filling defects [20]. *Barium enema is contraindicated in patients with acute severe inflammation because of the risk of perforation.*

Chronic disease presents with luminal narrowing, strictures, and a featureless colon with loss of haustrations, also known as *lead pipe colon* (Fig. 29.14). A patulous Ileocecal vale (IC) valve with granular terminal ileum is indicative of backwash ileitis (Fig. 29.15). *There is associated widening of the presacral space because of increased perirectal fat deposition* (Fig. 29.16). Longstanding disease also leads to formation of dysplastic nodules manifesting as nodular filling defects indistinguishable from pseudopolyps. *Colitis carcinomas usually present as annular narrowing and strictures* [20].

CT and MRI enterography: Features are divided into active and chronic phase. The active phase is characterized by mural hyperenhancement, concentric mural thickening, and stratification (Fig. 29.17). On MRI, submucosal edema presents T2 hyperintensity, best appreciated on fat-saturated T2 sequences. Actively inflamed segments show diffusion restriction. Pseudopolyps demonstrate contrast enhancement (Table 29.2) [13].

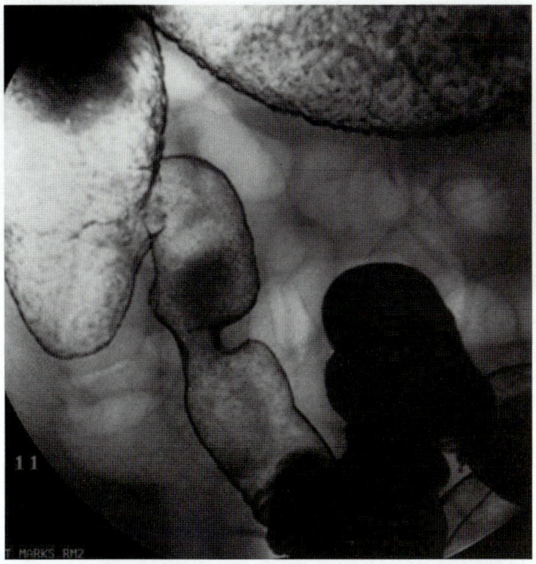

Figure 29.15 Double contrast barium enema shows patulous ileocecal valve with granular mucosa of the terminal ileum due to backwash ileitis.

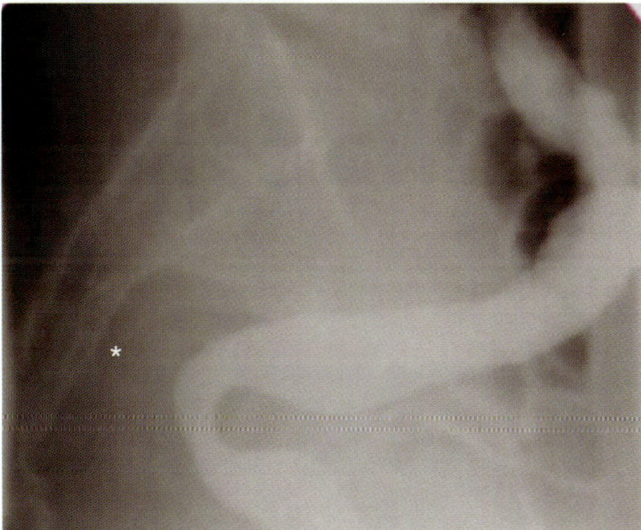

Figure 29.16 Barium enema shows widening of the presacral space (*asterisk*) in chronic ulcerative colitis.

TABLE 29.2 Histopathologic and CT/MRI Features of Active and Chronic Phases of Ulcerative Colitis

Pathology	CT/MRI Features
Active Phase	
Inflammatory infiltration causing cryptitis, crypt abscess, mucosal ulceration, and inflammatory pseudopolyp.	▪ Mural hyperenhancement ▪ Concentric mural thickening ▪ Submucosal edema. ▪ Mucosal ulceration and pseudopolyps
Chronic Phase	
Fibrosis causing a featureless, thickened, and shortened colon with luminal narrowing	▪ Mural thickening with luminal narrowing ▪ Increased submucosal fat ▪ Increased perirectal fat deposition causing widening of presacral space ▪ Postinflammatory pseudopolyps

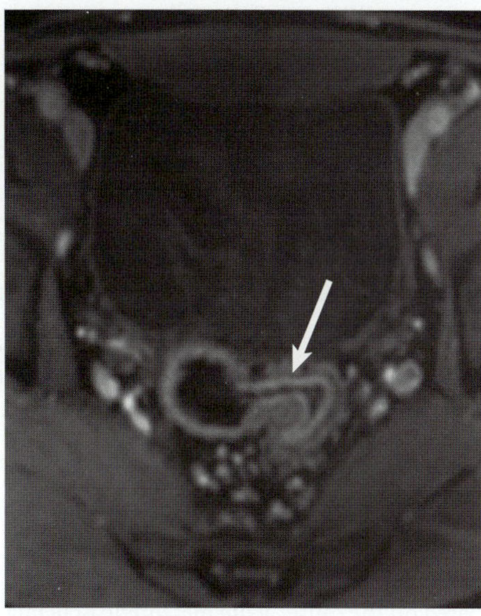

Figure 29.17 Axial T1-weighted magnetic resonance imaging of the pelvis from a 36-year-old woman shows concentric mural thickening and enhancement of the rectosigmoid colon in active ulcerative colitis (*white arrow*).

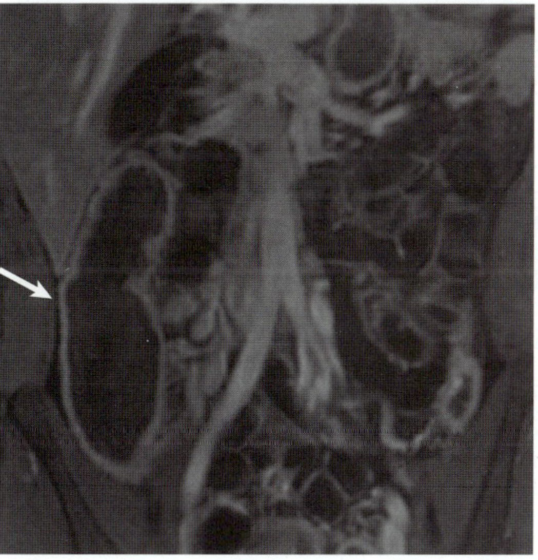

Figure 29.18 Coronal T1-weighted magnetic resonance imaging of the abdomen and pelvis from a 48-year-old man with chronic ulcerative colitis shows a featureless ascending colon and cecum demonstrating loss of haustration and mural thickening (*white arrow*).

The chronic phase leads to concentric mural thickening with luminal narrowing, strictures, a featureless lead pipe colon (Fig. 29.18), submucosal fat deposition, and widening of presacral space. Postinflammatory pseudopolyps may show contrast enhancement (Table 29.2) [13].

Differential diagnosis: The differential diagnosis includes Crohn's disease and infective, ischemic, and radiation colitis.

Certain differentiating imaging features between Crohn's disease and ulcerative colitis are summarized in Table 29.3.

Mesenteric Ischemia

Mesenteric ischemia can be into acute and chronic and is further subdivided into occlusive and nonocclusive types. Acute mesenteric ischemia is a life-threatening condition with a mortality rate of as high as 50–69%. Chronic mesenteric ischemia is relatively less common and is considered imminent acute mesenteric

TABLE 29.3 Differentiating Features Between Crohn's Disease and Ulcerative Colitis

Crohn's Disease	Ulcerative Colitis
▪ Skip lesions with predominant involvement of the ileum and caecum and relative sparing of the rectum ▪ Transmural inflammation leads to ulceration, fissure, and abscess formation ▪ Perianal disease present ▪ Marked bowel wall thickening ▪ Bowel wall may be affected asymmetrically with sacculations	▪ Continuous involvement of the colon with rectal involvement in 95% of cases; small bowel disease is not common ▪ Fissure and abscess are not common ▪ Perianal disease is not seen ▪ Bowel wall thickening is less compared with Crohn's disease ▪ Circumferential bowel wall symmetry is usually maintained

ischemia. Based on the cause, acute mesenteric ischemia is categorized into

- Mesenteric arterial embolism
- Mesenteric arterial thrombosis
- Mesenteric venous thrombosis
- Nonocclusive mesenteric ischemia [21,22]

Clinical Features

Acute mesenteric ischemia presents with abdominal pain, classically described as out of proportion to the clinical examination; nausea; vomiting; diarrhea; and hematochezia. Severe ischemia and bowel necrosis manifest with signs of peritonitis. Chronic mesenteric ischemia has a more gradual course with chronic postprandial pain (described as abdominal angina), weight loss, and early satiety. The overall incidence is higher in the older adult population in the seventh decade of life [21].

Pathophysiology and General Imaging Features

The severity of ischemia damage depends on the degree and extent of flow reduction, duration of ischemia, and degree of collateralization. Early-phase ischemia is characterized by spastic bowel contraction, which proceeds to adynamic ileus caused by ischemia of the muscles and nerves. Complete occlusion of more than 6 hours leads to irreversible injury with mucosal and mural infarction, transmural infarction, and perforation. Beyond a critical level of ischemia, reperfusion also leads to damage because of mucosal barrier disruption, bacterial invasion, and septicemia [22].

Multidetector CT with acquisition of noncontrast and biphasic contrast-enhanced phases (arterial–venous) with maximum intensity projection (MIP) and volume rendering is the most sensitive and specific technique for evaluation. General imaging features of mesenteric ischemia are as follows (Figs. 29.19–29.21) [21,22]:

1. **Bowel wall thickening:** Occurs because of edema, hemorrhage, or superimposed infection. *The target sign is produced by consecutive halos of hypo and hyperattenuation caused by submucosal edema and hemorrhage.* Hemorrhage also imparts high attenuation to the bowel on unenhanced CT.
2. **Abnormal wall enhancement:** Mural hyperenhancement is produced by congestion or reperfusion injury. *Mural hypoenhancement is more specific for cessation of arterial supply and implies severe or irreversible ischemia.*
3. **Bowel wall thinning:** This may relate to adynamic ileus or loss of tissue in irreversible ischemia and infarction.
4. **Bowel dilation:** This indicates loss of muscle tone or adynamic ileus caused by ischemia of the muscles and nerves.

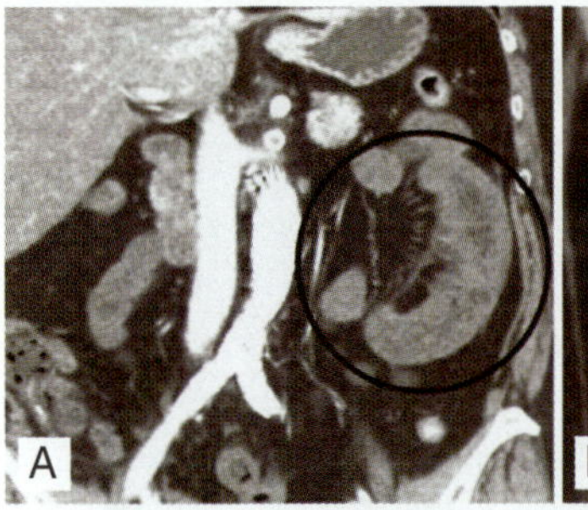

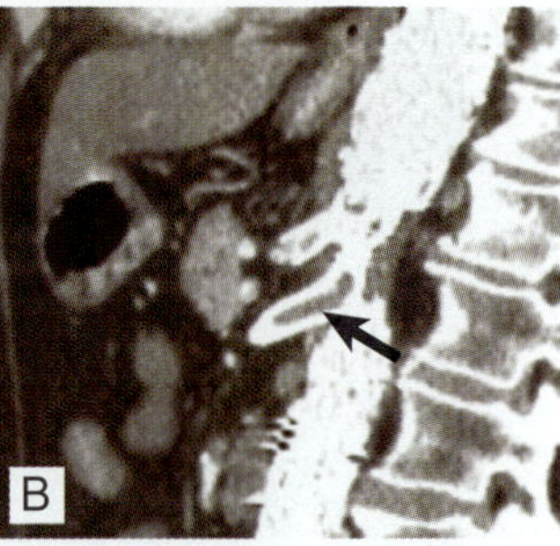

Figure 29.19 An 85-year-old man with aortomesenteric stent graft complained of acute abdominal pain and vomiting. (A) Coronal contrast-enhanced computed tomography of the abdomen and pelvis shows circumferential thickening of proximal jejunal loops with relative mural hypoenhancement and trace perienteric stranding indicating ischemia (*ellipse*). (B) A hypodense thrombus is identified within the superior mesenteric artery stent (*black arrow*).

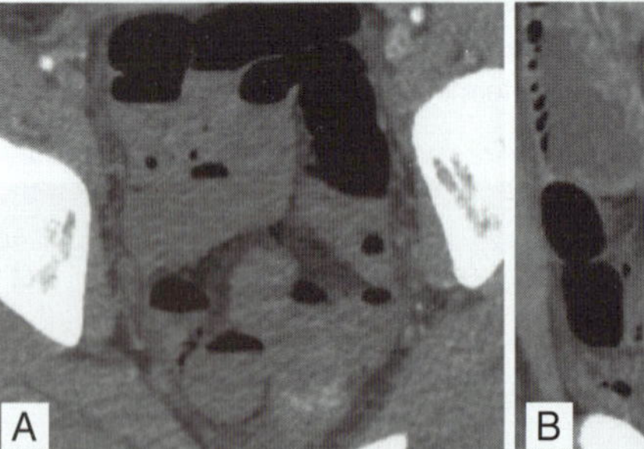

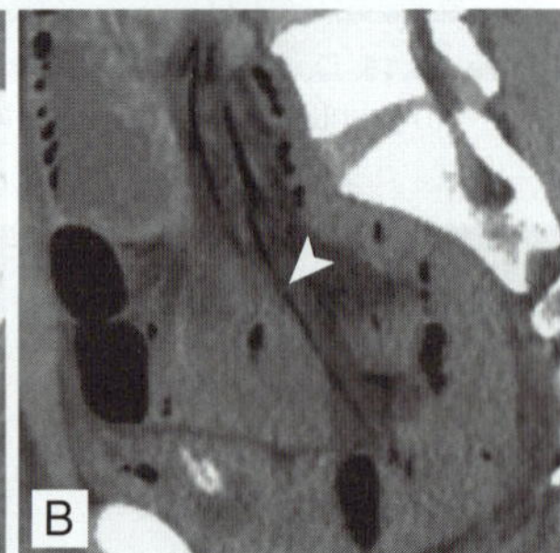

Figure 29.20 Contrast-enhanced computed tomography axial and coronal images from a 39-year-old man with closed-loop obstruction demonstrates hypoenhancing, dilated small bowel loops in the pelvis, consistent with severe ischemia (A). There is extensive associated mesenteric air (*white arrowhead*) (B).

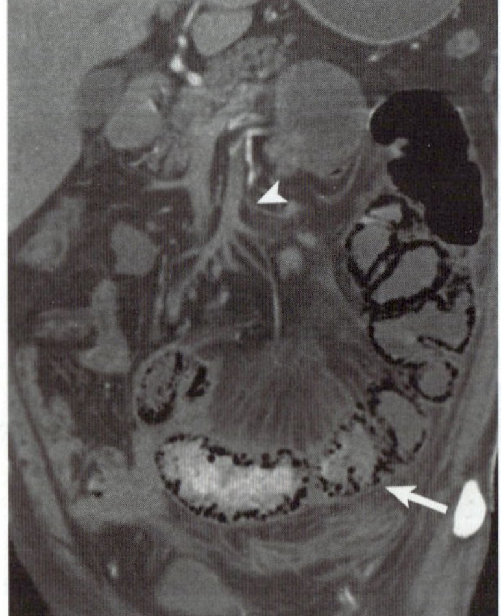

Figure 29.21 Contrast-enhanced coronal computed tomography of the abdomen and pelvis shows extensive small bowel pneumatosis (*white arrow*) from superior mesenteric artery thrombosis (*white arrowhead*). Note the associated extensive perienteric stranding.

5. **Pneumatosis, portal venous gas, and pneumoperitoneum:** These are hallmarks of irreversible ischemia and bowel infarction.
6. **Associated nonspecific mesenteric findings** are engorgement of the vessels, interbowel fluid, fat stranding, and ascites.

Certain specific features of different types of acute mesenteric ischemia are further described.

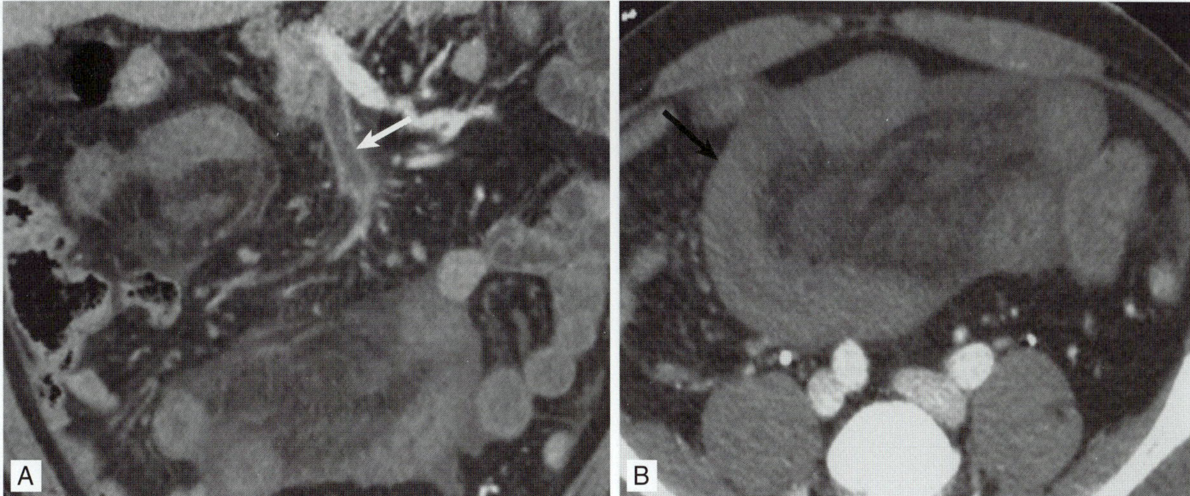

Figure 29.22 Contrast-enhanced coronal and axial computed tomography of the abdomen from a 54-year-old-man with superior mesenteric vein thrombosis (*white arrowhead*) (A) shows ischemic changes in the draining bowel loops, which demonstrate extensive circumferential wall thickening, submucosal edema, mesenteric standing, and interbowel fluid (*black arrow*) (B).

Mesenteric Arterial Embolism

This group constitutes approximately 40–50% of cases and is associated with emboli of cardiac origin from conditions such as atrial fibrillation and myocardial infarction. The SMA is most commonly involved, with typically emboli lodging around 6–8 cm distal to the origin, near the branching of middle colic artery. Proposed factors for a higher incidence of SMA embolism are an inherent high flow rate and a narrow branching angle with the abdominal aorta. Emboli are identified as a hypoattenuating filling defect with associated vascular expansion on contrast-enhanced CT. *Cessation of arterial flow leads to diminished or absent contrast enhancement. Mural thickening is rarely present.* Severe ischemia leads to wall thinning, pneumatosis, and perforation [22].

Mesenteric Arterial Thrombosis

This accounts for about 25% of cases. This group demonstrates the worst prognosis because it is associated with a broader territory of bowel ischemia because of the presence of preexisting atherosclerosis and occlusion of SMA origin [21]. Major risk factors are atherosclerosis, antiphospholipid syndrome, and estrogen therapy. On CT, there is evidence of generalized atherosclerotic disease and vascular calcifications in the celiac trunk, SMA, and IMA with superimposed stenosis or occlusion. Dissection may be detected. Collateral vessels can be observed in long-standing ischemia [22].

Mesenteric Venous Thrombosis

This group accounts for 5–15% of cases and is associated with hypercoagulable states such as oral contraceptive pills, pregnancy, sickle cell disease, and protein C/S deficiency. There is involvement of superior mesenteric vein (SMV) (70%–95%), inferior mesenteric vein, and portal vein. On CT, thrombus is identified as intraluminal filling defects in the veins. *Characteristic findings are prominent bowel wall thickening (with the halo or target sign), engorgement of the vessels, interbowel fluid, ascites, and mesenteric fat stranding* (Fig. 29.22). Mesenteric findings are more pronounced in this group because of the higher hydrostatic pressure in the bowel wall produced by venous obstruction, although the degree of mesenteric abnormality does not correlate with the ischemia severity [3,21,22].

Nonocclusive Mesenteric Ischemia

This refers to bowel ischemia caused by reflex mesenteric vasoconstriction occurring in the setting of decreased cardiac output states, such as hemorrhage or cardiogenic shock, myocardial infarction, and aortic insufficiency, which leads to shock bowel. Ischemic bowel lacks contrast enhancement and demonstrates a broader area of involvement of small and large bowel in a discontinuous manner. The typical finding on angiography is multifocal narrowing of the SMA branches with alternating dilation [22]. Characteristic findings of shock bowel are diffuse small bowel wall thickening and hyperenhancement with associated mesenteric fluid and relative sparing of the colon. It is commonly associated with additional signs of hypovolemia such as collapsed inferior vena cava (IVC) and hyperenhancing adrenal glands (Fig. 29.23) [3].

Chronic Mesenteric Ischemia

Duplex USG is indicated to evaluate SMA stenosis in chronic ischemia, with a peak systolic velocity of 275 cm/sec or greater suggestive of more than 70% stenosis. However, there are several limitations to the examination such as operator dependance, overlying bowel gas, and body habitus. Multidetector CT angiography performs better in evaluation of vascular stenosis, collateral vessels, and associated changes of bowel ischemia [23].

Differential Diagnosis

The differential diagnosis includes bowel wall thickening and mural hyperenhancement caused by infectious, inflammatory, and neoplastic processes; radiation injury; and graft-versus-host disease. Intramural bowel gas can be seen in benign pneumatosis [3].

Bowel Infections

Pathophysiology and Clinical Features

Infective enteritis and colitis are caused by bacterial, viral, fungal, and parasitic etiologies. Certain organisms have a predilection for specific bowel segments; for example, tuberculosis and amebiasis affect the distal ileum and cecum, *Giardia* involves the proximal small bowel, and *Salmonella* and *Shigella* involve the distal small bowel. Gonorrhea, herpesvirus, and chlamydia predominately affect the rectum and sigmoid colon. *Clostridium* and cytomegalovirus (CMV) are associated with pancolitis [24,25].

Imaging Features

On contrast-enhanced CT, general features of enterocolitis are circumferential bowel wall thickening and hyperenhancement,

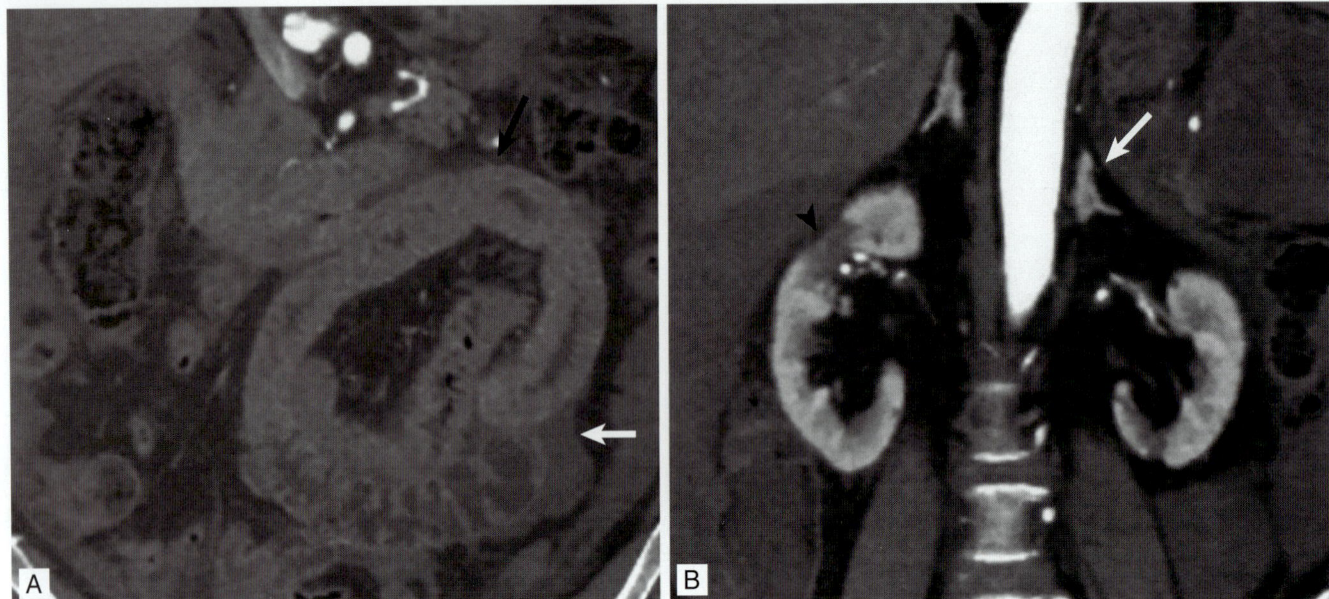

Figure 29.23 Coronal computed tomography angiography of the abdomen and pelvis from a 61-year-old man on Coumadin with history of fall demonstrate shock bowel with diffuse small bowel thickening (*black arrow*), hyperenhancement, and interbowel fluid (*white arrow*) (A). Associated signs of hypoperfusion include hyperenhancing adrenal glands (*white arrow*) and right renal infarct (*black arrowhead*) (B).

submucosal edema, perienteric and pericolonic fat stranding, lack of formed stool with air-fluid levels, interbowel fluid, and ascites.

Characteristic features of certain common bowel infections are discussed next.

Tuberculosis

Pathophysiology and Clinical Presentation: Tubercular bacilli can enter the GI tract through ingestion of infected sputum or milk. The bacilli then invade the mucosa and submucosa with formation of epithelial tubercle in the submucosal lymphoid tissue followed by caseous necrosis and ulceration. *The ileocecal region is the most common site of involvement because of abundant lymphoid tissues.* Isolated colonic involvement is seen in approximately 10% of cases, which has increased incidence in immunocompromised patients. Tubercular lesions are morphologically classified into ulcerative, hypertrophied, and ulcer-hypertrophied subtypes. Spread of infection through direct, lymphatic, and hematogenous routes leads to multisystemic disease, with the lymph nodes and peritoneum being the most common sites of involvement in the abdominal cavity. Clinical manifestations of ileocecal tuberculosis include chronic abdominal pain, fever, weight loss, and altered bowel habits. The most common complications are bowel obstruction and perforations [26].

Imaging Features

Radiographs: These may depict enteroliths, bowel obstruction as air-fluid levels, and signs of pneumoperitoneum in perforation.

Fluoroscopy: On small bowel follow-through, acute to subacute disease presents as spasm and edema involving the ileocecal valve and terminal ileum, which eventually thickens and ulcerates. *The Stierlin sign refers to rapid emptying of barium in the inflamed segments of the ileum and cecum with the presence a normal column of barium in the adjacent uninvolved segments.* There can be hypersegmentation of the barium column *(chicken intestine)*, flocculation, and precipitation, with thickening of the mucosal folds. Progressive infection can lead to fistula (e.g., enteroenteric, enterocolonic), bowel matting, or localized mass formation. Chronic infection leads to fibrosis with distorted pulled-up cecum, a fixed gaping ileocecal valve, and annular stenosis of the terminal ileum leading to *goose neck deformity*. The *Fleischner or inverted umbrella sign* refers to gaping and thickened lips of the ileocecal vale with a narrowed terminal ileum (Figs. 29.24 and 29.25) [26–28]

Contrast-enhanced CT: CT demonstrates circumferential thickening of the terminal ileum and caecum with asymmetric thickening of the ileocecal valve. Associated mesenteric adenopathy is pathognomonic. *Involved lymph nodes demonstrate characteristic central low-attenuation caused by caseous necrosis* (Figs. 29.26 and 29.27). The chronic stage results in formation of multifocal short segment strictures superimposed on diffuse narrowing of the ileum.

Differential diagnosis: The differential diagnosis includes Crohn's disease, lymphoma, amoebiasis, and cecal malignancy [26,27].

Amoebiasis

This is a type of infectious colitis caused by protozoa *Entamoeba histolytica*. The infection is endemic in tropical and subtropical countries and is acquired through ingestion of contaminated food

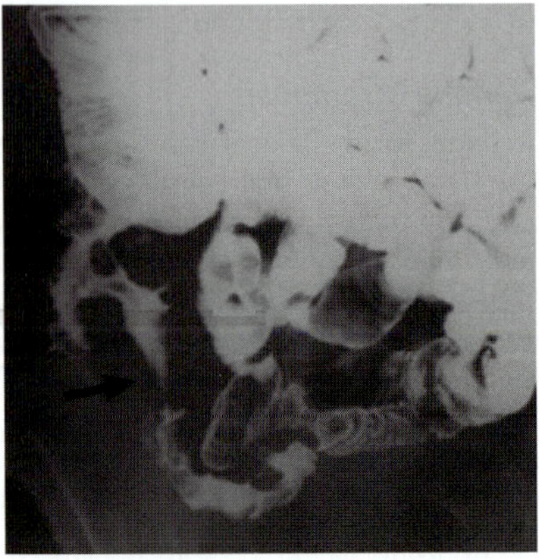

Figure 29.24 Small bowel enteroclysis demonstrates nodular fold thickening and irregular narrowing of the terminal ileum, with loop separation and deep mucosal ulceration (*black arrow*) caused by tuberculosis. The cecum is pulled up contracted (*black arrowhead*) with a wide ileocecal valve (goose neck deformity).

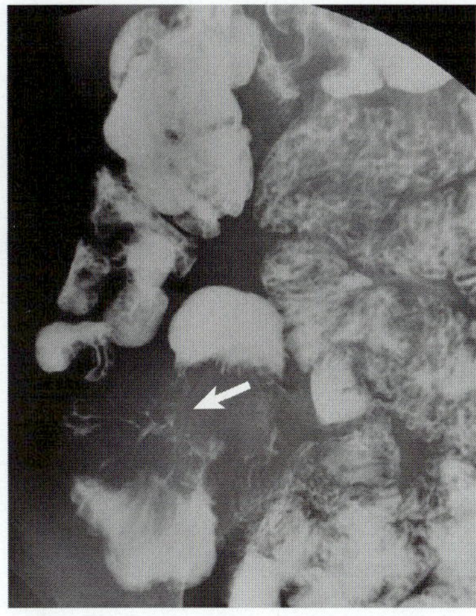

Figure 29.25 Small bowel follow-through demonstrates irregular narrowing of the terminal ileum, contracted cecum with a wide ileocecal valve (*white arrow*) (Fleischner sign).

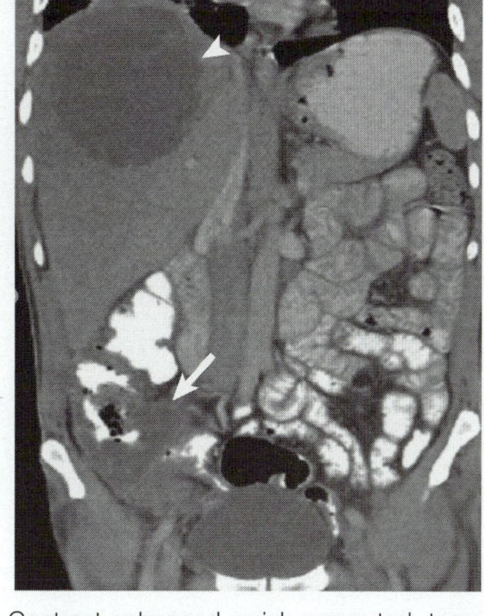

Figure 29.28 Contrast-enhanced axial computed tomography of the abdomen and pelvis from a patient with amoebic colitis demonstrates asymmetric thickening of the cecum (*white arrow*). There is an associated solitary amoebic liver abscess (*white arrowhead*).

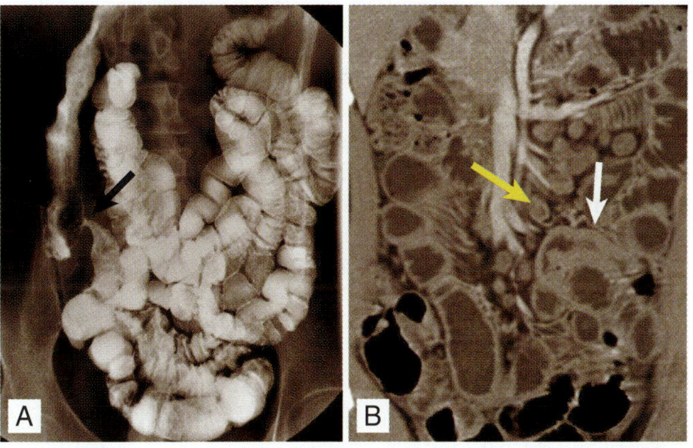

Figure 29.26 Small bowel follow-through demonstrates irregular narrowing of the terminal ileum (*black arrow*) and cecum caused by tuberculosis (A). Contrast-enhanced coronal computed tomography of the abdomen and pelvis in another patient (B) shows multiple enlarged mesenteric nodes with central low attenuation (*yellow arrow*) and a stricture of the mid small bowel (*white arrow*).

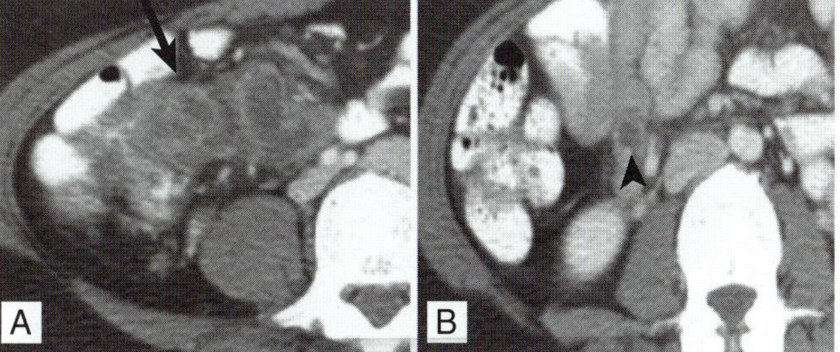

Figure 29.27 Contrast-enhanced axial computed tomography of the abdomen and pelvis from a 28-year-old woman with ileocecal tuberculosis demonstrates masslike thickening of the ileocecal valve and terminal ileum (*black arrow*) (A). Associated enlarged mesenteric nodes show central low attenuation caused by caseous necrosis (*black arrowhead*) (B).

or water. However, symptomatic disease seen in only 10% of the infected population with clinical manifestations of fever, bloody diarrhea, abdominal pain, and weight loss. Spectrum of disease varies from acute proctocolitis or dysentery, fulminant colitis with bowel perforations, chronic colitis, and amoeboma formation. *The most common extraintestinal manifestation is hepatic abscess secondary to the hematogenous spread of infection through the portal circulation.* On CT, amoebic colitis presents as circumferential or asymmetric bowel thickening with a predilection for cecal and ascending colonic involvement (Fig. 29.28). Transmural extension of infection in fulminant colitis leads to deep mucosal ulceration causing intramural dissection of contrast, marked colonic distension, and perforations. Skip bowel involvement may be seen. Amoeboma involves formation of large tumefactive lesions simulating colon cancer. Differential diagnoses are tuberculosis, Crohn's disease, ulcerative colitis, and colon cancer [29,30].

Ascariasis

Ascariasis involves intestinal infection with roundworm *Ascariasis lumbricoides*. Humans become infected after ingestion of embryonated eggs passed in the feces of infected individual. On small bowel series, worms are identified as tubular intraluminal filling defects associated with an internal linear collection of barium (Fig. 29.29). On real-time USG, adult worms are seen as mobile hypoechoic tubular structures with an echogenic wall. Major complications are mechanical bowel obstruction, volvulus, and intussusception [31].

Giardiasis

Giardiasis is caused by water borne protozoan *Giardia lamblia*. The most common sites of involvement are the proximal jejunum and duodenum. The pathogenesis involves invasion of the bowel mucosa by the organism inciting acute and chronic inflammatory changes, crypt hyperplasia, and villous atrophy with resultant malabsorption. Spectrum of findings on small bowel follow-through are mucosal thickening, indistinctness of mucosal folds, flocculation, and rapid transit of barium caused by bowel irritation and spasm [32].

Whipple Disease

Whipple disease is a multisystemic disease caused by infection with actinobacteria *Tropheryma whipplei*. GI manifestations are with symptoms of malabsorption such as weight loss, diarrhea, abdominal pain, and steatorrhea. The pathogenesis involves macrophagic infiltration of lamina propria infected with *T. whipplei*, leading to swelling and thickening of the intestinal villi. On small bowel follow-through, there is nodular thickening of the

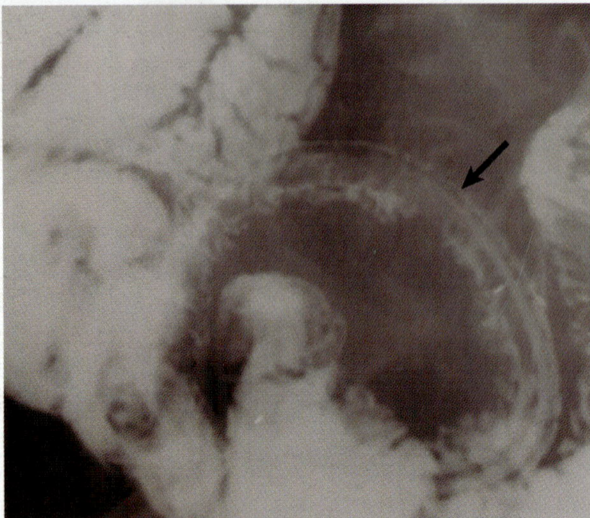

Figure 29.29 Small bowel follow-through demonstrates an ascaris worm in the ileum as an intraluminal filling defect with an internal linear column of barium (*black arrow*).

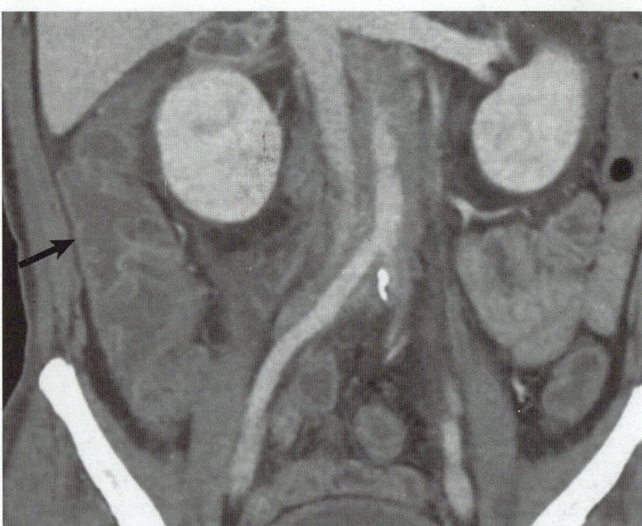

Figure 29.30 Contrast-enhanced coronal computed tomography of the abdomen and pelvis from a 64-year-old man with myeloid leukemia shows concentric ascending colonic thickening and mural enhancement secondary to typhlitis (*black arrow*).

valvulae conniventes with a normal small bowel caliber. There is a predilection for jejunal involvement. Mesenteric adenopathy is a predominant finding on CT, with involved lymph nodes demonstrating characteristic central low or fat attenuation [33].

Certain specific infections in immunocompromised hosts are as follows.

Typhlitis

Typhlitis, also known as neutropenic enterocolitis, most commonly occurs in patients undergoing treatment for malignancy. Summative effects of infection (particularly with CMV) and ischemia are proposed as the potential etiology. It is characterized by inflammation of the cecum, ascending the colon, and less commonly the terminal ileum. Severe cases demonstrate mucosal hemorrhage, transmural necrosis and perforation [28]. Contrast-enhanced CT demonstrates circumferential thickening involving the cecum and ascending colon with submucosal edema, pericolonic fluid, and stranding (Fig. 29.30). Pneumatosis and perforation are present in severe cases.

HIV-related Enterocolitis

Although opportunistic infections are the predominant cause of GI disease in HIV, primary HIV infection of the mucosa is known, particularly in the colon. Myriad of HIV-related opportunistic infections include CMV, cryptosporidiosis, *Mycobacterium avium, Shigella* spp., *Salmonella* spp., *Campylobacter* spp., *Clostridium difficile,* and *Strongyloides* spp. [34,35].

Cytomegalovirus GI disease develops in approximately 30% of patients with AIDS, particularly with a CD4 lymphocytes below 100/mm^3. Presenting symptoms include persistent diarrhea, fever, weight loss, severe abdominal pain, and hematochezia. The infection leads to endothelial involvement with occlusive vasculitis, tissue edema, and necrosis. CT features of CMV colitis are colonic wall thickening, which is predominantly asymmetric with a mean mural thickness of 15 mm; mural edema; and deep ulcerations. There is a predilection for involvement of the rectum, descending colon, and cecum. The small bowel is involved in approximately 42% of cases. Bowel involvement can be in a diffuse or segmental pattern. Lymphadenopathy is not common. A major complication is bowel perforation [36].

Clostridium Difficile–Associated Pseudomembranous Colitis

It usually follows administration of antibiotic and chemotherapy in hospitalized patients and carries significant morbidity. On CT, there is marked colonic wall thickening with characteristic *accordion sign, which refers to trapping of enteric contrast between markedly thickened and edematous haustral folds resembling an accordion* (Fig. 29.31) [24].

Radiation Injury

Small bowel mucosa is the most radiosensitive tissue in the GI tract caused by rapid cell turnover. The rectum is the least radiosensitive

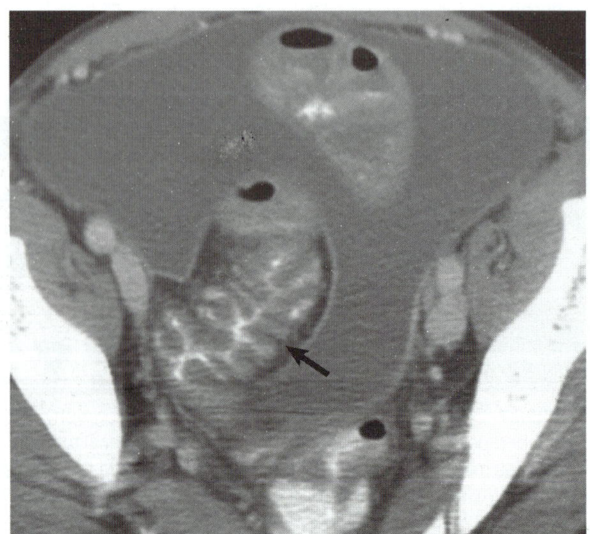

Figure 29.31 Contrast-enhanced axial computed tomography of the pelvis from a 56-year-old woman with *Clostridium difficile* colitis demonstrates marked thickening of rectosigmoid colon with the *accordion sign* (*black arrow*). Also seen are large-volume ascites and diffuse peritoneal thickening secondary to underlying peritoneal carcinomatosis from carcinoma of the ovary.

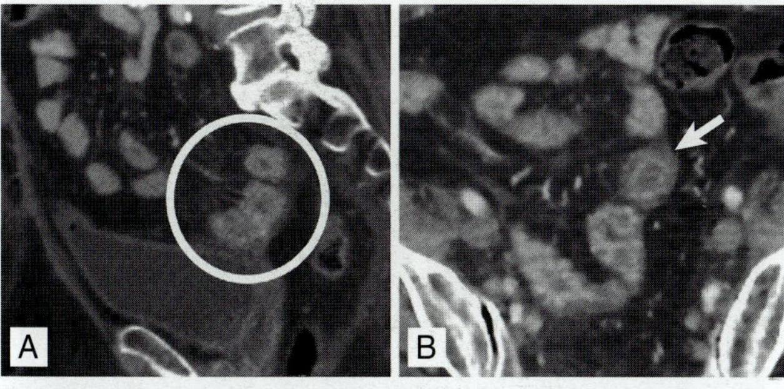

Figure 29.32 Contrast-enhanced sagittal computed tomography of the pelvis from a 68-year-old woman with endometrial cancer and history of recent radiation to the pelvis demonstrates circumferential thickening, mucosal hyperenhancement, and trace interbowel fluid involving few small bowel loops in the pelvis indicative of radiation enteritis (*circle*) (A). Axial image delineates the submucosal edema in the affected loops (*white arrow*) (B).

part commonly affected by radiation damage because of the proximity to radiosensitive organs such as the prostate and cervix. Radiation injury has been divided into acute and chronic subtypes.

- Acute radiation injury occurs within first few days or weeks of treatment, typically presenting with self-limited symptoms of malabsorption and short-term nonspecific CT findings such as focal circumferential bowel wall thickening, submucosal edema, and mucosal hyperenhancement (Fig. 29.32)
- Chronic radiation injury presents months to years after exposure because of progressive mural fibrosis and microvascular damage. CT features of this stage are circumferential bowel thickening, strictures, adhesions, and fistulations [37]

Specific Small Bowel Abnormalities

Small Bowel Obstruction

Pathophysiology and Clinical Features

Small bowel obstruction can be mechanical or functional, preventing normal transit of intraluminal contents. Causes of mechanical obstruction are divided into extrinsic, intrinsic, and intraluminal causes [38].

- **Extrinsic:** adhesions (*most common*), hernia, endometriosis, and vascular compressions
- **Intrinsic:** Crohn's disease, tuberculosis, neoplasm, intussusception, hematoma, and radiation enteritis
- **Intraluminal:** foreign body, gallstone ileus, bezoars, and distal intestinal obstruction syndrome. Distal intestinal obstruction syndrome is a manifestation of cystic fibrosis involving intestinal obstruction caused by inspissated feculent material and secretions in the distal ileum and right colon (Fig. 29.33)

Small bowel obstruction is further subclassified into high- and low-grade types, *with high-grade obstruction indicating no passage of bowel contents beyond the point of obstruction.* Clinical features are nausea, vomiting, colicky abdominal pain, distension, and high-pitched or absent bowel sounds. Associated leukocytosis and elevated lactate levels indicate strangulation or ischemia [39]. Management ranges from conservative with bowel decompression to surgery depending on the etiology and severity of obstruction.

Imaging Features

Radiographs: Supine and upright radiographs are the initial screening tests in symptomatic patients with overall low diagnostic accuracy (diagnostic in only 50–60% of cases). Detection sensitivity is relatively higher for high-grade obstruction. Normal, equivocal, and findings of low-grade obstruction necessitate further evaluation with multidetector CT [38,40].

Small bowel loops are identified because of the presence of valvulae conniventes, with a normal diameter of less than 3 cm. Obstructed small bowel has a diameter exceeding 3 cm (Fig. 29.34). The differential diagnosis is ileus, which presents as generalized gaseous distension of small and large bowel loops without a distinct transition zone or as focally distended sentinel loop.

Certain radiographic predictors of high-grade obstructions are

- Caliber of dilated small bowel loop more than 50% of caliber of largest visible colon
- Air-fluid levels with width greater than 2.5 cm
- Presence of air-fluid levels with height difference of more than 2 cm within the same loop [38,40]

The number of air-fluids levels proportionately increase with more distal obstruction (Fig. 29.35). Paucity of bowel gas or *gasless abdomen* occurs when bowel loops are predominately fluid

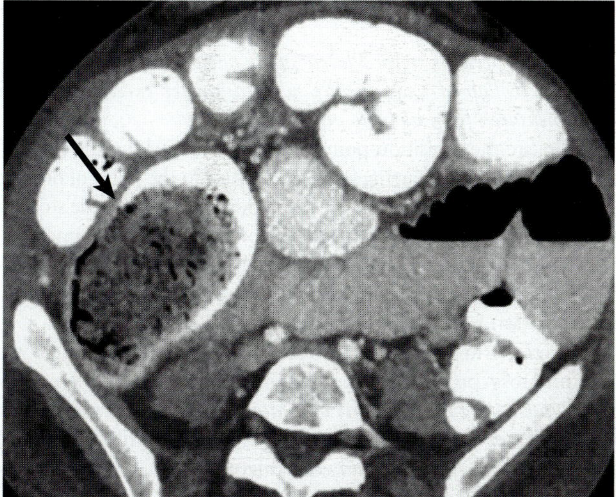

Figure 29.33 Contrast-enhanced axial computed tomography of the abdomen and pelvis from a 31-year-old man with cystic fibrosis and distal intestinal obstruction syndrome demonstrates large obstructive stool ball in the distal ileum (*black arrow*).

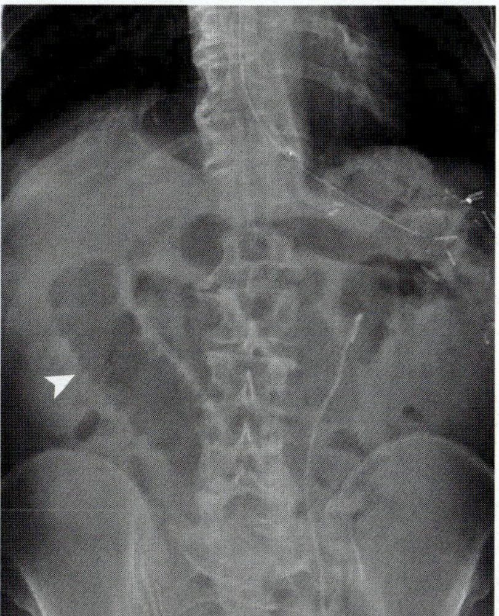

Figure 29.34 Supine abdominal radiograph from a 56 years-old-man with obstructive small bowel gas pattern. Small bowel loops are identified caused by valvulae conniventes (*white arrowhead*) and measure up to 3.5 cm in diameter.

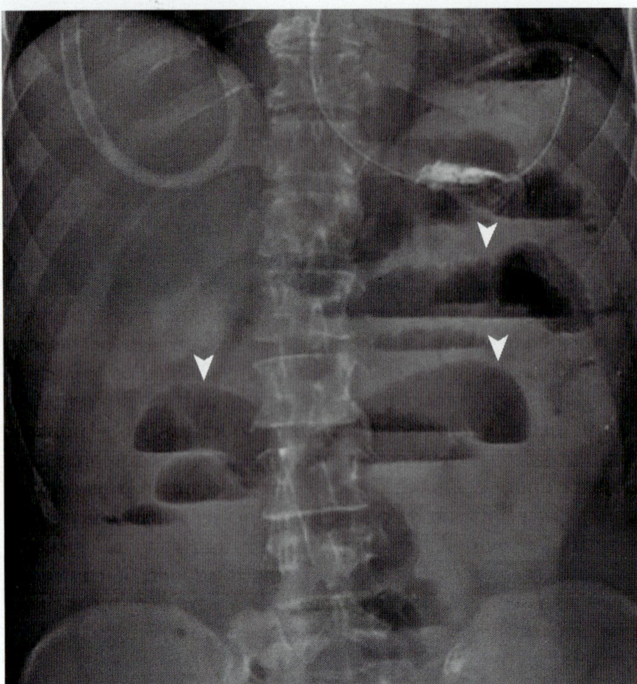

Figure 29.35 Erect abdominal radiograph shows obstructive small bowel gas pattern with numerous air-fluid levels. The presence of multiple air fluid levels with width greater than 25 mm (*white arrowheads*) and height difference exceeding 2 cm indicates high-grade obstruction.

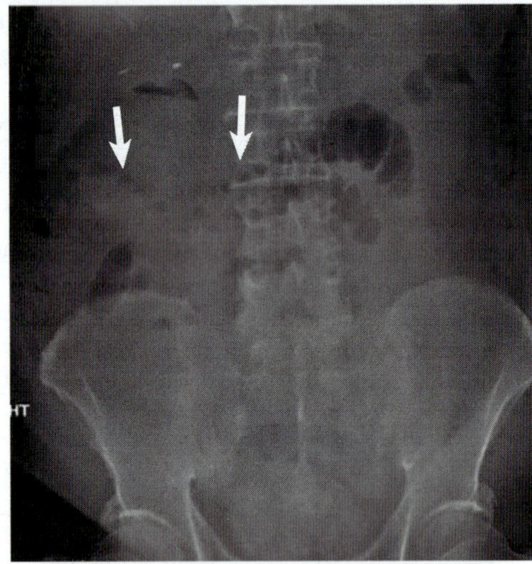

Figure 29.36 Upright abdominal radiograph shows "string of bead signs" in high-grade small bowel obstruction (*white arrows*).

filled, most commonly seen in the setting of high-grade or closed-loop obstruction. Upright abdomen radiographs in such cases can demonstrate the *"string of beads sign" secondary to air trapping between the valvulae conniventes* (Fig. 29.36) [39].

Ultrasonography: It is not usually indicated because of inherent technical limitations in evaluating gas containing structures. Findings are dilated fluid and gas-filled bowel demonstrating increased whirling or to-and-fro peristalsis. The loops may show a thickened wall and valvulae conniventes. The presence of inter-bowel fluid, wall thickness exceeding 3 mm, and aperistalsis are indicative of ischemia [38].

Computed Tomography: It is the technique of choice to evaluate the presence, degree, transition point, etiology of obstruction, and complications. IV contrast is imperative to detect ischemia unless contraindicated. Although oral contrast was previously routinely

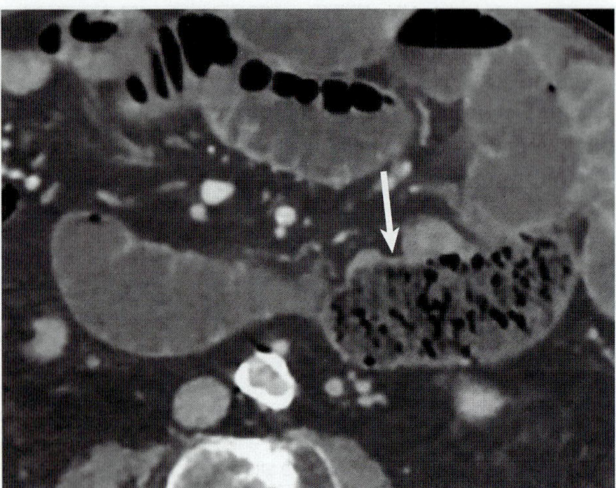

Figure 29.37 Contrast-enhanced axial computed tomography of the abdomen and pelvis from a 76-year-old man with small bowel obstruction caused by adhesions shows a fecalized small bowel (*small bowel feces sign*) at the transition point in left abdomen (*white arrow*).

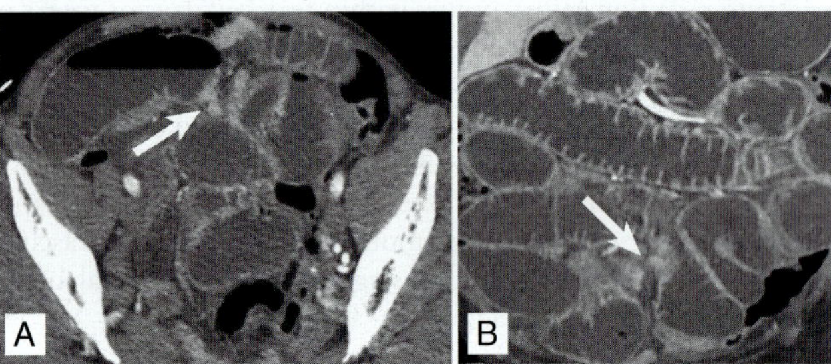

Figure 29.38 Axial (A) and coronal (B) contrast-enhanced computed tomography of the abdomen and pelvis shows high-grade small bowel obstruction caused by adhesion, with transition point in the central abdomen (*white arrow*).

administered to exclude high-grade obstruction, routine administration is debated in current clinical practice because of

1. Risk of aspiration in patients with vomiting
2. Retained intraluminal fluid serving as natural negative contrast
3. Contrast material rarely opacities bowel just proximal to transition point in high-grade obstruction
4. Elimination of the time delay in performing the CT examination [39]

Obstruction presents with dilated small bowel leading to a normal caliber or collapsed loop distally, with diameter exceeding 2.5 cm when measured from outer to outer wall [38].

To locate the transition point, we advocate tracking the bowel in a retrograde manner starting from the rectum to the point of obstruction, confirming with further anterograde tracking from the stomach down, and subsequent correlation on coronal and sagittal images.

It is also helpful to locate any fecalized segment *(small bowel feces sign)*, which is typically present immediately proximal or near the transition point (Fig. 29.37).

Adhesions are bands of fibrous tissue formed secondary to inflammatory process. *They are overall the most common cause of bowel obstruction in both early and late postoperative periods.* Adhesions are not directly visualized on CT but manifest as abrupt transition or tapering between dilated and collapsed bowel (Fig. 29.38) [39].

Gallstone ileus presents with an obstructing stone at or near the ileocecal junction (Fig. 29.39).

Findings of strangulation are wall thickening, abnormal wall enhancement (hyperenhancement caused by slow perfusion and

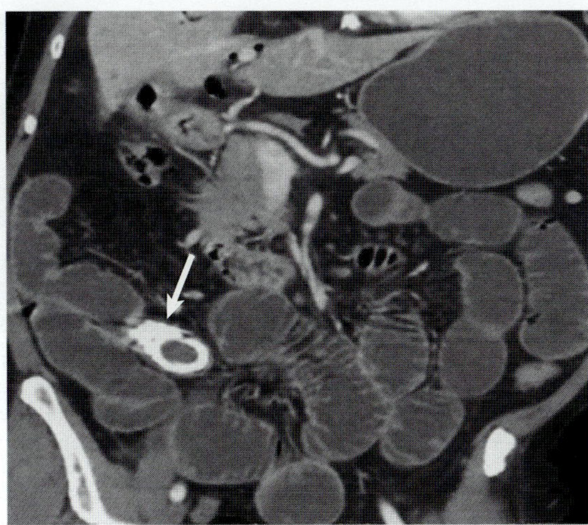

Figure 29.39 Coronal contrast-enhanced computed tomography of the abdomen and pelvis from a 44-year-old man with gallstones ileus demonstrates obstructive stone in the distal ileum (*white arrow*).

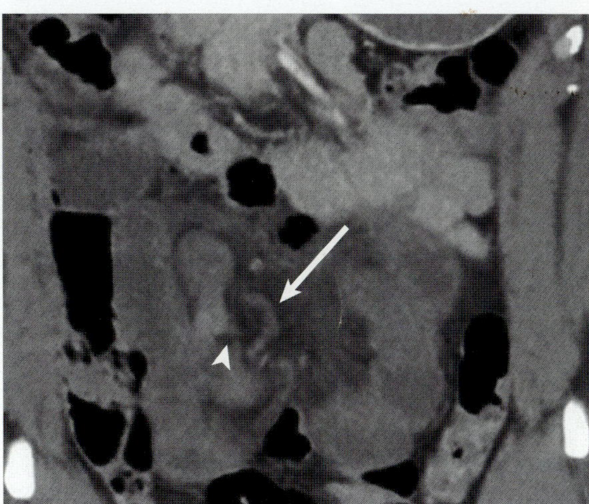

Figure 29.40 Coronal and axial contrast-enhanced computed tomography of the abdomen and pelvis from a 60-year-old man with closed-loop bowel obstruction caused by internal hernia. Small bowel loops are radially distributed in the central abdomen with beaking at the transition point (*white arrowhead*) and mesenteric vessel swirl (*white arrow*).

congestion, progressing to hypoenhancement in severe ischemia), interbowel fluid, mesenteric edema and hyperemia, pneumatosis, and mesenteric and portal venous air [38,39,41].

Closed-loop obstruction is a complex small bowel obstruction with a high risk of strangulations. It is characterized by obstruction of a segment of bowel at two points in a manner precluding any outlet for lumen decompression. Progressive buildup of secretions leads to increased intraluminal pressure and venous obstruction. Common causes are adhesive bands, internal hernias, umbilical hernia, and Roux-en-Y gastric bypass. *It presents as U- or C-shaped, radially distributed small bowel loops, double beak sign caused by tapering of at least two loops at the transition point, and whirl sign secondary to mesenteric twisting* (Fig. 29.40) [39,42]. Blood lactate levels can be normal with ischemia in closed loop because of simultaneous twisting and occlusion of both the supplying mesenteric artery and vein.

Certain reported imaging predictors of success of conservative treatment include the presence of the feces sign, anterior parietal adhesion (refers to close proximity of transition zone to the anterior peritoneum), and lack of the beak sign. The presence of two or more beak signs, whirl sign, and C- or U-shaped configuration of bowel loops are associated with failure of nonsurgical treatment [43].

Superior Mesenteric Artery Syndrome

This is a rare acquired vascular compression disorder involving duodenal obstruction from compression of the third portion between the SMA and aorta. Normally, the third portion of the duodenum passes between the aorta and SMA at L3 level and is surrounded by retroperitoneal fat. Major causes include rapid and severe weight loss and wasting conditions such as immunodeficiency, cancer cachexia, and malabsorption, which lead to loss of the retroperitoneal fat cushion. The incidence is higher in women presenting with symptoms such as postprandial epigastric pain, nausea, and vomiting. On barium studies, there is dilation of the stomach and proximal duodenum with a vertical extrinsic impression on the third portion of the duodenum. The obstruction decreases with postural change. *Mesenteric angiography demonstrates acute angulation of the SMA and reduction in the aortomesenteric angle and distance, with reported aortomesenteric angle ranging from 6 to 22 degrees and aortomesenteric distance of 2–8 mm (normal aortomesenteric angle, 28–65 degree, aortomesenteric distance, 10–34 mm)* (Fig. 29.41) [44].

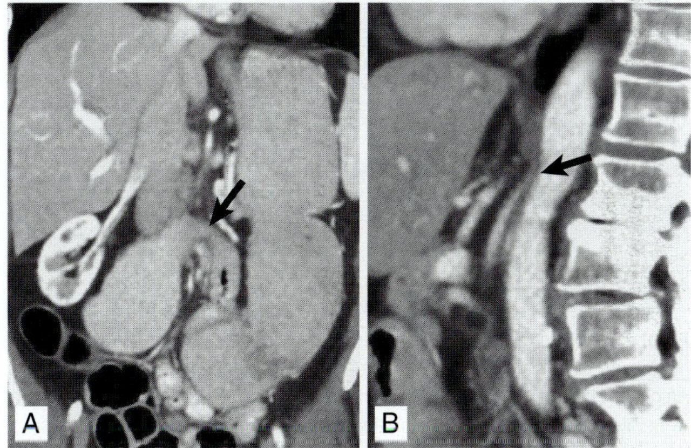

Figure 29.41 Coronal contrast-enhanced computed tomography of the abdomen and pelvis from a 62-year-old woman with chronic abdominal pain shows massive distension of the stomach and proximal duodenum with narrowing of third portion of duodenum where it crosses between the aorta and superior mesenteric artery (SMA) (*black arrow*) (A). Sagittal image shows an abnormal aortomesenteric angle and distance (6 degrees, 3 mm), consistent with SMA syndrome (*black arrowhead*) (B).

Internal Hernias

Pathophysiology and Clinical Features

Internal hernias are abnormal protrusion of abdominal viscera through the peritoneum or mesentery into a compartment of the abdominal cavity. The orifices of herniation can be congenital or acquired secondary to trauma, previous surgery, or inflammation.

Internal hernias can be classified based on the hernial orifices, as shown in the Table 29.4 [45,46].

The clinical presentation is with symptoms of bowel obstruction such as nausea, vomiting, abdominal pain, and distension. Intermittent abdominal pain and weight loss may accompany recurrent, spontaneously reducing internal hernias [45].

Imaging Features

Multidetector CT is the technique of choice for evaluation. Multiplanar and 3D volume-rendered reconstructions increase the

TABLE 29.4 Categories of Internal Hernia

Hernial Orifice	Hernia Type
Normal foramen	Foramen of Winslow
Unusual peritoneal fossa or retroperitoneal recess	Paraduodenal, pericecal, and intersigmoid hernia
Abnormal opening in mesentery or peritoneal ligament	Hernia through mesentery, omentum, transverse mesocolon, sigmoid mesocolon, falciform ligament, or broad ligament and Roux-en-Y anastomosis–related hernia

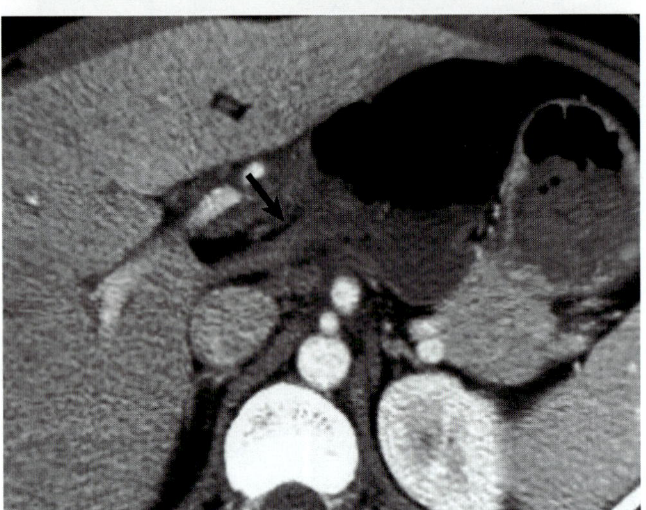

Figure 29.42 Axial contrast-enhanced computed tomography of the abdomen and pelvis from a 79-year-old woman with acute abdominal pain shows herniation of the cecum and terminal ileum in the foramen of Winslow. Note the beaklike pointing of the hernia toward the foramen of Winslow (*black arrow*).

diagnostic accuracy and help in surgical planning. Use of IV contrast is essential to evaluate the vascular relationships and identify signs of ischemia [45]. Imaging features of the most common subtypes of internal hernia are described.

Foramen of Winslow Hernia

Anatomy: The foramen of Winslow is an approximately 3-cm vertical slitlike communication between the lesser sac and peritoneal cavity. The foramen is located cephalad to the duodenal bulb, inferior to the caudate lobe, anterior to the IVC, and posterior to the hepatoduodenal ligament. These represent approximately 8% of internal hernias with hernia contents consisting of small bowel, cecum, ascending colon, transverse colon, and gallbladder [46].

Computed Tomography Features: These include the presence of a herniated sac in the lesser sac with beak-shaped projection of the hernial sac pointing toward the foramen of Winslow, the presence of mesentery between the IVC and portal vein, absence of the ascending colon in the right paracolic space, and two or more bowel loops in the high subhepatic space (Fig. 29.42) [45,46].

Paraduodenal Hernia

These constitute approximately 53% of the internal hernia and are divided into left and right subtypes.

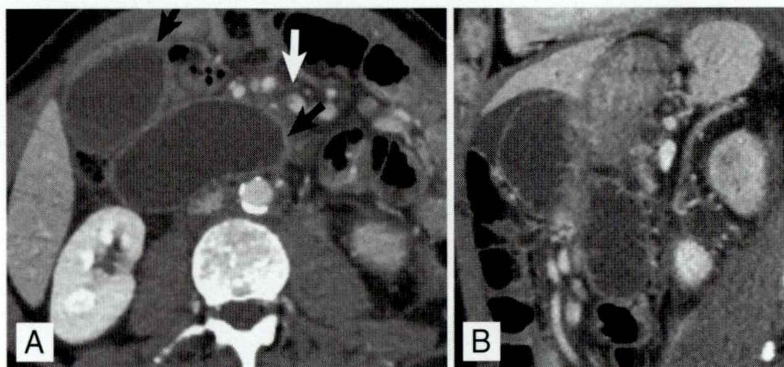

Figure 29.43 Axial (A) and sagittal (B) contrast-enhanced computed tomography of the abdomen and pelvis from a 61-year-old man demonstrates left paraduodenal hernia. Note the inferior mesenteric vein is located anterior and medial (*white arrow*) to the herniated bowel loops (*black arrows* in A).

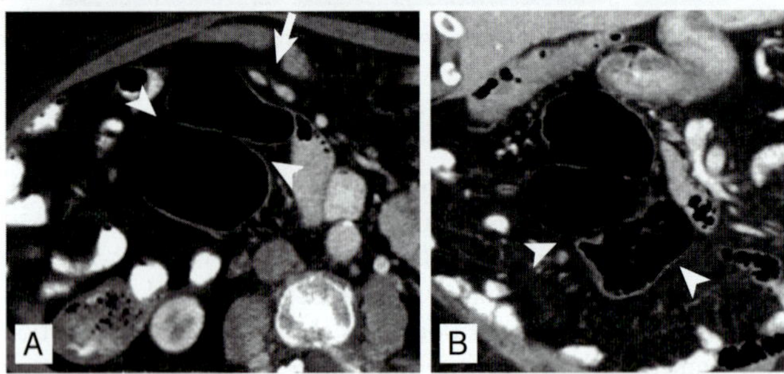

Figure 29.44 Axial and coronal contrast-enhanced computed tomography of the abdomen and pelvis from a 54-year-old man demonstrates right paraduodenal hernia containing sigmoid colon (*white arrowheads*) (A and B). Note the superior mesenteric artery and vein are located anterior and medial to the hernia sac (*white arrow* in A).

Left Paraduodenal Hernia

Anatomy: Hernia occurs through the *fossa of Landzert*, which is a congenital peritoneal recess formed by failure of fusion of the descending colon with the posterior parietal peritoneum. *The inferior mesenteric vein and ascending left colic artery* are situated at the anteromedial edge of this fossa [45,46].

Computed tomography features: These include saclike clustering of small bowel loops in the left anterior pararenal space with the *inferior mesenteric vein located anterior and medial to the hernial sac* (Fig. 29.43).

Right Paraduodenal Hernia

Anatomy: Hernia occurs through the *fossa of Waldeyer*, located inferior to the third portion of the duodenum and just behind the root of the small bowel mesentery. *The SMA and SMV* are situated at the anteromedial edge of this fossa. The recess is formed by failure of fusion of part of the ascending colon with the posterior parietal peritoneum. The hernia most commonly occurs in the setting of small bowel nonrotation [45–47].

Computed tomography features: *The SMA and SMV are located anterior and medial to the hernial sac.* As the fossa of Waldeyer extends to the right and downward into the ascending mesocolon, *the right colic vein is displaced anteriorly by the hernial sac.* In the setting of intestinal nonrotation, the SMV is more left and ventral relative to SMA with absence of normal horizontal duodenum (Fig. 29.44) [45–47].

Pericecal Hernia

Anatomy: Unusual recesses around the caecum are superior ileocecal recess, inferior ileocecal recess, retrocecal recess, and paracolic sulci.

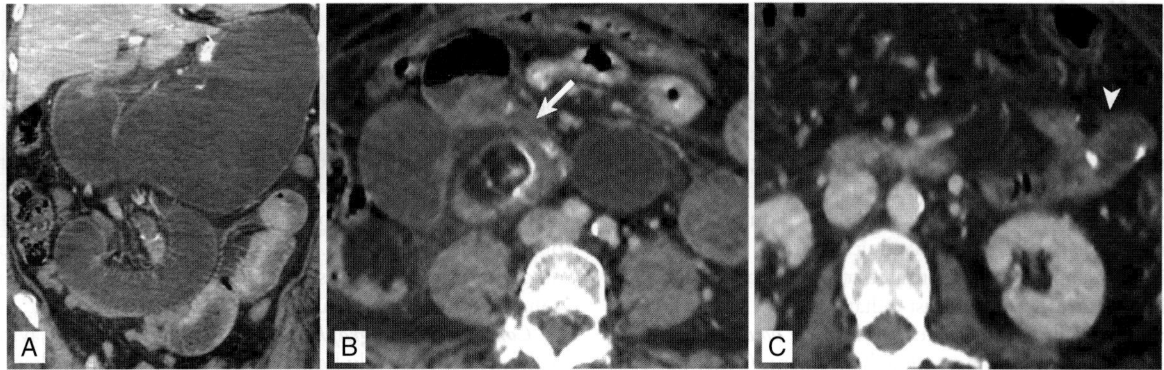

Figure 29.45 Coronal contrast-enhanced computed tomography of the abdomen and pelvis from a 46-year-old woman with Roux-en-Y gastric bypass demonstrates massive dilation of the excluded stomach and pancreaticobiliary limb secondary to internal hernia through the jejuno-jejunostomy mesenteric defect (A). On axial images, note the altered location of the jejuno-jejunostomy in midabdomen caused by internal hernia (*white arrow*) (B) compared with left hemiabdomen on the prior exam (*white arrowhead*) (C).

Acquired adhesions may also cause these hernias [45].

Computed Tomography Features: These include anterior or medial displacement of the cecum and ascending colon by the hernia sac.

Sigmoid Mesocolon Hernia

Anatomy: These account for approximately 6% of internal hernias and are classified into transmesosigmoid, intramesosigmoid, and intersigmoid subtypes. Transmesosigmoid and intramesosigmoid hernias occur through an abnormal defect within the sigmoid mesocolon, involving both peritoneal layers in the former and only one peritoneal layer in the latter. Intersigmoid hernia involve herniation into a congenital retroperitoneal fossa (intersigmoid fossa) located just above and behind the root of sigmoid mesocolon [45].

Computed Tomography Features: The hernia orifice is located between sigmoid colon and left psoas muscle in all the subtypes. Splaying of the sigmoid vessels is present in the intramesosigmoid hernia. *There is characteristic absence of a distinct hernial sac in transmesosigmoid hernias* [45].

Transmesenteric Hernia

Anatomy: These account for approximately 8% of internal hernias. These are most commonly congenital with a higher incidence in the pediatric population. The mesenteric defect is typically 2–5 cm in size and is located near the ligament of Treitz or ileocecal valve. In adults, the hernia is mostly acquired from trauma, surgery, or inflammation [46].

Computed Tomography Features: This presents with dilation of clustered small bowel loops with a transition zone of obstruction. There are engorgement, stretching, and crowding of the mesenteric vascular pedicle and displacement of the main mesenteric trunk with the mesenteric vessels converging at the hernia orifice [46].

Roux-en-Y Anastomosis–related Hernia

Anatomy: These hernias are related to Roux-en-Y anastomosis with three subtypes: transmesocolic, jejunojejunostomy mesenteric, and Petersen hernias. Transmesocolic hernias occur through a surgical defect in the transverse mesocolon. Jejunojejunostomy mesenteric hernia occurs through a small bowel mesenteric defect at the jejunojejunostomy site (Fig. 29.45). Peterson hernia occurs through the Peterson defect, located between the jejunal mesentery of Roux limb and transverse mesocolon [45,48].

Computed Tomography Features: The hernia is suggested by displacement of Roux limb, biliopancreatic limb, and transverse colon. Effects of herniation are mesenteric swirl, clustering of small bowel loops, and mesenteric edema. The *mushroom sign* (mushroom-shaped mesenteric root as it passes through a narrow opening between the vessels at the base of mesentery) and the *hurricane eye sign* (distal tubular mesentery fat surrounded by small bowel loops) have been described [45,49].

Small Bowel Neoplasms

Benign Neoplasms

Hemangiomas: These are rare congenital benign vascular malformations, classified into cavernous (most common), capillary, and mixed subtypes. The jejunum is the most common site of involvement. On contrast-enhanced CT, hemangiomas demonstrate nodular arterial phase and homogeneous delayed phase enhancement. Complications are GI bleed, obstruction, and intussusception, although the vast majority are detected incidentally [50].

Lipomas: These are incidental solitary tumors most commonly located in the duodenum and distal ileum. Complications are intussusception and GI bleed. On CT, lipomas are identified as circumscribed ovoid lesions with fat attenuation (Fig. 29.46). Larger tumors can present with necrosis, calcifications, and cystic degenerations [51].

Leiomyomas: These are usually solitary tumors with a predilection for the jejunum. The tumor originates from the muscle layer and can be submucosal, intramural, or subserosal. On CT, leiomyomas are circumscribed lesions with homogenous enhancement. Larger lesions may show calcifications [51].

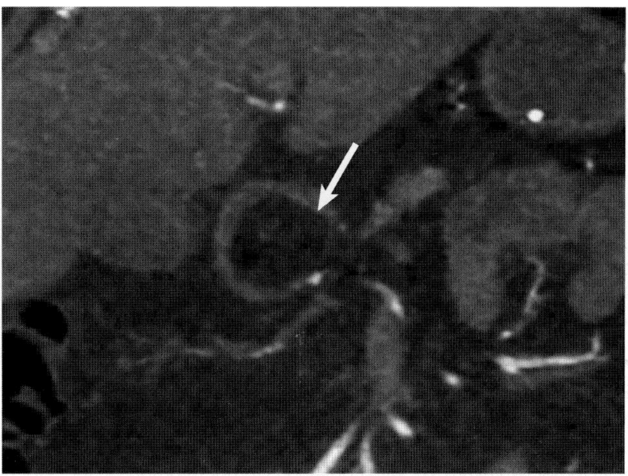

Figure 29.46 Contrast-enhanced coronal computed tomography of the abdomen and pelvis shows an incidental lipoma in the second portion of duodenum (*white arrow*).

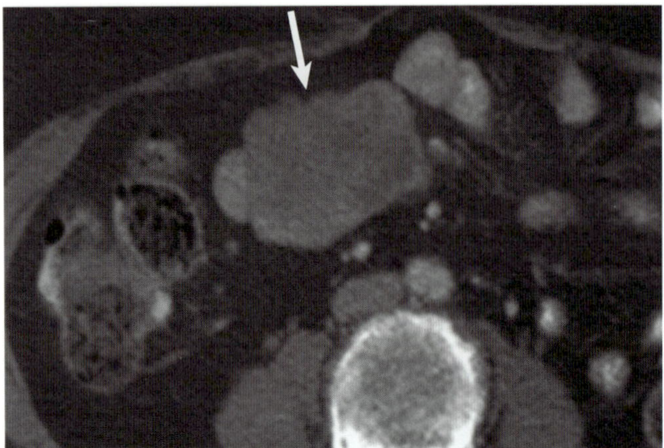

Figure 29.57 Contrast-enhanced axial computed tomography of the abdomen and pelvis from a 76-year-old woman with leiomyosarcoma of the ileum (*white arrow*) shows an exophytic, lobulated solid tumor with heterogeneous postcontrast enhancement.

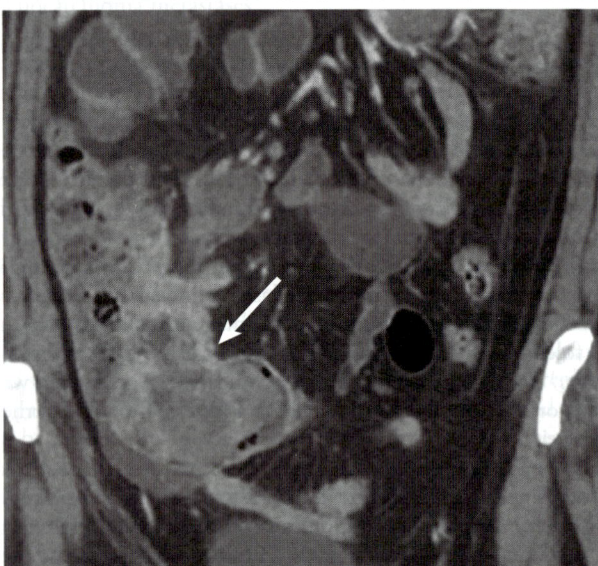

Figure 29.58 Contrast-enhanced coronal computed tomography of the abdomen and pelvis from a 41-year-old woman shows terminal ileal metastasis from ocular melanoma (*white arrow*). The intraluminal mass is a lead point for associated ileocolic intussusception.

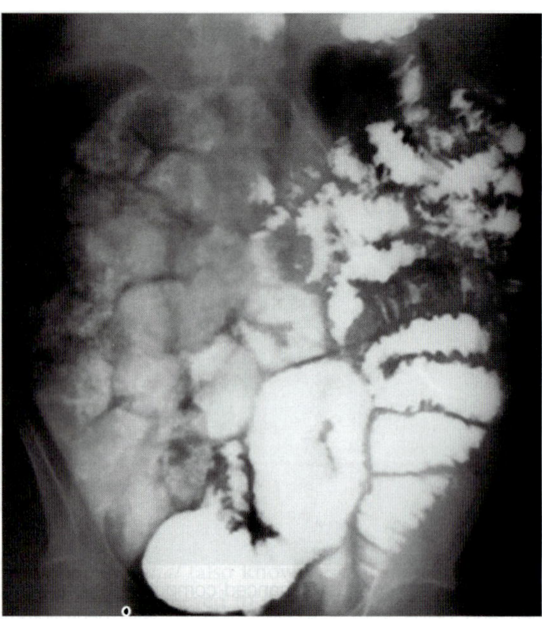

Figure 29.59 Small bowel follow-through from a 36-year-old woman with celiac disease demonstrates increased jejunal and ileal caliber, with increased intraluminal fluid diluting the barium and producing poor coating (flocculation).

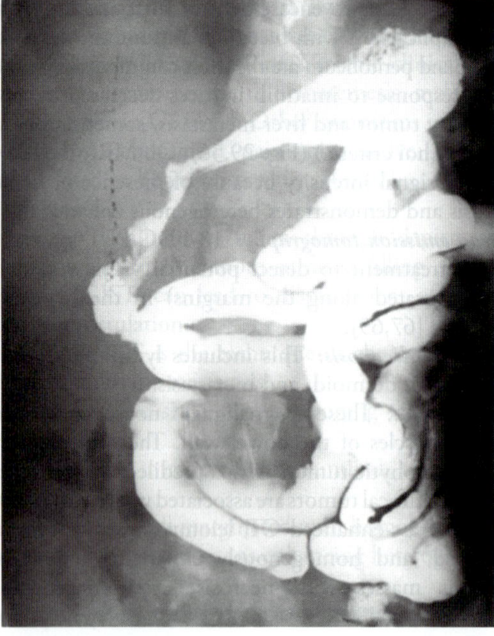

Figure 29.60 Small bowel follow-through from a 56-year-old man with celiac disease shows a mildly dilated jejunum with complete loss of the mucosal pattern (Moulage sign).

nodes and engorgement of mesenteric vessels may be present (Fig. 29.61) [70,72]

Complications are transient small bowel intussusceptions caused by uncoordinated peristalsis, multiple jejunal ulcerations, enteropathy-associated T-cell lymphoma, and small bowel adenocarcinoma [70].

Lymphangiectasia

Lymphangiectasia is a rare disorder characterized by dilation of small bowel lymphatics secondary to lacteal blockage, with resultant loss of lymph in the lumen. It can be primary or congenital or caused secondary to inflammatory damage, trauma, or neoplastic process. The bowel can be involvement in a localized or generalized pattern. Clinical manifestations include protein-losing enteropathy, ascites, and pleural effusions. On CT, there is circumferential bowel wall thickening of varying degree with characteristic submucosal hypoattenuating halo caused by lymphatic congestion *(halo sign)*. Broad differentials include bowel ischemia, inflammation, and neoplasms such as lymphoma [73].

Eosinophilic Enteritis

This is a rare inflammatory disease involving focal or diffuse eosinophilic infiltration in the GI tract, with predilection for involvement of the proximal small bowel and distal gastric body. Allergic or immunologic dysfunctions are proposed as causative factors, although the exact cause is unclear. The imaging

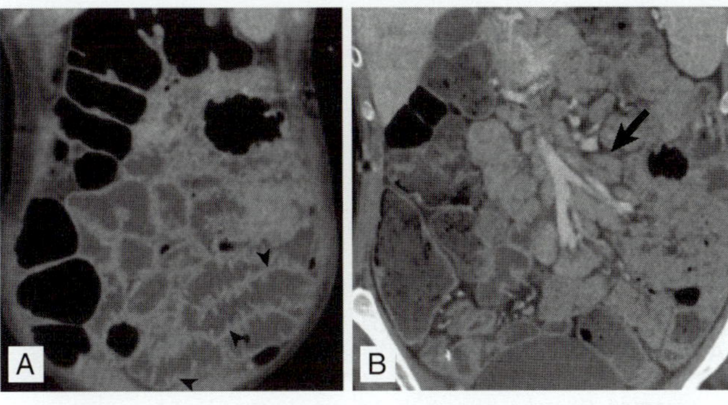

Figure 29.61 Contrast-enhanced coronal computed tomography from a 31-year-old woman with celiac disease shows increased mucosal folds in the ileum (ileal jejunization) (*black arrowheads*), with associated extensive mesenteric adenopathy (*black arrow*) (B).

appearance varies with the predominance of mucosa, muscularis, or serosal infiltration. CT features are mucosal fold thickening, intraluminal polyp, bowel wall thickening with layering or stratification, and luminal narrowing [74].

Small Bowel Diverticulosis

Jejunoileal diverticulosis or jejunal diverticulosis is characterized by herniation of mucosa through the weakened bowel wall along the mesenteric border. The jejunum is more commonly affected than the ileum. It is an acquired condition with increased incidence beyond the fourth decade of life. On fluoroscopy, jejunal diverticulosis is recognized by multiple rounded, contrast-filled outpouchings along the bowel with a relatively narrow neck. On CT, these present as round or oval, air- or contrast-filled outpouchings along the bowel wall (Fig. 29.62). Air-fluid levels or debris can be present. The diverticula have barely discernable wall and lack valvulae conniventes. Underlying communication with the adjacent bowel lumen is frequent delineated. Superimposed diverticulitis leads to bowel wall thickening, perienteric stranding and fluid, localized collections, or rarely free air. Other complications include stasis-related bacterial overgrowth causing diarrhea and malabsorption, hemorrhage, pseudo-obstruction, and less commonly perforation [75].

The duodenum is the second most common site of diverticular disease after the colon. Its occurrence has no specific gender or age predilection. The condition can be congenital or acquired. The less common congenital type contains all the bowel layers and is subdivided into intraluminal and extraluminal subtypes. The acquired type is a pulsion diverticula formed by an outpouching of mucosa or submucosa through foci of weakened duodenal wall, most commonly involving the second portion. On CT, duodenal diverticulum is recognized as a saccular outpouching containing air, air-fluid levels, debris, or contrast, frequently interposed between the duodenum and pancreas (Fig. 29.63). Compared with jejunoileal diverticulum, the incidence of complications such as inflammation and perforation is significantly less in duodenal diverticulum [76].

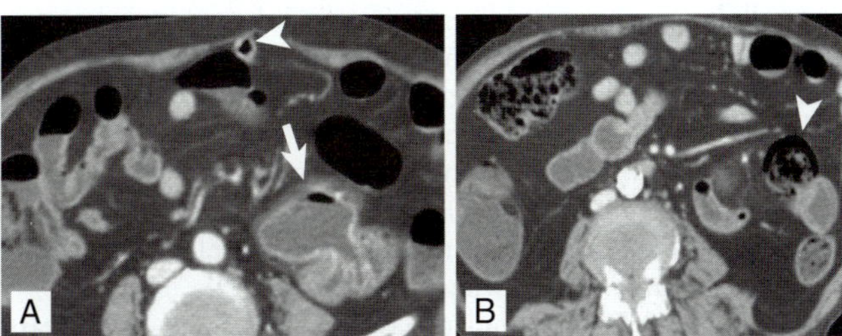

Figure 29.62 Contrast-enhanced coronal axial computed tomography of the abdomen shows jejunal diverticulosis (*white arrowheads*) (A and B). There is a larger diverticulum showing wall enhancement and subtle haziness of the surrounding fat indicating diverticulitis (*white* arrow in A).

Specific Large Bowel Abnormalities

Large Bowel Obstruction

Pathophysiology and Clinical Features

Acute large bowel obstruction carries high morbidity and mortality rate; however, the presentation is relatively gradual compared with small bowel obstruction. It commonly affects the older adult population [77]. Causes are colon cancer *(most common)*, volvulus, diverticulitis, intussusception, intraluminal obstruction by foreign body, fecal impaction, hernias, and strictures in ischemic and IBD. Adhesions and extrinsic compression are rare causes [77]. Clinical features are abdominal pain, distension, constipation, and obstipation. Ischemia and perforation are the major complications, *with higher risk associated with a combination of competent ileocecal valve and rapid obstruction leading to closed-loop physiology.*

Colonic pseudo-obstruction *(Ogilvie syndrome)* is characterized by diffuse colonic dilation without associated mechanical obstruction (Fig. 29.64). The incidence is relatively higher in male patients after the sixth decade of life. The proposed cause is autonomic system dysfunction causing impaired bowel motility and dilation; however, the exact etiopathogenesis is unclear. The condition is associated with myriad medical conditions such as metabolic (hypokalemia, hypocalcemia), cardiopulmonary disease (congestive heart failure, myocardial infarction, chronic obstructive pulmonary disease), systemic infection, malignancies, medications (anticholinergic, narcotics), and diabetes. Major complications are bowel ischemia and perforation [77,78].

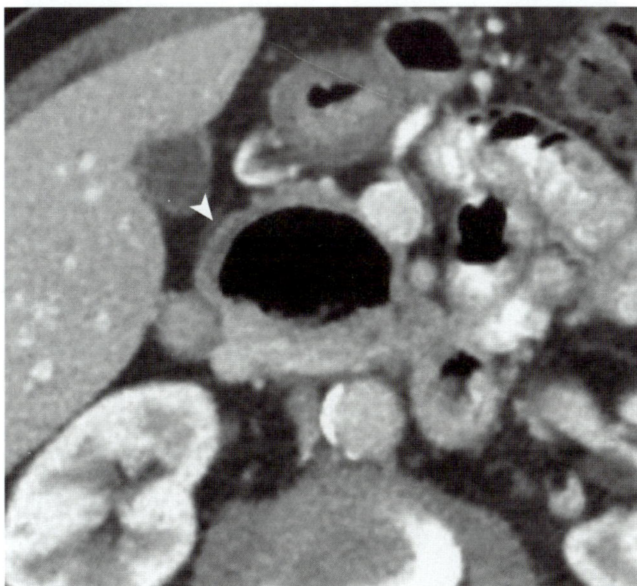

Figure 29.63 Contrast-enhanced coronal axial computed tomography of the abdomen shows a large duodenal diverticulum (*white arrowhead*).

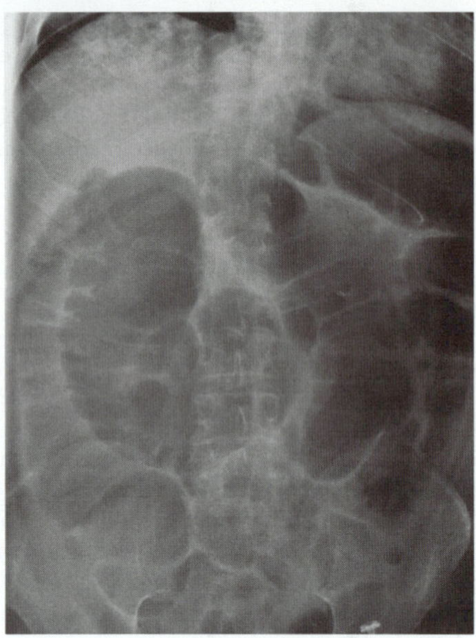

Figure 29.64 Supine abdominal radiograph demonstrates diffuse gaseous distension of large bowel in Ogilvie syndrome.

Imaging Features

Radiographs: Supine and upright abdomen radiographs demonstrate dilation of the colon up to the level of obstruction with a collapsed distal colon. Dilated segments show air-fluid levels. *Cut-off calibers are 9 cm for the cecum and 6 cm for the rest of the large bowel* [77]. Sigmoid volvulus is characterized by coffee bean-shaped configuration of the dilated sigmoid colon *(coffee bean sign)* (Fig. 29.65), with cranial extension above the level of transverse colon *(Northern exposure sign)*. The *Frimann-Dahl sign* refers to convergence of three dense white lines (representing the wall of the sigmoid colon) to the site of obstruction combined with an absence of rectal air [79,80].

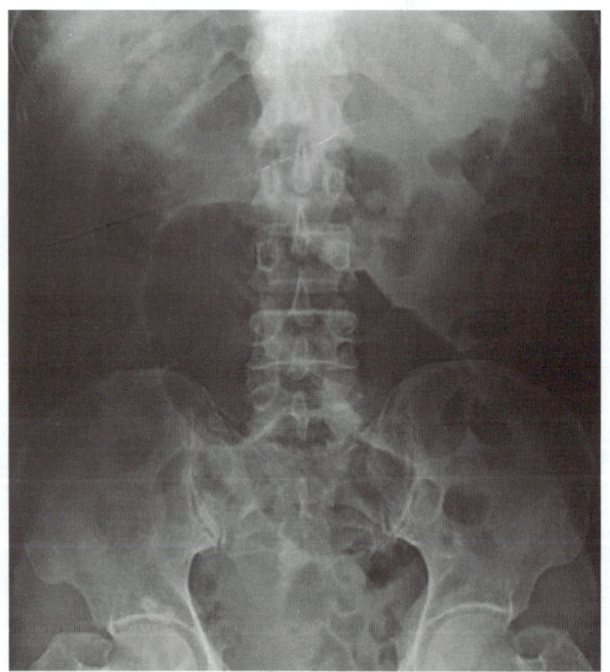

Figure 29.65 Supine abdominal radiograph shows coffee-bean sign in sigmoid volvulus.

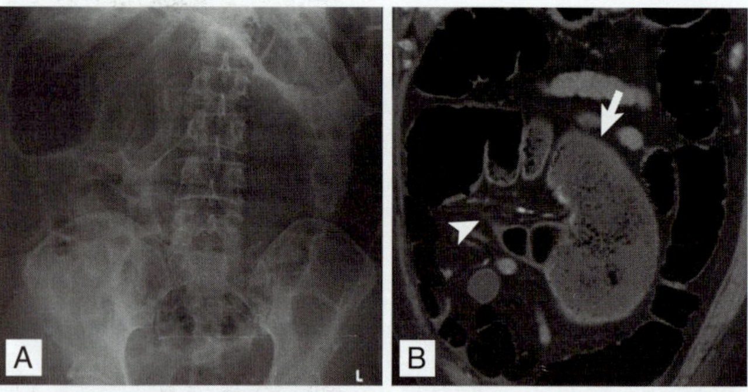

Figure 29.66 Supine abdominal radiograph from a 54 year-old man shows a gas-filled, dilated cecum in the central abdomen, suggesting volvulus (A). Subsequent contrast-enhanced coronal computed tomography demonstrates dilated cecum in the central abdomen (*white arrow*) with beaking at the transition point caused by volvulus (*white arrowhead*) (B).

Cecal volvulus presents with a gas-filled dilated cecum ectopically located in the left upper quadrant or midabdomen (Fig. 29.66). It can be confused with cecal bascule, which refers to a gas-filled, dilated cecum folded upward on itself without twisting, commonly located in the midabdomen [79].

Computed Tomography: This is the technique of choice to evaluate the obstructive cause and complications and exclude pseudo-obstruction, which presents with lack of an abrupt transition point or mechanical cause. Large bowel obstruction presents with colonic dilation up to the transition point with collapsed distal bowel. Associated small bowel dilation is seen in patients with incompetent ileocecal valve or severe or long-standing obstruction. Mural thickening, abnormal wall enhancement, pneumatosis, and portal venous air indicate ischemia.

In sigmoid volvulus, there is an abnormally positioned sigmoid colon with beaking of the bowel at the transition point and mesenteric swirl *(whirl sign)* (Fig. 29.67]. Cecal volvulus is recognized by an abnormally positioned cecum in the left upper or midabdomen, with associated swirling of the bowel and mesenteric vessels at the transition point (see Fig. 29.66) [79].

Differential Diagnosis

This includes small bowel obstruction, pseudo-obstruction, and toxic megacolon.

Colorectal Cancer

Pathophysiology

Colorectal cancer is the most common cancer of the GI tract and the second most common cause of cancer-related deaths globally. Ninety percent of colorectal cancers are adenocarcinomas. Mucinous adenocarcinoma as a subtype is characterized by pools of extracellular mucin, a more aggressive clinical course, and certain distinct imaging features. Other rare types are neuroendocrine, squamous cell, spindle cell, and undifferentiated carcinomas [81]. Precursor lesions and risk factors are

1. Adenomas: Most colon cancers develop from adenoma (adenoma–carcinoma sequence). Subtypes include tubular, villous, and tubulovillous. Risk of malignant degeneration of an adenoma depends on following factors [82,83]:
   - Duration: 2.5% cumulative risk at 5 years, 8% at 10 years, and 24% at 20 years
   - Size: Polyps larger than 2 cm are at 40% risk of malignancy; those that are smaller than 0.5 cm have no risk
   - Type: increased risk with villous architecture

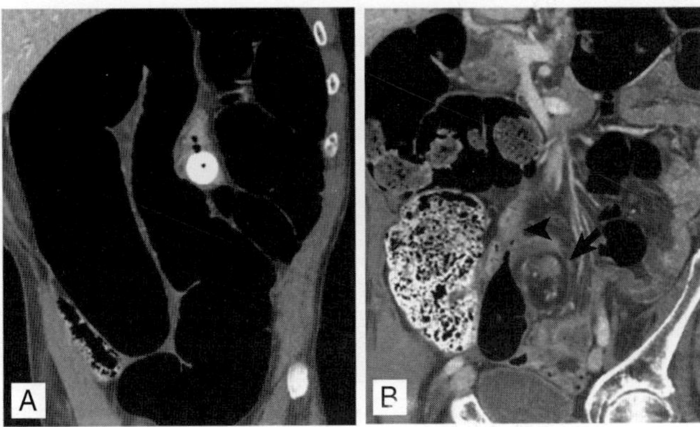

Figure 29.67 Contrast-enhanced coronal computed tomography from a 79-year-old man with sigmoid volvulus shows massively dilated sigmoid colon (A) with beaking at the transition point (*black arrowhead*) (B) and mesenteric swirl (*black arrow*).

2. Hyperplastic or serrated polyps
3. Dysplasia in IBD
4. **Lynch or hereditary nonpolyposis colorectal cancer syndrome:** This is an autosomal dominant syndrome characterized by mutation in DNA mismatch repair genes, with increased risks of several GI and gynecologic malignancies; colorectal and endometrial cancers are the most common [81].
5. **Familial adenomatous polyposis:** Autosomal dominant syndrome characterized by germline mutation in adenomatous polyposis gene, causing development of hundreds to thousands of adenomatous polyps in the colon and rectum. Imaging usually underestimates the disease burden because most polyps are subcentimeter in size. *Polyps typically develop around puberty with nearly 100% of cases progressing to colon cancer in the third and fourth decades of life*, necessitating total colectomy and ileoanal pouch creation as a prophylactic or definitive management (Fig. 29.68). Variants are *Gardner syndrome* characterized by development of desmoid tumors, epidermoid cyst, and osteomas and *Turcot syndrome* associated with medulloblastomas [81].
6. **Peutz-Jeghers syndrome:** This is an autosomal dominant syndrome characterized by mutation in the *LKB1/STK11* gene. It is characterized by multiple hamartomatous polyps in the GI tract (most commonly in the small bowel), colorectal cancers, and pigmented mucocutaneous lesions [81].
7. **Juvenile polyposis syndrome:** This is an autosomal dominant syndrome associated with germline mutations in the *SMAD4* or *BMPR1A* genes. It is characterized by formation of juvenile polyps throughout the GI tract with associated malignant transformation [81].
8. Obesity and low-fiber and high-fat animal protein–based diets are additional risk factors.

Cancer frequency according to the location: sigmoid, 30%; rectum, 25%, cecum and ascending colon, 25%; and transverse and descending colon, 20% [83].

Clinical Features

The incidence is higher in sixth and seventh decades of life. Clinical features are alteration in bowel habits, iron-deficiency anemia, weight loss, abdominal pain, hematochezia, and symptoms related to bowel obstruction.

Imaging Features

Fluoroscopy: Double-contrast barium enema has a higher sensitivity (48%) for detection of polyps more than 1 cm compared

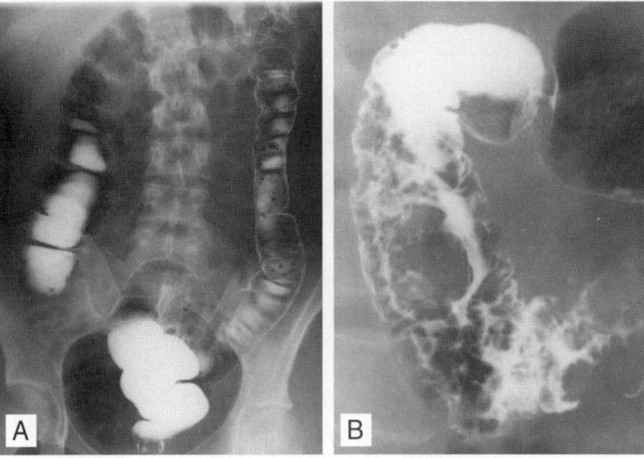

Figure 29.68 Double-contrast barium enema from a 24-year-old woman with familial adenomatous polyposis (FAP) shows several polypoidal and sessile mucosal filling defects in the colon and rectum (A). Double-contrast upper gastrointestinal examination from a different patient with FAP shows numerous duodenal polyps (B).

with single-contrast enema. Both examinations have low sensitivity for detection of smaller and early-stage lesions (35% detection sensitivity of double-contrast enema for lesions <1 cm). Detection sensitivity further decreases with severe diverticulosis and for lesions located in the region of ileocecal valve. Fecal material can lead to false-positive results [84,85]

Colonic polyps present as sessile or pedunculated filling defects. Villous tumors demonstrate a fine nodular or reticular surface pattern without a discrete mass *(carpet lesion)* (Fig. 29.69). Morphologic patterns of colon cancers are plaquelike, polypoidal, semiannular, and annular *(apple core)* (Fig. 29.70) [84].

Computed Tomography: This is the technique of choice for staging (Table 29.6) and follow-up.

- Primary tumor can present as focal wall thickening (circumferential or nodular asymmetric) with luminal narrowing, a

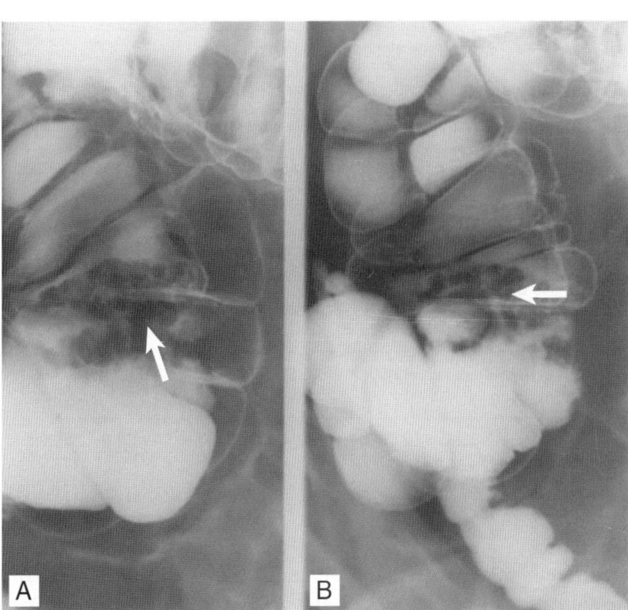

Figure 29.69 (A and B), Double-contrast barium enema shows a broad-based cauliflowerlike lesion with numerous polypoidal protrusions in the cecum (*arrows*). Biopsy demonstrated villous adenoma.

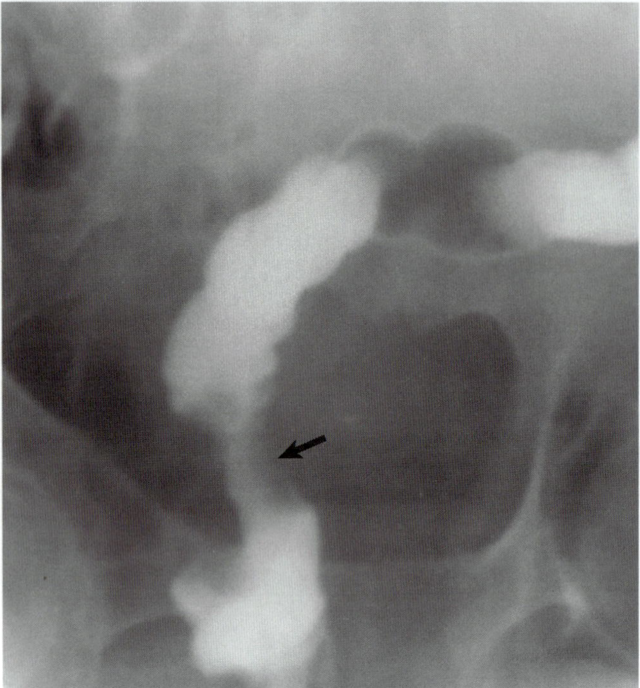

Figure 29.70 Single contrast barium enema shows annular stricture (apple core narrowing) in rectosigmoid carcinoma (*black arrow*).

TABLE 29.6 TNM Staging of Colorectal Cancer (8th Edition) [105]

Tx	Primary tumor cannot be assessed
T0	No evidence of primary tumor
Tis	Carcinoma in situ
T1	Tumor invades the submucosa
T2	Tumor invades the muscularis propria
T3	Tumor invades the muscularis propria into the pericolonic tissues
T4a	Tumor invades the visceral peritoneum
T4b	Tumor directly invades or is adherent to other organs or structures
Nx	Regional lymph nodes cannot be assessed
No	No regional lymph nodal metastasis
N1	Metastasis to 1-3 regional lymph nodes
N2	Metastasis in 4 or more regional lymph nodes
M0	No distant metastasis
M1	M1a: Metastasis to one site or organ without peritoneal metastasis
	M1b: Metastasis to two or more sites or organs without peritoneal metastasis
	M1c: Metastasis to the peritoneal surface alone or with metastasis to other sites or organs

discrete soft tissue mass, or large masses with necrosis and ulcerations (see Figs. 29.71 and 29.72) [86]

- Mucinous adenocarcinomas show a relatively higher degree of eccentric wall thickening, heterogenous mass formation with areas of necrosis, calcifications, and variable enhancement in the solid portions [87]

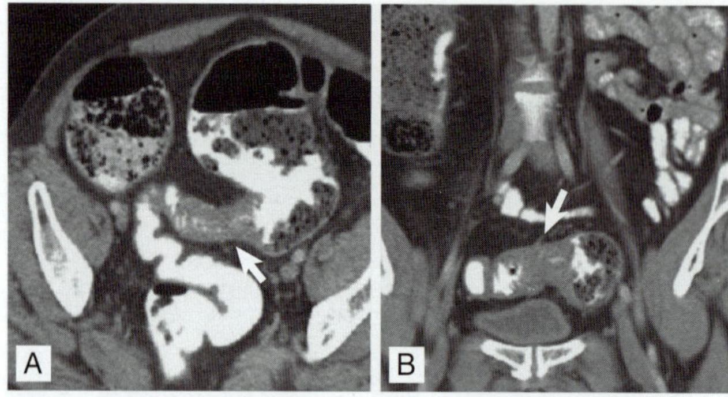

Figure 29.71 Contrast-enhanced axial and coronal computed tomography of the abdomen and pelvis shows sigmoid colon adenocarcinoma (*white arrow*) (A and B).

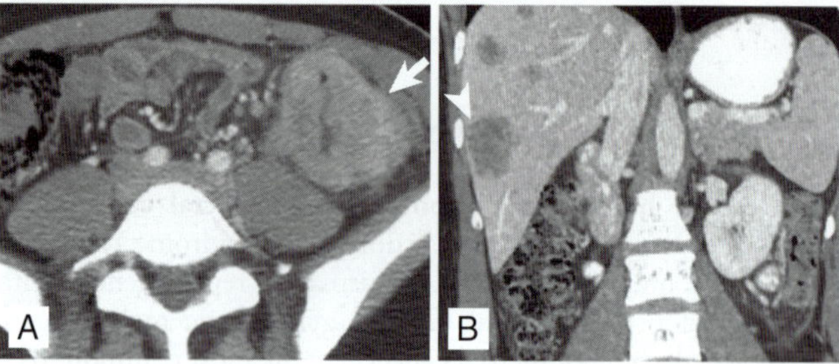

Figure 29.72 Contrast-enhanced axial computed tomography of the abdomen and pelvis from a 46-year-old woman with colonic adenocarcinoma shows marked irregular thickening of descending colon (*white arrow*) (A). Coronal image demonstrates several hypoattenuating liver metastases (*white arrowhead*) (B).

- Local spread leads to soft tissue infiltration into pericolic fat with or without invasion of adjacent structures
- Nodal involvement is characterized by node enlargement and rounded or irregular morphology
- The liver and lungs are the most common sites of metastasis. Liver metastases are hypoattenuating on the portal venous phase (Fig. 29.72)
- Complications are bowel obstruction, perforation, fistula, and intussusception [86]

Magnetic Resonance Imaging:

- This is the technique of choice for local rectal cancer staging and posttreatment response assessment. It provides accurate tumor localization, measurement of tumor length and distance between the tumor and anorectal junction, assessment of mesorectal fascia involvement, relationship to peritoneal reflection, involvement of anal sphincters, and extramural venous invasion. All these findings are evaluated on axial, sagittal, and coronal high-resolution T2-weighted imaging with scan planes along the tumor axis [88]. Whereas tumor demonstrates T2 intermediate signal, mucinous and signet carcinomas have high T2 signal. The T2 intermediate tumors respond to treatment by shrinkage or by developing T2 dark fibrosis or T2 bright mucinous change (which is acellular mucin). Viable tumor may remain T2 intermediate in signal intensity and show diffusion restriction
- Assessment of mesorectal fascia involvement is an essential component of staging (Fig. 29.73). Normally, mesorectal fat is surrounded by mesorectal fascia, which is identified as a thin line of low T2 signal. The fascia is only circumferential in the low rectum and does not apply to the anterior peritonealized surface of the mid and high rectum, which are covered by the anterior peritoneal reflection. *Mesorectal fascia (MRF) guides the circumferential*

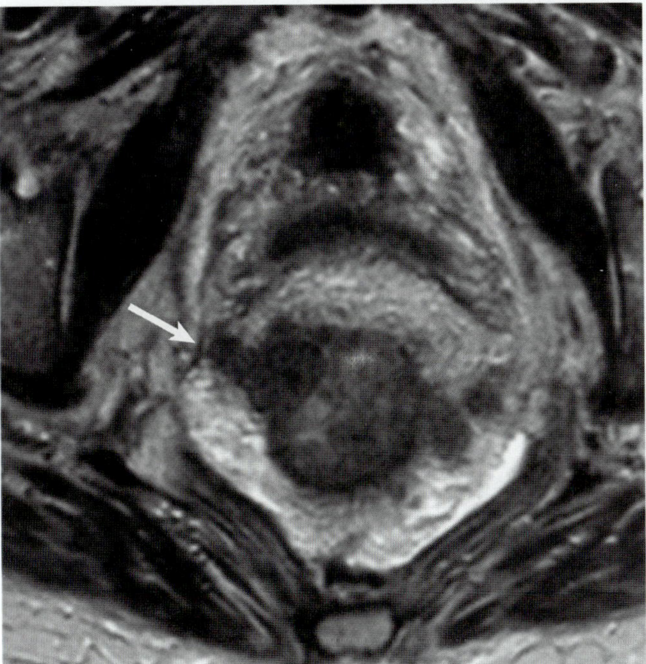

Figure 29.73 High-resolution axial T2-weighted magnetic resonance imaging from a 68-year-old woman with low rectal cancer shows tumor infiltration reaching the mesorectal fascia (*white arrow*).

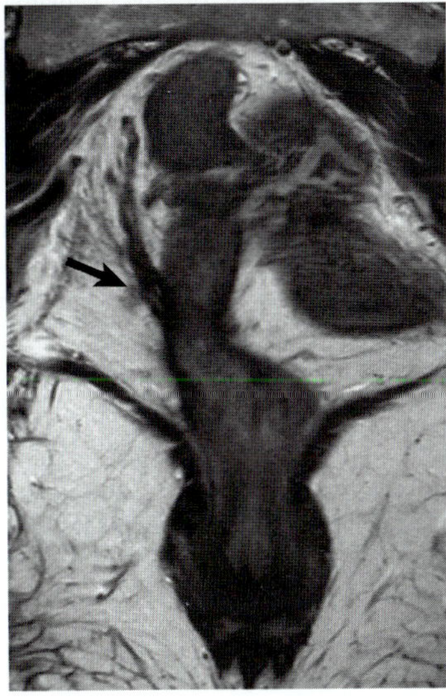

Figure 29.74 High-resolution coronal T2-weighted magnetic resonance imaging shows Extramural vascular invasion (EMVI) as irregularity and expansion of right mesorectal vein (*black arrow*).

resection margin, which refers to the standard plane of excision for total mesorectal excision. Circumferential resection margin status is obtained by measuring the outermost part of the rectal tumor and MRF, with tumor–MRF distance greater than 1 mm as a reliable predictor of negative margins after total mesorectal excision [88]

- Extramural vascular invasion (EMVI) refers to the extension of the tumor in the mesorectal vessels, identified as T2 intermediate signal in the vessel, with associated focal vascular enlargement or expansion and wall irregularity (Fig. 29.74)
- Suspicious nodal features are enlarged size and altered morphology in the form of rounded shape, heterogeneous signal intensity, or irregular borders. As per the Society of Abdominal Radiology criteria, a short-axis diameter of 9 mm or greater or a short-axis diameter of 5–9 mm with at least two abnormal morphologic features is considered metastatic
- Gadolinium enhancement is not currently used in routine clinical practice; however, there is an emerging role of dynamic contrast-enhanced MRI in assessment of tumor vascularization, degree of angiogenesis, and tumor aggressiveness and predicting response to adjuvant chemoradiation [88]

The pneumonic DISTANCE is useful to remember all important points which need to be reported in a rectal MRI: DIStance from anal verge, T stage, Anal complex involvement, N stage, CRM status, and EMVI.

Positron Emission Tomography: There is insufficient evidence regarding recommendation of FDG-PET in lieu of contrast-enhanced CT for disease surveillance because FDG-PET may produce false-positive results in the areas of inflammation. Hence, the utility of FDG-PET is limited for specific indications such as detection of extrahepatic or extrapulmonary metastases, especially in patients with high tumor markers or patients on surveillance with rising markers, and differentiating between benign and malignant lesions [89].

Differential Diagnosis: This includes diverticulitis, IBD, tuberculosis, and lymphoma. The presence of pericolonic adenopathy with acute diverticulitis should raise suspicion for an underlying colon cancer, warranting further evaluation with colonoscopy after resolution of acute inflammation.

Neoplasms of the Appendix

Pathophysiology and Clinical Features

Primary and secondary tumors of the appendix are uncommon neoplasms of the GI tract. This group consists of epithelial neoplasms; NETs; and rare neoplasms such as lymphoma, mesenchymal tumors, and metastasis. *Epithelial adenocarcinomas, with mucinous and nonmucinous histology, are the most common malignant tumors of the appendix.* These tumors demonstrate a higher incidence in the fourth and fifth decades of life. NETs are seen in approximately in 0.3–0.9% of appendectomy specimens and affect relatively younger patients in the fourth decade of life with a female predilection [60,90,91].

Benign tumors can be asymptomatic or incidental on appendectomy. Symptomatic patients can present with features of acute appendicitis (most common), palpable mass, GI bleed, or abdominal distension from associated peritoneal disease or pseudomyxoma [91].

Mucinous Neoplasms

These comprise approximately 70% of the epithelial tumors of the appendix and are divided into four subtypes: adenoma, low-grade appendiceal neoplasm, high-grade appendiceal neoplasm, and mucinous adenocarcinoma. The tumors have a propensity to form mucin with two characteristic radiologic manifestations as mucocele and pseudomyxoma peritonei.

Mucocele refers to distension of the appendix caused by abnormal accumulation of mucin. It can be caused by non-neoplastic entities such as appendicolith and hyperplastic poly or neoplasms, with neoplastic mucocele being typically larger [91].

Nonmucinous Neoplasms

The less common nonmucinous group includes colonic-type neoplasms consisting of polyps, adenoma, and adenocarcinoma.

Goblet Cell Tumors

Goblet cell tumors are rare usual tumors containing components of both adenocarcinoma and carcinoid tumors. The increased histologic ratio of adenocarcinoma to carcinoid inversely correlates with prognosis. The tumor occurs exclusively in the appendix as an infiltrative mass involving the entire appendix circumferentially [60,91].

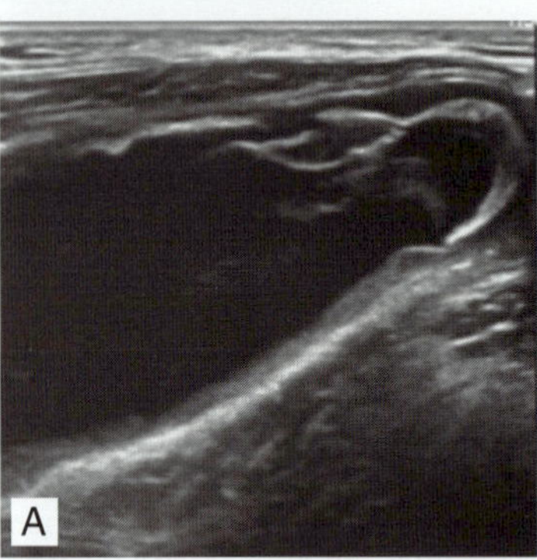

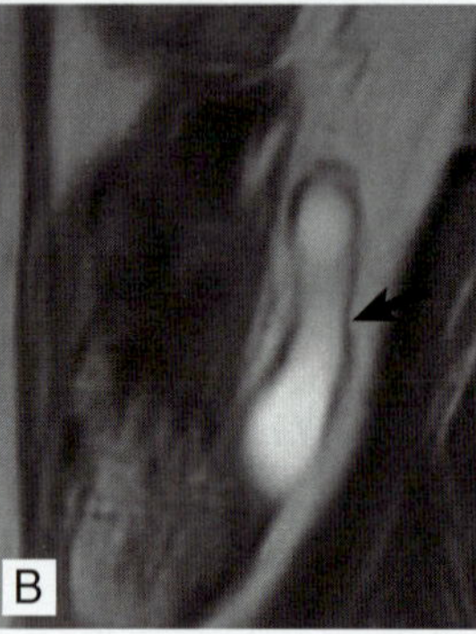

Figure 29.75 Longitudinal ultrasonography of the right lower quadrant shows appendiceal mucocele as dilated, noncompressible tubular structure in the right lower quadrant (A). Sagittal T2-weighted magnetic resonance imaging from a different patient demonstrates mucocele as T2 hyperintense structure arising from the caecum (*black arrow*) (B).

Mucoceles

Imaging Features

Radiographs: Radiographs may suggest a soft tissue mass in the right lower quadrant. The presence of associated curvilinear calcifications increases the diagnostic specificity; however, it is seen in fewer than 50% of cases [60].

Ultrasonography: This shows ovoid cystic mass in the right lower quadrant with variable internal echotexture; however, low-level internal echoes are typical (Fig. 29.75). Associated curvilinear mural calcifications produce posterior acoustic shadowing. Identification of the ovary is important to exclude pathologies such as cystic neoplasms, which can mimic mucoceles [60].

CT and MRI: Mucocele presents as circumscribed tubular structure originating from the base of the cecum. Lesions demonstrate homogenously low luminal attenuation and curvilinear mural calcifications. There is absence of mural hyperenhancement, periappendiceal stranding, and fluid unless there is associated inflammation. Superimposed infection may lead to intraluminal gas and air-fluid levels. Mural nodules and irregular wall enhancement are seen in malignant mucoceles. On MRI, mucoceles show high internal T2 and low T1 signal because of mucin (see Fig. 29.75) [60,91].

Differential diagnosis: This includes ovarian neoplasm, periappendiceal abscess, hydrosalpinx, enteric duplication cyst, and mesenteric cyst.

Appendiceal Adenocarcinoma

Imaging Features: CT is the technique of choice for staging and follow up. The primary tumor can present as an ill-defined soft tissue mass or soft tissue infiltration involving the entire appendix, without mucocele formation (Fig. 29.76). Periappendiceal fat stranding may relate to tumor extension or superimposed inflammation. The tumor spreads by direct invasion of adjacent organs, nodal involvement, and peritoneal metastasis commonly manifesting as pseudomyxoma [91].

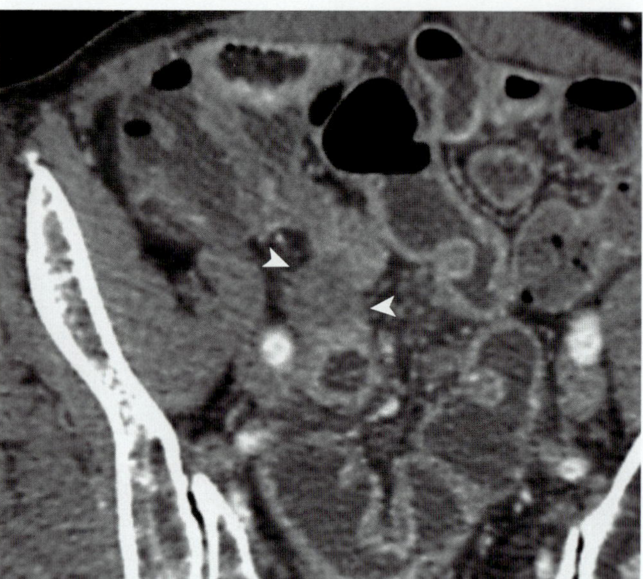

Figure 29.76 Contrast-enhanced axial and coronal computed tomography of the abdomen and pelvis from a 67-year-old man with appendiceal adenocarcinoma demonstrates soft tissue thickening involving the entire appendix (*white arrowheads*).

Imaging of Lower Gastrointestinal Tract Bleeding

Pathophysiology

Lower GI tract bleeding is defined as GI bleed occurring below the ligament of Treitz. Causes are diverticular disease (*most common*), IBD, neoplasm, infectious, ischemic and radiation colitis, coagulopathy, vascular malformations and angiodysplasia, aortoenteric fistula, Meckel diverticulitis, rectal ulcers, varices, and hemorrhoids. Although the lesser gastric curvature is the classic site for Dieulafoy lesion, which is characterized by dilated tortuous submucosal artery eroding into the mucosa, involvement of the small and rectum is known [92–94].

Clinical Features

The incidence is higher in the older adult population with a male predilection. It is a potentially life-threatening condition presenting with hematochezia or melena. Anemia and signs of hypovolemic shock may be present.

Imaging Features

Imaging techniques of choice for the evaluation of active lower GI bleed include multidetector CT angiography, technetium-99m–labeled red blood cell (^{99m}Tc-RBC) scan and catheter angiography. *Active bleeding detection rates are 0.3–0.5 mL/min for CT angiography, 0.5 mL/min for catheter angiography, and greater than 0.1 mL/min for ^{99m}Tc-RBC scan* [93].

Multidetector CT Angiography

This helps in localization of the bleeding source and evaluating any associated bowel pathology. CT is performed in three phases (unenhanced, arterial, and portal venous phases), with multiplanar and maximum intensity projection reconstructions. Oral contrast is not administered in the emergency setting. Multiphase CT enterography with administration of neutral oral contrast is indicated for stable patients and patients with occult bleed.

False-negative results can be seen in intermittent bleed, dilution of contrast in fluid-filled bowel, and collapsed bowel. False-positive results can be secondary to mucosal enhancement of collapsed bowel, hypervascular tumors, foreign bodies, fecalith, surgical clips, and sutures [93].

Lower GI bleed presents as intraluminal contrast blush on the arterial phase that expands and moves distally in the venous phase (Fig. 29.77). The venous phase shows extravascular blush

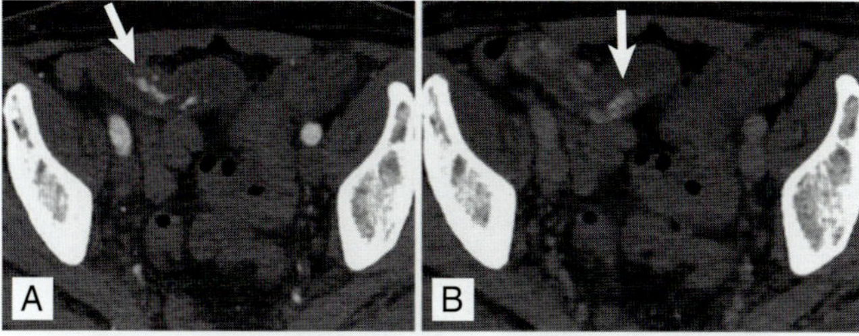

Figure 29.77 Contrast-enhanced axial and coronal computed tomography of the abdomen and pelvis from a 65-year-old woman with an ileocolic territory gastrointestinal bleed. Bleed in the distal ileum presents as intraluminal contrast blush on arterial phase (A) that expands and progresses distally on the portal venous phase (*white arrow*) (B).

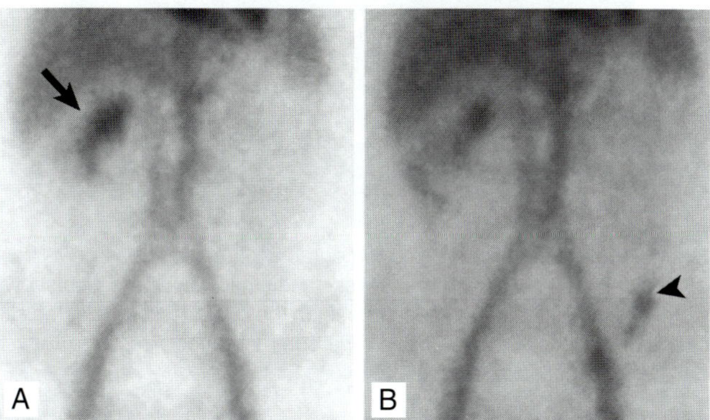

Figure 29.78 (A and B), Technetium-99m–labeled red blood cell (^{99m}Tc-RBC) scan demonstrates active gastrointestinal bleeding caused by angiodysplasia. There is concentration of radiolabeled RBCs in the hepatic flexure (*black arrow*), which progresses into the descending colon (*black arrowheads*).

with higher sensitivity because of greater accumulation of contrast with time. Unclotted extravascular blood and clotted blood less than 48 hours old are hyperattenuating on the unenhanced phase (except in patients with low hematocrit levels). MIP reconstructions acquired from arterial phase datasets depict detailed vascular anatomy and vascular malformations [92,93].

Radionuclide Scan

RBCs are labeled with ^{99m}Tc, and serial scintigraphy is performed. Active bleeding presents as areas of increased tracer accumulation along the bowel, with activity increasing over time in an antegrade or retrograde pattern (Fig. 29.78) [92]. Scintigraphy is only recommended for evaluation of active and overt GI bleed. Chronic occult bleed is usually evaluated with capsule enteroscopy.

Imaging of Postoperative Bowel

Imaging plays a vital role in evaluation of postsurgical bowel pathologies, and familiarity with the normal postoperative anatomy is essential to diagnose complications. Several bowel disorders such as IBD, ischemia, and obstructions and various benign and malignant tumors are treated with surgical management, requiring various types of resection and anastomosis depending on the severity and extent of bowel involvement. Three main types of bowel anastomosis include [95].

1. End to end: when there is sufficient luminal diameter on both sides
2. End to side: when there is size discrepancy between the two bowel segments
3. Side to side: used in creation of large anastomosis

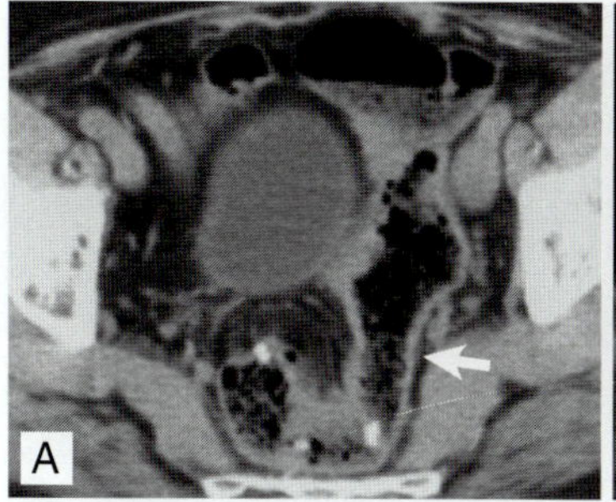

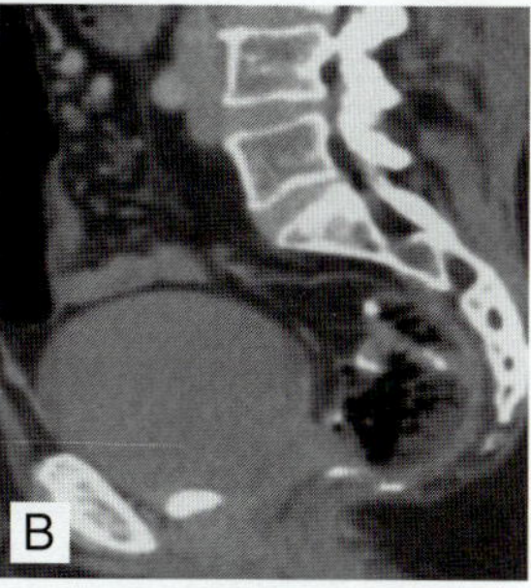

Figure 29.79 Axial (A) and sagittal (B) computed tomography of the pelvis from a 31-year-old man with history of Lynch syndrome shows the ileoanal pouch creation (*white arrow*).

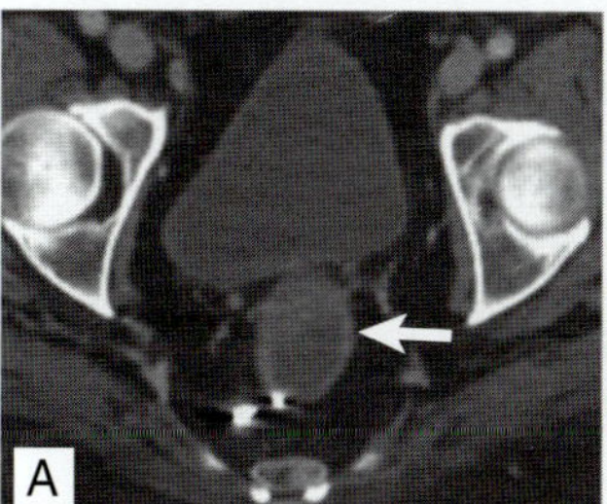

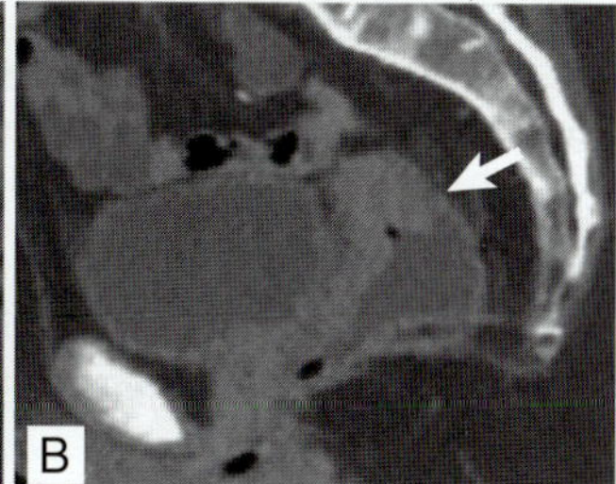

Figure 29.80 Axial (A) and sagittal (B) computed tomography of the pelvis from a 60-year-old man with perforated sigmoid cancer, after colectomy, shows the fluid-filled Hartmann pouch (*white arrow*).

Features of certain common bowel surgeries are as follows:

Ileal Pouch–Anal Anastomosis

Also known as ileoanal pull-through, this surgical technique allows fecal continence after total proctocolectomy, such as in patients with ulcerative colitis or familial adenomatosis polyposis. It involves colectomy, mucosal proctectomy, and creation of an ileal pouch via a side-to-side anastomosis (Fig. 29.79) [96].

Hartmann Procedure

The procedure involves creation of a blind-ending rectal stump with a temporary diverting colostomy. It is usually indicated in patients requiring bowel resection on an emergent basis or when there are contraindications for primary anastomosis such as suboptimal bowel preparation or associated peritonitis, for example, in complicated diverticulitis, obstructive or perforated colon cancer, and trauma (Fig. 29.80) [95].

Low Anterior Resection

This involves resection of the distal left colon, sigmoid, and proximal rectum with creation of a low colorectal or coloanal anastomosis in patients with tumors of rectosigmoid junction or rectum more than 5 cm from the anal border (Fig. 29.81) [97].

Abdominoperineal Resection

This is indicated for low rectal lesions less than 5 cm from the anal border and involves resection of the distal left colon, sigmoid colon, rectum, and entire anus with creation of permanent end colostomy [97].

Postoperative complications are classified into early and late ones. Early complications are anastomotic dehiscence, paralytic

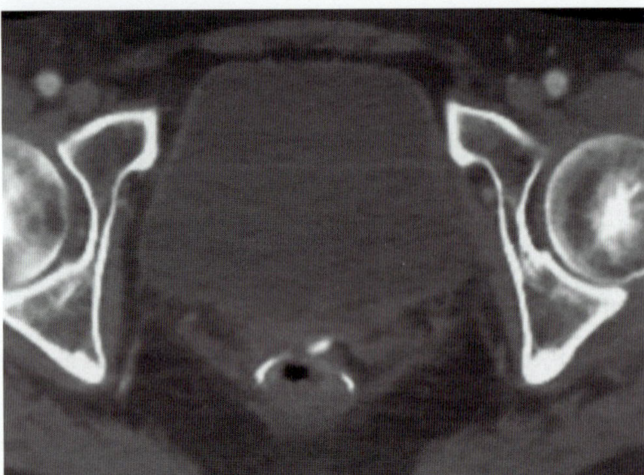

Figure 29.81 Axial computed tomography of the pelvis from a 60-year-old man with rectosigmoid cancer shows postsurgical changes of low anterior resection.

ileus, mechanical bowel obstruction, and abscess. Late complications include anastomotic strictures, fistulas, and pouchitis.

Imaging Techniques

Radiographs

Radiography is the initial study in postoperative patients with abdominal symptoms. Findings detected are air-fluid levels and pneumoperitoneum. Radiographs also help in evaluation of stapler location and assess the integrity of anastomotic ring [97].

Fluoroscopy

Water-soluble enemas and single-contrast studies are recommended in the initial postoperative weeks. Single- or double-contrast studies are performed in the late postoperative period (~3 months) to assess the new anatomy and evaluate anastomotic complications such as strictures and disease recurrence (Fig. 29.82).

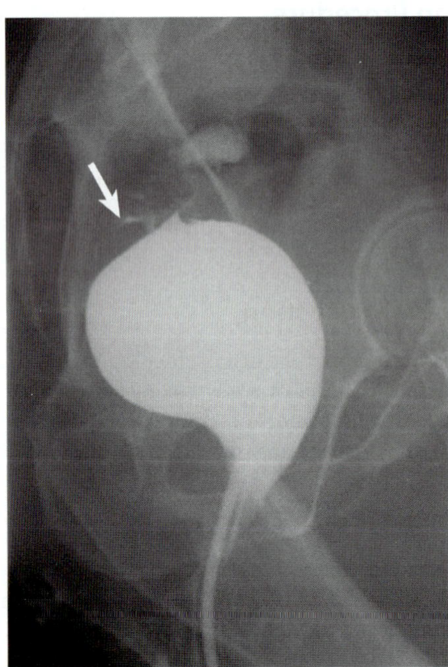

Figure 29.82 Single-contrast barium enema shows a high-grade anastomotic stricture involving the low anterior resection with a small presacral leak (*white arrow*).

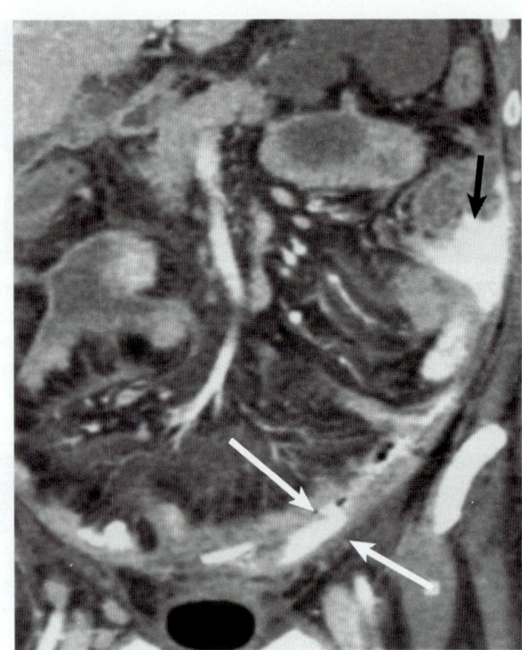

Figure 29.83 Coronal computed tomography of the abdomen pelvis from a 42-year-old man with Crohn's disease and small bowel resection shows extravasation of positive enteric contrast in the peritoneal cavity at the site of anastomotic leak (*white arrow*). The contrast percolates along the left paracolic space (*black arrow*).

Computed Tomography

Computed tomography with positive oral contrast helps in accurate identification of the anastomosis and perianastomotic complications such as leaks, abscess, fistula, or disease recurrence. It is the preferred technique in both the early and late postoperative periods (Fig. 29.83).

Perianal Fistulas

Anatomy of Anal Sphincters

The anal canal is surrounded by two muscular layers, the internal and external sphincters. The internal sphincter contains smooth muscle and is continuous with circular muscle of the rectum. The external sphincter contains striated muscles and merges proximally to the puborectalis muscle. The two sphincters are separated by the intersphincteric plane containing fat, areolar tissue, and longitudinal muscle (Fig. 29.84) [98].

Etiopathogenesis

Causes are idiopathic *(most common)*, Crohn's disease, tuberculosis, diverticulitis, pelvic infection, malignancy, and radiation therapy. The proposed pathogenesis in idiopathic cases is infection of the intersphincteric gland with formation of intersphincteric fistula track or abscess caused by obstruction of the draining duct. Chronic infection leads to persistently discharging fistula and recurring abscess. Surgical and radiologic classifications of perianal fistula are described in Tables 29.7 and 29.8 (Fig. 29.85).

Imaging

Conventional Fistulography

This involves catheterization of the external fistula opening with injection of water-soluble contrast (Fig. 29.86). The technique is

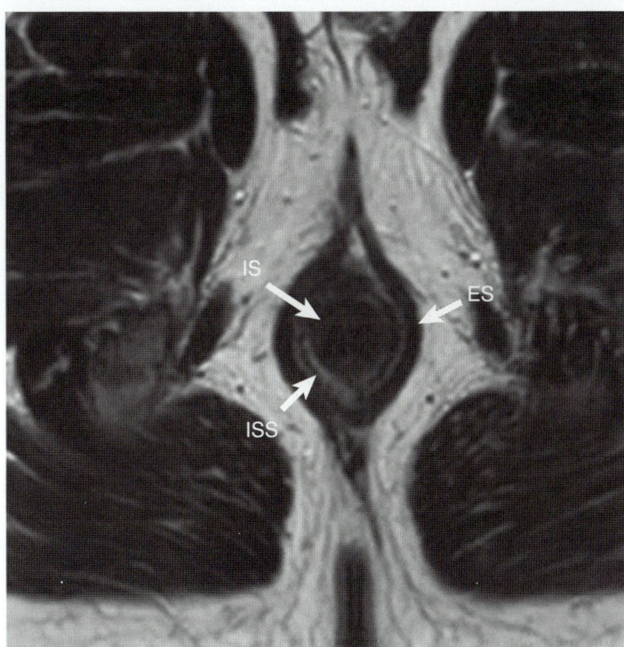

Figure 29.84 Axial T2-weighted magnetic resonance imaging image demonstrates the anatomy of the anal sphincters. *ES,* external sphincter; *IS,* internal sphincter; *ISS,* intersphincteric space.

TABLE 29.7 Park Classification of Perianal Fistulae

Intersphincteric	Fistula crosses intersphincteric space but does not cross external sphincter
Transsphincteric	Fistula crosses intersphincteric space and external sphincter into the ischiorectal fossa
Suprasphincteric	Fistula tracks upward into intersphincteric space, over the top of puborectalis muscle, then descends into the levator plate and ischiorectal fossa and then to the skin
Extrasphincteric	Fistula is outside the external sphincter; it crosses from the perineal skin through the ischiorectal fossa and levator muscle complex into the rectum

TABLE 29.8 St. James's University Hospital Classification of Perianal Fistulae

Grade 1	Simple linear intersphincteric
Grade 2	Intersphincteric with abscess or secondary tract
Grade 3	Transsphincteric
Grade 4	Transsphincteric with abscess or secondary tract in the ischiorectal or ischioanal fossa
Grade 5	Supralevator and translevator disease

inaccurate with major drawbacks of (1) lack of proper contrast filling, which leads to difficulty in assessment of secondary extensions, and (2) nonvisualization of the anal sphincter and its relation to the fistula [98].

Magnetic Resonance Imaging

MRI is the technique of choice because it delineates complex anatomy of the anal sphincters. The techniques involve acquisition of oblique axial and coronal images oriented orthogonal and

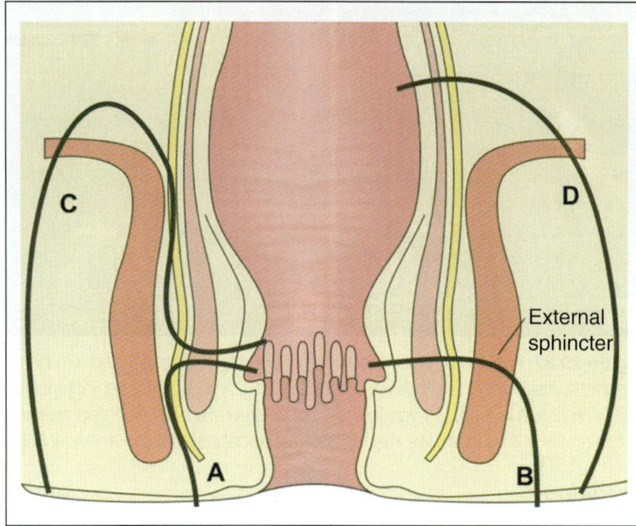

Figure 29.85 Parks classification. Illustration of the anal canal in the coronal plane shows the Parks classification of perianal fistulas. The external sphincter is the keystone of the Parks classification. *A,* intersphincteric; *B,* transsphincteric; *C,* suprasphincteric; *D,* extrasphincteric.

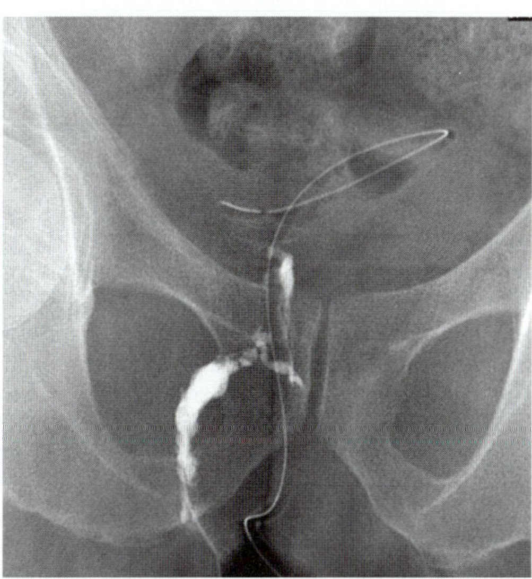

Figure 29.86 Conventional fistulogram delineates a right-sided transsphincteric fistula.

parallel to the anal canal. It is essential to describe the point of origin of the perianal fistula in the anal canal using the anal clock scheme. The fistula path is then described with respect to the pelvic anatomic boundaries. Active fistula demonstrates high T2 signal, isointense T1 signal, and intense contrast enhancement on fat-suppressed T1-weighted imaging (Fig. 29.87). Associated abscess show rim enhancement. Chronic fistula demonstrates low signal on both T1- and T2-weighted imaging [98].

Defecography

Fluoroscopic Defecography

Indications

These include constipation, anal incontinence, rectal prolapse, and pelvic floor abnormalities. Use of fluoroscopic defecography has substantially declined over the years because of the advent of MRI defecography.

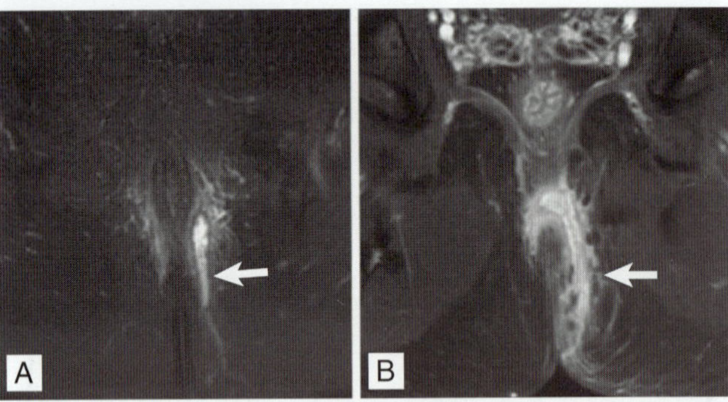

Figure 29.87 A 39-year-old man with history of rectal pain and firmness. Magnetic resonance fistulogram demonstrates complex transsphincteric fistula. The fistulous tract is hyperintense on fat-saturated T2-weighted imaging (*white arrow* in A) and shows intense contrast enhancement (*white arrow* in B).

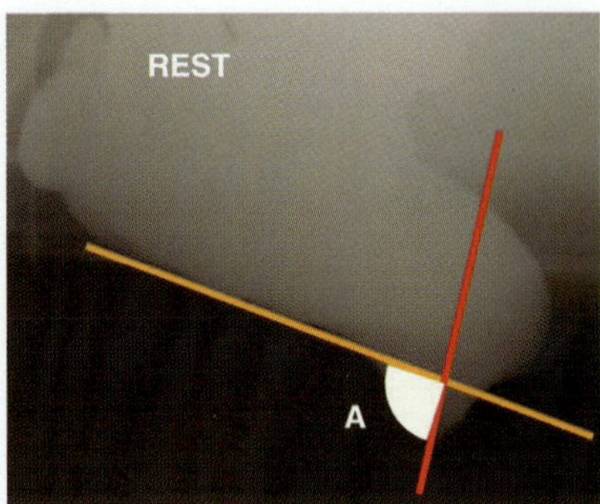

Figure 29.88 Conventional defecogram image illustrates the measurement of the anorectal angle.

Technique

Bowel preparation with laxatives is usually not necessary. The procedure involves injection of about 200–300 mL of thick barium paste into the rectum with the patient in the left lateral decubitus position until the point of a stimulus to evacuate. In women, the vagina is opacified with barium or water-soluble contrast agents. In patients with suspected enterocele, the small bowel should be opacified using 400–600-mL barium suspension given over 45–60 minutes before the procedure. Images are acquired with patient in the right lateral projection on a commode, with acquisition of spot films during the rest, squeeze, strain, and defecation phases. The patient is then asked to defecate completely followed by acquisition of postevacuation images [99].

Parameters and Normal Findings

The anorectal angle is measured between the longitudinal axis of the anal canal and posterior rectum (Fig. 29.88), with physiologic range of 65–100 degrees at rest and without much variability between men and woman. The second parameter for evaluation is the shift of the anorectal junction during straining, which indirectly indicates the function of the puborectalis muscle, using the tip of the coccyx as the fixed bony landmark. At rest, the puborectalis sling forms a visible impression on the posterior rectal wall. During the squeeze phase, the anorectal angle decreases to about 75 degrees with cranial migration of the anorectal junction. During the strain phase, there is partial or complete loss of puborectalis impression, an increase in the anorectal angle, and pelvic floor decent of less than 3.5 cm. The evacuation phase leads to a further increase in anorectal angle, complete loss of puborectalis impression, and wide opening of the anal canal [99–101].

Magnetic Resonance Imaging Defecography

MRI defecography is now the predominant technique for assessment of pelvic floor abnormalities and defecation disorders, with advantages of detailed assessment of the pelvic floor anatomy and higher sensitivity. A 1.5- or 3-T MRI unit is used with the patient in a supine position. The distal rectum is filled with about 120–150 mL of ultrasound gel mixed with gadolinium using a syringe. Sequences include T1-weighted localizer and T2-weighted images along the sagittal, axial, and coronal planes with thin sections. For dynamic study, a steady state or rapid T2-weighted sequences in the midsagittal plane is acquired.

Parameters and Normal Findings

Although there are several reference points and lines proposed for complete evaluation of the pelvic floor, only the parameters pertinent to the middle and posterior compartments are discussed here. The pubococcygeal line (PCL) is drawn from the inferior border of the inferior border of the pubic symphysis to the last coccygeal joint (not to be confused with the inferior tip of the last coccyx). The midpubic line (MPL) is drawn along the long axis of the pubic symphysis (Fig. 29.89). Normal measurements of anorectal angle are 108–127 degree at rest, decreasing by about 15–20 degree during squeezing and increasing by about 15–20 degree during straining and defecation [102].

Disorders

Rectoceles: An anterior rectocele is an abnormal bulge of the anterior rectal wall into the posterior vaginal wall caused secondary to weakness or damage of intervening rectovaginal fascia. On MRI, it is measured by extension of rectal wall beyond the expected margin of the anterior anorectal wall and is graded as small (<2 cm), medium (2–4 cm), or large (>4 cm). On fluoroscopy, anterior rectocele bulge displaces the opacified vaginal lumen during straining and evacuation (Fig. 29.90). Posterior rectoceles are less common [99,102].

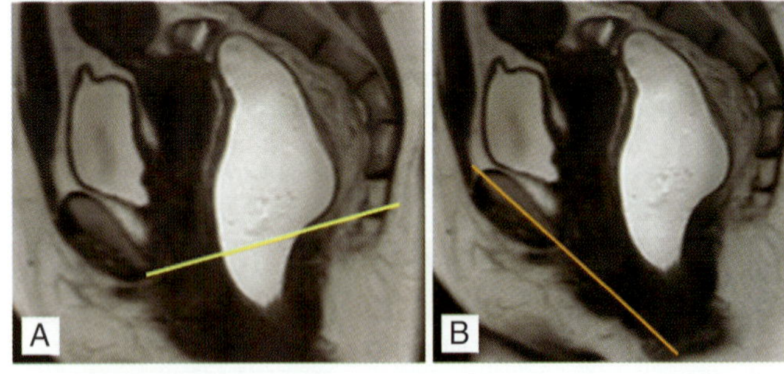

Figure 29.89 Midsagittal T2-weighted magnetic resonance imaging illustrates the pubococcygeal line (A) and midpubic line (B).

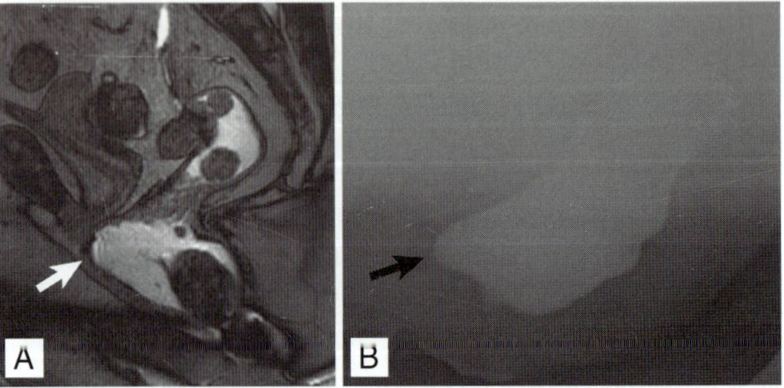

Figure 29.90 Magnetic resonance imaging defecogram from a 61-year-old woman demonstrates a large anterior rectocele (*white arrow*) (A). Conventional defecography from another patients shows moderate anterior rectocele (*black arrow*) (B).

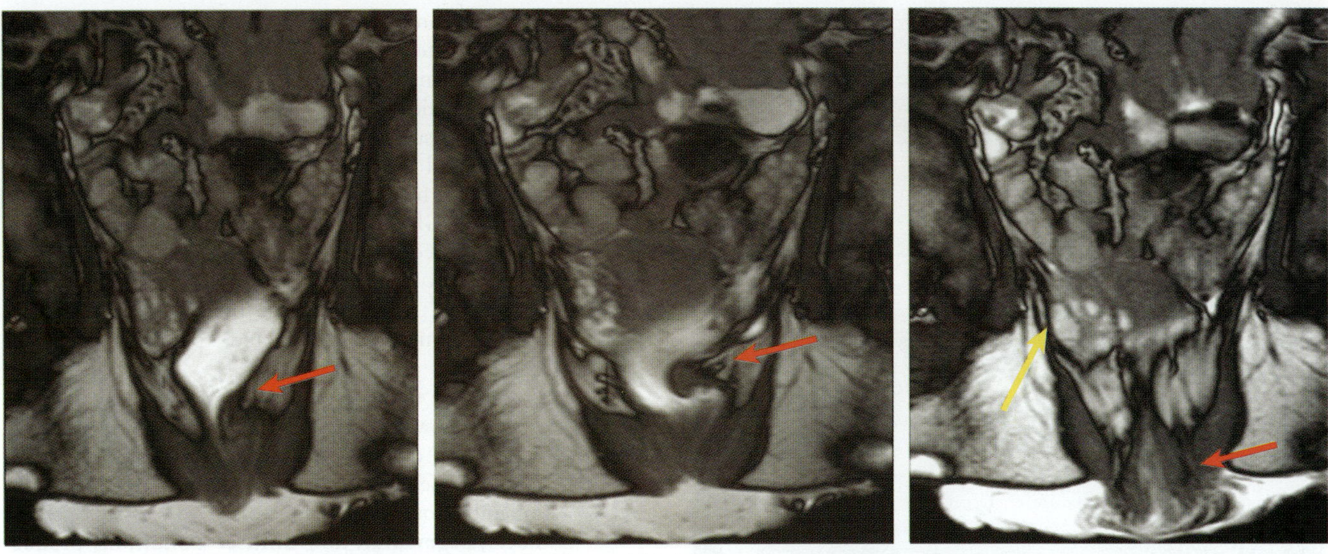

Figure 29.91 Serial coronal acquisitions obtained during defecation on MRI defecogram shows rectal prolapse (*red arrow*) and ovariocele (*yellow arrow*).

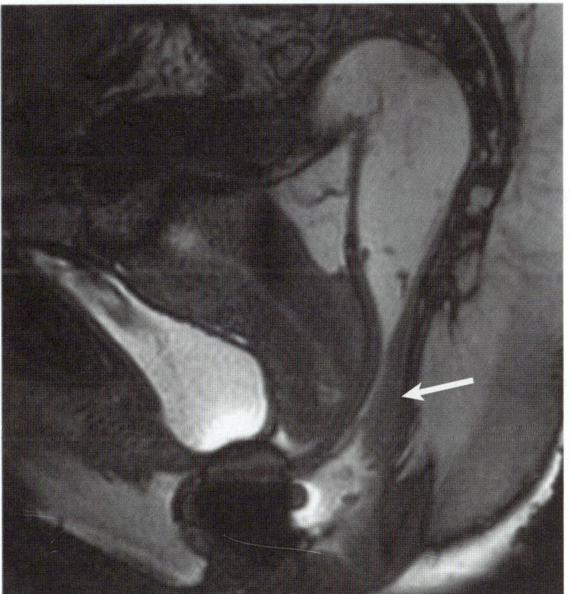

Figure 29.92 Magnetic resonance imaging defecogram from a 64-year-old woman with tricompartmental prolapse demonstrates intrarectal prolapse (*white arrow*).

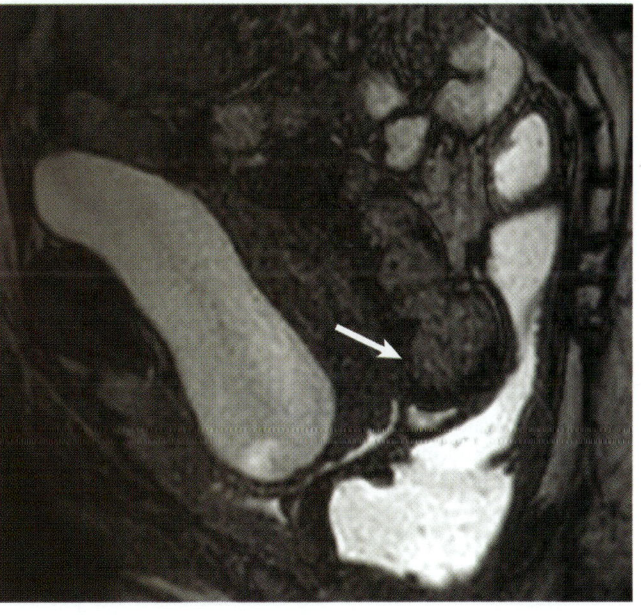

Figure 29.93 Magnetic resonance imaging defecogram from a 58-year-old woman with severe tricompartmental prolapse shows enterocele (*white arrow*) and a small peritoneocele.

Rectal Prolapse and Intussusception: There can be prolapse of only the rectal mucosa or intussusception involving infoldings of the full thickness of the rectal wall into the rectum, anal canal, or beyond the anus (complete rectal prolapse) (Figs. 29.91 and 29.92). On fluoroscopy, intussusception is identified as a transverse or oblique infoldings of the rectal wall of more than 3-mm thickness [99,102].

Enterocele and Sigmoidocele: This is herniation of the small bowel or sigmoid colon into an abnormally widened rectovaginal space caused by defects in the supporting fascia or musculature (Fig. 29.93).

Dyssynergic Defecation or Anismus: This is a functional disorder involving paradoxical, involuntary contraction of the puborectalis muscle, preventing normal evacuation. On MRI and fluoroscopy, there is prolonged and incomplete evacuation with failure of descent of pelvic floor during defecation and failure of the anorectal angle to open with a prominent puborectalis impression (Fig. 29.94) [102].

Descending Perineum Syndrome: This involves descent of the entire pelvic floor at rest, during evacuation, or both. Causes include damage to the pudendal nerve secondary to chronic straining or obstetric injury. On MRI, it is assessed by measuring the descent of the posterior aspect of the anorectal junction from the PCL, with an abnormal value of 2.5 cm or more. Descent of the anterior aspect of anorectal junction can be measured from the PCL or MPL. On fluoroscopy, there is more than 3.5 cm descent of the anorectal junction during straining [99,102].

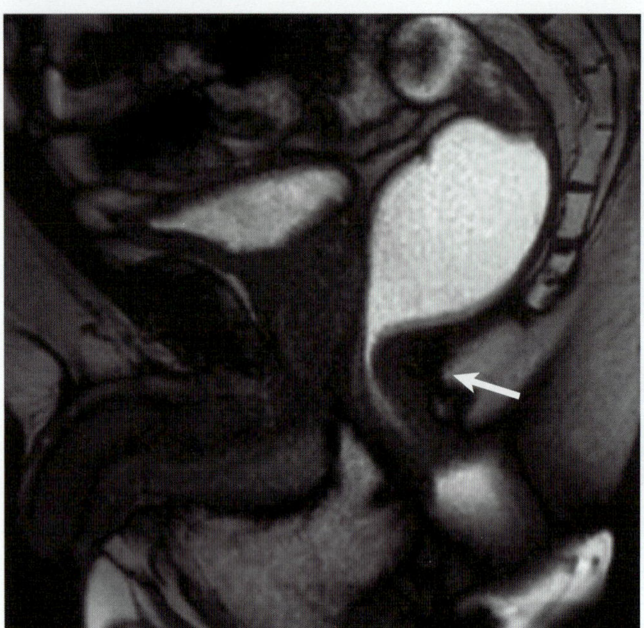

Figure 29.94 Magnetic resonance imaging defecogram from a 41-year-old man with dyssynergic defecation shows failure of relaxation of anorectal angle with a prominent puborectalis impression (*white arrow*).

Systematic Approach to Small and Large Bowel Evaluation on Contrast-enhanced Computed Tomography

A systematic stepwise approach for evaluation of the small and large bowel on contrast-enhanced CT is categorized into the following parts:

1. Evaluation for altered bowel location, caliber, intraluminal contents, wall thickening, mural enhancement, submucosal infiltration, and mucosal abnormalities
   a. **Altered bowel location:** This can be secondary to surgeries (such as Roux-en-Y reconstructions, diverting colostomy, J pouch creation), internal hernias, or cecal and sigmoid volvulus. Congenital abnormalities such as midgut volvulus and rotation anomalies are discussed under the pediatric section.
   b. **Caliber:** The upper limits of bowel caliber can be remembered as 3-6-9, with more than 3 cm diameter for the small bowel, 6 cm for the colon, and 9 cm for the cecum [38,77].
   c. **Intraluminal contents:** Fecalized contents in the small bowel indicate slow transit with the *small bowel feces* sign usually present at or near the transition point of the obstruction. A large colonic stool burden can be seen in the setting of constipation and obstruction. Hyperdense intraluminal contents can be seen with hemorrhage, foreign bodies, and fecalith formation. Excessive fatty intraluminal contents may indicate malabsorption. Several benign and malignant intraluminal masses serve as a lead point for intussusception.
   d. **Wall thickening:** Wall thickening is further divided into
      i. **Mild, moderate, and marked:** Small bowel mural thickening is classified as mild, 3–4 mm, moderate, 5–9 mm; and marked, more than 10 mm in an adequately distended loop [8]. Mild small bowel thickening is present with early Crohn's disease and infectious and ischemic enteritis. Crohn's disease, ischemia, and neoplasms such as adenocarcinoma demonstrate moderate mural thickening. Marked mural thickening is present with lymphoma (with associated aneurysmal dilation), GIST, leiomyosarcoma, and Crohn's disease. Ulcerative colitis, infections, and ischemic and radiation colitis demonstrate mild to moderate colonic thickening. Marked colonic thickening is associated with colon carcinoma and pseudomembranous colitis.
      ii. **Symmetric versus asymmetric:** Major causes of asymmetrical bowel thickening are neoplasms, tuberculosis, and Crohn' disease. Symmetric thickening is predominantly present with the rest of the bowel infections, inflammation, and ischemia.
      iii. **Focal, segmental, and diffuse:** Conditions producing focal bowel thickening include neoplasms, tuberculosis, Crohn' disease, and diverticulitis. Segmental involvement is present with Crohn's disease, ulcerative colitis, infections, ischemia, local radiation, diverticulitis, and lymphoma. Ischemia (shock bowel), vasculitis, angioedema, and infections can affect the entire small bowel. Involvement of the entire colon is seen in advanced-stage ulcerative colitis. Portal enteropathy and colopathy also demonstrate diffuse involvement [8].
   e. **Wall enhancement:** The degree of bowel wall enhancement ranges from mild, moderate, marked, or diminished to absent. Mild homogenous enhancement is present in chronic Crohn's disease and ulcerative colitis, ischemia, and neoplasms such as lymphoma. Active inflammatory bowel, shock bowel, infections, and neoplasms such as carcinoid demonstrate moderate to marked mural enhancement. Diminished and absent enhancements are indicative of ischemia [8].
   f. **Submucosal infiltrations:** This includes edema, hemorrhage, fat, and pneumatosis. Submucosal edema is present in active Crohn's disease, ulcerative colitis, ischemia, and infections. Submucosal hemorrhage is most commonly seen in the setting of ischemia. Submucosal fat deposition can be a normal finding, associated with obesity or celiac disease, or occur as a sequela of chronic bowel infection and inflammation [103].
      Pneumatosis or air in the wall can be secondary to life-threatening or benign causes. Life-threatening causes include ischemia, obstruction, infections, and toxic megacolon. There are myriad benign causes for pneumatosis, with common causes including drugs (steroid and chemotherapy), iatrogenic procedures, and organ transplantation [104].
   g. **Mucosal abnormalities:** This includes mucosal ulceration and pseudopolyps, predominantly seen in patients with Crohn's disease and ulcerative colitis. Abnormalities of mucosal folds such as reversal of the fold pattern and ileal jejunization are present in patients with celiac disease.
2. Evaluation for perienteric and pericolonic abnormalities such as hyperemia, stranding, adenopathy, fistula, abscess, and air

and mesenteric swirling. Perienteric and pericolonic hyperemia and stranding are present in vast majority of acute infective, inflammatory, and ischemic disorders. *Comb sign* is described for mesenteric hyperemia in Crohn's disease. Mesenteric air is associated with ischemic bowel. Complicated diverticulitis shows pericolonic air and abscess secondary to microperforation. Internal hernia and cecal and sigmoid volvulus demonstrate mesenteric swirl.

Suggested Readings

- MD Sugi, CO Menias, MG Lubner, et al., CT findings of acute small-bowel entities, Radiographics 38 (5) (2018 Sep-Oct) 1352–1369.
- JM Frye, SL Hansel, SG Dolan, et al., NSAID enteropathy: appearance at CT and MR enterography in the age of multimodality imaging and treatment, Abdom Imaging 40 (5) (2015 Jun) 1011–1025.
- KM Elsayes, MM Al-Hawary, J Jagdish, HS Ganesh, JF Platt, CT enterography: principles, trends, and interpretation of findings, Radiographics 30 (7) (2010 Nov) 1955–1970.
- G Masselli, G Gualdi, MR Imaging of the small bowel, Radiology 264 (2012) 2, 333–348.
- J Wittenberg, MG Harisinghani, K Jhaveri, J Varghese, PR Mueller, Algorithmic approach to CT diagnosis of the abnormal bowel wall, Radiographics 22 (5) (2002 Sep-Oct) 1093-107; discussion 1107–1109.

30

Liver Anatomy and Variants

RUCHI RASTOGI

Introduction

The liver has an enormous regenerative capacity, a fact mentioned even in 7th century BCE in Hesiod's Theogony, aiding the form of punishment Zeus inflicted upon Prometheus for his defiance against the gods. This ability of the liver allows for complex resections and subsequently transplantation surgeries; the first successful liver transplantation being performed by Starzl in 1967 [1,2]. The regenerative capacity of the liver is attributable to its unique lobar and segmental anatomy with exclusive vascular and biliary connections, which form the basis of various hepatic surgical advancements. Therefore, it is imperative to have a clear understanding of liver anatomy to provide an accurate roadmap before any surgical or interventional procedure.

Imaging Techniques

The choice of imaging technique depends on the clinical history, patient characteristics, availability, and expertise of interpreting radiologists. Ultrasound (USG) usually serves as the first line of investigation whereas multidetector computed tomography (CT) is the investigation of choice for vascular anatomical assessment. Magnetic resonance imaging (MRI) of the liver is an excellent technique to diagnose and characterize any parenchymal lesion, besides providing a good vascular assessment. Digital subtraction angiography has been superseded by CT and MR angiographies for serving as a diagnostic tool and is now largely reserved for therapeutic purposes.

Abdominal radiographs provide limited information in evaluation of solid organs in abdomen. The liver is seen as a relatively homogenous area of radiopacity bounded superiorly by the right hemidiaphragm, laterally by the properitoneal fat and inferiorly by the right kidney and perinephric fat.

Plain radiographs may provide an estimation of hepatomegaly, perihepatic abscesses, calcified parenchymal lesions, or diffuse siderosis revealed by increased density of the organ. Air in the portal venous system can be diagnosed by peripheral distribution of linear branching radiolucencies overlying the liver shadow. It should be differentiated from pneumobilia which is more central in location. The history of any recent biliary intervention or acute abdomen also aids in distinguishing the two conditions.

Ultrasonography is the most cost effective imaging technique to evaluate hepatic or perihepatic disorders and is a valuable technique in cases requiring repeated follow-up imaging. USG elastography helps to quantify liver parenchymal stiffness. Contrast-enhanced USG serves to evaluate lesional vascularity without any adverse effect of radiation exposure or nephrotoxic contrast. *Color Doppler imaging* is used to assess patency, flow volume, direction of flow, and spectral waveforms of hepatic vessels and portal vein. These studies are especially useful in the intraoperative and postoperative setting for early identification of any significant vascular insufficiency.

Computed tomography has the advantage of being less expensive (compared to MRI) and more easily available technique with higher spatial resolution images. Besides providing a fast and comprehensive abdominal assessment, CT is the best imaging technique for performing accurate vascular assessment and volumetry, especially while evaluating surgical feasibility. The images being isotropic are very well suitable for postprocessing softwares generating exquisite multiplanar reformats, maximum intensity projections, and volume-rendered images for analysis of course and branching pattern of hepatic vessels.

Magnetic resonance imaging is best suited for liver parenchymal and biliary system assessment, besides providing reasonably good vascular analysis. The lack of ionizing radiation, safer gadolinium-based contrast, and excellent soft tissue resolution more than compensates for the relatively stringent technical requirements and increased scanning time needed for a good liver MRI. Improvements in MR technique and contrast agents, especially addition of hepatobiliary contrast agents, help for better lesional characterization along with biliary and vascular assessment. Moreover, comprehensive evaluation of diffuse liver parenchymal steatosis, fibrosis, and iron deposition adds to the value of this technique.

On T1-weighted images, normal liver parenchyma is relatively hyperintense, compared to muscle, spleen, and kidney, aiding identification of pathological lesions which are usually T1 hypointense due to their higher water or cellular density. Presence of fat or iron infiltration in liver increases and decreases, respectively, the T1 in phase MR signal of dual in-opposed phase T1-weighted MRI of liver, when compared with the opposed phase image.

The normal liver signal on T2-weighted images is hypointense compared to spleen, kidney, and pancreas, helping in detection of lesions which are usually hyperintense on T2-weighted images.

The detailed technical protocols of these imaging technique are included in subsequent chapters.

External Anatomy

Located predominantly in the right upper abdominal cavity, with extension in mid and left upper abdomen, the liver is the largest gland and solid organ of the body. It is externally covered by a fibrous capsule, *Glisson's capsule*, which provides attachment to various ligaments on its outer surface (Fig. 30.1A and B). The largest of these is the *falciform ligament*, attaching the anterior aspect of the liver to the anterior abdominal wall and dividing it into anatomical left and right lobes. Its free edge contains ligamentum teres which is the remnant of the umbilical vein [3]. The

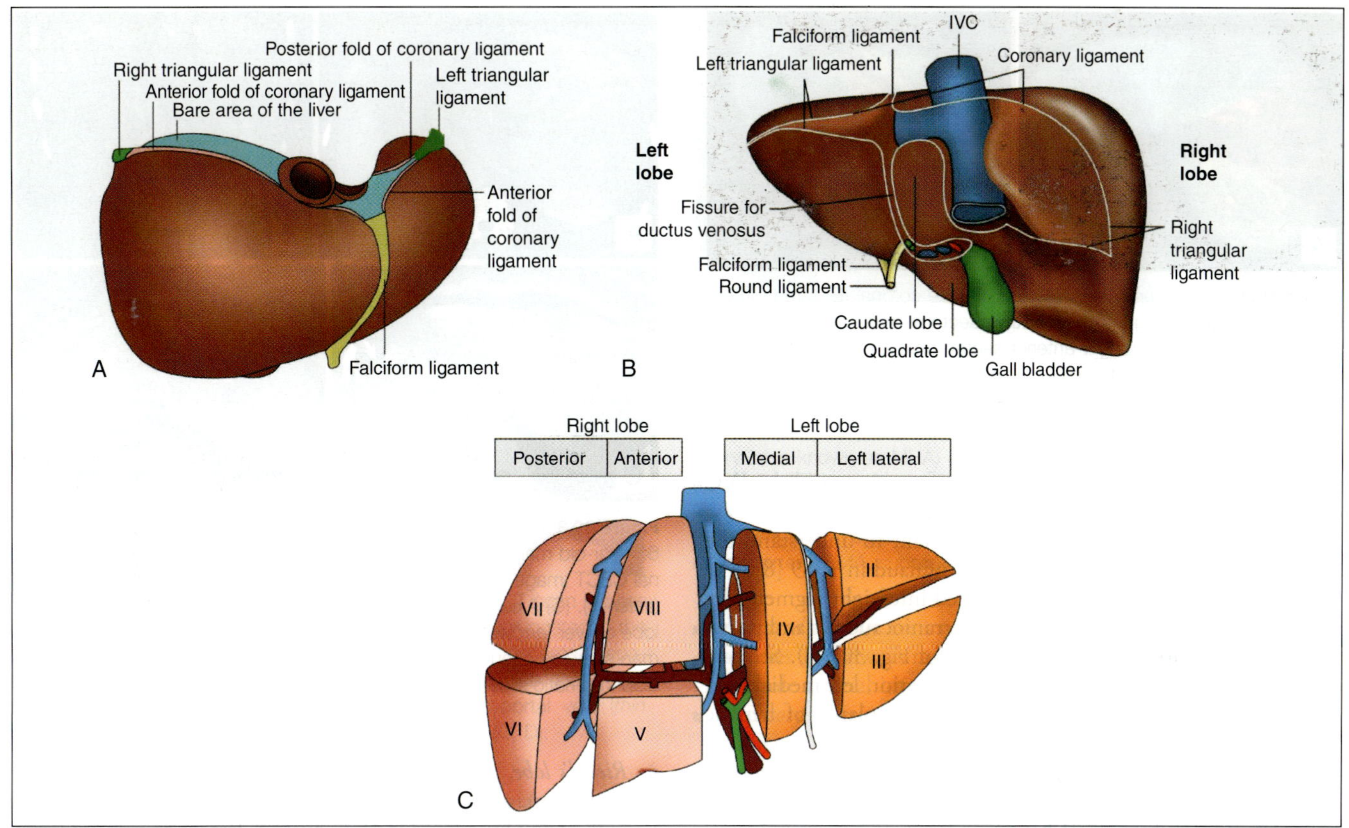

Figure 30.1 External morphology of liver. Anterior view (A) and posterior view (B) show attachment of falciform ligament and ligamentum teres, dividing liver in anatomical right and left lobe. (C) Segmental division of liver according to Couinaud classification.

two other smaller lobes of liver described historically include caudate lobe and quadrate lobe, which are part of the anatomical right lobe [4,5]. The other ligaments include *coronary ligaments*, whose anterior and posterior folds condense to form *triangular ligaments* on both right and left sides of liver, suspending it with right and left under surfaces of diaphragm, respectively. The bare area located in between the twofolds of coronary ligament on the posterior aspect of the diaphragmatic surface of the liver may sometimes demonstrate abnormal signal intensity or contrast enhancement due to its unique vascular connections apart from the hepatic artery and portal venous system [6].

Additionally, lesser omentum, spanning between the liver, lesser curvature of stomach and the first part of the duodenum condenses to form hepatogastric and hepatoduodenal ligaments, respectively, the latter containing the main portal vein, hepatic artery, and common bile duct, besides lymphatics, lymph nodes, and nerves.

The functional lobar division of the liver differs from the anatomical lobar division by inclusion of caudate and quadrate lobe in the functional left lobe of liver. The line of demarcation is the relatively avascular plane between right and left portal venous territories, known as Cantlie's line, extending through

TABLE 30.1 Segment Number, Location, Sector, Functional Lobe, Boundary

Segment	Location	Sector	Lobe	Boundary
I	Central	–	Caudate	Posterior to portal vein and anterior to IVC
II	Left lateral	Left lateral	Left	Medial to the left hepatic vein and superior to the left portal vein
III	Left lateral	Left lateral	Left	Lateral to the left hepatic vein and inferior to the left portal vein
IV (A and B)	Left paramedian	Left medial	Left	Between the middle and left hepatic veins and is further divided by the portal vein into segments IVA superiorly and IVB inferiorly
V	Right anteroinferior	Right anterior	Right	Between the right and middle hepatic veins inferior to the right portal vein branch
VI	Right posteroinferior	Right posterior	Right	Lateral to the right hepatic vein and inferior to the right portal vein branch
VII	Right posterosuperior	Right posterior	Right	Lateral to the right hepatic vein and superior to the right portal vein
VIII	Right paramedian anterosuperior	Right anterior	Right	Between the middle and right hepatic veins superior to the right portal vein branch

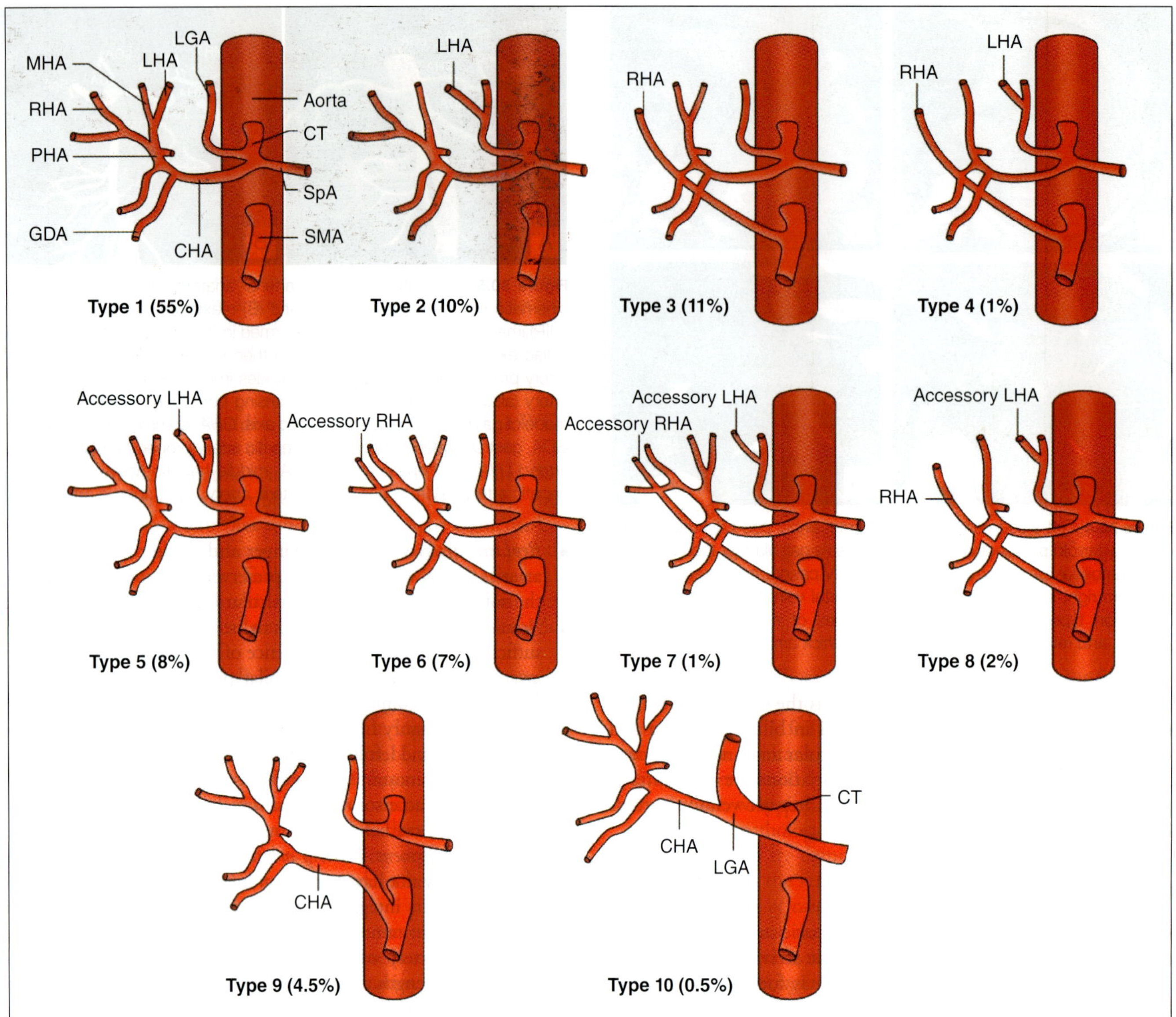

Figure 30.6 Mitchell's classification and incidence of hepatic arterial anatomic variations: Type I: RHA, MHA, and LHA arise from the CHA. Type II: RHA and MHA arise from the CHA; replaced LHA from the LGA. Type III: RHA and MHA arise from the CHA; replaced RHA from the SMA. Type IV: Replaced RHA and LHA from LGA and SMA, respectively. Type V: RHA, MHA, and LHA arise from the CHA; accessory LHA from the LGA. Type VI: RHA, MHA, and LHA arise from the CHA; accessory RHA from SMA. Type VII: Accessory RHA and LHA. Type VIII: Replaced RHA and accessory LHA or replaced LHA and accessory RHA. Type IX: Entire hepatic trunk arises from the SMA. Type X: Entire hepatic trunk arises from the LGA. *CHA*, common hepatic artery; *CT*, celiac trunk; *GDA*, gastroduodenal artery; *LGA*, left gastric artery; *LHA*, left hepatic artery; *MHA*, middle hepatic artery; *PHA*, proper hepatic artery; *RHA*, right hepatic artery; *SMA*, superior mesenteric artery; *SpA*, splenic artery.

supply caudate lobe. The LPV runs a longer extrahepatic course to the left before entering the liver along the falciform ligament. It has a horizontal segment supplying caudate lobe followed by an arch-like umbilical segment in its intrahepatic course, supplying segment II, III, and IV in this order (Fig. 30.8A and B).

Variants and clinical implications: The branching pattern of the main portal vein may be variable in 20–35% of the population [31–33]. These were classified in five types (A–E) by Nakamura et al. in 2002 (Fig. 30.9) [34]. Other classification schemes have also been proposed by various authors [31].

- While performing living donor liver transplantation (LDLT) surgery, conventional *type A* portal branching pattern is most suitable with single anastomotic requirement, minimizing the surgical complexity. In *type B* portal venous anatomy, it is still possible to achieve a single portal venous anastomosis due to close apposition of right anterior and posterior portal vein branches, while in type C anatomy, two separate portal venous anastomosis have to be made, increasing surgical complexity and risk of postoperative complications. This becomes even more complex when the right anterior portal vein–LPV stump is longer, requiring an extension graft for anastomosis in recipient. This anatomy is more suitable for right posterior sectoral donor hepatectomy (Fig. 30.10A–D)
- Intrahepatic origin of RPV branches in *type D and* separate segmental origin of RPV branches from LPV in *type E* are absolute contraindications for performing donor hepatectomy
- *Crossover branches* may exist between right and left lobes of liver which may be responsible for bleeding complications in intraoperative and postoperative period (Fig. 30.11A and B)

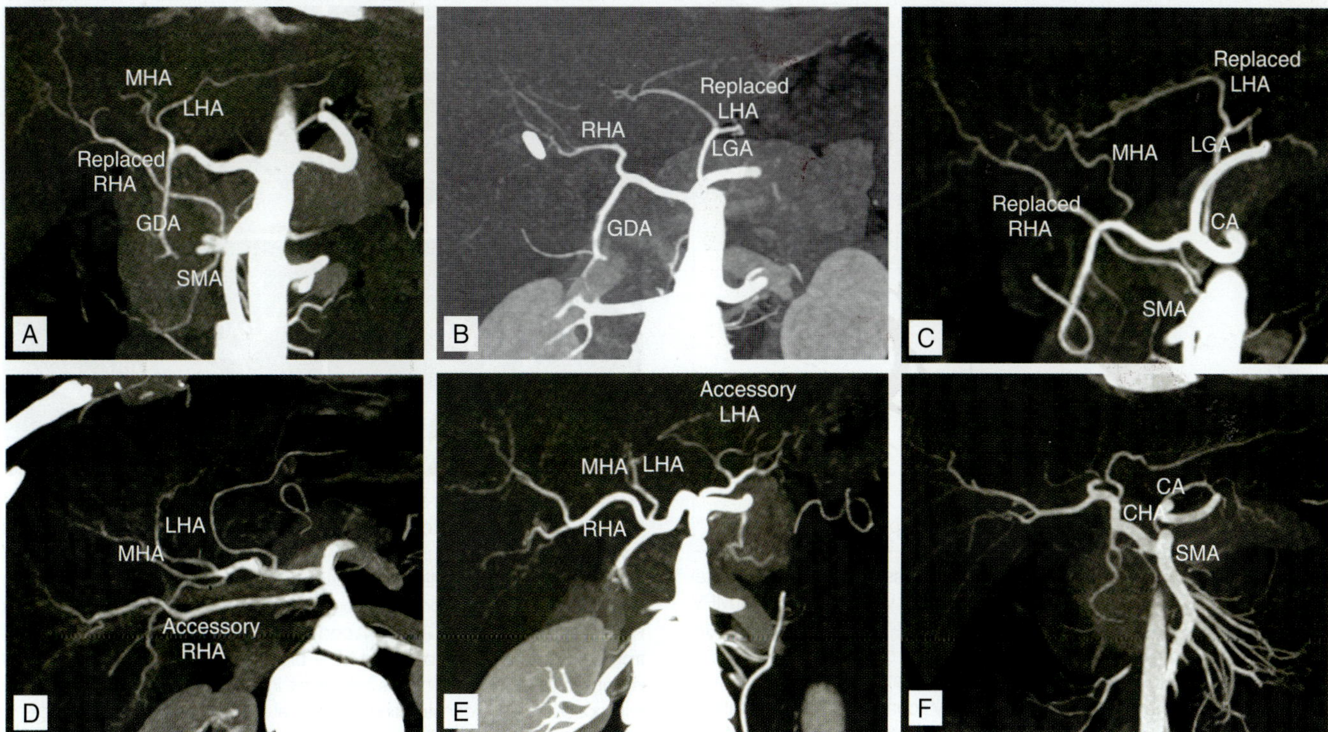

Figure 30.7 Variant arterial anatomy. Coronal oblique MIP images of CT angiograms performed in prospective living related liver donors reveal replaced RHA originating from SMA (A), replaced LHA arising from LGA (B), replaced RHA and replaced LHA arising from SMA and LGA, respectively (C), accessory right posterior hepatic artery branch arising from celiac axis (D), accessory LHA arising from LGA (E), and replaced CHA arising from SMA (F). *CA*, celiac axis; *CHA*, common hepatic artery; *GDA*, gastroduodenal artery; *LGA*, left gastric artery; *LHA*, left hepatic artery; *MHA*, middle hepatic artery; *RHA*, right hepatic artery; *SMA*, superior mesenteric artery.

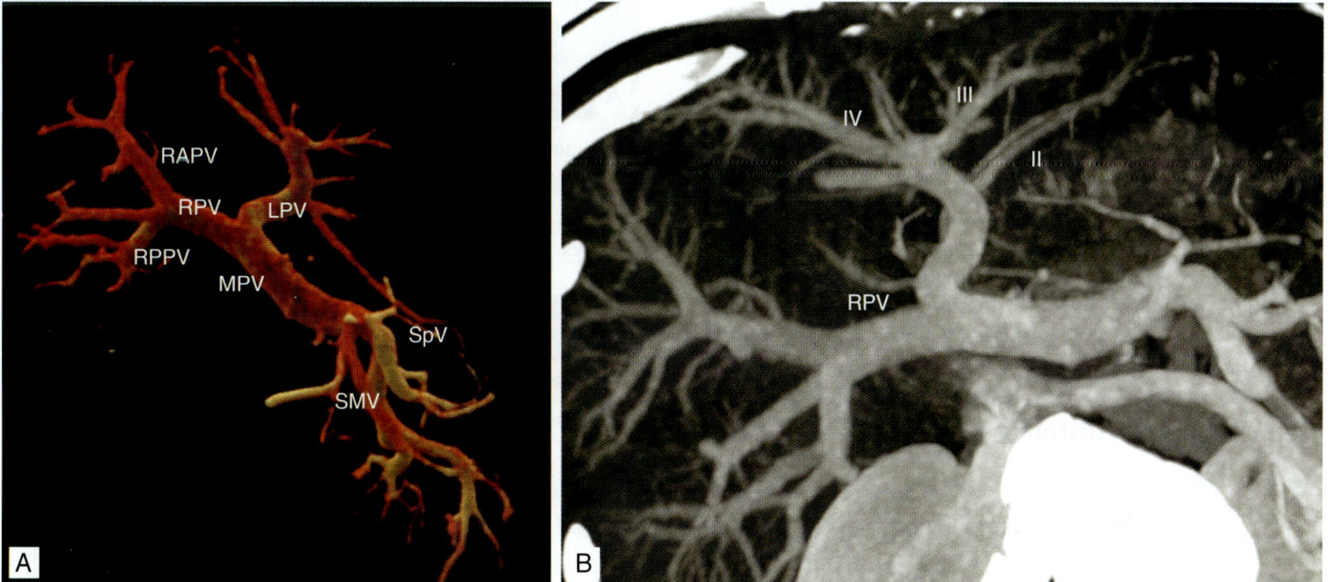

Figure 30.8 Normal portal vein anatomy. Coronal oblique cinematic volume-rendered image (A) and axial oblique MIP image of CT angiogram performed in a 34-year-old prospective liver donor. The main portal vein (MPV) divides into right portal vein (RPV) and left portal vein (LPV). The RPV divides into anterior and posterior segmental branches. The left portal vein (LPV) divides into three branches, one for each segment of the left lobe. *LPV*, left portal vein; *MPV*, main portal vein; *RPV*, right portal vein; *SMV*, superior mesenteric vein; *SpV*, splenic vein; II, segment II portal vein branch; III, segment III portal vein branch; IV, segment IV portal vein branch.

- Significant discrepancy in right and left portal venous diameters may indicate insufficient remnant liver volumes in a prospective liver donor [35,36]
- An acute angle of portal vein branching predisposes the liver graft for future ischemia due to post liver regeneration venous engulfment and narrowing
- Variations pertaining to portal venous system should also alert the radiologist to look for any variable biliary anatomy [37]
- Detailed portal venous anatomical analysis is an essential prerequisite before performing transjugular intrahepatic portosystemic shunt procedure

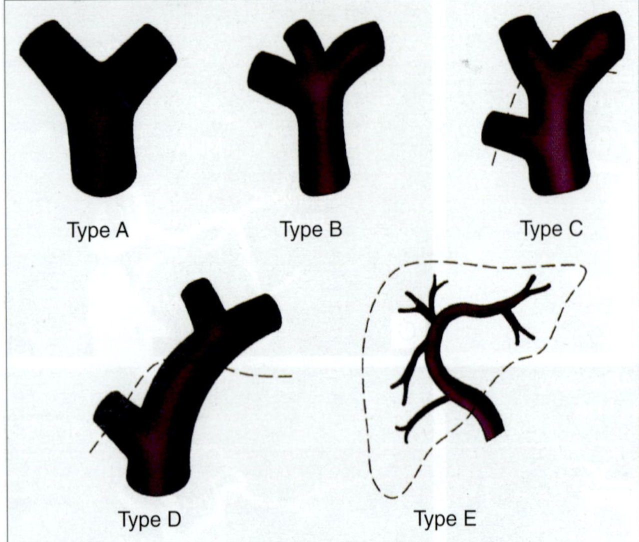

Figure 30.9 Portal vein variations. Nakamura classification: Type A portal venous anatomy indicates conventional anatomy with bifurcation of MPV in RPV and LPV seen in 92.5% population; Type B portal venous anatomy indicates trifurcation pattern with separate origins of RAPV, LAPV, and LPV found in 2.5% population; Type C portal venous anatomy indicates extrahepatic origin of RAPV from LPV found in 2.5% population; Type D portal venous anatomy indicates intrahepatic origin of RAPV from LPV found in 1.7% population; Type E portal venous anatomy indicates undivided main portal vein trunk with individual segmental branches arising from the MPV. It is an absolute contraindication for living donor hepatectomy. *LPV*, left portal vein; *MPV*, main portal vein; *RAPV*, right anterior portal vein branch; *RPPV*, right posterior portal vein branch; *RPV*, right portal vein.

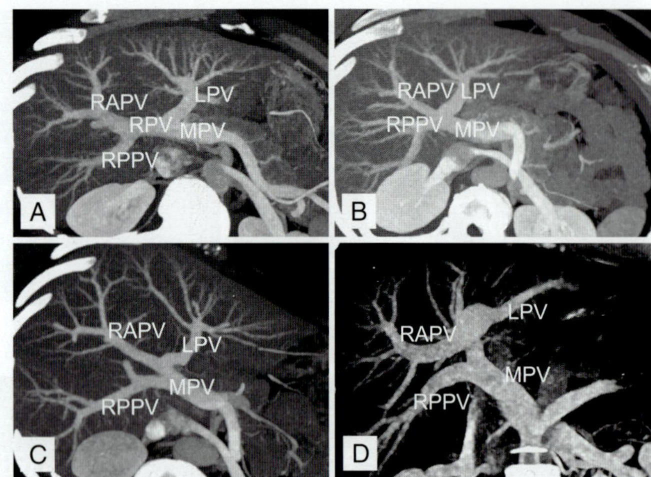

Figure 30.10 Portal vein anatomical variations. Axial oblique MIP images of CT angiogram study performed in prospective liver donors. (A) Type A portal venous anatomy with bifurcation of MPV in RPV and LPV. The length of RPV stump before its bifurcation in anterior and posterior branches should be measured. (B) Type B portal venous anomaly with trifurcation of MPV in RAPV, RPPV, and LPV. (C) Type C portal venous anatomy with RPPV arising from LPV. The distance between MPV bifurcation and RAPV–LPV junction is important. If this distance is longer as in (D), a venous graft has to be interposed while reconstructing the portal vein anastomosis in recipient. *LPV*, left portal vein; *MPV*, main portal vein; *RPV*, right portal vein; *RAPV*, right anterior portal vein branch; *RPPV*, right posterior portal vein branch.

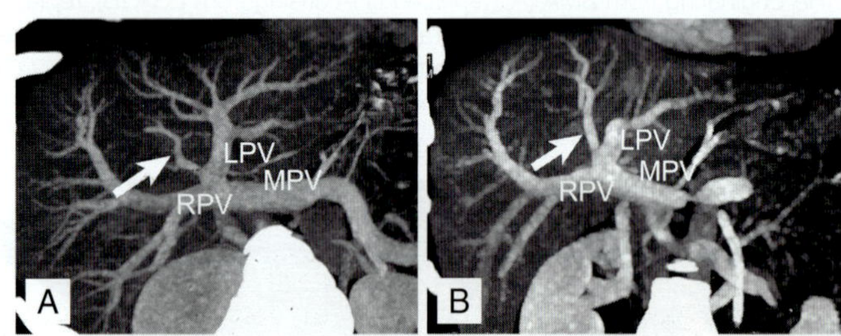

Figure 30.11 Axial oblique MIP image of CT angiogram study in a prospective liver donor reveals origin of one of the segment 8 branch (*arrows*) from LPV. Failure to identify this branch during donor hepatectomy surgery may result in bleeding complication. *LPV*, left portal vein; *MPV*, main portal vein; *RPV*, right portal vein.

Few *congenital anomalies* may also be encountered in the portal venous system. These include agenesis or hypoplasia of portal vein branches leading to inadequate lobar development, abnormal course of portal vein in prepancreatic location instead of normal retro pancreatic location, *double portal vein* and presence of *congenital portosystemic shunts*. These shunts may be extrahepatic (Abernathy type) or intrahepatic in location and are subclassified based on the level of communication (Table 30.3) [38–40]. These shunts may present with a plethora of systemic symptoms or may lead to formation of hypervascular liver masses such as hepatic adenoma and hepatocellular carcinoma (Fig. 30.12).

TABLE 30.3 Classification of Congenital Portosystemic Shunts

Congenital Portosystemic Shunts	
Extrahepatic	
Type I	Absence of intrahepatic portal branches with complete diversion of portal blood to systemic circulation
Type II	Intact portal vein with side-to-side communication between intrahepatic portal vein and systemic vein
Intrahepatic	
Type I	Single large communicating channel between right portal vein and IVC
Type II	Single or multiple peripheral communication between segmental portal vein branch and hepatic vein involving a single segment
Type III	Peripheral aneurysmal communication between portal vein branch and hepatic vein
Type IV	Multiple communicating channels between portal vein and hepatic vein in more than one segment

Hepatic Venous System

Conventional anatomy: The liver parenchyma is drained by three hepatic veins coursing in craniocaudal direction, responsible for its sectoral division. A typical right hepatic vein drains segment VI and VII, middle hepatic vein drains segment V, VIII and major part of segment IV, and the left hepatic vein drains segment II, III, and remaining part of segment IV. The RHV opens directly in IVC while the MHV and LHV unite with each other to form a common channel before opening into the IVC in 60–70% population [41] (Fig. 30.13A). Segment I vein is usually a separate short vein draining directly in IVC.

Variants and Clinical Implications

The course of middle hepatic vein corresponds to the Cantlie's line and serves as an important landmark at the time of harvesting liver graft for right donor hepatectomy. Similarly,

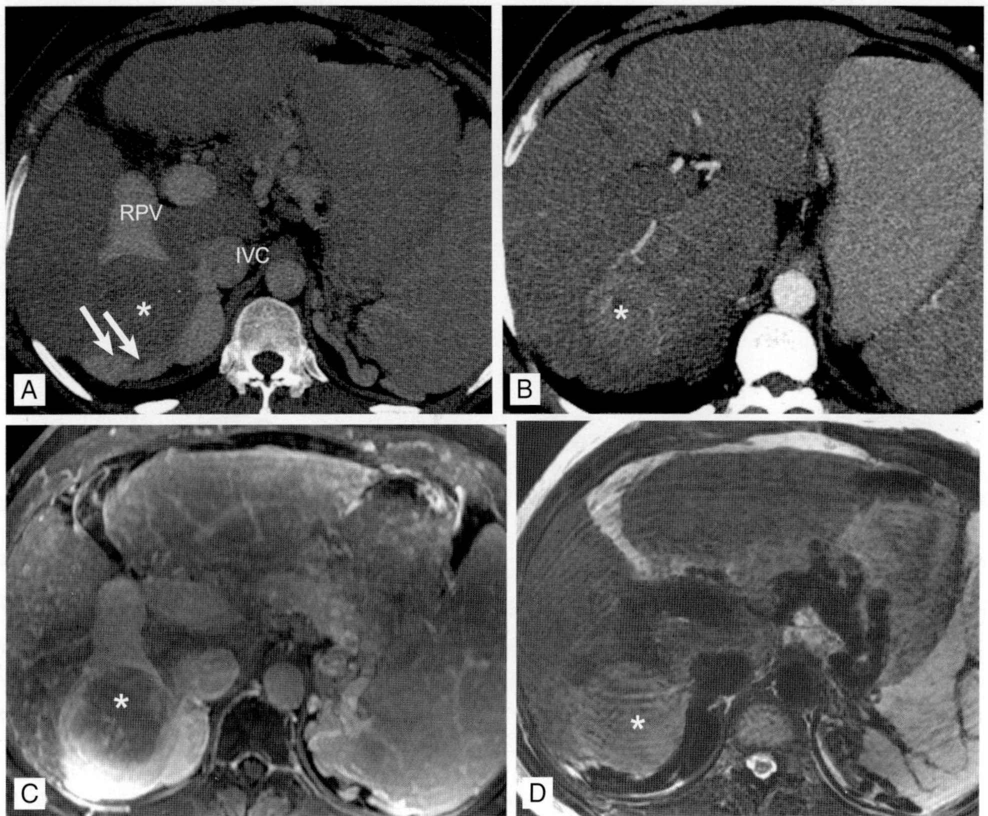

Figure 30.12 Abernathy malformation. Axial CT angiogram MIP image in venous phase demonstrates Type I extrahepatic portosystemic shunt with single large communicating channel between RPV and IVC (*arrows*). A rounded mass is seen splaying this channel, showing enhancement on arterial phase (*asterisk*) (B). The mass is demonstrating washout on venous phase of contrast-enhanced axial MR images (C) and hyperintense signal on T2-weighted images (D). The patient underwent liver transplantation surgery and the mass turned out to be hepatic adenoma on explant liver. *IVC*, inferior vena cava; *RPV*, right portal vein.

falciform ligament serves as a landmark for harvesting left lateral segment graft.

- The hepatic venous drainage may be RHV dominant or MHV dominant in different people (Fig. 30.13B and C), reflected in the caliber and tributaries of these veins and has been classified by Varotti et al. [42] (Fig. 30.14). RHV dominant graft gives an advantage in performing donor hepatectomy during LDLT surgery
- Rarely, MHV can be duplicated with two parallel veins draining segment V, VIII, and segment IV, respectively

Inferior/accessory hepatic veins may be present in 48% of population and their caliber and distance from MHV ostium should be noted. If they are >3 mm in diameter and opening in IVC at a distance of >40 mm from MHV ostium, then they need to be anastomosed separately with the IVC of liver transplant recipient, thus increasing surgical complexity (Fig. 30.15) [43].

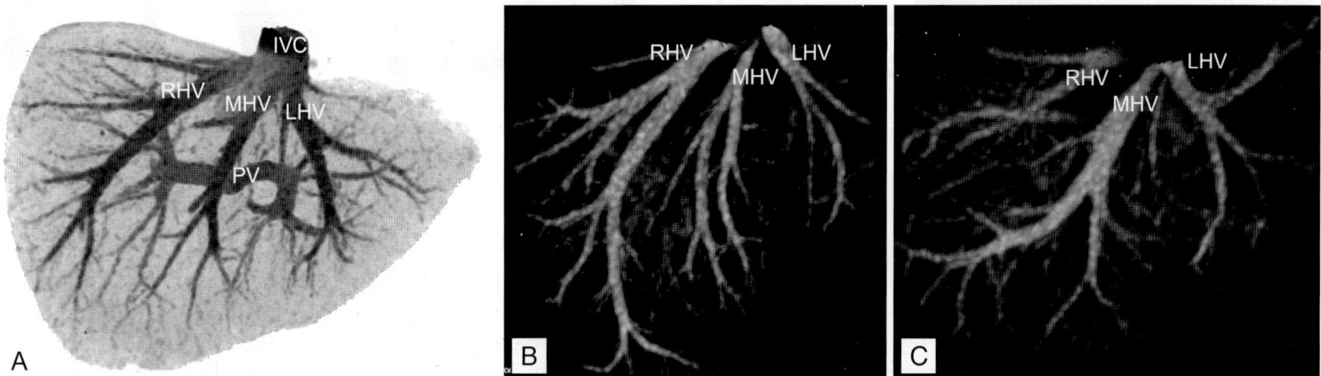

Figure 30.13 Oblique MIP images of CT angiogram study in prospective liver donors showing hepatic veins and venous confluence in IVC. (A) The LHV and MHV are joining to form a common channel before opening in IVC. RHV has a separate opening in IVC. The venous drainage of liver may be RHV dominant (B) or MHV dominant (C) in different people, and the former is preferred for right liver lobe donor hepatectomy. *LHV*, left hepatic vein; *MHV*, middle hepatic vein; *PV*, portal vein; *RHV*, right hepatic vein.

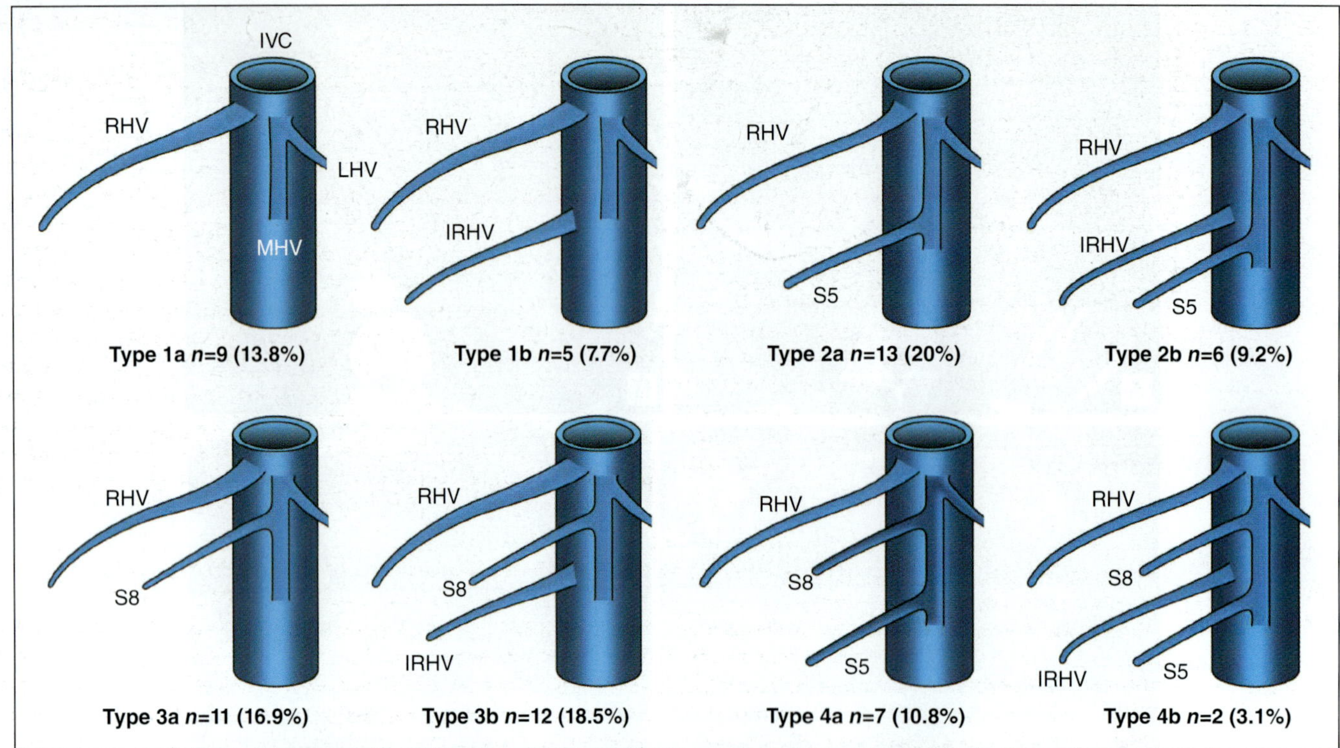

Figure 30.14 Classification and incidence of the right liver hepatic venous anatomy. Type Ia: Conventional anatomy with right hepatic vein represents the main venous outflow of the right hemiliver. Type Ib: Inferior right hepatic vein draining right posterior segment of liver to IVC. Type 2a: Segment 5 vein draining in MHV. Type 2b: Inferior right hepatic vein draining right posterior segment of liver to IVC and segment 5 vein draining in MHV. Type 3a: Segment 8 vein draining in MHV. Type 3b: Inferior right hepatic vein draining right posterior segment of liver to IVC and segment 8 vein draining in MHV. Type 4a: Both segment 5 and 8 veins draining in MHV. Type 4b: Inferior right hepatic vein draining right posterior segment of liver to IVC and segment 5 and 8 veins draining in MHV. *IRHV*, inferior right hepatic vein; *IVC*, inferior vena cava; *LHV*, left hepatic vein; *MHV*, middle hepatic vein; *RHV*, right hepatic vein.

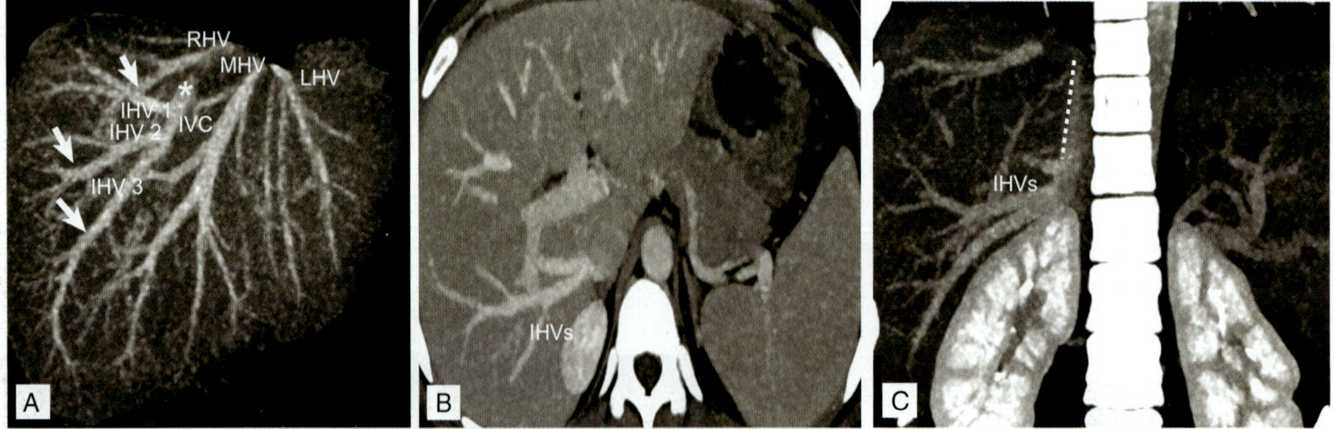

Figure 30.15 3D MIP image of CT angiogram in a 32-year-old prospective liver donor (A) reveals small caliber RHV (*curved arrow*) with the presence of three prominent IHVs draining segment VI and VII (*arrows*), opening in IVC (*asterisk*). The axial (B) and coronal (C) venous phase images of CT angiogram are useful for measuring luminal caliber of IHVs and the distance from hepatic venous confluence, respectively. *IHV*, inferior hepatic vein; *LHV*, left hepatic vein; *MHV*, middle hepatic vein; *RHV*, right hepatic vein.

Pseudolesions

Various pseudolesions may be seen in unenhanced or contrast-enhanced images of liver due to the presence of focal fatty infiltration/focal fat sparing or third inflow vascular connections, respectively. The focal fat pseudolesions are the result of altered hemodynamics and are best resolved using dual in-opposed phase MR images (Fig. 30.16A and B). Third inflow supply refers to hepatic vascular supply other than usual hepatic arterial or portal venous sources. The third inflow veins may arise from splanchnic circulation, draining directly into the hepatic veins after bypassing the portal venous system, or from the systemic circulation, draining directly into the liver parenchyma or into the umbilical or paraumbilical vein of Sappey

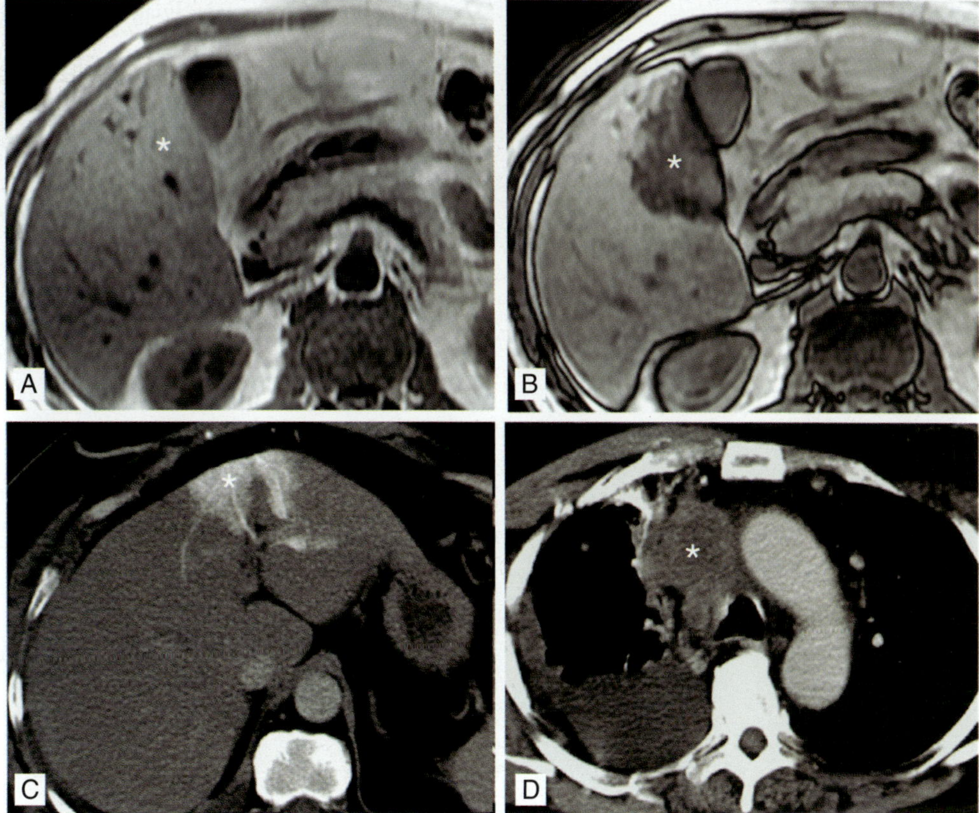

Figure 30.16 Focal fatty and vascular pseudolesions in two different patients. Axial in phase (A) and opposed phase (B) T1 W MR images of liver demonstrate pseudolesion (*asterisk*) in segment V of liver due to the presence of focal fat deposition showing signal drop on opposed phase images compared to in phase images. Contrast-enhanced CT images in another patient showing postcontrast hyperenhancement of liver through the third inflow vascular supply (C, *asterisk*) secondary to collateral development after malignant superior vena cava obstruction (D, *asterisk*).

[44]. The splanchnic vessels draining directly into the hepatic veins arise from parabiliary venous plexus draining in segment IV vein, cystic vein draining in segment IV/V vein, and the gastric veins draining in segment I and IV. Lesser diluted contrast agent coming from these venous communications lead to early and intense enhancement of hepatic parenchyma on early postcontrast images (Fig. 30.16C and D) [45].

To summarize, the hepatic vascular anatomy may be complex and variable in different people, which may affect procedural/surgical feasibility and postsurgical outcomes. Therefore, it should be carefully studied and mentioned in a meaningful radiology report after understanding the surgeon's or interventionist's perspective. A simplified structured reporting format for liver vasculature evaluation of a prospective LDLT donor is attached herewith (Table 30.4).

TABLE 30.4 A Simple Structured Reporting Format for Cross-Sectional Angiographic Study of Liver for Prospective LDLT Donor

Liver morphology	RPV diameter
Angiographic observations	RPV length
Arterial phase	LPV diameter
Hepatic arterial anatomy (origin of CHA, diameter, branching)	Crossover branches—present/absent
RHA diameter	Hepatic venous phase
RHA length	Common LHV–MHV ostium
LHA diameter	RHV diameter
Segment 4 artery arises from	MHV diameter
Any aberrant arteries	LHV diameter
Portal venous phase	MHV drainage
Portal vein anatomy type	IHVs (number, diameter, distance from hepatic vein ostium)
MPV diameter	Ancillary findings

Suggested Readings

- OA Catalano, AH Singh, RN Uppot, PE Hahn, CR Ferrone, DV Sahani, Vascular and biliary variants in the liver: implications for liver surgery, Radiographics 28 (2) (2008) 359–378.
- RP Mathew, SK Venkatesh, Liver vascular anatomy: a refresher, Abdom Radiol (NY) 43 (8) (2018) 1886–1895.
- AM Cahalane, A Mojtahed, DV Sahani, N Elias, AR Kambadakone, Pre-hepatic and pre-pancreatic transplant donor evaluation, Cardiovasc Diagn Ther 9 (Suppl 1) (2019) S97–S115.
- C Carneiro, J Brito, C Bilreiro, et al., All about portal vein: a pictorial display to anatomy, variants and physiopathology, Insights Imaging 10 (1) (2019) 38.
- K Yoshimitsu, H Honda, T Kuroiwa, H Irie, H Aibe, K Shinozaki, K Masuda, Unusual hemodynamics and pseudolesions of the noncirrhotic liver at CT, Radiographics 21 (Suppl_1) (2001) S81–S96.

31

Noncirrhotic Liver

KRISHNA SHANBHOGUE, LUKE GINOCCHIO, VENKAT KATABATHINA, SRINIVASA R. PRASAD

Introduction

There is a wide spectrum of congenital, infectious, parasitic, and neoplastic conditions that may affect the liver. Focal liver lesions may be broadly categorized based on imaging findings into cystic, fat-containing, and enhancing soft-tissue masses. Congenital disorders such as Caroli's disease and biliary hamartomas, as well as abscesses and parasitic infections, present as cystic lesions of variable complexity. Fat-containing liver lesions include angiomyolipomas (AMLs), hepatocellular adenomas (HCAs), and carcinomas. Benign neoplasms of the liver include hepatocellular lesions such as adenomas and focal nodular hyperplasias (FNHs), as well as mesenchymal tumors such as hemangiomas and AMLs. A variety of malignant neoplasms such as hepatocellular carcinomas (HCCs), cholangiocarcinomas, metastases, angiosarcomas, and solitary fibrous tumors (SFTs) occur in the liver. Cross-sectional imaging techniques such as ultrasonography (USG), computed tomography (CT), and magnetic resonance imaging (MRI) play an integral role in the diagnosis, localization, and characterization of a broad spectrum of non-neoplastic and neoplastic conditions of the liver [1]. Imaging studies help distinguish benign incidental findings from focal lesions that warrant prompt treatment. Imaging findings of a plethora of focal lesions that occur in a noncirrhotic liver will be discussed in this chapter.

Imaging Techniques

Ultrasonography (USG) is often the first-line investigation used in clinical practice to diagnose liver diseases and assess focal liver lesions. USG is widely used as the initial screening technique given its availability, lower cost, and noninvasive nature; however, it has an overall limited diagnostic accuracy in the characterization of liver lesions [1–3]. Contrast-enhanced USG significantly improves diagnostic accuracy in differentiating benign and malignant focal liver lesions [1]. Contrast-enhanced CT and MRI are preferred techniques to characterize focal liver lesions in the noncirrhotic liver [1]. MRI, in particular, is a problem-solving tool used for indeterminate lesions on CT or USG, particularly in the setting of diffuse hepatic steatosis (Fig. 31.1) [4]. A sample protocol for CT of the liver for the detection and characterization of focal liver lesions in the noncirrhotic liver is shown in Table 31.1. Unlike the cirrhotic liver, a 2–3 minutes delayed/equilibrium phase is often unnecessary in the noncirrhotic liver for evaluation of focal liver lesions. Several dose reduction techniques are now available and include automatic exposure control by tube current (mA) modulation, selection of lower tube potential (kVp), adaptive dose shielding to minimize over scanning in the *z* axis, iterative reconstruction, and dual-energy CT [5,6].

A sample protocol for MRI of the liver is shown in Table 31.2. Although specific acquisition sequences and the total scan time can vary by manufacturer, patient compliance, and the clinical scenario, the advent of parallel imaging and robust MRI sequences have significantly reduced the overall scan time. The introduction of multiband diffusion-weighted imaging (DWI) and 3D-DIXON techniques have further reduced the total scan time to as little as 15 minutes. Table 31.3 highlights the role of each MRI sequence in the detection and characterization of focal liver lesions. Dynamic gadolinium contrast-enhanced sequences

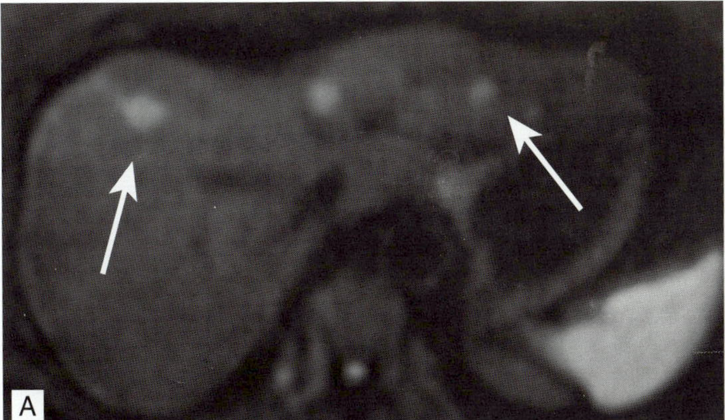

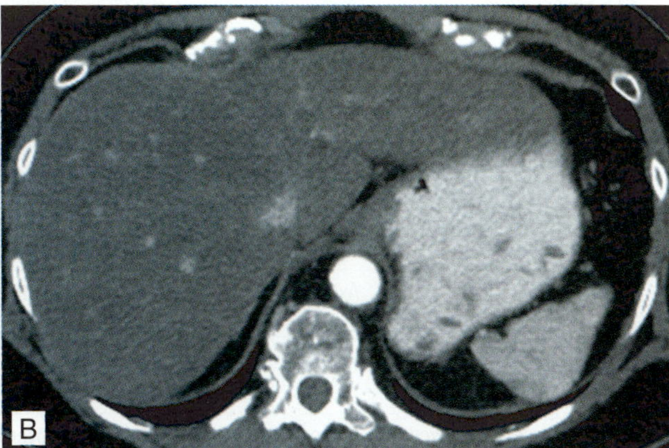

Figure 31.1 Role of MRI in the evaluation of focal liver lesions. MRI is superior to CT in the evaluation of focal lesions against diffuse hepatic steatosis. Diffusion-weighted MRI (A) shows multiple metastases in a patient with breast cancer (*arrows* in A). These focal liver lesions are not seen on contrast-enhanced CT (B) due to diffuse steatosis.

TABLE 31.1 Sample Multiphase CT Liver Protocol for the Detection and Evaluation of Focal Liver Lesions in the Noncirrhotic Liver on a 128-Slice Scanner

Oral contrast	500 cc water
IV contrast volume	Weight based—1.5 mL/kg (standard-120 cc of nonionic contrast)
Injection rate	4–5 cc/s
Acquisition phase	Unenhanced, arterial (bolus triggered level of T12, 150 HU), portal venous (70-second delay), delayed (180 seconds) if evaluating for HCC
Respiration phase	Inspiration
Anatomical coverage	Diaphragm through iliac crests
kVP	Ref. 120 (care KV on)
mAs	Ref. 150
Slice thickness	3–4 mm
Detector collimation	128 × 0.6 mm
Pitch	0.6
Window	450W/30C ST

are the cornerstone for the diagnosis and characterization of focal liver lesions on liver MRI. In addition, contrast-enhanced sequences are crucial in evaluating tumor response and recurrence after locoregional and systemic therapy. Hepatobiliary-specific MR contrast agents such as gadoxetic acid play a crucial role in characterizing focal liver lesions in the noncirrhotic liver given their ability to distinguish hepatocellular tumors from nonhepatocellular neoplasms. Gadoxetic acid is the most widely used hepatobiliary-specific contrast agent, given its significantly higher hepatobiliary excretion (50%) compared with gadobenate dimeglumine (4–5%), allowing for hepatobiliary phase imaging at 20 minutes after contrast administration. Gadoxetic acid-enhanced MRI is very helpful in differentiating FNH from HCAs and also improves the detection of hepatic metastases [7–9] (Fig. 31.2). For patients with breathing issues during the MRI, free-breathing sequences such as non-Cartesian radial T1-weighted imaging sequences can be performed [10]. DWI relies on the Brownian motion of water (microscopic mobility of water), which in turn depends on tissue cellularity, tissue organization, the integrity of cellular membranes, and extracellular space tortuosity. Apparent diffusion coefficient (ADC) maps are generated from two or more diffusion-weighted acquisitions (with at least two different *b* values). Although DWI has been found to be helpful in the detection of solid liver lesions, there is substantial overlap in ADC values between the benign and malignant solid liver lesions, somewhat limiting their role in the evaluation of focal liver lesions in the noncirrhotic liver [11].

Focal Hepatic Lesions

Benign Lesions

Simple Cysts

Simple hepatic cysts are the most common benign incidentalomas of the liver. Simple cysts are developmental lesions, do not communicate with the biliary tree, and can be single or multiple. On USG, cysts appear as well-circumscribed, round, or ovoid anechoic lesions with a thin imperceptible wall [12]. Associated posterior acoustic enhancement (increased through transmission) is also a characteristic feature (Fig. 31.3). Occasionally, these cysts may show a few septa or layering debris. On color Doppler interrogation, there is no internal vascularity. On CT, simple cysts appear as well-circumscribed, nonenhancing, hypoattenuating lesions (water attenuation 0–10 HU). On MRI, simple cysts demonstrate

TABLE 31.2 Sample MRI Liver Protocol for the Detection and Evaluation of Focal Liver Lesions in the Noncirrhotic Liver on a 1.5T. Patients Are Scanned in Supine Position With Phase Array Coil Over the Abdomen

Sequence	Plane of Imaging	Anatomic Coverage/Breathing Instructions	TR (ms)/TE (ms)/Slice Thickness (mm)/ FOV (mm)/Base Resolution/Phase Resolution (%)
Single shot T2 nonfat suppressed (HASTE)	Coronal	BH, straight coverage through the entire liver; skin to skin	1200/92/5/350/256/95
T2 fat suppressed	Axial	BH, straight coverage through the entire liver	3500/90/4/350/256/75
T1 in/out of phase	Axial	BH, straight coverage through the entire liver	170/2.2 and 4.4/5/350/256/95
Multiband diffusion	Axial	Instruct patient to breath lightly, straight coverage through the entire liver	2100/60/8/350/134/100
T1 fat-suppressed precontrast	Axial	BH, straight coverage through the entire liver; 2–3 mm	2.84/1.38/3/350/256/60
Timing run	Axial	Center through the mid-liver	
T1 fat-suppressed postcontrast	Axial	Copy Ax vibe precontrast – take 4 phases (two arterial phases, 60, 180 seconds) BH, straight coverage through the entire liver; 2–3 mm	2.84/1.38/3/350/256/60
T1 fat-suppressed delayed postcontrast	Coronal	BH, straight coverage through the entire liver same coverage as Cor HASTE	3.04/1.33/38/3/350/256/60

BH, breath holding.

TABLE 31.3 Role of Various MRI Sequences in the Detection and Characterization of Liver Lesions. The Sequences Are Acquired in the Axial Plane Except for the Single Shot Non–fat-Suppressed T2-Weighted Sequence (*), Which Is Obtained in the Coronal Plane

Sequence	Role in the Detection and Characterization Liver Lesions
Single shot T2 nonfat suppressed*	Localization
T2 fat suppressed	Differentiation of cysts and hemangiomas (markedly hyperintense) from malignant lesions (T2-intermediate signal)
T1 in/out	Intravoxel fat, intralesional iron, detection of hepatic steatosis, and iron overload
Multiband diffusion	Increased sensitivity for detection—more lesions detected Differentiate benign from malignant lesions
T1 fat-suppressed precontrast	Intralesional hemorrhage, melanoma metastases
T1 fat-suppressed postcontrast	Enhancement characteristics (hypervascular, hypovascular, washout on delayed phase)

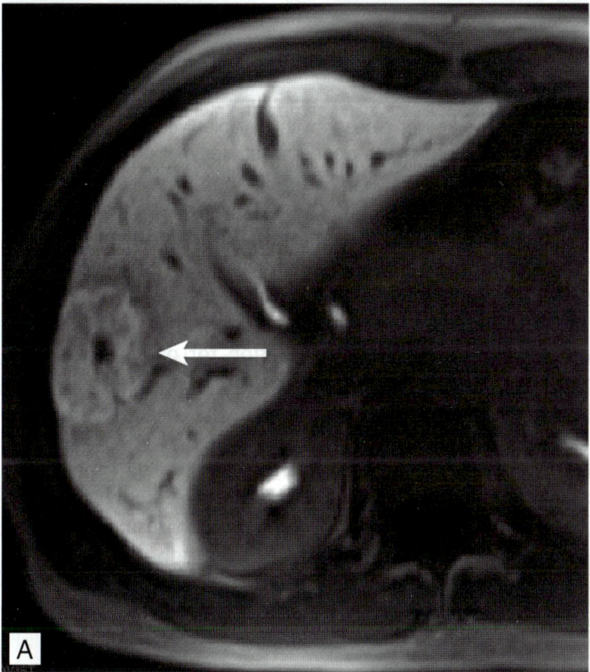

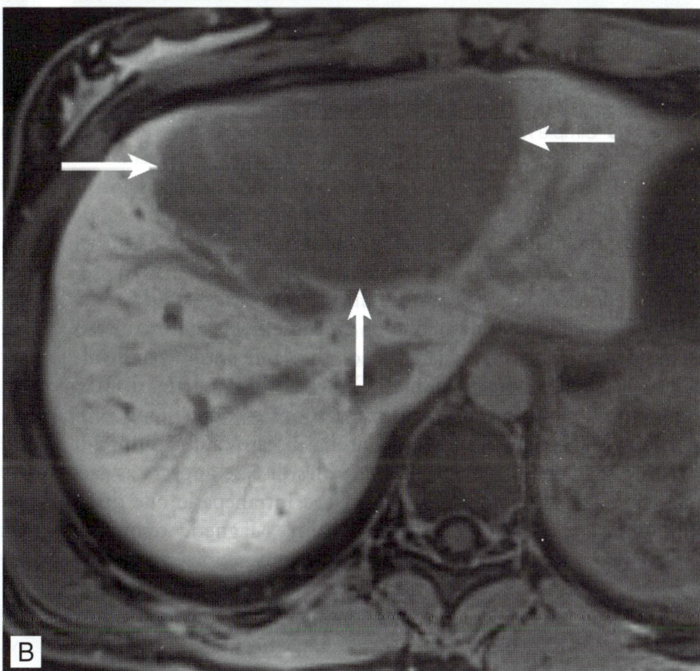

Figure 31.2 Role of gadoxetic acid-enhanced MRI in the evaluation of focal lesions in the noncirrhotic liver. Axial T1-weighted images obtained 20 minutes after administration of gadoxetic acid (hepatobiliary phase) demonstrates homogeneous uptake of contrast in focal nodular hyperplasia which appears hyperintense to the liver in the hepatobiliary phase (*arrow* in A) and no uptake or retention of contrast in hepatocellular adenoma which appears hypointense to the liver on hepatobiliary phase (*arrows* in B).

homogeneous low signal intensity on T1WI, high signal intensity on T2WI, and no contrast enhancement. High T1 signal intensity can occasionally be seen with proteinaceous or hemorrhagic content. Asymptomatic simple hepatic cysts do not require imaging follow-up or treatment. Large symptomatic cysts can be managed with surgical resection, drainage, or sclerotherapy.

Congenital Cystic Lesions of the Liver

Biliary Hamartoma/Von Meyenberg Complex: Biliary hamartomas (von Meyenberg complex) are benign congenital lesions that occur due to embryonic duct plate malformation and manifest as small cystic lesions that represent small dilated bile ducts with fibrous stroma [13]. The vast majority of the biliary hamartomas are asymptomatic and incidentally detected on imaging [14]. On imaging, biliary hamartomas appear as innumerable, small (5–15 mm), uniform, round cysts scattered throughout the liver (Fig. 31.4). Given the small size of the cysts, occasionally, these may appear hyperechoic and show reverberation artifact due to close proximity of the cyst interface [14,15].

Polycystic Liver Disease: Polycystic liver disease (PCLD) is a type of fibropolycystic liver disease arising from congenital ductal plate malformations and manifests as multiple, variably sized liver cysts in intrahepatic and peribiliary distribution [16,17]. PCLD is an autosomal dominant condition; up to 50% of patients have associated autosomal dominant polycystic kidney disease. Although most patients are asymptomatic, PCLD can progress to advanced liver disease with portal hypertension or become symptomatic due to hepatomegaly, cyst rupture, hemorrhage, or infection [18] (Fig. 31.5). Increased wall thickening, fluid level, and gas within the cysts imply superimposed infection. Symptomatic cysts can be treated with percutaneous aspiration with/without injecting sclerosing agents or resection. Advanced chronic liver disease secondary to PCLD may require liver transplantation [18]. On imaging, it is essential to differentiate PCLD from the other entities that belong to the fibropolycystic liver disease

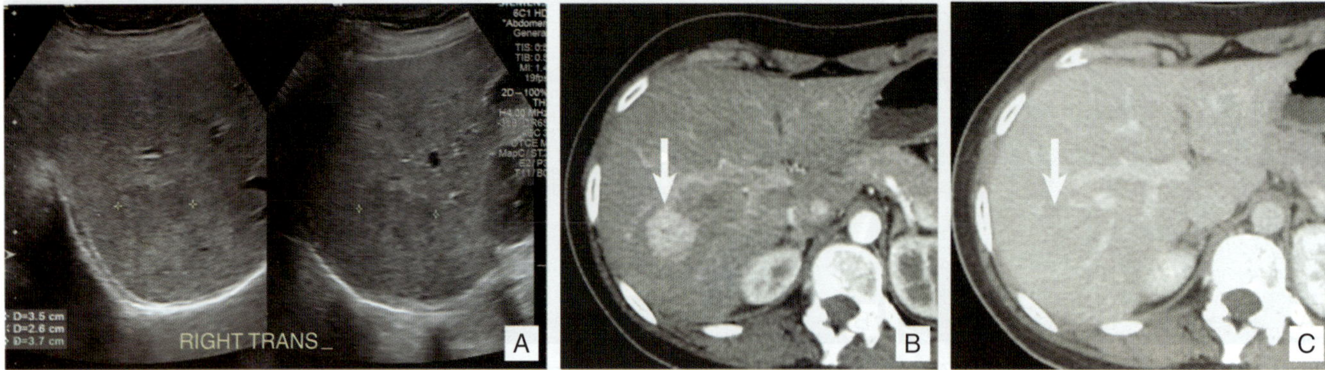

Figure 31.22 Focal nodular hyperplasia ultrasonography and CT appearance. Ultrasonography image (A) demonstrates an isoechoic to mildly hypoechoic lesion in the right lobe. Axial contrast-enhanced CT image during the hepatic arterial (B) and portal venous phase (C) shows a homogeneous enhancing mass in the arterial phase which becomes isodense to the liver on venous phase (*arrows* in B and C). A central scar is visible in the arterial phase.

MRI

- Iso- to mildly hypointense on T1WI, iso- to mildly hyperintense lesion on T2WI with a T2-hyperintense (due to the aberrant vessels) central scar (Fig. 31.23)
- Intense early arterial phase enhancement. Persistent enhancement (often isointense to the liver) on portal venous and delayed phase
- Similar to CT, the central fibrotic scar retains contrast on delayed scans
- FNHs can have atypical imaging appearances in up to 20% of cases, including lack of central scar, pseudocapsule, lesion heterogeneity, nonenhancement of the central scar, and intralesional fat
- Hepatobiliary contrast agents (gadoxetic acid) are often used to distinguish FNHs from other focal hepatic lesions. FNHs retain gadoxetic acid due to the presence of normal hepatocytes, and abnormal bile ductules, and increased expression of

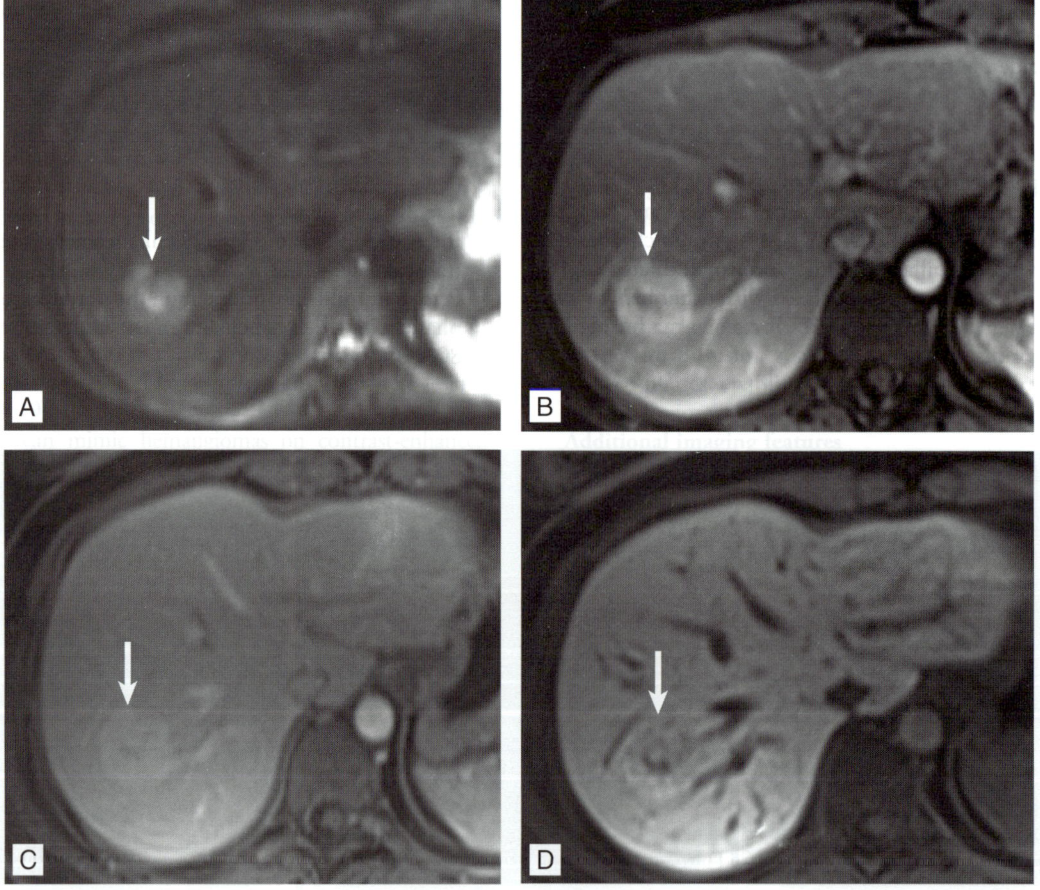

Figure 31.23 Focal nodular hyperplasia. Classical MRI appearance of focal nodular hyperplasia (*arrows*). Axial T2-weighted fat-suppressed image demonstrates a right hepatic lesion with mildly hyperintense T2 signal, with a T2 hyperintense central scar (A). The lesion demonstrates homogeneous arterial phase enhancement (B), with persistent enhancement in the venous phase (C) and appears isointense to mildly hyperintense to the liver on delayed hepatobiliary phase image, 20 minutes after administration of gadoxetic acid (D).

organic-anion-transporting polypeptides transporter. FNH appears as a hyperintense to isointense (to the liver) mass on the hepatobiliary phase images (Fig. 31.23) [36–38]

Hepatocellular Adenoma

Pathophysiology and Clinical Presentation: HCAs are uncommon benign hepatic neoplasms usually seen in young women with a history of long-standing oral contraceptive use (M:F ratio of 1:9) [34]. Other known risk factors for HCA include the use of anabolic steroids, glycogen storage disease (types Ia, III, and VI), hemochromatosis, androgen therapy, and medications (barbiturates, clomiphene) [34,39]. Unlike FNH, HCAs have increased proclivity to bleed and rupture as well as the propensity to undergo malignant change [40]. On pathology, HCAs are well-circumscribed lesions, often subcapsular with a yellow color (abundant fat and lack of bile) and frequent hemorrhagic change. There is a proliferation of pleomorphic hepatocytes without normal lobular architecture, near-complete lack of bile ducts, and Kupffer cells. Recently, many distinct genotypes of HCAs have been described [41,42] (Table 31.4). Although the inflammatory subtype, the most common subtype, occurs in young, obese women with alcohol use, hedgehog-mutated HCAs show a marked tendency to hemorrhage. HNF-1α-mutated HCA, the second most common subtype, shows intracellular and/or macroscopic fat. β-Catenin-mutated HCAs show the highest risk for malignant transformation and occur in men on anabolic steroids and in glycogen storage disease. Hepatic adenomatosis, the presence of more than 10 adenomas, is more common in women and not necessarily associated with the classic risk factors mentioned earlier [43]. Histology is similar to that of typical hepatic adenomas and although to develop secondary to abnormal vascularization of the liver [44]. Individual adenomas within the same patient may demonstrate different imaging features from one another.

Clinically, HCAs may manifest with right upper abdominal quadrant fullness or discomfort due to mass effect. Spontaneous rupture can lead to acute abdominal pain; rarely, rapid bleeding into the peritoneal cavity can lead to massive exsanguination. HCAs uncommonly undergo malignant transformation to HCC. Management of HCA depends on histological subtype, size, presence of the β-catenin mutation, and other complications (rupture or hemorrhage; Flowchart 31.1). HCAs with β-catenin mutation and all HCAs in male patients should be resected, given the risk of malignant transformation. Ruptured or bleeding HCAs can be treated with embolization, with or without subsequent surgical resection.

Imaging Features

Ultrasonography

- Solitary, well-defined, heterogeneous masses with variable echogenicity (Fig. 31.24)
- Hyperechoic foci due to fat or hemorrhage may be seen
- Perilesional sinusoids may be present on color Doppler [45]

CT

- Heterogeneous due to variable hemorrhage and macroscopic fat
- Arterially enhancing lesions, with persistent enhancement on delayed phase (typical; Fig. 31.25). Washout is rare and can suggest β-catenin mutation or HCC (Fig. 31.26)

MRI

- Exquisitely demonstrates the presence of hemorrhage and macroscopic or microscopic fat
- Imaging findings of HCA vary depending on the histological subtype (Table 31.4)
- Diffuse signal drop on in- and out-of-phase images secondary to microscopic fat helps distinguish HCA from FNH and is a distinctive feature of *HNF-1*α-mutated HCAs (Fig. 31.27) [46]
- Inflammatory HCAs show marked hyperintensity on T2WI due to sinusoidal dilatation, and heterogeneous enhancement (Fig. 31.28)
- *Atoll sign* described as a T2 hyperintense rind, which typically enhances in the delayed contrast-enhanced phase, likely corresponding to regions of sinusoidal dilatation (with hyperintense T2 signal reflective of high water content; Fig. 31.28)
- Many HCAs typically do not retain hepatobiliary contrast agents on delayed hepatobiliary phase [40,41,47]

TABLE 31.4 Genotype–Phenotype Classification of Hepatocellular Adenoma, With Their Salient Pathological, Clinical, and Imaging Features

Subtype	Genotype	Pathological Features	Clinical Features	Imaging Features
Inflammatory HCA (35–45%)	Gain of function mutation of IL6ST gene, coexistent β-catenin gene mutation in 10%	Inflammation, sinusoidal dilatation and pseudoportal tracts. Overexpression of CRP and SAA on immunohistochemistry	Associated with high BMI, background hepatic steatosis, and alcohol consumption. Increased risk of bleeding. Malignant transformation if coexistent β-catenin mutation	Moderate T2 hyperintense signal, Atoll sign, hypervascular in arterial phase with persistent enhancement on delayed phase imaging
HNF-1 alpha HCA (30–40%)	Somatic inactivating mutation of TCF1 (HNF1 alpha) gene, germline mutation of CYP1B1 (<5%)	Steatosis or clear cells. Lacks LFABP expression on immunohistochemistry	Small increased risk of bleeding, malignant transformation extremely rare, associated with familial adenomas	Contains bulk fat, enhancement in the arterial phase with or without washout on delayed phase; may demonstrate avidity on FDG-PET CT
β-Catenin HCA (20%)	β-Catenin gene (CTNNB1) activating mutations	Cytological atypia, small cell change, pseudoglandular architecture. Diffuse and strong expression of glutamine synthetase on IHC	Malignant transformation to HCC in up to 40%. Requires surgical resection. Adenoma in men, and androgen use	Enhances and washes out, indistinguishable from HCC
Sonic hedgehog HCA (4%)	Activation of sonic hedgehog pathway (GLI1 activation)	Hemorrhage, vessel abnormalities; ASS1 and PGTDS overexpression on IHC	More frequent in women with high BMI. Higher rate of clinically significant bleeding	No specific imaging features. Usually hemorrhagic HCA
Unclassified HCA (5–10%)	No identified mutation	No specific features	No specific features	No specific features

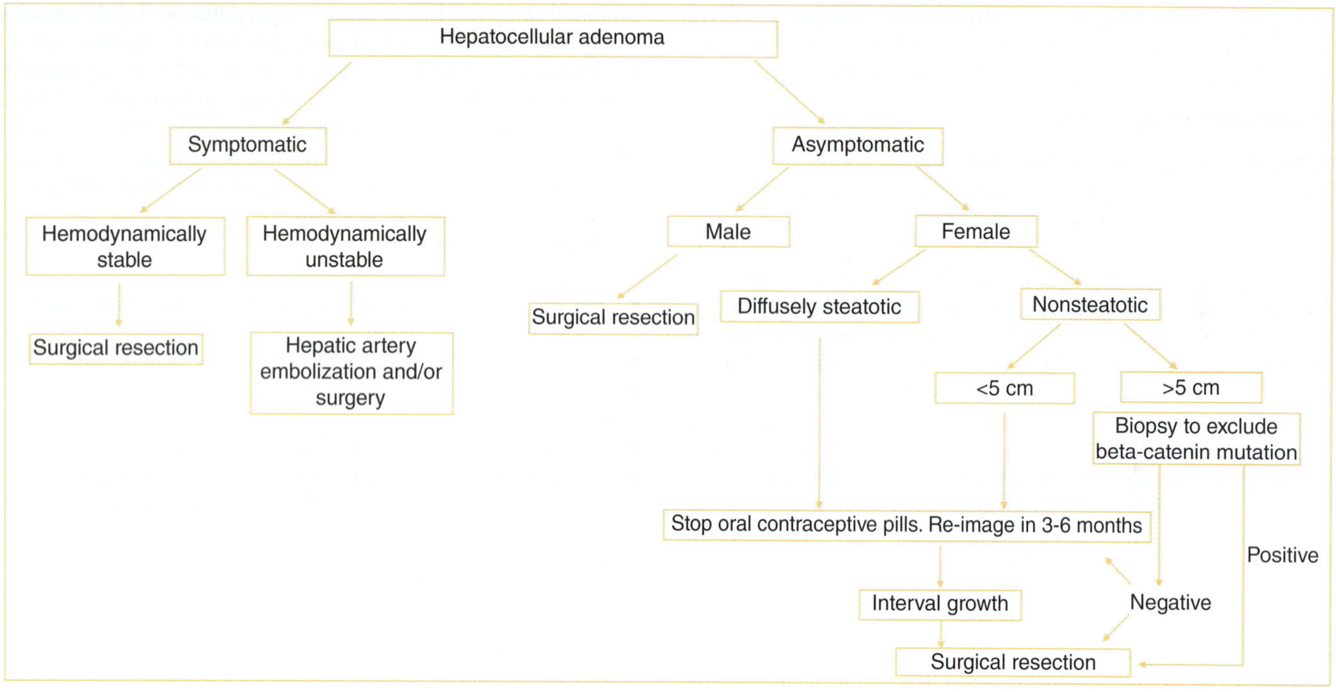

Flowchart 31.1 Management of hepatocellular adenomas.

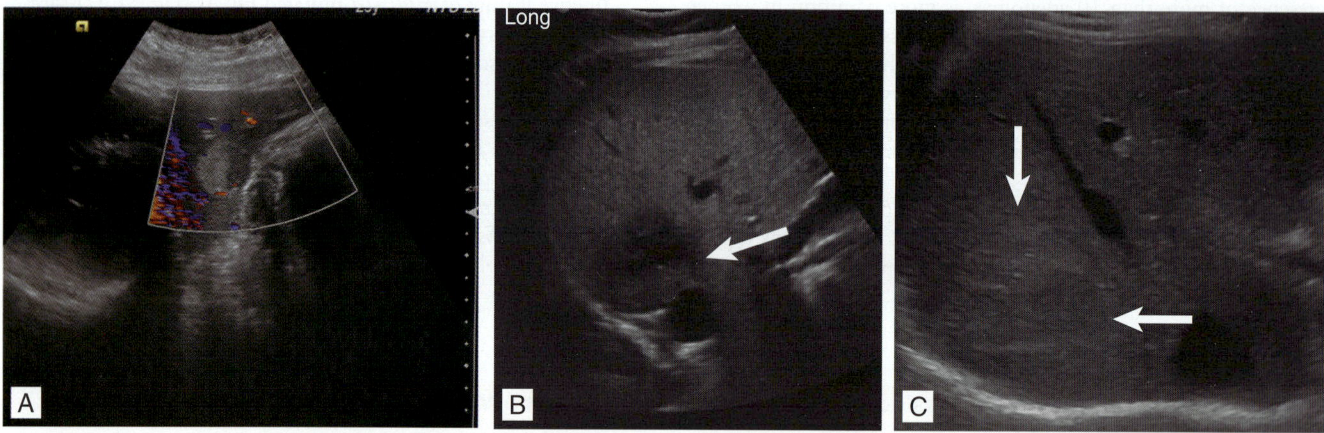

Figure 31.24 Ultrasonography appearance of hepatocellular adenoma. (A) Heterogeneous focal lesion is seen in the left lobe without visible internal vascularity on Doppler evaluation. (B) Hypoechoic mass in the right lobe (*arrow*), (C) isoechoic mass in the right lobe (*arrows*).

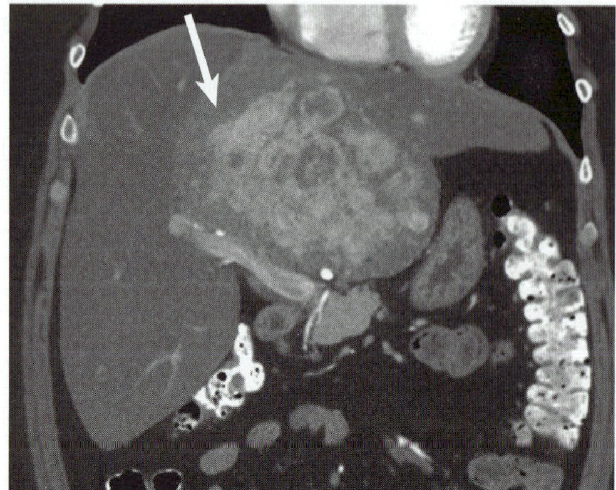

Figure 31.25 Hepatocellular adenoma CT. Coronal contrast-enhanced CT demonstrates a large heterogenously enhancing mass in the left lobe (*arrow*).

- Some inflammatory and β-catenin-mutated HCAs may appear as hyperintense masses on hepatobiliary phase images, and usually this is heterogeneous compared with the homogeneous uptake seen in FNH. Also, the presence of fat, hemorrhage, T2 hyperintense signal (intralesional as well as peripheral "atoll" sign) can help in differentiating FNH from HCA. Biopsy may be required for definitive diagnosis, subtyping, and detection of β-catenin mutation and is usually reserved for lesions larger than 5 cm in size

Mucinous Cystic Neoplasm

Pathophysiology and Clinical Presentation: Hepatic mucinous cystic neoplasm (MCN, formerly labeled biliary cystadenoma) is a rare, premalignant cystic tumor of the liver, which usually occurs as a solitary mass commonly within the left hepatic lobe. MCNs are almost exclusively seen in middle-aged women (over 85% cases), and over 50% of the lesions are seen in the hepatic segment IV [48]. On pathology, MCNs are lined by columnar, cuboidal, or flattened mucus-secreting epithelial cells with an ovarian type of mesenchymal stroma. MCNs are thought to originate from epithelial cells

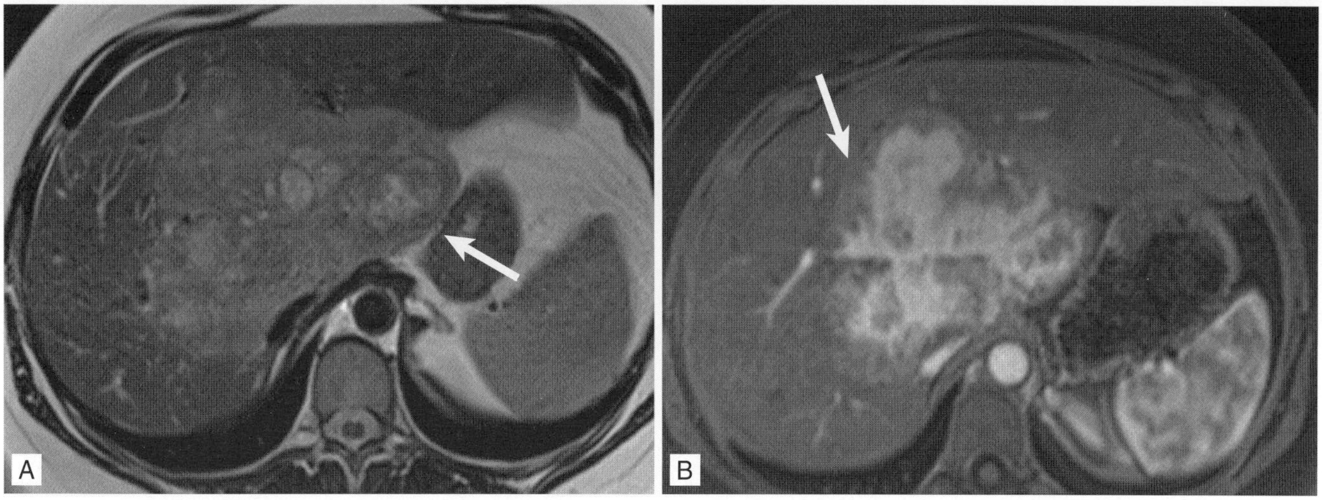

Figure 31.26 β-Catenin-mutated HCA. (A) Axial T2-weighted MR image shows a heterogenous, expansile mass (*arrow*) with high signal intensity foci. (B) Arterial phase postcontrast T1-weighted image depicts heterogeneous enhancement (*arrow*).

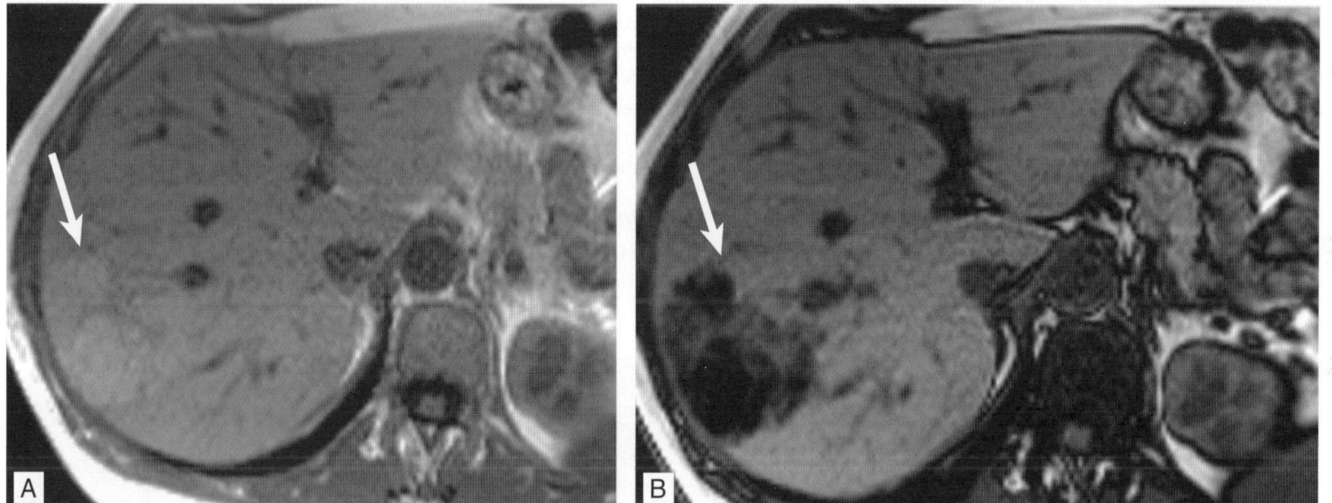

Figure 31.27 *HNF-1α*-mutated HCA with microscopic fat. In-phase (A) and opposed-phase T1-weighted (B) MR images show diffuse signal loss on out-of-phase image (*arrows* in A and B) consistent with the presence of intracellular lipid.

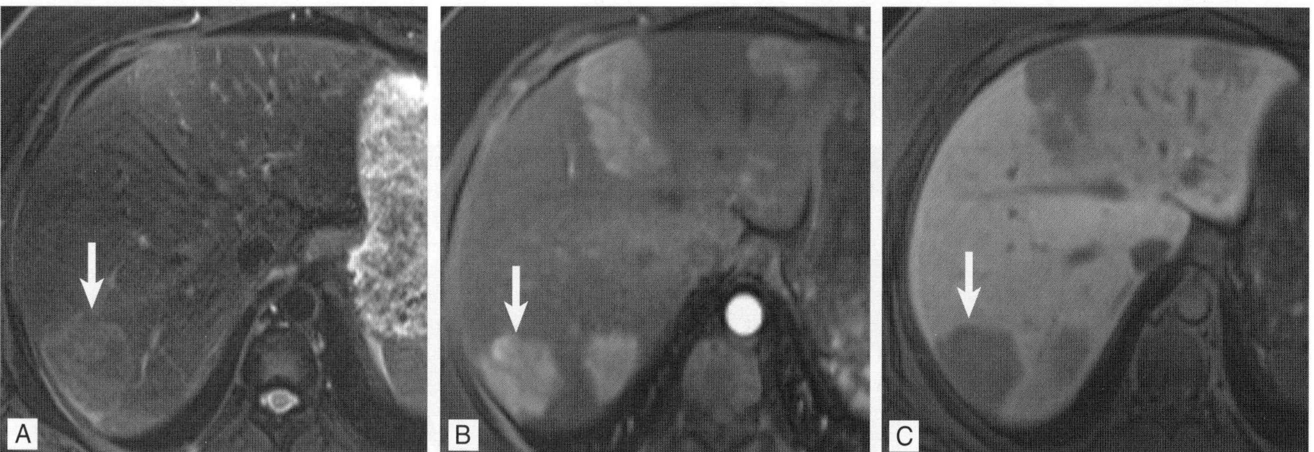

Figure 31.28 Inflammatory HCA. Axial T2 weighted image (A) shows a heterogeneous T2 hyperintense lesion in the right lobe (*arrow*) with peripheral T2 hyperintense signal ('Atoll' sign) and homogeneous arterial phase enhancement (B). Axial T1 weighted hepatobiliary phase image (C) 20 minutes after administration of hepatobiliary contrast agent shows lack of uptake/retention of the contrast agent (*arrow*). Multiple additional hepatocellular adenomas were also seen.

covering the embryonic gonads in early fetal life. Malignant transformation within the MCN is extremely rare. Clinically, MCNs may present with abdominal pain, cholangitis, biliary obstruction, or jaundice or present as an incidental finding. Surgery is the treatment of choice and usually curative for MCN.

Imaging Features

Ultrasonography

- Complex cystic lesions with internal septations on ultrasonography

CT (Fig. 31.29)

- Multilocular cystic lesions with enhancing septae
- Mural calcification
- Septal or mural nodules

MRI

- Multilocular cystic lesion
- Hypointense T1 signal, heterogeneous hyperintense T2 signal with enhancing septae [49] (Fig. 31.29)
- The individual locules within the lesion may demonstrate a variable T2 signal depending on the protein/mucin content
- Enhancing solid components or papillary projections indicate malignancy

Hepatic MCNs can be differentiated from simple biliary cysts with fair degree of accuracy using the following features [50]:

- The presence of septations (unilocular cyst indicates a simple biliary cyst with 95.2% positive predictive value)
- Septae arising directly from the wall (100% sensitive and 60% specific for MCN). Septae arising from macrolobulation is 100% specific for simple biliary cyst
- Septal enhancement (100% sensitive for MCN)

Angiomyolipoma

Hepatic AML is a rare benign mesenchymal tumor composed of blood vessels, smooth muscle cells, and adipocytes in varying proportions [51]. Hepatic AMLs are derived from perivascular epithelioid cells and hence are classified as PEComas according to the World Health Organization classification of liver tumors. Mostly sporadic, up to 15% of hepatic AMLs occur in the setting of tuberous sclerosis [52]. Hepatic AMLs are predominantly seen in women in the fifth to sixth decade [51,53].

On ultrasonography, AMLs are echogenic and may mimic hemangioma or other fat-containing lesions. On CT and MRI, hepatic AMLs are indistinguishable from other lesions such as HCC or HCA, warranting a biopsy for confirmation [51,53] (Fig. 31.30). Hepatic AMLs can be managed conservatively. Surgical resection is reserved for symptomatic patients, enlarging lesions, and inconclusive biopsy. Large tumor size (>5 cm), infiltrative growth pattern, necrosis, and vascular invasion predict malignant PEComas [53].

Tumor-Like Conditions

Nodular Regenerative Hyperplasia

Nodular regenerative hyperplasia (NRH) is a rare condition characterized by multiple small nodules in the absence of fibrosis. These are commonly seen in patients with myeloproliferative and lymphoproliferative syndromes, chronic vascular disorders, rheumatological disorders, systemic lupus erythematosus, steroids, and after chemotherapy. NRH may lead to portal hypertension. On imaging, NRH is characterized by multiple, small, solid nodules that show mild to moderate contrast enhancement (Fig. 31.31). Management of NRH involves the evaluation and treatment of the underlying condition.

Inflammatory Pseudotumor

Hepatic inflammatory pseudotumors (xanthogranulomas or plasma cell granulomas) are rare benign liver lesions. It commonly

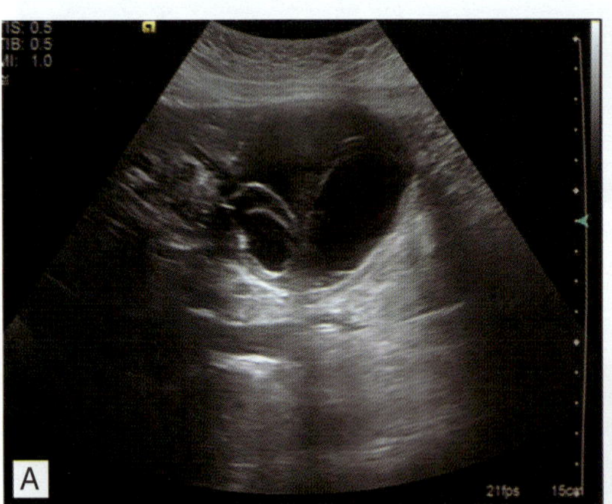

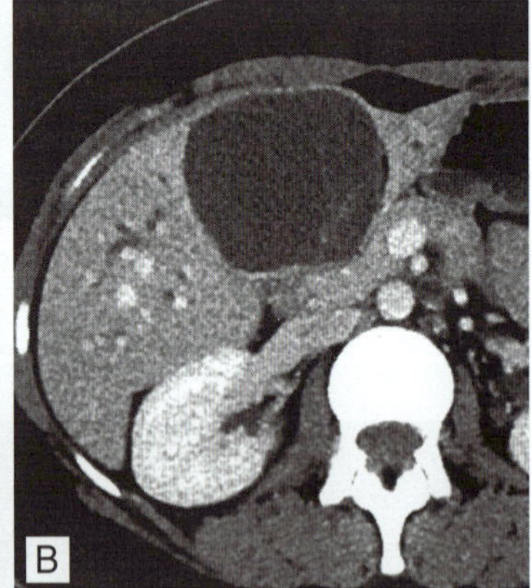

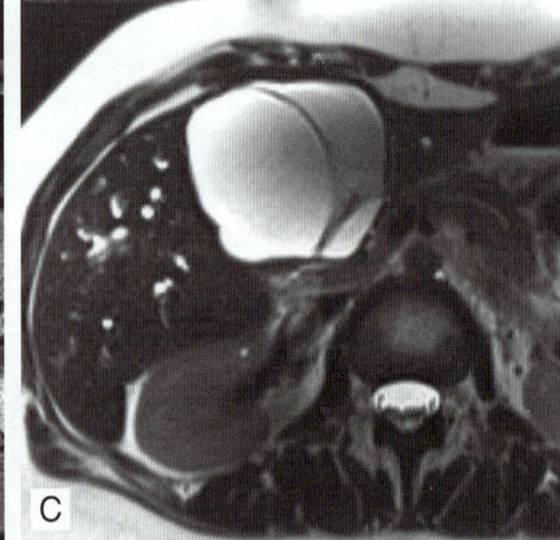

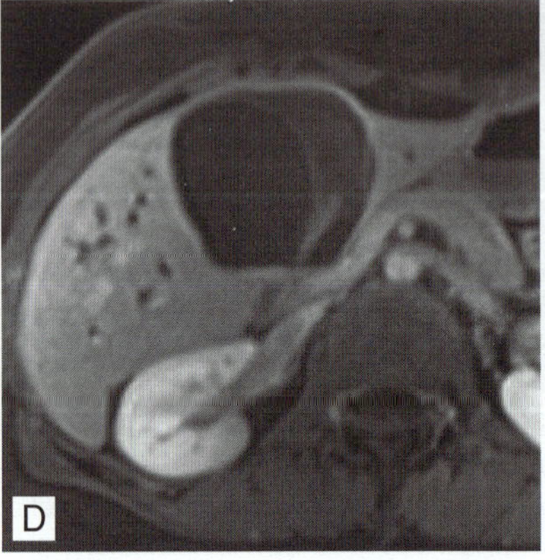

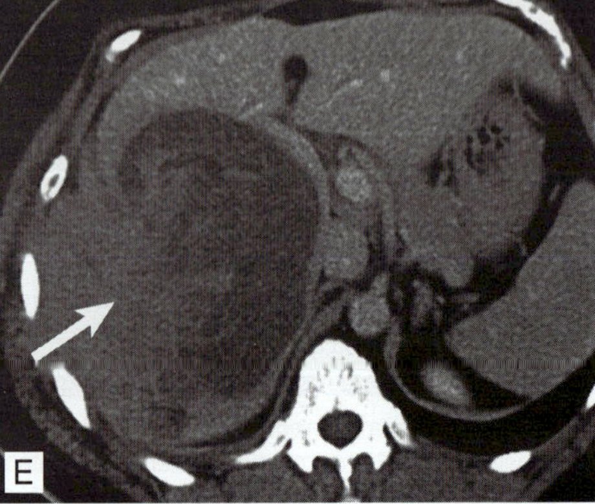

Figure 31.29 Mucinous cystic neoplasm (MCN) of the liver in a 45-year-old female (A–D), and mucinous cystic neoplasm with malignant change in a 55-year-old female (E). (A) A cystic lesion is seen in the left lobe of the liver with internal septations. Axial contrast-enhanced CT image (B), axial T2-weighted MR image (C), and axial contrast-enhanced T1-weighted image (D) demonstrates a cystic lesion in the left lobe with multiple internal septations. (E) Axial contrast-enhanced CT image of the liver in a 55-year-old woman shows a large, complex cystic liver mass with eccentric soft-tissue component (*arrow*), which on surgical pathology was a mucinous cystic neoplasm with cholangiocarcinoma.

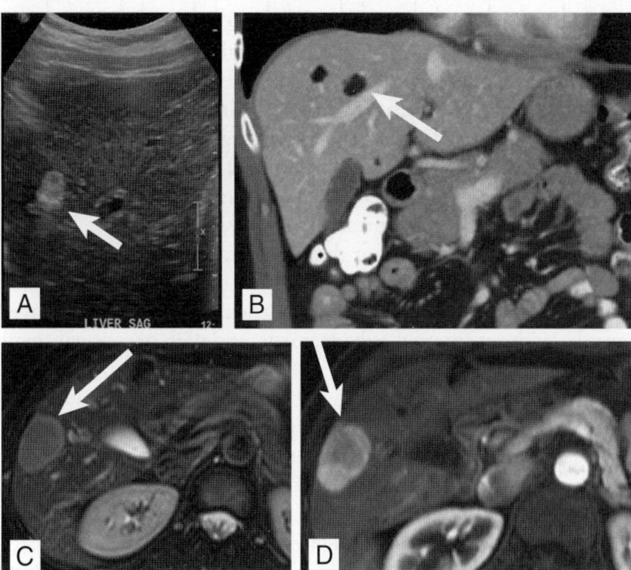

Figure 31.30 Hepatic angiomyolipomas in two different patients. (A and B) Ultrasonography image (A) shows a hyperechoic liver lesion (*arrow*). Axial contrast-enhanced CT image of the liver (B) shows macroscopic fat-density lesions in the liver consistent with angiomyolipomas (*arrow*). (C and D) Hepatic epithelioid angiomyolipoma. Fat-suppressed T2-weighted image of the liver shows a uniformly intermediate signal intensity mass. Arterial phase postcontrast T1-weighted MR image demonstrates heterogeneous enhancement (*arrow*).

affects young adults, with a slight male predilection [54]. On pathology, pseudotumors are well-circumscribed, encapsulated inflammatory masses; plasma cells with a variable amount of fibrosis, foamy histiocytes, and chronic inflammatory cells are seen. Clinically, these are often asymptomatic; and may occasionally present with right upper quadrant abdominal fullness or pain. Inflammatory pseudotumors are hypoattenuating masses on unenhanced CT with variable enhancement after administration of intravenous contrast [55]. On MRI, inflammatory pseudotumors are hypointense on T1WI and hyperintense on T2WI with heterogeneous enhancement after administration of gadolinium (Fig. 31.32). Definitive diagnosis requires needle biopsy or surgery [55].

Focal Steatosis

The risk factors for focal nodular steatosis or focal fatty change include diabetes mellitus, obesity, alcohol abuse, exogenous steroids, drugs (amiodarone, methotrexate, chemotherapy), and IV hyperalimentation. The classic location is the medial segment of the left lobe of the liver (segment IV), either adjacent to the falciform ligament or anterior to the porta hepatis. Focal steatosis is thought to be related to variations in vascular supply. Focal hepatic steatosis appears on USG as regions of increased hepatic echogenicity with geographic borders, minimal or no mass effect, absence of distorted vessels, and inability to visualize the portal vein walls. On unenhanced CT, focal steatosis appears as a hypoattenuating lesion with wedge-shaped margins (decrease by 1.6 HU per mg of fat in each gram of the liver). Signal drop on out-of-phase sequence without diffusion restriction or abnormal enhancement clinches the diagnosis on MRI [56,57] (Fig. 31.33). Multinodular hepatic steatosis is characterized by multiple foci of fat deposition throughout the liver parenchyma. Hepatic steatosis is a reversible condition with treatment.

Other

Vascular Shunt: Intrahepatic arterioportal shunts represent abnormal connections between the hepatic arterial system and portal venous system, and can broadly be characterized into tumorous and nontumorous shunts. Although small shunts are often asymptomatic, large shunts may cause portal hypertension. On dynamic contrast-enhanced CT and MRI, these lesions typically appear as small peripherally located wedge-shaped areas of arterial enhancement which become isodense/isointense to the liver on subsequent phases and are not visible on unenhanced sequences (Fig. 31.34). Occasionally, these may present similar to an enhancing nodule, mimicking HCC [58]. Small arterioportal shunts appear isointense to the liver on unenhanced MRI sequences; the larger portovenous shunts typically show T2 hypointense signal (flow void), enabling differentiation from other focal lesions.

Transient hepatic attenuation differences are areas of parenchymal enhancement seen on the hepatic arterial phase of CT, although to occur secondary to a localized mismatch in hepatic arterial versus portal venous blood supply [59]. The MRI equivalent to transient hepatic attenuation differences is transient hepatic intensity differences, which are secondary to the same phenomenon (Fig. 31.34).

Hot Quadrate Sign: Focal enhancement in the medial segment of the left hepatic lobe (segment IV) may be seen in the setting of superior vena cava obstruction, which is known as the "focal hepatic hot spot sign" or "hot quadrate sign." This occurs as a

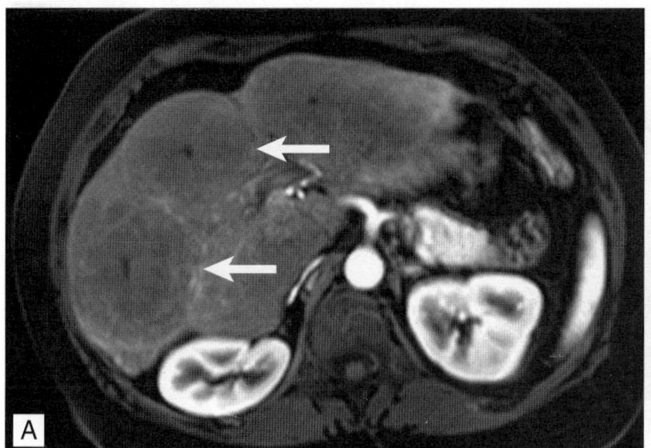

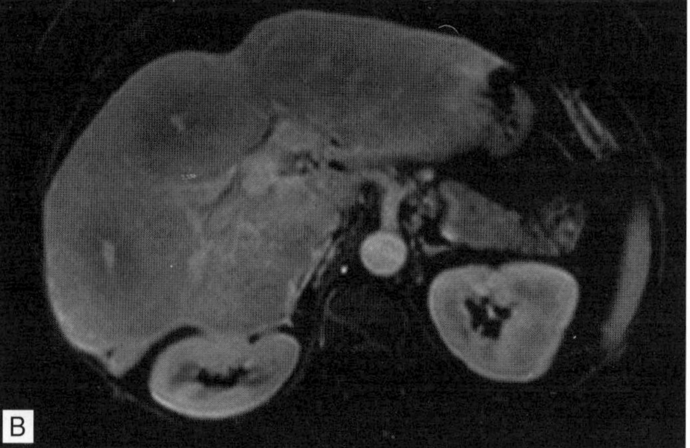

Figure 31.31 Nodular regenerative hyperplasia. Axial contrast-enhanced T1-weighted MR image in a patient with nodular regenerative hyperplasia demonstrates multiple large nodules, which are isointense to the liver on the arterial (*arrows* in A) and venous phase (B).

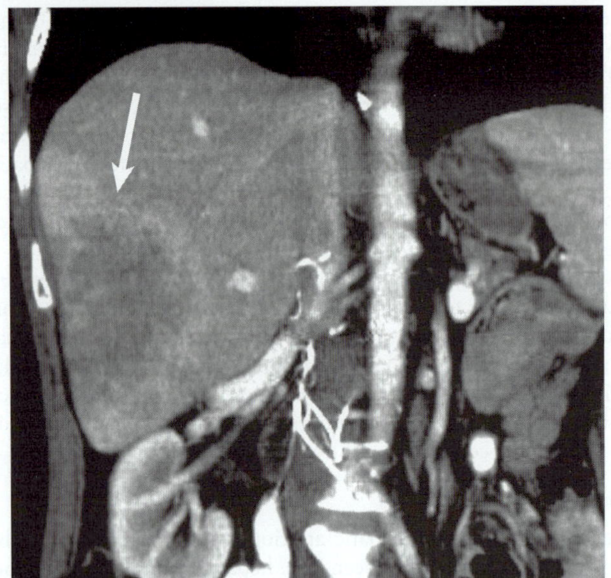

Figure 31.32 Inflammatory pseudotumor. Coronal contrast-enhanced CT image of the liver shows a large, heterogeneously enhancing liver mass (*arrow*) mimicking malignancy.

result of portosystemic venous shunting between the superior vena cava and the left portal vein through the internal thoracic and paraumbilical veins [60]. An equivalent finding can be seen on Technetium 99m sulfur colloid scan, in which there is a focal area of increased radiotracer uptake in segment IV (Fig. 31.35).

Psuedolipoma of the Glisson Capsule: Pseudolipoma of the Glisson capsule is a rare congenital anomaly, in which colonic epiploic fat becomes ectopically located within the liver capsule. Pseudolipoma can also occur due to a detached epiploic appendage that migrates to the perihepatic space. On CT and MRI, this appears as a well-circumscribed, fat-density lesion along the liver capsule, without internal enhancement, and with occasional small calcifications [61] (Fig. 31.36).

Other Vascular Entities: Hepatic infarcts are uncommon secondary to the liver's dual blood supply; however, the most common setting is after liver transplantation. On CT, infarcts will appear as ill-defined wedge-shaped hypodense areas, which are mostly peripheral without mass effect [62]. On MRI, these lesions will be hypointense on T1-weighted images, with hyperintensity on T2-weighted images.

Hepatic peliosis is a rare, benign vascular abnormality in which there is hepatic sinusoidal dilatation. On CT, multiple hypodense lesions of variable size are seen, which demonstrate globular

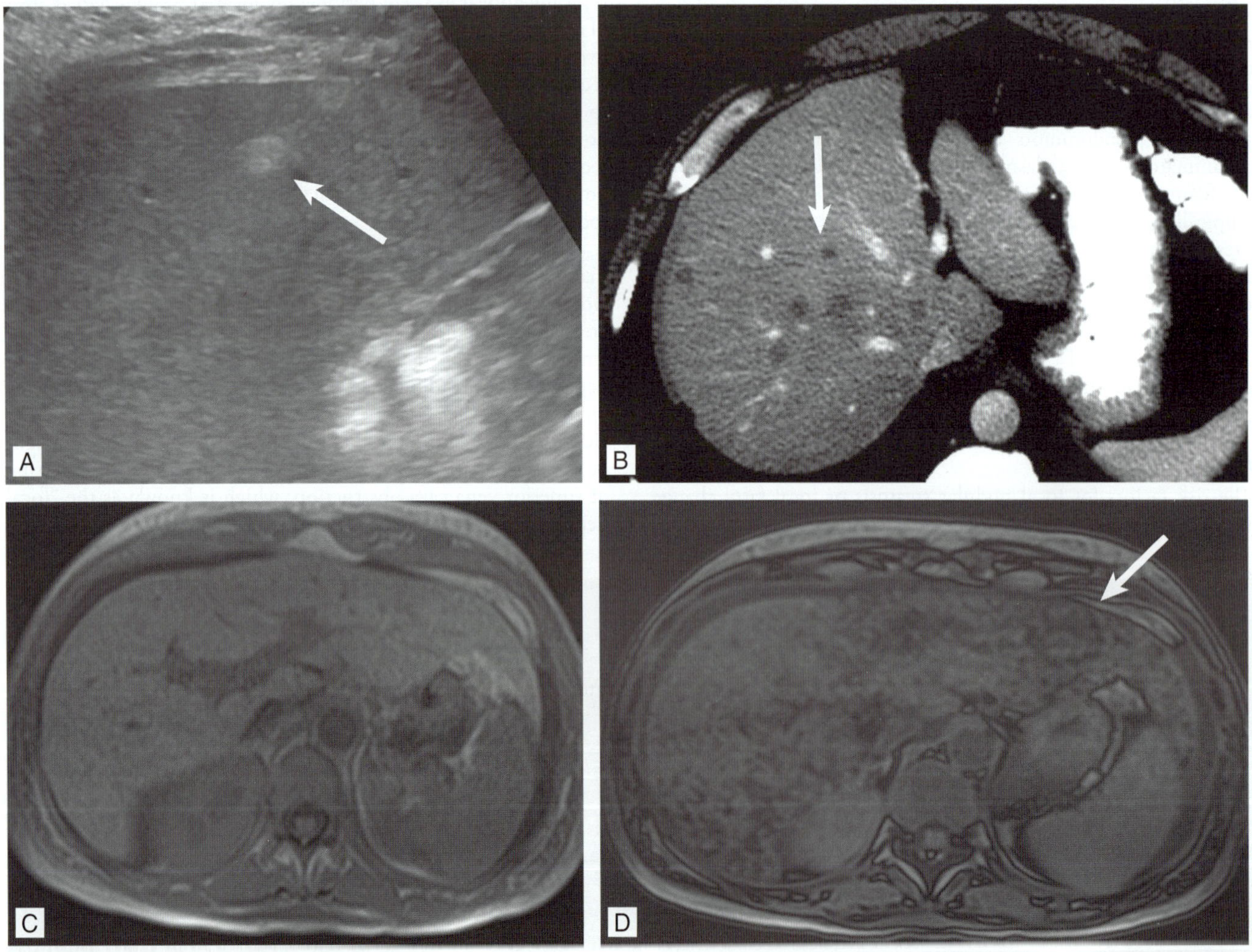

Figure 31.33 Focal steatosis and multinodular steatosis. Focal/multifocal fat in the liver. (A and B) USG image of the liver (A) shows a focal hyperechoic lesion (*arrow*). (B) Axial contrast-enhanced CT image of the liver shows multiple nonenhancing hypodense liver lesions (*arrow*), that were proven to be focal fat on biopsy. (C and D) Axial T1-weighted in-phase and opposed-phase MR images of the liver show multiple ill-defined lesions in the liver that demonstrate signal loss on opposed-phase image consistent with multifocal hepatic steatosis (*arrow*).

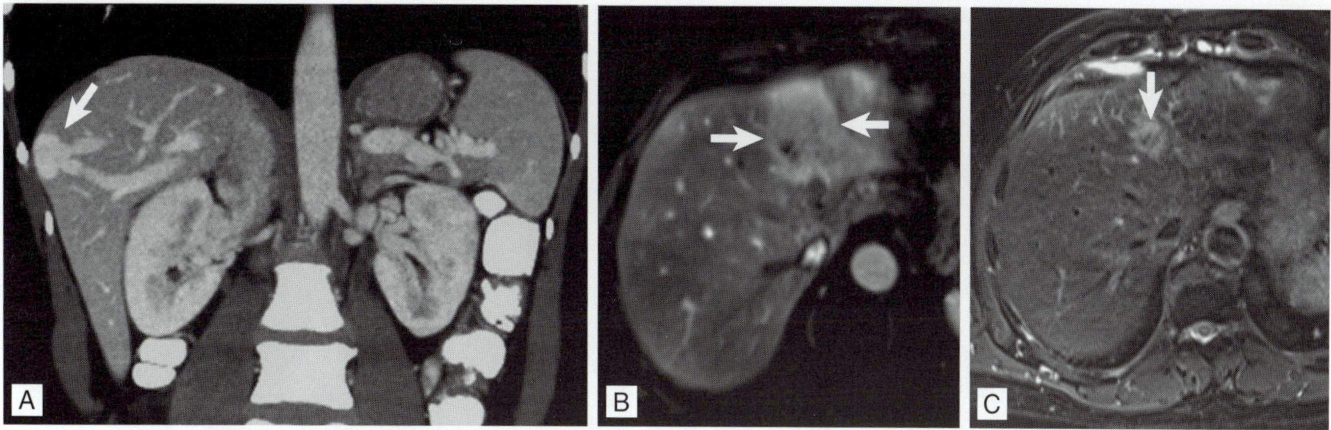

Figure 31.34 Vascular shunt and transient hepatic attenuation difference. Coronal contrast-enhanced CT (A) demonstrates a portovenous shunt. Axial contrast-enhanced MRI in the hepatic arterial phase (B) and axial fat-suppressed T2-weighted MR image (C) demonstrate intense transient enhancement in the left lobe of the liver (*arrows* in B) surrounding a small liver abscess (*arrow* in C).

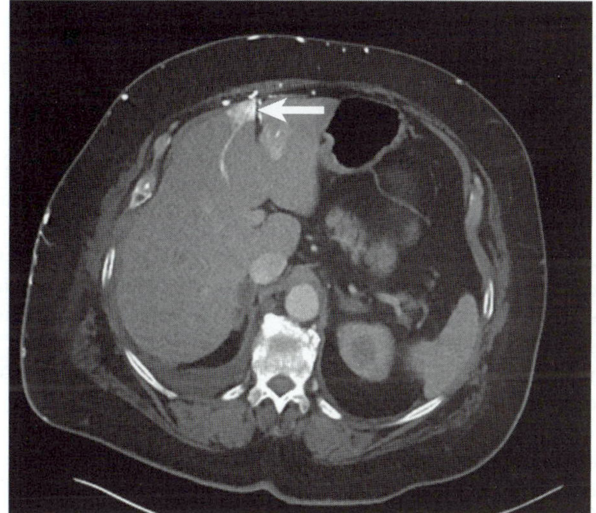

Figure 31.35 Hot quadrate sign. Axial contrast-enhanced CT image demonstrates pseudoenhancement within the hepatic segment 4 along the falciform ligament in a patient with SVC obstruction (*arrow*). Multiple venous collaterals are seen in the anterior abdominal wall.

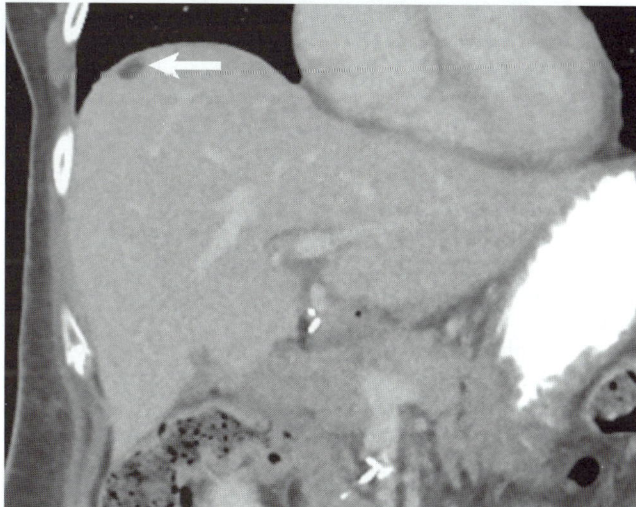

Figure 31.36 Pseudolipoma of Glisson's capsule. Coronal contrast-enhanced CT image demonstrates a fat-density lesion along the subcapsular aspect of the hepatic dome (*arrow*).

centrifugal or centripetal arterial enhancement without washout (Fig. 31.37) [63]. These lesions can be distinguished from hemangiomas, since enhancement is usually continuous.

Malignant Neoplasms

Hepatocellular Carcinoma

Pathophysiology and Clinical Presentation: HCC is the most common primary hepatic malignancy, usually occurring in patients with cirrhosis (alcohol and hepatitis B/C infection). HCC can arise de novo in an otherwise normal or noncirrhotic liver. Up to 20% of HCCs are thought to occur in a noncirrhotic liver [64]. Noncirrhotic HCCs occur more frequently in men, with a bimodal age distribution (second and seventh decades of life) [65]. The most common underlying etiology of noncirrhotic HCC is hepatitis B infection. Entities that result in HCC in the setting of cirrhosis, such as hepatitis C infection, alcoholism, and nonalcoholic fatty liver disease, can also result in HCC without underlying cirrhosis. Other rare entities contributing to hepatocarcinogenesis in the noncirrhotic liver include aflatoxins, hemochromatosis, chemical/industrial carcinogens, and inherited diseases such as alpha-1-antitrypsin deficiency, Wilson's disease, and type 1 glycogen storage disease [65,66]. Alpha-fetoprotein levels can be elevated in up to two-thirds of noncirrhotic HCCs [65].

Advanced stage HCCs can present with vascular invasion, satellite lesions, extrahepatic metastases (lymph nodal or distant metastases). Malignant thrombus can be distinguished from bland thrombus based on enhancement in the arterial phase and enhancement within the vein, similar to the primary tumor. HCCs do not retain hepatobiliary-specific contrast agents in the delayed hepatobiliary phase due to a lack of organic-anion-transporting polypeptides receptor expression or overexpression of the MMR receptor. Surgical resection is the treatment of choice for small HCCs in a noncirrhotic liver with a reported 5-year survival of up to 58%. Locoregional therapy, including transarterial chemoembolization, ablative procedures (RFA, cryoablation, or microwave ablation), selective internal radiation therapy, and systemic chemotherapy or immunotherapy are other treatment options [67].

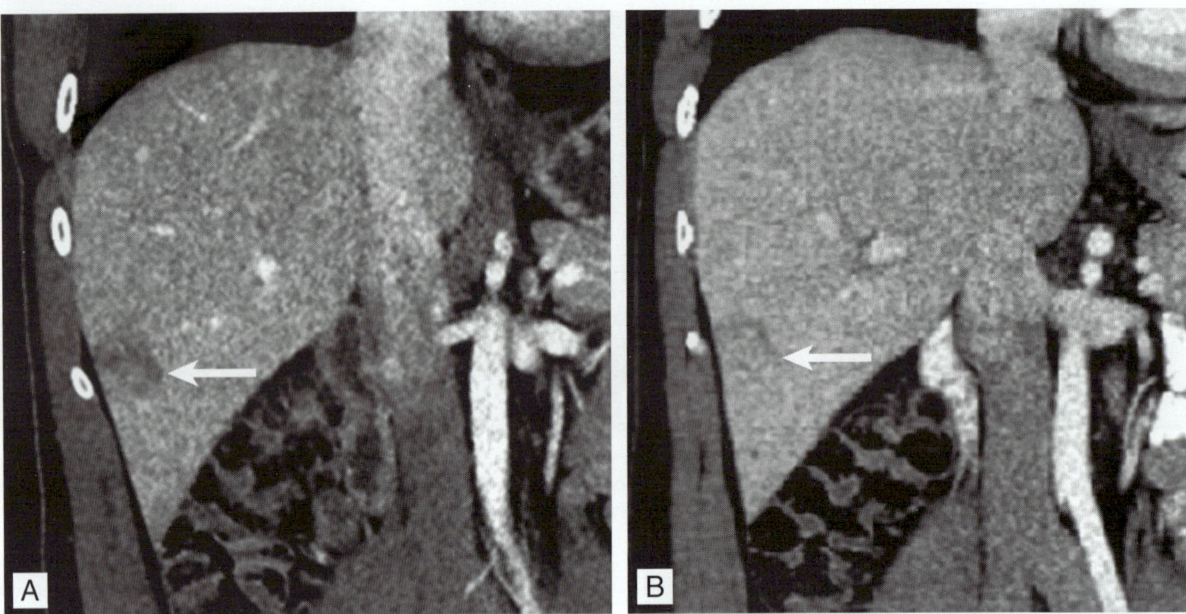

Figure 31.37 Peliosis hepatis. Axial contrast-enhanced CT in the late arterial phase (A) and portal venous phase (B) shows a predominantly centrally enhancing lesion in the arterial phase, with complete enhancement in the portal venous phase (*arrows* in A and B, respectively).

Imaging Features

Ultrasonography

- Heterogeneous lesions with varying degree of echogenicity related to the presence of fibrosis, fatty change, and necrosis (Fig. 31.38)

CT

- Arterial phase hyperenhancement with washout and/or pseudocapsule on portal venous/delayed phases [68,69], similar to HCC in cirrhotic livers (Fig. 31.38)
- Transient perfusion abnormalities can be seen surrounding the HCC in the arterial phase ("corona" enhancement) due to arterioportal shunting

MRI

- Iso- to hypointense to the liver on T1WI, moderately hyperintense/intermediate signal on T2WI, with enhancement characteristics similar to that seen on CT [66] (Fig. 31.39)

Fibrolamellar Hepatocellular Carcinoma

Pathophysiology and Clinical Presentation: Fibrolamellar HCC (FL-HCC) is a histological variant of HCC that typically occurs in young adults (second or third decade) without any gender predilection. FL-HCCs have no association with cirrhosis or other known risk factors for HCC described earlier; serum alpha-fetoprotein levels are normal. On pathology, FL-HCCs are well-differentiated and well-circumscribed masses with dense fibrotic background, with tumor cells arranged in cords and separated by sheet-like fibrous bands arranged in a parallel or lamellar distribution. Clinically, FL-HCCs present with a nonspecific presentation, including constitutional symptoms or gynecomastia (elevated estrogen levels); hepatomegaly is also common [70]. They usually present with advanced stage disease at the time of diagnosis. Resection is the treatment of choice with a 76% 5-year survival [71].

Imaging Features

Ultrasonography and CT

- FL-HCCs have variable echogenicity on ultrasonography
- On CT, FL-HCCs appear as a well-circumscribed mass with the central scar (about 75%) and calcifications
- FL-HCCs demonstrate rapid heterogeneous enhancement with delayed washout and persistent enhancement of the central scar (Fig. 31.40)

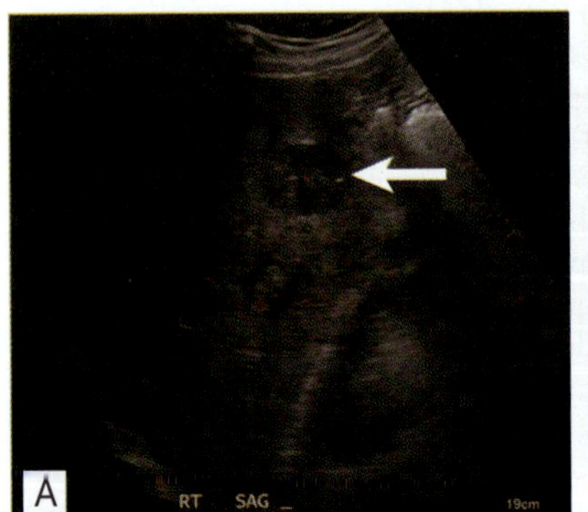

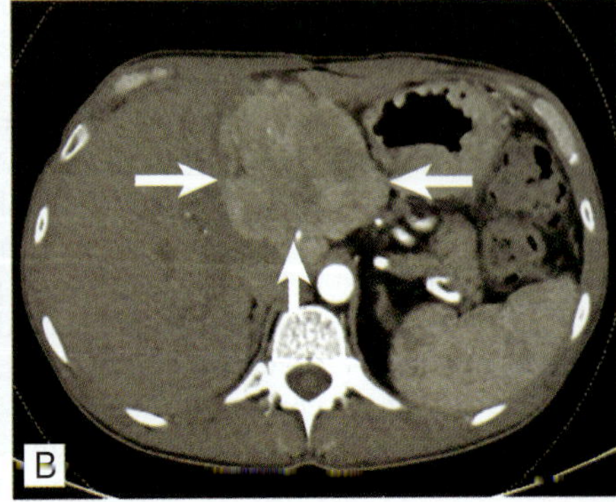

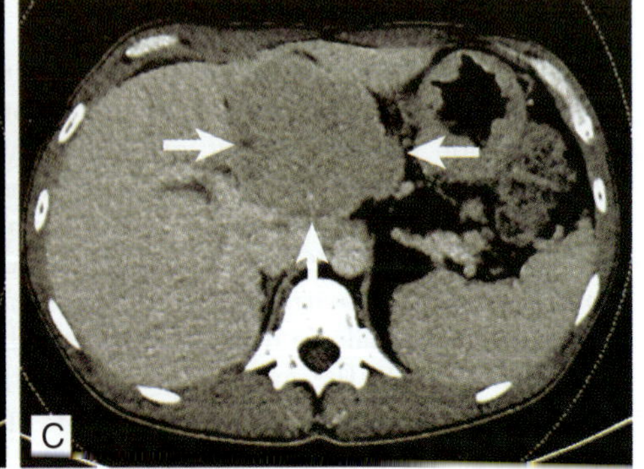

Figure 31.38 Hepatocellular carcinoma (*arrows*) in different patients. (A) Grayscale ultrasonography image demonstrates a hypoechoic mass within the left lobe. (B) Axial contrast-enhanced CT in the hepatic arterial phase and 3-minute delayed phase (C) demonstrates a large left hepatic mass with arterial phase hyperenhancement and delayed washout.

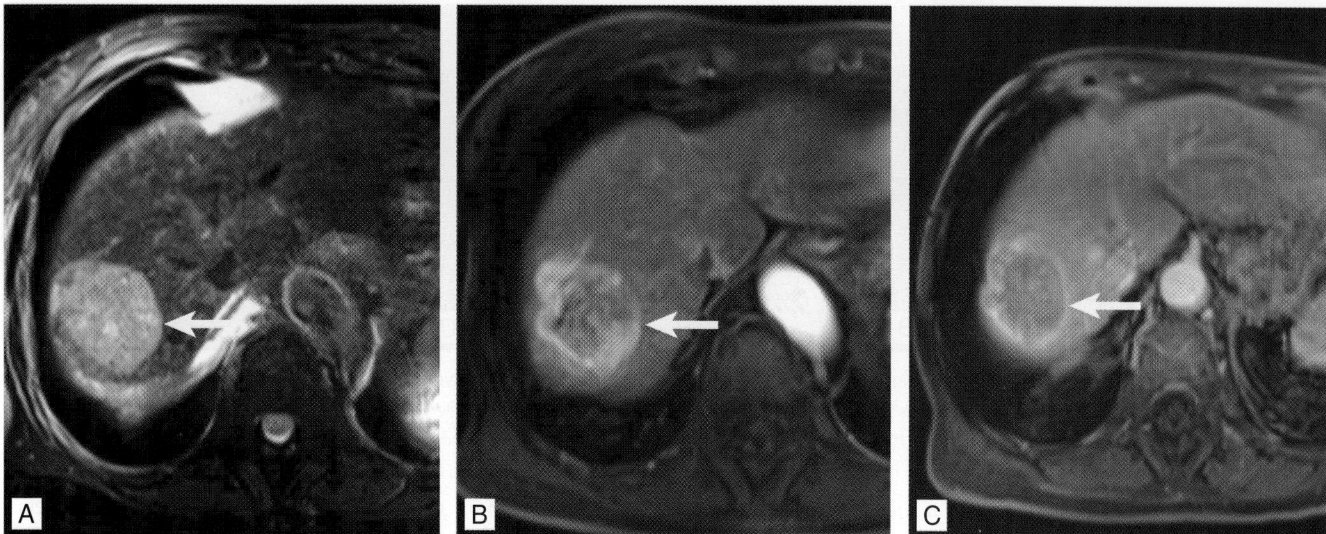

Figure 31.39 Hepatocellular carcinoma on MRI (*arrows*). Axial fat-suppressed T2-weighted MR image (A), axial contrast-enhanced T1-weighted image in the hepatic arterial (B), and 3-minute delayed phase (C) shows a T2-intermediate liver lesion in the hepatic dome with arterial phase hyperenhancement (B) and delayed washout with pseudocapsule (C).

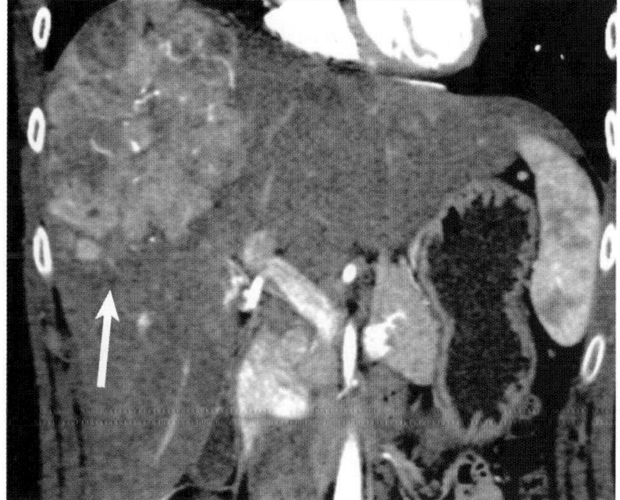

Figure 31.40 Fibrolamellar carcinoma in a 21-year-old woman. Coronal contrast-enhanced CT image demonstrates a large, heterogeneously enhancing liver mass (*arrow*).

MRI

- Iso- to hypointense to the liver on T1WI with a hypointense central scar
- Hypo- to slightly hyperintense to the liver with a hypointense central scar on T2WI (compared with a hyperintense central scar in FNH)
- Heterogeneous arterial enhancement and iso- to hypointense on portal venous/delayed phases [72]
- FL-HCCs do not retain contrast on the delayed hepatobiliary phase

Hepatic Lymphoma

Pathophysiology and Clinical Presentation: Hepatic lymphomas can be primary or secondary. Secondary lymphomas (secondary hepatic involvement in patients with lymphoma, most commonly non-Hodgkin lymphoma) are significantly more common than primary hepatic lymphoma. There is a slight male predominance with a typical age of presentation around 55 years. Primary lymphomas constitute <1% of all non-Hodgkin lymphomas, and by definition, should not show evidence for distant lymphadenopathy, splenic or bone marrow involvement or leukemic blood profile for at least 6 months after the onset of hepatic disease [73]. Secondary lymphomas are usually diffuse large B-cell lymphomas. Risk factors for liver lymphomas include HIV/AIDS (25–46%), hepatitis C (commonly in NHL, 15%), organ transplant (2–12%), and immunosuppression.

Secondary hepatic involvement is more common at the presentation in non-Hodgkin lymphoma (~20% of cases) than in Hodgkin lymphoma (~5% of cases). Clinically, patients manifest abdominal pain, jaundice, and weight loss; liver enzymes are commonly elevated. On imaging, primary hepatic lymphomas appear as single or multiple focal liver lesions (53–65% and 35–50%, respectively) and secondary lymphomatous involvement of the liver, presents as multiple liver lesions or diffusely infiltrating neoplasm. Lymphomas can also manifest as ill-defined periportal/porta hepatis infiltrative mass. Primary hepatic lymphoma is treated with chemotherapy; radiation therapy or surgery may also be considered.

Imaging Features

- On ultrasonography, hepatic lymphomas appear as hypoechoic with increased peripheral vascularity on color Doppler
- On CT, lymphoma typically appears as hypoattenuating lesions, hypoenhancing to the liver on all phases after administration of contrast [74]
- On MRI, the lesions are hypointense on T1WI, moderately hyperintense on T2WI, and hypoenhancing after administration of gadolinium (Fig. 31.41). Marked diffusion restriction is classical
- Avid 18F Fluorodeoxyglucose (FDG) uptake on FDG PET (positron emission tomography) study is also a characteristic finding
- Features that may help in suspecting lymphoma in patients with new onset liver lesions include no known history of primary malignancy, B symptoms, splenomegaly and splenic lesions, or distant lymphadenopathy (mediastinal, mesenteric, or retroperitoneal) [73]

Hepatic Metastases

Pathophysiology and Clinical Presentation: Hepatic metastases are 30–40 times more common than primary liver tumors [75].

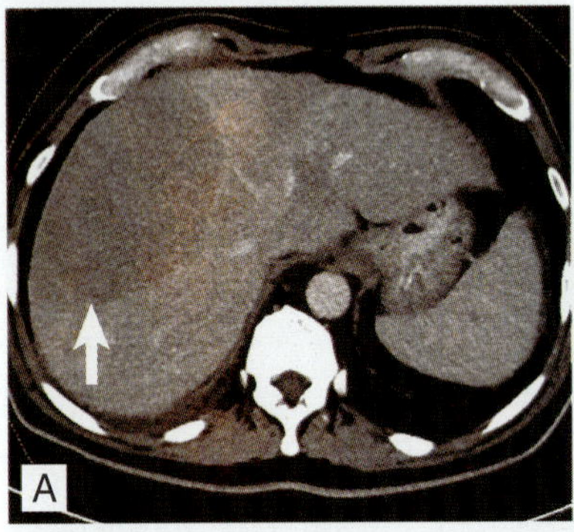
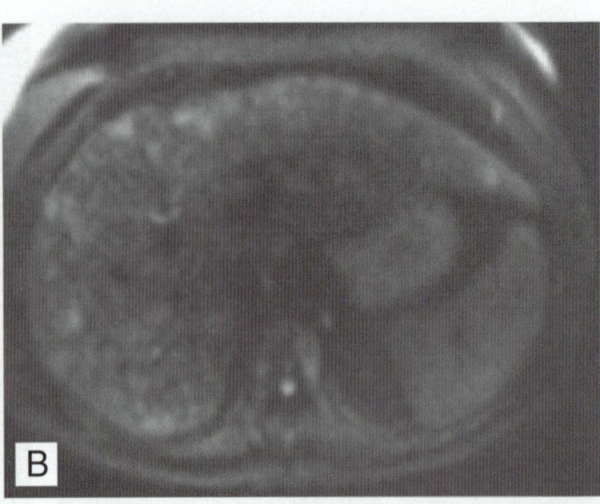
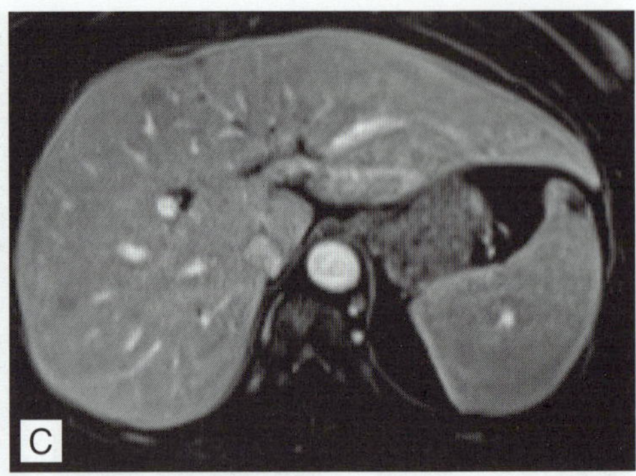

Figure 31.41 Hepatic lymphoma. (A) Axial contrast-enhanced CT of a patient with primary hepatic lymphoma, presenting as a large dominant hypoenhancing liver mass (*arrow*). (B and C) Secondary lymphomatous involvement of the liver presenting as diffuse signal abnormality best seen on diffusion-weighted images (B). Axial contrast-enhanced T1-weighted MR image (C) shows multiple small hypoenhancing lesions.

The most common primary tumors that metastasize to the liver are the gastrointestinal tract, breast, lung, genitourinary tract, melanoma, sarcomas, and testicular malignancies. The incidence of metastases increases with age. Clinical manifestations depend on the tumor burden and primary neoplasm. Patients with significant metastatic burden can present with symptoms such as right upper quadrant pain, altered liver metabolic function, ascites, or low-grade fever.

Imaging Features

- Hepatic metastases have a variable appearance on ultrasonography; however usually appear as round, well-circumscribed, hypoechoic masses with hypoechoic halo. Hepatic metastases can present with cystic change, calcification, or have an infiltrative appearance
- On CT, typically, liver metastases are hypoattenuating and hypoenhancing with peripheral arterial phase enhancement (Fig. 31.42). Hypervascular metastases from primaries such as renal cell carcinoma, thyroid carcinoma, neuroendocrine tumors, melanoma, and sarcoma appear as arterially enhancing lesions with or without washout
- MRI is generally more sensitive and specific for the detection of hepatic metastases [76]. Although the MRI appearance may vary depending on the primary neoplasm, metastases are generally hypointense on T1WI, moderately hyperintense on T2WI (follows the signal intensity of the spleen) and demonstrate diffusion restriction (Fig. 31.43). Most hepatic metastases are hypoenhancing to the liver with a peripheral rim of enhancement in the arterial phase. Peripheral washout on delayed phases has also been described to be a specific finding seen with liver metastases (both hypervascular and hypovascular metastases) [76]. T1 hyperintense signal may indicate hemorrhage (renal cell carcinoma, lung cancer) or melanin pigment (melanoma)
- DWI is the most sensitive sequence for evaluation of liver metastases, particularly the neuroendocrine and melanoma metastases (Fig. 31.44). Careful evaluation of diffusion-weighted images is therefore recommended in the evaluation of liver metastases, particularly from neuroendocrine tumors and melanomas
- Metastases do not retain contrast on the delayed hepatobiliary phase imaging
- Management of hepatic metastases depends on the underlying primary neoplasm [77]. Surgical resection is curative for colorectal cancer metastases. Transarterial chemotherapy and radioembolization are other evolving options for treatment for hepatic metastases

Hepatic angiosarcoma: Hepatic angiosarcoma is a rare, mesenchymal malignancy that comprise up to 2% of all primary liver neoplasm. It demonstrates variable clinical, pathological, and imaging characteristics. Angiosarcoma typically manifest in the sixth and seventh decades of life with a male preponderance. Although traditionally associated with Thorotrast, arsenic, or vinyl chloride exposure, 40% of angiosarcomas occur in the cirrhotic liver [78]. Most angiosarcomas appear as multifocal masses of variable size. A plethora of enhancement patterns have been described, including nodular, peripheral rim, and diffuse infiltrative patterns [78] (Fig. 31.45). Hemangioma-like centripetal enhancement and reverse hemangioma pattern of early central enhancement have also been described [79]. Although imaging findings can suggest a diagnosis of angiosarcoma, surgical pathology or biopsy is required for the definitive diagnosis. Biopsy can be safely performed, but carries an increased risk of bleeding due to vascular nature of these tumors. Hepatic angiosarcomas are highly aggressive tumors with frequent metastatic disease to the spleen, peritoneum, lungs, and bone marrow in 45–60% of patients [78].

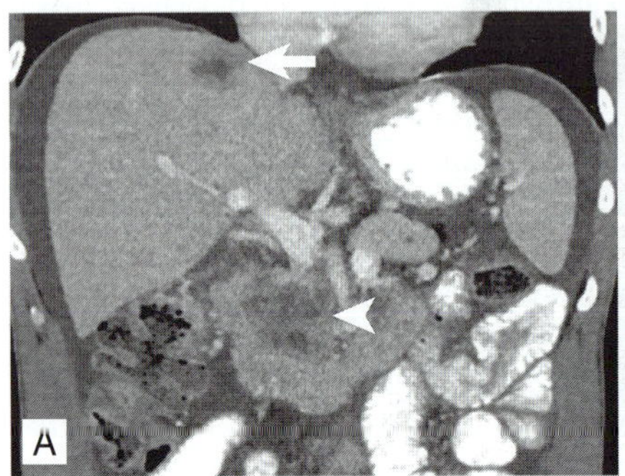
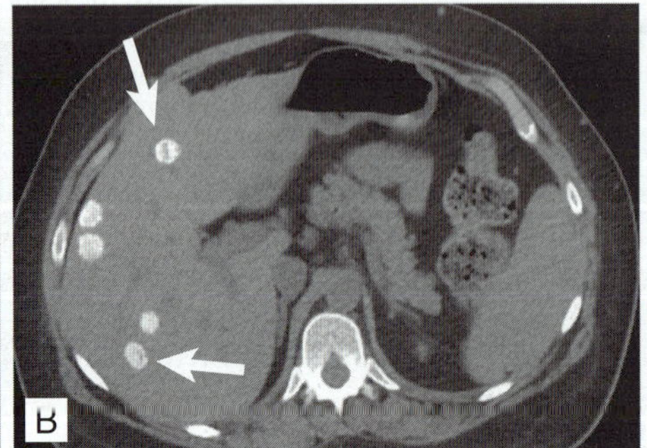
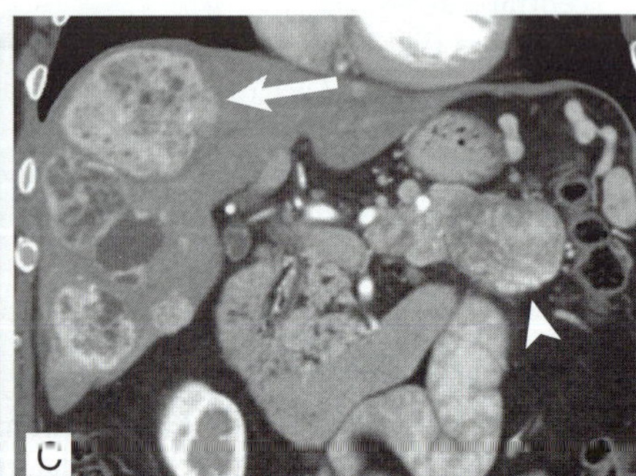

Figure 31.42 CT appearance of liver metastases. (A) Coronal contrast-enhanced CT image demonstrates a hypodense hepatic lesion with thick peripheral enhancement (*arrow*) in a patient with pancreatic cancer (*arrowhead*) compatible with metastases. (B) Unenhanced CT shows multiple, calcified, liver metastases from a pelvic chondrosarcoma (*arrows*). (C) Coronal contrast-enhanced CT image shows hypervascular and heterogeneous liver metastases (*arrow*) from a pancreatic tail neuroendocrine tumor (*arrowhead*).

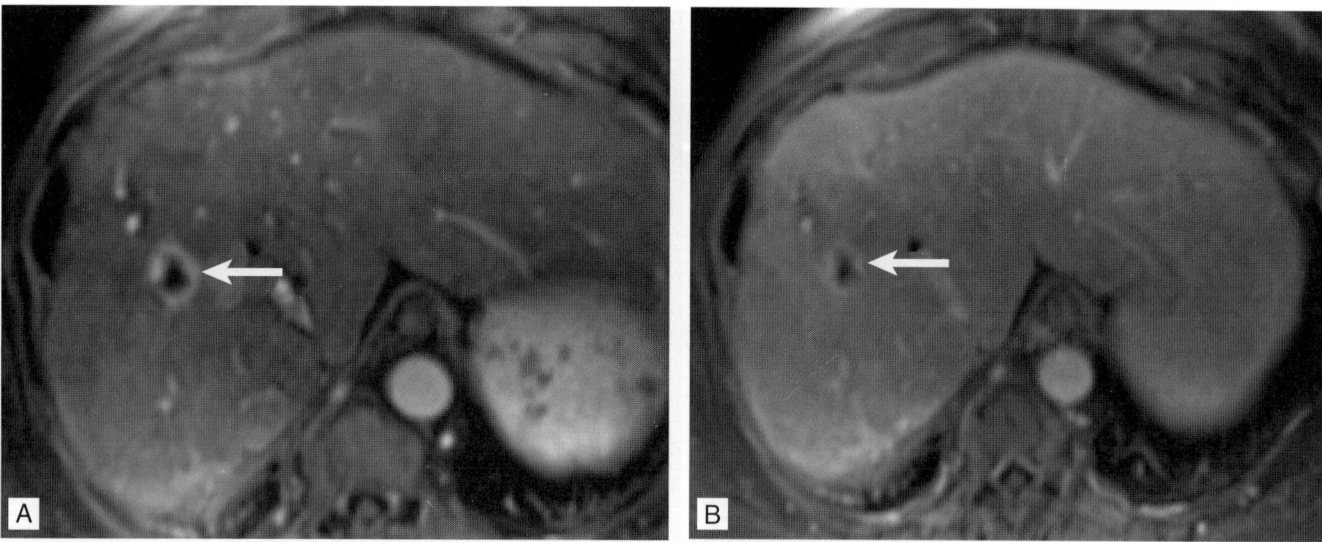

Figure 31.43 MRI liver metastases. Axial contrast-enhanced T1-weighted MRI in the late arterial (A) and 3-minute delayed phase (B) shows a peripherally enhancing lesion compatible with metastases from breast cancer (*arrows* in A and B).

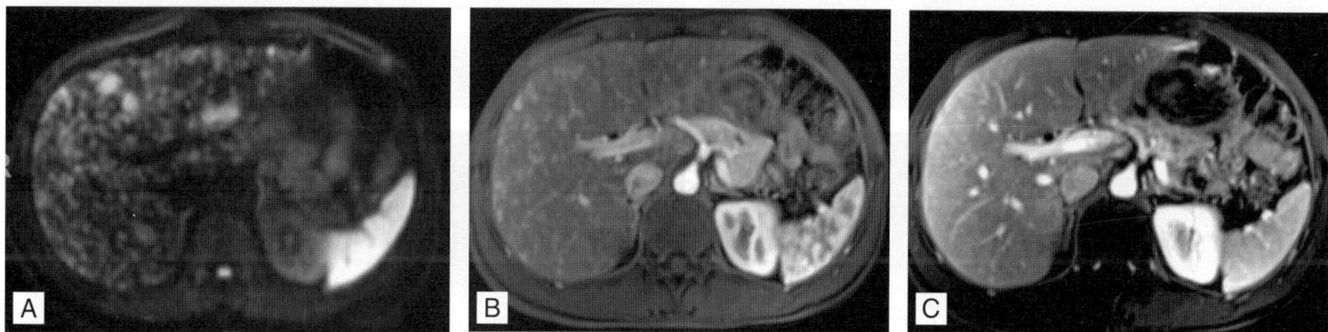

Figure 31.44 Value of diffusion-weighted MRI in the detection of hepatic metastases in neuroendocrine tumor. Axial diffusion-weighted (A), contrast-enhanced T1-weighted images in the hepatic arterial (B), and portal venous phases (C) demonstrate innumerable hepatic metastases best seen on diffusion-weighted images. The lesions are nearly isointense to the liver on venous phase.

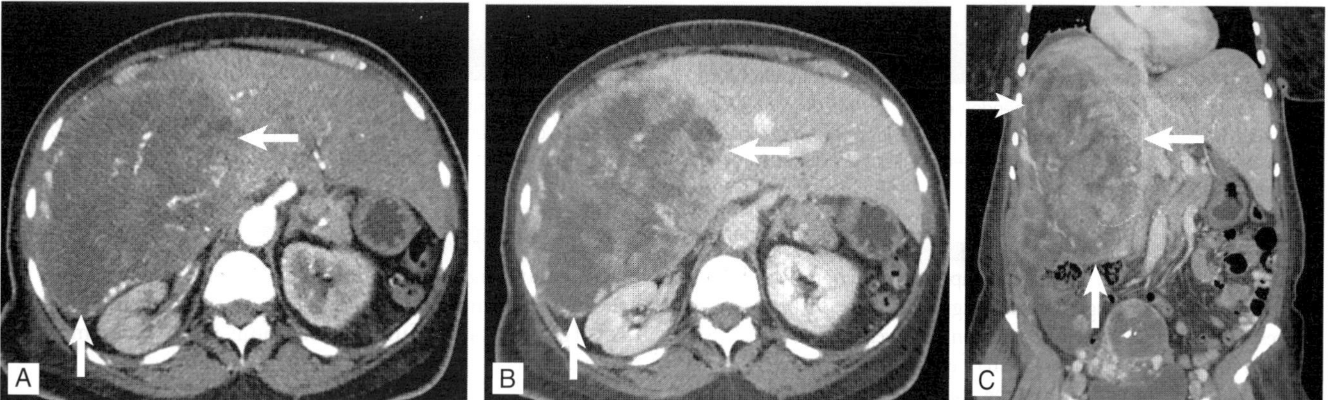

Figure 31.45 Hepatic angiosarcoma. Axial and coronal contrast-enhanced CT image demonstrates a large mass in the liver (*arrows*) with neovascularity in the arterial phase (A) and progressive enhancement in the venous and delayed phase (B and C).

Hepatic Epithelioid Hemangioendothelioma

Hepatic epithelioid hemangioendothelioma is an extremely rare, distinctive primary vascular tumor that is commonly seen in women [80]. Epithelioid hemangioendothelioma variably appears as multifocal nodules or as diffusely infiltrative masses with characteristic capsular retraction [78]. On CT, the tumors typically manifest as multifocal heterogeneously enhancing hypoattenuating lesions. These lesions may coalesce to form larger confluent masses in the peripheral

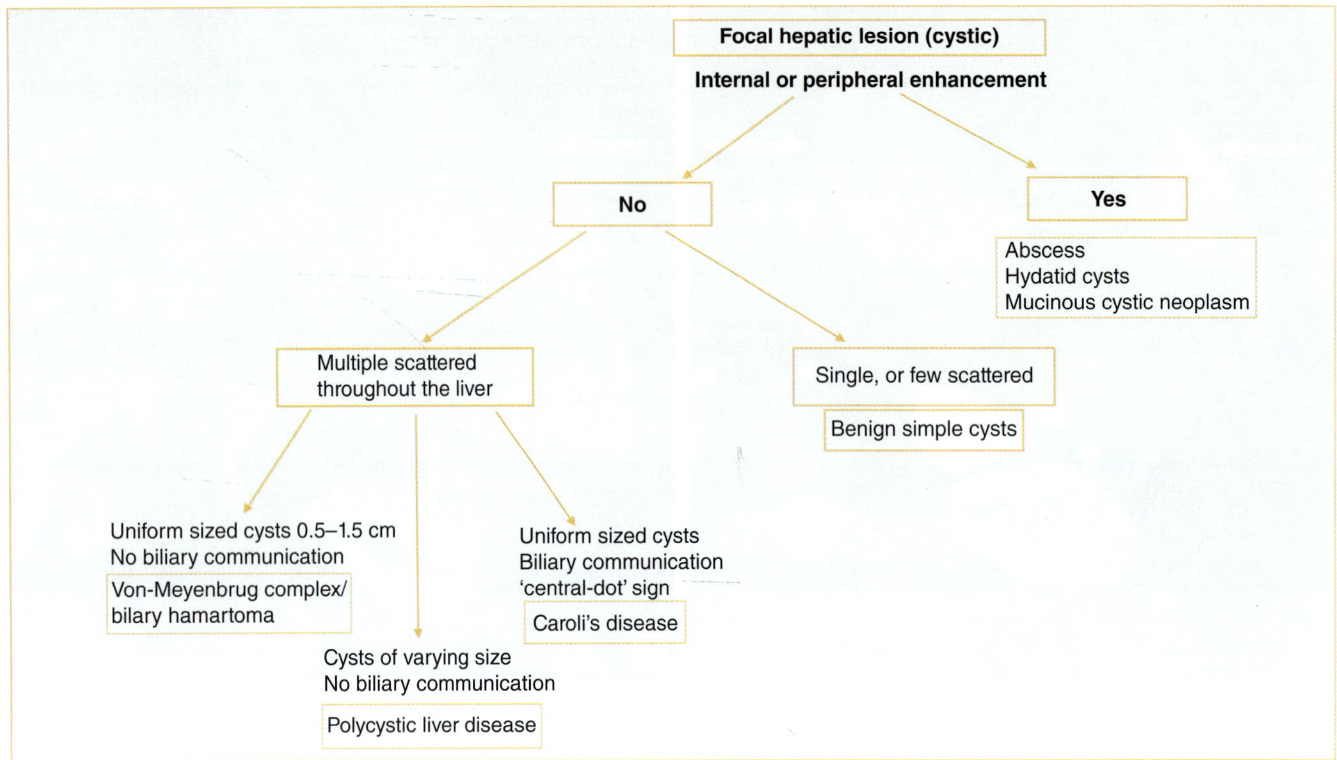

Flowchart 31.3 Flowchart illustrating an approach to imaging diagnosis of cystic focal hepatic lesions in noncirrhotic liver.

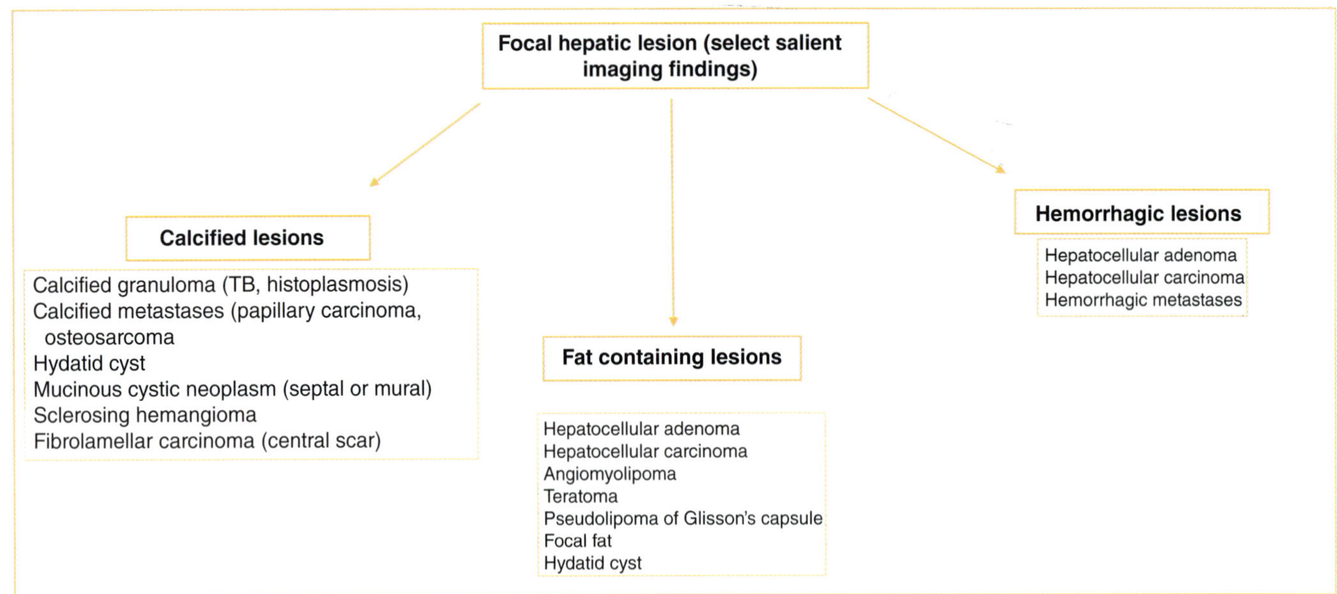

Flowchart 31.4 Flowchart illustrating an approach to imaging diagnosis of focal hepatic lesions in noncirrhotic liver.

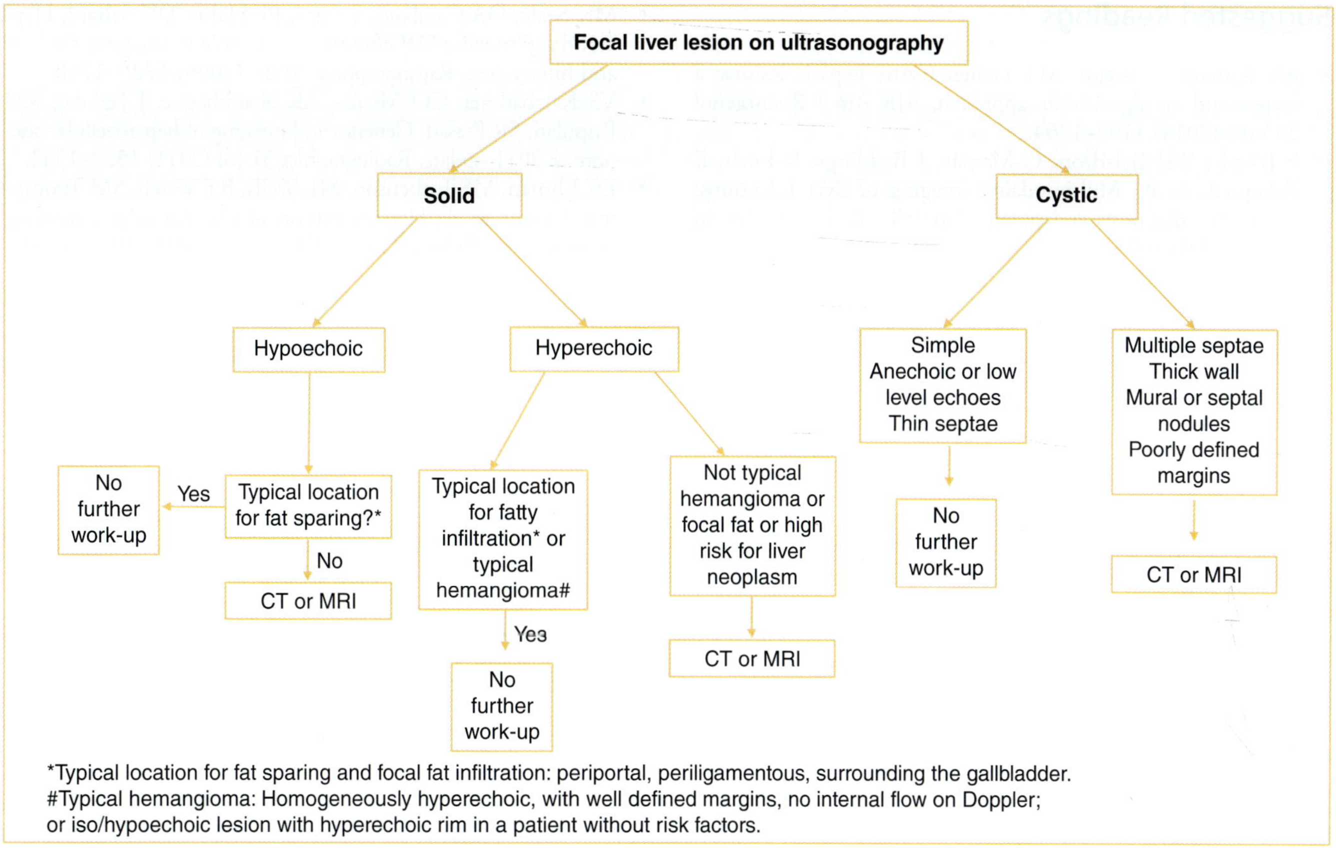

Focal liver lesion on ultrasonography

- **Solid**
  - Hypoechoic
    - Typical location for fat sparing?*
      - Yes → No further work-up
      - No → CT or MRI
  - Hyperechoic
    - Typical location for fatty infiltration* or typical hemangioma#
      - Yes → No further work-up
    - Not typical hemangioma or focal fat or high risk for liver neoplasm → CT or MRI
- **Cystic**
  - Simple: Anechoic or low level echoes, Thin septae → No further work-up
  - Multiple septae, Thick wall, Mural or septal nodules, Poorly defined margins → CT or MRI

*Typical location for fat sparing and focal fat infiltration: periportal, periligamentous, surrounding the gallbladder.
#Typical hemangioma: Homogeneously hyperechoic, with well defined margins, no internal flow on Doppler; or iso/hypoechoic lesion with hyperechoic rim in a patient without risk factors.

Flowchart 31.5 Flowchart illustrating an approach to an incidental focal hepatic lesion on ultrasonography.

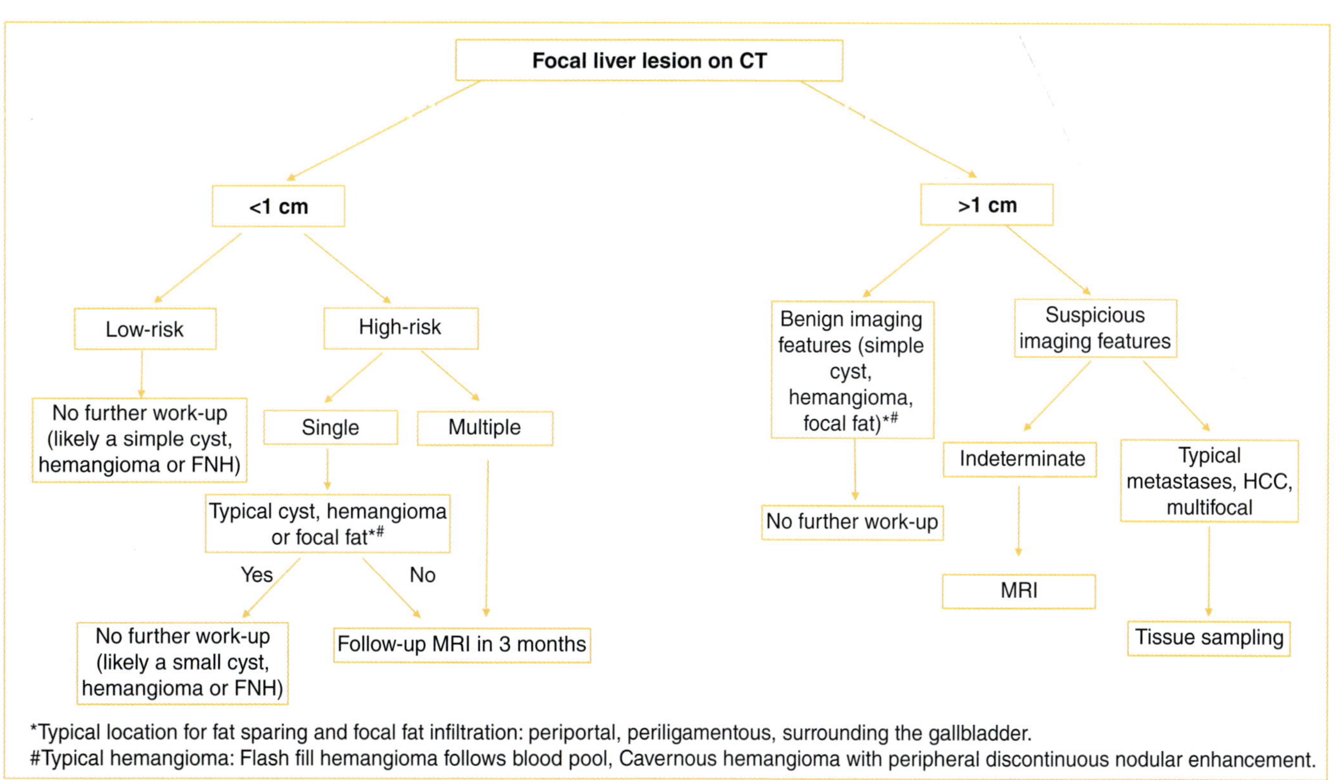

Flowchart 31.6 Flowchart illustrating an approach to an incidental focal hepatic lesion on CT.

Suggested Readings

- AA Borhani, A Wiant, MT Heller, Cystic hepatic lesions: a review and an algorithmic approach, AJR Am J Roentgenol 203 (6) (2014) 1192–1204.
- P Bächler, MJ Baladron, C Menias, I Beddings, R Loch, E Zalaquett, et al., Multimodality imaging of liver infections: differential diagnosis and potential pitfalls, Radiographics 36 (2016) 1001–1023.
- MK Seale, OA Catalano, S Saini, PF Hahn, DV Sahani, Hepatobiliary-specific MR contrast agents: role in imaging the liver and biliary tree, Radiographics 29 (6) (2009) 1725–1748.
- VS Katabathina, CO Menias, AK Shanbhogue, J Jagirdar, RM Paspulati, SR Prasad, Genetics and imaging of hepatocellular adenomas: 2011 update, Radiographics 31 (6) (2011) 1529–1543.
- EC Ehman, MS Torbenson, ML Wells, BT Welch, SM Thompson, I Garg, et al., Hepatic tumors of vascular origin: imaging appearances, Abdom Radiol (NY) 43 (8) (2018) 1978–1990.

32
Diffuse Liver Disease

VENKATESWAR R. SURABHI, CHARISSA KIM, VENKAT S KATABATHINA, SRINIVASA R. PRASAD

The liver is susceptible to a plethora of metabolic, toxic, immune-mediated, circulatory, infectious, and neoplastic disorders. A multitude of insults causes reversible degenerative changes such as steatosis and cholestasis and irreversible hepatocyte necrosis and apoptosis. When the injury is chronic, cumulative, and irreversible, it leads to scar formation. A complex inflammatory cascade orchestrated by Kupffer cells and lymphocytes activates myofibroblasts (transformed stellate cells), resulting in liver fibrosis. Chronic liver diseases (CLDs) result in cirrhosis and its associated complications, including hepatic failure. As such, early diagnosis and monitoring of hepatic fibrosis is of paramount importance. Serum enzyme panels and metabolic tests do not reliably quantify hepatic parenchymal injury [1,2], and liver biopsy is the gold standard to diagnose diffuse liver diseases [3]. However, a liver biopsy has limitations related to its invasiveness, sample variability, and intra- and interobserver variability [4]. Imaging plays an important role in the noninvasive evaluation of diffuse liver diseases; and multidetector computed tomography (CT), magnetic resonance imaging (MRI), and ultrasonography (USG) are routinely used to assess morphological changes of cirrhosis and for evaluating its complications, including portal hypertension, ascites, and hepatocellular carcinoma [5]. However, routine USG, CT, and MR are not sensitive for detecting early hepatic fibrosis [6,7]. Quantitative imaging techniques with MR for quantification of hepatic steatosis, iron overload, and hepatic fibrosis, and USG elastography for assessment of hepatic fibrosis are most useful for early detection [6,7]. MRI is ultimately the most promising technique for quantification of hepatic steatosis, iron overload, and hepatic fibrosis.

Hepatic Steatosis

The diagnosis of hepatic steatosis, which occurs due to excessive parenchymal accumulation of triglycerides, is made when >5% of hepatocytes show the fatty change [8]. Based on histopathological grading, steatosis is further classified into mild (<30%), moderate (30–60%), and severe (>60%) categories [9,10]. Alcoholic and nonalcoholic fatty liver disease (NAFLD) are common causes of hepatic steatosis. NAFLD refers to a spectrum of acquired metabolic disorders that are characterized by steatosis, inflammation, and fibrosis [8]. NAFLD, associated with obesity and metabolic syndrome, is now the most common cause of the CLD and a leading cause of liver transplantation next to hepatitis C [11]. Although the diagnosis of NAFLD is currently based on liver biopsy findings, noninvasive detection, and quantification of hepatic fat by imaging studies are important.

Imaging Features

Ultrasonography

Steatosis manifests as diffuse increased echogenicity of the liver parenchyma on USG. However, this is a nonspecific finding, and quantification of fatty changes with the grayscale USG has limited accuracy. USG grading of fatty infiltration in the liver uses USG features such as liver brightness, contrast between the liver and the kidney, intrahepatic vessels, liver parenchyma, and diaphragm [12].

- A normal echotexture is given a score of 0,
- slight/diffuse increase of liver echogenicity with normal visualization of the diaphragm and the portal vein wall is given a score of 1,
- moderate increase of liver echogenicity with slightly impaired appearance of portal vein wall and diaphragm is given a score of 2, and
- marked increase of liver echogenicity with poor/no visualization of portal vein wall, diaphragm, and posterior part of the right liver lobe is given a score of 3 [12].

CT

CT is a useful noninvasive tool to assess hepatic steatosis; the spleen is used as an important reference organ for comparison with the liver. The attenuation of the liver parenchyma on unenhanced CT ranges from 50 to 65 Hounsfield units (HU), 8–10 HU more than the spleen, and denser than the hepatic veins [13,14].

Several criteria have been developed for the diagnosis of hepatic steatosis on both unenhanced and enhanced CT scans. On an unenhanced CT scan, hepatic steatosis can be diagnosed when

- the liver measures <40 HU,
- the liver/spleen attenuation ratio of <0.9, or
- the spleen–liver attenuation difference is >10 HU,
- a spleen–liver attenuation difference of >20 HU on CECT (scan delay of 80–100 seconds) has also been used to diagnose steatosis [13] (Figs. 32.1 and 32.2).

Clinical studies have validated the use of dual-energy CT (80 and 140 kVp) for liver fat quantification by generating percentage fat volume fraction images using a multimaterial decomposition algorithm [15]. However, due to the risks associated with ionizing radiation exposure and its relative diagnostic inferiority compared with MRI, CT is not recommended for evaluating hepatic steatosis.

MRI

MRI is a comprehensive technique for evaluating hepatic steatosis. Three different techniques are predominantly used for this purpose.

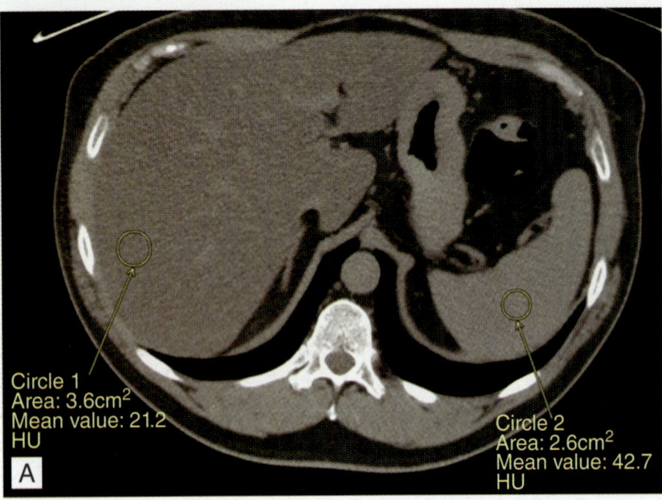

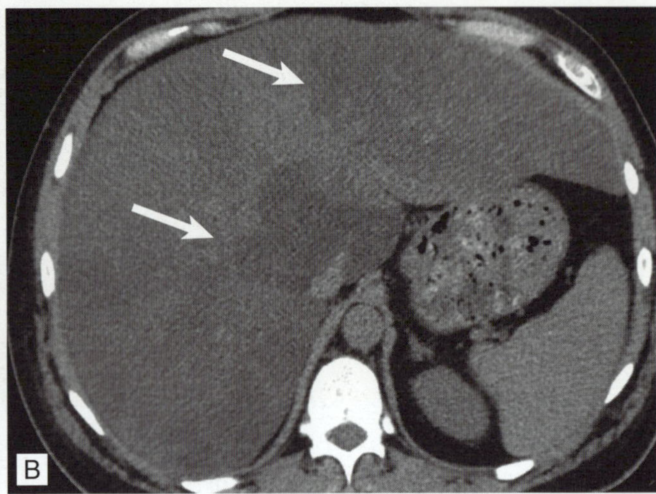

Figure 32.1 Unenhanced CT appearance of hepatic steatosis in two different patients. (A) Axial unenhanced CT image of the abdomen shows liver attenuation of 21 HU and splenic attenuation of 43 HU, consistent with diffuse hepatic steatosis. (B) Multifocal hepatic steatosis: Axial unenhanced CT image of the abdomen shows multiple scattered hypodense areas (*arrows*), consistent with multifocal hepatic steatosis.

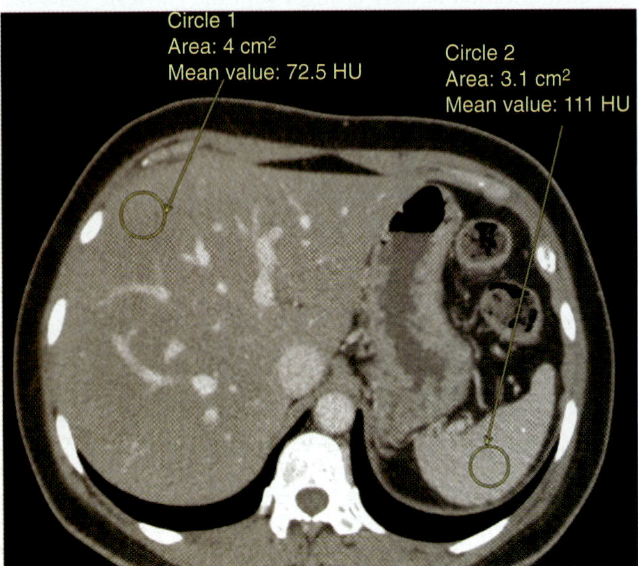

Figure 32.2 Contrast-enhanced CT appearance of hepatic steatosis. Axial contrast-enhanced CT image of the abdomen shows liver attenuation of 72 HU and splenic attenuation of 111 HU, consistent with diffuse hepatic steatosis.

The main sequence used in routine clinical practice is the T1W gradient-echo in-phase/opposed-phase imaging [16]. The cumulative signal from both water and fat protons contributes to liver signal intensity on in-phase imaging, whereas on opposed-phase imaging, the signal from fat protons cancels with that of water protons leading to signal drop of the liver in the presence of hepatic steatosis (Fig. 32.3) [16]. The range of hepatic steatosis that can be quantified with this technique is only 0–50%. In addition, the sequence is easily influenced by iron and other paramagnetic substances.

Other techniques for detecting and quantifying hepatic steatosis are chemical shift imaging and magnetic resonance spectroscopy (MRS) [17]. Recently developed proton density fat fraction (PDFF) sequencing using chemical shift-encoded methods allow coverage of the entire liver in less than 20 seconds with a single-breath hold. They also allow quantification of fatty deposition through drawing regions of interest (ROIs) over the liver parenchyma and demonstrate a good correlation with histopathological data (Figs. 32.4 and 32.5) [15]. In addition to the creation of IP and OP images and water and fat images, the main advantage of PDFF estimation using multipoint Dixon techniques is the generation of R2* and T2* maps, thereby allowing quantification of iron overload. PDFF-based quantification is optimized to decrease the effects of magnetic field inhomogeneity and T2* effects. Moreover, PDFF estimation using multipoint Dixon techniques has been shown to reproducible across readers and vendor imaging platforms and magnetic field strengths in a study conducted by Serai et al. [18].

MRS, by measuring protons in acyl groups of liver tissue triglycerides, is the most accurate imaging technique for the quantification of steatosis. However, MRS evaluates a small portion of the liver parenchyma and therefore can be affected by geographical differences in fatty deposition. It also requires postprocessing and technical expertise (Figs. 32.4 and 32.5).

The advantages and disadvantages of various MRI techniques for the quantification of fat are summarized in Table 32.1.

Hepatic Iron Deposition

Although hepatic parenchyma stores physiological amounts of iron, an abnormal accumulation of iron in the hepatocytes, reticuloendothelial system, or both leads to a toxic condition [19]. Hepatic iron deposition may be due to primary (hereditary) or secondary disorders. Hereditary hemochromatosis is characterized by markedly excessive absorption of iron from the gastrointestinal tract and involves liver, pancreas, and myocardium. Hemosiderosis results from nongenetic causes of iron accumulation, such as transfusion-related iron overload and is related to chronic liver pathologies and involves liver, spleen, and bone marrow. The signs and symptoms of iron overload are highly nonspecific. Hepatic biopsy remains the gold standard method for diagnosis, but it is an invasive procedure with potential risks. Imaging, particularly MRI, helps provide accurate quantifiable information on hepatic iron deposition.

Imaging Features

- USG may show diffuse hyperechogenicity of the liver parenchyma with iron deposition but it does not differentiate it from other pathologies such as steatosis and fibrosis

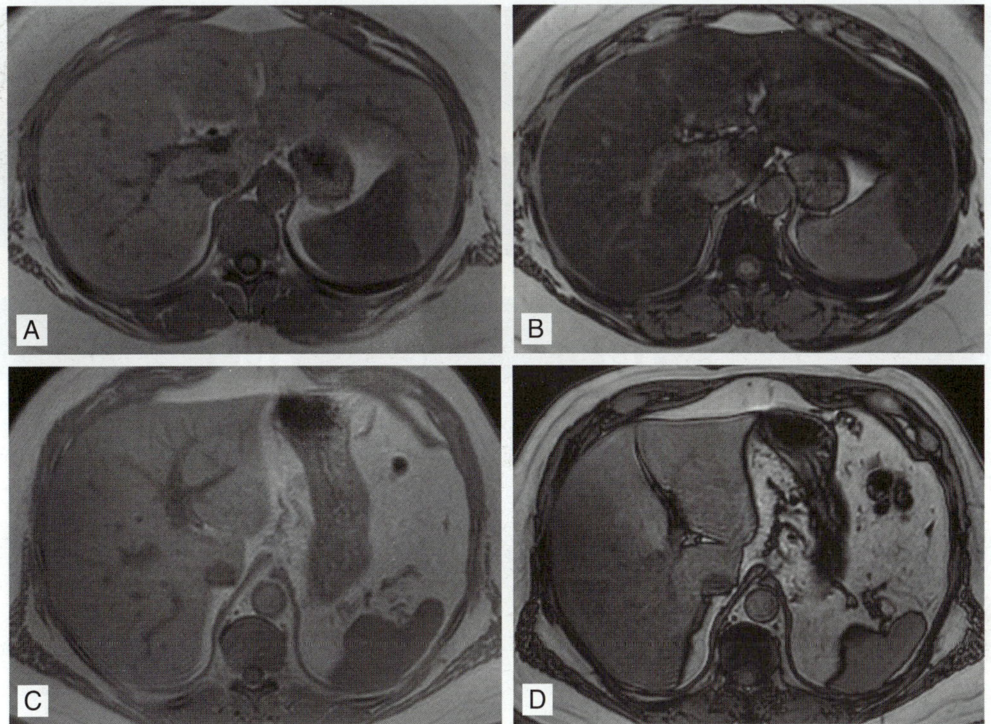

Figure 32.3 MRI appearance of hepatic steatosis in two different patients. (A and B) Axial T1-weighted in-phase (A) and opposed-phase (B) images of the liver demonstrate diffuse signal of the liver parenchyma in the opposed-phase image, consistent with diffuse hepatic steatosis. (C and D) Geographic hepatic steatosis: Axial T1-weighted in-phase (C) and opposed-phase (D) images of the liver demonstrate signal loss of the right hepatic lobe parenchyma in the opposed-phase, consistent with geographic hepatic steatosis involving the right hepatic lobe.

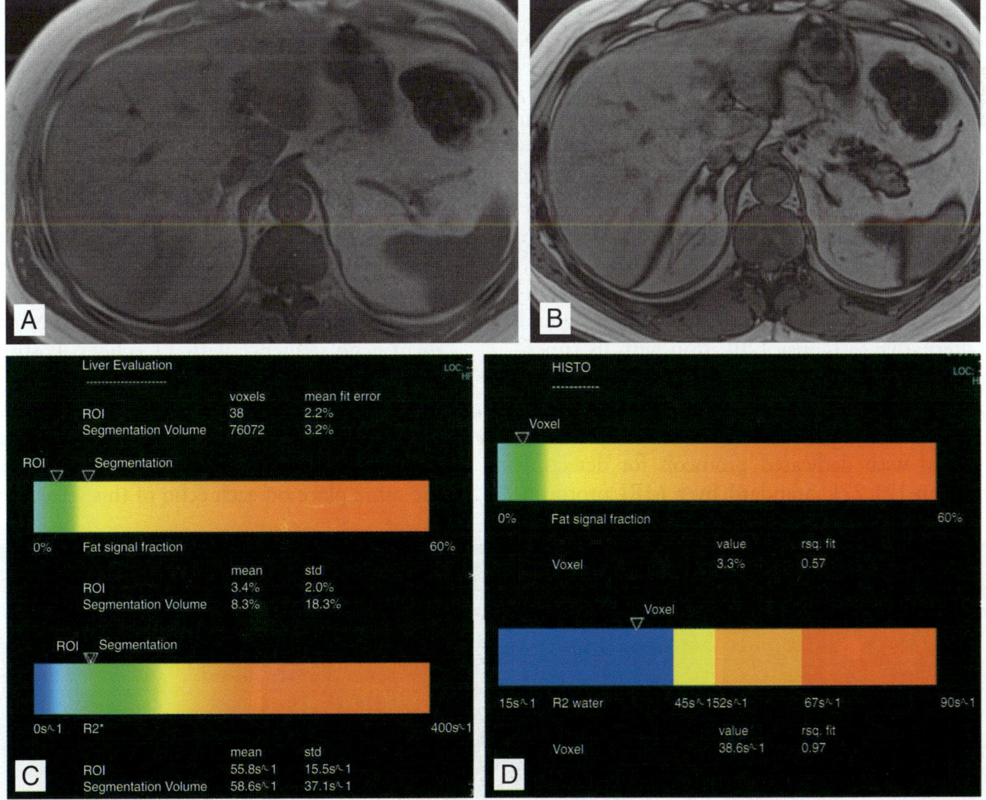

Figure 32.4 Normal MRI appearance of the liver on proton density fat fraction (PDFF) and MR spectroscopy (MRS) sequences with normal fat fraction. (A and B) Axial T1-weighted in-phase (A) and opposed-phase (B) images of the liver do not demonstrate significant signal loss on opposed-phase images and do not suggest hepatic steatosis. (C) Proton density fat fraction (PDFF) and R2 star values show the hepatic fat signal fraction of 3.4%, suggestive of normal parenchyma (<5% is normal). Also, note normal R2* values are suggestive of an absence of hepatic parenchymal iron deposition. (D) MR spectroscopy map (HISTO) shows the fat signal fraction of 3.4%. Also note, R2 water value within the normal limits suggest an absence of hepatic parenchymal iron deposition.

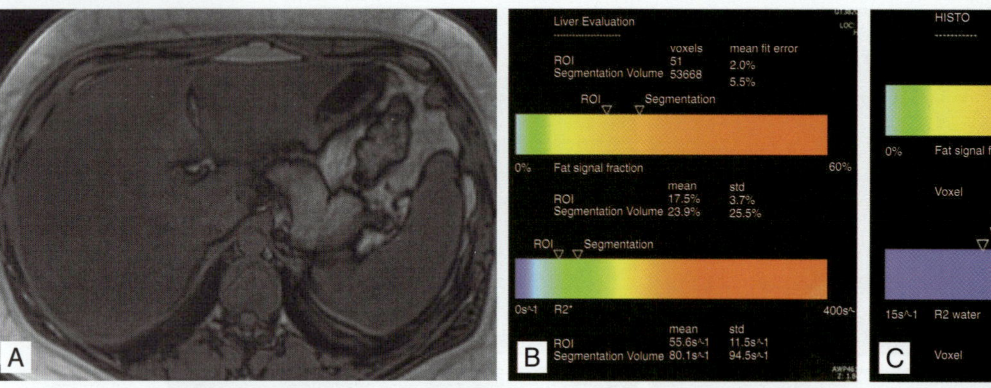

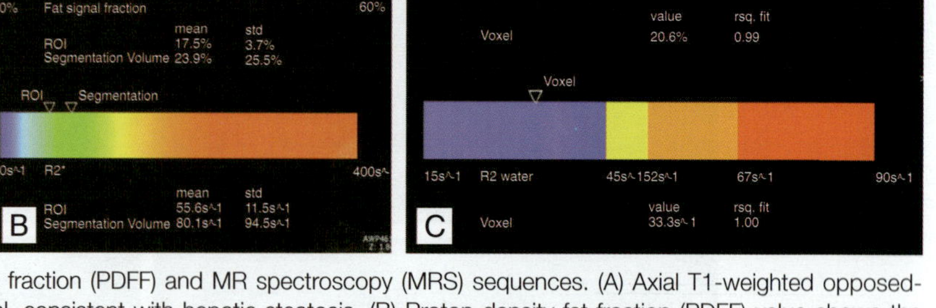

Figure 32.5 Diffuse hepatic steatosis on proton density fat fraction (PDFF) and MR spectroscopy (MRS) sequences. (A) Axial T1-weighted opposed-phase image of the liver demonstrates diffuse loss of signal, consistent with hepatic steatosis. (B) Proton density fat fraction (PDFF) value shows the hepatic fat signal fraction of 18–23%, suggestive of mild hepatic steatosis. (C) MR spectroscopy map (HISTO) shows the fat signal fraction of 21%, suggestive of mild hepatic steatosis.

TABLE 32.1 MRI Techniques for the Quantification of Hepatic Fat

Method	Characteristics	Advantages/Disadvantages
In-phase	Signal from both water and fat protons contributes to liver signal intensity	Range of steatosis that can be quantified is only 0–50%. Sequence is confounded by iron and other paramagnetic substances
Opposed-phase	Signal from fat protons cancels that of water protons	Same as with in-phase imaging
PDFF	Allows coverage of the entire liver and quantification of fatty deposition	Fast method <20 seconds with single-breath hold. Optimized to decrease the effects of magnetic field inhomogeneity and T2* effects
MRS	Proton measurement in acyl groups of liver tissue triglycerides	Accurate technique but only evaluates a small segment of the liver parenchyma. Affected by the heterogeneity of fatty deposition

MRS, magnetic resonance spectroscopy; *PDFF*, proton density fat fraction.

- Iron overload results in an increased liver density on noncontrast CT. However, CT cannot differentiate iron deposition from other causes of increased liver density, such as Wilson disease, colloidal gold treatment, and amiodarone treatment. In addition, coexistent hepatic steatosis can reduce the sensitivity of CT. Hence, CT is not considered a reliable technique for the diagnosis and quantification of liver iron overload
- MRI is the most sensitive tool for assessing liver iron concentration (LIC) for the diagnosis and treatment monitoring and is an excellent alternative to biopsy [20]. Iron with its superparamagnetic property causes shortening of T1, T2, and particularly of the transverse relaxation time of T2* [21,22]. Therefore, T2*-weighted images have higher sensitivity and are more routinely used with dedicated protocols for detecting and quantifying iron [21,22]. Standard liver MRI protocols with IP/OP images can also detect iron overload incidentally by detecting a signal drop on IP images compared with OP images (Fig. 32.6)
- The two methods used in quantifying liver iron overload are signal intensity ratio (SIR) between the liver and paraspinal muscles and relaxometry, which have been extensively validated with histology and thus are now used in routine clinical practice to diagnose, quantify, and monitor iron overload [20,23]
- MR technique includes the acquisition of one multiecho gradient echo sequence with 11 echoes. Postprocessing to assess LIC by SIR includes drawing three ROIs (on the selected images) in the right liver, two ROIs in the right and left paraspinal muscles, and one ROI in the air outside of the body for noise measurement. All ROIs will be automatically copied to the same place on each echo of this selected location

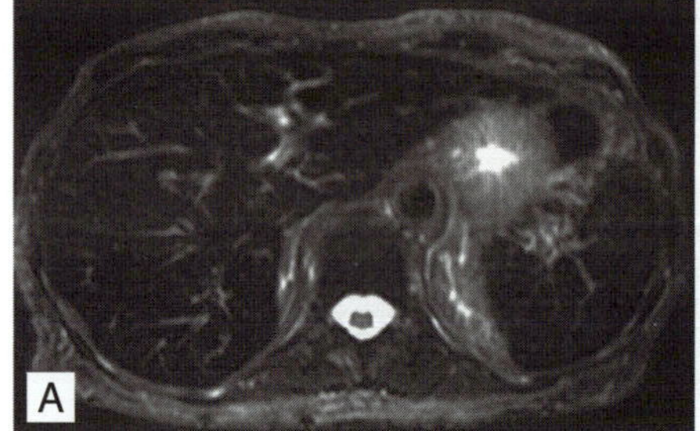

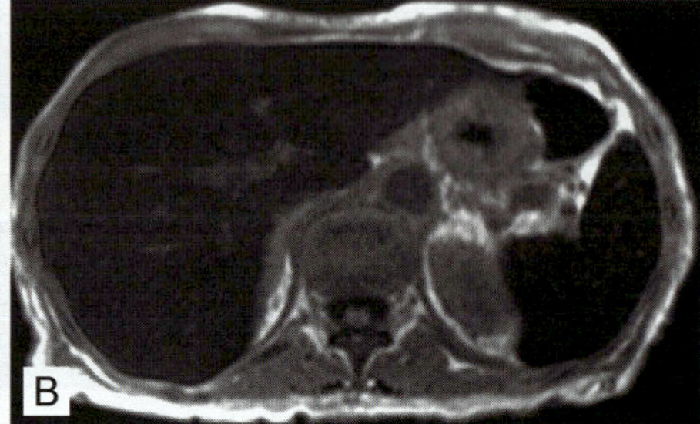

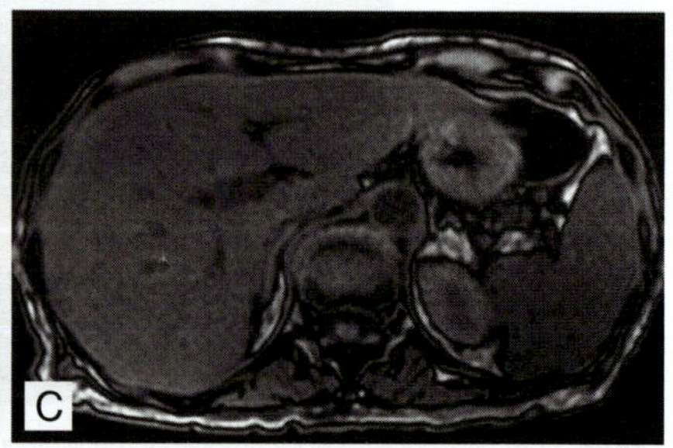

Figure 32.6 MR imaging appearance of diffuse hepatic parenchymal iron deposition in a patient with multiple blood transfusions. (A–C) Axial T2-weighted (A), T1-weighted in-phase (B), and opposed-phase (C) images of the abdomen show that the liver and the spleen are diffusely T2 hypointense and have a loss of signal on in-phase images when compared with opposed-phase images, consistent with hepatic and splenic parenchymal iron deposition. These findings are consistent with secondary hemochromatosis.

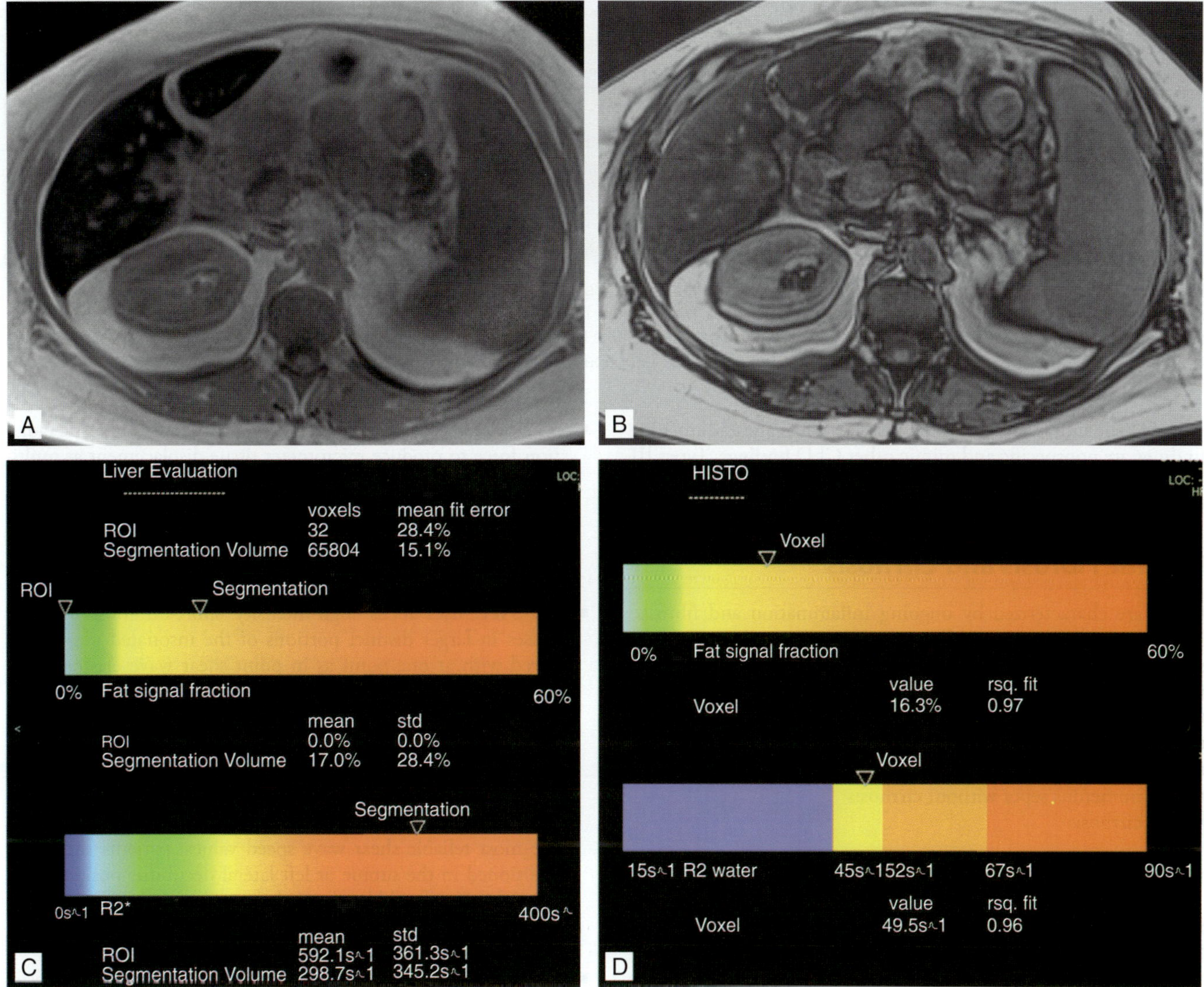

Figure 32.7 Primary hemochromatosis. Diffuse hepatic parenchymal iron deposition on proton density fat fraction (PDFF) and MR spectroscopy (MRS) sequence. (A and B) Axial T1-weighted in-phase (A) and opposed-phase (B) images of the abdomen demonstrate diffuse signal loss of the liver on in-phase images, consistent with hepatic parenchymal iron deposition. The spleen has normal signal intensity. (C) Proton density fat fraction (PDFF) and R2 star values show increased R2* values, consistent with hepatic parenchymal iron deposition. Given the high iron content, the fat fraction could not be evaluated on PDFF. (D) MR spectroscopy map (HISTO) shows mildly increased R2 water value indicating hepatic parenchymal iron deposition. This sequence is more helpful to assess hepatic fat fraction in patients with hepatic parenchymal iron deposition.

- T2* and R2* values can be obtained using standard formulae and can be used to calculate the LIC. Note that while T2* values are inversely related to iron concentration, R2* values are directly related to iron concentration
- Limitations of SIR include its inability to quantify LIC >350 μmol Fe/g and the tendency to overestimate LIC. High field strength MR has an advantage in the quantification of low iron overload. However, the susceptibility to artifacts reduces the sensitivity for the detection and quantification of severe iron overload
- In relaxometry, multipoint Dixon technique that automatically generates PDFF and R2* maps for fat and iron quantification, respectively, are useful for clinical practice without the need for additional postprocessing (Fig. 32.7) [18]. MRS sequence generates R2 water maps for hepatic iron quantification

Genetic and Metabolic Diseases

Wilson Disease

Wilson's disease is a rare autosomal-recessive disease resulting in the accumulation of copper in the liver parenchyma. It can manifest as fatty changes, acute and even fulminant hepatitis with rapid progression into mostly macronodular type cirrhosis, whereas malignant transformation into hepatocellular carcinoma rarely occurs. Imaging findings are nonspecific and mimic other CLD findings [24].

Glycogen Storage Diseases

Glycogen storage diseases (GSDs) are autosomal-recessive diseases. Different subtypes of GSD involving the liver are types Ia (von Gierke), Ib, II (Pompe), III (Forbes), IV (Anderson), VI, and

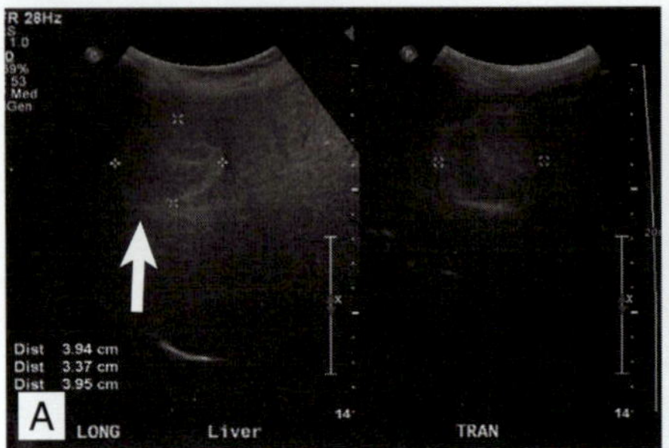

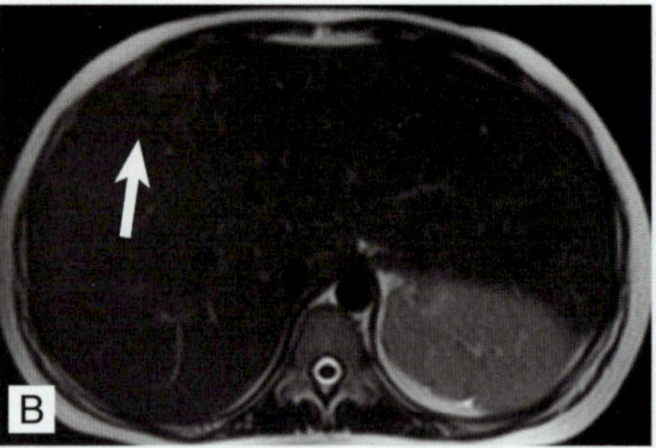

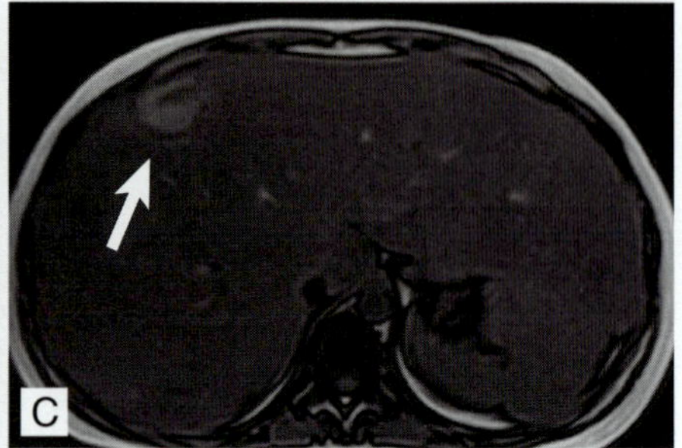

Figure 32.8 Hepatocellular adenoma in a patient with glycogen storage type 1a. (A) Longitudinal and transverse grayscale images of the liver demonstrate diffusely hyperechoic liver and a well-circumscribed hyperechoic liver lesion (*arrow*). (B and C) Axial T2-weighted (B) and T1-weighted opposed-phase (C) images of the abdomen show hepatomegaly and diffuse hepatic steatosis. There is a mildly T2- and T1-hyperintense focal lesion in the right hepatic lobe (*arrows*). This was proven to be an unclassified hepatic adenoma on surgical resection.

IX [25]. The most frequent finding is hepatomegaly, and imaging findings are nonspecific and mimic other CLD findings. Types III and IV GSD can lead to cirrhosis, whereas types Ia, Ib, and III have a tendency to develop hepatocellular adenomas (Fig. 32.8).

Hepatic Fibrosis and Cirrhosis

CLDs are characterized by ongoing inflammation and fibrosis. Early fibrosis can be potentially reversible; however, hepatic fibrosis, when untreated, progresses to irreversible cirrhosis. Hepatic fibrosis can be staged from F0 to F4:

- F0: no fibrosis
- F1: portal fibrosis without septa
- F2: portal fibrosis with few septa
- F3: numerous septa without cirrhosis
- F4: cirrhosis

Imaging Features

Ultrasonography

Imaging detection and staging of hepatic fibrosis are essential in the management of CLDs. Grayscale USG can identify a cirrhotic liver in CLD; however, it is unreliable in identifying mild changes of fibrosis and often unable to differentiate between mild and severe fibrosis [26].

USG-based elastography is useful for evaluating early fibrosis of CLD and follows the disease evolution during treatment [27]. USG-based elastography methods include vibration-controlled transient elastography (VCTE), point shear wave elastography (pSWE), and 2D-shear wave elastography (2D-SWE) [28–30].

- VCTE technique uses a low-frequency point-of-care mechanical actuator (50 Hz), which generates a shear wave that propagates through the tissue and is tracked with USG [29,30]. Shear wave propagation velocity is proportional to tissue stiffness. Higher stages of fibrosis are associated with increased tissue stiffness, permitting fibrosis staging with VCTE [30]
- Several VCTE probes are available, including the M probe (3.5 MHz), generally used in adults, the XL probe (2.5 MHz) for obese and morbidly obese patients, and the S probe (5.0 MHz) for use in children [29]. VCTE has been shown to be highly accurate for the diagnosis of cirrhosis (stage F4 fibrosis) and to have intermediate accuracy for the differentiation of liver fibrosis ≥ METAVIR stage F2 from F0 and F1 fibrosis [29–31]. VCTE does not produce images of the underlying liver anatomy. However, VCTE is limited in patients with ascites and morbid obesity due to the failure of transmission of the mechanical or USG pulse through a thickened body wall
- pSWE is a recently developed technique that uses acoustic radiation force to produce micrometer tissue displacement at multiple points [32,33]. Propagation of the shear wave is measured and depicted as a quantitative elasticity colorized map termed an elastogram. Quantitative elastography data can be presented as the estimated tissue Young's modulus in kilopascals (kPa) or as the estimated shear wave speed in meters per second (m/s)
- 2D-SWE uses focus high-intensity short-duration intensity pulses in larger distinct portions of the insonated area (compared with at one point as in point shear wave elastography) AND is useful in CLD, where it can be used to stage liver fibrosis and risk stratify patients with hepatitis C virus liver disease and NAFLD. Splenic 2D-SWE may also be used to detect portal hypertension secondary to liver fibrosis. Unlike transient elastography, 2D-SWE can be successfully performed in patients with ascites. As in other types of elastography, to get the most reliable shear wave speed values, patients should be positioned in the supine or left lateral decubitus position, and the right arm should be elevated above the head. When placing the ROI, vessels, bile ducts, rib shadows, and focal lesions should be avoided
- 2D-SWE imaging is best performed through an intercostal acoustic window, typically the right seventh or eighth intercostal spaces. Measurements should only be obtained after a minimum of 4 hours of fasting [33]. Obesity may reduce measurement quality
- SWE is more accurate for the diagnosis of cirrhosis than for the intermediate stages of liver fibrosis, and its use should be more focused on the former indication

USG elastography characteristics are summarized in Tables 32.2 and 32.3 [34] (Figs. 32.9 and 32.10).

CT

CT diagnosis of advanced fibrosis and cirrhosis is based on the identification of morphological changes, such as nodular liver surface, fissural widening, segmental atrophy and hypertrophy, and features of portal hypertension like esophageal varices and ascites (Fig. 32.11) [5]. Similar to USG, CT sensitivity is low for the diagnosis of early occult fibrosis and is not the preferred technique because of the risk of radiation.

MRI

Parenchymal heterogeneity due to underlying fibrosis or inflammation can be better appreciated on MRI sequences, particularly on diffusion-weighted images, which helps to detect earlier stages of fibrosis compared with CT [35]. However, conventional MRI is also limited in the detection of early hepatic fibrosis, making it unreliable for early detection of fibrosis and disease follow-up.

TABLE 32.2 Ultrasonography Elastography Characteristics

Use Method	Characteristics	Disadvantages	Confounding Factors
VCTE	Portable and point of care (liver clinic) Rapid (less than 5 minutes)	No real-time imaging guidance and no anatomical information Successful measurements within a defined interquartile range to obtain a valid result Obesity Ascites	Hepatic steatosis without inflammation effect on liver stiffness remains controversial Inflammation can lead to an increase in elasticity and viscosity Right heart failure is associated with increased liver stiffness Hepatic venous congestion can also increase liver stiffness
pSWE	Anatomical information and ROI selection Follow-up with ROI in the same spot/segment Real-time imaging Less impact from obesity and ascites compared with VCTE	More expertise required than VCTE	Postprandial state can increase liver stiffness; hence, liver stiffness should be measured preferably in the fasting state
2D-SWE	Larger ROI Real-time color map of tissue viscoelastic properties Confidence map to accurately place ROI in the color box to avoid vessels Less impact from obesity and ascites	More expertise required than VCTE Needs more validation	

pSWE, point shear wave elastography; *ROI*, regions of interest; *SWE*, shear wave elastography; *VCTE*, vibration-controlled transient elastography.

TABLE 32.3 Liver Stiffness Measurement Values Obtained With ARFI Techniques in Patients With Viral Hepatitis and NAFLD (Modified From [34])

Liver Stiffness Value	Recommendation
<5 kPa (1.3 m/s)	Normal
<9 kPa (1.7 m/s)	In the presence of other known clinical signs, may need further test for confirmation In the absence of other known clinical signs, rules out chronic liver disease
9–13 kPa (1.7–2.1 m/s)	Suggestive of chronic liver disease but need further test for confirmation
13 kPa (2.1 m/s)	Rules in chronic liver disease
17 kPa (2.4 m/s)	Suggestive of portal hypertension

NAFLD, nonalcoholic fatty liver disease.

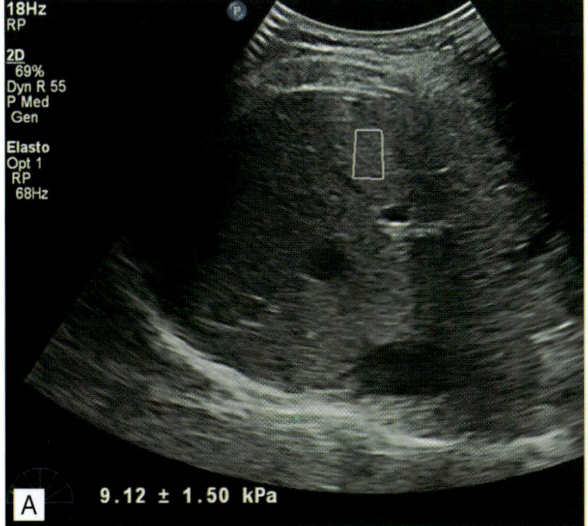

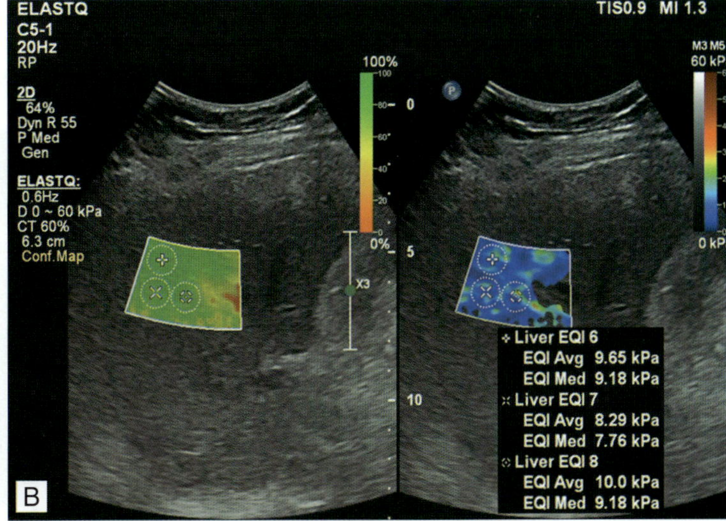

Figure 32.9 USG-based elastography techniques: point shear wave elastography (pSWE) and shear wave elastography (2D-SWE). (A) Cursor placement while the acquisition of liver stiffness using pSWE. (B) Liver stiffness measurement using 2D-SWE. Split-screen USG image shows a confidence map on the left side of the screen, and the right side of the screen shows the color box for ROI placement for measurement of hepatic stiffness in kPa.

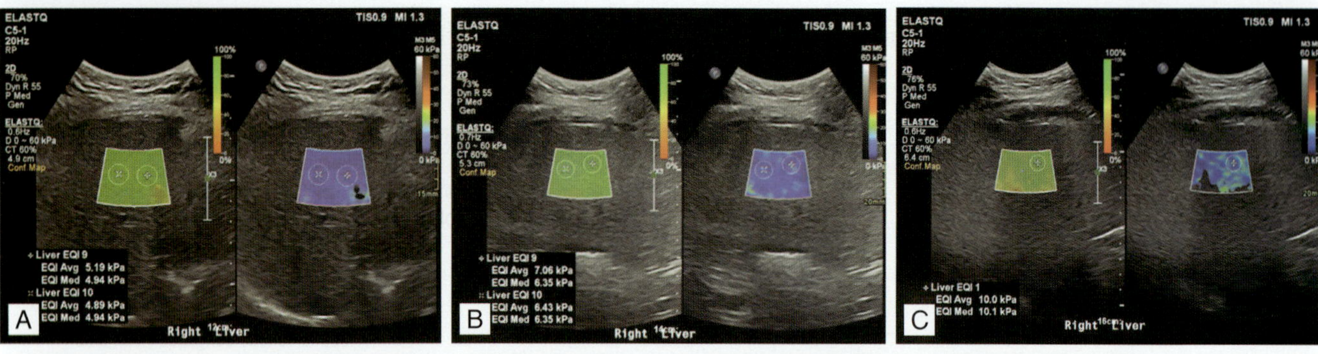

Figure 32.10 2D-SWE measurement of liver stiffness in three different patients with varying degrees of hepatic fibrosis. (A) The median liver stiffness value of 4.9 kPa (less than 5) is normal. (B) The median liver stiffness value of 7.1 kPa is indeterminate. Clinical signs and other tests are required for confirmation. (C) The median liver stiffness value of 10.1 kPa is suggestive of chronic liver disease, but further tests are required for confirmation.

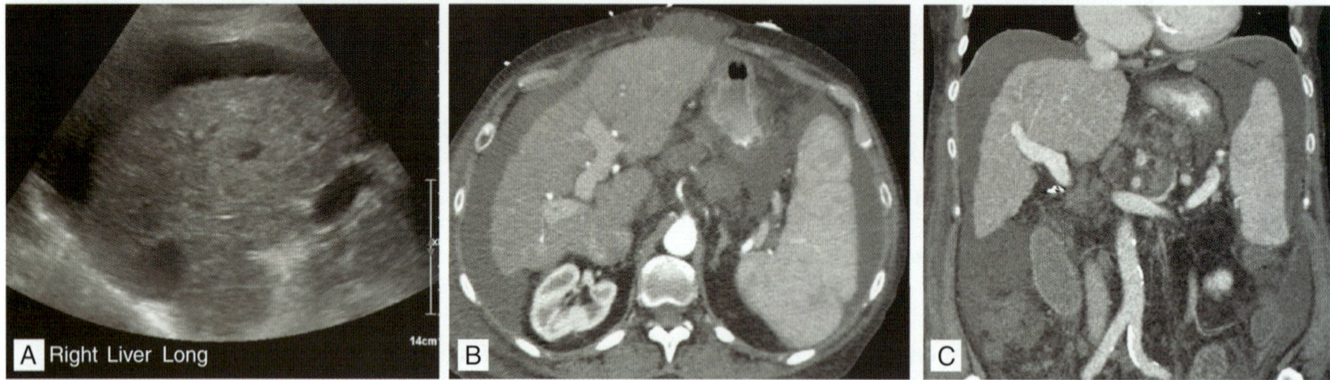

Figure 32.11 USG and CT appearance of the cirrhotic liver. (A) USG of the liver shows coarsened echogenicity of the liver with surface nodularity and perihepatic ascites. (B and C) Contrast-enhanced CT image of the liver in the arterial phase (B) and portal venous phase (C) images demonstrate cirrhotic liver with sequelae of portal hypertension, including ascites and splenomegaly. Also, note the patent portal venous system.

Magnetic resonance elastography (MRE) is a relatively recent technique used to evaluate liver tissue stiffness and early changes of fibrosis. Similar to ultrasonography SWE, MRE utilizes compression waves continuously generated outside the patient's body at a frequency of 60 Hz and is transmitted through a flexible tube to a vibrating passive driver placed over the liver. These waves are then imaged with a special phase-encoded MRI sequence. The wave information is automatically processed with software and produces maps for liver stiffness measurement (Table 32.4).

The healthy liver parenchyma presents liver stiffness values less than 2.5 kPa, whereas fibrosis and cirrhosis cause increased stiffness (Fig. 32.12) (Table 32.4). MRE has 98% sensitivity and 99% specificity detection of hepatic fibrosis

TABLE 32.4 Liver Stiffness Measurement Cut-offs With MRE

MRE Stiffness (kPa)	Fibrosis Stage
<2.5	Normal
2.5–2.9	Normal or inflammation
2.9–3.5	Stage 1–2
3.5–4.0	Stage 2–3
4.0–5.0	Stage 3–4
>5.0	Stage 4 or cirrhosis

MRE, magnetic resonance elastography.

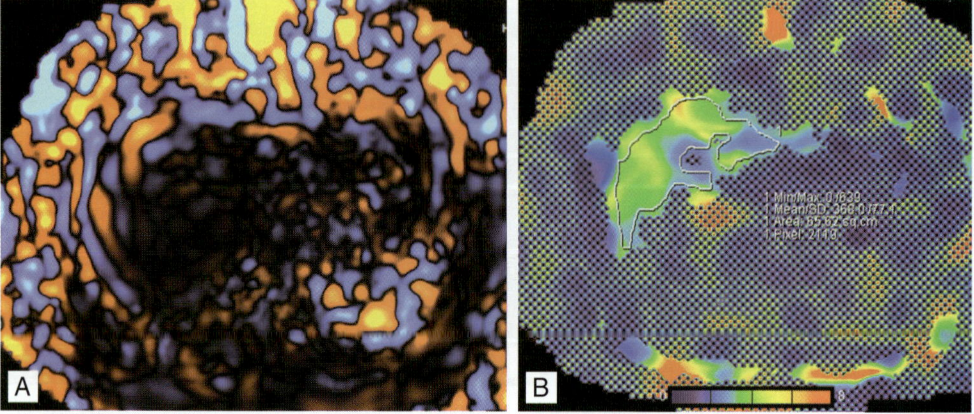

Figure 32.12 MR elastography technique. (A) Wave image and (B) elastography image with mean MRE stiffness value. Proper image acquisition is key for a good interpretation of MRE liver stiffness values.

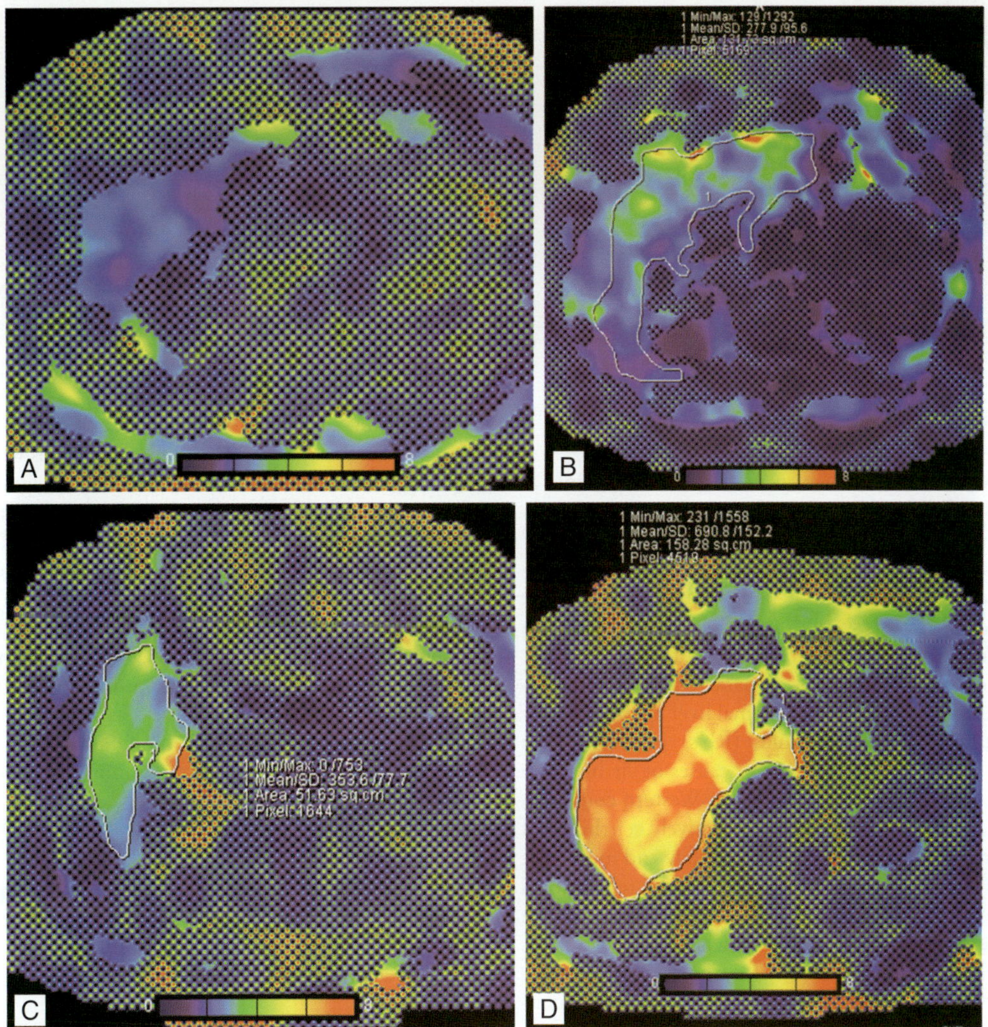

Figure 32.13 Magnetic resonance elastography (MRE) measurement of liver stiffness in four different patients with varying degrees of hepatic fibrosis. Liver stiffness value is calculated from mean stiffness value from at least four different areas of the liver. Different venders use different methods to calculate mean stiffness value. (A) MRE liver stiffness value of 2.0 kPa (less than 2.5) is normal. (B) MRE liver stiffness value of 2.8 kPa is normal or inflammation. The image demonstrates a mean value of 277, which is equal to about 2.77 kPa. (C) MRE liver stiffness value of 3.6 kPa is suggestive of stage 2–3 fibrosis. (D) MRE liver stiffness value of 6 kPa is suggestive of stage 4 fibrosis or cirrhosis.

and is considered an alternative gold standard for liver biopsy (Fig. 32.13). MRE assesses a larger area of the liver, is not affected by ascites, obesity, or hepatic steatosis, and has high intra- and interobserver agreement for measurement of stiffness. However, limitations of MRE include potential failure in patients with moderate-to-severe iron overload, lack of availability at all centers, and additional time required for positioning the driver.

Conclusion

Recent advances in MRI-based quantification of liver fat, iron, and fibrosis and increased availability of USG as the point of care have led to early and improved detection of diffuse liver diseases. MRI is the primary technique for imaging diffuse liver diseases.

Suggested Readings

- DT Boll, EM Merkle, Diffuse liver disease: strategies for hepatic CT and MR imaging, Radiographics 29 (6) (2009) 1591–1614.
- IS Idilman, I Ozdeniz, M Karcaaltincaba, Hepatic Steatosis: Etiology, Patterns, and Quantification, Seminars in ultrasound, CT, and MR 37 (6) (2016) 501–510.
- CB Sirlin, SB Reeder, Magnetic resonance imaging quantification of liver iron, Magn Reson Imaging Clin N Am 18 (3) (2010) 359–381, ix.
- RG Barr, SR Wilson, D Rubens, G Garcia-Tsao, G Ferraioli, Update to the Society of Radiologists in Ultrasound Liver Elastography Consensus Statement, Radiology 296 (2) (2020) 263–274.

33

Cirrhotic Liver

KANTHAN AMIN, BENJAMIN STRNAD

Introduction

Cirrhosis of the liver has been known to Western medicine since at least the 5th century BCE, when it was described by Hippocrates. Its name derives from the Greek word kirros, meaning "yellowish" or "tawny" after the appearance of the jaundiced patient. Thousands of years later, care of the cirrhotic patient remains a challenge for multiple medical specialists, including radiologists, who play an increasingly important role in both diagnosis and management.

Cirrhosis is a chronic liver disorder characterized by progressive distortion and replacement of the normal liver architecture by fibrotic tissue and regenerative nodules (RNs) in response to injuries of varied etiology [1]. The primary causes of cirrhosis are viral hepatitis, alcohol use, and increasingly in Western countries, nonalcoholic steatohepatitis (NASH). Collectively, cirrhosis of viral, alcoholic, or NASH etiology imposes a heavy and increasing burden on global health, accounting for 2.4% of total global deaths in 2017 compared with 1.9% in 1990, as shown in a recent global systemic analysis [2]. The same analysis also affirms that NASH is a rapidly growing cause of cirrhosis, with the age-standardized global prevalence of compensated and decompensated cirrhosis due to NASH having doubled, and more than tripled, respectively, from 1990 to 2017. In general, cirrhosis in Western countries is more often caused by alcohol use and NASH, whereas in Asia it is primarily caused by hepatitis B and C viral infection. A number of other less common chronic sources of liver injury can also lead to cirrhosis (Table 33.1).

Imaging Diagnosis and Staging of Fibrosis

There are a variety of tests which may indicate the presence of developing fibrosis or cirrhosis in the liver beyond a suggestive clinical presentation. Liver biopsy is the gold standard for diagnosing and staging fibrosis and provides valuable prognostic information, but is limited by cost and risk to the patient. It is also subject to sampling error in earlier stages where fibrosis is not yet diffuse. Thus, noninvasive means of diagnosing and staging fibrosis are desirable, and include both laboratory and imaging assessment. Laboratory assessment can help rule in the presence of advanced fibrosis, but is generally not reliable in the detection or differentiation of the earlier stages of fibrosis [3,4].

The primary strategies for the assessment of liver fibrosis with imaging can be broadly categorized as focused on

i. detection and quantification of its morphologic features,
ii. quantification of liver stiffness as a physical property proportional to fibrosis, that is, elastography, or
iii. detection of the stigmata of portal hypertension, such as enlarged portosystemic collateral veins.

TABLE 33.1 Etiologies of Chronic Liver Injury Which Can Progress to Cirrhosis

Etiology	Example
Cholestasis	Primary sclerosing cholangitis
Autoimmune	Autoimmune hepatitis
Vascular congestion	Heart failure, Budd–Chiari, sinusoidal obstruction syndrome
Metabolic	Hemochromatosis, Wilson's, α1-antitrypsin deficiency

Imaging the Morphology of Cirrhosis

In general, fibrosis and cirrhosis results in

i. hypertrophy of the left lateral section of the liver (segments II and III),
ii. hypertrophy of the caudate lobe (segment I), and
iii. atrophy of the left medial section and right hemiliver (segments IV–VIII).

All of these changes are appreciable with ultrasonography (USG), computed tomography (CT), or magnetic resonance imaging (MRI). As fibrosis advances, liver surface nodularity develops, which can also be seen with CT or MRI but which is often best and earliest appreciated with USG due to its higher spatial resolution (Fig. 33.1).

Although assessment of liver morphology can be subjective and qualitative, various imaging signs have been proposed for confident recognition of fibrosis. These include [5,6]

i. periportal space widening due to medial left section atrophy,
ii. expanded gallbladder fossa due to medial left section atrophy, and
iii. posterior right liver surface notching due to both right hemiliver atrophy and caudate lobe hypertrophy.

Overt morphologic changes in the liver are usually seen in more advanced stages of fibrosis or cirrhosis, and their absence on imaging does not exclude clinically significant fibrosis. Various measurements intended to reflect these morphologic changes while allowing more standardized assessment have also been proposed (Fig. 33.2) and are listed in Table 33.2.

In addition to such measurements, there is ongoing investigation of more advanced image postprocessing, including volume segmentation and textural analysis, in more accurate noninvasive staging of fibrosis that can be performed retrospectively. For example, semiautomated CT liver segmentation and segmental volume calculation enables determination of a liver segmental volume ratio (i.e., volume of segments I–III/segments IV–VIII),

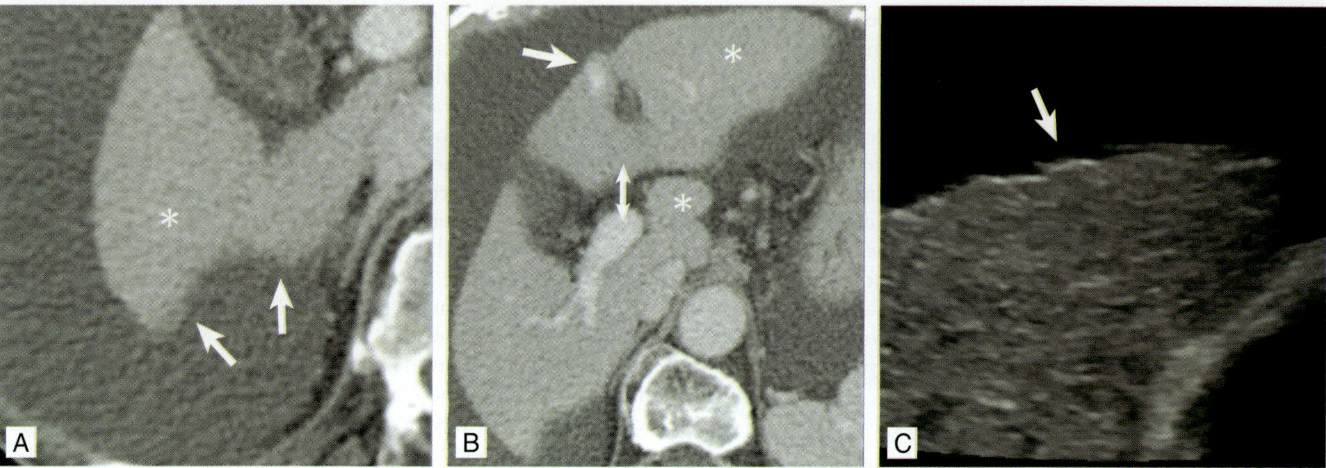

Figure 33.1 A 79-year-old man with hepatitis B and cirrhosis with typical morphologic changes. (A) Axial CT image showing right hemiliver atrophy (*asterisk*) and associated notching of the posterior liver surface (*arrows*). (B) Periportal space widening, indicated by a distance greater than 1 cm from the anterior wall of the right portal vein to the posterior surface of the left medial section (*double-headed arrow*). Also note relative hypertrophy of the left lateral section and caudate lobe (*asterisk*) and enhancement of a recanalized umbilical vein (*arrow*). (C) Although surface nodularity can be difficult to detect with confidence on CT or MRI, ultrasound in this case shows it clearly (*arrow*).

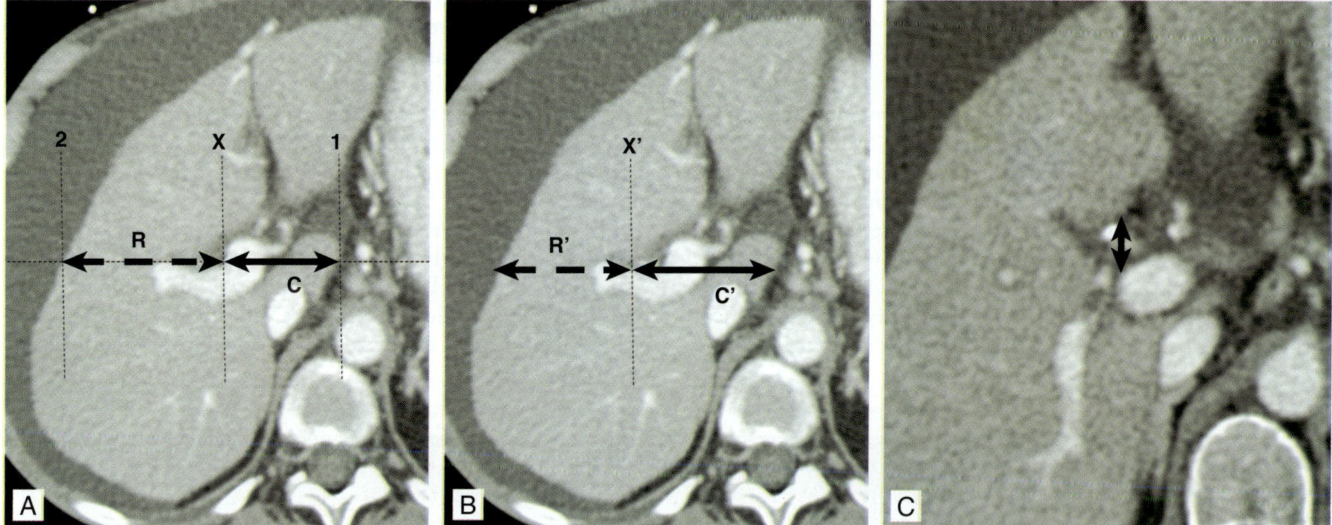

Figure 33.2 A 55-year old with known alcoholic cirrhosis. (A) Calculation of the caudate to right hepatic lobe ratio (C/R) is performed in the axial plane at which the most lateral margin of the main portal vein is identified (x, vertical dashed line). The distance from this margin to the medial surface of the caudate (1, vertical dashed line) along a horizontal line midway between the portal vein and vena cava is "C" (*solid double-headed arrow*), and the distance to the most lateral margin of the right hepatic lobe along the same line is "R" (*dashed double-headed arrow*). (B) Calculation of the modified caudate to right hepatic lobe ratio (C'/R') is similar but uses the most lateral margin of the right portal vein (x', vertical dashed line) as the reference for measurement. (C) Measurement of the periportal space is performed along a vertical line between the anterior wall of the main portal vein and the posterior surface of the left medial section (*double arrow*).

TABLE 33.2 Measurements Reflecting the Morphologic Changes of Fibrosis and Cirrhosis

Measurement	Method	Abnormal Threshold
Periportal space width [7]	Distance from anterior wall of RPV to posterior edge of segment IV	>1 cm
Caudate to right lobe ratio: C/R [8]	Caudate width (C) = distance from medial edge of caudate to lateral edge of PV at main bifurcation Right lobe width (R) = distance from lateral edge of PV at main bifurcation to lateral edge of liver	>0.55
Modified caudate to right lobe ratio: C'/R' [9]	C' = distance from medial edge of caudate to lateral edge of the right PV bifurcation R' = distance from lateral edge of right PV bifurcation to lateral edge of liver	>0.90

PV, portal vein; *RPV*, right portal vein.

which more accurately reflects the global morphologic change within the liver than ratios of two-dimensional (2D) measurements [10]. Semiautomated quantification of liver surface nodularity by CT has shown potential in discriminating earlier stages of fibrosis and may have prognostic value in prediction of decompensation or death in patients with compensated cirrhosis [10].

Overall, image-based morphologic assessments for liver fibrosis remain limited by relatively low sensitivity for the earlier stages of fibrosis and by their inability to accurately distinguish the stages of fibrosis, but they are useful to keep in mind when evaluating the liver in a patient with clinically suspected fibrosis. More advanced retrospective image analyses show promise in the detection and staging of earlier fibrosis, but are not yet widely available in clinical practice.

Morphology of Cirrhosis: Pearls to Remember

- Results in left lateral section and caudate hypertrophy
- Results in left medial section and right hemiliver atrophy
- Signs of cirrhosis include the posterior right hepatic surface notch, the expanded gallbladder fossa, and liver surface nodularity
- Morphologic changes are usually late indicators of fibrosis

Liver Elastography

Elastography is a method by which tissue deformation in response to a stress, or its stiffness, can be measured. Stiffness has been shown to correlate with degree of hepatic fibrosis, although there are several confounding factors in this determination which must be controlled, such as liver congestion in the setting of heart failure or even the recently fed state. The most widely used USG-based elastography applications for quantifying liver stiffness employ shear wave elastography—they quantify stiffness by measuring the velocity of shear waves through the liver which are created either by USG-induced vibration in the tissue or by mechanical vibrations from an external source [11]. The earliest elastography method to be widely adopted in clinical practice, single dimension transient elastography (FibroScan; Echosens, Paris, France) uses an external mechanical vibrating device to create shear waves in the liver and a point source A-mode transducer to measure the velocity of shear waves along a single dimension. This method is commonly used by referring doctors in the office and is both fast and inexpensive. However, it is limited by the inability to correlate measurement with real-time imaging of the liver. A newer method, known as 2D shear wave elastography, allows for simultaneous B-mode imaging with a conventional diagnostic USG transducer for selection of a region of interest in the liver and uses the USG transducer to create the tissue vibration and shear waves. A map of liver stiffness values is superimposed on the B-mode image, allowing for real-time assessment of the sample adequacy and any necessary adjustments to be made before each measurement (Fig. 33.3) [11,12].

MRI elastography is similar conceptually to USG methods, and uses an external device to create mechanical vibrations within the patient. Phase-contrast MR sequences are used to detect and measure the velocity of the resulting shear waves in the liver, allowing for creation of a liver stiffness map or elastogram that encompasses the majority of the liver (Fig. 33.4) [13]. Although similarly accurate compared with USG techniques, MR elastography is more expensive and less widely available [14]. It can be added to conventional MR sequences in high-risk patients who already require MRI for liver surveillance or can be used in patients for whom USG electrography is technically difficult.

Liver stiffness values obtained from elastography have shown strong correlation with liver fibrosis stage, although threshold values differ between USG and MR methods due to differences in the way these are calculated and are difficult to compare, especially as liver stiffness increases [13]. The discrepancy in calculated

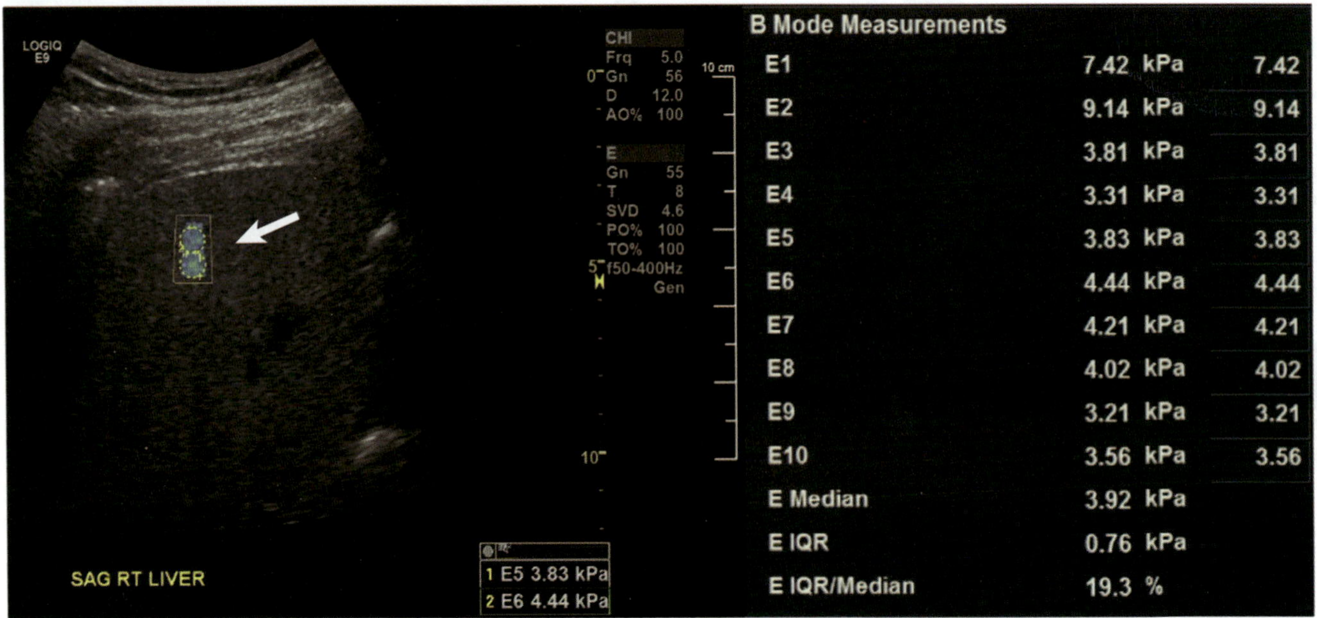

Figure 33.3 Normal 2D ultrasound elastography. Left: Shear wave velocity is measured within a region of interest (ROI) box ideally placed 2 cm deep to the liver surface (*arrow*), enabling automatic calculation of liver stiffness in kPa. Right: A series of measurements and kPa calculations is made for quality control. The median value (3.9 kPa) is compatible with stage 1–2 fibrosis. The interquartile range/median ratio (IQR/median) indicates the range of variation across measurements. A ratio of less than 30% is considered acceptable.

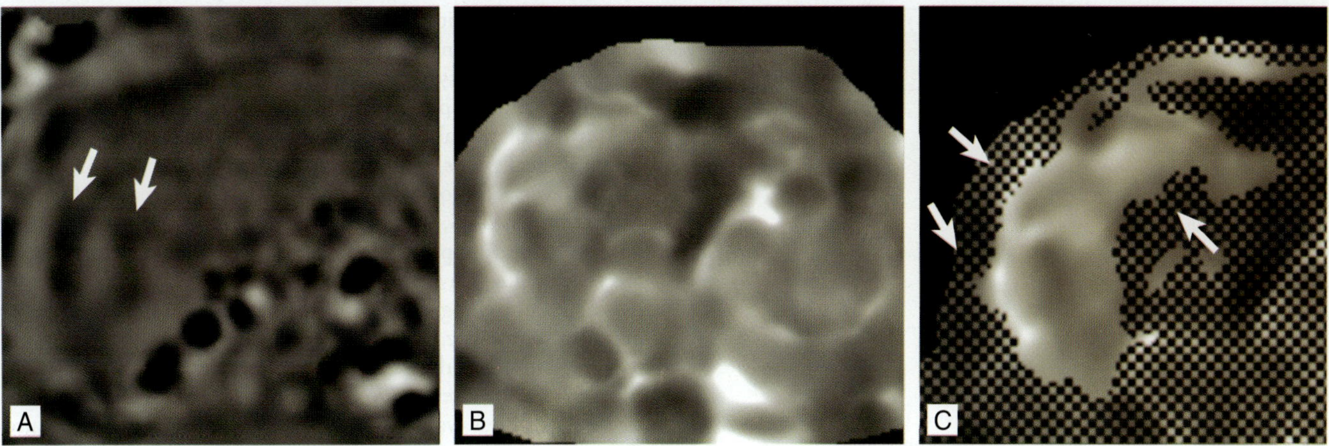

Figure 33.4 MR elastography in a 62-year-old man with chronic hepatitis C and fibrosis. (A) Phase-contrast sequence obtained during application of external mechanical vibration to the patient, showing shear waves propagating through the liver (*arrows*). (B) The velocity of these waves is determined and used to generate an elastogram of the liver at each slice. (C) A checkered mask (*arrows*) is applied to include only measurements with an acceptable range of variation, within which ROIs can be used to measure liver stiffness. This patient's average liver stiffness was 4.1k, compatible with stage 3 fibrosis.

liver stiffness between USG and MR currently prevents interchange of these techniques in follow-up of fibrosis stage in the same patient. Cut-off values for liver stiffness with corresponding METAVIR fibrosis stage (F0–F4) for 2D shear wave and MR elastography are listed in Table 33.3.

Elastography: Pearls to Remember

- Transient elastography fast and available in office, but lacks real-time imaging correlation
- 2D USG and MR elastography allow imaging correlation, wider sampling of the liver
- USG and MR elastography liver stiffness values are not interchangeable
- Best available noninvasive technique for staging fibrosis

Complications of Cirrhosis

As discussed earlier, noninvasive imaging techniques, particularly USG or MR elastography, can help in the detection and staging of fibrosis before the development of cirrhosis. The clinical focus in these patients is on the determination of the etiology of liver injury in hope of either reversing or preventing progression of fibrosis (e.g., with eradication of chronic hepatitis C or with cessation of alcohol use) to irreversible cirrhosis. Once the diagnosis of cirrhosis is made, the clinical focus shifts toward the prevention and treatment of decompensated cirrhosis and the complications of clinically significant portal hypertension, as well as the surveillance, diagnosis, and treatment of hepatocellular carcinoma (HCC).

Portal Hypertension

Diagnosis

Portal hypertension occurs in the setting of cirrhosis and is defined as an increased portal-systemic pressure gradient >5 mm Hg. In cirrhotic portal hypertension, this gradient is equivalent with the hepatic venous pressure gradient (HVPG) [17]. Clinically significant portal hypertension, which presages development of decompensated cirrhosis with associated complications, is defined as a HVPG >10 mm Hg [18]. The HVPG is determined by obtaining the hepatic vein wedge pressure (approximating the hepatic sinusoidal pressure) and the free hepatic vein pressure through a transjugular catheter transducer. The wedge pressure is calculated by occluding the proximal hepatic vein with a balloon and then measuring the resulting pressure within the vein, which is equilibrated with the sinusoidal pressure. The balloon is then deflated and a second measurement is made of the free hepatic vein pressure. The difference between the two pressures is the gradient.

In the setting of cirrhosis, the HVPG is the most accurate method for grading portal hypertension and for quantifying

TABLE 33.3 Liver Stiffness Cut-Off Values for the Stages of Liver Fibrosis Using Ultrasound and MR Elastography

Stage	Histologic Description	2D USG Stiffness Value (kPa)	MR Stiffness Value (kPa)
F0	No fibrosis	<5.8	<2.9
F1	Mild, portal fibrosis without bridging septa	5.8–6.8	2.9–3.5
F2	Moderate, portal fibrosis with rare bridging septa	6.8–9.1	3.5–4.0
F3	Severe, numerous bridging septa without cirrhosis	9.1–10.3	4.0–5.0
F4	Cirrhosis	>10.3	>5.0

Ultrasound stiffness values are from Lu et al. [15]; MR stiffness values are from Venkatesh and Ehman [16].

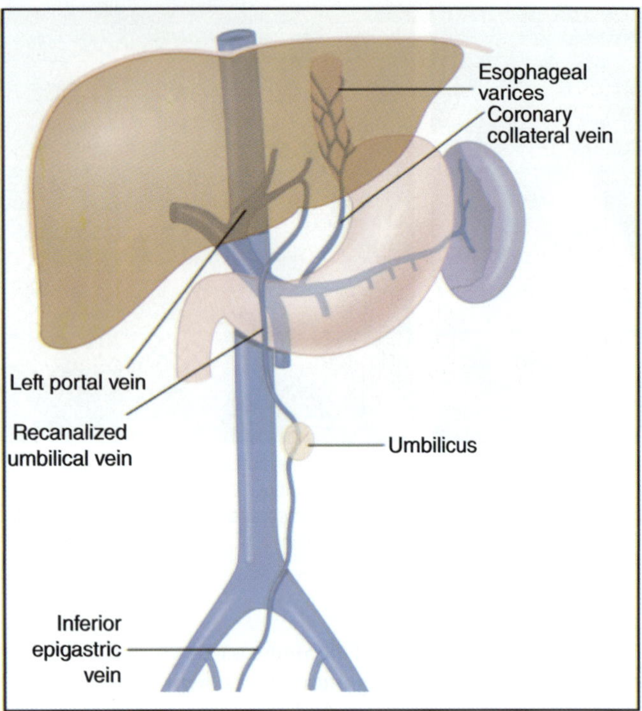

Figure 33.5 Diagram illustrating portosystemic collateral pathways, including esophageal varices, the coronary vein, and the umbilical vein. Although there are many sites of portosystemic collateralization, these are the most commonly identified ones at imaging, and are all identifiable with Doppler USG.

response of portal hypertension to treatment [19]. Given that this technique is invasive and relatively expensive, noninvasive imaging can be a helpful adjunct in the detection of clinically significant portal hypertension.

The most specific finding of clinically significant portal hypertension on any noninvasive imaging technique is the identification of portosystemic collateral formation. This includes identification of esophageal varices or a recanalized umbilical vein, which should be sought on any imaging performed for a patient with suspected chronic liver disease or fibrosis (Figs. 33.5 and 33.6). The first-line examination for the detection of vascular manifestations of portal hypertension is Doppler USG of the liver. This can assess patency and direction of flow within the portal-venous system, and can detect collateral formation. The most common portosystemic collaterals detected by USG in the setting of portal hypertension are recanalized umbilical or paraumbilical veins, and the coronary vein (Figs. 33.7 and 33.8). Reversal of flow within the coronary vein, readily detected with Doppler USG, is another specific finding of clinically significant portal hypertension. Short of collateral formation, reversal, or sluggish within the portal vein is also highly suggestive of clinically significant portal hypertension [20]. Splenomegaly also often accompanies the development of portal hypertension, although the size of the spleen does not necessarily correlate with the severity of portal hypertension [21].

Liver stiffness values obtained by elastography have also shown value in the noninvasive prediction of clinically significant portal hypertension, with a transient elastography value greater than 15 kPa considered highly suggestive of compensated portal hypertension in an asymptomatic patient. Liver stiffness values greater than 20 kPa, and platelet counts of less than 150,000 mm^{-3} predict a high risk for clinically significant portal hypertension with the development of esophageal varices or other complications [22]. These patients require surveillance with endoscopy for the detection and treatment of varices in primary prevention of variceal bleeding. Patients with clinically significant portal hypertension can also develop refractory ascites or, as more spontaneous portosystemic shunts develop, hepatic encephalopathy.

Other Causes of Portal Hypertension (Noncirrhotic Portal Hypertension)

The most common cause of portal hypertension is cirrhosis. However, there are other (noncirrhotic) etiologies of portal hypertension for which radiologists play an important role in the diagnosis and management.

Budd–Chiari Syndrome

Budd–Chiari syndrome encompasses a variety of conditions which result in obstruction of the large hepatic veins or of the IVC between the hepatic venous confluence and the right atrium. Obstruction of hepatic venous outflow at these levels results in

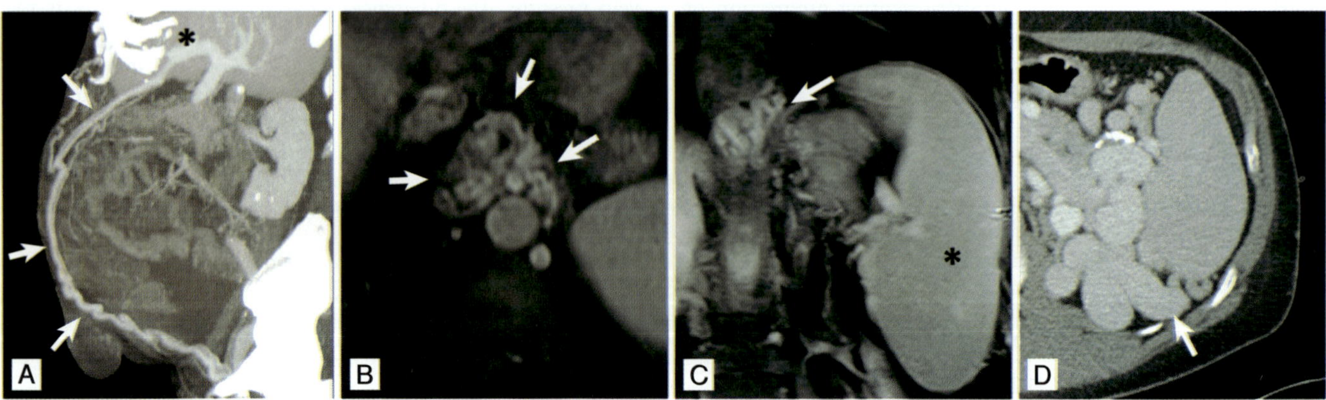

Figure 33.6 Examples of portosystemic collateral pathways. (A) Maximum intensity projection of a sagittal CT image shows a recanalized umbilical vein with dilated periumbilical and epigastric vein collaterals (*arrows*). The recanalized umbilical vein is identified at the terminus of the left portal vein umbilical segment at the base of the falciform ligament (*asterisk*). Postcontrast T1 sequences in a patient with cirrhosis and portal hypertension show tortuous and engorged esophageal varices (*arrows*, B and C) and marked splenomegaly (*asterisk*, C). Axial CT image with contrast shows a dilated, tortuous collateral vein extending from the splenic hilum to the left renal vein—a spontaneous splenorenal shunt (*arrow*, D).

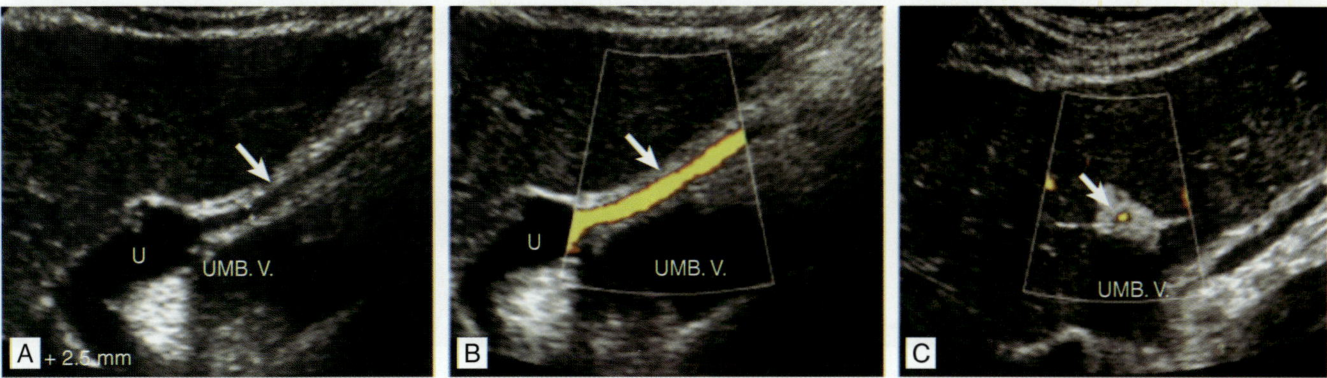

Figure 33.7 Recanalized umbilical vein collateral in two different patients. Longitudinal grayscale (A) and power Doppler (B) views of the left hemiliver show an umbilical collateral (UMB. V. - *arrow*) seen as a small, 2.5-mm, central vessel in the ligamentum teres. Note that the umbilical vein collateral communicates with the umbilical segment of the left portal vein (U). (C) Transverse power Doppler view of the left hemiliver shows the umbilical collateral (*arrow*) in the middle of the echogenic ligamentum teres.

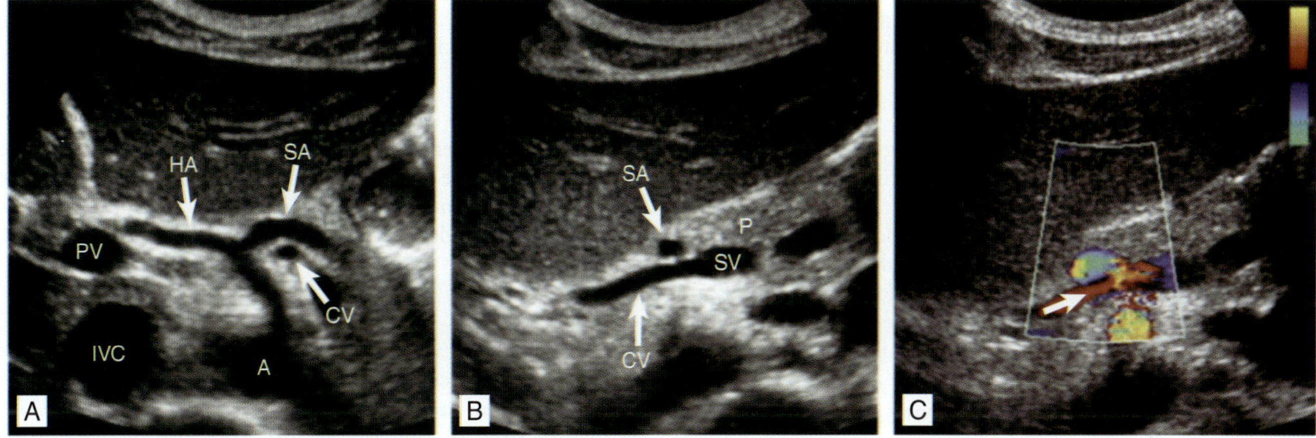

Figure 33.8 Normal coronary vein. (A) Transverse view shows the aorta (A) and the celiac axis. The coronary vein (CV) is seen immediately posterior to the splenic artery (SA). The hepatic artery (HA), portal vein (PV), and inferior vena cava (IVC) are also seen. (B) Longitudinal view shows the splenic vein (SV) immediately posterior to the body of the pancreas (P). The CV is seen arising from the SV and passing under the SA. (C) Longitudinal color Doppler view similar to B shows flow (*arrow*) in the coronary vein directed toward the splenic vein, as expected.

congestion and venous stasis of the liver, ultimately causing progressive liver injury, fibrosis, portal hypertension, liver failure (which can be fulminant or chronic), and cirrhosis. The most common cause of large hepatic venous occlusion is an underlying hematologic disorder which results in hypercoagulopathy and spontaneous venous thrombosis. Any process obstructing the hepatic veins or suprahepatic vena cava, including extrinsic compression by an adjacent mass, can also result in a secondary Budd–Chiari syndrome. It is important to recognize and distinguish the features of hepatic congestion, fibrosis, and portal hypertension associated with Budd–Chiari from those of cirrhotic portal hypertension, because the underlying etiologies and management differ substantially (Fig. 33.9). Apart from demonstrating occlusion or stenosis of the IVC or the hepatic veins, imaging often demonstrates the presence of venovenous collaterals in the liver, which can be distinguished from a normal hepatic vein or its tributary (which are straight) by their tortuous curvilinear appearance. Treatment involves identifying and correcting the underlying predisposition to thrombosis and relief of the venous outflow obstruction—with thrombectomy or angioplasty when possible, or with bypass of the obstruction with a portosystemic venous shunt, as discussed later [23].

Sinusoidal Obstruction Syndrome (Previously Veno-occlusive Disease)

Previously known as "veno-occlusive disease," sinusoidal obstruction syndrome (SOS) is distinguished from Budd–Chiari by venous outflow obstruction at the level of the hepatic sinusoids and venules, and is caused by toxic endothelial injury of the sinusoids. The most common etiology is the conditioning phase of bone marrow transplantation, during which endothelial injury throughout the body is common and can produce a variety of organ-specific syndromes in addition to SOS. Another increasingly recognized etiology is oxaliplatin-based chemotherapy, such as in patients being treated for metastatic colorectal cancer. Most patients with sinusoidal endothelial injury do not progress to SOS—this occurs in a minority of patients, usually within 30 days after transplant. The diagnosis is primarily clinical, with liver failure and toxicity manifesting with fluid retention/ascites, tender hepatomegaly, and jaundice occurring within a suggestive time frame after bone marrow transplantation.

Most of the imaging findings in SOS, as in other causes of acute liver failure, are nonspecific, but can suggest the correct diagnosis in the appropriate clinical context. Gadoxetate-enhanced

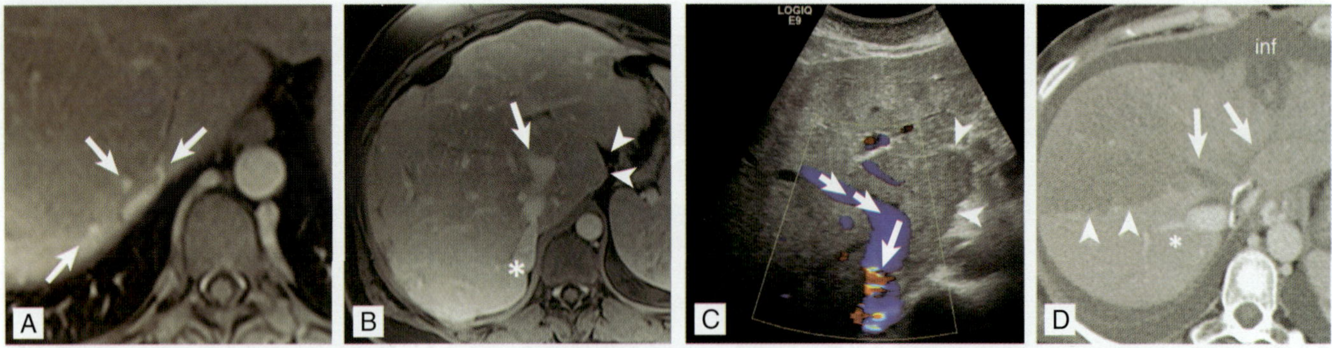

Figure 33.9 A 42-year-old woman with JAK2 mutation and related hypercoagulopathy with recurrent, spontaneous thrombosis of the hepatic veins and features of chronic Budd–Chiari. Axial MRI T1 vibe postcontrast image at the level of the hepatic venous confluence (A) shows a narrowed, atretic IVC, and diminutive hepatic vein remnants (*arrows*). Another MR image inferior to this plane (B) shows a large, tortuous collateral vein (*arrow*) draining from the caudate lobe (*arrowheads*) into the IVC (*asterisk*). The liver is nodular, with relative hypertrophy of the central liver and caudate lobe (*arrowhead*). Color Doppler image (C) of the same collateral vein shows flow in the expected direction (*arrows*) toward the vena cava. (D) A 50-year-old woman with polycythemia vera and features of acute Budd–Chiari syndrome after liver transplantation for previous chronic Budd–Chiari and associated end stage liver failure. Axial CT image with contrast at the level of the hepatic vein confluence shows thrombosis of the left and middle hepatic veins (*arrows*) and a patent right hepatic vein (*asterisk*). Relative hypoenhancement is noted in the left and anterior right hemiliver, secondary to hypoperfusion, and edema (*arrowheads*). Superimposed liver infarction ("inf") is seen in the periphery of the left lateral section. This patient went on to develop features of chronic Budd–Chiari and recurrent fibrosis within her transplant liver despite multiple interventions (not pictured).

MRI with delayed hepatobiliary phase imaging is relatively specific for SOS in the appropriate clinical setting, demonstrating a characteristic peripherally predominant, reticular pattern of hypoenhancement (Fig. 33.10) [24]. Treatment is primarily supportive, with cessation of any implicated therapy or exposures which might have triggered the toxic endothelial injury [25]. Prompt recognition and removal of the offending agent is crucial to avoiding irreversible liver damage, liver failure, and death.

Management of Portal Hypertension

TIPS

Transjugular intrahepatic portosystemic shunt (TIPS) is a treatment for the complications of portal hypertension, which entails placement of a stent through the liver between a portal and hepatic vein, or the vena cava, allowing portal-venous inflow to bypass the liver into systemic circulation, thus lowering the portal and sinusoidal pressure and the likelihood of associated complications.

Indications

The primary indications for TIPS placement in the setting of cirrhosis are for secondary prevention of bleeding varices after failed first-line medical and endoscopic therapy, and for refractory large volume ascites. TIPS can also be used in the setting of life-threatening variceal bleeding if first-line therapy is unsuccessful (Fig. 33.11). TIPS can serve as a bridge to definitive management with liver transplant in any of these

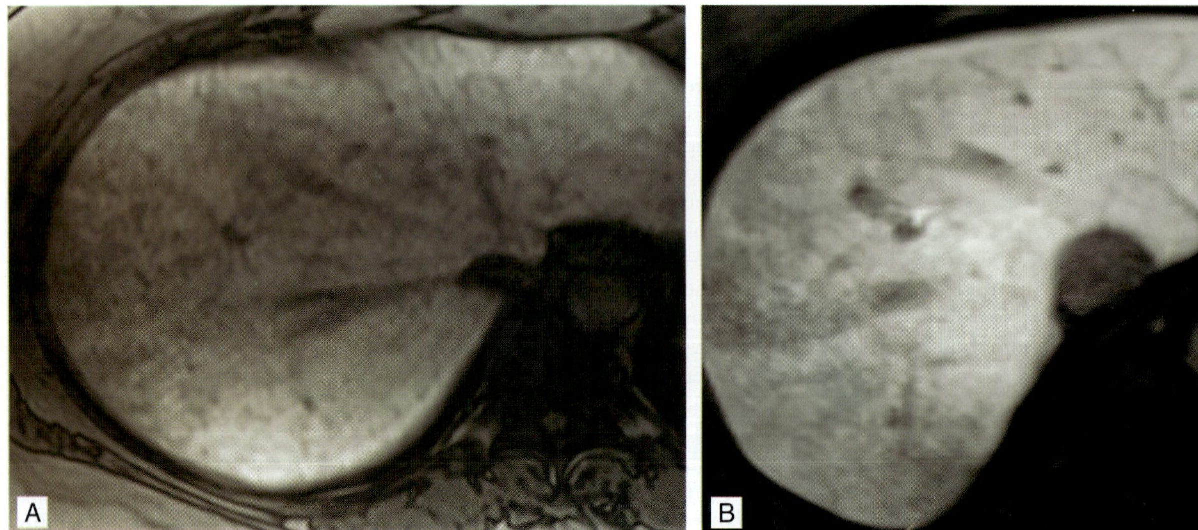

Figure 33.10 Two different patients with sinusoidal obstruction syndrome (SOS). Imaging findings are generally nonspecific and may include heterogenous liver enhancement or edema, ascites, and splenomegaly. A reticular pattern of hypoenhancement on the delayed hepatobiliary phase of gadoxetate-enhanced MRI has been reported as a relatively specific finding of SOS. (A) T1 gadoxetate enhanced axial MRI image of a 47-year-old woman with rectal cancer being treated with a oxaliplatin, which is known to cause hepatotoxicity and SOS. (B) Similar image in a 27-year-old man who recently underwent bone marrow transplant for leukemia.

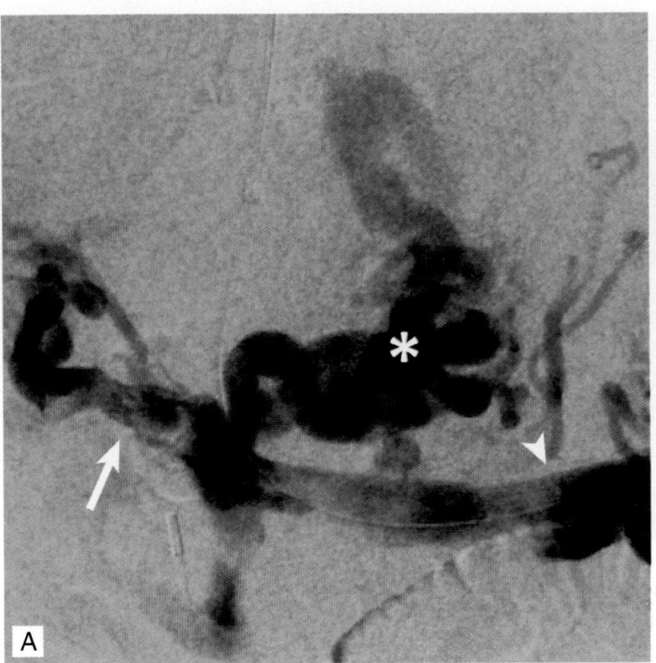

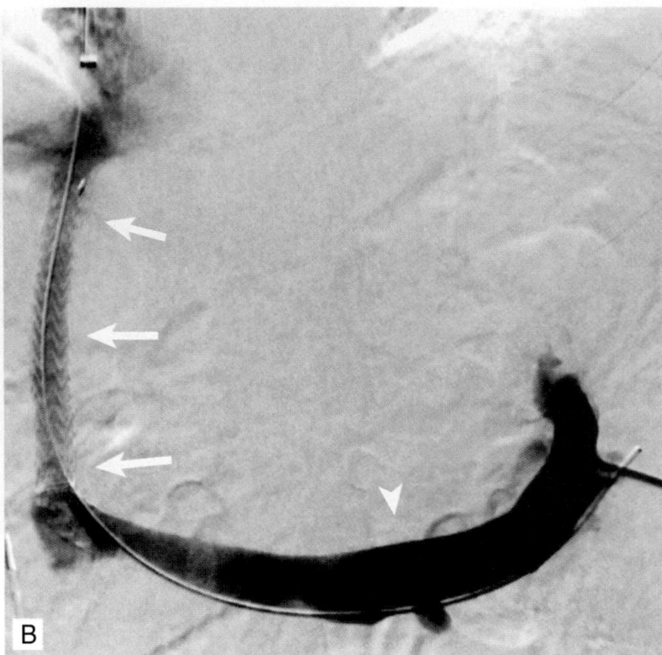

Figure 33.11 Flouroscopic digital subtraction angiography images obtained during placement of a TIPS device in a patient with cirrhosis, chronic portal-venous occlusion with cavernous transformation, and refractory bleeding of esophageal varices. Cavernous transformation necessitated cannulation of the portal system through transplenic puncture to access the splenic vein (*arrowheads*). (A) Initial contrast injection from the splenic vein shows the remnant portal vein (*arrow*) and multiple dilated, tortuous portal collaterals as well as dilated esophageal varices (*asterisk*). (B) Repeat injection after placement of the TIPS (*arrows* in B) from the right hepatic vein to the portosplenic confluence/portal vein remnant shows no filling of the varices.

scenarios. TIPS is also indicated in the setting of Budd–Chiari syndrome, when direct relief of venous outflow obstruction (e.g., with thrombectomy or angioplasty) have failed or are impossible.

TIPS has shown benefit in multiple randomized trials and meta-analyses, with overall reported success of portal decompression in over 95% of cases [26]. One of the main risks of TIPS placement is the development of hepatic encephalopathy, which occurs as ammonia and other toxins within the portal blood are shunted into systemic circulation. Other risks include heart failure from increased preload from blood shunted into the systemic circulation, and progressive liver ischemia and failure if the liver's arterial supply is insufficient.

Post-TIPS Imaging

- Once a TIPS has been placed, it is commonly monitored for patency and evidence of failure—1 year patency rates for modern, covered stents range from 80% to 90%. USG with Doppler imaging is a noninvasive and relatively low-cost method for surveilling the TIPS device, although there is a lack of strong consensus on how it should be used [27]. At the author's institution, Doppler is performed at 24–48 hours for baseline assessment and followed up at 3 months, 6 months, and 12 months after placement, with annual follow-up thereafter
- Doppler findings suggestive of TIPS malfunction can prompt transjugular venography and pressure gradient measurement for more precise assessment and treatment
- The normal appearance of the TIPS on Doppler imaging includes detectable flow throughout the stent, the absence of focal aliasing artifact within the stent, flow velocities throughout the stent ranging from 90 cm/s to 190 cm/s,

Portal Hypertension: Pearls to Remember

- It is important to recognize and distinguish noncirrhotic causes of portal hypertension, including Budd–Chiari syndrome and SOS, from cirrhotic portal hypertension
- HVPG measurement is the most accurate method for grading cirrhotic portal hypertension
- Portal hypertension = HVPG > 5 mm Hg; Clinically significant portal hypertension = HVPG > 10 mm Hg
- Liver stiffness value >20 kPa and platelet count <150,000 mm^{-3} predict clinically significant portal hypertension
- Patients with clinically significant portal hypertension require endoscopic surveillance for gastric and esophageal varices
- Varices and other portosystemic collateral vessels are specific noninvasive imaging findings of clinically significant portal hypertension
- TIPS indicated for secondary prevention of varices, variceal bleeding unresponsive to medical/endoscopic therapy and refractory ascites
- TIPS may also be used to bypass hepatic venous outflow obstruction in Budd–Chiari syndrome
- Doppler findings of TIPS stenosis include focal aliasing, velocities >190 cm/s at site of stenosis, velocities <190 cm/s elsewhere in the stent, portal vein velocity <30 cm, and portal flow direction away from the stent
- Multiple abnormal Doppler parameters are expected in the setting of real TIPS malfunction

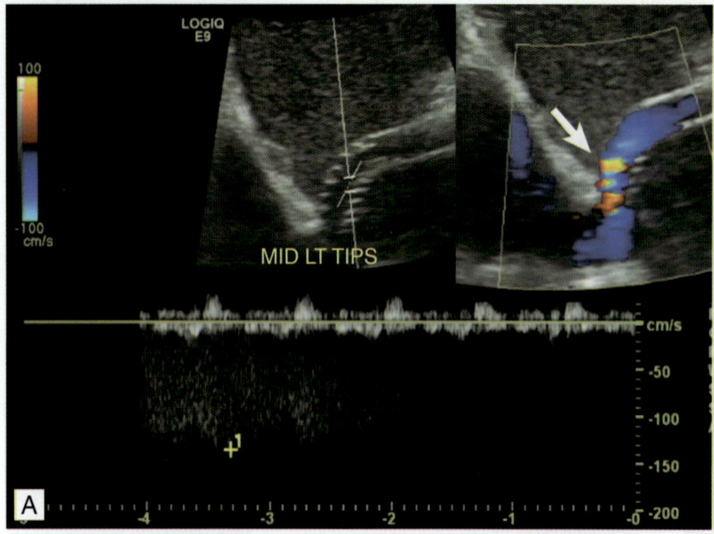

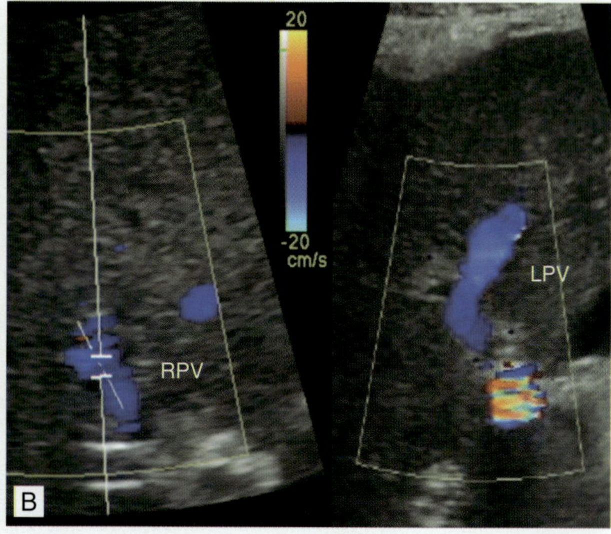

Figure 33.12 Doppler surveillance of the TIPS device. (A) Spectral Doppler analysis of a TIPS device showing flow throughout the stent. Apparent focal aliasing within the distal stent (*arrow*) results from the higher frequency shifts at steeper Doppler angles. The velocity measured at this point is normal (between approximately 90 and 190 cm/s) and reassuring that no stenosis is present. (B) Confirmation that flow persists in the expected retrograde direction toward the stent in the RPV and LPV is also reassuring. *LPV*, left portal vein; *RPV*, right portal vein.

retrograde flow in the right and left portal veins toward the stent and flow velocity in the main portal vein >30 cm/s (Fig. 33.12) [28]. Conversely, findings at TIPS USG which are suggestive of a tips stenosis include focal aliasing within the stent, increased velocities (>190 cm/s) at the site of suspected stenosis, and reduced velocity (<90 cm/s) elsewhere within the stent

- The reduced intrahepatic vascular resistance that occurs after successful bypass of the hepatic sinusoids accounts for the normally elevated portal vein velocity, and significant reduction in velocity below 30 cm/s is another suggestive finding of stent malfunction
- It is important to note that mild deviations from normal in any one of these parameters alone are not likely to represent TIPS malfunction. Rather, multiple Doppler abnormalities should be observed before venography or intervention is considered [28]
- Other findings highly suggestive of TIPS malfunction include reversal in portal-venous flow direction from toward the stent to away from it, or a visible filling defect within the stent or flow void on color Doppler. Complete absence of detectable flow within the stent is suggestive of thrombosis (Fig. 33.13)

Hepatocellular Carcinoma

Introduction

Primary liver cancers are the fourth leading cause of cancer deaths worldwide, the majority (~75%) of which are HCC [29]. East Asian countries have the highest incidence but have seen a recent decrease in the rates of disease. North America and Europe have a more modest number of cases, but have seen an increase over time in incidence, likely related to cirrhosis from a higher burden of hepatitis C virus in the population born in between 1945 and 1965, and also the increased rate of nonalcoholic fatty liver disease (NAFLD) [30]. In the United States, the incidence of primary liver cancers increased between the years of 2012 and 2016 at an average annual rate of 2.5% and 3.7% for men and women, respectively. This was the largest increase in incidence of the analyzed cancers, including melanoma, breast, lung, prostate, pancreatic, and renal carcinomas [31]. Recent reports delineate a possible peak in the United States, with a slight decline in HCC cases in the last few years [32]. Nonetheless, HCC remains a prevalent disease that can greatly benefit from early diagnosis and treatment. Uniquely, radiology has a central role in the surveillance, diagnosis, and treatment of HCC.

Risk Factors

There are several risk factors that influence the development of HCC, but they predominantly revolve around the central premise of chronic liver injury. The majority (80–90%) of HCC cases occur in the setting of cirrhosis [33–35]. In the same line of thought, the risk of developing HCC in a cirrhotic liver is much higher than a noncirrhotic liver (2.7–45 fold) [36].

Worldwide, the predominant chronic liver diseases leading to HCC are from viral hepatitis and alcohol use. Hepatitis B virus globally is the number one cause of HCC and carries a 10–25% lifetime risk of developing the cancer, despite widespread vaccination programs. It is also unique in that HCC frequently develops with hepatitis B infection even without underlying cirrhosis (up to 30%) [37,38]. Hepatitis C-related HCC, in contrast, almost exclusively develops in the setting of cirrhosis, and rarely, in the setting of advanced fibrosis. Dual infections with hepatitis C and B have a synergistic effect and increase the risk of HCC [35,39,40]. Use of antiviral therapies for HBV and HCV have reduced the subsequent risk of developing HCC; however, the risk is not eliminated even if a sustained viral response is attained.

The risk of developing HCC related to alcohol use is linearly proportional to the amount of alcohol consumption. The greater the intake of alcohol, the greater the risk of developing the liver cancer. In one study, the odds ratio (OR) was significantly increased (8.3) in those who consumed greater than 80 mL of ethanol per day [40]. Other studies have also demonstrated similar elevated risks of HCC with increasing alcohol intake. Alcohol use in the setting of viral hepatitis and other chronic liver diseases, also synergistically increases the risk for HCC [40,41].

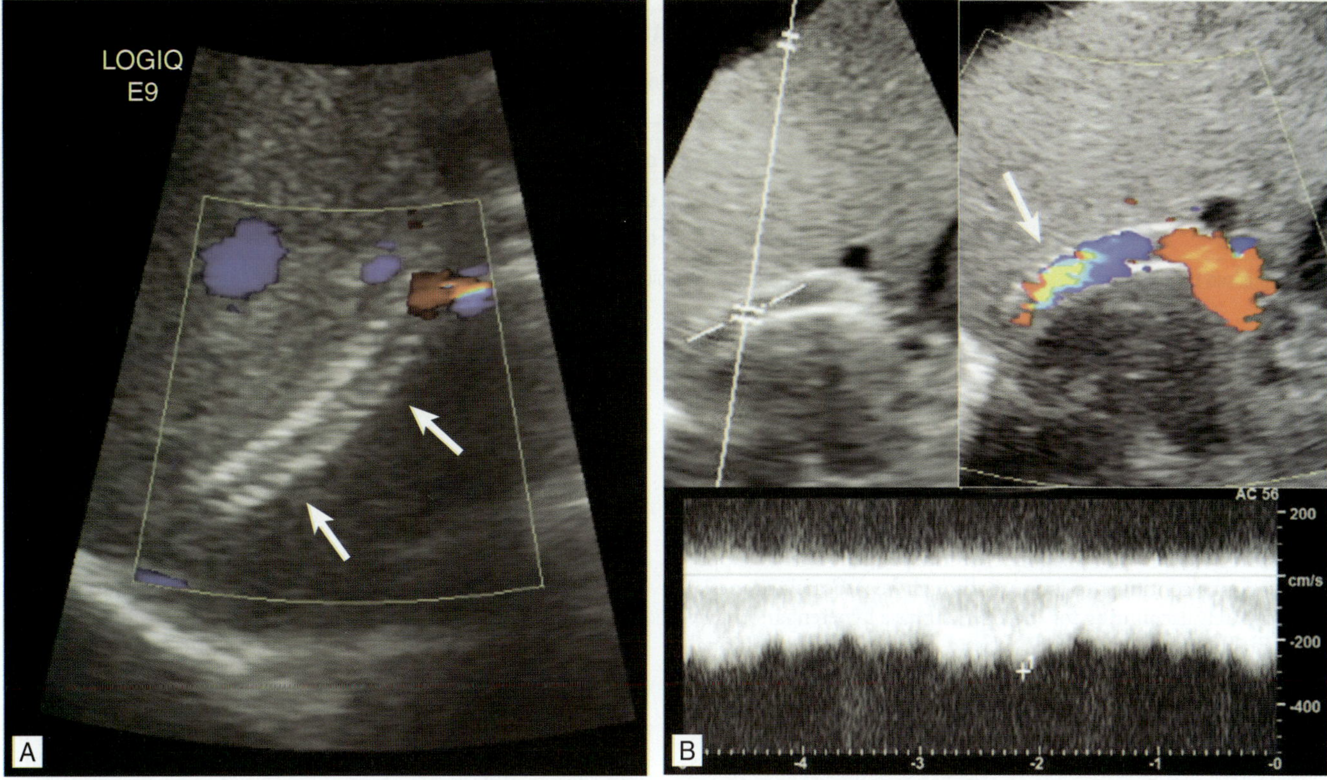

Figure 33.13 TIPS occlusion and stenosis. (A) Doppler evaluation of the tips shows no flow within the stent, new from the previous assessment and consistent with stent occlusion. This required stent revision. (B) Focal aliasing in the mid-distal stent with a corresponding elevation in velocity at this location to nearly 300 cm/s. Velocity within the proximal stent had also lowered from previous exam. Transjugular venography confirmed a stenosis within the stent and elevation of the HVPG above 14 mm Hg. After stent revision, the gradient lowered to 10 mm Hg.

In the United States and other developed nations, NAFLD is becoming a larger portion of the underlying cause of cirrhosis and HCC, as its prevalence continues to increase in the population [42]. Although it was previously though that HCC does not occur without NAFLD progressing to cirrhosis, recent studies demonstrate a number of cases occurring in the setting of NAFLD without cirrhosis or advanced fibrosis present [38,43]. NAFLD is associated with obesity and type 2 diabetes, each of which are also independent risk factors for HCC. Although confounding factors make it difficult to accurately predict the individual contribution of increased risk from these entities, it is estimated that diabetes has a 2.5-fold increased risk, and obesity has an approximately 1.5-fold increased risk of developing HCC [39,44–46].

Pathogenesis

- The pathogenesis of HCC varies on a molecular level depending on the underlying risk factors. For example, mutations in TP53 and TERT promoter genes are most frequent with HBV-associated HCC, whereas activation of IL-6-Janus kinase signal transducer and activator of transcription (JAK/STAT) is predominantly found in the setting of NAFLD/NASH [47,48]. These differences lead to varying histological and even clinical presentations and outcomes. Further discussion of the molecular and genetic profile of HCC is outside the scope of this text; however, the future exploration in this realm may call for correlation of the genetic make up to imaging features, leading to a more precise noninvasive diagnosis of the subtype of HCC
- In terms of imaging characteristics, HCC is the last stage along a spectrum ranging from RN, to dysplastic nodules and finally to HCC. RNs occur in the presence of repeated injury and repair. In the setting of chronic liver disease, there is continuous inflammation and cell damage leading to cell death and subsequent cellular division and replacement. This is also the process that in parallel leads to intrahepatic fibrosis and eventual cirrhosis [49]. In this constant process, there is repeated DNA damage, leading to genetic mutations, some of which are malignant, resulting in heterogeneous cell types throughout the liver depending on where and when the genetic mutations occurred [50]
- Grossly and microscopically, RNs are indistinguishable from each other and even from normal hepatocytes. There is no visible atypia in these cells even on histology, although a number of underlying genetic mutations may already be present [51]. For this reason, RNs are generally considered "benign"
- Atypical cells can be found within the RNs or in single lobules if there is no cirrhosis present. A group of these cells is referred to as "dysplastic foci" and can be seen on histology but are not distinguishable on current diagnostic images. These are thought to grow larger into dysplastic nodules, which measure greater than 1 cm, and differ in size, color, and/or consistency from the other cirrhotic nodules and the background liver parenchyma, and are visible on imaging. Depending on the histological features, these can be classified as either low-grade or high-grade dysplastic nodules [49]. Dysplastic nodules contain precancerous cells, which ultimately develop into HCC

TABLE 33.4 Imaging Characteristics of Nodules on the HCC Parthenogenesis Spectrum

Nodule	CT Density	T1 Intensity	T2 Intensity	Fat	Arterial Phase Enhancement	Venous/Delayed Phase	Hepatobiliary Phase
RN	Iso	Iso; rarely hyper	Iso; rarely hypo	–	Iso	Iso	Iso, rarely hyper
LGDN	Iso	Iso or hyper	Iso or hypo	+/–	Iso or hypo	Iso	Iso
HGDN	Iso	Iso or hyper	Iso or hypo	+/–	Iso or hypo: rarely hyper	Iso or hypo	Iso or hypo
Early HCC	Iso/hypo	Iso or hyper	Iso, hypo, or hyper	++/–	Iso or hypo: rarely hyper	Iso or hypo	Iso or hypo
Progressed HCC	Iso/hypo	Iso, hypo or hyper	Iso, hypo or hyper	+/–	Typically hyper	Typically hypo	Hypo

HGDN, high-grade dysplastic nodule; *LGDN*, low-grade dysplastic nodule; *RN*, regenerative nodule.

- Angiogenesis first occurs in these dysplastic nodules, which demonstrate internal unpaired arteries, that is, arteries outside the portal triad (nontriadal arteries), again best appreciated on histology rather than imaging. The independent arterial supply this forms continues to increase through hepatocarcinogenesis, ultimately accounting for the arterial phase hyperenhancement (APHE), a long-established, classic feature, of the traditional HCC lesion [52]
- Stromal invasion (tumor cells invading into the surrounding fibrous tissue) is the key feature distinguishing HCC from dysplastic nodules [53]. This is indistinguishable on gross pathology and can even be difficult to assess on histology. However, there are certain stains for biomarkers which can be utilized to help in the differentiation
- As the HCC grows larger and increases in surrounding invasion, the blood supply transitions to almost solely arterial supply. There is also increase in cell number, which causes displacement of the surrounding parenchyma leading to the additional classic feature of tumor capsule. Vascular and biliary invasion as well as intrahepatic metastases also become more frequent with progressed HCC
- Lastly, larger HCCs (>2 cm) are correlated to a higher grade, more aggressive behavior, and higher frequency of vascular invasion and intra/extrahepatic metastases. These lesions may have internal areas of hemorrhage, necrosis, and occasionally fatty metamorphosis [49,52]
- Venous drainage during hepatocarcinogenesis is variable as well. Initially, venous drainage is through the hepatic veins for RNs, dysplastic nodules, and early HCC. As the HCC progresses, there is transition to venous drainage through the sinusoids. Progressed HCC with fibrous capsule drains through the portal veins. This may explain the predilection of metastatic dissemination through the portal system rather than the hepatic venous system and may also explain the feature of "corona enhancement" in progressed disease [46]
- Fat and iron content also show distinct patterns throughout carcinogenesis. Initially, fat content increases as the lesion progresses from RNs to dysplastic nodules and to early HCC. Steatosis within the lesions peaks in early HCC measuring approximately 1.5 cm, and progressively declines as the size and grade of the tumor increase. Iron similarly is present within low-grade dysplastic nodules and some high-grade nodules. However, most high-grade nodules and HCC are devoid of iron content, likely related to utilization by the neoplastic cells [46]
- The imaging features of these nodules are listed in Table 33.4. These can be well predicted based on the pathophysiology discussed earlier

Surveillance

As described earlier, HCC is a major public health problem. A method to combat this problem is to detect and offer early treatment, which is associated with decreased mortality, while detection at an advanced stage is associated with a dismal prognosis. It has been previously identified that an adequate screening program benefits overall mortality rates in HCC. For example, a 2014 meta-analysis found HCC surveillance was associated with significantly prolong survival (OR 1.90, 95% CI 1.67–2.17) [54]. This was also found to be beneficial when taking into account the lead time bias (found to be approximately 6.5 months) associated with the surveillance test [55]

A successful surveillance program balances the cost and benefits of the detection test and progression of the disease process. A previous study of cirrhotic patients in Italy found a cost-effective benefit of both semiannual and annual surveillance in high-risk patients [56]. In congruence with this frequency, many of the leading hepatic medicine societies, such as the American Association for the Study of Liver Diseases (AASLD), recommend USG surveillance every 6 months in cirrhotic patients, and also in noncirrhotic patients with HBV infection with specific demographics (Asian male >40, Asian female >50, African or African-American, family history of HCC, etc.) [57,58]. As mentioned earlier, cases of HCC have been seen in the setting of other disease process without cirrhosis, such as NAFLD; however at this time, incidence rates do not meet surveillance criteria.

USG is a quick, cost-effective, and relatively harmless method for screening. Sensitivities for detecting HCC at any stage have been found to be in the low 90% range while sensitivity for early stage tumors is in the low 60% range. This increases to 70% when performing surveillance every 6 months as opposed to annually [58]. The addition of alpha-feto protein has been proposed; however, evidence supporting the benefit of AFP screening has been inconsistent as not all HCCs secrete AFP, and AFP can be elevated without HCC as well. It is recommended by the Asian professional liver societies in addition to USG, however, it is presented as an optional addition to USG by the AASLD.

CT and MRI are not utilized currently in the surveillance setting given the paucity of data on their efficacy and cost-effectiveness, despite their high diagnostic performance. Abbreviated MRI examinations may play an important role in surveillance in the future as the cost and accessibility of these exams becomes more reasonable as a surveillance technique. This is especially true in situations where USG is difficult, such as truncal obesity or marked parenchymal heterogeneity.

Ultrasound LI-RADS: The interpretation of surveillance US *in high-risk patients* can be guided by the US Liver Imaging-Reporting and Data System (LI-RADS) algorithm established in 2017. An "observation" is defined as any focal area distinct from background hepatic parenchyma and is preferred over the term "lesion," as it does not imply a level of suspicion. There are three diagnostic categories which can be applied to each US screening examination, US-1 (negative), US-2 (subthreshold), and US-3 (positive). It is important to remember that the categorization is applied to the entire exam and not individual lesions.

- If no observations are present, or the observation perceived is definitely benign, such as calcification, simple cyst, or previously identified hemangioma, then US-1 would be applied to this exam (Fig. 33.14)
- If the observation detected is less than 10 mm in diameter, and not definitely benign, then US-2 would be utilized (Fig. 33.15)
- Lastly, if the observation is larger than 10 mm in diameter and not definitely benign, or if there is a new thrombus identified in a vein, then exam would be categorized as US-3 (Fig. 33.16)

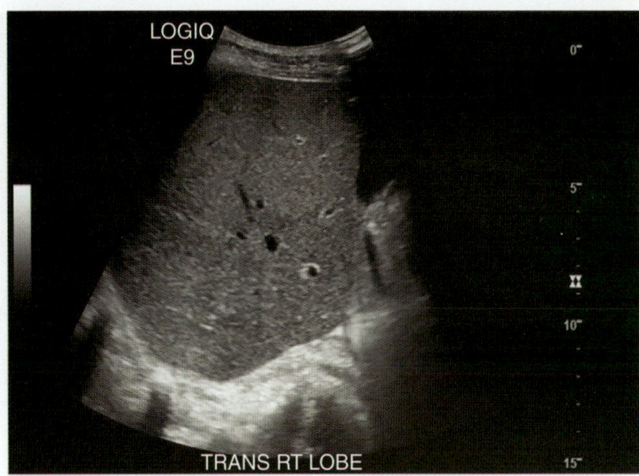

Figure 33.14 Ultrasound image from a patient with hepatitis B virus, who underwent HCC screening exam. There are no focal lesions in the liver, hence US-1.

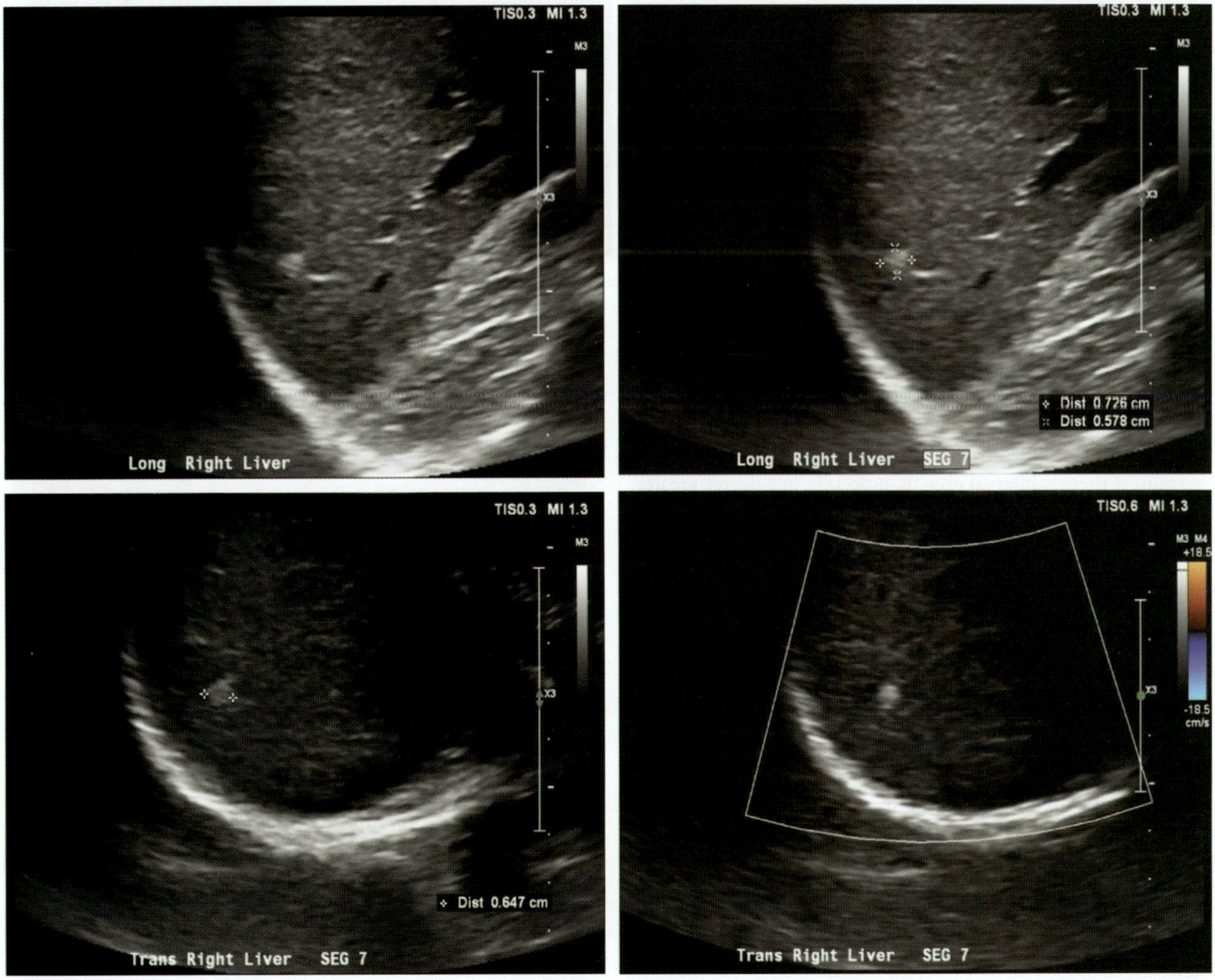

Figure 33.15 Hyperechoic lesion identified in the posterior right hepatic lobe (segment 7) on HCC screening exam. The lesion measures up to 7 mm, consistent with US-2 lesion.

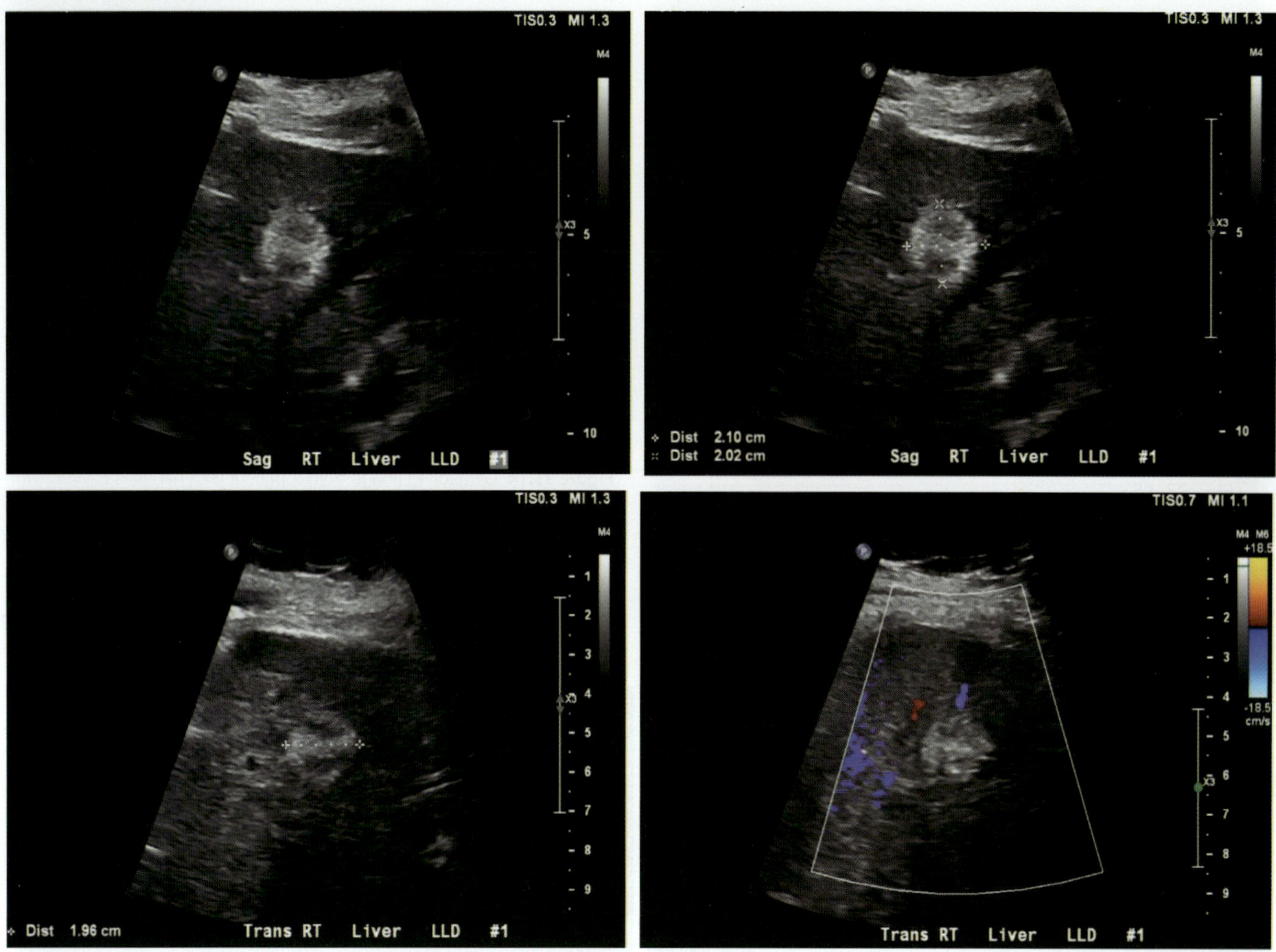

Figure 33.16 Slightly heterogenous, predominantly hyperechoic lesion identified on HCC screening ultrasound, measuring up to 21 mm, classified as US-3.

The threshold of 10 mm is applied between US-2 and US-3 because observations that are less than 10 mm are common, often benign, and difficult to characterize definitively on contrast-enhanced imaging. Therefore, observations resulting in US-2 categorization should be followed with a short interval US to determine if there is interval growth, especially to a degree greater than 10 mm in diameter, at which point it would warrant further evaluation with contrast-enhanced imaging. If an observation is stable and smaller than 10 mm over 2 years, it can be considered benign [59].

Management for the three categories is as follows:

- US-1 (negative): routine 6-month surveillance US
- US-2 (subthreshold): short interval (3–6 months) surveillance US recommended
- US-3 (positive): observation warrants multiphase contrast-enhanced exam (MR, CT, or USG)

In addition to a categorization, the exam will also receive a visualization score, ranging from A (no or minimal limitations) to C (severe limitations). With a score of A, limitations, if any are unlikely to meaningfully affect sensitivity. A score of B, moderate limitations, is applied when the limitation may obscure small masses. Finally, a score of C deems that the limitations significantly lower sensitivity for focal liver lesions. This is generally applied in situations when a majority of the liver or diaphragm is not visualized, or if there is severe heterogeneity of the liver, beam attenuation, or shadowing.

Key Pearls of Surveillance

- Surveillance USG every 6 months recommended in anyone with cirrhosis or select noncirrhotic patients with chronic HBV infection.
- Categories of US-1, US-2, and US-3 are given for all surveillance USG exams according to the LI-RADS criteria.
- Visualization scores of A, B, and C are applied, depending on the amount of liver and diaphragm that is visualized and how limited the exam is in detecting liver lesions.
- US-2 (observations <10 mm) exams are recommended to have short interval (3–6 months) follow-up to monitor for growth, while US-3 (observations >10 mm) should be further evaluated with multiphasic contrast-enhanced exam.

Diagnosis

Background and Technical Considerations

HCC is unique in that it is predominantly diagnosed by imaging features only, without the requirement of tissue sampling. Histopathologic confirmation of the diagnosis is avoided due to high specificity of the diagnosis through imaging and the risks and costs associated with biopsy. These include complications with the invasive procedure, as well as the low, but nonetheless concerning risk of biopsy tract seeding of approximately 2.7% [60].

First established in 2011, the LI-RADS aims to standardize imaging and reporting of studies used for the diagnosis of HCC in high-risk patients (namely, those with cirrhosis or chronic HBV, excluding a few select patients, for example, those under the age of 18 and patients with cirrhosis due to vascular causes). This classification system was initially established to be more specific in diagnosing HCC from imaging features alone and provide a high positive predictive value. A high specificity was desired because the definitive and preferred treatment in the United States for HCC is transplant, which is a great burden to undertake for the patients, providers, and healthcare system. Other countries, including Eastern countries, prefer early intervention over transplantation, likely related to the higher incidence of HBV-related HCC and better baseline liver function even in individuals presenting with HCC. Additionally, transplantation networks, resources, and coordination are often not as robust worldwide. For the early intervention treatment pathway, early detection is desired, thus exams with higher sensitivity are more prevalent often leading astray from the strict LI-RADS recommendations.

Subsequent updates to LI-RADS have occurred in 2013, 2014, and 2017 with advances in knowledge and technology. In 2018, the AASLD adopted LI-RADS into their clinical practice patterns, after alterations to the system were made for it to be in line with AASLD and Organ Procurement and Transplantation Network definitions and criteria. As such, LI-RADS was updated again in 2018, with anticipated updates occurring every 3–4 years in the future.

After detection of a liver lesion on surveillance USG larger than 10 mm (US-3), or as an incidental finding on other imaging techniques, a diagnostic algorithm is initiated, resulting in a multiphase CT or MRI examination. In some cases, CT or MRI imaging examination may be used as an alternative to USG surveillance (such as difficulty with USG exams due to body habitus), in which case the screening and diagnostic exam is the same. Liver protocol multiphase contrast-enhanced exams are performed with the following technical specifications guided by LI-RADS:

- CT (eight rows of detectors or greater)
  - Required: Arterial phase (late-arterial phase preferred ~35 seconds), portal-venous phase (~75 seconds), and delayed phase (3–5 minutes)
  - Optional: Precontrast if patient had locoregional treatment previously, multiplanar reformats
- MRI (1.5 or 3T with phased array torso coil)
  - Required: Unenhanced T1 in and out of phase imaging, T2-weighted imaging, T1-weighted arterial phase (late-arterial phase preferred), portal-venous phase, and delayed phase
  - Optional: Diffusion-weighted imaging, subtraction images, multiplanar acquisitions

The late-arterial phase is defined by the enhancement of the hepatic arteries and partial enhancement of the portal vein. Early arterial phase is when the hepatic arteries are the only vasculature opacified with contrast. The late-arterial phase is preferred to early arterial phase, as HCC enhances most avidly in the late-arterial phase where most of the contrast material has accumulated in the lesion. Subtraction imaging can help, especially with MRI, as intrinsic T1 signal can be separated from subtle enhancement within the lesion, which may be difficult on the raw images. Portal-venous phase subtraction can also be helpful in detecting subtle washout in the lesion, compared with background liver parenchyma, especially in lesions that have intrinsic T1 signal, perhaps from post-treatment change or internal hemorrhage. However, care must be taken when evaluating subtraction images to ensure that the lesions line up and there is no significant motion between the pre- and postcontrast images.

Imaging Interpretation

LI-RADS consists of several descriptive terms that an imaging abnormality in the liver can be defined with, as mentioned earlier. "Observation," "lesion," "mass," and "nodule" are terms used hierarchically to describe these abnormalities. A nodule is a type of mass, a mass is a type of lesion, and a lesion is a type of observation. Thus, all nodules are observations; however, not all observations are nodules. For example, an artifact or perfusion defect in the liver would be categorized as an "observation" as there is an imaging abnormality. It would however not be further classified as a lesion, mass, or nodule as there is no pathologic abnormality appreciated. Lesions would be further categorized as mass lesions, or nonmass lesions, which include focal fat or iron deposition. Masses are space-occupying such as infiltrative cholangiocarcinoma. Nodules are masses that have spherical or ovoid margins, such as typical HCC, which would also classify as a "mass," "lesion," and "observation." As a result, "observation" is used most often and is preferred to describe most imaging abnormalities in the liver [61].

Each observation is evaluated for the presence of certain features to determine the likelihood that the observation represents HCC. The major criteria (Figs. 33.17 and 33.18) that are used to favor HCC are as follows.

Major criteria

- *Arterial phase hyperenhancement*—Nonrim-like enhancement in arterial phase unequivocally greater in whole or in part than liver. The enhancing part must be higher in attenuation or intensity than background liver in arterial phase
- *Enhancing capsule*—Smooth, uniform, sharp border around most or all of an observation, unequivocally thicker or more

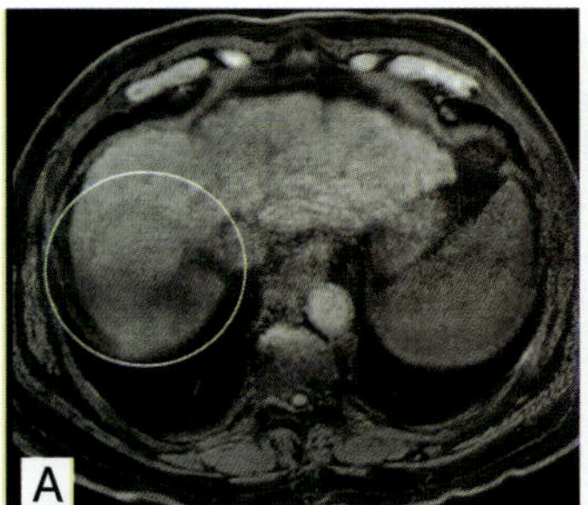

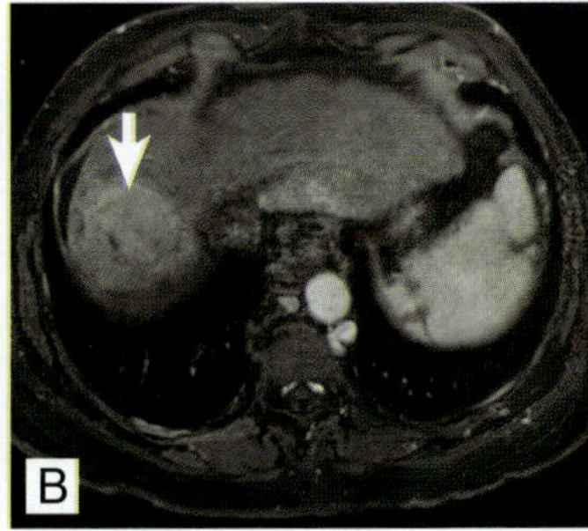

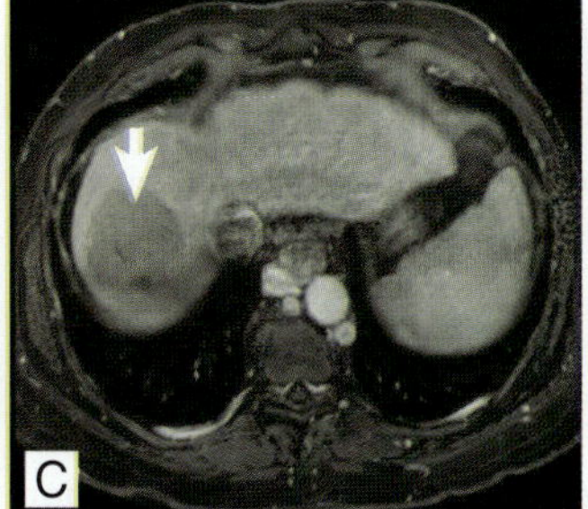

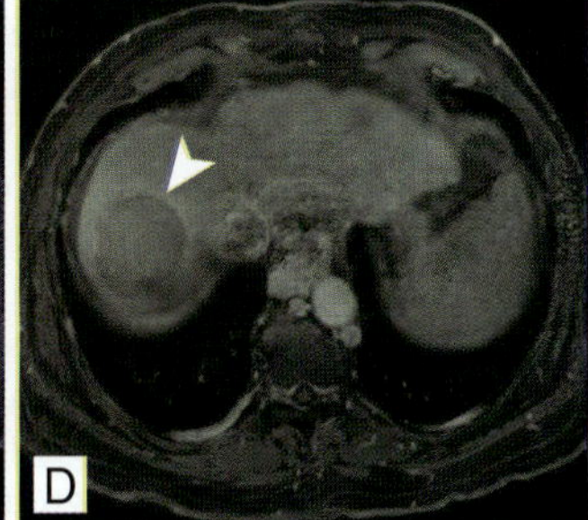

Figure 33.17 MRI of the abdomen with T1 precontrast (A), T1 arterial phase (B), T1 portal-venous phase (C), and T1 delayed phase images (D). Classic HCC near the dome of the liver with arterial phase hyperenhancement (*arrow*), washout on portal-venous phase (*thick arrow*), and enhancing pseudocapsule best seen on delayed phase (*arrowhead*). Note that the lesion is barely visible on the precontrast portion of the exam (*circle*). This lesion demonstrates the classic major features.

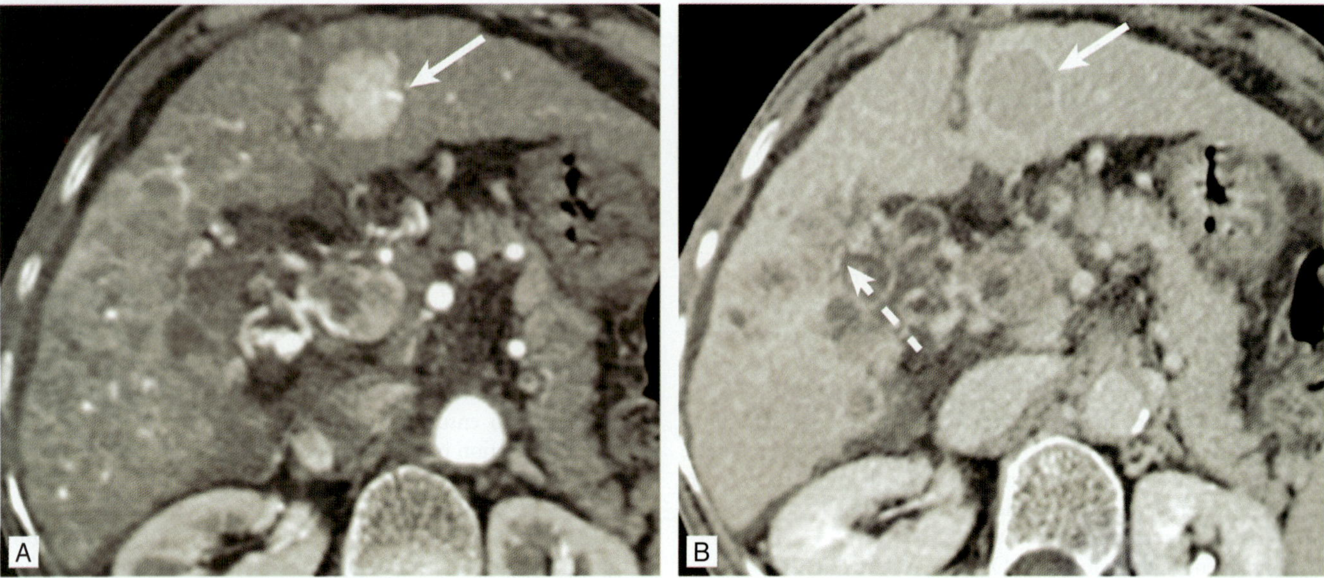

Figure 33.18 Late-arterial and delayed phase images demonstrate a segment III arterial hyperenhancing nodule (*arrow* in A) with washout and enhancing capsule (*solid arrow* in B), consistent with a LIRADS 5 lesion. Note an additional area of heterogeneity in segment IVb/V demonstrating washout on the delayed images (*dashed arrow* in B) without arterial hyperenhancement or enhancing capsule; LIRADS 4. (Courtesy: Akshay Baheti, Department of Radiodiagnosis, Tata Memorial Hospital.)

conspicuous than fibrotic tissue around background nodules, and visible as enhancing rim in portal-venous phase or delayed phase

- *Nonperipheral washout*—Nonperipheral, visually assessed, temporal reduction in enhancement in whole or in part relative to composite liver tissue from earlier to later phases (with gadoxetic acid, hypointensity must be present in portal-venous phase)
  - If a nodule does not have APHE, but demonstrates reduced enhancement from earlier to later phases (i.e., on delayed phase), this would be deemed as "washout." This feature in combination with APHE is much more specific for HCC rather than either feature alone
  - A nodule which enhances on arterial phase and has reduction in enhancement, but not below adjacent parenchyma would only be deemed as APHE, and have no "washout"
- *Threshold growth*—Size increase of a mass by ≥50% in ≤6 months
  - Only applied if observation is a mass. Do not apply if lesion can be a pseudolesion such as a perfusion abnormality
  - Only applicable when comparing to a sufficient quality previous CT or MRI. Not applicable when comparing to previous contrast-enhanced ultrasound (CEUS)
  - Measure on same phase, sequence, and plane if possible

The observations are then classified into categories of LR-1 to LR-5, based on likelihood of it being HCC, with LR-1 being definite certainty of benignity and LR-5 being definite certainty of HCC (Fig. 33.19).

- LR-1 (definite benign)—Definite cyst, hemangioma, vascular anomaly, perfusion alteration, focal scar, etc.
- LR-2 (probably benign)—Similar to LR-1 but the appearance is highly suggestive instead of diagnostically certain. For example, atypical hemangioma. A distinctive nodule without malignant features (solid nodule <20 mm distinctive compared with background nodules and with no major or ancillary features) is categorized as LR-2. This includes T2 hypointense, and T1 hyperintense, siderotic, or hepatobiliary phase hyperintense nodules
- LR-3 (indeterminate)—Not definitely benign and not definitely HCC. Nodules with ONE OR MORE ancillary features favoring malignancy and no features favoring benignity would be excluded from LR-2 and categorized as LR-3 (steatotic nodule, T2 hyperintense nodule, diffusion restricting nodule, HBP hypointense nodule, etc.). In a high-risk patient, nodules with features suggestive of focal nodular hyperplasia or hepatocellular adenoma usually should be LR-3, as these are diagnoses of exclusion in these patients. Performing an MRI with a hepatobiliary phase-contrast agent may significantly increase the specificity of identifying an FNH; such lesions may be categorized as LR-2 on these exams with caution
- LR-4 (probably HCC)—At least one major criteria is present. Depending on the size and presence of other major criteria, other observations can also fall into this category (Fig. 33.19)

CT/MRI Diagnostic Table

Arterial phase hyperenhancement (APHE)		No APHE		Nonrim APHE		
Observation size (mm)		< 20	≥ 20	< 10	10–19	≥ 20
Count additional major features: • Enhancing "capsule" • Nonperipheral "washout" • Threshold growth	None	LR-3	LR-3	LR-3	LR-3	LR-4
	One	LR-3	LR-4	LR-4	LR-4 / LR-5	LR-5
	≥ Two	LR-4	LR-4	LR-4	LR-5	LR-5

LR-4 / LR-5: Observations in this cell are categorized based on one additional major feature:
- LR-4 – if enhancing "capsule"
- LR-5 – if nonperipheral "washout" **OR** threshold growth

If unsure about the presence of any major feature: characterize that feature as absent

Figure 33.19 From the LI-RADS manual, this table is an easy reference to categorizes LR-3 to LR-5 observations based on the size and presence of certain imaging features [34]. In general, increase in the size and presence of major features results in a higher LR category. Note that LR-5 cannot be applied without APHE.

- LR-5 (definite HCC)—Observations 10 mm in size or larger and demonstrate APHE with at least one additional major feature
  - Exception: if the observation is between 10 and 19 mm in size and demonstrates APHE with only an enhancing capsule, then it would be categorized as LR-4

In addition to the major criteria, there are also additional ancillary features which can be used at radiologist discretion to improve detection, increase confidence, or adjust the final category up or down by 1, between LR-1 and LR-4. These features are grouped as in favor of HCC (Figs. 33.20–33.23), in favor of malignancy (not HCC in particular) (Fig. 33.24), or in favor of benignity (Fig. 33.25). It is important to remember that ancillary features can never upgrade an observation to LR-5 (Fig. 33.26) [61].

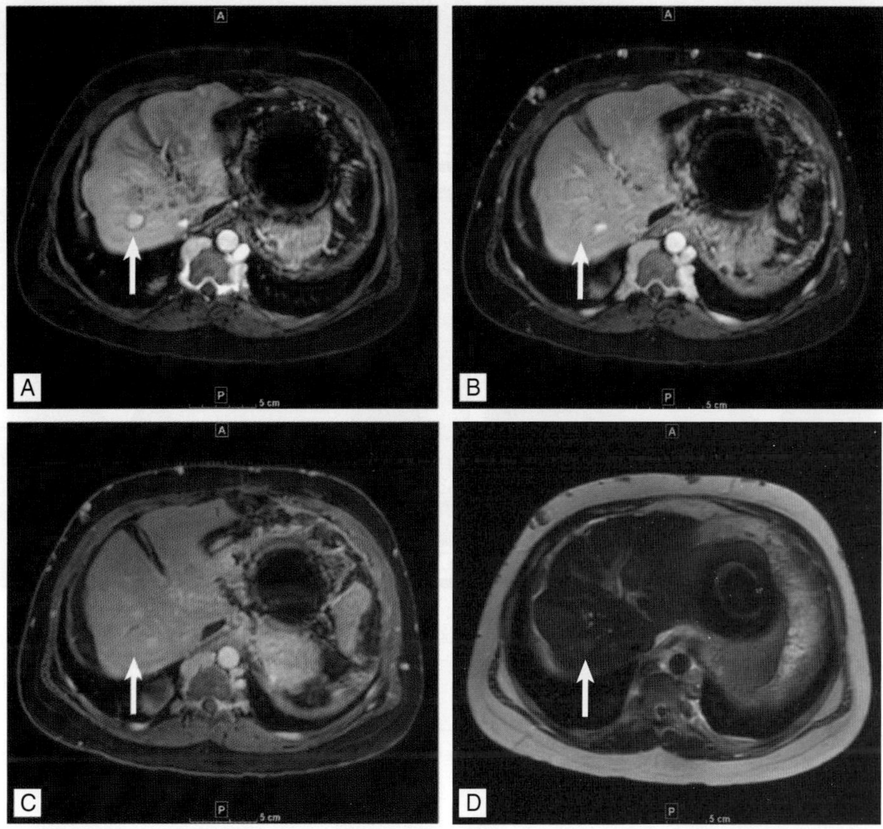

Figure 33.20 Nonenhancing capsule around a focal hepatic lesion (*arrows*). There is arterial phase hyper enhancement (A), without definitive washout (B and C), but T2 moderate hyperintensity (D). The lesion measures approximately 14 mm, categorizing it as LR-3; however, the nonenhancing capsule, an ancillary feature favoring HCC, can be used to upgrade this lesion to LR-4.

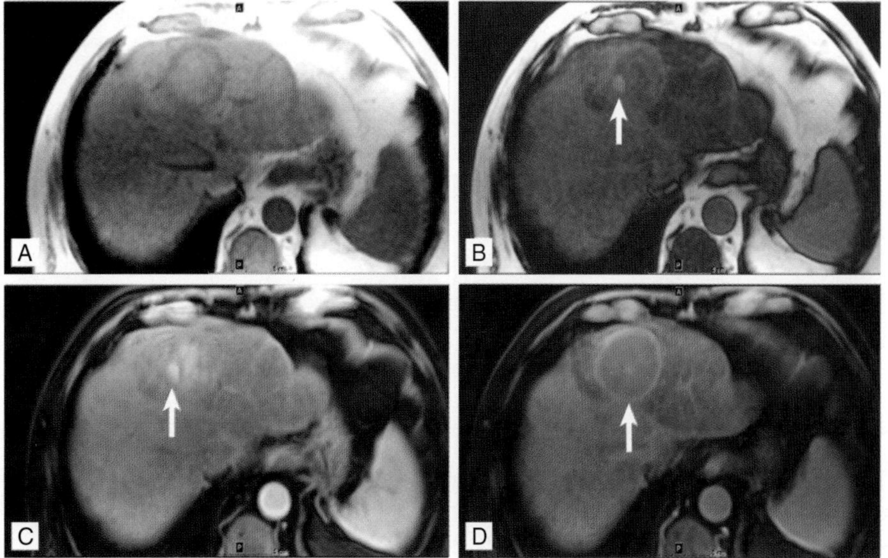

Figure 33.21 In and out of phase images (A and B) demonstrate loss of signal in majority of the mass, except of one nodule within (*arrow*, B). This nodule also demonstrates avid arterial phase hyperenhancement (*arrow*), while mild patchy arterial phase enhancement in the rest of the mass (C). The entire mass demonstrates an enhancing capsule (*arrow* in D). This nodule-in-nodule characteristic is indicative of HCC. Given that other signs of HCC are also present, this mass would be classified as LR-5.

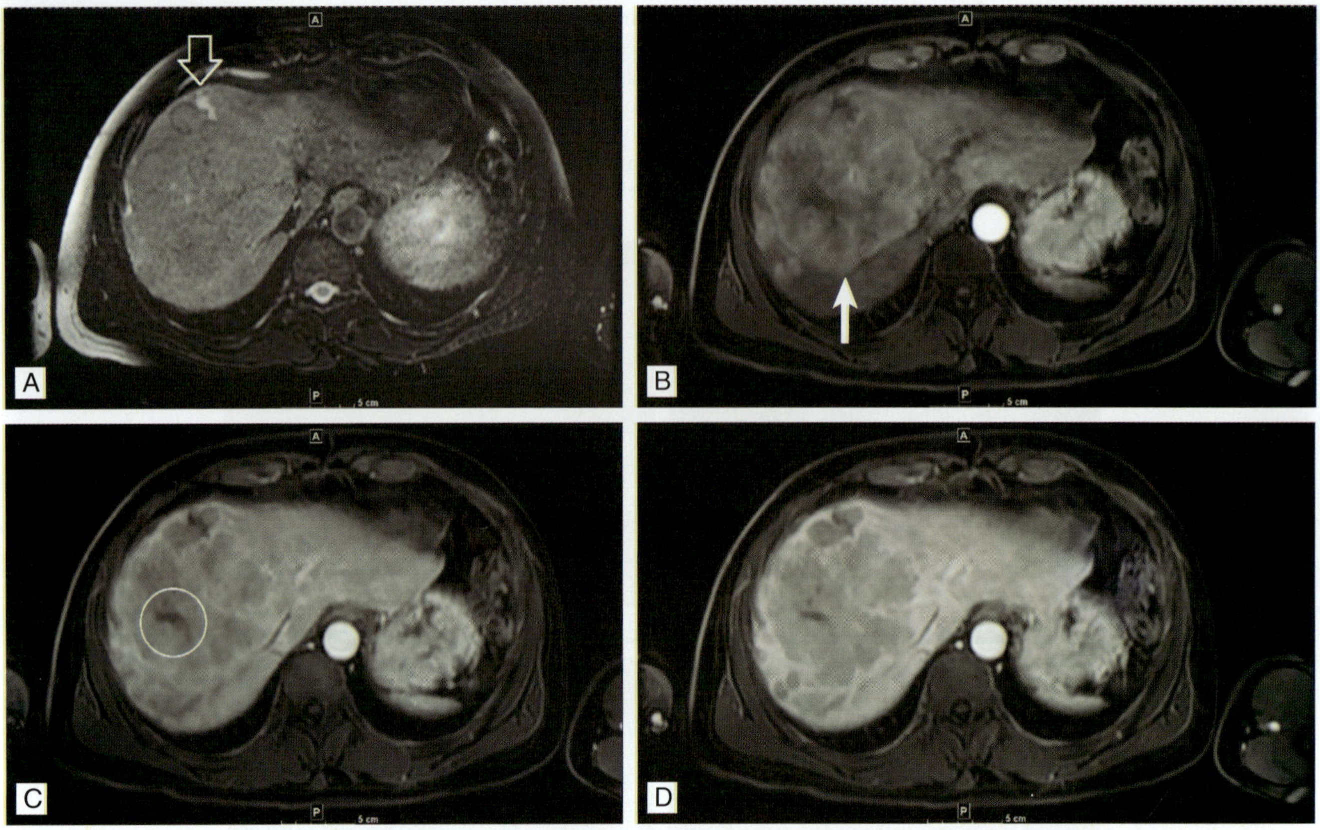

Figure 33.22 Large HCC in the right hepatic lobe demonstrating mosaic architecture. Note that the T2 signal in image (A) demonstrating more cystic portions of the mass (*hollow arrow*), in addition to arterially enhancing portions (*arrow* in B), as well as T1 hypointense central portions (*circle* in C). The mass demonstrates washout on the delayed phase (D). These varying features are suggestive of underlying HCC.

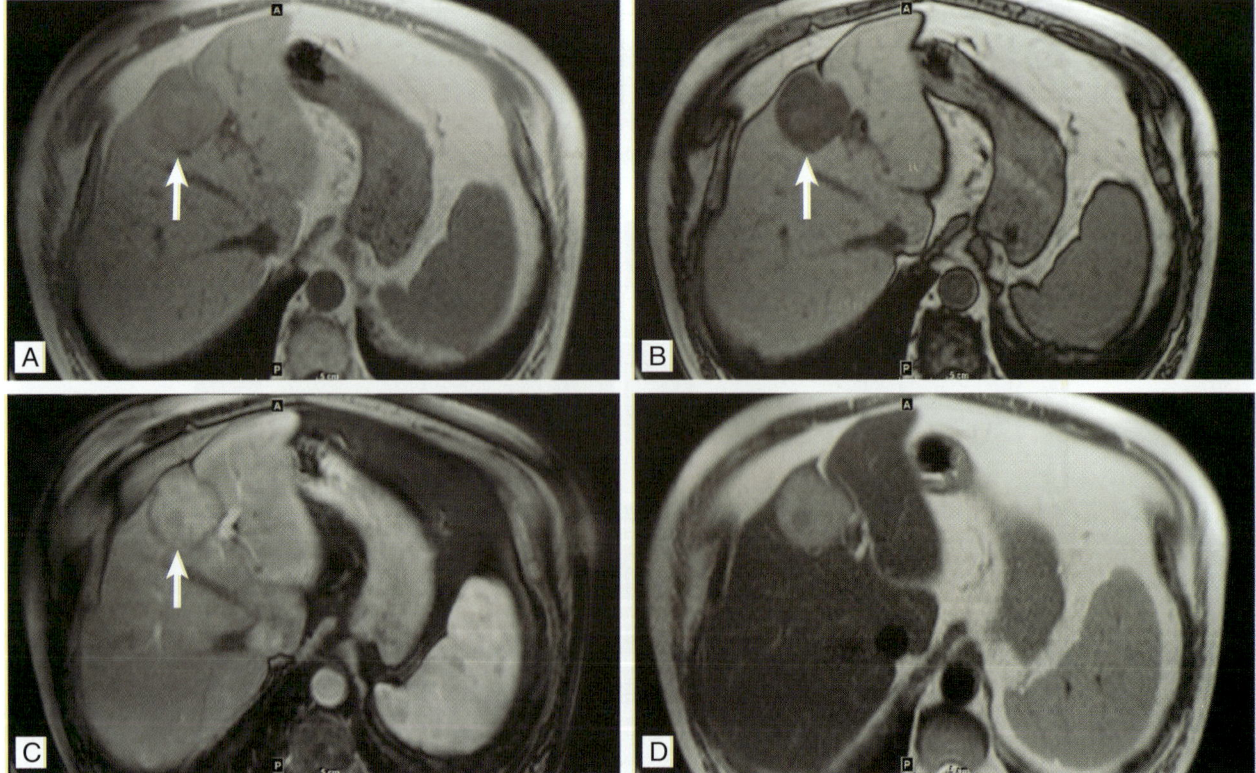

Figure 33.23 The mass in segment 4a demonstrates drop in signal on the in and out of phase images (*arrows* in A and B respectively), indicative of fat within the lesion, a sign suggestive of underlying HCC. Additional feature of nodule within nodule, nonenhancing capsule (*arrow* in C), and moderate T2 hyperintensity (*arrow* in D) also favor HCC and malignancy, respectively.

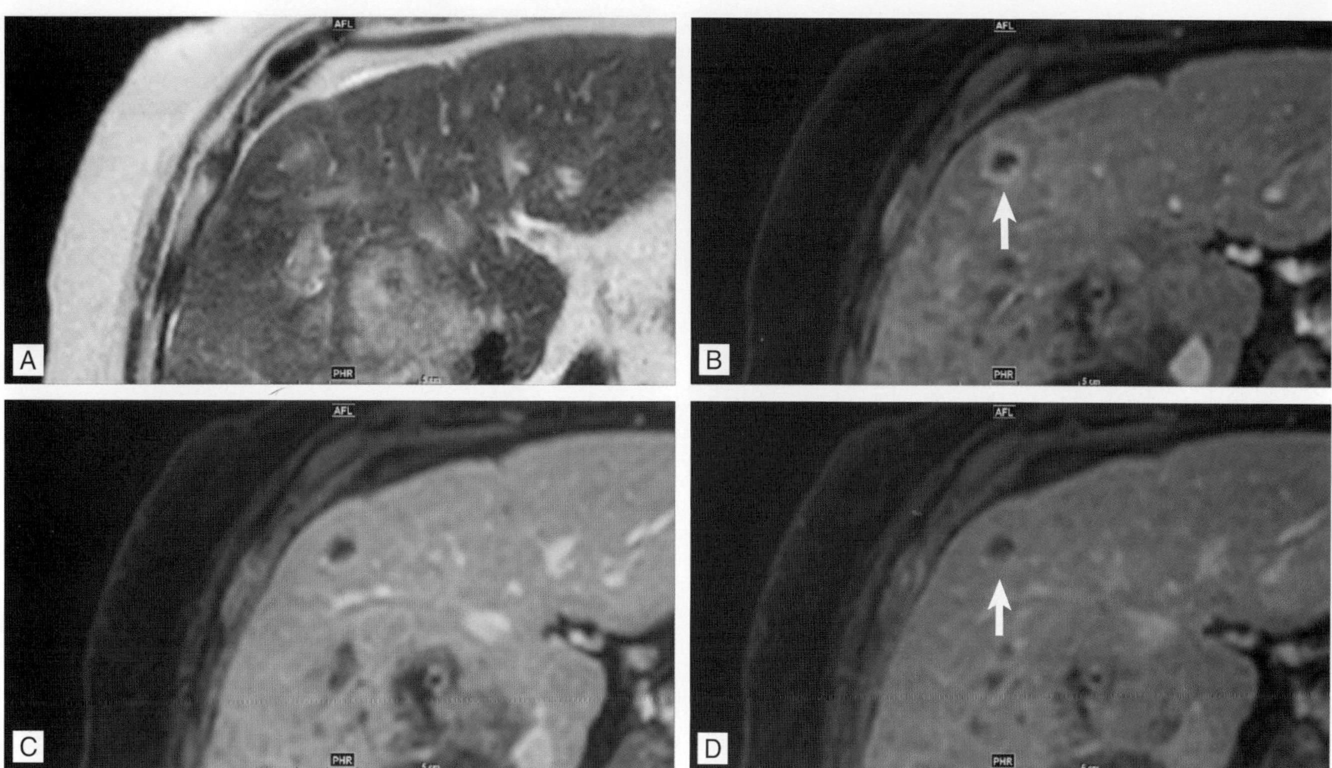

Figure 33.24 Note that the slightly ill-defined, thicker corona enhancement surrounding the lesion, which is only seen in arterial phase (*arrow*, B). This is not seen on the delayed phase images (*arrow* in D). The enhancement is due to early sinusoidal drainage from the lesion. This lesion is LR-M.

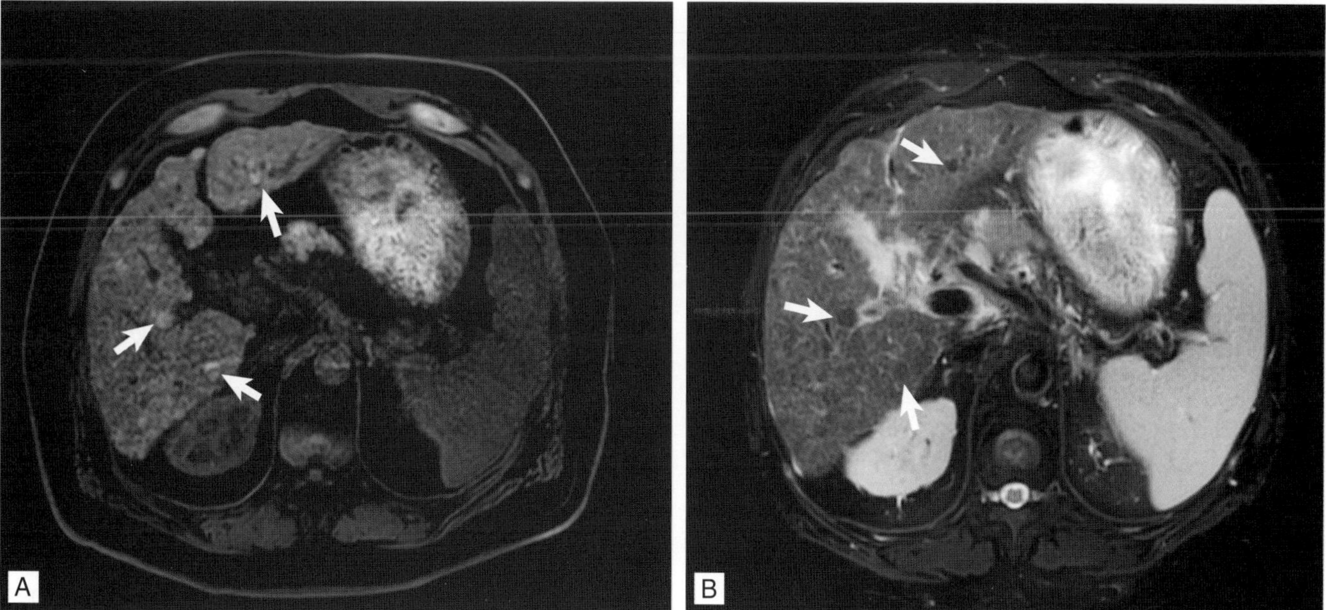

Figure 33.25 Numerous T1 hyperintense (A) and T2 hypointense (B) nodules are identified in the liver indicative of siderotic nodules, which would be classified as LR-2. Iron accumulation generally favors a benign process. If there is presence of iron sparing in a lesion (less iron than background liver), it is presumed that the cells within the lesion are utilizing the available iron stores, an indication of malignant growth.

Ancillary Features Favoring HCC

- Nonenhancing capsule (Fig. 33.20)
- Nodule-in-nodule (Fig. 33.21)
  - Smaller inner nodule within and having different imaging features than larger outer nodule, consistent with the pathophysiology of HCC of gradual dedifferentiation of nodules
- Mosaic architecture (Fig. 33.22)
  - Randomly distributed internal nodules or compartments usually with different imaging features
- Blood products in mass
- Fat in mass, more than adjacent liver (Fig. 33.23)
  - Relative ischemia in transition from dysplastic nodule to early HCC with transition from portal venous to arterial supply contributes to fatty change. The presence of fat indicates a hepatocytic process (and not say a cholangiocellular process). Thus this is a specific, yet not very sensitive feature of HCC

Ancillary Features Favoring Malignancy

- USG visibility as discrete nodule
- Subthreshold growth
- Diffusion restriction
  - Highly sensitive for detections of additional lesions
- Mild–moderate T2 hyperintensity
- Corona enhancement (Fig. 33.24)
  - Periobservational enhancement in late-arterial or early portal-venous phase due to accumulation of contrast in hepatic sinusoids.
- Fat sparing in solid mass
- Iron sparing in solid mass
  - Hypothesized that malignant cells will use free iron in growth thus relatively decrease
- Transitional phase hypointensity
- Hepatobiliary phase hypointensity

Features Favoring Benignity

- Size stability >2 years
- Size reduction
- Parallels blood pool
- Undistorted vessels
- Iron in mass, more than liver (Fig. 33.25)
  - Siderotic nodule will collect iron before transitioning to malignancy
- Marked T2 hyperintensity
  - Suggests cystic lesion if marked T2 hyperintensity. Moderate T2 hyperintensity is an ominous sign, usually signaling malignant pathology.
- Hepatobiliary phase isointensity.

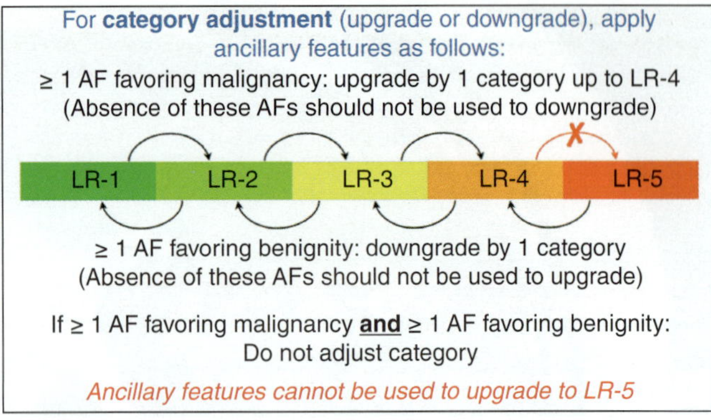

Figure 33.26 Application of LIRADS ancillary features for category adjustment. Categories can be upgraded or downgraded based on ancillary feature favoring malignancy or favoring benignity. Ancillary features can never upgrade a lesion the LR-5.

There are also three categories outside the LR-1 to LR-5 categories listed earlier, which are special categories.

- LR-NC (not categorizable)—The technical quality of the imaging study does not allow for adequate evaluation of the major features
- LR-TIV (tumor in vein)—Unequivocal enhancing soft tissue in vein, regardless of visualization of parenchymal mass. This finding is a contraindication to liver transplantation, thus important to identify and report. Differentiating bland versus tumor thrombus can be difficult; however, some clues which may hint at TIV, but are not diagnostic, include an occluded vein with ill-defined walls, diffusion restriction, or contiguity with a malignant parenchymal mass. In these cases, scrutinize carefully for enhancing thrombus (Fig. 33.27). After TIV is identified, the most probable etiology should be determined and reported. If the TIV is contiguous with a targetoid mass then it should be reported as "LR-TIV, may be due to non-HCC malignancy." If it is contiguous with LR-5 mass then it would be deemed "LR-TIV, definitely due to HCC." Otherwise, it is to be reported as "LR-TIV, probably due to HCC"
- LR-M—Probably or definitely malignant observation that is not necessarily HCC; more than half of these are intrahepatic cholangiocarcinomas or mixed tumors, while approximately 42% are diagnosed as HCCs (atypical HCCs)
  - Targetoid mass—For example, arterial phase enhancement is most pronounced in the periphery with peripheral washout and delayed central enhancement. This can also be seen as a targetoid mass on DWI with restricted diffusion in the periphery
  - Nontargetoid mass with infiltrative appearance, marked diffusion restriction, necrosis or severe ischemia, or any other appearance that in the radiologist's judgment suggests malignancy
    - HCC can sometimes also have an infiltrative appearance (Fig. 33.28). This type of HCC is more likely to cause TIV

Each observation should be evaluated with the LI-RADs system above. If there is uncertainty in imaging characteristics of any observation, then the category reflecting less certainty should be chosen as the philosophy of LIRADS is to be more specific and have a high positive predictive value. For example, an observation demonstrating APHE measuring 15 mm with possible but uncertain enhancing capsule, should be deemed LR-3, rather than LR-4 unless there is any suspicious ancillary feature present. Similarly, if there is uncertainty about a lesion being definitely benign, then LR-2 should be selected over LR-1 [61].

Based on the LI-RADS classification of each lesion, follow-up recommendations will guide management of the patient. Probabilities of the lesion being HCC and the progression to

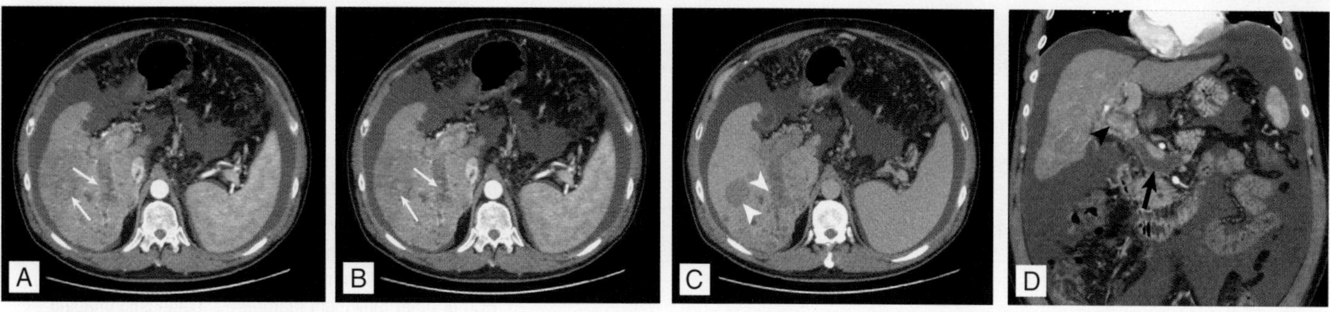

Figure 33.27 Axial CT of the abdomen in arterial (A), portal venous (B), and delayed phase (C), as well as coronal reformat in the arterial phase (D). There is arterially enhancing nodular foci in the right portal vein and in the hepatic parenchyma (*white arrows*), which demonstrate progressive washout on portal-venous phase (*thick white arrows*), and delayed phase imaging (*white arrowheads*). The lesion in the parenchyma is consistent with LR-5 categorization; however, the tumor in vein is more relevant in this patient and would be deemed LR-TIV. The coronal image demonstrates the difference in appearance between bland *nonenhancing* thrombus (*black arrow*) near the portal confluence and tumor thrombus (*black arrowhead*) near the portal bifurcation.

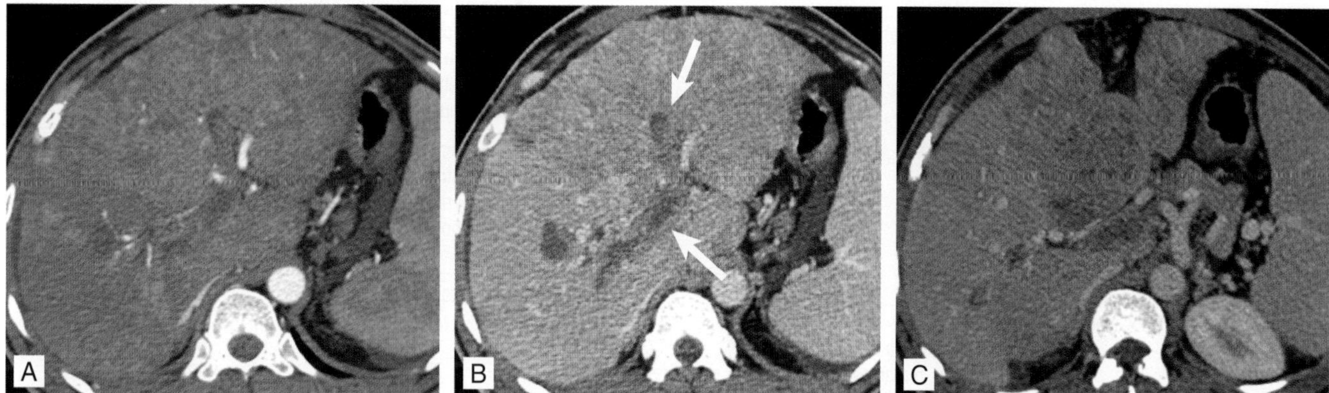

Figure 33.28 Late-arterial (A) and delayed phase (B and C) images demonstrate diffuse ill-defined patchy arterial hyperenhancement without a well-defined measurable nodule along with washout which is better appreciable on an inferior section (C). Tumor thrombus is present in the right and left portal veins (*arrows*). Findings are consistent with an infiltrative HCC. (Courtesy: Akshay Baheti, Department of Radiodiagnosis, Tata Memorial Hospital.)

malignancy of each category of LI-RADS has also been quantified using historical data and classification. A summary of these data is provided in Table 33.5.

Contrast-Enhanced Ultrasound

CEUS has also been proposed as a method used to diagnose HCC. A recent meta-analysis showed a pooled sensitivity and specificity of 85% and 91%, respectively [62].

A LI-RADS CEUS manual was also developed in 2017. This system also relies predominantly on the classic APHE and washout pattern of HCC as the backbone for categorization. A recent study showed that the LI-RADS CEUS categorization had a sensitivity of 73% and a specificity of 97% in diagnosing HCC in nodules less than 20 mm in high-risk patients [63].

Because of the way the contrast material behaves, however, there is also APHE and washout in other malignant lesions as well. HCCs demonstrate mild and late washout (≥60 seconds), while other malignancies have early (<60 seconds) and/or marked washout (Fig. 33.29). Therefore, the radiologist should have confidence in their ability to accurately evaluate the timing and degree of the washout characteristics when using CEUS. Other challenges include that image acquisition is user dependent, requires visualization of the observation on precontrast images, and cannot adequately evaluate the rest of the liver for other lesions. Also, there is not adequate imaging information for accurate staging from this study, for example, lymphadenopathy and metastatic disease.

Due to these current limitations, the AASLD has not adopted CEUS as a recommended study for the diagnosis of HCC. Organ Procurement and Transplantation Network also does not accept HCC diagnosis currently from only CEUS examinations. Overall, this method can be useful as a supplement to troubleshoot difficult observations. Further evaluation and prospective studies are needed to establish the utility of CEUS in the diagnosis and management of HCC.

Key Pearls of Diagnosis

- HCC is predominantly diagnosed with imaging only, rarely needing tissue biopsy for confirmation.
- LI-RADS aims to standardize imaging and diagnosis of HCC in high-risk patients. The term "observation" is preferred to describe imaging abnormalities in the liver. This system has been adopted by the AASLD recently as part of their clinical practice guidelines.
- LR-1 to LR-5 categories are applied predominantly based on the size and presence of major features of HCC. Ancillary features can help increase or decrease the LR category by 1. Each observation receives its own LR score.
- LR-5 observations require the presence of APHE.
- CEUS can also be used to diagnose HCC, although at this time it is not recommended as a primary tool by the major societies.

TABLE 33.5 LI-RADS Summary

Category	Meaning	Probability of HCC [30]	Progression to Malignancy on 24-Month Follow-Up	Example	Follow-Up
LR-1	Definitely benign	0%	None	▪ Definite cysts, hemangioma, perfusion anomaly, focal fat, etc.	Return to 6 month surveillance
LR-2	Probably benign	11%	0–6%	▪ Probably cyst, hemangioma, perfusion anomaly, focal fat, etc. ▪ Solid nodule <20 mm without HCC or other malignant features	Return to 6 month surveillance Consider repeat diagnostic imaging in ≤6 months
LR-3	Indeterminate probability of malignancy	33%	6–15%	▪ 12 mm observation with APHE only ▪ 17 mm observation with only enhancing capsule	Repeat alternative diagnostic imaging in 3–6 months
LR-4	Probably HCC	80%	46–68%	▪ 25 mm observation with APHE ▪ 15 mm observation APHE and enhancing capsule ▪ 23 mm observation without APHE, but has nonperipheral washout and threshold growth	Multidisciplinary discussion for tailored workup May include biopsy
LR-5	Definitely HCC	96%	N/A	▪ >10 mm observation with APHE and either enhancing capsule, nonperipheral washout or threshold growth	HCC confirmed Multidisciplinary discussion for consensus management
LR-M	Malignancy, but not HCC specific	42% HCC 57% other (ICC, combined HCC and ICC, lymphoma, metastases, etc.)	N/A	▪ Targetoid mass	Multidisciplinary discussion for work up. May include biopsy
LR-TIV	Tumor in vein	N/A	N/A	▪ Enhancing tumor in the portal vein	Multidisciplinary discussion for work up. May include biopsy
LR-NC	Not categorizable	N/A	N/A	▪ Significant breathing motion artifact or deficient contrast timing	Repeat alternative diagnostic imaging in ≤3 months

Staging and Treatment

Once a diagnosis of HCC has been established, either as an LR-5 observation, through biopsy, or presumptive diagnosis with multidisciplinary consultation in a LR-4 or LR-TIV observation, staging is the next step. The most commonly used and endorsed staging system is the Barcelona Clinic Liver Cancer (BCLC) algorithm [57,64–67], which takes into account the degree of liver disease to balance the benefits and harms of treating the tumor.

In the BCLC algorithm, patients are stratified based on the degree of tumor burden, defined by the number and size of HCC nodules, vascular invasion, and extrahepatic spread. In addition, the liver dysfunction is also measured to help categorize the patients into an appropriate treatment regimen. Traditionally, the Child–Turcotte–Pugh classification has been used, which assess the total bilirubin, serum albumin, INR, presence of ascites, and presence of hepatic encephalopathy to grade the severity of liver disease. Unfortunately, this does not take into account significant factors that could signal end-stage liver disease such as bacterial peritonitis, renal failure, hyponatremia, etc [66]. Thus other scores, such as the albumin–bilirubin grade, and model for end-stage liver disease (MELD) are also taken into account to assess liver function in these patients [67]. In addition, the Eastern Cooperative Oncology Group score is also assessed to gauge the patient's general well-being and ability to perform activities of daily living to help in stratification.

Patients in very early stage (0) and early stage (A) are defined as having a solitary HCC nodule ≤2 cm, or up to 3 nodules ≤3 cm, respectively (Fig. 33.30). They also have preserved liver function and fully active performance status. These patients can benefit from resection, ablation, or transplantation based on varying factors affecting each treatment and outcome, such as portal pressures, bilirubin, and other associated diseases. Optimal candidates for surgical resection are those that have relatively preserved liver function, and thus can tolerate resection of parenchyma and endure the stress of the surgery and postsurgical recovery. These candidates are classified as Child–Pugh A, without clinically significant portal hypertension or elevated bilirubin [68,69]. It is important to remember that the size of the solitary nodule in early stage disease does not exclude the patient from resection.

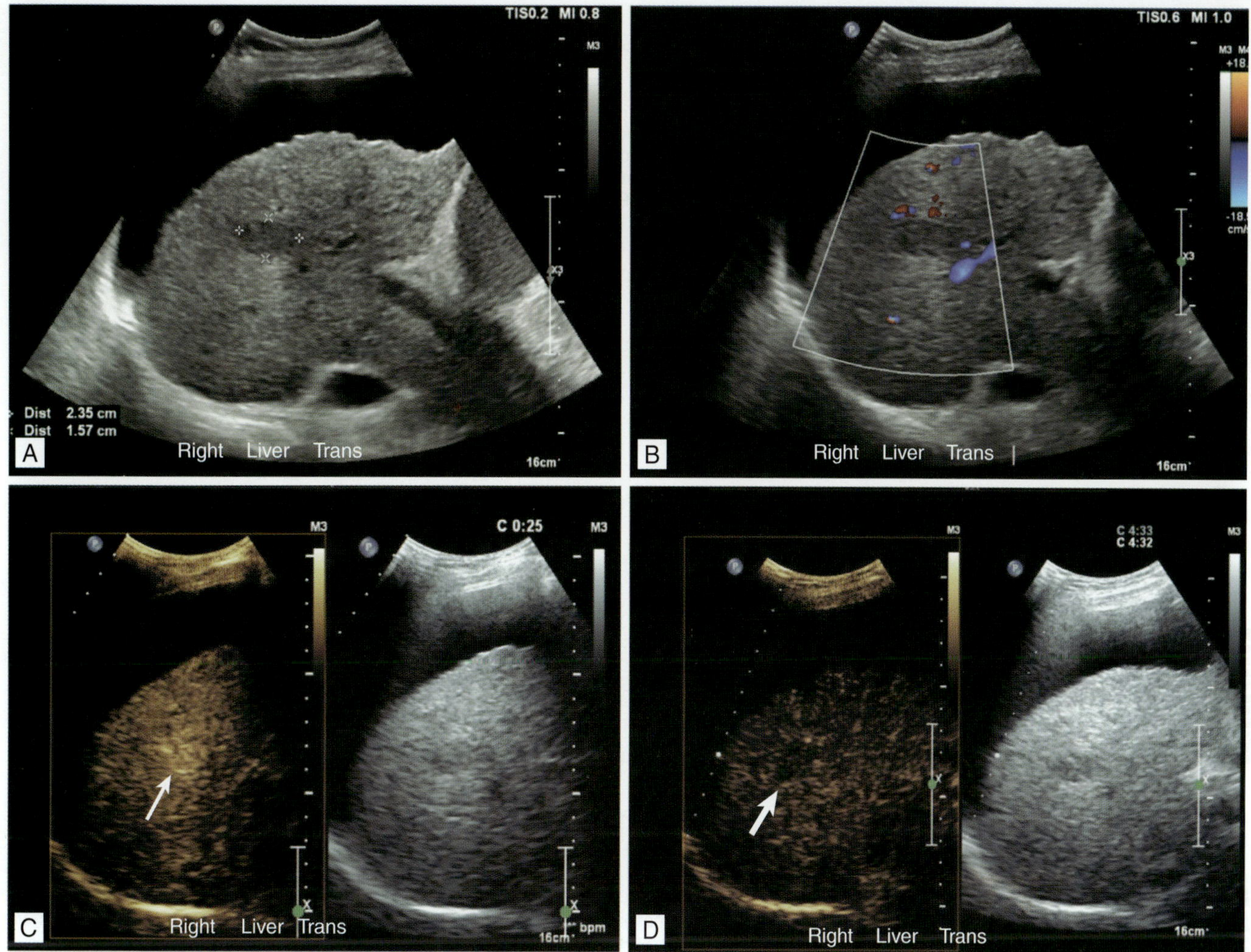

Figure 33.29 Contrast-enhanced ultrasound with precontrast images (A), color Doppler (B), arterial phase images (C), and delayed phase images (D). The observation is hypoechoic on precontrast images without evidence of internal vascularity, and subsequently shows arterial phase enhancement (*white arrow*), and delayed phase washout (*thick white arrow*). This is consistent with an LR-5 lesion, HCC.

The Milan criteria are generally accepted as guidance for liver transplantation in patients with cirrhosis and HCC who are not candidates for resection. The criteria state that patients with a single nodule ≤5 cm, or up to 3 nodules less ≤3 cm, with no extrahepatic involvement and no major vessel involvement are deemed suitable transplant candidates [67]. Patients may receive neoadjuvant treatments, including ablation and transarterial therapies, to reduce tumor progression or even make previously ineligible candidates eligible for transplantation.

Patients with stage 0 or A disease who are not eligible for resection or transplant are recommended to undergo ablation. The main method is image guided, percutaneous radiofrequency ablation, which increases intratumoral temperature, thereby inducing necrosis. Alternatives include microwave ablation, cryoablation, and ethanol injection. Ablation has been found to be comparable to resection in smaller sized tumors (less than 2 cm) in favorable locations. However, local control of larger tumors is not as beneficial [67].

Intermediate stage (B) has large multinodular disease, defined as greater than three HCC nodules or ≥2 nodules if any are larger than 3 cm without vascular invasion or extrahepatic spread. These patients still have preserved liver function and fully active performance status. The only treatment that shows a survival benefit in these patients is transarterial chemoembolization (TACE) predominantly performed by interventional radiologists. Bland embolization without the chemotherapeutic agents is a more controversial treatment. Transarterial radioembolization, or selective internal radiation therapy, is a similar and promising option to TACE using the radioisotope yttrium-90 (Y90) infused microspheres as the antitumoral agent rather than a chemical agent. Although initial investigation has shown effectiveness of this method, further research is needed to establish this as a viable treatment option [69].

Patients with advanced stage (C) demonstrate extrahepatic spread, portal invasion, and/or mild cancer-related symptoms (Eastern Cooperative Oncology Group- Performance Score (ECOG-PS 1-2)). These patients have a median overall survival without treatment of 4–10 months and are recommended to undergo systemic therapy to prolong survival times. Sorafenib a multikinase inhibitor with antiangiogenic and antiproliferative effects has been shown to increase median survival from 7.9 months to 10.7 months when compared with placebo [70]. Recently, Levatinib has also been approved for use as a first-line systemic therapy agent. Options as second-line agents, if first-line therapy fails, include regorafenib, cabozantinib, and ramucirumab.

Terminal stage (D) patients are patients that are not transplant candidates with end-stage liver disease and/or patients with severe cancer-related symptoms (EGOG >2). These patients do not benefit from current therapies and the best option is to offer supportive care [69].

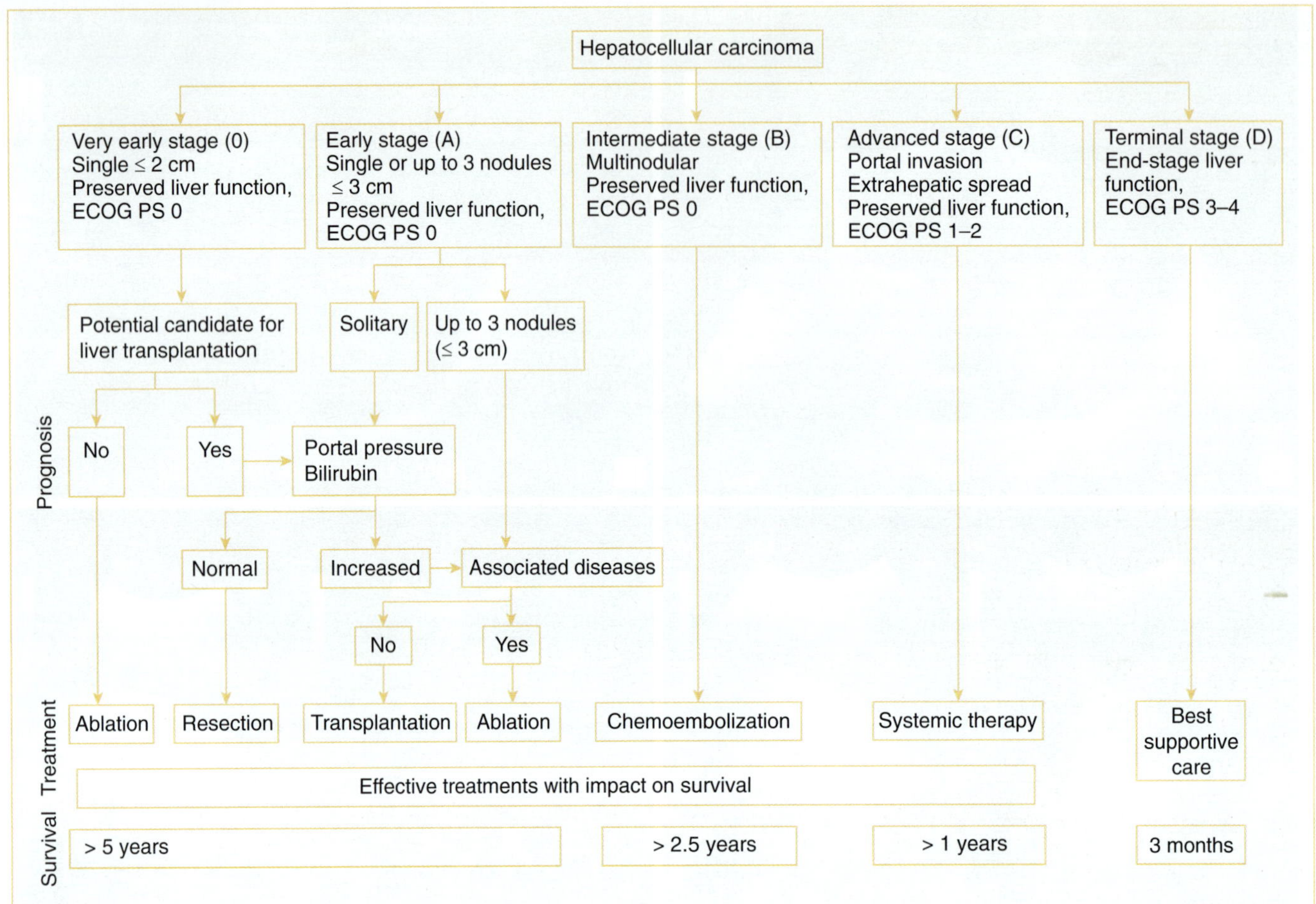

Figure 33.30 The BCLC is used to help stratify patients into different stages, which help in prognostication and guiding therapy. The criteria take into account both the degree of tumor burden and the liver function of the patient as both will affect the patients' ability to tolerate specific treatments. Very early and early stage patients will be able to undergo resection, ablation, and transplantation treatments, while these may not be feasible options for later stage patients. (Redrawn from Forner et al. [66].)

Key Pearls of Staging and Treatment

- Staging should consider the tumor burden as well as the liver function and functional status of the patient. The BCLC uses these to stratify patients into different stages.
- Best prognosis is for patients who have very early disease, who meet criteria to undergo tumor resection.
- For intermediate disease, TACE is the only therapy which has demonstrated improved outcomes.
- Advanced stage disease has a median survival of approximately 8 months increased to 11 months with systemic therapies.
- Terminal stage patients are those with end-stage liver disease that cannot undergo transplantation, which can be offered best supportive care.

Post-Treatment Follow-Up

After patients undergo local treatment, they receive repeat imaging to evaluate for residual or recurrent disease, usually every 3 months. Upon repeat CT/MRI imaging, LI-RADS has an algorithm for the treatment response, which can be used to stratify patients in different categories, based on imaging findings, and provide guidelines for follow-up and management. For each observation that is treated, the following categories they can either be classified as LR-TR nonviable, LR-TR equivocal, LR-TR viable, or LR-TR nonevaluable. Table 33.6 summarizes the definitions and follow-up for each.

Normal post-treatment findings include T1 hyperintensity or increased density throughout the lesion, predominantly related to post-treatment hemorrhage, and coagulative necrosis within the lesion. Liquified portions within the treated lesion may also demonstrate T2 hyperintensity. On postcontrast imaging, a thin peripheral enhancement along the ablation margin and subtle adjacent parenchymal enhancement may be normally present in the first 6 months due to reactive hyperemia.

Similar to the de novo evaluation of a lesion, if there is uncertainty between two categories, the one reflecting lower certainty should be selected (LR-TR nonviable → LR-TR equivocal, and LR-TR viable → LR-TR equivocal). Often, immediately post-treatment, enhancement can be variable, and difficult to differentiate viable tumor from post-treatment enhancement changes. This is a common scenario that is reported as LR-TR equivocal. Over time, the atypical pattern of enhancement should reduce or stabilize, demonstrating higher likelihood of benignity.

Once it is determined that a patient indeed has viable tumor, the size of this viable region should be obtained as the longest dimension through the enhancing area of the treated lesion, not traversing the nonenhancing area. These patients will be followed

TABLE 33.6 LI-RADS Treatment Categories

LR-TR Category	Definition	Follow-Up
Nonviable (Fig. 33.31)	There is no lesion enhancement or there is expected treatment-related enhancement.	Continue monitoring in ≤3 months with same or different technique.
Equivocal (Fig. 33.32)	Enhancement is present and atypical for a treatment-related pattern, however, it does not meet criteria for probably or definitively viable.	Continue monitoring in ≤3 months with same or different technique.
Viable (Fig. 33.33)	Nodular, mass-like, or thick irregular tissue in or along the treated lesion demonstrating either APHE, washout, OR enhancement similar to the pretreatment pattern.	Multidisciplinary discussion for consensus management. Often includes retreatment.
Nonevaluable	The treatment response cannot be evaluated due to image degradation or omission.	Continue monitoring in ≤3 months with same or different technique.

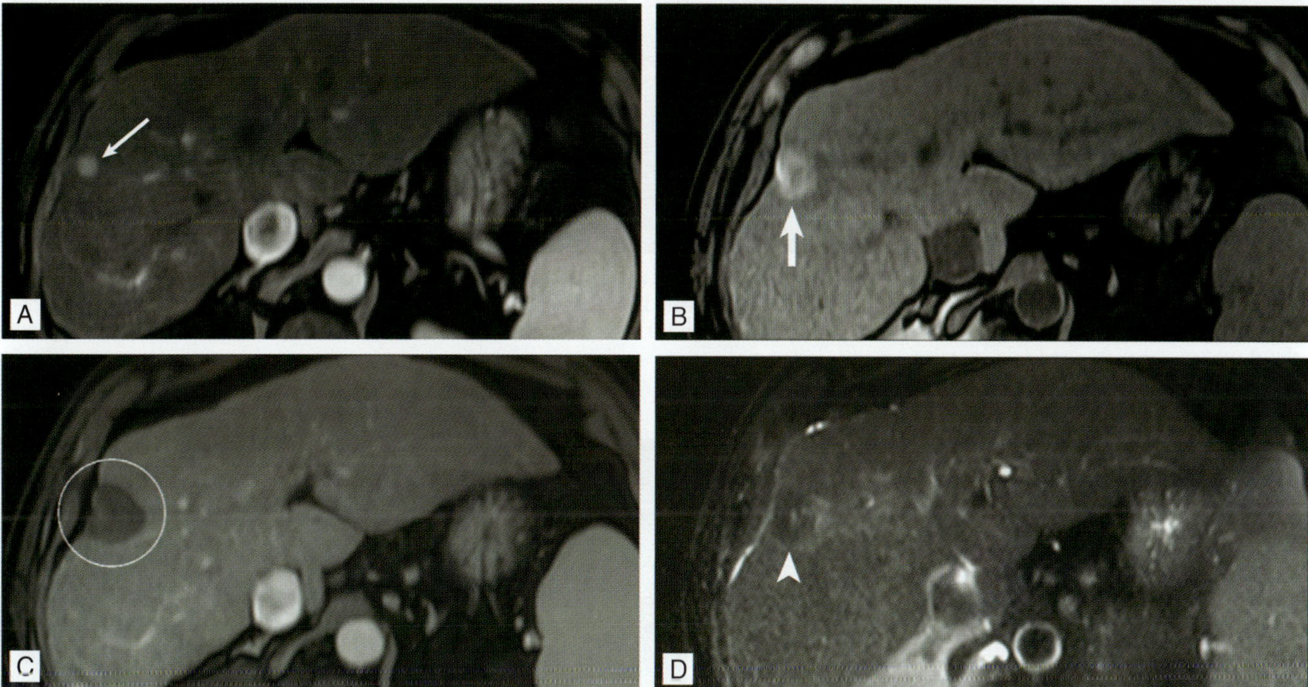

Figure 33.31 Arterially enhancing lesion which demonstrated washout (*thin arrow*, A) was ablated. There is new T1 hyperintensity, likely a combination of blood products and increased protein from necrosis (*arrow*, B). No areas of enhancement are identified (*circle* in C). There is also subtle T2 hyperintensity centrally (*arrowhead*, D), likely related to fluid centrally from necrosis. The ablation zone also demonstrates T2 hypointensity (D). LR-TR nonviable.

up with multidisciplinary discussion and often will receive retreatment [61].

Liver Transplant

Indications

Ultimately, the only cure for end-stage liver failure is liver transplant. Indications for liver transplant in the setting of cirrhosis are listed in Table 33.7 [71].

In general, a patient's place on the waiting list for a liver transplant is determined by the severity and acuity of their hepatic dysfunction. This is reflected by the presence of one of the above index complications as well as by the patient's MELD score, which is a predictor of 3-month short-term survival in patients with advanced liver disease, acute hepatitis and acute liver failure [72]. Scores range from 6 to 4, corresponding with 3-month survival likelihood of 90% and 7%, respectively [71]. The score is calculated based on INR, serum creatinine level, and serum bilirubin, and is regularly recalculated to update the patient's priority on the transplant list. Generally, the risks of liver transplantation still exceed the risks of hepatic dysfunction in patients with MELD scores <15 [73].

In the United States, there are also MELD "exception points" which may be added to the patient's score to increase their priority on the waiting list. These exception points allow additional factors which may bear on the urgency of transplant (e.g., the development of hepatopulmonary syndrome) to be considered in the patient's priority on the waiting list. Another important qualification for exception points in the United States is the diagnosis of HCC in a patient on the transplant waiting list, as discussed previously.

Due to various religious and cultural factors, Asian countries rely much more heavily on living donor liver transplantation when compared with Western countries, and because the rates of HCC are

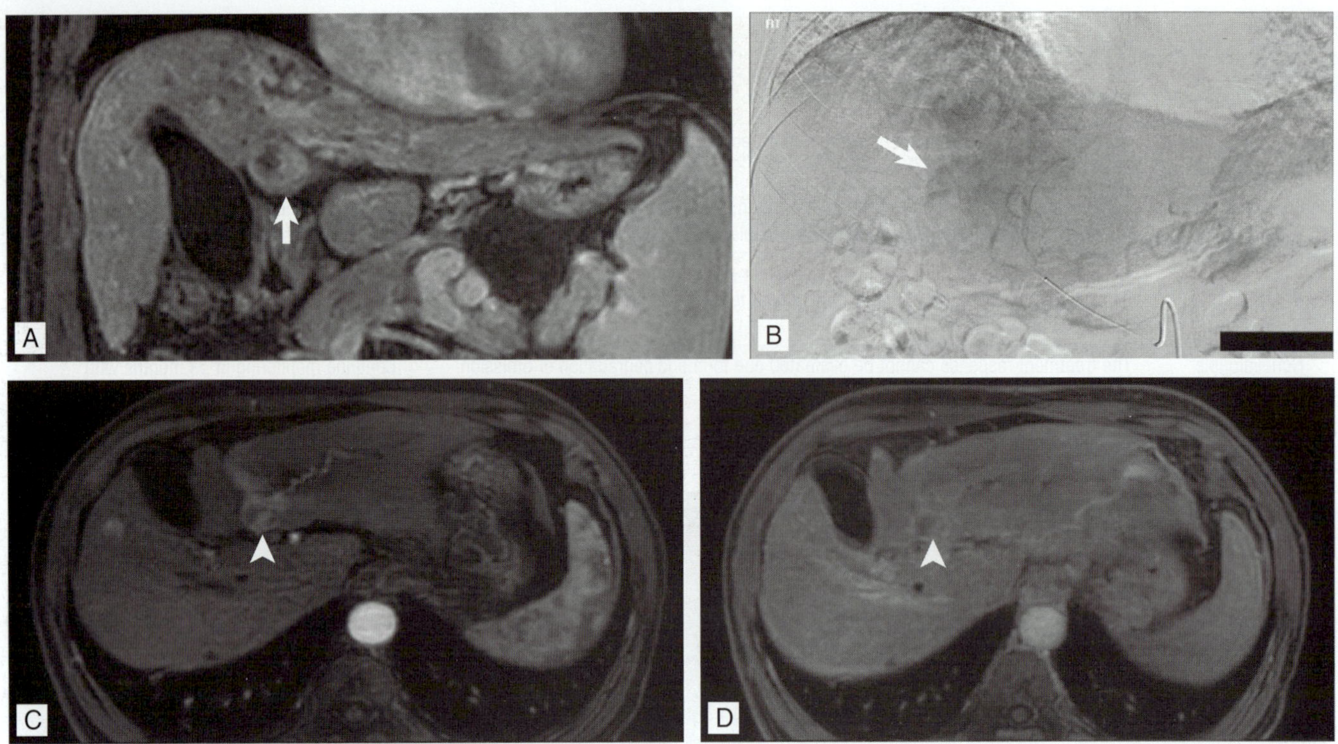

Figure 33.32 There is an arterially enhancing lesion referenced in figure 33.33 (C) and 33.33 (D) here seen in the coronal portal-venous phase (A). There was subtle late-arterial phase enhancement seen on DSA, which was treated with chemoembolization at the same time (B). Subsequent imaging demonstrated small nodularity, but no significant washout (*arrowhead* in C and D respectively). This lesion was characterized as LR–TR equivocal given the residual arterially enhancing nodularity, but without other features.

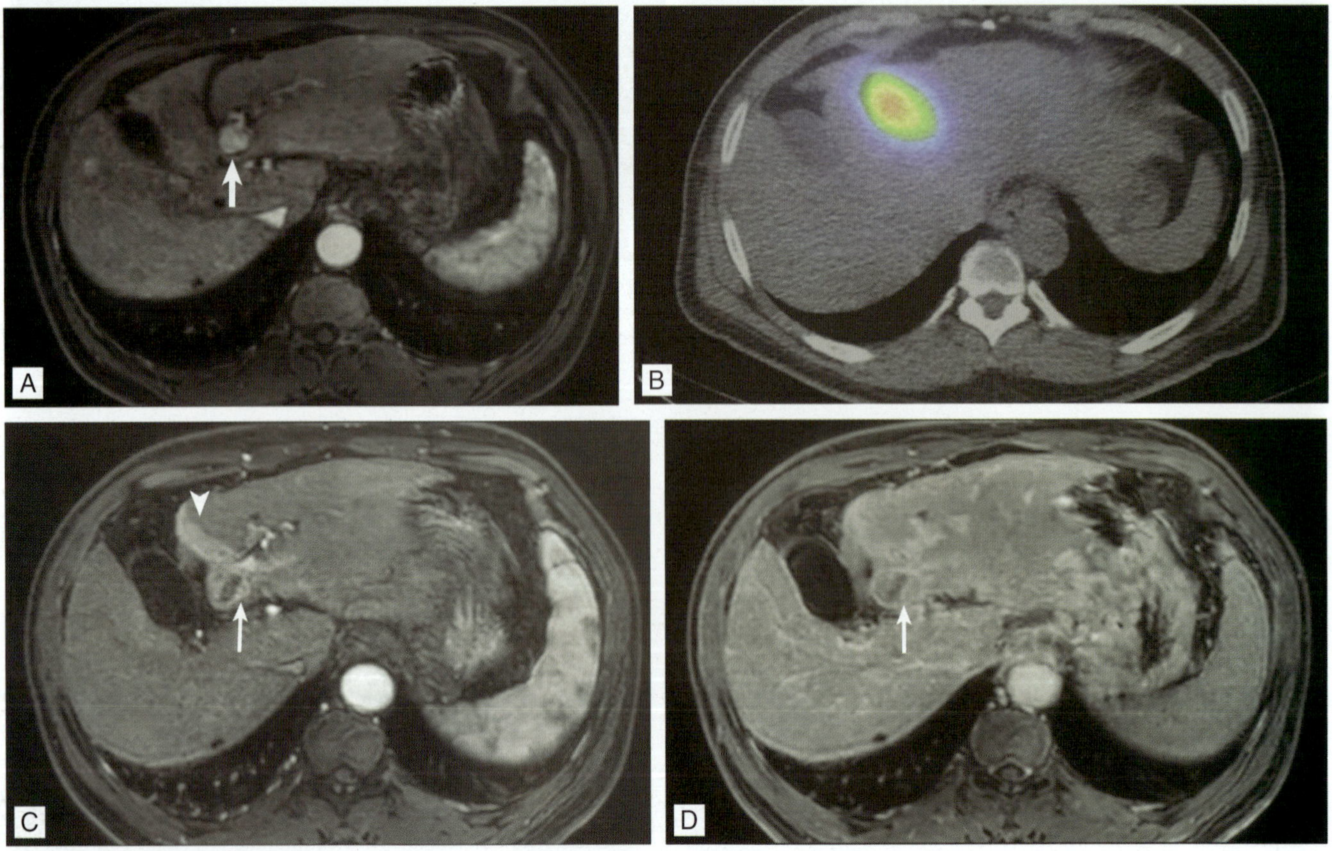

Figure 33.33 LR-5 lesion in segment 4 (A). The patient underwent Y-90 treatment (B). However, there was residual arterially enhancing nodularity at the periphery of the lesion with washout (*thin arrow*, C and D). Given the classic features, this is deemed as a viable treated lesion (LR-TR viable). The patient underwent subsequent treatment for the viable lesion which is demonstrated in figure 33.32. In addition, perfusion changes are noted in the treatment zone (*arrowhead*, C).

TABLE 33.7 Indications for Liver Transplant in the Setting of Cirrhosis [71]

Refractory ascites
Chronic gastrointestinal blood loss due to portal hypertensive gastropathy
Encephalopathy
Liver cancer
Refractory variceal hemorrhage
Synthetic dysfunction of liver

higher in patients waiting for liver transplant in Asia due to endemic hepatitis, HCC does not grant exception points in Asia as it does in the United States [74,75]. Instead, Asian countries focus on bridging to transplant with liver-directed therapy for newly diagnosed HCC.

Surgical technique

- Deceased liver donor transplantation, the most common procedure performed in Western countries, entails four surgical anastomoses—donor vena cava to recipient vena cava, donor portal vein to recipient portal vein, donor hepatic artery to recipient hepatic artery, and donor bile duct to recipient bile duct (Fig. 33.34). These connections are all sites of potential complication, and are the most frequently interrogated sites on post-transplant imaging
- The cavocaval anastomosis can either be created using an interposition technique, with the donor vena cava connected end-to-end between the upper and lower segments of the recipient vena cava, or using a "piggy-back" technique (Fig. 33.34). The piggy-back technique is now typically used because it is associated with lower ischemia time and less often requires venovenous bypass [76]. It is formed by tying off the donor vena cava inferiorly and connecting it superiorly end-to-side with the recipient vena cava
- The hepatic arterial anastomosis can be formed in a variety of ways depending on donor and recipient anatomy [77]. The most common methods are creation of a Carrel patch using the donor aortic wall around the celiac origin, or using the donor hepatic–celiac artery bifurcation to form a "fish-mouth" anastomosis with the recipient hepatic artery (Fig. 33.35). An

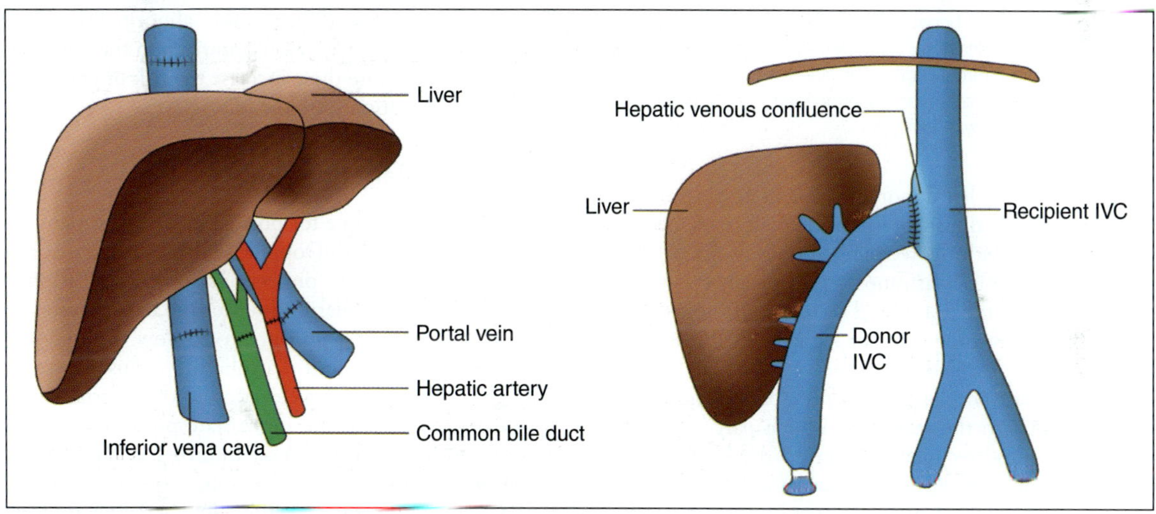

Figure 33.34 Diagrams showing the conventional vascular and biliary anastomoses of a liver transplant (left) and the more modern "piggy-back" cavocaval anastomosis (right). *IVC*, inferior vena cava.

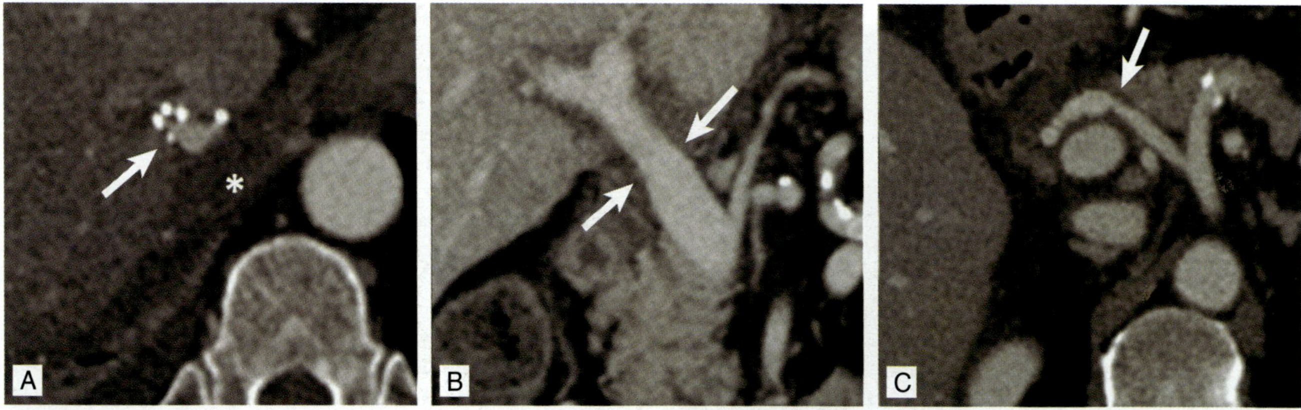

Figure 33.35 Normal postoperative CT appearance of the transplant liver vascular anastomoses. (A) Axial image at the level of inferior cavocaval anastomosis (*arrow*). Mild narrowing at this location in the postoperative setting is normal. Also note the retrohepatic hematoma (*asterisk*), which is an expected finding. (B) Coronal image showing the end-to-end portal-venous anastomosis (*arrows*). There is a subtle caliber difference between the donor and recipient veins. (C) Axial image at the level of the hepatic arterial "fish mouth" anastomosis, showing a transition in caliber between donor and recipient vessels and the expected focal bulbous appearance, which should not be confused with an aneurysm. The appearance of the arterial anastomosis will vary depending on donor and recipient hepatic arterial anatomy.

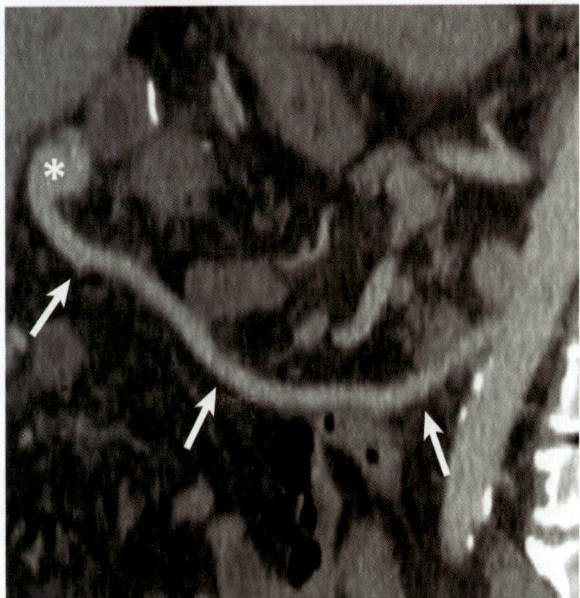

Figure 33.36 Arterial anastomosis with an iliac artery conduit. Attempted conventional arterial anastomosis was unsuccessful due to inadequate flow through a small native common hepatic artery. The donor artery was connected through side-to-side anastomosis (*asterisk*) with a deceased iliac arterial graft (*arrows*) to the infrarenal aorta. The side-to-side anastomosis is large in diameter and easily mistaken for a pseudoaneurysm without knowledge of how the anastomosis was formed.

alternative method if either donor or recipient artery is insufficient is to use an external iliac interposition graft to connect the donor hepatic artery with the recipient aorta (Fig. 33.36)

- Biliary and portal-venous anastomoses are typically end-to-end anastomoses between the donor and recipient. If the recipient bile duct is diseased or otherwise inadequate, a choledochojejunostomy can be performed
- In living-donor liver transplantation, only a part of the donor's liver is transplanted to the recipient. Which part is donated depends on donor and recipient anatomy. Care is taken both to leave the donor with adequate functional remnant liver volume, as well as to transplant a sufficient liver volume to the recipient. Careful preoperative imaging assessment of the donor and recipient vascular and biliary anatomy, as well as calculation of the donor liver and segmental volumes, is therefore crucial (Figs. 33.37 and 33.38). Postoperative imaging appearance of the living donor transplant will vary with the type of transplant performed (Fig. 33.39). Detection and quantification of diffuse liver abnormalities (particularly hepatic steatosis in Western countries) in the donor liver is also important because these increase the risk of graft loss and may preclude donation [78]

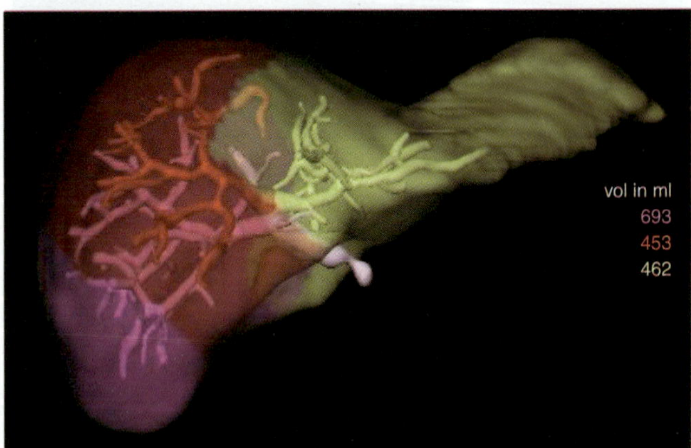

Figure 33.37 Liver volumetry based on hepatic vein territories. Volume rendered image showing colored territories based on the left (*green*), middle (*red*), and right (*pink*) hepatic vein drainage territories. (Courtesy: Abhishek Agarwal, Max Hospital, New Delhi.)

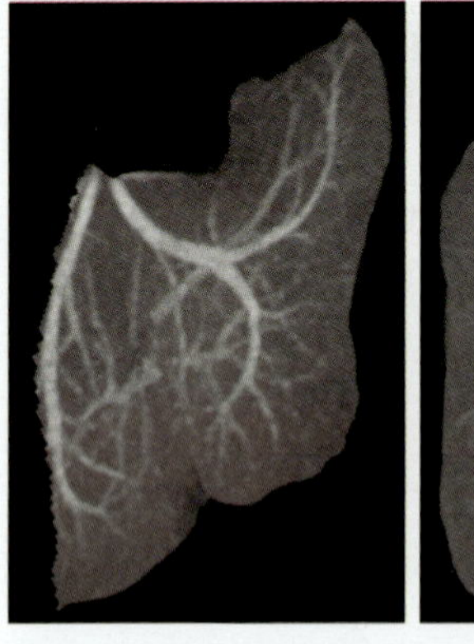

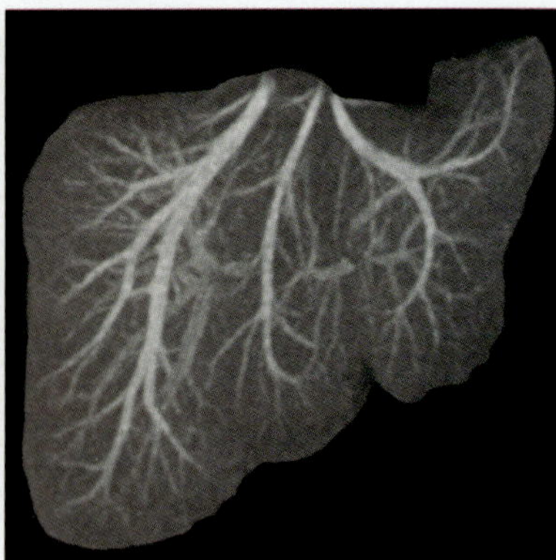

Figure 33.38 Standard volumetry for adult liver transplantation. Transection plane is planned from the GB fossa, along the lateral aspect of the middle hepatic vein up to the IVC. The remnant volume is calculated along with the MHV, which remains with the donor in most cases. (Courtesy: Abhishek Agarwal, Max Hospital, New Delhi.)

Post-Transplant Imaging

The first-line technique for postoperative assessment of the liver transplant is USG with Doppler, which is capable of assessing all of the above vascular connections for complications. Normal post-transplant Doppler findings of the hepatic artery include a brisk systolic upstroke and preserved flow throughout diastole. Decreased or even absent diastolic flow, caused by anastomotic site edema, with resulting elevation in the arterial resistive index is not uncommon in the immediate postoperative period and usually resolves in 1–2 weeks. Blunting of the hepatic arterial waveforms, with reduced systolic upstroke and relatively increased diastolic flow yielding low resistive indices <0.5, is worrisome for hepatic arterial stenosis and should prompt further investigation with CT or conventional angiography (Fig. 33.40) [79]. The absence of detectable flow within the hepatic arteries raises concern for hepatic artery thrombosis and should also prompt further assessment with CT or conventional angiography (Fig. 33.41). A rarer arterial anastomotic complication, which is usually asymptomatic and detected incidentally, is a hepatic arterial pseudoaneurysm. Its appearance on USG and Doppler is typical of pseudoaneurysms elsewhere, and may also require confirmation with additional imaging (Fig. 33.42).

The portal vein waveform may initially exhibit pulsatility and increased flow velocity related to anastomotic edema, which typical resolves in the weeks after transplant. The hepatic venous waveform is biphasic or monophasic in the immediate postoperative period due to edema, and also tends to normalize. Portal and hepatic vein anastomotic stenosis are rare. Reported USG Doppler criteria for portal vein stenosis include narrowing of the portal vein to <2.5 mm and peak systolic velocity at the site of narrowing >125 cm/s, or a ratio of maximum peak systolic velocity to prestenotic velocity of 2.5:1 to 3:1 [27]. Stenosis of the hepatic vein or IVC at the anastomosis is suggested by a threefold to fourfold increase in flow velocity [27].

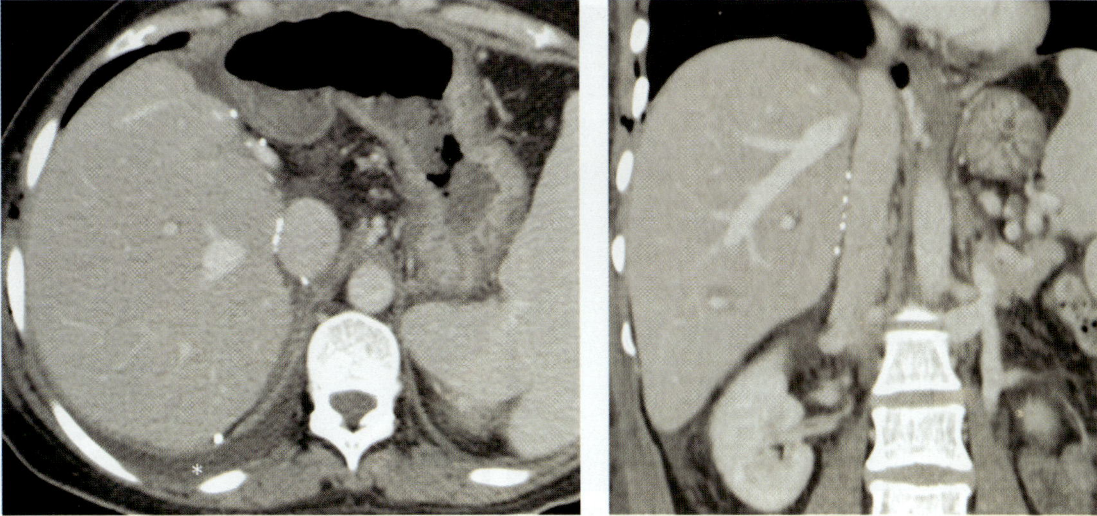

Figure 33.39 Axial and coronal images showing normal appearance of the transplanted right lobe of liver in an adult. The mild right pleural effusion (*asterisk*) is reactive and common finding post-transplantation. (Courtesy: Abhishek Agarwal, Max Hospital, New Delhi.)

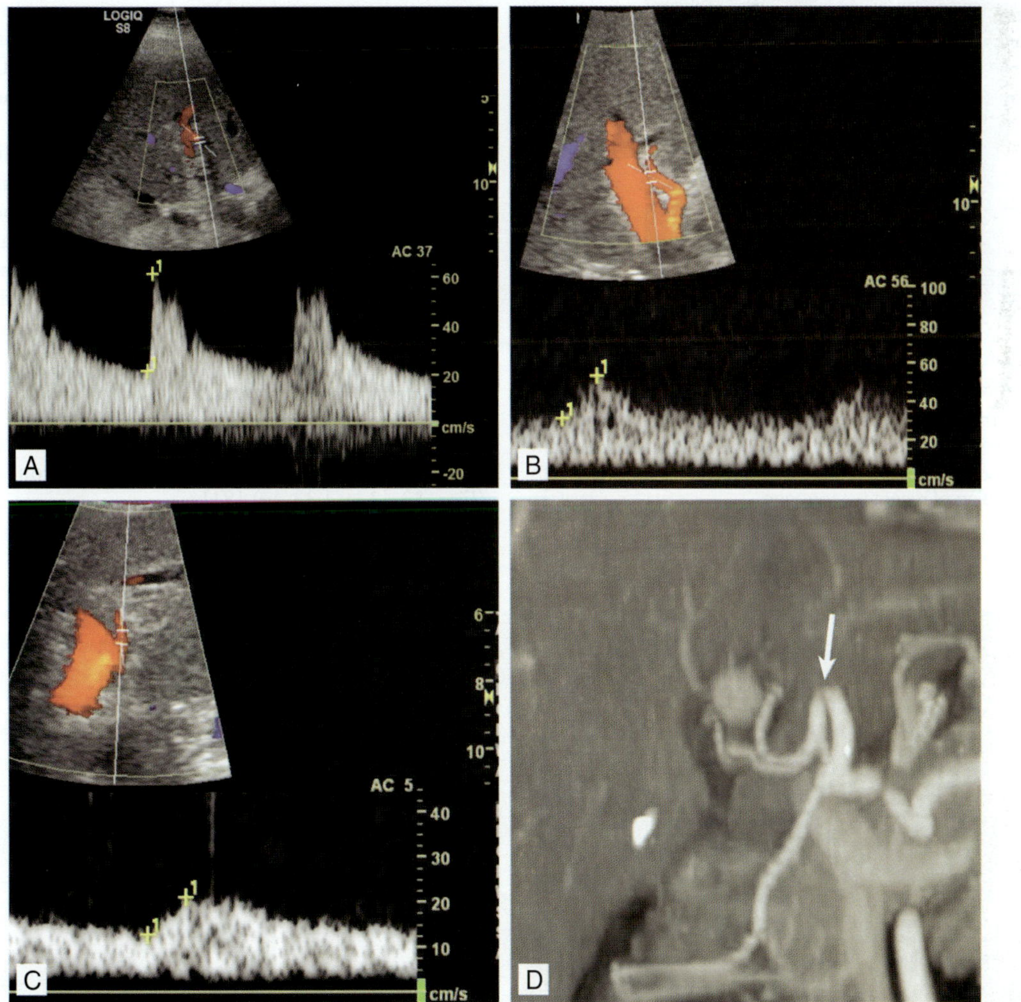

Figure 33.40 Hepatic arterial anastomotic stenosis. (A) Normal hepatic arterial waveform at baseline assessment 48 hours after liver transplantation, with brisk systolic upstrokes and preserved diastolic flow. Another patient with worsening liver function tests after transplant whose follow-up Doppler assessment showed new deterioration of the hepatic artery waveform. The right (B) and left (C) hepatic artery waveforms are blunted with decreased slope of the systolic upstrokes, decreased peak systolic velocities from baseline, and relatively increased diastolic compared with systolic flow velocities yielding low resistive indices of 0.42 and 0.41, respectively. These changes in the arterial waveform are highly suspicious for a proximal stenosis. Coronal maximum intensity projection images from the subsequent CT angiogram (D) confirm severe focal narrowing in the proximal hepatic artery (*arrow*) due to kinking of the vessel.

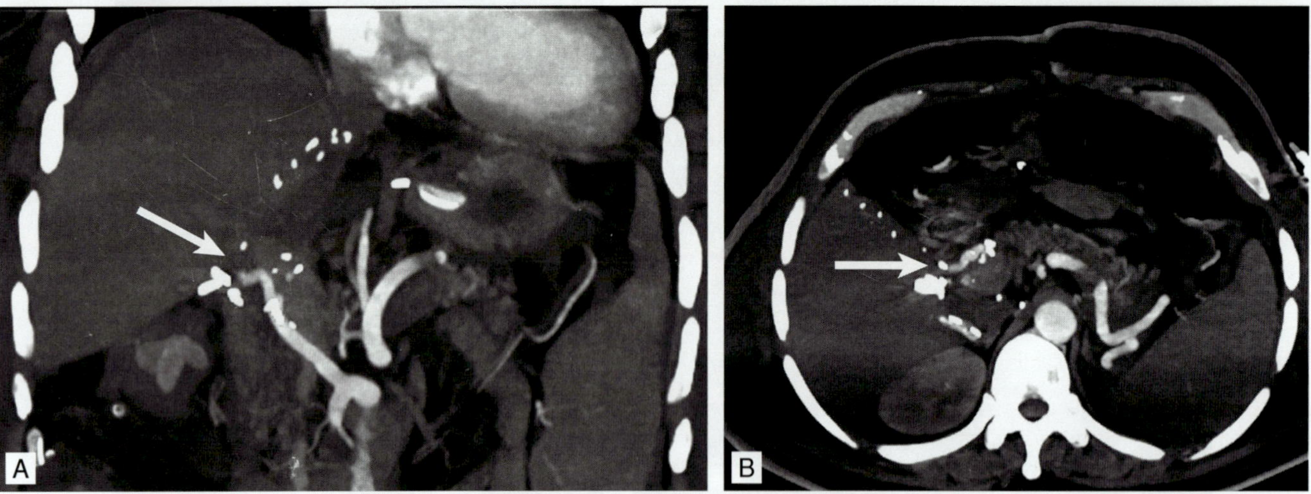

Figure 33.41 Coronal and axial MIP projections (A and B respectively) post-LDLT in adult. Arrows denote complete nonvisualization of the hepatic artery beyond the anastomosis suggesting hepatic artery thrombosis (HAT). (Courtesy: Abhishek Agarwal, Max Hospital, New Delhi.)

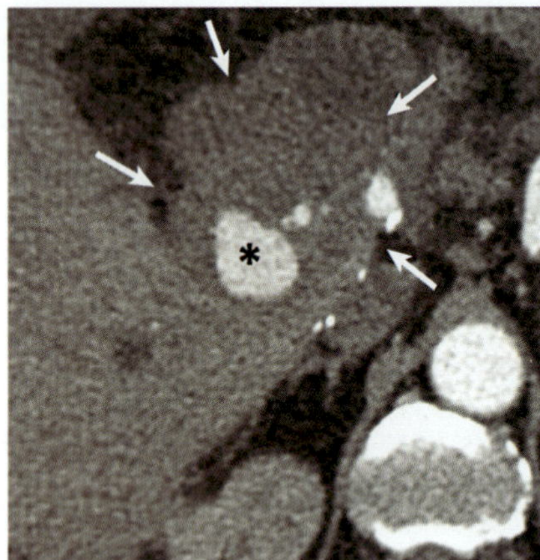

Figure 33.42 Bleeding anastomotic pseudoaneurysm in a patient after liver transplantation. Globular enhancement within the pseudoaneurysm (*asterisk*) is surrounded by high attenuation material, consistent with hematoma in the setting of recent hemorrhage.

Overall, the postoperative appearance of the vascular anastomoses on post-transplant Doppler assessment can be variable, and it is important to compare follow-up examinations with the immediate postoperative study as a baseline. Deterioration or significant changes at any of the vascular anastomoses should raise concern for a complication.

USG findings which suggest vascular complications may be more definitively characterized with CT angiography as necessary or, where available, CEUS [80]. USG is less specific for biliary complications of liver transplantation. Bile leak and bilomas may appear similarly on USG to ascites or postoperative hematoma/seroma. Moreover, an anastomotic biliary stricture does not always result in intrahepatic biliary dilation which could otherwise be detected with USG. These factors favor magnetic resonance cholangiopancreatography, which can be performed with a hepatobiliary MR contrast agent, when there is concern for bile leak, or endoscopic retrograde cholangiopancreatography for workup of a suspected biliary complication after transplant (Figs. 33.43 and 33.44) [81].

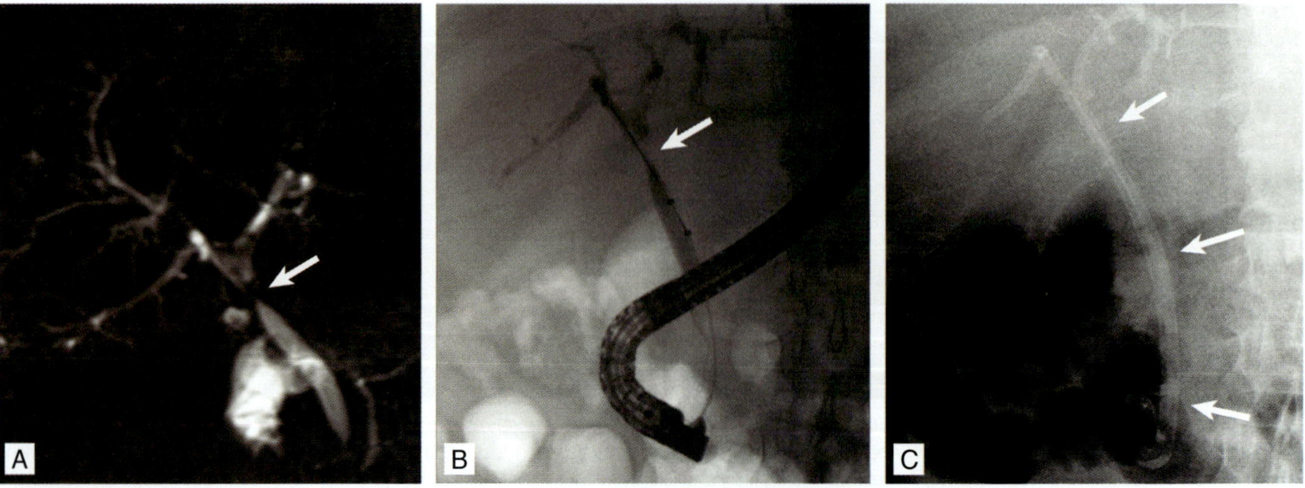

Figure 33.43 Biliary anastomotic stricture. Thick slab MRCP image (A) showing short segment narrowing of the extrahepatic bile duct at the anastomosis (*arrow*). This finding was confirmed at endoscopic retrograde cholangiography (*arrow* in B), and managed with stent placement across the stenosis (C).

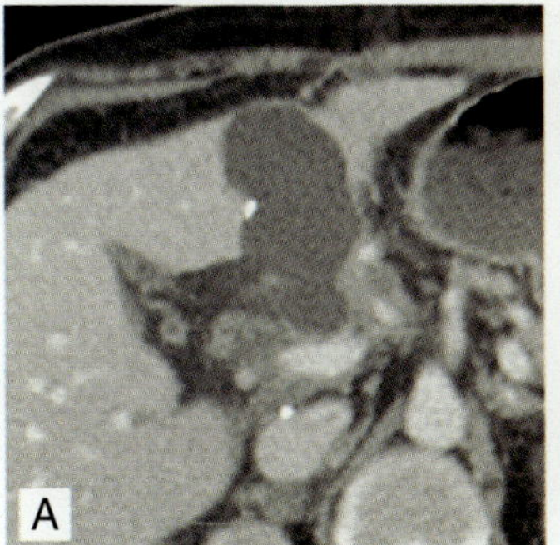

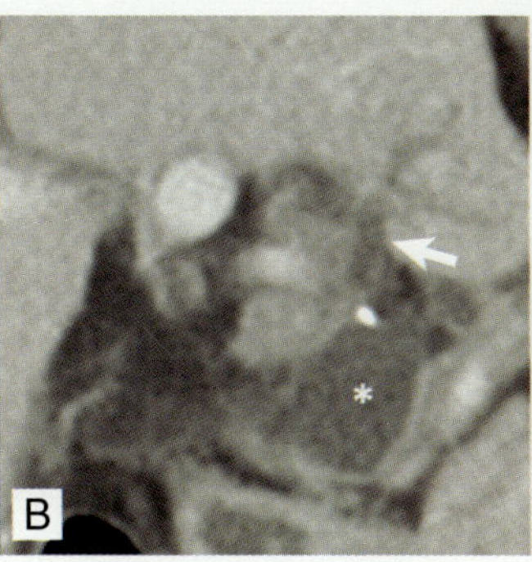

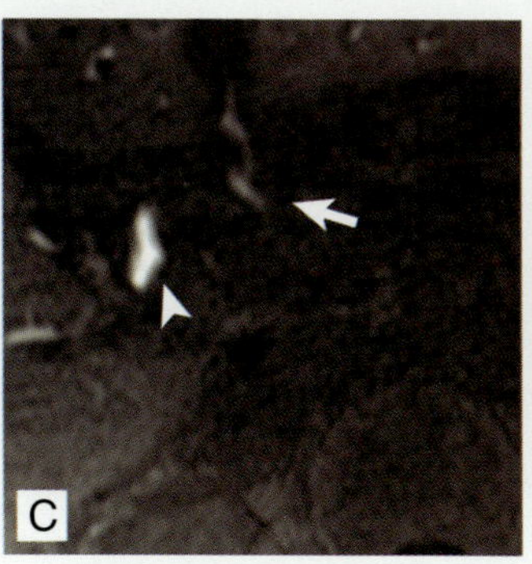

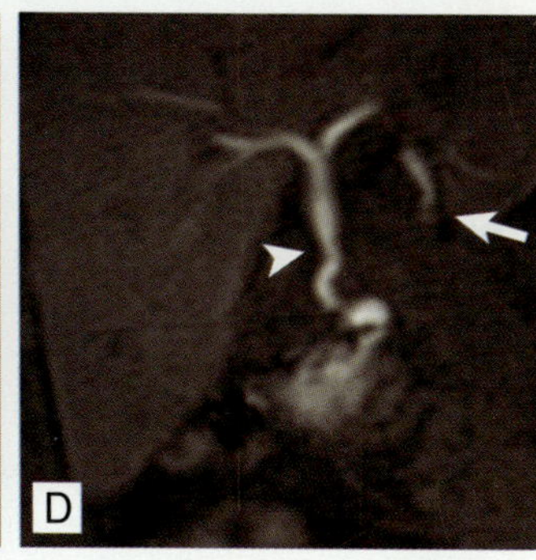

Figure 33.44 Post-transplant bile leak and biloma. Axial (A) and coronal (B) CT images show a lobulated fluid collection (*asterisk*) closely related to the liver hilum. The coronal image shows focal biliary dilation in the transplant caudate lobe, with close approximation of a caudate duct (*arrow*) with the fluid collection. Gadoxetate disodium (Eovist, Bayer AG) enhanced MR with hepatobiliary excretory phase imaging (C and D) shows excretion of contrast through the intact biliary anastomosis (*arrowhead*), and confirms a bile leak from a disconnected caudate lobe duct (*arrow*), resulting in a biloma.

Pearls to Remember for Postoperative Imaging of the Liver Transplant

- Knowledge of the surgical anatomy and anastomotic technique is important
- Doppler ultrasound is the first-line technique for postoperative evaluation
- Deterioration or significant deviation from baseline on Doppler should prompt confirmatory imaging
- General increases in vessel flow velocity and reduction or absence of diastolic hepatic arterial flow with high resistive indices are expected and usually resolve over 1–2 weeks
- IVC and PV stenosis are rare complications
- Biliary complications are often best imaged with magnetic resonance cholangiopancreatography or endoscopic retrograde cholangiopancreatography

Conclusion

Radiologists are critical in the evaluation and management of the patient with cirrhosis. As diagnostic imaging and image-guided intervention technologies evolve, they will play an increasingly important role in the detection and staging of hepatic fibrosis, and in the surveillance and management of cirrhotic patients who develop portal hypertension and HCC. For patients who underwent invasive procedures for these complications of cirrhosis, including TIPS placement, liver-directed therapy, or liver transplantation, radiologists also play a critical role in the follow-up assessment of those interventions.

Suggested Readings

- BS Hertzberg, WD Middleton, Liver, in: Ultrasound: The Requisites, third ed., Elsevier, Philadelphia, PA, 2016, pp. 51–88. [Internet][cited 2020 Sep 8]. Available from: https://www.clinicalkey.com/#!/content/book/3-s2.0-B9780323086189000031?scrollTo=%23hl0002085.
- WD Middleton, "Ultrasound assessment of the hepatic vasculature," in: *Introduction to vascular ultrasonography.*
- P A, B Ek, W Km, Surveillance for portal hypertension in the course of liver cirrhosis [Internet], Clin Exp Hepatol 4 (2018). [cited 2020 Sep 15]. Available from: https://pubmed.ncbi.nlm.nih.gov/29904721/.
- V Chernyak, KJ Fowler, A Kamaya, AZ Kielar, KM Elsayes, MR Bashir, et al., Liver Imaging Reporting and Data System (LI-RADS) version 2018: imaging of hepatocellular carcinoma in at-risk patients, Radiology 289 (3) (2018) 816–830.
- T Hibi, AK Wei Chieh, A Chi-Yan Chan, P Bhangui, Current status of liver transplantation in Asia, Int J Surg 82S (2020) 4–8.

34 Spleen

AKSHAY BAHETI, APARNA KATDARE, PUNEET BHARGAVA

Normal Anatomy

The spleen normally lies in the left upper quadrant of the abdomen. Its length varies with age, height, gender, and ethnicity, with a median length between 10.1 and 10.7 cm in adult females and between 10.2 and 12 cm for adult men with heights between 150 and 200 cm; albeit it reaches 13.5 cm for adults >200 cm tall [1]. Given the different factors affecting splenic length, it is not possible to have a single cutoff for splenomegaly on ultrasonography (USG), as the radiologist has to weigh in all of these. Practically, in average height individuals, a size less than 12 cm is generally considered normal, between 12 and 13 cm is considered indeterminate or borderline, while a spleen greater than 13 cm in length is considered enlarged.

The spleen is formed embryologically by the fusion of multiple embryonic buds within the dorsal mesogastrium. The spleen may thus normally have lobulations or clefts due to incomplete fusion (Fig. 34.1). Splenic clefts are usually present on the medial or superior aspect of the spleen but can be located anywhere. These should not be confused with lacerations in trauma patients, given their uniform well-defined contour and the lack of perisplenic fluid or hematoma. Similarly, rib notching may also be normally present on the splenic surface.

The spleen is a peritonealized structure, with the phrenicocolic, splenorenal (lienorenal), and gastrosplenic ligaments holding it in place. The splenorenal ligament contains the pancreatic tail and splenic vessels within it, while the phrenicocolic ligament connects the lower pole of the spleen to the splenic flexure and diaphragm.

Imaging Techniques

USG and computed tomography (CT) remain the most common tools used to evaluate the spleen. On USG, the spleen is best scanned with the patient lying in the right lateral decubitus position. Intercostal scanning is usually necessary to demonstrate the normal-sized spleen. Due to the presence of overlying ribs, the patient may need a deep inspirational breath-hold to optimally visualize the spleen. The splenic size (length) is usually taken in the right lateral decubitus position, measured from upper to lower pole. On CT, the portal venous phase (60–70 seconds) is usually sufficient for splenic imaging. A delayed phase may be taken for trauma patients. For splenic lesion characterization, noncontrast and late-arterial phase images (30 seconds) should also be obtained [2]. Magnetic resonance imaging (MRI) may be performed in select cases for splenic lesion characterization, and for iron deposition assessment. Positron emission tomography (PET-CT) and nuclear scintigraphy have specific roles in the splenic evaluation as well, discussed in more detail in the chapter on nuclear medicine.

Normal Imaging Appearance

On USG, the spleen has homogeneous echotexture and is more echogenic than the liver and kidney [3]. The noncontrast CT density of normal spleen is 40–60 HU, about 5–10 HU less than that of normal liver [3]. Diffuse increased splenic attenuation is abnormal and can be seen in hemosiderosis, Fanconi's anemia,

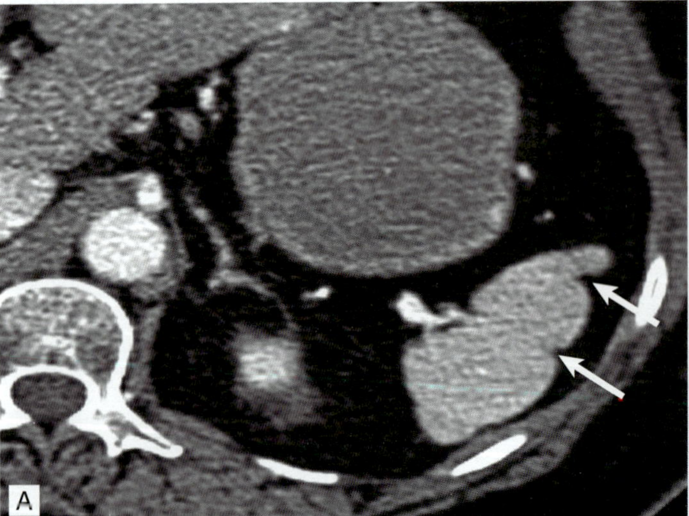

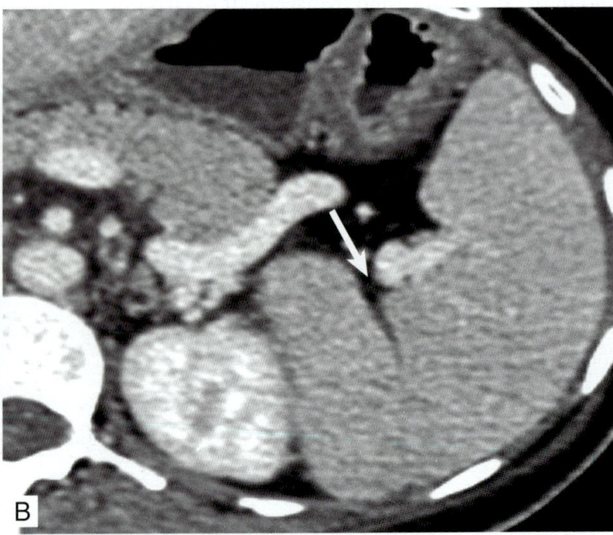

Figure 34.1 (A and B) Surface lobulations (*arrows*) along the lateral surface of the spleen (A) and splenic cleft along the medial margin of the spleen (B); these are seen normally in some patients and should not be confused for lacerations.

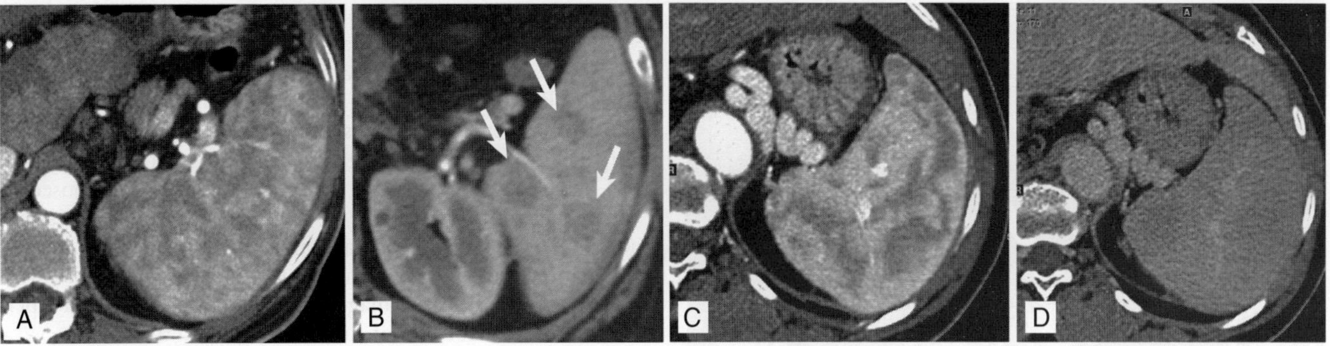

Figure 34.2 The different normal appearances of the spleen in arterial phase, including a mottled appearance (A), a pseudomass-like appearance (B), and an arciform pattern of enhancement (C). Delayed phase (D) of the patient with arciform pattern shows the expected homogeneous appearance of the spleen.

sickle cell disease hemochromatosis, and amiodarone toxicity [4,5]. The spleen has a larger fractional heme content, leading to longer T1 and T2 relaxation times compared with the liver. Thus, the normal spleen is hyperintense to the liver on T2WI, and hypointense on T1WI. Being the largest organ of the lymphatic system, microscopically, the spleen contains the age-variable amount of lymphatic follicles and reticuloendothelial cells on one hand along with vascular sinusoids on the other, namely white and red pulp, respectively. Due to differential enhancement of the white and red pulp, the spleen appears heterogeneous on arterial phase images, with a variety of enhancement patterns described, including an arciform pattern (zebra or psychedelic pattern consisting of alternating bands of low and high attenuation), a diffuse mottled pattern, and more focal heterogeneity, which may also simulate a mass [6]. In the delayed phase, the splenic parenchyma demonstrates a homogeneous appearance (Fig. 34.2).

Splenic Abnormalities and Diseases

Anomalies

Accessory Spleen (Supernumerary Spleen/Splenule/Splenunculus)

Accessory spleen (also called supernumerary spleen, splenule, or splenunculus) is formed due to failure of fusion of one of the embryonic splenic buds. It can also be considered a normal variant given its ubiquity. It can be single or multiple and has been described to be present in 10–30% of normal individuals in autopsy studies and in 11–16% of patients in CT studies [7]. The accessory tissue is usually supplied by a branch of the splenic artery with venous drainage into splenic veins. In total, 88% of patients have a single focus, with 9% having two foci, and 3% having multiple foci which are usually clustered together. The splenic hilar and perisplenic region is the most common site, followed by the pancreatic tail region (in up to 16% cases) (Fig. 34.3) [8]. However, a splenunculus can be found anywhere in the peritoneal cavity, including the gastric wall, colon, omentum, mesentery, the retroperitoneum, and even the pelvis and scrotum. Typically less than 2–3 cm in diameter, it follows splenic attenuation and signal characteristics on all imaging techniques and phases. A splenunculus may hypertrophy after splenectomy [9].

Given the lack of clinical significance in most cases, an accessory spleen may not be reported at all if it has a classic location and appearance (unless it can potentially confuse the referring physician). However, it may mimic a neuroendocrine tumor (particularly if intrapancreatic in location) or other neoplasms if in an atypical location and need further evaluation. An MRI or Tc-99m-labeled heat-damaged RBC scintigraphy can be used to identify it as an accessory spleen.

Wandering Spleen

This refers to a normal spleen located outside the left upper quadrant, due to congenital laxity of ligaments. Usually asymptomatic, it may present as a palpable lump, be more susceptible to trauma, and may present as acute abdomen with torsion/infarction. The diagnosis is made by its spleen-like appearance clubbed with

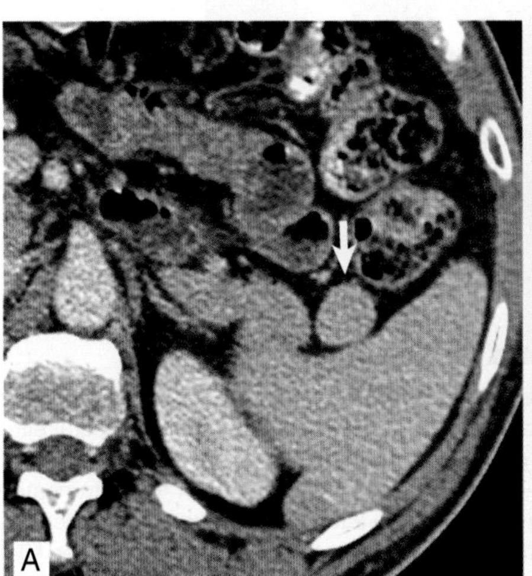

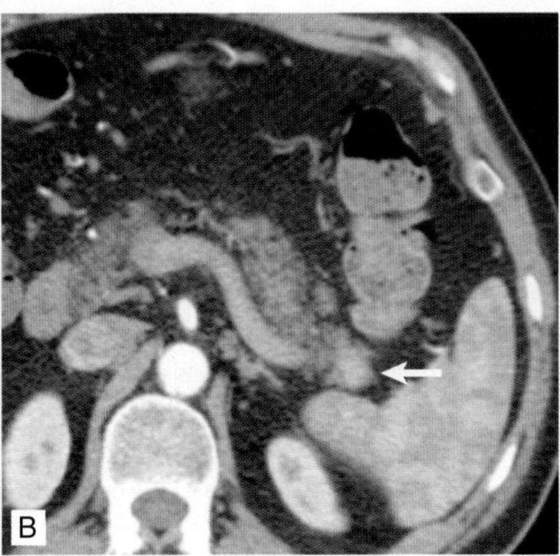

Figure 34.3 (A) An incidental splenunculus at the splenic hilum, seen as a well-defined isoattenuating nodule (*arrow*) with enhancement mirroring that of the spleen. (B) A 50-year-old man with an enhancing lesion in the pancreatic tail, with similar attenuation as the spleen. Histopathology revealed an accessory intrapancreatic spleen. (Source: https://www.ncbi.nlm.nih.gov/pmc/articles/PMC4898223/).

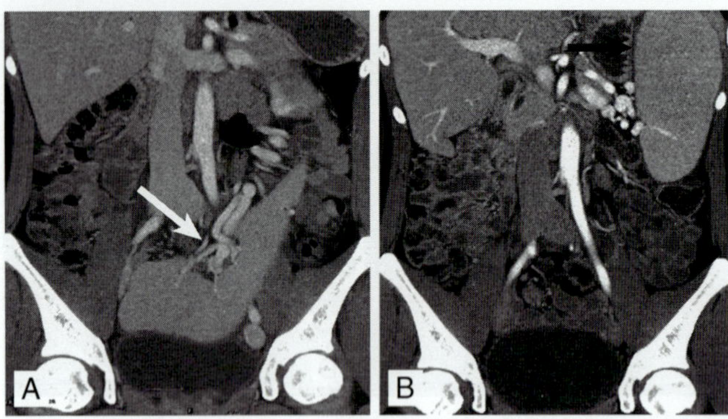

Figure 34.4 A 37-year-old man with vague abdominal pain. (A) CT revealed the spleen to be in the left lower quadrant, with splenic vessels supplying it (*white arrow*), consistent with wandering spleen. (B) There was no infarct or torsion. CT performed 1 year later reveals normal position of the spleen in the left upper quadrant (*black arrow*).

the lack of the spleen in normal location and the blood supply by the splenic vessels (Fig. 34.4).

Heterotaxy Syndromes

Asplenia syndrome: Situs ambiguus with asplenia involves duplication of the right-sided structures with an absent spleen. It is almost always accompanied by other malformations as well, especially cardiovascular (in 85–95% patients) [10]. CT demonstrates a symmetric and midline liver with an absent spleen. Bowel malrotation is present, with inversion of the superior mesenteric artery–superior mesenteric vein relationship (Fig. 34.5). Both lungs are trilobed, and the aorta and IVC characteristically have a common course, juxtaposed to each other on the same side of the spine. There may be stomach on either side, gall bladder agenesis, horseshoe kidney, imperforate anus, and a host of other anomalies as well. Tc-99m-labeled heat-damaged RBC scintigraphy may be performed to look for foci of functional splenic tissue.

Polysplenia syndrome: Situs ambiguus with left isomerism entails duplication of left-sided structures and has a lower incidence of cardiac abnormalities (50–90%), which are lesser in severity as well. Individuals with polysplenia can present incidentally as well due to lower incidence and severity of the abnormalities. Cross-sectional imaging demonstrates multiple (2–16) splenic nodules in the left and right upper quadrants (Fig. 34.6). Some may have poor function, and Tc-99m-labeled heat-damaged RBC scintigraphy may be performed to identify functional splenic tissue. Associated abnormalities which can be seen include stomach dextroposition (about 45% cases), gut malrotation (27%), biliary atresia (20%), interrupted inferior vena cava (IVC) between renal and hepatic veins, with azygos continuation of the

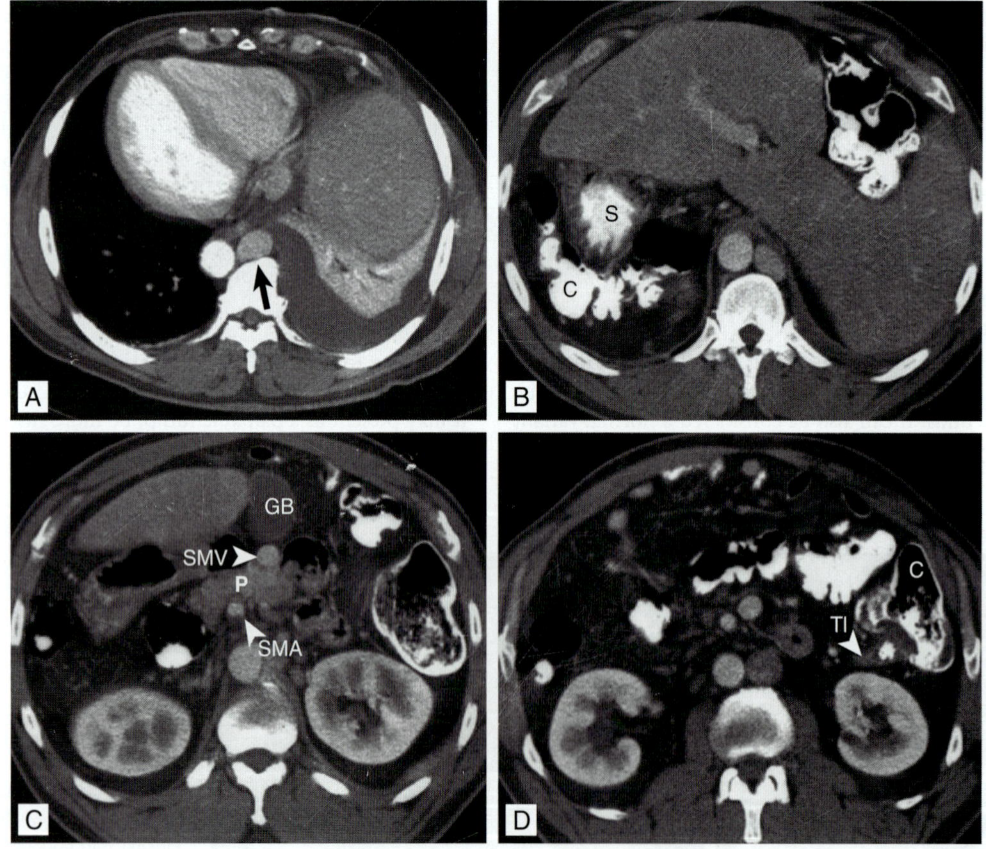

Figure 34.5 Axial CECT sections of a 48-year-old man with situs ambiguus with asplenia. Note dextrocardia and azygos continuation of the inferior vena cava (A). The aorta is located to the right of the enlarged azygos vein (*arrow*). There is also a left lower lobe collapse and a left pleural effusion. The stomach (S) and colon (C) lie in the expected location of the spleen (B). Hypoplasia of the anterior segment of the right hepatic lobe allows cephalic migration of the colon. The gallbladder (*GB*) lies in the midline (C). The superior mesenteric vein (*SMV*) lies anterior to the truncated pancreas (P), whereas the superior mesenteric artery (*SMA*) lies posterior to it. The cecum (C) is located in the left lower quadrant (D). Notice the terminal ileum (*TI*) entering the colon. Image obtained from Richard Gore and Mark Levine's Textbook of Gastrointestinal Radiology, Chapter 104: Anomalies and Anatomic Variants of the Spleen.

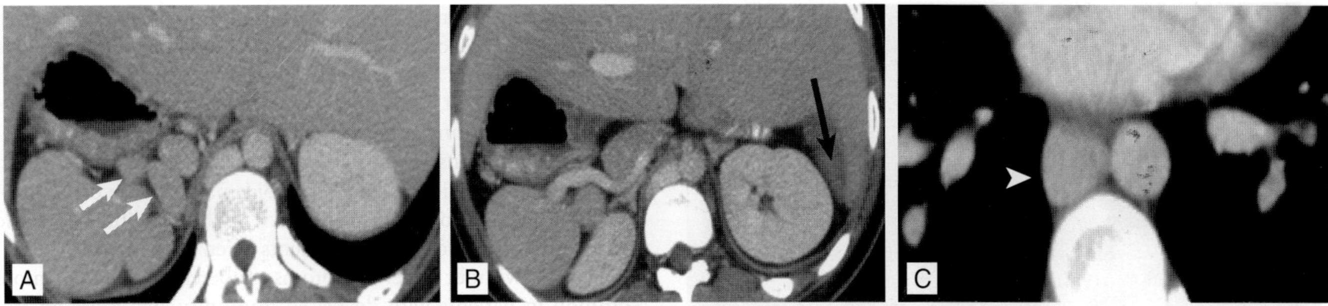

Figure 34.6 Polysplenia with situs inversus. (A) Multiple splenic nodules in the right upper quadrant (*white arrows*): (B) absence of dorsal spleen (*black arrow*): and (C) IVC interruption with azygos continuation (*white arrowhead*).

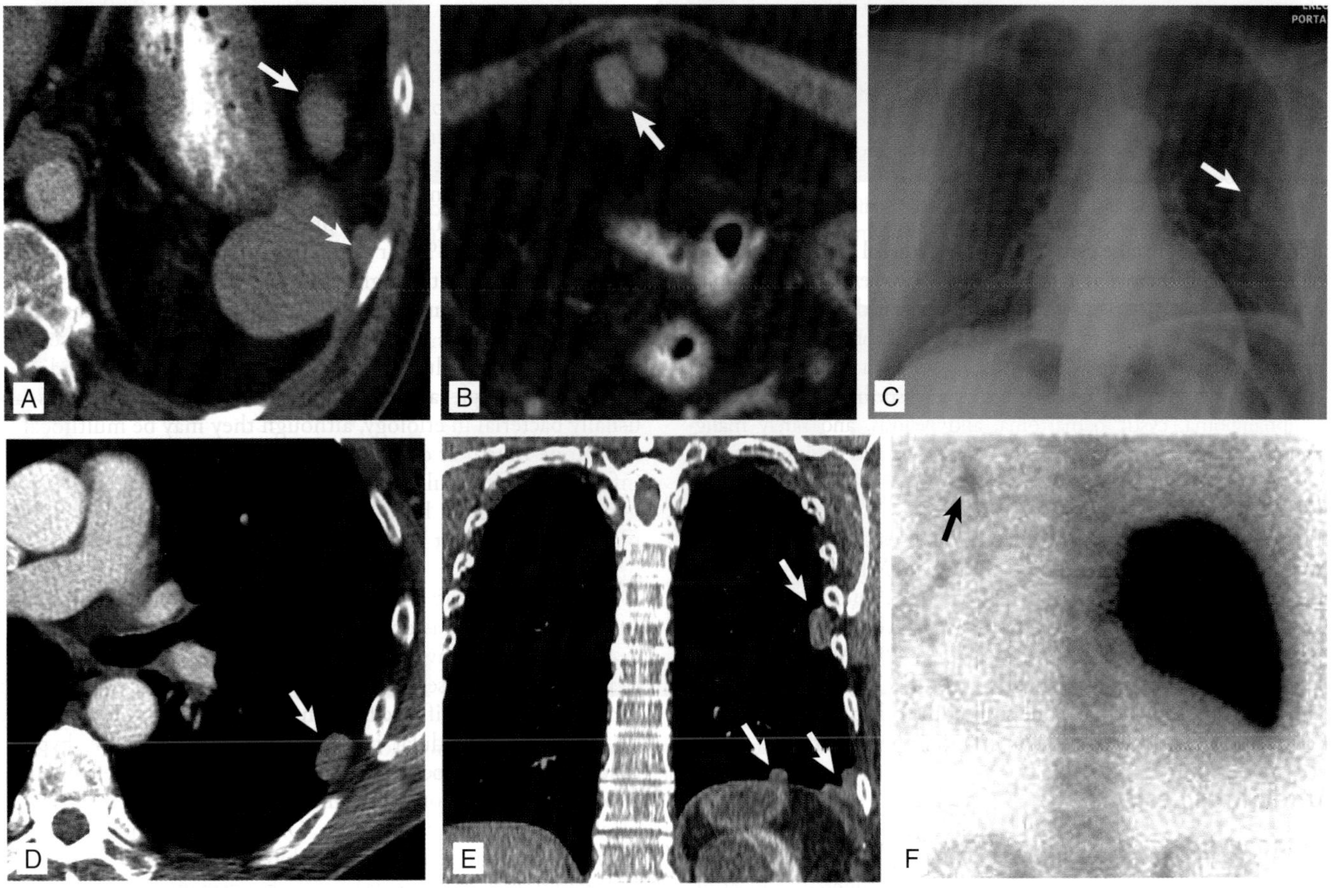

Figure 34.7 (A and B) A 42-year-old man with a history of high-speed motor vehicle collision a decade ago. CT shows post-traumatic splenosis, with splenic tissue (*arrows*) in the left upper quadrant (A) and midline omental region (B). (C–F) A 32-year-old man with a history of road traffic accident and left rib pain. Chest radiograph (C) reveals a solitary pulmonary nodule in the left mid zone, and an absent splenic shadow. CT (D and E) shows the left intrathoracic splenosis (*arrows*), with absent spleen. Planar Tc-99m-labeled heat-damaged RBC scintigraphy (posterior view) (F) confirms the splenosis (*black arrow*).

IVC, and independent drainage of the hepatic veins into the right atrium [10].

Splenosis: Unlike the above congenital anomalies, splenosis is acquired. It represents benign heterotopic autotransplantation of splenic tissue post splenic injury (traumatic or surgery). These tissues hypertrophy and present as single or multiple homogenous lesions in the abdomen (or even chest if there was penetrating diaphragmatic injury). Clinically, the diagnosis is suspected if there are no Howell–Jolly bodies on peripheral blood smear after splenectomy, indicating the presence of functional splenic tissue [11]. Splenosis may be detected incidentally even 1–2 decades after the inciting event (Fig. 34.7). Tc-99m-labeled heat-damaged RBC scintigraphy is diagnostic.

Focal Splenic Lesions

Given the known heterogeneous enhancement of the spleen in arterial phase, it is first important to confirm the presence of a true splenic lesion in the patient on the portal venous or (if needed) delayed phase.

Cystic Lesions

Pathophysiology and Clinical Presentation

Cystic lesions in the spleen can be due to a variety of causes, and are often incidental in nature. The most common etiology (75–80%) is a post-traumatic cyst, secondary to previous hemorrhage, infarct, or

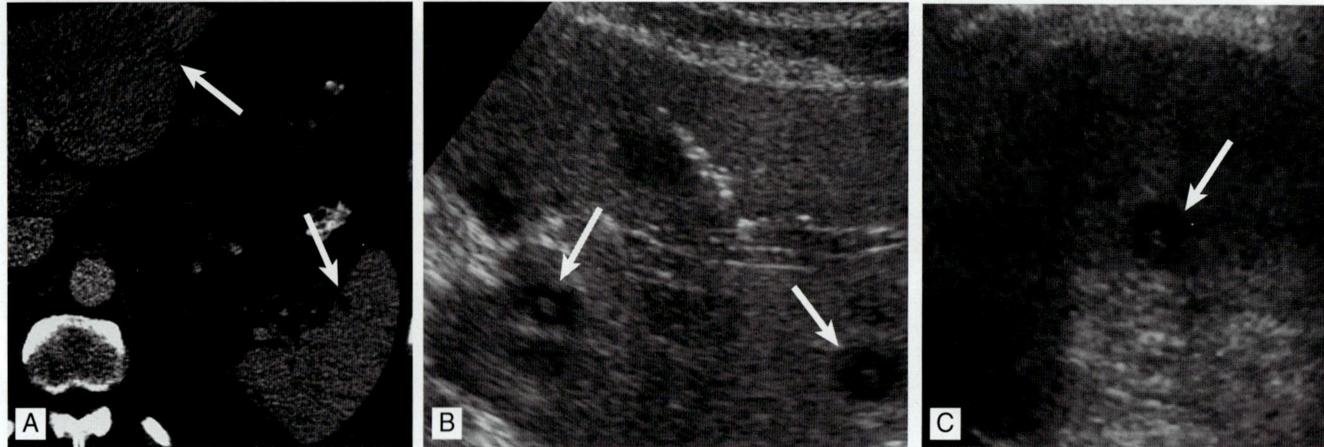

Figure 34.12 A 46-year-old man with bone marrow transplantation with multiple small hypodense microabscesses in liver and spleen on CECT (*arrows* in A). On USG, the hepatic (B) and splenic (C) lesions show a typical "bull's eye" appearance (*arrows*). Ultrasound-guided sampling from the liver lesion (B) confirmed candidiasis.

They are, however, less commonly detected on imaging, and usually as an incidental finding. They are usually cavernous, although capillary and mixed types may also occur in the spleen. Infarction, thrombosis, and fibrosis may occur in splenic hemangiomas, similar to hemangiomas elsewhere. Usually single and small (<2 cm), they may be multiple and large and may be associated with generalized angiomatosis syndromes like Klippel–Trénaunay–Weber syndrome [2,21].

Clinical Presentation

Usually asymptomatic, they may however grow slowly and cause the left upper quadrant pain and fullness. They may however also present acutely with rupture, or develop anemia and coagulopathy (Kasabach–Merritt syndrome) [2,22].

Imaging Features

Ultrasonography. It usually presents as a small well-defined echogenic lesion, sometimes with posterior acoustic enhancement. If incidental, this can be assumed to be benign [23,24]. However, atypical features such as hypoechoic appearance, cystic changes, and calcifications may be present in some, making accurate diagnosis more challenging. Contrast-enhanced ultrasound (CEUS) may be helpful, and demonstrate persistent late-phase enhancement, appearing isoechoic with the normal spleen [25]. However, some atypical hemangiomas may remain hypoechoic and difficult to characterize as benign. Capillary hemangiomas show marked homogeneous enhancement both on CEUS as well as contrast-enhanced CT/MRI.

CT and MRI. Hemangiomas are usually solid homogeneous lesions that are iso-hypodense on CT, and demonstrate low signal on T1WI and high signal on T2WI (including long TE sequences). However, larger hemangiomas may appear more complex with cystic components and may show central punctate or peripheral curvilinear calcifications [4,12,25]. On postcontrast images, they demonstrate peripheral enhancement with centripetal filling in. It is important to note that the classic peripheral nodular discontinuous enhancement seen in hepatic hemangiomas is uncommon. A peripheral rim of variable thickness with irregular inner margins is more commonly seen [4,12,21,25]. Homogeneous diffuse enhancement can also be seen. They may have a uniform or mottled hyperattenuating appearance on the delayed images; the latter due to cystic degeneration or fibrotic changes within the hemangioma. A central enhancing scar has also been described [20,26]. If it remains indeterminate, follow-up imaging or rarely a biopsy may be needed for diagnosis. Tc-99m-labeled heat-damaged RBC scintigraphy may also be used. It demonstrates increased activity on the delayed images (Figs. 34.13 and 34.14).

Hemangioma: Pearls to Remember

- Usually asymptomatic and a leave-alone lesion.
- Presents as a small well-defined echogenic lesion, sometimes with posterior acoustic enhancement. Can be assumed benign if incidental.
- Demonstrates peripheral rim enhancement with centripetal filling-in; the classic liver hemangioma type of nodular discontinuous enhancement pattern is however very uncommon.
- May be atypical on imaging and remain indeterminate on imaging, in which case follow-up imaging may be needed.

Lymphangioma

These are rare asymptomatic lesions and usually occur in children. Usually solitary, they may present as part of a generalized lymphangiomatosis spectrum. USG demonstrates a single or multiple well-defined cystic lesions, with thin septae, calcifications, low-level internal echoes, and internal vascularity. CT and MRI reveal well-defined multiloculated nonenhancing (usually) subcapsular lesions following water attenuation/intensity (Fig. 34.15). Uncommonly,

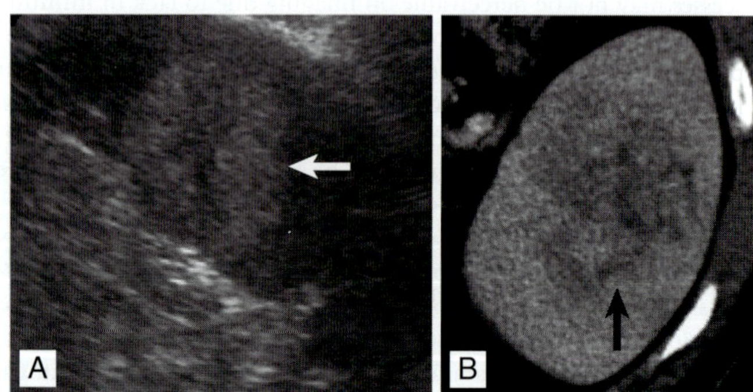

Figure 34.13 A 50-year-old man with an incidental splenic mass on USG. The lesion was echogenic with minimal heterogeneity on USG (*white arrow* in A) and was heterogeneously hypodense on CT (*black arrow* in B) with focal areas of contrast enhancement. It was proved to be a hemangioma on Tc-99m RBC scan (image not shown).

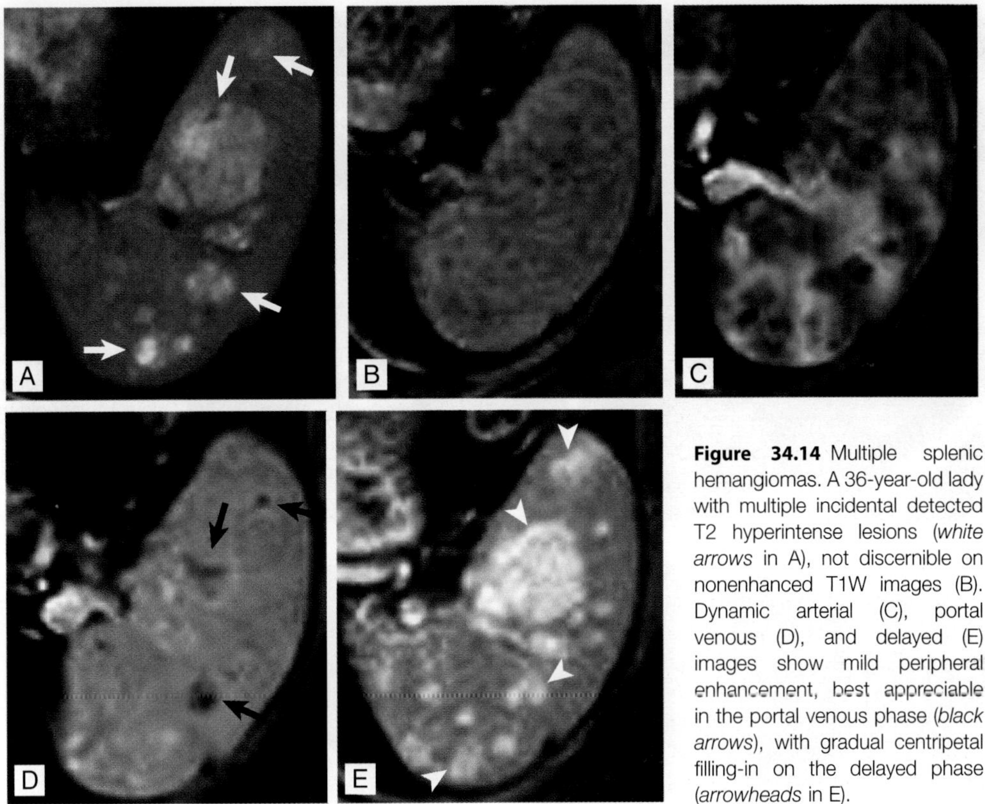

Figure 34.14 Multiple splenic hemangiomas. A 36-year-old lady with multiple incidental detected T2 hyperintense lesions (*white arrows* in A), not discernible on nonenhanced T1W images (B). Dynamic arterial (C), portal venous (D), and delayed (E) images show mild peripheral enhancement, best appreciable in the portal venous phase (*black arrows*), with gradual centripetal filling-in on the delayed phase (*arrowheads* in E).

the lesions may be T1 hyperintense on MRI if there are hemorrhagic or proteinaceous contents. Peripheral calcifications may be present [2,4,21]. They are managed conservatively, unless they are large and symptomatic, in which case splenectomy is performed.

Hamartoma

Pathophysiology and Clinical Presentation

Splenic hamartomas are rare (incidence of 0.024–0.13% in autopsy studies) benign neoplasms consisting of malformed splenic tissue. Pathologically, they can be white pulp or red pulp or mixed lesions. Usually asymptomatic, they may rarely cause splenomegaly or cytopenias if large. Multiple hamartomas may be present in tuberous sclerosis or Wiskott–Aldrich syndrome [21]. It can be difficult, particularly on cytology, to differentiate them from malignant lesions, and a partial or total splenectomy may sometimes be needed to make the diagnosis.

Imaging Features

On USG, hamartomas are well-defined lesions of variable but usually increased echogenicity, and may demonstrate internal vascularity [20,23,27]. Hamartoma is generally iso to minimally hypodense on noncontrast and venous phase CT, making it difficult to appreciate them on routine scans, where they may present only as a subtle contour abnormality. They demonstrate prolonged enhancement on delayed images, while larger lesions might have heterogeneous enhancement. The delayed enhancement is due to contrast retention within the red pulp of the hamartoma [14,20,21,25]. Calcifications, cystic or necrotic changes, and macroscopic fat may be present as well [14,20,25].

On MRI, hamartomas are T1 isointense and T2 hyperintense (although T2 hypointense lesions have also been reported rarely), and do not retain the T2 hyperintensity on long TE (TE=120–150 ms) sequences, unlike hemangiomas. On postcontrast imaging, they reveal diffuse heterogeneous arterial enhancement that either becomes homogeneous or can show prolonged enhancement on the delayed images (Fig. 34.16).

Given the variable imaging findings, differentiation with a hemangioma is often not possible, but it does not matter clinically. However, ruling out malignancy may sometimes be difficult as well (although the presence of delayed enhancement may help), especially in cases with cystic/necrotic changes, and a biopsy/splenectomy may be needed for confirmation.

Littoral Cell Angioma

Pathophysiology and Clinical Presentation

These are rare vascular neoplasms arising from the Littoral cell, which lines the red pulp sinuses. Majority are benign, but some may be malignant (the low-grade Littoral cell hemangioendothelioma or higher-grade angiosarcoma). Usually asymptomatic, patients may present with cytopenias or pain; splenomegaly is usually present in the symptomatic patients [2,13,21,26].

Imaging Features

Littoral cell angiomas present as multiple nonspecific lesions of variable echogenicity on USG. CECT reveals hypodense lesions of variable sizes and shapes, with delayed enhancement given their vascular nature (Fig. 34.17). Calcification and cystic changes are generally absent. Littoral cell angiomas contain hemosiderin due to the hemophagocytic capacity of the Littoral cells. Accordingly, they appear T1 and T2 dark on MRI due to siderosis [2,13,21,24,26,27].

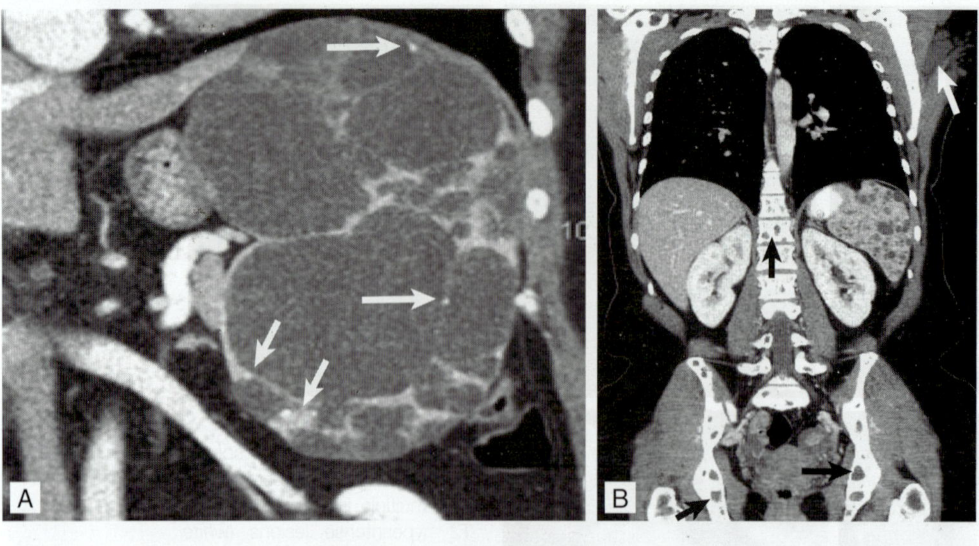

Figure 34.15 (A) Splenic lymphangioma in a 5-year-old boy. Coronal reconstructed CT image reveals multiple confluent thin-walled nonenhancing cystic lesions, predominantly subcapsular in location. Note subtle specks of septal calcifications. (B) Coronal reconstructed CT image in a 14-year-old boy with lymphangiomatosis. Note the multiple cystic splenic lymphangiomas, along with lesions in the left axilla (*white arrow*) and multiple bones (*black arrows*).

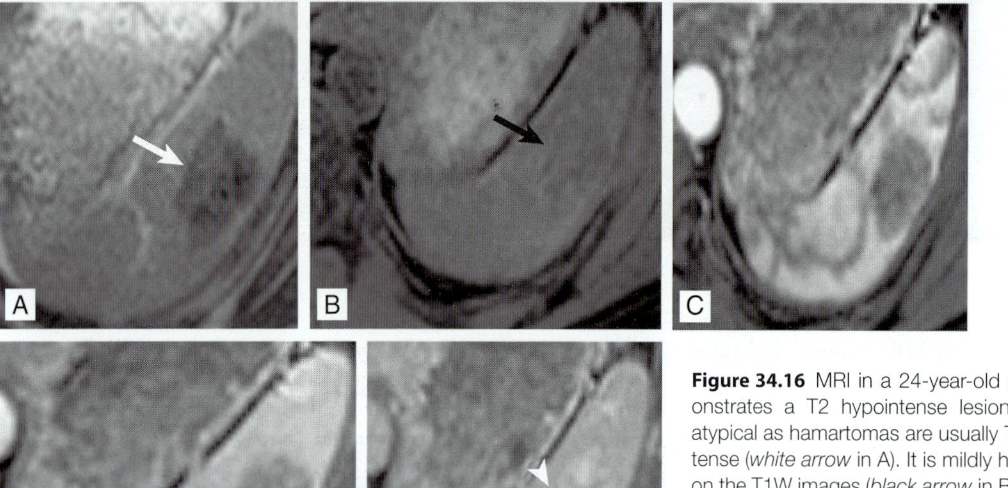

Figure 34.16 MRI in a 24-year-old male demonstrates a T2 hypointense lesion, which is atypical as hamartomas are usually T2 hyperintense (*white arrow* in A). It is mildly hypointense on the T1W images (*black arrow* in B). Dynamic late arterial, portal venous, and delayed images (C–E, respectively) show lack of early enhancement (again an atypical finding) but with delayed mildly heterogeneous filling in (*arrowhead* in E). A biopsy was performed given the atypical findings, which confirmed a splenic hamartoma.

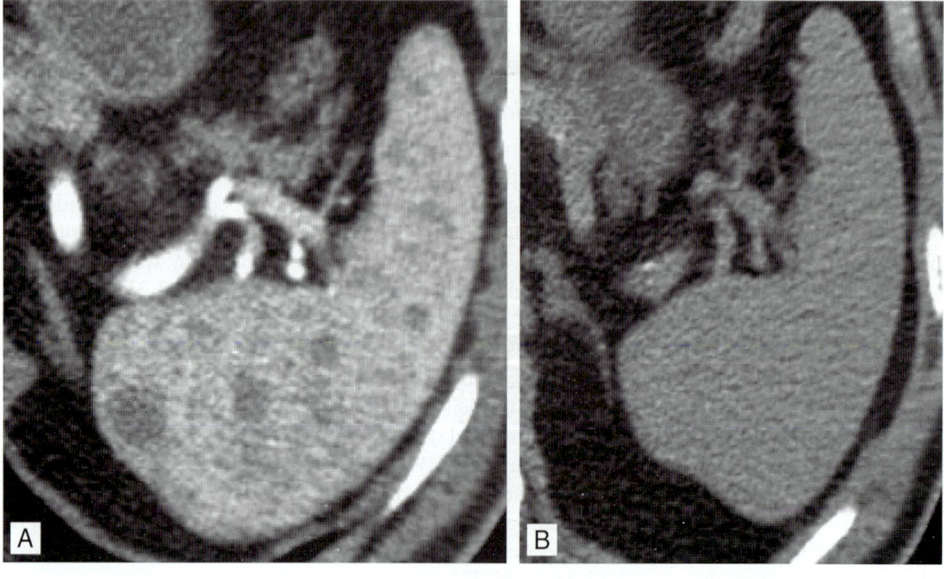

Figure 34.17 Late arterial (A) and delayed (B) phase CT images in a 23-year-old lady being investigated for hypersplenism show multiple hypodense lesions in the spleen which retain contrast and become isoattenuating to the splenic parenchyma in the delayed phase. These were proved to be Littoral cell angiomas on splenectomy.

Peliosis

Pathophysiology and Clinical Presentation

Splenic peliosis is a rare condition in which there is sinusoidal dilatation with multiple cyst-like blood-filled cavities present involving the spleen. It is usually associated with hepatic peliosis. Risk factors include infections (including bacillary angiomatosis), hematologic disorders, anabolic steroids usage, and immunocompromised state. Patients are generally asymptomatic, but can rarely present with rupture.

Imaging Features

USG reveals multiple hypoechoic cystic splenic lesions. Peliosis presents as multiple well-defined hypodense cyst-like lesions on CECT. Fluid–fluid levels and hyperattenuating content may be present occasionally depending on the presence of recent hemorrhage. On MRI, peliosis commonly presents as T2 hyperintense and T1 iso-hypointense nonenhancing or hypoenhancing lesions in most cases, although the intensity is variable depending on the stage of the blood components (Fig. 34.18). Various patterns of enhancement have been described, including hypoenhancing lesions, peripheral enhancement, and centripetal filling in [2,21].

The cystic nature of the lesions is helpful to differentiate them from more solid neoplasms like lymphoma, especially in association with relevant history. However, the lesions are often indeterminate, and a biopsy or a splenectomy may be performed.

Sclerosing Angiomatoid Nodular Transformation

This is an uncommon benign vascular neoplasm having multiple vascular nodules surrounded by fibrous bands that often become centrally coalescent to form a scar. It is usually asymptomatic and detected incidentally. It is hypoechoic on USG and hypodense on CT, with progressive delayed enhancement. Given the presence of both vascular and sclerosed elements, it is often heterogeneous and overall T2 hypointense on MRI due to the sclerotic component and chronic hemorrhage. It may demonstrate T2 hypointense radiating fibrotic bands or/and a T2 hyperintense central scar which is hypoenhancing (Fig. 34.19). There may be the presence of old hemorrhage and iron deposition, with foci of increased signal on the T1 in-phase images [4,28]. Peripheral radiating enhancing lines with a "spoke-wheel" appearance of sorts have been described as common, corresponding to fibrous bands. Other forms of enhancement like rim enhancement may be present.

The imaging features of benign vascular splenic neoplasms are summarized in Table 34.1.

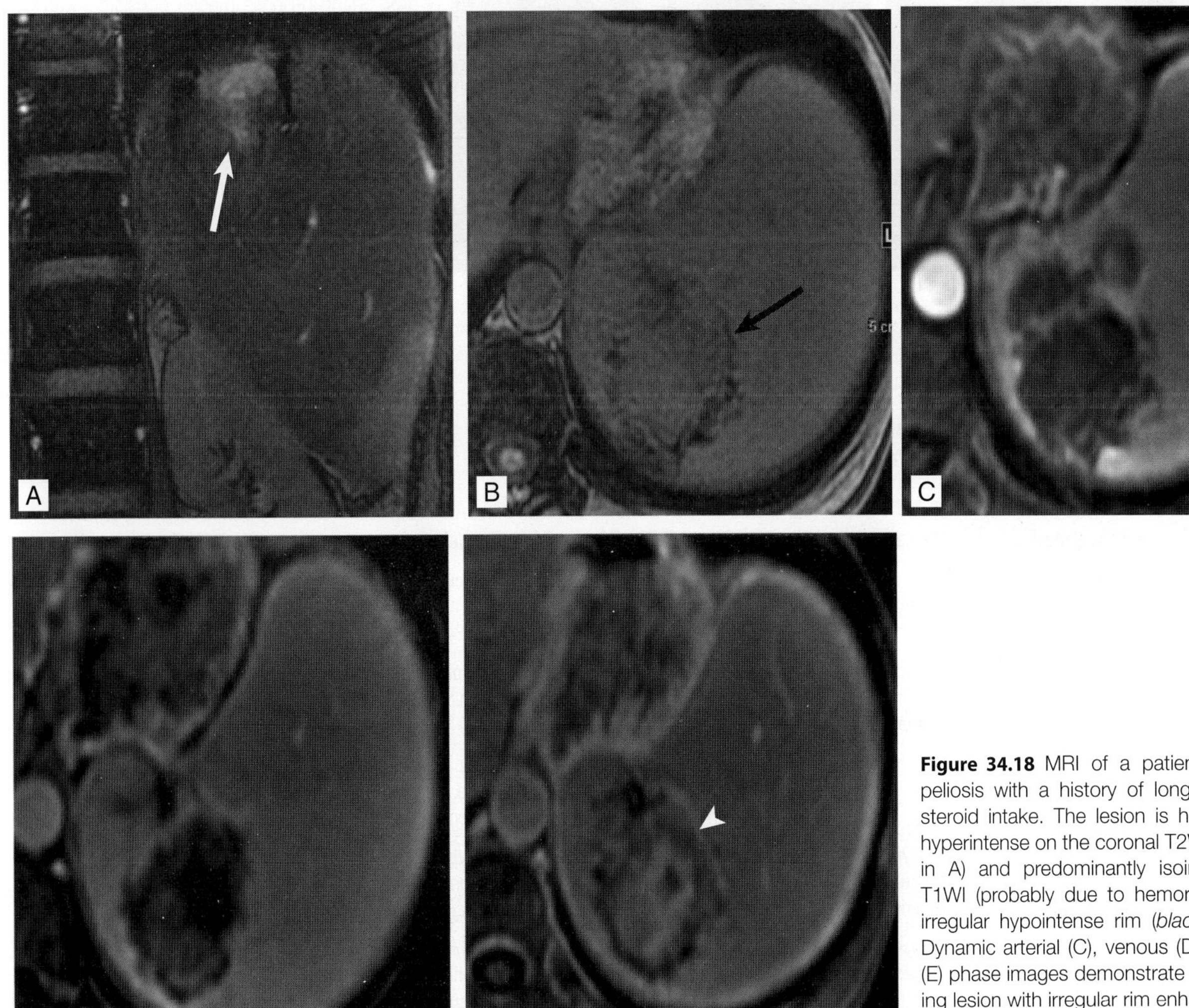

Figure 34.18 MRI of a patient with splenic peliosis with a history of long-term anabolic steroid intake. The lesion is heterogeneously hyperintense on the coronal T2WI (*white arrow* in A) and predominantly isointense on the T1WI (probably due to hemorrhage) with an irregular hypointense rim (*black arrow* in B). Dynamic arterial (C), venous (D), and delayed (E) phase images demonstrate a hypoenhancing lesion with irregular rim enhancement, with heterogeneous progressive enhancement on the delayed phase (*arrowhead* in E).

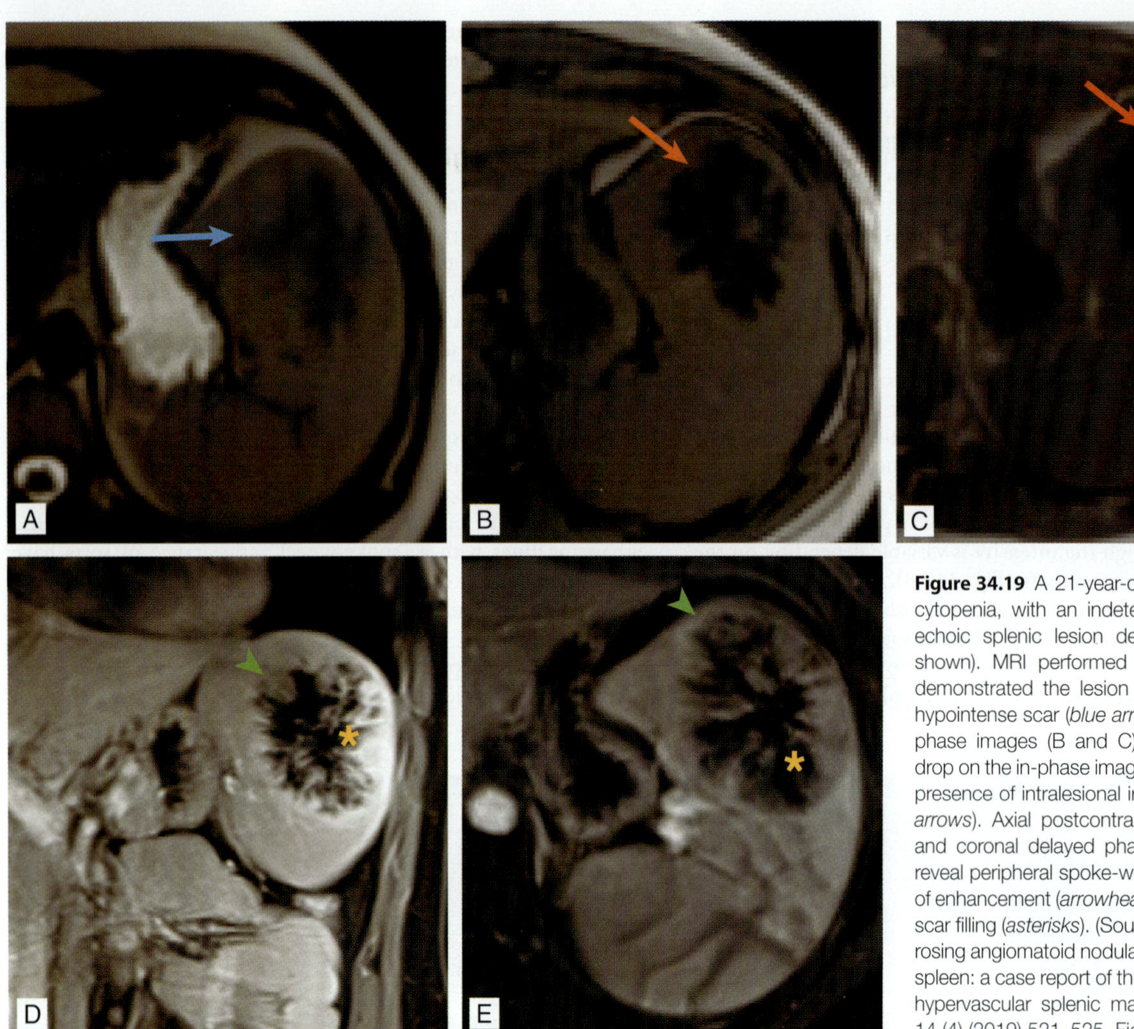

Figure 34.19 A 21-year-old lady with thrombocytopenia, with an indeterminate mildly hyperechoic splenic lesion detected on USG (not shown). MRI performed for further evaluation demonstrated the lesion to have a central T2 hypointense scar (*blue arrow* in A). In and out of phase images (B and C) demonstrated signal drop on the in-phase images, consistent with the presence of intralesional iron deposition (*orange arrows*). Axial postcontrast axial arterial phase and coronal delayed phase images (D and E) reveal peripheral spoke-wheel like radiating lines of enhancement (*arrowheads*) and lack of central scar filling (*asterisks*). (Source: Gooch et al. Sclerosing angiomatoid nodular transformation of the spleen: a case report of thrombocytopenia and a hypervascular splenic mass, Radiol Case Rep 14 (4) (2019) 521–525. Figs are Figs. 1C–E,G,I.)

TABLE 34.1 Imaging Features of Benign Vascular Neoplasms

	Hemangioma	Hamartoma	Littoral Cell Angioma	Peliosis	Sclerosing Angiomatoid Nodular Transformation
Pathophysiology	Commonest benign neoplasm	Rare, usually asymptomatic	Rare and usually asymptomatic, but may present with cytopenias or pain	Associated with risk factors	Contains both vascular and fibrous tissue
USG	Well-defined echogenic lesion, but can be heterogeneous	Well-defined lesions of variable but usually increased echogenicity	Nonspecific lesions of variable echogenicity	Multiple hypoechoic cystic splenic lesions	Hypoechoic
CT	Iso-hypodense	Isodense	Hypodense	Cystic lesions; fluid–fluid levels and hyperattenuating content may be present	Hypodense
MRI	T2WI hyperintense, retain hyperintensity on long TE	T2 hyperintense, but do not retain the hyperintensity on long TE	T2 dark on MRI due to hemosiderin content	T2 hyperintense and T1 iso-hypointense	T2 hypointense due to fibrous component and old blood products
Enhancement pattern	Peripheral enhancement with centripetal filling-in	Delayed enhancement present	Delayed enhancement present	Variable— hypoenhancement, peripheral enhancement, centripetal filling	"Spoke-wheel" appearance of radiating enhancing lines; scar remains hypoenhancing

Malignant Neoplasms

Angiosarcoma

Pathophysiology

Angiosarcoma, although very rare, is the commonest nonhematolymphoid primary splenic neoplasm. It is an aggressive malignancy arising from the endothelium of the splenic sinuses, with most patients dying within a year of presentation. Unlike hepatic angiosarcomas, there is no proved correlation with a history of vinyl chloride, arsenic, or thorium exposure [21,29–31].

Clinical Presentation

The average age of presentation is over 55 years, although younger patients can be affected as well. Most patients present with abdominal pain (~70%), with splenomegaly and cytopenias often present. Spontaneous rupture is relatively common (~25%), and most patients have metastases (most commonly to the liver) at the time of presentation.

Imaging Feature

Imaging usually reveals splenomegaly along with single or (more commonly) multiple heterogeneous splenic masses (Fig. 34.20) with variable amount of cystic, necrotic, and hemorrhagic areas. Diffuse splenic involvement has also been described. There may be associated hemoperitoneum. The solid components generally show increased vascularity. Given the presence of hemorrhage, T2 hypointense siderotic nodules may be seen on MRI. Calcifications may rarely be present.

Imaging differentials for lesions limited to the spleen include benign vascular neoplasms, as well as other malignancies such as lymphoma, Kaposi sarcoma, and metastasis; biopsy is needed for the final diagnosis. Care must be taken before biopsying, a possible angiosarcoma as it is a very vascular neoplasm and may cause life-threatening hemorrhage.

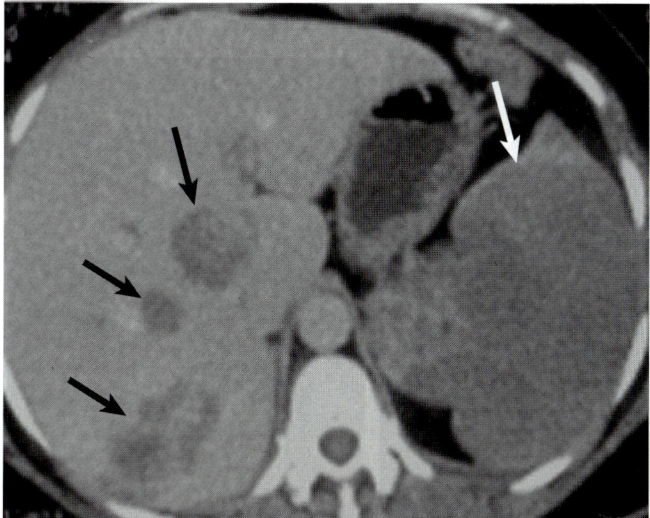

Figure 34.20 A 43-year-old man with abdominal pain. CT demonstrates a large heterogeneous hypodense mass replacing most of the spleen (*white arrow*), with multiple heterogeneous hepatic metastases (*black arrows*), confirmed to be primary splenic angiosarcoma on biopsy.

Lymphoma

Pathophysiology

Lymphomatous involvement is the most common malignancy involving the spleen. Although primary splenic lymphoma is rare (<2% of all lymphomas), the spleen is commonly involved secondarily with lymphoma and other hematological malignancies. The spleen is involved in about 30–40% patients of non-Hodgkin's lymphoma (NHL), and in about one-third patients with Hodgkin's disease. Splenic involvement is considered nodal in both NHL and Hodgkin's disease.

Clinical Presentation

Lymphomas generally present as painless enlargement of one or more groups of peripheral nodes, with or without constitutional symptoms like fever, weight loss, and night sweats. Patients with abdominal disease may manifest with vague abdominal pain and fullness. Primary splenic lymphoma may present with the left upper quadrant pain and splenomegaly.

Imaging Features

PET-CT is the imaging technique of choice for baseline evaluation and response assessment of FDG-avid lymphomas as per the Lugano classification, as it is more sensitive and specific than CECT alone [32–34]. Visual assessment is considered sufficient for evaluation. The CT component of the PET-CT may be a diagnostic full-dose CECT or a lower dose noncontrast CT. CECT can help improve more accurate evaluation of nodal size, bulk (differentiating an aggregate of small discrete nodes from confluent nodes), differentiating bowel from nodes, and assessing vascular compression (as in SVC syndrome). CECT is recommended for evaluation of nonavid or less-avid lymphomas, like CLL or cutaneous lymphomas.

The Lugano classification for staging lymphomas recommends a cutoff of 13 cm in vertical length for splenomegaly [33,34]. The splenic vertical length should be measured in the coronal image (coronal reconstructed CT image or coronal MIP image of a PET study) (Fig. 34.21). If only axial CT sections are used for measurement, the vertical length can be calculated by multiplying the number of splenic slices (axial sections on which the spleen is visible) with the slice thickness [33]. However, the cutoff of 13 cm is not very specific, with a study demonstrating sensitivity and specificity of 74% and 48%, respectively [34]. This is because almost 30% of enlarged spleens may be uninvolved in patients with lymphoma, while almost one-third patients can have splenic involvement without splenomegaly.

On PET, splenic involvement presents as diffusely increased or focal splenic uptake. High-grade lymphomas have significantly more FDG-avid involvement than lower-grade lymphomas. Deauville score is used for defining involvement.

Splenic Lymphoma: Pearls to Remember

- Commonly involved secondarily by lymphoma
- PET-CT is the investigation of choice for FDG-avid lymphomas
- The Lugano classification recommends a cutoff of 13 cm in splenic vertical length for splenomegaly
- Four patterns of involvement on CT:
  1. homogenous splenomegaly without an appreciable focal lesion,
  2. diffuse involvement by tiny miliary nodules,
  3. multiple larger splenic lesions, and
  4. a solitary splenic mass

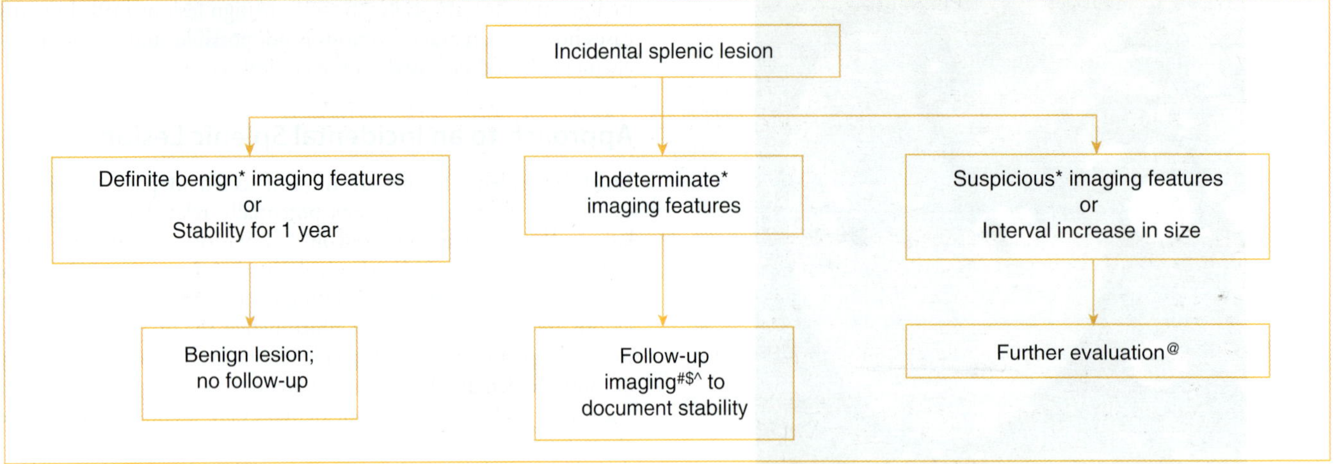

Figure 34.33 Suggested management algorithm for patients with incidental splenic lesions.
*Defined as per the ACR White Paper guidelines described in the preceding text.
#ACR White Paper on splenic incidentalomas on CT and MRI (2013) suggests follow-up MRI at 6–12 months.
$If lesion is visible on ultrasonography, ultrasonography follow-up should be considered.
^Recent data (Siewert B et al., Radiology 2018) suggest that no follow-up is also a reasonable option.
@Further evaluation by MRI, PET-CT or histopathology as clinically relevant.

(2018) retrospective CT review revealed that only 2/201 (1%) of incidental splenic lesions were malignant, and the diagnosis of malignancy was evident in both these cases as synchronous tumors were also identified on the CT [54]. Of the 205 patients, 167 (81%) were indeterminate, while 36 (18%) were cysts. Furthermore, 49/145 (34%) of splenic lesions in cancer patients were malignant. The authors concluded that incidental splenic lesions need not be worked-up or followed-up further.

The take-home point is that an incidental splenic lesion should be considered benign even if not cystic, unless there are specific imaging or clinical findings to suggest otherwise, and follow-up (if recommended) should be kept to a minimum (Fig. 34.33).

Further Evaluation of an Indeterminate/ Suspicious Splenic Lesion

- At the time of writing this chapter, there are no ACR Appropriateness Criteria or other society guidelines recommending imaging options. The options available for evaluating indeterminate or suspicious splenic lesions include CEUS, MRI, PET-CT, biopsy, or surgery
- It must be remembered that the point of the study is not to necessarily diagnose the exact etiology, but to simply label the lesion benign or malignant
- Often, the lesion is detected on a single-phase CECT study, If the patient has no known malignancy, an MRI would be a reasonable option to evaluate indeterminate splenic lesion, instead of repeating a multiphase CT as it may help definitively characterize benign lesions [49,55]. CEUS is another possible option to help differentiate benign and malignant lesions [56–58]
- If the patient has a known malignancy, the ACR White Paper suggests performing immediate further evaluation if the splenic lesion is >1 cm in these cases, while a follow-up MRI is recommended at 6 and 12 months if <1 cm [52]. However, this must be taken in a relevant clinical context
- For a patient of known hematolymphoid malignancy, classic splenic lesions can be considered to be due to lymphomatous involvement without needing further imaging. These patients anyway often undergo PET-CT routinely for staging
- For other malignancies, the chances of an isolated splenic metastasis are rare. The splenic lesion is likely metastatic only if the patient has other sites of metastases as well [2]
- Further evaluation will be warranted only if it will lead to a change in patient management. For example, if the patient of melanoma has hepatic and pulmonary metastases and an indeterminate splenic lesion, the patient will receive chemotherapy irrespective of the etiology of the splenic lesion; hence there is no reason to further evaluate the splenic lesion. However, in the case of an isolated splenic lesion which needs to be characterized as patient management will depend on it (say for example an operable breast cancer patient with an indeterminate splenic lesion), a PET-CT is usually preferred over MRI, as lack of FDG uptake associated with an FDG-avid primary will resolve the question without needing any further follow-up imaging or biopsy
- A direct conversation with the referring physician may often help in deciding the appropriate next step
- Lesions which remain indeterminate on MRI can either be followed up on USG or CT, or be biopsied for a definitive diagnosis [55]. Symptomatic indeterminate lesions may often be operated directly in this scenario
- Splenic biopsy has an increased risk of bleeding due to the normal splenic vascularity, a thin capsule, and a possible vascular lesion. However, several studies have demonstrated the safety of splenic biopsy, and it should be considered when the only other option for diagnosis is a splenectomy for an asymptomatic lesion [2,59,60]. FNAC has a lower complication rate but also a lower yield compared with a core biopsy [60]. *Having a back-up team ready while performing a splenic biopsy would be advisable*

Splenic Lesions in Immunocompromised Patients

- HIV-positive patients or immunocompromised patients on chemotherapy with fever and multiple hypodense subcentimeter splenic lesions can be assumed to have fungal or mycobacterial microabscesses. Pinpointing the causative organism is not possible on imaging

- A concomitant CT chest may demonstrate a classic fungal or mycobacterial infection, which could help guide treatment. Splenic sampling may sometimes be needed, if the clinical picture is uncertain and there are no other sites for obtaining the tissue for culture
- Lymphoma is also more common in immunocompromised patients and should be kept in mind for afebrile patients with larger more heterogeneous lesions. Associated adenopathy is usually present
- Kaposi's sarcoma may affect HIV patients with very low CD4 levels but again is disseminated by the time it involves the spleen
- Apart from these etiologies, any of the common benign splenic lesions may also present in this patient subset as well; comparison with previous imaging (these patients usually undergo imaging multiple times) is useful in this regard

Suggested Readings

- S Ahmed, KM Horton, EK Fishman, Splenic incidentalomas, Radiol Clin North Am 49 (2011) 323–347.
- RM Abbott, AD Levy, NS Aguilera, L Gorospe, WM Thompson, From the archives of the AFIP: primary vascular neoplasms of the spleen: radiologic-pathologic correlation, Radiographics 24 (2004) 1137–1163.
- SS Saboo, KM Krajewski, KN O'Regan, et al., Spleen in haematological malignancies: spectrum of imaging findings, Br J Radiol 85 (2012) 81–92.
- RK Kaza, S Azar, MM Al-Hawary, IR Francis, Primary and secondary neoplasms of the spleen, Cancer Imag 10 (2010) 173–182.
- KJ Mortele, B Mortele, SG Silverman, CT features of the accessory spleen, AJR Am J Roentgenol 183 (2004) 1653–1657.
- ST Lake, PT Johnson, S Kawamoto, RH Hruban, EK Fishman, CT of splenosis: patterns and pitfalls, AJR Am J Roentgenol 199 (2012) W686–W693.

35

Gallbladder and Biliary Tree

ARGHA CHATTERJEE, ANISHA GEHANI, ALIREZA B. ABADI, SAUGATA SEN

Anatomy

The entire biliary system is derived from the ventral outpouching of the primitive foregut. The hollow outpouching undergoes solidification and subsequent recanalization. Like most structures derived from foregut, the gallbladder is lined by columnar epithelium, mucus secreting glands, and few enteric endocrine glands. *There are multiple intramural diverticula lined by mucosal epithelium in the gallbladder wall called the **Rokitansky–Aschoff sinuses**, hyperplasia of which leads to adenomyomatosis.*

Gallbladder Anatomy

- The gallbladder lies in the right hypochondrium along the inferior surface of the liver, between hepatic segments IV and V (Fig. 35.1)
- It is divided into the fundus (most anterior and inferior portion), body, and neck. The neck joins the common hepatic duct (CHD) through the cystic duct to form the common bile duct (CBD)
- At the region of the neck, there is a small outpouching called the *Hartmann's pouch* (or *infundibulum*), which is a common location for impaction of gallstones
- The gallbladder stores bile and releases it into the duodenum in response to ingestion of fatty foods

Intrahepatic Bile Duct Anatomy

- The right hepatic duct is formed by the fusion of right anterior sectoral duct (RASD) draining segments V and VIII and right posterior sectoral duct (RPSD) draining segments VI and VII. RASD runs a more vertical course. RPSD runs a more horizontal course and characteristically forms a "U"-shaped bend before joining the RASD
- Bile duct branches from segment II to IV unite to form the left hepatic duct (LHD)
- The right and left hepatic ducts then unite to form the CHD. Duct from segment I drains to either the right or left hepatic ducts. However, this classic anatomy is thought to be present in only a little more than half of the population [1]

Extrahepatic Biliary Duct Anatomy

- At the hilum, the CHD lies anterior to the bifurcation of the portal vein. It is joined by the cystic duct to form the CBD. The CBD lies anterior to the portal vein and to the right and anterior to the common hepatic artery (CHA). In upper abdominal ultrasound along the long axis of the CBD, the CHA is seen in cross section between the portal vein and the CBD
- A triangular space called the cystohepatic space or Calot's triangle is formed at the porta hepatis between the cystic duct, CHD, and the inferior surface of the liver. This space is important as it contains the cystic artery, right hepatic artery, and cystic node of Lund. This requires careful dissection at the time of cholecystectomy to avoid inadvertent ductal/vascular injuries
- The CBD courses inferiorly posterior to the first portion of duodenum and head of pancreas and then pierces the parenchyma of the pancreatic head. Then it fuses with the main pancreatic duct (MPD) to form a common short channel at the ampulla of Vater that enters duodenum through the major papilla. The sphincter of Oddi is a circular band of smooth muscle which surrounds the distal end of the CBD and MPD union at the ampulla

Vascular Supply

Most of the supply to the intra- and extrahepatic bile ducts comes from the peribiliary plexus arising from hepatic artery proper and gastroduodenal arteries, both branches of CHA [2,3]. Hence, the

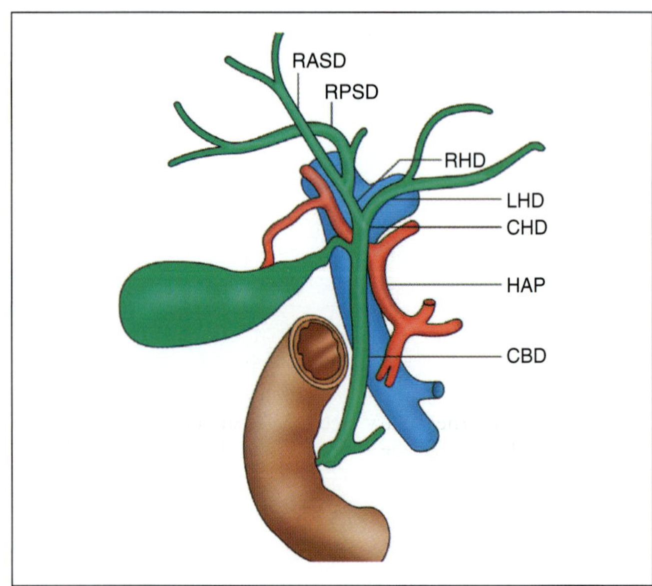

Figure 35.1 Diagram of the gallbladder and the biliary tree. Note that the RASD is more vertical and medial whereas the RPSD is more horizontal and lateral, when seen in frontal view. Usually, the RPSD loops posterior to the RASD and joins it from the medial side to form the RHD. Also, note that the right hepatic artery passes posterior to the CBD. *CBD*, common bile duct; *CHD*, common hepatic duct; *HAP*, hepatic artery proper; *LHD*, left hepatic duct; *RASD*, right anterior sectoral duct; *RHD*, right hepatic duct; *RPSD*, right posterior sectoral duct.

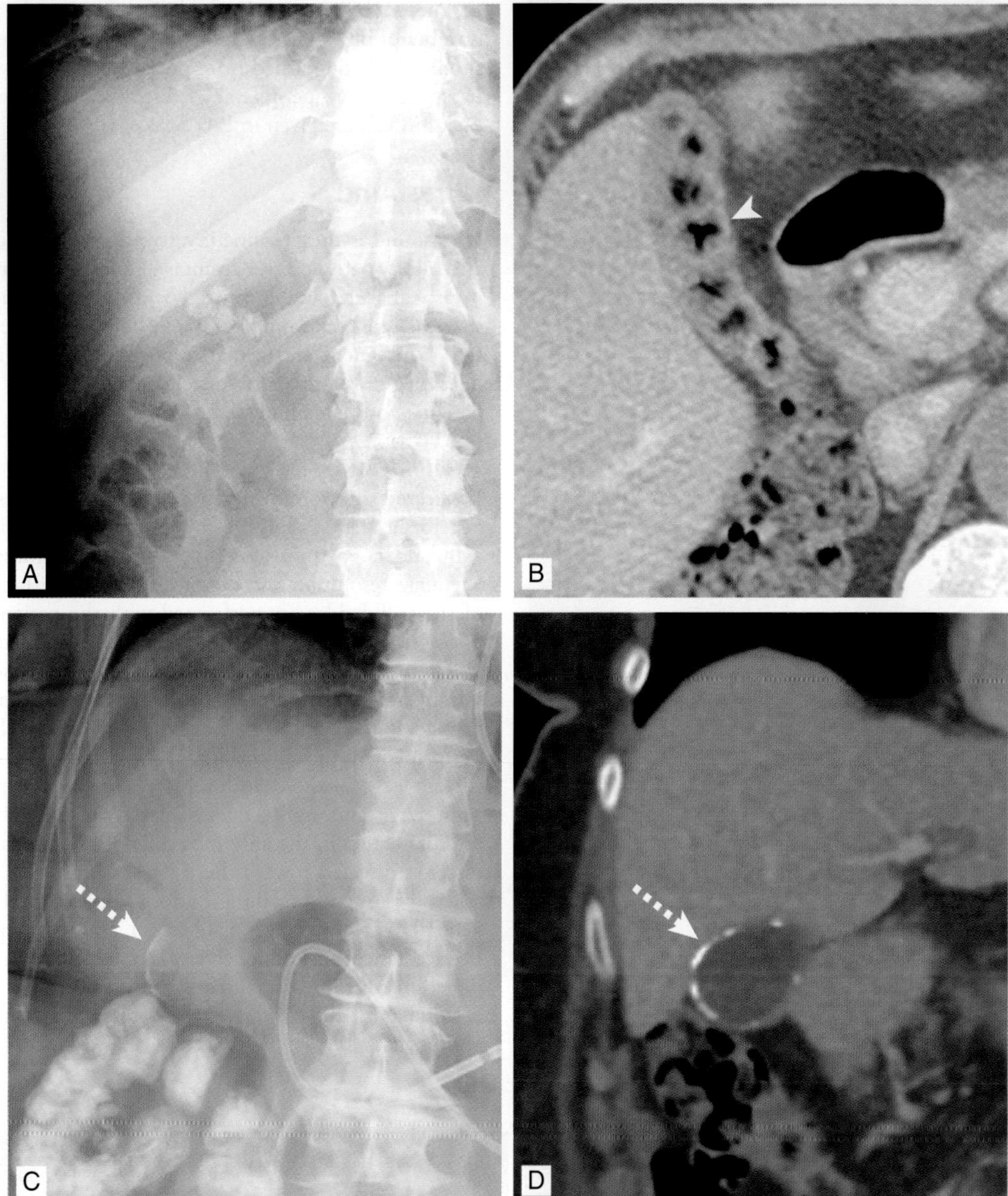

Figure 35.2 Appearance of gallstones on imaging. (A) Calcium carbonate ("mulberry") stones in the gallbladder. (B) "Mercedes Benz" stone; characteristic appearance (*arrowhead*). (C and D) Calcified ("porcelain") gallbladder (*dotted arrows*) in plain radiograph (C) and coronal reformat CECT (D).

blood supply of the biliary tract and gallbladder comes entirely from the CHA and not from the portal vein. Therefore, transection of CHA during surgery will result in biliary necrosis, unlike the liver parenchyma. The biliary tree is also susceptible to ischemic changes after cholecystectomy or liver transplantations resulting in biliary strictures (see ischemic injury of the bile duct) [4]. The veins of the peribiliary plexus drain into tributaries of portal vein. This may dilate in extrahepatic portal venous occlusion and give rise to pericholedocal varices.

Methods of Investigation

Plain Radiograph

Plain radiograph has minimal usage in biliary pathologies. However, incidental biliary pathologies may be identified on an abdominal radiograph obtained for other indications.

Calcified Gallstones

Only 15–20% gallstones contain enough calcium to be visible on plain radiograph [5]. Pure calcium carbonate stones are most radiopaque (mulberry stones) (Fig. 35.2A). Gallstones are often lamellated with a central lucency. Sometimes, gallstones can trap gas, which can appear as a central triradiate lucency (Mercedes Benz sign) (Fig. 35.2B). Calcification is less common in bile duct stones.

Limey bile, also known as milk of calcium of the gallbladder, represents layering of calcium carbonate in the dependent portions due to bile stasis. This is sometimes seen in patients in intensive care units or after prolonged parenteral feeding. This should not be confused with biliary sludge seen on ultrasound.

Calcification of the gallbladder wall results in porcelain gallbladder (Fig. 35.2C). This condition can predispose to gallbladder adenocarcinoma [6]. Gas in the gallbladder wall may be seen in emphysematous cholecystitis (Fig. 35.3).

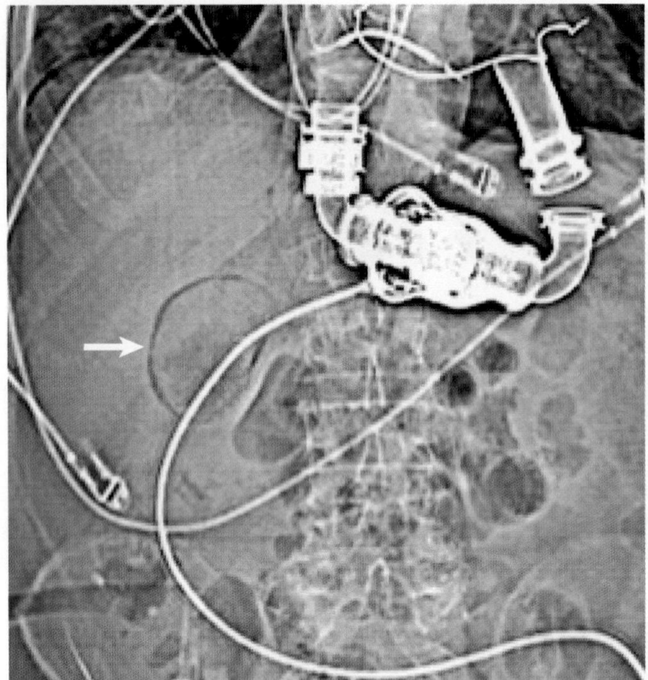

Figure 35.3 Emphysematous cholecystitis. CT scout image of upper abdomen shows gas in the wall of the gallbladder. (Courtesy: Dr. Frank H. Miller, Northwestern University Feinberg School of Medicine, Chicago, USA.)

BOX 35.1 Causes of Pneumobilia

- Instrumentation of bile duct (ERCP or stent insertion)
- Fistulous communication of the biliary tree with small bowel or colon
- Incompetent sphincter of Oddi (due to sphincterotomy or passage of stone)
- After hepaticojejunostomy

Pneumobilia or gas in the biliary tree can be attributed to a number of physiological and pathological processes (Fig. 35.4). It should be distinguished from portal venous gas, which is characteristically more peripheral in distribution. Important causes of pneumobilia are given in Box 35.1.

Ultrasound

Ultrasound is the first-line investigation in suspected gallbladder and biliary pathologies. Advantage includes wide availability, noninvasive nature, and effectiveness in differentiating medical from surgical causes of jaundice. It can be done at the bedside and is safe in pregnant and pediatric populations. Limitations include high degree of operator dependence and poor penetration in patients with large body habitus.

Technique and Views

Dedicated ultrasound for the gallbladder requires the patient to fast for at least 4–6 hours to allow maximum distension of the gallbladder. For most patients, a 3–7 MHz transducer provides adequate resolution and depth. Standard sagittal and axial views of the gallbladder are performed with the patient in the supine position. In case of nonvisualization of the gallbladder, the patient is asked to lie in the left lateral decubitus position or sit up in semirecumbent posture and bend forward. These positions help in displacing the colonic gas from the field of view. Scanning is also performed by the subcostal axial oblique view. In this position, the left edge of the transducer is placed more cephalad than the right edge and right edge is placed in the subcostal location approximately in the anterior axillary line. The face of the transducer is directed toward the right shoulder. The patient may be asked to suspend breathing in deep inspiration. This view gives a general overview of liver, gallbladder, and intrahepatic bile ducts. Intercostal coronal oblique view is obtained by putting the transducer in lower intercostal spaces at the mid-axillary line. This view is suitable for the entire sweep of gallbladder fossa, CHD, CBD, and porta.

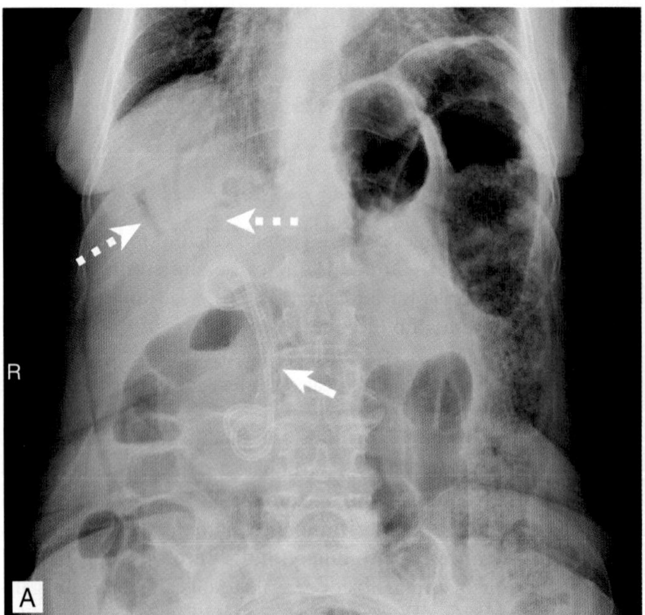

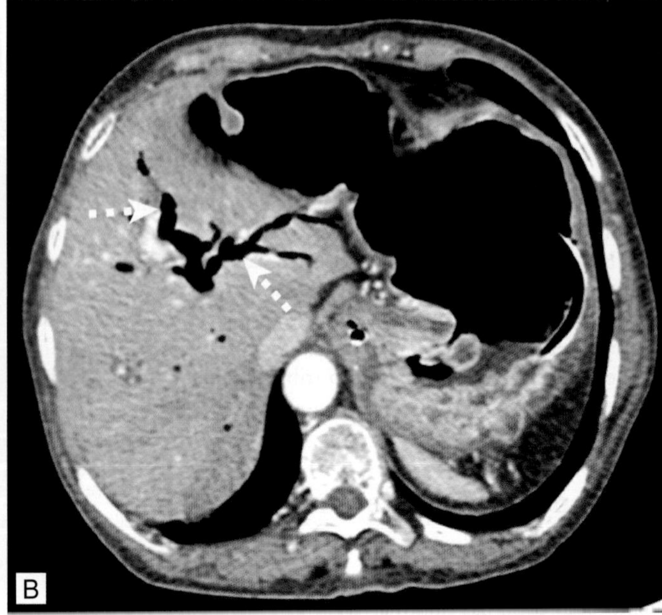

Figure 35.4 Pneumobilia. (A) Plain radiograph of abdomen shows air within the biliary tree (*dotted arrows*). The reason of pneumobilia is placement of stents within the common bile duct (*solid arrow*). (B) Contrast CT of upper abdomen demonstrated air within the left hepatic ducts (*dotted arrows*).

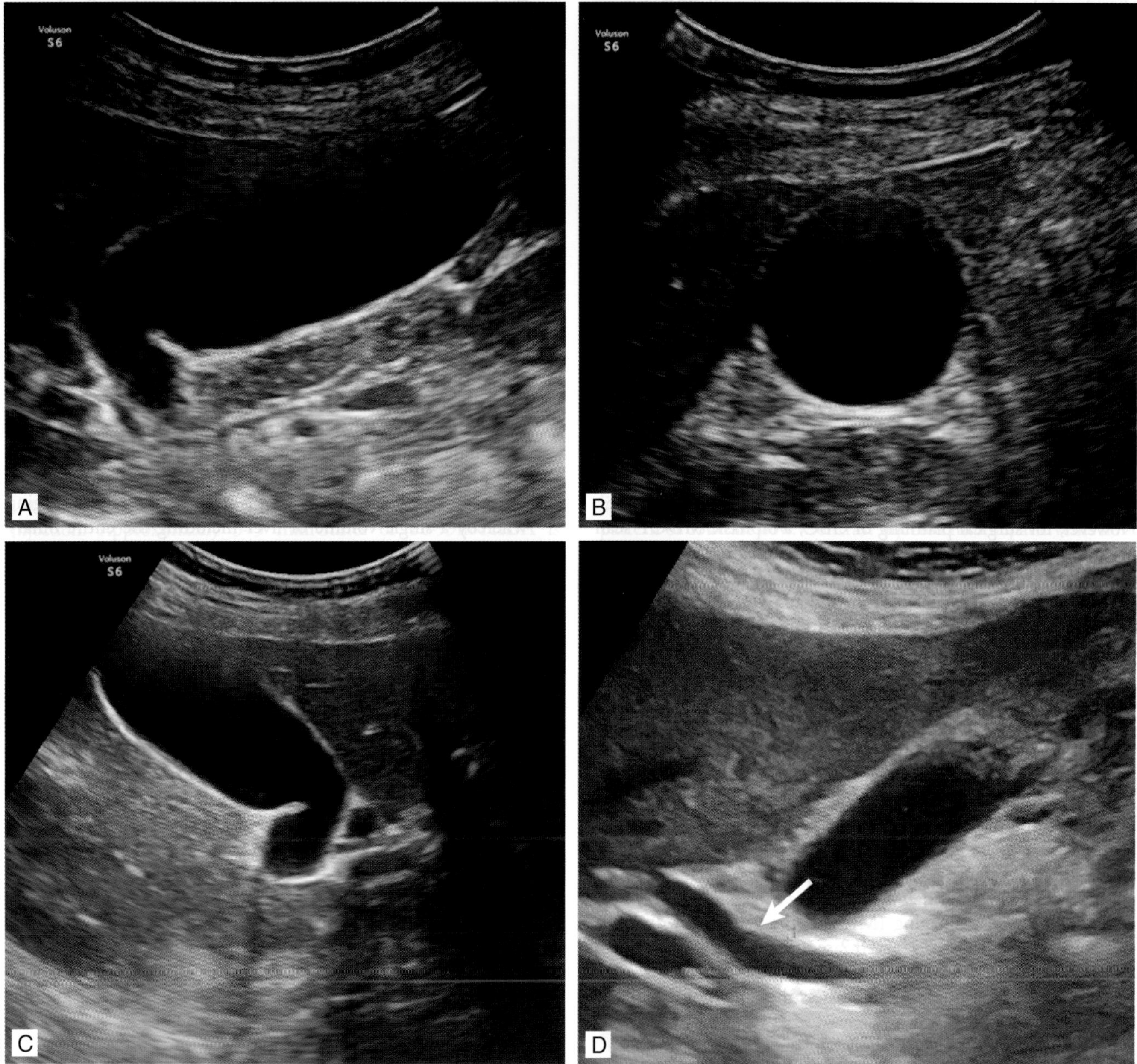

Figure 35.5 Standard ultrasound views of the gallbladder and CBD. (A) Sagittal view of the gallbladder. (B) Axial view of the gallbladder. (C) Subcostal axial oblique view of the gallbladder. (D) Intercostal coronal oblique view shows the common bile duct in long axis (*arrow*).

Additionally, color Doppler may be used to assess the vascularity of gallbladder walls or polyps. Use of tissue harmonic imaging can improve the contrast between the ductal system and surrounding structures making the visualization of ductal lumen and wall pathologies easier.

Normal Appearance

The normal gallbladder, in the fasting state, is a sonolucent pear-shaped structure with thin smooth walls (measuring <3 mm in thickness) with a length of approximately 7 cm and AP diameter of 4 cm (Fig. 35.5). Intrahepatic bile ducts are rarely seen unless they are dilated and usually measure up to 1–2 mm. Dilated intrahepatic ducts course parallel to portal venous tributaries and can be differentiated from them by means of their echogenic walls and by color flow Doppler. The CHD measures up to 4–5 mm normally. Proximal CBD can be readily identified on ultrasound however, visualization of the distal CBD may be difficult due to overlying duodenal gas. Proximal CBD can measure up to 7 mm in normal individuals. CBD diameter may increase with age and after cholecystectomy; however, this fact is contested and there is no standardized upper limit according to age [7,8]. All cases with a CBD diameter of 8 mm or more should be investigated for ductal dilatation [9,10].

Endoscopic Ultrasound

Endoscopic ultrasound incorporates a high-frequency ultrasound transducer at the tip of the endoscope which can acquire radial or linear images depending upon the type of probe and can also help in guided procedures such as fine needle aspirations and endoscopic retrograde cholangiopancreatography (ERCP). Due to the high frequency of the probe used, penetration and visualization of deeper structures is limited and the use of endoscopic

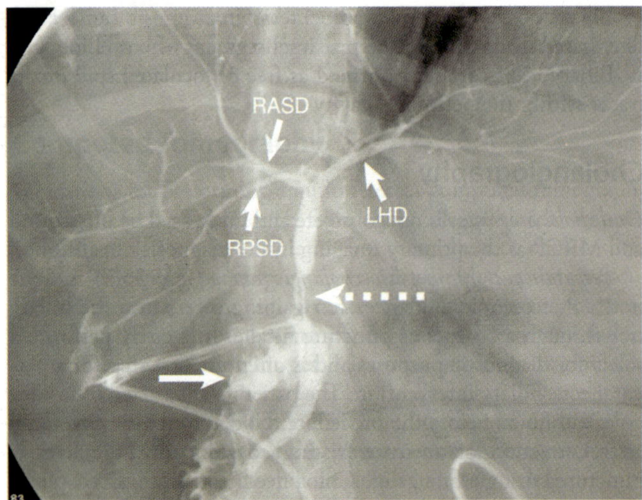

Figure 35.8 Normal T-tube cholangiogram, right anterior oblique projection. Contrast injected through the T-tube (*dotted arrow*) positioned in the common bile duct has opacified the entire biliary tree and shows free passage of contrast in the duodenum (*solid arrow*). *LHD*, left hepatic duct; *RASD*, right anterior sectoral duct; *RPSD*, right posterior sectoral duct. Note the hook-like configuration of the RPSD before it joins the RASD.

Operative cholangiography is performed at the time of cholecystectomy to detect any obscure CBD stones. A cannula is placed directly in the CBD during the surgery and 5–10 mL of contrast is injected. This procedure is not only used to detect stones but can also be used at the time of surgery to demonstrate anomalous duct anatomy, and defining developmental disorders of the biliary tree, such as biliary hypoplasia and biliary atresia before surgical drainage if the preoperative investigations are equivocal.

Postoperative cholangiography or T-tube cholangiography is performed through the T-tube placed in the CBD after CBD exploration to look for retained stones (Fig. 35.8). If stones are found at the time of postoperative cholangiogram, they can be removed *through* the endoscopic route. A T-tube cholangiogram is considered optimum when both intrahepatic and extrahepatic biliary ducts are opacified. Stones should be differentiated from gas bubbles as the latter would rise to nondependent parts on changing the patient's position to reverse Trendelenburg.

Developmental Anomalies

Knowledge of the common variants and anomalies is important to avoid chances of inadvertent intraoperative injuries resulting in bile leaks and cholangitis.

Intrahepatic Anomalies

1. The most common anomaly in terms of insertion site includes drainage of the RPSD into the LHD (13–19% of the population) [1,16].
2. Right lateral insertion of RPSD into RASD (10–12% of the population).
3. "Triple confluence" of RPSD, RASD, and LHD (11% population).
4. Uncommon variants include aberrant RPSD draining into CHD (Fig. 35.9A), RASD draining into LHD and accessory hepatic ducts (2–6% of the population).

Extrahepatic Anomalies

1. Anomalies of the gallbladder number—duplication with separate cystic ducts, agenesis.
2. Anomalies of the gallbladder position—ectopic gallbladder (left sided, intrahepatic, or retroplaced).
3. Anomalies of the gallbladder shape—folds (Phrygian cap deformity) (Fig. 35.9B), septated gallbladder (bilobed, with single cystic duct), and diverticulum.
4. Anomalies of cystic duct insertion—low cystic duct insertion at the distal third of the CBD, medial cystic duct insertion at the left side of CHD, and parallel course of cystic duct with the CHD (for at least 2 cm; Fig. 35.9C).
5. Anomalous pancreatico biliary junction involves formation of a long common channel (>1.5 cm) outside the duodenal wall by early fusion of CBD and MPD.

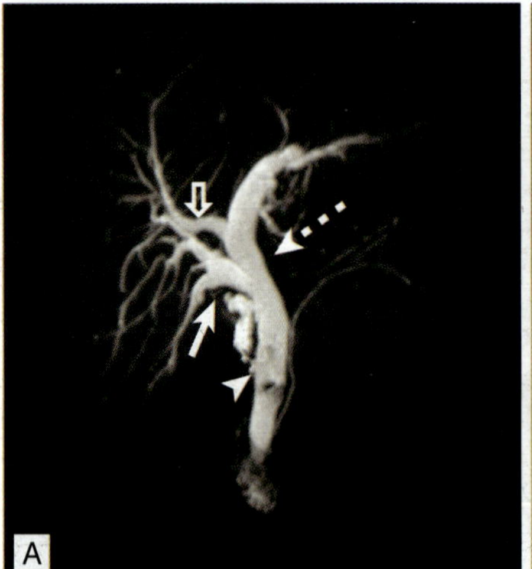

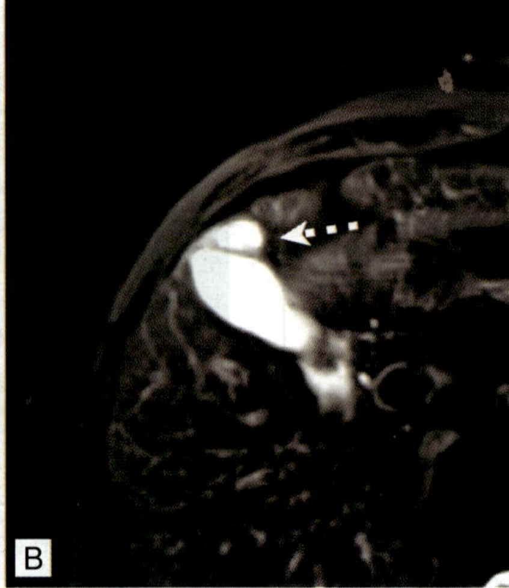

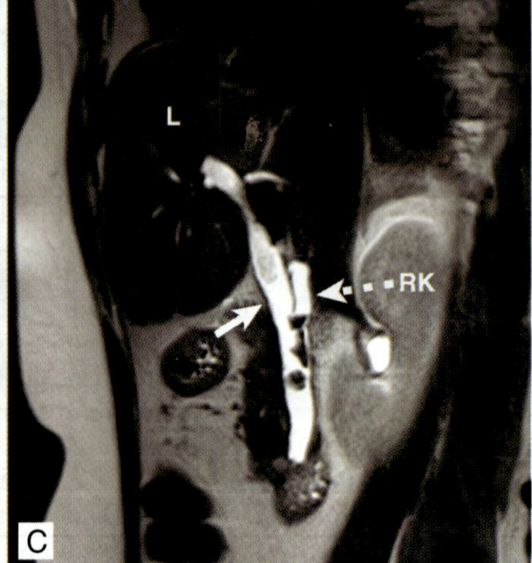

Figure 35.9 (A) 3D maximum intensity projection MRCP shows right posterior sectoral duct (*solid arrow*) meeting the common hepatic duct (CHD) (*dotted arrow*) and CHD is formed by the union of right anterior sectoral duct (*open arrow*) and left hepatic duct. The biliary system is dilated due to the presence of a common bile duct calculus (*arrowhead*). (B) Axial fat-suppressed T2-weighted images show Phrygian cap deformity at gallbladder fundus. (C) Sagittal T2-weighted image shows long cystic duct (*dotted arrow*) inserting posteriorly into the common hepatic duct (*solid arrow*). Note multiple calculi within the bile duct. *L*, liver; *RK*, right kidney.

TABLE 35.1 Types of Gallstone [17,18]

Types	Constituent	Comment
Cholesterol	>90% cholesterol with calcium bilirubinate	Rare. Caused by high fat diet, high serum lipid
Mixed	At least 50% cholesterol with calcium bilirubinate	Most common (75–80%)
Black pigment	<25% cholesterol. Rest calcium bilirubinate with bilirubin polymers and mucin glycoproteins	About 20% of stones. Associated with hemolysis, cirrhosis, malabsorption
Brown pigment	<25% cholesterol with calcium salts of unconjugated bilirubin and variable amounts of protein	About 4.5% of stones. Associated with infection (e.g., bacterial infection, clonorchis)

Gallbladder

Gallstone Disease

Gallstones are solid particles composed of cholesterol and bile pigment (Table 35.1). Gallstones form within the gallbladder but can pass to different parts of the biliary tree and gastrointestinal tract.

Epidemiology and Risk Factors

Gallstone is one of the most common ultrasound findings in daily practice. In the United states, North American Indians have the highest reported rates of cholelithiasis [19]. Common risk factors are increasing age, female gender, obesity, diabetes, and pregnancy.

Gallstone-Related Diseases

Gallstone-related diseases can be classified as:

- Asymptomatic cholelithiasis: About 80% cases of gallstones are asymptomatic and may be discovered incidentally
- Symptomatic cholelithiasis: About 20% cases with gallstones have intermittent dull aching pain in right hypochondrium, often precipitated by a fatty meal and accompanied by sweating, nausea, and vomiting (biliary colic). It usually subsides within an hour. An episode lasting for more than 6 hours indicates acute cholecystitis
- Complicated cholelithiasis: Symptomatic patients have a risk of 1–2% per year of developing complications [20] (Box 35.2)

Imaging Features

Ultrasound is the imaging technique of choice in suspected gallstone disease. CECT is indicated only when complications are suspected. MRCP is necessary when choledocholithiasis or CBD stone is suspected.

Ultrasound: Ultrasound has a sensitivity of 84% and a specificity of 99% for the diagnosis of gallstones [21]. Whereas, the sensitivity of the CT scan for detecting gallstones ranges from 55% to 80% [22].

BOX 35.2 Complications of Gallstone Disease

- Acute cholecystitis
- Bile duct stone (choledocholithiasis) and cholangitis
- Gallstone pancreatitis
- Mirizzi syndrome
- Gallstone ileus

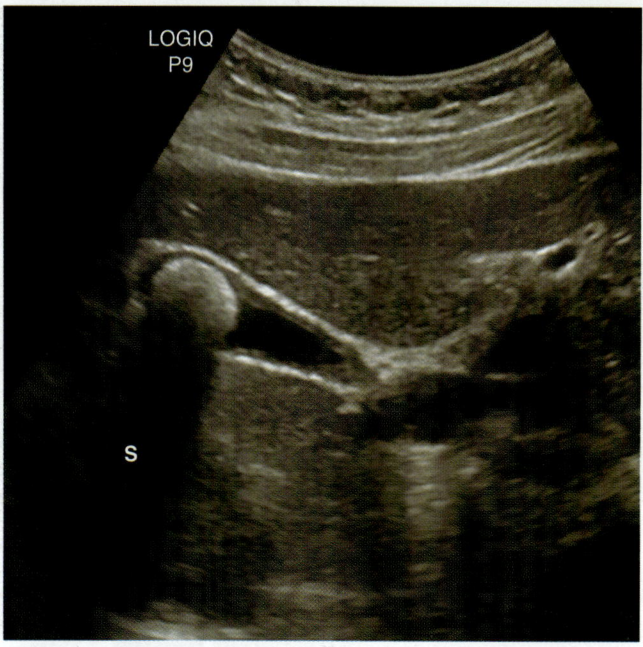

Figure 35.10 Large gallstone is noted in the fundus of the gallbladder shown in ultrasound, right subcostal oblique view. Note the dense acoustic shadow (S).

On ultrasound, gallstones appear as echogenic foci with posterior acoustic shadow (Fig. 35.10). The shadow is detected irrespective of the composition of the gallstones. On color Doppler ultrasound, small stones may be detected by *twinkling artifacts* which look like foci of alternating colors behind the calculus. The position of the stone changes as the patient is turned ("rolling stone" sign). Multiple small stones are called *gravel*. With too many stones, the posterior wall of the gallbladder may be obscured by acoustic shadow. In such cases the gallbladder wall is visualized in the near field, followed by the bright echo of the stones, which is followed by the acoustic shadowing. This finding is called the wall–echo–shadow complex (Fig. 35.11). This can mimic gas in the duodenal bulb.

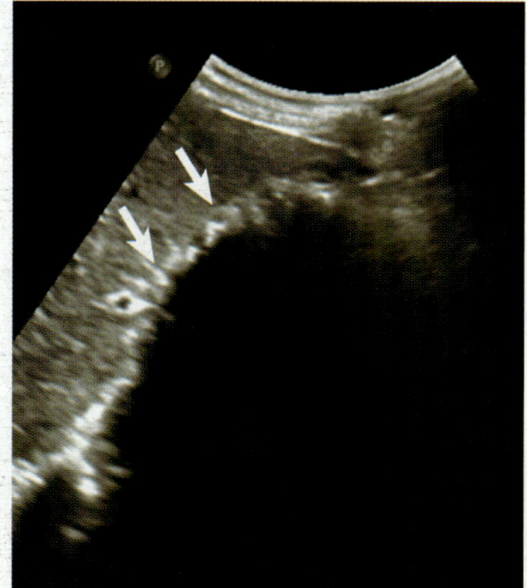

Figure 35.11 "Wall–echo–shadow" complex. Ultrasound shows strong echoes within the gallbladder lumen (*arrows*) followed by dense acoustic shadows which obscures further detail. (Courtesy: Dr. Mousam Dey, Indian Institute of Liver and Digestive Sciences, Kolkata.)

Biliary sludge is composed of lithogenic bile that contains cholesterol monohydrate crystals, bilirubin granules, and a mucus glycoprotein gel (Fig. 35.12). It is commonly seen in pregnancy, critically ill patients and in patients who are on parenteral nutrition (Table 35.2). Sludge can become organized and immobile to form tumefactive sludge and mimic a gallbladder polyp [23]. Unlike a true polyp, tumefactive sludge does not show internal vascularity on color Doppler or contrast enhancement on CECT (Fig. 35.13) [24].

Ultrasound examination should focus on ruling out complications, especially choledocholithiasis (Box 35.3). A dilated bile duct (≥8 mm) in a case of cholelithiasis should raise suspicion of a CBD stone (Fig. 35.14A). Examining the lower end of the CBD is of utmost importance.

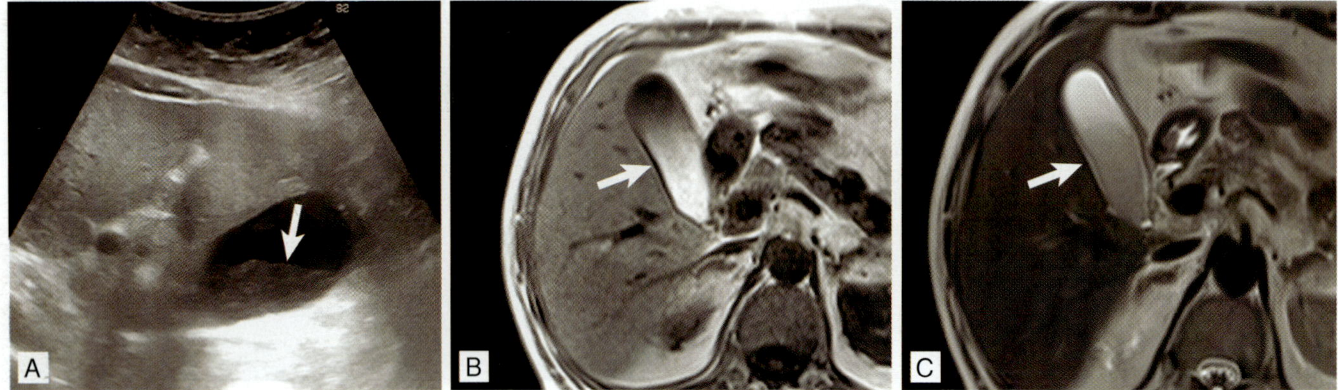

Figure 35.12 Gallbladder sludge. (A) Ultrasound shows nonshadowing dependent low-level echo within the lumen of the gallbladder (*arrow*). (B and C) T1-weighted (B) and T2-weighted (C) axial images show altered signal intensity content in the gallbladder lumen (*arrow*). Note sludge can be hyperintense on T1-weighted images.

TABLE 35.2 Lithogenic Bile: Spectrum of Ultrasound Appearance

Type	Number	Echogenicity	Mobility	Posterior Shadow	Clinical Significance
Sludge	Fluid	Low	Slow	No	Indicate stasis, can cause symptomatic gallstone disease
Limey bile	Fluid	High	Slow	Yes	Indicate stasis, can cause symptomatic gallstone disease
Gravel	Multiple	Very high	Fast	Yes	Can be missed as WES
Calculus	Few	Very high	Fast	Yes	Can cause symptoms and complications
Tumefactive sludge	Single	Low	Nil	No	Up to 15% cases may be malignancy, follow-up is necessary

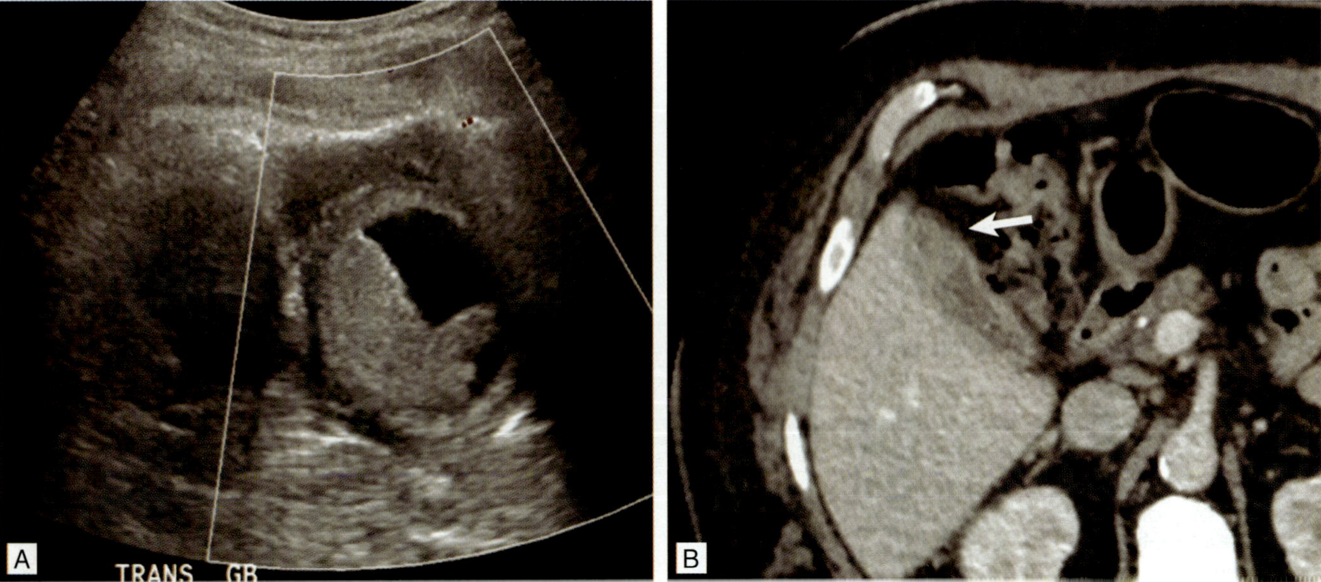

Figure 35.13 Tumefactive sludge. (A) Ultrasound in axial view of the gallbladder shows echogenic immobile polypoid lesion within the gallbladder lumen without any Doppler signals. (B) Axial CECT shows nonenhancing polypoid lesion at the fundus of the gallbladder (*arrow*).

BOX 35.3 Minimum Ultrasound Reporting Standard in Gallstone

Gallstone: size and number.
Mobility.
Gallbladder wall thickness (in mm) and other signs of acute or chronic cholecystitis, if any.
Common bile duct diameter (in mm). If dilated, exclude choledocholithiasis.
Other causes of upper abdomen discomfort (fatty liver, pancreatitis).

Magnetic Resonance Cholangiopancreatography: CBD stone is found in 10–20% cases with symptomatic gallstone disease [25]. Presence of CBD stone requires a CBD exploration during cholecystectomy. CBD stone may be detected at surgery or follow-up in 3–17% patients with a normal ultrasound. If ultrasound shows a dilated bile duct or intraductal echoes, the probability of the presence of a CBD stone increases to 45–85% [26]. Therefore, in patients with an intermediate probability of CBD stone (raised serum alkaline phosphatase and dilated CBD on ultrasound), preoperative MRCP is indicated.

Gallstones typically appear as low-signal intensity structures or "filling defects" surrounded by hyperintense bile (Fig. 35.14B). MRCP has a high sensitivity of 90–94% and specificity of 95–99% for the detection of CBD stone [27].

Computed Tomography: The size and extent of matrix calcification determines the visibility of gallstones on CT. However, most pure cholesterol stones can also be visualized by narrowing the window settings on noncontrast acquisitions. Gallstones sometimes appear lamellated with a lucent center and concentric calcified rims.

Complications

Mirizzi Syndrome: Mirizzi syndrome is caused by extrinsic compression of the CHD by a gallstone impacted within the cystic duct, gallbladder neck, or Hartmann's pouch. The obstruction can result in jaundice, repeated cholangitis, and acute cholecystitis. With prolonged pressure, the common duct wall can erode and a fistula may form with the gallbladder (cholecystocholedochal fistula). Mirizzi syndrome is often confused with cholangiocarcinoma (CCA) or GBC.

- On ultrasound, the gallbladder shows an impacted stone at the neck. Intrahepatic biliary radicles and proximal CHD are dilated. However, diagnosis is difficult solely based on ultrasound
- MRCP shows smooth gradual tapering of the CHD suggesting an extrinsic obstruction rather than a malignant stricture. The impacted calculus and cholecystocholedochal fistula can be demonstrated. MRCP also helps in ruling out distal CBD stones
- ERCP shows the classical appearance of smooth stricture of the CHD with concavity to the right
- CT findings are similar (Fig. 35.15)

It is important to remember that GBC cannot be ruled out with certainty and up to 6–28% of patients with a preoperative diagnosis of Mirizzi syndrome are later found to have GBC [28].

Cholecystoenteric Fistula and Gallstone Ileus

Chronic irritation and inflammation caused by a large gallstone can create a fistula into the small bowel resulting in the passage of the stone into the small bowel. Sufficiently large stones can cause intestinal obstruction, most commonly at the level of the ileocecal valve and the ensuing obstruction is called gallstone ileus. It is more common in the elderly and has a high mortality rate. The classical finding in abdominal radiograph consists of the Rigler's triad; pneumobilia in the right upper quadrant (RUQ), dilated small bowel loops, and the gallstone in the right iliac fossa. CT can demonstrate the obstructing gallstone even when it is not radiopaque (Fig. 35.16). CT can demonstrate even small cholecystoenteric fistula, especially with multiplanar reconstruction (Fig. 35.17). Uncommonly, gallstone may obstruct the duodenum causing gastric outlet obstruction (Bouveret's syndrome).

Acute Cholecystitis

Acute cholecystitis is a clinical syndrome of RUQ pain, fever, and leukocytosis that is caused by acute gallbladder inflammation. It is most commonly associated with gallstone disease, however, a

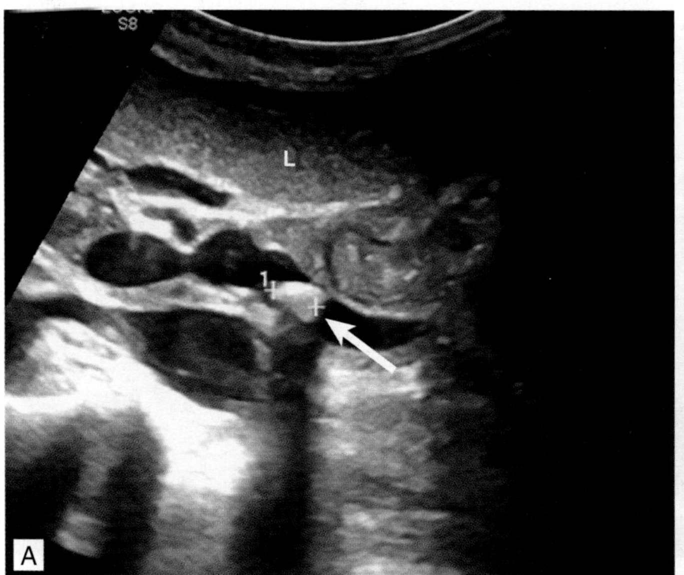

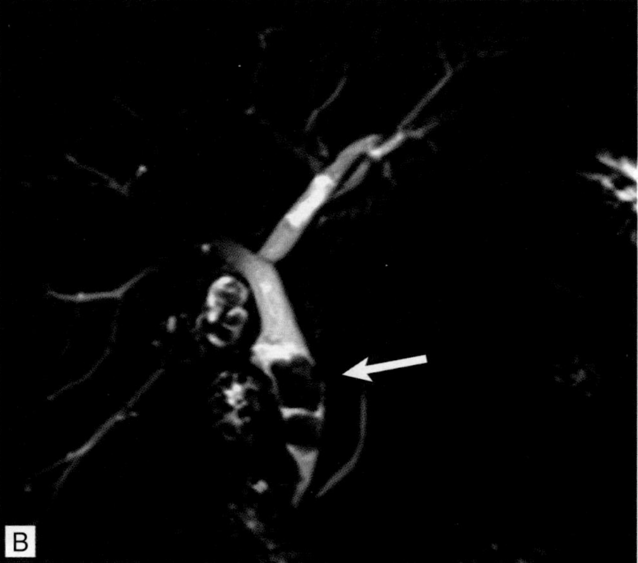

Figure 35.14 Choledocholithiasis. (A) Long-axis ultrasound image of the common bile duct shows large calculus within the dilated duct. (B) 3D coronal MRCP in a different patient shows multiple calculi (*arrow*) within the common bile duct. *L*, liver.

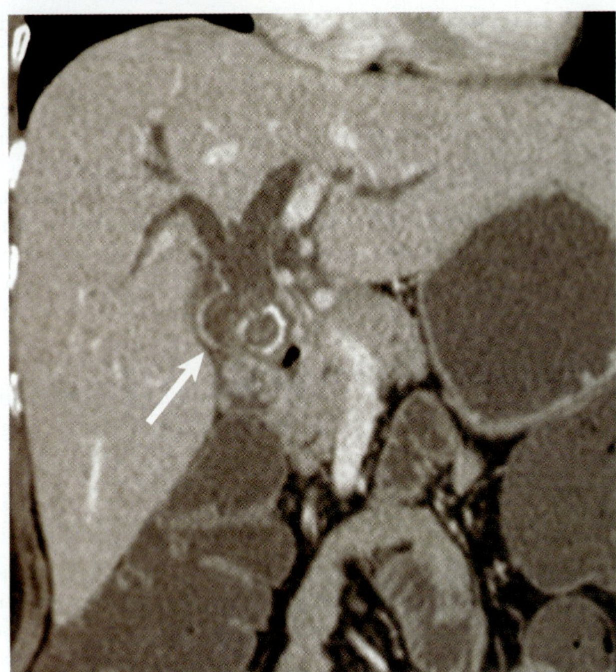

Figure 35.15 Mirizzi syndrome. Coronal reformat of contrast CT shows dilated biliary tree with a large calculus impacted at the junction of cystic duct (*arrow*) and common hepatic duct. Note wide communication between the two ducts.

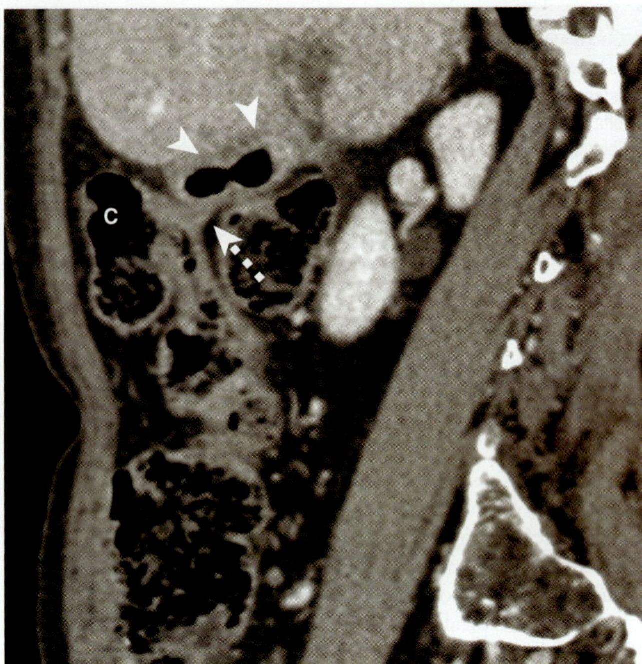

Figure 35.17 Cholecystocolic fistula. Oblique sagittal reformat of CECT shows a small fistulous tract (*dotted arrow*) between colon (C) and gallbladder (*arrowheads*). Note air within the gallbladder lumen.

small proportion of cases occur in the absence of gallstones and are called acalculous cholecystitis.

Epidemiology

Acute cholecystitis develops in about 6–11% cases of symptomatic gallstone disease [29]. It is more common after the age of 50 years [30]. Acute cholecystitis is twice as common in women, but it tends to be more severe in men [31]. Other risk factors for acute cholecystitis include obesity, diabetes mellitus, and certain drugs such as oral contraceptives and hormone replacement therapy.

Pathophysiology

Central to the pathogenesis of acute cholecystitis is cystic duct obstruction, which is most commonly caused by a stone. Obstruction due to tumor, helminthic infection, or extrinsic compression by tumor or nodes may also lead to acute cholecystitis. Infection of the stagnant bile can also be a contributing factor to the inflammation but it is not always present [32].

Clinical Features

- RUQ or epigastric pain: It may radiate toward the right shoulder or back and lasts for more than 6 hours

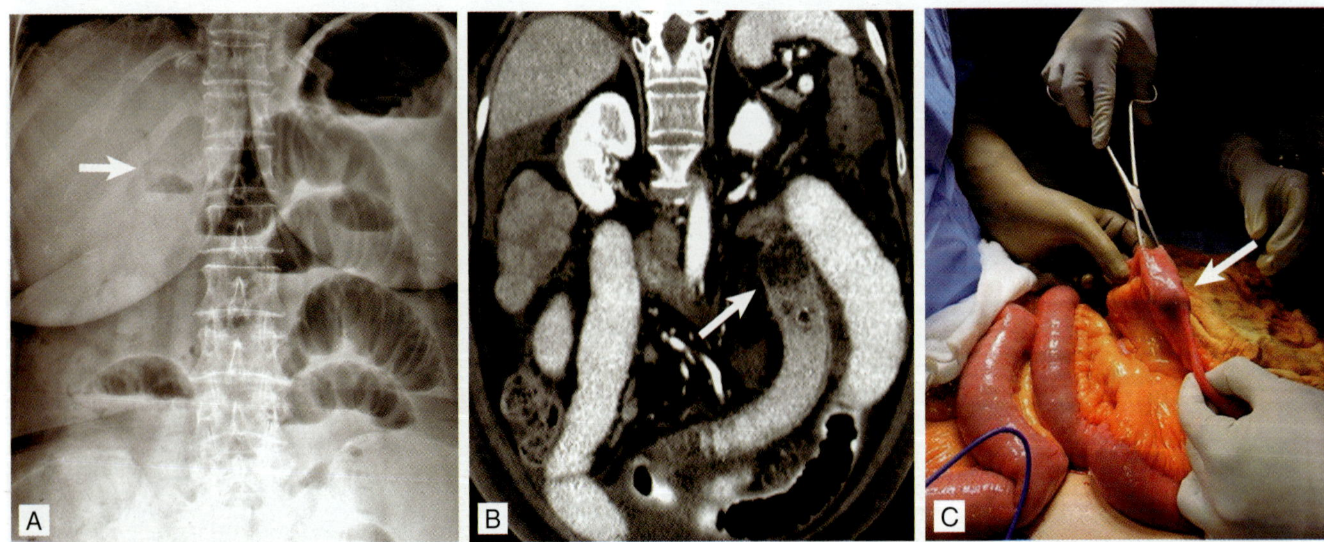

Figure 35.16 Gallstone ileus. (A) Straight radiograph of abdomen in erect posture shows dilated small bowel loops and pneumobilia (*arrow*). The gallstone is not visible. (B) Oblique coronal reformat of contrast-enhanced CT shows dilated bowel loops and low attenuation radiolucent gallstone at the zone of transition of the proximal obstructed small bowel and distal collapsed bowel loops (*arrow*). (C) Operative photograph shows the gallstone within small bowel (*arrow*). (Courtesy: Dr. Bharat Aggarwal, Max Healthcare, New Delhi, India.)

- Fever
- Nausea, vomiting, and anorexia

On examination, RUQ tenderness, guarding, and Murphy's sign are present. Murphy's sign is described as an arrest in inspiration while palpating the right subcostal region during a deep breath due to tenderness.

Blood leukocytosis is usually seen. Frank jaundice and elevated alkaline phosphatase should raise suspicion of bile duct obstruction.

Imaging

Imaging confirmation of the clinical diagnosis of acute cholecystitis is necessary [33]. The imaging investigation of choice is ultrasound. Technetium-99m HIDA scan is performed when ultrasound is equivocal. The CECT scan or MRI is performed only when complication is suspected.

Ultrasound: The ultrasound diagnosis of acute cholecystitis requires at least one of the two features [33]:

- Gallbladder wall thickening of more than 5 mm
- Sonographic Murphy sign: When the ultrasound probe is pressed on the distended gallbladder, pain is elicited. This is more accurate than clinical "Murphy's sign" as the gallbladder is directly visualized

There are other ancillary findings which may be detected on ultrasonography.

- Gallstones: Ultrasound detects gallstone in up to 98% cases of acute cholecystitis
- Enlarged gallbladder (long axis >8 cm, short axis >4 cm)
- Pericholecystic fluid
- Gallbladder wall edema, showing a triple layer appearance with a sonolucent middle layer
- Increased Doppler signals from the gallbladder wall

Sensitivity and specificity of ultrasound for the diagnosis of acute cholecystitis are 88% and 80%, respectively [21]. Caution should be exercised in cases of acute hepatitis which may also cause subserosal edema of the gallbladder and present as an acute RUQ pain; this should not be diagnosed as cholecystitis on ultrasound. Other findings of acute hepatitis should be an indicator to the diagnosis. Edema of the gallbladder wall is also seen in the presence of ascites and hypoproteinemia of any cause and should be differentiated from cholecystitis.

Hepatic Iminodiacetic Acid Scan: In the absence of cystic duct obstruction, the gallbladder is usually visible within 30 minutes of injection of radiotracer. If the gallbladder is not visualized within 30 minutes, Morphine injection is given that contracts the sphincter of Oddi and increases intrabiliary pressure. If the gallbladder is not visible even after 30 minutes of morphine injection, acute cholecystitis is diagnosed. The false-negative rate of HIDA scan is less than 0.5% [34]. Pericholecystic increase in radiotracer activity is sometimes noted ("rim sign").

Magnetic Resonance Cholangiography: Some referring surgeons may prefer MRCP before elective cholecystectomy to rule out CBD stone (Fig. 35.18).

CT Scan: The CT scan is often requested in the emergency department for the evaluation of acute abdominal pain and it can show features of acute cholecystitis.

- Diffuse wall thickening of the gallbladder (>4 mm)
- Calculus, if it is radiopaque
- Blurring of interface between the gallbladder and liver and pericholecystic fat stranding, representing pericholecystic edema.

Complications

Development of signs of sepsis (increased respiratory rate, systolic blood pressure <100 mm Hg, and altered mental status) should raise concern for complicated acute cholecystitis and a CECT scan is indicated (Box 35.4).

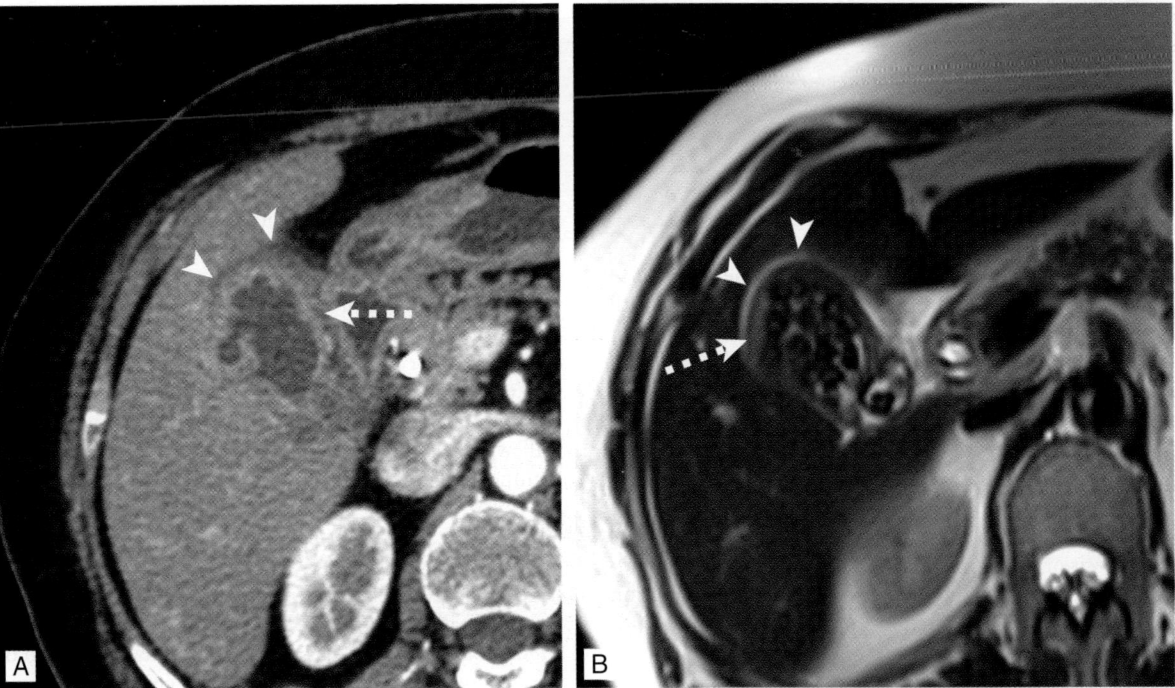

Figure 35.18 Acute calculous cholecystitis. (A) Contrast CT scan shows wall thickening of the gallbladder with continuous enhancing mucosa (*dotted arrow*). Note no calculus is visible. (B) T2-weighted axial MRI shows that the gallbladder is packed with calculi. Note thin bright line within the gallbladder wall suggesting edema (*dotted arrow*). Note pericholecystic edema (*arrowheads* in A and B).

BOX 35.4 CT in Acute Cholecystitis

When to order CT?

- Clinical suspicion of complicated acute cholecystitis
- Nonvisualization of the gallbladder on ultrasound (can be due to air in the gallbladder wall)
- Presence of pericholecystic fluid or ascites
- Clinical suspicion of an alternative diagnosis (especially acute pancreatitis)

What kind of CT to order?

- Contrast-enhanced single phase CT of whole abdomen

What are the danger signs to look for?

- Absence of the gallbladder wall enhancement
- Presence of air in the gallbladder lumen, wall, or peritoneal cavity
- Pericholecystic or peritoneal localized collection

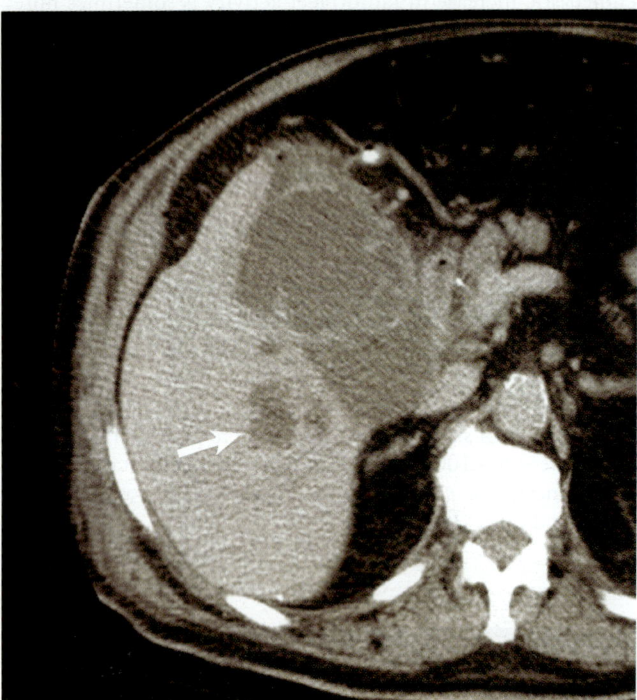

Figure 35.19 Empyema gallbladder. Axial CECT shows a distended gallbladder, with irregular walls and high-density intraluminal content. Adjacent hepatic abscess is noted (*arrow*).

Mucocele (Gallbladder Hydrops)

In the presence of chronic cystic duct obstruction, the pigment in the bile gets absorbed and the gallbladder is distended with mucoid material. Patients usually present with mild upper abdominal discomfort. Ultrasound shows overdistended gallbladder and the obstructing calculus. CT is sometimes ordered to rule out an obstructing tumor. Treatment is by cholecystectomy.

Empyema Gallbladder

In rare occasions, the gallbladder lumen may be filled with pus. Imaging diagnosis of intraluminal pus is difficult. Rest of the findings resemble that of acute cholecystitis. Percutaneous aspiration of pus may be diagnostic but often is not necessary (Fig. 35.19).

Gangrenous Cholecystitis

Prolonged distension of gallbladder can lead to ischemia and necrosis of the gallbladder wall and in up to 20% cases of acute cholecystitis, a gangrenous cholecystitis may develop [35]. Elderly patients and diabetics are at a higher risk. On ultrasound, the presence of wall striations and intraluminal membranes are suspicious of the development of gangrene. Sonographic Murphy's sign may not be present in these cases [36]. This may be due to ischemic death of the visceral afferent nerves responsible for eliciting gallbladder tenderness on palpation [37]. On noncontrast CT, the gallbladder wall can show hyperattenuation due to mucosal hemorrhage. CECT characteristically shows discontinuous or absent mucosal enhancement (Fig. 35.20). Perforation is a common complication. It is important to remember that imaging cannot rule out gangrene and only about 9% cases of gangrenous cholecystitis are diagnosed preoperatively [38].

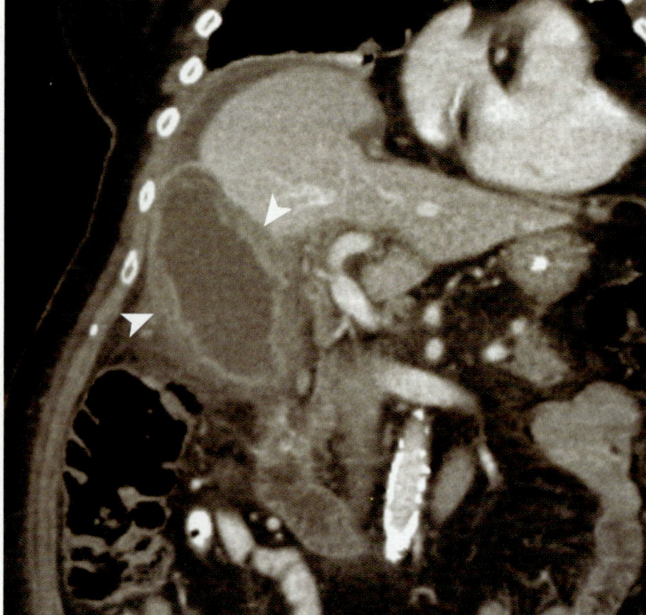

Figure 35.20 Gangrenous cholecystitis. Coronal reformat of CECT shows a distended gallbladder with irregular appearance of the GB wall with brisk GB wall enhancement suggestive of gangrenous cholecystitis.

Gallbladder Perforation and Rupture

Perforation is usually a result of ischemia in a distended gallbladder and can occur both in cases of calculous and acalculous cholecystitis. Fundus of the gallbladder is the most common site of perforation because of its poor blood supply. Niemeier categorized perforation into three types:

- Type 1: Perforation with free peritoneal spillage
- Type 2: Subacute perforation with localized pericholecystic collection or abscess
- Type 3: Biliobiliary or bilioenteric fistula

Perforation is indicated by the discontinuity in the gallbladder wall with pericholecystic collection. Type 2 perforation is more common (Fig. 35.21) [39].

Emphysematous Cholecystitis

Emphysematous cholecystitis is caused by secondary infection of the gallbladder with gas-forming organisms (such as *Clostridium welchii*). It is more common in elderly and diabetics. Ultrasonography shows highly echogenic air foci within the lumen with low-level posterior shadowing and reverberation artifact ("dirty shadowing"). Small air foci may be seen rising from the dependent portion of the lumen in real-time

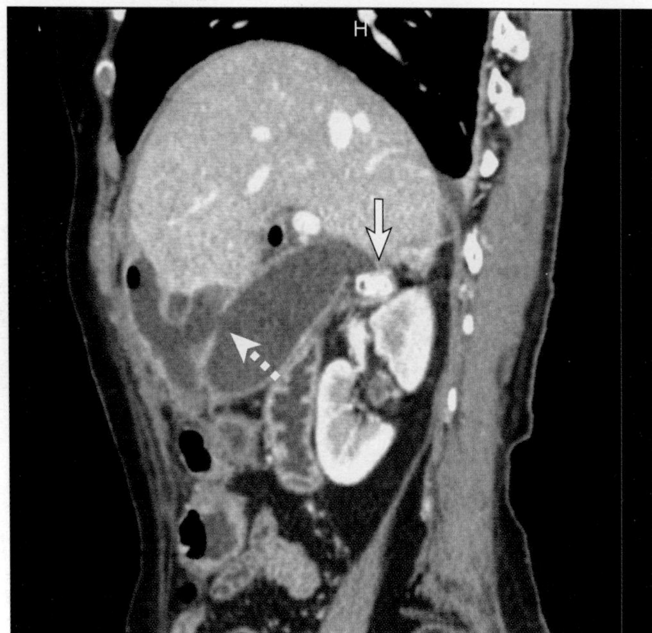

Figure 35.21 Gallbladder perforation. Sagittal reformatted contrast CT shows distended gallbladder with a calculus impacted at its neck (*solid arrow*) and a small rent in the fundus of the gallbladder (*dotted arrow*). Localized collection is noted in the gallbladder fossa with foci of air inside.

(*"champagne sign"*). CT demonstrates the air in the gallbladder lumen or wall better than ultrasound does (Fig. 35.22).

Management

Mild cases of acute cholecystitis are treated with supportive care and antibiotics. In emphysematous cholecystitis, treatment also includes blood glucose control in addition to the usual management of acute cholecystitis. Cholecystectomy is, however, indicated for nearly all patients, especially for those who require hospitalization. Early cholecystectomy (within 7 days of symptom onset) is preferred to delayed cholecystectomy (within 1–6 weeks) [40]. Emergency cholecystectomy is indicated when there is a clinical or imaging suspicion of a complicated cholecystitis or symptom progression on conservative management. In some surgically high-risk but critically ill patients, the gallbladder drainage is indicated.

Percutaneous Cholecystostomy: Percutaneous cholecystostomy (PCC) involves the introduction of an 8F pigtail catheter to decompress the gallbladder lumen and drain infected contents. This is usually done under ultrasound guidance with or without fluoroscopic guidance (Fig. 35.23). Indications include both calculous and acalculous cholecystitis, mucocele, and empyema gallbladder. Both Seldinger and direct trocar techniques are used, however, a trocar technique is easier to perform in an ICU. A transhepatic route is preferred to a transperitoneal route as there is less risk of free bile leak. If surgery is not performed, the catheter is kept in situ for 2–3 weeks and removed only after a mature tract is formed. PCC alone resolves acute cholecystitis in approximately 85% of patients but the chance of recurrent symptoms is high [41].

Acalculous Cholecystitis

Acute acalculous cholecystitis accounts for about 5–10% cases of acute cholecystitis.

Epidemiology

It is more commonly seen in men and in hospitalized and critically ill patients. Other risk factors include diabetes, major trauma, severe burns, total parenteral nutrition, recent bone marrow transplantation, and major vascular surgery.

Pathophysiology

It results from prolonged gallbladder stasis and increased viscosity of bile causing gallbladder ischemia and eventual necrosis. Perforation may occur.

Clinical Features

In critically ill patients, unexplained fever may be the only clinical feature. In outpatients, the presentation is similar to that of acute calculous cholecystitis. Jaundice may develop due to biliary stasis by infection or phlegmon. Gangrenous cholecystitis and perforation are more common in acalculous cholecystitis.

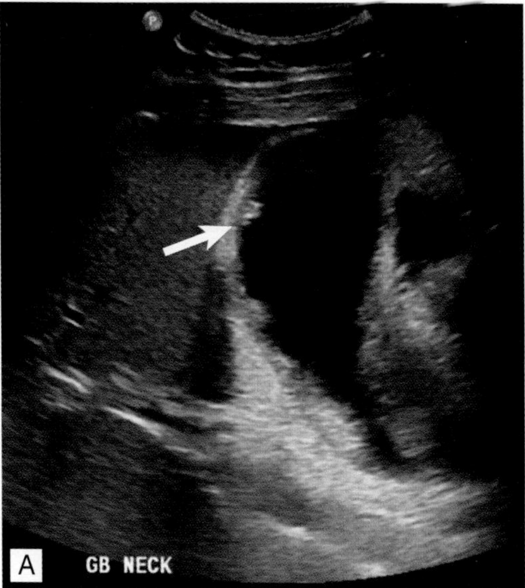

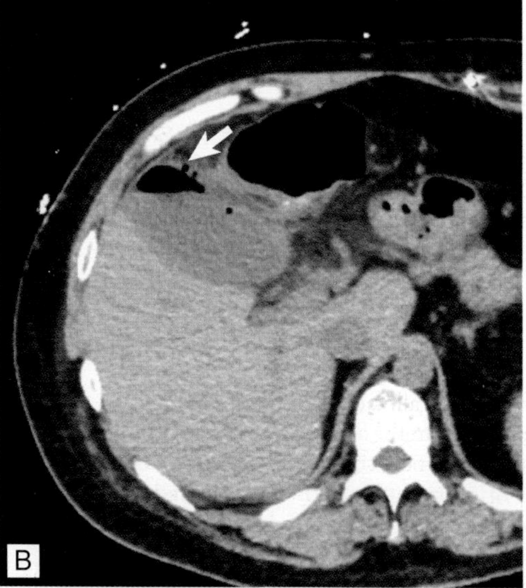

Figure 35.22 Emphysematous cholecystitis. (A) Ultrasound shows distended gallbladder with debris in the lumen, wall thickening, and intramural gas (*arrow*). (B) Axial CT shows intraluminal gas and intramural gas (*arrow*) in the gallbladder.

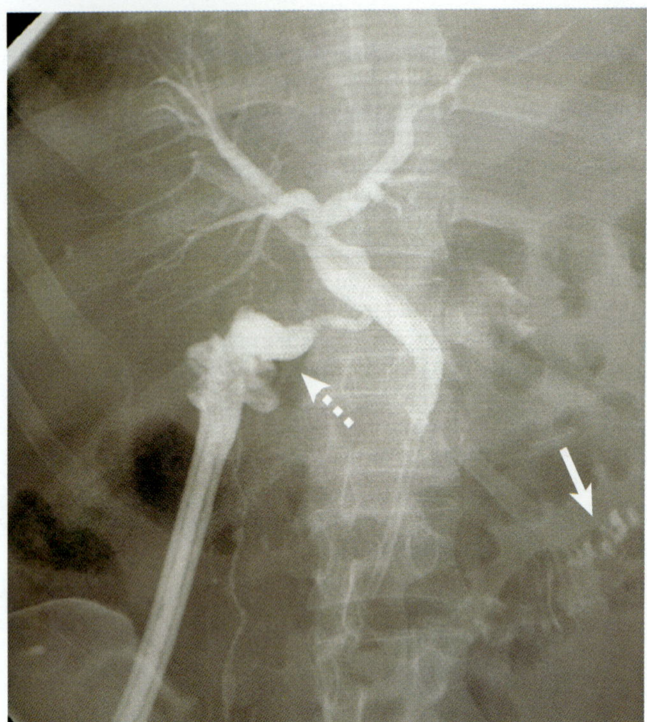

Figure 35.23 Percutaneous cholecystostomy (PCC). PCC catheter is places within the gallbladder lumen in a case of acute cholecystitis associated with the common bile duct (CBD) stone. CBD stones are removed endoscopically and stent is placed. Check cholecystogram through PCC catheter shows free passage of contrast from the gallbladder (*dotted arrow*) to the small bowel (*solid arrow*).

Imaging Features

Ultrasound shows features of acute cholecystitis without calculus. However, intraluminal sludge is often detected. In HIDA scan, nonvisualization of the gallbladder even after 60 minutes of radiotracer injection is indicative of acute cholecystitis.

Management

Poor surgical risk patients are treated with the gallbladder drainage. As there is no true cystic duct obstruction, subsequent cholecystectomy is often not required after drainage. Other patients may be treated with early cholecystectomy.

Chronic Cholecystitis

Chronic cholecystitis is defined by infiltration of the gallbladder wall by chronic inflammatory cells and is often diagnosed on imaging in asymptomatic patients.

Epidemiology

Chronic cholecystitis is the most common disorder of the gallbladder. It is more common in women in the fifth or sixth decades of life.

Pathophysiology

Chronic cholecystitis is almost always associated with cholelithiasis. It is a result of chronic irritation of the gallbladder wall by recurrent attacks of acute cholecystitis. The gallbladder is usually small and fibrosed. Long-standing chronic cholecystitis may cause mural calcification, also known as a porcelain gallbladder.

The porcelain gallbladder is associated with GBC, however, the strength of association may be less than what traditionally believed and prophylactic cholecystectomy is not always necessary [42–44].

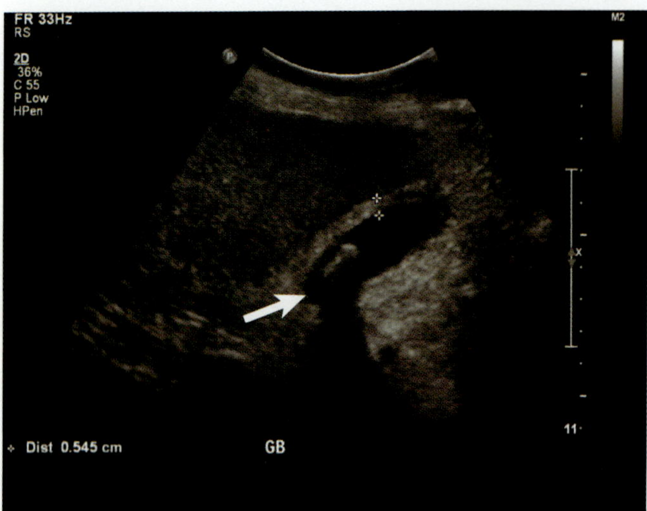

Figure 35.24 Chronic cholecystitis. Sagittal view ultrasound of the gallbladder shows small, contracted gallbladder with wall thickening (between calipers), and intraluminal calculus (*arrow*).

Clinical Features

Dull intermittent right upper abdominal or epigastric pain that is precipitated by a heavy or fatty meal is the most characteristic symptom. Other symptoms such as nausea, flatulence, and upper abdominal fullness are commonly present.

Imaging Features

Ultrasound is the imaging investigation of choice. The most common findings are (Fig. 35.24):

- Thickening of the gallbladder wall (>4 mm)
- Small, contracted gallbladder
- Cholelithiasis

MRCP shows small, contracted gallbladder and cholelithiasis. Pericholecystic edema is uncommon. MRCP is more commonly ordered to detect clinically silent concurrent CBD stones, which can be seen in 4–26% cases [45,46]. CT has no role.

Differential Diagnosis

Although the clinical differential diagnoses include peptic ulcer disease, irritable bowel syndrome, chronic pancreatitis, and gastroesophageal reflux disease; the imaging differential diagnosis includes causes of diffuse gallbladder wall thickening (Box 35.5).

Management

Medical methods aimed at dissolving the gallstones may be tried (ursodeoxycholic acid) but definitive management is elective laparoscopic or open cholecystectomy.

BOX 35.5 Diffuse Gallbladder Wall Thickening: Differentials and Mimics

Causes of the gallbladder wall thickening:

- Acute and chronic cholecystitis
- Ascites
- Hypoproteinemia
- Heart failure
- Acute hepatitis

Mimics of the gallbladder wall thickening:

- Intraluminal sludge
- Nonshadowing calculi

Xanthogranulomatous Cholecystitis

Xanthogranulomatous cholecystitis (XGC) is commonly confused with the gallbladder carcinoma, both clinically and on imaging.

Epidemiology

XGC is uncommon but not rare, accounting for up to 1–5% of surgically resected gallbladder specimens. It is more commonly seen in women in their sixth and seventh decades, although some studies have shown male preponderance. About 80% cases are associated with gallstone, often impacted at the neck [47–49].

Pathogenesis

Proposed pathogenesis of XGC involves extravasation of bile in the gallbladder wall resulting in a xanthogranulomatous response. Bile extravasation can be due to mucosal ulceration or rupture of Rokitansky–Aschoff sinus caused by calculous obstruction of the cystic duct. The mural nodules that are characteristic of XGC on imaging studies are probably lipid-containing xanthogranulomas or abscesses. Inflammation and fibrosis can involve surrounding structures which mimic gallbladder carcinoma. Carcinoma often coexist with XGC [50].

Clinical Features

Clinical features are similar to acute or chronic cholecystitis. Serum tumor marker carbohydrate antigen 19-9 (CA 19-9) can be elevated in up to 46% cases of XGC [51].

Imaging Features

- One ultrasound, XGC shows segmental or diffuse wall thickening and hypoechoic or mixed echogenicity mural nodules are seen. Coexistent gallstones are usually seen
- On CT, wall thickening and poorly enhancing mural nodules are seen. On contrast enhancement, the mucosa enhances and is seen as a thin, continuous layer with hypodense outer submucosal and subserosal layer. Stranding of pericholecystic fat and loss of fat plane with liver and other surrounding structures are common (Fig. 35.25)
- On MRI, findings similar to CT are seen. Additionally MRI demonstrates the intraluminal calculus. As the mural nodules in XGC represent lipid, signal drop on opposed phase chemical shift T1-weighted images can be seen, however, this is not a common feature [52]
- Differentiation from GBC is the biggest challenge and often the diagnosis is not made preoperatively [53]. A thick, interrupted layer of inner mucosal enhancement is more often noted in GBC. Diffuse wall thickening, presence of mural nodules and a thin, continuous mucosa is more common in XGC [52]. Image-guided fine needle aspiration may be helpful in the differentiation [50]

Management

Laparoscopic cholecystectomy is difficult in cases of XGC and sometimes avoided because of suspicion of cancer. Open cholecystectomy can also be difficult due to dense adhesions and more extended resection of surrounding structures is often necessary. Since XGC is difficult to diagnose either preoperatively or intraoperatively, intraoperative frozen-section examination should be carried out to differentiate XGC from carcinoma of the gallbladder. The plan of resection is decided based on the result of the frozen section.

Hyperplastic Cholecystosis

Hyperplastic cholecystoses are noninflammatory pathologies of the gallbladder associated with hyperplastic thickening of the wall. It comprises cholesterolosis and adenomyomatosis of the gallbladder.

Cholesterolosis

Cholesterolosis is caused by diffuse deposition of cholesterol esters in macrophages of the lamina propria of the gallbladder wall that form yellowish excrescences. When it is associated with hyperemia,

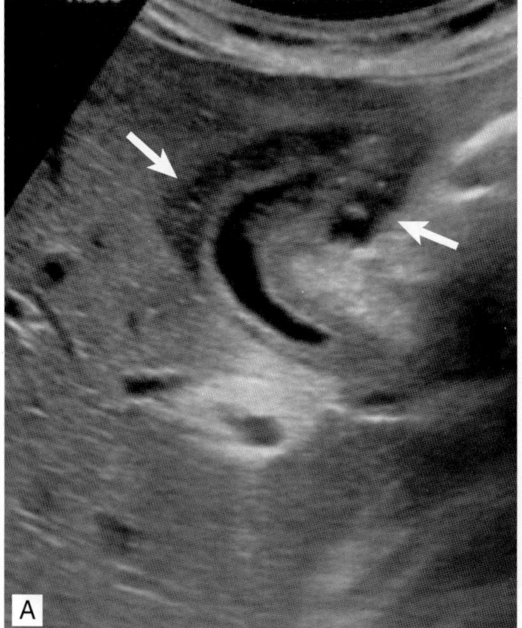

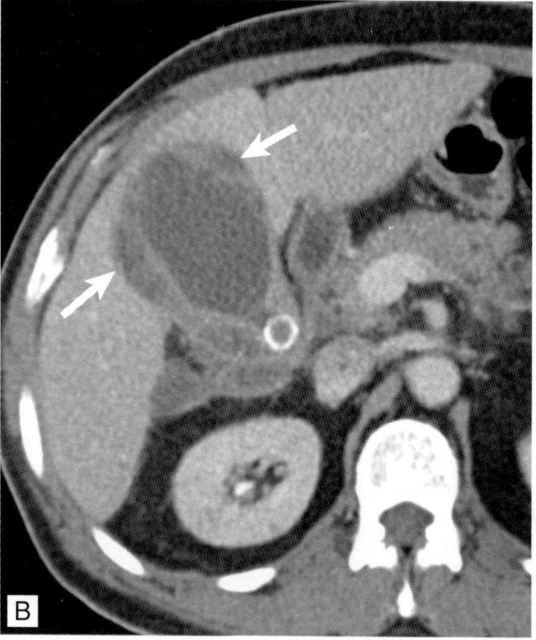

Figure 35.25 Xanthogranulomatous cholecystitis. (A) Oblique coronal view of upper abdomen shows thickened gallbladder wall. Note low-density areas within the gallbladder wall (*arrows*). (B) Axial contrast CT shows distended gallbladder with an impacted calculus at the neck and gross wall thickening. Small low attenuation areas are noted within the thickened walls (*arrows*). (Courtesy: Dr. Akshay Baheti, Tata Memorial Hospital, India.)

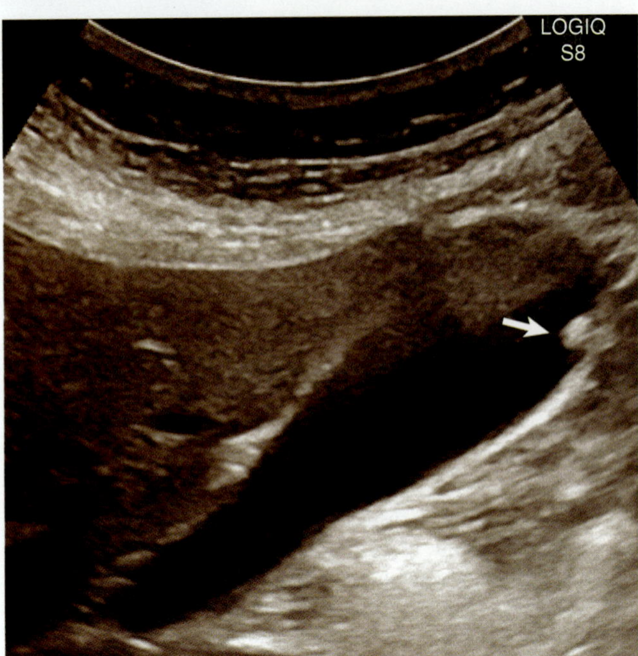

Figure 35.26 Cholesterol polyp. Hyperechoic polypoid lesion noted within gallbladder fundus without posterior acoustic shadow (*arrow*).

the mucosa resembles the skin of a strawberry (strawberry gallbladder). The diffuse form cannot be diagnosed on imaging. When cholesterol deposition forms focal polypoid lesions of size 2–10 mm, it gives rise to a cholesterol polyp and can be detected on imaging.

Cholesterol polyps are the most common polypoid lesion of the gallbladder. These have no malignant potential. These polyps typically manifest as multiple small (usually 1–2 mm, always <10 mm) smooth-walled hyperechoic intraluminal lesions with no posterior acoustic shadowing (Fig. 35.26).

Gallbladder Adenomyomatosis

Gallbladder adenomyomatosis is a common condition that has a characteristic imaging appearance. It accounts for approximately 25% of polypoid lesions of the gallbladder [54]. It is caused by hyperplastic thickening of the gallbladder wall caused by deposition of cholesterol crystals or calculi in the Rokitansky–Aschoff sinuses. These sinuses appear as anechoic cystic spaces around the gallbladder lumen at ultrasound. When these sinuses contain cholesterol crystals, or calculi, they appear hyperechoic with twinkling or a comet-tail artifact. On MRI, these spaces appear as multiple round T2-hyperintense foci around the gallbladder lumen (*"pearl necklace" sign*). Three morphologic types of adenomyomatosis are recognized.

- Focal adenomyomatosis causes thickening of the fundus of the gallbladder and mimics a GBC
- The segmental form results in thickening of the body of the gallbladder and results in the appearance of a characteristic "hourglass gallbladder"
- Diffuse adenomyomatosis involves the whole gallbladder (Fig. 35.27)

Gallbladder Carcinoma

Epidemiology and Risk Factors

GBC accounts for 1.2% of all global cancer diagnoses and 1.7% of all cancer deaths [55]. However, there is significant geographical variation in GBC incidence. Incidence is the highest in East Asia, Latin America, and Eastern Europe, whereas it is relatively uncommon in North America and Western Europe. The average 5-year survival in the United States for GBC is 18% [56]. It is more common in women and it is diagnosed commonly after the age of 60 years. Risk factors for GBC include gallstone disease, porcelain gallbladder, gallbladder polyp, primary sclerosing cholangitis (PSC), chronic biliary infection with *Salmonella* and *Helicobacter*, anomalous pancreaticobiliary junction, and obesity.

Pathophysiology

Most GBCs are adenocarcinomas. Adenocarcinomas involving the gallbladder progress from dysplasia to carcinoma in situ, and then to invasive cancer. Chronic irritation of gallbladder mucosa by gallstones and repeated cholecystitis is thought to predispose to carcinogenesis.

Gallbladder carcinoma spreads through direct invasion, lymphatic or hematogenous metastasis, perineural invasion, intraperitoneal spread, or intraductal invasion. Lymphatic tumor cell spread occurs at first to lymph nodes along the biliary tract and hepatic artery followed by pancreaticoduodenal lymph nodes and CHA and finally, to lymph nodes along the celiac axis and para-aortic region. Involvement of posterior superior pancreaticoduodenal nodes are considered a sign of inoperability by some surgeons, whereas others consider it to be a regional node. Involved lymph nodes along the left side of the celiac axis, superior mesenteric artery, and retroperitoneum are considered inoperable. Preoperative mapping of the extent of nodal involvement is therefore crucial. Gallbladder carcinoma has a predisposition to involve the liver bed because of its venous drainage, predominantly into segments IVb and V. The serosa of gallbladder is absent on the hepatic side and the perimuscular connective tissue adherent to the liver. Therefore, partial liver resection including removal of portions of segments IVb and V is necessary for complete resection of tumors that have invaded the muscularis layer and beyond. Radiologists should comment on whether the primary tumor is present on the free peritoneal (T2a) or the hepatic side (T2b) of the gallbladder, as tumors on the hepatic side have worse prognosis [57]. Tumor may directly invade the liver hilum, infiltrate along the cystic duct to the extrahepatic bile duct or spread within the duct and cause biliary obstruction [58]. Cholangiography, most commonly MRCP, is necessary in cases with biliary involvement to evaluate level and extent of biliary involvement.

Clinical Features

Only about 50% of patients with GBC are diagnosed preoperatively [59,60]. Other cases are diagnosed incidentally during cholecystectomy or on histopathological examination after gallbladder surgery done for other reasons. Incidentally detected GBC may present with metastases to the peritoneum or the abdominal wall that occurs due to intraoperative tumor seeding. If suspicion of GBC exists, the specimen should always be removed in a bag to prevent tumor seeding.

Symptomatic patients present with pain, anorexia, nausea, vomiting, and weight loss. Some patients present with obstructive jaundice due to obstruction of bile duct by tumor or enlarged node. On examination, gallbladder may be palpable. Liver enlargement may be seen in the presence of diffuse liver metastasis.

Imaging Features

- Morphologically, gallbladder carcinoma can present as a gallbladder fossa mass, intraluminal polyp or irregular gallbladder wall thickening, the last being the least common. Most lesions

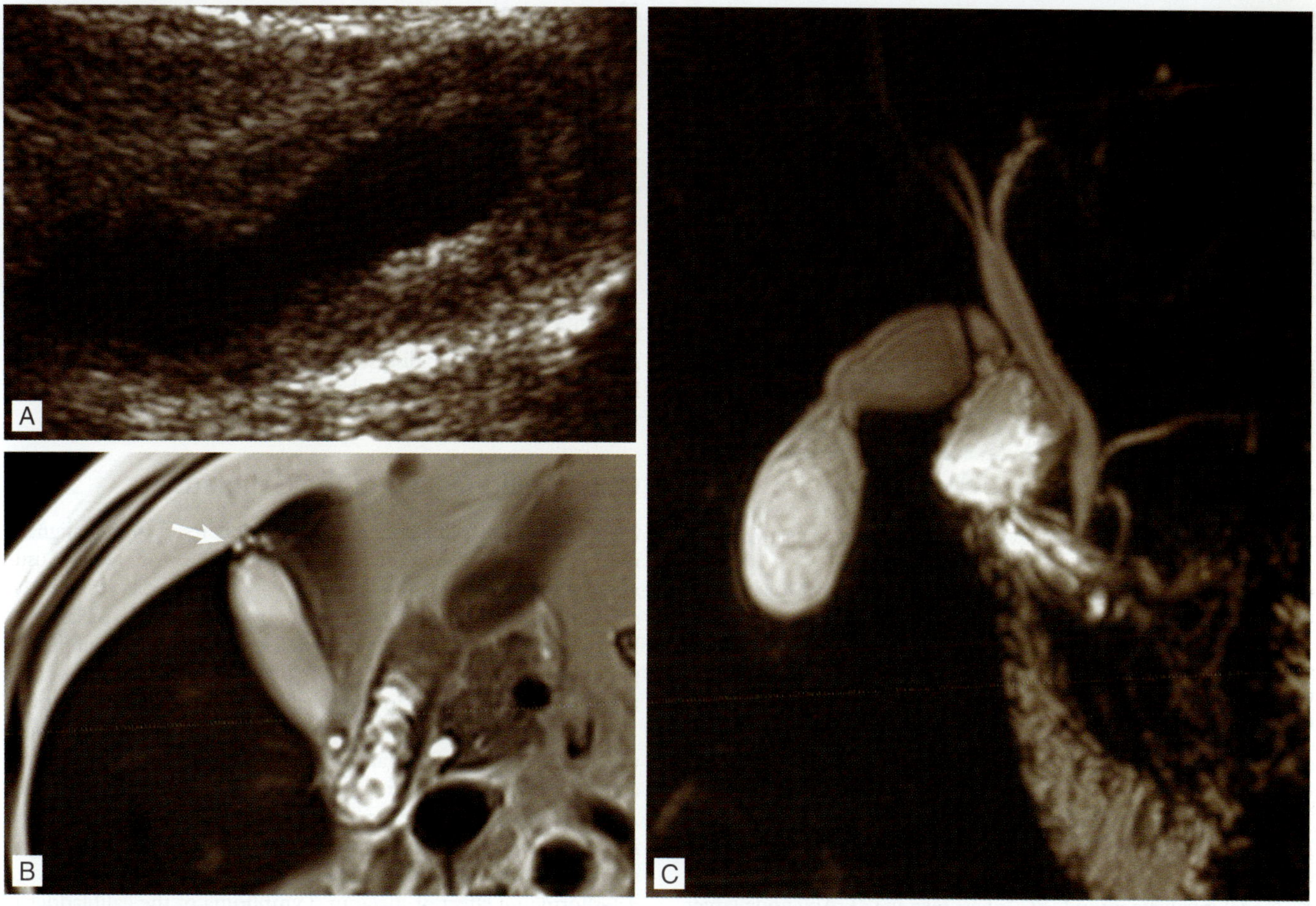

Figure 35.27 Adenomyomatosis of the gallbladder. (A) Long-axis ultrasound image of the gallbladder showing focal wall thickening of fundus of the gallbladder with small hypoechoic areas within the wall. (B) Axial T2-weighted MRI shows focal thickening of fundus of the gallbladder with multiple hyperintense cystic spaces within. (C) 3D maximum intensity projection MRCP shows hourglass morphology of the gallbladder. (Courtesy: Dr. Frank H. Miller, Northwestern University Feinberg School of Medicine, Chicago, USA.)

present as a mass replacing the gallbladder and most lesions arise in the fundus and body of the gallbladder (Fig. 35.28) [58]

- Ultrasound can detect GBC with up to 85% sensitivity [61]. However, its utility is limited in the primary staging and pre-operative evaluation. Features on ultrasound that are suspicious of GBC are given in Box 35.6
- Biphasic CT scan with arterial and portal venous phase is the imaging technique of choice for primary staging in a suspected or proved case of GBC [12]. In some centers, a hepatic venous phase is also acquired. Arterial phase imaging is necessary for the delineation of the arterial anatomy and determination of encasement of arteries by the tumor. Portal venous anatomy and

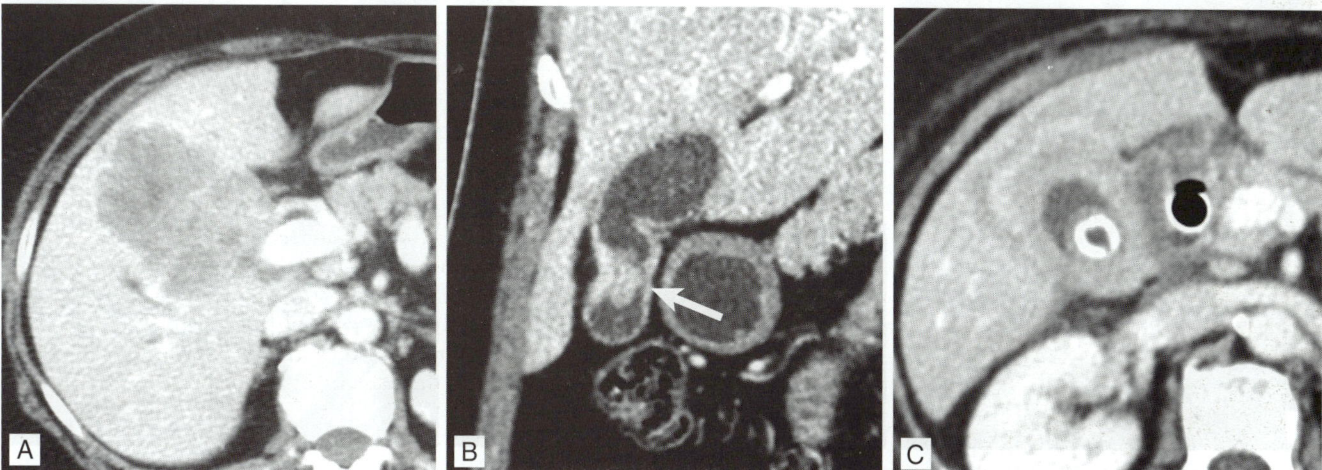

Figure 35.28 Gallbladder carcinoma, different morphological types. (A) Gallbladder fossa mass. (B) Polypoid intraluminal mass associated with wall thickening (*arrow*). (C) Diffuse wall thickening. Note intraluminal calculus.

BOX 35.6 Ultrasound Features Suspicious of Gallbladder Malignancy

- Nonvisualization of the gallbladder in the absence of a history of cholecystectomy
- "Embedded stone"—gallstone surrounded by soft tissue
- Irregular or nodular gallbladder wall thickening >4 mm
- Gallbladder polyp >10 mm
- Sessile polyp
- Presence of irregular enlarged nodes in porta or close to celiac artery origin

BOX 35.7 Reporting a Gallbladder Cancer in Cross-Sectional Imaging: What the Referring Surgeon Wants to Know? (Fig. 35.29)

- Primary gallbladder mass (size in at least two dimensions)
- Liver invasion (segments involved, fissure for ligamentum teres involved or not)
- Surrounding organ invasion (transverse colon, duodenum, antrum, and pancreas)
- Biliary involvement (level of obstruction, patency of biliary confluences)
- Vascular involvement (right and common hepatic artery, right and main portal vein)
- Nodal involvement (operable: portal nodes, inoperable: retroperitoneal nodes)
- Peritoneal metastases (omental nodule or caking, peritoneal nodule)
- Other metastases (liver, adrenal, and lung)

tumor extent is best seen in portal venous phase. Hepatic venous phase is necessary for delineation of hepatic venous anatomy which is crucial for surgical planning and liver volumetry

- Nodal involvement in GBC is best seen in CT. Any node larger than 1 cm in the short axis is regarded as a pathological node
- The minimum reporting requirement of GBC is given in Box 35.7
- MRCP is sometimes done in cases of GBC to map the biliary anatomy and determine the level and extent of biliary involvement before biliary intervention and surgery

Management

Definitive surgery is the only curative option, but only few patients present early enough to be operable. Radical cholecystectomy is necessary in all cancers involving muscularis propria. For tumors involving surrounding organs, liver resection and pancreaticoduodenectomy is often necessary as well. Inoperable cancers need to be palliated by biliary drainage and chemotherapy. Up to 47% patients are diagnosed with early GBC incidentally at or after gallbladder surgery for other indications [60]. Incidentally detected GBCs are often evaluated by CT to look for residual tumor, nodal involvement, and distant metastases before undergoing completion surgery. Nodes, liver, abdominal wall, and peritoneum (including ovaries) are common sites of metastatic disease. Radiologists need to be aware of this imaging indication beforehand as, in this case, the gallbladder itself will be absent.

Other Malignancies of the Gallbladder

Metastases to the gallbladder most commonly result from malignant melanoma, gastric carcinoma, or renal cell carcinoma. These are usually asymptomatic but may manifest with acute cholecystitis if the cystic duct is obstructed. Metastases from malignant melanoma, hepatocellular carcinoma, or renal cell carcinoma may manifest as polypoid lesions whereas that from gastrointestinal tract adenocarcinomas usually present as irregular gallbladder wall thickening [62].

Squamous cell carcinomas of the gallbladder are rare. Risk factors for these tumors are gallstones and parasitic infection. Biliary and bowel obstructions are common because of direct extension. *Primary gallbladder melanoma* is extremely rare, unlike metastatic melanoma. Primary or metastatic melanomas may show high-signal intensity on T1-weighted MR images because of the T1-shortening effect of melanin. Lymphoma of the gallbladder is also extremely rare. Low-grade lymphomas manifest as mild thickening of the gallbladder wall, and high-grade lymphomas manifest as a solid mass within the gallbladder or irregular wall thickening. A characteristic finding of lymphoma is the presence of intact mucosa with infiltration of the submucosal layer. It may be associated with periportal and para-aortic lesions [63].

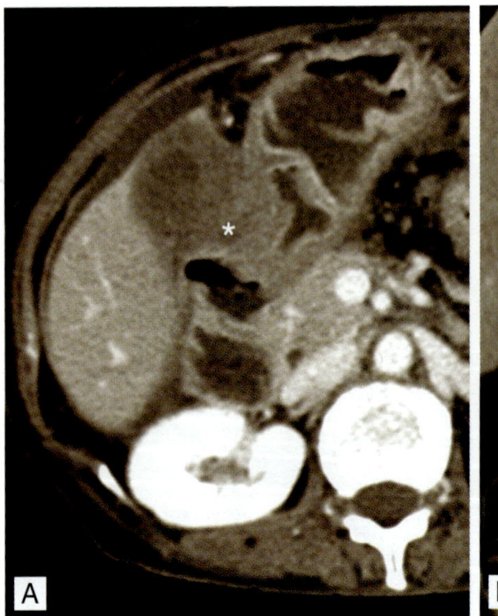

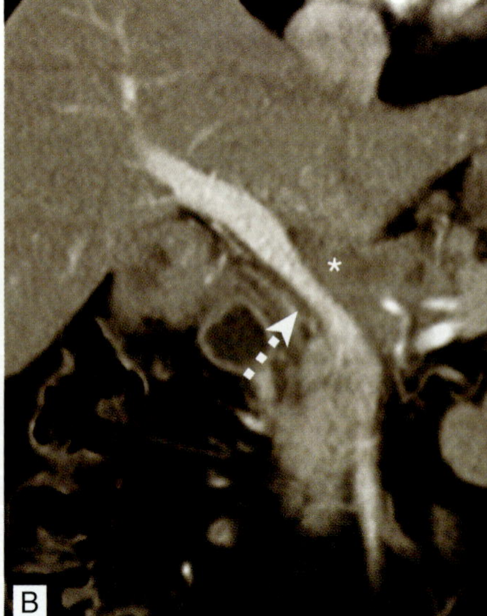

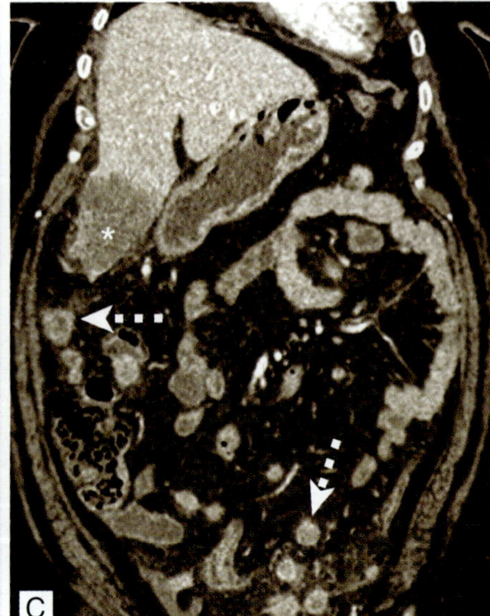

Figure 35.29 Gallbladder carcinoma, staging. (A) Gallbladder mass infiltrating the lateral wall of antrum of stomach (*asterisk*). (B) Gallbladder cancer with portal lymphadenopathy (*asterisk*) that is causing stenosis of the main portal vein (*dotted arrow*). (C) Gallbladder mass (*asterisk*) with multiple peritoneal metastases (*dotted arrows*).

BOX 35.8 Differential Diagnosis of a Gallbladder Polyp

Common
- Cholesterol polyps
- Adenomyomatosis
- Gallbladder adenocarcinoma

Uncommon
- Gallbladder adenoma
- Metastases

Mimics
- Tumefactive sludge
- Adherent gallstone

BOX 35.9 High-Risk Factors Associated With Gallbladder Polyp (Apart From Size >1 cm)

- Sessile polyp (including focal wall thickening >4 mm)
- Presence of symptoms related to gallbladder
- Age >50 years
- Primary sclerosing cholangitis
- Indian ethnicity

(Modified from Wiles et al. [67].)

Approach to a Case of Gallbladder Polyp

A mass in the gallbladder wall that projects into the lumen is called a gallbladder polyp. The prevalence of gallbladder polyps detected at ultrasound of abdomen is approximately 0.3–9% [64]. Only 0.6% of these polyps turn out to be malignant [65]. A gallbladder polyp can be neoplastic in nature, or it can be a pseudotumor related to cholesterol deposition, adenomyomatosis, or inflammation (Box 35.8). A true polyp of the gallbladder is characterized by an intraluminal mass without any posterior acoustic shadowing or comet-tail artifact in ultrasound. Presence of a comet-tail artifact indicates the diagnosis of adenomyomatosis.

The most important task of the radiologist is to assess the risk of malignancy of the polyp. A surgical consult for a potential cholecystectomy is recommended for polyps >1 cm in diameter, for polyps associated with symptoms of gallbladder disease, and for polyps between 6 and 9 mm if associated with other risk factors [66,67]. The high-risk factors for malignancy associated with a polyp is given in Box 35.9. Polyps between 6 and 9 mm without risk factors should be followed up with ultrasound at 6 months and then yearly up to 5 years. The American College of Radiology does not recommend follow up for asymptomatic polyps ≤6 mm [66]. However, according to the joint guidelines of European Society of Gastrointestinal and Abdominal Radiology, European Association for Endoscopic Surgery and other Interventional Techniques, and International Society of Digestive Surgery—European Federation, all polyps <6 mm should be followed up with ultrasound at 1 year, 3 years, and 5 years. Polyps that are stable at 5 years do not need further follow-up. Any growth in size during follow-up by 2 mm should warrant cholecystectomy [67].

Cholesterol polyps are the most common polypoid lesion of the gallbladder. Gallbladder adenomyomatosis accounts for approximately 25% of polypoid lesions of the gallbladder [54].

Gallbladder adenoma accounts for 3–7% of intraluminal polypoid lesions of the gallbladder and can display premalignant behavior [68]. Adenomas usually range in size from 5 to 20 mm. Internal vascularity at color Doppler imaging is reported. Differentiation of adenoma and adenocarcinoma is not possible with imaging studies alone.

Intracholecystic papillary neoplasms are premalignant lesions. These lesions are analogous to intraductal papillary mucinous neoplasm (IPMN) of the pancreas. It is rare with no strong association with gallstones. An associated invasive cancer is often present [69].

Bile Ducts

Inflammatory Diseases of Bile Ducts

Acute Bacterial Cholangitis and Cholangitic Abscess

Pathophysiology: Acute bacterial cholangitis occurs as a result of biliary obstruction and stasis, most commonly due to calculus, postoperative stricture, and malignancy. It is also called ascending cholangitis as the infecting organisms typically ascend from duodenum, most commonly *E. coli*, *Klebsiella*, and *Enterococcus sp*.

Clinical Features: The classic Charcot's triad (fever, abdominal pain, and jaundice) is not present in all patients. Only about 60–70% of patients have jaundice at presentation [70]. Laboratory features include leukocytosis, hyperbilirubinemia, and raised alkaline phosphatase. Most centers require imaging evidence of biliary obstruction for the diagnosis of acute cholangitis.

Imaging Features

- Ultrasound is the first and often the only imaging technique necessary for evaluation. Ultrasound shows biliary dilatation, circumferential thickening of the wall of the CBD along with the cause, and the level of obstruction. Ultrasound can also detect hepatic abscesses (cholangitic abscesses). These appear as grouped hypoechoic round lesions, often confined to a segment or a lobe of liver
- CT is only necessary when ultrasound is unequivocal. CT shows dilated bile ducts with thickening and enhancement of the wall. Cholangitic abscesses appear as grouped centrally hypoattenuating lesions ("cluster sign"). The affected segment of liver may show perfusion abnormalities showing diffuse enhancement in arterial phase that becomes isoattenuating to the rest of the liver in portal venous phase. Individual lesions show a central low attenuation suppurative area which may contain gas, an inner enhancing hyperattenuating rim of granulation tissue, and an outer hypoattenuating rim of edema ("double rim sign") (Fig. 35.30) [71]

Management: Acute bacterial cholangitis is a medical emergency and requires immediate biliary drainage on antibiotic cover. In the presence of pancreaticobiliary malignancy with bile duct obstruction, abscesses can simulate metastases. Presence of fever, leukocytosis, and rim of edema surrounding the abscess on imaging are helpful features favoring an abscess.

Recurrent Pyogenic Cholangiohepatitis

Recurrent pyogenic cholangiohepatitis (hepatolithiasis, oriental cholangiohepatitis) is characterized by chronic biliary obstruction, stasis, and pigment stone formation, leading to recurrent episodes of acute cholangitis. Chronic inflammation may lead to atrophy of the affected liver segment and multifocal biliary stricture. Its incidence is highest in Southeast and East Asia. The etiology is unclear. Left lateral segment of the liver is affected the most.

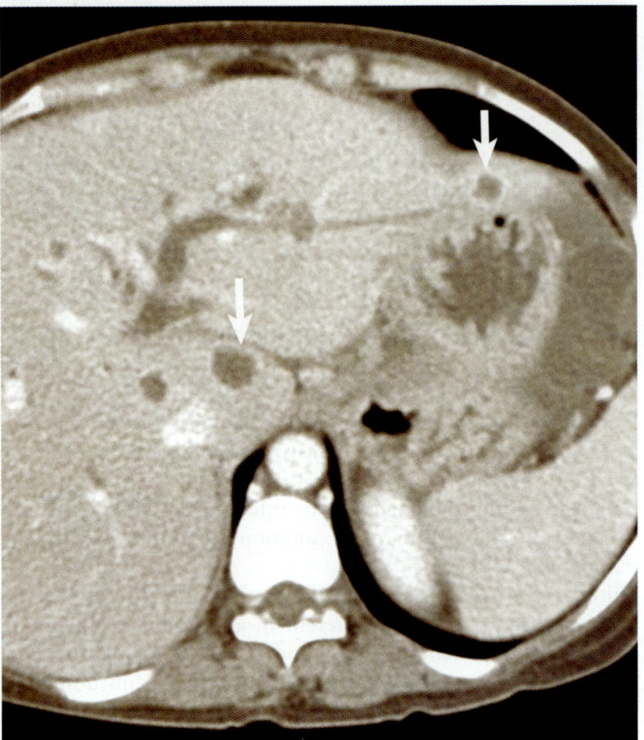

Figure 35.30 Cholangitic abscess. Multiple rim-enhancing hypoattenuating rounded lesions are noted in liver (*arrows*). Note dilated left hepatic duct indicating biliary obstruction.

Ultrasound shows dilated intrahepatic ducts filled with sludge and stones, confined to one or more segments of the liver. The CT scan localizes the disease better and shows dilated ducts as well as intrahepatic calculi, when they are radiodense. MRCP demonstrates the multifocal stricture involving the bile ducts and intraductal calculi with greater detail. Abrupt distal tapering of peripheral bile ducts with decreased arborization ("arrowhead sign") and complete occlusion ("absent duct sign") are seen in cholangiography (Fig. 35.31) [72,73].

AIDS Cholangiopathy

Opportunistic infection of the bile duct, with *Cryptosporidium* sp., Cytomegalovirus, or *Pneumocystis jirovecii,* results in an obliterative cholangiopathy with a picture similar to sclerosing cholangitis. Abdominal pain and cholangitis are the predominant presenting feature and endoscopic sphincterotomy may result in symptomatic and biochemical improvement.

Parasitic Infection

Fasciola hepatica infection is caused by consumption of water or raw vegetables contaminated with the larva of the *F. hepatica* fluke. In the acute phase of the infection, the immature larvae migrate through the bowel wall into the peritoneal cavity and enter the liver through the liver capsule. Patients may present with acute abdominal pain, hepatomegaly, and prolonged fever. This migratory tract in the liver can be demonstrated in CT or MRI as a specific finding manifested by small cyst-like clusters ("cluster of grape" sign) or serpiginous tracks ("Fasciola tunnel" sign) in the peripheral subcapsular portion of the liver [74] (Fig. 35.32). In the chronic phase, the larva finally reaches the biliary tree. The mature *Fasciola* can be directly seen within the bile ducts on ultrasound. Living flukes can be shown within the gallbladder or bile ducts as moving structures [75].

Clonorchis sinensis, *Opisthorchis viverrini,* and *Opisthorchis felineus* are endemic in East and Southeast Asia. The infection is acquired by ingestion of raw fish contaminated by the larvae that migrate up the bile duct, mature and live within the intrahepatic bile ducts. Ultrasound shows dilation of the peripheral portion of the intrahepatic bile ducts with normal appearing central and extrahepatic ducts. Other findings include periportal edema and sludge within the gallbladder. Chronic infection by these parasites is linked to CCA [76].

Ascaris lumbricoides infection is extremely common, predominantly involving the small bowel in children in developing countries. It may enter the biliary tree retrogradely through the ampulla of Vater, causing acute biliary obstruction. Generally, infected patients are asymptomatic but may present with biliary colic, cholangitis, or acalculous cholecystitis. On ultrasound, most often a single worm is seen. It appears as a tube or as parallel

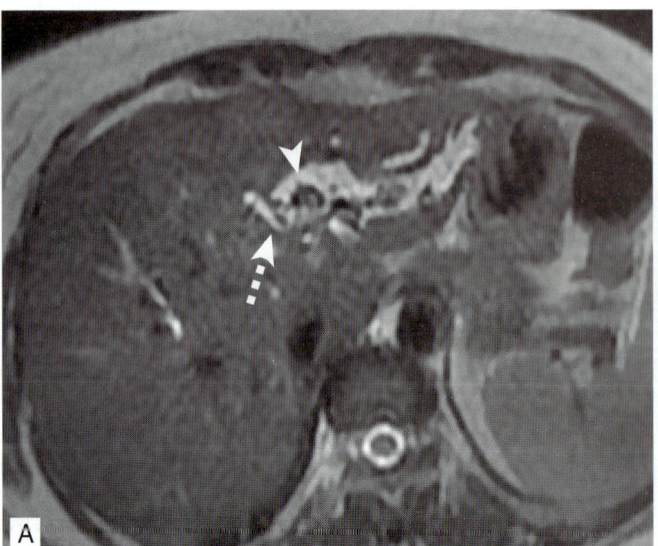

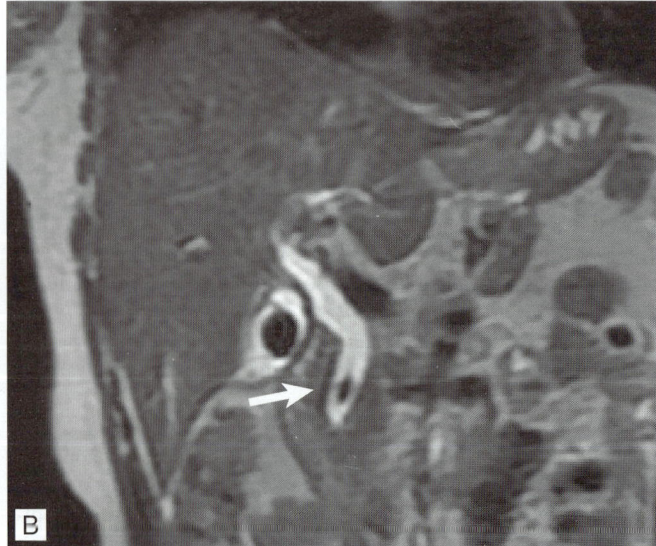

Figure 35.31 Recurrent pyogenic cholangitis. (A) Axial T2-weighted image of liver shows atrophy of left lobe of liver with focal dilatation of left hepatic duct with downstream stricture (*dotted arrow*) and intraductal calculi (*arrowhead*). (B) Coronal T2-weighted image shows calculus within the common bile duct (*arrow*).

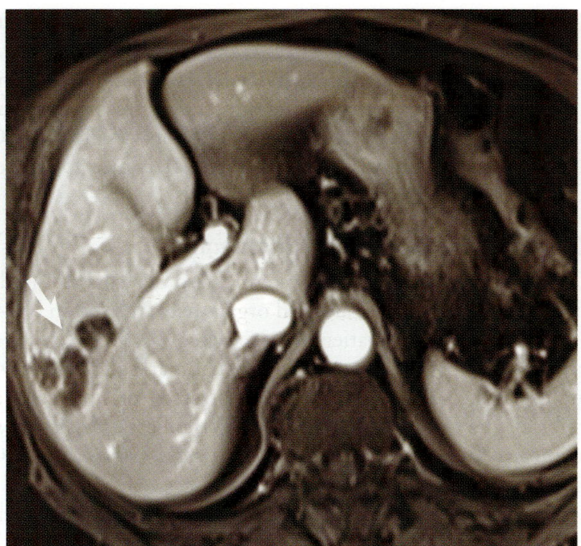

Figure 35.32 *Fasciola hepatica* infection. Serpiginous tract (*arrow*) extending from the peripheral subcapsular portion of the liver to the central portal radicles.

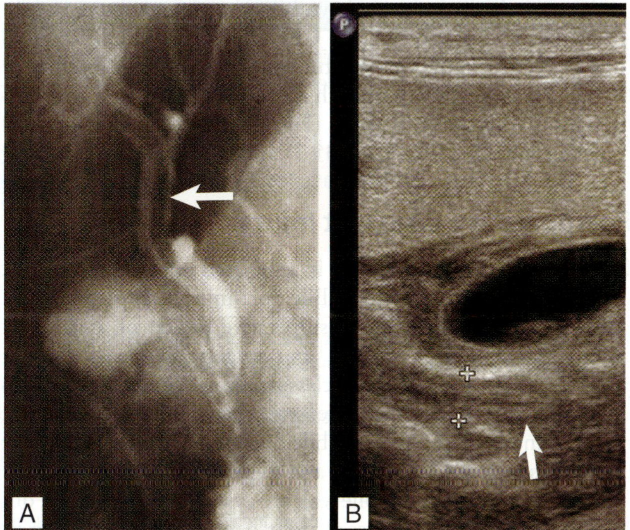

Figure 35.33 Biliary ascariasis. (A) Percutaneous cholangiogram shows elongated filling defect suggestive of worm within the bile duct (*arrow*). (B) High-resolution ultrasound in a different case shows the worm in the common bile duct (between calipers) as a tubular structure simulating a tube or a stent (*arrow*).

echogenic lines within the bile ducts, simulating a biliary stent. On cross section, the worm gives a target appearance. With heavy infestation, multiple worms may be seen (Fig. 35.33).

Hydatid cyst of liver is caused by the parasites *Echinococcus granulosus* and *Echinococcus multilocularis.* Humans are usually infected by ingesting the ova of the parasite through contact with a dog or ingestion of food or water contaminated with a dog's feces. The ova releases the hexacanth embryo in the duodenum which is taken up by the portal circulation into the liver. On ultrasound, hydatid cysts appear as unilocular or multilocular cystic lesions with a characteristic double layer in the wall. The cyst may contain dependent and mobile amorphous echogenic foci (hydatid sand), detached endocyst ("floating membrane" sign), or several daughter cysts. The daughter cysts may give rise to a "honeycomb" or "wheel spoke" pattern on ultrasound. On CT, calcification of the cyst wall is commonly seen. Daughter

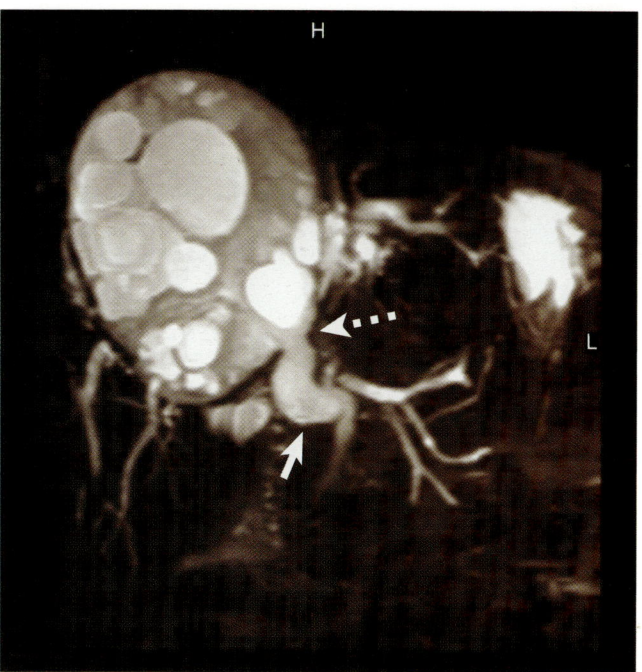

Figure 35.34 Biliary rupture of hydatid cyst. Maximum intensity projection coronal MRCP image shows multilocular hydatid cyst with a large communication (*dotted arrow*) with a dilated bile duct (*solid arrow*).

cysts are seen on CT as relatively lower attenuation structures (compared with the fluid in the mother cyst) positioned peripherally within the mother cyst. Occasionally, hydatid cyst may rupture in the biliary tree. Patients may present with jaundice and fever with chills due to ensuing cholangitis. A cyst wall defect may be visible on ultrasound, CT, or MRI showing communication with a dilated bile duct (Fig. 35.34). Cyst material escaping into the bile ducts may be seen on ultrasound as echogenic linear structure without posterior acoustic shadowing.

Immunological Diseases of Bile Ducts

Primary Biliary Cholangitis (Primary Biliary Cirrhosis)

Primary biliary cholangitis (PBC) is a chronic cholestatic liver disease of possible autoimmune etiology characterized by slow progression of cholestasis and the development of liver fibrosis, eventually cirrhosis. It is commonly seen in females in their fifth to sixth decade.

Patients usually present with fatigue and pruritus. On examination, jaundice and clubbing may be found. Laboratory investigations reflect cholestasis and chronic liver disease along with elevated serum antimitochondrial antibodies.

The bile ducts involved in the disease are too small to be resolved by imaging and hence most findings in PBC are secondary to the development of liver fibrosis. Imaging shows changes of cirrhosis, periportal lymphadenopathy, splenomegaly, and portal hypertension. A sign described for PBC is the presence of a hypointense halo around a small portal venous branch in T1-weighted, T2-weighted, and postcontrast T1-weighted images ("periportal halo sign") [77]. However, this is not a very sensitive sign and it may also be seen in autoimmune hepatitis [78].

Primary Sclerosing Cholangitis

Pathophysiology and Clinical Presentation: PSC is a rare chronic progressive disorder characterized by inflammation and fibrotic stricture of medium and large caliber bile ducts ultimately resulting in cholestasis and liver failure. Most cases involve both intrahepatic and extrahepatic bile ducts. Up to 54% cases are

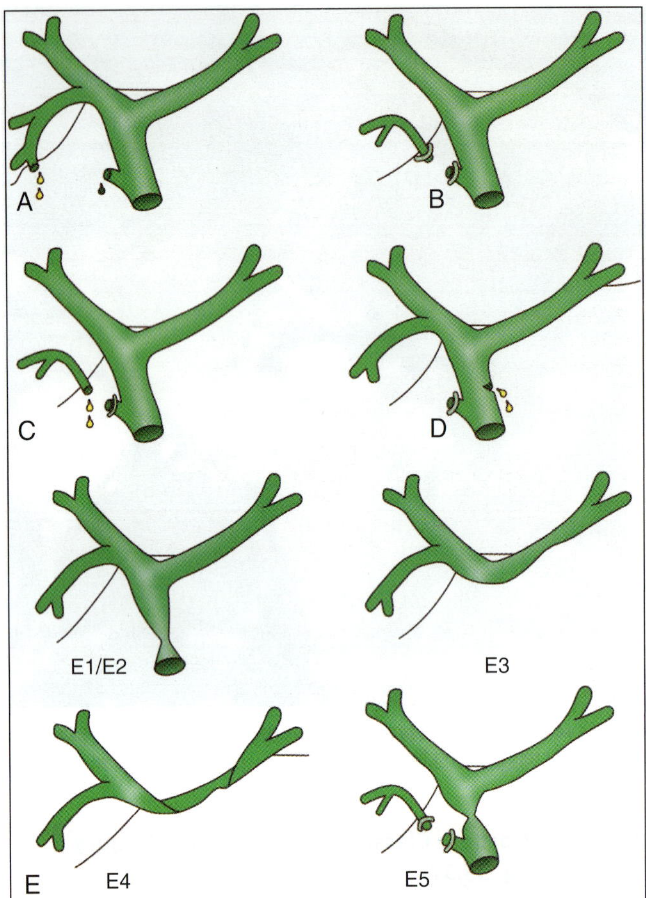

Figure 35.37 Strasberg classification of bile duct injury. See the text for description. Note in type A injury, continuity between the bile leakage site and main CBD is maintained while there is no continuity in type C injury.

Figure 35.39 Strasberg type B bile duct injury after laparoscopic cholecystectomy. 3D MRCP shows focal dilatation of right posterior sectoral duct (RPSD) with abrupt cutoff. The RPSD was aberrant and was inadvertently ligated during surgery.

within the wall of the CBD. Biliary obstruction may be secondary to obstruction by dilated collaterals or due to ischemia of the bile duct wall resulting in fibrosis. Characteristic imaging features include smooth wavy stenosis and acute kinking of the CBD at the site of stenosis. Pericholedochal collaterals are usually demonstrated in Doppler ultrasound or CECT. Dilated epicholedochal collaterals appear as thickening and enhancement of the CBD wall (Fig. 35.40) [94].

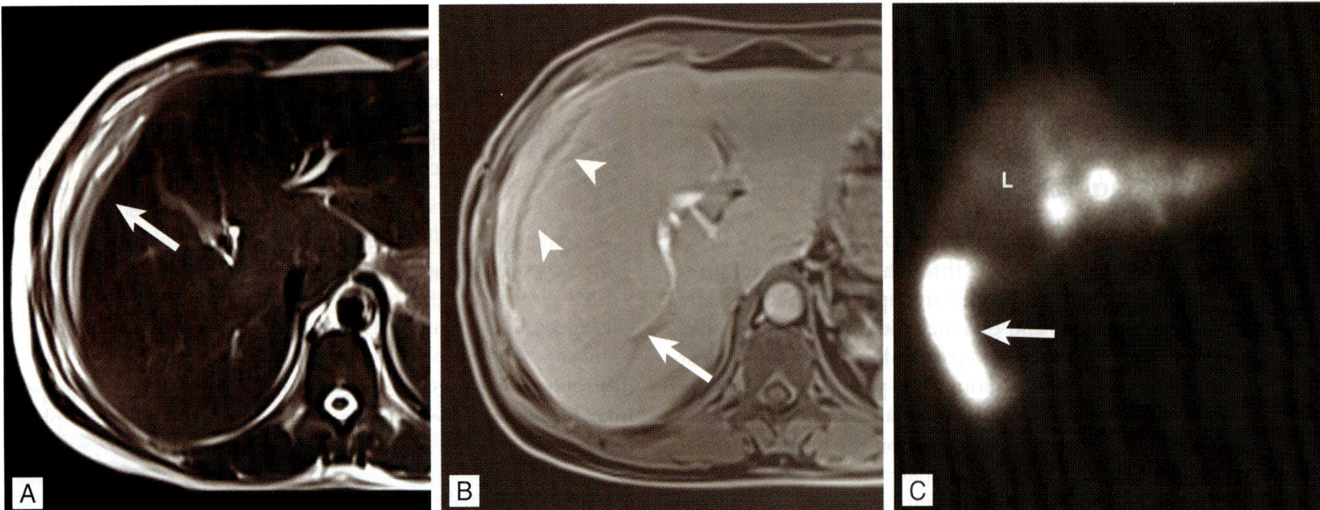

Figure 35.38 Postoperative bile leak. (A) T2-weighted axial MR shows small perihepatic collection (*arrow*). (B) Axial postcontrast T1-weighted hepatobiliary phase image (90 minutes after injection of gadobenate) shows accumulation of contrast in the collection (*arrowheads*) with a faint tract extending from right posterior sectoral duct (*arrow*) suggesting a leak. (C) Tc-99m-HIDA scan in anteroposterior projection shows accumulation of radiotracer in the perihepatic space (*arrow*) confirming the bile leak. *L*, liver.

BOX 35.11 Bile Duct Injury—What the Referring Surgeon Wants to Know?

- Is there evidence of bile leak? (Ascites, biloma)—localization and amount
- Is there evidence of bile duct stricture? (Focal biliary dilation—especially in the right hepatic lobe) (Fig. 35.38)
- Site and extent of injury (contrast extravasation; stricture location, number, and length)
- Presence of aberrant bile duct (most commonly right posterior hepatic segment)
- Any evidence of complication (cholangitis)

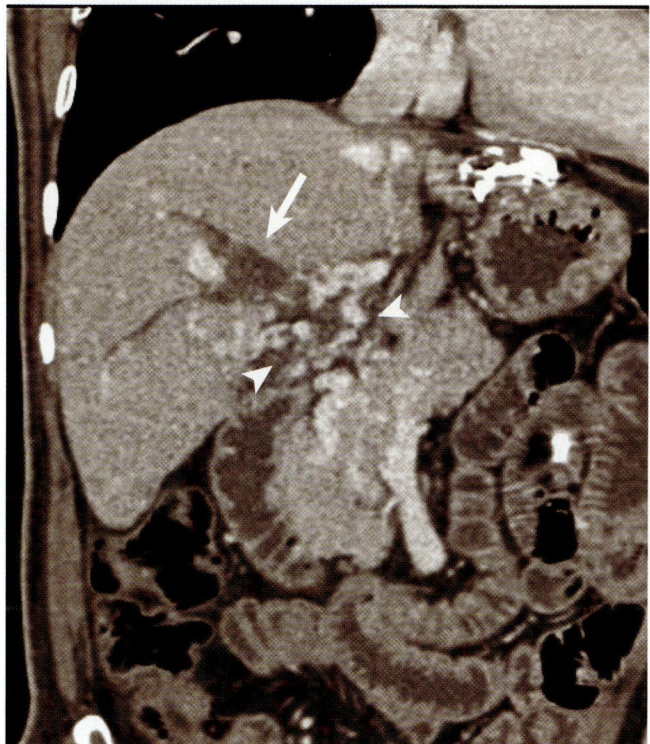

Figure 35.40 Portal biliopathy. Oblique coronal reformatted contrast CT shows multiple dilated tortuous venous channels replacing the main portal vein suggesting portal cavernoma formation (between *arrowheads*). Dilated bile ducts are also noted (*arrow*).

Cholangiocarcinoma

CCAs are usually adenocarcinomas arising from biliary epithelium. Based on its location it is classified into intrahepatic and extrahepatic CCA. Extrahepatic CCA is much more common, accounting for about 90% of the CCA [95].

Classification

1. According to site (Fig. 35.41):
   a. Intrahepatic: Tumors that arise peripheral to the secondary bifurcation of the left or right hepatic duct are considered intrahepatic CCA.
   b. Extrahepatic:
      i. Perihilar cholangiocarcinoma (pCCA): Tumors that arise anywhere from the bifurcation of right and left CHD up to the insertion of the cystic duct are called perihilar CCA. It can be further classified according to the extent of involvement of primary and secondary biliary confluence based on the Bismuth–Corlette classification (Fig. 35.42). When the tumor involves the CHD bifurcation, they are called Klatskin tumors.
      ii. Distal CCA: Cancers arising between cystic duct insertion and the ampulla, but not including the ampulla.

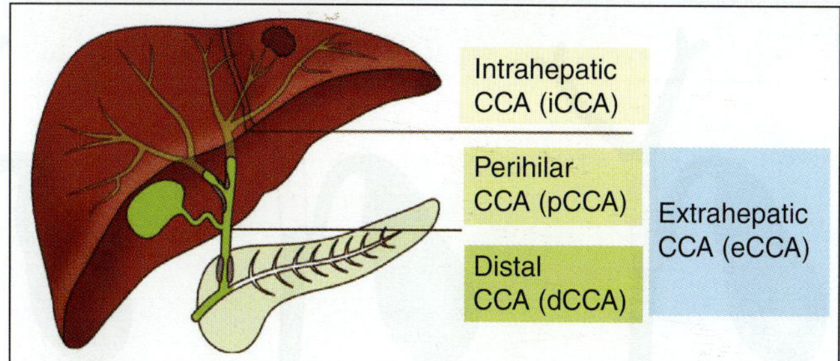

Figure 35.41 Classification of cholangiocarcinoma (CCA) according to site of origin. *dCCA*, distal CCA; *eCCA*, extrahepatic CCA; *iCCA*, intrahepatic CCA; *pCCA*, perihilar CCA. See the text for description.

2. According to morphology: CCA is also traditionally divided into three macroscopic subtypes:
   a. Mass-forming: Frequently shows satellite nodules, spread by venous and lymphatic invasion and often shows fibrosis and central necrosis. Most intrahepatic CCA are mass-forming.
   b. Periductal infiltrating: Grows along the wall of the bile ducts; associated with dense fibrosis that causes biliary stricture and vascular encasement. Hilar and mid-bile duct CCA are commonly of this type.
   c. Intraductal growing type: May spread along the mucosa and cause partial biliary obstruction. Distal CCA is commonly of this type.

Epidemiology and Risk Factors

CCA is the second most common cancer of the hepatobiliary system worldwide after HCC. It is slightly more common in men, usually diagnosed within 50–70 years of age. About 90% patients diagnosed with CCA do not have any identifiable risk factors, but commonly recognized risk factors are PSC, hepatolithiasis, liver fluke infestation, choledochal cyst, and abnormal pancreaticobiliary junction [96].

Pathology

There are two precursors to CCA: IPMN of the bile duct (IPN-B) and biliary intraepithelial neoplasia [68]. Biliary intraepithelial neoplasia is often seen in the vicinity of invasive CCA in microscopic examination but it is not visible on imaging [97]. IPN-B is similar to IPMN of pancreas. IPN-B appears as solitary or multiple papillary lesions within the bile duct lumen (Fig. 35.43). These tumors produce a variable degree of mucin. About half of all cases of IPN-B are associated with an invasive cancer [98]. It is seen more commonly in male patients between the ages of 40 and 80 years and may cause symptoms due to biliary obstruction by the tumor or thick mucin. Since the ductal dilatation may be due to overproduction of mucin, bile ducts both distal and proximal to the tumor may be dilated in case of IPN-B.

CCAs are characterized by slow growth, local invasion, and intense desmoplastic reaction. Metastases are not common. Based on histology, CCAs can be of three types.

1. Sclerosing: Most common type. It invades bile ducts early with low resection rate.
2. Nodular: Highly invasive with low resection and cure rate.
3. Papillary: Intraductal masses that cause early biliary obstruction; highest cure rate.

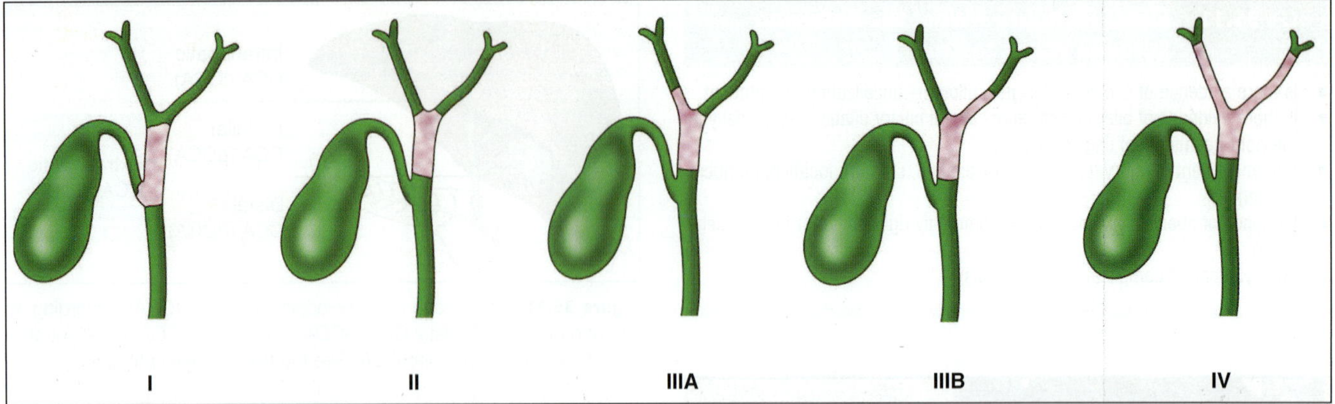

Figure 35.42 Bismuth–Corlette classification for malignant biliary stricture. Type I, primary confluence is not involved with maintained communication between right and left hepatic ducts. Type II, primary confluence is involved with separation of right and left hepatic ducts. Type IIIA, involvement of the right hepatic duct or right secondary confluence. Type IIIB, involvement of the left hepatic duct or left secondary confluence. Type IV, involvement of both secondary confluences with separation of right anterior and posterior sectoral duct and segment 2 and segment 3 ducts.

Combined hepatocellular-CCA (also called biphenotypic primary liver cancer) is a distinct type of CCA with histologic features of both cancers [99]. It is postulated to arise from a common hepatic progenitor cell.

It is important to remember that CCA, GBC, and liver metastases from pancreatic cancer and gastric nonsignet cell cancer are all adenocarcinomas and may look similar under microscope without immunohistochemistry. Imaging may help in the differentiation of these lesions by localizing the primary.

Clinical Features

Patients with extrahepatic CCA present with painless progressive jaundice, which may be associated with abdominal pain and weight loss. Intrahepatic CCA presents with a liver mass and jaundice is uncommon. Laboratory tests in extrahepatic CCA show elevated direct bilirubin. Both intrahepatic and extrahepatic cancers may have elevated alkaline phosphatase and gamma-glutamyl transpeptidase. Elevated serum CA 19-9 and low alpha-fetoprotein provide clues to the diagnosis and help to differentiate it from HCC. Note that elevated CA 19-9 may be seen in biliary, gallbladder, and pancreatic cancers and these other primary sites need to be ruled out as well. Also, absence of raised CA 19-9 does not rule out a pancreaticobiliary neoplasm.

Imaging Features

Ultrasound is the initial imaging technique of choice. Triphasic CT (late arterial, portal venous, and delayed phase) is indicated if a malignant obstruction of the biliary tract is suspected by initial ultrasound. In case of an intrahepatic mass, some centers may prefer multiphasic MRI for better characterization of the mass (see section on primary liver cancer). ERCP and percutaneous cholangiography is reserved when biliary drainage or stenting is necessary. Sometimes, these procedures are also used to take a brush cytology of the lesion for diagnosis. The PET scan has a limited role.

Intrahepatic Cholangiocarcinoma: Mass-forming ICC appears as an irregular but well-defined mass on gross pathology (Fig. 35.44). Upstream peripheral biliary dilatation is often seen. It can invade the portal vein and adjacent liver-forming satellite nodules. On ultrasound, it appears as a mass with mixed echogenicity. The typical triphasic CT finding of a mass-forming ICC is a hypoattenuating mass that shows irregular continuous rim-like enhancement in the hepatic arterial phase with gradual centripetal enhancement on portal venous and delayed phases [100]. Differentiation from hemangioma is done by demonstration of peripheral discontinuous nodular ("puddle-like") enhancement that matches the aortic attenuation in all

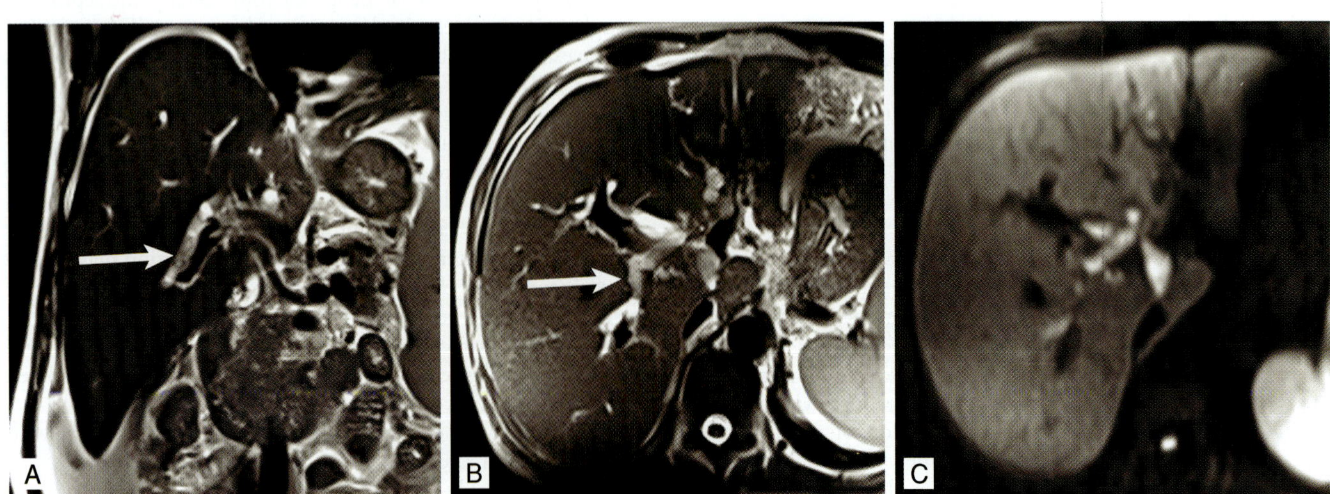

Figure 35.43 Intraductal papillary mucinous neoplasm of bile duct (IPN-B). Coronal (A) and axial (B) T2-weighted MRI show dilated intrahepatic bile duct with intraductal low-signal mass (*arrow*). (C) Diffusion-weighted image shows diffusion restriction within the mass.

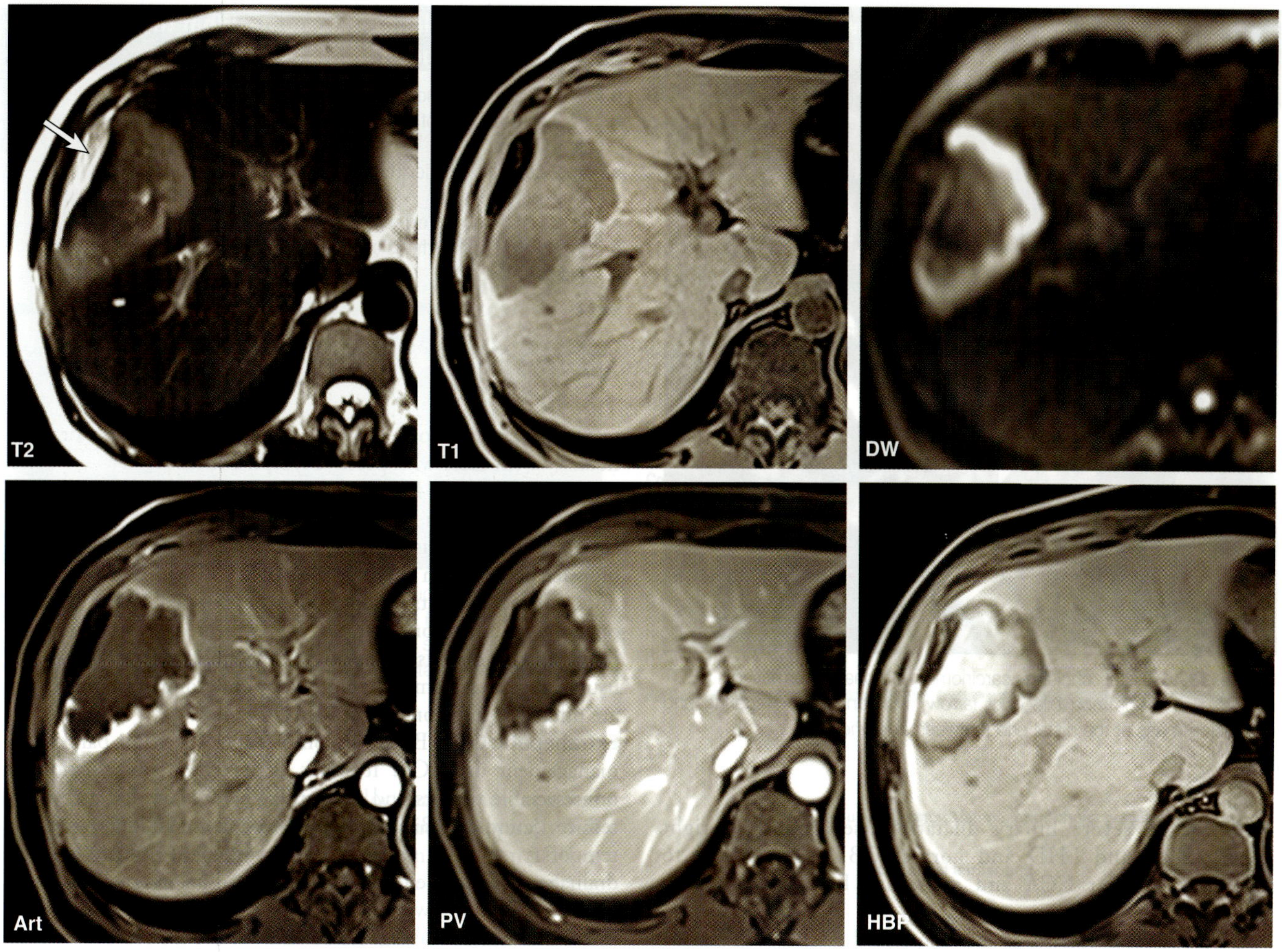

Figure 35.44 Intrahepatic mass-forming cholangiocarcinoma. T2-weighted (T2) and T1-weighted fat suppressed VIBE images show a well-defined lobulated mass in right lobe of liver. Note capsular retraction (*arrow* in T2). Diffusion-weighted (DW) images show peripheral hyperintensity suggestive of diffusion restriction. Postcontrast T1-weighted VIBE in arterial phase (Art) shows peripheral rim-like enhancement which shows gradual centripetal filling on portal venous phase (PV). Hepatobiliary phase (HBP) shows contrast washout from the peripheral portion of the mass but retention is noted at the center.

phases. The peripheral portion of the tumor enhances early because it has viable malignant cells. The central portion has necrosis and fibrous stroma that accumulate the contrast in the delayed phase. Multiphasic MRI shows the same finding. Additionally, MRI with a hepatobiliary contrast agent shows peripheral hypointensity with contrast retention at the center in the hepatobiliary phase. The peripheral rim of malignant cells is also responsible for the rim-like diffusion restriction characteristic of these lesions. Another useful finding is overlying liver capsular retraction [101]. Although iCCA usually presents as a hepatic mass with or without satellite lesions, it can also present with multiple hypoenhancing liver lesions with or without a dominant mass (akin to metastases from unknown primary). In the absence of a primary elsewhere in the body and with corresponding histopathology, the radiologist can help make the accurate diagnosis.

Extrahepatic Cholangiocarcinoma: Extrahepatic CCAs are often not seen on ultrasound or even on CT due to the periductal infiltrating morphology, but identified by indirect signs of biliary dilatation. Klatskin tumor presents as bilobar biliary dilatation with nonunion of right and left hepatic ducts. A focal mass at liver hilum may sometimes be appreciated (Fig. 35.45]). Therefore, in the presence of

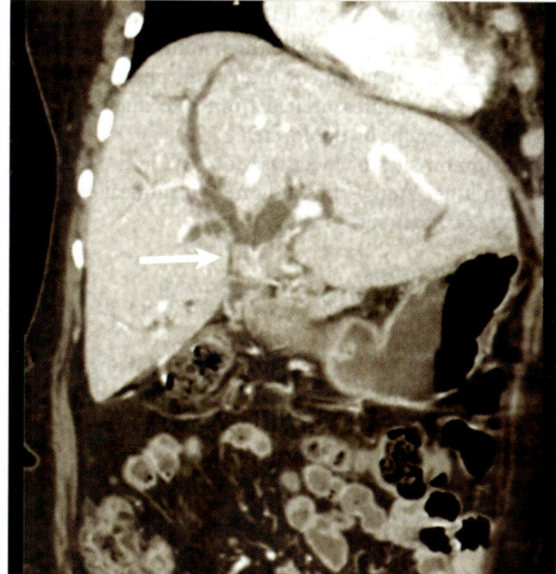

Figure 35.45 Hilar cholangiocarcinoma (Klatskin tumor). Oblique coronal reformatted contrast CT shows enhancing mass (*arrow*) at the junction of the right and left hepatic duct.

Suggested Readings

- RM Gore, V Yaghmai, GM Newmark, JW Berlin, FH Miller, Imaging benign and malignant disease of the gallbladder, Radiol Clin North Am 40 (6) (2002) 1307–1323.
- M Yokoe, J Hata, T Takada, SM Strasberg, HJ Asbun, G Wakabayashi, et al., Tokyo Guidelines 2018: diagnostic criteria and severity grading of acute cholecystitis (with videos), J Hepatobiliary Pancreat Sci 25 (1) (2018) 41–54.
- A Furlan, JV Ferris, K Hosseinzadeh, AA Borhani, Gallbladder carcinoma update: multimodality imaging evaluation, staging, and treatment options, AJR Am J Roentgenol 191 (5) (2008) 1440–1447.
- R Wiles, RF Thoeni, ST Barbu, YK Vashist, SR Rafaelsen, C Dewhurst, et al., Management and follow-up of gallbladder polyps: joint guidelines between the European Society of Gastrointestinal and Abdominal Radiology (ESGAR), European Association for Endoscopic Surgery and other Interventional Techniques (EAES), International Society of Digestive Surgery-European Federation (EFISDS) and European Society of Gastrointestinal Endoscopy (ESGE). Eur Radiol 27 (9) (2017) 3856–3866.
- G Joshi, KA Crawford, TN Hanna, KD Herr, N Dahiya, CO Menias, US of right upper quadrant pain in the emergency department: diagnosing beyond gallbladder and biliary disease, Radiographics 38 (3) (2018) 766–793.

36 Pancreas

VENKAT KATABATHINA, MADELEINE SERTIC, ABRAHAM FOURIE BEZUIDENHOUT, AVINASH KAMBADAKONE, ATIF ZAHEER, SRINIVASA R. PRASAD

Introduction

The pancreas (derived from the Greek word "*Pankreas*" meaning "all flesh") is an important retroperitoneal gland with exocrine and endocrine components. Anatomically, the pancreas is divided into the uncinate process, head, neck, body, and tail regions and is located within the anterior pararenal space. The pancreatic head is nestled within the C-loop of the duodenum, the tail extends to the splenic hilum (Fig. 36.1) [1]. The head of the pancreas is the thickest part that lies to the right of superior mesenteric artery (SMA) and superior mesenteric vein (SMV), the neck is the thinnest part that lies anterior to the SMA and SMV. The uncinate process is an extension of the head and lies anterior to the aorta and inferior vena cava and posterior to SMA and SMV. The SMA is the boundary between the uncinate process and the neck. The main pancreatic duct measures between 3.5 mm at the head to 1.5 mm at the tail region. The body of the pancreas is the main part that lies to the left of SMA and SMV and anterior to the lumbar spine. Tail of the pancreas lies anterior to the left kidney, abutting the splenic hilum, and splenic flexure of the colon (Fig. 36.1) [1].

The common bile duct joins the main pancreatic duct to form the ampulla of Vater, which opens into the second portion of the duodenum through the major duodenal papilla. The pancreas receives its blood supply from branches of the splenic, superior mesenteric, and gastroduodenal arteries; pancreatic veins drain into superior mesenteric and splenic veins. The acinar cells constitute the exocrine component of the pancreas (80–85% of the organ), whereas approximately 1 million clusters of endocrine cells, the islets of Langerhans (1–2% of the organ), form the endocrine component [1]. The acinar cells synthesize and secrete proenzymes and enzymes that aid in digestion. The islet cells secrete hormones such as glucagon and insulin that mainly regulate body and blood glucose levels. The pancreas is an unencapsulated organ; this facilitates the spread of infection or tumor into the surrounding viscera and anatomical compartments [1]. Given the retroperitoneal location, the pancreas is not easily accessible for physical examination. Imaging studies play a pivotal role in the evaluation, characterization, and staging of a plethora of pancreatic diseases and thus influence management decisions. A wide spectrum of pancreatic pathologies, including developmental anomalies, congenital diseases, pancreatitis, and pancreatic neoplasms, will be discussed.

Overview of Imaging Techniques

Plain radiography plays a limited role in the evaluation of pancreatic disorders. Radiographs allow the detection of calcifications (chronic pancreatitis [CP] and calcifications within a tumor) and focal ileus (acute pancreatitis [AP]) (Fig. 36.2).

Ultrasonography (USG) permits diagnosing pancreatitis and its attendant complications (pseudocysts, vascular thrombosis, and aneurysms) and the distinction of solid from cystic

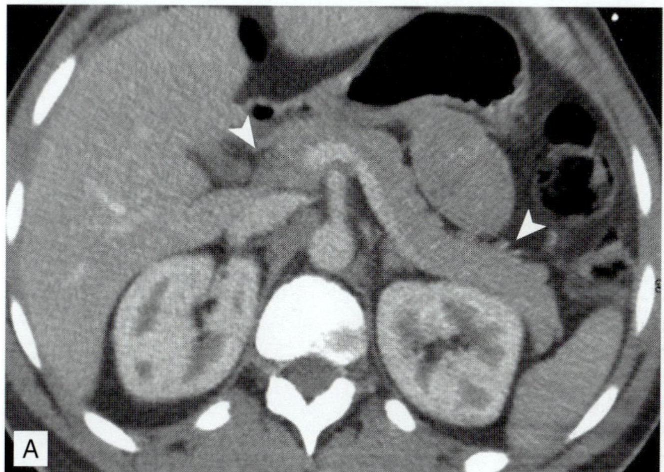

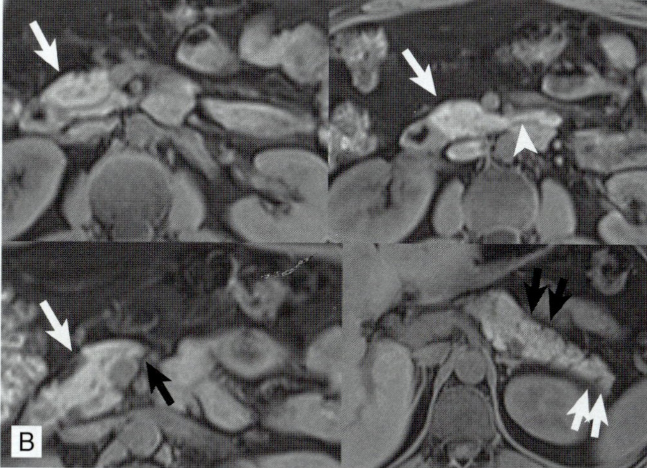

Figure 36.1 Normal CT and MRI appearance of the pancreas. (A) Axial CT image of the abdomen demonstrates normal pancreas with lobulated surface (*arrowheads*). (B) Multiple unenhanced T1-weighted images of the abdomen show uncinate process (*white arrowhead*), head (*single white arrow*), neck (*single black arrow*), body (*double black arrows*), and tail (*double white arrows*) of the pancreas.

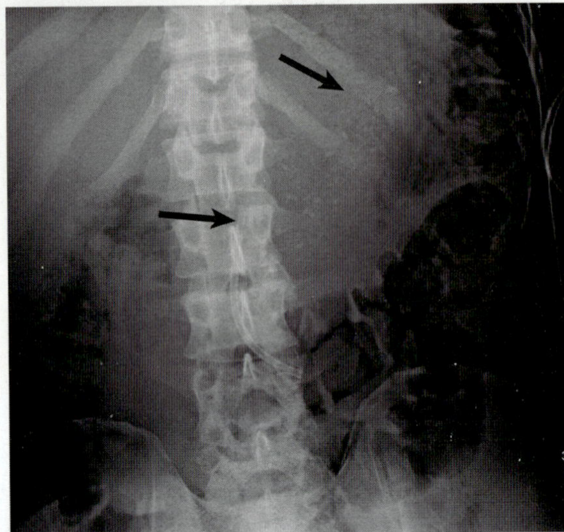

Figure 36.2 Chronic pancreatitis. Plain radiograph demonstrates multiple calcifications in the expected location of the pancreas (*arrows*).

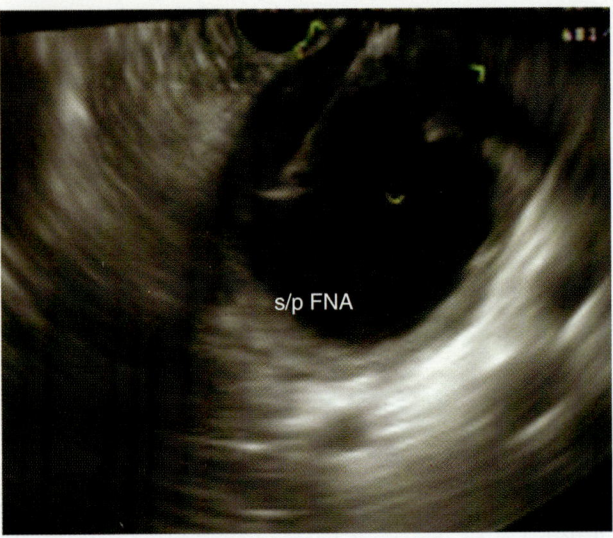

Figure 36.4 Role of endoscopic USG (EUS) in the evaluation of the pancreatic pathologies. EUS image obtained during aspiration of a cystic pancreatic neoplasm. *EUS*, endoscopic ultrasound; *USG*, ultrasonography.

neoplasms. On account of universal availability, real-time, inexpensive, and noninvasive scanning technique by a portable machine without the routine need for intravenous contrast, USG may be considered as the technique of choice in the initial assessment of the pancreas (Fig. 36.3). However, USG has limited value in the evaluation of pancreatic disorders, particularly in the context of patient factors such as obesity and increased bowel gas as well as operator dependence. Endoscopic ultrasound (EUS) is invaluable in the evaluation of pancreatic neoplasms and serving to direct interventional techniques, including targeted biopsies and/or cyst aspiration (Fig. 36.4).

Multiphasic CT is the preferred primary technique for a detailed assessment of a wide array of pancreatic disorders. Multiparametric MRI and Magnetic resonance cholangiopancreatography (MRCP) are equivalent or superior to CT scans in evaluating diseases of the pancreas, particularly in the assessment of cystic pancreatic neoplasms (Fig. 36.5). Endoscopic retrograde cholangiopancreatography (ERCP) helps identify pancreatic ductal abnormalities and image-guided biopsy (Fig. 36.6). Functional imaging with positron emission tomography (PET) using 18F-fluorodeoxyglucose (FDG) plays a major role in the staging evaluation of pancreatic cancer. Gallium-68 DOTATATE scans are invaluable in the diagnosis and staging of pancreatic neuroendocrine neoplasms (Fig. 36.7).

Multidetector CT allows faster acquisition of volumetric imaging data in a short breath-hold, thereby permitting thin section, high-resolution, dynamic, multiphasic CT images, as well as multiplanar reconstructions [1,2]. Multiphasic CT scan is the primary workhorse in the evaluation of pancreatic disorders. Noncontrast images of the abdomen permit detection of calcifications, fatty changes, and fluid collections. The postcontrast images are obtained after administration of iodinated contrast medium (1.8–2 mL of contrast/kg or 550 mg Iodine/kg) injected at a rate of 3–5 mL/s. Approximately 35–40 seconds

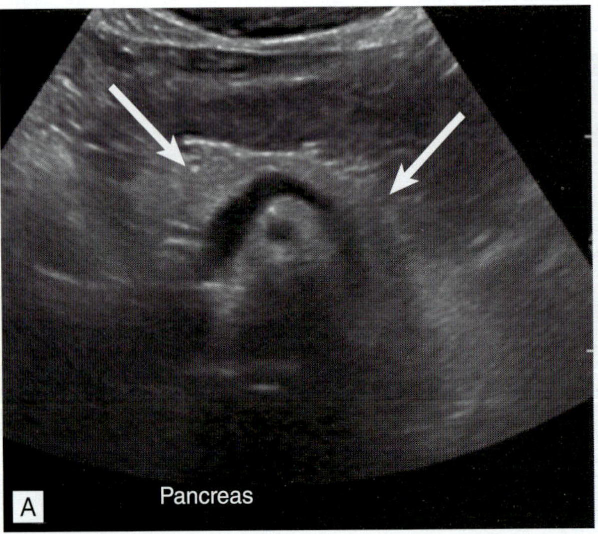

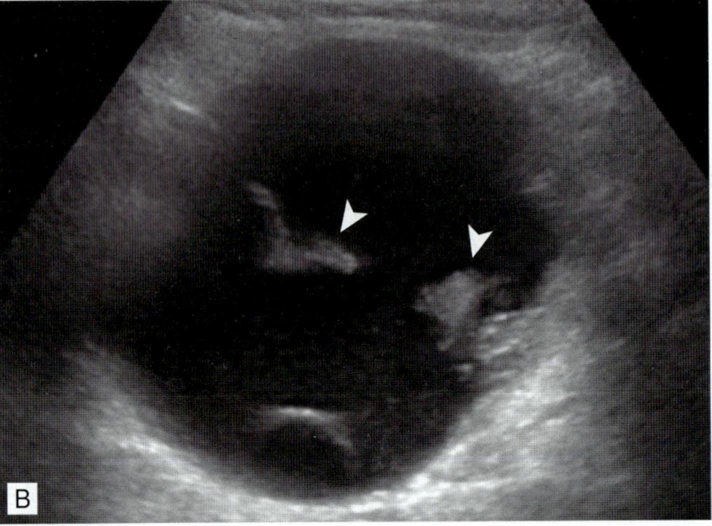

Figure 36.3 Role of transabdominal USG in the evaluation of the pancreas. (A) USG image demonstrates normal pancreas anterior to the splenic vein (*arrows*). (B) Axial USG image of the pancreas demonstrates a large cystic mass in the pancreas with a few thickened septations and solid components (*arrowheads*). This mass is proved to be a mucinous cystic neoplasm on pathology. *USG*, ultrasonography.

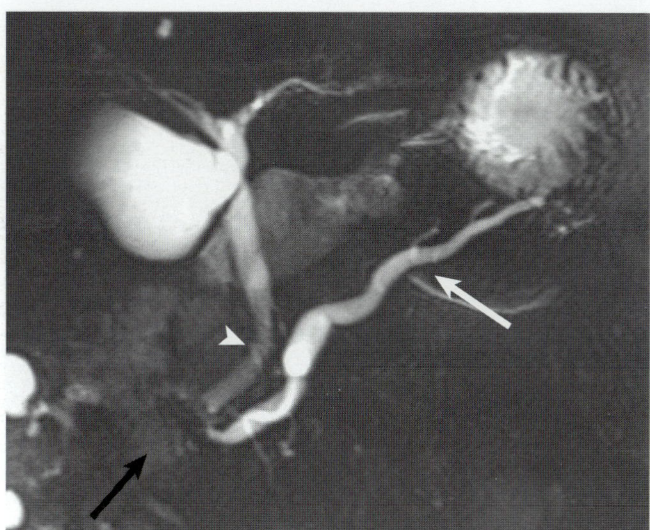

Figure 36.5 Role of MRI and MRCP in the evaluation of the pancreas. MRCP is the most commonly used noninvasive imaging test for the evaluation of pancreatic ducts. Coronal 3D MRCP image demonstrates dilated main pancreatic duct (*white arrow*) and dilated common bile duct (*white arrowhead*) secondary to a partially seen duodenal diverticulum (*black arrow*).

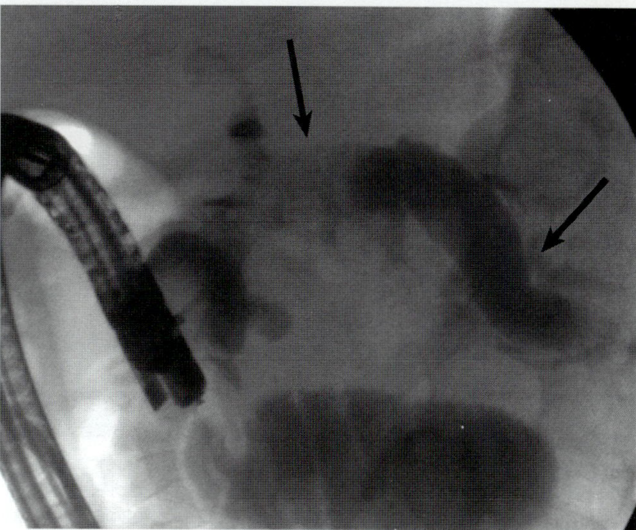

Figure 36.6 Role of ERCP in the evaluation of pancreatic pathologies. ERCP image shows a dilated main pancreatic duct (*arrows*) in this patient with main duct IPMN. *ERCP*, endoscopic retrograde cholangiopancreatography; *IPMN*, intraductal papillary mucinous neoplasm.

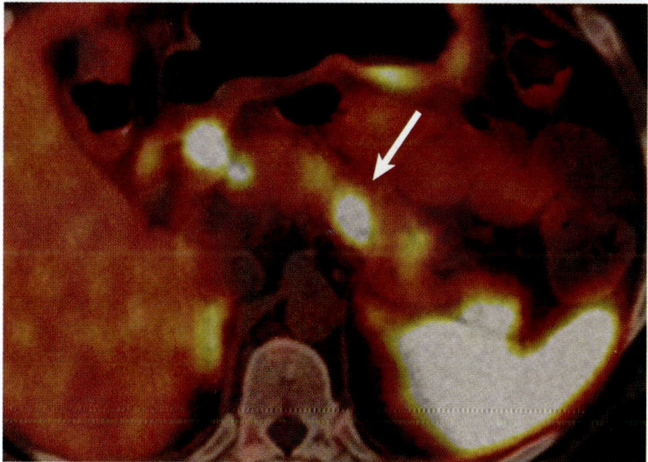

Figure 36.7 Role of gallium-68 DOTATATE PET/CT for the evaluation of pancreatic neuroendocrine tumors. Axial gallium-68 DOTATATE PET/CT image in a MEN1 syndrome patient depicts multiple focal lesions of the pancreas with increased uptake (*arrow*) consistent with pancreatic neuroendocrine tumors. *PET*, positron emission tomography.

after contrast administration, the pancreatic parenchyma shows peak enhancement (pancreatic phase), allowing for maximal contrast between normal parenchyma and diseased tissue. A number of dynamic postcontrast images may be obtained that include early arterial phase (20–25 seconds delay), pancreatic parenchymal phase/late arterial phase (35–40 seconds delay), portal venous phase images (60–70 seconds delay), and equilibrium phase images (100–120 seconds delay) [1,2].

- For suspected pancreas tumor, including ductal adenocarcinoma, a triple-phase CT study that includes a noncontrast study, pancreatic parenchymal phase, and portal venous phase images should be obtained (pancreatic CT protocol). Portal venous phase images help to assess porto-mesenteric venous system and liver metastases
- If there is suspicion of a hypervascular pancreatic lesion such as pancreatic neuroendocrine tumor or hypervascular metastases from renal cell carcinoma or thyroid carcinoma, one can replace the pancreatic parenchymal phase with arterial phase
- Pancreatitis: Only portal venous phase images should be acquired
- Neutral enteric oral contrast such as water is administered before the CT

Multiphasic MRI protocols incorporate precontrast T1WI and T2WI as well as fat-suppressed 3-D T1WI after administration of gadolinium chelates while scanning during different phases as discussed with dynamic contrast-enhanced CT scans. Normal pancreatic parenchyma demonstrates high signal intensity on fat-suppressed T1-weighted images due to high content of aqueous protein and appears abnormally hypointense on T1W images in conditions such as AP (Fig. 36.8).

Pseudotumors

Intrapancreatic Splenule

Accessory spleens/splenules are formed due to the failure of fusion of an embryonic splenic bud. The pancreas is the site of the accessory spleen in up to 16% of cases, the third most common site after the splenic hilum and perisplenic region. Intrapancreatic splenule can pose diagnostic dilemmas. *As they follow the enhancement pattern of the spleen*, the intrapancreatic splenule will demonstrate mild hyperenhancement to the background pancreatic parenchyma on a portal venous phase CT and may be mistaken for an enhancing primary pancreatic tumor (such as a well-differentiated neuroendocrine tumor) or metastasis [3]. On MRI, the intrapancreatic splenule will follow the splenic signal on all sequences (Fig. 36.9). Tc-99m sulfur colloid scan or Tc-99m RBC scintigraphy may be performed to confirm the diagnosis, although EUS-guided biopsy is needed in select cases.

Duodenal Diverticulum

A duodenal diverticulum is a common finding, seen in up to 23% of asymptomatic patients [4]. Duodenal diverticula are readily

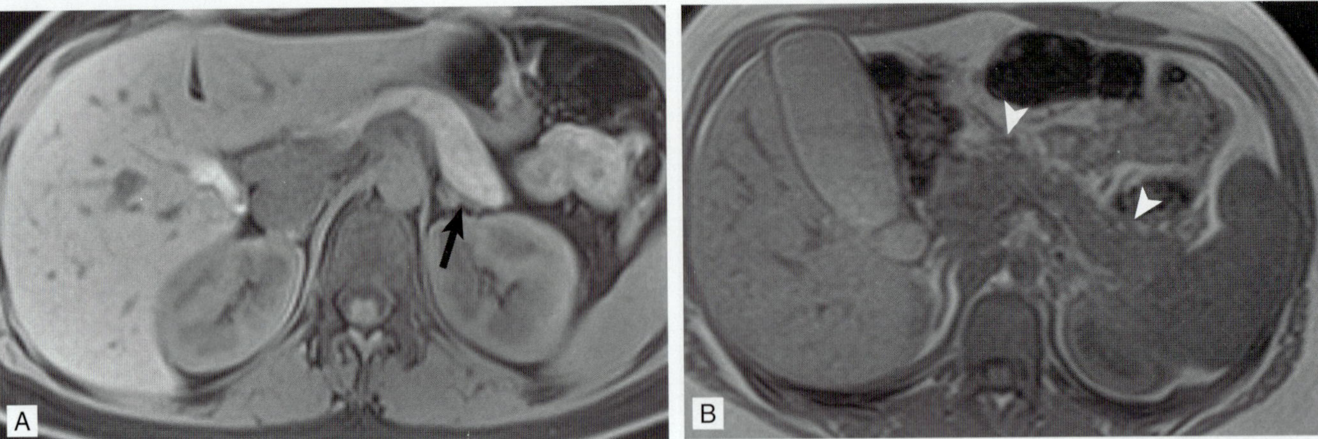

Figure 36.8 Role of MRI in the identification of normal and abnormal pancreatic parenchyma. (A) Axial T1-weighted fat-suppressed MR image shows high signal intensity of the normal pancreatic parenchyma due to high content of aqueous protein. (B) Axial T1-weighted MR image shows diffusely low signal intensity of the abnormal pancreatic parenchyma in this patient with acute pancreatitis (*arrowheads*).

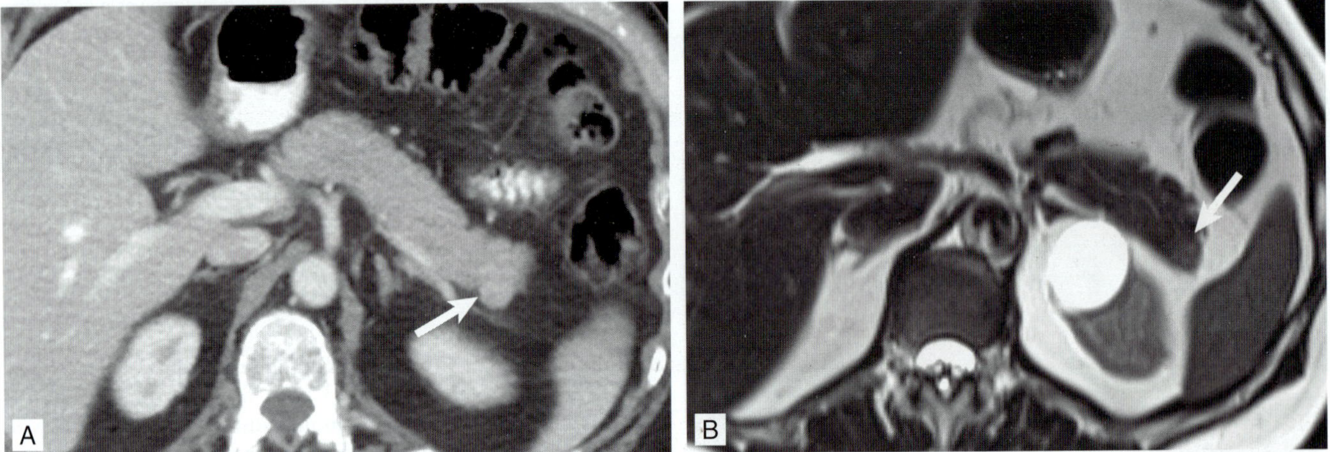

Figure 36.9 A pancreatic splenule mimics a neoplasm. (A) Axial contrast-enhanced CT image of the pancreas shows a small homogenously enhancing focal lesions in the pancreatic tail (*arrow*). (B) Axial T2-weighted MR image of the pancreas in the same patient shows a mildly T2 hyperintense focal mass in the tail (*arrow*). This mass was proved to be a splenule on pathology.

identified by the presence of intraluminal gas. When the lumen is fluid-filled, a diverticulum may be mistaken for a cystic lesion of the pancreatic head. Mixed density ingested contents or dilute enteric contrast may further confound the imaging findings and mimic a solid or enhancing pancreatic mass. The key to the diagnosis is recognizing the characteristic location of a duodenal diverticulum and identifying intraluminal gas when present. On CT, utilization of a wide window such as a typical lung window may be helpful. On MRI, the careful scrutinization of gradient-echo sequences for blooming artifacts can help in the detection of small locules of intraluminal gas. Follow-up imaging with positive enteric contrast can be performed to confirm the diagnosis (Fig. 36.10) [5].

Congenital Anomalies

The adult pancreas is formed by embryological rotation as well as the fusion of ventral and dorsal primordia (derived from the foregut diverticulum). The ventral anlage contributes to the posterior and inferior parts of the pancreatic head, while the dorsal primordium gives rise to the remainder of the organ. The fusion of the fetal ducts of both primordia leads to drainage of most of the pancreas through the duct of Wirsung into the major papilla. The accessory duct of Santorini drains into the minor papilla [6].

Pancreas Divisum

Pancreas divisum, characterized by variable fusion anomalies of the ducts of the ventral and dorsal pancreatic primordia, is the *most common congenital anomaly of the pancreas*, being seen in 3–10% of the population [6,7]. There is predominant drainage of most of the exocrine pancreas through the dorsal pancreatic duct into the minor papilla (smaller caliber). The ventral duct is either absent, separate, or connected to the dorsal duct by a thin filamentous channel.

- MRCP is a highly sensitive and specific noninvasive examination for pancreas divisum and demonstrates noncommunicating dorsal and ventral pancreatic ducts, independent drainage sites, a dominant dorsal duct, and a short, narrowed ventral duct (Fig. 36.11) [7].
- On axial CT/MR image, pancreatic duct is seen anterior to the common bile duct (Fig. 36.11).
- CT/MRI helps in detecting associated findings such as santorinicele and choledochal cyst and acute/CP.

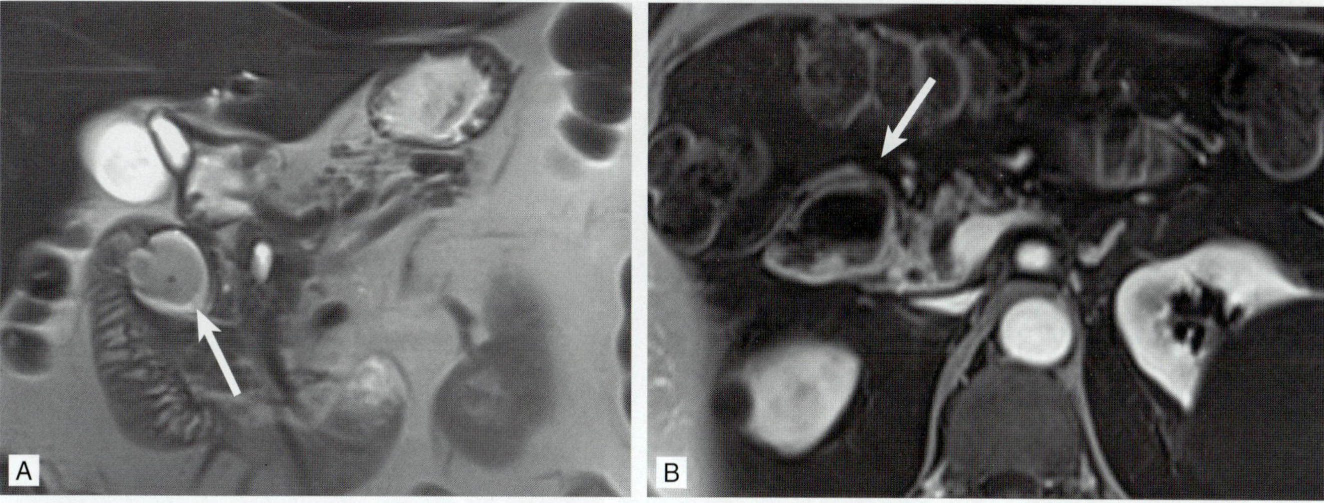

Figure 36.10 A duodenal diverticulum mimics a cystic pancreatic neoplasm (A and B). Coronal T2-weighted (A) and contrast-enhanced T1-weighted (B) MR images of the pancreas show a T2 hyperintense cystic lesion in the region of head of the pancreas that shows mild wall enhancement after contrast administration, mimicking a cystic pancreatic neoplasm (*arrows*). On further investigation, this was proved to be a duodenal diverticulum.

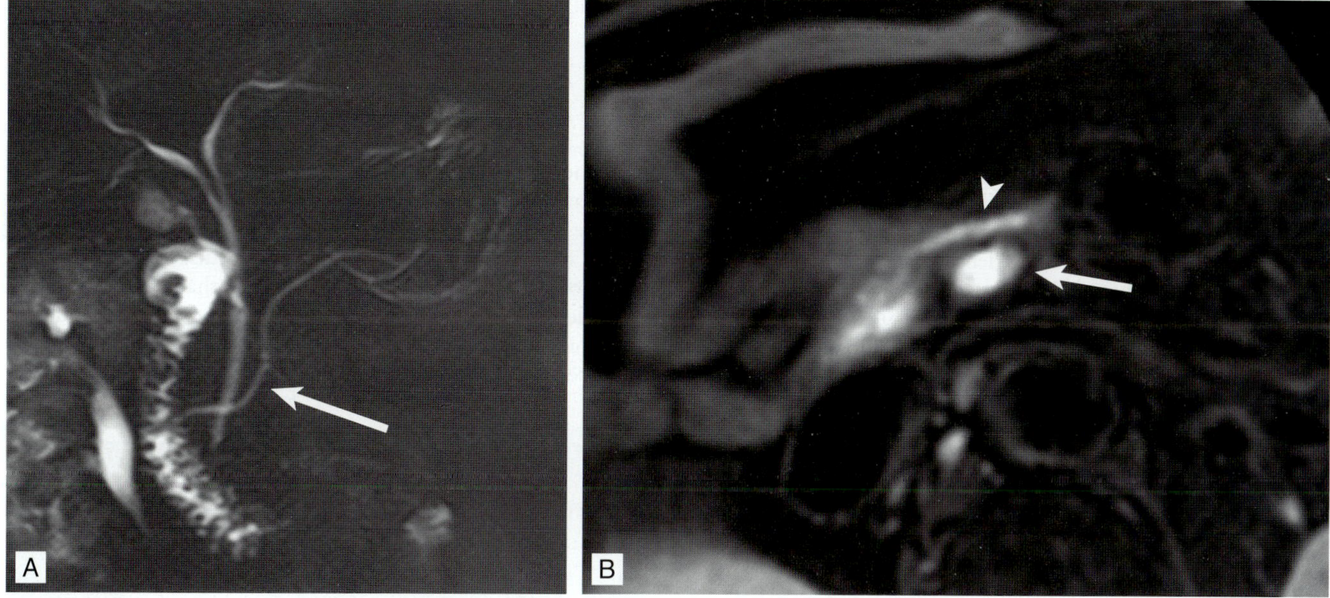

Figure 36.11 Pancreas divisum in two different patents. (A) 3D MRCP image demonstrates crossing of the main pancreatic duct and the common bile duct in the region of the pancreatic head/uncinate process with main pancreatic duct opening at the minor papilla (*arrow*). (B) Axial T2-weighted MR image of the pancreas shows that the main pancreatic duct (*arrowhead*) is seen anterior to the common bile duct (*arrow*). Both MR appearances are consistent with pancreas divisum.

- ERCP is the gold standard examination and shows only ventral duct opacification with standard cannulation of the major papilla.
- Pancreas divisum is thought to predispose to acute/CP due to presumptive relative outflow obstruction.

Annular Pancreas

Annular pancreas is the result of either persistent pancreatic primordium or a rotational anomaly that leads to partial or complete encasement of the second portion of the duodenum by pancreatic tissue [7]. Associated duodenal anomalies, including atresia or stenosis, and pancreatic anomalies such as pancreas divisum may be seen. Annular pancreas is commonly diagnosed in children because of upper gastrointestinal tract obstruction. Most often, this anomaly is asymptomatic in adults, being incidentally found on imaging. Pancreatitis or peptic ulcer disease may be seen in symptomatic adult patients [7].

- The upper gastrointestinal series shows a filling defect or focal concentric narrowing involving the second part of the duodenum.
- On CT, a complete ring of pancreatic tissue is seen around the duodenum in the case of complete type. Partial annular pancreas is characterized by the extension of pancreatic tissue posterolateral to the second portion of duodenum or "crocodile-jaw" configuration of the pancreatic parenchyma in relation to the duodenum (Fig. 36.12) [6,7].
- MRCP is the best noninvasive test to assess the ductal anatomy in the annual pancreas that typically shows annular duct on the lateral aspect of the duodenum (Fig. 36.12).

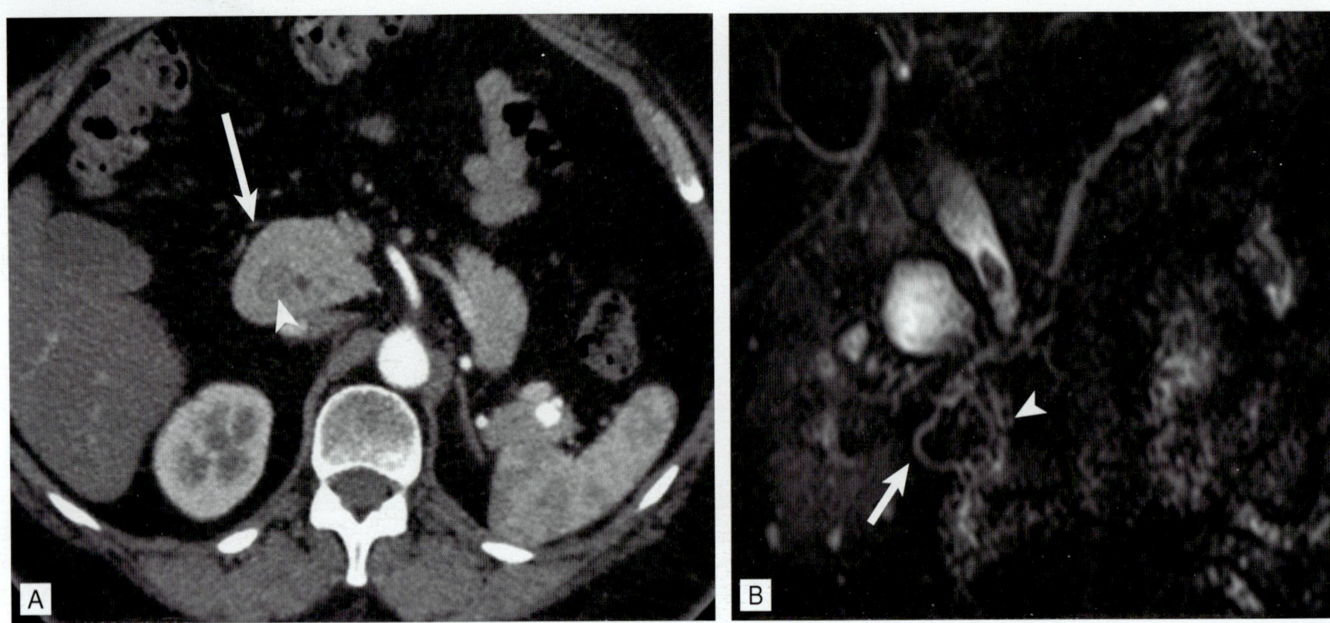

Figure 36.12 Annular pancreas. (A) Axial contrast-enhanced CT image of the pancreas shows pancreatic parenchyma (*arrow*) completely encircling the second part of the duodenum (*arrowhead*) consistent with annular pancreas. (B) MRCP image shows the main pancreatic duct (*arrow*) lateral to the second part of the duodenum (*arrowhead*), consistent with annular pancreas.

Ectopic Pancreas

Pancreatic tissue may be seen outside of the pancreas, most often in the stomach and duodenum. These embryological rests are incidental findings that may be discovered at endoscopy or imaging. An oval or round soft-tissue density masses in the intestinal wall with attenuation and signal intensities similar to pancreatic parenchyma is seen on CT/MRI (Fig. 36.13) [6,7]. The ectopic pancreas may lead to inflammation or rarely mucosal bleeding.

Diffuse Changes Within the Pancreas

Pancreatic parenchyma may demonstrate changes in attenuation (CT) or signal intensity changes (MRI) due to fat deposition, calcifications, or iron deposition. Macroscopic fat within the pancreas may be focal, segmental, or diffuse. A focal area of fatty change in the pancreas can be mistaken for mass or focal inflammation (Fig. 36.14) [6,7]. Lipomatous pseudohypertrophy of the pancreas is characterized by a focal or diffuse enlargement of the pancreas due to significant increase in intraparenchymal adipose tissue and may be seen in patients with cystic fibrosis. Cystic fibrosis is an autosomal recessive disease secondary to mutations of the CFTR gene (ch7q31) that cause abnormal chloride ion transport resulting in multiple exocrine gland dysfunction, including the pancreas. In cystic fibrosis patients, the most common abnormality seen on CT and MRI is the fatty

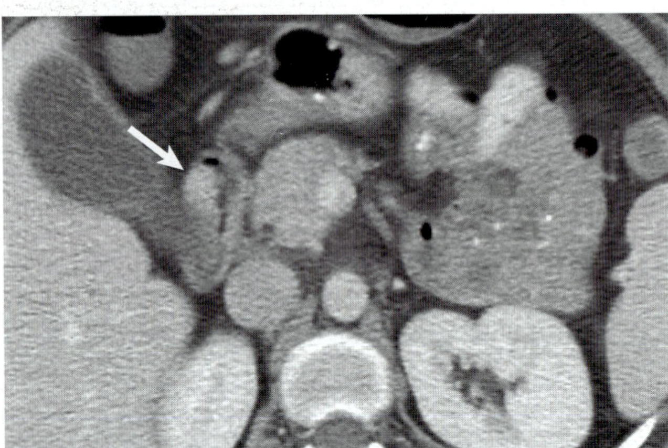

Figure 36.13 Ectopic pancreas. Axial contrast-enhanced CT image of the pancreas shows ectopic pancreatic tissue in the lateral wall of the second part of the duodenum (*arrow*), without any connection with the main pancreatic parenchyma.

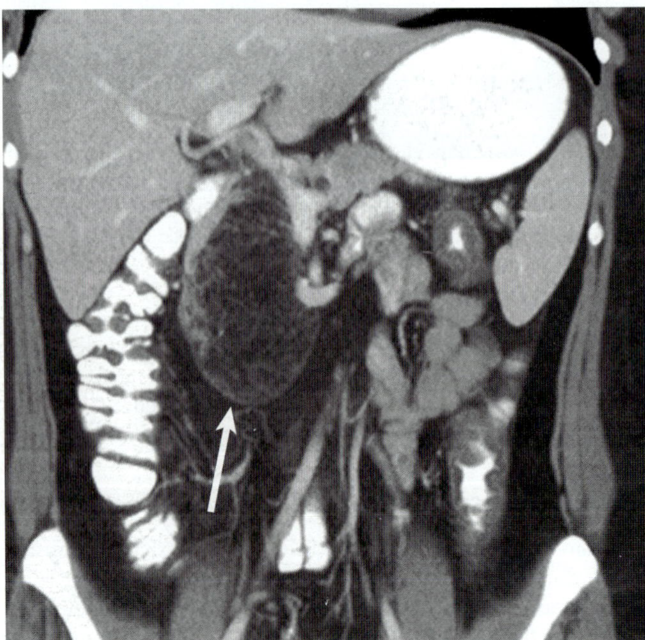

Figure 36.14 Lipomatous hypertrophy of the pancreas. Coronal contrast-enhanced CT image of the pancreas shows fatty replacement and hypertrophy of the head and uncinate process of the pancreas (*arrow*).

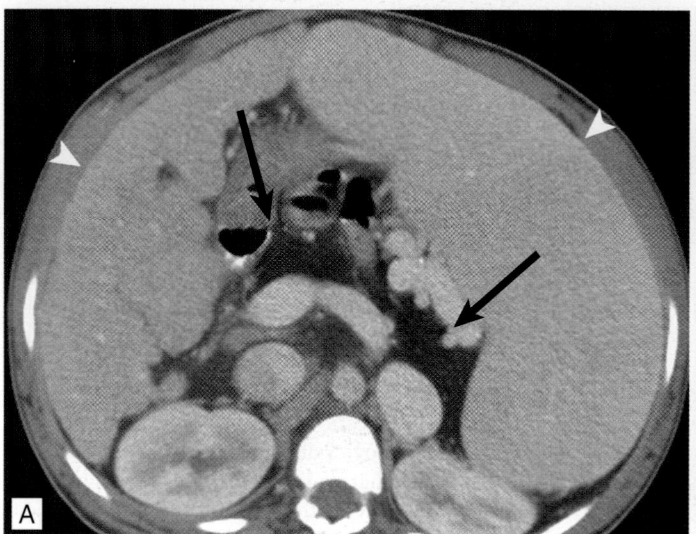

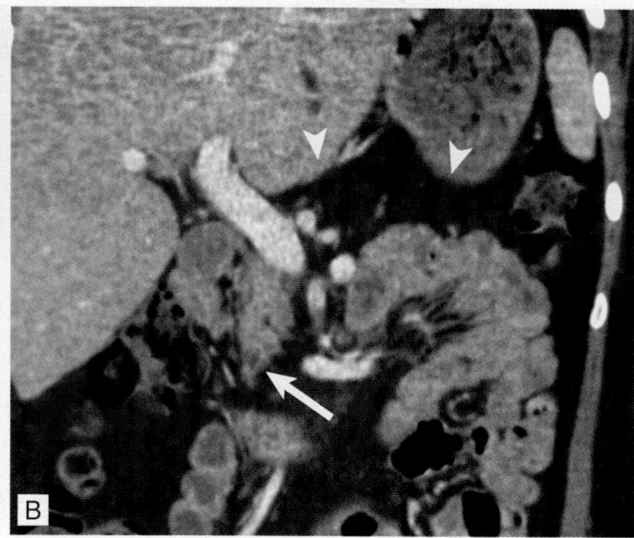

Figure 36.15 Imaging of cystic fibrosis in two different patients. (A) Axial contras-enhanced CT image of the pancreas shows complete fatty replacement of the pancreas (*black arrows*). Also, note cirrhotic liver with splenomegaly (*white arrowheads*). (B) Coronal contrast-enhanced CT image of the pancreas shows fatty replacement of the body and tail of the pancreas (*arrowheads*) with fatty sparing of the pancreatic head and the uncinate process (*arrow*).

replacement of the pancreas, which may be diffuse leading to glandular hypertrophy or limited to the distal pancreas with focal fatty sparing of the pancreatic head (Fig. 36.15) [6,7]. Diffuse, variable fatty replacement of the pancreas may also be seen in cystic fibrosis, diabetes mellitus, or in elderly patients (Fig. 36.16). No follow-up is needed in the diffuse or focal fat deposition of the pancreas in noncystic fibrosis patients.

Diffuse punctate calcifications may be seen in patients with CP. Diffuse parenchymal atrophy frequently manifests as a sequela of CP. Pancreatic parenchymal iron deposition seen in patients with primary hemochromatosis is exquisitely demonstrated on MRI. Diffuse parenchymal iron deposition is characterized by diffuse loss of signal intensity on in-phase T1-W gradient-echo images as well as marked hypointensity on fat-saturated T2-W images (Fig. 36.17) [7].

Pancreatic manifestations in von Hippel–Lindau (VHL) disease include simple cysts, serous microcystic adenomas, and neuroendocrine tumors; among them, multiple cysts are the most common finding (Fig. 36.18).

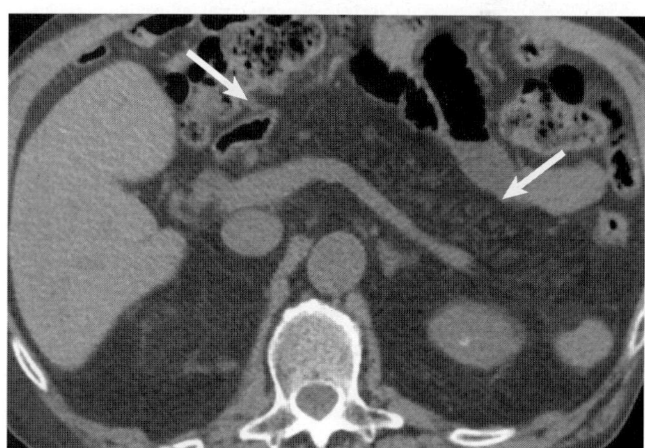

Figure 36.16 Diffuse fatty replacement of the pancreatic parenchyma in a patient with chronic type 2 diabetes mellitus. Axial CT image of the abdomen shows diffuse fatty replacement of the pancreatic parenchyma (*arrows*).

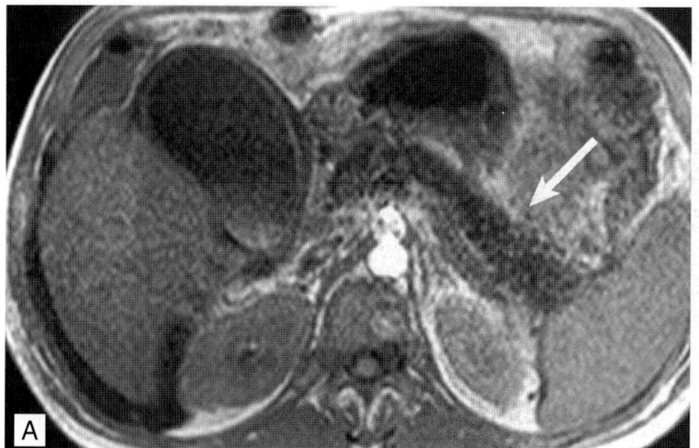

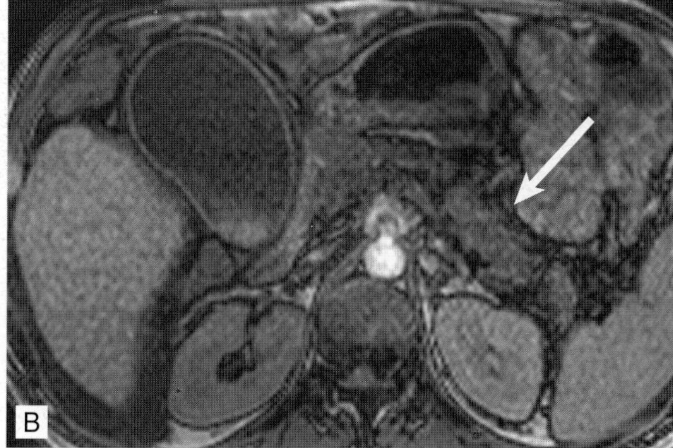

Figure 36.17 Primary hemochromatosis. Axial T1-weighted in-phase (A), and out-of-phase (B) MR images of the pancreas demonstrate diffuse signal loss of the pancreas on in-phase images (*arrows*) compared with out-of-phase images consistent with iron deposition in this patient with primary hemochromatosis. Note that the spleen is normal without any iron deposition, which is typically seen in secondary hemochromatosis.

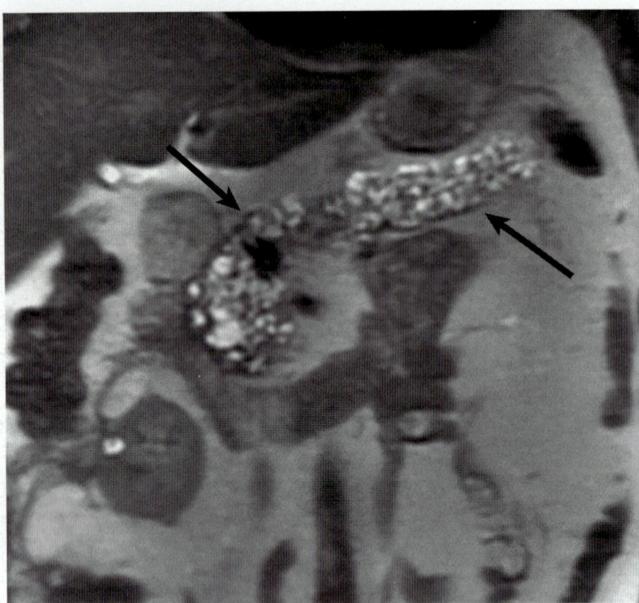

Figure 36.18 Pancreatic involvement in von Hippel–Lindau (VHL) disease. Coronal T2-weighted MR image shows multiple pancreatic cysts (*arrows*) consistent with VHL.

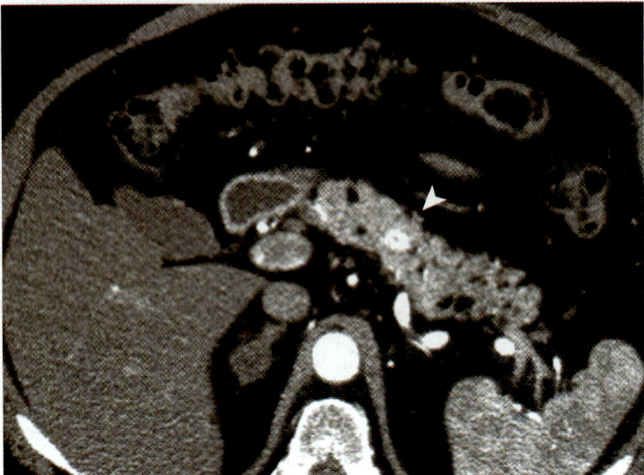

Figure 36.19 Pancreatic involvement in multiple endocrine neoplasia 1 (MEN1) syndrome. Axial contrast-enhanced CT image of the pancreas shows a focal enhancing mass in the body of the pancreas (*arrowhead*). This was proved to be a neuroendocrine tumor (gastrinoma) on pathology.

Pancreatic neuroendocrine tumors (PanNETs) are the most common pancreatic manifestation of multiple endocrine neoplasia 1 (MEN 1) syndrome; gastrinomas and nonfunctional tumors are commonly seen. PanNETs appear as single or multiple enhancing masses on imaging; somatostatin receptor scintigraphy using gallium-68 DOTATATE scan is very useful (Fig. 36.19).

Acute Pancreatitis (AP)

Pathophysiology and Clinical Presentation

AP is an acute inflammatory condition of the pancreas which ranges in severity from a mild self-limiting episode to a severe life-threatening condition. The diagnosis of AP as defined by the revised Atlanta classification requires at least two of the following three criteria:

- acute abdominal pain characteristic of pancreatitis,
- elevated amylase and lipase levels (>3 times the upper limit of normal), and
- characteristic findings on diagnostic imaging [8].

Elevated serum amylase and lipase levels are 95% specific for the diagnosis of AP. Imaging is only required to establish the diagnosis if the first two criteria are not met and simultaneously to exclude alternative etiologies. Imaging plays a major role in the detecting late complications, helps guide treatment decisions, and elucidates the underlying cause. The two morphologic subtypes of AP include interstitial edematous pancreatitis (~80–90%); and necrotizing pancreatitis that is characterized by pancreatic and/or peripancreatic necrosis [8].

The most common etiologies of AP are gallstones and alcohol consumption (~80%); other causes include hypertriglyceridemia, hypercalcemia, post-ERCP, trauma, infection, toxins, medication, tumors, congenital anomalies (pancreas divisum), and idiopathic causes [9]. The underlying pathophysiology mechanisms consist of premature activation of pancreatic enzymes with associated inflammation and autodigestion of pancreatic tissue, disruption of small pancreatic ducts, and leakage of enzymes. The unencapsulated pancreas facilitates the spread of inflammation and enzyme-induced autodigestion in multiple anatomical compartments [10–12].

Imaging Classification of Acute Pancreatitis

AP is divided into interstitial edematous and necrotizing morphologic subtypes based on imaging [8,13].

- In interstitial edematous pancreatitis, the pancreas is swollen, but the pancreatic microcirculation is intact with resultant homogenous contrast enhancement. Mild peripancreatic fat stranding and fluid are often seen.
- Necrotizing pancreatitis is characterized by disruption of the microcirculation leading to nonenhancement of the necrotic pancreatic parenchyma. Pancreatic and peripancreatic inflammatory and necrotic changes are dependent on the severity of the episode; the imaging appearance is thus time-dependent. The degree of gland necrosis is predictive of the development of organ failure, superimposed infection, morbidity, and mortality.

Early CT within the first few days may fail to show morphological changes of necrosis and underestimate the severity of AP. Early heterogeneous pancreatic enhancement from edema may be difficult to distinguish from pancreatic necrosis, leading to the recommendation that CT should ideally be performed at least 72 hours after onset of pain [8].

In an attempt to eliminate ambiguity and improve communication between providers, the *revised Atlanta classification* was published to introduce a standard lexicon and terminology for AP imaging findings [8,12,14] (Table 36.1).

Based on the absence or presence of necrosis, acute collections in the first 4 weeks are called acute fluid collections or acute necrotic collections, respectively. The natural course of acute fluid collections varies; they can either be resorbed or persist/enlarge to become encapsulated typically over 4 weeks when fluid collections are referred to as pseudocysts, and necrotic collections are named as walled-off necrosis.

All collections can be sterile or become infected, with the gas formation being the best imaging clue to suggest infection. Infected pancreatic necrosis is a severe condition that results

TABLE 36.1 Revised Atlanta Classification of Morphologic Subtypes of Acute Pancreatitis

Morphologic Subtypes	Distribution	Collection Within the First 4 Weeks	Collection After the Fourth Week
Interstitial edematous pancreatitis		Acute peripancreatic fluid collection (nonencapsulated) (sterile or infected)	Pseudocyst (encapsulated) (sterile or infected)
Necrotizing pancreatitis	Combined pancreatic and peripancreatic necrosis (75%) Peripancreatic necrosis only (20%) Pancreatic necrosis only (5%)	Acute necrotic collections (nonencapsulated) (sterile or infected)	Walled-off necrosis (encapsulated) (sterile or infected)

when infection spreads from the pancreas to the peripancreatic tissues, retroperitoneum, and peritoneum in patients with acute necrotizing pancreatitis. Mimickers of an abscess include fistulization to the gastrointestinal tract and introduction of gas from previous interventions. In the absence of gas, differentiation of infected from noninfected collections is only possible by sampling. The revised Atlanta classification also advocates that ambiguous terms such as pancreatic abscess, acute pseudocyst, and intrapancreatic pseudocyst should be avoided; other authors have advocated for the use of a structured reporting template [12].

Imaging of Acute Pancreatitis

Imaging is not required to make the diagnosis of AP. CECT is the first-line technique and considered the primary workhorse for comprehensive, initial assessment of AP [15].

Radiography

Radiographs play a limited role in the evaluation of AP. Abdominal radiographs may demonstrate a sentinel bowel loop due to localized small bowel ileus or the colon cut-off sign due to spasm of the left hemi-colon. Chest radiographs may demonstrate pleural effusions (typically on the left), elevation of the left hemidiaphragm, basal atelectasis, and in severe cases, noncardiogenic edema in the setting of acute respiratory distress syndrome.

Ultrasonography

Ultrasonography (USG) imaging of AP is of limited value. Imaging findings range from normal to focal or diffuse enlargement of the pancreas with hypoechoic changes because of edema or necrosis. USG allows for visualization of complications of AP such as peripancreatic fluid collections, ascites, and vascular thrombosis or pseudoaneurysm. However, the main role of USG is to evaluate for alternative etiologies of an acute abdomen in equivocal cases, and in the presence of AP, to identify gallstones as a possible etiology, and to evaluate for choledocholithiasis, which would prompt referral to ERCP. USG could be used to monitor peripancreatic fluid collections, differentiate fluid-filled collections, and could aid as guidance for diagnostic or therapeutic interventions [16].

Computed Tomography

Interstitial edematous pancreatitis may demonstrate mildly heterogeneous enhancement of the pancreas, which should not be mistaken for pancreatic necrosis [12] (Fig. 36.20). In more severe cases, pancreatic necrosis develops in the form of distinctly hypoenhancing areas, often with surrounding acute necrotic fluid collections (Fig. 36.21). The fluid typically tracks along fascial planes and accumulates in the anterior and posterior pararenal space and in the lesser sac. CECT is the technique of choice for the evaluation of AP and its complications, which includes superinfection of collections, vascular complications, fistula formation, disconnected or disrupted duct secondary to necrosis, and

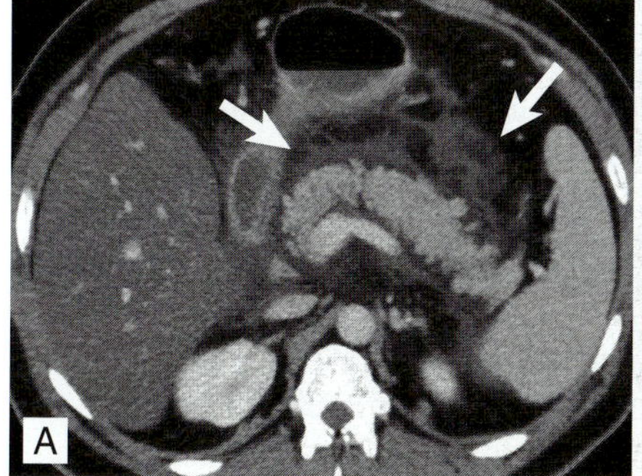

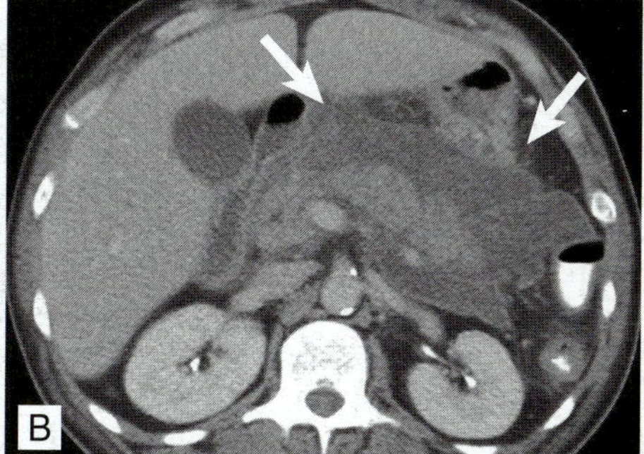

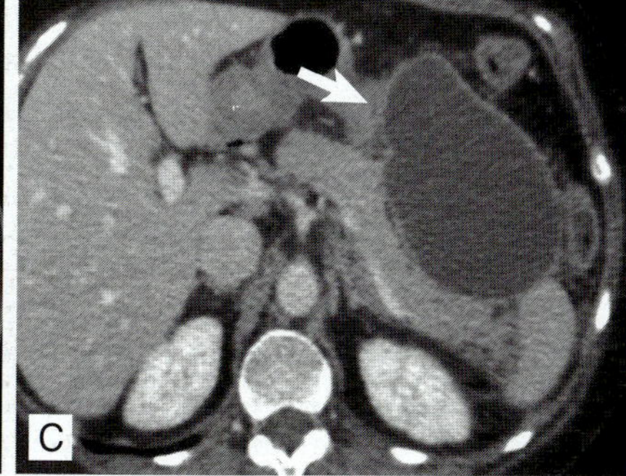

Figure 36.20 Acute interstitial edematous pancreatitis in three different patients. (A) Axial contrast-enhanced CT image of the pancreas shows mildly bulky pancreas with significant peripancreatic stranding (*arrows*). The pancreas is normally enhancing, and the splenic vein is patent. The modified CT severity index is 2, suggestive of mild pancreatitis. (B) Axial contrast-enhanced CT image 2 days after onset of symptoms demonstrates a heterogeneously enhancing pancreatic parenchyma with peripancreatic fluid collection (*arrows*). The modified CT severity index is 4 suggestive of moderate pancreatitis. The subsequent CT studies (not shown here) demonstrated normal enhancement of the pancreas with complete resolution of the peripancreatic fluid. These findings are consistent with acute peripancreatic fluid collection in a patient with interstitial edematous pancreatitis. (C) Axial contrast-enhanced CT image of the pancreas obtained 7 weeks after the symptom onset shows a well-defined peripancreatic fluid collection (*arrow*) consistent with a pseudocyst.

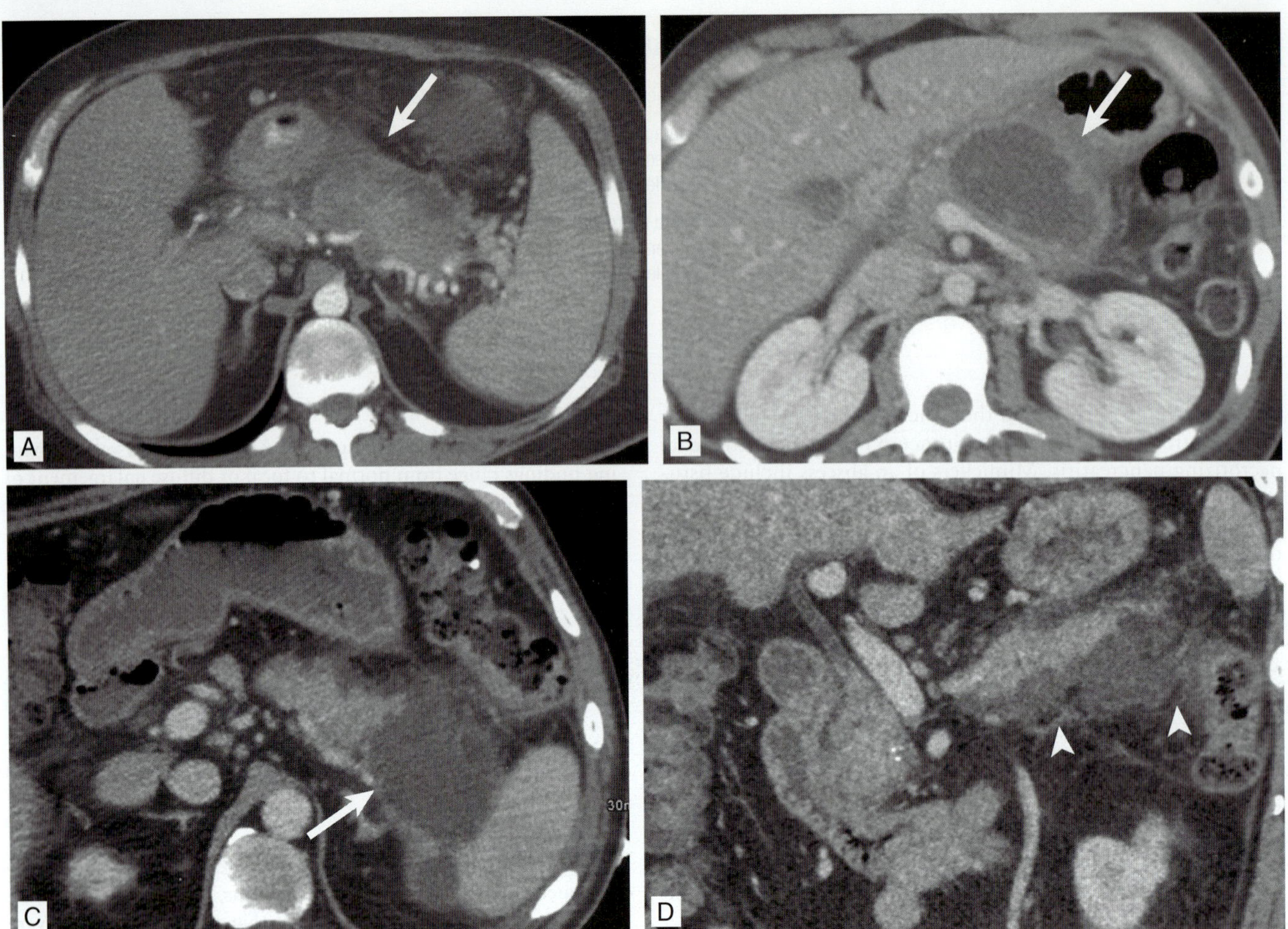

Figure 36.21 Necrotizing pancreatitis in four different patients. (A) Axial contrast-enhanced CT image 3 days after onset of symptoms demonstrates necrotizing pancreatitis with heterogenous appearance of the pancreas with predominant peripancreatic necrosis (*arrow*). (B) Axial contrast-enhanced CT image 10 days after onset of symptoms demonstrates a heterogeneously hypodense fluid collection in the body of the pancreas (*arrow*) in keeping with predominant pancreatic parenchymal necrosis resulting in an acute necrotic collection in the setting of necrotizing pancreatitis. (C and D) Necrotizing pancreatitis with combined pancreatic and peripancreatic necrosis. Axial (C) and coronal (D) CT images of the abdomen 20 days after onset of symptoms demonstrate combined pancreatic and peripancreatic necrosis with acute necrotic collections in the tail of the pancreas (*arrow*) and in the peripancreatic region (*arrowheads*). The modified CT severity index is 6 suggestive of moderate pancreatitis.

additional extrapancreatic complications such as splenic and renal infarcts (Figs. 36.22–36.27) (Table 36.2). Hemosuccus pancreaticus is defined as bleeding from the pancreatic duct into the gastrointestinal tract through the ampulla of Vater and is commonly caused by the rupture of the pseudoaneurysm of a peripancreatic vessel into pancreatic duct or pancreatic pseudocyst in the context of pancreatitis or pancreatic tumors.

CT is also useful in monitoring peripancreatic collection and can guide intervention. Limitations of CT include limited ability to characterize internal content of peripancreatic collections, the ability to detect gallstones, and ionizing radiation. In an attempt to limit radiation exposure, CT should only be repeated in case a patient demonstrates pyrexia which may indicate superinfection of collections or bowel perforation, sudden clinical deterioration (in the setting of circulatory shock for example which may indicate hemorrhage), and when intervention is planned [17].

The CT severity index (CTSI) was developed to assess the severity of AP and is based on findings from a CECT by evaluating the Balthazar score (grading of pancreatitis) and the extent of pancreatic necrosis [18]. This has been updated to the modified CT severity index (MCTSI) in 2004 to include pancreatic and peripancreatic inflammation, pancreatic necrosis as well as extrapancreatic complications, which includes one or more of the following: pleural effusion, ascites, vascular complications, and/or gastrointestinal involvement [19]. These indices are used to grade AP into mild, moderate, and severe forms and have been shown to correlate well with patients' clinical outcomes and can assist the clinician by providing valuable prognostic information (Table 36.3).

Modified CTSI 0-2: Mild pancreatitis.
Modified CTSI 4-6: Moderate pancreatitis.
Modified CTSI 8-10: Severe pancreatitis.

Magnetic Resonance Imaging

MRI can also be utilized to evaluate for the presence of pancreatic inflammation and/or necrosis, disease severity, the extent of retroperitoneal involvement as well as the underlying cause. MRI can detect more subtle cases of interstitial edematous pancreatitis as well as better characterize hemorrhage and necrosis due to its multiparametric nature compared with CT. Pancreatic edema and hemorrhage are best depicted on unenhanced T1-W images

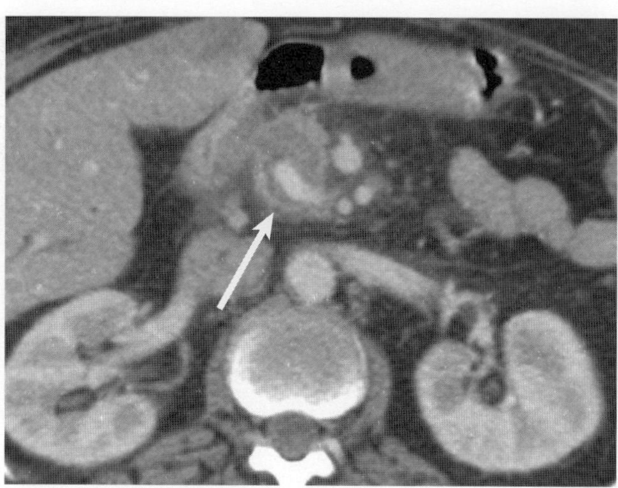

Figure 36.22 Pseudoaneurysm as a complication of necrotizing pancreatitis. Axial contrast-enhanced CT image of the pancreas shows an acute necrotic collection in the pancreatic uncinate process with a pseudoaneurysm arising from the gastroduodenal artery (*arrow*).

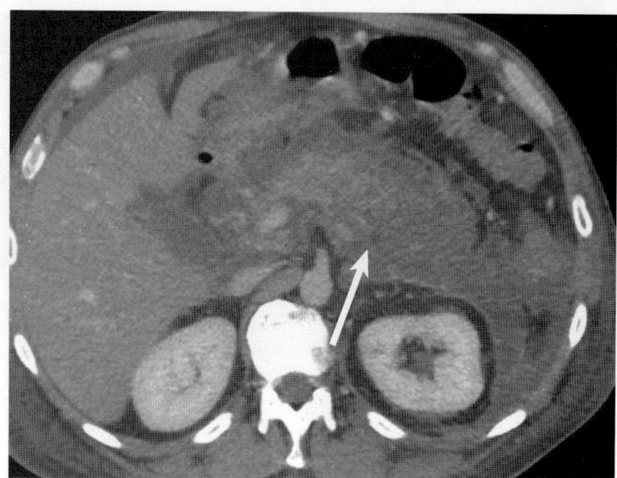

Figure 36.23 Splenic vein thrombosis as a complication of necrotizing pancreatitis. Axial contrast-enhanced CT image of the pancreas shows thrombosis of the splenic vein (*arrow*) secondary to extensive necrotizing pancreatitis and peripancreatic necrosis.

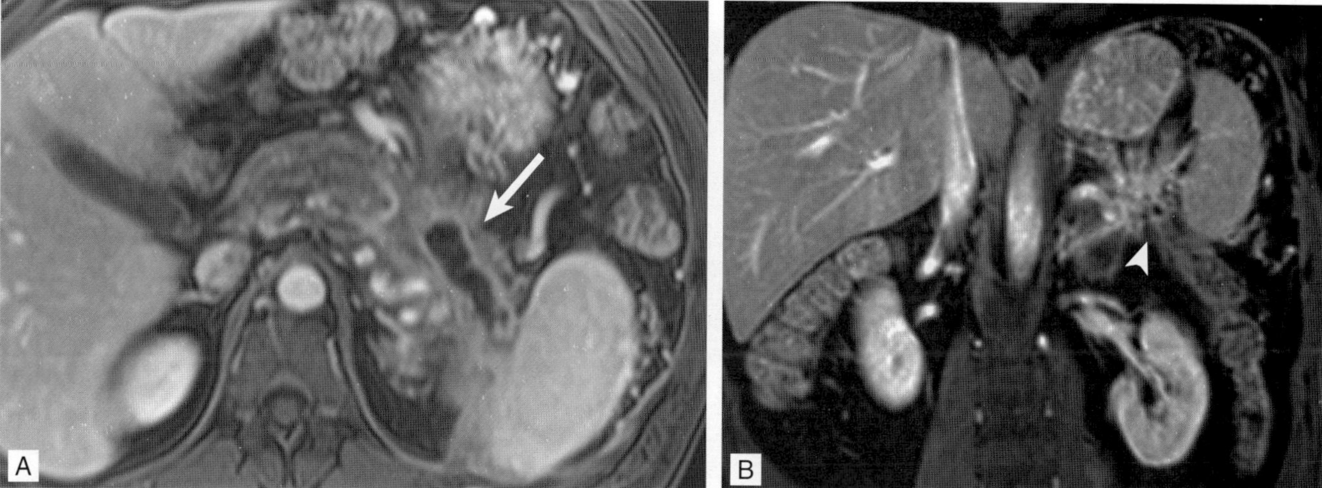

Figure 36.24 Colonic fistula as a complication of acute necrotizing pancreatitis (A and B). Axial (A) and coronal (B) contrast-enhanced MR images of the abdomen demonstrate necrotizing pancreatitis with walled-off necrosis in the tail (*arrow*) and fistulous communication with splenic flexure of the colon (*arrowhead*).

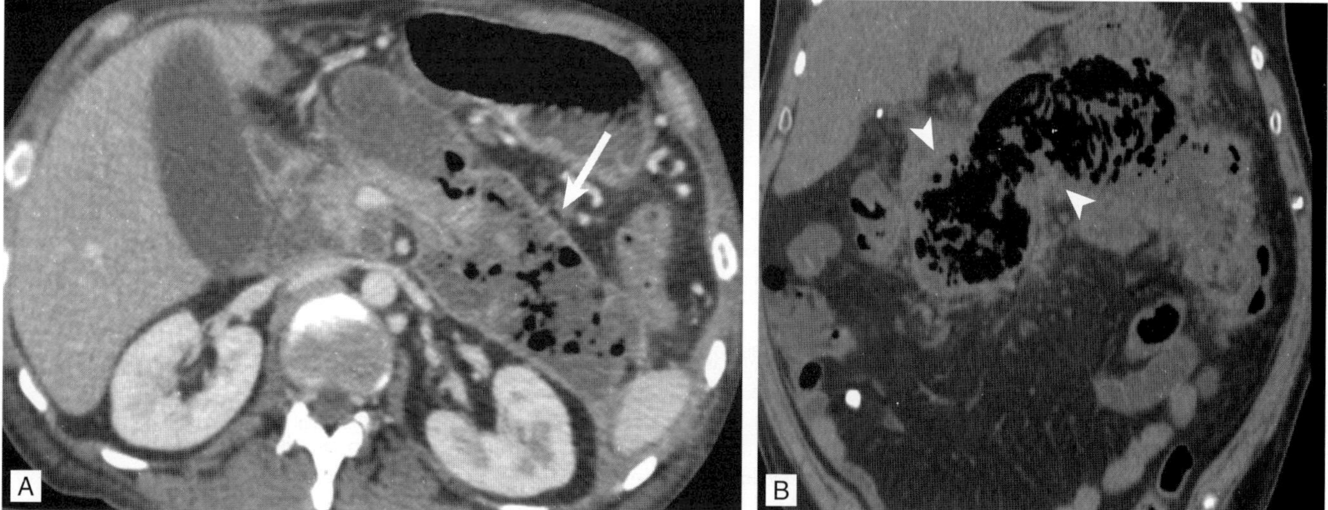

Figure 36.25 Infected pancreatic necrosis and emphysematous pancreatitis in two different patients. (A) Axial contrast-enhanced CT image of the abdomen shows significant pancreatic and peripancreatic necrosis with multiple air locules (*arrow*). Note that there is no fistulous communication with the bowel loops, which is the other possible differential for the presence of air. These findings are consistent with infected pancreatic/peripancreatic necrosis. (B) Coronal unenhanced CT image of the abdomen shows significant amount of air replacing the pancreatic parenchyma (*arrowheads*) consistent with emphysematous pancreatitis.

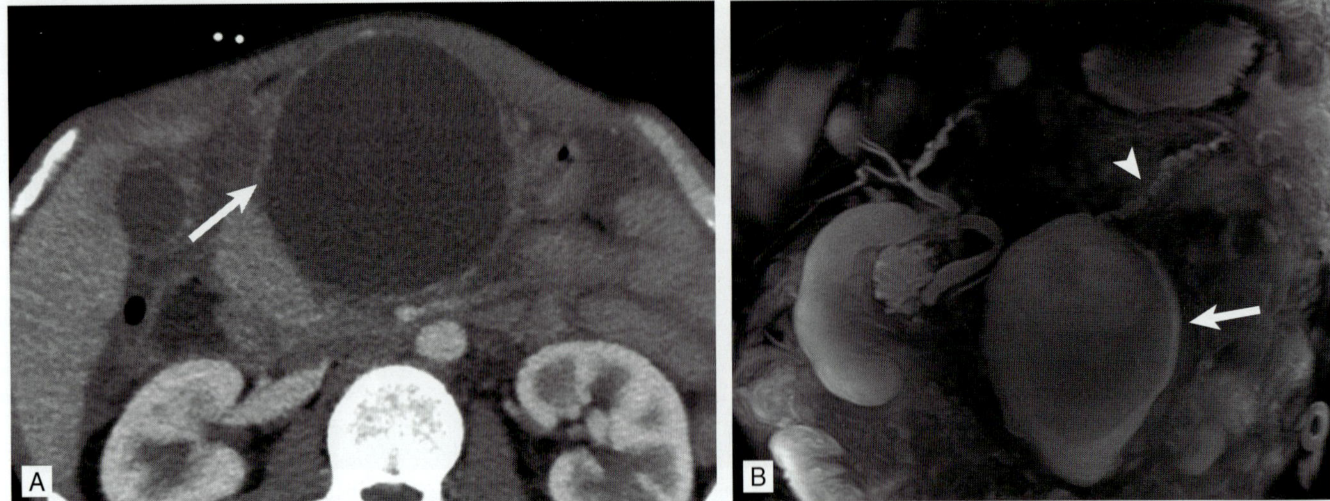

Figure 36.26 Pancreatic duct disruption in patient with acute necrotizing pancreatitis. (A) Axial contrast-enhanced CT image of the abdomen shows a large cystic lesion (*arrow*) in the body of the pancreas. (B) Coronal 3D MRCP images depict a large cystic lesion in the body of the pancreas (*arrow*) with associated dilated main pancreatic duct in the tail and body of the pancreas (*arrowhead*). These findings are consistent with duct disruption due to necrotizing pancreatitis.

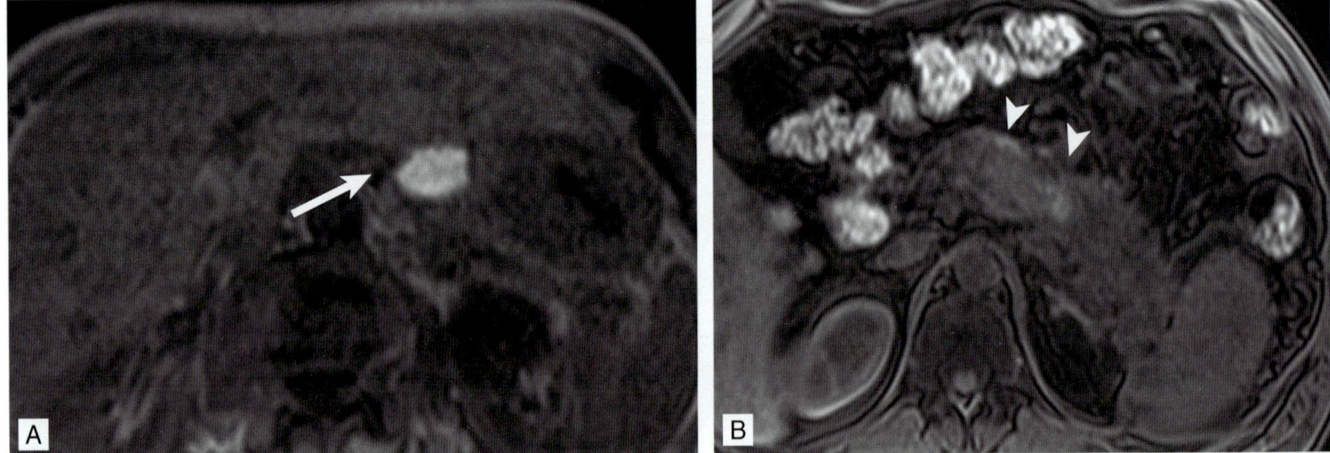

Figure 36.27 Hemorrhagic pancreatic pseudocyst and hemorrhagic pancreatitis in two different patients. (A) Axial T1-weight MR image of the pancreas shows a T1 hyperintense cystic lesion in the pancreatic body (*arrow*) suggestive of hemorrhagic pancreatic pseudocyst. (B) Axial T1-weight MR image of the pancreas shows diffusely T1 hypointense pancreas with heterogenous T1 hyperintense areas (*arrowheads*) suggestive of hemorrhagic acute pancreatitis.

TABLE 36.2 Complications of Acute Pancreatitis

- Superinfection of collections (typically in the setting of necrotic collections)
- Vascular complications
  - Hemorrhage
  - Pseudoaneurysm
  - Hemosuccus pancreaticus (wirsungorrhagia)
  - Splenic vein thrombosis and secondary perigastric varices
- Disconnected/disrupted duct secondary to necrosis
- Fistula formation
- Extrapancreatic infarcts and ischemia (spleen, kidneys, and bowel loops)

(Fig. 36.27) [20]. T2-W images are superior to CT in evaluating the internal content of peripancreatic fluid collections by demonstrating necrotic debris, which would typically necessitate necrosectomy at the time of the drainage procedure, possibly justifying an ancillary role for MRI to CT when intervention is

TABLE 36.3 Modified CT Severity Index

Prognostic Indicator		Points
Pancreatic inflammation	Normal pancreas	0
	Intrinsic pancreatic abnormalities with or without inflammatory changes in peripancreatic fat	2
	Pancreatic or peripancreatic fluid collection or peripancreatic fat necrosis	4
Pancreatic necrosis	None	0
	Equal to less than 30%	2
	More than 30%	4
Extrapancreas complications	One or more of the following: pleural effusion, ascites, vascular complications, and/or gastrointestinal involvement	2

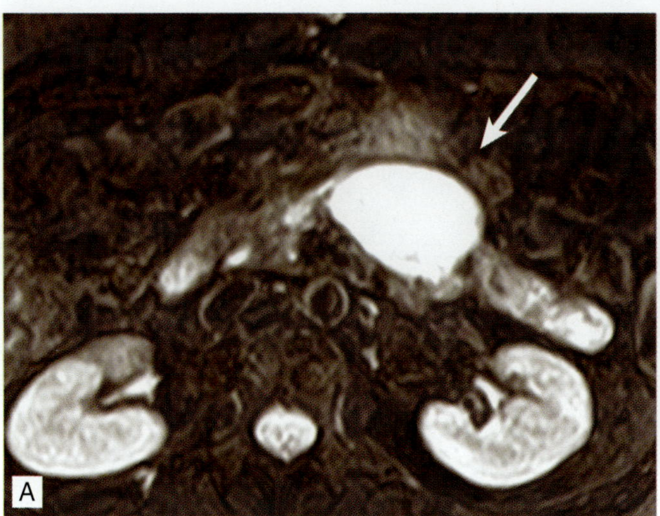

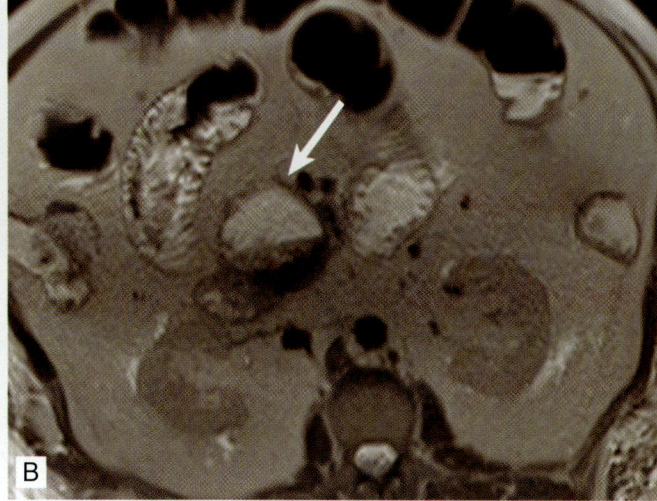

Figure 36.28 Role of MRI in differentiating pseudocyst from walled-off necrosis. (A) Pseudocyst: axial T2-weighted image of the pancreas shows a well-defined, uniformly T2 hyperintense cystic lesion in the peripancreatic region (*arrow*) without any identifiable T2 hypointensity. (B) Walled-off necrosis: axial T2-weighted MR image demonstrates T2 hypointense necrotic debris (*arrow*) with greater conspicuity in a postpancreatitis collection. The presence of necrotic debris may influence treatment decision-making (endoscopic cystogastrostomy with or without necrosectomy).

contemplated (Fig. 36.28). Hemorrhage indicates a worse prognosis and is best depicted as a high signal on T1 images (Fig. 36.27). Both MRI and CT are helpful in characterizing different fluid collections in AP. Both acute peripancreatic fluid collection and pseudocyst develop in peripancreatic region and contain homogenous fluid density, the former has no fully definable wall, and the latter contains a well-defined wall. In a similar fashion, acute necrotic collection, and walled-off necrosis both have heterogenous internal contents with hemorrhagic/necrotic debris; however, the former has no fully definable wall, and the latter has well-defined wall (Figs. 36.20, 36.21, 36.27, and 36.28). On MRCP, ductal disruption should be suspected when there is a discontinuity of the duct in an area of ≥2 cm pancreatic necrosis and viable upstream pancreatic tissue (Fig. 36.26) [21]. This can be confirmed with the extravasation of contrast on ERCP. MRI is particularly useful in pregnant and young patients as well as patients requiring multiple imaging studies. ACR appropriateness criteria discuss the role and timing of different imaging techniques in the evaluation of AP [22]. Although USG is usually appropriate as the initial examination in suspected AP with elevated lipase/amylase early on (less than 48–72 hours of symptom onset), CECT abdomen and pelvis or MRI abdomen with MRCP are useful in patients with equivocal symptoms/laboratory findings, more than 72 hours of symptoms onset and critically illpatients [22]. In addition, CECT/MRI is helpful for follow-up, assessing complications, and treatment response [22].

Prognosis and Management of Acute Pancreatitis

Predicting the severity of AP is critical for patient management. The two principal forms differ greatly in terms of mortality, being less than 1% in patients with interstitial edematous pancreatitis and range from 15% to 30% in patients with necrotizing pancreatitis, emphasizing the importance of early clinical identification of these subgroups to start an aggressive therapeutic approach to prevent mortality [23]. The therapy of interstitial edematous pancreatitis is mainly supportive with fluid resuscitation to maintain vital functions often being successful. The management of severe necrotizing pancreatitis is more complex requiring a multidisciplinary approach [23]. Prophylactic antibiotics are not indicated unless there are signs of infection. During the late phase, starting around days 7–10, patients with clinical suspicion of superinfection of peripancreatic collection should undergo percutaneous sampling to evaluate for infection [23]. Patients with infected necrosis require treatment with the appropriate antibiotics and debridement of infected necrosis. The timing of debridement is dependent on the clinical condition of the patient. There is a trend to delay debridement until it has been walled-off with debridement options including percutaneous and endoscopic techniques, minimally invasive and laparoscopic surgical techniques, and sometimes even traditional surgery to deal with the complications of the disease process. Lastly, it is recommended that patients with gallstones found on imaging undergo cholecystectomy before discharge [23].

Chronic Pancreatitis (CP)

Pathophysiology and clinical presentation. CP is a progressive and prolonged inflammatory disease characterized by irreversible parenchymal fibrosis and atrophy, leading to endocrine and exocrine pancreatic dysfunction. The most common cause of CP is a long history of moderate to heavy alcohol consumption [9]. Additional causes include malnutrition, hyperparathyroidism, hyperlipidemia, trauma, cystic fibrosis, autoimmune diseases, smoking, pancreas divisum, and recurrent AP. In approximately a third of cases, no cause is identified, and CP is considered idiopathic [24]. The chronically inflamed pancreas becomes fibrotic and demonstrates loss of acinar tissue, which manifests over time in the form of morphologic changes such as ductal dilation, ductal irregularity, parenchymal atrophy, and intraductal stones and calcifications [25]. Clinical manifestations include chronic abdominal pain, weight loss, malabsorption (exocrine dysfunction), and type 3c diabetes mellitus (endocrine dysfunction). Tropical pancreatitis is a type of CP that usually occurs in young individuals in tropical countries and involves the main pancreatic duct resulting in multiple large ductal calculi. Although etiology is not well understood, environmental factors, and *SPINK1* gene mutation [26]. Steatorrhea, abdominal pain, and diabetes are commonly seen, and malignant transformation is more frequent than in CP.

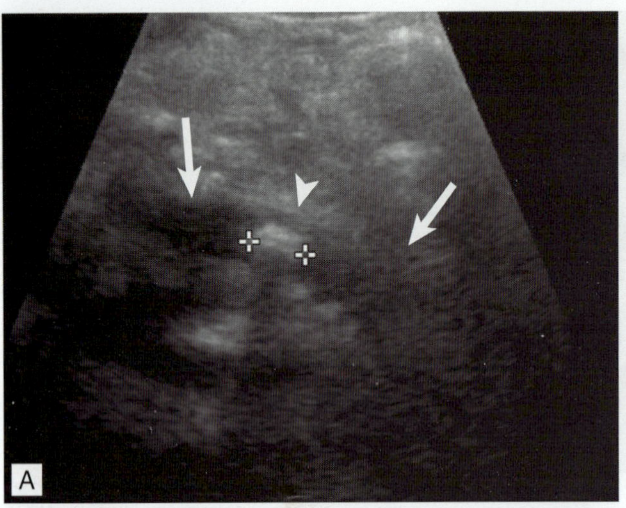

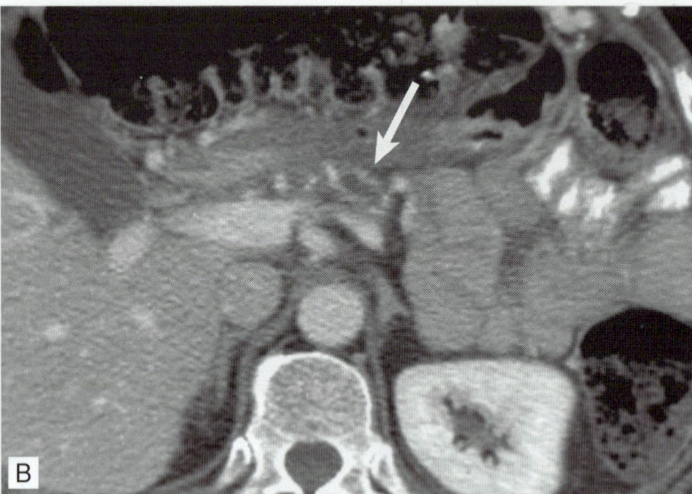

Figure 36.29 USG appearance of chronic pancreatitis. (A) Transabdominal grayscale USG image of the abdomen shows atrophic pancreatitis with dilated main pancreatic duct (*arrows*) and a large intraductal stone (*arrowhead*). (B) Corresponding axial CT image shows severely atrophic pancreas with dilated main pancreatic duct (*arrow*). These findings are consistent with chronic pancreatitis. *USG*, ultrasonography.

Imaging Features

Radiography. Abdominal radiographs may reveal pancreatic calcifications projecting over the mid-abdomen at the L1-L2 level in the expected location of the pancreas (Fig. 36.2).

Ultrasonography. USG may demonstrate parenchymal atrophy, hyperechoic changes indicating fibrosis, pancreatic calcifications, pancreatic ductal irregularity, and dilation (Fig. 36.29). Sequelae of CP such as pseudocysts, pseudoaneurysms, thrombosis as well as ascites may be seen with ultrasound.

Computed Tomography

Although CT is limited in the early diagnosis of CP, it is useful to diagnose advanced disease and its complications.

- CT findings of CP include changes in size, shape, contour, dilatation, and irregularity of the main pancreatic duct, pancreatic calcifications, and pseudocysts (Fig. 36.30) [27].
- Pancreatic calcifications develop due to calcium carbonate deposition in inspissated intraductal protein plugs predominantly located in peripheral side branches [28,29].

Tumefactive CP (mass-forming CP) is reported in up to 30% of patients with CP and is most common in the head of the pancreas [30]. Features that favor an inflammatory process over cancer are evidence of CP (pancreatic calcifications and pseudocysts), lack of displacement of calcifications, and the absence of abrupt duct cutoff discussed under MRCP later [29]. As the incidence of pancreatic cancer is higher in CP, the differentiation between cancer and CP is even more difficult. FDG PET/CT may be helpful in select patients to identify pancreatic cancer in the background of CP [31].

Magnetic Resonance Imaging

MRI exceeds other imaging techniques in its sensitivity of the diagnosis of early CP while accomplishing morphologic (parenchymal and ductal) and functional imaging [32]. Loss of acinar cells, which precede ductal changes in CP, is best seen as decreased T1 signal on T1-W fat-saturated precontrast images. Recently T1 mapping has been introduced as a quantitative technique for the evaluation of suspected mild CP, and it may be a more reliable method compared with conventional T1WI. Other advanced MRI techniques such as MR extracellular volume fraction calculation and MR elastography have also shown promising results in the early detection of CP.

- MRCP allows for a detailed evaluation of the ductal manifestations of CP, including duct ectasia of side branches, main duct dilatation, strictures, and irregularities (chain-of-lake appearance), intraductal stones, and intraparenchymal cyst formation, which could be graded using the Cambridge classification (Figs. 36.31 and 36.32). This classification is used clinically in some institutions and is based on abnormal side branches and main pancreatic duct and has five grades. Note that dilated main pancreatic duct indicates moderate to severe CP [29].
- The Consortium for the Study of CP, diabetes, and pancreatic cancer published a consensus document with new cross-sectional imaging feature definitions and standardized reporting recommendations for CP in an attempt to standardize the approach to diagnosis and disease severity assessment, which could also assist in longitudinal assessment in clinical trials [29,33].
- The important imaging findings to comment in CP patients include parenchymal thickening/contours, parenchymal calcifications, main pancreatic duct caliber/contour/strictures and intraductal calculi, side ductal morphology and dilatation, T1 signal intensity ratio, parenchymal enhancement ratio, and secretin enhanced MRCP observations [29].

Ductal changes could be augmented by hormonal stimulation of the pancreas by intravenous secretin administration [34]. Secretin stimulates the secretion of bicarbonate-rich fluid into the pancreatic ductal system and induces spasm of the sphincter of Oddi. Secretin simulation allows for the assessment of the exocrine function of the pancreas by evaluating duodenal filling by quantitative and semiquantitative methods (Fig. 36.33). Improved duct visualization with MRCP has led to the description of additional imaging features to assist in the previous conundrum of differentiating mass-forming CP from pancreatic cancer.

- In addition to CT imaging features discussed earlier, the described MRCP features favoring mass-forming CP include the "duct penetrating sign" (referring to an unobstructed pancreatic duct penetrating a mass-like lesion; however, the

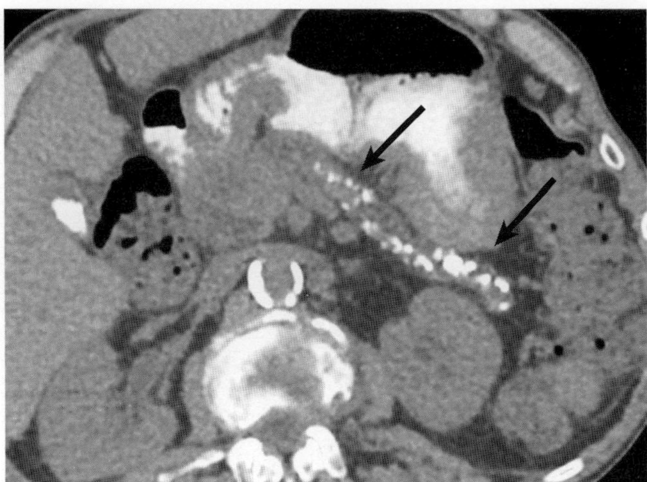

Figure 36.30 Chronic pancreatitis. Axial unenhanced CT demonstrates extensive coarse pancreatic calcifications (*arrows*) in an atrophic pancreas, typical of chronic pancreatitis.

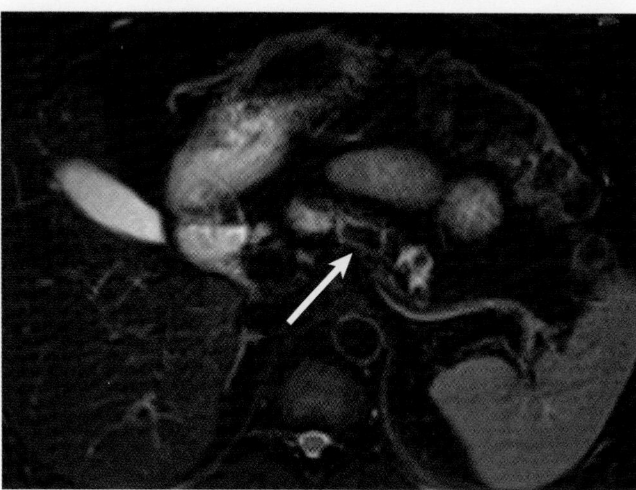

Figure 36.32 Chronic pancreatitis with intraductal calculi. Axial T2-weighted MR image of the pancreas demonstrates changes of chronic pancreatitis with multiple T2 hypointense intraductal calculi (*arrow*).

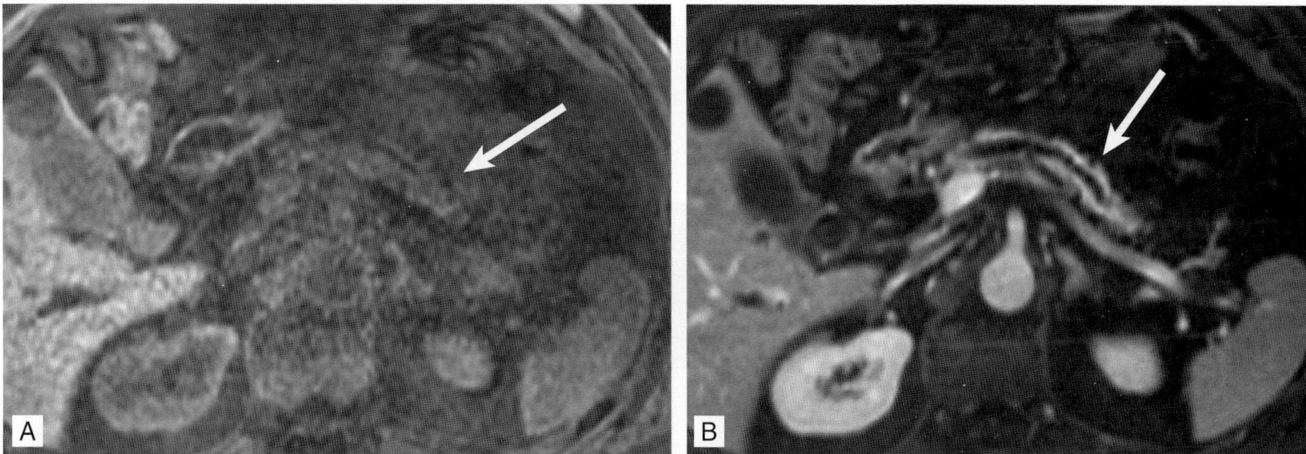

Figure 36.31 Chronic pancreatitis. (A) Axial T1-weighted fat-saturated MR image demonstrates decreased intrinsic T1 signal of the pancreas in keeping with chronic pancreatitis (*arrow*). (B) Axial T1-weighted postcontrast fat-saturated MR image during delayed phase demonstrates increased enhancement (*arrow*) secondary to underlying fibrosis.

duct often has mild smooth tapering) and the "attraction sign" (referring to the CBD being attracted or pulled into the inflammatory mass, if located in the pancreatic head). In contrast, the "corona sign" (referring to obstructed side branches being displaced by the pancreatic mass) and the well-known "double duct sign" (simultaneous dilation of the CBD and pancreatic duct) favor pancreatic cancer [35] (Fig. 36.34).

Variants of Chronic Pancreatitis

Autoimmune Pancreatitis

Pathophysiology and clinical presentation. Autoimmune pancreatitis (AIP) is characterized by chronic, relapsing, tumefactive, and steroid-responsive pancreatitis associated with immune dysregulation. AIP shows typical clinical, imaging, laboratory, and histopathology findings. Two subtypes have been described: type 1 AIP (lymphoplasmacytic sclerosing pancreatitis) and type 2 AIP (idiopathic duct-centric pancreatitis or granulocytic epithelial lesion- positive pancreatitis). These two subtypes are fundamentally two different diseases that display significant differences in demography, serology, multiorgan involvement, and disease relapse rates [36]. Type 1 AIP is a prototype IgG4-related disease with elevated serum/tissue IgG4 levels, whereas type 2 AIP lack definitive serologic markers. Patients typically present with obstructive jaundice. Diagnostic criteria were proposed by the International Association of Pancreatology in 2010, which includes five cardinal features of AIP: imaging of the pancreatic parenchyma, serology, other organ involvement, pancreatic histology, and an optional criterion of response to corticosteroid therapy [37].

Imaging of Autoimmune Pancreatitis

- On imaging, pancreatic involvement can be focal, multifocal, or diffuse (more common). A diffusely "swollen" pancreas resembling a "sausage" and associated peripancreatic fibroinflammatory "halo" are characteristic findings of AIP (Fig. 36.35).

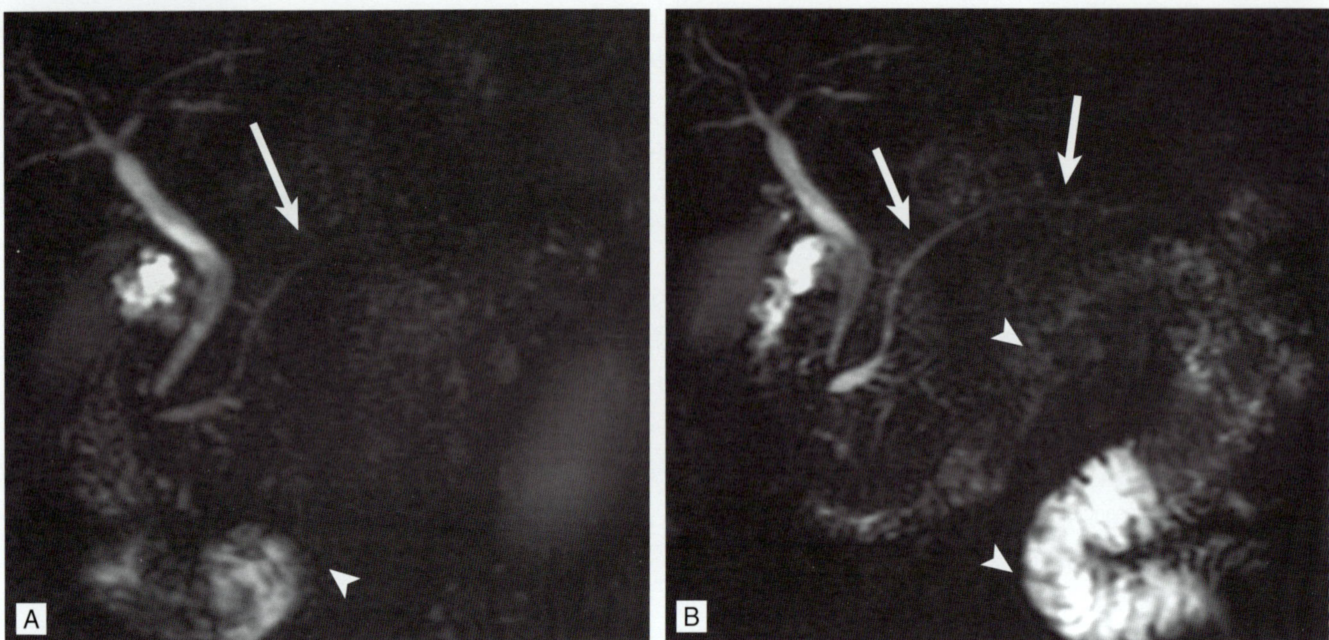

Figure 36.33 Role of secretin MRCP in the evaluation of chronic pancreatitis. (A) Presecretin MRCP image demonstrates mildly prominent main pancreatic duct with a few dilated side branches (*arrow*) which is equivocal for chronic pancreatitis. Also, note fluid is seen in the third part of the duodenum (*arrowhead*). (B) Delayed postsecretin MRCP 10 minutes after the secretin administration demonstrates the main pancreatic duct and the dilated side branches with more conspicuity (*white arrows*) and pancreatic secretions reach the fourth part of the duodenum and beyond (*arrowheads*) consistent with chronic pancreatitis with good pancreatic exocrine reserve.

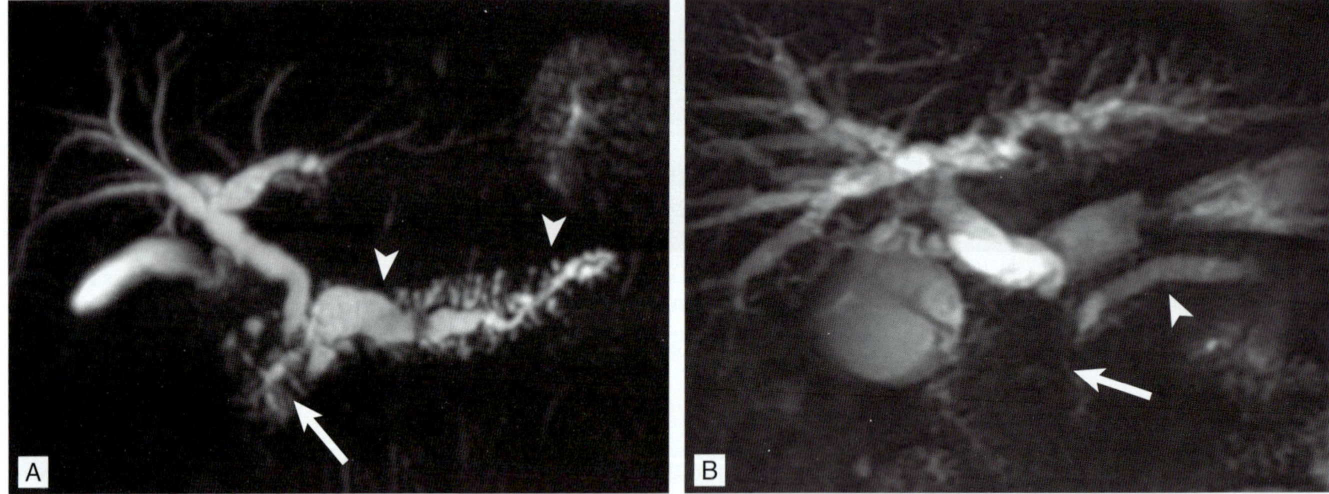

Figure 36.34 Role of MRI and MRCP in differentiating chronic pancreatitis from pancreatic ductal adenocarcinoma (*PDAC*). (A) MRCP image demonstrates the "duct penetrating sign," which refers to the pancreatic duct penetrating a mass-like lesion with smooth tapering (*white arrow*) with dilated main pancreatic duct with side branch ectasia (*arrowheads*) and the "attraction sign" which refers to the common bile duct being attracted or pulled into an inflammatory mass in the pancreatic head. These findings favor chronic pancreatitis. (B) MRCP image demonstrates the "double duct sign," which refers to simultaneous dilation of the main pancreatic duct (*arrowhead*) and common bile duct due to a mass in the head of the pancreas (*arrow*). Other MRCP sign that favors malignancy is the "corona sign," which refers to obstructed pancreatic side branches being displaced by the pancreatic mass (image not shown).

- AIP demonstrates progressive and delayed enhancement on CT and MRI as well as restricted diffusion on diffusion-weighted images [38].
- The focal form of AIP most commonly occurs in the head of the pancreas and may be difficult to distinguish from pancreatic cancer.
- Imaging features favoring AIP over cancer include the "duct penetrating sign," milder upstream main duct dilation, skipped duct strictures, delayed enhancement of pancreatic parenchyma, low ADC values on MRI, and presence of another organ involvement [38] (Fig. 36.36).

Paraduodenal Pancreatitis

Pathophysiology and clinical presentation. Previously known as groove pancreatitis and cystic dystrophy of the duodenal wall, paraduodenal pancreatitis is a distinct variant of CP that involves the groove

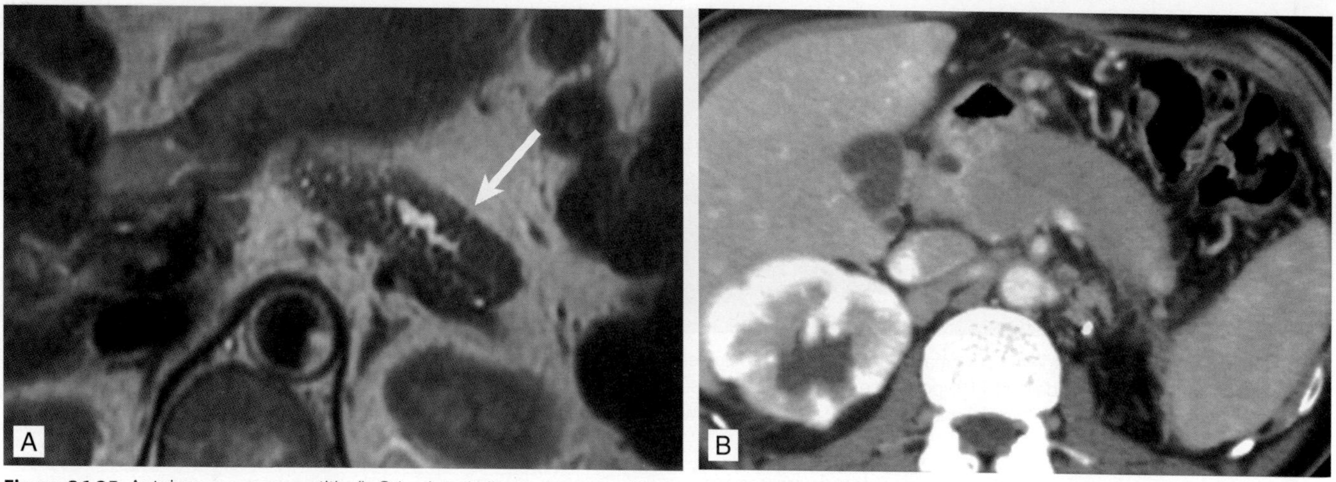

Figure 36.35 Autoimmune pancreatitis (IgG4-related disease) in two different patients. (A) Axial T2-weighted MR image demonstrates an edematous sausage-shaped pancreas with peripancreatic T2 hypointense rim and mildly dilated main pancreatic duct (*arrow*). These findings are diagnostic of autoimmune pancreatitis. (B) Axial contrast-enhanced CT image of the abdomen shows a diffusely hypodense, sausage-shaped edematous pancreas consistent with autoimmune pancreatitis.

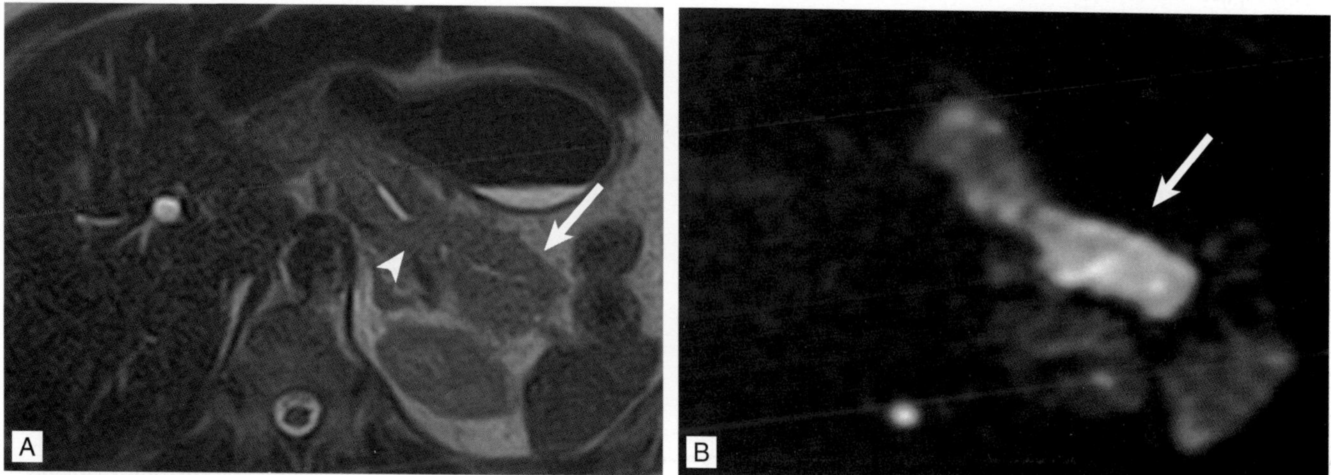

Figure 36.36 Autoimmune pancreatitis (IgG4-related disease). (A) Axial T2-weighted MR image demonstrates mildly hyperintense appearance of the pancreas (*arrow*) and a stricture (*arrowhead*) in the pancreatic duct. (B) There is marked restricted diffusion restriction, predominantly in the pancreatic tail region on DWI (*arrow*). These findings are diagnostic of autoimmune pancreatitis.

between the head of the pancreas, the duodenum, and the common bile duct [39,40]. Presumed increased viscosity of pancreatic secretions caused by excessive alcohol consumption leads to stone formation and duct obstruction. Two forms of paraduodenal pancreatitis have been described: a "pure form" that exclusively involves the groove and a "segmental form" which involves the groove with spillage into the adjacent pancreatic head.

Imaging of Paraduodenal Pancreatitis

- On CT/MRI, the most characteristic finding is a sheet-like, curvilinear soft-tissue mass centered in the pancreaticoduodenal groove, often with typical adjacent duodenal wall thickening and cystic change (Fig. 36.37) [39,40]. The soft tissue appears as a hypoenhancing mass on CT with occasional calcifications.
- On MRI, the soft tissue centered in the groove is typically hyperintense on T2-WI in the acute or subacute phase due to edema and may become more hypointense on T2-WI as fibrosis sets in. Thickening of the duodenal wall with the associated cystic change, when present, is well depicted on T2-WI (Fig. 36.38) [39,40].

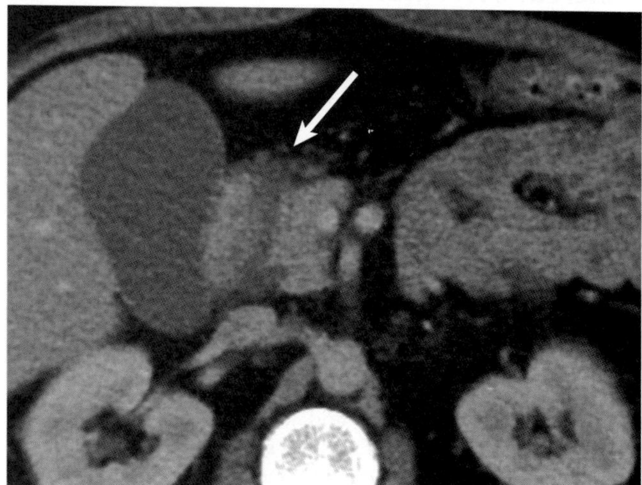

Figure 36.37 Paraduodenal ("Groove") pancreatitis. Axial contrast-enhanced CT image of the pancreas demonstrates sheet-like, curvilinear soft-tissue thickening in the pancreaticoduodenal groove (*white arrow*) consistent with paraduodenal or groove pancreatitis.

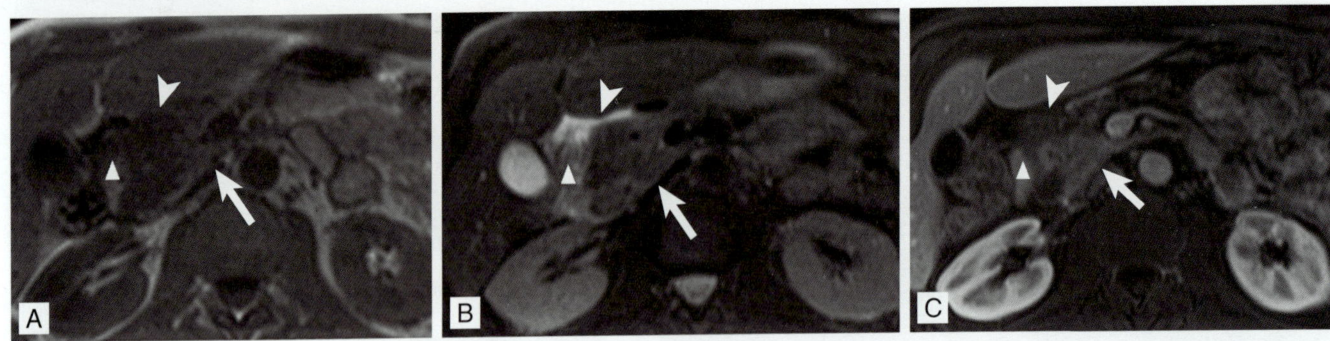

Figure 36.38 Paraduodenal ("Groove") pancreatitis. (A–C) Axial T1-weighted (A), T2-weighted (B), and contrast-enhanced T1-weighted (C) MR images of the pancreas demonstrate an ill-defined T1 hypointense and T2 hyperintense lesion with associated fat stranding in the pancreaticoduodenal groove (*arrowheads*) in between the duodenum (triangle) and head of the pancreas (*arrows*). These findings are consistent with paraduodenal or groove pancreatitis.

- On postcontrast imaging, the soft tissue demonstrates initial peripheral enhancement with gradual centripetal enhancement on more delayed imaging. There may be narrowing of the CBD and pancreatic duct with a widening of the space between the CBD and duodenal lumen best depicted on MRCP images. It is important to differentiate the segmental form of paraduodenal pancreatitis that involves the pancreatic head from pancreatic cancer, with abrupt CBD cutoff and vascular invasion favoring malignancy [39,40].

Hereditary Pancreatitis

HP refers to genetic disorders that are characterized by mutations involving *PRSS1* or *SPINK1* genes that predispose patients to early onset (before 20 years of age) and symptomatic pancreatitis [9]. *PRSS-1*-related disease typically presents with recurrent idiopathic AP in childhood with frequent progression to CP. The hallmark of the disease is large ductal calcifications with resultant ductal dilation seen in adolescent patients, often with a positive family history. There is an associated 50–70-fold increased risk of pancreatic adenocarcinoma; about 30–40% of patients with HP will develop cancer by the age of 70 years, particularly among smokers [9].

Pancreatic Neoplasms

Pancreatic neoplasms can be subclassified into solid and cystic pancreatic tumors. Solid tumors can be further categorized into exocrine tumors, endocrine tumors, mesenchymal, and miscellaneous tumors (Fig. 36.39).

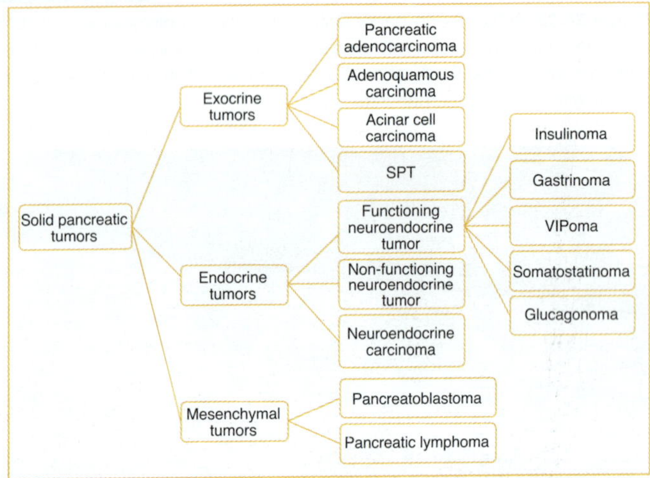

Figure 36.39 Classification of solid pancreatic neoplasms. *SPT*, solid pseudopapillary tumor.

Pancreatic Ductal Adenocarcinoma

Pathophysiology and clinical presentation. Pancreatic ductal adenocarcinoma (PDAC) is the most common type of pancreatic cancer, a highly lethal malignancy with a 5-year survival rate of 4% [41]. Risk factors include hereditary syndromes (HP, Peutz–Jeghers syndrome, Familial atypical mole and melanoma syndrome, Hereditary nonpolyposis colon cancer [Lynch syndrome], Hereditary breast and ovarian cancer syndromes, Ataxia-telangiectasia, Li–Fraumeni syndrome), smoking, CP, obesity, and long-standing diabetes mellitus. The high mortality rate of PDAC is attributed to the aggressive phenotype, combined with an indolent presentation. PDAC most commonly presents with nonspecific symptoms, including weight loss, abdominal pain, back pain, jaundice, and nausea; PDAC may also present with a new diagnosis or exacerbation of diabetes mellitus [42]. Over 90% of cases are diagnosed in stage III or stage IV with local invasion or distant metastases, limiting the treatment options [42].

The National Comprehensive Cancer Network (NCCN) classification into resectable, borderline resectable, and unresectable disease (Table 36.4) combined with the tumor/node/metastases staging system, determines the treatment options and prognosis. Surgical resection with negative margins is the only potentially curative treatment option [43]. The tumor marker CA19-9 (carbohydrate antigen 19.9) is frequently elevated in PDAC with a sensitivity of 80% and a specificity of 73%. The marker is used to assess treatment response in known cases and for surveillance, as opposed to as a screening tool.

Imaging Features

- Pancreatic protocol CT is the primary technique for diagnosis and staging of PDAC. PDAC commonly appears as an infiltrative hypoattenuating mass with associated ductal obstruction and frequent stenosis/thrombosis of adjacent veins (Fig. 36.40) [44]. Extrapancreatic spread around the neighboring veins and arteries determines the feasibility of satisfactory surgical resection.
- The remarkable proclivity of PDAC for perineural involvement and invasion of small veins are postulated to be a major determinant of advanced local disease, frequent liver

TABLE 36.4 National Comprehensive Cancer Network Criteria Defining Resectability Status of Pancreatic Adenocarcinoma [43]

	Arteries		Veins	Other
Resectable	No contact with the CA, SMA, or CHA		No contact with the SMV, PV, or venous abutment without contour irregularity	
Borderline resectable	Head or uncinate process	Abutment of the CHA without extension to the CA or HA. Abutment of SMA	SMV/PV encasement or contour deformity (e.g., tear drop) or tumor thrombus, allowing for safe resection and reconstruction. IVC abutment	
	Body or tail	Abutment of CA Encasement of CA without the involvement of aorta or GDA (permitting modified Appleby procedure)		
Unresectable/locally advanced	Encasement of SMA or CA Tumor contact with CA and aortic involvement		Tumor involvement or occlusion of SMV/PV that cannot be reconstructed	Distant metastases

CA, celiac axis; *CHA*, common hepatic artery; *GDA*, gastroduodenal artery. Abutment: tumor/vascular contact ≤180°, encasement: tumor/vascular contact >180° or vascular deformity; *PV*, portal vein; *SMA*, superior mesenteric artery; *SMV*, superior mesenteric vein.

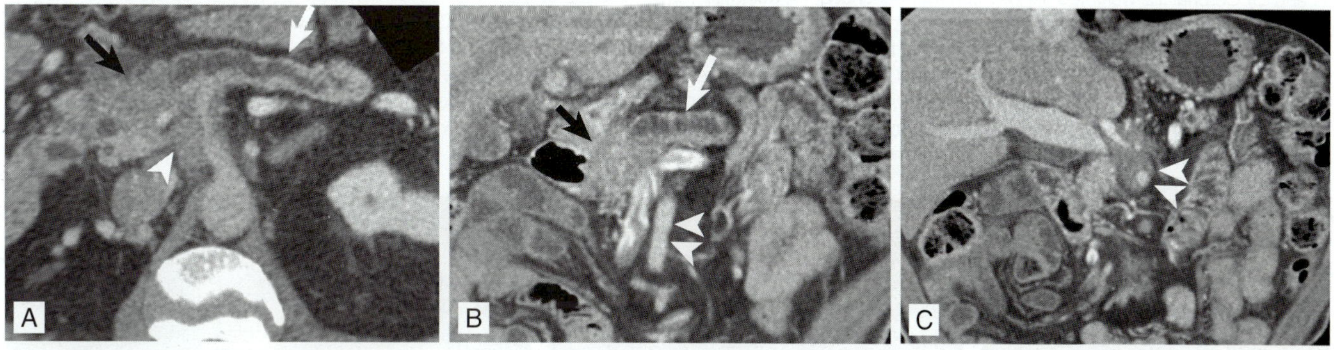

Figure 36.40 Role of CT in the evaluation of pancreatic ductal adenocarcinoma (*PDAC*). (A–C) Axial and coronal contrast-enhanced CT images of the pancreas demonstrate an ill-defined hypoenhancing mass in the pancreatic head (*black arrows*). There is upstream parenchymal atrophy, pancreatic duct dilatation (*white arrows*), and encasement of the celiac axis, and the superior mesenteric artery and vein (*arrowheads*). Note that the involvement of the vessels can be better assessed on coronal images. As per NCCN classification, the disease is unresectable given the encasement of SMA and celiac axis. *NCCN*, National Comprehensive Cancer Network; *SMA*, superior mesenteric artery.

metastases, and high rates of local disease recurrence. Delayed enhancement of the tumor is attributed to its characteristic dense desmoplastic stroma.

- However, CT is inferior to multiphasic MRI in the evaluation of tumors that are "isodense" to the parenchyma as well as small (<1.5 cm) tumors (Fig. 36.41). Although EUS assists in local staging and biopsy, PET/CT allows for staging of PDAC with a sensitivity and specificity that are superior to CECT (Fig. 36.42) [31].
- Given the infiltrative nature of the PDAC with associated desmoplastic reaction in the adjacent fat and fat stranding, it is difficult to differentiate between the real tumor and desmoplastic reaction on CT/MRI.
- Careful attention should be paid to the relation between the PDAC and the vessels to establish resectability. *As per the NCCN, there are three categories:* resectable, borderline resectable, and unresectable (Fig. 36.43) (Table 36.4). CT has a sensitivity of 70–96% and specificity of 82–100% in assessing vascular invasion in PDAC; as vascular involvement is major deciding factor in differentiating borderline resectable tumors from resectable tumors, CT plays a pivotal role in PDAC patients. Features that make a tumor unresectable include encasement of the SMA or celiac axis or common hepatic artery (defined as more than 180 degrees of tumor/vessel contact), unreconstructible venous involvement, or distant metastases [43].
- It is important to look at vessels in both coronal and axial planes to assess vascular encasement versus abutment because some tumors may appear as abutting on axial images, but actually demonstrate complete encasement on the coronal images (Fig. 36.44). Care should also be taken to identify variant arterial anatomy, which may have implications for surgical management.
- Multiplanar/multisequence MRI is recommended as an adjunct technique in the work-up of PDAC when CT findings are indeterminate or when contrast-enhanced CT is not possible. MRI is mainly useful in staging of PDACs with minimal or no visibility at CT and assessing liver

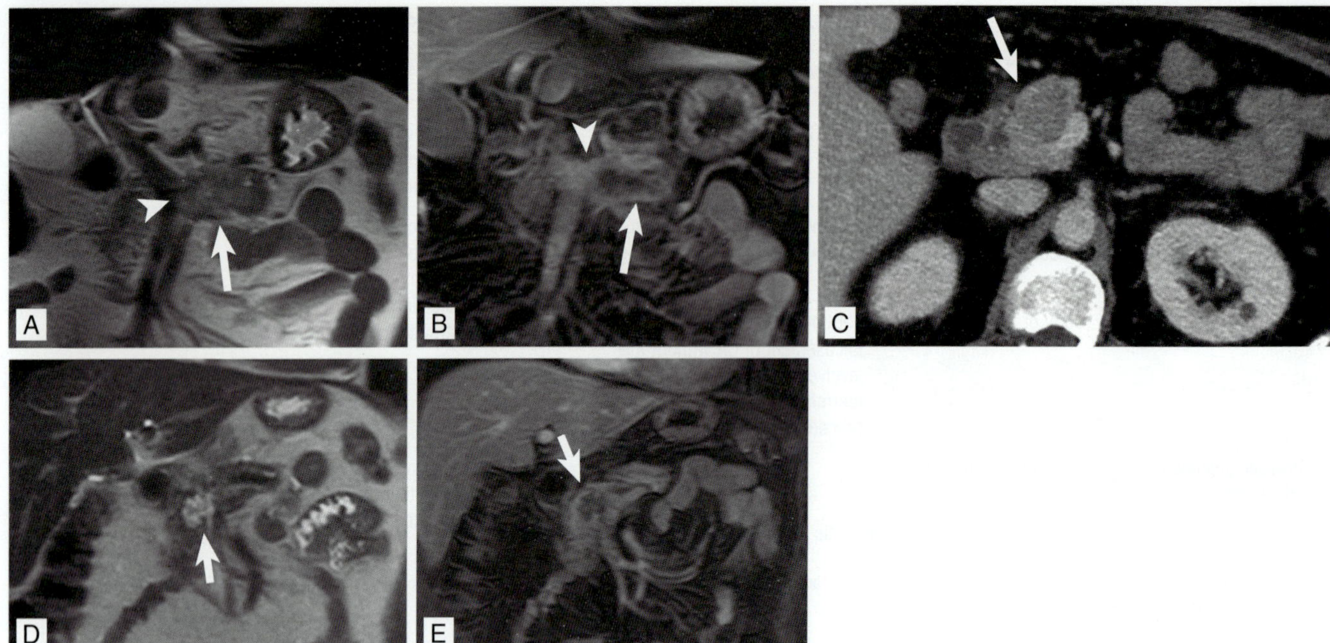

Figure 36.41 MR imaging appearance of pancreatic ductal adenocarcinoma (*PDAC*) and the role of MRI in the evaluation of small relatively isodense PDAC. (A and B) Coronal T2-weighted (A) and contrast-enhanced T1-weighted (B) MR images of the pancreas demonstrate a T2 intermediate signal intensity pancreatic mass, which is hypoenhancing on the postcontrast images (*arrows*). The mass is seen encasing the confluence of the SMV and splenic vein and SMA (*arrowhead*). As per NCCN classification, the disease is unresectable given the encasement of SMA. (C–E) A small iso- to mildly hypodense PDAC initially missed on CT. (C) Axial contrast-enhanced CT image of the pancreas shows a mildly hypodense pancreas mass (*arrow*), which was missed on this CT examination. (D and E) Coronal T2-weighted (D) and contrast-enhanced T1-weighted (E) MR images of the pancreas demonstrate a T2 mildly hyperintense pancreatic mass, which is hypoenhancing on the postcontrast images (*arrows*). This was proved to be a PDAC on pathology. *NCCN*, National Comprehensive Cancer Network; *SMA*, superior mesenteric artery.

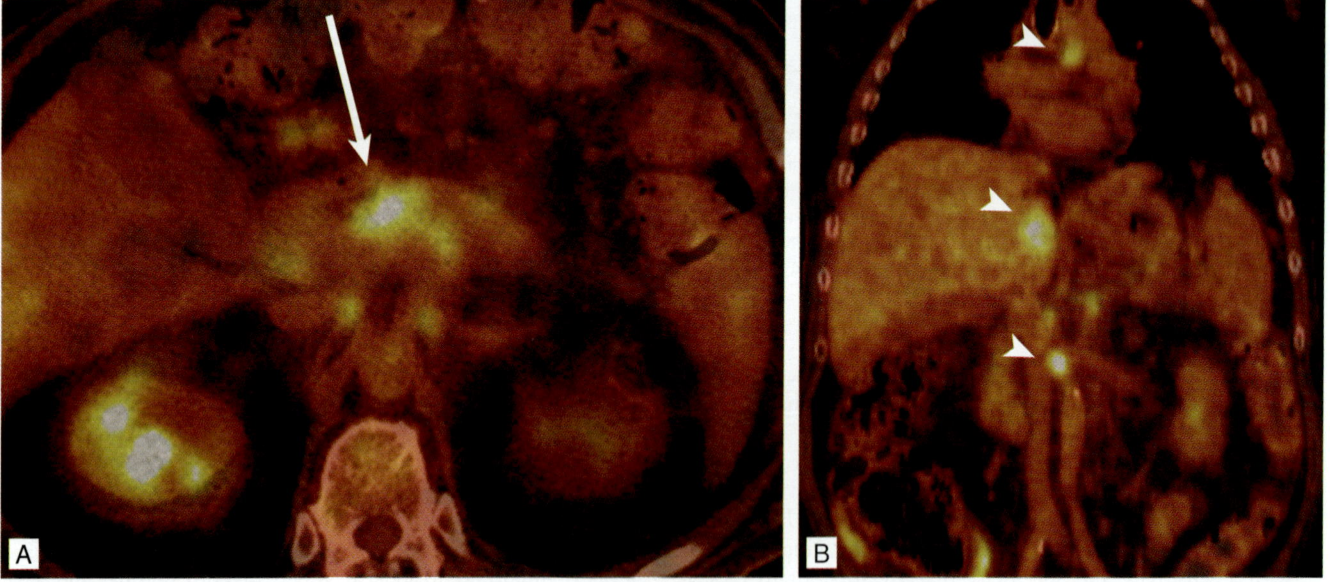

Figure 36.42 Role of FDG PET/CT in the evaluation pancreatic ductal adenocarcinoma (*PDAC*). (A and B) Axial (A) and coronal (B) FDG PET/CT images of the chest and abdomen demonstrate a hypermetabolic pancreatic mass (*arrow*) with hypermetabolic liver metastases, retroperitoneal, and mediastinal lymph adenopathy (*arrowheads*). *PET*, positron emission tomography.

metastases. MRI is also helpful in assessing response to neoadjuvant therapy as CT has a tendency to underestimate it. MRI and MRCP permits detection of subtle ductal changes and small tumors while facilitating local staging (Fig. 36.45).

- PET/CT is normally not indicated in the initial assessment of PDAC and is helpful in assessing distant metastatic disease, especially in bones.

Pancreatic Adenocarcinoma—Diagnostic Pearls

- Double duct sign is a clue to a pancreatic head/ampullary mass
- Cutoff of the pancreatic duct, absence of the duct penetrating sign, suggests a tumor over a focal region of pancreatic inflammation
- Multiphase imaging is important; tumors may be isoenhancing on the portal venous phase, but are often hypoenhancing on the pancreatic phase
- Establish tumor/vessel relation to determine resectability

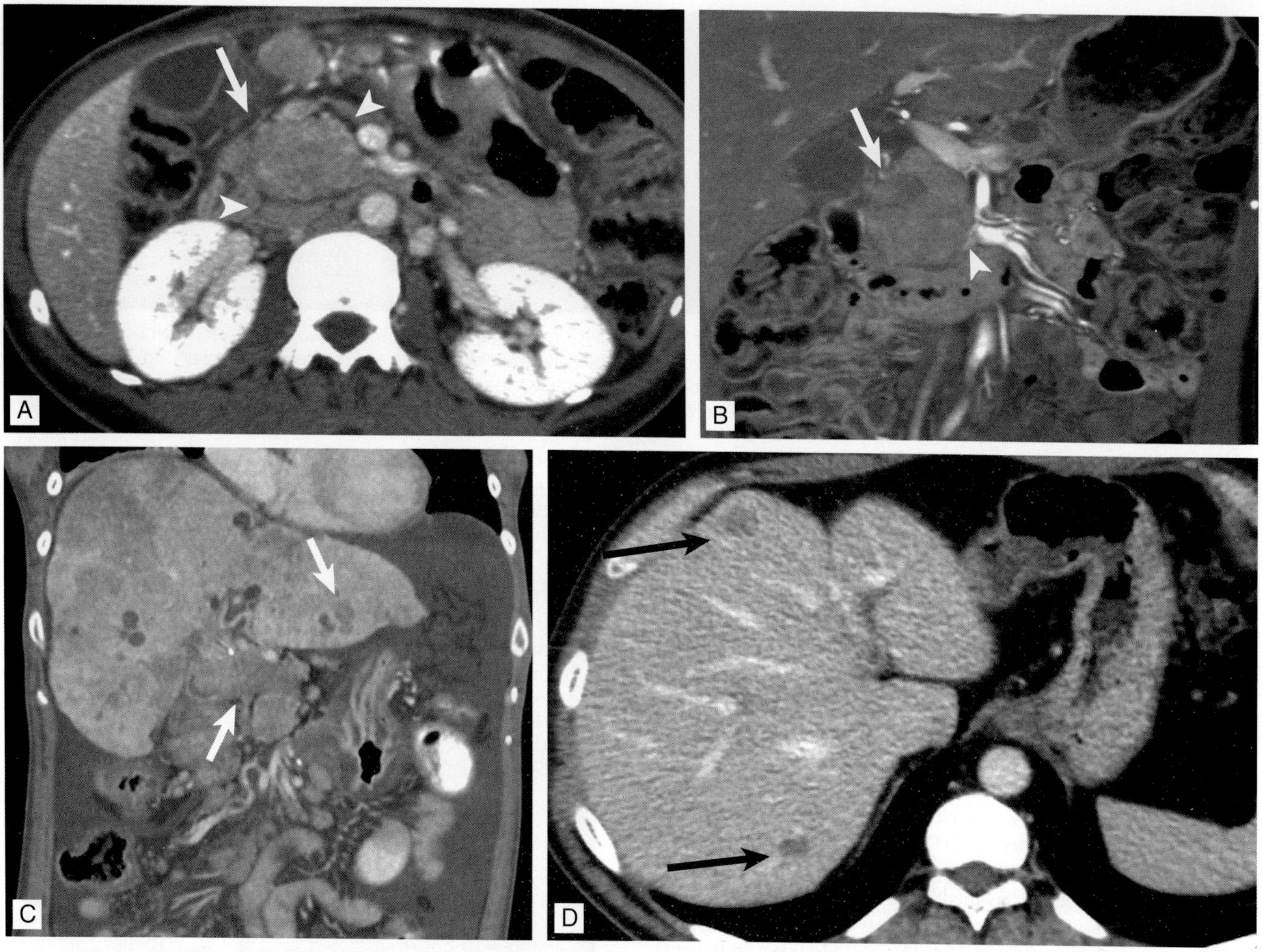

Figure 36.43 (A–C) Borderline resectable pancreatic ductal adenocarcinoma (*PDAC*) with recurrent/metastatic disease 2 years after surgical resection. Axial (A) and coronal (B) contrast-enhanced CT images of the pancreas show a PDAC in the head/uncinate process of the pancreas (*arrows*) abutting the SMV and compressing on the IVC (*arrowheads*). This mass is borderline resectable as per NCCN classification. (C) Coronal contrast-enhanced CT image of the abdomen 2 years after Whipppleʼs surgery demonstrates recurrent mass in the surgical bed and multiple liver metastases (*arrows*). (D) Pancreatic ductal adenocarcinoma (PDAC) with liver metastases. Axial contrast-enhanced CT image of the abdomen demonstrates multiple hypodense liver metastases in this patient with PDAC (images not shown). The presence of metastases in PDAC patients, commonly liver, indicates unresectable disease. *NCCN*, National Comprehensive Cancer Network.

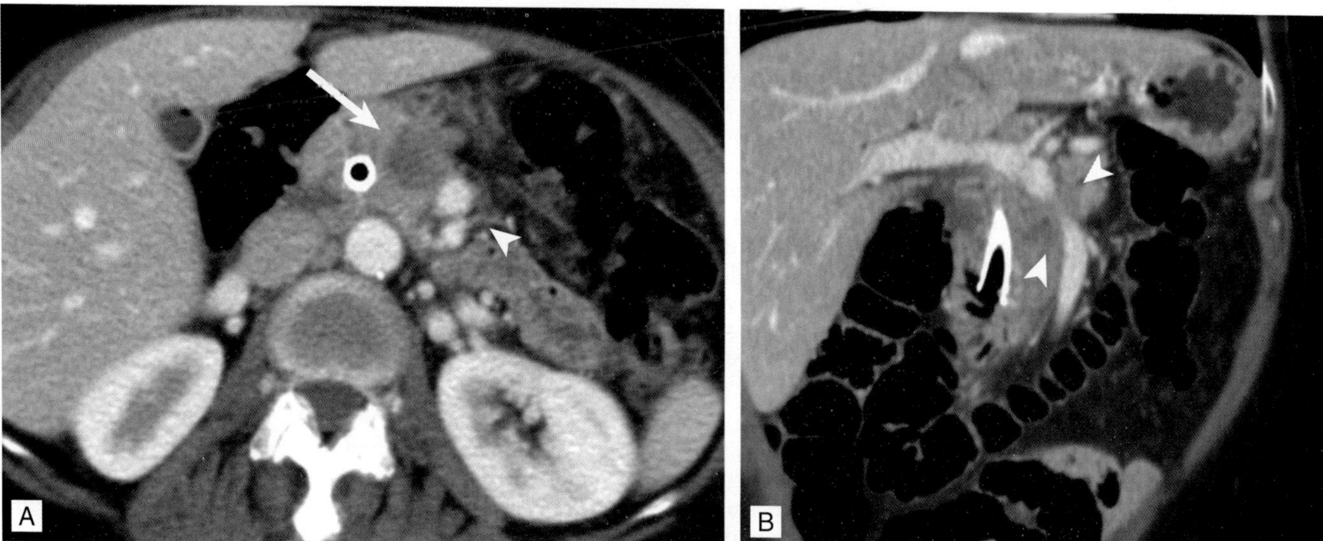

Figure 36.44 Importance of coronal CT/MR images in the assessment of vascular involvement in pancreatic ductal adenocarcinoma (*PDAC*). (A) Axial contrast-enhanced CT image of the pancreas shows a PDAC in the uncinate process of the pancreas (*arrow*) abutting the SMV that appears less than 180-degree involvement (*arrowhead*). (B) Coronal contrast-enhanced CT image of the pancreas shows near-complete encasement of the SMV (*arrowheads*). It is important to use coronal images in the assessment of vascular involvement.

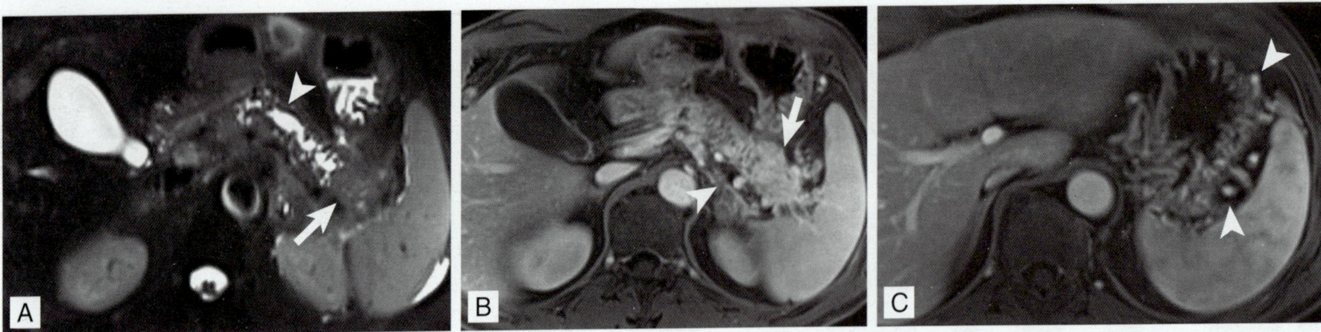

Figure 36.45 MR imaging appearance of pancreatic ductal adenocarcinoma (*PDAC*) involving the tail with associated splenic vein thrombosis. (A–C) Axial T2-weighted (A) and contrast-enhanced T1-weighted (B and C) MR images of the pancreas demonstrate a heterogeneously enhancing, T2 intermediate signal intensity pancreatic tail mass (*arrows*) with associated splenic vein thrombosis (*white arrowhead* in B) resulting in multiple perigastric collaterals (*arrowheads* in C). Also, note changes of chronic pancreatitis in the visualized pancreas with irregular main pancreatic duct dilatation (*arrowhead* in A).

Pancreatic Neuroendocrine Tumor

Pathophysiology and clinical presentation. Pancreatic neuroendocrine tumors (PanNETs) account for 1–2% of pancreatic neoplasms [45]. Historically referred to as "islet cell tumors," the term is no longer used, as PanNETs arise from pancreatic ductal pluripotent stem cells as opposed to islets of Langerhans [45,46]. They can manifest at any age but most often occur in the fourth–sixth decade of life [45]. Although most PanNETs are sporadic, approximately 10% are associated with hereditary syndromes, including multiple endocrine neoplasia type 1 (MEN1), VHL syndrome, neurofibromatosis type 1, and tuberous sclerosis. Patients with hereditary syndromes are more likely to have multiple PanNETs, and they tend to manifest at an earlier age [45,46]. Approximately half of the PanNETs are functioning, and half are nonfunctioning [45]. Functioning tumors can be subclassified based on the hormones that are produced. Insulinoma, the most common type of functioning PanNETs, accounts for 35–40% of cases [45,46]. However, in patients with MEN1, more than 50% of tumors are gastrinomas, while insulinomas account for one-third of tumors [46]. Most of the gastrinomas (90%) develop in "gastrinoma triangle," which is formed by joining the three points: (1) Medially: junction of the neck and the body of the pancreas. (2) Superiorly: confluence of common bile duct and cystic ducts. (3) Inferiorly: junction of second and third portions of the duodenum. Pathologically, on the basis of proliferative activity (Ki-67 index and mitotic index), PanNETs are classified into three grades (grades 1, 2, and 3), which demonstrate increasing aggressiveness. PanNECs (pancreatic neuroendocrine carcinomas) are always grade 3 and carry a worse prognosis.

In general, nonfunctioning PanNETs are larger on diagnosis than functioning PanNETs. Because insulinomas are present earlier, they are typically small and localized to the pancreas at diagnosis. They have the best prognosis of all PanNETs, with an overall long-term survival rate similar to the general population [45]. Noninsulinoma PanNETs recur or metastasize in 50–80% of patients. The 3-year survival rate for patients with PanNETs without hepatic metastases is 82% and is 56% for patients with hepatic metastases [45,46].

Imaging Features

- PanNETs are solid, circumscribed masses. Although smaller tumors are homogenous, larger tumors are more likely to demonstrate cystic change, necrosis, and calcifications (Fig. 36.46). PanNETs classically show hyperenhancement on arterial and portal venous phases. Even necrotic and cystic PanNETs will typically maintain a hypervascular rim, which can help distinguish them from other cystic pancreatic neoplasms [45].
- Metastases to lymph nodes and the liver also tend to be hypervascular and are often best appreciated in the arterial phase (Fig. 36.47). Typically, there is no associated pancreatic duct dilatation [47], although it may be seen secondary to mass effect from large tumors [46,48].
- On MRI, PanNETs are hypointense on T1-WI and hyperintense on T2-W sequences. Certain tumors with increased collagen content may be intermediate or hypointense on T2-W sequences (Fig. 36.48) [45,46]. In a patient with a specific clinical syndrome associated with functioning PanNETs, nuclear medicine studies may be helpful in localizing the tumor and evaluate for metastatic disease.
- Poorly differentiated and nonfunctioning neuroendocrine tumors may demonstrate uptake on 18-fluorodeoxyglucose (FDG) PET. Functioning PanNETs usually do not demonstrate increased activity on FDG PET [45]. However, Gallium gallium-68-DOTATATE/PET labeled with octreotide has a high affinity for somatostatin receptors and is useful in the work-up of functioning PanNETs.

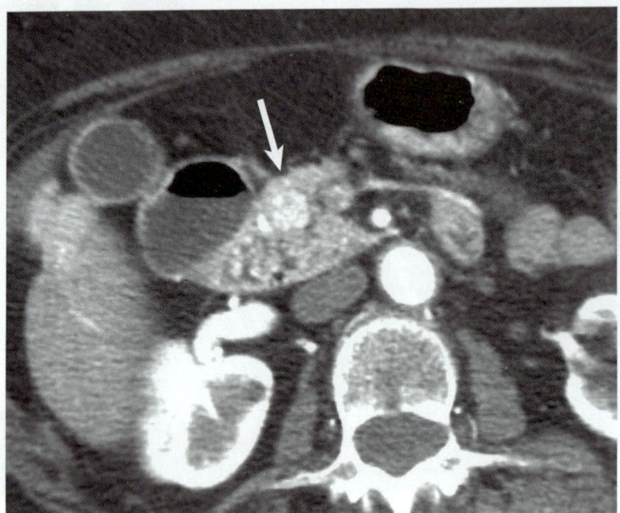

Figure 36.46 Well-differentiated pancreatic neuroendocrine tumor (panNET). Axial contrast-enhanced CT image of the pancreas demonstrates an arterially enhancing focal lesion in the uncinate process of the pancreas (*arrow*).

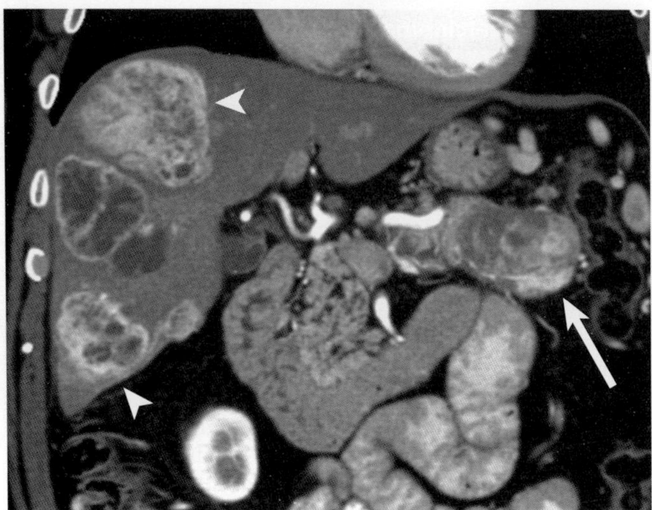

Figure 36.47 A moderately differentiated pancreatic neuroendocrine tumor (panNET) with liver metastases. Coronal contrast-enhanced CT image of the upper abdomen demonstrates tumor thrombus in the splenic vein (*arrow*) with multiple enhancing liver metastases (*arrowheads*).

- Although well-differentiated PanNETs are avid on DOTATATE scan and low on FDG PET, poorly differentiated PanNETs and all PanNECs show the opposite imaging phenotype. This is known as "flip-flop" phenomenon. Note that this pattern may not be seen in all tumors as some well-differentiated tumors, especially insulinomas, may not express somatostatin receptors and all aggressive tumors may not use glucose for their metabolism. Gallium scans may also be of value for the detection of small metastases in the liver, lymph nodes, and bones [45,46].

Pancreatic Neuroendocrine Carcinoma

Pancreatic neuroendocrine carcinomas (panNECs) are poorly differentiated neuroendocrine neoplasms. They account for 2–3% of all pancreatic neuroendocrine neoplasms. Most patients manifest nonspecific symptoms [45]. Unlike PanNETs, panNECs commonly demonstrate mutations in TP53 and RB1 genes. As most cases are locally advanced at the time of diagnosis, the first-line treatment is chemotherapy and radiation. Prognosis is poor, and most cases are fatal within 1 year of diagnosis [45,46].

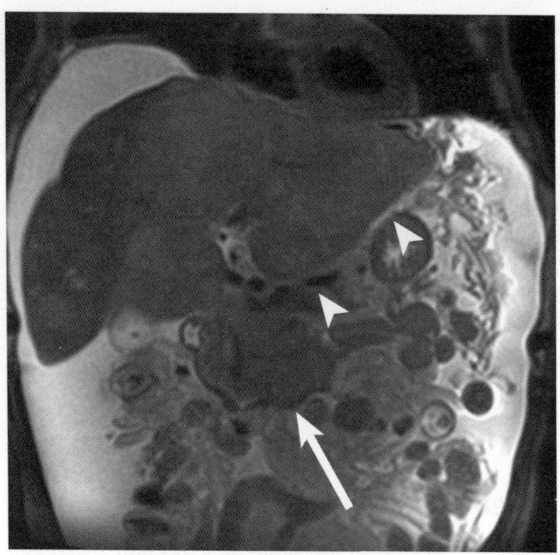

Figure 36.49 MR imaging appearance of a pancreatic neuroendocrine carcinoma (panNEC). Coronal T2-weighted MR image of the abdomen demonstrates an ill-defined pancreas mass (*arrow*) with extensive hepatic metastatic disease (*arrowheads*). This mass was proved to be a poorly differentiated panNEC on pathology.

Imaging Features

- PanNECs are typically large at presentation (mean diameter 5.8 cm) and demonstrate heterogeneous enhancement (Fig. 36.49) [45,46]. Most cases are locally invasive at presentation, with obstruction of the common bile duct and invasion of the duodenum. On MRI, panNEC is hypointense on T1-W sequences and mildly hyperintense on T2-W sequences (Fig. 36.49) [46].
- Unlike with PanNETs, gallium-68-DOTATATE/PET is not commonly used, as poorly differentiated panNEC tumors lack sufficient somatostatin receptors. 18-FDG PET plays an important role in local and distant staging [46].

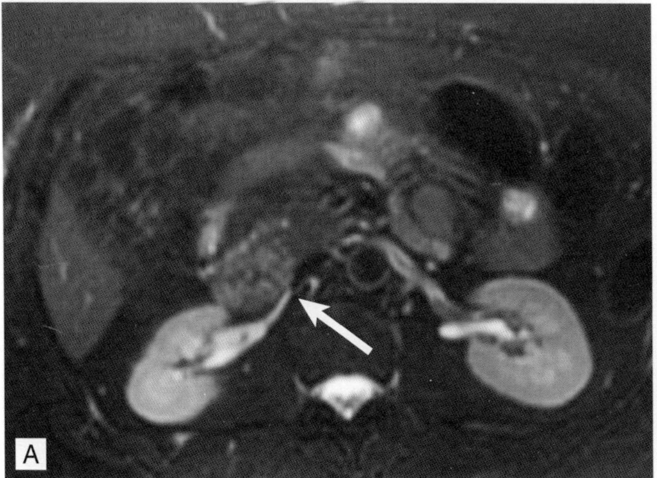

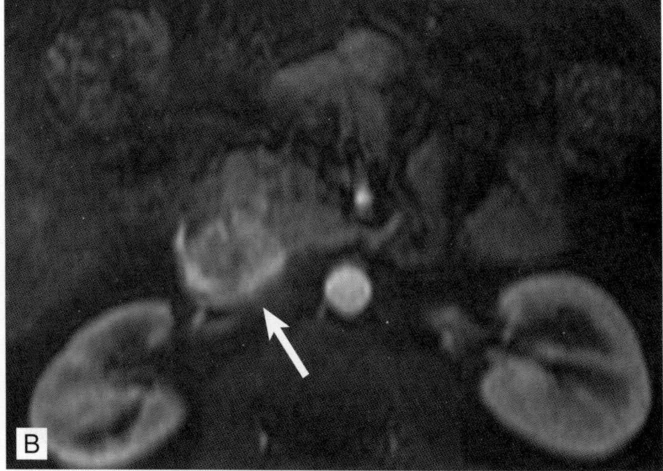

Figure 36.48 MR imaging appearance of a well-differentiated pancreatic neuroendocrine tumor (panNET) (A and B). Axial T2-weighted (A) and contrast-enhanced T1-weighted (B) MR images of the pancreas demonstrate a T2 intermediate signal intensity pancreatic mass that shows homogenous enhancement after contrast administration (*arrows*).

Pancreatic Neuroendocrine Tumor (PanNET) and Neuroendocrine Carcinoma (PanNEC)—Diagnostic Pearls

- Multiple endocrine neoplasia type 1 (MEN1) and VHL are the two most common genetic syndromes with panNETs and panNECs
- Well-differentiated panNETs appear as homogenously enhancing tumors and increased activity on DOTATATE and low activity on FDG PET
- Poorly differentiated panNETs appear as heterogeneously enhancing and necrotic tumors with decreased activity on DOTATATE and increased activity on FDG PET

Acinar Cell Carcinoma

Pathophysiology and clinical presentation. Although acinar cells comprise the majority of the pancreatic parenchyma, acinar cell carcinomas (ACCs) are rare, accounting for approximately 1% of exocrine pancreatic tumors [49]. ACCs may result in increased serum lipase, which can precipitate Schmid's Triad or lipase hypersecretion syndrome: subcutaneous fat necrosis, eosinophilia, and bone infarcts resulting in polyarthralgia [49]. ACCs demonstrate less aggressive growth and better long-term survival than PDAC.

Imaging Features

- Imaging features of ACCs are variable. ACCs are large, with a mean diameter of 10 cm at diagnosis [50]. Smaller tumors less than 5 cm are more likely to be homogenous and solid, while larger tumors are more likely to show cystic changes. ACCs tend to be less locally invasive than PDACs.
- On CT, ACCs may be iso- to hypodense to pancreatic parenchyma on noncontrast imaging [51]. Similar to PDAC, ACC demonstrates hypoenhancement on pancreatic and portal venous phases (Fig. 36.50) [51].
- Calcification is seen in one-third to one-half of cases, which can help distinguish the tumor from PDAC [50]. However, imaging features are often nonspecific, and histology is often required for definitive diagnosis.

Acinar Cell Carcinoma—Diagnostic Pearls

- Large size, mean diameter 10 cm
- Exophytic
- Central necrosis
- Calcifications

Pancreatoblastoma

Pancreatoblastoma (PB) is a rare tumor of childhood, typically diagnosed within the first decade of life [50]. The most common presenting complaint is a painless abdominal mass.

Most cases of PBs are sporadic; congenital cases of PB are associated with Beckwith–Wiedemann syndrome, a syndrome characterized by macrosomia, macroglossia, omphalocele, and visceromegaly [52].

PB is often large at presentation. Due to the soft composition of the tumor, biliary obstruction is rare.

- On CT, PB is a large, lobulated, well-marginated mass that demonstrates heterogenous and septal enhancement, with internal areas of necrosis (Fig. 36.51) [52]. Small foci of calcifications may be seen.
- On USG, PB demonstrates heterogeneous echogenicity, with internal foci of hypoechoic cystic change and echogenic septa [52].
- On MRI, PB is hypo to isointense on T1-W sequences and heterogeneously hyperintense on T2-W sequences. Internal heterogeneity is due to tumoral necrosis and hemorrhage.

The primary treatment is surgical resection. However, metastases to lymph nodes and the liver are diagnosed in 35% of cases at presentation [50].

Pancreatic Lymphoma

Pathophysiology and clinical presentation. Primary pancreatic lymphoma is rare; less than 2% of cases of extranodal non-Hodgkin's lymphoma occur in the pancreas [53]. Secondary involvement of the pancreas is much more common and occurs

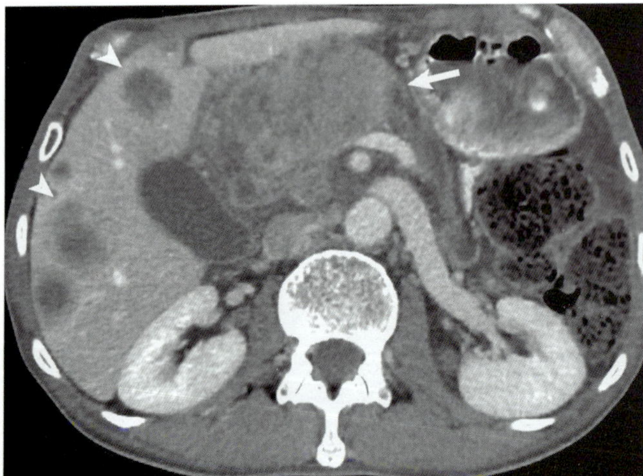

Figure 36.50 Acinar cell carcinoma. Axial contrast-enhanced CT image of the abdomen shows a large, exophytic mass in the pancreatic head with internal necrosis (*white arrow*) and multiple hypoenhancing liver metastases (*arrowheads*). This was a biopsy-proved pancreatic acinar cell carcinoma.

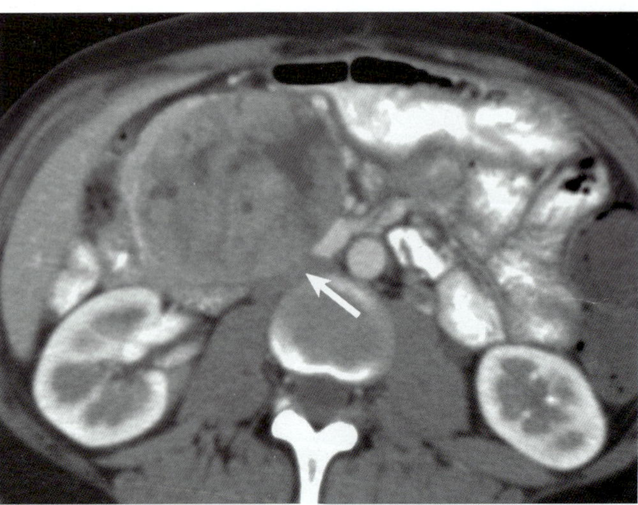

Figure 36.51 Pancreatoblastoma. Axial contrast-enhanced CT image of the abdomen shows a large, well-encapsulated mass in the pancreatic head with internal necrosis (*white arrow*).

Pancreatic Lymphoma—Diagnostic Pearls

- Focal and diffuse forms
- Focal form = homogenous, mildly enhancing mass
- Mild or no pancreatic duct dilatation, no calcifications
- Look for lymphadenopathy below the level of the renal veins; excludes the diagnosis of pancreatic adenocarcinoma
- No pancreatic ductal dilatation

in up to 30% of cases with non-Hodgkin's lymphoma [53]. This is typically secondary to invasion from the peripancreatic nodal disease. There is an increased incidence of primary pancreatic lymphoma in patients with HIV. Patients range from age 35 to 75 years at diagnosis, with a median age of 55 years [54]. Diagnostic criteria for primary pancreatic lymphoma include predominant pancreatic mass, only peripancreatic nodal involvement with no palpable superficial lymphadenopathy or no mediastinal lymphadenopathy, no splenic/hepatic involvement, and normal leukocyte count. Pancreatic lymphoma has a better prognosis than PDAC, with cure rates of up to 30%. The first-line treatment is chemotherapy [54].

Imaging Features

- There are two patterns of primary pancreatic lymphoma: the focal form and the diffuse form. The focal form involves the pancreatic head 80% of the time. It presents as a large, well-circumscribed mass with a mean diameter of 8 cm (Fig. 36.52) [54]. The mass is homogenously hypointense on CT.
- On MRI, the focal form demonstrates hypointensity on T1-W sequences, in intermediate signal to mild hyperintensity on T2-W sequences [54]. There is mild homogeneous contrast enhancement on CT and MRI. Calcifications are not seen in untreated cases. Peripancreatic lymphadenopathy is often seen [53].
- The diffuse form presents as an infiltrative, poorly defined mass, which may cause diffuse pancreatic enlargement. There is low signal intensity on both T1- and T2-W sequences. There is typically homogenous contrast enhancement [54]. This pattern may be mistaken for AP on imaging. However, the clinical and biochemical picture should indicate an alternative diagnosis.
- Like other forms of lymphoma, pancreatic lymphoma does not respect anatomic boundaries and may infiltrate into the adjacent upper abdominal and retroperitoneal solid organs or gastrointestinal tract. A key finding is a lymphadenopathy below the level of the renal veins. This is extremely rare in pancreatic adenocarcinoma [53].

Metastases

Metastases to the pancreas are seen in 2–11% of autopsies [54]. The most common sources of metastases include renal cell carcinoma, lung carcinoma, breast carcinoma, colorectal carcinoma, melanoma, and leiomyosarcoma. Metastases from renal cell carcinoma typically present 6–12 years and up to 20 years after nephrectomy [54]. Up to 80% of patients with renal cell carcinoma metastases to the pancreas will have no other sites of metastatic involvement [54]. Most patients with metastases to the pancreas are asymptomatic. When present, clinical symptoms are nonspecific [54]. Surgical resection may be considered

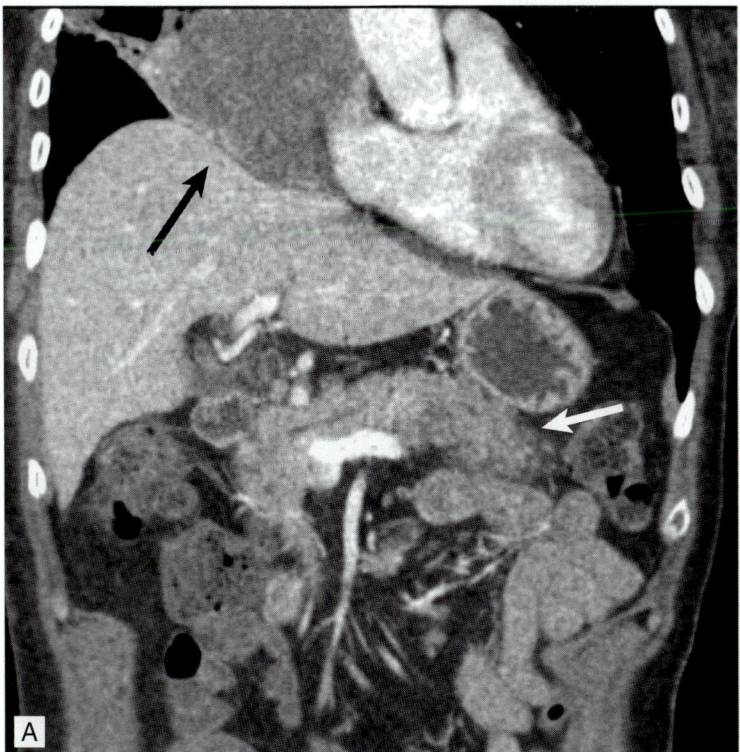

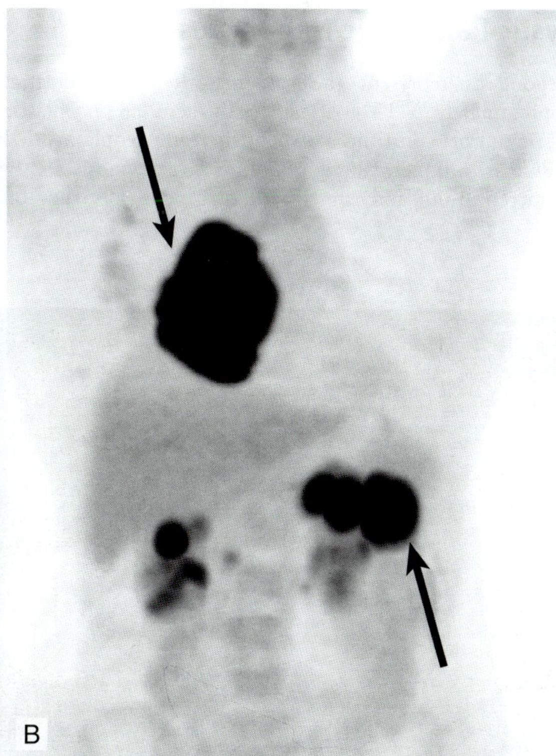

Figure 36.52 Pancreatic lymphoma (A and B). (A) Axial and coronal contrast-enhanced CT images of the abdomen show an infiltrative poorly defined hypoenhancing mass in the pancreatic tail, causing diffuse pancreatic enlargement without ductal dilatation and a large mediastinal mass (*black arrow*) (*white arrow*). (B) Coronal MIP image from an FDG-PET demonstrates radiotracer uptake in the pancreatic and mediastinal nodal masses (*arrows*). *PET*, positron emission tomography.

Pancreatic Cystic Lesions

- Pseudocyst
- Serous cystic neoplasm
- Mucinous cystic neoplasm
- Solid pseudopapillary tumor
- Intraductal mucinous cystic neoplasm
  - Main duct type
  - Branch duct type
- Cystic pancreatic neuroendocrine neoplasms
- Metastases with extensive necrosis

in patients who have metastatic disease confined to the pancreas or those who had a long disease-free period between the primary malignancy and the development of the pancreatic metastases [54].

Imaging Features

- There are three morphologic patterns of metastatic disease to the pancreas. Solitary metastasis is the most common and occurs in 50–70% of cases. A diffuse pattern occurs in 15–44% of cases. The least common pattern is multifocal, occurring in 5–10% of cases [54]. In most cases, the imaging characteristics of metastases follow those of the primary malignancy.
- Typically, smaller metastases (less than 1.5 cm in diameter) demonstrate homogenous enhancement, and larger lesions demonstrate peripheral enhancement on both CT and MRI (Fig. 36.53) [54]. Hypervascular metastases, for example, renal cell carcinoma, will demonstrate arterial phase hyperenhancement. Larger lesions may demonstrate central necrosis.

Cystic Pancreatic Neoplasms

Pseudocysts represent the vast majority of pancreatic cysts. Approximately 5–15% of pancreatic cysts are neoplastic [55]. Cystic tumors constitute <5% of pancreatic neoplasms. MRI and MRCP are uniquely suited for noninvasive diagnosis, localization, characterization, and surveillance of a wide spectrum of cystic pancreatic neoplasms, particularly in younger patients due to lack of nonionizing radiation [55,56].

Serous Cystic Neoplasm

Pathophysiology and clinical presentation. Serous cystic neoplasms constitute up to a third of cystic pancreatic neoplasms. Serous cystic neoplasms are overwhelmingly benign, although isolated case reports of serous "cystadenocarcinomas" showing aggressive growth patterns and metastases exist in the literature. Most serous cystadenomas (SCAs) are sporadic in etiology; 80% of tumors occur in women in the sixth-seventh decades (grandmother tumors) [55–58]. Multiple SCAs can coexist with pancreatic neuroendocrine tumors and epithelial cysts in patients with VHL disease. Approximately 80% of patients with SCAs are asymptomatic. Patients may manifest variable symptoms, including abdominal pain, weight loss, palpable mass, or rarely, jaundice.

Imaging Features

- Approximately 40% of SCAs arise within the pancreatic head and uncinate process. SCAs typically consist of innumerable small cysts leading to polycystic (70%) or honeycomb (20%) morphology [55–58].
- On USG, CT, and MRI, SCAs appear as large, lobulated, multilocular, and expansile microcystic masses with thin enhancing septations. There is no associated pancreatic ductal dilatation. A characteristic central, stellate scar that may calcify is seen in 30% of tumors (Fig. 36.54) [55,56]. Serous SCAs may show macrocystic or oligocystic morphology in 10% of cases. Some hypervascular SCAs with innumerable microcysts may be mistaken for solid neoplasms.
- High VEGF-A levels are characteristically seen on cyst fluid analysis [58].
- Most sub-4 cm serous SCAs are asymptomatic; surgical resection may be warranted in patients with symptomatic SCAs.

Mucinous Cystic Neoplasm

Pathophysiology and clinical presentation. Mucinous cystic neoplasms (MCNs) occur almost exclusively (98%) in perimenopausal women

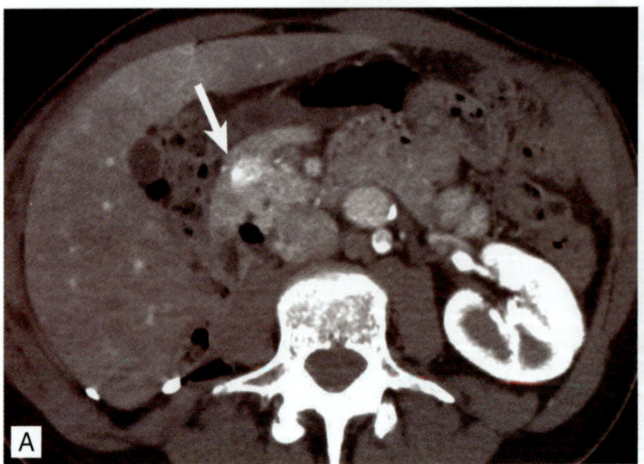

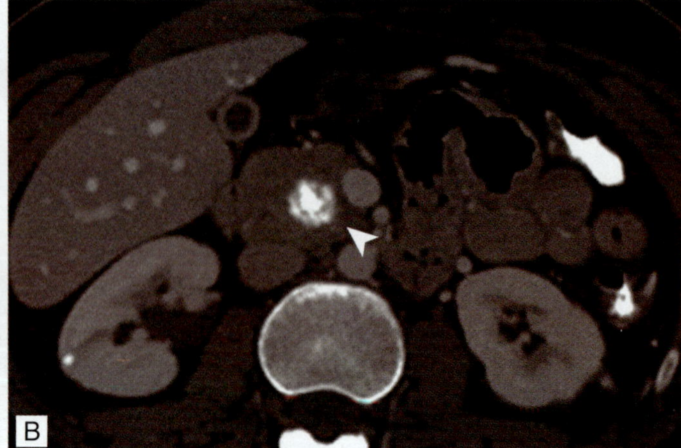

Figure 36.53 Pancreatic metastases in two different patients. (A) Metastases from renal cell carcinoma. Axial contrast-enhanced CT image of the abdomen shows an enhancing mass in the uncinate process of the pancreas (*arrow*) in this patient with right nephrectomy for renal cell carcinoma. (B) Metastases from osteosarcoma (*arrowhead*). Axial contrast-enhanced CT image of the abdomen shows a calcified mass in the uncinate process of the pancreas in this patient with extremity osteosarcoma.

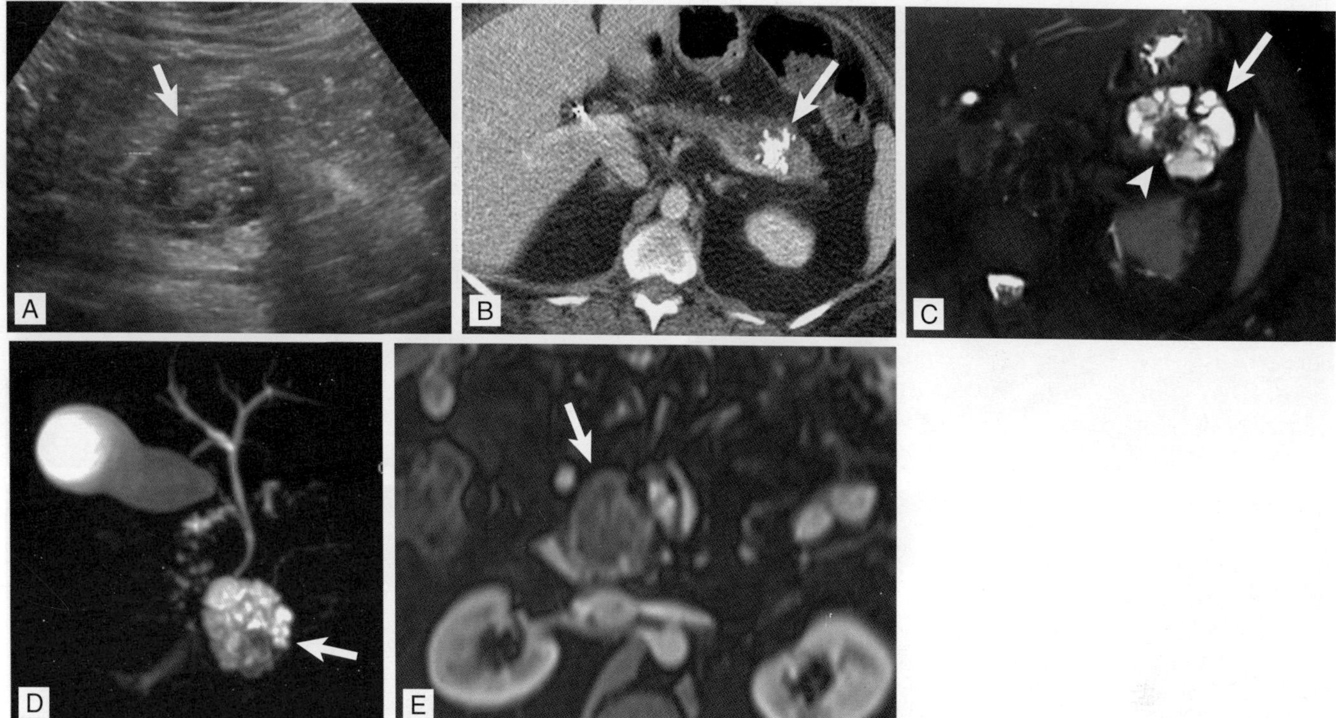

Figure 36.54 Multimodality imaging findings of serous cystadenoma (*SCA*) in different patients. (A) Grayscale USG image of the pancreas in a 52-year-old man shows a focal mass in the pancreas with multiple small, peripheral cystic foci (*arrow*). (B) Axial contrast-enhanced CT image of the pancreas in a 77-year-old woman shows a hypodense mass in the pancreatic tail with central stellate calcification (*arrow*). (C) Axial T2-weighted MR image of the pancreas in a 59-year-old man shows a cystic lesion in the pancreatic tail that demonstrates multiple small cysts with septations giving to a "honeycomb" appearance (*arrow*) and a central T2 hypointense stellate scar (*arrowhead*). (D and E) 3D MRCP image and axial contrast-enhanced T1-weighted MR image of the pancreas shows a cystic lesion with multiple small internal cysts (*arrows*) giving to a "honey-comb" appearance. The microcystic appearance and central scar with stellate calcifications are characteristic imaging features of pancreatic SCA. *USG*, ultrasonography.

(40–60 years—mother tumor); >90% of tumors occur in the tail region [56–58]. MCNs are large, complex, macrocystic tumors filled with thick/tenacious mucus, are lined by columnar mucinous epithelium, and show pathognomonic ovarian-type, spindle cell stroma [55–57]. MCNs are associated with invasive malignancy in 16% of cases; they commonly undergo transformation to a tubular variant of PDAC. Given this increased risk of malignancy, MCNs are typically considered surgical lesions and should be removed.

Imaging Features

- On imaging studies, MCNs typically manifest as large, multilocular, and macrocystic, complex cystic masses with variable densities and signal intensities due to mucin, hemorrhage, and peripheral calcifications, unlike the central calcifications in SCNs.
- Thick septations (normally more than 3 mm in thickness) and enhancing mural nodules herald malignant transformation [56–58] (Fig. 36.55). MRI and MRCP exquisitely demonstrate internal characteristics and solid components of MCNs.
- Surgical resection is warranted in MCNs >4 cm, MCNs with aggressive features on imaging studies, and in symptomatic patients. Long-term surveillance may be indicated in asymptomatic patients with smaller MCNs. Surveillance protocols vary from different institutions. However, annual imaging with either CT/MRI is commonly performed if the lesion is not resected.
- EUS-guided biopsy is recommended in patients with suspicious findings and interval increase in size. Faster growth rates of MCNs have been observed in pregnant women that may prompt close monitoring in this patient cohort.
- The prognosis of malignant MCNs is better than PDAC; 5-year survival rates vary from >60% in patients with invasive cystadenocarcinomas to 100% in patients with noninvasive tumors [55–57].

Solid Pseudopapillary Tumor of the Pancreas

Solid pseudopapillary tumor (SPT), also called solid pseudopapillary epithelial neoplasm, is an uncommon solid cystic neoplasm, accounting for 1–2% of all exocrine tumors [58]. Also referred to as the "daughter tumor," it predominantly occurs in young women in the second and third decades of life [47], with a mean age of 25 years [56,59]. MCN ("mother tumor") affects middle-aged women, and SCA ("grandmother tumor") occurs in older women [59]. SPT shows a predilection for Asian and African-American women [58,60]. Clinically, SPT is often asymptomatic; nonspecific symptoms such as abdominal pain and mass may be seen [55,60].

Imaging Features

- SPT typically presents as a large, well-encapsulated pancreatic mass, with an average diameter of 8 cm [58]. On CT, it manifests as a heterogeneous mass with solid and cystic components, frequently containing foci of hemorrhage and necrosis. The pancreatic duct is typically not dilated (Fig. 36.56) [56,58,61].
- Peripheral calcifications may be present. On MRI, signal intensity is variable; foci of hyperintensity on T1-W sequences suggest hemorrhage or high protein content. Fluid/fluid levels are identified in up to 18% of cases (Fig. 36.56) [57,59]. There

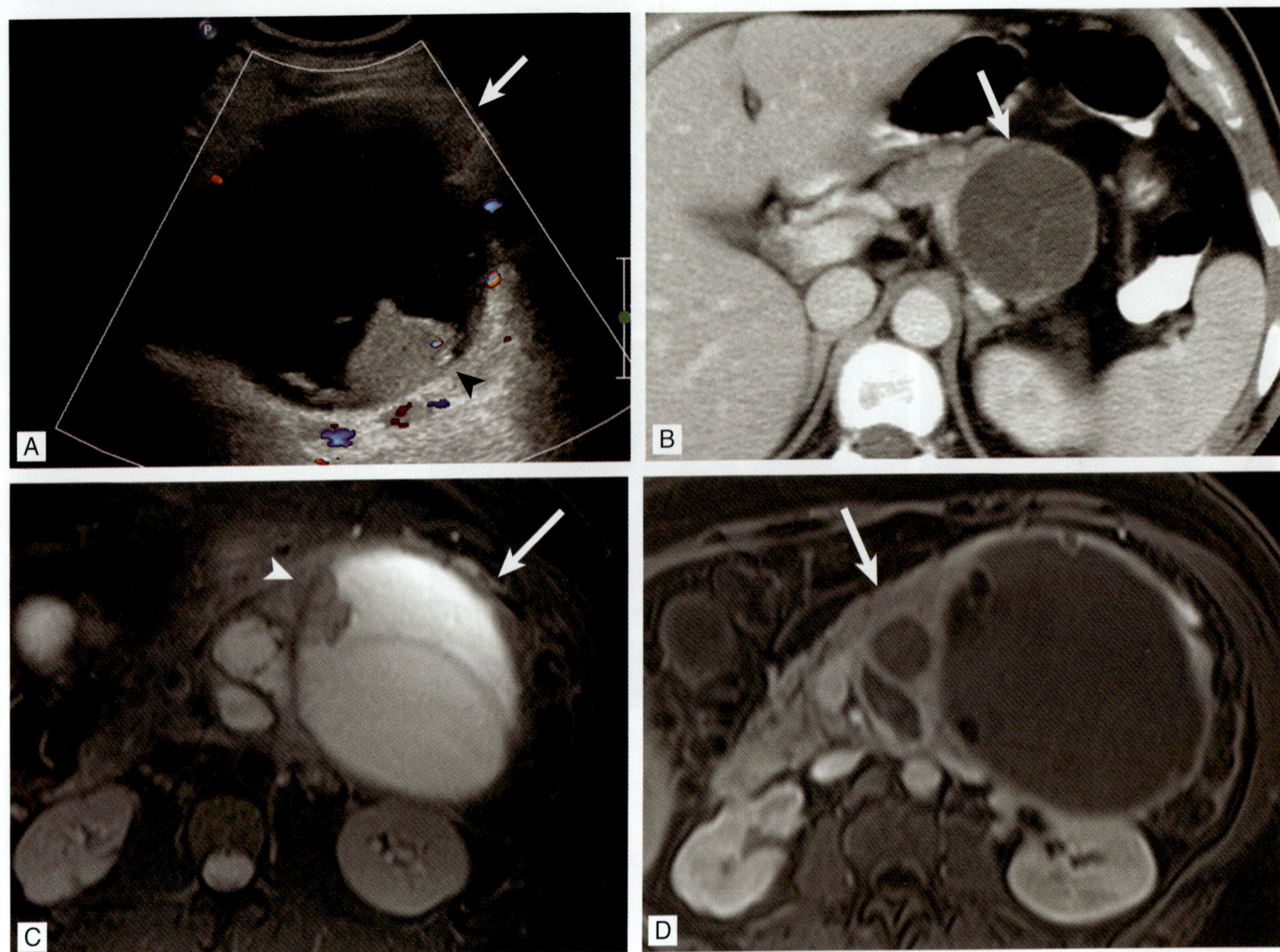

Figure 36.55 Multimodality imaging findings of mucinous cystic neoplasms (*MCNs*) of the pancreas in different patients. (A) Color Doppler image of the pancreas in a 44-year-old woman shows a well-defined cystic lesion in the pancreas that demonstrates echogenic debris (*arrow*) and peripheral solid components with increased vascularity. (B) Axial CT image of the pancreas in a 39-year-old woman shows a pancreatic cystic lesion with multiple internal septations (*arrow*). (C and D) Axial T2-weighted (C) and contrast-enhanced T1-weighted MR images of the pancreas in a 49-year-old woman show a cystic pancreatic lesion (*arrow*) with multiple septations (*arrowheads*) and a peripheral solid component (*arrowheads*). These features are somewhat characteristic of pancreatic MCN.

is typically early heterogenous and slowly progressive enhancement with gadolinium contrast [61].

- SPT has a good prognosis, with low malignant potential. Surgical resection is curative in more than 80% of cases [58,59]. However, up to 15% of cases are malignant at presentation [55,58,60]. Malignant tumors are more likely to affect older and male patients.

Intraductal Papillary Mucinous Neoplasm

Pathophysiology and clinical presentation. Intraductal papillary mucinous neoplasms (IPMNs) are characterized by intraductal papillary growth, abundant mucin production, and variable malignant potential [56–58]. IPMN is the most common macroscopic precursor for PDAC.

IPMNs differ from MCNs on the following features:

- Proclivity to involve the pancreatic head (two-thirds of tumors)
- Origin within the larger ducts
- Male preponderance
- The absence of dense "ovarian" stroma at pathology [55–57]
- Contradistinction to solitary MCNs, IPMNs are multifocal in 20–40% of cases

IPMNs may be broadly categorized based on anatomic distribution into the main duct, branch duct, or mixed types. IPMNs may also be classified based on the predominant epithelial cell type or histologic criteria. Gastric type IPMNs are frequently multifocal that commonly involve branch ducts within the uncinate process and have a lower risk of malignancy [55–58]. Colloid carcinomas (intestinal type) and oncocytic subtype of malignant IPMNs demonstrate indolent behavior compared with tubular PDACs associated with pancreaticobiliary type IPMNs [56–58]. IPMNs comprise 25–50% of resected cystic tumors occurring mainly in men during the seventh decade (mean age: 65 years). Most patients are asymptomatic; symptomatic patients often present with nonspecific abdominal pain, jaundice, or diabetes mellitus.

Imaging Features

- MRI/MRCP exquisitely demonstrate cyst features such as septations, mural nodules, and wall thickening, as well as depict communication of the cysts with the ducts [56–58]. On CT/MRI, branch duct IPMNs manifest as unilocular or complex multilocular cystic lesions that communicate with the main pancreatic duct (Fig. 36.57).

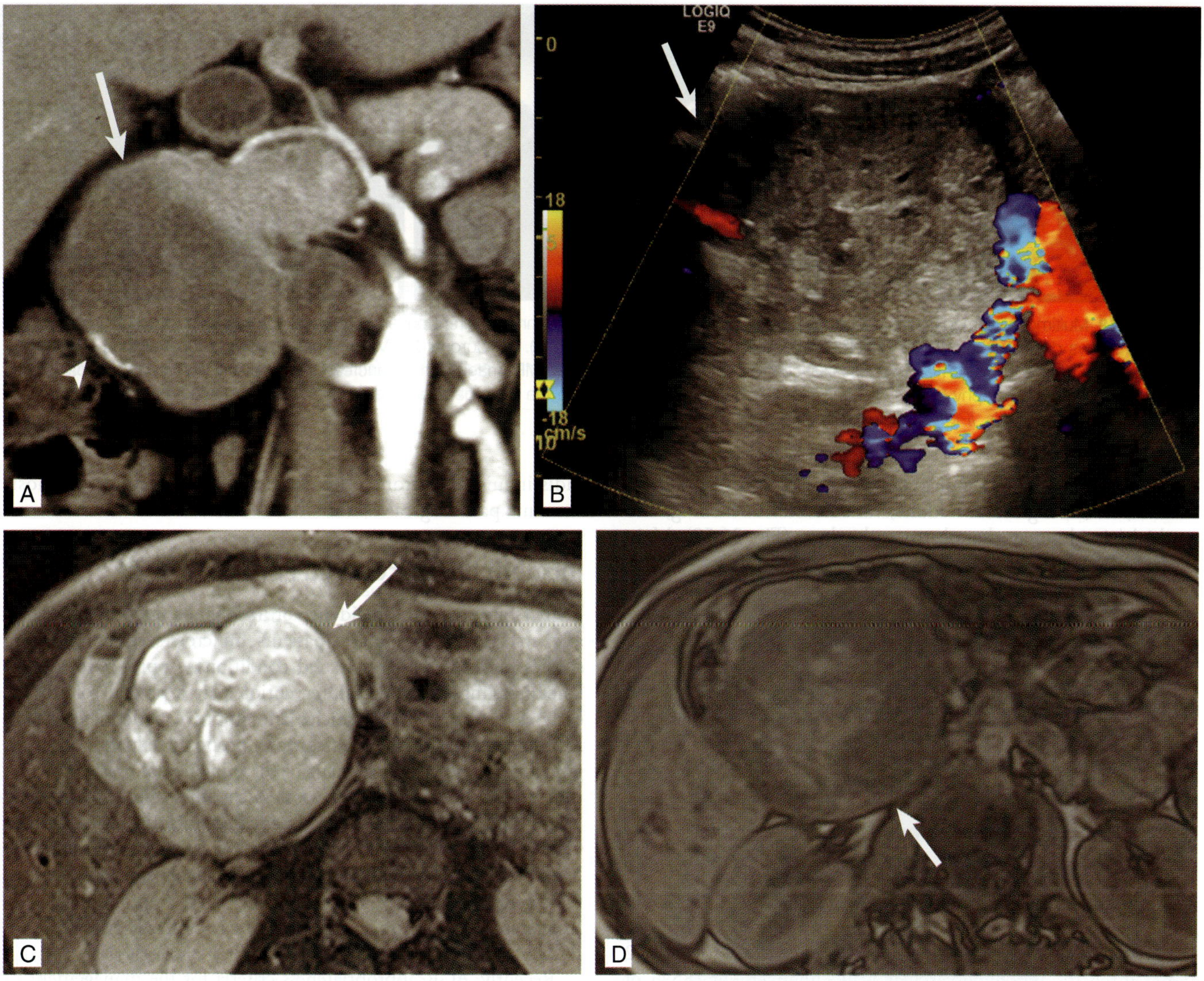

Figure 36.56 Solid pseudopapillary tumor (SPT) of the pancreas in two different patients. (A) Coronal contrast-enhanced CT image of the pancreas in a 24-year-old woman shows a mixed solid cystic mass arising from the head/uncinate process of the pancreas (*arrow*) with peripheral calcifications (*arrowhead*). (B–D) Color Doppler image (B), axial T2-weighted (C), and T1-weighted (D) MR images of the pancreas in a 27-year-old woman show a predominantly solid, isoechoic mass with mixed signal intensities on T1- and T2-weighted images (*arrows*). These findings are consistent with SPT of the pancreas.

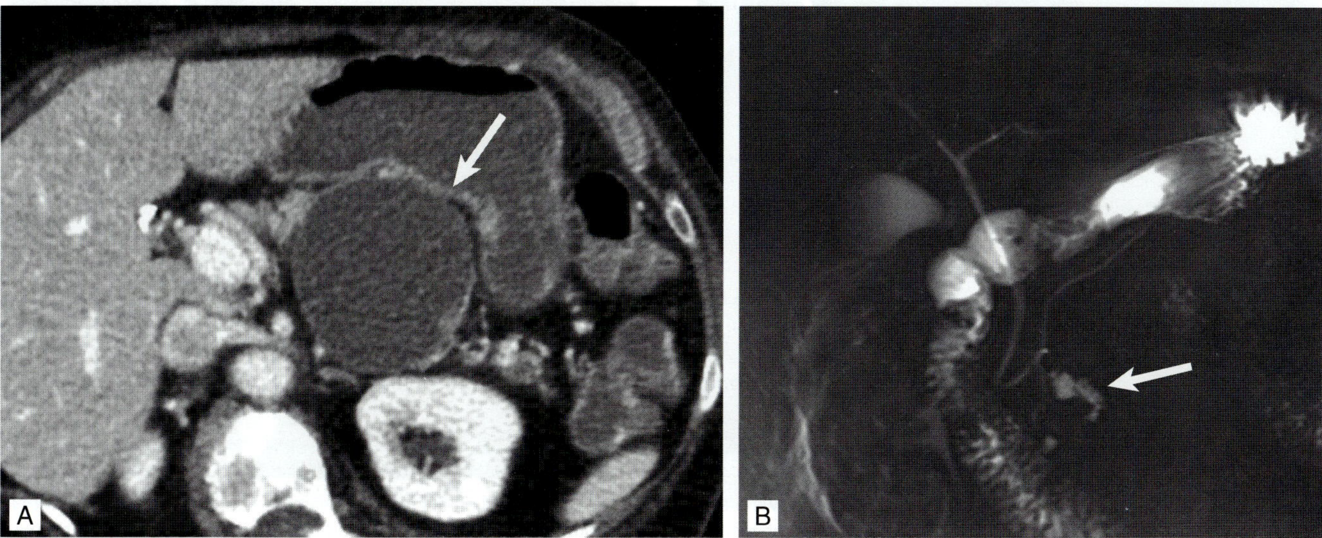

Figure 36.57 Side duct IPMNs of the pancreas in two different patients. (A) Axial contrast-enhanced CT image of the pancreas shows a well-defined cystic lesion of the pancreas without any septations or solid components (*arrow*). (B) Coronal 2D MRCP image shows a few small cystic lesions in the uncinate process (*arrow*) that communicates with main pancreatic duct. *IPMNs*, intraductal papillary mucinous neoplasms.

gene abnormalities, MCNs and IPMNs contain mucinous fluid with elevated CEA levels and abnormal *KRAS*. *GNAS* is elevated in IPMNs and *CTNNB1* mutation is seen in SPTs. *PIK3CA* and *MEN1* mutations are seen in cystic panNETs.

Cysts without worrisome features or high-risk stigmata are stratified based on the size and are followed-up on surveillance imaging. As per the ACR White Paper, the important points in managing incidental pancreatic cysts include management of cysts as mucinous unless proved otherwise, broad use of EUS and cyst fluid analysis for more refined characterization, specific definition of cyst measurement and growth criteria, follow-up periods of 9–10 years in most patients, and modified management for patients older than 80 years. The main reason for follow-up imaging is to identify PDAC when it is confined to the cyst or within the pancreas. The integration of biochemical/molecular profile of the cyst fluid, along with imaging features, risk of malignancy, comorbidities, and surgical candidacy, will ultimately govern the decision to operate on any incidental pancreatic cyst [62,65].

Suggested Readings

- Pancreatitis Disease Focus Panel. Society of Abdominal Radiology. Teaching Series 2020: Atlas of Pancreatitis. Available from: https://cdn.ymaws.com/www.abdominalradiology.org/resource/resmgr/education_dfp/pancreatitis/atlas/pancreatitis_dfp_atlas_2020-.pdf.
- AK Shanbhogue, N Fasih, VR Surabhi, GP Doherty, DK Shanbhogue, SK Sethi, A clinical and radiologic review of uncommon types and causes of pancreatitis, Radiographics 29 (4) (2009) 1003–1026.
- VS Katabathina, OY Rikhtehgar, AK Dasyam, et al., Genetics of pancreatic neoplasms and role of screening, Magn Reson Imaging Clin N Am 26 (3) (2018) 375–389.
- NM Kulkarni, DM Hough, PP Tolat, EV Soloff, AR Kambadakone, Pancreatic adenocarcinoma: cross-sectional imaging techniques, Abdom Radiol (NY) 43 (2) (2018) 253–263.
- L Khanna, SR Prasad, A Sunnapwar, et al., Pancreatic neuroendocrine neoplasms:2020 update on pathologic and imaging findings and classification, Radiographics 40 (5) (2020) 1240–1262.
- DV Sahani, R Kadavigere, A Saokar, et al., Cystic pancreatic lesions: a simple imaging-based classification system for guiding management, Radiographics 25 (6) (2005) 1471–1484.
- Expert Panel on Gastrointestinal I Gastrointestinal, K Fabrega-Foster, IR Kamel, JM Horowitz, et al., ACR appropriateness criteria(R) pancreatic cyst, J Am Coll Radiol 17 (5S) (2020) S198–S206.

37

Peritoneum, Retroperitoneum, and Abdominal Wall

PRIYA PATHAK, PUNEET BHARGAVA

Anatomy of Peritoneum, Omentum, and Mesentery

Peritoneum is a complex serous membrane consisting of parietal peritoneum lining the abdominal wall, and visceral peritoneum covering the viscus. It is lined by a single layer of mesothelial cells, and encloses the peritoneal cavity containing a thin film of serous fluid (approximately 50–100 mL). The cavity is a closed space in males. In females, the peritoneal cavity is open through the fallopian tubes [1].

To briefly review the peritoneal embryology, primitive gut is suspended by two primitive mesenteries in the abdominal cavity, which subsequently divide into dorsal and ventral portions. Development of various organs within these mesenteries leads to the creation of peritoneal ligaments. Anteriorly, development of liver within the ventral mesentery forms the gastrohepatic ligament (between liver and stomach), hepatoduodenal ligament (between liver and duodenum), and falciform ligament (between liver and abdominal wall). Posteriorly, development of spleen within the dorsal mesentery leads to the formation of the gastrosplenic ligament between stomach and spleen. Dorsal mesentery containing the pancreas fuses with subperitoneal tissues anterior to the kidney to form the splenorenal ligament (Fig. 37.1). Mid and hindgut develop within the dorsal mesentery to form the small bowel mesentery and mesocolon, respectively [2].

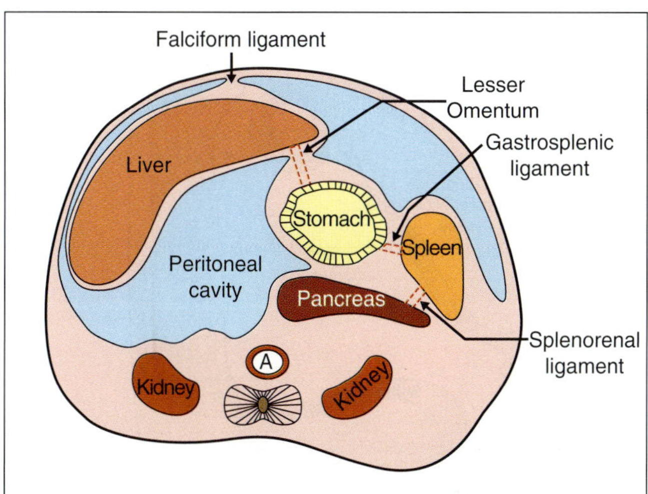

Figure 37.1 Illustration demonstrates the location of various peritoneal ligaments in the supramesocolic peritoneal compartment.

Peritoneal Ligaments

Many infectious, inflammatory, neoplastic, and traumatic processes help delineate the peritoneal folds and ligaments that are normally not visible. These ligaments can be identified by recognizing the vessels traversing them (Table 37.1).

Peritoneal ligaments around the liver consist of the following:

a. Right and left triangular ligaments formed by the fusion of superior and inferior coronary ligaments. Right triangular ligament is relatively long and separates the right subphrenic space from right subhepatic space. Left triangular ligament is shorter and poorly compartmentalizes the left subphrenic space.
b. Falciform ligament, containing obliterated umbilical vein, partially separates right subphrenic from left subphrenic space (Fig. 37.2) [1].

The greater and lesser omenta are double layers of visceral peritoneum attaching stomach and duodenum to the adjacent structures. Greater omentum hangs from the greater gastric curvature like an apron (Figs. 37.2 and 37.3). Gastrocolic ligament, as a component of the greater omentum, extends from the greater gastric curvature to the transverse colon and forms the anterior wall of the lesser sac. Lesser omentum consists of gastrohepatic ligament containing coronary veins and left gastric artery; and hepatoduodenal ligament containing portal vein, common hepatic artery, and common hepatic duct. Additional ligaments around stomach and spleen are gastrosplenic and splenorenal ligaments, the latter contains the tail of the pancreas [1,2].

The peritoneal ligaments around the bowel are the small bowel mesentery, transverse colon, sigmoid mesocolon, and phrenicocolic ligament. Small bowel mesentery attaches the small bowel to the retroperitoneum and extends from ligament of Treitz to ileocecal valve; it contains the superior mesenteric vessels. Transverse and sigmoid mesocolon attach transverse colon and sigmoid colon to the posterior abdominal wall, respectively. The phrenicocolic ligament extends from splenic flexure of colon to the diaphragm, separating the left paracolic gutter from the left supramesocolic space (Figs. 37.4 and 37.5) [1].

The visceral peritoneum reflects over the bladder, uterus, and rectouterine spaces forming the folds of broad ligament, which further divides into mesometrium, mesosalpinx, and mesovarium [2].

TABLE 37.1 Attachments and Contents of the Peritoneal Ligaments

Ligaments	Organ Associated	Vascular Contents
Falciform ligament	Between liver and anterior abdominal wall	Obliterated left umbilical vein. Recanalized umbilical vein in portal hypertension
Gastrohepatic ligament	Between lesser gastric curvature and hepatic hilum	Coronary veins and left gastric artery. Replaced left hepatic artery
Hepatoduodenal ligament	Between first portion of duodenum and hepatic hilum	Portal vein and common hepatic artery
Gastrosplenic ligament	Between greater gastric curvature and splenic hilum	Short gastric vessels. Venous collaterals in splenic vein thrombosis
Splenorenal ligament	Between splenic hilum and left kidney	Splenic artery and vein. Splenorenal shunts in portal hypertension
Small bowel mesentery	Between duodenojejunal junction and ileocecal valve	Superior mesenteric artery and vein
Transverse mesocolon	Between transverse colon and posterior abdominal wall	Middle colic vessels
Sigmoid mesocolon	Between sigmoid colon and posterior abdominal wall	Sigmoid and superior rectal vessels

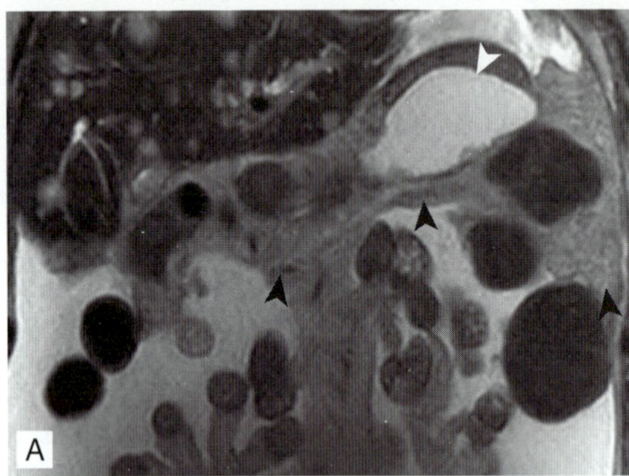

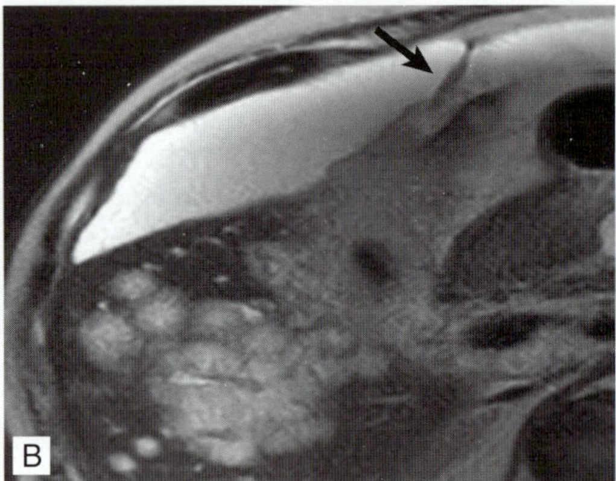

Figure 37.2 (A) T2 W Coronal MR abdomen from a 58-year-old man with pancreatic cancer, multifocal hepatic metastasis, peritoneal carcinomatosis and large volume ascites delineates the thickened omentum (*black arrowheads*). Note the loculated fluid in the lesser sac causing mass effects on the stomach (*white arrowhead*). (B) T2 W axial image shows the involvement of the falciform ligament by the tumor implant (*black arrow*).

Peritoneal Spaces

The transvers mesocolon divides the peritoneal cavity into supra and larger inframesocolic spaces (Fig. 37.4) (Flowchart 37.1). Supramesocolic space is further divided into the right compartment containing right subphrenic, subhepatic spaces, and lesser sac; and left compartment containing the left subphrenic, perihepatic, and perisplenic spaces (Fig. 37.5). Of all the supramesocolic spaces, right subhepatic space (also known as Morrison's

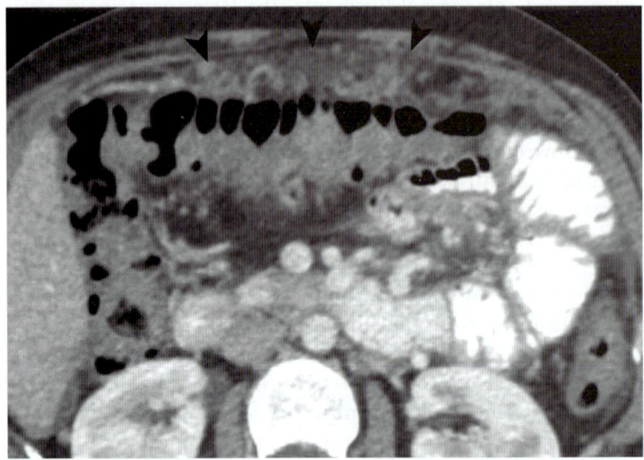

Figure 37.3 Contrast-enhanced axial CT abdomen from a 52-year-old man with pancreatic cancer and peritoneal carcinomatosis shows reticulonodular tumor implants in the greater omentum (*black arrowheads*).

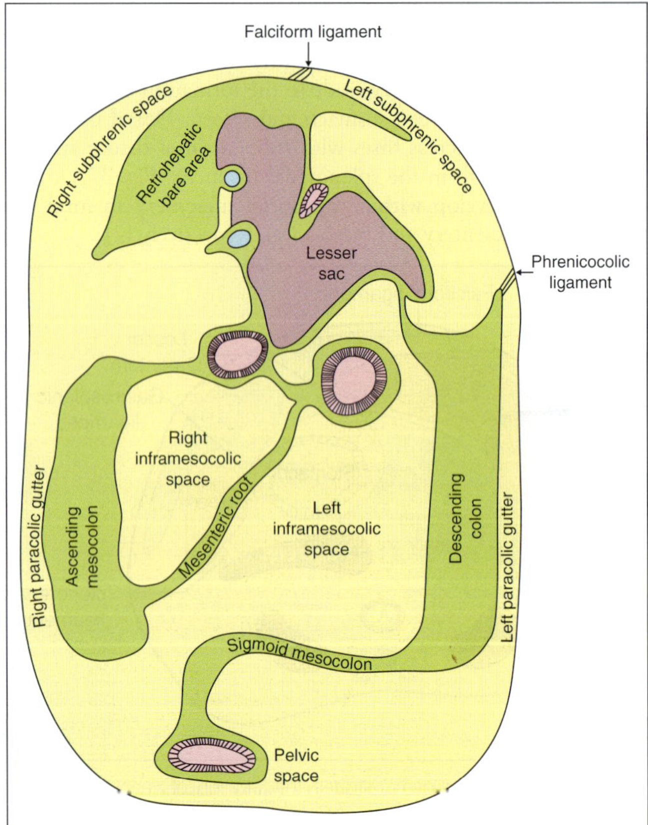

Figure 37.4 Illustration demonstrates the compartments of peritoneal cavity and locations of the peritoneal ligaments.

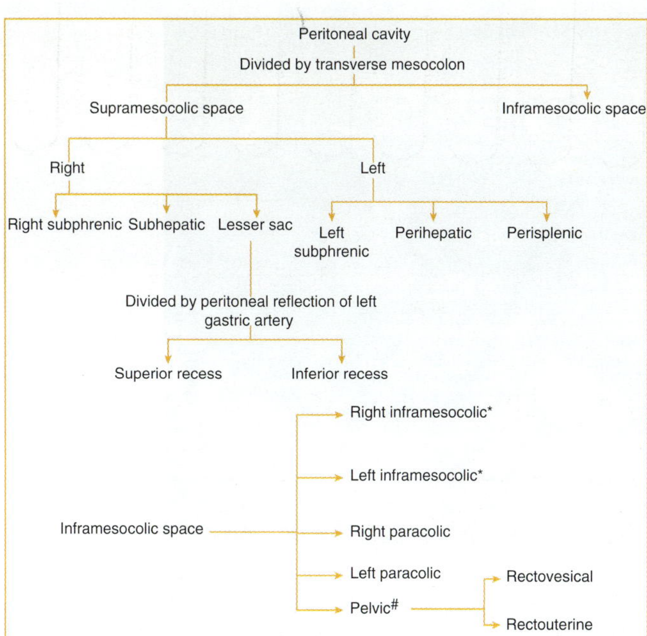

Flowchart 37.1 Compartments of the peritoneal cavity.
*Right inframesocolic space is closed by attachment of mesentery to caecum. Left inframesocolic space freely communicates with pelvis.
#Pelvic space is divided by medial umbilical ligament into medial and lateral compartments. Lateral compartment is further divided into medial and lateral inguinal fossa [1].

hepatorenal pouch) is the most gravity dependent in a supine position and serves as a site for early ascites and fluid collections resulting from the liver injury. Lesser sac is divided into the superior and inferior recesses by the peritoneal reflection of the left gastric artery (Fig. 37.6); the inferior recess communicates with the right subhepatic space through the foramen of Winslow. Inframesocolic space is divided into right and left inframesocolic, right and left paracolic and pelvic spaces. Smaller right inframesocolic space is limited inferiorly due to the attachment of the small bowel mesentery to the caecum, whereas the larger inframesocolic space communicates freely with the pelvis (Fig. 37.7). Paracolic spaces are present lateral to the peritoneal reflections of the right and left colon, respectively (Figs. 37.5, 37.6, and 37.7). Pelvic space consists of the rectovesical space in males, and vesico-uterine and rectouterine spaces (also known as pouch of Douglas) in females; the latter is the most gravity-dependent site (Fig. 37.8) [1].

Role of peritoneal ligaments in tumor spread:

The peritoneal ligaments can serve as both a barrier or as a conduit for spread of disease across the abdominal cavity. For example, the pancreas is situated in the anterior pararenal space but sits at the base of several mesenteries. The spread of pancreatic cancer occurs through the peritoneal ligaments along distinct pathways as follows (Flowchart 37.2) [2].

Other examples are spread of gastric carcinoma to the liver through the gastrohepatic and hepatoduodenal ligaments. Liver and gall bladder tumors spread to the peripancreatic nodes via the hepatoduodenal ligament. Phrenicocolic ligament serves as a barrier to tumor spread between left paracolic space and left subphrenic space [2,3].

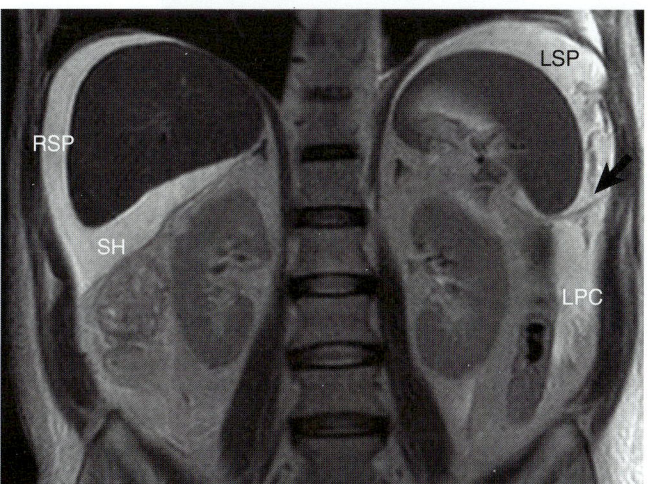

Figure 37.5 T2 W Coronal MR abdomen and pelvis from a 50-year-old man with alcoholic cirrhosis delineates various peritoneal compartments and phrenicocolic ligament in the left upper abdomen (*black arrow*). *RSP*: Right subphrenic space, *LSP*: Left subphrenic space, *SH*: Subhepatic space, *LPC*: Left paracolic space.

Pattern of Peritoneal Fluid Spread and Potential Areas of Stasis

Flow of peritoneal fluid is described as circulatory and "preferential" (Fig. 37.9). Initially, fluid is present in the gravity-dependent areas with upward ascent in certain preferred pathways (Fig. 37.10) [1–3].

Sites of peritoneal fluid stasis and hence hotspots for tumor seeding are rectouterine pouch, inframesocolic compartment, and paracolic spaces. Areas of peritoneal fluid reabsorption such as right subdiaphragmatic space and greater omentum serve as additional hot spots (Fig. 37.11) [4].

Imaging Techniques

Ultrasonography (USG), CT, MRI, and PET are the technique for the assessment of peritoneal pathologies. USG is predominantly used in detection of ascites, differentiation of simple from complex ascites, and guided paracentesis. Although it is easily available and lacks ionizing radiation, it is limited in evaluation of peritoneal anatomy or detection of tumor implants, with added technical difficulties in obese patients. Contrast-enhanced CT with a single venous phase (60–70 s) is the technique of choice to assess most peritoneal pathologies. Administration of neutral or positive oral contrast helps in better delineation of serosal implants [1].

Typical MRI protocol includes T1 and T2WI, DWI, and dynamic contrast sequences. Dynamic contrast sequences are essential as most peritoneal pathologies demonstrate slow enhancement with gadolinium. Antiperistalsis agents aid in decreasing motion artifacts. Although MRI provides better tissue characterization, its overall utility in peritoneal imaging is largely limited due to motion artifacts, fat interface artifacts, dielectric artifacts produced by ascites, and increased scan time [1,5]. It is however evolving as a tool for the detection of subtle peritoneal disease and quantification of peritoneal carcinomatosis index.

Developmental Lesions

Congenital Cysts

Pathophysiology and clinical features: Congenital cysts include enteric duplication cysts, enteric cysts, and mesothelial cysts. These are most frequently present within the ileal mesentery [6].

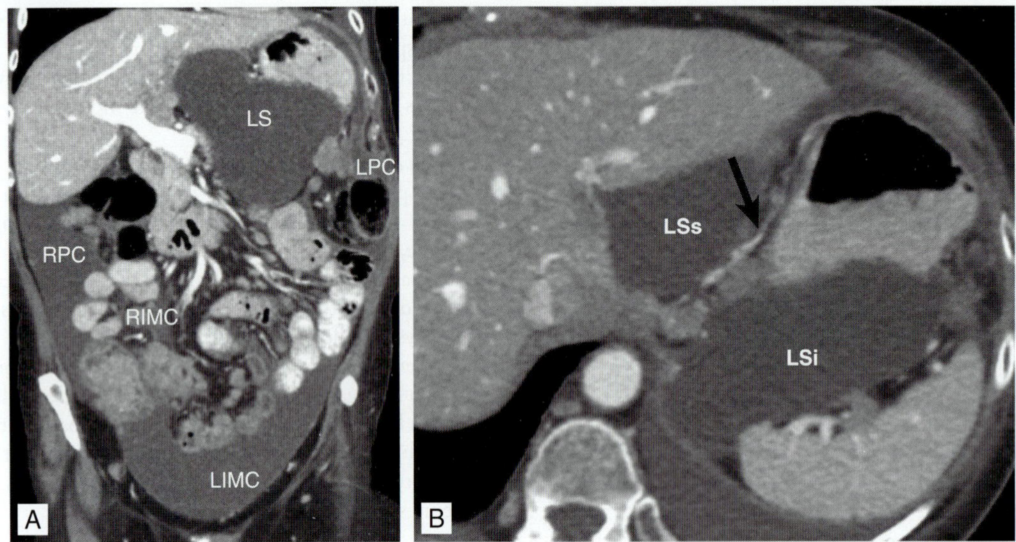

Figure 37.6 Contrast-enhanced coronal (A) and axial (B) CT abdomen and pelvis from a 62-year-old woman with ovarian cancer, peritoneal carcinomatosis, and moderate volume ascites demonstrate various peritoneal compartments. *LS*: Lesser sac, *RPC*: Right paracolic space, *LPC*: Left paracolic space, *RIMC*: Right inframesocolic space, *LIMC*: Left inframesocolic space. Note the thickened peritoneal reflection along the left gastric artery (*black arrow*) separating the superior (LSs) and inferior (LSi) lesser sac recesses (B).

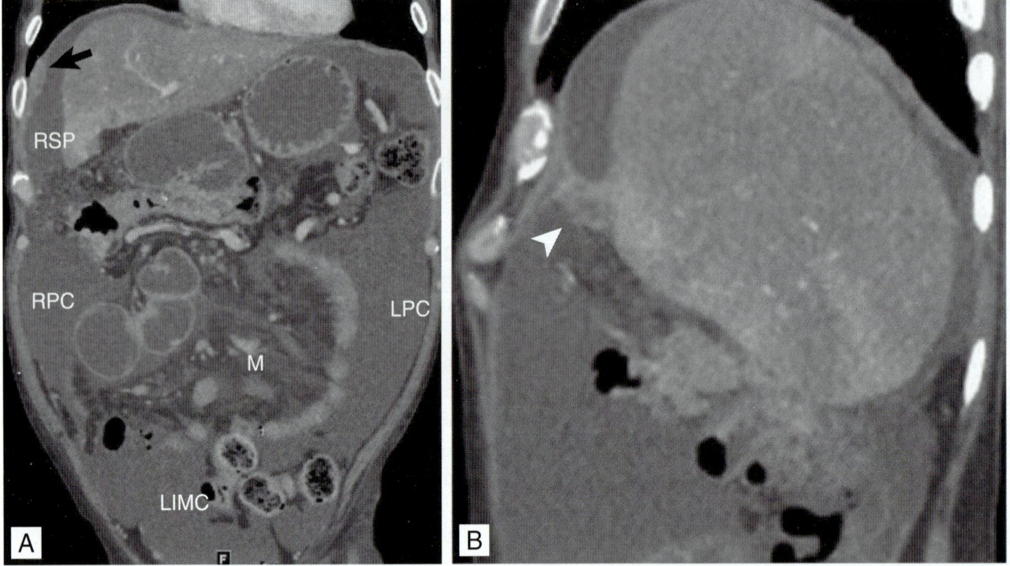

Figure 37.7 Contrast-enhanced coronal (A) and sagittal (B) CT abdomen and pelvis from a 78-year-old woman with ovarian cancer, peritoneal carcinomatosis and large volume ascites demonstrate various peritoneal compartments and thickened mesentery due to tumor implants (M). *RSP*: Right subphrenic space, *RPC*: Right paracolic space, *LPC*: Left paracolic space, *LIMC*: Left inframesocolic space. Note the enhancing tumor implant in the right subphrenic space (*black arrow*) (A) and nodular thickening of the falciform ligament (*white arrowhead*) (B).

Although a pediatric diagnosis, congenital cysts may remain undetected till adulthood. The cysts can be incidentally detected on imaging or present with complications secondary to infection, perforation, bowel obstruction, intussusception, or malignant degeneration [7]. On pathology, enteric duplication cysts are thick walled containing the entire gut lining from mucosa to muscularis layers. Enteric cysts are thin-walled cysts containing only the mucosal layer; these are formed secondary to migration of bowel diverticulum into the mesentery. Mesothelial cysts are thinned walled containing a single layer of mesothelial cells, and are formed secondary to incomplete fusion of mesothelial lined peritoneal surfaces [6,8].

Imaging Features

USG: Enteric duplication cysts are thick-walled anechoic lesions with inner echogenic mucosal layer and outer hypoechoic muscle layer, and demonstrate the gut signature sign (Fig. 37.12). Complexities in the cyst result from calcification, hemorrhage, or fecolith formation. Enteric and mesothelial cysts are thin-walled unilocular lesions within the mesentery [8].

CT and MRI: Uncomplicated duplication cysts demonstrate simple fluid attenuation without solid components or enhancement on contrast-enhanced CT. On MRI, cysts follow fluid signal, that is low T1 and high T2 signal. Complex cysts demonstrate variable T1 and T2 signal secondary to

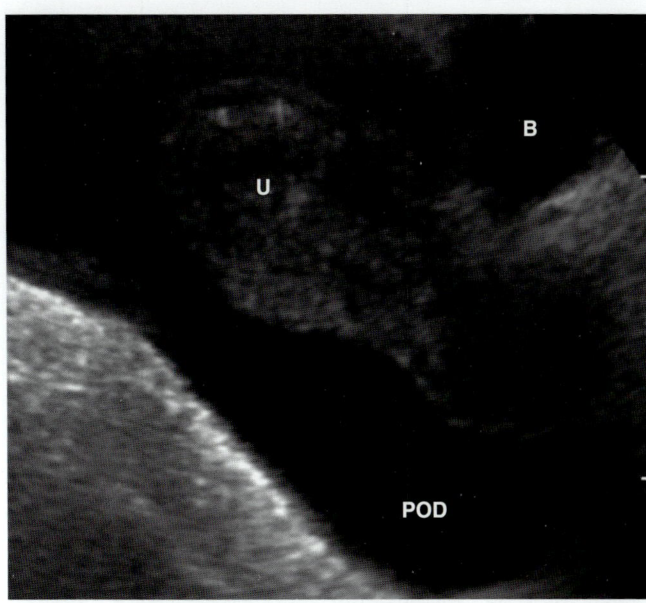

Figure 37.8 Longitudinal transvaginal USG from a 64-year-old woman with large volume ascites demonstrates fluid in the rectouterine pouch or pouch of Douglas (POD). Vesico-uterine pouch is present between the uterus (U) and bladder (B).

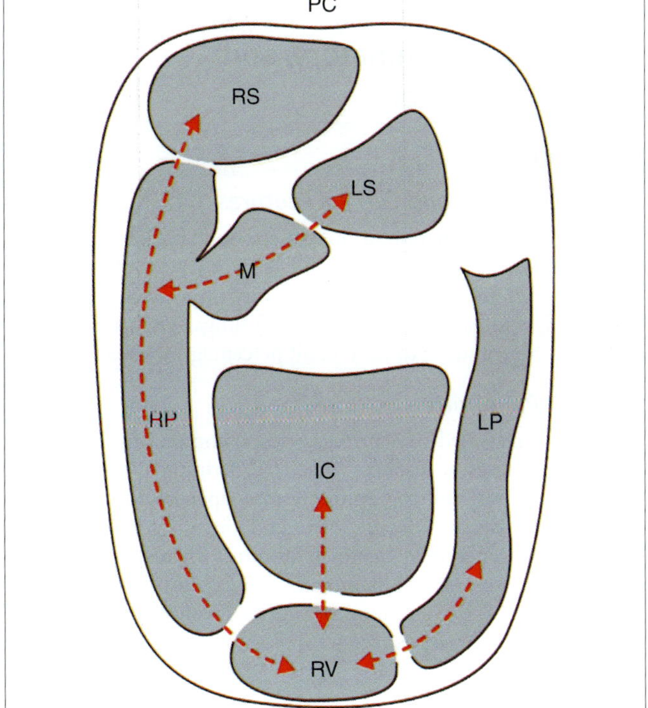

Figure 37.9 Illustration demonstrates the circulatory flow of peritoneal fluid in various peritoneal compartments. *PC*: Peritoneal Cavity, *RS*: Right subphrenic space, *LS*: Lesser sac, *M*: Morison's pouch, *RP*: Right paracolic space, *LP*: Left paracolic space, *IC*: Inframesocolic compartment, *RV*: Rectovesical space.

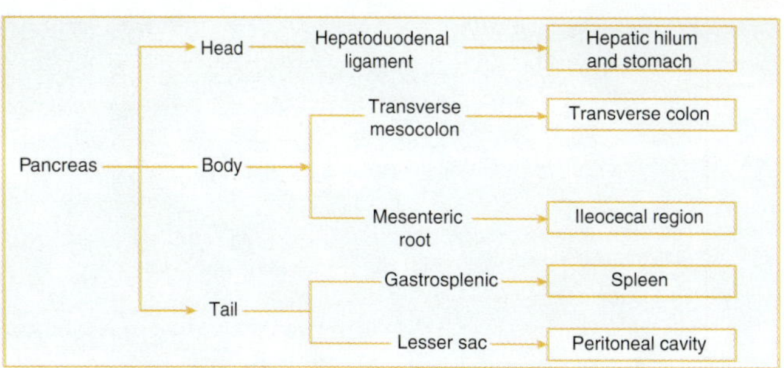

Flowchart 37.2 Routes of pancreatic cancer spread through the peritoneal ligaments.

calcifications and internal proteinaceous or hemorrhagic contents (Fig. 37.13).

Lymphatic Malformations

Pathophysiology and clinical features: Previously known as lymphangioma, these are rare benign vascular malformations with lymphatic differentiation; typically described as slow-growing insinuating multicompartmental masses that do not respect fascial planes [9,10].

On histopathology, lymphatic malformations are thin walled cystic masses with either large macroscopic interconnecting cysts or microscopic cysts containing dilated lymphatics lined by flattened endothelial cells [9]. Abdominal lymphatic malformations most commonly occur in mesentery, followed by omentum, mesocolon, and retroperitoneum; with retroperitoneal lymphatic malformation accounting for only 1% of cases [10]. The lesions can be asymptomatic or present with abdominal distention, palpable mass, or pain, often secondary to complications such as hemorrhage, infection, or rupture.

Imaging Features

USG: Circumscribed multilocular cystic masses, anechoic or with layering internal debris. Avascular internal septae show variable thickness (Fig. 37.14) [11].

CT and MRI: Contrast enhanced CT (CECT) demonstrates multilocular or multiseptated cystic mass with thin wall and septae showing mild or absent enhancement (Figs. 37.15 and 37.16). Areas of high attenuation could reflect hemorrhage or less commonly calcification [9]. On MRI, the mass follows fluid signal, that is, homogenously low T1 and high T2 signal, unless complicated by infection, hemorrhage or rare stromal myxoid degeneration and fibrosis, in which case it may present as a multilocular mass with solid components [12].

Lymphatic Malformations: Pearls to Remember

- Slow-growing insinuating multicompartmental masses that do not respect fascial planes.
- Most commonly occur in mesentery, followed by omentum, mesocolon, and retroperitoneum.
- On CECT, multilocular multiseptated cystic mass with thin enhancing wall and septae.

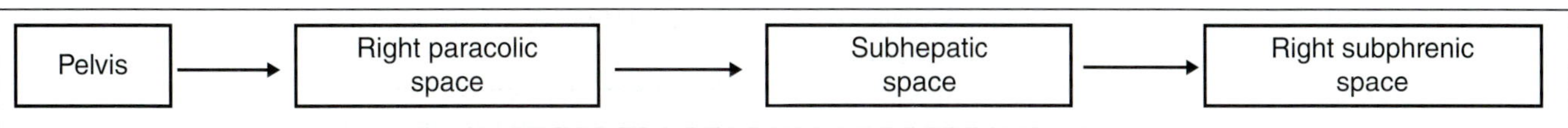

Figure 37.10 Preferential pathway for peritoneal fluid circulation.

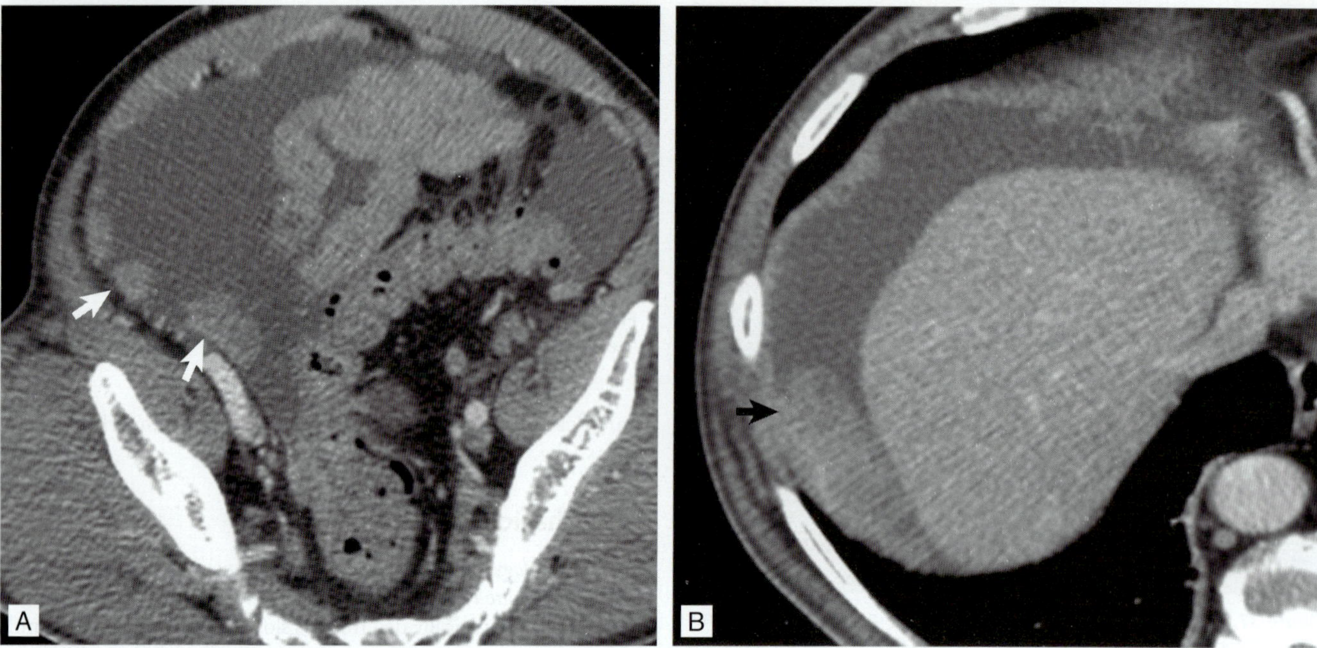

Figure 37.11 Contrast-enhanced axial CT abdomen and pelvis from a 68-year-old woman with metastatic ovarian cancer and peritoneal carcinomatosis. Although there is large burden peritoneal disease and ascites, tumor implants are most numerous at the site of peritoneal fluid stasis such as right paracolic space (*white arrows*) (A) and site of peritoneal fluid reabsorption at the right subphrenic space (*black arrow*) (B).

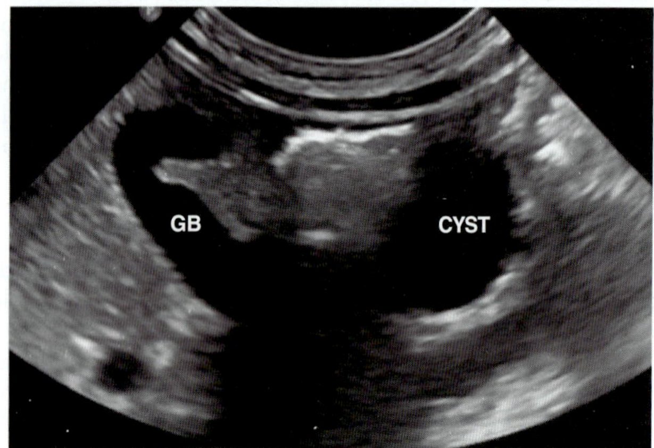

Figure 37.12 Transabdominal USG from a 1-year-old male shows an enteric duplication cyst associated with duodenum. No calcifications or solid components are present.

Differential diagnosis: Cystic peritoneal and retroperitoneal lesions such as pseudocysts, lymphocele, hydatid cysts, cystic teratoma and peritoneal inclusion cysts [9,10].

Nonpancreatic Pseudocysts

Pathophysiology and clinical features: These are rare, acquired and incidental mesenteric and retroperitoneal cysts unrelated to pancreatitis. Proposed etiologies are as a sequela of infection or unresolved hematoma. Retroperitoneal nonpancreatic pseudocysts arise from the fatty tissues of retroperitoneum. The cyst may have serous, purulent, hemorrhagic, or chylous internal contents [10,13].

Imaging features: On USG, these are unilocular or multilocular cysts, anechoic or with internal echogenic debris. CECT demonstrates well-defined cyst with internal fluid or fat attenuation, and a thin or thick enhancing wall (Fig. 37.17). Fluid-fluid or fat-fluid levels can be present. Calcification may be seen [10,13].

Infectious, Inflammatory, and Ischemic Disorders

Peritonitis

Pathophysiology and Clinical Features

Peritonitis is inflammation of the parietal and visceral peritoneum. It is classified into acute and chronic secondary to infectious and noninfectious etiologies. The vast majority of peritoneal infections are secondary to bacterial etiologies, with fungal, viral, and parasitic infections contributing to only small percentage of cases [14].

Bacterial Peritonitis

It is further classified into primary (less common) and secondary types [14]. Causes of secondary bacterial peritonitis include bowel perforation, diverticulitis, Crohn's disease, appendicitis, and pelvic inflammatory disease. Small bowel and peptic ulcer perforation present with generalized acute peritonitis, whereas appendicitis, diverticulitis, and pelvic inflammatory disease usually cause localized peritonitis. Most common organisms involved are Gram-negative bacilli and anaerobes [5,14,15].

Tuberculous Peritonitis

It can be secondary to reactivation of latent tuberculous foci or lymphohematogenous spread, with only 14% of the patients having associated radiological evidence of pulmonary tuberculosis [14]. It is classified into (1) wet type with ascites and loculated collections; (2) dry or plastic type characterized by mesenteric thickening, caseous nodules, and adhesions; and (3) Fibrotic type with formation of omental, mesenteric masses and matting of bowel loops [15,16].

Spontaneous Bacterial Peritonitis

It is a subtype of primary infective peritonitis involving diffuse bacterial infection of the peritoneum in patients with cirrhosis

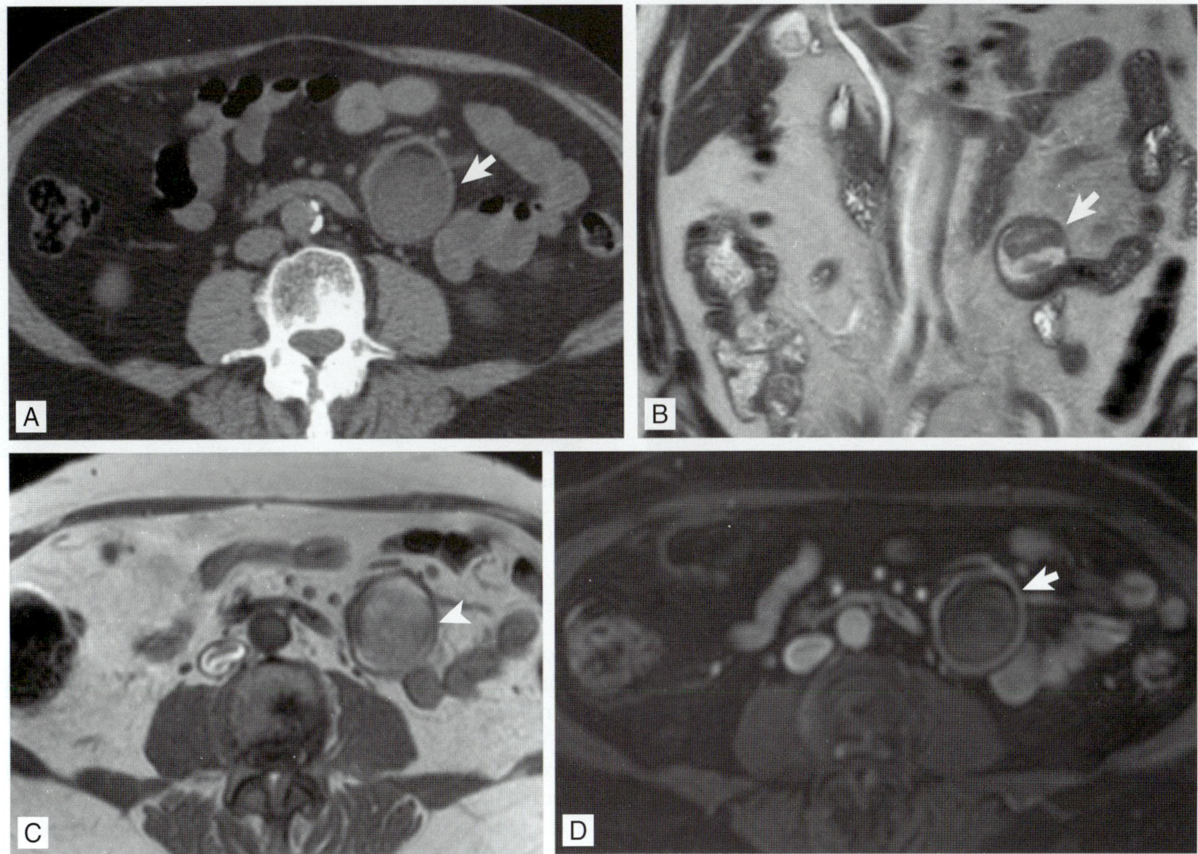

Figure 37.13 (A) Contrast-enhanced axial CT abdomen from a 72-year-old man with an incidental left enteric duplication cyst. The cyst demonstrates hyperdense internal contents (*arrow*). (B) On MR, the cyst shows hyperintense areas on single-shot FSE T2WI (*arrow*), (C) intrinsic T1 hyperintensities indicative of hemorrhagic/proteinaceous contents (*arrowhead*), and thin enhancing wall on venous phase T1WI (*arrow* in D). No discrete solid components are present.

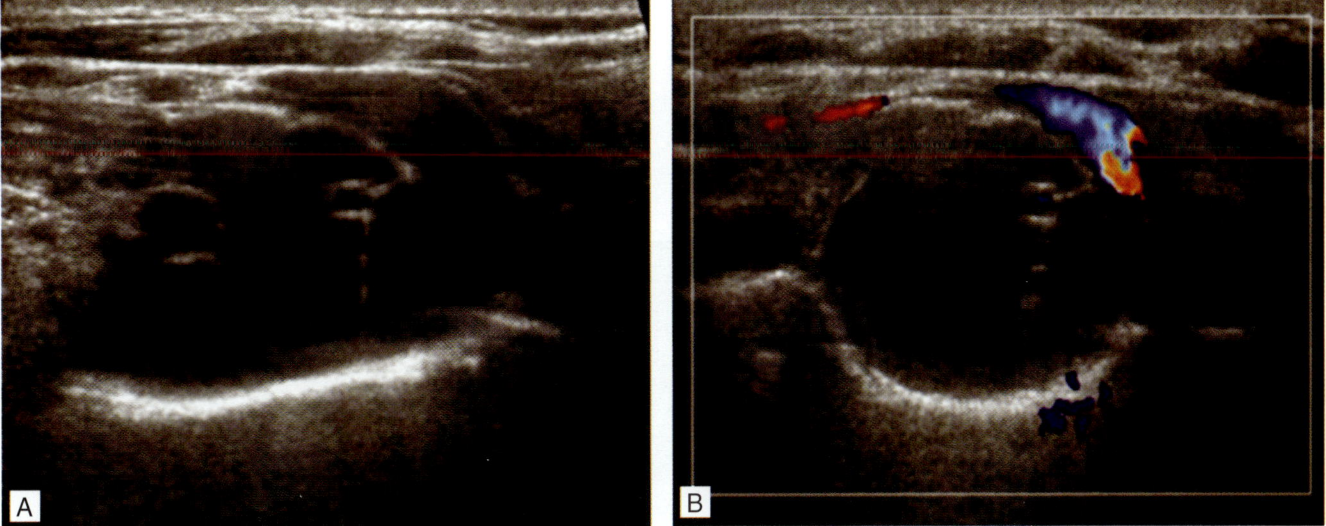

Figure 37.14 Longitudinal USG (A) with Doppler (B) of right lower quadrant shows a multiloculated multicystic lymphatic malformation. The mass shows no mural or septal vascularity or solid components.

or a nephrotic syndrome. Pathogenesis involves hematogenous spread of infection to peritoneum due to impaired filtration and neutrophil function. Typically, only one type of bacteria, most commonly *Escherichia coli*, is found in the ascitic fluid [14].

Less common noninfectious peritonitis includes chemical peritonitis (such as biliary peritonitis), granulomatous peritonitis (secondary to foreign body), and eosinophilic peritonitis [5].

Imaging Features

Radiographs: These help in detection of free air under the diaphragm (pneumoperitoneum) due to bowel perforation. Large volume ascites can lead to centralization of the bowel loops.

USG: Bacterial peritonitis presents as particulate ascites or loculated intraperitoneal collection containing gas seen as posterior reverberation artifacts, echogenic debris, and septations

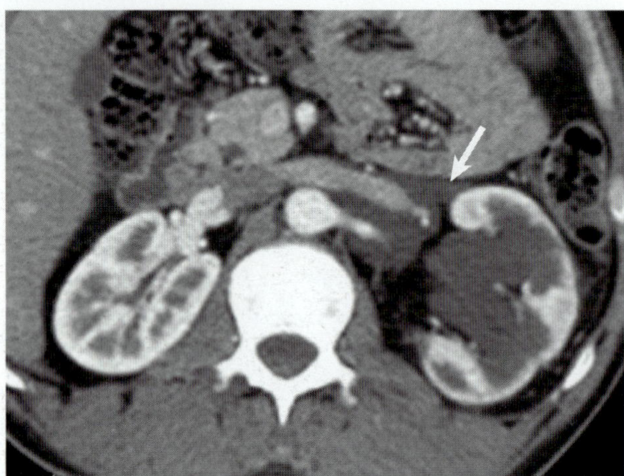

Figure 37.15 Contrast-enhanced axial CT abdomen shows left para-aortic lymphatic malformation (*white arrow*), which is insinuating between renal vasculature and extending into the renal hilum. The mass shows no enhancement.

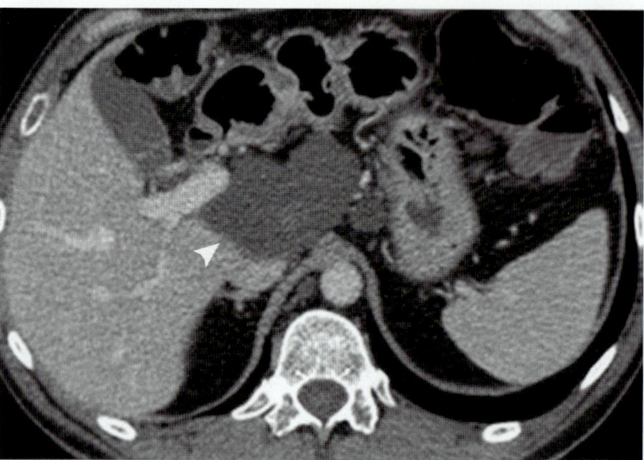

Figure 37.16 CT abdomen shows a lymphatic malformation located in the porto-caval region, as a circumscribed hypoattenuating structure with lack of enhancement (*white arrowhead*). The mass is insulating between the involved structures without substantial mass effects.

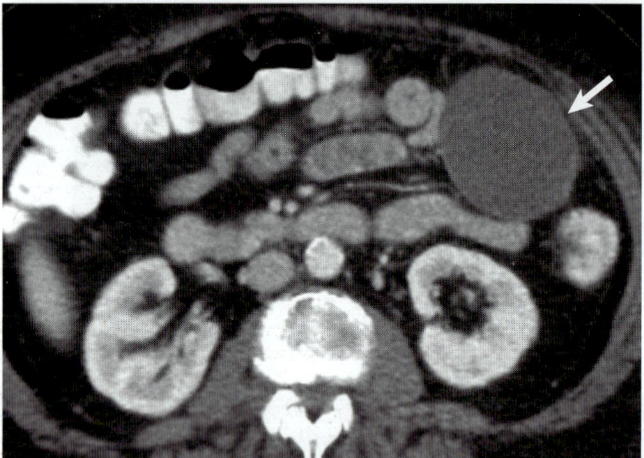

Figure 37.17 Contrast-enhanced axial CT abdomen from a 60-year-old man shows an incidental left mesenteric cyst with a thin nonenhancing wall and homogenous internal hypoattenuation (*white arrow*). Differential considerations are enteric cyst, mesothelial cyst, and nonpancreatic pseudocyst.

associated with peritoneal thickening (Fig. 37.18) [14]. USG more accurately depicts ascites characteristics (simple vs complex) and guides diagnostic and therapeutic paracentesis.

Wet-type tuberculous peritonitis presents with simple or complex particulate ascites with loculations containing lattice-like floating internal septations composed of fibrin [14]. Dry and fixed types demonstrate irregular or nodular hypoechoic omental and mesenteric thickening and masses. Bowel and mesentery can be matted. Associated abdominal and retroperitoneal adenopathy is frequent [16,17].

CT and MRI: General features of both infective and noninfective peritonitis are smooth peritoneal enhancement (in contrast to carcinomatosis where peritoneal enhancement is nodular) (Fig. 37.18), ascites, and sometimes loculated intraperitoneal collections or abscess. Intraperitoneal free air is present in peritonitis secondary to bowel perforation.

Wet-type tubercular peritonitis can present as high attenuation free ascites, loculated collections, or abscess (Figs. 37.19 and 37.20). Adhesions in dry-type peritonitis can lead to clumping

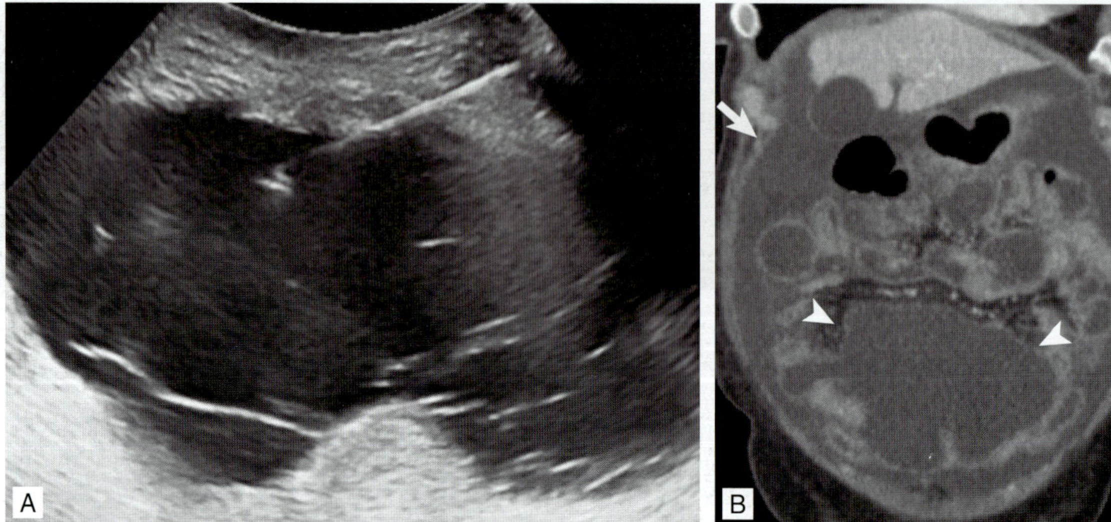

Figure 37.18 Longitudinal USG abdomen (A) in a 64-year-old woman with bacterial peritonitis undergoing therapeutic paracentesis shows particulate ascites with internal septations. Contrast-enhanced coronal CT abdomen and pelvis (B) demonstrates large volume ascites, subtle diffuse peritoneal enhancement (*arrow*), and a loculated component in the mid abdomen (*arrowheads*).

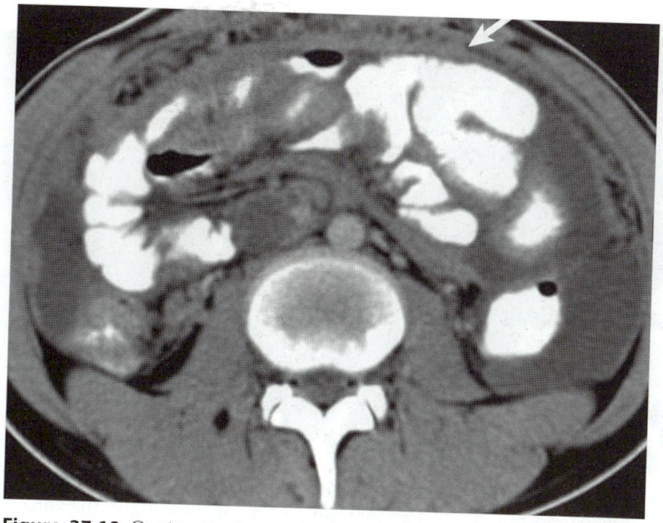

Figure 37.19 Contrast-enhanced axial CT abdomen shows wet-type tuberculous peritonitis with ascites and peritoneal thickening (*white arrow*).

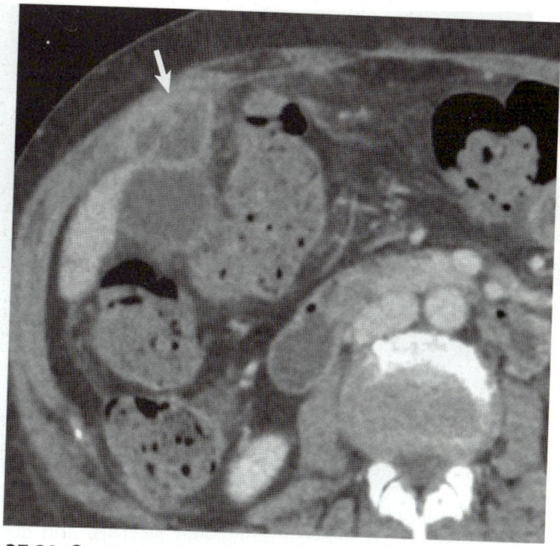

Figure 37.20 Contrast-enhanced axial CT abdomen from a 44-year-old woman with tubercular peritonitis demonstrates a rim-enhancing perihepatic abscess (*arrow*).

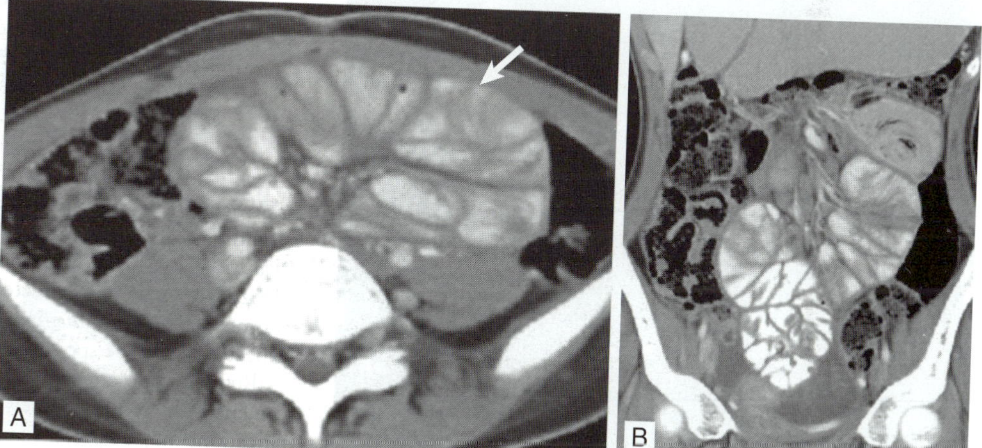

Figure 37.21 Contrast-enhanced CT abdomen and pelvis from a 17-year-old girl with abdominal pain and fever shows localized clumping of the bowel loops in the mid abdomen (abdominal cocoon formation) from tuberculous peritonitis (*white arrow*) (A and B).

of bowel loops and cocoon formation (Fig. 37.21). Caseous nodules demonstrate soft tissue attenuation and contrast enhancement. Associated necrotic abdominal and retroperitoneal adenopathy is frequently seen. Involvement of ileocecal junction with thickening commonly occurs in conjunction with peritonitis (Fig. 37.22). Dry and fibrotic type tubercular peritonitis shows extensive fibrous adhesions and cake-like omental thickening [15].

MRI has a limited role in routine evaluation. Dynamic enhanced MRI shows diffuse smooth peritoneal enhancement in both infective and noninfective peritonitis (Fig. 37.23).

Differential Diagnosis

Peritoneal carcinomatosis is the major differential consideration, especially with dry and fibrotic types of tubercular peritonitis containing omental and mesenteric masses. Definitive diagnosis is such cases necessitates tissue sampling/omental biopsy, unless there is an active focus of tuberculosis elsewhere in the body as well to help clinch the diagnosis.

Sclerosing Mesenteritis

Pathophysiology and Clinical Features

Sclerosing mesenteritis is a spectrum of idiopathic inflammatory disorder of the mesentery and peritoneum. Known associations are other idiopathic inflammatory conditions such as retroperitoneal fibrosis, sclerosing cholangitis, Riedel thyroiditis, and orbital pseudotumor [18]. It involves the mesenteric root (most common), mesocolon, omentum, and retroperitoneum. Proposed etiologies are autoimmune disorder, vasculitis, infection, trauma, and previous abdomen surgery. It is also associated with several malignancies such as lymphoma, melanoma, gastric, breast, lung and colon cancer [18,19].

Pathologically, three stages of sclerosing mesenteritis are described.

- The first stage of mesenteric lipodystrophy involves replacement of mesenteric fat by foamy macrophages.
- The second stage is mesenteric panniculitis consisting of infiltration of polymorphonuclear leukocytes, plasma cells, and foamy macrophages.
- The third stage is retractile mesenteritis involving fat necrosis followed by fibrosis [20].

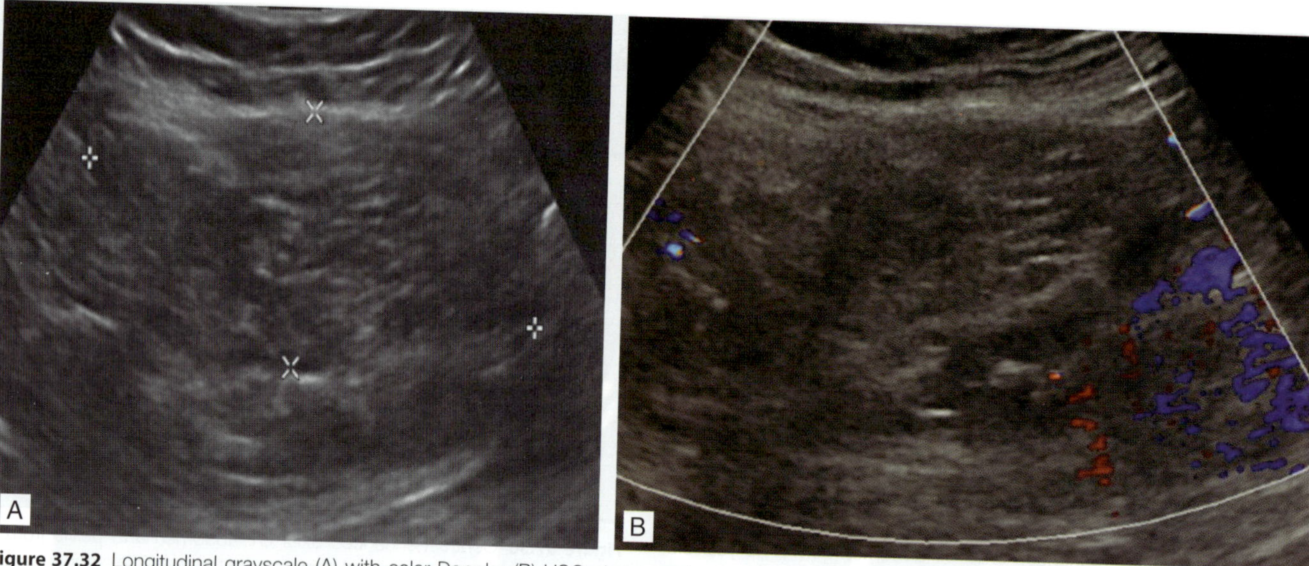

Figure 37.32 Longitudinal grayscale (A) with color Doppler (B) USG abdomen from a 24-year-old man with abdominal pain shows a large ill defined, heterogenous, incompressible and avascular lesion in the right upper quadrant representing omental infarction (calipers) (A).

enhancement (Fig. 37.33). Smaller infarct demonstrates central soft tissue attenuation with a peripheral halo. Early or developing infarction can manifest as an area of fat haziness or mild stranding (Fig. 37.34). Common location is anterior to the transverse colon or anteromedial to the ascending colon. There is swirling of the omental vasculature in omental torsion. Contiguous extension of inflammation may lead to focal colonic thickening. Rare instance of superimposed infection presents as rim enhancement, fat fluid, or air-fluid levels [27,28].

Differential Diagnosis

Epiploic appendagitis, acute appendicitis, acute diverticulitis, and mesenteric panniculitis. Differentiation from epiploic appendagitis can be suggested by the size (epiploic appendagitis are usually less than 5 cm) and location (along the sigmoid colon in epiploic appendagitis and transverse or ascending colon in omental infarction). Infected omental infarction can mimic an abscess [28].

Intraperitoneal Collections

Pneumoperitoneum

Pathophysiology and Clinical Features

Pneumoperitoneum is air within the peritoneal cavity. Etiologies are disruption of bowel secondary to peptic ulcer perforation, ischemia, neoplasm, appendicitis, diverticulitis, trauma, foreign body, iatrogenic such as endoscopy, peritoneal dialysis, cardiopulmonary resuscitation, mechanical ventilation, vaginal aspiration, and insufflation and postoperative, peritoneal infection with gas-forming organism, and secondary to pneumomediastinum and

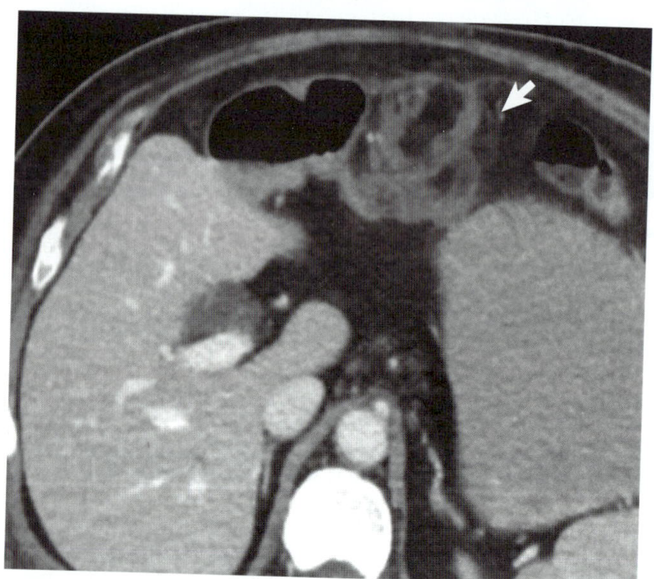

Figure 37.33 Contrast-enhanced axial CT abdomen shows an omental infarct abutting the distal gastric body. The lesion demonstrates heterogeneous attenuation with scattered fat and soft tissue densities and absent contrast enhancement (*white arrow*).

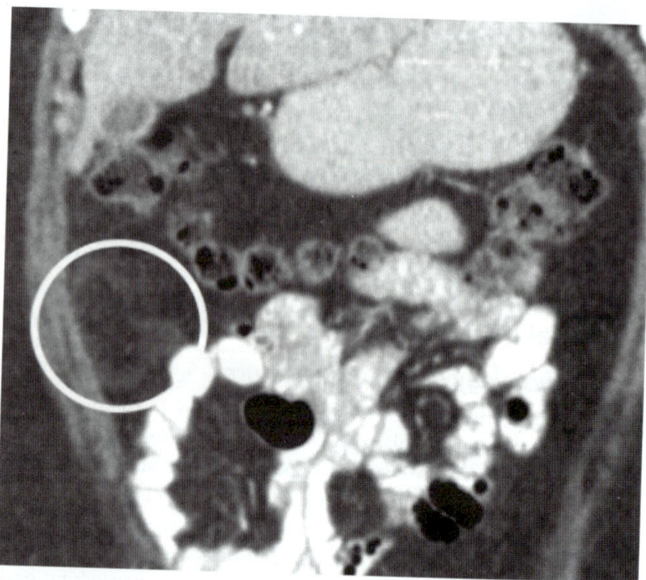

Figure 37.34 Contrast-enhanced axial CT abdomen from a 54-year-old man demonstrates early omental infarction as mild circumscribed stranding in the right upper abdomen (ellipse).

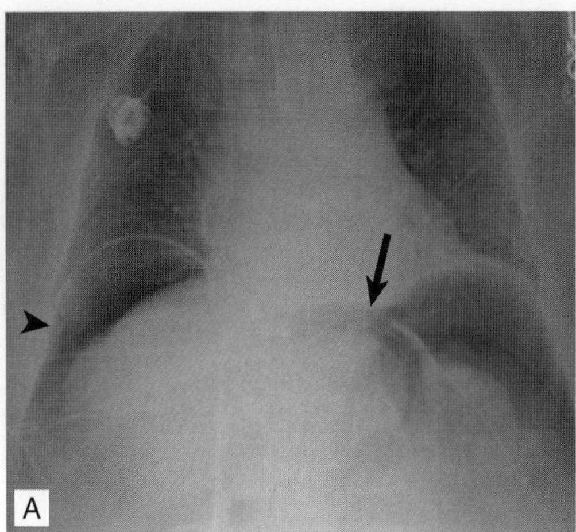

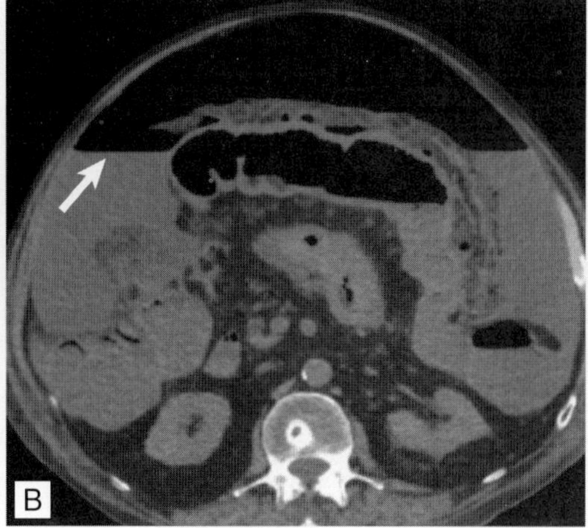

Figure 37.35 Pneumoperitoneum from peptic ulcer perforation. Supine abdomen radiograph (A) shows free air under the diaphragm (*black arrowhead*) and cupola sign (*black arrow*). Subsequent noncontrast axial CT abdomen (B) demonstrates large volume pneumoperitoneum (*white arrow*).

pneumothorax with air dissecting into the peritoneal cavity [31,32]. Clinical symptoms are abdominal distention, tenderness, guarding, tachycardia, fever, and signs of shock.

Imaging Features

Radiograph: Pneumoperitoneum on upright chest and abdominal radiograph presents as subdiaphragmatic free air. Supine abdominal radiographs are less sensitive in detection unless there is large volume of air. Following radiographic signs are described [31,33]:

a. Central abdomen:
   - Cupola, saddlebag, or mustache sign: Air collection below the central diaphragmatic tendon (Fig. 37.35).
   - Football sign: Massive pneumoperitoneum outlining the peritoneal cavity.

b. Around the liver:
   - Falciform ligament sign: Air outlining the falciform ligament (Fig. 37.36).
   - Lucent liver sign: Lucent appearance of liver secondary to air anteriorly (Fig. 37.36).
   - Doge's cap sign: Triangular air collection in the Morrison pouch.

c. Around the bowel:
   - Rigler's or double wall sign: Air outlining both sides of the bowel wall (Fig. 37.36).
   - Telltale triangle sign: Triangular air collection between three bowel loops.

d. Pelvis:
   - Inverted V sign: Air along the lateral umbilical ligaments.
   - Urachus sign: Air along the median umbilical ligament.

USG: Sonographic detection is based on distortion of USG waves by air present in atypical location. A liner array transducer (10–12 MHz) is more sensitive than a curvilinear transducer. Reverberation of ultrasonic waves between transducer and air results in high amplitude linear echoes causing increased echogenicity of underlying peritoneum, known as peritoneal enhancement (Fig. 37.37). It is accompanied with posterior reverberation and ring down artifacts, best observed between liver and anterior abdominal wall where there is usually no intervening bowel. Extensive reverberation artifacts in large volume pneumoperitoneum can sometimes completely obscure the underlying viscera [32, 34]. A study conducted by Jones et al. showed sensitivity of plain radiographs at 79%, specificity at 64% and a positive predictive value at 96% for pneumoperitoneum detection. USG demonstrated a higher sensitivity at 93%, specificity at 64%, and positive predictive value at 97% [35]. However, operator dependency limits the overall utility of USG in actual clinical practice as detection is technically challenging even for an experienced sonographer and in obese patients.

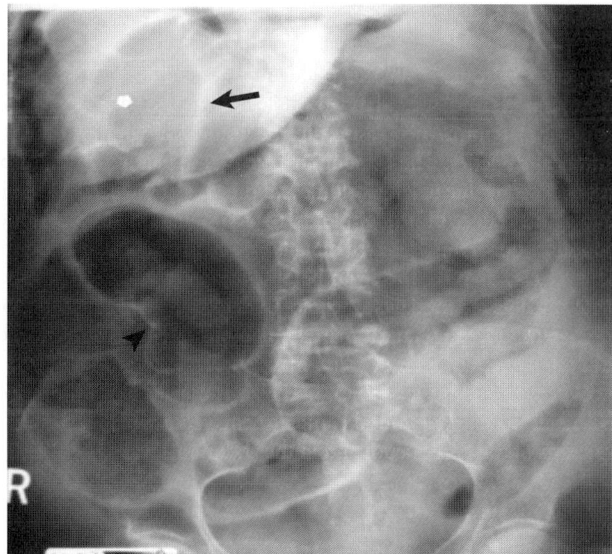

Figure 37.36 Pneumoperitoneum from perforated sigmoid diverticulum. Supine abdomen radiograph shows Rigler's sign (*black arrowhead*), lucent liver sign (white polygon), and falciform ligament sign (*black arrow*).

CT and MRI: CT is the modality of choice to detect the presence, volume, location, and etiology of intraperitoneal free air. It helps in evaluation of complex postsurgical abdomen and patients with suspected anastomotic leak. MRI is rarely used for evaluation. Intraperitoneal air produces signal loss on T1 and T2WI with dephasing artifacts on gradient sequences [5].

Differential diagnosis: Chilaiditi Syndrome (Hepato-diagrammatic interposition of colon) (Fig. 37.38), linear basilar atelectasis, skin folds, properitoneal fat stripe and subdiaphragmatic lipomatosis producing false-positive lucencies on radiographs and pneumoretroperitoneum [31].

Pneumoretroperitoneum refers to the presence of air in the retroperitoneal space. The gas most often originates from perforation of

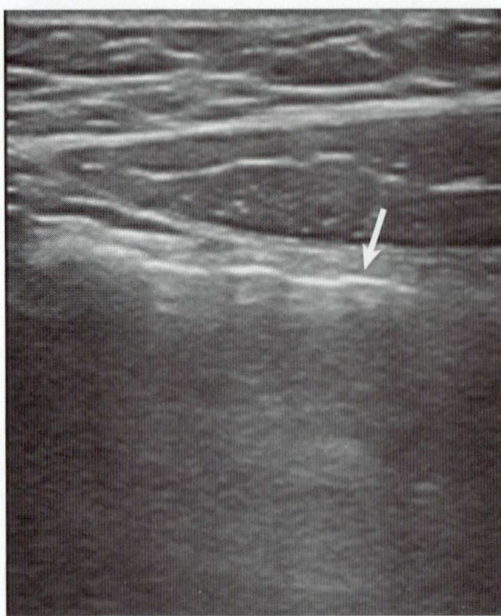

Figure 37.37 Linear array transducer USG image shows echogenic peritoneal stripe (*white arrow*) with reverberation artifacts in pneumoperitoneum. (Courtesy of Dr Amit Sahu, Consultant, Max Hospital, Saket, India.)

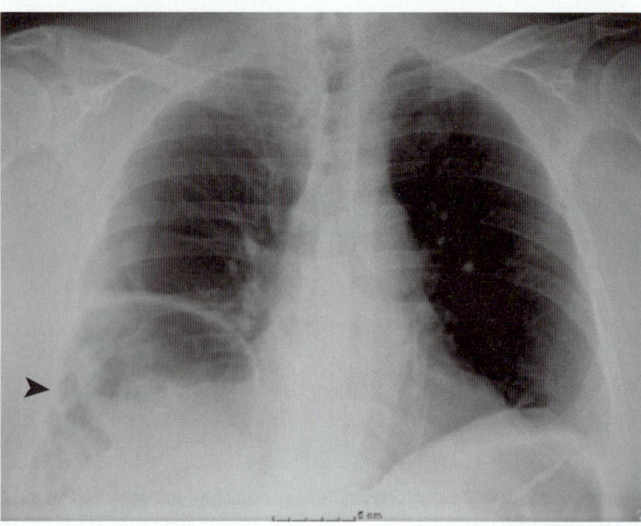

Figure 37.38 Upright chest radiograph shows hepato-diagrammatic interposition of colon in Chilaiditi syndrome (*black arrowhead*).

retroperitoneal organs such as duodenum, ascending or descending colon, and rectum secondary to etiologies such as duodenal ulcer perforation, trauma, neoplasm, diverticulitis, endoscopy, and retroperitoneal surgeries. The extraluminal air is particularly high-volume post endoscopy due to large volume and pressure of the insufflated air. Cranial dissection of the air leads to accumulation in the upper abdominal quadrants, detected on radiographs as lucencies around the kidneys (Fig. 37.39). There can be obscuration of the normal psoas shadow. CT is the modality of choice in detection and differentiation from pneumoperitoneum. It may also demonstrate focal collection of extraluminal fecal matter or "dirty mass," which is a specific indicator of colorectal perforations [36, 37]. The air is usually seen in multiple pockets in the extraperitoneal compartments, occasionally within the ligaments of the peritoneum and in the abdominal wall (Fig. 37.40).

Hemoperitoneum

Pathophysiology and Clinical Features

Hemoperitoneum refers to the presence of blood within the peritoneal cavity. Etiologies are trauma (penetrating and blunt), neoplasm rupture (such as hepatic adenoma, hepatocellular carcinoma, ovarian cysts), rupture of vascular aneurysms, ruptured ectopic pregnancy, hemorrhagic pancreatitis, coagulopathy, and iatrogenic such as post biopsy and surgery [38].

Imaging Features

USG: Sonographic appearance varies from hypoechoic to echogenic fluid in the peritoneal cavity with occasional blood-fluid levels [39].

CT and MRI: CT appearance depends on the age, extent, and location of hemorrhage with following attenuation values [38]:

a. Unclotted extravascular blood: 30–45 HU, except in patients with low hematocrit (attenuation usually less than 30 HU).
b. Clotted blood: 45–70 HU.
c. Bleed more than 48 h and old blood products: Usually less than 30 HU.

Sentinel clot sign refers to higher attenuation of bleed near the organ of injury (Figs. 37.41 and 37.42) [40]. Blood in the peritoneal cavity produces hematocrit effects with layering densities and blood-fluid levels.

On MRI, signal intensity varies as bleed evolves with acute blood (deoxyhemoglobin) isointense on T1 and hyperintense on T2WI. Subacute bleed is T1 hyperintense and T2 hypointense (intracellular methemoglobin) and later T2 hyperintense (extracellular

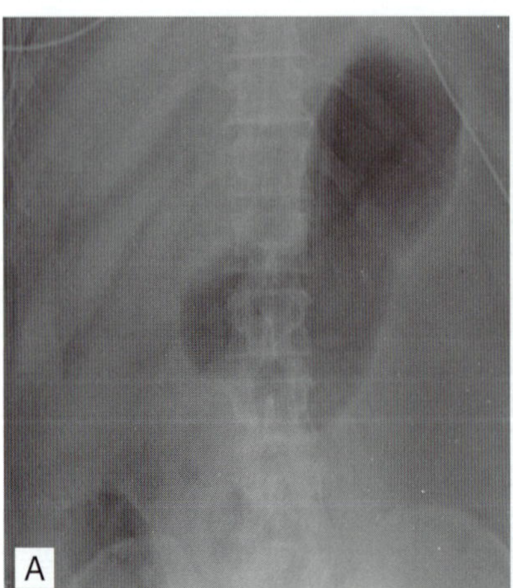

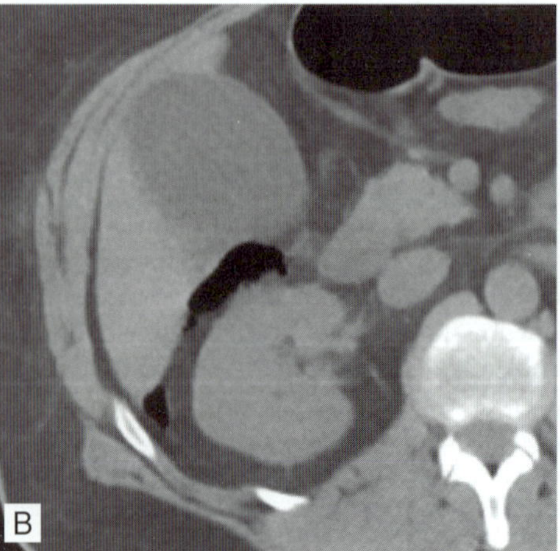

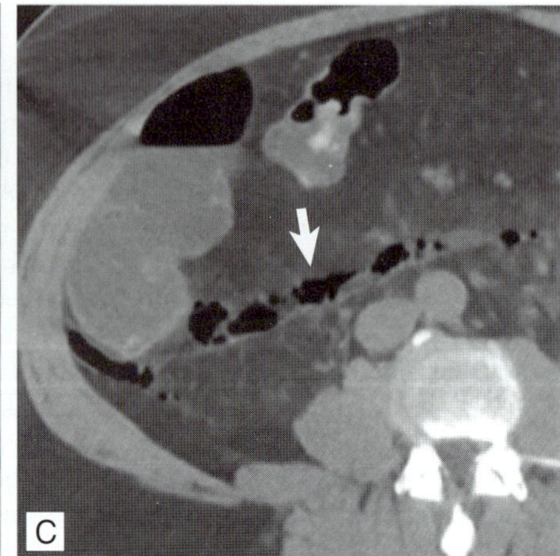

Figure 37.39 (A) Upright abdomen radiograph from a patient with colonic perforation shows pneumoretroperitoneum as curvilinear air in the right renal fossa. (B) Subsequent noncontrast CT demonstrates retroperitoneal air around the kidneys, (C) retromesenteric (*white arrow*), and lateral conal planes.

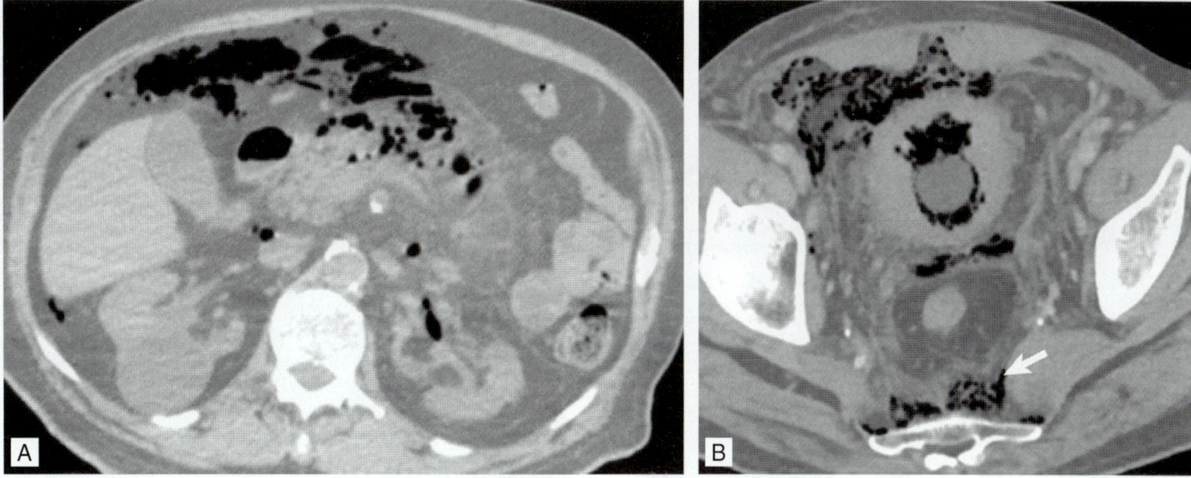

Figure 37.40 Pneumoretroperitoneum. (A) CT abdomen from a patient with complicated sigmoid diverticulitis shows scattered air in the retroperitoneum including peripancreatic fat and greater omentum. (B) CT pelvis from a different patient with extra peritoneal bladder rupture shows scattered air in the pelvic retroperitoneum and presacral space (*white arrow*).

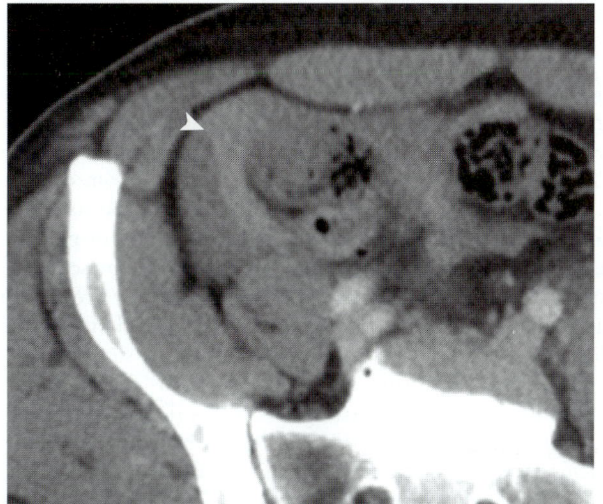

Figure 37.41 Contrast-enhanced axial CT abdomen and pelvis from a 35-year-old man involved in motor vehicular accident shows small volume free fluid in the right lower quadrant, with an associated hyperdense component along the caecum (*white arrowhead*) indicating the sentinel clot. Mesenteric hematoma was detected intraoperatively.

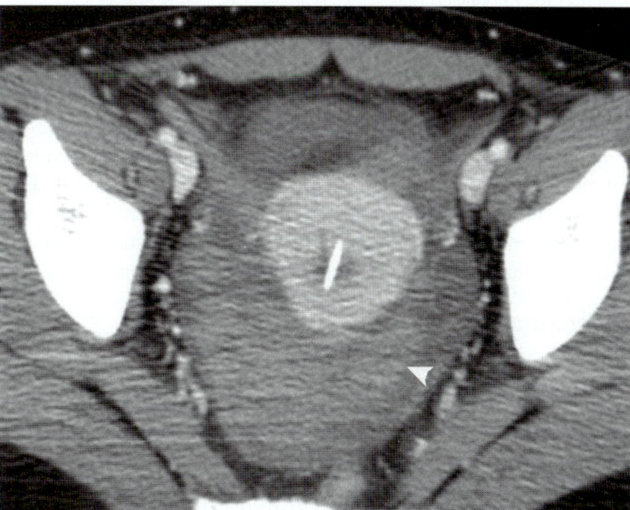

Figure 37.42 Contrast-enhanced axial CT pelvis from a 31-year-old woman with ruptured hemorrhagic ovarian cyst and free fluid in the pelvis. Focal hyperdensity in the rectouterine space indicates the sentinel clot (*white arrowhead*).

methemoglobin). Old hemorrhage is T1 and T2 hypointense (hemosiderin). Hemosiderin and deoxyhemoglobin demonstrate susceptibility dephasing on gradient echo sequences [5].

Neoplastic Disorders

Mesothelioma

Pathophysiology

These are rare tumors derived from the mesothelial cells. Pathological subtypes are the aggressive malignant mesothelioma, and the lower-grade well-differentiated papillary mesothelioma and cystic mesothelioma. Debate and confusion persists about cystic mesothelioma and peritoneal inclusion cyst (described above) being the same entity due to similar reported imaging features and common etiologies such as endometriosis, pelvic inflammatory disease, and prior surgery [41,42]. Asbestos exposure is the etiology in vast majority of malignant mesothelioma, with usually higher exposure level compared to pleural mesotheliomas. Papillary mesothelioma is not linked to asbestos exposure [41–43].

Clinical Features

Malignant mesotheliomas are aggressive neoplasms occurring in older men in fifth to sixth decades. Papillary mesothelioma demonstrates low-grade malignant potential with higher incidence in women of reproductive age [41,42]. Patients present with nonspecific symptoms such as abdominal pain, weight loss, distention, or a palpable mass.

Imaging Features

CT: Malignant mesotheliomas present as dry versus wet types in a focal or diffuse pattern. Dry type demonstrates peritoneal plaques and enhancing masses without associated ascites (Fig. 37.43). Peritoneal plaques do not commonly show calcification unlike the pleural counterpart. Extensive disease presents with rinds of tumor encasing intraabdominal organs. Wet type demonstrates free or loculated ascites and enhancing peritoneal masses indistinguishable

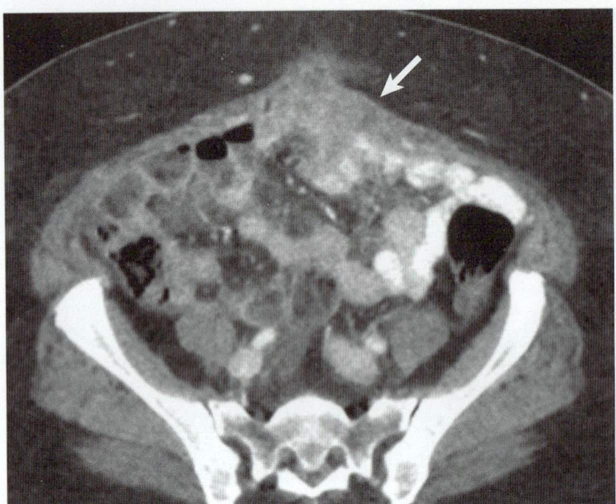

Figure 37.43 Contrast-enhanced axial CT abdomen and pelvis from a 57-year-old woman with peritoneal mesothelioma shows irregular enhancing mass at the level of umbilicus infiltrating into the anterior abdominal wall and the underlying bowel (*white arrow*). Ascites is absent.

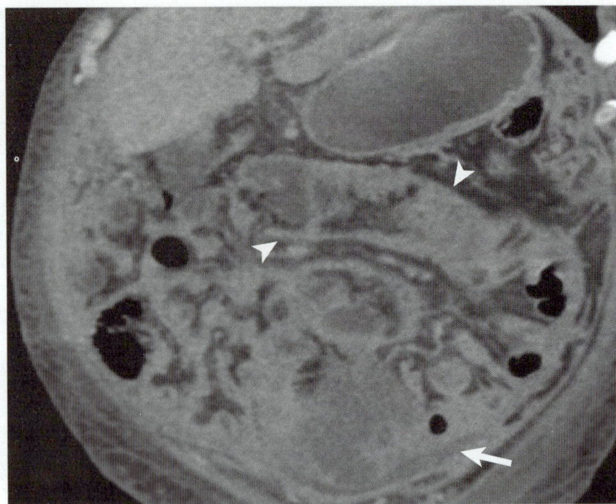

Figure 37.44 Contrast-enhanced coronal CT abdomen and pelvis from a 41-year-old man with peritoneal mesothelioma shows extensive peritoneal disease with multifocal peritoneal plaques, thickening and masses (*white arrow*). Note that only trace loculated ascites is present in the background of large burden peritoneal disease (*white arrow*).

from peritoneal carcinomatosis (Fig. 37.44]. Scalloping of visceral organs may be seen. Nodal metastasis is uncommon [41–43].

Well-differentiated papillary mesothelioma demonstrates multifocal calcified peritoneal plaques without substantial associated soft tissue component. There is predilection for omental involvement with caking and extensive calcification. The absence of adnexal or ovarian mass helps to exclude metastasis from ovarian serous carcinoma [41,42].

Differential Diagnosis

Peritoneal carcinomatosis, lymphomatosis, and tuberculosis [42].

Peritoneal Carcinomatosis

Pathogenesis and Clinical Features

Peritoneal carcinomatosis implies peritoneal metastasis from malignant tumors of the epithelial origin. Common primaries are carcinoma of the ovary, stomach, colon, appendix, pancreas, gallbladder, uterus, breast, and lung [3,4,44]. Metastasis occurs by direct extension or by hematogenous and lymphatic routes, by which tumor cells invade the peritoneal surfaces and grow along the subperitoneal connective tissues. Histological characteristic vary with tumor type [3,45]. Patients can be initially asymptomatic but progressively develop abdomen pain and distention. Nausea, vomiting and constipation accompany bowel obstruction.

Imaging Features

USG: Ascites is the hallmark and is frequently complex with the presence of echoes indicating proteinaceous or hemorrhagic contents or septations. Peritoneal deposits present as hypoechoic nodules or irregular masses. Omental caking involves replacement of omental fat by malignant cells producing echogenic, free floating or fixed masses. Mesentery and small bowel loop are thickened, matted, and fixed with associated adenopathy in extensive disease. Ascites helps in better delineation these findings [14].

CT: It is the modality of choice for staging, restaging, and surveillance. It is imperative to pay dedicated attention to areas of peritoneal fluid stasis such as pouch of Douglas, right subhepatic, subphrenic, paracolic spaces, and right lower quadrant to detect early disease presenting as subtle abnormal peritoneal enhancement, thickening, or nodularity (Fig. 37.45). Patterns of carcinomatosis can be plaque-like, reticulonodular, formation of soft tissue nodules or large masses (Fig. 37.46) [4]. Soft tissue nodules may show calcification, particularly from serous carcinoma from ovary and mucinous carcinoma of the rectum. Mucinous deposits are typically low attenuating (Fig. 37.47) [46]. Infiltration of mesenteric fat leads to a pleated, radiating appearance of the mesentery [3]. Extent of secondary bowel involvement can vary from serosal thickening to endoluminal masses producing bowel obstruction.

MRI: Peritoneal implants have low T1, mixed T2 signal with slow enhancement, increasing in conspicuity after about 5 min of gadolinium administration (Fig. 37.46) [44]. Implants demonstrate diffusion restriction (Fig. 37.48), with the exception of the mucinous variant due to low cellularity [46].

F18-Fluorodeoxy glucose PET: It can complement CT/MRI. Findings vary from focal increased F18-Fluorodeoxy glucose (FDG) uptake to diffuse uptake along the peritoneal and serosal surfaces. Limitations are nonvisualization of subcentimeter nodules, no uptake in mucinous tumor, physiological activity in the bowel obscuring serosal implants, and low spatial resolution [3,44,45].

Differential Diagnosis

Mesothelioma, tuberculosis, peritoneal lymphomatosis, and sarcomatosis [3]. Extensive peritoneal fat saponification and necrosis in pancreatitis can also mimic carcinomatosis (Fig. 37.49).

Peritoneal Carcinomatosis: Pearls to Remember

- Metastasis occurs by direct extension, hematogenous, and lymphatic routes.
- Sonographic findings are complex ascites, hypoechoic nodules, irregular masses, omental caking, mesenteric, and small bowel matting.
- Patterns of carcinomatosis on CECT are plaque-like, reticulonodular, formation of soft tissue nodules and large masses.
- Mucinous deposits are typically low attenuating.
- Peritoneal implants demonstrate slow enhancement with intravenous gadolinium.

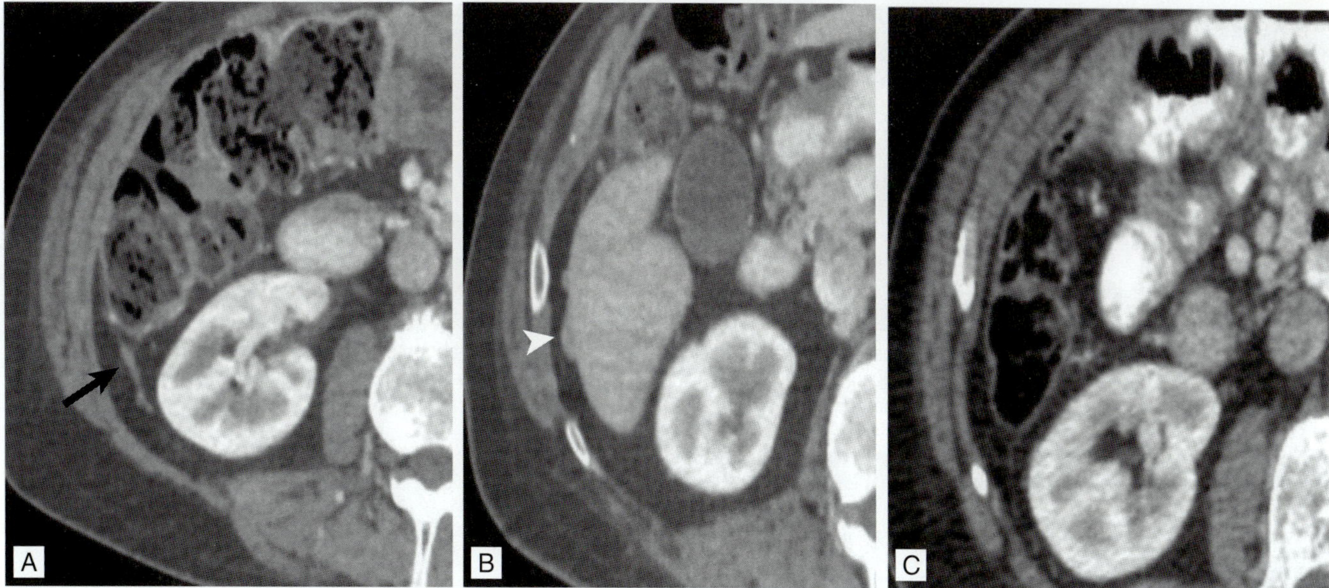

Figure 37.45 Contrast-enhanced axial CT abdomen from a 57-year-old man with colorectal cancer shows early peritoneal carcinomatosis with subtle nodular peritoneal thickening in the right paracolic space (*black arrow*) (A) and tiny implants along the hepatic surface (*white arrowhead*) (B). Note the unremarkable appearance of upper right paracolic space in the same patient 1 year ago (C).

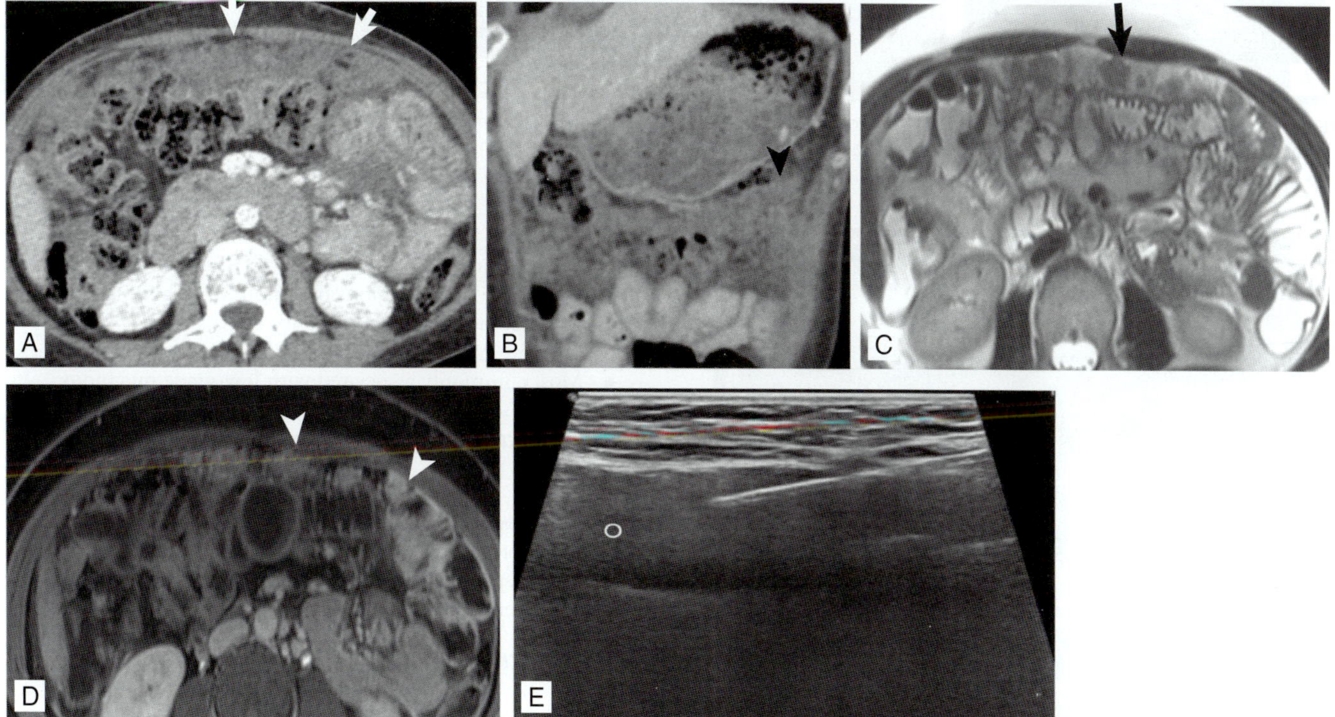

Figure 37.46 A 35-year-old woman with metastatic clear cell ovarian carcinoma. Contrast-enhanced axial and coronal CT abdomen and pelvis demonstrate large burden peritoneal carcinomatosis with numerous soft tissue nodules and omental caking (*white arrow*, *black arrowhead*) (A and B). On single-shot T2WI MR, the peritoneal masses show intermediate signal (*black arrow*) (C), with enhancement on delayed phase T1WI (*white arrowheads*) (D). The patient underwent subsequent USG-guided biopsy of the hypoechoic omental cake (O) (E).

Pseudomyxoma Peritonei

Pathophysiology

Pseudomyxoma is characterized by accumulation of copious mucinous or gelatinous material in the peritoneal cavity. Histological classification divides pseudomyxoma into low- and high-grade variants. Low-grade pseudomyxoma shows pools of mucin, sparse tumor cells with bland cytological features, and generally no invasion of subperitoneum or lymphatics. High-grade pseudomyxoma demonstrates high-grade malignant cells, invasion, and overall poorer prognosis [3,47]. The majority of low-grade pseudomyxoma arises from low-grade mucinous tumor of the appendix, commonly secondary to appendiceal

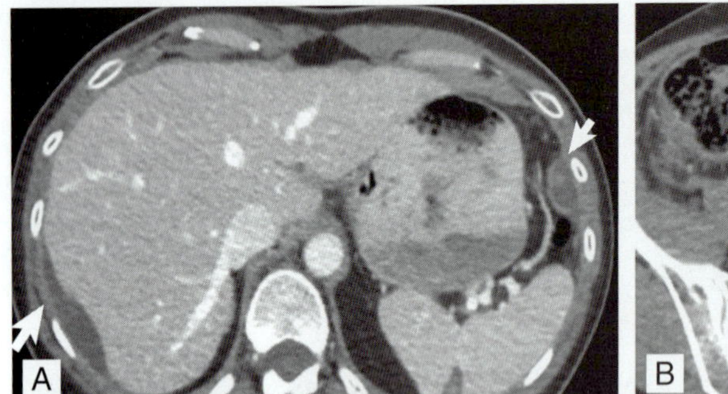

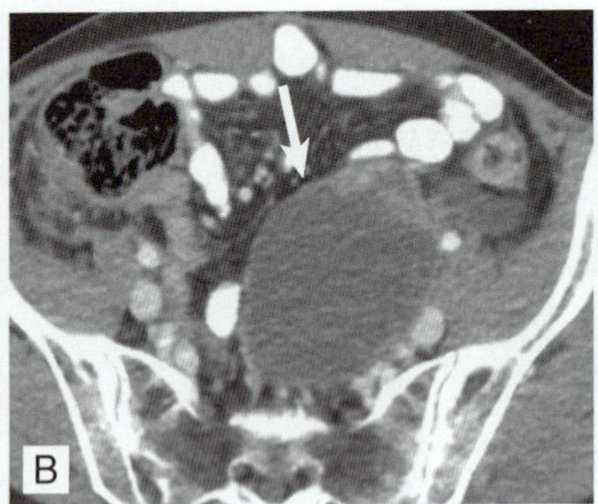

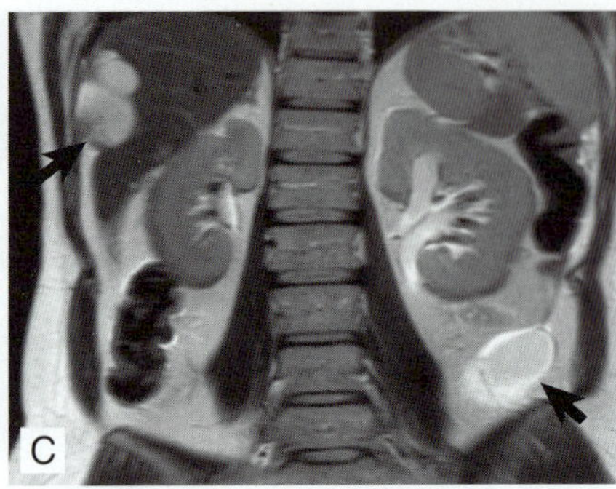

Figure 37.47 A 62-year-old woman with mucinous ovarian cancer. Contrast-enhanced axial CT abdomen and pelvis demonstrate hypoattenuating implants in the right perihepatic space, left upper quadrants (*white arrows*) (A), and left pelvis (*white arrow*) (B). On single-shot T2WI MR, the peritoneal masses show high signal indicative of mucinous composition (*black arrows*) (C).

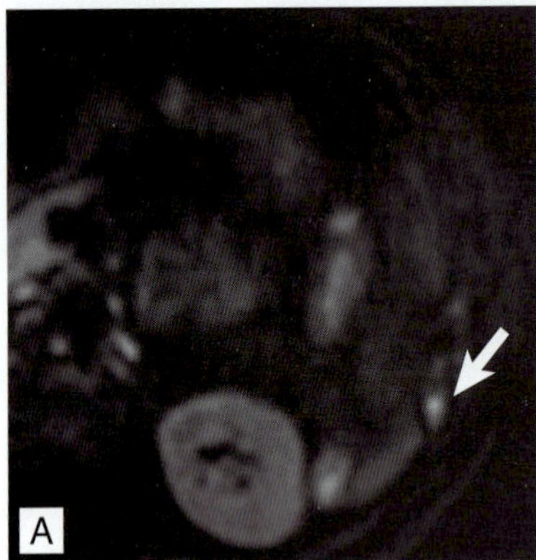

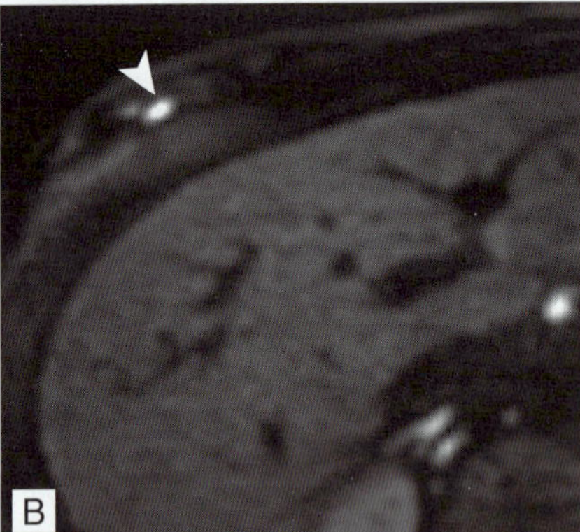

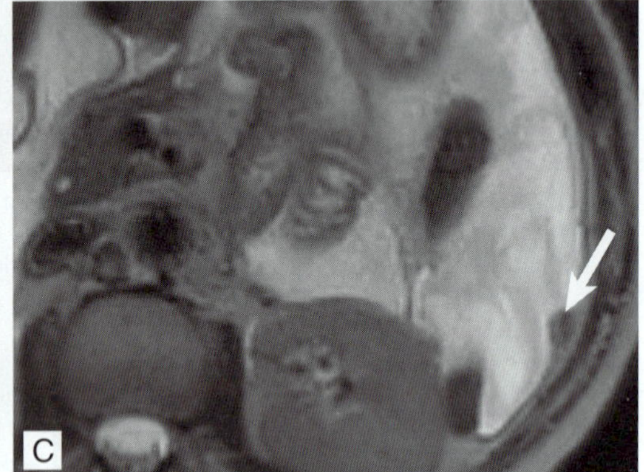

Figure 37.48 A 57-year-old woman with metastatic fallopian tube cancer. Axial diffusion MR abdomen at b = 800 (A, B) demonstrates high signal of small peritoneal implants in left paracolic (*white arrow*) (A) and right perihepatic spaces (*white arrowhead*) (B). Note that the implants are much less conspicuous on single-shot T2WI (*white arrow*) (C).

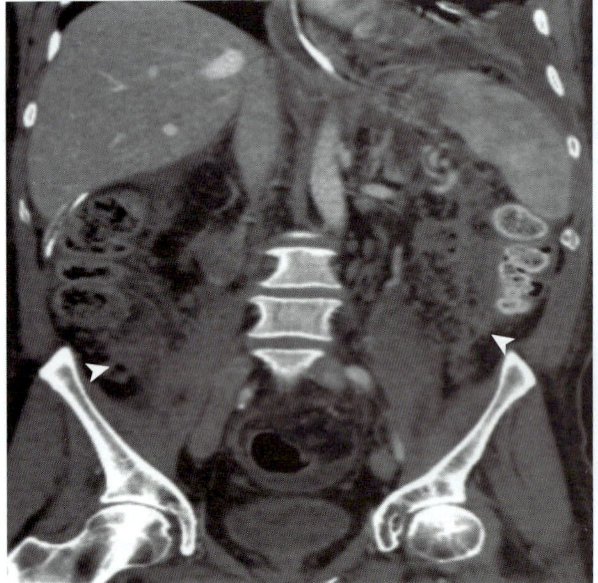

Figure 37.49 Contrast-enhanced coronal CT abdomen and pelvis from a 36-year-old man with necrotizing pancreatitis demonstrates widespread fat saponification mimicking peritoneal carcinomatosis (*white arrowheads*).

rupture. Occurrence with ovarian tumors is proposed secondary to be due to ovarian metastasis from an appendiceal primary rather than primary ovarian tumors [3,48]. High-grade pseudomyxoma is associated with carcinoma of rectum, ovary, stomach, and urachus [47].

Pseudomyxoma Peritonei: Pearls to Remember

- Accumulation of copious mucinous or gelatinous material in the peritoneal cavity.
- Divided into low- and high-grade variants.
- Most commonly associated with low-grade mucinous tumor of the appendix.
- Scalloping of hepatic and splenic surfaces on CT.

On pathology, there is jelly-like covering on the peritoneum with predilection for accumulation under the right diaphragm, right subhepatic spaces, paracolic and rectouterine spaces, with relative sparing of the bowel serosa due to constant displacement by peristalsis [3].

Clinical Features

Incidence is higher in females, presenting with progressive abdominal distention and weight loss.

Imaging Features

Radiograph: Abdominal radiographs simulate the appearance of massive ascites in large volume pseudomyxoma, with centralization of bowel loops, diffuse ground glass opacification, and displacement of properitoneal fat. Faint curvilinear calcifications may be detected [3].

USG: It demonstrates echogenic ascites with nonmobile echoes and septations. Echogenic peritoneal and omental masses can be present [14].

CT and MRI: Mucinous ascites causes scalloping of visceral surfaces of intraperitoneal organs, a diagnostic finding on CT

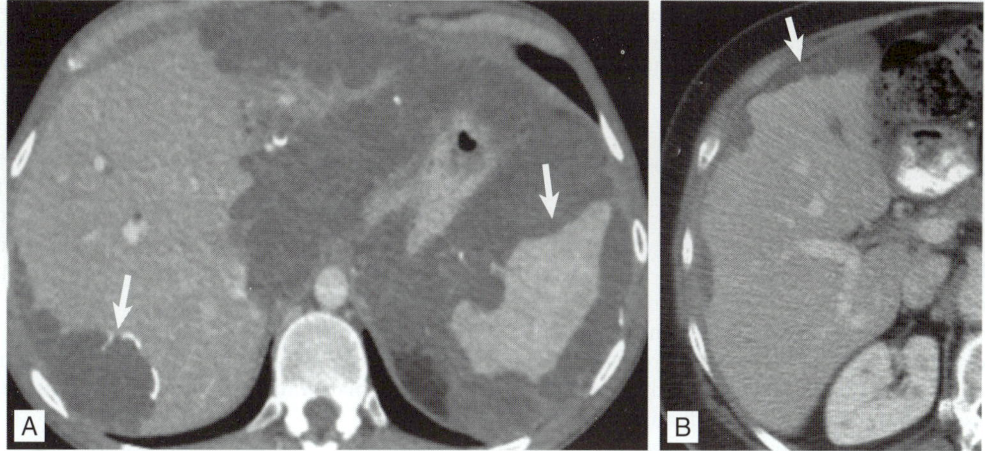

Figure 37.50 (A) Contrast-enhanced axial CT abdomen shows widespread hypoattenuating implants causing scalloping of hepatic and splenic surfaces in pseudomyxoma peritonei (*white arrows*). Few areas of thin curvilinear calcifications are also noted. (B) CT image from a different patient with adenocarcinoma of the appendix with pseudomyxoma shows scalloping of the liver surface (*white arrow*).

best appreciated along the hepatic and splenic surfaces. Low attenuating ascites may show septations, loculations, and occasionally solid elements. Curvilinear calcifications may be present (Fig. 37.50) [3].

Close inspection of appendix is warranted in all cases, which may demonstrate nodular or irregular wall thickening and periappendiceal soft tissues. High-grade pseudomyxoma demonstrates aggressive features such as abdominal and retroperitoneal adenopathy, omental caking, invasion of solid organs, and chest metastasis [3]. The peritoneal implants are hyperintense on T2WI due to mucin.

Desmoid Tumor

Pathophysiology and Clinical Presentation

Desmoids are locally aggressive tumors with a high rate of recurrence and no potential for distant metastasis. The most common location is rectus abdominis and internal oblique musculatures. Other locations include mesentery, extra-abdominal sites such as shoulder, extremities, and chest wall. Risk factors are trauma, prior surgery, pregnancy (pregnancy-associated desmoids almost always involve the abdominal wall), oral contraceptive pills, familial adenomatous polyposis, and Gardner syndromes [49,50]. On microscopy, the tumor contains fascicles of spindle cells and fibroblasts in a dense collagen stroma [49]. There is slightly higher incidence in females in third and fourth decades. Most common presentation is with a palpable mass.

Imaging Features

USG: Presents as a well-circumscribed or infiltrative hypoechoic mass with variable vascularity (Fig. 37.51).

CT and MRI: CECT demonstrates a circumscribed or infiltrative soft tissue mass with variable attenuation and enhancement depending on the degree of necrosis and degeneration. On MRI, the tumor shows variable T2 signal ranging from intermediate or high (due to increased cellularity) as seen in the active or growth phase of the disease (Fig. 37.51), and hypointense (indicating a high degree of collagen) seen in the later plateau or burnt-out phase of the disease, with heterogonous postcontrast enhancement [49,51]. The same tumor may demonstrate both components, which must be identified and reported accordingly.

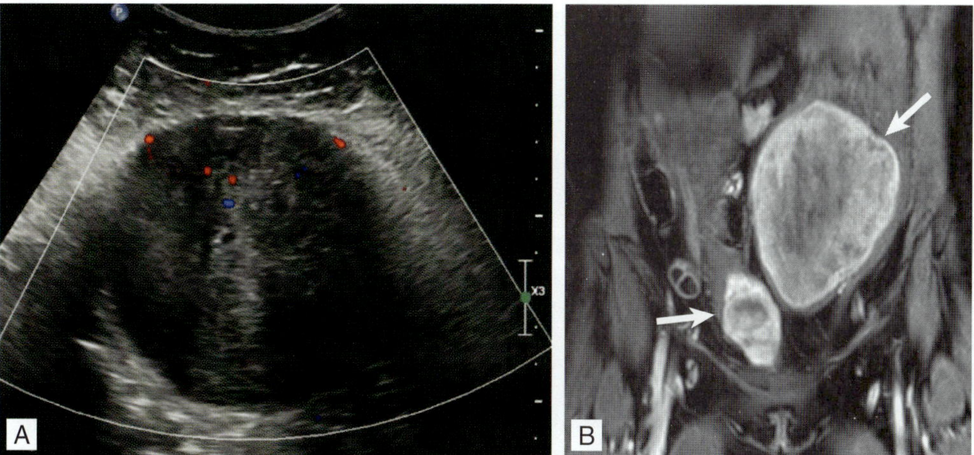

Figure 37.51 (A) Transverse USG of left anterior abdominal wall desmoid shows a circumscribed hypoechoic mass with minimal vascularity. (B) Delayed phase T1WI coronal MRI demonstrates two lobulated anterior abdominal desmoids with heterogeneous enhancement (*white arrows*).

Differential diagnosis: Abdominal wall hematoma, abscess, hernia, sarcoma, and metastasis. When it occurs in the mesentery, carcinoid, lymphoma and sclerosing mesenteritis are in the differential consideration.

Miscellaneous

Peritoneal Inclusion Cyst

Pathogenesis and Clinical Features

Also known as peritoneal pseudocyst or benign cystic mesothelioma, peritoneal inclusion cysts are slow-growing, nonneoplastic cystic pelvic masses occurring exclusively in the premenopausal women [52]. Pathogenesis involves initial peritoneal damage secondary to etiologies such as endometriosis, abdominal or pelvic surgery, trauma and pelvic inflammatory disease, with resultant defective absorption and adhesions. This leads to focal retention and gradual accumulation of ovarian secretion in the pelvis associated with reactive mesothelial proliferation [52,53]. The cyst can be incidental or present with pelvic pain and mass effects.

Imaging Features

USG: It is the mainstay diagnostic exam. Peritoneal inclusion cyst presents as a uni- or multilocular cystic adnexal mass of variable size, ranging from a few millimeters to several centimeters, occupying the entire pelvis or lower abdomen (Fig. 37.52]. The cyst can be anechoic or complex with internal debris. Complex cysts demonstrate internal septations with color flow. The lesion can be unilateral or bilateral [52,53]. Ovaries can be present within or along the wall of the cyst.

CT and MRI: CT depicts a uni or multilocular cystic pelvic mass with fluid attenuation, thin enhancing wall, and with no solid components. Internal septations are often present. On MRI, hemorrhage may be present with variable signal intensities in the cyst components depending on the bleed chronicity (Fig. 37.52) [53].

Differential Diagnosis

Hydrosalpinx, paraovarian cysts, cystic ovarian neoplasms, lymphatic malformations, and loculated ascites [52].

Peritoneal Inclusion Cyst: Pearls to Remember

- Nonneoplastic cystic pelvic masses occurring exclusively in the premenopausal females.
- Etiologies are endometriosis, abdominal or pelvic surgery, trauma and pelvic inflammatory disease.
- Uni or multilocular cystic adnexal mass of variable size.
- On CT, cysts have fluid attenuation, thin enhancing wall, internal septations, and no solid components.

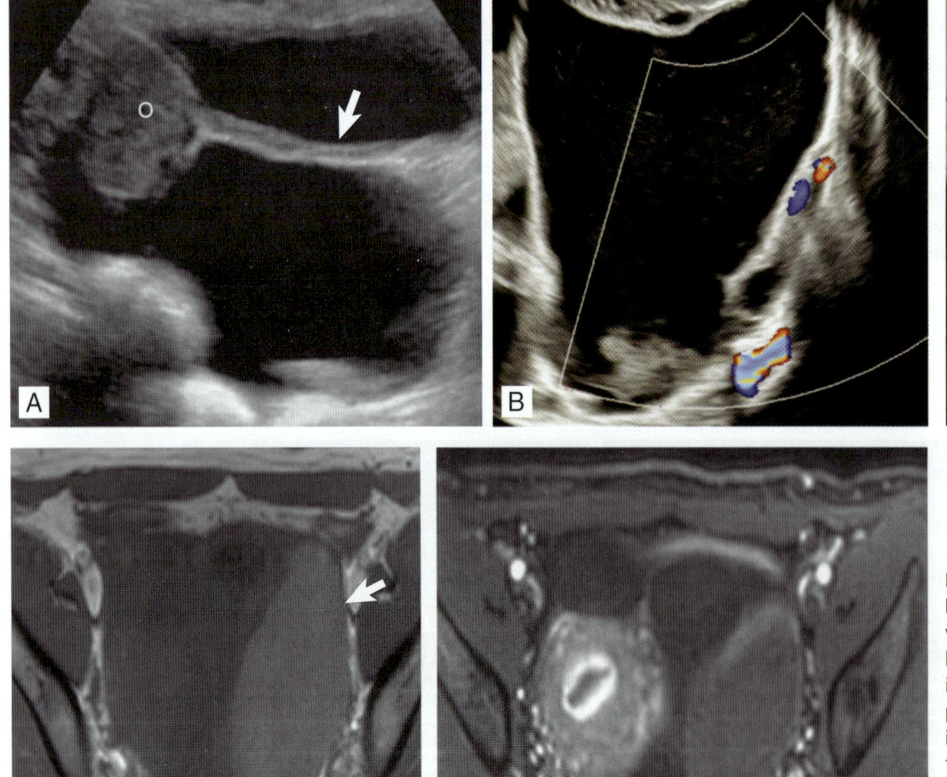

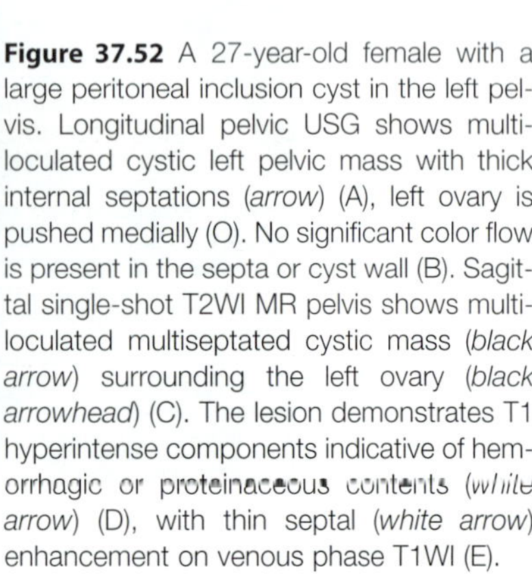

Figure 37.52 A 27-year-old female with a large peritoneal inclusion cyst in the left pelvis. Longitudinal pelvic USG shows multiloculated cystic left pelvic mass with thick internal septations (*arrow*) (A), left ovary is pushed medially (O). No significant color flow is present in the septa or cyst wall (B). Sagittal single-shot T2WI MR pelvis shows multiloculated multiseptated cystic mass (*black arrow*) surrounding the left ovary (*black arrowhead*) (C). The lesion demonstrates T1 hyperintense components indicative of hemorrhagic or proteinaceous contents (*white arrow*) (D), with thin septal (*white arrow*) enhancement on venous phase T1WI (E).

Overall Clinical Approach for Diagnosis of Peritoneal Lesions

A systematic approach for diagnosis of peritoneal masses requires categorization into cystic and solid lesions. Cystic lesions are further divided into simple cysts, complex cysts without solid elements, and lesions with solid elements. All the imaging features need correlation with clinical presentation.

Cystic lesions:

- Simple cystic lesions are enteric cysts, enteric duplication cysts, mesothelial cysts, seromas, and lymphoceles.
- Complex cysts without solid elements include complex duplication cysts, nonpancreatic pseudocyst, lymphatic malformations, peritoneal inclusion cysts, abscess, and hydatid cysts. Peritoneum is an uncommon location for echinococcal cyst. Distinct imaging and clinical features of these lesions are summarized in Table 37.2. Cystic lesions with solid elements include pseudomyxoma and mucinous carcinomatosis. The differentiating feature of pseudomyxoma is scalloping of the liver and splenic surfaces.

Solid lesions: This includes tuberculosis, carcinomatosis, mesothelioma, sclerosing mesenteritis, carcinoid, desmoid and lymph nodal masses/lymphoma.

Retroperitoneum

Anatomy

The retroperitoneum is divided into three major compartments (Fig. 37.53):

Perinephric space: It is a cone-shaped space containing kidneys and adrenal glands. It is bound anteriorly by anterior renal fascia (Gerota's fascia), and posteriorly by posterior renal fascia (fascia of Zuckerkandl). The posterior renal fascia consists of two layers; the anterior layer is continuous with anterior renal fascia. The posterior layer of posterior renal fascia forms the lateral conal fascia, which fuses with peritoneum anteriorly. The perinephric space is usually closed inferiorly by fusion of anterior and posterior renal fascia [1,2].

Anterior pararenal space: It is present between the posterior surface of the parietal peritoneum and the anterior renal fascia. The space contains the pancreas, duodenum, ascending, and descending colon [2].

Posterior pararenal space: It is situated between posterior renal fascia and fascia transversalis. The space contains only fat and is continuous with the properitoneal fat [1,2].

- The small midline space between the perinephric spaces encloses the aorta and Inferior Vena Cava (IVC) and is contiguous superiorly with the posterior mediastinum.

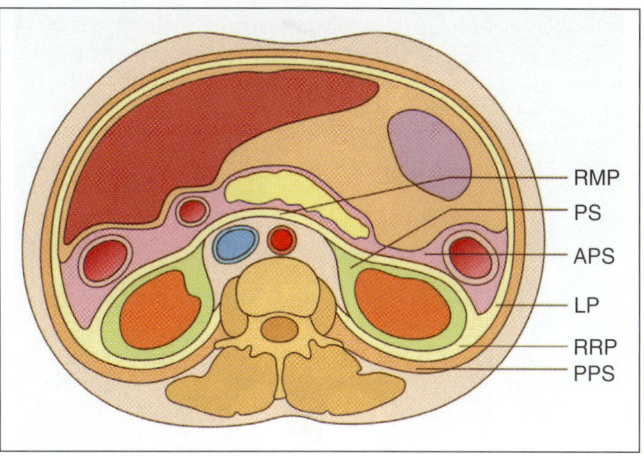

Figure 37.53 Illustration demonstrating the retroperitoneal anatomy. *RMP*: Retromesenteric plane, *PS*: Perirenal space, *APS*: Anterior pararenal space, *LP*: Lateral conal plane, *RRP*: Retrorenal plane, *PPS*: Posterior pararenal space.

- The intervening spaces between the three compartments form the interfascial planes, consisting of retromesenteric plane, retrorenal plane, and lateral conal plane (Fig. 37.53). These expansile planes serve as additional routes of spread of pathologies such as tumor and infection [54].
- The retromesenteric and retrorenal planes communicate inferiorly with the pelvic retroperitoneum; pathological processes can also spread across the midline via retromesenteric space. Lateral conal plane is present between the layers of the lateral conal fascia. All three interfascial planes communicate at the fascial trifurcation [1].
- Grey turner sign in acute pancreatitis (manifesting as flank discoloration) is caused by spread of pancreatic enzymes from anterior pararenal to posterior pararenal space and then to lateral edge of the quadratus lumborum [55].

Nonneoplastic Disorder

Retroperitoneal Fibrosis

Pathophysiology: Retroperitoneal fibrosis is rare spectrum of disorders characterized by aberrant fibrotic reaction causing encasement of the retroperitoneal organs. It is classified into primary or idiopathic (two-third of cases) and secondary forms. It is also divided into benign and malignant subtypes depending on the prognosis, with malignant type commonly associated with retroperitoneal neoplasms [56].

Etiologies of secondary retroperitoneal fibrosis are drugs such as ergot, hydralazine, beta-blockers, methyldopa, and neoplasms such as lymphoma, sarcoma and carcinoid, infections (histoplasmosis,

TABLE 37.2 Imaging and Clinical Features of Complex Cystic Peritoneal Lesions

Complex Duplication Cyst	Nonpancreatic Pseudocyst	Lymphatic Malformation	Peritoneal Inclusion Cysts	Abscess
▪ Thick walled, containing bowel layers on USG ▪ Commonly incidental	▪ Fat-fluid levels ▪ Commonly incidental	▪ Multilocular multiseptated insinuating masses ▪ Mesentery is the most common location in the abdomen	▪ Multilocular multiseptated masses in pelvis ▪ Exclusively seen in premenopausal females with history of endometriosis, surgery, trauma and pelvic inflammatory disease	▪ Rim enhancement, the presence of air ▪ Usually associated with additional features of peritonitis and initiating etiology such as diverticulitis, appendicitis, pelvic inflammatory disease

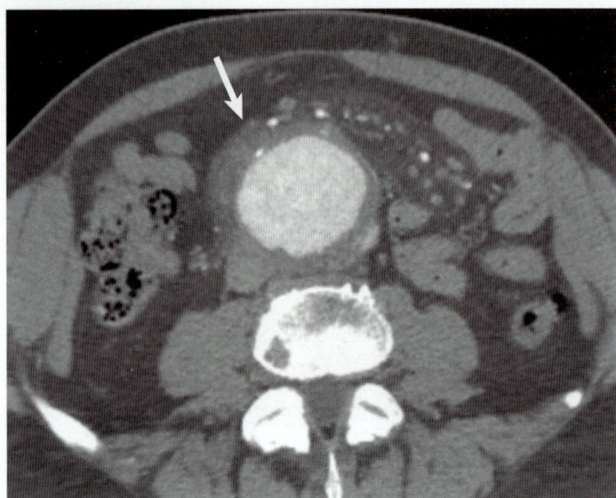

Figure 37.54 Contrast-enhanced axial CT abdomen from a 65-year-old woman with abdominal aortic aneurysm shows perianeurysmal retroperitoneal fibrosis (*white arrow*).

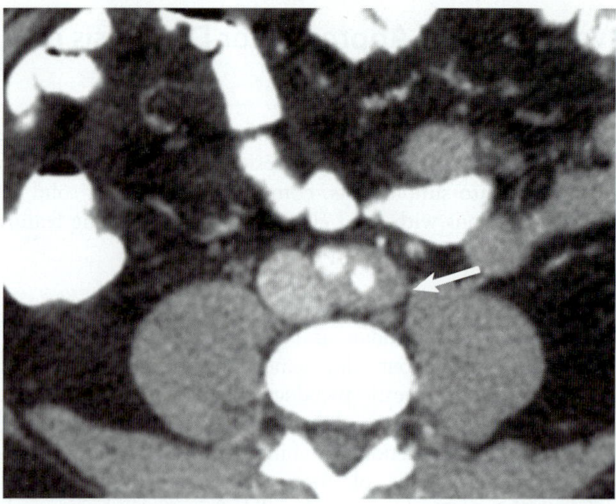

Figure 37.55 Contrast-enhanced axial CT abdomen from a 37-year-old man with idiopathic retroperitoneal fibrosis shows soft tissue encasing the common iliac arteries (*white arrow*).

tuberculosis), Ig4 disease, radiation, and hemorrhage [56,57]. Perianeurysmal retroperitoneal fibrosis, as a subtype of retroperitoneal fibrosis spectrum, is associated with inflammatory aortic aneurysms (Fig. 37.54) [58].

Clinical features: Incidence is higher in males. Nonspecific presentation includes malaise, weight loss, pain, fevers, and features of renal failure secondary to obstructive uropathy [56,59].

Imaging Features

USG: It has poor sensitivity to visualize retroperitoneal soft tissues, hence the utility is limited to detect and follow up hydronephrosis.

CT: It is the modality of choice to evaluate the extent of disease and complications. Retroperitoneal fibrosis presents as ill-defined soft tissue encroaching and encasing retroperitoneal structures such as ureters, aorta, IVC and kidneys depending on the disease severity; with initial epicenter of the disease typically located near the distal aortic bifurcation or proximal iliac arteries (Fig. 37.55) [59]. The degree of enhancement varies with the stage, with avid enhancement seen in early disease and minimal to no enhancement in chronic fibrosis. The soft tissue is present anterior and lateral to the aorta, relatively sparing the posterior aspect and without associated aortic displacement; unlike lymphomas. Concomitant reactive retroperitoneal adenopathy can be present [56,59].

MRI: It has better tissue characterization, with fibrosis demonstrating low signal on T1WI. On T2WI, signal intensity varies

Retroperitoneal Fibrosis: Pearls to Remember

- Spectrum of disorders characterized by aberrant fibrotic reaction causing encasement of the retroperitoneal organs.
- On CECT, ill-defined soft tissue encroaching and encasing retroperitoneal structures such as ureters, aorta, IVC, and kidneys.
- Avid enhancement in early disease and minimal to no enhancement in chronic fibrosis.
- The soft tissue is present anterior and lateral to the aorta, relatively sparing the posterior aspect and without aortic displacement.

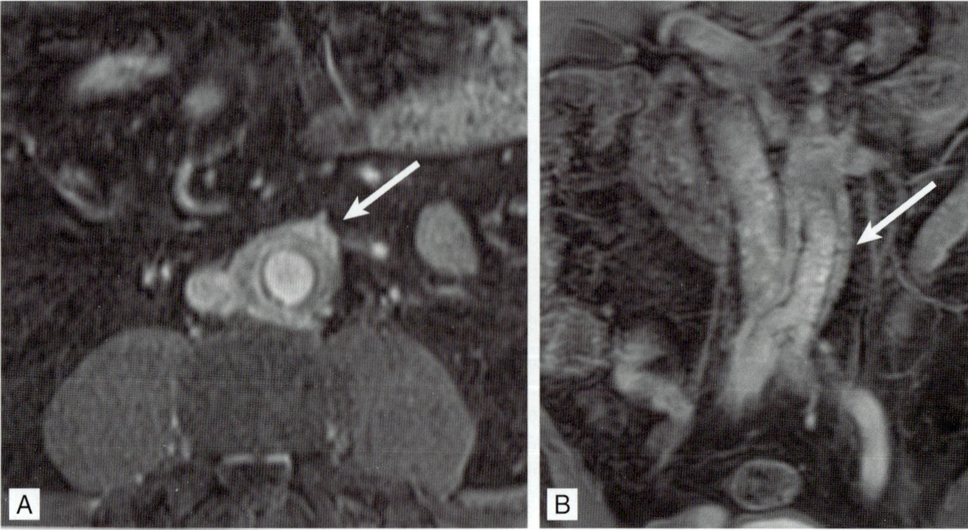

Figure 37.56 Delayed phase axial and coronal T1WI MR abdomen and pelvis demonstrate ill-defined enhancing soft tissue encasing the distal abdominal aorta in active idiopathic retroperitoneal fibrosis (*white arrow*) (A and B).

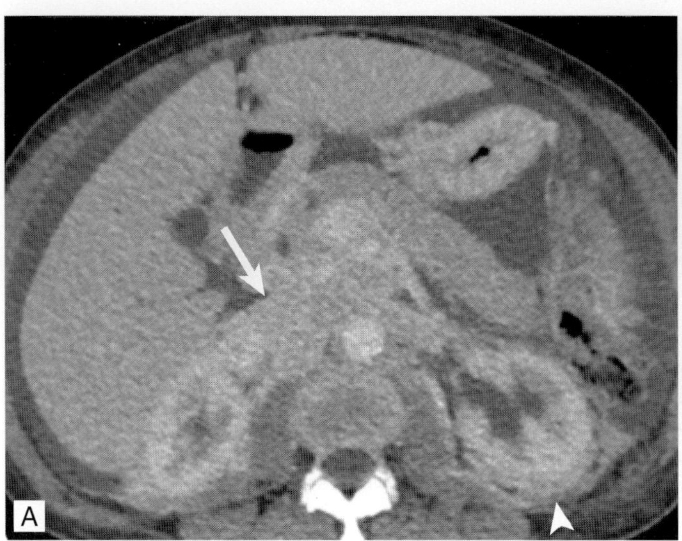

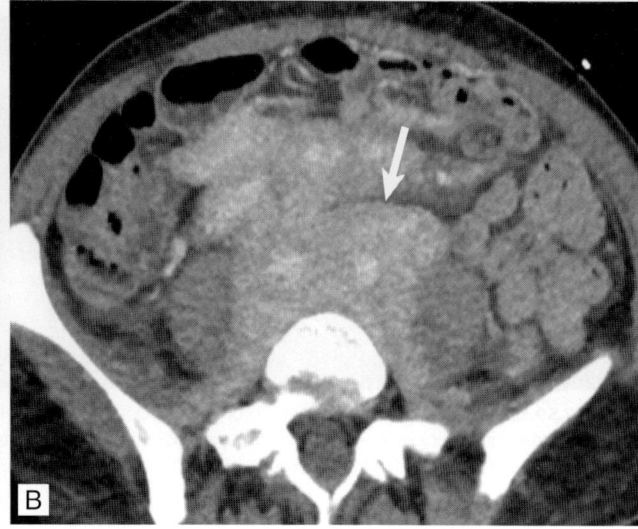

Figure 37.57 Contrast-enhanced axial CT abdomen and pelvis from a 56-year-old woman with breast cancer demonstrates enhancing retroperitoneal soft tissue metastasis simulating retroperitoneal fibrosis (*white arrow*) (A and B). Note that the soft tissue encases both kidneys (*white arrowhead*), aorta, and extends into the pelvic retroperitoneum.

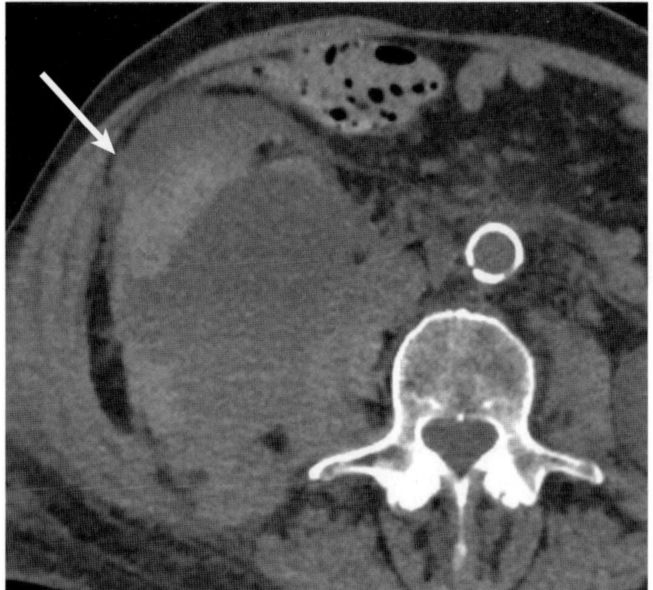

Figure 37.58 Noncontrast axial CT abdomen shows a large right retroperitoneal hematoma, with mixed densities, blood-fluid levels, and hyperdense components indicative of active bleed (*white arrow*).

with the stage of fibrosis; early fibrosis shows high T2 signal due to edema and late fibrosis shows T2 dark signal. The degree of contrast enhancement usually parallels T2 signal, with avid enhancement in active inflammation (Fig. 37.56) [56,59].
Differential diagnosis: Lymphoma, retroperitoneal sarcoma, tuberculosis, and metastasis (Fig. 37.57).

Retroperitoneal Bleed

Etiologies of retroperitoneal bleed are trauma, blood dyscrasias, anticoagulation therapy, rupture of abdominal aortic aneurysm, and surgery. Appearance varies with the bleed chronicity, with acute and subacute blood hyperdense on CT (Fig. 37.58). Chronic hematoma has low attenuation. Major differential consideration is retroperitoneal sarcoma; with bleed characterized by temporal evolution/resolution time [60].

Neoplastic Disorder

Retroperitoneal Liposarcomas

Pathophysiology and clinical features: These are the most common primary malignant retroperitoneal tumors of mesenchymal origin. Retroperitoneal liposarcomas are classified into (1) Well differentiated with or without dedifferentiation, (2) myxoid and round cell, and (3) pleomorphic subtypes. Well-differentiated liposarcomas are the most common subtypes [61]. Incidence is higher in fifth to sixth decades with no specific sex predilection. The tumor is frequently asymptomatic, often detected as a large mass [60,61].

Imaging Features

CT and MRI: Well-differentiated liposarcomas present as lobulated fat–containing retroperitoneal masses, with typically large volume fat composition (Fig. 37.59). The mass demonstrates septae and may have solid components <1 cm in size [62]. Fat component has high signal on T1WI and low signal on T2WI. Well-differentiated liposarcomas almost always recur after resection, and may undergo dedifferentiation over time. Unlike the former, dedifferentiated liposarcomas have metastatic potential. They can be identified on imaging by the presence of nodular nonlipomatous component >1 cm. Nonfatty areas are hypointense on T1WI and iso to hyperintense on T2WI. Myxoid liposarcoma is a more aggressive tumor presenting as a hypoattenuating mass due to its myxoid component. On MRI, the tumor shows high T2 signal with a variable degree of contrast enhancement (Fig. 37.60) [61]. Macroscopic fat forms a relatively small component of the tumor.

Pleomorphic liposarcoma is the most aggressive subtype presenting as a predominantly nonlipogenic mass with none or little fat. The tumor shows extensive necrosis and hemorrhage due to anaplasia [63]. Unlike the other subtypes that may be prospectively diagnosed on imaging, pleomorphic liposarcoma cannot be differentiated radiologically from other soft tissue sarcomas in most cases.
Differential diagnosis: Fat containing retroperitoneal lesions such as lipoma, angiomyolipoma, teratoma, myelolipoma and sarcomas such as leiomyosarcoma [61,64].

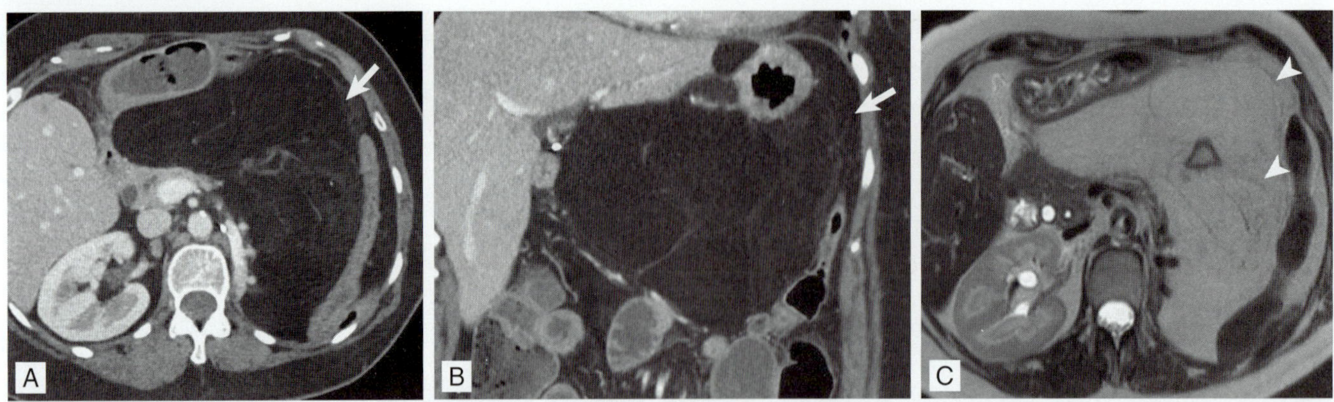

Figure 37.59 Contrast-enhanced axial and coronal CT abdomen shows a large, well-differentiated left retroperitoneal sarcoma displacing the small bowel loops and descending colon (A and B). The mass demonstrates fat attenuation without solid components or calcifications. On single-shot T2 W MR, the mass shows fat signal with thin internal septations (*white arrowheads*) (C). Note that the patient status is post left nephrectomy.

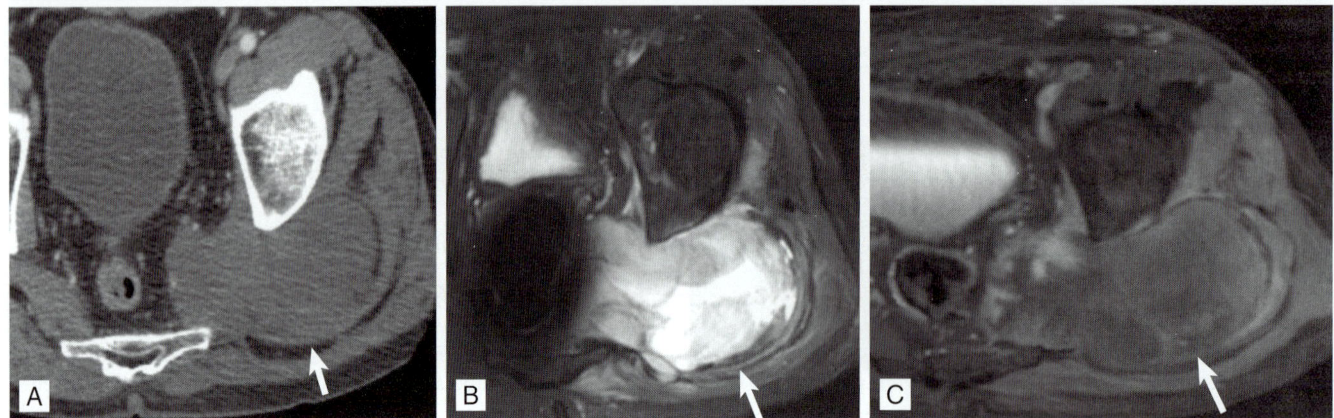

Figure 37.60 Contrast-enhanced axial CT pelvis (A) from a 42-year-old man with biopsy-proven left pelvic myxoid liposarcoma of the left gluteal region (*white arrow*) (A). The lobulated, hypoattenuating mass is extending into the greater sciatic foramen. On MR, the mass is T2 hyperintense (B), and shows heterogeneous enhancement on venous phase T1WI (C).

Leiomyosarcoma

Pathophysiology and clinical features: Retroperitoneal leiomyosarcoma is a malignant neoplasm with smooth muscle differentiation. The tumor originates from smooth muscle of the retroperitoneum or more commonly from the wall of large vasculature such as IVC and renal veins. On histology, the tumor is composed of fascicles of spindle cells with occasional fibrosis, myxoid change, or coagulative necrosis. Cellular atypia and mitotic figures are common. Most affected patients are in the fifth or sixth decades with a female predilection. The mass can be asymptomatic, which leads to the formation of large masses till diagnosis, or present with compressive symptoms due to pain. Intraluminal tumors tend to present early due to associated IVC obstruction and symptoms of the Budd Chiari syndrome such as hepatomegaly, jaundice, ascites, and leg edema [65].

Imaging Features

USG: USG demonstrates lobulated, heterogeneous solid mass with scattered cystic areas and internal vascularity. Intravascular tumor shows expansile growth and best appreciated with color Doppler [65].

CT: The tumor is typically large lobulated solid mass with occasional scattered cystic components, areas of necrosis, and heterogeneous contrast enhancement (Fig. 37.61). Calcifications are uncommon. Perirenal and posterior pararenal spaces are common locations for extravascular tumors. Intravascular tumors can be classified based on the location as present caudal to renal vein (segment 1), caudal to hepatic veins (segment 2, most common), and cranial to the hepatic veins (segment 3, least common). Bland thrombus can be present (Fig. 37.62). The spread is by direct invasion to adjacent organs such as kidneys, adrenals, pancreas, or stomach or by distant metastasis. Sites of metastasis include the lungs (most common), peritoneum, liver, bones and lymph nodes, with overall higher incidence in intravascular tumors due to hematogenous dissemination [65–67].

MRI: The solid tumor components demonstrate low to iso T1 and high T2 signal with heterogeneous contrast enhancement. Associated hemorrhage can impart high T1 signal to the tumor components. Black blood imaging helps in delineation of intravascular tumors, which are usually hyperintense, and to evaluate the tumor extent [66].

Differential diagnosis: Major differentials include other retroperitoneal neoplasms such as liposarcoma, lymphoma, metastasis, germ cell, and neurogenic tumors. Hematoma and retroperitoneal fibrosis are the most common nonneoplastic entities in the differential consideration [65].

Lymphomas

Retroperitoneum is a common site of involvement by both Hodgkin and non-Hodgkin lymphomas. Findings on CECT are para-aortic lymphadenopathy and mass formation with mild homogenous

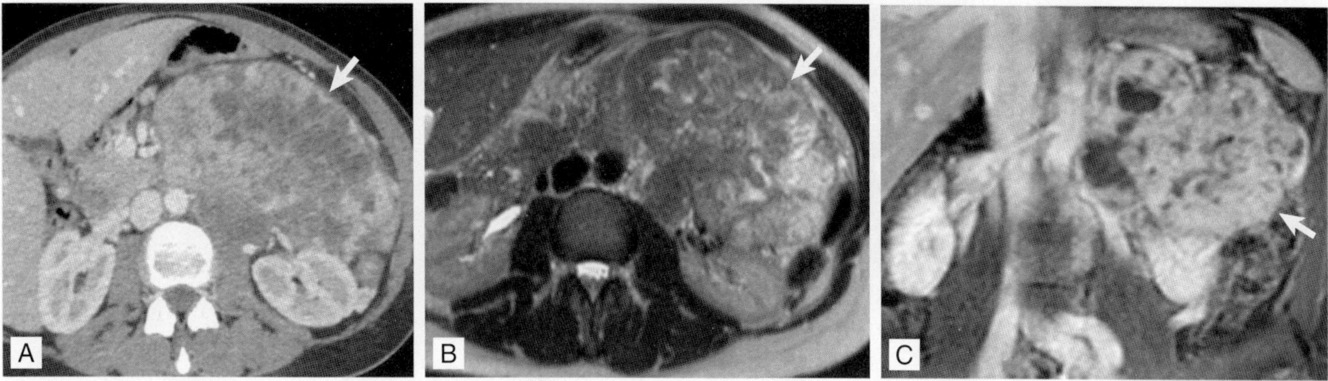

Figure 37.61 Contrast-enhanced axial CT abdomen demonstrates retroperitoneal leiomyosarcoma as a large heterogeneous solid mass with scattered cystic areas (*white arrow*) (A). The mass is encasing the left renal vasculatures and extending along the right paraspinal musculature. On MRI, the mass shows hyperintense cystic areas on T2 WI (B), with heterogeneous post contrast enhancement (C).

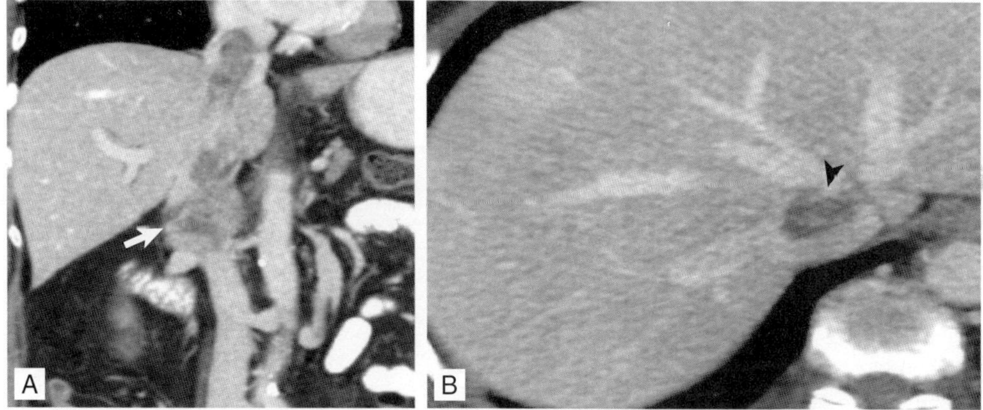

Figure 37.62 (A) Contrast-enhanced coronal CT abdomen demonstrates IVC leiomyosarcoma as heterogeneously enhancing, expansile mass within the IVC (*white arrow*). (B) Axial CT image shows a bland thrombus present superior to the mass in the intrahepatic IVC segment (*black arrowhead*).

enhancement. Calcification and necrosis are usually present post-treatment. Floating aorta sign refers to anterior displacement of aorta and IVC by extensive retroperitoneal adenopathy (Fig. 37.63). On MRI, lymphomatous masses are T1 isointense, iso to hyperintense on T2WI, with moderate homogenous or heterogeneous enhancement [60].

Neurogenic Tumor

These are tumors of variable malignant potential with higher incidence in younger age groups. The tumors can arise from nerve sheath (schwannoma, neurofibroma, malignant nerve sheath tumors), ganglionic (ganglioneuroma, neuroblastoma), and paraganglionic cells (paraganglioma, pheochromocytoma) [60]. Schwannomas represent 6% of retroperitoneal neoplasms. These are well-defined masses with homogenous (Fig. 37.64), or heterogeneous attenuation and variable enhancement. Internal calcifications and cystic changes may be present [60,68].

Teratomas

These are germ cell tumor with higher incidence in females and early adulthood. Classified into benign or malignant types; benign teratoma is further divided into mature and immature subtypes. Mature teratoma (also known as dermoid cyst) is predominately cystic and contains fat with sometimes fat-fluid level, cystic changes (Fig. 37.65), calcifications and occasional tooth formation. Differential diagnosis includes fetus *in fetu,* a rare anomaly occurring secondary to abnormal embryogenesis in diamniotic, monochorionic twins in which a vertebrate fetus is enclosed within the normally developing fetus (Fig. 37.66). It presents as a calcified mass with some identifiable fetal components such as vertebral column and limbs on CT. Retroperitoneum serves as the most common location for this anomaly

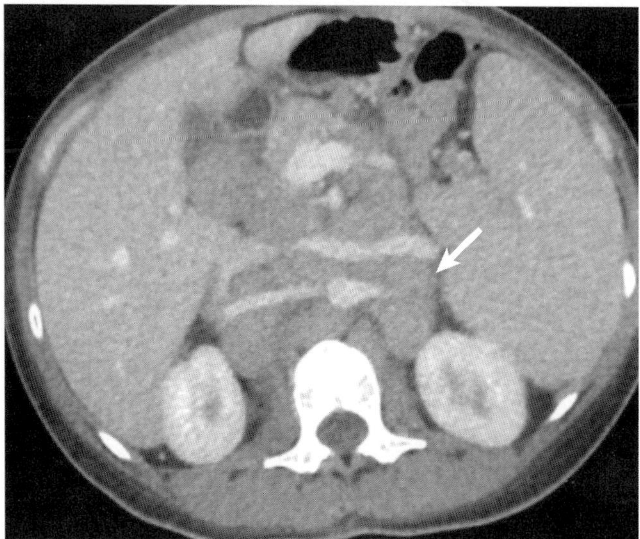

Figure 37.63 Contrast-enhanced axial CT abdomen from a 36-year-old man with non-Hodgkin's lymphoma shows bulky retroperitoneal adenopathy (*white arrow*). The adenopathy is lifting the abdominal aorta producing "floating aorta sign".

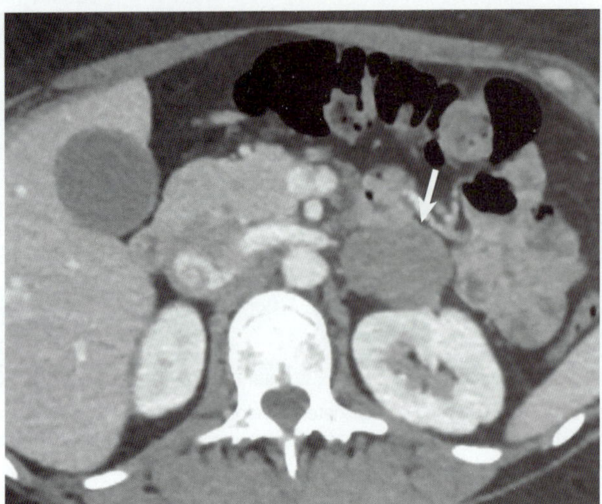

Figure 37.64 Contrast-enhanced axial CT abdomen from a 31-year-old-female with left retroperitoneal Schwannoma (*white arrow*). The circumscribed solid mass demonstrates mild homogenous enhancement.

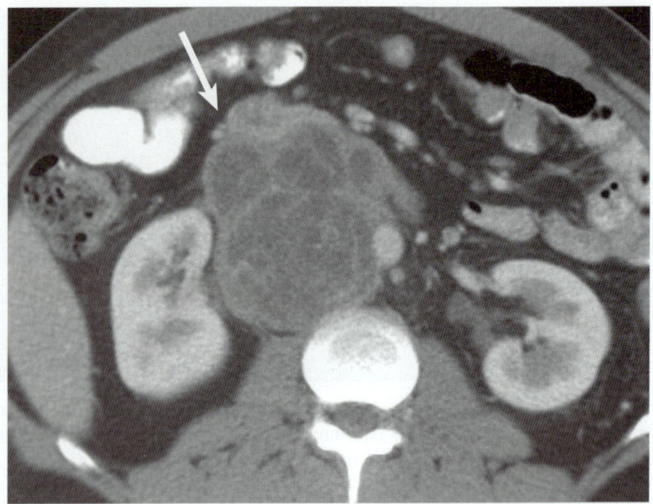

Figure 37.65 Contrast-enhanced axial CT abdomen from a 56-year-old woman with right retroperitoneal mature teratoma (*white arrow*). The lobulated mass demonstrates multifocal cystic areas, heterogeneous enhancement, and is inseparable from the aorta.

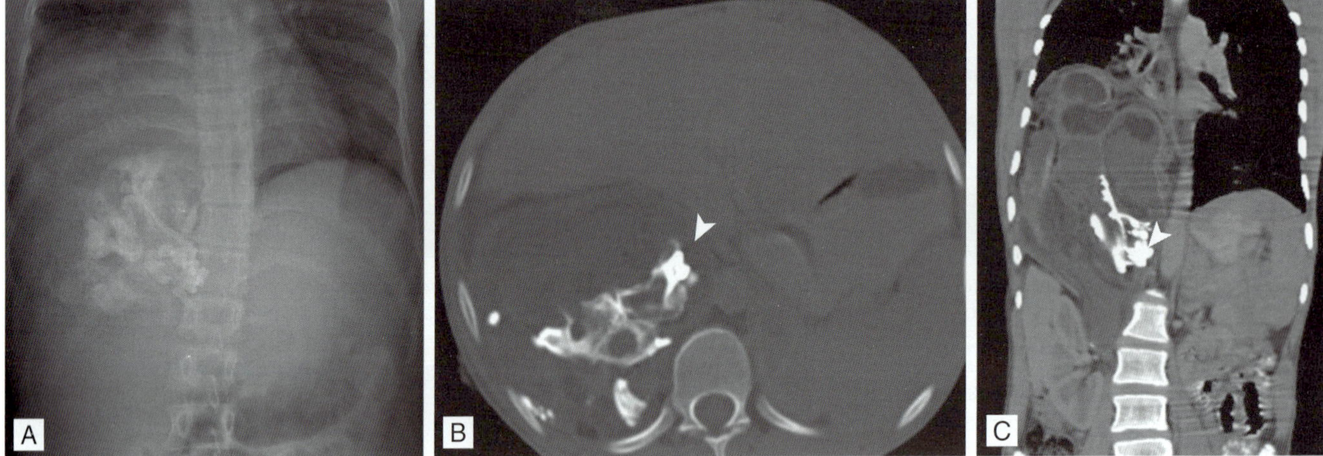

Figure 37.66 Patient with fetus *in fetu*. On abdominal radiograph, there is elevation of the right diaphragm with an ill-defined soft tissue density and coarse calcifications in right upper quadrant (A). Subsequent CT abdomen shows a large mass in the right retroperitoneum with internal coarse calcifications, tooth formation, and fat densities in fetus *in fetu* (*white arrowhead*) (B and C). (*Source:* Chadha M, Aggarwal B. Foetus in Foetus: CT findings in two cases; Abdominal Imaging 27:595-599, September 2002.)

[69]. Immature teratomas are commonly solid. Malignant transformation is associated with invasion of adjacent organs and vascular involvement; however, incidence is low in the retroperitoneum [60].

Abdominal Wall

Anatomy: The layers of the abdominal wall (from superficial to deep) include the skin, subcutaneous fat, deep subcutaneous membranous tissue (also known as Scarpa fascia), muscle layer, extraperitoneal fat, and parietal peritoneum. The muscle layer can be further divided into anterior, lateral, and posterior compartments (Fig. 37.67). Anterior compartment includes two longitudinally oriented rectus abdominis muscles extending from the xiphisternum to pubis. Lateral compartment (from superficial to deep) consists of external oblique, internal oblique, and transverse abdominis muscles. Rectus abdominis is enclosed by a fascial sheath formed by aponeurosis of three lateral abdominis muscles; this fascial sheath is deficient posteriorly below the arcuate line. Curvilinear tendinous intersection at the junction of the anterior and lateral muscle groups forms the semilunar line. The posterior compartment includes the latissimus dorsi, quadratus lumborum, and erector spinae muscles; these muscle groups are lined by the thoracolumbar fascia. The major vascular supply of the anterior abdominal wall is through the superior and inferior epigastric vessels running along the posterior border of rectus abdominis [70].

Abdominal Wall Hernia

Pathophysiology and clinical features: Abdominal wall hernias (also known as external hernia) are abnormal protrusions of intrabdominal contents through the weakened musculofascial layers. They can be congenital or acquired. Their incidence is higher in males, with highest frequency being of inguinal hernias. Females

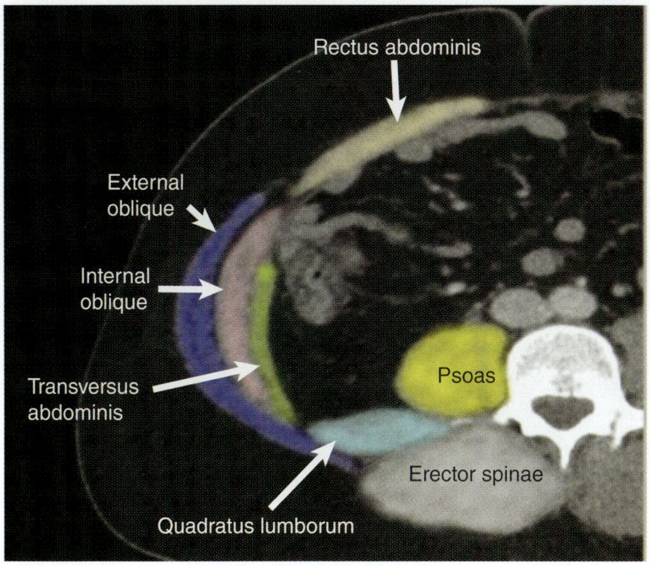

Figure 37.67 Axial CT abdomen with colored illustration of the abdominal wall anatomy.

have an increased tendency to develop femoral and umbilical hernias due to anatomic predispositions [71].

The diagnosis is made on clinical examination in patients presenting with abdominal bulge, mostly accompanied with pain and discomfort that increases with straining or cough. Clinical detection is limited in patients with obesity and in postoperative abdomen, warranting need for imaging.

Imaging techniques

USG: It is the modality of choice for detection, size measurement of the defect, delineation of the hernia contents, and real-time evaluation of reducibility and incarceration. Color Doppler helps in detection of flow abnormalities related to bowel ischemia [71].

CT: CT helps in preoperative planning, detection of hernia complications, in obese and postsurgical patients. Applications of maneuvers such as Valsalva or straining and scanning in decubitus positions aid in detection and evaluation of small hernias. CT also helps to distinguish hernia from other abdominal wall pathologies such neoplastic masses and hematomas.

Classification of Abdominal Wall Hernias

1. *Groin hernias*: Inguinal (direct and indirect) and femoral hernia.
   a. Indirect inguinal hernia: Most common subtype involving herniation through the internal inguinal ring via a patent process vaginalis. The hernia sac is present lateral to the inferior epigastric vessels (Fig. 37.68). Inguinal hernia containing appendix is known as Amyand's hernia (Fig. 37.69). Littre hernia is inguinal hernia containing Meckel's diverticulum. Pantaloon hernia is a combination of adjacent hernia sacs of inguinal and femoral regions [72–74].
   b. Direct inguinal hernia: Involves herniation through the posterior wall of inguinal canal due to acquired weakness in the transversalis fascia. The sac is present medial to the inferior epigastric vessels (Fig. 37.70) [71,72].
   c. Femoral hernia: Involves herniation through the femoral ring into the femoral canal present posteroinferior to inguinal ligament and medial to femoral veins. It has increased incidence in females as broader pelvis predisposes herniation into the femoral canal. Narrow neck of the sac increases risk of complication such as obstruction and incarceration (Fig. 37.71). De Garengeot hernia is a femoral hernia containing appendix [71,75].
2. *Ventral hernias*: Include hernia through the anterior, lateral, and posterior abdominal wall. Midline hernias include umbilical, paraumbilical, epigastric, and hypogastric. Spigelian hernia involves the lateral ventral wall. Lumbar hernia occurs through the posterior wall.
   a. Umbilical hernia: Most commonly acquired in adults. Predisposing factors are pregnancy, obesity, and ascites (Fig. 37.72) [72].
   b. Paraumbilical hernia: Occurs through linea alba at the level of umbilicus secondary to rectus diastasis (Fig. 37.73) [72].
   c. Epigastric and hypogastric hernia: Occurs along the linea alba above and below the level of umbilicus, respectively. Contents usually include properitoneal fat and rarely viscera. Obesity is a predisposing factor [76].
   d. Spigelian hernia: Involves herniation along the linea semilunaris (fibrous union of rectus and oblique muscle aponeuroses) due to acquired weakness or prior surgery (Fig. 37.74) [71,72].

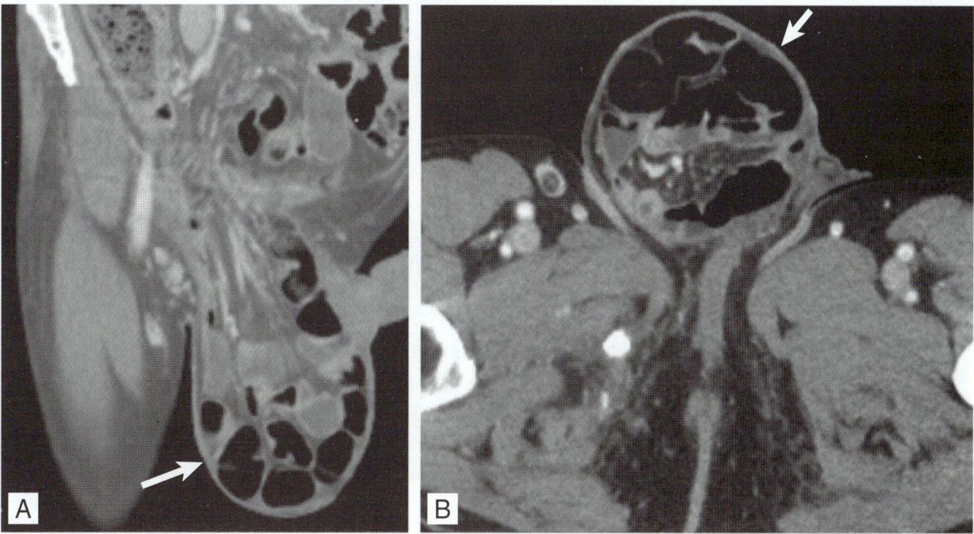

Figure 37.68 Contrast-enhanced coronal (A) and axial (B) CT pelvis shows right indirect inguinal hernia containing small bowel and mesentery, occupying the scrotal sac (*white arrow*). No signs of obstruction or strangulation are present.

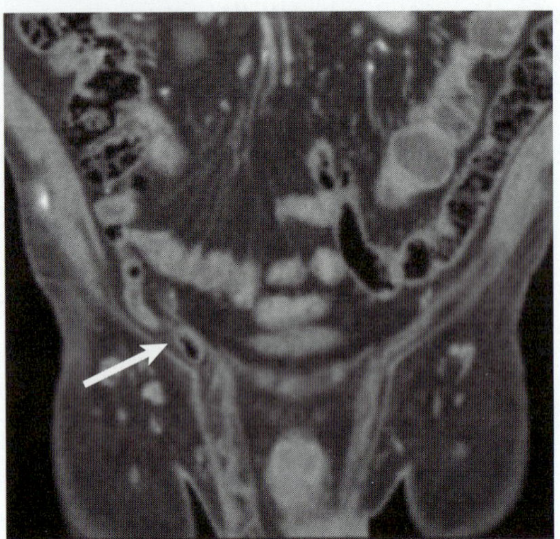

Figure 37.69 Contrast-enhanced coronal CT abdomen and pelvis shows Amyand's hernia containing appendix (*white arrow*).

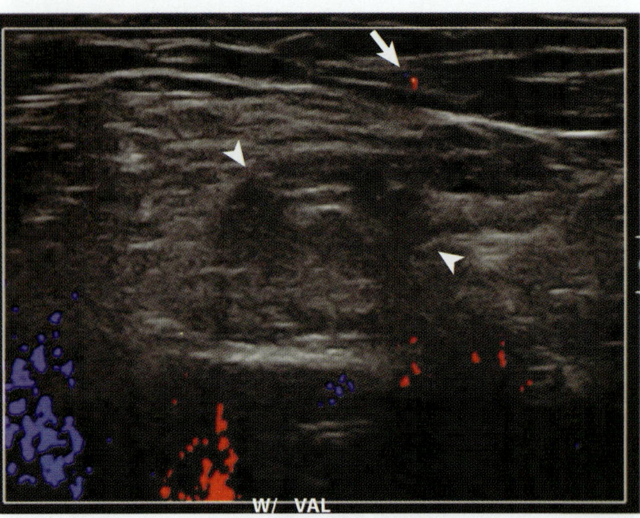

Figure 37.70 Transverse USG of right groin shows a small fat containing direct inguinal hernia (*white arrowheads*). Note that the hernia sac is located medial to the inferior epigastric vessels (*white arrow*).

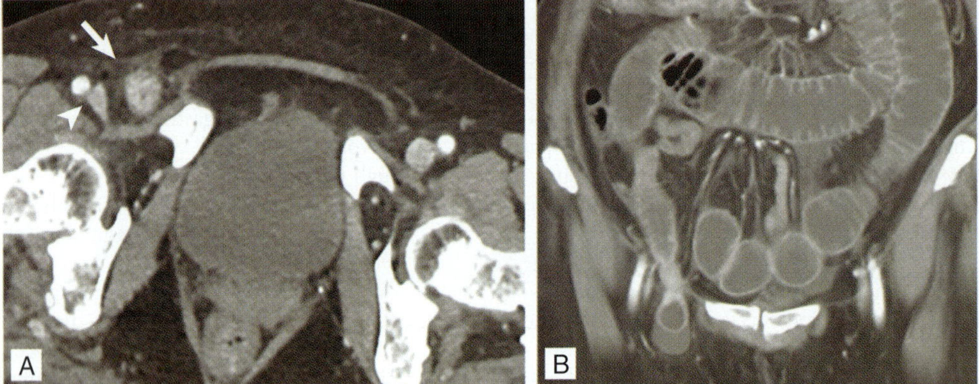

Figure 37.71 Contrast-enhanced axial and coronal CT pelvis shows an obstructed right femoral hernia containing small bowel (*white arrow*) (A and B). Note the upstream bowel obstruction (B). Note compression and flattening of the right femoral vein (*arrowhead* in A).

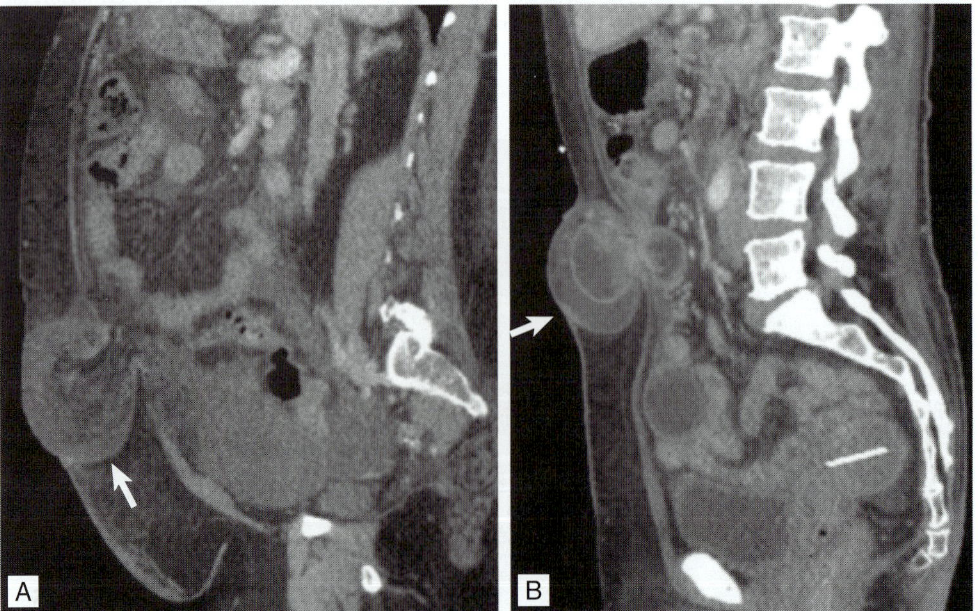

Figure 37.72 Contrast-enhanced sagittal CT abdomen and pelvis shows a moderate sized nonobstructed umbilical hernia containing fluid and mesenteric fat (*white arrow*) (A). Contrast enhanced sagittal CT abdomen and pelvis from a different patient shows a moderate sized small bowel containing umbilical hernia with closed-loop obstruction (*white arrow*) (B). The involved bowel shows dilatation and mural hyperenhancement. The presence of fluid and stranding in this hernial sac (with absent abdominal ascites) is related to strangulation.

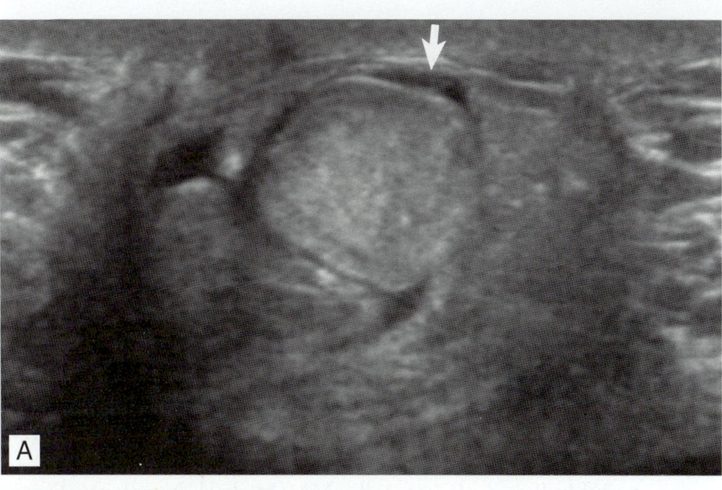

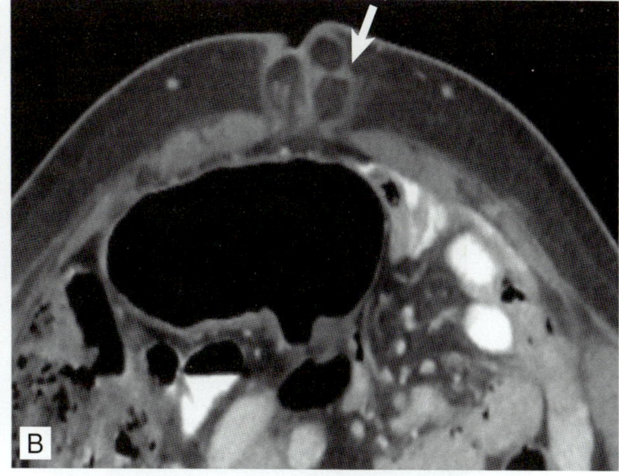

Figure 37.73 (A) Transverse USG of umbilical region shows a nonreducible fat containing left paraumbilical hernia, with trace fluid in the hernia sac (*white arrow*). (B) Subsequent contrast-enhanced axial CT abdomen demonstrates left paraumbilical hernia with surrounding subcutaneous stranding related to underlying incarceration (*white arrow*).

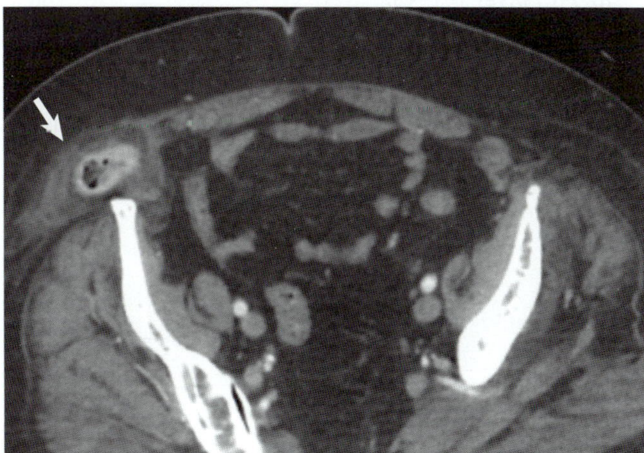

Figure 37.74 Contrast-enhanced axial CT pelvis shows ascending colon containing right Spigelian hernia (*white arrow*). The presence of fluid and stranding in the hernia sac is related to underlying incarceration.

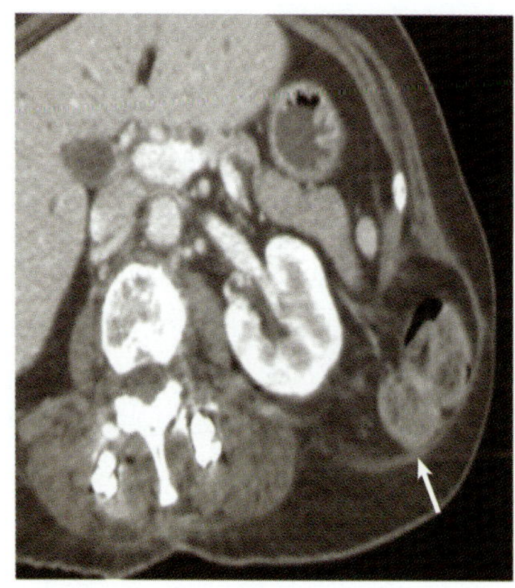

Figure 37.75 Contrast-enhanced axial CT abdomen shows a moderate-sized, nonobstructed left lumbar hernia containing descending colon (*white arrow*).

   e. Lumbar hernia: Occurs through the defect in the musculature of superior (Grynfelt–Lesshaft) or inferior lumbar triangles (Petit's) located between 12th rib and iliac crest. It can be posttraumatic, postsurgical (especially after renal surgeries), or spontaneous (Fig. 37.75) [72].
3. Incisional hernia: These occur as a complication of abdominal surgeries, more commonly with vertical than transverse incisions. Parastomal and port site hernias are included in this subtype [72].
4. Miscellaneous: Includes interparietal (between the fascial planes of abdominal muscles), Richter (herniation of partial circumference of the bowel wall), sciatic (through the sciatic foramen), obturator (through obturator canal), and perineal hernias (through the pelvic floor). All these are highly prone to incarceration [77].

Table 37.3 summarizes the abdominal wall hernias with specific names.

Complications are incarceration (implying nonreducibility), strangulation, and bowel obstruction. Strangulation refers to compromise of vascular supply, which presents as thickening of the hernia sac, fluid within the sac, mesenteric fat stranding, bowel wall edema, hypoenhancement or pneumatosis. Post hernia repair complications include recurrence, infections, fluid collections, and mesh related issues such as extrusion and infection [77].

Differential diagnosis: Abdominal wall hematomas, abscess, lipoma, desmoid, hydrocele, and varicocele.

TABLE 37.3 Hernias With Specific Names

Amyand's hernia	Inguinal hernia containing appendix
Littre hernia	Inguinal hernia containing Meckel diverticulum
Pantaloon hernia	Combination of adjacent hernia sacs of inguinal and femoral regions
De Garengeot hernia	Femoral hernias containing appendix
Richter hernia	Herniation of partial circumference of the bowel wall

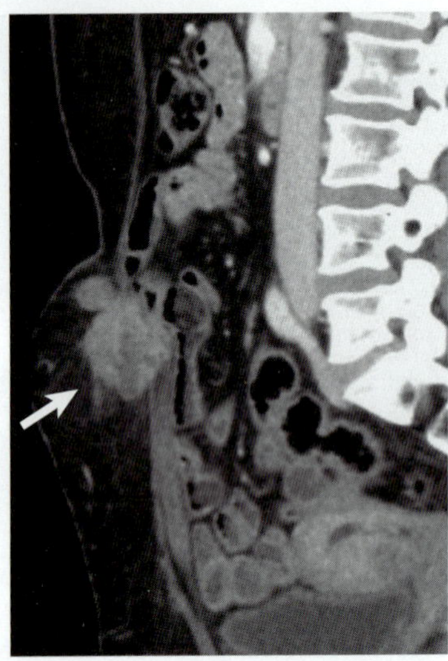

Figure 37.76 Contrast-enhanced sagittal CT abdomen and pelvis from a 56-year-old man shows metastatic nodules at the umbilicus (Sister Mary joseph nodules; *arrow*) from carcinoma of GE junction (not shown).

Neoplastic Disorder

Desmoid tumors are the most common primary neoplasms of the anterior abdominal wall. These are discussed under the section on neoplastic disorders of the mesentery and peritoneum.

Abdominal wall metastasis: These are the most common malignant lesions of the anterior abdominal wall. Abdominal wall metastases are usually associated with advanced stage malignancy with widespread metastasis, except in the instances of postsurgical, laparoscopic port site or needle tract seeding. Imaging features resembles the primary. Characteristic example is Sister Mary Joseph's nodule from cancers of the gastrointestinal tract and ovary [78]. This is an eponymous name given to a metastatic nodule at the umbilicus from these tumors. Gall bladder cancers and ovarian tumors in particular have a propensity for abdominal wall metastasis (Fig. 37.76).

Suggested Readings

- R Diab, M Virarkar, M Saleh, et al., Imaging spectrum of mesenteric masses, Abdom Radiol 45 (2020) 3618–3636.
- DMc Patrick, F Antonella, MM Michael, Neoplastic diseases of the peritoneum and mesentery, Am J Roentgenol 200 (5) (2013) W420–W430.
- A Coffin, I Boulay-Coletta, D Sebbag-Sfez, M Zins, Radioanatomy of the retroperitoneal space, Diagn Interv Imaging 96 (2) (2015) 171–186.
- Rajiah P, Sinha R, Cuevas C et al. Imaging of uncommon retroperitoneal masses, Radiographics 31 (4) (2012) 949–976.
- HB David, M Parisa, CO Daniel, GL Meghan, OM Christine, JP Perry, DM William, M Vincent, Mellnick. Imaging of abdominal wall masses, masslike lesions, and diffuse processes, RadioGraphics 40 (3) (2020) 684–706.

38

Urinary Tract: Anatomy, Conventional Radiology, and Ultrasonography

SMITA ESTHER RAJU, SHALINI GOVIL

Introduction

We begin the section on urinary tract imaging by focusing on the basics. We discuss the anatomy of the urinary tract viscera along with conventional imaging and ultrasonography (USG) techniques in the first half of the chapter. We subsequently focus on the basics of intravenous urography (IVU) interpretation, while advanced cross-sectional techniques and their interpretation are discussed in the chapters ahead.

Anatomy

Kidneys and Ureters

- The kidneys are bean-shaped organs with their concave edges pointing medially. The right kidney is placed lower than the left, owing to the presence of the liver above. In quiet respiration, the kidneys move up and down ~2–3 cm but can move twice that distance on deep inspiration
- The hilum of the kidney is a vertical opening on the medial aspect that contains the renal pelvis. The renal vein and one or two branches of the renal artery pass through the hilum to enter the kidney anterior to the renal pelvis, with a further branch of the renal artery passing through the hilum posterior to the renal pelvis. The hilum also contains fat, sympathetic nerve fibres, and lymphatic channels that drain into the para-aortic lymph nodes around the origins of the renal arteries from the aorta
- Renal tissue is divided into a peripherally placed cortex and the central medulla. The cortex contains the glomeruli and the proximal and distal convoluted tubules. The medulla consists of 8–16 pyramids and contains the Loop of Henle and the collecting ducts. The apex of each pyramid projects into a calyx as a renal papilla. The medullary collecting ducts converge into central, papillary ducts (of Bellini) near the tip of each medullary pyramid and drain into a minor calyx through tiny orifices in the renal papillae (Fig. 38.1)
- The superior end of the ureter expands to form the renal pelvis which divides into 2–4 major calyces, each of which divide into 2–4 minor calyces. Each calyx is indented by a papilla, which is the apex of a medullary pyramid. The calyces therefore have a characteristic shape with a well-defined extension around the convexity of the papilla (the fornices). The minor calyces drain into a major calyx via a neck (infundibulum). Often at the renal poles (especially the upper pole) several papillae drain into one large calyx. These are referred to as compound calyces and are particularly vulnerable to damage from reflux nephropathy
- The ureter runs in the retroperitoneum along the anterior aspect of the psoas muscle, separated from it by the transversalis fascia. As it enters the pelvis, it crosses over the anterior aspect of the common iliac artery bifurcation immediately in front of the sacroiliac joint. It descends along the lateral pelvic wall, just medial to the obturator internus, to the level of the ischial spine, from where it runs anteromedially until it enters the superolateral angle of the bladder base. The vas deferens crosses over the ureter, separating it from the bladder just before the ureters enter the bladder wall (Fig. 38.2). The ureters run obliquely through the bladder wall for around 2 cm
- A fibrous capsule is closely applied to the renal cortex over the entire kidney apart from the hilum. The kidney is surrounded by perinephric fat and lies within a space partly enclosed by layers of fascia: the perinephric space (Fig. 38.3)
- During embryological development, as the kidneys ascend from the pelvis, the surrounding perinephric fascia forms a cone, with its apex inferiorly. The perinephric fascia anterior to the kidney is often referred to as Gerota's fascia, the posterior fascia as Zuckerkandl's fascia and the enclosed space as the perinephric space. It contains the kidney, the adrenal gland (anteromedial to the kidney on the left, superomedial to the kidney on the right), the upper ureter and the perinephric fat

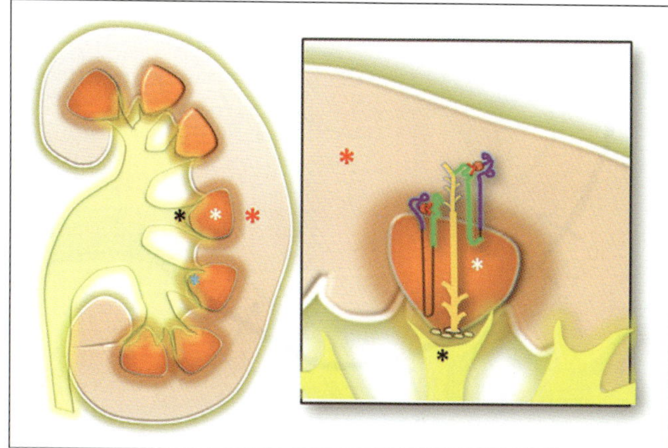

Figure 38.1 Kidney: anatomy. Cortex (*red asterisk*); Medulla (*white asterisk*); Papilla (*blue asterisk*); Calyx (*black asterisk*); Bowman's capsule (brown); Proximal convoluted tubule (*blue*); Loop of Henle (*black*); Distal convoluted tubule (*green*); Collecting duct (*yellow*).

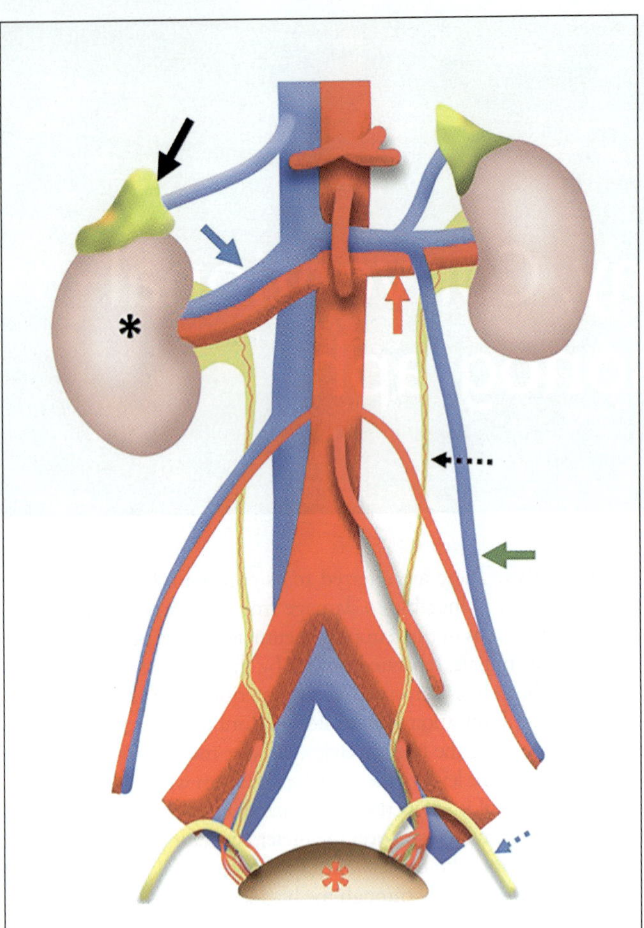

Figure 38.2 Urinary tract: anatomy. Adrenal gland (*black arrow*); Renal vein (*blue arrow*); Renal artery (*red arrow*); Kidney (*black asterisk*); Ureter (*black dashed arrow*); Gonadal vein (*green arrow*); Vas deferens (*blue dashed arrow*); Bladder (*red asterisk*). (Courtesy: Dr. Karthikumar.)

- The anterior interfascial or retromesenteric space is a potential space within the laminated anterior perinephric fascia that can eventually transmit disease processes across the midline. The posterior interfascial or retrorenal space is also laminated and contains a potential space. Fluid in either of these potential spaces may track to the other and also via the fascial trifurcation into the lateroconal fascia. Fibrous septae are found within the perinephric space running from the renal capsule to the perinephric fascia and act as potential conduits between the perinephric and interfascial potential spaces
- Posteriorly, the kidneys lie over the psoas, paraspinal muscles, 12th rib on the right and 11th rib on the left. Anterosuperiorly, the kidneys are in contact with the adrenal glands and anteroinferiorly with the jejunum. Anterolaterally, the kidneys abut the liver and hepatic flexure on the right; the spleen and splenic flexure on the left. The right kidney is related anteromedially to the duodenum and the left kidney is related to the pancreas and stomach anteromedially (Fig. 38.4)
- The arterial supply and venous drainage of the kidneys are both extremely variable. The renal arterial supply is most commonly provided by a single lateral branch of the aorta, the renal artery, originating at the level of the first lumbar disc. The right renal artery has the longer course and runs posterior to the inferior vena cava. The renal arteries run posterior to their respective renal veins. The renal artery gives off the inferior adrenal and the renal capsular arteries and then classically divides into three branches as it enters the renal sinus, two running anterior to the renal pelvis, and one posterior. The main renal branches subsequently divide into the interlobar arteries, which run centrifugally within the cortical tissue between the medullary pyramids. At the level of the base of the pyramids the interlobar arteries give off the arcuate arteries, which run along the line of the corticomedullary junction
- The venous drainage mirrors the arterial tree except that the kidneys are drained by five or six major venous branches, which most commonly combine to form a solitary renal vein that drains into the inferior vena cava, also around the level of the first lumbar disc. The lymphatic drainage of the kidneys is to the para-aortic lymph nodes around the origin of the renal arteries

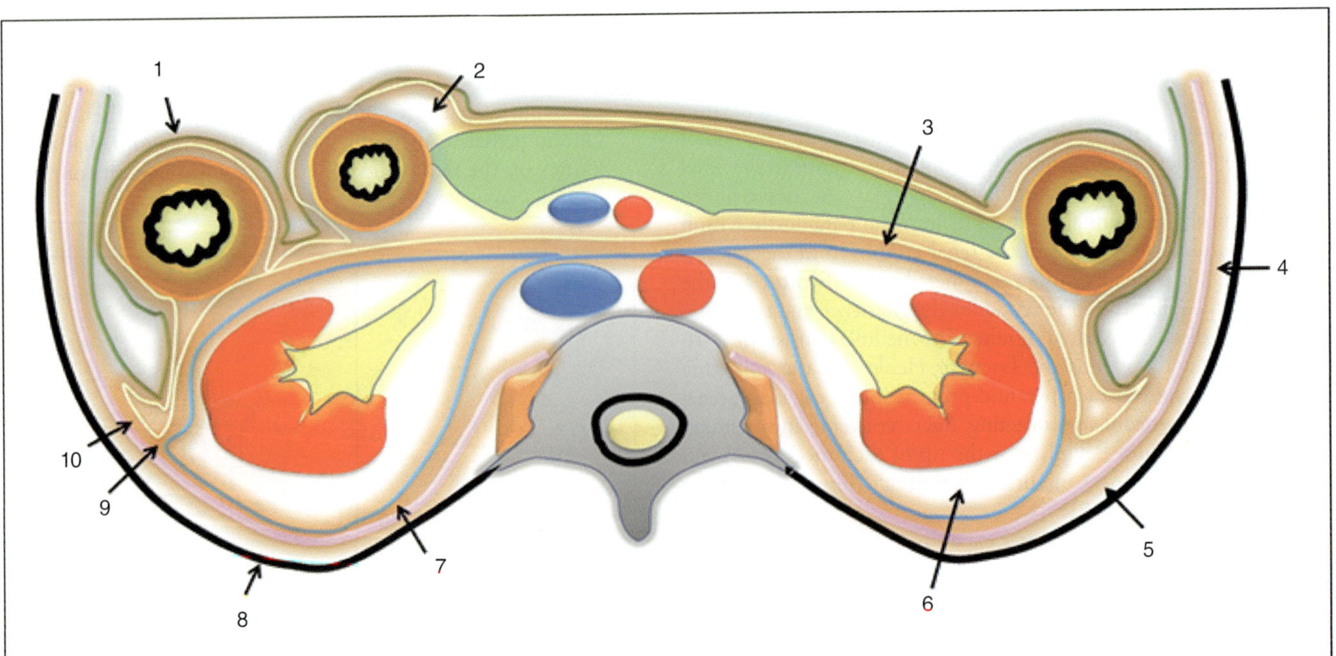

Figure 38.3 Retroperitoneal fascial spaces. 1. Parietal peritoneum; 2. Anterior pararenal space; 3. Anterior perinephric (Gerota) fascia; 4. Properitoneal fat line; 5. Posterior pararenal space; 6. Perinephric space; 7. Posterior perinephric (Zuckerkandl) fascia; 8. Transversalis fascia; 9. Fascial trifurcation; 10. Lateroconal fascia.

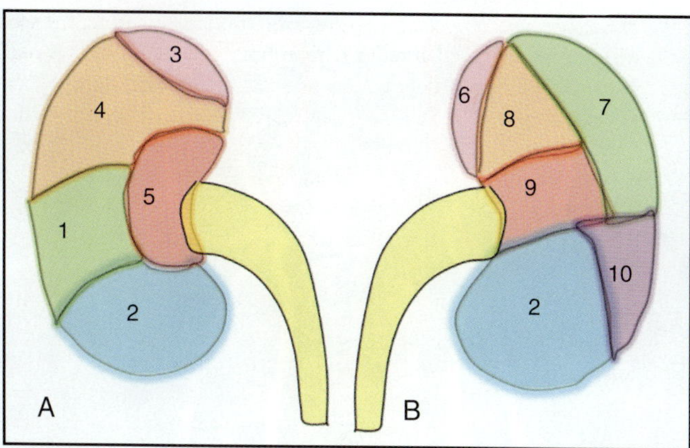

Figure 38.4 Anterior relations of (A) the right kidney and (B) the left kidney. 1. Hepatic flexure; 2. Small intestine; 3. Right adrenal gland; 4. Liver; 5. Duodenum; 6. Left adrenal gland; 7. Spleen; 8. Stomach; 9. Pancreas; 10. Splenic flexure.

Bladder and Pelvis

- The urinary bladder lies immediately posterior to the pubic bones. When full, it is roughly spherical but when empty, it approximates to a pyramidal shape, having an apex and four roughly triangular surfaces: posterior (base), superior and two inferolateral. The apex lies immediately behind the upper margin of the symphysis pubis and gives rise to the urachus, which is the fibrous remnant of the allantois. The urachus runs superiorly in the extraperitoneal fat to the umbilicus as the median umbilical ligament
- The superior surface of the bladder is covered by parietal peritoneum and loops of ileum and sigmoid colon. The inferolateral surfaces relate anteriorly to retropubic fat and pubic bones and posteriorly to the obturator internus (superiorly) and the levator ani (inferiorly). In males, the bladder base receives the ureters at its superolateral angles, gives rise to the urethra at its inferomedial angle and rests inferiorly on the prostate. Muscle fibres of the bladder wall run continuously into the prostate and are thickened around the origin of the urethra as the internal sphincter vesicae at the bladder neck
- The bladder mucosa is thrown into folds when the bladder empties, except over the base where it is firmly adherent to the underlying muscle layers as the trigone. The superior border of the trigone is defined by a muscular ridge running between the ureteric orifices (the interureteric ridge). The upper part of the base is covered by peritoneum and lies anterior to the rectovesical pouch (uterovesical pouch in the female), the lower part is subperitoneal and separated from the rectum by the vasa deferentia and seminal vesicles (vagina in the female)
- Lymphatic drainage of the bladder is into the internal and external iliac lymph nodes lying along the course of the respective arteries. These in turn drain into the common iliac nodes. The medial chains of the external iliac lymph nodes (obturator nodes) lie between the external and internal iliac vessels along the pelvic side wall. They are frequently involved early in metastatic spread of bladder or prostatic cancers and are therefore often referred to as sentinel nodes
- The transversalis fascia that lines the inside of the abdominopelvic cavity extends from the inferior surface of the diaphragm, along the inner surface of the abdominal wall musculature to cover the superior surface of the pelvic diaphragm or levator ani. It then continues inferiorly as the pelvic fascia, lining the obturator internus laterally and the pelvic diaphragm inferiorly
- The parietal peritoneum of the abdomen also continues inferiorly and is reflected over the pelvic viscera and fat-containing spaces of the pelvis, leaving most of the pelvic organs outside the peritoneal cavity
- The umbilicovesical fascia is a large triangular fascia with its apex at the umbilicus that extends inferiorly, dividing the prevesical space anteriorly from the perivesical space posteriorly and centrally. The cave of Retzius is the part of the prevesical space immediately posterior to the pubis. The prevesical space continues posterolaterally into the paravesical spaces (Fig. 38.5). These spaces are continuous superiorly with the properitoneal fat stripes or lateral extraperitoneal spaces of the abdomen and the posterior pararenal spaces
- The perivesical space contains the bladder, the urachus and the seminal vesicles and is limited posteriorly by the rectovesical septum in males and rectovaginal septum in females

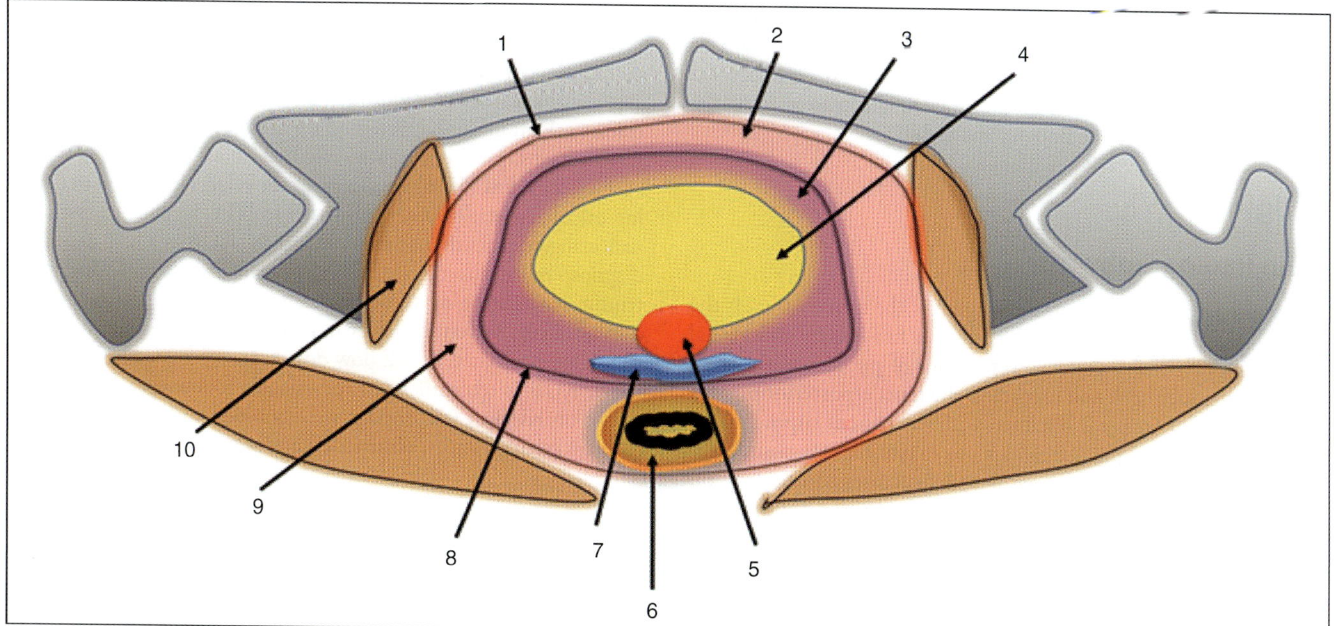

Figure 38.5 Extraperitoneal spaces of the pelvis. 1. Transversalis fascia; 2. Prevesical space (cave of Retzius); 3. Perivesical space; 4. Bladder; 5. Prostate; 6. Rectum; 7. Seminal vesicles; 8. Rectovesical septum; 9. Paravesical space; 10. Obturator internus.

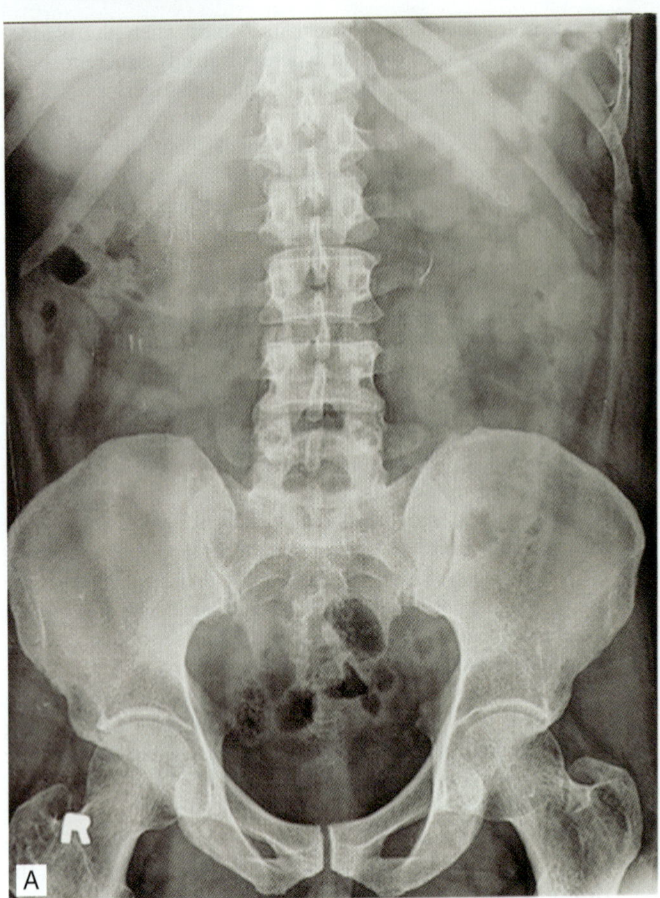

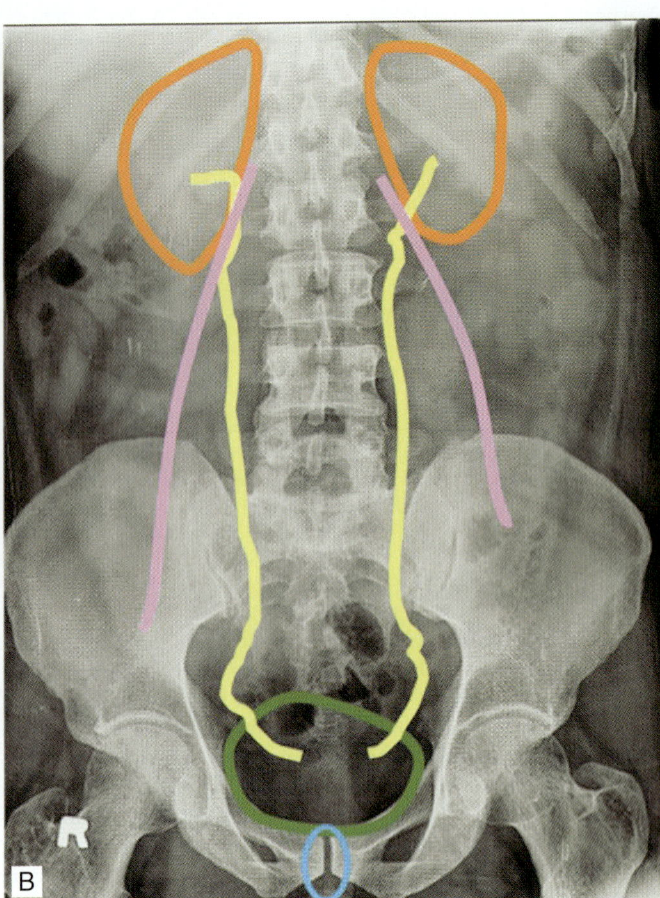

Figure 38.6 Normal KUB radiograph. (A) Supine x-ray AP view: kidney-ureter-bladder. (B) Color-key diagram: kidneys (*brown line outline*), psoas muscles (*pink outline*), the anticipated line of the ureters (*yellow line*), bladder (*green outline*) and anticipated line of the urethra (*blue outline*).

- The pelvic organs are supported by the pelvic floor, which is formed by the pelvic diaphragm that separates the pelvic cavity superiorly from the perineum inferiorly. The pelvic diaphragm consists of the large levator ani and the small coccygeus muscles and their covering fascia. The puborectalis sling is a prominent part of the levator ani which runs around the lateral and posterior aspects of the anorectal junction and sweeps forward along the lateral margins of the prostate and inserts into the posterior aspect of the body of the pubis

Imaging

Plain Radiography

The standard plain radiographic imaging of the urinary tract is the "KUB" (kidneys, ureters, and bladder), a full-length abdominal film extending down to the lower border of pubic symphysis to cover the bladder neck and urethra in the female/posterior urethra in the male. The image is obtained with the patient supine, using a low voltage technique (60–65 kV) to maximize soft-tissue contrast. The outline of several anatomical structures can be seen on the KUB, including kidneys, bladder, psoas muscles, lumbosacral spine, bony pelvis, bowel, and lung bases. Therefore, a wide range of pathology may be incidentally evident on a KUB radiograph taken for urinary calculi or as a 1st "scout"/precontrast image of an intravenous urography (IVU) (Fig. 38.6).

Sensitivity of KUB for ureteric calculi is dependent on many factors including stone location, size, composition, patient habitus and overlying bowel contents. Notably, the KUB is extremely limited in the detection of small calculi (<5 mm) and those located in the ureter distal to the iliac vessel crossing. While the commonest stones are calcium-containing and radiopaque in nature, there are radiolucent calculi (uric acid, ammonium urate, xanthine, cystine, Indinavir stones) which cannot be detected on radiography. Nonenhanced CT (NECT), in comparison, is able to detect all radiolucent calculi except Indinavir stones [1]. Moreover, there are multiple causes of abdominal and pelvic calcifications that can mimic calculi in the KUB region on a radiograph, such as vascular calcifications, phleboliths, and calcified nodes (Box 38.1).

Given the low (57%) sensitivity of the KUB radiograph in detecting calculi, especially when compared to NECT (95%), most international guidelines do not recommend the KUB as a first step in the diagnosis of calculus disease [2]. Many patients with calculus disease require repeat imaging to determine passage, migration or progression of calculi. Given the lower radiation dose of a KUB radiograph (0.8 mSv) compared to CT (low dose CT: 3–4 mSv, NECT: 10–12 mSv), KUB is recommended for calculus follow-up when initially visible on KUB or CT Topogram, combined with ultrasonography to assess calculus status, obstruction and stent position [3,4].

Intravenous Urography

The IVU was originally developed by Leonard Rowntree of the Mayo Clinic in the 1920s [5]. Until the 1990s, IVU was the test of choice for diagnosing ureteric obstruction, but was replaced by CT because of its greater specificity regarding etiology of obstruction (Box 38.2) [6]. The IVU consists of a standard KUB, a nephrotomogram and series of films taken after administration of

BOX 38.1 Calcification on the KUB Radiograph

Urinary Tract

Calculi

Ureteral:
- uniform (vs central lucency in phlebolith)
- steinstrasse/"stone street" (post ESWL): collection of stones
- stent encrustation

Renal, bladder calculi:
- laminated, faceted, spiculated, seedlike
- dumbbell: stone in diverticulum extending into bladder lumen

Urethral: pubic symphysis

Nephrocalcinosis
- Cortical nephrocalcinosis
- Medullary nephrocalcinosis

Dystrophic

Cyst:
- Mural: curvilinear
- Intracystic: "eggshell"
- Luminal: milk of calcium

Tumor:
- RCC: central or rim
- TCC: stippled or linear
- Metastases: serous cystadenocarcinoma ovary, osteosarcoma

Vascular origin: incomplete ring, tramline
- Diabetic vascular calcification
- Artery aneurysm
- AVM

Sloughed papilla: triangular/ring-shaped
Urachal carcinoma: bladder dome
Schistosomiasis: thin, arcuate mural calcification
Tuberculosis: "putty kidney"
Abscess: "parenchymal stone"
Prostatic calcification

Outside the Urinary Tract

Musculoskeletal: costal cartilage calcification
Hepatobiliary: gallstones, hepatic granuloma
Pancreas: chronic pancreatitis
Adrenal: TB, Addison's disease
Spleen: granuloma
Aorta: atheroma, aneurysm
Venous: phlebolith
Uterine: fibroid
Lymphatic: calcified lymph nodes

BOX 38.2 IVU (Historical) Indications

1. Calculi: size, location
2. Obstruction: level, effects on renal excretion
3. Functional versus mechanical obstruction (post diuretic IVU)
4. Ureteric fistula
5. Ureteric stricture
6. GU Tuberculosis
7. Collecting system integrity: trauma/intervention
8. Congenital anomalies
9. Upper tract urothelial lesion

Cheaper, readily available alternative to CT in resource-limited settings

iodinated intravenous contrast to observe renal excretion and evaluate the collecting system.

Although both IVU and CT are subject to the risks of exposure to IV contrast and ionizing radiation, CT is faster, unaffected by body habitus, more sensitive, more specific and provides information about structures outside the urinary tract. However, in resource-limited settings, the low cost and wide availability of IVU makes it a viable alternative to CT for many indications [7].

Technique

- Patient preparation in terms of bowel cleanse, dietary restrictions and dehydration has been largely dispensed with [8], although avoidance of food 2–4 hours before the procedure is still thought reasonable should there be a severe contrast reaction with the need for cardiovascular/cardiopulmonary support
- A preliminary postmicturition, plain film, or "scout" KUB is performed to check exposure factors, centering and obvious pathology, particularly urinary tract calcification
- IV iodinated contrast is then instilled relatively rapidly by hand. The standard dose is 50 mL of 350–370 mg organic iodine per mL water-soluble iodinated contrast through an indwelling cannula or needle that can be secured into place for the duration of the investigation, allowing for further injection of contrast if opacification is seen to be inadequate. A doctor should be available in the department throughout the investigation since most adverse events occur within the first few minutes after the injection. Emergency drugs, oxygen, and resuscitation equipment should also be readily available
- A cross-kidney radiograph is taken immediately after contrast injection and at 5 minute after the injection. Abdominal compression is applied as soon as the 5 minute radiograph has been taken (via a compression device such as a binder) to inhibit ureteric drainage and promote distension of the pelvicalyceal systems, optimizing their visualization. A further cross-kidney radiograph is taken at 15 minute to demonstrate this. Compression is routinely omitted in children and should be avoided in a number of situations including acute painful abdomen, aortic aneurysm, or a recent abdominal surgery
- If the 15 minute radiograph is satisfactory, the compression is removed and a full-length KUB radiograph is taken immediately to offer the best opportunity of demonstrating the ureters.
- When the bladder is poorly filled on the release film (as is often the case) delayed films of the fuller bladder may be performed. The patient is then asked to empty the bladder and a further full-length KUB radiograph is taken to demonstrate drainage of the upper tract and the postmicturition bladder volume
- When there is significant acute obstruction, usually due to calculi, there is a delay in opacification of the collecting system. The delay may be considerable, up to 24 hours or more. It is then necessary to perform the minimum number of additional radiographs. The time interval between is traditionally doubled, with radiographs taken at 0.5, 1, 2, 4, 16, and 24 hours, as necessary; however, to minimize the radiation exposure, if there is no opacification of an acutely obstructed kidney at 30 minute it is usually unhelpful to perform the next radiograph before around 4 hours after contrast injection. A further maneuver to minimize radiation dose in patients with a strong clinical suspicion of ureteric colic is to omit all exposures after contrast until a full-length 15 minute radiograph is performed
- Patients with proven or suspected ureteric calculus may require one or more follow-up IVUs. These should have the minimum number of exposures required to answer the specific question, for example a full-length plain and 15 minute postcontrast radiograph may be sufficient

Modifications to the IVU technique are outlined in Table 38.1.

TABLE 38.1 **Modifications of IVU**

Radiography	Modification	Purpose
Plain films	Additional obliques or tomograms	To assist the location of potentially intrarenal opacities Rarely required; ultrasonography and other imaging manoeuvers usually preferable
Nephrogram	Thick slice tomogram Omit along with the 5 minutes film and take a solitary 3 minutes film	To improve definition of the renal outlines To reduce radiation dose
5 minutes film	Second injection of contrast	To improve opacification of the pelvicalyceal systems if inadequate
15 minutes compression film	Series of 1 cm thick tomograms	To differentiate between overlying shadows and filling defects within the collecting systems To delineate the renal outlines when inadequately seen (better done with ultrasonography)
15 minutes release film	Additional bladder views	When the bladder is poorly filled on the release film (as is often the case) delayed films of the fuller bladder may be performed When equivocal filling defects are seen in the bladder area oblique films may be performed The above additional bladder views are rarely indicated as they increase the radiation burden to the patient and the relevant clinical problems are better answered by ultrasonography or cystoscopy. However, occasionally a small suspected calculus in the distal ureter may be confirmed with the appropriate oblique
Full-length postmicturition film	Bladder area only	If the upper tracts have already been adequately imaged then imaging the bladder area alone will reduce the patient's radiation burden
	Omit	The preceding films may have already provided all the information required from the investigation
Prone full-length film	Additional view	Where the renal pelvis is dilated, contrast may be slow to pass into the ureter; this can be accelerated by positioning the patient prone when the heavier contrast will run anteroinferiorly into the ureter, often to the level of the obstruction. Simply asking the patient to sit or stand for a few minutes first may improve the result
Erect images	Additional radiograph or fluoroscopy	If it is difficult to determine whether or not there is a small ureteric calculus, an erect oblique radiography of the ureter or screening the ureter in this position may be useful on rare occasions
Furosemide IVU	Administration of 20 mg of Furosemide intravenously after the 15 minutes film with a further film 15 minutes later	If suspected pelviureteric junction obstruction is being investigated and there is no evidence of this on the standard IVU, this manoeuvre can be performed. It may provoke hydronephrosis and pain. It is rarely necessary if the patient is to be investigated with radionuclide renography, as is often the case in this situation

Normal Appearances

- The typical appearances of the normal IVU are as follows: it takes approximately 12–20 seconds for contrast to reach the renal arteries following its intravenous injection. At this stage, its concentration is maximal in the vascular compartment; however, this falls rapidly as the contrast medium begins to escape into the extracellular compartment and also undergoes rapid glomerular filtration and enters the renal tubules
- In the first minute of the IVU, healthy kidneys (assuming a normal cardiovascular system) show diffuse enhancement. This is referred to as the nephrogram. During the nephrogram or nephrographic phase, the renal size (normally at least three vertebrae in length but no more than four) and outlines are best seen (Fig. 38.7)
- In the 1st 30 seconds, contrast is within the arterial system and causes greater enhancement of the cortex than the medulla, a differentiation rarely visible on the 1-minute IVU nephrogram but clearly demonstrated on CT
- In the 2nd 30 seconds, contrast density increases within the tubules and results in diffuse renal enhancement, with contrast appearing within the calyces at ~1 minute. In high quality images, pyelotubular stasis of contrast in the collecting ducts may be seen as fine linear opacities within the medullary pyramids running towards the calyces, known as the "medullary pyramidal blush," a normal phenomenon
- Contrast in normal calyces will begin to drain immediately into the pelvis and ureter and this phase is referred to as the pyelogram. The successful application of compression impedes ureteric drainage and distends the pelvicalyceal system, producing optimal visualization of the pelvicalyceal system at around 15 minutes. After compression is released, there is a transient increase in flow down the ureters and the release radiograph offers the best chance of demonstrating the ureters. The normal ureters exhibit continual peristalsis and with a single exposure it is uncommon to demonstrate the entire length of both ureters (Figs. 38.8 and 38.9)
- The ureters will often demonstrate smoothly narrowed areas at the pelviureteric junction and as they cross the iliac vessels in the pelvis but also some more relaxed, capacious areas. This is normal and how vigorously further efforts are made to demonstrate the entire length of the ureter depends on the clinical situation
- In most situations, partial visualization of a nonobstructed but otherwise normal ureter is acceptable. In limited-resource settings where CT may not be available or even affordable, further efforts to demonstrate the ureter can be made with prone films, fluoroscopy (spot films/recordings) or retrograde pyelography.
- On the postmicturition full-length KUB radiograph, there will be drainage of contrast from the upper tracts as well as emptying of the bladder

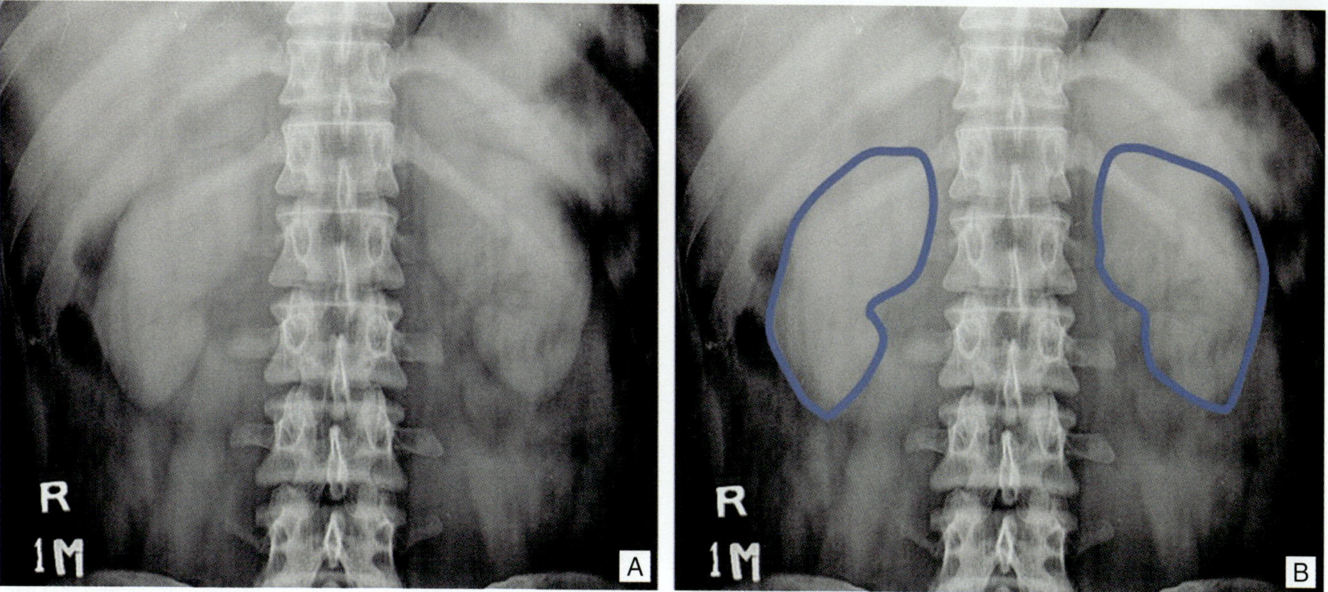

Figure 38.7 Normal IVU: 1-minute nephrotomogram. (A) X-ray tomogram of kidneys 1 minute after IV contrast. (B) Color-key diagram: normal kidney (*blue outline*) size, location, and contour with nephrogram demonstrating bilateral, symmetric, diffuse, homogeneous renal opacification. (Courtesy: Dr. Anu Eapen.)

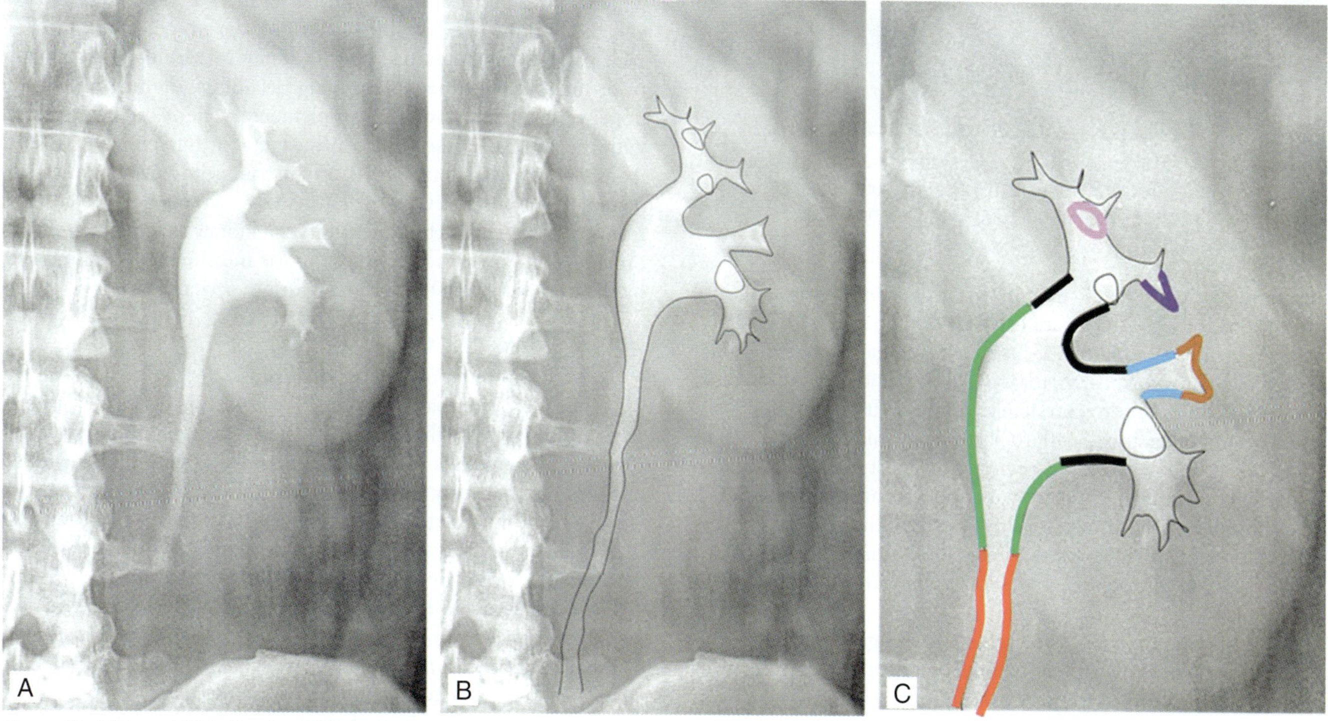

Figure 38.8 Normal IVU: 15-minute binder tomogram. (A) X-ray tomogram 15 minutes after IV contrast and application of pelvic binder. (B) Pencil outline: pelvicalyceal system and proximal ureter. (C) Color-key diagram: ureter (*red*), pelvis (*green*), major calyx (*black*), infundibulum (*blue*), minor calyx (*brown*), fornix in profile (*purple*), fornix end-on (*pink*).

Ultrasonography

Gray Scale Ultrasonography

Routine gray scale ultrasonography (USG) of the urinary tract consists of examination of the kidneys and the full urinary bladder. Assessment of the postmicturition bladder volume is often also performed as part of the same examination. USG is noninvasive, radiation free, lower cost than CT/MRI, and widely available, making it the most utilized renal imaging technique. This includes the use of POCUS (point of care ultrasonography) in emergency rooms and urological practices. Advanced software, portability, affordability, faster order-to-image turnaround times, fast-tracking triage, and management have all popularized POCUS.

Indications

According to the American College of Radiology (ACR) appropriateness criteria 2020, renal ultrasonography is the most appropriate technique in the evaluation of renal impairment of any

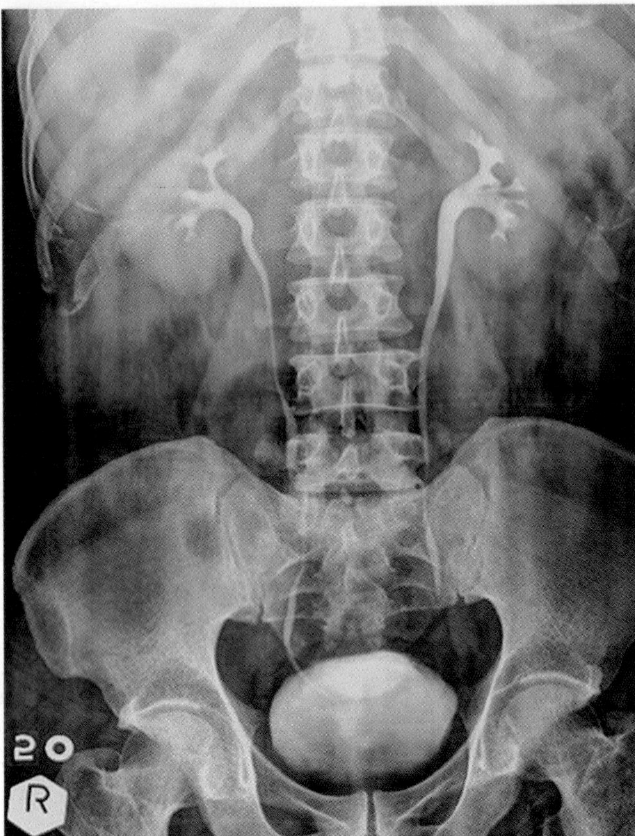

Figure 38.9 Normal kidneys, pelvicalyceal systems, ureters, bladder. IVU: 15-minute release-binder KUB. X-ray KUB 15 minutes after IV contrast and release of binder compression. (Courtesy: Dr. Anu Eapen.)

duration, with greatest value in the exclusion of obstruction. Indications for USG KUB are listed in Box 38.3.

- USG is indispensable as the first line investigation in the evaluation of genitourinary symptoms in children and pregnant women
- In the evaluation of acute flank pain and suspected stone disease, ultrasonography is appropriate as an initial imaging technique, although NECT is preferred in most guidelines due to its high accuracy, especially with the advent of low dose CT techniques with similar sensitivity to routine NECT in the detection of calculi. For the detection of ureteric calculi, the sensitivity of ultrasonography is low (24%) compared to NECT (57%) [9]
- Ultrasonography is not the first line investigation when evaluating painless hematuria as its sensitivity for detection of urothelial malignancy is poor. An exception is made in the case of a pregnant woman with microhematuria, where the chance of malignancy is low
- Ultrasonography is generally of low efficacy in the diagnosis and management of acute pyelonephritis, given its low sensitivity in the detection of diffuse parenchymal inflammation, perinephric extension and foci of gas in emphysematous pyelonephritis. However, USG is useful in identifying complications such as renal abscess and pyonephrosis; evident as mobile echoes within a hydronephrosis
- Ultrasonography is frequently used to guide diagnostic and therapeutic procedures; real-time capability enables the tracking, accurate and safe insertion of percutaneous needles, guidewires, biopsy instruments, and drainage tubes
- USG with Doppler is utilized in the evaluation of renovascular hypertension and in suspected vascular injury related to abdominal trauma
- USG with Doppler assessment is an integral part of renal transplant imaging of both donor and recipient, pre- and post-transplant

BOX 38.3 Indications for Ultrasonography KUB Region

1. Renal impairment of any duration
2. Exclusion of obstruction
3. Identification of "small echogenic kidneys": chronic renal disease
4. Urinary symptoms in children/pregnant women
5. Evaluation of indeterminate renal mass on CT
6. Acute flank pain/suspected stone disease
7. Recurrent urinary symptoms
8. Pregnant woman with microhematuria
9. Renal abscess/pyonephrosis
10. Guided diagnostic and therapeutic procedures

Technique

Most modern probes emit a broad band of ultrasonography that can be biased towards high or low frequency, usually within the 2–6 MHz range for abdominal and pelvic work. Higher frequency with attendant low penetration and high resolution are useful in thin, asthenic patients. The position of the normal kidneys is extremely variable and the optimal window for visualization has to be determined for each patient. Conventionally, each kidney is examined sub-costally from the loin with the patient lying decubitus, the side of interest uppermost. Often, however, complementary views can be obtained with the patient supine with a more lateral or intercostal approach. An unconventional, but surprisingly useful technique, is to turn the patient decubitus and view the kidney closer to the bed sub-costally from the loin. This technique splints the kidney against the bed and provides sagittal views for ease of bipolar measurement, unhindered by the foreshortening that occurs with other views.

Normal Appearance

- On ultrasonography, the normal renal cortex appears slightly hypoechoic compared to the liver and spleen and forms a peripheral rim with normal invaginations (columns of Bertin) projecting inwards between the medullary pyramids. The pyramids are markedly hypoechoic compared to the cortex in the first 6 months of life, becoming less hypoechoic with ageing and in some disease states. Corticomedullary differentiation is therefore most obvious in young adults and children, and the hypoechoic pyramids are occasionally mistaken for the dilated calyces of a hydronephrosis
- Arcuate arteries can be identified in 25% of the adult population as focal hyperechoic areas at the corticomedullary junction
- The centrally placed renal sinus contains the calyces, infundibula, part or all of the renal pelvis, blood vessels, lymphatics, fibrous tissue, and fat. It is the most hyperechoic part of the kidney, owing to the presence of fat (Fig. 38.10)
- The normal renal pelvis may be seen within the sinus fat as an echo-free structure, especially with a full bladder in the female that will often decrease in size when the bladder is emptied. This, and the absence of dilated calyces separating the sinus fat, allows differentiation from hydronephrosis. Dilatation of the collecting system in absence of obstruction may also be observed in patients with reflux, recent previous obstruction or those on diuretic medication
- Most normal adult kidneys have a maximum length of 10–12.5 cm, although a substantial number of normal kidneys

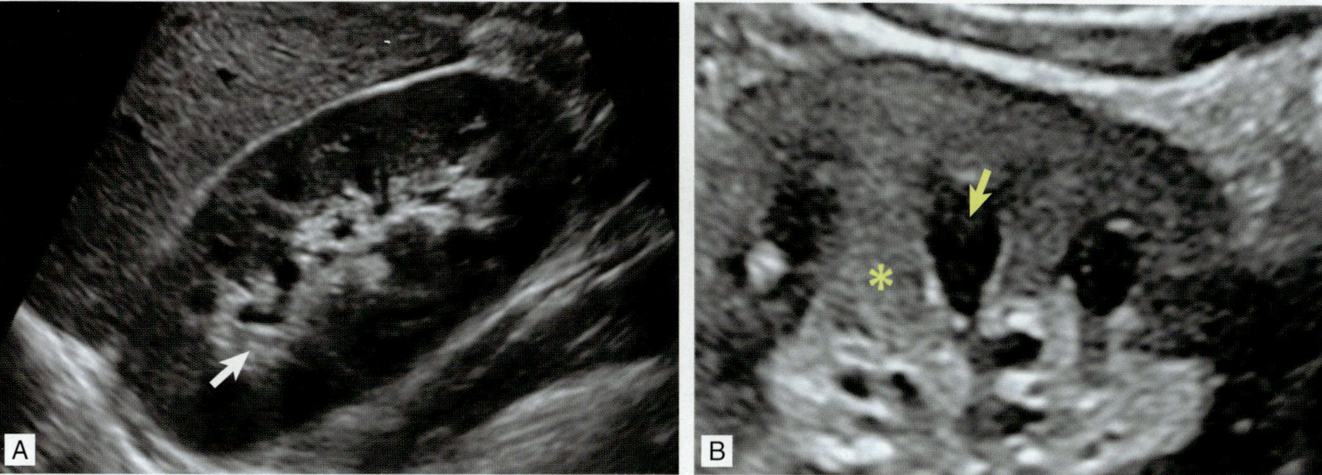

Figure 38.10 Normal kidney. Ultrasonography. (A) Longitudinal scan right kidney Normal renal parenchyma: hypoechoic to liver parenchyma, surrounding echogenic central renal sinus (*white arrow*). (B) Longitudinal scan lower pole left kidney. Normal, pyramid-shaped medulla (*yellow arrow*), hypoechoic to surrounding cortex. Normal variant: column of Bertin (*yellow asterisk*)—a cortical invagination between two medullary pyramids, extending to the central sinus.

are within the 9–13.5 cm range. Kidney length is largely related to patient size with some decrease in length as age progresses beyond 80 years. A 2 cm or more difference in length between the two kidneys raises the possibility of unilateral disease

- Cortical thickness is measured from the renal capsule to the base of the triangular medullary pyramids (Fig. 38.11A). In a young healthy adult, cortical thickness measures 7–10 mm but varies within the kidney and is thicker at the poles. This decreases with age and can be associated with an increase in the central sinus fat. In addition to reduced renal size, cortical thinning has been shown to be a reliable predictor of chronic renal disease [10,11]. When the corticomedullary differentiation is not defined, parenchymal thickness is best measured from the outer edge of the renal sinus to the renal capsule (Fig. 38.11B); parenchymal thickness is usually 1.5–2 cm in adults [12]
- Tissue echogenicity is the collective backscatter from numerous microscopic tissue interfaces and is determined by the micro-architecture of the structure being insonated. Increased renal cortical echogenicity lacks specificity and in histological studies has been correlated with interstitial fibrosis, tubular atrophy, inflammation, and glomerulosclerosis. Other than fibrosis and inflammatory infiltrates, proteinaceous casts may also increase reflectivity. Most causes of chronic renal disease show increase in echogenicity; small and echogenic kidneys (Fig. 38.12) being a hallmark of the condition with the exception of diabetic nephropathy, HIV, and amyloid nephropathy. Some causes of acute renal impairment can also show increased cortical echogenicity, for example, acute interstitial nephritis, glomerulonephritis, acute tubular necrosis (ATN), multiple myeloma and HIV nephropathy. Reduced cortical echogenicity is typically seen in acute

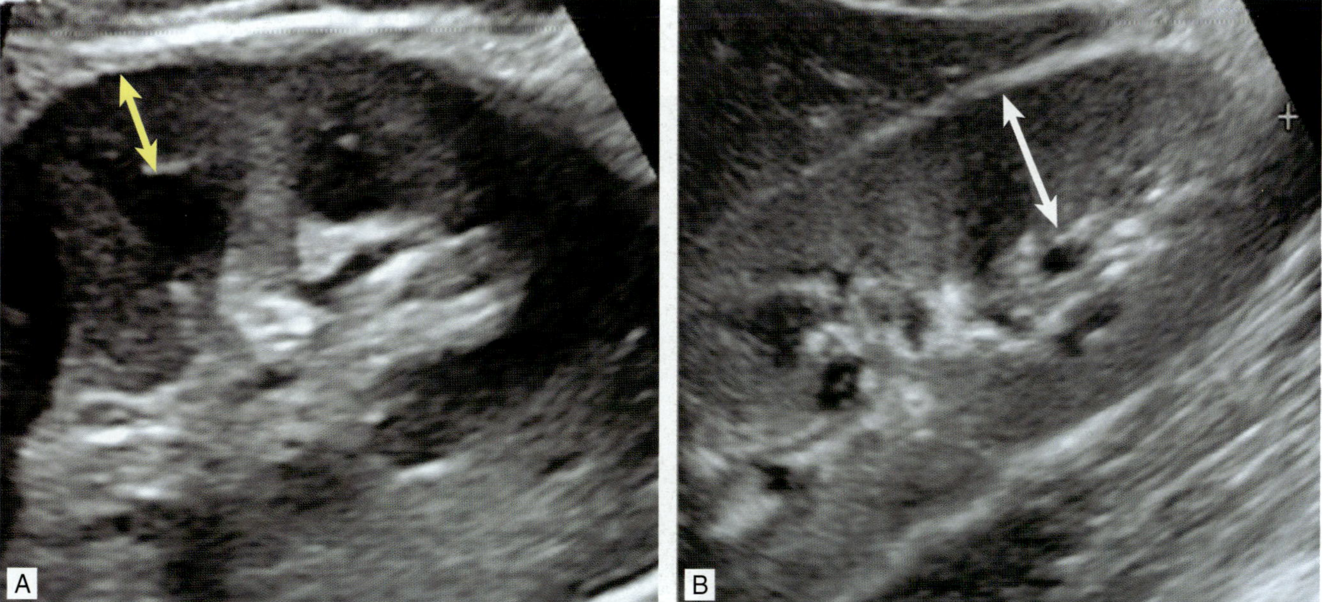

Figure 38.11 Normal renal parenchymal and cortical thickness. Longitudinal scans section of the kidney in two different patients. (A) Cortical thickness: distance from renal capsule to base of the triangular medullary pyramid (*yellow double arrow*). (B) Parenchymal thickness: distance from capsule to outer edge central sinus echoes (*white double arrow*).

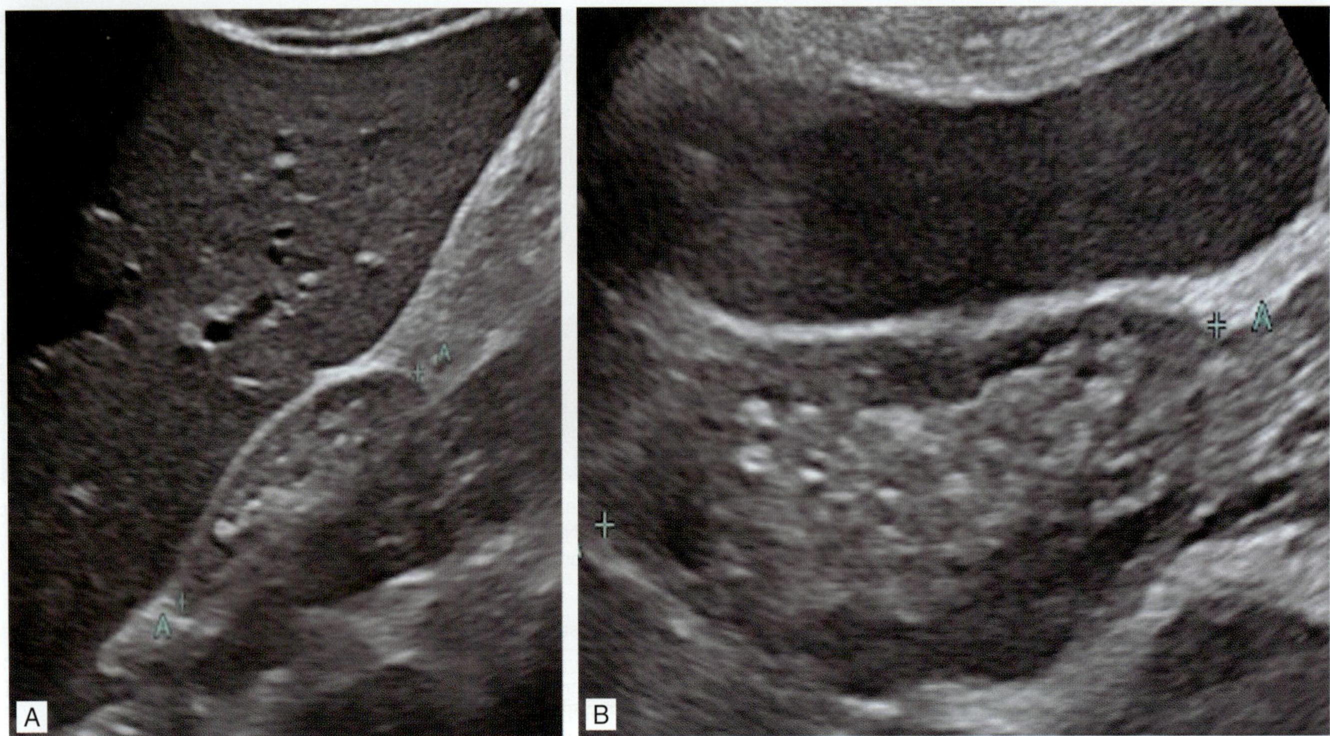

Figure 38.12 Chronic renal disease. Ultrasonography. (A) Right kidney. (B) Left kidney. Bilateral small, echogenic kidneys with diffuse parenchymal thinning and loss of corticomedullary differentiation.

cortical necrosis. Increased medullary echogenicity can be seen in medullary nephrocalcinosis (Fig. 38.13) as part of medullary sponge kidney, hyperparathyroidism, renal tubular acidosis, Vitamin D toxicity and sickle cell disease [13–16]

- Routine examination of the bladder requires it to be moderately full. The normal bladder has a triangular shape in the sagittal plane, and that of a square with the corners rounded off in the transverse plane. The normal wall thickness is 2–3 mm when the bladder is moderately full (Fig. 38.14)
- An assessment of postmicturition residual volume is usually calculated by multiplying the transverse, sagittal, and craniocaudal dimensions with the mathematical constant for an ellipse volume (0.533). No particular threshold has been assigned for diagnosis of bladder outflow obstruction. A measurable post void residue may be seen with both bladder outflow obstruction and decreased detrusor function
- In males, the prostate is routinely identified at the bladder base, especially when enlarged, with seminal vesicles above seen posterior to the bladder

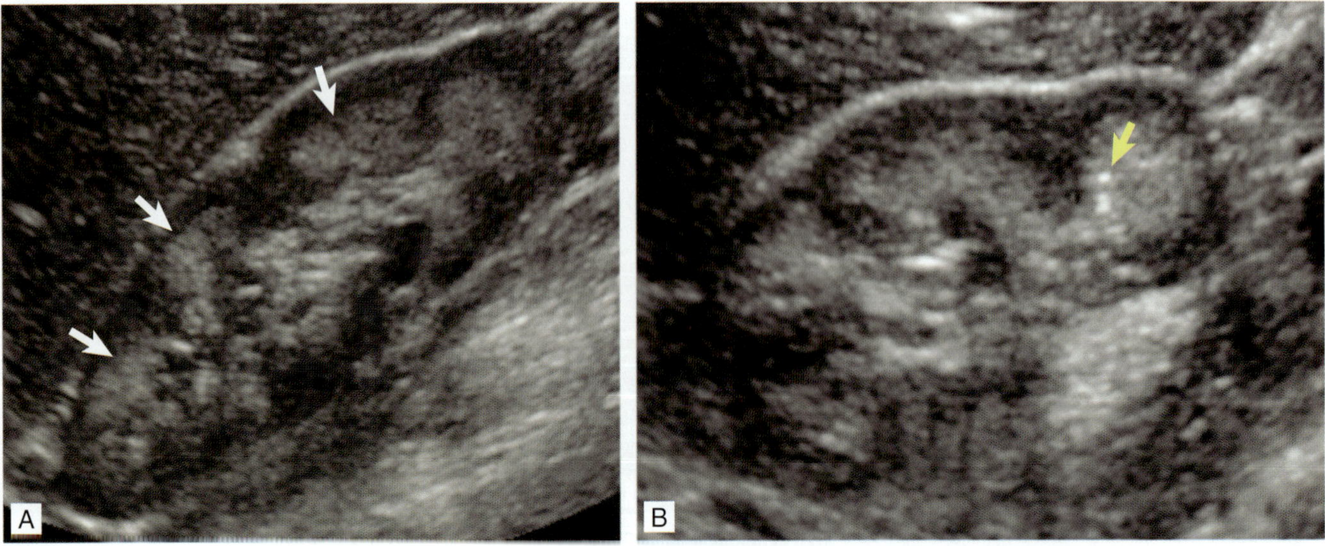

Figure 38.13 Medullary nephrocalcinosis. Ultrasonography. (A) Right kidney longitudinal scan. (B) Right kidney transverse scan. Diffusely echogenic medullary pyramids (*white arrows*) and shadowing medullary calcification (*yellow arrow*).

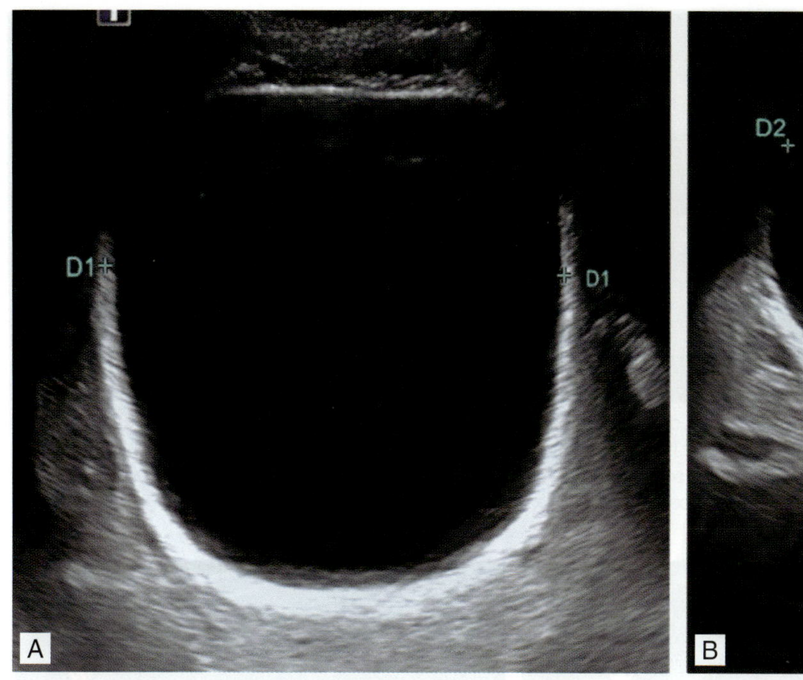

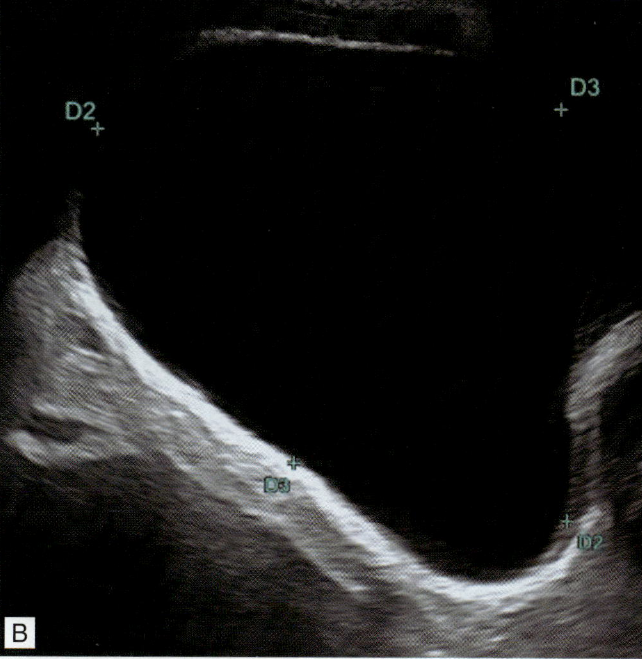

Figure 38.14 Normal bladder. Ultrasonography. (A) Sagittal scan bladder. (B) Transverse scan bladder. Normal anechoic, moderately distended lumen and smooth, thin 2–3 mm wall.

Doppler Ultrasonography

Doppler assessment of the kidney is performed to assess renal arterial and venous blood flow. Compared to other methods of imaging the vascular system such as CTA and DSA, Doppler USG is radiation free, devoid of contrast related toxicity and less expensive. The technique is, however, challenging due to the depth and small caliber of renal vessels and operator expertise has a significant role in the adequacy of assessment. Patient factors such as large habitus, poor compliance with breath hold instructions and overlying bowel add to these technical difficulties [17].

In addition to vascular assessment, demonstration of color/spectral flow within a lesion provides confirmation of a solid vascular nature. For instance, distinction between a urothelial bladder lesion and an adherent clot, a bland or tumor venous thrombus, a complicated cyst and a solid lesion can all be achieved with a Color Doppler assessment (Boxes 38.4–38.5) (Fig. 38.15).

Twinkle Artifact

Color Doppler can improve the specificity of ultrasonography in differentiating calculi from other echogenic structures. Twinkle artifact is a mosaic of colors induced by Doppler on rough reflective surfaces and is related to intrinsic noise/jitter within the Doppler circuitry of the USG machine (Fig. 38.16). For all categories of stone sizes, B-mode USG was more sensitive, but the Twinkle artifact was more specific. Addition of color Doppler scanning with the Twinkle artifact improves sensitivity from 48–66% to 55–99% [19,20].

Doppler Technique

A standard Doppler assessment starts with the morphological assessment of the kidneys on gray scale, after an overnight fast. Renal arterial assessment is performed along its entire length from aortic origin to intrarenal segmental and interlobar arteries. Periaortic segments of the renal arteries are best assessed in a transverse plane perpendicular to the aorta. The right renal artery arises from the anterolateral aspect of the aorta just below the superior mesenteric artery origin and runs deep to the right renal vein and IVC. The left renal artery is shorter and originates below the right renal artery from the posterolateral aspect of the aorta and runs deep to the left renal vein.

Spectral tracings are taken from the renal artery at the para-aortic, mid and perihilar segments with one trace from the prerenal aorta. In a renal transplant artery, tracings are taken at and around the anastomosis with the iliac artery. The insonation angle is set at 60 degrees and the gate placed to include the central one-half to one-third of the lumen on a longitudinal section of the vessel. The intrarenal traces are obtained at both poles and the interpolar region. The insonation angle is not critical for these intrarenal traces.

BOX 38.4 Indications for Color Doppler Renal Artery [18]

1. Suspected renovascular hypertension (RVH)
2. Poor renal function (eGFR <30 mL/min/1.73 m^2)
3. Post renal artery angioplasty, stent placement/surgical bypass
4. Abdominal or flank bruit
5. Suspected aneurysm, pseudoaneurysm, dissection, thrombosis, arteriovenous malformation, arteriovenous fistula
6. Suspected vascular etiology of renal insufficiency/renal length discrepancy
7. Exclude renal vein compression ("nutcracker" syndrome), thrombosis/intravenous tumor extension
8. Suspected vascular injury related to abdominal trauma
9. Renal transplant imaging of both donor and recipient, pre and post-transplant

BOX 38.5 Indications for Color Doppler Renal Vein

1. Renal vein bland thrombus: *dehydration, sepsis, sickle cell disease, nephrotic syndrome, SLE*
2. Renal vein tumor thrombus: extent

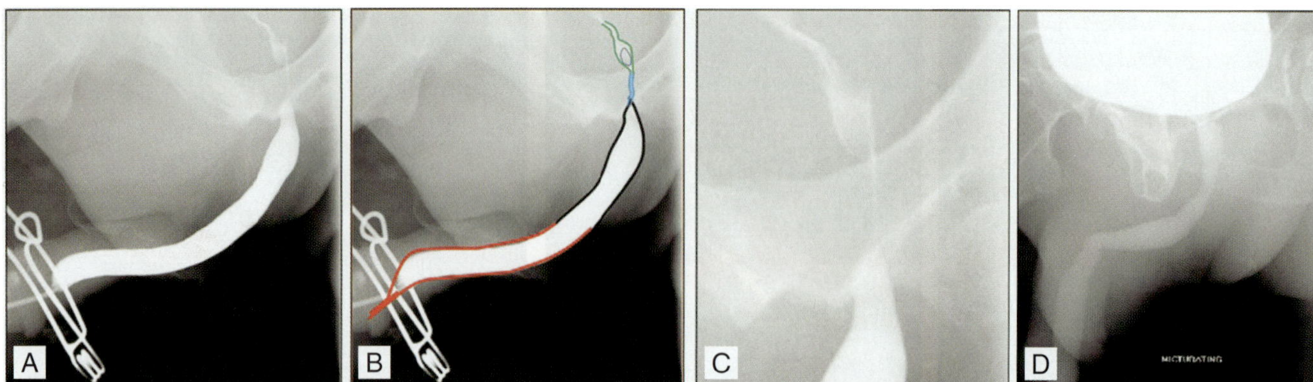

Figure 38.19 Normal male urethra. Ascending/retrograde urethrogram (RGU). Voiding or micturating cystourethrogram (VCUG/MCU). (A) RGU: supine oblique view. (B) RGU: color-key diagram. (C) RGU: magnified view of bulbomembranous junction. Anterior urethra: red—penile urethra, black—bulbar urethra. Posterior urethra: blue—membranous urethra, green—prostatic urethra, gray ring—verumontanum. Normal membranous urethra: narrowest, shortest, 10 mm segment, at the level of the urogenital diaphragm/external sphincter. Normal cone-like configuration of bulbomembranous junction. (D) MCU: erect oblique view. Normal funnel-shaped bladder neck and open membranous urethra during micturition.

Voiding/Micturating Cystourethrogram (VCUG/MCU)

MCU is performed for bladder and urethral assessment—the entire female urethra and the posterior urethra in males. The bladder is filled by advancing a transurethral catheter into the bladder or via an indwelling suprapubic catheter; bladder images are obtained when in full capacity, allowing for the demonstration of contour, filling defects, diverticuli, leaks or fistulous tracts. Supine and oblique views are typically obtained to ensure demonstration of vesicoureteric reflux. For the voiding phase, the transurethral catheter is removed unless a pericatheter study is desired and any indwelling suprapubic catheter clamped. The patient voids in a standing position under fluoroscopy (Fig. 38.19D).

The posterior urethra in male patients is composed of a 3.5 cm long prostatic urethra and a 1–1.5 cm long membranous urethra that ends at the inferior aspect of the urogenital diaphragm. On voiding, the bladder neck has a funnel-shaped configuration. A small, oval filling defect due to the indentation of the verumontanum is seen in the midline of the prostatic urethra, with its lower end at the superior aspect of the urogenital diaphragm/membrane. The membranous urethra is the narrowest segment. The female urethra is 4 cm long and extends from bladder neck to the vestibule where it ends in the external meatus between the labia minora.

Periurethral structures that may opacify and be mistaken for pathology include prostatic ducts and reflux into ejaculatory ducts or seminal vesicles; this could be a normal variant or occur with distal obstruction. Cowper's ducts are paired in nature and their opacification appears as small wisps of contrast adjacent to the bulbar urethra into which they drain. The Cowper's gland has a frond-like appearance and is located at the level of the membranous urethra. The opacification is rare and usually associated with a posterior urethral abnormality/stricture and should not be mistaken for a leak. Littré's glands opacification is usually associated with urethral inflammation or stricture and are seen as tiny outpouchings of contrast along the penile urethra in the shaft.

Introduction to IVU Interpretation

In 1976, Howard M. Pollack [24,25], widely considered the "moving spirit behind the creation and development of the specialty of Uroradiology", devoted a whole review in The Journal of Urology to: "Some Limitations and Pitfalls of Excretory Urography". At that time, ultrasonography was still a "new concept" and IVU "...the most important x-ray examination of the urinary tract." With a handful of x-rays, a vial of contrast, some ingenuity and extraordinary perception, radiologists discovered and recorded subtle signs that enabled complex diagnosis of urinary tract pathology. Conventional imaging was as much art as science.

Today, the IVU is an uncommon investigation having been supplanted by more detailed and expensive cross-sectional imaging. Yet, despite this shift away from conventional imaging, their low cost, wide availability and dynamic capability keeps them relevant, especially in limited-resource settings.

"Looking Through IVU Eyes..."

IVU is essentially a planar projection of an abdominal CECT. Signs described on IVU are identifiable on CT and vice versa. It is therefore imperative that we safeguard and pay forward the repository of IVU signs that have been carefully crafted, curated, and handed down to us.

IVU Interpretation

When reviewing an IVU, the images should always be viewed in the temporal sequence they were acquired. Understanding the movement of contrast from peripheral vein to renal artery, through cortex and medulla, calyx, pelvis, ureters, and bladder will ease recognition of deviations from normal physiology.

Scout/Plain Radiograph KUB Region

The plain radiograph of the abdomen or KUB region is a 2D grayscale depiction of complex 3D abdominal anatomy that is a challenge to interpret. A structured review system is essential to avoid errors of perception; "Stones, Bones, Solids, Liquids, Gases," given below, is one such memory aid. A systematic review ensures reading of all structures and avoids "satisfaction of search", a common cause for perceptual error in imaging.

"Stones"

Review the anticipated line of the urethra, ureters, and renal shadows for calculi.

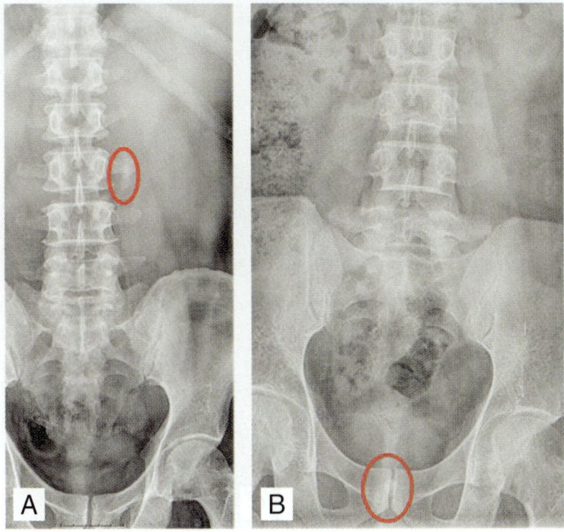

Figure 38.20 (A) Left ureteric calculus at L3 (*red circle*). (B) Urethral calculus (*red circle*).

Starting inferiorly, check the line of the urethra behind the pubic symphysis, inspect the bladder within the perivesical fat plane and identify the vesicoureteric junction (VUJ) located ~1.5–2 cm lateral to the sacrococcygeal junction at the level of the ischial spine. From here, trace the anticipated line of the ureter as it curves laterally and upward, medial, and parallel to the inlet of the pelvis until the sacral ala where it abruptly straightens and continues vertically upward along the outer half of the transverse processes up to L3. Here, it courses laterally across the psoas to the renal hilum, acutely and with an abrupt right angle into the right hilum, oblique and more gradually into the left renal hilum, located at a slightly higher level. The renal shadows are located on either side of the spine, and extend from T12 to L3 (Figs. 38.20 and 38.21).

"Bones"

Review the bony pelvis, femora, ribs, vertebrae for fractures, joint abnormality, focal or diffuse alterations in density that may have a bearing on the etiology of KUB pathology, such as fractures, metastases, spine infection, femoral head AVN, spinal dysraphism and sacroiliitis. Alongside the bones, review soft tissues for subcutaneous emphysema, calcification, deformities, and masses.

"Solids": Solid Viscera

Review the liver, spleen, psoas, and kidneys for air, calcification, enlargement, and collection.

"Liquids": Fluid-Containing Hollow Viscera

Review the bladder, Post-cholecystectomy syndrome (PCS), gall bladder and biliary tree for air and calculi. Air in the bladder could indicate infection, recent instrumentation or a fistula and while aerobilia may not be related to KUB pathology, it is nonetheless a significant finding (Fig. 38.22).

"Gases": Air-Containing Hollow Viscera

Review the lung bases below the diaphragm for lung lesions (Fig. 38.23A) and search for pneumoperitoneum, retropneumoperitoneum, intramural gas and signs of an abnormal intraluminal bowel gas pattern. Fig. 38.23B illustrates a case where dilated small and large bowel distracted attention from a large, obstructing right ureteric calculus at L1-2 near the right hilum; systematic review of "stones" before "gases" circumvents these distractions.

1-Minute Nephrogram: Kidney

On the immediate 1-minute image, the nephrograms will be visible if there is normal arterial supply, venous and urinary drainage.

Density, size, symmetry: The nephrograms should be of similar, normal size and an enhanced, discernible, similar density. The kidney normally ranges in size from 9 to 13 cm, with the left kidney being 0.5 cm longer than the right kidney. Kidney size is considered abnormal if the right kidney is 1.5 cm longer than the left kidney or the left kidney is 2 cm longer than the right kidney. Generally, renal length is >3 vertebral bodies and <4 vertebral bodies in length and the renal axis is parallel to the psoas muscle margin, with the upper pole lying medial to the lower pole.

Contour: The normal reniform shape has a smooth contour; any indentations or bulges need to be correlated with the uniformity of renal parenchymal thickness on the 15-minute pyelogram.

Position: The upper poles are located above the 12th rib with the right kidney positioned lower than the left due to the large space occupied by the liver.

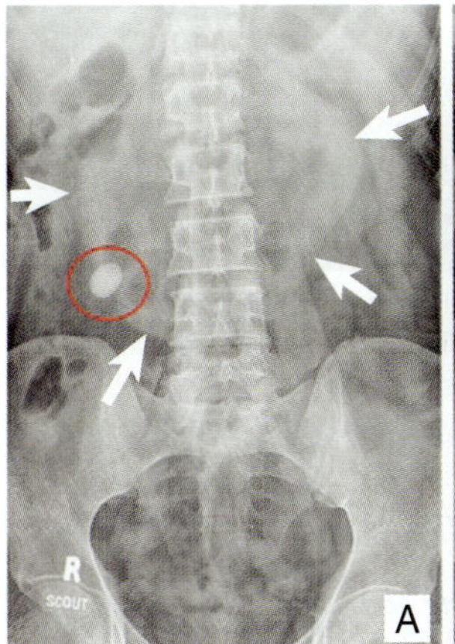

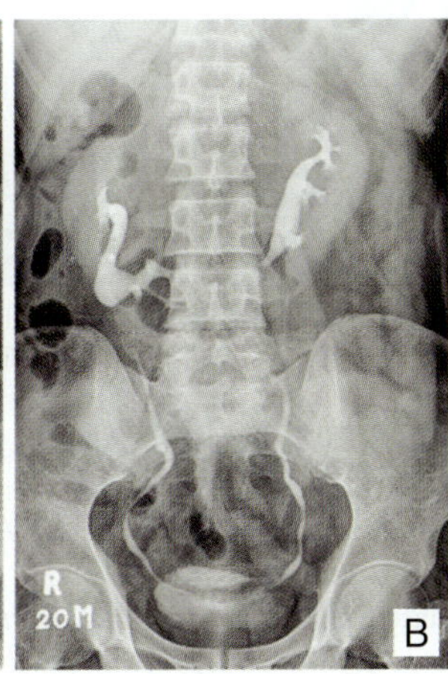

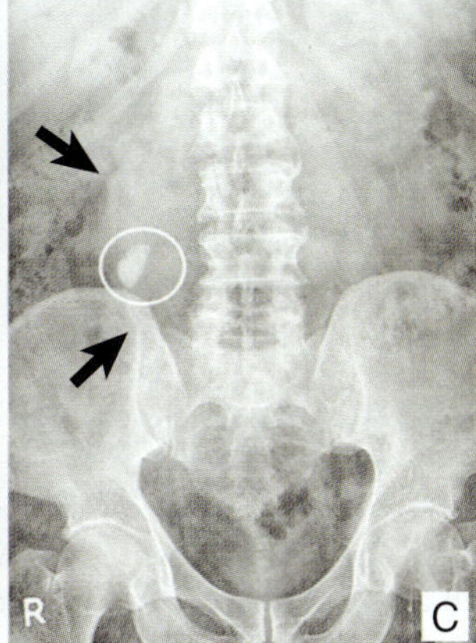

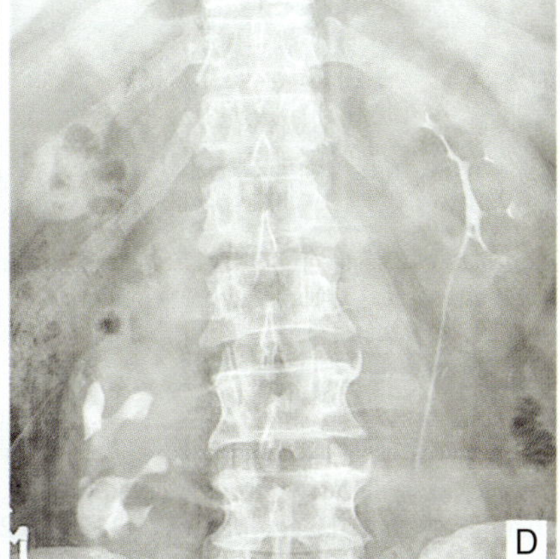

Figure 38.21 Ectopic calculus: outside the anticipated line of the ureter. (A) (C) Plain x-ray KUB. (B) (D) IVU postcompression release KUB. Horseshoe kidney (*white arrows*) with right moiety pelvic calculus (*red circle*) outside the anticipated line of the ureter. Right ectopic, malrotated kidney (*black arrows*) with pelvic calculus (*white circle*) outside the anticipated line of the ureter.

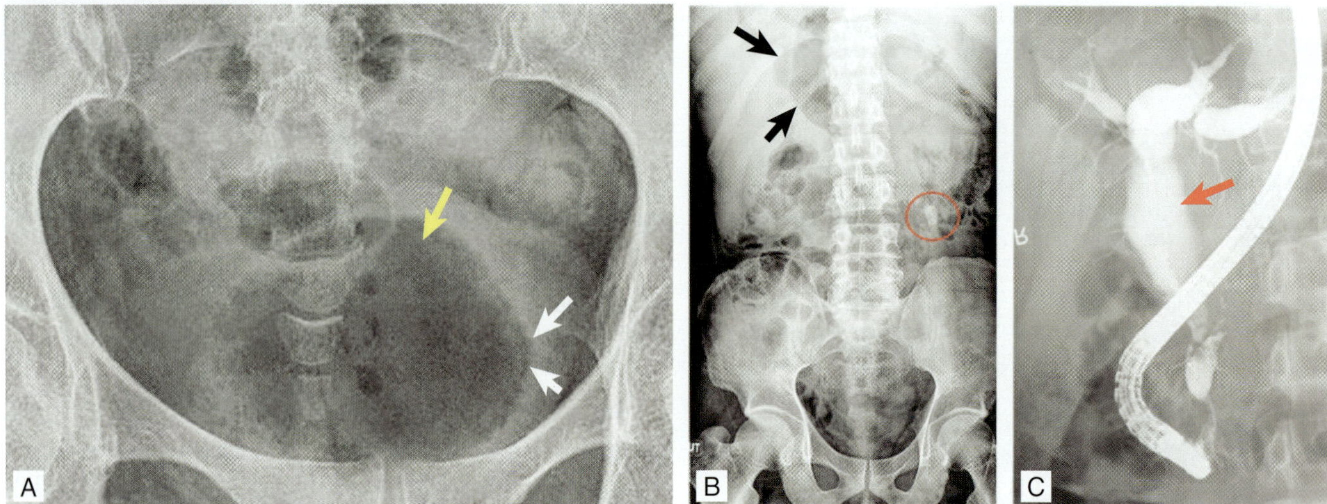

Figure 38.22 Abnormal locations of air. (A) Supine x-ray AP view: bladder: Bubbles of contained air in bladder wall (*white arrows*). Air in bladder lumen (*yellow arrow*). Findings are consistent with emphysematous cystitis. (B) Supine x-ray AP view: KUB: Aerobilia within dilated CBD and intrahepatic bile ducts (*black arrows*). Note left ureteric calculus within anticipated location (*encircled in red*). (C) ERCP correlation of findings in (B): Contrast opacification of fusiform dilated CBD (*red arrow*), intrahepatic bile ducts and abnormal pancreaticobiliary junction, indicating a type 1 choledochal cyst.

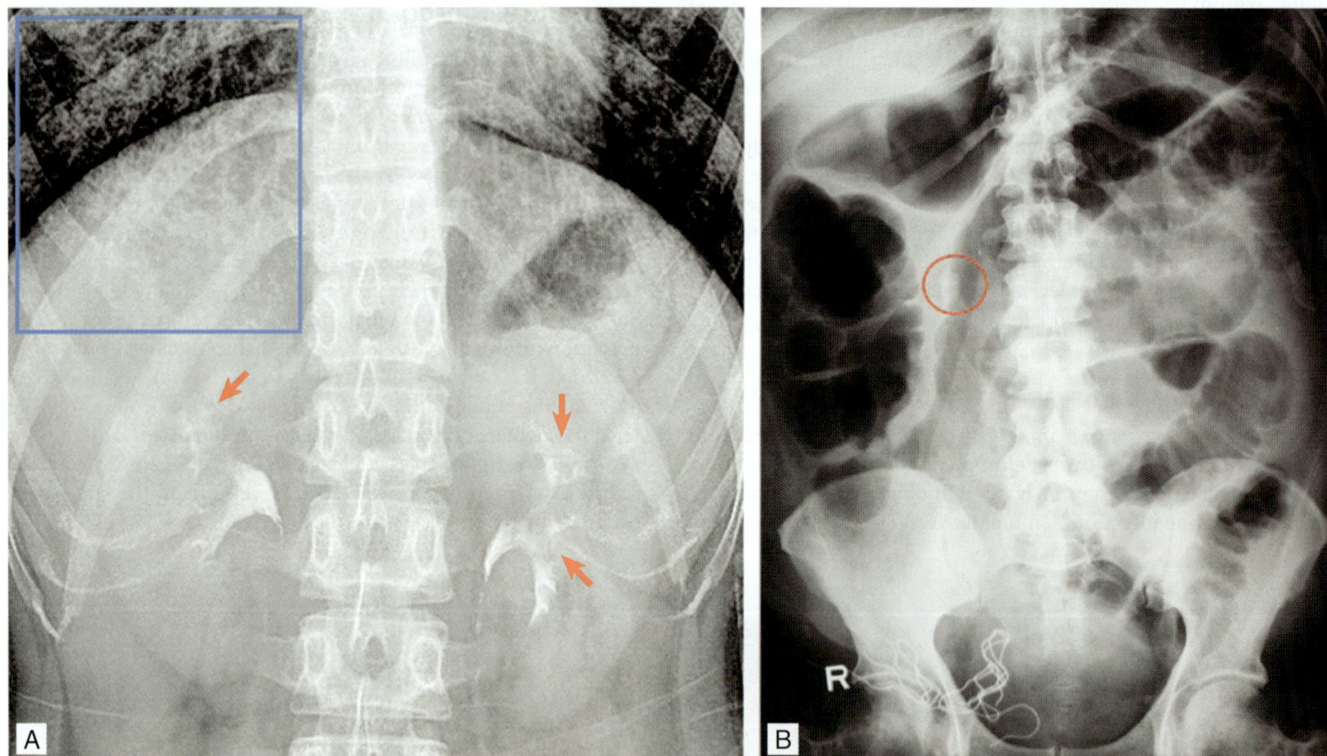

Figure 38.23 Systematic review of lung base and bowel: avoiding "diversions." (A) IVU 5-minute: Miliary TB. Bilateral moth-eaten calyces (*red arrows*) divert the eye away from extensive miliary mottling in both lung bases (*blue rectangle*). (B) Supine x-ray AP view KUB: Ileus diverts attention from a large, obstructing right ureteric calculus (*red circle*) at L1-2.

Axis: The vertical axis is parallel to the upper 1/3 of the psoas major muscle; any alteration in axis and position could indicate a mass, change in size, renal ectopia/fusion (Fig. 38.21B and D).

Pattern: When the nephrogram is abnormal, recognizing the nephrographic pattern will provide a clue to the cause.

- Faint persistent nephrogram: *hypotension, impaired function*
- Increasing dense nephrogram: *obstruction, Renal artery stenosis (RAS), Renal vein thrombosis (RVT)*
- Immediate dense nephrogram: Acute tubular necrosis *(ATN), Acute papillary necrosis (APN)*
- Striated nephrogram: *APN, acute obstruction, Autosomal recessive polycystic kidney disease (ARPKD), Medullary sponge kidney (MSK)*
- Patchy nephrogram: *Vasculitis*
- Cortical rim nephrogram: *Infarction*

5 and 15-Minute Pyelogram

By the 15-minute image, contrast has transited through the parenchyma and been excreted into the collecting system. Consequently, the nephrographic density is reduced while the PCS appears as the dominant opacity. PCS opacification and filling can be augmented by applying a binder on the lower abdomen and pelvis, between the 5- and 15-minute exposures. The PCS as displayed on a 15-minute "binder" image has a high spatial resolution and provides an excellent depiction of the urothelium-lined surfaces (Fig. 38.9).

Temporal symmetry: Contrast opacification of the parenchyma and excretion into the PCS should be similar, indicating bilateral equal and normal arterial supply, venous and urinary drainage. Any dissimilarity, however subtle, could indicate significant pathology: an asymmetric unilateral persistent, dense nephrogram with delayed excretion into the PCS suggests an acute high-grade obstruction.

Papillae

Papillary contrast: A papillary blush can be seen on the 5-minute image as a prominent papillary opacity without resolvable tubular structures that gradually decreases in density on the 15-minute compression image and the later compression release image. This differs from tubular ectasia and medullary sponge kidney where the papillary opacity shows resolvable linear striations. In papillary necrosis, linear or pool-like extensions of contrast are seen extending from the fornices into the renal substance of the papilla. An aberrant papilla appears as a filling defect in the middle of the infundibulum with a rim of contrast at the margin of the angular defect.

Interpapillary line and parenchymal thickness: The interpapillary line is a line drawn through the papillae that normally runs parallel to the renal outline. The distance between the interpapillary line and the renal outline is the parenchymal thickness, a uniform thick rind of renal cortical and medullary tissue that envelops the fatty sinus and its contents, including the PCS and vessels.

Contour bulges/indentations: Bulges and indentations noted on the nephrogram can be analyzed in relation to the uniformity of the parenchymal thickness. The normal parenchymal thickness at the poles is 3–3.5 cm poles and 2–2.5 cm at the interpolar region. Parenchymal thickness can help differentiate the causes of renal contour bulges and indentations (Box 38.7).

Collecting system: Once filtration occurs at the level of the glomerulus, urine flows through a continuous lumen extending from the tubules and collecting ducts through tiny papillary orifices into the calyces, infundibuli, renal pelvis, ureter, and bladder.

BOX 38.7 Contour Indentations/Bulges

Congenital anatomic variation:
- uniform PT + indentations between normal calyces = fetal lobulation
- uniform PT + predictable location = dromedary hump/hilar lip/column of Bertin

Pathology:
- focally thinned PT
  - + abnormal underlying calyx = scar (VUR/stone)
  - – abnormal calyx = renal infarction
- focally thickened PT
  - + calyceal extrinsic impression = mass
  - + focal filling defect = simple cyst (low density)
  - + parenchymal "beaking" = cyst/solid mass
  - + "double contour" = solid enhancing mass (high/equal density)

PT = parenchymal thickness.

BOX 38.8 Grading of Hydronephrosis on IVU

Grade 1: blunting of fornices
Grade 2: dilated fornices + preserved papillary impressions
Grade 3: rounding of calyces + loss of papillary impressions
Grade 4: ballooning of calyces + marked parenchymal thinning

Calyx: When drainage is obstructed, the calyceal fornices lose their sharpness and with increasing obstruction, balloon and evert into the clubbed calyx of severe hydronephrosis (Box 38.8).

Apart from simple dilatation, calyceal deformities can occur that provide clues to the diagnosis.

- Tuberculosis (TB) and transitional cell carcinoma (TCC) can give rise to "phantom" calyces that are so filled with inflammatory/cancerous tissue that they do not opacify or when partially opacified, appear "moth-eaten" or enlarged and tumefactive like the "oncocalyx" of TCC
- Clustered calculi near a calyx can indicate a calyceal diverticulum communicating with a calyx that will slowly fill and enlarge with contrast (Fig. 38.24A)
- Calyces can be splayed or spread apart by cysts and solid masses that have an SOL effect (Fig. 38.24B and C)
- The normal number of calyces ranges from 7–14; an increased number could indicate a congenital polycalycosis while a decreased number could indicate the presence of "phantom" calyces or, if localized to one part of the kidney, could suggest a duplex kidney with an obstructed nonfunctioning upper moiety (Fig. 38.25)

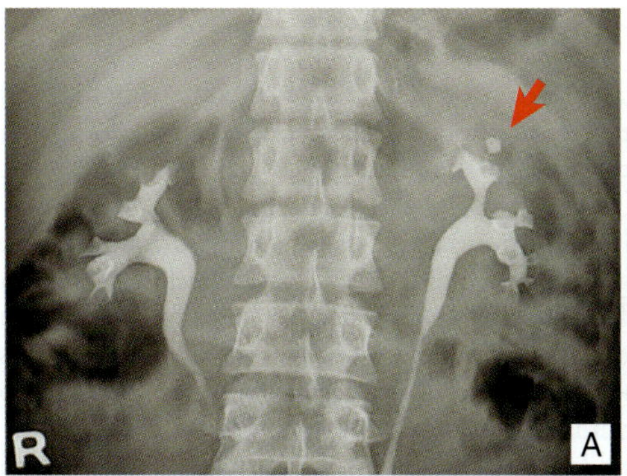

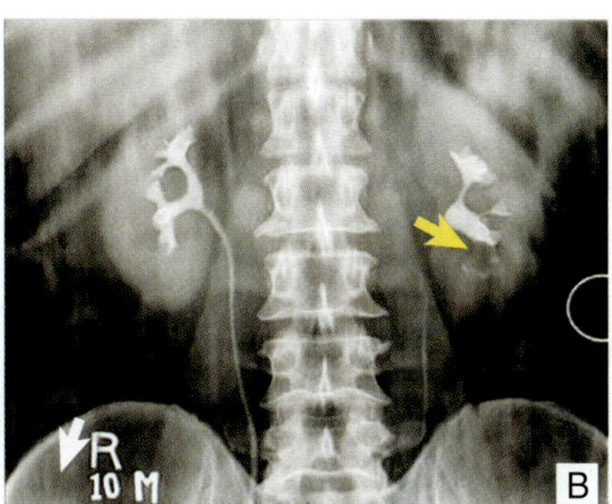

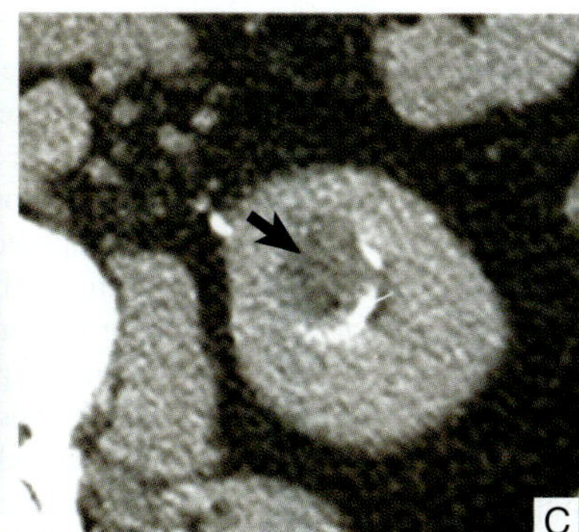

Figure 38.24 Calyceal abnormality. IVU 10-minute: (A) Left upper pole calyceal diverticulum (*red arrow*). (B) Left lower pole smooth, extrinsic filling defect (*yellow arrow*). (C) Correlative CECT delayed axial section through left renal lower pole: simple cyst causing extrinsic impression seen in (B).

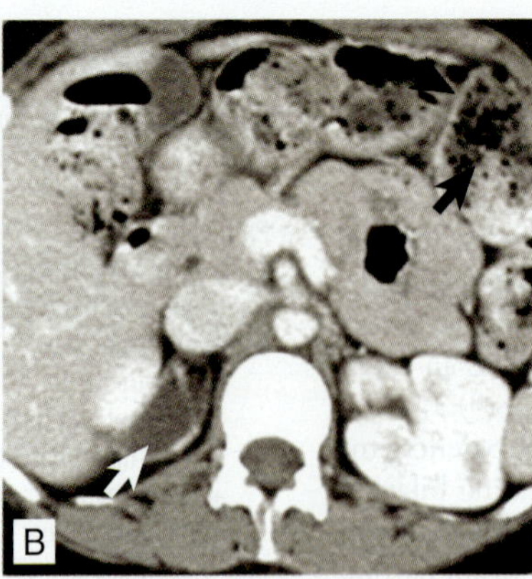

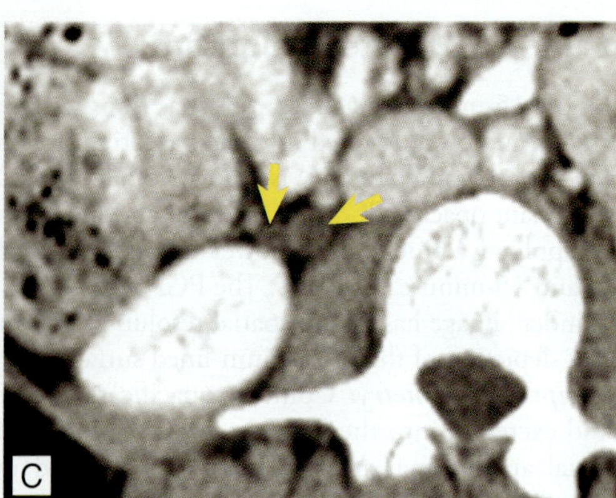

Figure 38.25 Duplex kidney: obstructed upper moiety. (A) IVU 10-minute: Bilateral duplex kidneys. Right upper pole obstructed moiety with delayed excretion (*red circle*) and lower moiety appearing like a "short" right kidney containing few calyces (*black arrow*). (B–C) Correlative CECT axial sections: right upper pole obstructed moiety seen in (A) with pencil-thin parenchyma (*white arrow*) and two ureters (*yellow arrows*).

Infundibulum: Normal vessels at the upper pole can cause vascular impressions that mimic stenosis or filling defects, especially when combined with the larger, compound calyx found at the upper pole. Vascular impressions are identified by their straight, smooth, band-like lucent appearance that becomes smaller on the 15-minute binder/compression image or on a prone image.

Pelvis: Variants include bifid renal pelvis and extra-renal pelvis, the latter mimicking PUJ obstruction, but lacking definitive calyceal dilatation and postfrusemide decompression. The pelvis is oriented medially unless malrotated when the pelvis appears end-on or oriented laterally. A disproportionately small renal pelvis in the presence of dilated calyces may be due to extrinsic compression by sinus lipomatosis/parapelvic cysts or pelvic wall fibrosis causing luminal stenosis. This "multi-infundibulo-pelvic" stenosis, is in fact, characteristic of urinary tract TB.

15-Minute Release-Binder KUB

Visualization: Contrast–laden urine that enters the ureters on release-compression image should be of equal density throughout the entire length. *Segmental nonvisualization* can be due to peristalsis and is usually overcome with compression release but may require a prone image or fluoroscopy guided spot views to definitively display these segments (Fig. 38.8).

Standing column: It is unusual to capture a full-length "standing" column of contrast within the ureter and its appearance should be treated with suspicion since it likely represents an obstruction such as a calculus or a ureteric "ileus" that is nonobstructive dilatation related to adjacent inflammation.

Medial deviation: The ureter may overlie or lie medial to the lumbar pedicle or be separated from the opposite ureter by <5 cm. This can be due to a normal variant such as the psoas muscle hypertrophy found in young, muscular males or abnormalities such as congenital retrocaval/circumcaval ureter or retroperitoneal fibrosis (RPF).

Lateral deviation: The ureter can also be deviated laterally >1 cm beyond the tip of the transverse process, due to an acute obstruction leading to a sudden increase in luminal pressure, making the ureter swing away from the spine. Lateral displacement can also occur from aortic aneurysm and para-aortic adenopathy or abrupt lateral angulation over an iliac artery aneurysm.

Caliber: Ureteric caliber >8 mm or more significantly, ureteric caliber asymmetry, indicates dilatation that could be obstructive or nonobstructive in etiology. Acute, high-grade obstruction causes minimal ureteral dilatation, while chronic, low-grade obstruction causes greater ureteral dilatation. Nonobstructive dilatation can be due to fluid diuresis, diabetes insipidus, chronic vesicoureteral reflux (VUR) or ileus related to an inflammatory process. Focal lower third ureteric dilatation is characteristic of congenital megaureter.

Anatomic narrowing: The ureter is physiologically and intrinsically narrowed at the ureteropelvic junction (UPJ) and vesicoureteric junction (VUJ) or extrinsically narrowed at the iliac vascular transition where it creates a proximal focal dilatation known as the ureteric "spindle" or where the gonadal vein crosses the ureter. Pathological causes of filling defects and narrowing can be single or multiple, luminal, mural or extrinsic. The "goblet" sign is typical of a polypoidal, intussuscepting mucosal filling defect that has enlarged the lumen of the ureter, creating a concave meniscus at the site of obstruction (Fig. 38.26).

Calculus not evident on scout image: When a calculus is not evident on the scout image, a standing column with a subtle difference in ureteric density can red-flag its location. Scrutinizing the inferior end of the standing column on the post void and looking back on the scout image can reveal a faint opacity that increases in density following the flow of luminal contrast over it that gives rise to a "growing calculus" effect. Often, these calculi are missed on the scout because they overlie complex bony sacral anatomy or are obscured by bowel gas.

Contour: Indentations or ureteral "notching" can occur from extrinsic vascular narrowing such as arterial or venous collaterals or a prominent gonadal vein. Tiny ulcerations due to inflammatory processes can give rise to pseudoverticulae.

Full Bladder and Post Void KUB

Normal: The full bladder is spherical and smooth with the wall appearing progressively less evident. It rests on the pelvic floor, with the bladder base projected over the superior margin of the pubic symphysis.

Wall: Perivesical fat can be seen as a thin lucency surrounding the bladder, enabling visualization of the bladder wall thickness. Smooth indentations at the bladder base from the prostate or superiorly from the uterine fundus can be visible especially when the bladder is under-filled. Inner surface irregularity, when diffuse, is likely due to trabeculation secondary to bladder outflow obstruction.

Contour: A bladder diverticulum is incidentally detected and congenital, while multiple sacculations between trabeculations are acquired secondary to bladder outflow obstruction and can

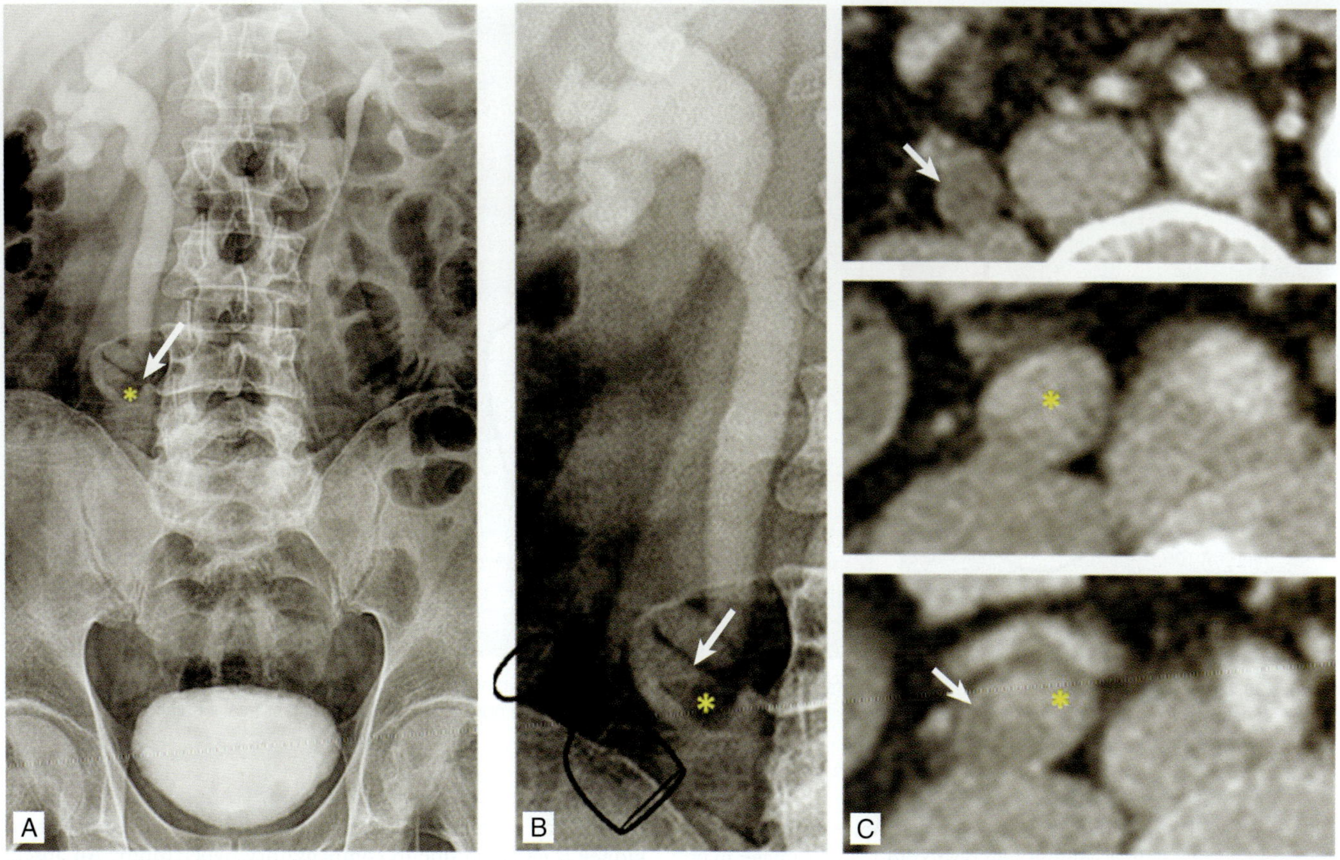

Figure 38.26 Goblet sign: TCC. IVU postcompression release: (A–B) Obstructing right mid ureteric, polypoid filling defect (*yellow asterisks*) focally dilating distal lumen (*white arrows*): Goblet sign. (C) Correlative CECT axial sections through right ureter: Focally dilated right ureter (*white arrows*) with intraluminal solid enhancing lesion (*yellow asterisks*) along medial wall seen as filling defect in (A) and (B).

alter the contour. Neurogenic bladder with detrusor hypertrophy and outflow obstruction related to detrusor-sphincter dyssynergia can give rise to a cone-shaped, highly trabeculated and sacculated bladder called a fir-tree bladder. Excess fat accumulation in the pelvis can laterally compress the bladder as can hypertrophy of the obturator internus muscles and give rise to a pear-shaped bladder.

Filling defects: Small filling defects can be obscured when the bladder is distended and may be better visualized on the early filling 15-minute KUB and the post void image. Stippling of contrast on the surface of a papillary filling defect, the "stipple" sign, is seen in TCC.

VUJ: A lucent filling defect at the VUJ could represent edema following the passage of a stone. A thick halo of mucosal edema can be seen around an impacted VUJ calculus (Fig. 38.27), while a thin halo of lucency around the submucosal ureterocoele is due to an overlying thin mucosal layer.

Post void KUB: The post void image is a full KUB to evaluate drainage of the upper tracts since nonobstructive and insignificant

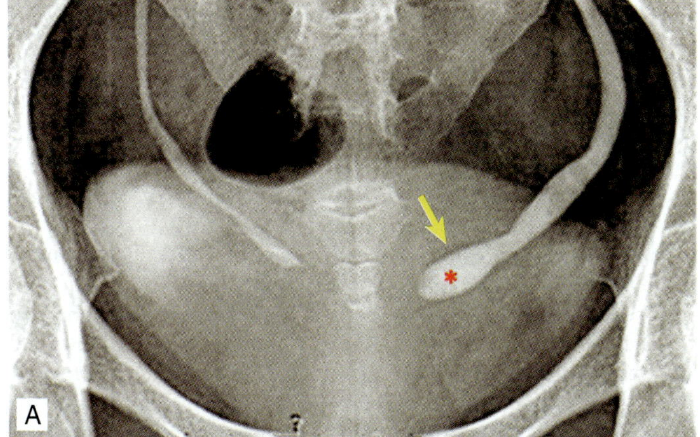

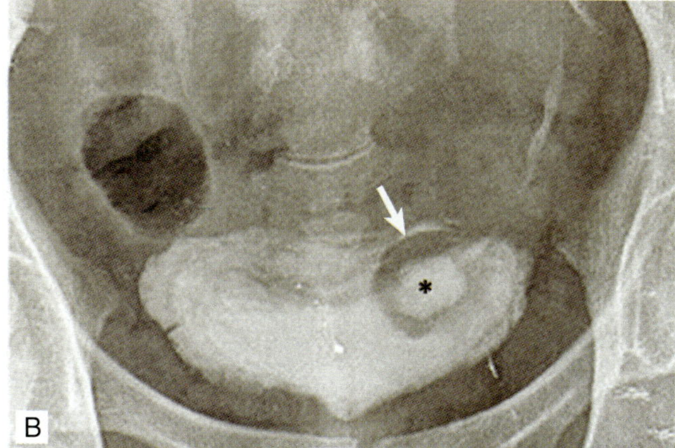

Figure 38.27 Halo at VUJ. IVU postcompression release (bladder): (A) Focally dilated terminal ureter (*red asterisk*) due to ureterocoele, with thin halo of normal overlying mucosa (*yellow arrow*). (B) Impacted VUJ calculus (*black asterisk*) with thick halo of surrounding mucosal edema (*white arrow*).

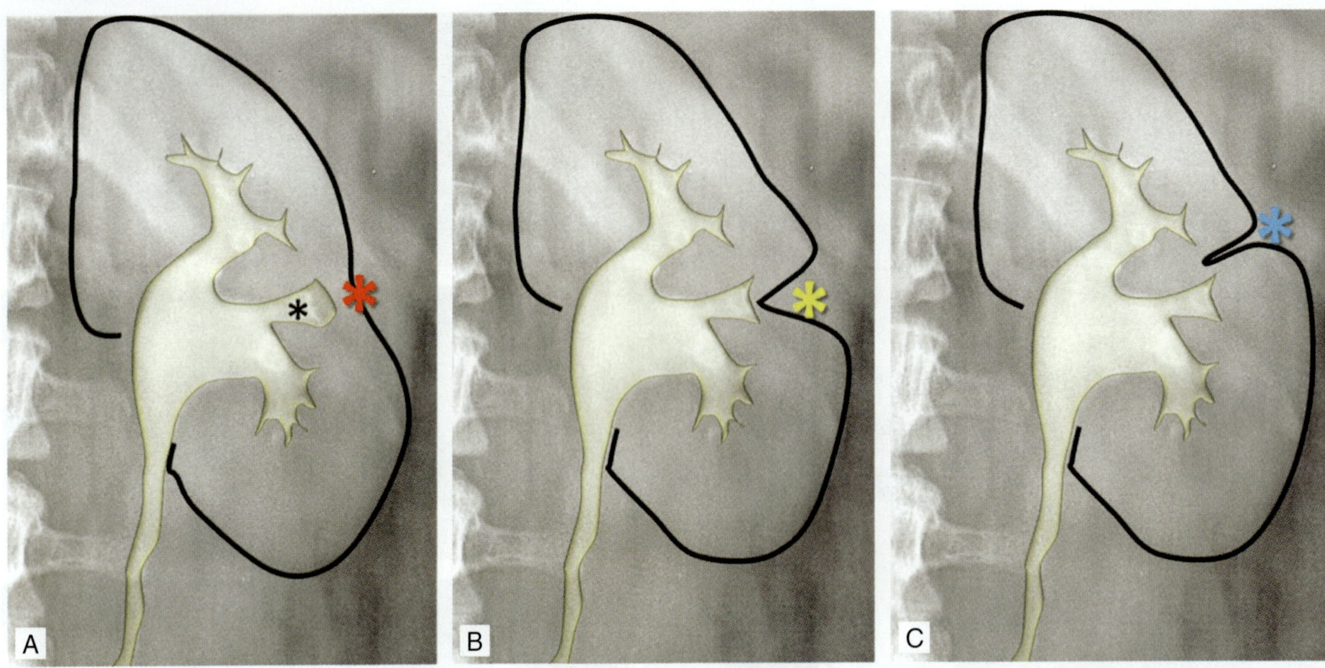

Figure 38.28 Contour indentations. Color-coded diagram of IVU 10-minute nephrogram with binder: (A) Scar (*red asterisk*): broad indentation overlying clubbed calyx (*black asterisk*). (B) Infarct (*yellow asterisk*): wedge-shaped indentation overlying normal calyx. (C) Persistent fetal lobulation (*blue asterisk*): acute indentation between normal calyces.

dilatation will have drained on this image. Apart from bladder emptying and residual volume, the post void bladder image may reveal small filling defects obscured on the full bladder image.

Congenital Lesions and Variants

Persistent Fetal Lobulations

These are due to the incomplete fusion of developing metanephric lobules. On IVU, the renal outline is smoothly and acutely indented at regular intervals between the calyces, with preserved, uniform parenchymal thickness. Renal scars, on the other hand, are seen as foci of parenchymal thinning with broad indentations at irregular intervals and overlying clubbed calyces, while renal infarcts are wedge-shaped indentations overlying normal calyces (Fig. 38.28).

Renal Pseudotumors

These are prominent foci of normal renal tissue that can mimic masses.

On IVU, a hypertrophied column of Bertin is a cortical prominence that splays calyces without bulging the contour and is continuous with renal cortex on USG. Dromedary humps are focal bulges caused by the normal splenic impression on the superolateral margin of the left kidney. The calyces underlying the hump extend further laterally into the hump than the other calyces, preserving a normal parenchymal thickness (Box 38.7).

Renal Agenesis

This is due to failure of the ureteric bud to reach the metanephros and is associated with an absent ipsilateral ureter and hemitrigone and, sometimes, features of the VATER anomaly (**V**ertebral, **V**entricular septal anomalies, **A**norectal/**T**racheal/**E**sophageal fistula/atresia, **R**adial bone). On IVU, the renal shadow is absent, replaced by air-filled splenic or hepatic flexure. The contralateral kidney is enlarged due to compensatory hypertrophy. An absent renal shadow may also be due to renal ectopia, nephrectomy or severe atrophy from VUR/multiple infarctions.

Renal Hypoplasia

This is due to an intrauterine vascular insult. On IVU, the hypoplastic kidney is seen as a functioning, small, smooth, normal shaped kidney with 5 (or <5) normal calyces. Hypoplastic kidneys may be supernumerary and are usually left-sided and caudally positioned, with ureteric drainage into the bladder or into the normal kidney's ureter.

Rotational Abnormalities and Renal Ectopia

- On IVU of an incomplete developmental rotation or malrotation, the PUJ points anteriorly, with the pelvis projected over medially oriented calyces. In the rare over-rotation, the PUJ points posteriorly
- In renal ectopia due to failure of complete ascent, there is a small pelvic kidney, prone to trauma, VUR, and calculus formation (Fig. 38.21C and D), which may be associated with contralateral agenesis, ectopia or midline fusion of both unascended kidneys as a "pancake" kidney. Renal ectopia due to over-ascent can occur through a localized eventration and result in an intrathoracic kidney
- **Horseshoe kidney,** connected by a fibrous or parenchymal isthmus, is arrested in its ascent by the IMA origin. On plain film and IVU, the characteristic horseshoe configuration may be seen although the isthmus is poorly visualized over the lower lumbar spine. The kidneys are low lying and malrotated, with upper poles at the same height, pointing superolaterally. The lower poles point inferomedially and the renal pelvis and ureters run anteriorly over the isthmus. PUJ obstruction (PUJO), calculi and Wilms' tumor may be associated with it,

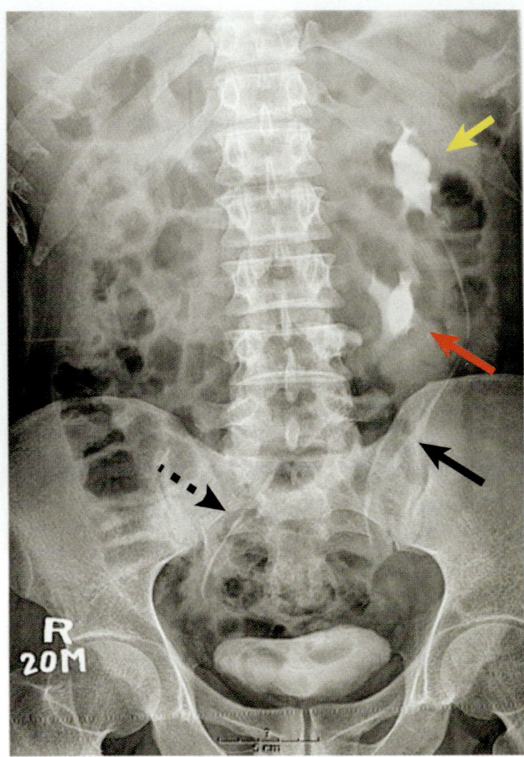

Figure 38.29 Crossed fused ectopia. IVU postcompression release: Crossed, fused kidney in the left renal fossa with distinct, malrotated upper (*yellow arrow*) and lower (*red arrow*) moiety pyelograms. Upper moiety ureter (*black arrow*) inserts ipsilaterally on the left. Lower moiety ureter (*dashed black arrow*) crosses midline to insert contralaterally on the right.

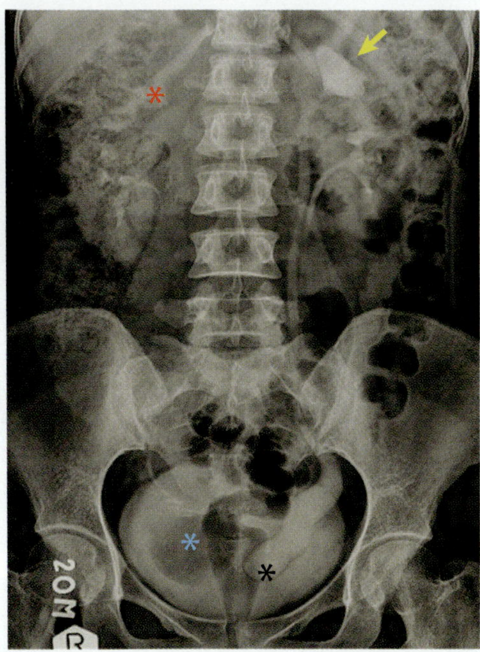

Figure 38.30 Bilateral duplex kidneys: drooping lily, ureterocoeles. IVU postcompression release-binder KUB: Right lower pole moiety displaced inferolaterally by unopacified, obstructed, hydronephrotic upper pole moiety (*red asterisk*)—"drooping lily" sign. Left mild upper moiety hydroureteronephrosis (*yellow arrow*). Right obstructing, ectopic, unopacified ureterocoele (*blue asterisk*) inferomedial to orthotopic lower moiety VUJ, causing a smooth, round, filling defect. Left partially obstructing, ectopic, opacified ureterocoele (*black asterisk*) with a thin mucosal halo, causing a cobra-head appearance.

as also anomalies of the GI tract and cyclic vomiting syndrome (CVS), and Turner's or Ellis–van Creveld syndromes (Fig. 38.21A and B)

- **Crossed fused ectopia** is a horseshoe kidney with both kidneys on the same side. On IVU, the left kidney usually crosses to the right forming an enlarged left renal shadow and an absent right renal shadow. Two distinct malrotated pyelograms are evident with the upper moiety ureter orthotopically inserting into the ipsilateral side of the bladder and the lower moiety ureter crossing the midline to insert orthotopically into the contralateral side of the bladder (Fig. 38.29) [26,27]

Duplication Abnormalities

These range from a bifid renal pelvis to completely duplicated pelvis and ureters.

- In incomplete duplication, there is a bifid ureter with ureteric fusion at varying points, forming a common distal ureter and orifice in the bladder. Yo-yo reflux can occur in bifid or Y-shaped ureters, detected on fluoroscopy or from ipsilateral renal scarring
- In complete duplication, the orthotopic lower moiety ureter refluxes while the ectopic upper moiety ureter is associated with a ureterocoele that obstructs (Weigert-Meyer rule)
- On IVU, the duplex is bilateral in 20% causing renal enlargement on plain radiograph. Evidence of lower moiety reflux nephropathy is seen in the form of cortical scarring over clubbed calyces, while upper moiety obstruction, marked hydronephrosis, parenchymal thinning and delayed excretion causes inferior displacement of the lower moiety ("drooping lily" sign) (Fig. 38.30) [30]
- In the bladder, ureterocoeles appear as submucosal, focal dilatations of the intramural terminal ureter that project into the lumen. Large ureterocoeles obstruct the contralateral ureter or urethral orifice and cause bilateral hydronephrosis. If obstructed with loss of upper moiety function, the ureterocoele will appear as a well-defined radiolucent mass within the opacified bladder. Simple ureterocoeles are contrast-filled structures with a thin smooth radiolucent wall ("halo") surrounded by contrast-containing urine resulting in a cobra-head appearance (Figs. 38.27 and 38.30)

Polycystic Kidneys

Autosomal recessive polycystic kidney disease (ARPKD) consists of bilateral enlarged kidneys containing numerous tiny (1–8 mm) cysts. Renal function improves with age but associated periportal fibrosis worsens and causes liver failure. On IVU, there are enlarged kidneys with a striated nephrogram caused by contrast within preserved functioning tubules, next to dilated nonopacified diseased tubules.

Autosomal dominant polycystic kidney disease (ADPKD) is a bilateral, progressive disease with numerous cysts of varying size that can grow extremely large, replace normal renal parenchyma and lead to renal failure. ADPKD is associated with cysts in the liver, pancreas, spleen and lung, berry aneurysms, coarctation, and valvular heart disease. On plain radiograph, curvilinear cyst calcification and enlarged kidneys are seen with multiple, well-defined, low density, round foci in the nephrogram ("Swiss cheese" nephrogram). On IVU, the kidneys are enlarged, with cysts splaying, thinning, and stretching the calyces, broadening the infundibula and give rise to a spider leg PCS deformity (Fig. 38.31).

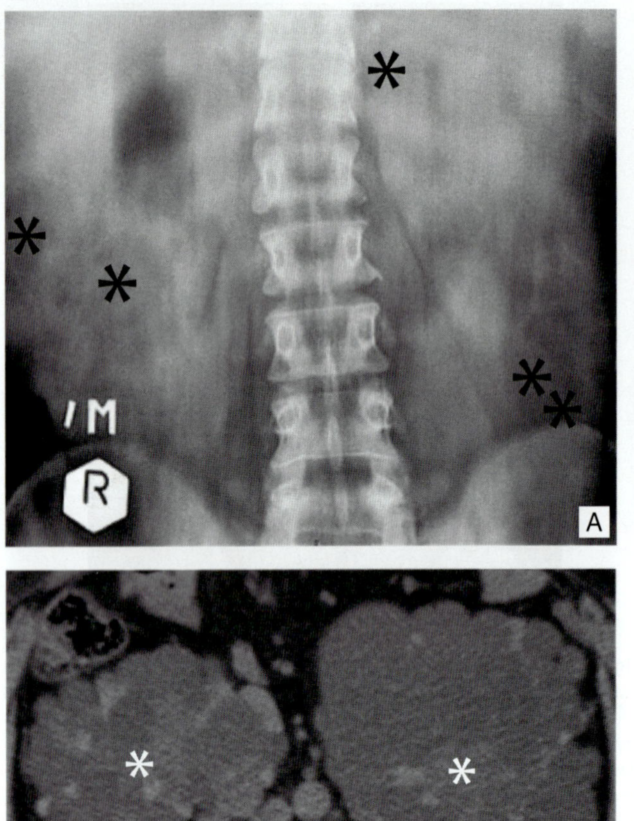

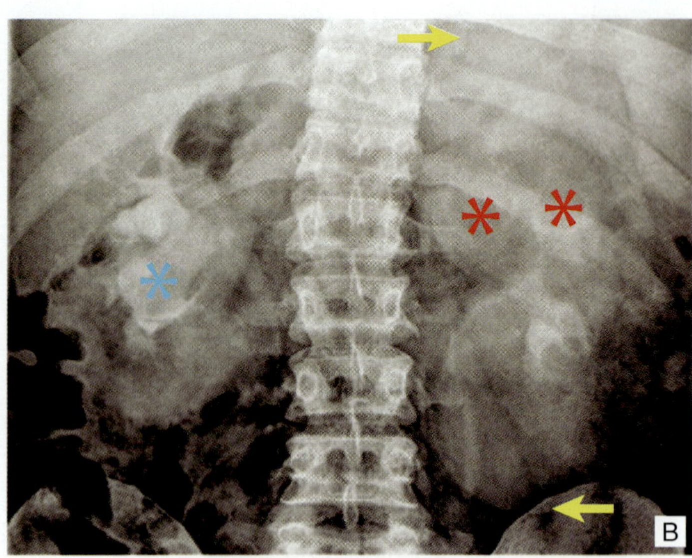

Figure 38.31 Autosomal dominant Polycystic Kidney Disease. (A) IVU 1-minute nephrotomogram: multiple lucencies (*black asterisks*) in bilateral enlarged kidneys, caused by numerous parenchymal cysts: "Swiss cheese" nephrogram. (B) IVU 10-minute pyelogram: multiple cysts causing bilateral lucencies (*red asterisks*), splaying calyces, broadening infundibula (*blue asterisk*) and enlarging kidneys (*yellow arrows*). (C) NECT axial sections through kidneys: numerous bilateral cysts, enlarged kidneys with paucity of normal intervening renal parenchyma (*white asterisks*).

Medullary Sponge Kidney

This is a congenital abnormality of tubules in the medullary pyramid, where concretions within fusiform and cystic ducts produce stippled and bristle medullary calcifications that can progress to medullary nephrocalcinosis. It can be associated with Caroli disease and Ehlers-Danlos syndrome.

On IVU, multiple linear, brush-like ("paintbrush" sign) and saccular contrast collections are seen within the medulla. This differs from the normal papillary blush where distinct and resolvable tubular structures are not evident. Small calculi within the ectatic tubules can progress to medullary nephrocalcinosis and the formation of ureteric calculi. Calculi within the papillae on the scout image appear to enlarge as the cavities fill: "growing calculus sign" (Fig. 38.32)

Calyceal Diverticulum

It is an intraparenchymal cavity lined with transitional epithelium, usually a few millimeters in size, that communicates with the minor calyx/fornix or less commonly with the

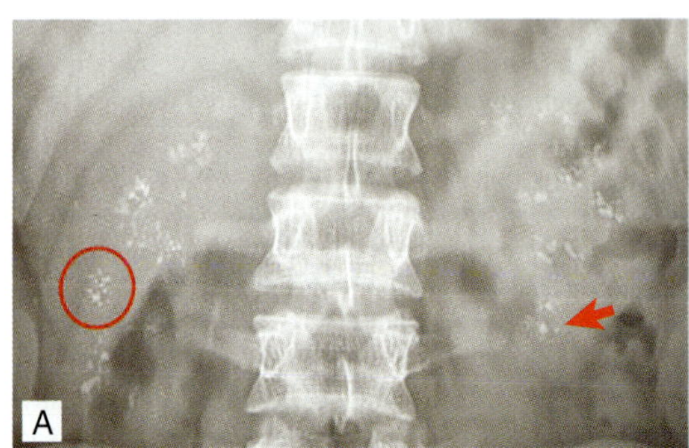

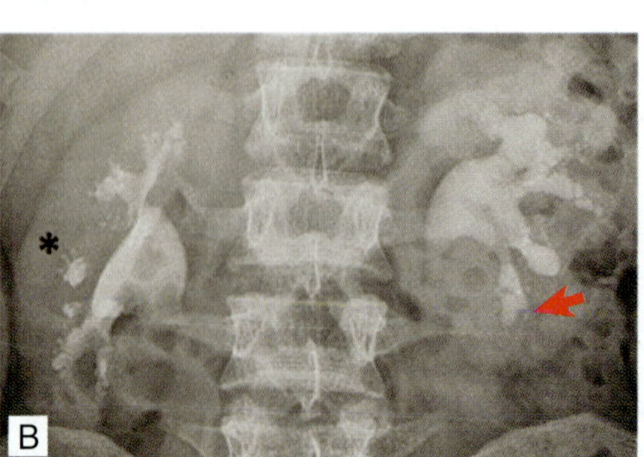

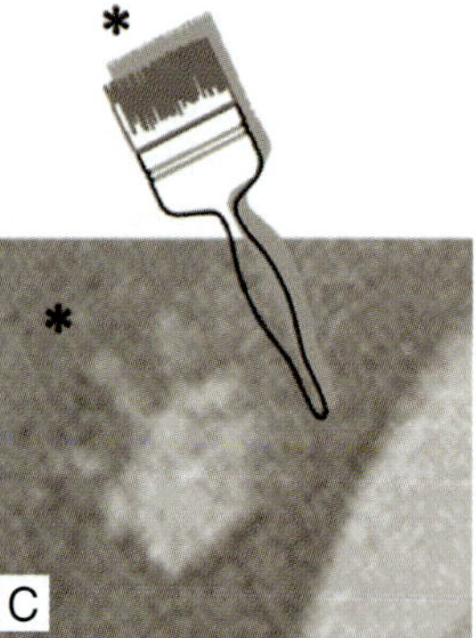

Figure 38.32 Medullary sponge kidney. (A) IVU scout view: Bilateral, tiny calculi within ectatic tubules (*red circle*) giving rise to medullary nephrocalcinosis (*red arrow*) (B–C) IVU 10-minute + zoomed-in right interpole medulla: Multiple, small, linear, "paintbrush" (*black asterisks*) and saccular contrast collections within the medulla. Calculi within the papillae on scout appear to enlarge as the cavities fill: "Growing calculus sign" (*red arrow*).

infundibulum/renal pelvis. The diverticulum does not receive drainage from nephrons and therefore, opacifies after the calyx. Infection and calculi can result from the stasis. On scout image, calculi are seen in clusters within the parenchyma with gradual contrast filling around the cluster within the diverticulum on delayed IVU images (Fig. 38.24A). Calculi that shift with change in position can also differentiate mobile calculi within a calyceal diverticulum from parenchymal calcification.

Pelvi-Ureteric Junction Obstruction (PUJO)

- PUJO is a congenital obstruction with a spectrum of severity ranging from severe antenatal hydronephrosis with global cortical loss to an adult asymptomatic PUJO. PUJO is bilateral in 20% and can be associated with multicystic disease of kidney, renal agenesis, renal duplication and VUR
- On plain radiograph, a massive hydronephrosis from PUJO can displace bowel, creating a paucity of bowel on the side of the abnormal kidney as well as reveal an absence of the renal shadow
- On IVU, there is severe acute obstruction with a delayed, increasingly dense nephrogram and delayed excretion resulting in a negative pyelogram: dilated PCS lucency within a dense nephrogram. The opacified PCS shows clubbed calyces, dilated pelvis and "crescents" peripheral to calyces due to stasis in displaced collecting ducts [29]. The PUJ appears tightly closed with ureter unopacified; the large round dilated pelvis, round dilated calyces and thin rim of parenchyma have the appearance of an elephant's foot
- In chronic obstruction, cortical loss, calculus formation and pyonephrosis can be demonstrated. Subtle PUJO presents as a large extra-renal pelvis that balloons following frusemide-induced diuresis

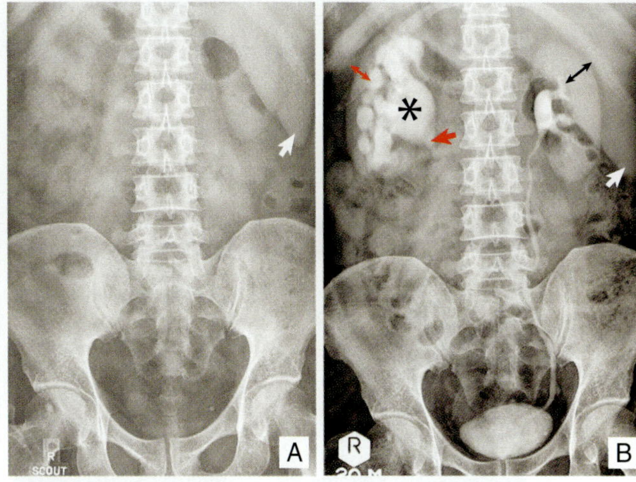

Figure 38.33 PUJ obstruction with Incidental situs inversus. (A) IVU scout: Incidental situs inversus, with liver on the left (*white arrow* in A and B) and left kidney lower than the right. (B) IVU postcompression release: Abrupt cutoff at the right PUJ (*red arrow*) with moderate hydroureteronephrosis (*black asterisks*), nonvisualization of the ureter and parenchymal thinning (*double red arrow line*) compared to the normal parenchymal thickness on the left (*double black arrow line*).

- Following pyeloplasty, IVU shows a characteristic straight vertical medial edge to the pelvis with the ureter arising from the inferomedial angle of the pelvis. Dilatation of the collecting system persists despite improvement of urinary drainage (Figs. 38.33 and 38.34)

Retrocaval or Circumcaval Ureter

This is due to an abnormality in the embryogenesis of the IVC, with persistence of the right posterior cardinal vein ventral to the ureter

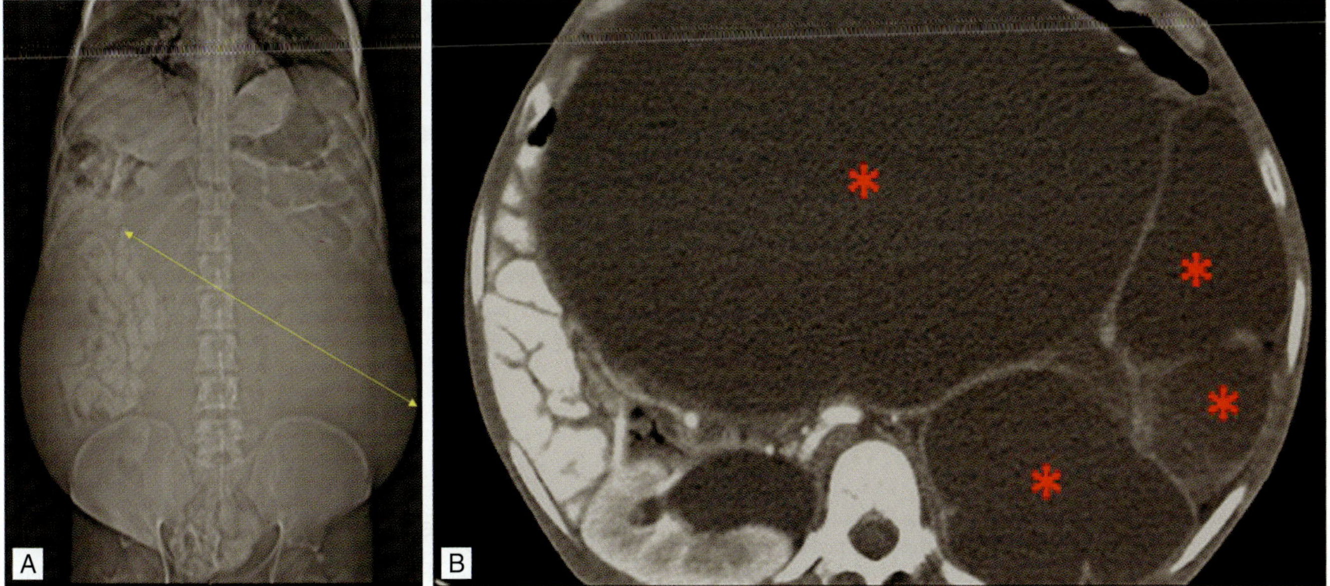

Figure 38.34 Massive PUJ obstruction: "Elephant foot" sign. (A) CT Topogram: Paucity of bowel on the left with bulging left flank and displacement of the bowel to the right (*double yellow arrow line*). (B) CECT axial section at the level of the kidneys: Massive left hydronephrosis accounting for the SOL effect in (A). "Elephant foot" sign—heel pad: pelvis + toes: calyces (*red asterisks*). Note the markedly thinned, imperceptible parenchyma. There is contralateral mild PUJ obstruction.

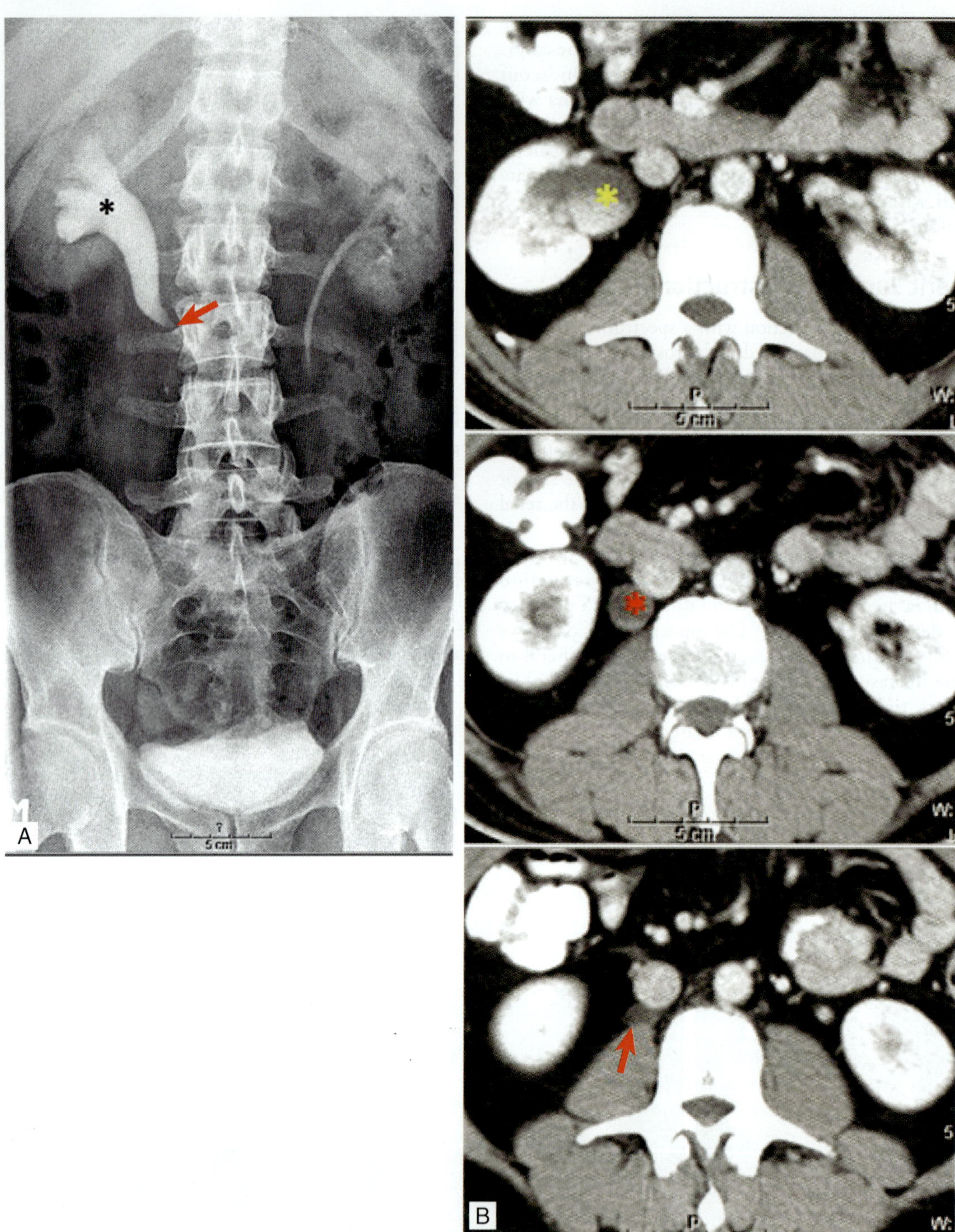

Figure 38.35 Retrocaval ureter. (A) IVU postcompression release KUB: Proximal right ureter swings medially over the L3 pedicle (*red arrow*). There is moderate right hydronephrosis (*black asterisk*). (B) CECT axial sections (correlative): Note the right hydronephrosis (*yellow asterisk*). The right ureter (*red asterisk*) passes behind the IVC (*red arrow*).

and failure of the right supracardinal system to develop. On IVU, the proximal right ureter swings medially over the L3-4 pedicle, where it passes behind the IVC and emerges to the right of the aorta to continue inferiorly towards the pelvis medial to the pedicles. Hydronephrosis can occur secondary to constriction of the retrocaval segment of the ureter by the IVC, with ensuing stasis, stone formation and infection (Fig. 38.35).

Primary Megaureter

It is due to congenitally abnormal musculature of the distal ureter that results in a focal failure of peristalsis. On IVU, the distal ureter just above the abnormal segment is dilated, but the proximal ureter caliber is normal and the calyceal fornices are sharp. The abnormality is bilateral in 20%. The urinary stasis results in urinary tract

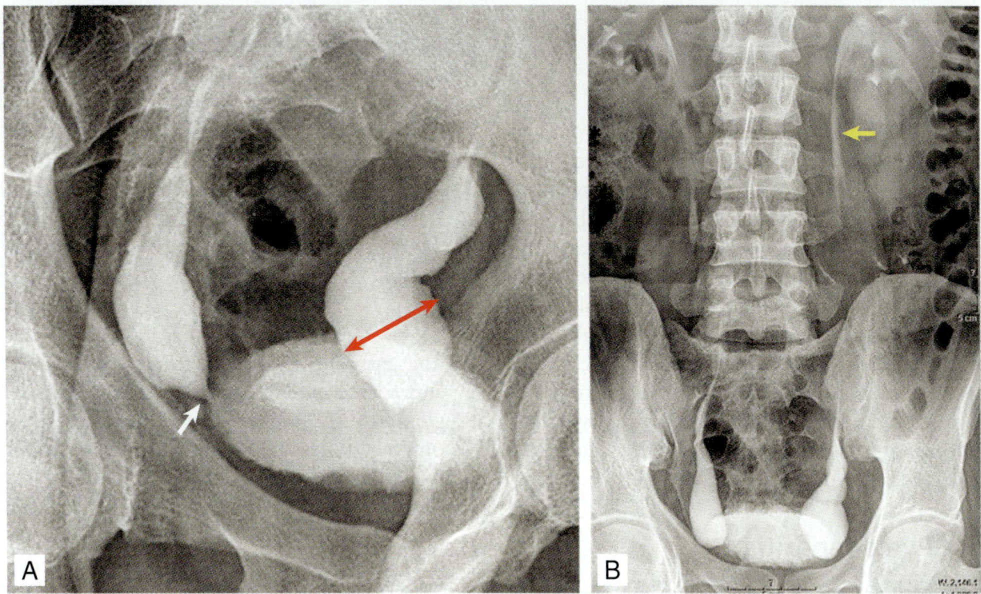

Figure 38.36 Primary megaureter. (A–B) IVU postcompression release KUB with bladder oblique: There is bilateral localized dilatation of the lower ureters (*double arrowed red line*) along with bilateral smooth juxtavesical ureteric narrowing (*white arrow*). Note the normal caliber upper ureter (*yellow arrow*).

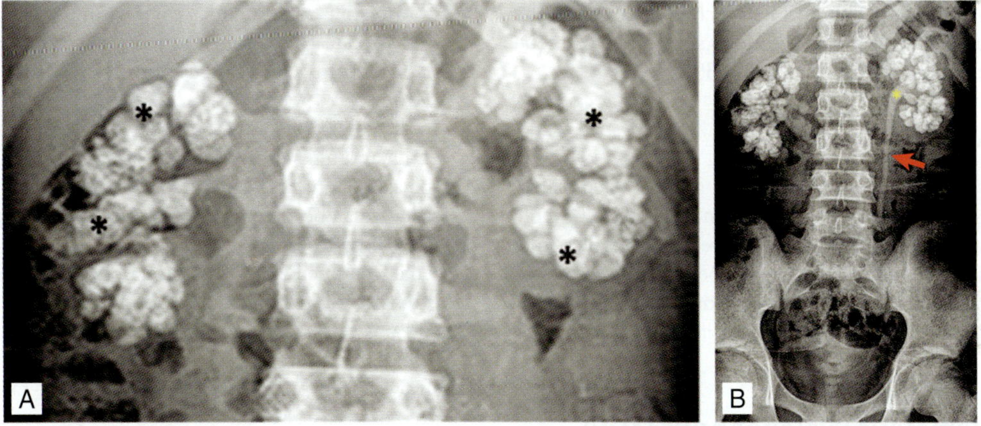

Figure 38.37 Congenital megapolycalicosis. (A) IVU scout: Numerous, extensive polygonal-shaped calculi (*black asterisks*) resembling the pyelogram (B) IVU postcompression release KUB: There are increased number of calyces >14 (polycalycosis), along with abnormal calyceal shape: enlarged, polygonal, and rounded with blunting of fornices. Note the normal caliber pelvis (*yellow asterisk*) and ureter (*red arrow*).

infections and calculi. In severe cases, the dilatation involves the whole ureter, pelvis, and calyces (Fig. 38.36).

Megacalycosis and Polycalycosis

On IVU, the number of calyces is increased to greater than 14 (polycalycosis) and the calyces are abnormal in shape, appearing polygonal or rounded with blunting of fornices (megacalycosis) and associated with megaureter. The scout radiograph can show extensive polygonal-shaped calculi resembling the pyelogram (Fig. 38.37).

Prune Belly Syndrome

It is a congenital abnormality seen in males related to bladder outflow obstruction in utero secondary to urethral valves causing hydroureteronephrosis. Eventually, the obstruction is overcome but during the obstructive phase, there is defective development of the anterior abdominal wall and ureteric musculature resulting in poor peristalsis, persistent nonobstructive dilatation, associated cryptorchidism, prostatic, and urethral valves (Fig. 38.38).

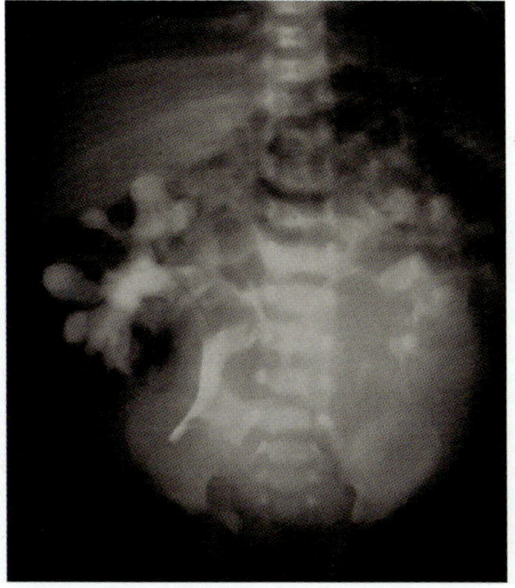

Figure 38.38 Prune belly syndrome. IVU in an infant with prune belly syndrome. There is gross overdistension of the bladder, bilateral hydronephrosis and hydroureters.

Inflammatory Disease

Acute Pyelonephritis (APN)

IVU can be normal in mild acute pyelonephritis. In the 30% that are severe, the kidney appears smoothly enlarged with a delayed striated nephrogram, the calyces being compressed by the swollen parenchyma with reduction in perfusion and function. Nonobstructive endotoxin-related ureteric ileus or true obstructive dilatation due to luminal inflammatory and necrotic debris can delay excretion for several hours. Focal pyelonephritis ("lobar nephronia") which has an SOL effect on the adjacent calyces can lead to an abscess. Although diabetics can develop APN spontaneously, IVU may reveal an underlying cause such as calculi, PUJO or bladder outlet obstruction. Pyonephrosis can occur within the obstructed system, causing an early, severe loss of renal function, although the dilatation is disproportionately less than the delay in excretion.

Emphysematous Pyelonephritis

It is a severe pyelonephritis caused by a gas-producing organism (e.g., *E. coli*) usually affecting elderly diabetics especially those with ureteric obstruction. On plain film, gas is seen within the renal shadow that can be branching and tubular when within the PCS or streaky and mottled when intraparenchymal or perinephric. Gas in the urinary tract can also be due to surgical instrumentation and enteric/cutaneous fistula (Fig. 38.39).

Perinephric Abscess

On IVU, there is a loss of the psoas shadow, a poorly delineated renal outline, reduced or absent renal function and delayed excretion. Intrarenal and perirenal air may be seen as "bubbles and streaks" of lucencies extending into the retroperitoneum, crossing the midline or into the lateral extraperitoneal space, lateral abdominal wall, transversalis fascia, psoas, quadratus, and iliacus muscles.

Xanthogranulomatous Pyelonephritis (XGP)

This is a chronic granulomatous disease resulting in a nonfunctioning kidney in the setting of recurrent UTI and struvite (staghorn) calculi. Lipid-laden histiocytes are seen invading and replacing normal renal parenchyma.

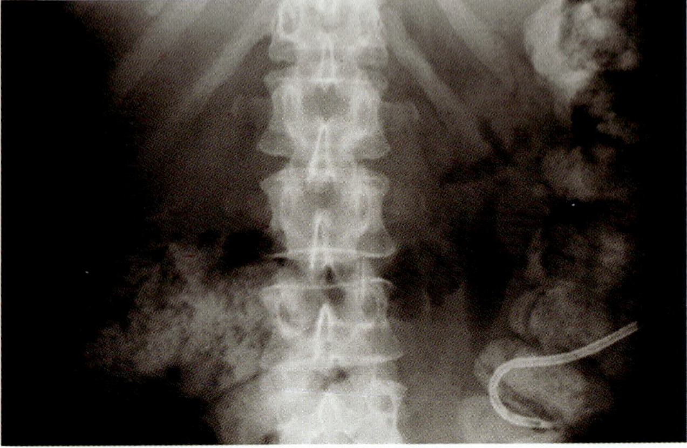

Figure 38.39 Emphysematous pyelitis. Plain radiograph: characteristic configuration of branching air in the left kidney collecting system. A drainage catheter is also seen in the left flank.

In the diffuse form, IVU shows a complete or partial staghorn, laminated, branching or fragmented calculus within an enlarged nonfunctioning kidney. The less common focal or tumefactive XGP presents as a focal mass within a nonfunctioning segment in an otherwise normal kidney or diffuse XGP involving one moiety of a duplex system. Complications of XGP include obstructive renal atrophy and obliteration of perinephric, psoas, and abdominal wall tissue planes and cutaneous/enteric fistula.

Urinary Tract Tuberculosis

- The pathophysiology of urinary tract TB is a game of "catch and release" where bacilli trapped at various bottlenecks in the glomerulus, loop of Henle, calyceal neck, PUJ and VUJ, unleash a destructive inflammatory response into the surrounding microenvironment
- Periglomerular caseating, cortical granulomas invade the medulla and cause a destructive, cavitating papillary necrosis that ruptures into the collecting system and results in a descending pyelonephritis, ureteritis, and cystitis. Subsequent fibrosis, calcification and stricturing causes obstruction, hydronephrosis/pyonephrosis and progressive renal dysfunction
- In the parenchyma, mass-forming caseous destruction, granuloma coalescence, cavitation, and liquefaction result in sequelae that range from parenchymal scarring to autonephrectomy: end-stage, nonfunctioning, calcified "putty" kidney
- In the collecting system, urothelial inflammatory mucosal thickening and ulceration occurs at sites of normal narrowing such as the calyceal neck, PUJ and VUJ that result in multiple fibrosing strictures, a beaded ureter, multi-infundibulo-pelvic stenosis and uneven hydrocalicosis. Renal failure occurs in 24% as a result of renal parenchymal inflammation, obliterative endarteritis, extensive dystrophic calcification, secondary renal amyloidosis and postobstructive atrophy
- On plain radiograph, only 10% of patients with renal TB show active pulmonary TB on chest x-ray. Plain radiography may also reveal calcified lymph nodes, psoas abscess, calcified granulomas in the adrenal glands, liver, spleen or evidence of TB spine. Calcification is unusual in the early stages but is seen in every end-stage urinary tract TB (Box 38.9)
- On IVU, urinary tract TB shows a gamut of findings depending on the stage and severity of disease. Box 38.10 lists the findings and Table 38.2 correlates the pathology with the IVU findings at different sites and stages of the disease (Fig. 38.40)

BOX 38.9 Calcification in Renal TB

Punctate, amorphous, granular, curvilinear
Triangular/ring-like: papillary necrosis
Lobar pattern of calcification:
  Calcific rims at the periphery of distorted renal lobes
'Putty kidney': *reniform cast of calcified caseous tissue*
Ureteral calcification
Renal or ureteric calculi (19%)
Soft-tissue calcification
Scarred calculus: *upward-pointing renal pelvis calculus*

BOX 38.10 IVU Findings in Urinary Tract TB

Swollen papilla indenting calyx
Calyceal fornix erosion
Papillary pools/horns of contrast
Fuzzy/ragged/feathery/moth-eaten calyx
Narrowed, irregular infundibulum
Amputated calyx/phantom calyx/hydrocalyx
Multi-infundibular stenosis
Asymmetric hydrocalicosis
SOL splaying calyx
Distorted, enlarged calyx
Pelvic narrowing/irregularity
Ureteric irregularity/notching
Pelvic stenosis
Kerr kink/hiked-up pelvis
Sawtooth ureter
Pipe-stem ureter
Beaded/corkscrew ureter
Bladder septations
Thimble bladder
Hydronephrosis/pyonephrosis
Renal scars
Renal atrophy
Pseudocalculi
Renal lobar calcification
Scarred stones
Autonephrectomy/putty kidney

Schistosomiasis

This is caused by a parasitic blood fluke that involves the bladder and distal ureters. On IVU, findings are bilateral, asymmetric with multiple small filling defects related to inflammatory polyps, ureteric strictures and linear ureteric and bladder calcification.

Hydatid Disease

Hydatid disease is a parasitic infection caused by the dog tapeworm Echinococcus granulosus that gives rise to a multiloculated cystic mass containing a dominant central cyst and multiple daughter cysts. On plain radiograph, a calcified cyst wall may be

TABLE 38.2 Urinary Tract Tuberculosis: *Pathology and Imaging*

		IVU					
Urinary Tract TB	**Pathology**	**Parenchyma**	**Calyx**	**Infundibulum**	**Pelvis**	**Ureter**	**Bladder**
Bacillary seeding via blood ≥ glomerulus	Periglomerular cortical granuloma						
Bacillary seeding via filtrate PCT ≥ loop of Henle	Peritubular: loop of Henle, medullary papilla Granuloma, caseation necrosis, ulceration, cavitation Papillitis, papillary necrosis	Swollen papilla indenting calyx Papillary pools/ horns of contract	Calyceal fornix erosion Fuzzy/ragged/ feathery/moth-eaten calyx				
Rupture into collecting system	Caseating papillary necrosis ruptures into calyx Coalescent granulomas, caseation liquefaction Caseous mass/abscess ruptures into collecting system		SOL splaying calyx Irregular cavity communicating with calyx				
Descending inflammation	Mucosal edema, granuloma, ulceration, caseous necrosis		Distorted, enlarged calyx	Infundibular narrowing and irregularity	Pelvis narrowing/ irregular filling defects	Ureteric notching	Irregular bladder wall
Stenosis strictures	Fibrosis		Calyceal deformity	Infundibular stenosis/multi-infundibular stenosis	Pelvic stenosis, Kerr kink, Hiked-up pelvis	Sawtooth ureter, Pipe-stem ureter, Beaded ureter, Corkscrew ureter	Bladder septations, Thimble bladder
Obstruction	Proximal dilatation		Amputated calyx/phantom calyx/ hydrocalyx/ asymmetric hydrocalicosis Hydronephrosis, caseous pyonephrosis: filling defects				

Continued

TABLE 38.2 Urinary Tract Tuberculosis: *Pathology and Imaging—cont'd*

		IVU					
Urinary Tract TB	**Pathology**	**Parenchyma**	**Calyx**	**Infundibulum**	**Pelvis**	**Ureter**	**Bladder**
Scarring	Focal parenchymal thinning	Contour indentation overlying abnormal calyx					
Atrophy	Diffuse parenchymal thinning	Reduced parenchymal thickness					
Calcification	Dystrophic calcification	Lobar pattern of calcification: calcific rims around the distorted renal lobes			"Scarred stone"	Pseudocalculi	
Renal dysfunction	Autonephrectomy		Putty kidney: small, calcified, irregular Reniform cast, Curvilinear peripheral rim, calcifications				

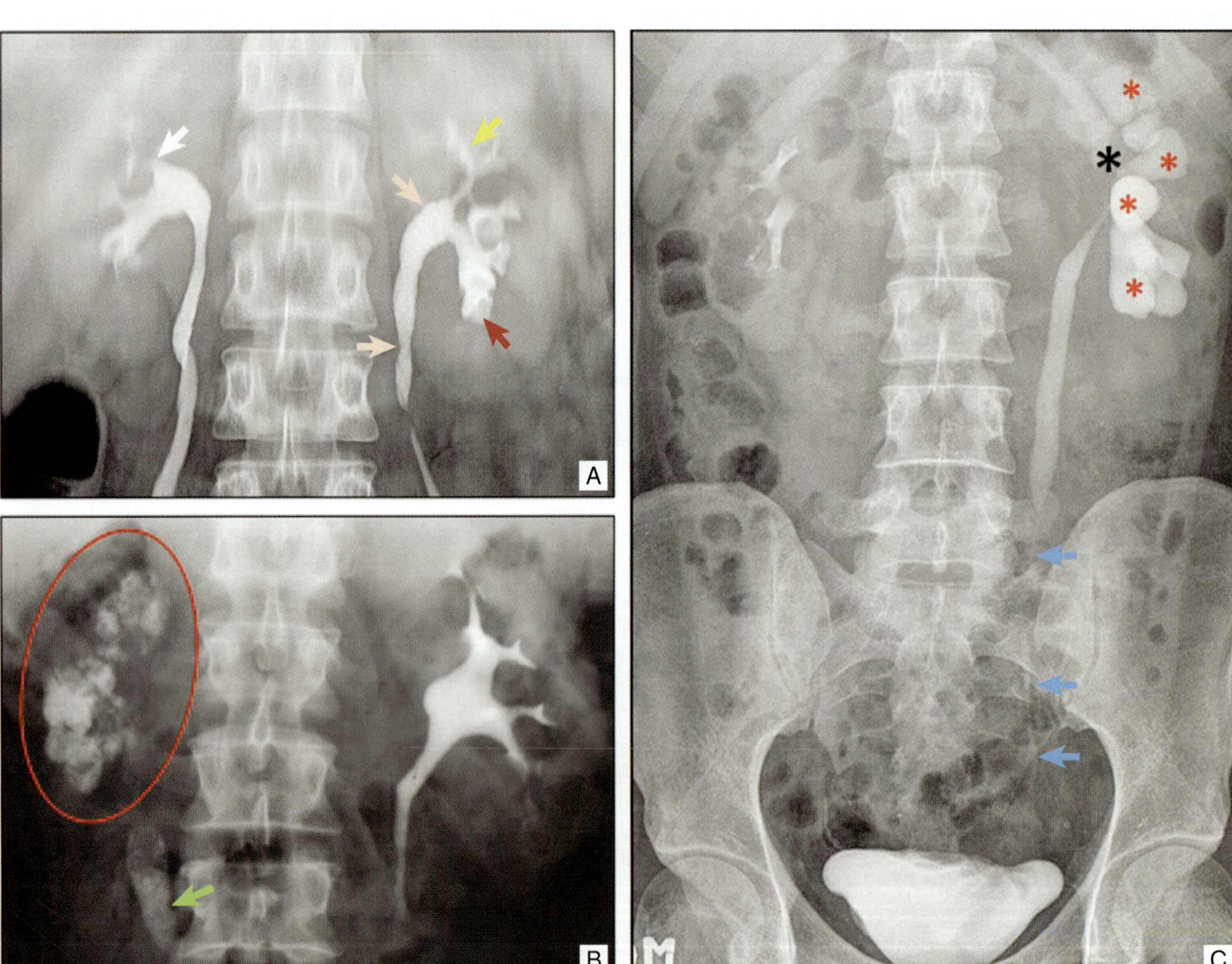

Figure 38.40 Urinary Tract Tuberculosis. (A) IVU 10-minute binder tomogram shows swollen papilla (*red arrow*), fuzzy/ragged calyx (*yellow arrow*), narrowed infundibulum (*white arrow*) and pyeloureteric irregularity (*pink arrow*). (B) IVU 10-minute shows autonephrectomy/putty kidney (*red circle*) and pseudocalculi (*green arrow*). (C) IVU postcompression release shows multi-infundibulo-pelvic stenosis (*black asterisk*), asymmetric hydrocalicosis (*red asterisks*) and pipe stem ureter (*blue arrows*).

seen within the renal perirenal space. On IVU, the cyst may cause a focal bulge of the renal contour and show an SOL effect in the form of splayed and compressed calyces. Rarely, the cyst may communicate with the collecting system and demonstrate delayed opacification outlining the inner cyst wall and daughter cysts as varying sized round lucencies.

Reflux Nephropathy

On IVU, renal cortical scarring is seen as indentations overlying dilated calyces and is indicative of severe VUR causing recurrent UTI especially in the absence of stone disease. Findings are asymmetrical and unilateral with cortical scarring over clubbed calyces at the renal poles, especially the upper pole compound calyces. The kidneys are small and show diffuse cortical loss, following severe continuing reflux in childhood. A dilated PCS and capacious ureters are evident with ureteric striations due to redundant mucosa and focal compensatory parenchymal hypertrophy between the scars that mimic tumor: "pseudotumor". IVU displays the anatomy and effectiveness of surgical treatments such as ileal conduit/ureteric reimplantation/ureterosigmoidostomy (Fig. 38.41). Grades of VUR on MCU have been described in the pediatric GUT Chapter 86.

Rare Inflammatory Conditions

Pyeloureteritis cystica is a rare inflammation of the ureter secondary to chronic obstruction and infection with the formation of subepithelial cysts in the pelvis and upper third of the ureter. On IVU/RGP, this gives rise to a distinctive appearance with multiple pyeloureteric filling defects that are usually 1–4 mm but can be as large as 20 mm.

Malacoplakia is an uncommon chronic granulomatous inflammatory disease due to defective cell-mediated immunity in the setting of recurrent urinary tract infection (*E. coli*). Malacoplakia involves the bladder most often, although plaques may also occur in the ureters. On IVU, malacoplakia appears as multiple, polypoid, solid filling defects or as narrowing with evidence of VUR and upper tract dilatation. These filling defects can range in size from a few millimeters to several centimeters. Rarely, malacoplakia can be locally invasive.

Leucoplakia is a premalignant squamous metaplasia of the urothelium secondary to chronic irritation, calculi, chronic urinary tract infection or schistosomiasis. They are multiple small flat plaques associated with squamous cell carcinoma. The bladder is involved more often than the PCS with the plaques seen on IVU as subtle, flat, filling defects.

Urinary tract cholesteatoma is due to chronic irritation from infection or calculus that results in squamous metaplasia and the formation and desquamation of masses of keratin.

IVU reveals nonspecific filling defects in the pelvis or bladder and is associated with stricturing chronic infections from TB/schistosomiasis and chronic UTI.

Fungal pyelonephritis is a rare, hematogenous infection occurring in reduced immune competence and associated with chronic indwelling central lines and catheters. Medullary and cortical abscesses result from destruction of renal parenchyma and papillae by fungal hyphae (*C. albicans*) in the renal pelvis, producing fungus balls in the ureters. On IVU, fungus balls produce multiple 1–4 cm filling defects associated with papillary necrosis, obstruction, renal abscesses splaying and distorting the calyces and reduced renal function. Fungal balls can also be found forming around long-term urinary catheters, resulting in a bizarre appearance of a partly calcified,

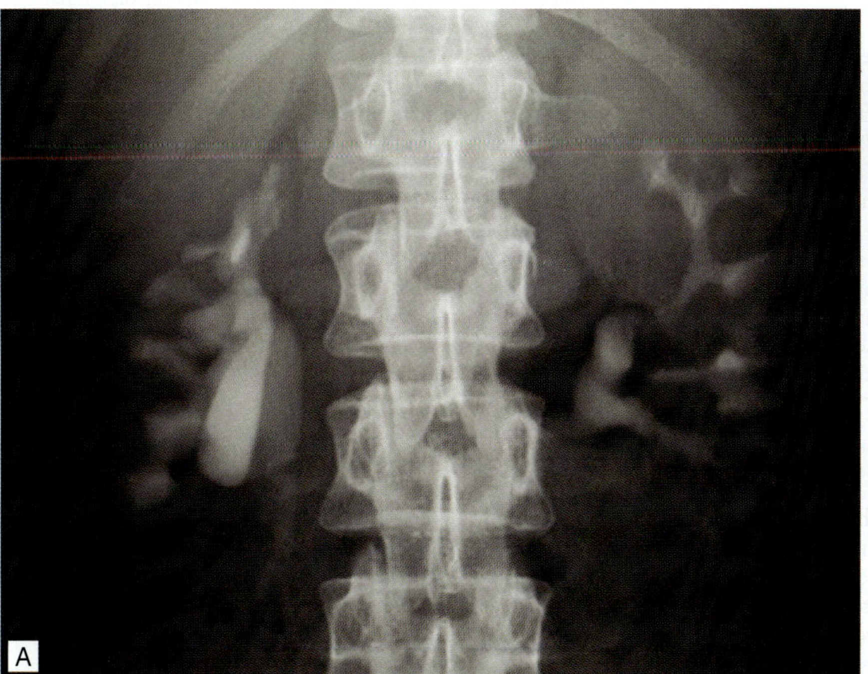

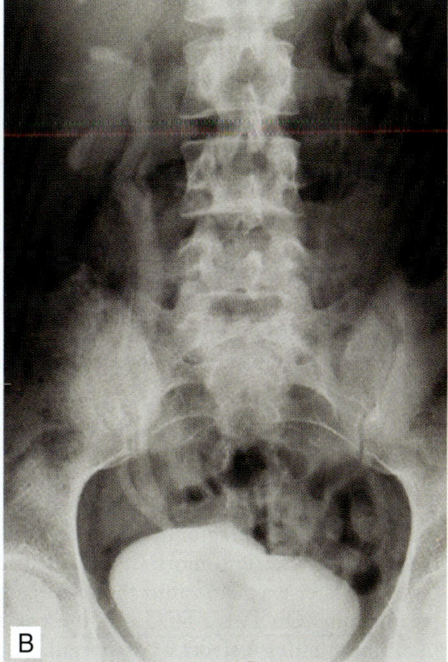

Figure 38.41 Reflux nephropathy. (A) IVU postcompression release kidneys: small right kidney, extensive parenchymal scarring and thinning, maximal at upper pole with clubbing of calyces. (B) IVU postcompression release KUB: Right duplex system. Lower moiety clubbing of calyces and parenchymal scarring/thinning. Lower moiety ureter: persistent dilatation due to severe VUR.

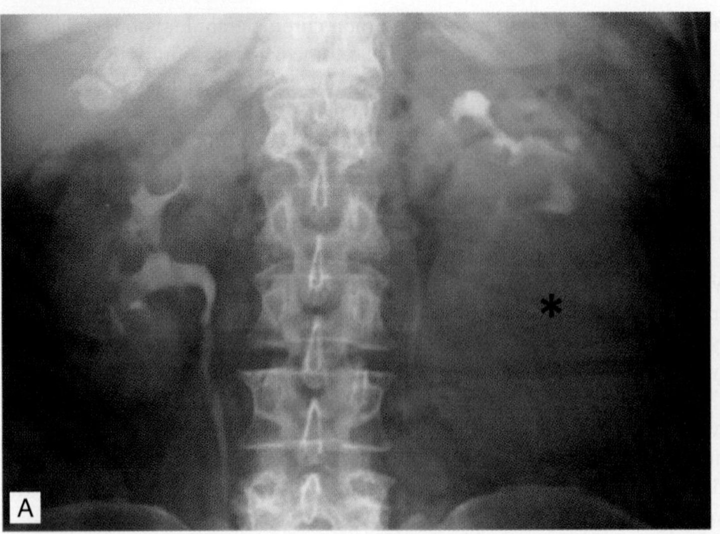

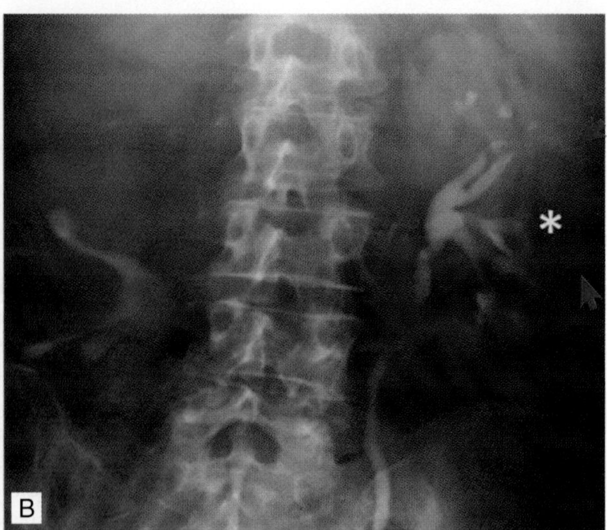

Figure 38.42 Renal masses. IVU 15-minute: (A) RCC left lower pole. Left lower pole mass (*black asterisk*) causing a focal bulge of the renal contour, superiorly displacing, compressing, and distorting the lower pole calyces and rotating the upper pole medially. Enhancing solid mass produces a "double density." (B) Simple cyst left interpole. Space-occupying effect on the interpole calyces. Low density defect in the parenchyma (*yellow asterisk*). Beaking of renal parenchyma compressed superiorly (*red arrows*).

ball-like, whorled filling defect around the catheter tip within the bladder.

Tumors

On IVU, a renal mass may be evident from curvilinear calcification, an SOL effect on the calyces, cortical "beaking" from a cyst or a "double density" from a solid mass (Fig. 38.42).

Renal Cell Carcinoma (RCC)

IVU is a traditional technique used to investigate hematuria; however, one-third RCCs are <3 cm and not visible on IVU. Larger tumors are seen on plain film as a soft-tissue mass, with dense, central, amorphous calcification in 10%. The SOL effect displaces calyces, bulges the contour with an enhancement density similar to normal renal tissue, resulting in a double density sign, although some poorly vascular tumors can be similar to simple cysts and demonstrate beaking. The axis of the kidney can change from the weight of a large mass at the upper or lower pole.

Unusual presentations of RCC on IVU include a renal mass with acute obstruction from ureteric clot secondary to RCC bleed, and a renal mass with nonfunctioning kidney secondary to renal vein tumor thrombus [30].

Transitional Cell Carcinoma

TCC can be synchronous (20%) or metachronous (20%) in the ipsilateral KUB region, or develop within the contralateral kidney in 6%. Early tumors are confined to the collecting system with later extension into the renal parenchyma and retroperitoneum. On IVU, TCC can present as annular, plaque-like, linear filling defects or as irregular, sessile or polypoidal masses projecting into the PCS, enlarging (oncocalyx) or obliterating (phantom calyx) the calyx. As the tumor enlarges, dilatation of the ureter distal to the lesion occurs secondary to chronic intussusception induced by ureteric peristalsis (goblet sign). Infiltrating, irregular strictures cause hydronephrosis or hydrocalyx and can result in a nonfunctioning kidney from extensive parenchymal invasion (Fig. 38.43) [31].

Box 38.11 lists the causes of a filling defect on IVU.

Other Renal Masses

- In ***renal sinus lipomatosis***, renal sinus fat increases significantly in response to age-related renal atrophy, severe infection or ischemia, Cushing's disease or steroid treatment, and causes narrowing and stretching of the calyces
- ***Cysts*** include simple cysts, parapelvic cysts, complex renal cysts and acquired cystic disease of dialysis. On plain radiograph and IVU, cysts can appear as large well-defined soft-tissue renal masses bulging the renal contour and on nephrogram as well-defined nonenhancing masses that distort the PCS. Parapelvic cysts are small, multiple, congenital, lymphatic cysts lying between the calyceal infundibula, stretching and compressing the calyces, similar in appearance to renal sinus lipomatosis. On USG, they can mimic hydronephrosis [32]
- ***Angiomyolipomas*** may present with a normal IVU when small; when large and fatty, plain film can reveal a low-density lesion arising from the kidney
- ***Renal lymphoma*** is usually secondary to extensive retroperitoneal lymphoma arising in the renal sinus and extending into the perinephric space or within the parenchyma as bilateral solid masses. On IVU, there is lateral displacement of the proximal ureters by para-aortic nodal masses and medial displacement of the distal ureters by iliac lymphadenopathy, causing hydronephrosis. Nonspecific focal masses can distort the renal outline and PCS
- ***Leukemia*** on IVU appears as bilateral symmetrical renal enlargement with renal insufficiency due to urate nephropathy. Urate calculi and blood clot filling defects may be seen within the collecting system
- ***Wilms' tumor*** on IVU presents as a nonspecific mass whose multicystic nature may be evident from multiple nonenhancing, low density defects within the nephrogram that characteristically bulge into the renal pelvis. Calcification is not a common feature

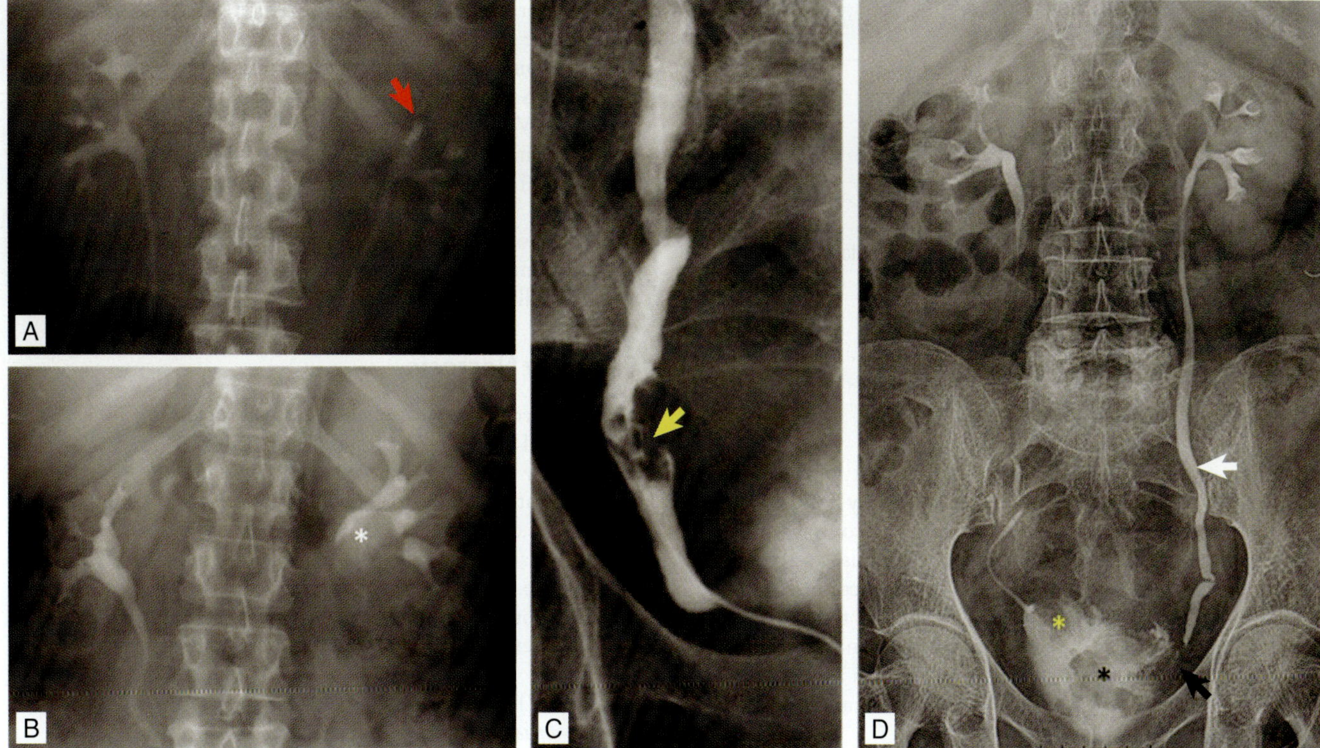

Figure 38.43 TCC. (A–B) IVU 10-minute: Subtle irregularity of the left upper pole infundibulum (*red arrow*) and calyceal cutoff. Large filling defect in the left renal pelvis (*white asterisk*). (C) RGU: Multiple, small, irregular, papillary, filling defects in the right distal ureter (*yellow arrow*). (D) IVU postcompression release: irregular filling defects in the bladder (*black, yellow asterisks*), involving the left VUJ and distal left ureter (*black arrow*) causing a standing column of contrast (*white arrow*).

BOX 38.11 Causes of a Filling Defect on IVU

1. RCC invading collecting system
2. TCC
3. Radiolucent calculus
4. Sloughed papilla
5. Fungus ball
6. Gas bubble
7. Clot
8. Pyeloureteritis cystica
9. Vascular notching

Renal Vascular Disease

- Renal arterial infarcts are due to thrombosis, trauma, renal artery dissection, arteritis, and embolus. On IVU, main renal artery occlusion results in a nonfunctioning kidney with no nephrogram or contrast excretion, while branch occlusion leads to a wedge-shaped defect in the nephrogram, with apex pointing towards the hilum. The infarcted renal tissue atrophies and creates a focal scar seen as an indentation overlying a normal calyx (Fig. 38.28)
- ***Renal artery stenosis*** presents on IVU with a small and smooth affected kidney showing reduced perfusion and a delayed nephrogram. Contrast-containing urine moves slowly within the tubules and concentrates more than the unaffected side, resulting in a dense nephrogram and delayed excretion. Notching of the ureter can occur from compensatory hypertrophy of ureteric artery branches of the lumbar arteries or from collateral arteries
- ***Renal vein thrombosis*** may be idiopathic or due to abnormal coagulation, connective tissue disease, amyloid, sepsis, trauma, pressure by lymph nodes/tumor, haemoglobinopathies or nephrotic syndrome. On IVU, acute, complete thrombosis results in a nonfunctioning swollen kidney, while subacute, partial thrombosis causes smooth renal enlargement with a delayed, hyperdense nephrogram and pyelogram showing calyceal compression from parenchymal swelling with associated notching of the ureter by dilated venous collaterals
- ***Shock nephrogram*** manifests on IVU with delayed onset dense nephrogram, disappearance of contrast from the pelvicalyceal systems and profound hypotension during an IVU. This is usually seen secondary to an adverse contrast reaction

Calculi and Obstruction

Renal and Ureteric Calculi

Box 38.12 lists the types of urinary tract calculi.

The plain radiograph displays renal calculi with reasonable reliability but can be false negative for ureteric calculi when obscured by bowel or sacrum and false positive when phleboliths are misdiagnosed as calculi. However, the dense persistent nephrogram indicates obstruction, even if the stone itself is not identified. This capability along with the lower cost keeps IVU relevant in the NECT era.

On IVU, there is a delay in the nephrogram and contrast excretion with mild HUN down to the calculus. A standing column of contrast, best demonstrated on prone views, is suspicious for a calculus. Review of the region where the standing column ends on

BOX 38.12 Types of Calculi

Radiopaque
- 75% calcium salts—mix of oxalate and phosphate
- 5–7% pure calcium phosphate

Less radiopaque
- 15% struvite (triple phosphate)

Radiolucent
- <10% radiolucent calculi due to abnormal metabolic states
- 5–8% urate calculi
- 1% cystine calculi—ground glass
- 1% xanthine (indinavir treatment)—radiolucent on CT

the scout image and comparison with the post void image may reveal a "growing" calculus—that is, a density that apparently increases in size with a coating of luminal contrast. Contrast extravasation from ruptured fornices, pyelosinus, and pyelolymphatic extravasation can be seen in acute obstruction. 95% calculi <4 mm in size pass spontaneously. Calculi tend to arrest over the sacrum, as the ureter crosses the iliac artery and in the VUJ. Mucosal edema around an impacted VUJ calculus can appear as a thick halo or pseudoureterocele (Figs. 38.27B, 38.44, and 38.45).

Upper Urinary Tract Trauma

Renal Trauma

IVU has been historically used in the evaluation of renal trauma. IVU in renal trauma is currently used in resource-limited settings. For the hemodynamically unstable patient who needs an emergency laparotomy, a single shot IVU (i.e., a full-length KUB 15 minutes after IV contrast), can confirm a functioning contralateral kidney and provide vital information about the injured kidney. Absence of excretion on a single side indicates major vascular injury such as a renal artery avulsion, while perirenal soft-tissue swelling or loss of the psoas margin indicate a large retroperitoneal hematoma. Disruption of the PCS is seen as extravasation of opacified urine. Shock kidneys due to significant hypotension will produce little or no secretion bilaterally [33].

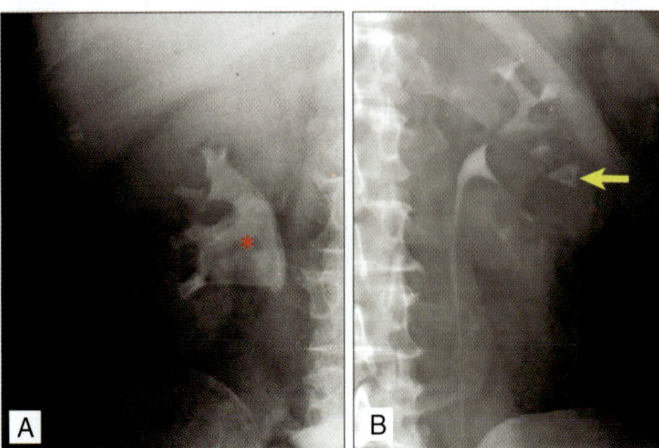

Figure 38.44 Calculi: staghorn and radiolucent urate. (A) IVU scout: Large, branching, laminated staghorn calculus occupying the entire right PCS (*red asterisk*). (B) IVU 10-minute: Radiolucent urate calculus in a left interpole calyx giving rise to a small, round filling defect (*yellow arrow*).

In ureteric trauma, a severe deceleration injury causes avulsion at the PUJ or the upper third of ureter. Trauma from hyperflexion in children, gynaecological surgery and other serious injuries can lead to ureteric trauma that can be overlooked [34]. On IVU, ureteric trauma results in contrast extravasation and urinoma with ureteric discontinuity and mild to moderate fullness of the PCS. The site of extravasation will indicate the site of the tear. In complete transection, the ureter fails to opacify below the level of transection and fistulation into other structures may be demonstrated such as a ureterovaginal fistula or UVF following hysterectomy (Fig. 38.46).

Papillary Necrosis

Papillary necrosis is an ischemic necrosis of the medullary pyramid tip and has many causes as listed in Box 38.13.

Papillary necrosis can be bilateral, asymmetric with parenchymal loss that results in small, smooth, poorly functioning kidneys. The papilla can necrose, separate, and slough into the PCS, leaving behind a papillary defect, a clubbed calyx and a calcified papillary triangle. On IVU, pools and horns of contrast are seen within small necrotic areas, which erode the tip of the papillae and irregularly excavate from the fornices into the pyramids.

Typical appearances on IVU include the following (Fig. 38.47):

- *Ball-on-tee*
- *Forniceal excavation*
- *Lobster claw*
- *Signet ring*
- *Sloughed papilla + clubbed calyx.*

Endometriosis

Up to 10% endometriosis involves the urinary tract with endometrial implants on the bladder, ureter or retroperitoneum. Bladder serosa implants are clinically less significant than the ureteric implants that lead to stricturing and obstruction; lesions are bilateral in 10%.

On IVU, endometriosis implants on the ureter produce short, smooth, abruptly tapered strictures in the distal third of the ureter at the level of the uterosacral ligaments, with associated medial angulation of the ureter.

Retroperitoneal Fibrosis (RPF)

RPF is composed of fibrosis and a chronic inflammatory cell infiltrate that can be caused by a variety of etiologies as listed in Box 38.14.

RPF starts just lateral to the aorta and sequentially involves the left ureter, right ureter, pericaval, and inter-aorto-caval areas. The ureter is involved from the PUJ to the bladder, L3 to L5, encased and hypoperistaltic with sparing of the mucosa and ureteric wall, resulting in a gradual HUN. Stents characteristically pass easily retrograde through the ureters. On IVU, there is variable medial deviation of the ureters at L3-5 (Fig. 38.48).

Miscellaneous Conditions

- ***Ischemic ureteric lesions*** can follow aortic or radical pelvic surgery, with acute ischemia seen as swollen, scalloped mucosa that can progress to a fibrous stricture
- ***Radiation*** strictures are a variant of ischemic stricturing with smooth abruptly narrowed segments seen within the port that appears 1 year after radiotherapy

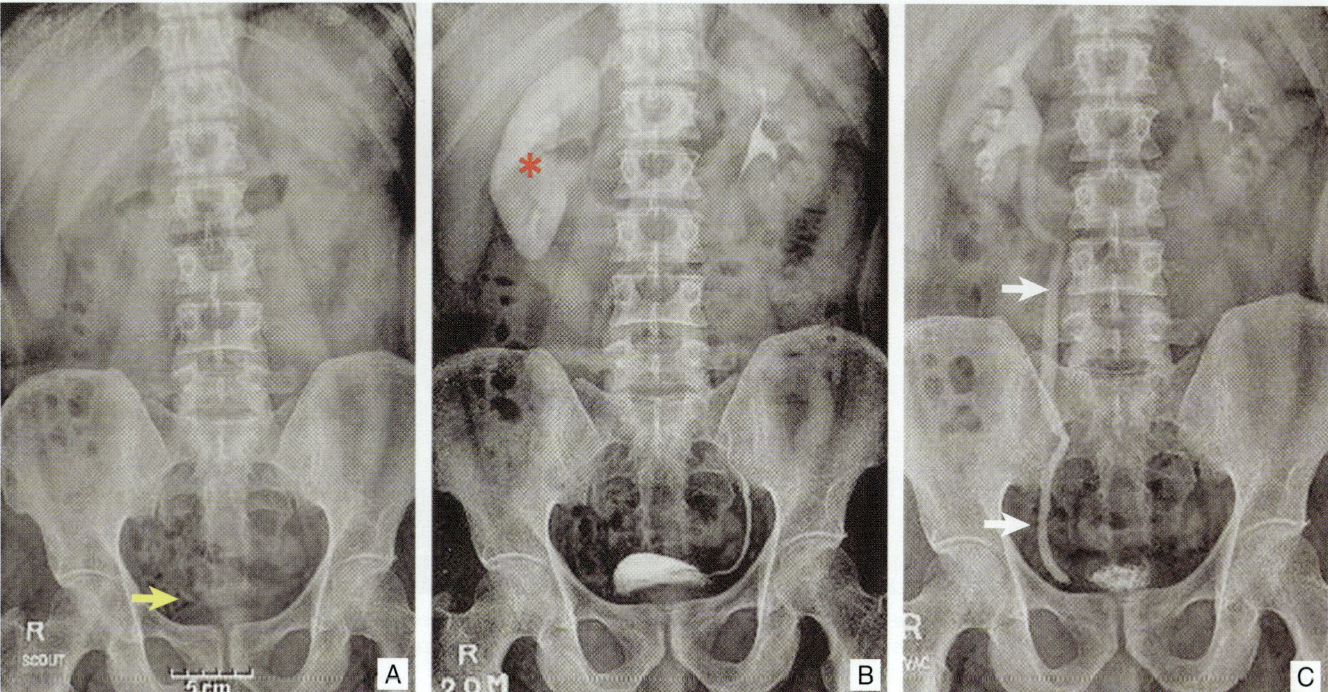

Figure 38.45 Acutely obstructing VUJ calculus: standing column. (A) IVU scout KUB: Poorly visualized right VUJ opacity (*yellow arrow*). (B) IVU postcompression release: Dense persistent right nephrogram (*red asterisk*) with delayed excretion. (C) IVU 45-minute: Standing column of contrast in the right ureter (*white arrows*) down to the right VUJ opacity seen in (A). This confirms site of obstruction and calculus at VUJ.

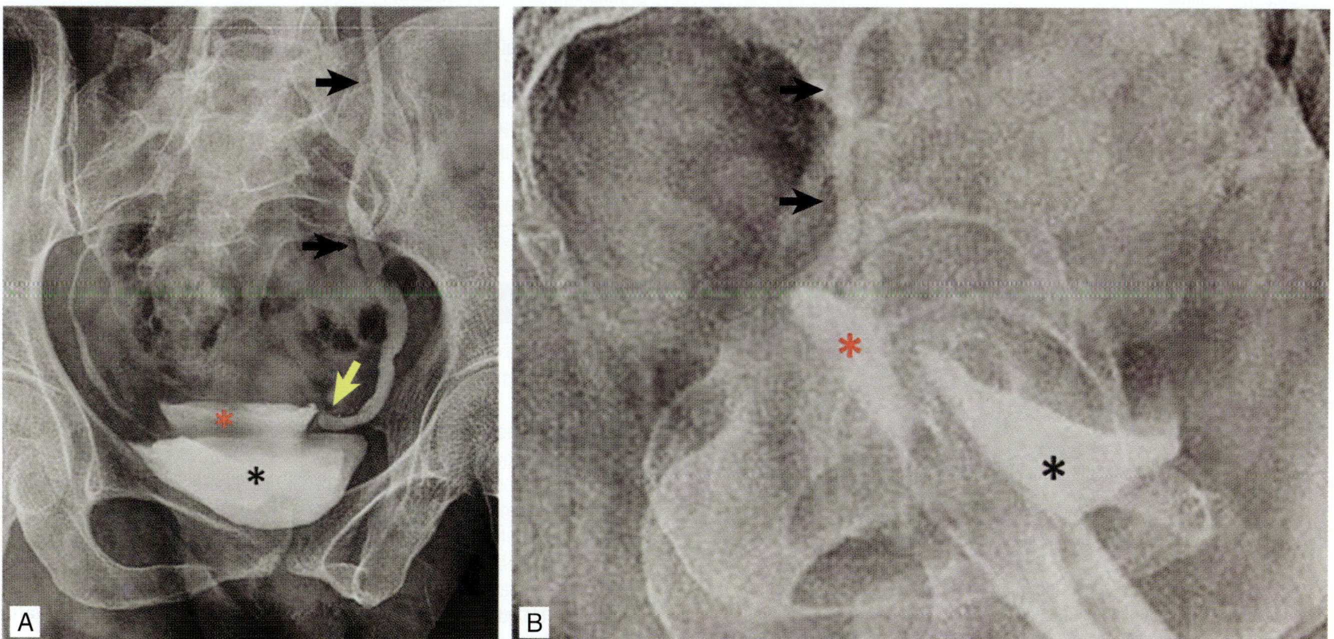

Figure 38.46 Ureteric trauma: ureterovaginal fistula post hysterectomy. IVU postcompression release (pelvis): (A) AP. (B) Lateral Contrast pooling in the vagina (*red asterisk*) behind the bladder (*black asterisk*). Standing column of contrast in the left ureter (*black arrows*). Altered course of left ureter in the pelvis with sharp medial angulation above and away from the VUJ (*yellow arrow*) and toward vaginal pool of contrast.

- ***Pelvic lipomatosis*** is an *idiopathic* condition found in overweight middle-aged men that causes proliferation of fat within the pelvis and can be asymptomatic, or produce lower tract symptoms and HUN. On plain radiograph, excess fatty lucency can be identified in the pelvis, which on IVU causes medial displacement of the distal ureters, upward displacement of the bladder and a laterally compressed, pear-shaped bladder that can cause HUN and rectosigmoid obstruction

Boxes 38.15–38.18 summarize and list the causes of nephrocalcinosis, urinary tract obstruction, ureteric narrowing, diffuse, and focal renal parenchymal disease.

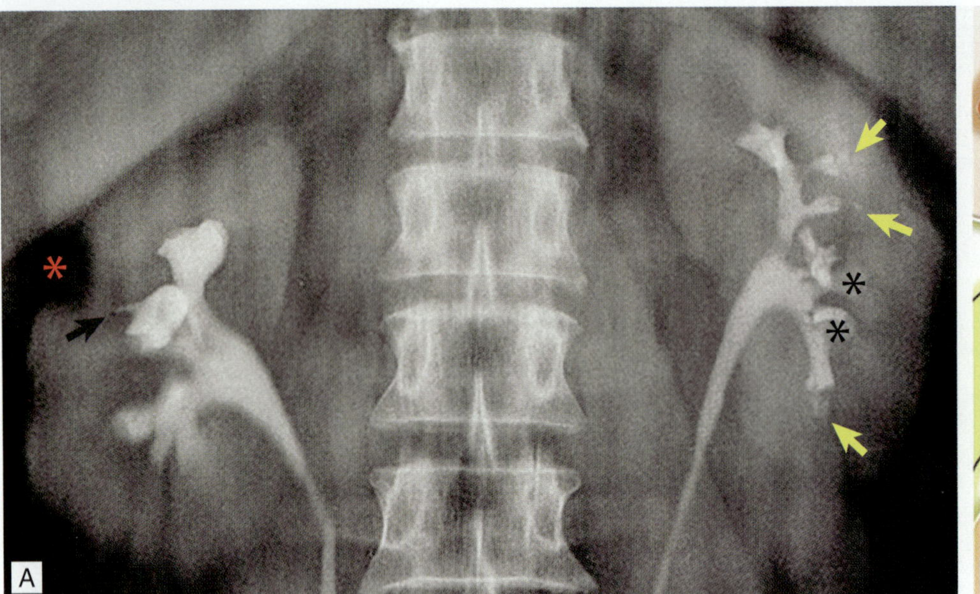

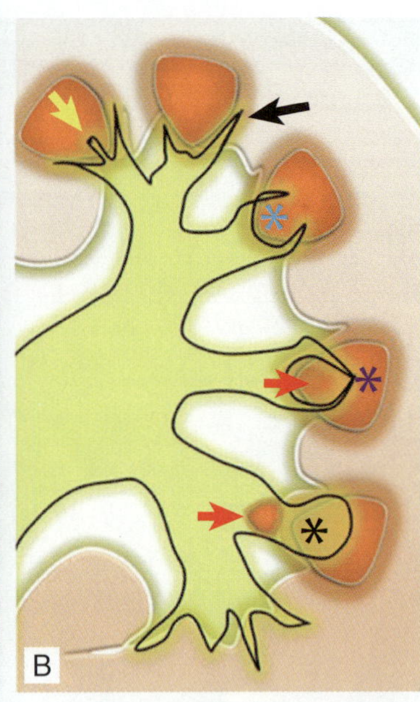

Figure 38.47 Papillary necrosis. (A) IVU 10-minute binder with tomogram (kidneys). (B) Diagrammatic representation: stages of papillary necrosis. Ball on tee (*yellow arrows*). Forniceal excavation/horn (*black arrow*). Lobster claw (*blue asterisk*). Signet ring (*purple asterisk*). Sloughed papilla (*red arrow*) with clubbed calyx (*black asterisk*) and right renal scar (*red asterisk*).

BOX 38.13 Papillary Necrosis: Causes

1. Analgesic nephropathy (phenacetin, aspirin, NSAID)
2. Sickle-cell disease
3. Diabetes mellitus
4. TB
5. Acute severe pyelonephritis
6. VUR-related infection
7. Renal vein thrombosis
8. Cirrhosis
9. CHF
10. Dehydration
11. Acidosis and respiratory distress

BOX 38.14 Causes of RPF

1. IgG4
2. IBD Crohn's disease
3. Inflammatory aortic aneurysm
4. Vascular grafts
5. Retroperitoneal metastases
6. Lymphoma, carcinoma breast/colon, carcinoid
7. Retroperitoneal hemorrhage
8. Inflammation: abscess, urinoma, diverticulitis, appendicitis
9. Drugs: ergot alkaloids, hydralazine

BOX 38.15 Nephrocalcinosis: Multiple Nondystrophic Parenchymal Calcifications

- Cortical nephrocalcinosis
  - Chronic renal failure
    - small kidneys
    - peripheral tramline/eggshell calcification
  - Acute cortical necrosis
    - hypotensive renal insult: perinatal/septic/hemorrhage
    - nephrotoxin: ethylene glycol
    - hyperoxaluria
    - Alport's syndrome (sensorineural hearing loss + congenital nephritis)
    - chronic transplant rejection
- Medullary nephrocalcinosis: calcification of the pyramids with sparing of the cortex
  - Medullary sponge kidney
  - Hypercalcaemia
    - metastatic soft-tissue calcification
    - hyperparathyroidism
    - disseminated malignancy causing hypercalcaemia
    - sarcoidosis hypercalcaemia
    - historical: milk–alkali syndrome, vitamin D overtreatment
    - rare: acromegaly, thyrotoxicosis
  - Metabolic causes
    - renal tubular acidosis: dense medullary nephrocalcinosis + calculi + renal failure
    - hyperoxaluria: cortical and medullary nephrocalcinosis

BOX 38.16 Causes of Urinary Tract Obstruction

- Calculi
- Pelviureteric junction obstruction
- Tumors
  - extrinsic compression: malignancy or large benign cysts/masses
  - intrinsic narrowing: urothelial tumor
- Inflammatory lesions: Crohn's disease/appendicular abscess/diverticular abscess
- Noncalculous ureteric strictures
- Noncalculous ureteric filling defects
- Retroperitoneal fibrosis
- Endometrial implant
- Pregnancy-related hydronephrosis and hydroureter
- *Causes of nonobstructive hydronephrosis and hydroureter:*
  - Severe VUR
  - Primary megaureter
  - Megacalycosis
  - Diabetes insipidus
  - Endotoxin-related ureteric ileus

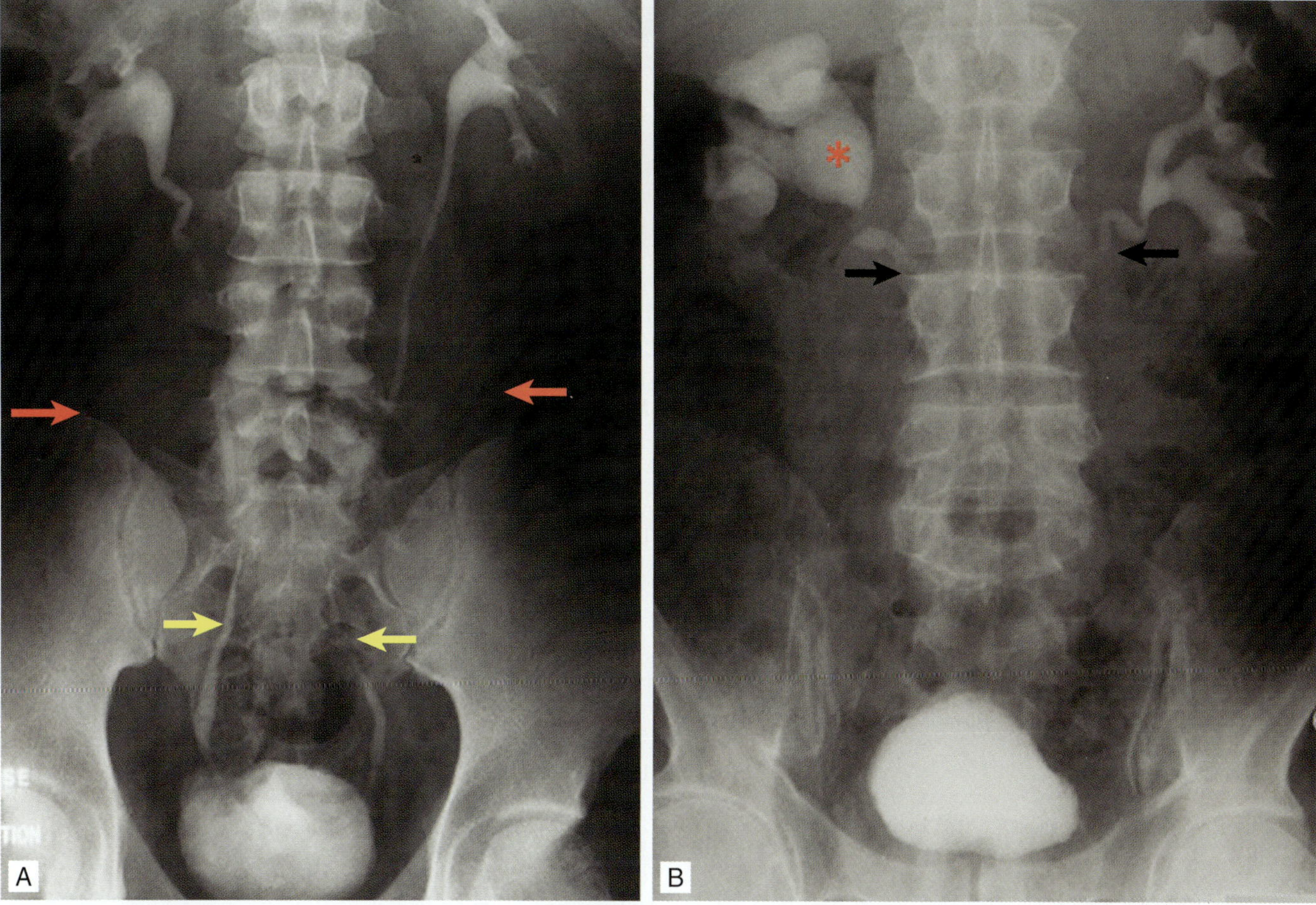

Figure 38.48 Medial deviation of ureters. (A) Physiological psoas muscle hypertrophy: Bilateral gradual, long segment, smooth medial deviation of the lower ureters (*yellow arrows*). Lateral margin of psoas muscles (*red arrows*). (B) Retroperitoneal fibrosis: Bilateral marked, abrupt medial deviation of both upper ureters (*black arrows*), causing right hydronephrosis (*red asterisk*).

BOX 38.17 Diffuse and Multifocal Renal Parenchymal Abnormalities

Small scarred kidneys
- reflux nephropathy: clubbed calyces opposite scars
- renal infarcts: scars between normal calyces
- papillary necrosis
- previous surgery
- previous renal vein thrombosis
- radiotherapy
- trauma with subcapsular hematoma

Bilateral small smooth kidneys
- renal arterial insufficiency: hypertensive nephrosclerosis, bilateral RAS
- chronic glomerulonephritis
- end-stage nephropathies: hereditary, analgesic-induced
- medullary cystic disease: small kidneys with cysts

Unilateral small kidney with clubbed calyces
- postobstructive atrophy
- reflux nephropathy

Unilateral small smooth kidney with normal calyces
- renal artery stenosis
- developmental hypoplasia

Bilateral smooth renal enlargement
- DM
- acute glomerulonephritis
- acute nephropathy: AIDS, urate-induced
- interstitial nephritis: SLE, Wegener's
- leukemia, occasionally lymphoma or myeloma
- amyloidosis, acromegaly, ARPKD, hereditary depositional diseases

Unilateral smooth renal enlargement
- acute obstruction
- acute pyelonephritis
- acute vascular disturbances: main arterial/venous occlusion, acute arteritis
- compensatory hypertrophy: increase in size and cortical thickness
- hemihypertrophy

BOX 38.18 Causes of Ureteric Obstruction

Intrinsic
- Luminal
  - calculi
  - clots
  - sloughed papillary necrosis
  - polypoidal tumor: TCC
  - sloughed tumor: TCC, RCC
  - inflammatory debris
  - viscid pus
  - fungal ball: Candida, Aspergillus
  - air bubbles: urinary diversions, fistula, infection
  - keratin
- Mural lesions
  - sessile tumor: TCC
  - edema
  - pyeloureteritis cystica
  - leukoplakia, malacoplakia
  - endometriosis
  - inflammatory: TB, schistosomiasis
  - hemorrhage
  - extrinsic prominent vessel (normal variant, collateral arteries or veins)
  - ischemic
  - radiation
  - trauma:
  - radical pelvic surgery
  - fistula: with vaginal stump after hysterectomy
  - passed calculus
  - instrumentation

Extrinsic
- collateral notching: arterial, venous
  - RAS
  - hypervascular renal tumors
  - AVM
  - occlusive aortoiliac disease
  - RVT
- enlarged gonadal veins
  - gonadal varices
  - ovarian vein syndrome
  - gonadal thrombophlebitis
  - iliac venous occlusion
- inflammation: Crohn's disease/appendix/diverticular abscess
- tumors: pelvic, lymph nodes, retroperitoneal
- iliac and/or para-aortic/paracaval lymph node metastases
  - lymphoma and malignant teratoma

Medial ureteric deviation:
- physiological psoas muscle/iliacus/obturator internis hypertrophy
- pelvic lipomatosis
- RPF
- retrocaval ureter

Lateral ureteric deviation
- renal malrotation
- horseshoe kidney
- tumors
- para-aortic/paracaval lymphadenopathy
- surgery—urinary diversions/post op RPF
- tumors lower pole kidney/RP/pelvis/iliac lymph nodes/pelvic walls
- iliac artery aneurysms
- post abdominoperineal resection of rectal tumors

Ureteric displacement
- into femoral or inguinal hernias
- into sciatic notch

Suggested Readings

- HM Pollack, BL McClennan, Clinical Urography: 3 Volume Textbook, Saunders, Philadelphia, PA, 2000.
- HM Pollack, Some limitations and pitfalls of excretory urography, J Urol 116 (5) (1976 Nov) 537–543.
- A Daneman, DJ Alton, Radiographic manifestations of renal anomalies, Radiol Clin North Am 29 (1991) 351–363.
- MP Federle, Evaluation of renal trauma, in: HM Pollack (ed.), Clinical Urography, Saunders, Philadelphia, PA, 1989, pp. 1422–1494.
- E Levine, Acute renal and urinary tract disease, Radiol Clin North Am 32 (1994) 989–1001.

39

Urinary Tract: Nontumorous Diseases

SHARAD MAHESHWARI

Introduction

This chapter discusses nontumor pathologies affecting the renal tract, radiologic findings with respect to various technique, and the role these findings play in management. Infections, inflammatory conditions, obstructive pathologies, calculi, and parenchymal diseases have been covered extensively. We also discuss the imaging associated with renal transplants in both the pre- and post-transplant periods. Genitourinary trauma is discussed at the end of the chapter because it will be covered in abdominal trauma extensively.

Infections and Inflammatory Conditions

Introduction

Urinary tract infection (UTI) is one of the most frequent infections worldwide. Clinical features and laboratory investigations can establish the diagnosis among uncomplicated cases, and radiologic investigations are seldom asked for.

Imaging is restrained for the assessment of complications of UTI such as pyelonephritis and abscess formation, especially among high-risk patients, and plays a vital role in the diagnosis and management of complications. Immunocompromised patients; patients with diabetes; and patients with renal stones, vesicoureteral reflux (VUR), and congenital urinary tract anomalies are at higher risk to develop complications secondary to UTI.

Renal involvement from the ascending infection from the lower urinary tract (LUT) is the most common route of spread.

Acute Pyelonephritis

Acute pyelonephritis is an acute infection involving the renal parenchyma and the collecting system without abscess formation. It may be focal or diffuse, with or without renal enlargement or focal swelling, and can be unilateral or bilateral.

Clinical Features

- High fever spikes
- Unilateral or bilateral flank pain
- Dysuria and urinary frequency and urgency [1]
- Leucocytosis with increased neutrophils increased C-reactive protein and erythrocyte sedimentation rate
- Urine examination showing pyuria, bacteriuria, positive urine culture, and presence of leucocyte casts [2]

Patients with diabetes are at risk because they may not manifest flank pain, making the clinical diagnosis difficult. Also, they are at higher risk to develop complications such as emphysematous pyelonephritis [1,3].

Pathophysiology

In most cases, the cause is an ascending spread of lower UTI by a microorganism, which in most cases is *Escherichia coli*. Other organisms include Enterobacteriaceae (*Klebsiella* spp. and *Proteus* spp.), *Pseudomonas* spp., enterococci, and staphylococci [4]. The bacterial endotoxins block ureteric peristalsis, causing urinary stasis. If the infection is not controlled, spread to the renal tubule and the interstitium occurs. Hematogenous spread to the kidneys is less common and occurs mostly in intravenous (IV) drug abusers and patients with endocarditis [2].

Indications for Imaging

Acute pyelonephritis is a clinical diagnosis, and most patients respond to antibiotics without imaging. However, diagnostic imaging might be warranted in specific scenarios:

- Patient risks such as immunocompromised patients, patients with diabetes, older adult patients, transplant recipients, and patients receiving chemotherapy
- If any anatomic or functional abnormality in the urinary tract is suspected
- When a patient fails to respond to antibiotics in the first 72 hours
- To rule out obstruction

Imaging

Intravenous Urography: Although intravenous urography (IVU) can delineate the pelvicalyceal anatomy, it is unable to characterize cysts, neoplasms, or abscesses and lacks fine parenchymal detail. Moreover, only 25% of patients with acute pyelonephritis have abnormal IVU findings [1]. Thus, IVU is not indicated in the initial evaluation of acute pyelonephritis [5].

Ultrasonography: The sensitivity of ultrasonography (USG) in diagnosing acute pyelonephritis is low because it fails to detect subtle interstitial nephritic changes and underestimates the severity of renal involvement and perinephric extension [1,2]. Color and power Doppler increase the sensitivity by showing altered blood flow in the affected region [6]. Recent techniques such as contrast-enhanced USG have improved the sensitivity by diagnosing hypoperfusion caused by acute pyelonephritis with comparable sensitivity and specificity with that of contrast-enhanced computed tomography (CT) [7].

Various imaging findings of acute pyelonephritis on USG are:

- Enlarged kidney with increased echogenicity of fat around the kidney and reduced echogenicity of the parenchyma (Fig. 39.1A)
- Dilated pelvicalyceal system either caused by bacterial endotoxins or mechanical obstruction

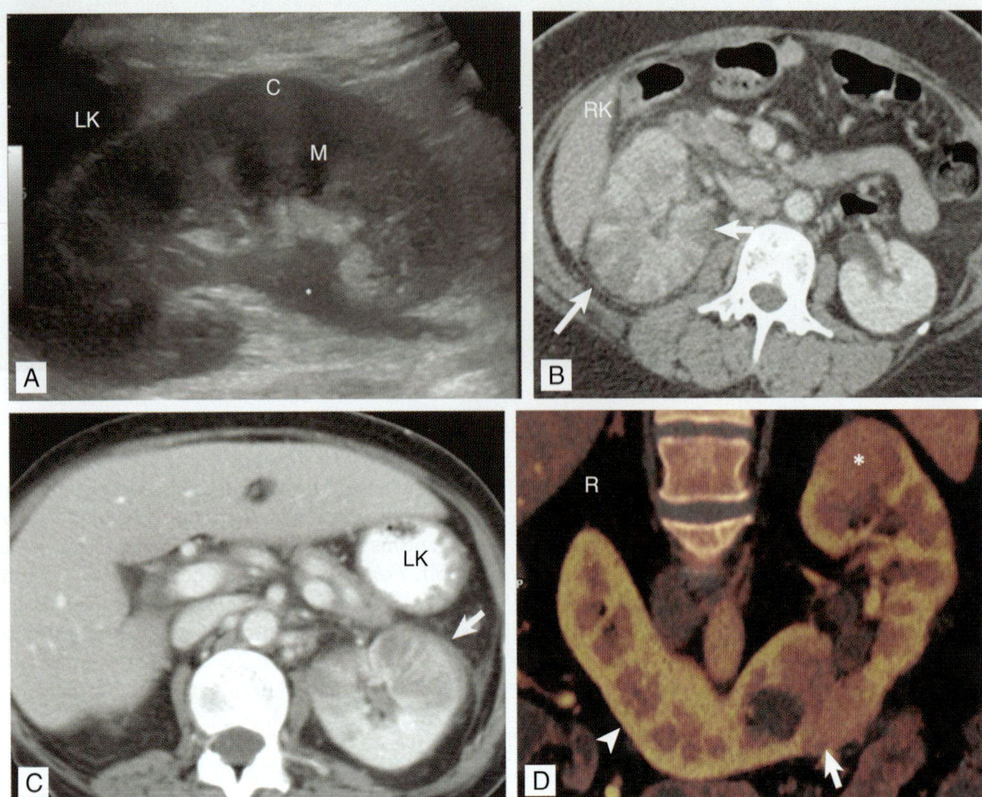

Figure 39.1 Acute pyelonephritis. (A) Two-dimensional B-mode ultrasound image of the kidney in longitudinal plane demonstrates hypoechogenicity of the renal cortex (c). The pelvicalyceal system is dilated. Echoes in the renal pelvis (*white asterisk*) represent infection (pyonephrosis). *M,* Medulla. (B) Contrast-enhanced computed tomography (CT) in the axial plane during the nephrographic phase demonstrates wedge-shaped, ill-defined, hypodense, and hypoenhancing areas in the kidney radiating from the papilla in the medulla and extending to the cortex (*small white arrow*). The *large white arrow* is thickened adjacent fascia. (C) Contrast-enhanced CT in the axial plane during the nephrographic phase demonstrates a focal area in the left kidney (LK) with multiple radial hypodensities involving both the medulla and cortex with alternate enhancing linear bands (*white arrow*). In the vicinity is seen fluid and fascial thickening. (D) Contrast-enhanced dual-energy CT scan, multiplanar reconstruction of mixed image (superimposed iodine image) during the nephrographic phase of a horseshoe kidney demonstrates multiple hypoenhancing focal regions involving the cortex and medulla representing lower iodine concentration (*white asterisk* and *white long arrow*). The right kidney (RK) shows normal iodine concentration (*white arrowhead*).

- Increased echogenicity in the collecting system and uroepithelial thickening [8]

Increased bladder wall thickness (wall thickness ≥2 mm in the distended bladder and ≥5 mm in nondistended bladder), significant postvoid residual volume, and the presence of any obstruction can also be demonstrated on USG.

Computed Tomography: Computed tomography scan is an excellent tool to evaluate for complications of acute pyelonephritis.

Indications

- For complicated presentations
- For patients who do not respond to antibiotic therapy
- To assess for abscesses, whether renal or perinephric, and for emphysematous pyelonephritis [1,5]

Scan protocol: The CT scan protocol is described in Table 39.1.

The nephrographic phase is preferred over the corticomedullary phase. In the corticomedullary phase, there is an intense enhancement of the renal cortex, and the medulla is less enhanced because of preferential arterial flow to the cortex and glomerular filtration of the contrast material, but in the nephrographic phase, tubular filtration of contrast material allows for a homogeneous enhancement of the renal parenchyma. The nephrographic phase is the best phase for detection of subtle parenchymal lesions such as streaky zones of hypoenhancement that extend from the papilla to the renal cortex in acute bacterial nephritis [9].

TABLE 39.1 Scan Protocol for Contrast-Enhanced Computed Tomography for Evaluation of the Renal System

Phase	Timing	Uses
Precontrast	Before contrast administration	Identifying calculi, gas in the urinary tract, any hemorrhage, renal enlargement, perinephric fat stranding, inflammatory masses, and obstruction
Nephrographic	90–100 sec after contrast injection	Best defines the abnormalities within the renal parenchyma
Excretory	7–9 min after contrast injection	To rule out urinary tract obstruction and anatomic anomalies

Whether to do the delayed excretory phase in every patient remains contentious as few authors suggest that the excretory phase be taken only when an obstruction is suspected [1,2]. However, the 2018 American College of Radiology (ACR) appropriateness criteria document states that more studies are needed to prove whether the nephrographic phase alone is enough to rule out urinary tract obstruction [5].

Imaging findings

- Thickened, and enhancing walls of the pelvicalyceal system and ureter can sometimes be the only finding
- Wedge-shaped, ill-defined, hypodense, and less enhancing areas in the kidney radiating from the papilla in the medulla and extending to the cortex (Fig. 39.1B), representing the affected region where there is obstruction of the tubules by the inflammatory debris, vasospasm, and interstitial edema [10]
- Striated nephrographic (Fig. 39.1C) is a common feature that refers to alternating bands of hypo- and hyperattenuating linear areas caused by the juxtaposition of obstructed and normal tubules
- Other conditions that need to be taken into consideration when encountered with striated nephrographic are ureteric obstruction, contusion, and renal vein thrombosis (RVT) in case of unilateral striated nephrographic and autosomal-recessive polycystic kidney disease, tubular obstruction, and systemic hypotension in case of bilateral striated nephrographic [11]
- Round and peripherally hypoattenuating lesions are seen within the renal parenchyma with hematogenous spread (Fig. 39.1D)
- In advanced stages, renal papillary necrosis might set in which shows small collections of contrast peripheral to calyces in the papillary region. The entire papillae might become necrotic and may slough off. The sloughed-off papilla sometimes is seen as a filling defect in the collecting system (Fig. 39.2)
- Other imaging findings are global enlargement of the kidney, thickening of Gerota's fascia, and perinephric fat stranding. Perinephric fat stranding can also be seen in the setting of trauma and previous infection and should be interpreted with caution

It is important to note that the healing process in CT lags behind clinical improvement by few weeks to months [1].

Magnetic Resonance Imaging: Magnetic resonance imaging (MRI) offers a radiation-free modality for imaging and is particularly helpful in pregnant females and young kids. The findings in the MRI follow that of in the CT, namely, increased renal size; perinephric fat stranding; and fluid, striated nephrograms [12] (Fig. 39.3). The various sequences useful in evaluation for pyelonephritis are described in Table 39.2.

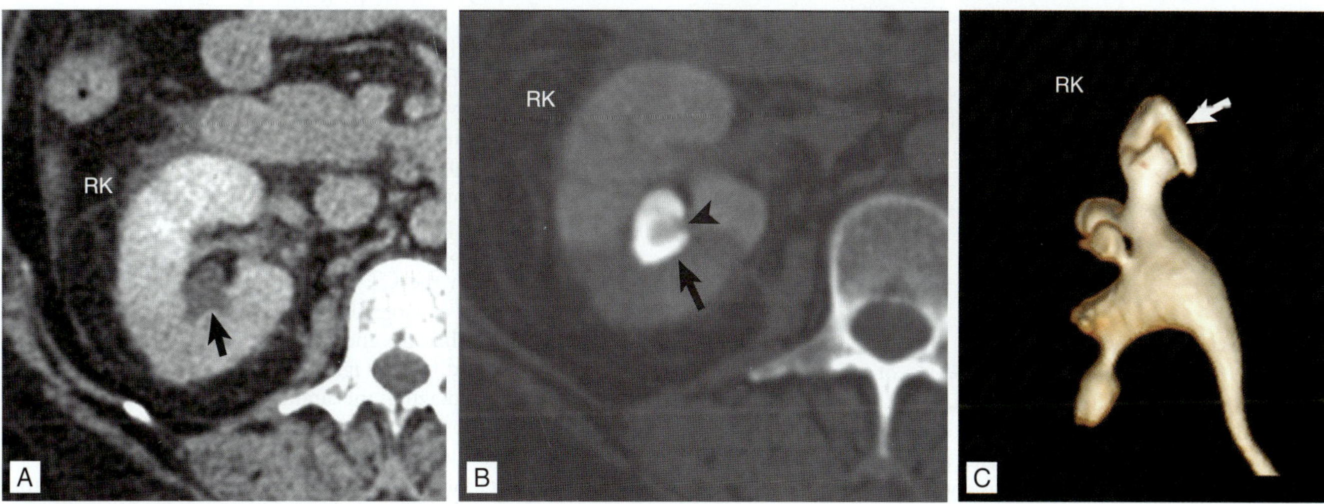

Figure 39.2 Acute pyelonephritis with papillary necrosis. (A) Contrast-enhanced computed tomography (CT) in the axial plane during the nephrographic phase demonstrates cavity formation with dilation of the upper pole calyx and blunting (*black arrow*) secondary to papillary necrosis and sloughing. (B) Contrast-enhanced CT in the axial plane during the excretory phase at the same level demonstrates contrast in the cavity formed by sloughing of the papilla (*black arrow*) with filling defect (*black arrowhead*). (C) Three-dimensional volume rendering technique of contrast-enhanced CT during the excretory phase demonstrates dilation of the calyx and blunting. There is communication with the cavity formed by the sloughed papilla (*white arrow*). *RK,* right kidney.

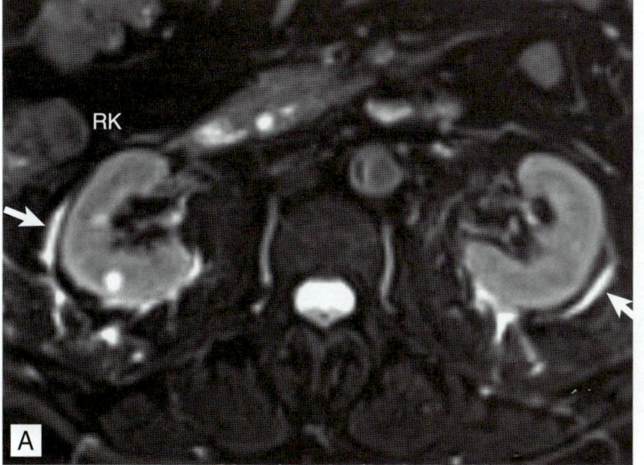

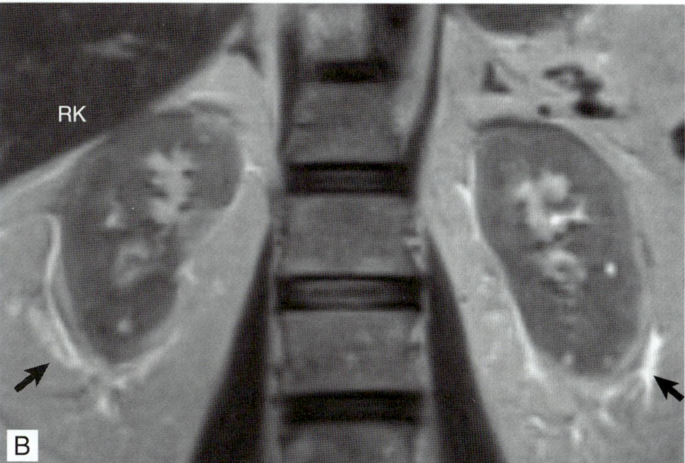

Figure 39.3 Acute pyelonephritis in chronic kidney disease. (A) T2-weighted turbo spin echo (TSE) fat-suppressed image in the axial plane through both kidneys demonstrates septal thickening running from cortex to cortex (*small white arrows*), which is probably due to underlying chronic inflammation. (B) T2-weighted half Fourier single shot turbo spin echo (HASTE) image in the coronal plane through both kidneys demonstrates irregular renal margin, septal thickening (same as *white arrow* in Fig. 39.3A) and perinephric edema (*short black arrows*), suggestive of acute inflammation. The signal intensity of the normal renal parenchyma is altered with the loss of corticomedullary differentiation. Findings suggest acute pyelonephritis in a background of chronic kidney disease. *RK,* right kidney.

TABLE 39.2 Various Magnetic Resonance Imaging Sequences That Can Be Used in Assessing Acute Pyelonephritis

Sequence	Description
Noncontrast	Affected regions in the kidney appear hyperintense on T2-weighted imaging and hypointense on the T1 sequence, reflecting edema within the renal parenchyma.
Postgadolinium-based contrast	Correctly depicts the regions of involvement. The findings on MRI follow those of CT, namely, increased renal size, perinephric fat stranding, and fluid, and striated nephrograms [13].
Gadolinium-enhanced inversion recovery	Because of tubular obstruction and stasis, less amount of gadolinium accumulates in the affected region of the kidney while the rest of the healthy kidney that is normally perfused shows a much higher signal drop, making the affected region stand out against a backdrop of a generalized signal drop [14].
MRU	Used when an obstruction is suspected.
Diffusion-weighted imaging	Areas of pyelonephritis show significantly lower apparent diffusion coefficient values than that of in the normal renal parenchyma [15].

CT, computed tomography; *MR*, magnetic resonance imaging; *MRU*, magnetic resonance urography.

Renal Scintigraphy: Scintigraphy using technetium-99m dimercaptosuccinic acid (Tc^{99m} DMSA) is of particular value in the pediatric population in which it can become difficult to differentiate between lower UTI and acute pyelonephritis [5]. It offers visualization of the renal cortex and areas of hypoperfusion associated with acute pyelonephritis and scar formation. However, it provides limited information on the extrarenal and perinephric spread of the disease.

Acute Lobar Nephronia

Acute lobar nephronia is a localized inflammatory, nonliquefactive renal bacterial infection that typically involves one or more lobes or lobules of the kidney. In the spectrum of inflammatory renal pathology, it falls in the middle, with acute pyelonephritis at one end and renal abscess at the other, with clinical features overlapping with both the diseases [13].

On USG, it appears as a renal mass-like lesion with altered echogenicity disrupting the corticomedullary differentiation (Fig. 39.4A) [14]. On color Doppler examination, no color flow is seen, which differentiates it from a neoplasm (Fig. 39.4B). On CT, it appears as a wedge-shaped parenchymal region with poor perfusion. Adjacent perinephric fat stranding might be seen (Fig. 39.4C).

Emphysematous Pyelonephritis

Emphysematous pyelonephritis is a fulminant, life-threatening, gas-producing, necrotizing infection of the kidney and sometimes perirenal tissue, carrying a very high mortality rate. Diabetes is present in around 80% of patients [15]. The causative organisms in most of the cases are *E. coli, Klebsiella pneumoniae,* and *Proteus mirabilis* [1].

Imaging

Ultrasonography: The imaging finding includes several nondependent echogenic foci within the renal parenchyma and collecting system with distal shadowing showing reverberations and low-level echoes often called “dirty shadowing.” However, adjacent calculi and bowel gas might create problems in diagnosis and reduce the sensitivity of USG.

Computed Tomography: This is the imaging modality of choice for diagnosis of emphysematous pyelonephritis [1,2]. CT can accurately depict the presence of air with the kidney and extra-renal extension of the disease.

The findings on the CT are multiple air bubbles within the parenchyma, renal enlargement, perinephric fat stranding, and sometimes perinephric gas and the presence of focal abscess sometimes with gas-fluid levels (Fig. 39.5) [16].

Based on the imaging appearance, emphysematous pyelonephritis has been classified into two groups [17] (Table 39.3).

Computed tomography-guided drainage along with proper antibiotic coverage can be used in the management. Renal scintigraphy can be used to assess the function of the kidney before surgical treatment. Patients having very poor renal function can benefit from total nephrectomy [18].

Renal and Perinephric Abscess

These most commonly develop on a background of pyelonephritis. However, hematogenous seeding may happen against a backdrop

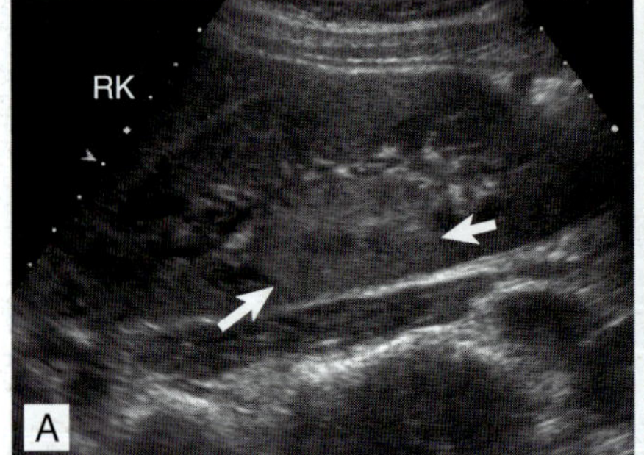

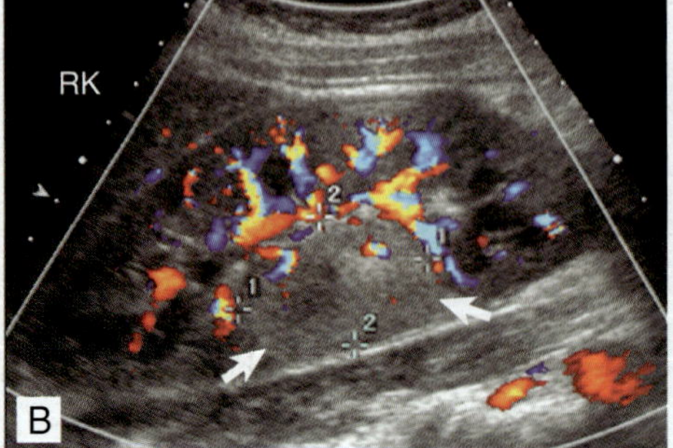

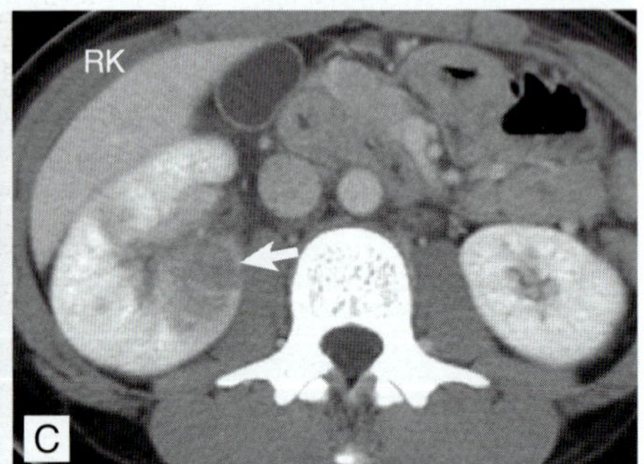

Figure 39.4 Focal pyelonephritis (nephronia). (A) Longitudinal section of the right kidney (RK) on two-dimensional ultrasound image, demonstrates a noncapsulated, focal hyperechoic corticomedullary lesion in the interpole region (*white arrows*). (B) The longitudinal section of the right kidney on color Doppler demonstrates a lack of vascularity in the lesion (*white arrows*). (C) Contrast-enhanced computed tomography in the axial plane during the nephrographic phase demonstrates corresponding focal and poorly enhancing lesion (*white arrow*) in the right kidney. The margins are ill defined, and adjacent perinephric fat stranding is seen.

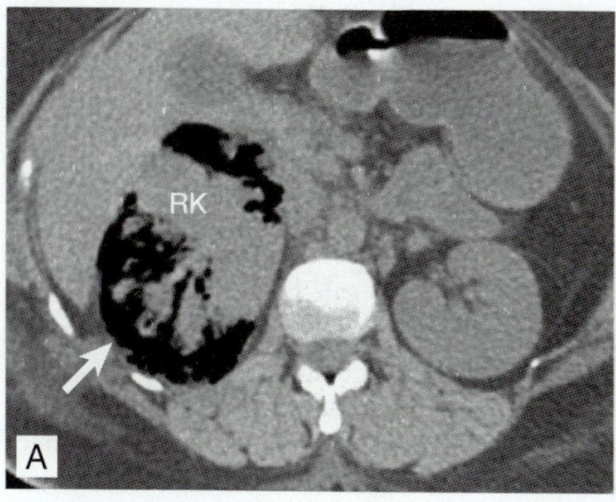

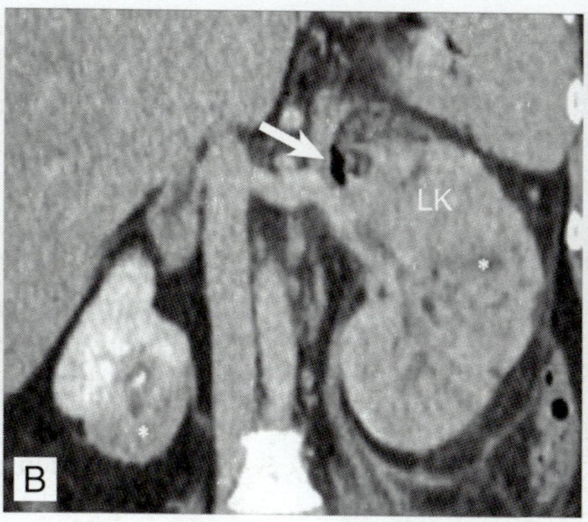

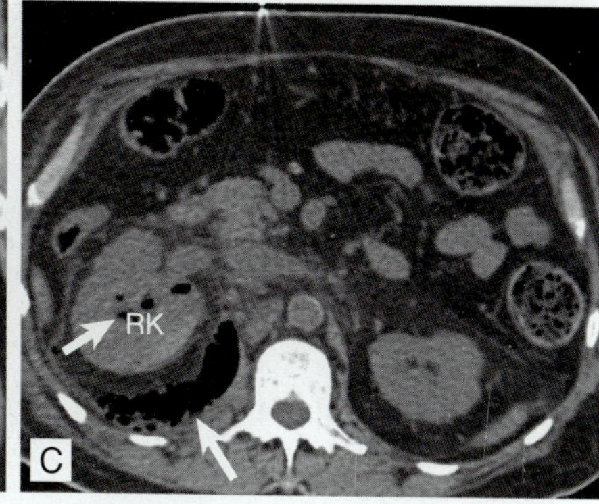

Figure 39.5 Emphysematous pyelonephritis. (A) Type 1: noncontrast computed tomography (CT) in the axial plane demonstrates extensive corticomedullary air (*white arrow*) in the right kidney (RK). (B) Type 2: contrast-enhanced CT in the coronal plane during the nephrographic phase demonstrates a bulky left kidney (LK) with diffuse changes of pyelonephritis. There are multiple small abscesses (*white asterisk*) and cortical air (*white arrow*) in the upper pole. Changes of focal pyelonephritis are seen in the lower pole of the right kidney (*white asterisk*). (C) Noncontrast CT in the axial plane demonstrates air in the pelvicalyceal system (*white arrow*) in the RK. The *long white arrow* is extensive air in the peri- and paranephric space. *L*, left; *R*, right.

TABLE 39.3 Types of Emphysematous Pyelonephritis Based on Imaging

Type 1	Type 2
▪ Fulminant course; high mortality rate (69%)	▪ Less mortality rate (18%)
▪ Mottled or streaky air bubbles without fluid collections	▪ Bubbly or loculated gas along with the presence of intrarenal and perirenal fluid collections

of staphylococcal bacteremia in IV drug abusers. The predisposing factors are diabetes; pregnancy; and anatomic abnormalities such as renal stone, VUR, obstructive tumor, papillary necrosis, and neurogenic bladder [19,20].

Renal abscess starts with focal renal parenchymal necrosis caused by infection. Soon liquefaction sets in, which convert into a walled-off abscess. In the case of a perinephric abscess, usually the necrosis occurs in perinephric fat because of the outward spread of the infection from the kidney. A perinephric abscess might rupture through the Gerota's fascia and lead to a paranephric abscess.

Imaging

Ultrasonography: The typical appearance of a renal abscess is of a hypoechoic lesion with internal debris and a thick irregular wall. On Doppler examination, no flow is seen within the lesion. A perirenal abscess appears as hypoechogenicity around the kidney with floating internal debris.

Computed Tomography: Computed tomography scan is the imaging modality of choice for the diagnosis of renal and perirenal abscesses. A contrast-enhanced CT scan is done, and images are acquired in the noncontrast, nephrographic, and excretory phases.

A mature renal abscess appears as a hypodense, nonenhancing lesion on noncontrast images. On postcontrast evaluation, it shows peripheral enhancement because of pseudocapsule formation (Fig. 39.6A). A halo of hypoenhancement is seen around the abscess in the nephrogram phase. Other associated findings that are seen are perinephric fat stranding and thickening of Gerota's fascia. It may also present as multiple small abscesses (Fig. 39.6B and 39.6C). A peripheral cortical abscess can rupture and form a subcapsular collection in the liver (Fig. 39.6D) or spleen.

Magnetic Resonance Imaging: Magnetic resonance imaging can be done in pregnant patients and those who are hypersensitive to iodinated contrast. MRI shows rounded or ovoid lesions with

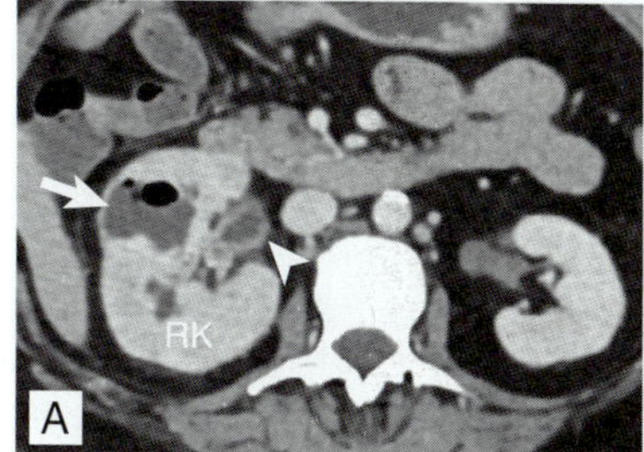

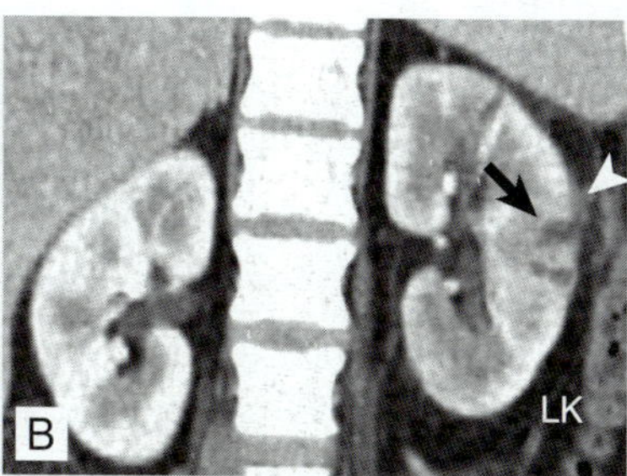

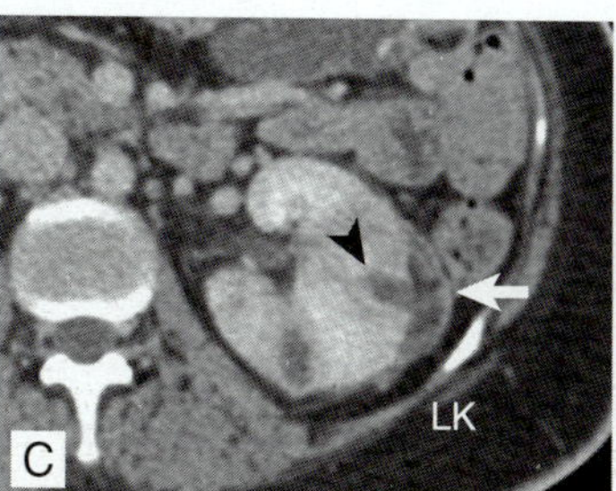

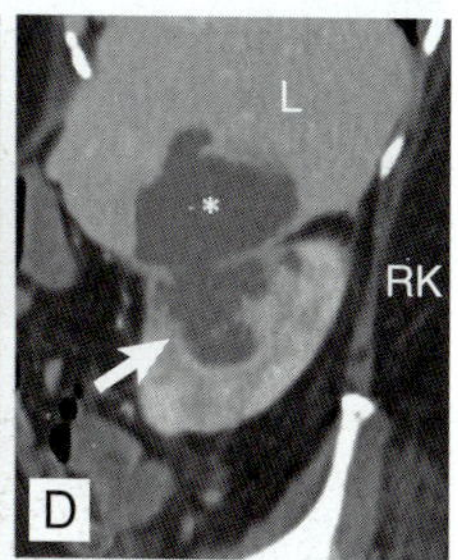

Figure 39.6 Renal abscess. (A) Contrast-enhanced computed tomography (CT) in the axial plane during the nephrographic phase demonstrates a renal abscess (*white arrow*) with air and fluid in the right kidney (RK). Uroepithelial thickening is seen in the renal pelvis (*white arrowhead*). (B) Contrast-enhanced CT in the coronal plane in a different patient demonstrates bulky left kidney and formation of small renal abscesses in the lateral cortex (*black arrow*). The *white arrowhead* is subcapsular fluid. (C) Contrast-enhanced CT in the axial plane in the same patient as in *B* demonstrates a ruptured abscess in the outer cortex (*black arrowhead*) with the formation of the subcapsular collection (*white arrow*). (D) Contrast-enhanced CT in the sagittal oblique plane in a different patient demonstrates a large abscess in the renal parenchyma (*white arrow*) that has ruptured beyond the paranephric space into the liver (*white asterisk*). *L*, liver.

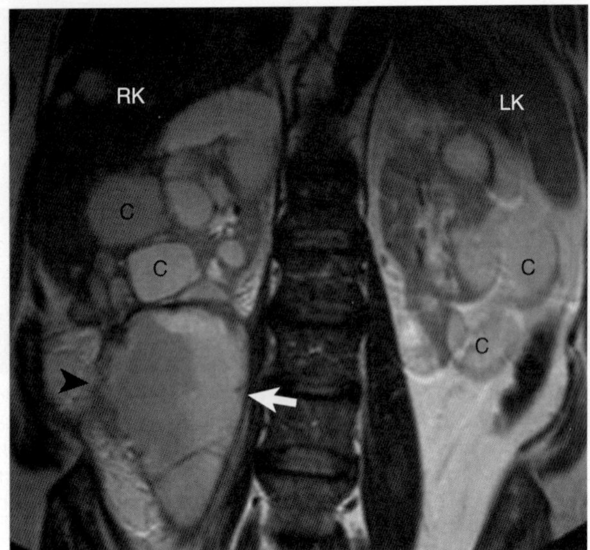

Figure 39.7 Autosomal dominant polycystic kidney disease with cyst infection. (A) T2-weighted magnetic resonance imaging (MRI) in the coronal plane demonstrates multiple cysts (C) of a varied signal. A large, complex cyst is seen in the lower pole (*white arrow*) demonstrating internal debris and irregular margin on the lateral aspect (*black arrowhead*).

increased T2 signal and decreased T1 signal depending on the amount of protein and cellular debris within the abscess. On diffusion-weighted imaging (DWI), diffusion restriction is seen within the abscess. Fluid-fluid levels and septations might be observed. Gadolinium-enhanced images can identify the extrarenal extension. Patients with autosomal dominant polycystic kidney disease (ADPKD) are prone to have cyst infection. In such a scenario, MRI can be appropriate (Fig. 39.7).

Pyonephrosis

Pyonephrosis is an infected pelvicalyceal system with a backdrop of obstructive uropathy, leading to the formation of pus within the collecting system. It is a urologic emergency that needs to be urgently drained [6]. If immediate measures are not taken, it might lead to permanent renal impairment and life-threatening sepsis. In adults, the obstruction arises from varied causes such as calculi, tumor, strictures, or sloughed papilla from acute pyelonephritis.

Imaging

Ultrasonography: Ultrasonography can be used for initial examination and shows a lack of a completely anechoic collecting system with moving echogenic debris within (Fig. 39.8A). Sometimes gas might be seen as well as "dirty shadows" [21,22]. The presence of dense echogenic debris is the most reliable sign of pyonephrosis [22].

Computed Tomography: Computed tomography diagnoses the pelvicalyceal dilation and determines the level of obstruction. The findings of pyonephrosis in CT are dilated and obstructed collecting system with high attenuation (Fig. 39.8B) than what is normally seen, thickened pelvicalyceal walls (>2 mm), perinephric and renal inflammatory changes, and layering of contrast media in the collecting system in the excretory phase images [21,23,24].

Magnetic Resonance Imaging: Significantly low apparent diffusion coefficient (ADC) values have been observed in the renal pelvis in pyonephrosis compared with hydronephrotic kidneys.

Xanthogranulomatous Pyelonephritis

Xanthogranulomatous pyelonephritis is a chronic granulomatous inflammation of kidneys with most cases occurring in a background of obstruction caused by renal stones [25,26]. It is almost always unilateral. Middle-aged women with a history of recurrent UTIs are most commonly affected in the adult population [26].

Clinical Features

The presenting symptoms are flank pain, fever, malaise, and weight loss. The physical examination often reveals a palpable unilateral renal mass. Urine analysis often shows pyuria and bacteriuria. The most commonly associated organisms are *E. coli*, *Proteus mirabilis*, *Pseudomonas* spp., *Enterococcus faecalis,* and *Klebsiella* spp. [27].

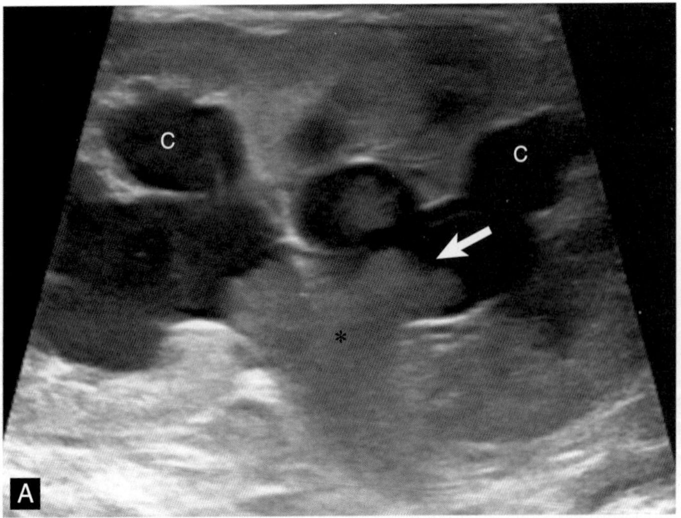

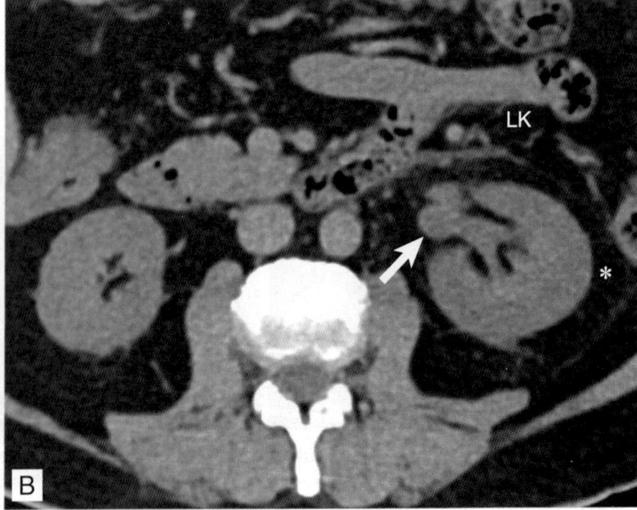

Figure 39.8 Pyonephrosis. (A) Two-dimensional B-mode ultrasound image in the longitudinal plane demonstrates a dilated pelvicalyceal system. Sludge (*black asterisk*) is seen in the renal pelvis extending into the infundibulum (*white arrow*). There is consequent dilation of the caliceal system (C). (B) Noncontrast computed tomography in the axial plane demonstrates mildly bulky and hypodense left kidney (LK) compared with the right kidney. The *white asterisk* is perinephric fat stranding. The *white arrow* demonstrates a dilated pelvicalyceal system with increased density in the dilated renal pelvis.

Pathophysiology

Xanthogranulomatous pyelonephritis is a chronic granulomatous response toward recurrent renal infection that leads to the destruction of renal parenchyma and its replacement by lipid-laden foamy macrophages. The inflammatory process starts in the renal pelvis and spreads into the medulla and cortex, causing gradual destruction. Usually, there is a staghorn calculus present in the pelvis, which is nondilated [28].

Imaging Findings

Ultrasonography: On USG, an enlarged kidney is seen typically with a large echogenicity in the center with posterior acoustic shadowing indicative of a staghorn calculus. Replacement of renal parenchyma with hypoechoic mass with internal echoes might be observed with loss of corticomedullary differentiation (Fig. 39.9A).

Computed Tomography: Computed tomography is the imaging modality of choice. It shows characteristic multiple, rounded, low-density areas surrounded by a rim of enhancement, replacing the normal renal parenchyma. These findings are similar to a fingerprint of a bear paw and is hence called the "bear paw" sign. The kidney is enlarged and nonfunctioning with the presence of staghorn calculus, a contracted renal pelvis, and expanded calyces (Fig. 39.9B).

Computed tomography scan accurately demonstrates the extrarenal involvement of the disease, which is vital in preoperative assessment [28]. Extension can be seen in the perinephric space, anterior and posterior pararenal spaces, psoas muscle, diaphragm, and the posterior abdominal wall. Failure to document extrarenal spread might lead to postoperative complications such as draining sinuses, delayed wound healing, and bowel fistulas [28].

Chronic Pyelonephritis

Chronic pyelonephritis results from a repeated insult to the kidney from recurrent or continuous infections, VUR, or obstruction, which results in fibrosis and scarring of the kidney. There is a chronic inflammation of renal tubules and interstitium with scarring and deformity of the renal pelvis and calyces. Obstruction to renal outflow predisposes to infection. Reflux nephropathy is the most common cause of chronic pyelonephritis.

The imaging findings are typical with renal scarring; shrinkage in size; cortical thinning; clubbing of the calyces, which happens secondary to retraction of the scar overlying; and calyceal dilation (Fig. 39.10A and 39.10B). Overall, there are renal architectural distortion and decreased function of the kidney. The decreased function can also be elicited on a DMSA scan, which will show areas of photopenia and scarring (Fig. 39.10C).

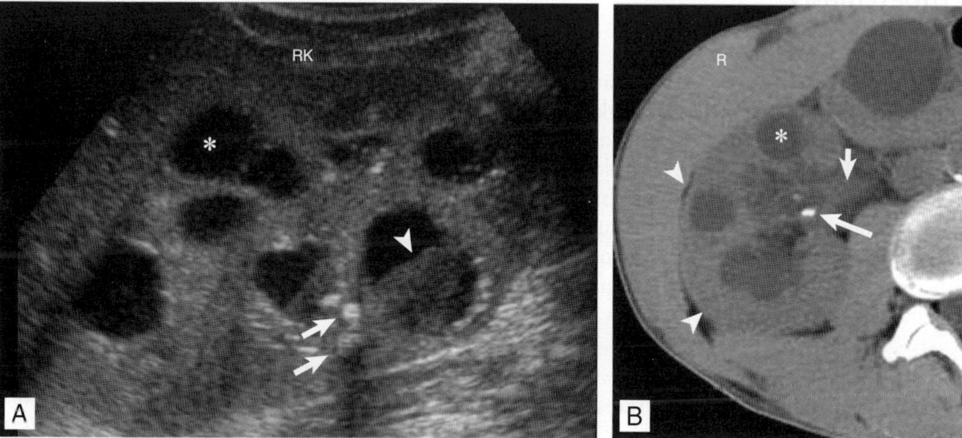

Figure 39.9 Xanthogranulomatous pyelonephritis. (A) Two-dimensional ultrasound image in the longitudinal plane demonstrates dilated calyces, giving a multiloculated appearance (*white asterisk*). Calculus is seen in the renal pelvis (*white arrows*). The *white arrowhead* is sludge in the calyces. (B) Noncontrast computed tomography in the axial plane demonstrates an enlarged kidney (*white arrowheads*) with dilated calyces, giving a multiloculated appearance (*white asterisk*). Calculus is seen in the renal pelvis (*long white arrow*). The *small white arrow* is a uroepithelial thickening of the renal pelvis. *RK,* right kidney.

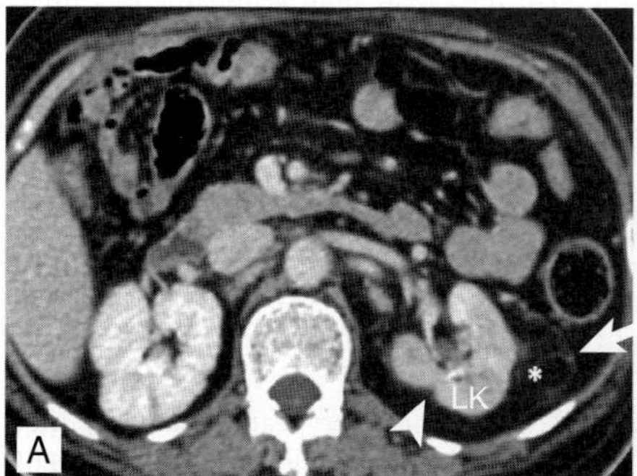

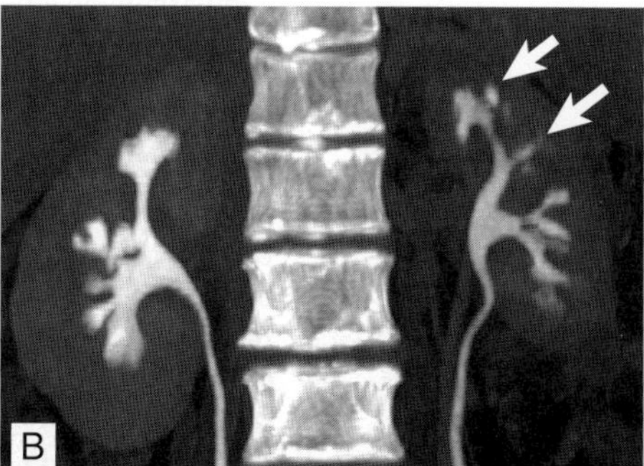

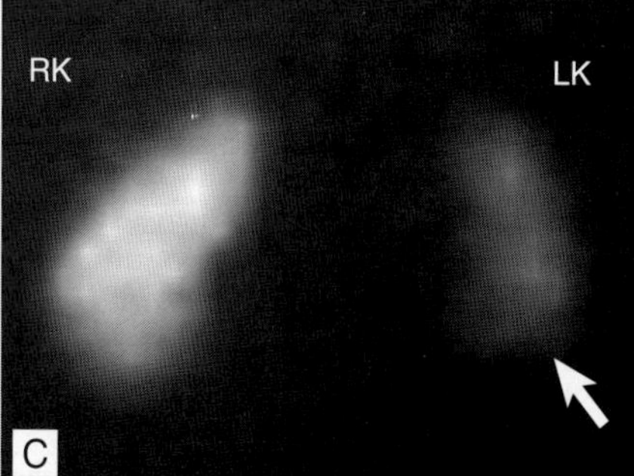

Figure 39.10 Chronic pyelonephritis. (A) Contrast-enhanced computed tomography (CT) in the axial plane during the nephrographic phase demonstrates a small left kidney (LK) with reduced enhancement compared with the right kidney (RK). A focal scar is seen with cortical thinning (*white arrowhead*). The *white asterisk* is hypertrophied perinephric fat. The *white arrow* is thickened perinephric fascia. (B) Contrast-enhanced CT thin maximum intensity projection, in the coronal plane during the excretory phase demonstrates a small left kidney. There is clubbing of the calyces (*white arrows*). (C) A dimercaptosuccinic acid (DMSA) nuclear scan demonstrates a small left kidney with photopenia and scarring (*white arrows*).

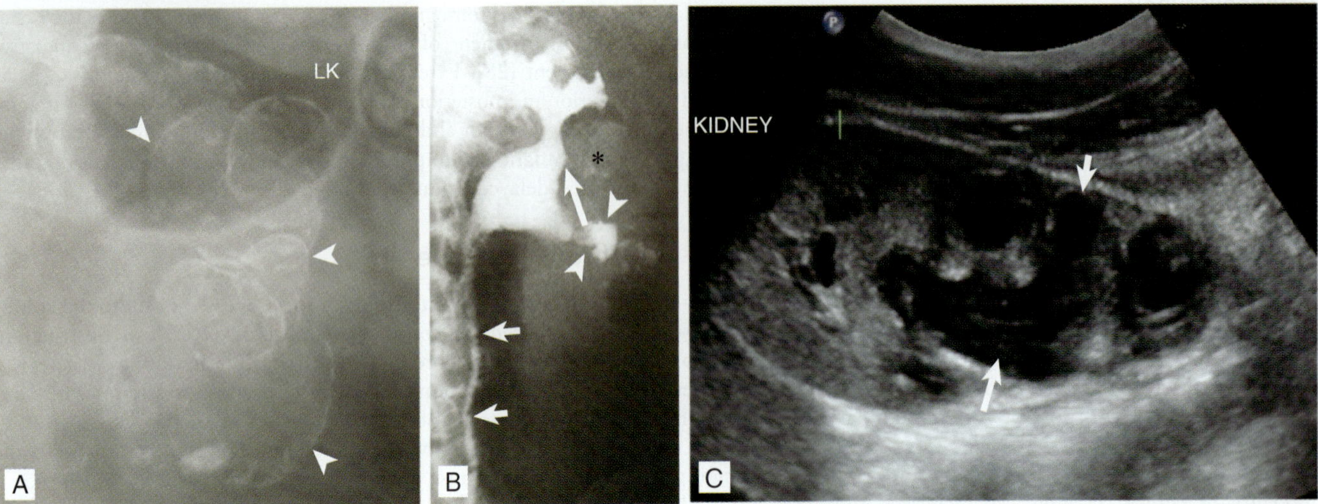

Figure 39.11 Urogenital tuberculosis. (A) Abdominal radiograph in anteroposterior view demonstrates lobulated left kidney (LK) with calcification of cortical surface (*arrowheads*), suggestive of chronic tuberculosis (putty kidney). (B) Intravenous urography during the excretory phase in a different patient demonstrates papillary necrosis with a deformed lower calyx and irregular margins "moth-eaten appearance" (*white arrowheads*). The inter pole calyx is faintly seen (*black asterisk*) because of infundibular stenosis (*long white arrow*), or "phantom calyx." The ureter is irregular and demonstrates multiple areas of narrowing (*small arrows*). (C) Two-dimensional B-mode ultrasound image demonstrates dilated calyces (*short white arrow*) and significant uroepithelial thickening in the pelvicalyceal system (*long white arrow*).

Genitourinary Tuberculosis

Clinical Features

The genitourinary tract serves as the most common site for the manifestation of extrapulmonary tuberculosis (TB), making up to 14–41% of total extrapulmonary TB cases [29]. However, in patients with genitourinary TB, only 50% have been detected to have pulmonary disease [1]. The spread of infection is through the hematogenous route. Commonly, bladder symptoms such as frequency, urgency, and dysuria are also seen. Approximately half patients present with gross hematuria, and low back pain is the manifestation in one-third of cases [30,31].

Pathophysiology

The pathogenesis of genitourinary TB involves the transfer of the mycobacterium to the genitourinary tract and reactivation of the mycobacterium. In the kidney, the bacilli reside in the periglomerular capillaries and form microscopic granulomas, which later develop into macroscopic granulomas [29]. The active infection spreads from the cortex into the medulla, the renal papilla, the collecting system, and further into the ureters and bladder.

Imaging Findings

Kidneys and the Pelvicalyceal System

Radiography: The most common manifestation on abdominal radiographs is the presence of renal calcifications, which are reported in 24–44% of the patients [32]. A lobar pattern of calcification, with calcific rims that outline the distorted renal lobes, is pathognomonic of TB [29]. *Putty kidney* is a term given to the appearance of calcified caseous necrotic tissue appearing homogenous and moderately dense on radiograph and seen in end-stage renal TB (Fig. 39.11A).

Intravenous urography: The earliest change is the loss of sharp outlines of the minor calyces. Other findings are calyceal dilatation, papillary necrosis, and initial cavitation. In further stages, stricturing can happen because of fibrosis at calyces, the pelviureteric junction (PUJ), and the ureter, which might lead to focal or diffuse hydrocalycosis. Infundibular stenosis with resultant failure of contrast excretion by involved parenchyma may happen and is called a phantom calyx. The renal pelvis may be dilated or may show filling defects caused by caseous debris and granulation tissue. The involvement progresses to fibrosis with scarring. The traction from strictured infundibulum and parenchymal fibrosis might result in kinking of the renal pelvis, which is known as *Kerr's kinks* [33]. A "hiked-up" pelvis might also be seen, which results from stricture at the inferior margin of the renal pelvis and its cephalic retraction [34]. Ureteral involvement is seen in the form of fibrosis and stricturing, which leads to a beaded or corkscrew appearance of the ureter [35]. In the later stages, severe thickening of the wall produces a rigid shortened ureter with narrow lumen termed "*pipe stem ureter*."

Bladder involvement in the advanced stage shows a thickened bladder wall with trabeculations. Later fibrosis and contracture result in a "thimble bladder" with reduced capacity. The fibrosis at the trigone can cause wide open ureterovesical junctions, causing VUR. Fig. 39.11B depicts the changes associated with genitourinary TB in the IVU.

Ultrasonography: The most frequently seen renal parenchymal abnormality is a focal renal lesion, which is a parenchymal granuloma seen as regions of hyper, mixed, or hypoechogenicity [29]. Papillary involvement may also be seen as an echogenic medullary mass adjacent to the calyx and, into which (calyx) it can fequently rupture. Focal caliectasis caused by infundibular stenosis can be seen as well. A pattern of diffuse, uneven caliectasis without renal pelvic dilation with associated urothelial thickening signals toward renal TB, especially when a renal calculus is absent [29] (Fig. 39.11C). Hydro-ureteronephrosis can be seen in the cases in which the ureters and urinary bladder are involved. A tubercular renal abscess also might develop, appearing as a hypoechoic cavity with thick, ill-defined walls.

Computed tomography: Except for very early changes, most findings on an IVU should be detectable on CT. CT is usually done to know the extent of renal and extrarenal spread of the disease. The findings on CT are as follows:

- Presence of parenchymal tuberculous granulomas, which are seen as solid masses with minimal to no postcontrast enhancement, accompanied by changes in the collecting system [36]. Large granulomas may show calcification

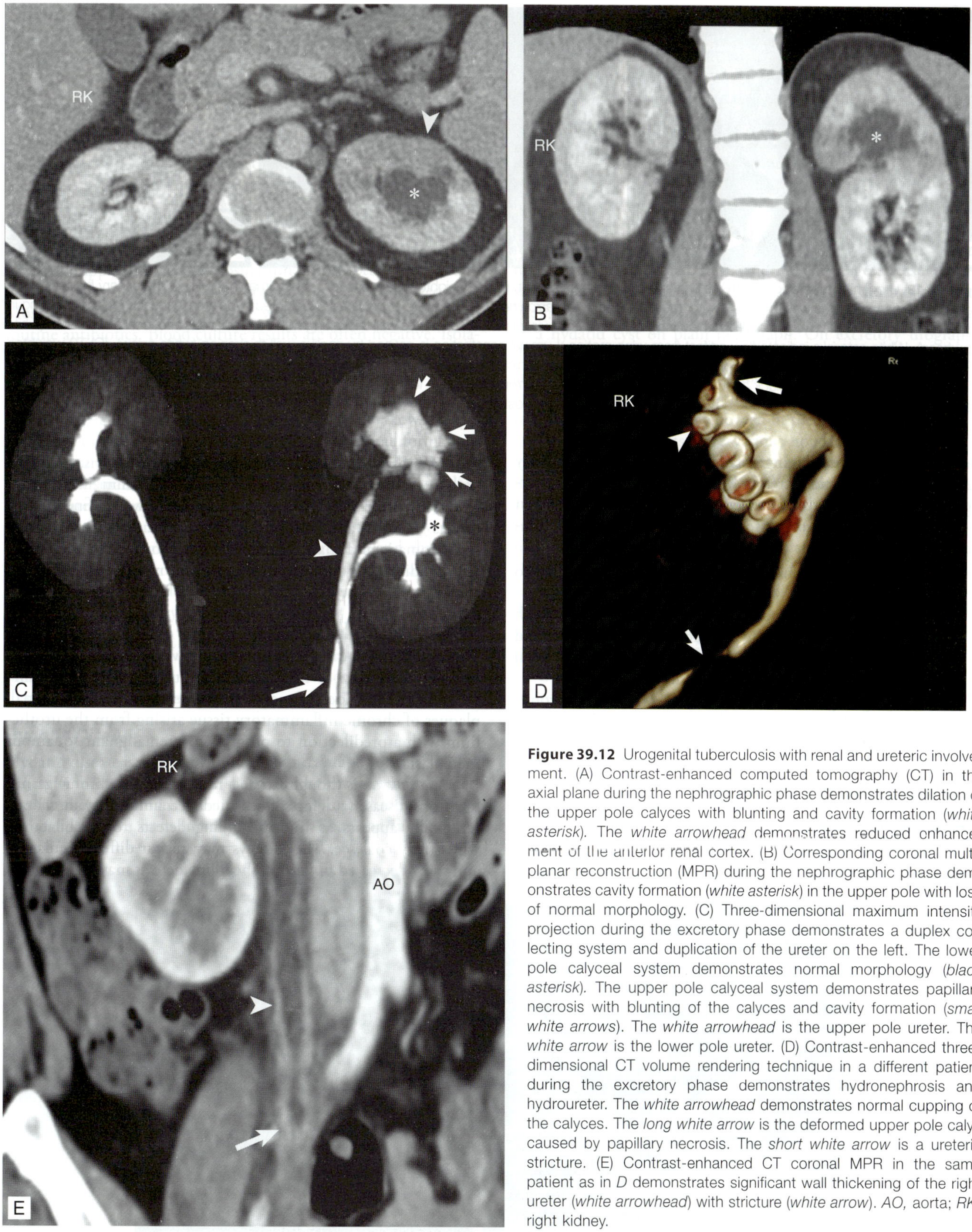

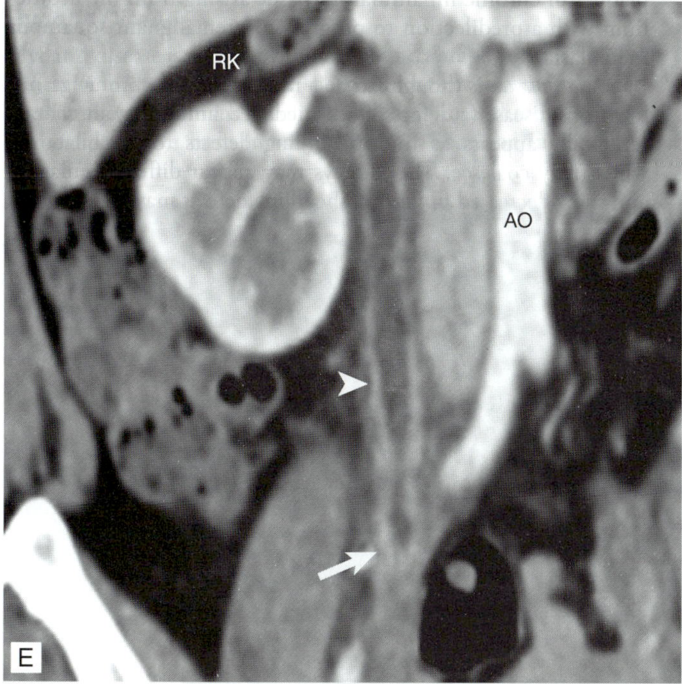

Figure 39.12 Urogenital tuberculosis with renal and ureteric involvement. (A) Contrast-enhanced computed tomography (CT) in the axial plane during the nephrographic phase demonstrates dilation of the upper pole calyces with blunting and cavity formation (*white asterisk*). The *white arrowhead* demonstrates reduced enhancement of the anterior renal cortex. (B) Corresponding coronal multiplanar reconstruction (MPR) during the nephrographic phase demonstrates cavity formation (*white asterisk*) in the upper pole with loss of normal morphology. (C) Three-dimensional maximum intensity projection during the excretory phase demonstrates a duplex collecting system and duplication of the ureter on the left. The lower pole calyceal system demonstrates normal morphology (*black asterisk*). The upper pole calyceal system demonstrates papillary necrosis with blunting of the calyces and cavity formation (*small white arrows*). The *white arrowhead* is the upper pole ureter. The *white arrow* is the lower pole ureter. (D) Contrast-enhanced three-dimensional CT volume rendering technique in a different patient during the excretory phase demonstrates hydronephrosis and hydroureter. The *white arrowhead* demonstrates normal cupping of the calyces. The *long white arrow* is the deformed upper pole calyx caused by papillary necrosis. The *short white arrow* is a ureteric stricture. (E) Contrast-enhanced CT coronal MPR in the same patient as in *D* demonstrates significant wall thickening of the right ureter (*white arrowhead*) with stricture (*white arrow*). *AO,* aorta; *RK,* right kidney.

- Focally, the renal cortex is hypodense compared with the normal parenchyma and is the result of hypoperfusion, as seen in acute pyelonephritis (Fig. 39.12A)
- Frank tubercular abscesses might be seen in the form of focal hypodense areas with peripheral enhancement (Fig. 39.12B)
- Uneven caliectasis is characteristic findings similar to that of IVU (Fig. 39.12C and 39.12D)
- Urothelial thickening in the pelvicalyceal system and the ureter with or without stricture is an important clue if identified (Fig. 39.12E)

TABLE 39.6 Subtypes of Renal Calculi

Type	Subtype	Urinary pH	Content	Risk Factors	Computed Tomography Density	Other
Calcium stones (70–80%)	Calcium oxalate	Acidic pH, 5–6.5	CA oxalate ▪ Calcium oxalate monohydrate (COM) ▪ Calcium oxalate dihydrate ▪ Mixed with calcium phosphate	Hypercalciuria, hyperoxaluria, and hypocitraturia	Radiodense	High recurrence rate COM is resistant to ESWL
	Hydroxyapatite	Alkaline pH, 7.5	Unbalanced proportion of calcium and phosphate	Hypercalciuria, hyperoxaluria, and hypocitraturia	Radiodense	Resistant to ESWL
	Brushite	Alkaline pH, 7.5	Equal mix of calcium and phosphate	Hypercalciuria, hyperoxaluria, and hypocitraturia	Radiodense	Resistant to ESWL
Uric acid (5–10%)		Acidic pH, 5.8	Uric acid	Metabolic syndrome (insulin resistance) Gout Hyperuricosuria (high-purine diet)	Radiolucent	Can be differentiated on Dual Energy (DE) from calcium stones
Struvite (10%)		Alkaline	Magnesium Ammonium Phosphate	Infection (*Proteus* spp. or *Klebsiella* spp.)	Radiodense	
Cystine (1%)		Normal	Cystine	Autosomal recessive Cystinuria	Radiodense	
Others	Matrix		Organic matrix with proteins	Recurrent urinary tract infections *Proteus mirabilis* and *Escherichia* spp.	Radiolucent	
	Drug		Indinavir	HIV	Radiolucent	
	Papilla		Necrosed papilla	Long-standing diabetes	Radiolucent	

ESWL, extracorporeal shockwave lithotripsy; *HIV*, human immunodeficiency virus.

Computed Tomography

Multidetector CT and dual-energy computed tomography (DECT) have enhanced the role of CT in stone disease management. It aids in treatment planning and post-treatment follow-up.

Nonenhanced Computed Tomography of the Kidneys, Ureters, and Bladder: Unenhanced helical CT is highly sensitive (>95%) and specific (>96%) for the diagnosis of urolithiasis and is the imaging investigation of choice for the initial assessment of patients with suspected urolithiasis [57]. Stone hardness can be predicted based on the Hounsfield unit (HU), which can be of help to consider extracorporeal shockwave lithotripsy (ESWL) versus surgical management [58]. *It has been observed that treatment success rates with ESWL were significantly higher for stones of average HU value of less than 815* [59].

In the emergency setting of acute flank pain, noncontrast, low-dose CT is a quick investigation and provides clear detail of the stone location, accurate measurement of the stone size, and CT density.

Computed tomography easily detects stones that are otherwise radiolucent on radiography. These include urate, xanthine, and cystine stones. Completely radiolucent stones on CT scan with soft tissue attenuation can be difficult to identify, such as matrix stones (Fig. 39.20), deposition of druglike indinavir (Fig. 39.21), and necrosed papilla (Fig. 39.22).

Dual-Energy Computed Tomography: Dual-energy CT scan or spectral imaging is simultaneous scanning of a body part and acquiring two different datasets using two different x-ray energy spectra. Typically ,the two energies used are 80 and 140 kVp [60]. DECT specifically plays a role in treatment planning by characterization of stone composition by differentiating non-uric calculi from UA calculi. It potentially allows patients with UA stones to avoid invasive interventional procedures for stone removal or ESWL. HU based differentiation of various materials using conventional single-energy has considerable overlap in material attenuation, leading to inaccurate differentiation [61]. *DECT allows characterizing different materials based on their elemental composition. It provides material-specific attenuation properties at different energy levels.*

The x-ray attenuation profile of UA and non-UA stones is different at multiple energies because of their unique chemical composition. Uric acid stones are composed of elements with low atomic numbers compared with that of non-UA stones, which are composed of elements with higher atomic numbers [62]. A CT number ratio (or index) is created for each material, which

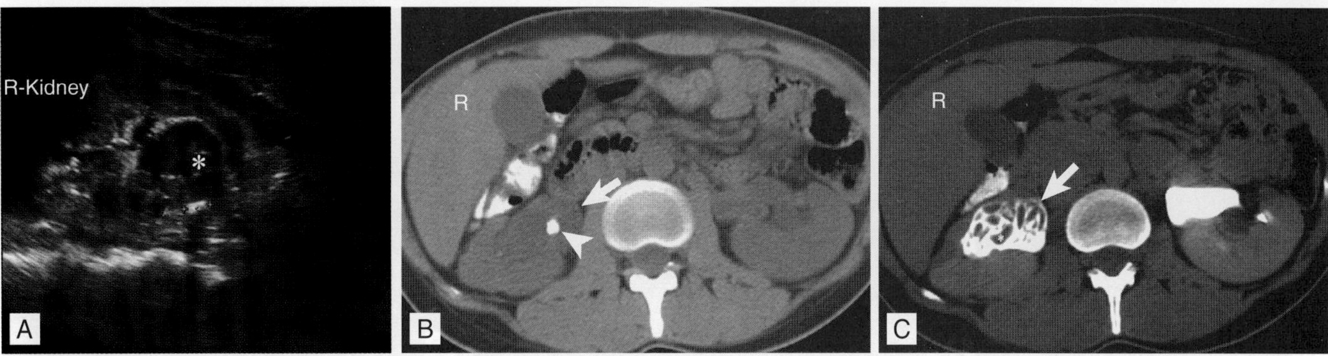

Figure 39.20 Matrix calculi. (A) Two-dimensional ultrasound image demonstrates a dilated renal pelvis with debris or sludgelike contents in it (*white asterisk*). Also seen is a hyperechoic calculus in the renal pelvis ("A" with markers). (B) Noncontrast computed tomography scan demonstrates the dilated renal pelvis (*white arrow*) with a hyperdense calculus (*white arrowhead*). The higher density of urine in the renal pelvis represents debris or sludge. (C) Contrast-enhanced computed tomography during the excretory phase demonstrates multiple filling defects in the renal pelvis representing noncalcified matrix calculi (*white arrow*). Calcified calculus is masked by excreted intravenous contrast.

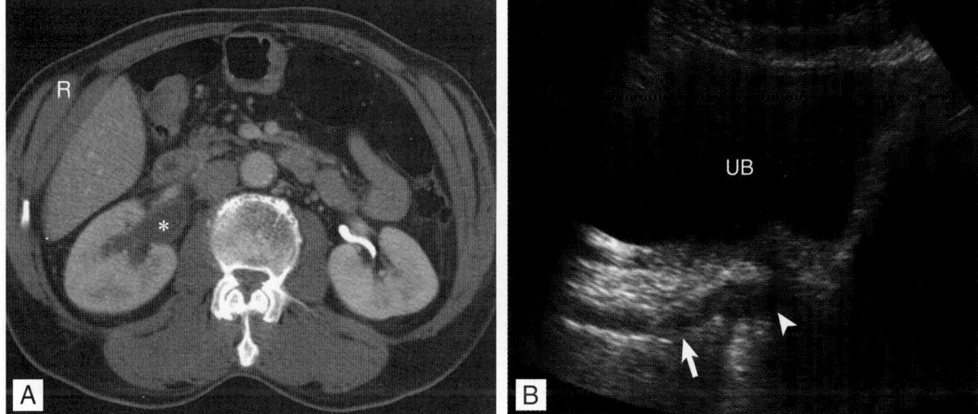

Figure 39.21 Renal obstruction caused by indinavir crystal deposits in an HIV-positive patient. (A) Split-bolus computed tomography urography demonstrates normal nephrogram and contrast excretion in the left kidney. The right kidney demonstrates reduced enhancement of renal parenchyma with hydronephrosis (*white asterisk*). There is no contrast excretion in the renal pelvis and the calyces. (B) Two-dimensional ultrasound demonstrates fine echogenic foci (*white arrowhead*) in the dilated juxta-vesical ureter (*white arrow*) and represent indinavir crystal deposition. *UB*, urinary bladder.

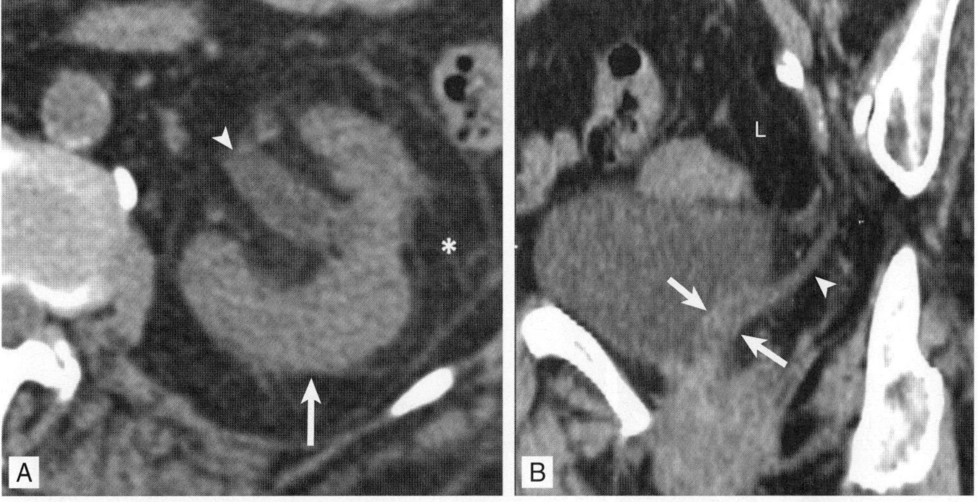

Figure 39.22 Renal obstruction caused by necrosed papilla. (A) Noncontrast computed tomography demonstrates a bulky left kidney (*white arrow*) with significant perinephric fat stranding (*white asterisk*). There is dilation of the renal pelvis (*white arrowhead*). (B) Noncontrast computed tomography demonstrates hydroureter (*white arrowhead*) and focal thickening at the vesicoureteric junction with soft tissue density (*white arrows*). On ureteroscopy, there was an impacted necrosed papilla.

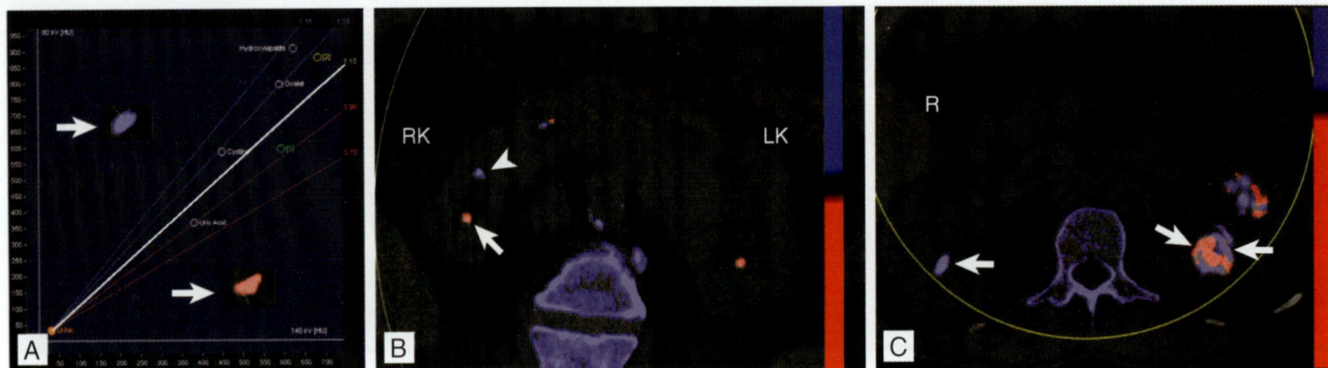

Figure 39.23 Dual-energy computed tomography (CT) number ratio and stone characterization. (A) A graphic representation of CT number ratio and stone characterization. The *x*-axis demonstrates Hounsfield unit values of calculus at higher energy (140 kVp), and the *y*-axis demonstrates Hounsfield units of the same calculus at lower energy (80 kVp). Images of two calculi have been superimposed. The *red color* signifies urate calculus (CT number ratio <1.15) and marked as a *green circle* on the graph. The *blue color* signifies nonurate calcium calculus (CT number ratio >1.15) and is marked as a *yellow circle* on the graph. (B) Concurrent calcium oxalate and urate calculi. Dual-energy oblique multiplanar reconstruction image in a horseshoe kidney demonstrates concurrent urate (*white arrow*) and oxalate (*white arrowhead*) calculi. (C) Mixed calcium oxalate and urate calculi. Dual-energy axial image demonstrates mixed calculi in the left kidney (LK) containing urate (*red color*) and calcium (*blue color*). *RK,* right kidney.

is defined as the ratio of the HU value on the low-energy image to the HU value of the same material on the high-energy image (spectral separation) [63] (Fig. 39.23A). The larger the spectral separation, the easier it is to discriminate between two materials.

$$\text{CT number ratio} = \frac{\text{HU value at 80 kVp}}{\text{HU value at 140 kVp}}$$

Single-energy CT has an accuracy of 64–81% in identifying the subtypes of calculi [64]. Dual-energy scanners have an accuracy of 90–100% in differentiating UA from non-UA calculi [65]. Color coding is done for the stones. Urate stones are red, and nonurate stones are blue (Fig. 39.23B). Stones can also be a combination of urate and calcium components (Fig. 39.23C).

Imaging of small stones adjacent to ureteric stent poses a diagnostic challenge because they are often missed. In DECT, the polyurethane-based stents are blue and stents composed of silicone are red. The colored stent–stone–contrast images can be displayed on DECT, which improves detection, especially of calculi smaller than 3 mm next to indwelling ureteral stents [66].

Computed Tomography Urography: Intravenous iodinated contrast can be administered selectively in certain situations such as detection of radiolucent stones on NCCT or differentiation of stone from phlebolith or renovascular calcification. It also gives additional functional information such as the enhancement characteristics of the kidney. Contrast excretion on delayed images helps in opacifying and delineating the entire urinary tract with intravenous urography (IVU)-like pictures. An additional benefit is to detect any anatomic abnormality (Fig. 39.24), ureteral stricture, PUJ obstruction caused by vascular compression (Fig. 39.25), and differentiation of urothelial thickening from tumors. In suspected calyceal rupture, it can demonstrate urinary leak and urinoma formation (Fig. 39.26).

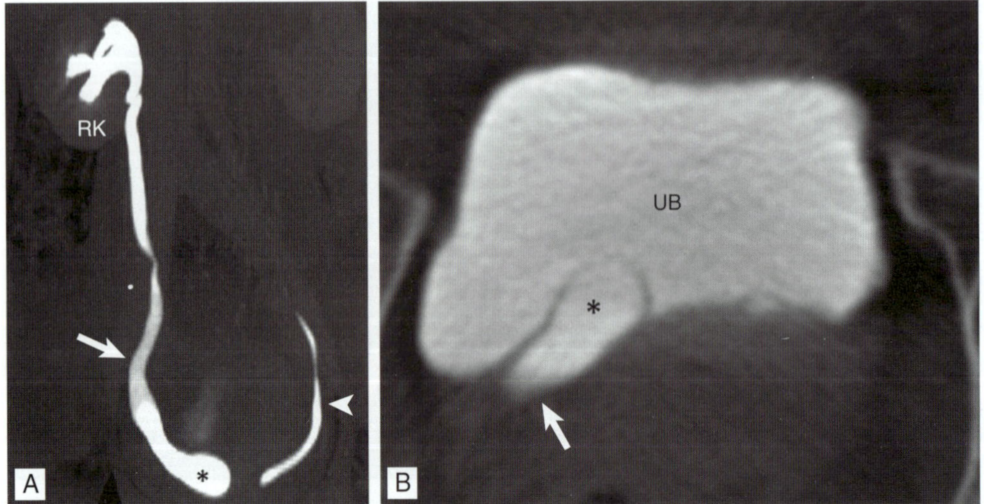

Figure 39.24 Computed tomography (CT) urography in a dilated right collecting system with a ureterocele. (A) Contrast-enhanced CT three-dimensional maximum intensity projection performed during the excretory phase demonstrates right hydronephrosis and hydroureter (*white arrow*). A ureterocele is seen at the vesicoureteric junction (*black asterisk*), normal left ureter (*white arrowhead*). (B) Contrast-enhanced CT axial image through the bladder during the excretory phase further demonstrates the ureterocele (*black asterisk*). *RK,* right kidney; *UB,* urinary bladder filled with contrast.

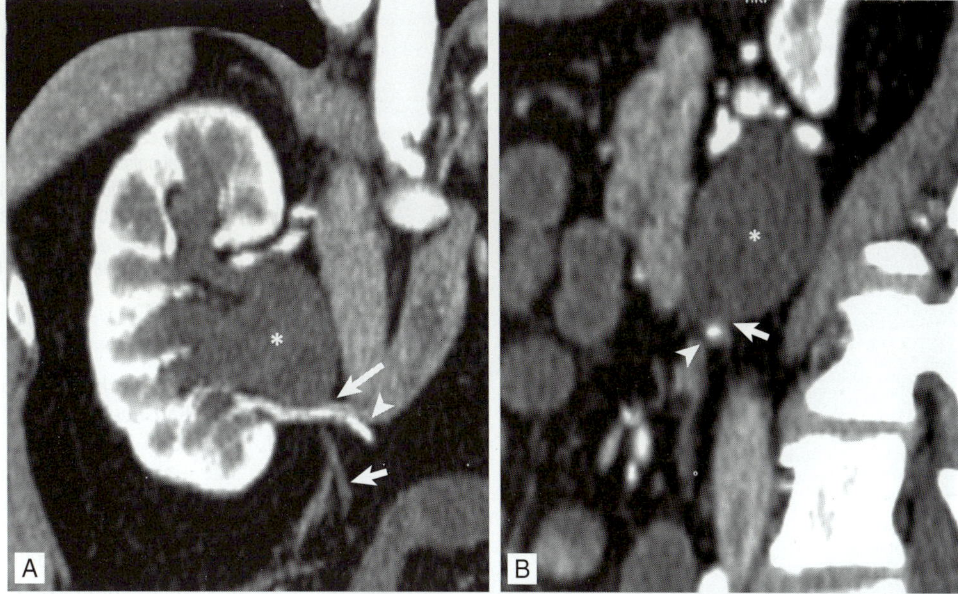

Figure 39.25 Pelviureteric junction (PUJ) obstruction caused by arterial compression. (A) Contrast-enhanced computed tomography (CT) coronal maximum intensity projection performed during the angiographic phase demonstrates a dilated collecting system and the renal pelvis (*white asterisk*). At the level of the PUJ (*white arrow*), there is compression caused by an accessory renal artery (*white arrowhead*). A *small white arrow* is the collapsed ureter. (B) Contrast-enhanced CT sagittal maximum intensity projection performed during the angiographic phase demonstrates a dilated renal pelvis (*white asterisk*). At the level of PUJ (*white arrow*), there is compression by an accessory renal artery (*white arrowhead*).

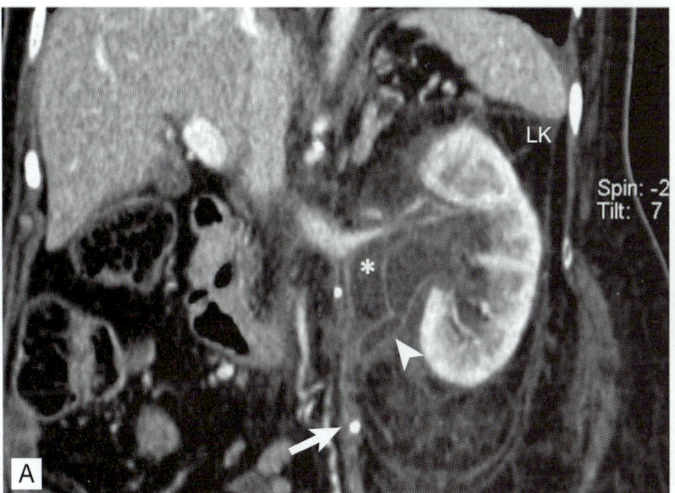

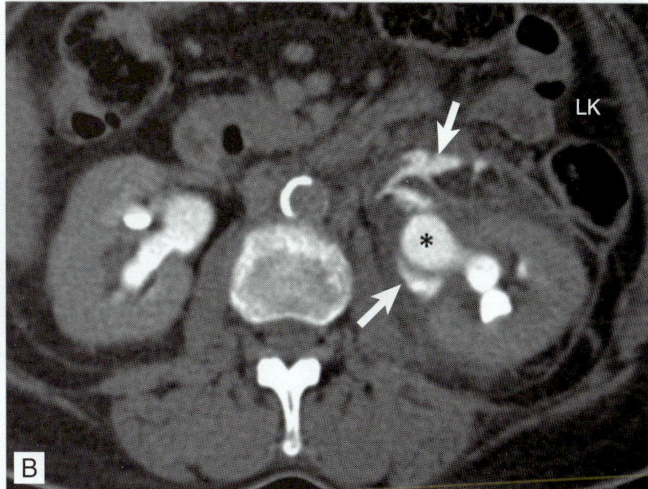

Figure 39.26 Calyceal rupture in acute renal obstruction. (A) Contrast-enhanced computed tomography (CT) coronal multiplanar reconstruction during the corticomedullary phase demonstrates dilated renal pelvis and proximal hydroureter with uroepithelial thickening (*white arrowhead*) secondary to an obstructing ureteric calculus (*white arrow*). Fluid and significant edema are seen in the perinephric space and around the renal pelvis (*white asterisk*). (B) Contrast-enhanced CT axial plane during the excretory phase demonstrates contrast leak with urinoma formation (*white arrows*). The *black asterisk* is the renal pelvis with contrast. *LK,* left kidney.

Computed Tomography Signs of an Obstructed System Caused by Ureteric Calculus: Table 39.7 lists the signs of an obstructed system caused by ureteric calculus.

Calculus Mimics: Calcifications along the course of ureters that may need differentiation are listed in Table 39.8.

Computed Tomography Scan Reporting: In an institutional or group practice, a unique reporting format that covers all the important points pertaining to management can be used across all the radiologists to reduce interobserver variability.

Important stone characteristics for treatment planning include the location, size, mean stone density (MSD), stone heterogeneity index (SHI), and dual-energy characterization if a dual-energy scanner is available. Careful evaluation should be done and documented for each stone. Thin maximum intensity projections are helpful for the detection of small stones and multiple stones, which may be missed on routine scans (Fig. 39.32A). Curved multiplanar reconstruction can create a

TABLE 39.7 Computed Tomography Signs of an Obstructed System Caused by Ureteric Calculus

Direct Signs

1. Identification of stone
2. Rim sign: thickening of urothelium in a circular fashion (Fig. 39.27)

Indirect Signs

1. Hydronephrosis and proximal hydroureter
2. Perinephric fat stranding, which is represented by the visualization of perirenal septa due to edema (perirenal cobwebs) [84] (Fig. 39.28A)
3. Perinephric fluid
4. Rupture of one of the fornices or pelvis in a high-pressure obstructed system (Fig. 39.26) (This is unrelated to the size of stone because even a small calculus measuring 3 or 4 mm can be responsible.)
5. Periureteral edema
6. Urothelial thickening
7. Pyelitis: inflammatory mural thickening caused by chronically impacted renal pelvis calculus (Fig. 39.29)
8. Reduced renal perfusion on the side of obstruction (Fig. 39.30)

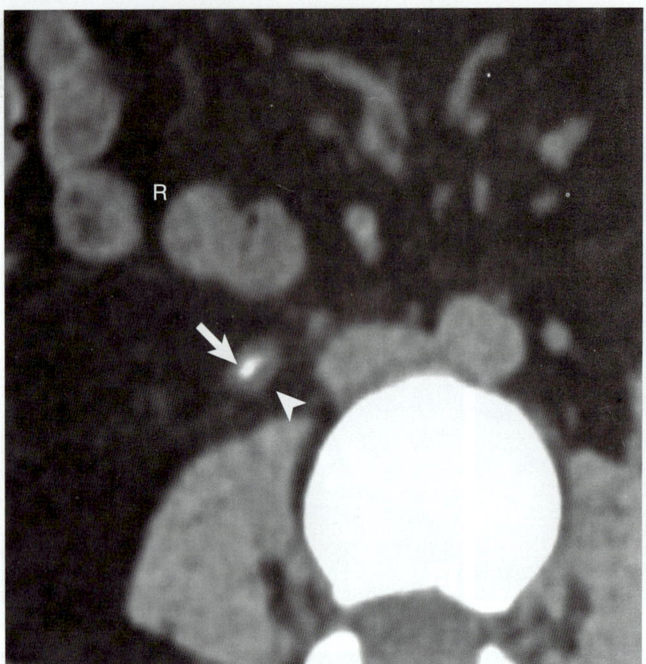

Figure 39.27 Noncontrast computed tomography in the axial plane demonstrates calculus in the abdominal ureter. The *white thin arrow* is calculus. The *white arrowhead* is a thickening of the ureteric wall (*rim sign*).

TABLE 39.8 Various Types of Ureteric Calculi Mimics

Calcifications along the course of ureters that may need differentiation

1. Arterial calcification in the renal hilum: contrast (Fig. 39.31A)
2. Arterial calcification in the iliac artery: contrast
3. Venous calcification in phlebolith: comet-tail appearance (Fig. 39.31B)
4. Calcifications of seminal vesicles: bilateral and symmetrical and central lucency
5. Calcified papilla (Fig. 39.31C)

single image of the entire urinary tract and show the exact location of the calculus (Fig. 39.32B).

1. Location
2. Size measurement is done in both axial and coronal planes after zooming the image in a bone window setting. The location of the calculus is marked in relation to the vertebral body level, which helps the referring physician to follow up on radiography and during the intervention. The bone window can also help in identifying multiple stones (Fig. 39.33)
3. The HU value is taken, preferably on a 120-kV scan. It is measured on a magnified, axial NCCT image in a bone window setting using an elliptical region of interest and includes

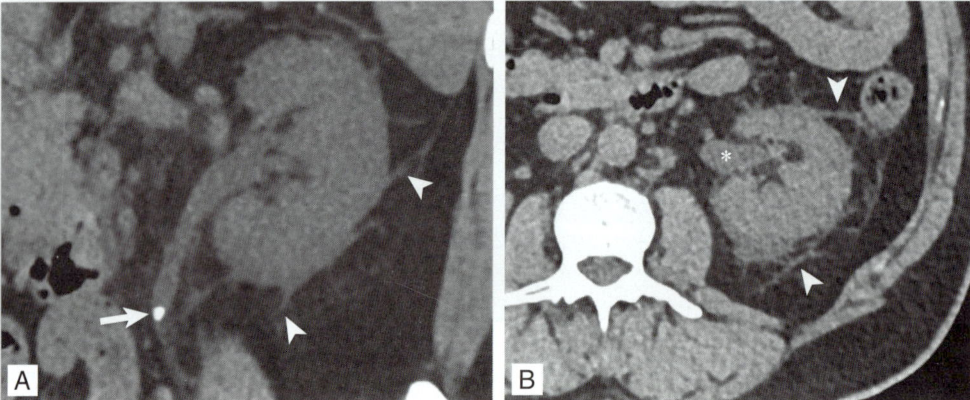

Figure 39.28 Acute ureteric obstruction. (A) Noncontrast computed tomography (CT) coronal multiplanar reconstruction demonstrates acute ureteric obstruction caused by calculus (*arrow*). Note the thickened and edematous perinephric septae (*white arrowheads*). (B) Noncontrast CT in the axial plane demonstrates a dilated renal pelvis (*white asterisk*). Note the perinephric edema and thickened septae (*white arrowheads*).

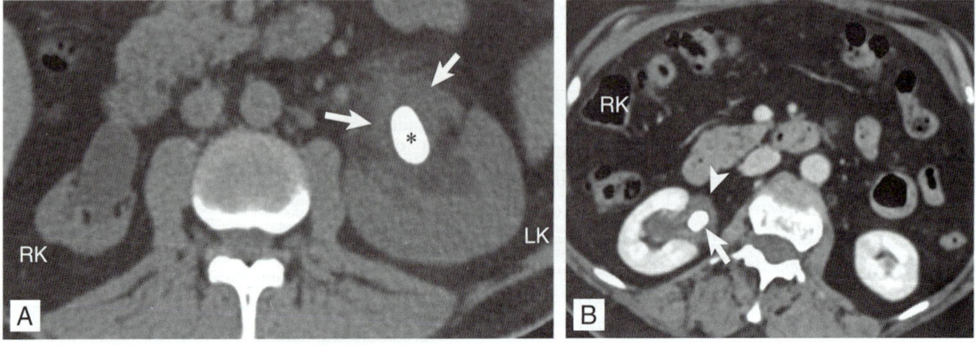

Figure 39.29 Chronic pelvic calculus with uroepithelial thickening. (A) Noncontrast computed tomography (CT) in the axial plane demonstrates calculus (*black asterisk*) in the left renal pelvis with significant uroepithelial thickening. The margins are blurred (*white arrows*). (B) Contrast-enhanced CT in the axial plane in a different patient during the nephrographic phase demonstrates a dilated right renal pelvis with calculus (*white arrow*). There are diffuse uroepithelial thickening and mucosal enhancement (*white arrowhead*). *RK,* right kidney.

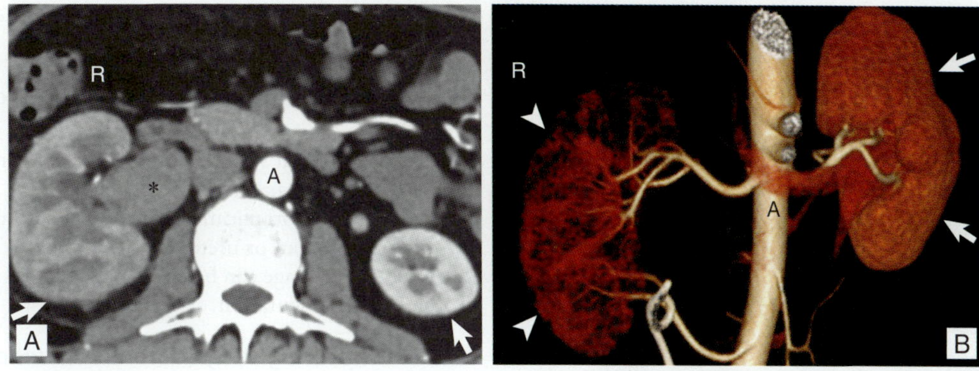

Figure 39.30 Reduced renal perfusion after obstruction. (A) Contrast-enhanced computed tomography (CT) axial image performed during the angiographic phase demonstrates reduced perfusion of the renal cortex (*white arrow*) compared with the left renal cortex (*white small arrow*) from obstruction caused by hemorrhage in the renal pelvis (*black asterisk*). (B) Contrast-enhanced CT 3D volume rendering technique of the angiographic phase demonstrates reduced perfusion of the right kidney (*white arrowheads*) compared with the left kidney (*white arrows*). *A,* aorta.

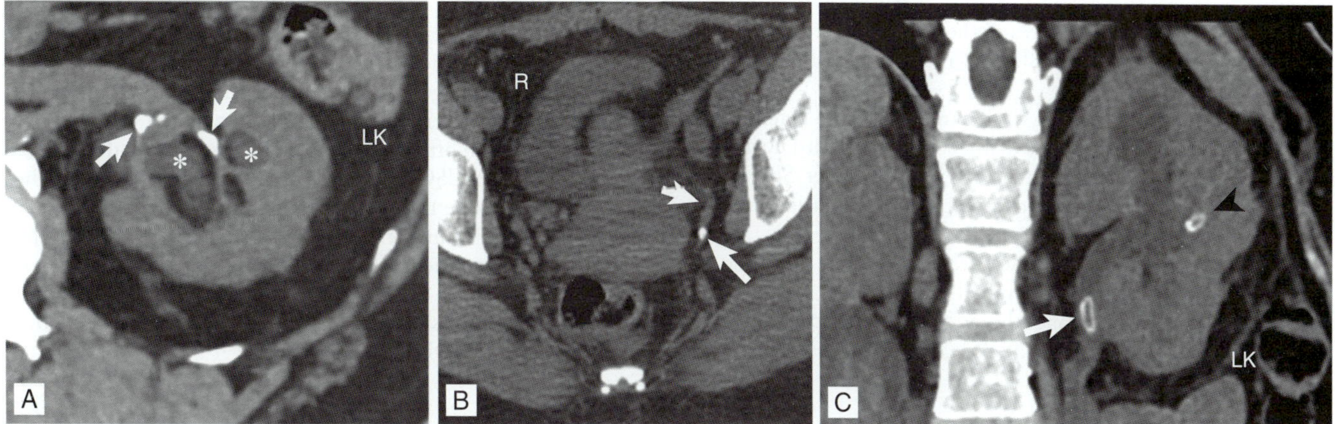

Figure 39.31 Mimics of calculus. (A) Vascular calcification mimicking calculus. Noncontrast computed tomography (CT) axial image through the left renal hilum demonstrates multiple vascular calcifications (*white arrows*). On careful observation, the branching of the vessel can be seen. The *white asterisk* is the collecting system, which is mildly prominent. (B) Phlebolith mimicking calculus. Noncontrast CT axial image through the renal pelvis demonstrates left calcific foci (*small white arrow*) along the expected course of the ureter. On careful observation, the phlebolith leads a vessel (*long white arrow*). This radiologic sign is called the "comet-tail appearance." (C) Noncontrast CT multiplanar reconstruction in the coronal plane demonstrates hydronephrosis caused by an obstructing chronic, necrosed papilla with peripheral calcification in the proximal ureter (*white arrow*). Another calcified papilla (*black arrowhead*) is seen in the collecting system. *LK,* left kidney; *RK,* right kidney.

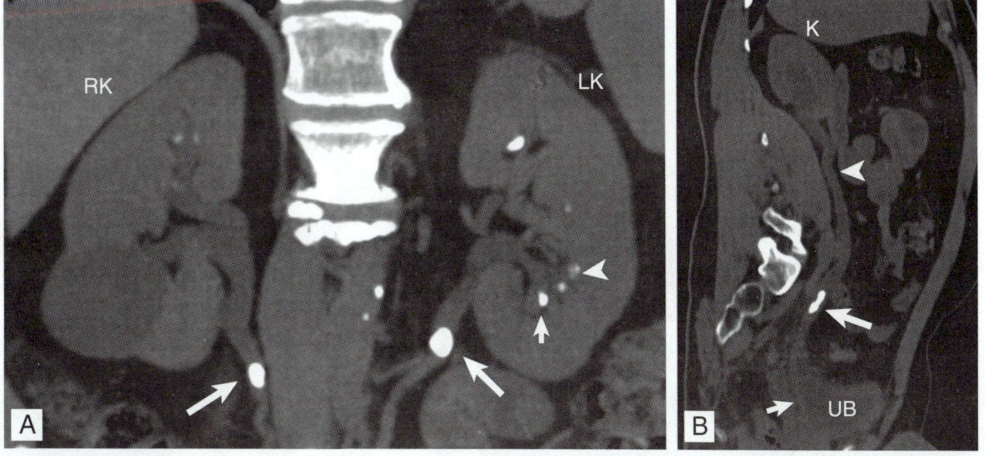

Figure 39.32 Multiplanar reconstructions. (A) Detection of multiple stones in a maximum intensity projection (MIP) image. Noncontrast computed tomography (CT) coronal oblique thin MIP image easily demonstrates multiple renal stones in both kidneys (*short white arrow*), including the medullary calcifications and early calculi formation (*white arrowhead*), which may be missed on routine thin images. Also, seen are bilateral ureteric stones (*long white arrows*). (B) Detection of multiple ureteric stones in a curved MPR, Noncontrast CT curved MPR demonstrates the entire course of the ureter (*white arrowhead*). The *large white arrow* demonstrates two ureteric calculi in tandem. The *small white arrow* is the vesicoureteric junction. *LK,* left kidney; *RK,* right kidney; *UB,* urinary bladder.

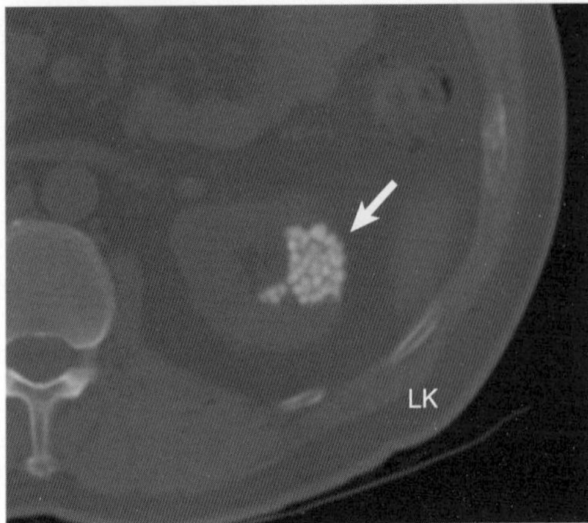

Figure 39.33 Detection of multiple stones using bone window (*white arrow*).

the largest cross-sectional area of the stone while excluding the adjacent soft tissue [67,68]. The mean HU value is documented as a MSD

4. Another important feature to document is stone heterogeneity, also called the SHI. It is defined as the standard deviation of HU in the same region of interest. A higher SHI is an independent predictor of treatment success during ESWL (Fig. 39.34)
5. The stone-to-skin distance measurement is from the stone to the posterior and lateral abdominal walls. It helps urologists in planning the distance and the angle used for percutaneous nephrolithotomy [68] (Fig. 39.35)

Key points to be documented during the stone evaluation on a NCCT KUB are outlined in Table 39.9

Role of Computed Tomography Scan in Follow-Up Imaging

1. Evaluate residual stones before removing stents (Fig. 39.37)
2. Follow up after medical management
3. Postoperative complications such as hematoma or injury to the collecting system or ureter (Fig. 39.38)
4. A CT scout image can be used if the calculus was identified on the initial presentation.

Role of Ultrasonography in Stone Evaluation

Ultrasonography is the often first investigation performed with suspected renal colic. The sensitivity of USG is around 61–90% in the setting of acute flank pain. Color Doppler demonstrates an intense multicolored signal behind a stone "twinkle artifact," which improves the ability of the detection of stones [69] (Fig. 39.39).

Additional features of the USG in obstructive uropathy are hydronephrosis, dilation of the ureter, and perinephric fluid.

The main challenges in USG are patient habitus, stone in the renal pelvis and ureter, and tracing the nondilated ureter. Stones smaller than 3 mm often do not produce posterior shadowing and can be missed on USG, especially in a nondilated system. Echogenic stones may be missed in the nondilated system because of echogenic central sinus fat [70]. The role of USG in follow up is present especially when calculus is present at the vesicoureteric junction (VUJ).

Ultrasonography signs of an obstructed system caused by a ureteric calculus are given in Table 39.10.

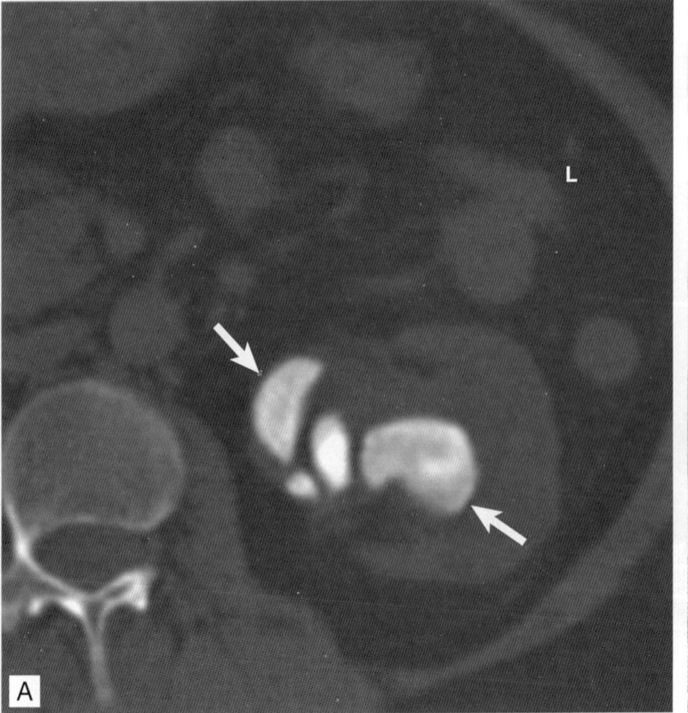

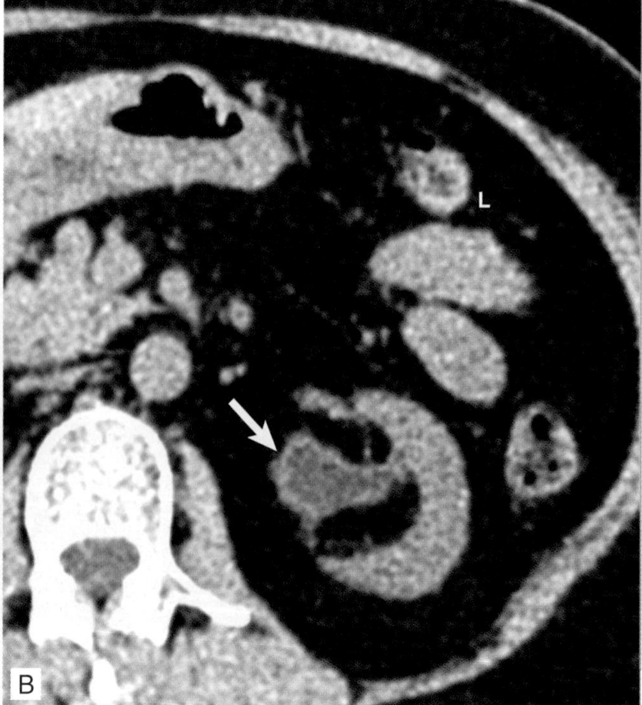

Figure 39.34 Predicting response to extracorporeal shockwave lithotripsy (ESWL) based on stone heterogeneity. (A) Noncontrast computed tomography (CT) axial image in the bone window through the left kidney demonstrates multiple large calculi in the renal pelvis and collecting system (*white arrows*). The calculi show heterogeneous attenuation. (B) Corresponding noncontrast CT axial image through the left kidney after ESWL demonstrates resolution of all stones despite the size and multiplicity (*white arrow*).

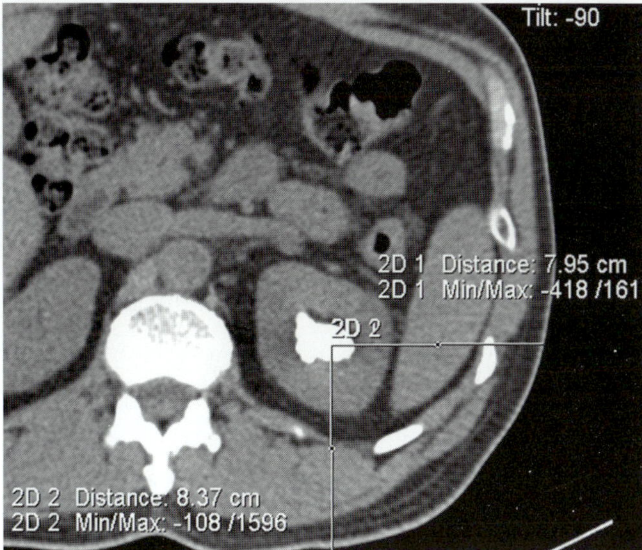

Figure 39.35 Stone-to-skin distance. Noncontrast computed tomography axial image through the left kidney demonstrates a large homogeneously dense calculus in the collecting system. Distance is measured from the center of the stone to the left lateral abdominal wall and the left posterior abdominal wall. This distance helps the treating urologist to plan the approach for percutaneous nephrolithotomy. *2D,* two-dimensional.

TABLE 39.9 Salient Points for Stone Evaluation in a Computed Tomography Report

Stones in Renal Tract: What a CT Report Must Contain?
Location and Measurements
■ Stone measurement
■ Exact location in relation to the renal poles and anterior and posterior calyx
■ Distance from the VUJ or PUJ in ureteric stones
■ Location in relation to the vertebral body level
■ Skin-to-stone distance for renal stone concerning the abdominal wall
Stone Characterization
■ Hounsfield value
■ Stone characterization using dual-energy scan
■ Stone heterogeneity
Other
■ Prone scan findings to differentiate stone in intramural part of the ureter at the VUJ from bladder calculus (Fig. 39.36A and B)
■ Mention any vascular calcification or phlebolith in the proximity of ureteric course of the calculus
■ Cortical scarring at the level of the stone

PUJ, pelviureteric junction; *VUJ*, vesicoureteric junction.

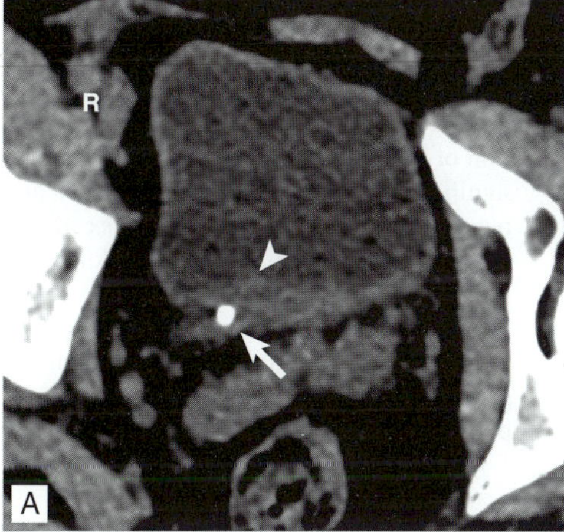

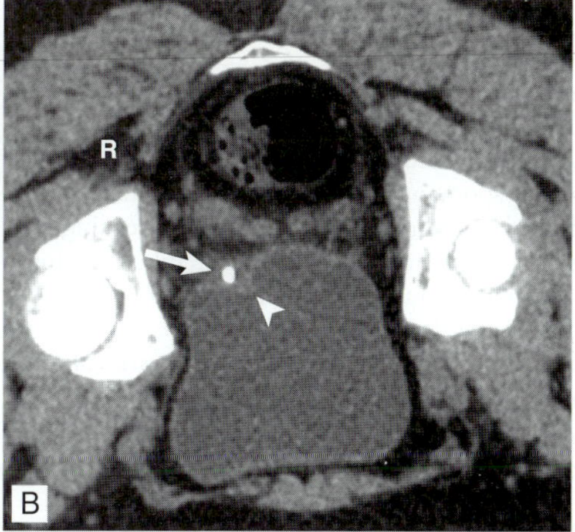

Figure 39.36 Vesicoureteric junction (VUJ) calculus and differentiation from bladder calculus. (A) Noncontrast computed tomography (CT) axial image through the urinary bladder at the level of the VUJ demonstrates impacted calculus (*arrow*) in the intramural portion with significant edema (*arrowhead*). (B) Noncontrast CT axial image through the urinary bladder at the level of the VUJ in the prone position demonstrates that the impacted calculus (*arrow*) in the intramural portion is not mobile. *Arrowhead* represents edema.

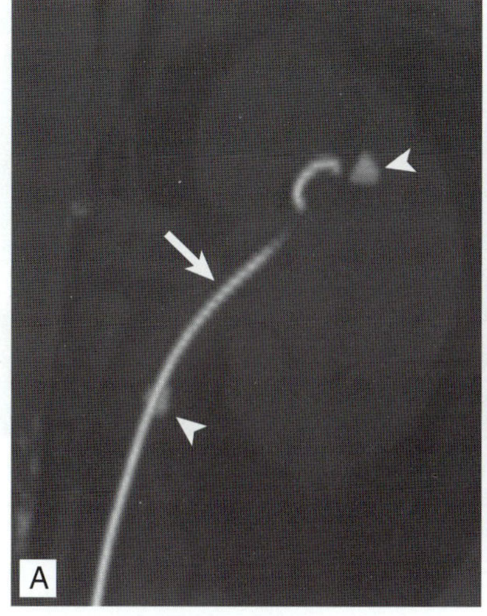

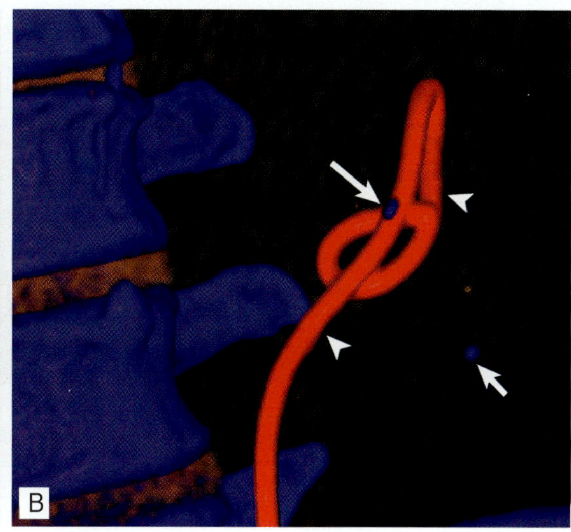

Figure 39.37 Calculus fragments along the double J stents after extracorporeal shockwave lithotripsy (ESWL). (A) Coronal oblique multiplanar reconstruction image in bone window demonstrates calculi fragments (*arrowhead*) along the double J stent (*arrow*), which are formed after ESWL. (B) Three-dimensional volume rendering technique image of the DJ stent in a dual-energy mixed image in a different patient demonstrates stent in red color (*arrowheads*) and oxalate calculus in blue color (*white arrow*). A *small white arrow* lateral to the double J stent is another calcium oxalate calculus.

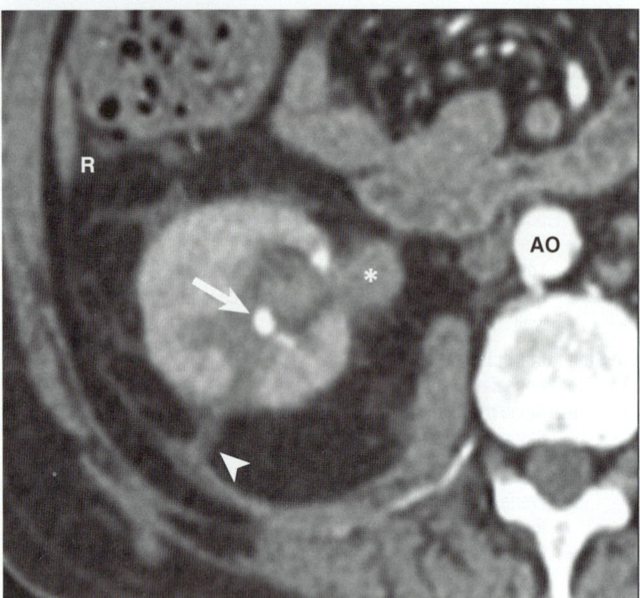

Figure 39.38 Pseudoaneurysm formation after percutaneous nephrolithotomy (PCNL). Contrast-enhanced computed tomography axial image through the right kidney during the angiographic phase demonstrates PCNL tract (*arrowhead*) reaching to the posterior cortex of the kidney. The calyceal system and the renal pelvis are distended because of hemorrhage (*white asterisk*). The *white arrow* is a small pseudoaneurysm. *AO*, aorta.

Special situation: hydronephrosis but no calculus in the kidney or ureter

1. **Recently passed out calculus:** In acute ureteric obstruction, a stone may have a spontaneous passage with residual mild hydronephrosis and hydroureter. This may be misleading to the radiologist because no calculus is seen. Careful evaluation of the ureterovesical junction, bladder, and urethra needs to be done to document any calculus.
2. **Necrosed and obstructing papilla:** Renal papillae are vulnerable to ischemia because of vascular disorders such as diabetes. After necrosis, it may slough and obstruct the ureter or the vesicoureteric junction (VUJ) (Figs. 39.22 and 39.40). In chronic cases, it may sometimes calcify in the periphery giving an appearance like a calculus(see Fig. 39.31C). On CT urography, a necrosed papilla can be seen as deformed calyx or filling defects. Long-standing diabetes, especially in older adult patients, and lack of stone identification in a setting of obstruction should raise suspicion and be communicated. A higher HU value of the fluid in the renal pelvis also indicates stasis and infection, typically seen with papillary obstruction.
3. **Pregnancy hydronephrosis and hydroureter:** Nonobstructive dilation of the ureter in pregnancy is known because of smooth muscle relaxation. It is pronounced (or exclusively) on the right because of compression of the ureter by the gravid uterus. If the patient presents with severe loin pain, the elevation of the resistive index on Doppler USG may help diagnose significant obstruction. In the case of acute flank pain and negative USG findings, if the index of suspicion for stone is high, further evaluation can be done by MRI or low-dose NCCT.
4. **Stones in children:** These present a unique situation for a treating physician and a diagnostic challenge for a radiologist. They may also require sedation and may need proper planning. Stone recurrence is common in children, and

TABLE 39.10 Ultrasound Signs of an Obstructed System Caused by Ureteric Calculus

Ultrasound Direct Signs
Echogenic foci
Acoustic shadowing
Color Doppler sign: twinkling and comet-tail artifact; shows a sensitivity of only 24% in identifying calculi; nearly 75% of calculi not visualized were <3 mm
Indirect Signs on Ultrasound
Hydronephrosis and hydroureter; early calyceal dilation is better depicted on ultrasonography
Weak or absent ureteric jets
Increased resistive index in the obstructed kidney

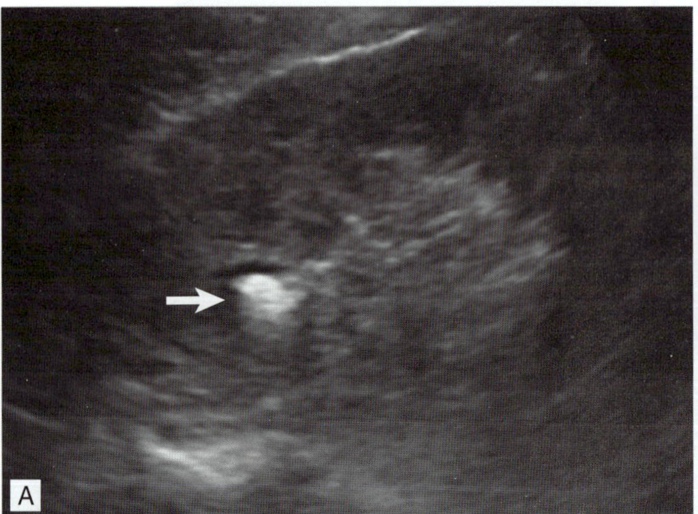

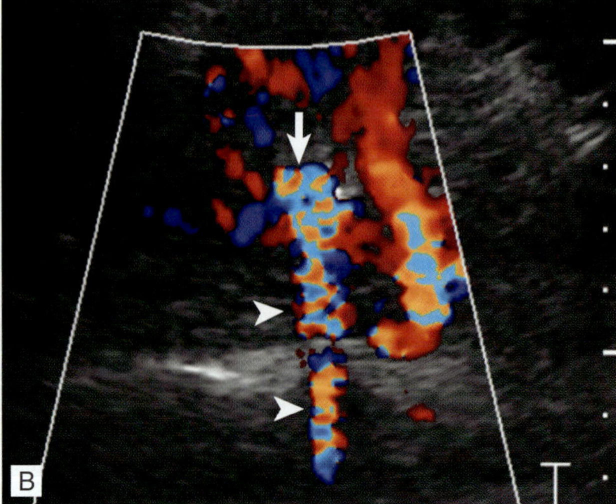

Figure 39.39 Renal calculus ultrasound appearance. (A) Two-dimensional ultrasound image in the longitudinal plane demonstrates an echogenic calculus in the calyceal system (*white arrow*). (B) Corresponding Doppler image demonstrates "twinkling artifact" (*white arrowheads*) arising from the calculus (*white arrow*).

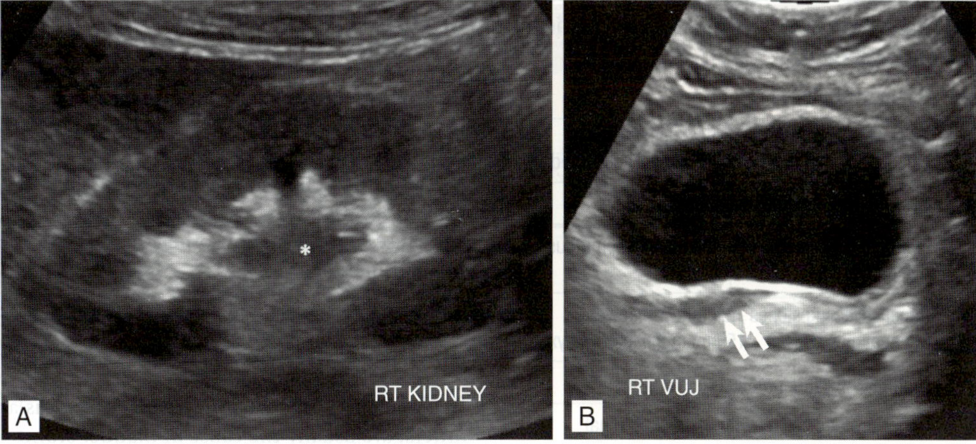

Figure 39.40 Necrosed papilla. (A) Two-dimensional ultrasound image in the longitudinal plane demonstrates a dilated collecting system with tiny echoes (*white star*) suggesting pyonephrosis. (B) Two-dimensional ultrasound image in the oblique plane demonstrates a dilated juxtavesiscal ureter with soft tissue echogenicity (*small white arrows*), which is necrosed papilla on ureteroscopy.

thorough metabolic evaluation and stone characterization is critical. In children with acute flank pain, USG is the investigation of choice at initial presentation. Careful evaluation of the kidney and ureter should be performed. A full bladder evaluation with visualization of ureteric jets should be done. NCCT could be considered if USG findings are negative and the index of suspicion is high. Other investigations are IVU, radiography, and voiding cystourethrography in the case of VUR.

Magnetic Resonance Urography

Magnetic resonance urography can evaluate the renal parenchyma and collecting system without ionizing radiation; however, it is less sensitive for renal tract stone evaluation. Renal calculi have low signal intensity in all sequences and thus can be distinguished from blood clots and cancers, which appear with high signal intensity on T1-weighted images and intermediate signal on T2-weighted imaging; clot and calculi show no postcontrast enhancement, but tumor shows postcontrast variable enhancement. Depending on the level of obstruction hydronephrosis and hydroureter, periureteral and perinephric fat stranding is seen proximal to the obstruction on T2-weighted imaging. Ureteric strictures can be better characterized by MRI.

The disadvantages of MRI for renal tract stone evaluation are low sensitivity for renal calculi detection, relatively long imaging times, sensitivity to motion, and lower spatial resolution compared with CT and radiography.

Stone Management

Treatment options for acute ureteric obstruction

1. **Conservative:** As per the new American Urological Association guidelines [71], uncomplicated stones smaller than 10 mm may be appropriate for conservative management. *However, patients with infectious symptoms, intolerable patient symptoms, or a threat to renal function need intervention.* In a study, it was found that stones smaller than 5 mm in size in the distal ureter have a more than 90% chance of spontaneous passage [72]. Those that are 5–7 mm in size have a modest chance (50%) of passage [73]. The axial diameter of the stone compared with the length is closely correlated with the stone passage rate [74].

TABLE 39.11 Predictors of Poor Extracorporeal Shockwave Lithotripsy Outcome

1. HU > 1000
2. Lower pole renal calculi
3. Nonheterogenous stone
4. Size >1.5 cm
5. Chemical composition: COM and brushite stones
6. Higher stone-to-skin distance (obesity)
7. Stone location: narrow infundibulopelvic angle with a long, narrow infundibulum
8. High stone volume

COM, calcium oxalate monohydrate; *HU,* Hounsfield units.

2. **ESWL:** This is a noninvasive way of treating stone. High energy shocks are delivered through the body to break the stones. There are many factors that determine the success of the procedure, and NCCT plays a crucial role. Attenuation values of urinary calculi on NCCT before ESWL helps to predict treatment outcome [75]. El-Nahas et al. [76] found that MSD greater than 1000 HU has a lower success rate. The success rate in ureteral stone cases is higher than that in renal stone cases. The stone-free rate in lower pole stone cases is lower than other sites [77]. It has been reported that stone volume is a better predictor of ESWL outcome than stone size [78]. Infundibular length of a calyx 25 mm or larger is the negative predictor for SWL outcome [79]. Factors determining poor outcome are outlined in Table 39.11.
3. **Surgical management:** Common surgical techniques are emergent double J stent, ureteroscopic retrieval of the calculus, and percutaneous nephrolithotomy (PCNL). Further details are outside the purview of this textbook.

Various treatment options are summarized in Table 39.12.

Treatment Plan for Surgical Management

It is based on multiple factors. Flowcharts 39.1 and 39.2 have been provided for detailed management based on the location of the stone in the kidney or ureter. *(Although treatment options vary, the flowcharts are basis an institutional practice in the geography where the author practices.)*

TABLE 39.13 Causes of Obstruction in the Renal Tract Other Than Calculus or Tumor

Causes	Etiology
PUJ or ureteric obstruction	Congenital or vascular (Fig. 39.41A)
Retroperitoneal fibrosis	Commonly idiopathic (Fig. 39.41B and 39.41C)
Inflammatory lesions	Appendicitis, diverticular abscess, or Crohn's disease
Pregnancy	Hormone related, more commonly on the right side
VUR	Neurogenic bladder, posterior urethral valve, developmental, prune-belly syndrome, and bladder outlet obstruction
Congenital	Primary megaureters

PUJ, pelviureteric junction; *VUR*, vesicoureteral reflux.

TABLE 39.14 Causes of Bladder Stones

- Outlet obstruction
- Infection
- Long-standing Foley bulb (foreign body)
- Neurogenic bladder

Urethral Calculus

This is a rare cause of obstruction and usually arises from the kidney or bladder. Most are impacted in the prostatic urethra (Fig. 39.43A) and some in the penile urethra (Fig. 39.43B). They need to be differentiated with prostatic calcification or vascular calcification in the anterior urethra. Prostate calcifications are seen in the paramedian region. Occasionally, calculus may get impacted in the penile urethra. Vascular calcifications are usually linear and on careful observation are seen outside the course of the urethra.

Diffuse Multifocal and Renal Parenchymal Abnormalities

Several pathological processes (some of which have already been discussed) produce global or multifocal changes in the imaging appearances of one or both kidneys. These appearances include changes in the size and outline of the kidneys and the presence of multiple calcified areas.

Small Kidneys

When evaluating for small kidneys, the following should be considered:

1. Renal contour: smooth or irregular (scarring)
2. Unilateral or bilateral

Small, Scarred Kidneys

The commonest causes of small and scarred kidneys are recurrent reflux nephropathy, lobar renal infarcts, analgesic nephropathy or renal papillary necrosis, recurrent infections, and stone disease (Figs. 39.44 and 39.45). Although renal infarction and renal papillary necrosis are discussed elsewhere in this section, we will briefly discuss reflux nephropathy here.

Various cause of small scarred kidneys are provided in Flowchart 39.3.

Reflux Nephropathy

Reflux nephropathy is usually unilateral and is caused by VUR of urine, which can be either sterile or infected. VUR happens in children and rarely persists in adulthood. However, long-standing VUR can cause focal or widespread renal parenchymal scarring, developing over a period of time.

Clinical Features

Presentation of reflux nephropathy in adults is usually associated with recurrent UTI (which may be associated with pyelonephritis). If the nephropathy is severe, patients may present with hypertension or renal insufficiency.

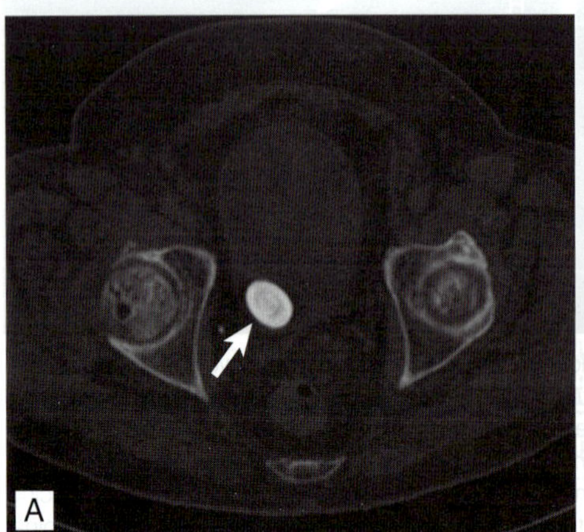

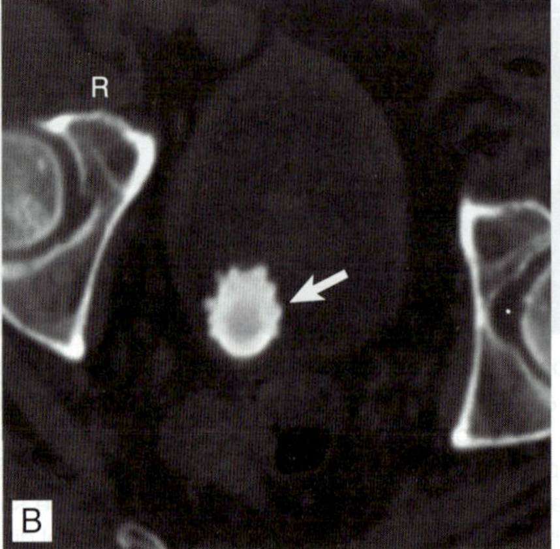

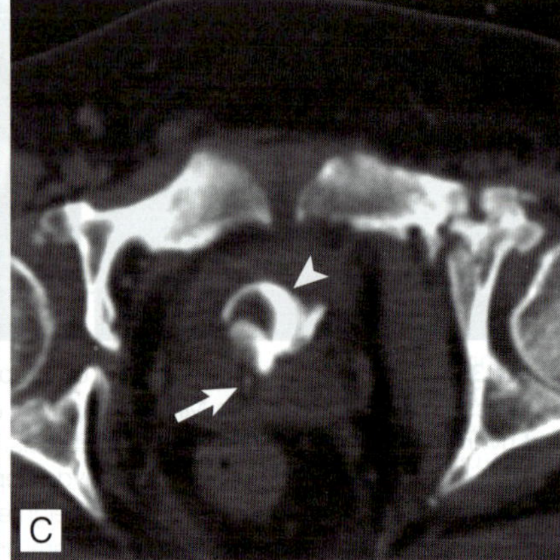

Figure 39.42 Urinary bladder calculus. (A) Noncontrast computed tomography (CT) scan demonstrates hyperdense calculus with laminated appearance (*white arrow*). (B) Noncontrast CT scan demonstrates hyperdense calculus with peripheral spikes (*white arrow*). (C) Noncontrast CT scan in a patient with long-term catheterization demonstrates hyperdense curvilinear calculi (*white arrowhead*) around the Foley bulb (the *white arrow* is the catheter).

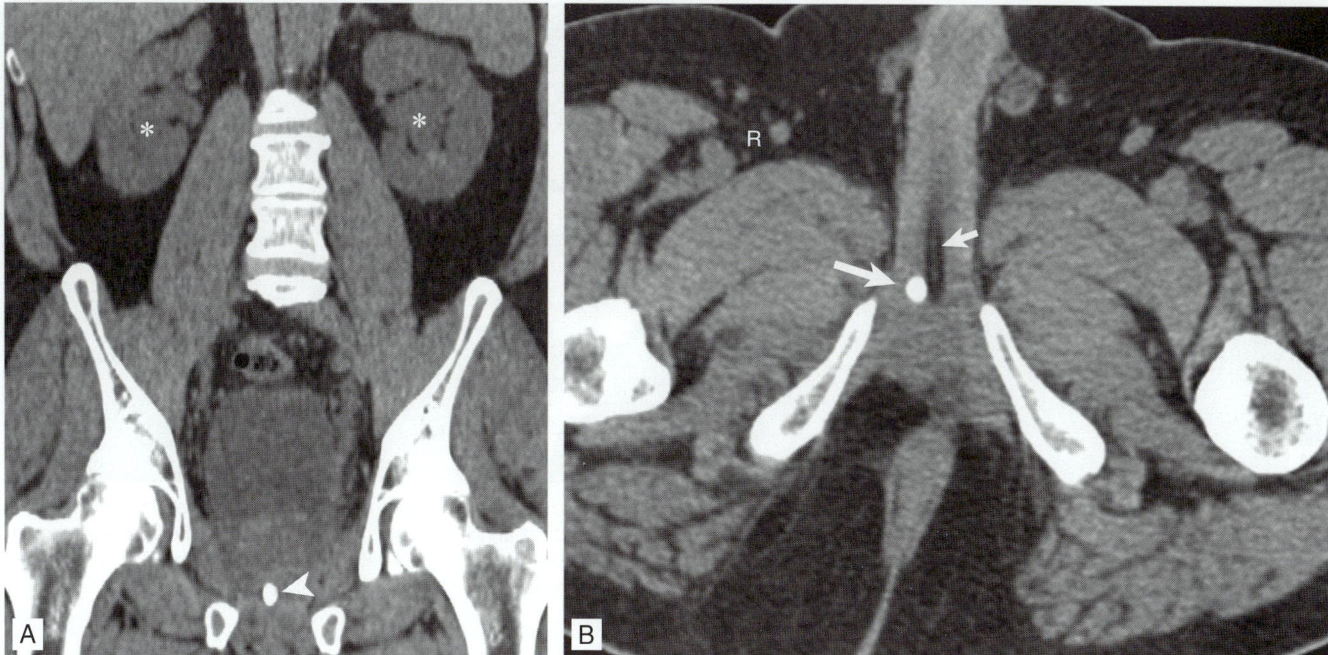

Figure 39.43 Urethral calculus. (A) Noncontrast computed tomography (CT) coronal multiplanar reconstruction demonstrates bilateral hydronephrosis (*white asterisk*). Obstruction secondary to calculus is seen in the prostatic urethra. (B) Noncontrast CT axial image demonstrates calculus in the penile urethra (*white arrow*) beside the catheter (*short white arrow*).

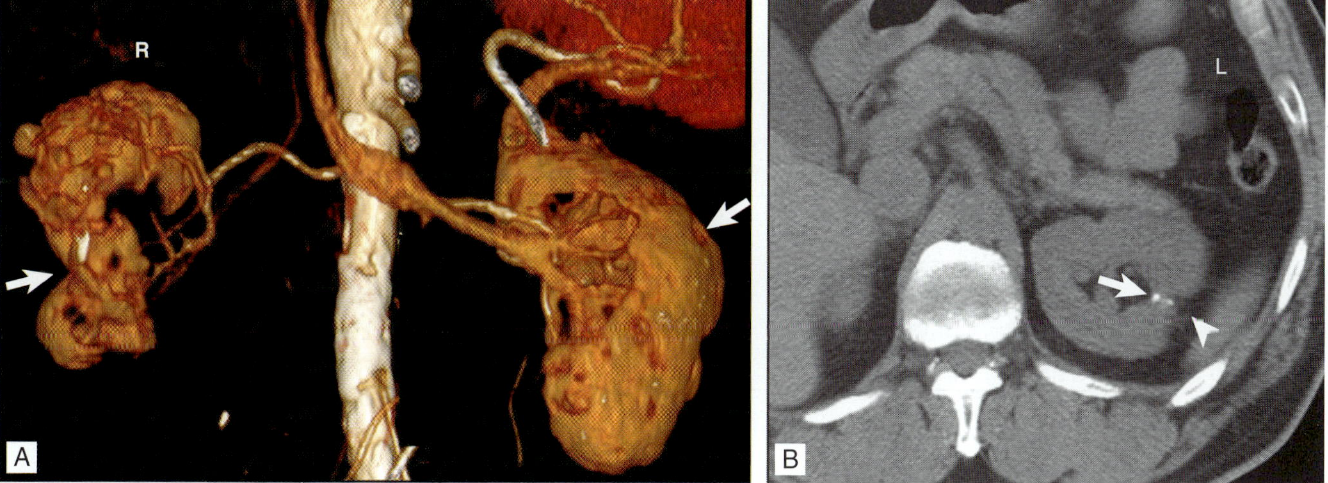

Figure 39.44 Chronic renal scarring. (A) Three-dimensional volume rendering technique reconstruction of the kidneys during the corticomedullary phase demonstrates multiple scars in both kidneys (*white arrow*). The right kidney is small in size. (B) Noncontrast computed tomography in an axial plane through the left kidney demonstrates calcific foci in the lateral cortex with scaring.

Imaging

Focal areas of compensatory parenchymal hypertrophy may occur between the scars and, if prominent, may give rise to concern about the presence of a tumor. On USG or CT, their appearance is of normal parenchyma. USG, CT, and radionuclide imaging (DMSA) all demonstrate the areas of scarring.

As a result of chronic reflux, the renal calyces lose their concave shape and balloon outward to become flat or convex (Fig. 39.46A). Cortical scars are present over these blunted calyces (in contrast to fetal lobulations or vascular scarring where the calyces are normal and cortical indentions are present between these normal calyces and not above them). The parenchymal scarring has a predilection toward renal poles because the ducts of Bellini at the poles are less effective in preventing intrarenal reflux. As the urinary reflux keeps on increasing with time, the entire kidney might get affected with parenchymal scarring leading to small, contracted, and scarred kidneys with blunted calyx and tortuous ureters seen on imaging (Fig. 39.46B).

Although reflux nephropathy does not develop in adult kidneys in the way it does in childhood, a related condition is seen in patients with some LUT surgical procedures that permit long-term significant reflux of potentially infected urine. The ureters and pelvicalyceal systems dilate, and there is a progressive

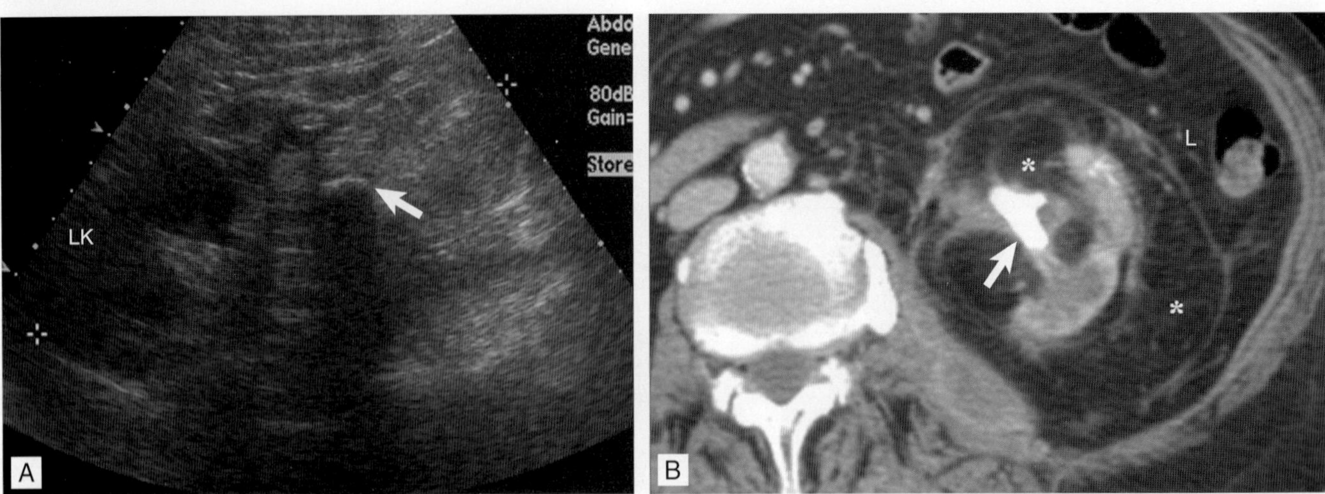

Figure 39.45 Chronic kidney disease caused by chronic renal stone disease. (A) Two-dimensional ultrasound image of the left kidney (LK) demonstrates calculus in the renal pelvis (*white arrow*) with poor corticomedullary differentiation. (B) Contrast-enhanced computed tomography in the axial plane through the left kidney demonstrates staghorn calculus (*white arrow*). The renal parenchyma is atrophic and demonstrates poor enhancement. The *white asterisk* is hypertrophied fat at the renal hilum (anterior to the calculus) and perinephric region secondary to chronic inflammation.

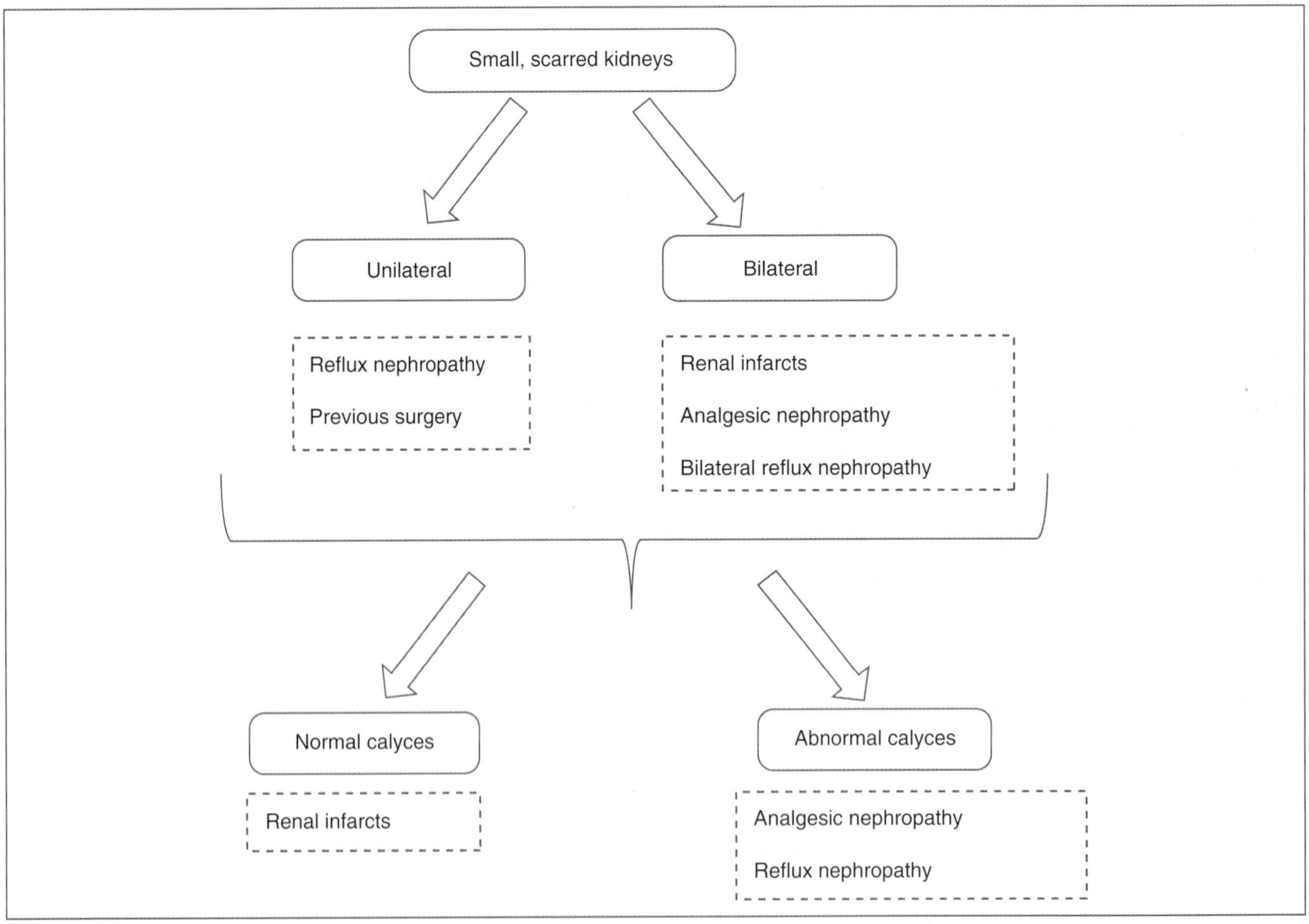

Small, scarred kidneys

- Unilateral
  - Reflux nephropathy
  - Previous surgery
- Bilateral
  - Renal infarcts
  - Analgesic nephropathy
  - Bilateral reflux nephropathy

- Normal calyces
  - Renal infarcts
- Abnormal calyces
  - Analgesic nephropathy
  - Reflux nephropathy

Flowchart 39.3 Small, scarred kidneys.

diffuse loss of renal cortex and function. The condition is usually bilateral, although it may show considerable asymmetry. It is most commonly seen with an ileal conduit but is also encountered in other procedures, especially those involving ureteric reimplantation, for example, ureterosigmoidostomy.

Small, Smooth Kidneys

The commonest cause of unilateral small and smooth kidney is long-standing renal artery stenosis (RAS) (Fig. 39.47). The imaging studies such as IVU, contrast-enhanced CT and MR, and

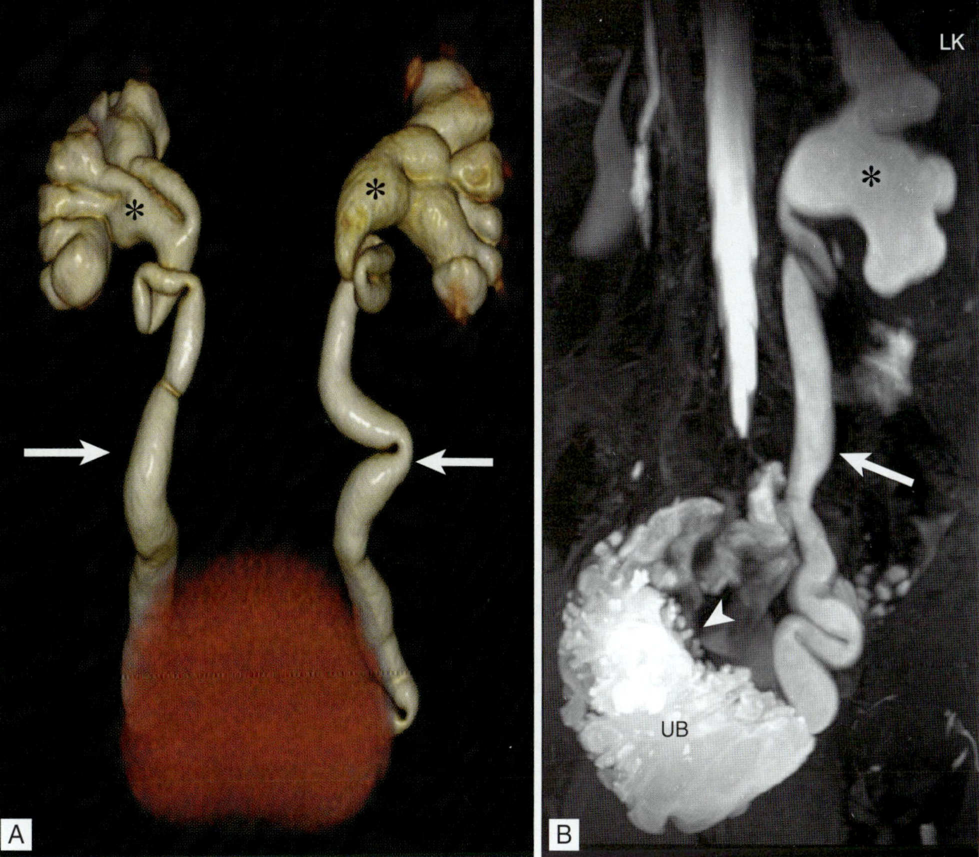

Figure 39.46 Vesicoureteral reflux. (A) Three-dimensional (3D) volume rendering technique contrast-enhanced computed tomography image during the excretory phase demonstrates bilateral dilated and tortuous ureters (*white arrow*) and hydronephrosis caused by reflux. The *black asterisk* is the dilated renal pelvis. (B) 3D volume rendering technique of a high time to echo (TE) T2-weighted magnetic resonance urogram in a patient with paraplegia demonstrates multiple diverticula and trabeculations (*white arrowhead*) in the urinary bladder (UB). There are gross hydronephrosis (*black asterisk*) and a dilated tortuous left ureter (*white arrow*). *LK,* left kidney.

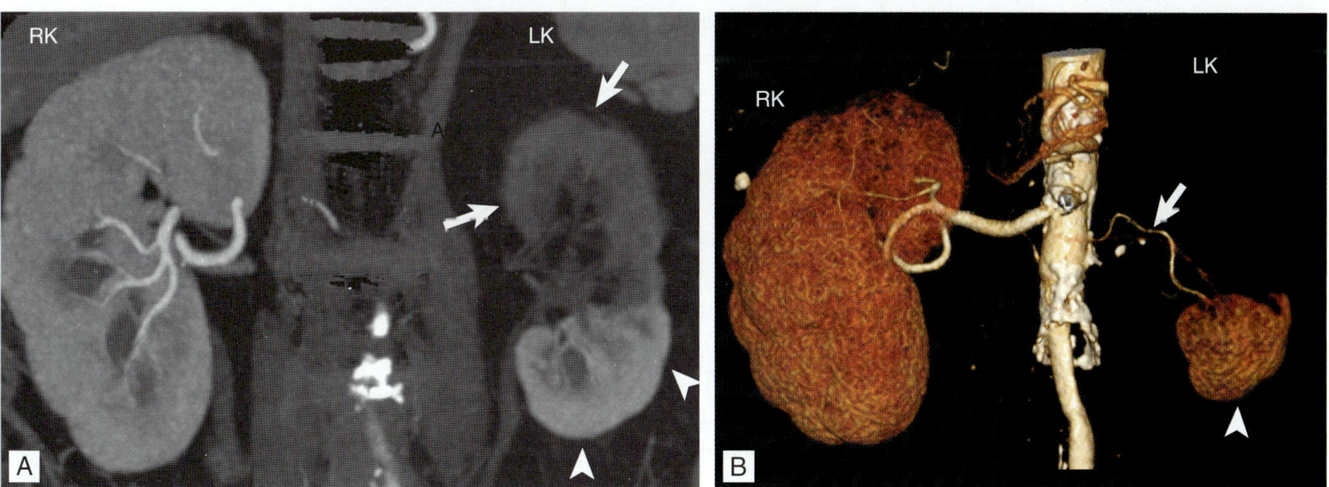

Figure 39.47 Unilateral small kidney caused by renal artery occlusion. (A) Contrast-enhanced computed tomography (CT) thin maximum intensity projection coronal image during the angiographic phase demonstrates a small left kidney (LK) with nonopacification of the upper and interpole regions (*white arrows*). The lower pole shows normal enhancement and is supplied by an accessory artery (*white arrowheads*). (B) Contrast-enhanced CT three-dimensional volume rendering technique in the same patient during the angiographic phase demonstrates enhancement of the lower pole only (*white arrowhead*). *RK,* right kidney.

renal scintigraphy show delayed nephrogram and delayed hyperdense pyelogram. Ureteral notching is also sometimes seen as a result of increased collateral vessels of which few become enlarged and create an impression on the ureter.

A unilaterally small kidney with clubbed calyces is likely to be caused by postobstructive atrophy (Fig. 39.48), although the appearances overlap with reflux nephropathy. (When the cortex is thin and the kidney particularly small, scars may not be evident.) Generally, at least 1 week of high-grade sterile obstruction is required to produce irreversible obstruction. There is associated renal pelvic and ureteric ectasia.

Bilateral small smooth kidneys are most commonly seen as a late stage of numerous pathological processes. The commonest is probably renal arterial insufficiency (hypertensive nephrosclerosis, bilateral renal artery stenoses, small vessel disease), although these may be associated with scarring. Chronic

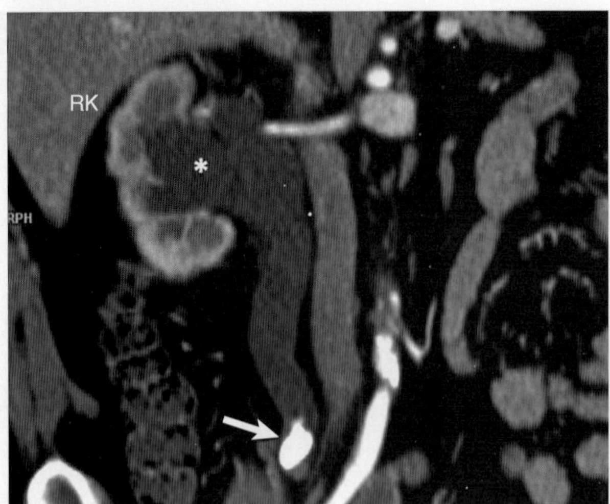

Figure 39.48 Small kidney caused by chronic ureteric obstruction. Post-contrast computed tomography in the coronal plane demonstrates small right kidney (RK) with hydronephrosis (*white asterisk*) caused by ureteric obstruction from an impacted calculus (*white arrow*). Note that there is no perinephric fat stranding suggesting chronic obstruction.

glomerulonephritis and the end stage of other nephropathies (hereditary, analgesic, etc.) also lead to small smooth kidneys. All of these processes lead to loss of the normal renal architectural pattern on USG, with a general increase in echogenicity. The medullary cystic disease is responsible for small kidneys with cysts.

Various cause of small smooth kidneys has been provided in Flowchart 39.4.

Large Kidneys

Unilateral Renal Enlargement

Causes

- Acute obstruction: Commonest cause. The diagnosis is usually obvious clinically and caused by imaging features (Fig. 39.49A)
- Acute pyelonephritis
- Acute vascular disturbances: main arterial or venous occlusion, acute arteritis including recent radiotherapy
- Infiltration with tumor (leukemia, lymphoma, transitional cell carcinoma, renal cell carcinoma, and metastases, especially squamous cell carcinoma) or an inflammatory process (tumefactive xanthogranulomatous pyelonephritis)
- Compensatory hypertrophy of a kidney after loss or longstanding disease of the other kidney (Fig. 39.49B)
- Enlarged kidney with paper-thin renal cortex in chronic PUJ obstruction (Fig. 39.49C)

Various cause of unilateral renal enlargement are provided in Flowchart 39.5.

Bilateral Renal Enlargement

Causes

- Diabetes: The commonest cause of bilateral smoothly enlarged kidneys is diabetes, often before it has become clinically apparent

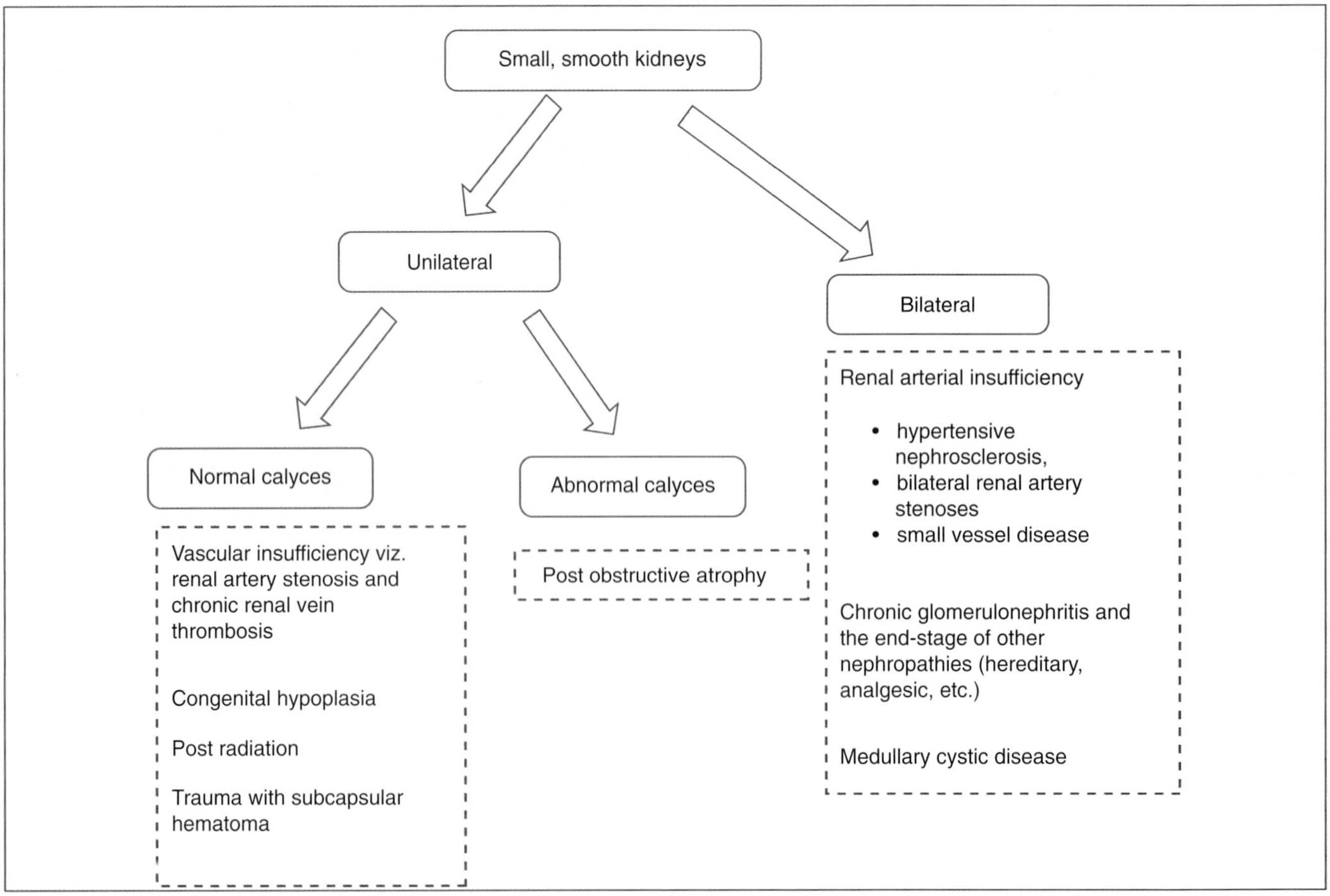

Small, smooth kidneys

Unilateral

Normal calyces

Vascular insufficiency viz. renal artery stenosis and chronic renal vein thrombosis

Congenital hypoplasia

Post radiation

Trauma with subcapsular hematoma

Abnormal calyces

Post obstructive atrophy

Bilateral

Renal arterial insufficiency

- hypertensive nephrosclerosis,
- bilateral renal artery stenoses
- small vessel disease

Chronic glomerulonephritis and the end-stage of other nephropathies (hereditary, analgesic, etc.)

Medullary cystic disease

Flowchart 39.4 Small, smooth kidneys.

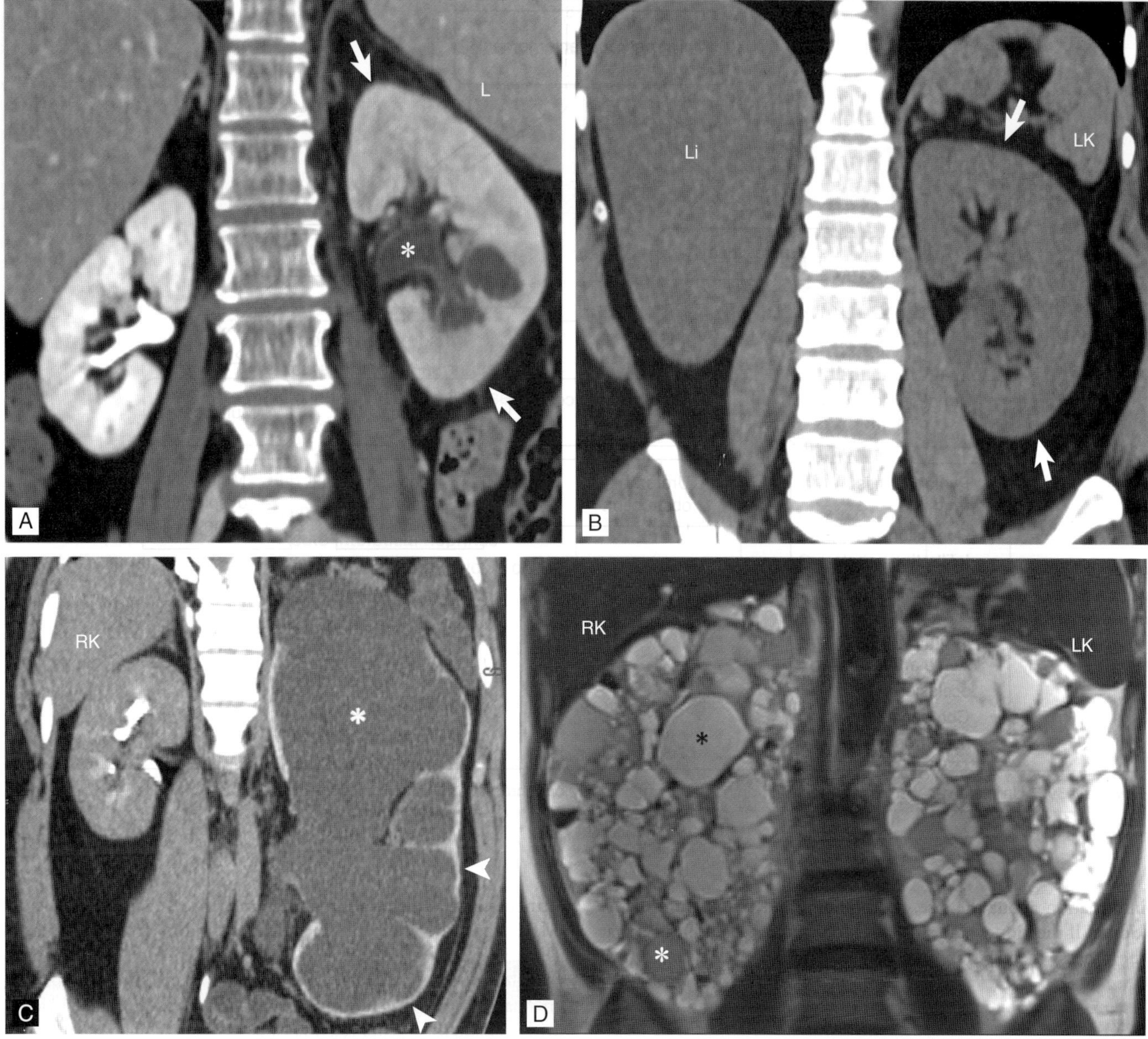

Figure 39.49 Enlarged kidneys. (A) Contrast-enhanced computed tomography (CT) in the coronal plane during the excretory phase demonstrates a smooth enlargement of the left kidney (*white arrows*) with delayed nephrographic and lack of contrast excretion in the collecting system. (B) Noncontrast CT in the coronal plane demonstrates compensatory hypertrophy of the LK (*white arrows*) caused by congenital absence of the right kidney (RK). (C) Postcontrast CT in the coronal plane demonstrates a smooth enlargement of the LK caused by chronic pelviureteric junction stricture. There is gross hydronephrosis (*white asterisk*) with a paper-thin renal cortex (*white arrowheads*). (D) T2-weighted magnetic resonance imaging in the coronal plane demonstrates enlarged bilateral kidneys with multiple cysts in the case of autosomal dominant polycystic kidney disease. These cysts are of varying signal intensities. The *black asterisk* is a simple cyst. The *white asterisk* is a complex cyst. *Li,* liver.

- Acute global renal insults: acute glomerulonephritis, acute nephropathy (e.g., AIDS, urate), interstitial nephritis, and renal involvement in connective tissue diseases (e.g., systemic lupus erythematosus, Wegener granulomatosis)
- Diffuse infiltration with tumors (leukemia, occasionally lymphoma or myeloma) also produces this appearance
- Rare causes include amyloidosis, acromegaly, ADPKD (Fig. 39.49D), and hereditary depositional diseases

Various cause of bilateral renal enlargement are provided in Flowchart 39.6.

Renal Insufficiency and Failure

Renal failure is defined as the inability of the kidney to maintain homeostasis, leading to azotemia or the accumulation of nitrogenous wastes. Even though obstruction is present in fewer than 10% of patients with renal failure, it is the most important condition to diagnose or exclude because it is very treatable. The ACR appropriateness criteria for imaging in renal failures recommend USG as the imaging modality of choice for evaluation of renal failure [1].

In a patient with previously undiagnosed renal failure, the most helpful initial diagnostic test is grayscale USG. It provides

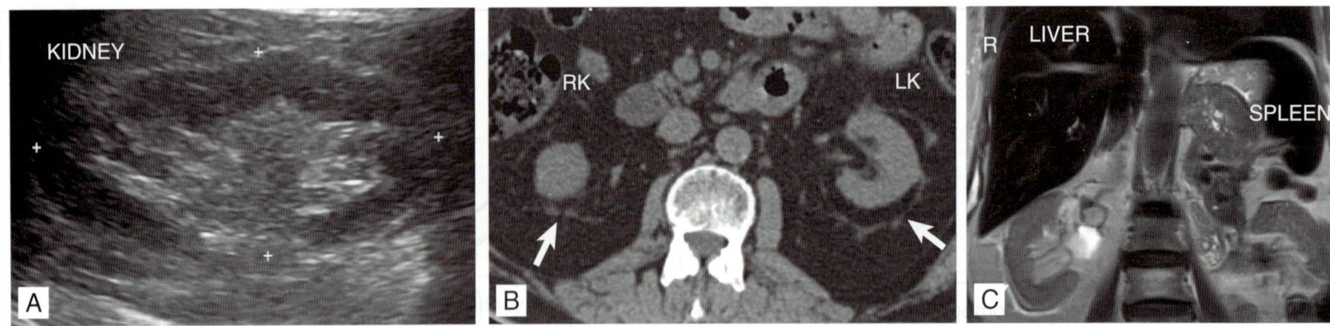

Figure 39.51 Chronic kidney disease. (A) Two-dimensional ultrasound image in the longitudinal plane demonstrates a small kidney with loss of corticomedullary differentiation and increased echogenicity of the renal parenchyma. (B) Noncontrast computed tomography in the axial plane shows thickening of the perirenal septae (*white arrow*) and pathologically represents chronic subclinical inflammation. (C) Magnetic resonance imaging T2-weighted coronal image in a different patient demonstrates a small right kidney with cortical thinning and loss of corticomedullary differentiation. Note that the left kidney is absent.

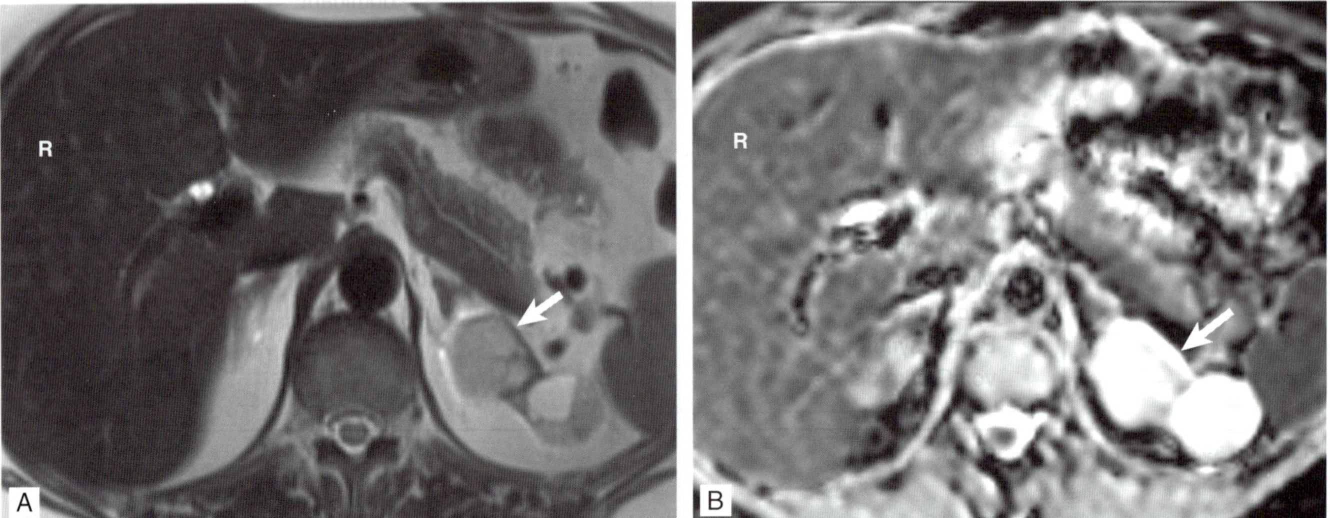

Figure 39.52 Pseudomass appearance on magnetic resonance imaging (MRI) in chronic kidney disease. (A) MRI T2-weighted in the axial plane demonstrates intermediate signal intensity mass (*white arrow*). The renal cortex is atrophic. (B) Apparent diffusion coefficient (ADC) in the axial plane demonstrates the mass (*white arrow*) is hyperintense (high ADC value), suggesting a benign cause, and represents renal tissue between atrophic areas.

The imaging features of cortical nephrocalcinosis are common between different causes and do not help in delineating the cause.

Medullary nephrocalcinosis: Medullary nephrocalcinosis (Fig. 39.53) is relatively common than the cortical variant and is characterized by calcification of the pyramids with sparing of the cortex.

Causes:

- Medullary sponge kidney: Pathologically, the calcification is in the form of tiny calculi within dilated collecting ducts. Radiologically, however, the calcification is seen in the region of the pyramids, and it is convenient and accepted to include it in this category
- Hypercalcemic states such as hyperparathyroidism and renal tubular acidosis: Any cause of hypercalcemia may produce medullary nephrocalcinosis
  - The most important cause is hyperparathyroidism
  - Disseminated malignancy causing hypercalcemia is fairly frequently seen, but it is unusual for it to persist long enough to cause medullary nephrocalcinosis
  - Sarcoidosis is worth bearing in mind as a cause of hypercalcemia
  - For completeness, there are some historical (milk-alkali syndrome, vitamin D overtreatment) and extremely rare (acromegaly, thyrotoxicosis) causes. Because of hypercalciuria, these patients have a higher incidence of urolithiasis
  - A final rare cause of medullary nephrocalcinosis is chronic furosemide use in premature infants with cardiovascular disease

Renal Papillary Necrosis

Renal papillary necrosis is characterized by ischemic necrosis of the papillae. The major causes are analgesic nephropathy (especially phenacetin but also aspirin and other nonsteroidal antiinflammatory agents), sickle cell disease, diabetes mellitus, TB, acute severe pyelonephritis, RVT, cirrhosis, chronic heart failure, and chronic obstruction (especially with infection). It is rarely seen in severely ill infants and neonates with dehydration, acidosis, and respiratory distress.

The presentation is usually insidious, with hematuria (usually microscopic), pyuria, frequency, polydipsia, and symptoms of

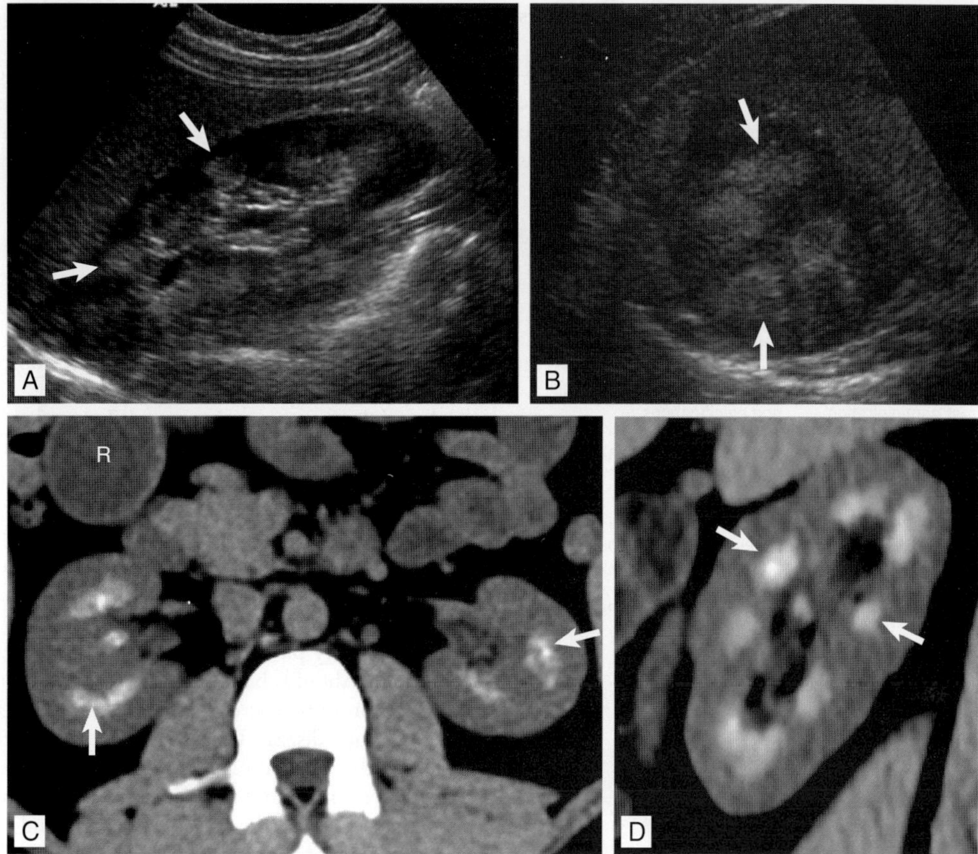

Figure 39.53 Medullary nephrocalcinosis. (A) Two-dimensional ultrasound image in the longitudinal plane demonstrates a hyperechoic rim of the renal medulla (*white arrows*). This is also known as "Anderson-Carr kidney." (B) Two-dimensional ultrasound image in the short axis demonstrates the hyperechoic rim of the renal medulla (*white arrows*). (C) Noncontrast computed tomography (CT) in the axial plane in a different patient demonstrates a cluster of calcifications in the medulla and papillary tips in both kidneys (*white arrows*). (D) Noncontrast CT in the sagittal multiplanar reconstruction demonstrates similar findings as image.

poor ability to concentrate the urine as medullary tissue is lost (frequency and polydipsia). Episodes of acute papillary necrosis are associated with flank pain, hematuria, and acute renal failure.

The classical features are described on IVU. Initially, there are small necrotic areas that are at the tip of the papillae and irregularly excavate from the fornices into the pyramids. As these excavations develop, the papilla becomes virtually surrounded by contrast (the so-called ball-in-cup appearance) and may slough into the pelvicalyceal system, pass into the ureter, and present with colic. The defect left behind appears as flattening or concavity of the pyramidal tip (clubbing of the calyx). The necrotic papillae often calcify (Fig. 39.54). The disease is typically bilateral but asymmetrical, and as it progresses, there is parenchymal loss, and the kidneys become small with smooth outlines and poorly functioning.

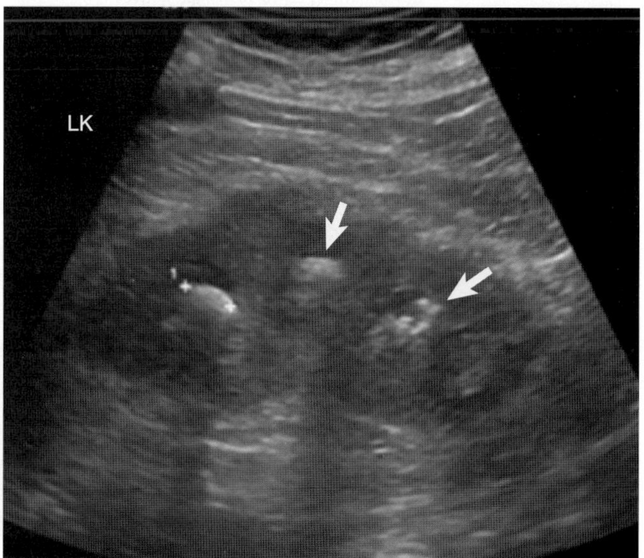

Figure 39.54 Chronic kidney disease with papillary necrosis in a patient with long-standing diabetes. Two-dimensional ultrasound image in the longitudinal plane demonstrates a small kidney with loss of corticomedullary differentiation and increased echogenicity. Multiple calcified papillae are seen at the medullary tips (*white arrows*). *LK*, left kidney.

Pretransplant Evaluation in Renal Donors

The primary aim in pretransplant imaging in kidney donors is to meticulously map the vascular anatomy along with visualizing the renal anatomy and look for associated pathologies. Multidetector computed tomography angiography (CTA) is the modality of choice for preoperative evaluation of living renal donors. CTA is more accurate than magnetic resonance angiography (MRA) and depicts more accessory renal arteries than MRA [83].

Typically, the arterial phase, nephrographic phase, and excretory phase are acquired. Additionally, a delayed arterial phase imaging (corticomedullary phase) can be acquired at a 25- to 30-second delay, which depicts some venous structures such as adrenal and gonadal veins well [84]. The protocol has been provided in detail in Table 39.15.

Postprocessing of the acquired images can help to generate an overview of the vascular anatomy for the surgeons to review. The postprocessing methods are summarized in Table 39.16, which can be applied for CT and MRI. Images from various reconstructions are demonstrated in Figure 39.55.

TABLE 39.15 Computed Tomography Protocol for Assessment of the Donor Renal System

Phase	Timing of Image Acquisition	Utility
Precontrast	Before intravenous contrast administration	For detection of renal calculi and calcifications
Arterial	Through bolus tracking	Assessment of arterial anatomy
Nephrogenic	100 sec postcontrast injection	Renal parenchymal assessment and venous anatomy assessment
Excretory	5–10 minutes postcontrast injection	Assessment of collecting system and urothelial pathologies

TABLE 39.16 Post-processing Methods

Method	Description
Multiplanar reconstruction (MPR)	For measurement of kidneys
Curved MPR	To depict bilateral renal vessels in a single image
Maximum intensity projection (MIP)	MIP excels at displaying vascular maps and small intraparenchymal vessels in enhancing organs, thus helping in the delineation of tiny accessory vessels because of inherent sensitivity to contrast density
3D volume rendering technique	Depicting small extraparenchymal vasculature, grading intraluminal stenosis with calcium, and demonstrating 3D relationships between structures; evaluation of complex venous anatomy because of excellent depth perception [84]

3D, three-dimensional.

Role of Imaging in Donor Selection

The selection of a donor kidney is dictated by the complexity of vascular anatomy with the less complex anatomy given precedence for transplant. If one kidney shows altered morphology compared with the other, the former should be selected.

- **Arterial anatomy variants and their role**

In cases with multiple renal arteries, the vessel with the largest diameter is considered the main renal artery, and the rest are considered accessory [85].

In the case of accessory arteries, interarterial distance is measured. The diameter of the main renal arteries is measured in a real orthogonal plane and should be at least 3 mm.

The various anatomical variants are discussed in Table 39.17.

- **Renal artery pathology**

Patients should be evaluated for renal artery pathologies, namely, fibromuscular dysplasia (FMD) (Fig. 39.56) and severe atherosclerotic disease. Calcified plaques in the renal artery should be reported. Calcified plaques do not allow a vessel to close properly when clamped and may cause laceration of the intima of both the renal artery and the aorta in the aorta and should be reported [86]. Significant atherosclerotic disease in renal arteries might require endarterectomy [87]. Patients with FMD involving both renal arteries are not eligible to become donors; however, unilateral renal artery involvement can be considered in selective cases [88].

- **Venous anatomy variants and their role** (Table 39.18 and Fig. 39.57)

Since venous bleeding is one of the most common complications leading to the conversion of laparoscopic procedure into an open one [84], a detailed evaluation of venous anatomy is necessary. The number, course, and length of renal veins and their tributaries must be detailed in the radiologist's reports.

Careful assessment of the vascular tributaries to the left and right renal veins should be done to help the surgeon to plan the surgery and thus avoid hemorrhagic complications.

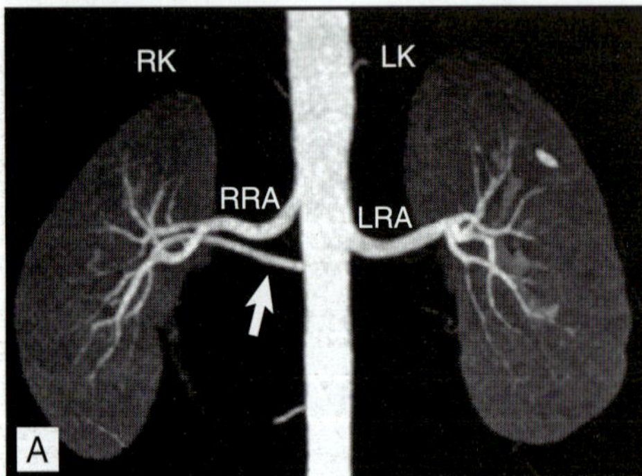

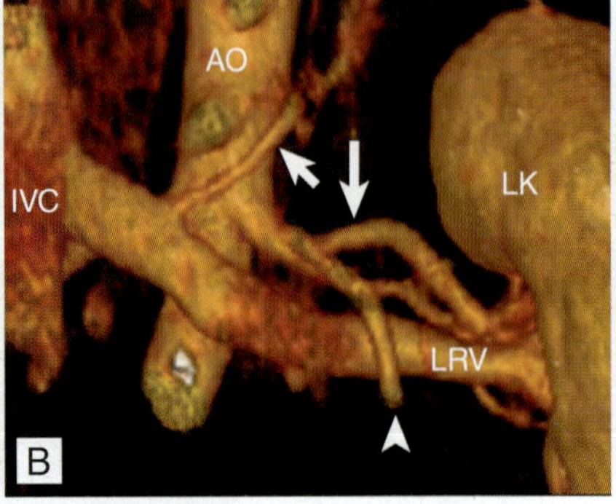

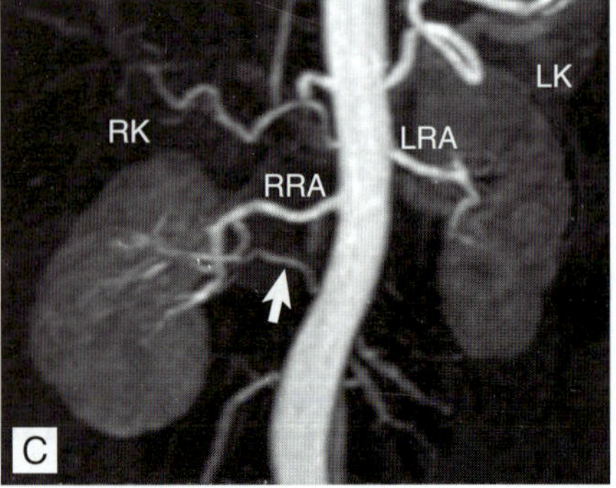

Figure 39.55 Renal artery anatomy. (A) Three-dimensional (3D) maximum intensity projection (MIP) computed tomography angiography image demonstrates a single renal artery on the left side and two renal arteries on the right side. The *white arrow* is an accessory right renal artery (RRA). (B) 3D volume rendering technique image demonstrates the relationship between the left renal artery (LRA) and the left renal vein (LRV). The *white arrow* is the superior branch of the left renal artery that courses superior to the LRV. The *white arrowhead* is a lower pole branch that courses anterior to the left renal vein. A *small white arrow* is an adrenal vein draining into the left renal vein. (C) 3D MIP MR angiography demonstrates a single renal artery on the left side and two renal arteries on the right side. The *white arrow* is an accessory right renal artery. *IVC,* inferior vena cava; *LK,* left kidney; *RK,* right kidney.

TABLE 39.17 Arterial Anatomy Variants and Their Roles

Variants		Description	Implications
Extrarenal arteries	Accessory arteries	They extend to the kidney through the hilum with the main renal artery [85]. Mostly arise from the aorta	The presence of accessory arteries increases the risk of thrombosis and intraoperative time [84]. The presence of more than two arteries within a kidney is a contraindication for donation [86].
	Aberrant arteries	They can be capsular arteries or polar arteries. Capsular arteries are thin vessels that course along with the renal capsule tangentially [86]. Polar arteries enter the kidneys through the superior or inferior pole.	Small upper polar and intracapsular arteries of caliber <2 mm can be sacrificed because the renal infarct produced is very small [87,88]. Lower polar arteries should be preserved because their excision can lead to ureteral complications because they may supply the ureter [89].
Early branching of renal artery		The first branch at <10–15 mm of its origin in the case of the left renal artery [86] Branching behind the IVC or within 1 cm of the right IVC margin in the case of the right renal artery [86].	Expert surgeons require at least 1 cm of the main renal artery to properly anastomose the artery in the recipient. Working posterior to the IVC is difficult because of the possibility of injuring a large vessel.

IVC, inferior vena cava.

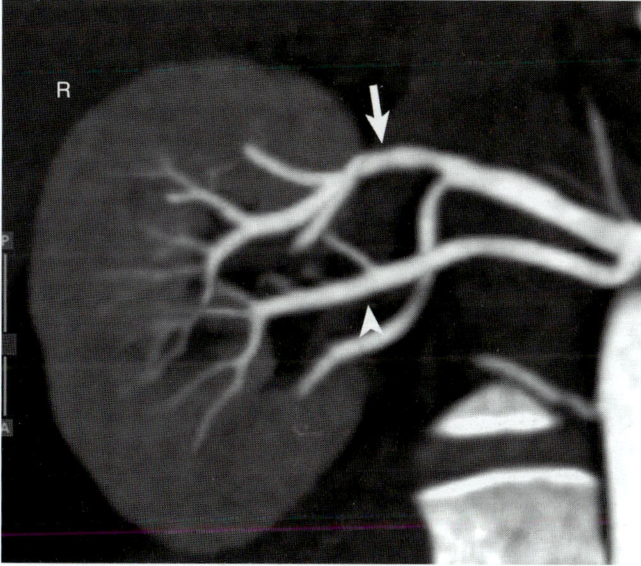

Figure 39.56 Incidental fibromuscular dysplasia of renal artery in a donor. Three-dimensional maximum intensity projection computed tomography angiography demonstrates beading of the upper pole branch of the right renal artery (*white arrow*), which was an incidental finding in a potential renal donor. There is an early branch that supplies the interpolar and the lower pole of the right kidney and demonstrates a normal smooth appearance (*arrowhead*). The kidney demonstrates normal enhancement.

- **Measurements to be made:**
  - Length of the right renal vein
  - Length of the left renal vein
  - The distance between the confluence of the left renal vein with the lumbar vein to the confluence of the left renal vein with the IVC

Nonvascular Assessment

1. **Calyceal and ureteric anatomy** (Fig. 39.58)
2. **Renal calculi**
   - In an asymptomatic patient, a kidney with a single renal calculus measuring less than 4 mm in absence of a history of a stone disease or metabolic disease [86,89]
   - A single renal calculus of size 5 mm and more or the presence of multiple renal calculi renders the kidney unfit for transplant donation
3. **Perirenal fat**

Perirenal fat has to be removed before the kidney is transplanted and is usually stripped while harvesting the kidney. The surgeon should be informed about the amount of perirenal fat because an increased amount leads to increased intraoperative time and makes the surgery difficult by obscuring anatomical landmarks.

4. **Cysts and masses**
   - Simple cysts may be excised, and then the kidney can be transplanted without increased morbidity [90].

TABLE 39.18 Venous Anatomy Variants and Their Importance

Variant	Description	Implications
Multiple renal veins	This the most common variant [91]. These supernumerary double or triple renal veins are more common on the right side.	In case of multiple renal veins inserting into the IVC, the insertions should be evaluated for circumferential and craniocaudal separation. Circumferential separation without craniocaudal separation creates difficulty for the surgeon in IVC repair.
Circumaortic and retroaortic renal veins	These are common on the left side [86]. Whereas circumaortic vein embraces the dorsal and ventral aorta and is more common, the lesser common retroaortic veins are present posterior to the aorta.	In the case of a circumaortic vein, if there is a significant discrepancy between the calibers of anterior and posterior veins or if one of the veins is significantly small, then the surgeon may completely ligate the smaller vein.

IVC, inferior vena cava.

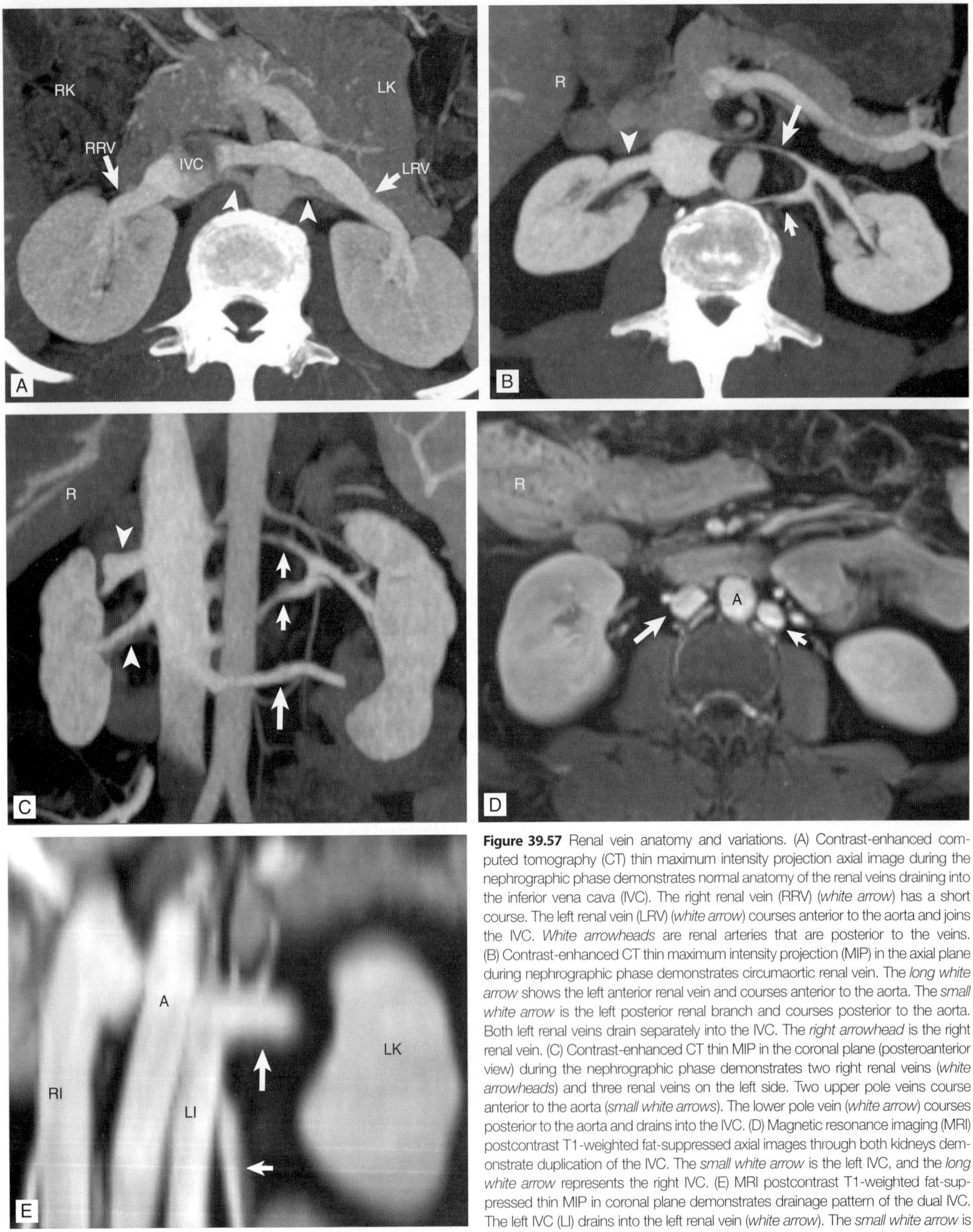

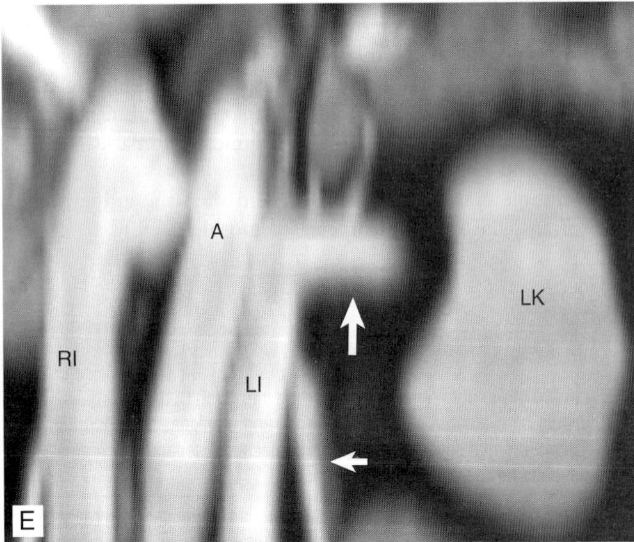

Figure 39.57 Renal vein anatomy and variations. (A) Contrast-enhanced computed tomography (CT) thin maximum intensity projection axial image during the nephrographic phase demonstrates normal anatomy of the renal veins draining into the inferior vena cava (IVC). The right renal vein (RRV) (*white arrow*) has a short course. The left renal vein (LRV) (*white arrow*) courses anterior to the aorta and joins the IVC. *White arrowheads* are renal arteries that are posterior to the veins. (B) Contrast-enhanced CT thin maximum intensity projection (MIP) in the axial plane during nephrographic phase demonstrates circumaortic renal vein. The *long white arrow* shows the left anterior renal vein and courses anterior to the aorta. The *small white arrow* is the left posterior renal branch and courses posterior to the aorta. Both left renal veins drain separately into the IVC. The *right arrowhead* is the right renal vein. (C) Contrast-enhanced CT thin MIP in the coronal plane (posteroanterior view) during the nephrographic phase demonstrates two right renal veins (*white arrowheads*) and three renal veins on the left side. Two upper pole veins course anterior to the aorta (*small white arrows*). The lower pole vein (*white arrow*) courses posterior to the aorta and drains into the IVC. (D) Magnetic resonance imaging (MRI) postcontrast T1-weighted fat-suppressed axial images through both kidneys demonstrate duplication of the IVC. The *small white arrow* is the left IVC, and the *long white arrow* represents the right IVC. (E) MRI postcontrast T1-weighted fat-suppressed thin MIP in coronal plane demonstrates drainage pattern of the dual IVC. The left IVC (LI) drains into the left renal vein (*white arrow*). The *small white arrow* is a gonadal vein draining into the left IVC (LI). The suprarenal IVC is formed by the confluence of the LRV (*white arrow*) and the right IVC (RI). *A,* aorta; *LK,* left kidney; *RI,* right inferior vena cava.

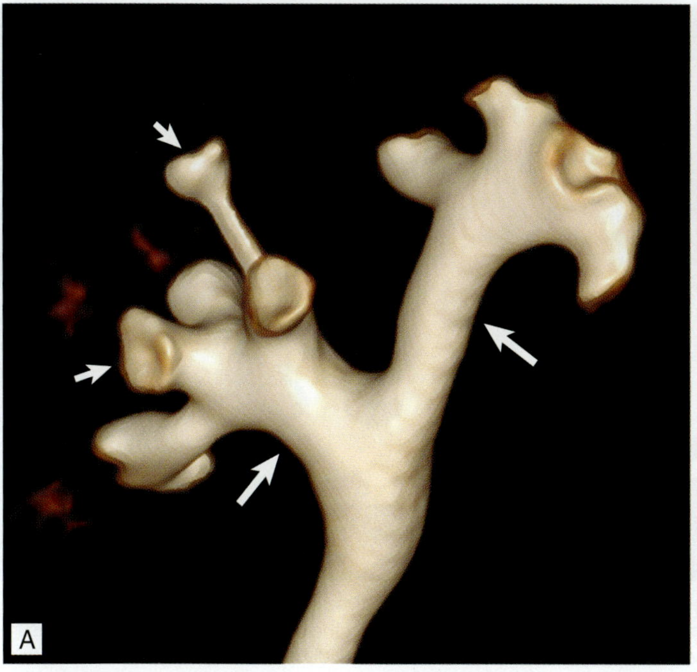

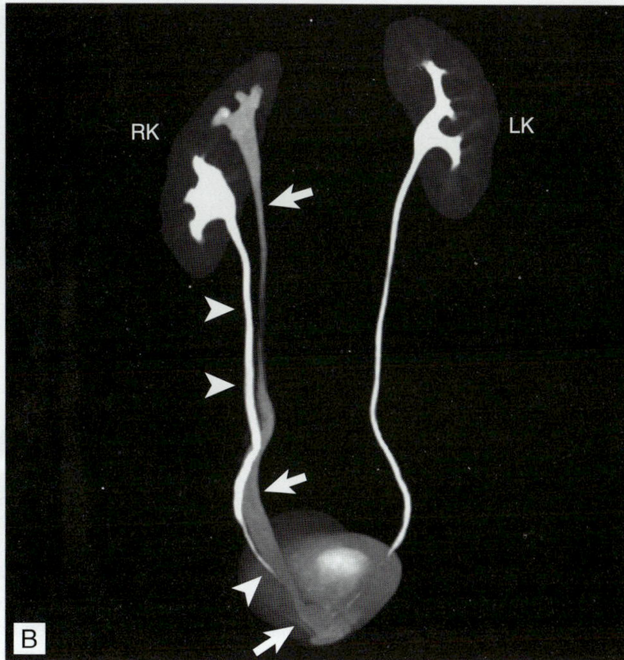

Figure 39.58 Computed tomography (CT) urography. (A) CT three-dimensional (3D) volume rendering technique demonstrates calyceal anatomy during the excretory phase. The *white arrows* represent infundibulum. The *small white arrows* represent calyceal fornices. (B) Contrast-enhanced CT 3D maximum intensity projection during the excretory phase demonstrates a dual collecting system in the right kidney (RK). The *white arrows* represent upper pole moiety which has lower density caused by delayed excretion and has an ectopic insertion in the bladder. The lower pole moiety is mildly dilated and has a higher density. The ureter (*white arrowheads*) of lower moiety has a normal insertion at the vesicoureteric junction. *LK,* left kidney.

TABLE 39.19 Computed Tomography Report for Renal Donor: What Must Be Reported

1. Renal morphology: location, length, and axis of kidneys
2. Amount of perirenal fat
3. Number, location, and size of cysts, calculi, and angiomyolipoma (if present)
4. Presence of any upper or lower urinary tract infection
5. Status of the renal pelvis and ureter
6. Several renal arteries and veins
7. Type of accessory renal arteries
8. Intervessel distance and separation of accessory arteries and veins
9. Vascular measurements (Fig. 39.59)
   a. Arterial measurements
      - The real orthogonal diameter of arteries
      - Location and measurement of first arterial segmentary bifurcation
      - The distance between the right arterial origin and the first segmentary bifurcation
      - The distance between the right IVC margin and the first segmentary bifurcation
      - The distance between the left arterial origin and the first segmentary bifurcation
   b. Venous measurements
      - Location and measurement of the segmentary confluence of renal veins
      - Renal vein tributaries: number, types, and caliber
      - Distance between lumbar vein confluence with left renal vein and the confluence of a left renal vein with IVC

IVC, inferior vena cava.

- Angiomyolipomas smaller than 5 mm need not be excised, and the kidney can be transplanted. Larger angiomyolipomas greater than 5 mm or fat poor angiomyolipomas masquerading as renal cell carcinoma may be locally excised [91].

What must be reported in the CT report for the renal donor is given in Table 39.19.

Postrenal Transplant Imaging

Introduction

Renal transplant is the treatment of choice for patients with chronic renal failure on dialysis. The graft is selected after matching the human lymphocyte antigen with the recipient.

The source of the graft can be can be

- Deceased-donor related transplantation, which is obtained from a cadaver with a life expectancy of around 7–10 years
- Living donor-related transplantation, which is obtained from a family member or as per guidelines in the individual country and has a life expectancy of 10–15 years

Clinical monitoring and periodic imaging are pivotal in the successful outcome of the renal transplant graft.

Surgical Procedure

Radiologists should be well versed with the surgical procedure of the transplant, including vascular and ureterovesical anastomosis.

The left renal vein is longer, and hence the left kidney is preferred for transplantation. In pediatric donors, both kidneys

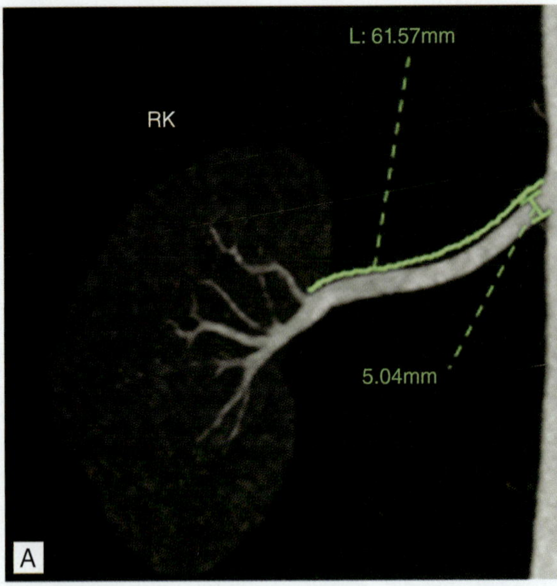

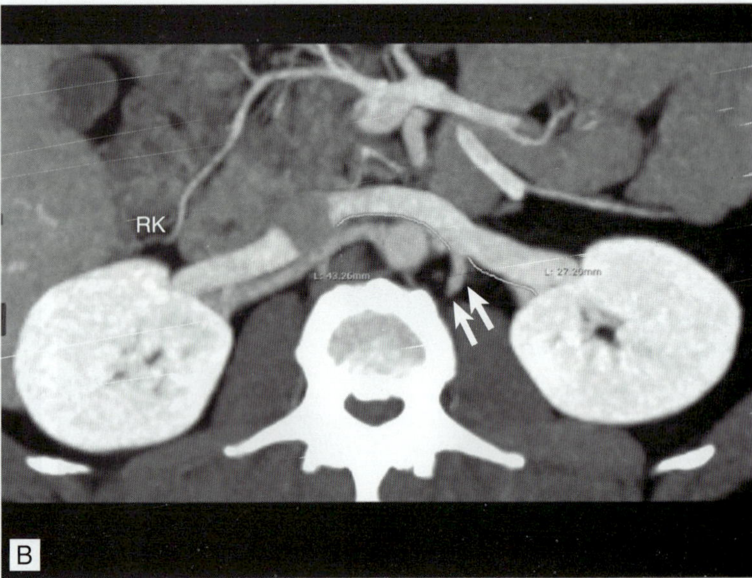

Figure 39.59 Vascular measurements. (A) Contrast-enhanced computed tomography (CT) three-dimensional maximum intensity projection of the right renal artery during the angiographic phase. The short-axis measurement made at the origin of the renal artery is the diameter. The longitudinal measurement is the distance of the first renal artery branch from the origin of the renal artery. (B) Contrast-enhanced CT during the nephrographic phase demonstrates the confluence of the lumbar vein with the left renal vein (*white arrows*). Measurement is made from lumbar vein confluence to the renal hilum and the confluence of the left renal vein to the inferior vena cava. *RK*, right kidney.

may be used (en bloc renal transplant). A renal transplant is a heterotopic transplant because the kidney is placed in a different location than the existing kidneys. The right iliac fossa is the preferred site for transplant because the right iliac vein is more superficial and horizontal and is easier for surgical anastomosis [92].

The arterial anastomosis depends on the deceased or living-related donor allograft, number, size, and presence of accessory renal arteries.

- In deceased-related allograft, end-to-side anastomosis of the donor artery along with a portion of the aorta (Carrel patch) to the external iliac artery is performed
- In living-donor transplants, the donor renal artery is anastomosed to the internal iliac artery (end to end) or the external iliac artery (end to side) of the recipient
- In the presence of more than one renal artery, the arteries are anastomosed as a Carrel patch, or individual arteries are separately anastomosed to the external iliac artery [92]

The donor renal vein is usually anastomosed end to side to the external iliac vein. In the case of multiple renal veins, smaller renal veins are ligated because multiple renal veins are associated with internal collateral vessels [92].

Various techniques are used for urinary tract reconstruction. Uretero-neocystostomy is the most popular technique. Uretero-ureterostomy or uretero-pyelostomy is usually reserved for the management of further complications.

Imaging Technique

Ultrasonography

Ultrasonography is the first investigation of choice, routinely performed within 24 hours of the transplant and during follow up. The superficial location of the transplanted kidney in the pelvis provides a good acoustic window for USG.

Grayscale USG (Fig. 39.60A)

- Size, shape
- The echogenicity of the renal parenchyma:
    - Loss of corticomedullary differentiation: increased or reduced renal parenchymal echoes and increased cortical echogenicity indicative of graft dysfunction
    - Reduction in renal sinus echogenicity
- Collecting system:
    - Obstructive dilation of collecting system, grading of hydronephrosis, cortical thinning
    - Ureteric stricture or thickening
    - Ureterovesical junction and bladder
- Calculi, clot, and renal masses are first detected on the grayscale USG
- Perigraft collection
- Ureteric stents and drainage tubes: for the location, kink, migration, and patency

Color Doppler and Spectra Analysis

- Assessment for patency, flow direction, vascular stenosis, thrombosis, and vascular anomalies for the abdominal aorta, aortoiliac axis, external iliac artery, and transplanted vessels)
- Assessment of the spectral waveform in the segmental and interlobar arteries: fast systolic upstroke with a subsequent slow decay in diastole with the forward flow until the next cardiac cycle
- Various Doppler indices to assess flow quantification, which includes resistivity index, pulsatility index, and systolic-to-diastolic ratio (Fig. 39.60B and C)
- Color Doppler and spectral analysis (Table 39.20)

Ultrasonography-Guided Drainage Procedures and Biopsy are routinely performed which can avoid complex surgeries with a low rate of complications.

Contrast-Enhanced USG

- Ultrasound contrast is not nephrotoxic
- For evaluation of renal graft perfusion and infarcts:
    - Chronic allograft nephropathy shows lower blood flow values
    - Confirm RAS and estimate the degree of stenosis
    - Vascularity of allograft masses
    - Confirmation of the presence of renal abscesses (Fig. 39.61)

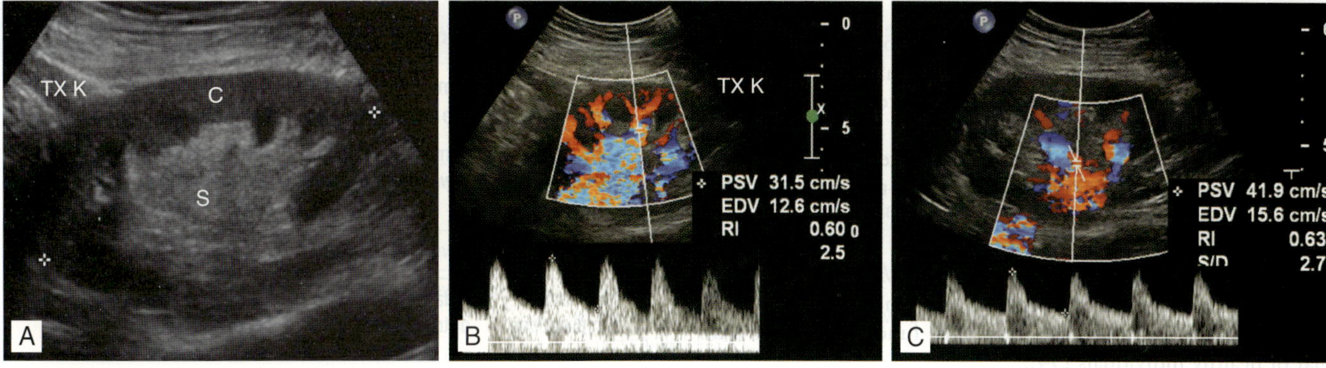

Figure 39.60 Normal transplant kidney. (A) Two-dimensional ultrasound image of a transplant kidney (TXK) in the longitudinal plane demonstrates normal anatomy. The medulla is seen as hypoechoic regions. (B) Color Doppler image of the transplanted kidney demonstrates normal segmental and interlobular arterial flow. Spectral Doppler from intrarenal artery demonstrates a normal wave with a sharp systolic upstroke, normal acceleration time, and good forward diastolic flow is seen. The resistive index (RI) is within the normal range. (C) Spectral Doppler from the renal artery demonstrates normal waveform with a sharp systolic upstroke, normal acceleration time (AT), and good forward diastolic flow. The RI is within the normal range. *C,* cortex; *S,* sinus fat.

TABLE 39.20 Color Doppler and Spectral Analysis in Transplanted Kidneys

	Where to Measure	Application	Values
Resistivity index	Renal segmental or interlobar artery measured by duplex Doppler USG	Differentiate a normal from abnormal allograft function	>0.80 associated with allograft dysfunction
Peak systolic velocity	In the renal artery	RAS	>200–300 cm/sec highly suggestive of RAS

RAS, renal artery stenosis; *USG,* ultrasonography.

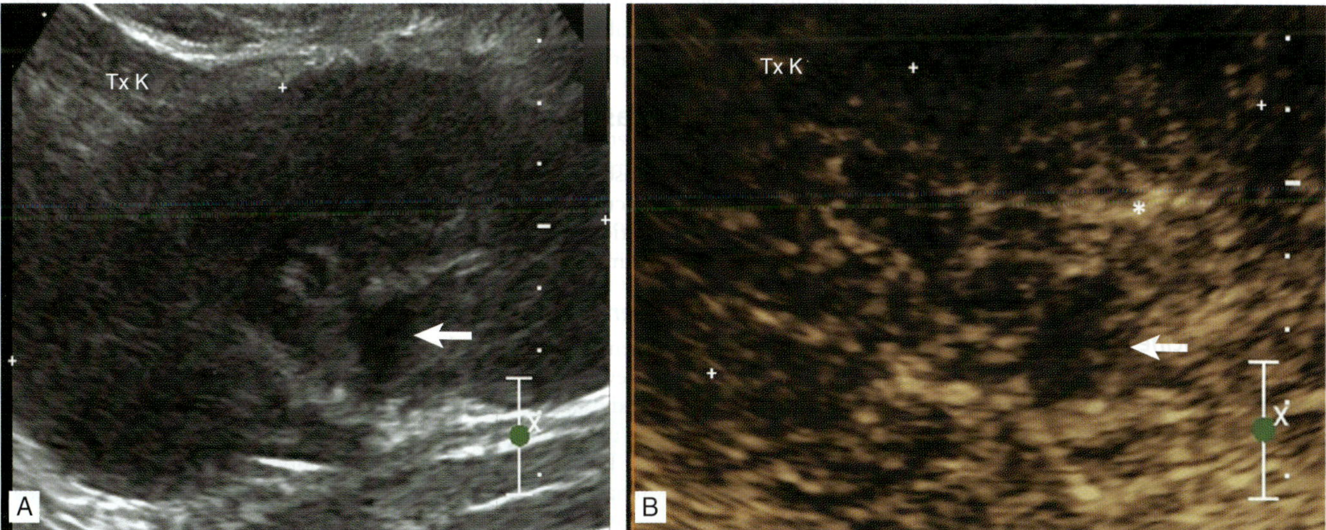

Figure 39.61 Renal abscess in a transplant kidney (TxK). (A) Two-dimensional B-mode ultrasound image demonstrates a hypoechoic area within the kidney in the parapelvic region (*white arrow*). (B) Contrast-enhanced ultrasound image demonstrates peripheral enhancement of the abscess (*white arrow*), renal enhancement (*asterisk*). (Courtesy: Dr. Rajas Chaubal, radiologist and director, Thane Ultrasound Centre, Thane, Mumbai, Maharashtra, India.)

- Not yet approved by the US Food and Drug Administration

US-Based Elastography:

- This is a recently introduced, promising technique
- Renal parenchymal stiffness is measured by the transient elastography technique correlates with histologic interstitial fibrosis associated with the diseased transplant kidney [93]

Computed Tomography and Computed Tomography Angiography

This is often performed when USG fails to demonstrate the pathology or before surgical or endovascular intervention.

Noncontrast CT: acute hemorrhage, nephrolithiasis

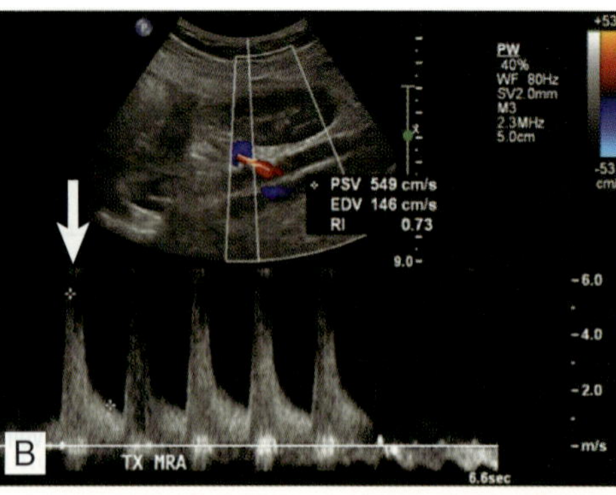

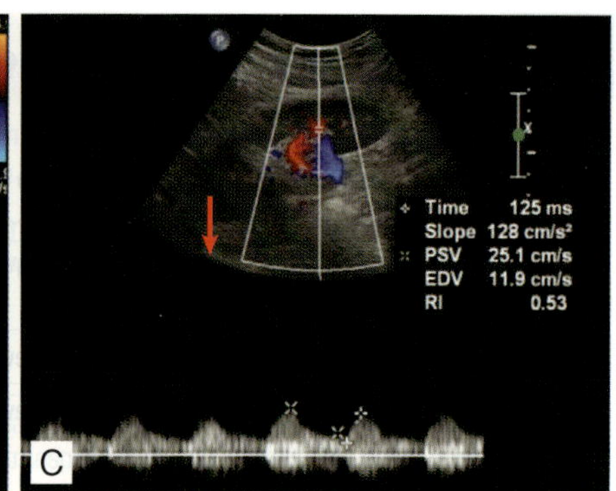

Figure 39.63 Renal artery stenosis of a transplant kidney. (A) Color Doppler ultrasound image demonstrates mosaic flow (*white arrow*) in the transplant renal artery at the anastomotic site. (B) Spectral imaging of the renal artery at the origin demonstrates a high systolic peak with aliasing (*white arrow*). (C) Spectral imaging of the intrarenal artery demonstrates tardus parvus waveform (*cursors*), with an increase in the acceleration time. *EDV*, end diastolic velocity; *PSV*, peak systolic velocity; *RI*, resistivity Index. (Courtesy: Dr. Rajas Chaubal, radiologist and director, Thane Ultrasound Centre, Thane, Mumbai, Maharashtra, India.)

Predisposing factors for RAS

- Donor or recipient related: atherosclerotic disease, infection, immunologic causes, older recipient or donor
- Recipient factors:
  - Rejection, delayed graft function (DGF), and ischemic heart disease
  - Extrinsic compression: polycystic kidney or an extrarenal PSA
- Surgical trauma

Renal artery stenosis may be focal or diffuse and may be seen at one location or multiple locations. Depending on the site, RAS is classified as preanastomotic (i.e., before the anastomosis associated with recipient atherosclerotic disease), anastomotic, or post-anastomotic seen in the main renal artery or segmental branches.

Ultrasonography:

- Aliasing at the stenotic site on color Doppler (Fig. 39.63A)
- Elevated peak systolic velocity: PSV greater than 200 to 300 cm/sec [105] (Fig. 39.63B)
- Tardus parvus waveform (small peak amplitude with delayed upstroke) at the stenosis with an elevated accelerated time of 0.1 sec [106] (Fig. 39.63C)
- Renal artery–to–external iliac artery ratio with a cutoff value of 1.8 and elevated PSV of more than 250 cm/sec in a transplant renal artery suggest significant RAS [107]

Computed tomography angiography or MRA is confirmatory and performed before endovascular intervention.

Renal Arteriovenous Fistula and Pseudoaneurysm

Laceration of the vessel wall with the communication of adjacent arterial and venous structures may lead to arteriovenous communication [108], and injury to all three layers of the arterial wall may result in contained blood leakage and pseudo-aneurysm (PSA) formation. In a series of 2824 renal transplant biopsies, arteriovenous fistulas (AVFs) were seen in 8.3% of cases [109].

Arteriovenous fistulas have a focal mosaic appearance on color Doppler because of tissue reverberation. The feeding artery demonstrates a high-velocity, low-resistance waveform, and the draining vein waveform shows a pulsatile or "arterialized" spectral wave pattern.

On grayscale USG, the PSAs appear as a simple or minimally complex cyst [110]. A "to-and-fro" flow pattern (also known as the "yin-yang sign") is seen in the aneurysm sac; a similar flow may be seen in the neck of the aneurysm.

Computed tomography angiography depicts the anatomic details such as a feeding vessel, draining vein, and size and extension of AVF and PSA. CTA is often performed before planning percutaneous endovascular therapy.

Large or symptomatic AVFs with persistent gross hematuria, significant hypertension, and high cardiac output failure, seen in 1–2% of cases, are at risk for graft dysfunction. These are treated with catheter embolization [111]. Larger (>2 cm) or progressively increasing PSAs warrant endovascular treatment [112]. PSAs are treated with endovascular technique; anatomically suitable PSAs can be treated with ultrasound-guided percutaneous thrombin injection.

Renal Parenchymal Complications

The role of imaging in the detection of renal parenchymal complications is limited and mainly used to exclude vascular and collecting system anomalies. Image-guided allograft biopsy is the gold standard.

Renal parenchymal complications include both acute and delayed.

- Allograft rejection (hyperacute, acute, or chronic)
- ATN
- DGF
- Infections
- Calculi
- Nephrotoxic drugs

Allograft Rejection

Types of rejections are described in Table 39.23.

Role of imaging:

- Grayscale USG shows an edematous, thickened cortex in the initial phase (Fig. 39.64A). Subsequently, the cortex becomes thinned out. There is a loss of corticomedullary differentiation, and medullary pyramids appear hypoechoic [113]
- Color Doppler USG and spectral analysis show diminished diastolic blood flow and resultant elevated resistive indices (Fig. 39.64B). An elevated resistive index between 0.75 and 0.80 has good sensitivity and specificity for the detection of acute rejection. However an elevated resistive index may be seen in other conditions such as ATN, nephrotoxicity secondary to toxic levels of tacrolimus or cyclosporine, obstruction, and extrinsic compression [107]

TABLE 39.23 Types of Allograft Rejection

Rejection	Features	Pathogenesis	Treatment
Hyperacute rejection	Irreversible and rapidly evolving complication secondary to nonperfusion of the graft followed by ischemia seen just after vascular anastomosis (few minutes to 48 hr post-transplant) rare because of efficient immunosuppressant therapy	The response of recipient cytotoxic antibodies to the graft tissue antigen	The nonviable graft is explanted
Acute rejection	The antibody-mediated reaction often seen among patients who are sensitized or received a prior blood transfusion or have organ transplantation within 1 week to 3 months post-transplant	Caused by T-cell activation	Efficient immunosuppressant therapy is available
Chronic rejection	Gradual progressive allograft dysfunction observed months to years after transplantation		

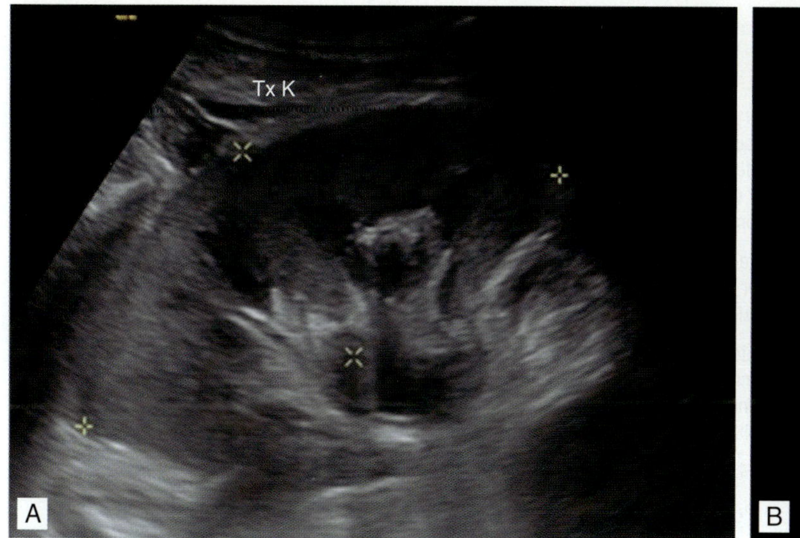

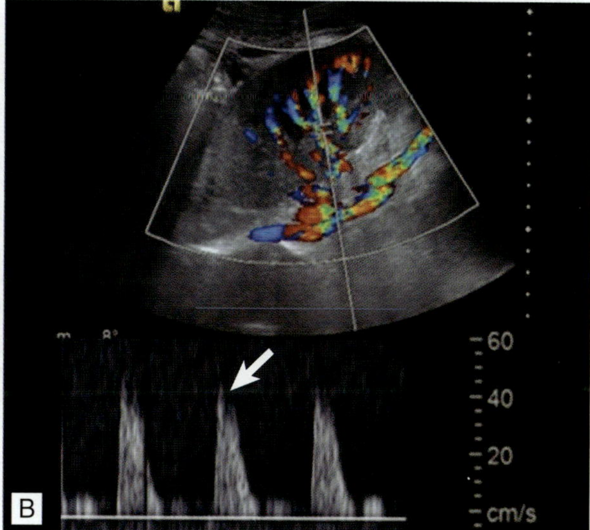

Figure 39.64 Acute rejection in a transplanted kidney (TxK). (A) Two-dimensional ultrasound image demonstrates an enlarged kidney with a hypoechoic cortex. (B) Color Doppler ultrasound image demonstrates a peripheral cut-off of vessels. On spectral Doppler, the waveform demonstrates a sharp upstroke of the systolic wave (*white arrow*). There is absent diastolic flow with an increase in the resistivity index. (Courtesy: Dr. Rajas Chaubal, radiologist and director, Thane Ultrasound Centre, Thane, Mumbai, Maharashtra, India.)

- Contrast-enhanced USG evaluates microvascular renal perfusion and predicts graft viability and an impending loss of renal function [114]. Delayed cortical perfusion is seen in acute rejection [115]
- CT scan shows an edematous, bulky kidney and patchy post-contrast enhancement. These findings are not specific for allograft rejection and can be seen in ATN [113]
- DWI has emerged as a noninvasive modality for graft function assessment. BOLD and arterial spin-labeling MRI techniques are reassuring and detect allograft oxygenation and perfusion function. An increased level of deoxyhemoglobin caused by hypoxia results in a decrease in intrarenal T2 signal [116]

Acute Tubular Necrosis

Acute tubular necrosis is one of the most common causes of acute renal failure within the first week of transplant, which usually progresses through the diuretic phase and shows a gradual recovery of renal function. It is relatively common in cadaveric transplants and infrequent among live donor transplants. Although the exact cause is unknown, it is believed to be caused by prolonged graft ischemia and compensated allograft perfusion.

- On grayscale USG, ATN shows enlarged kidneys with loss of corticomedullary differentiation. Cyclosporine toxicity and rejection show similar features [117]. Reversal of blood flow seen during diastole is also seen in RVT, acute rejection, and occasionally nephrosclerosis [118] (Fig. 39.65)
- MRI BOLD imaging has emerged as a noninvasive way to detect intrarenal oxygenation and can distinguish acute rejection from ATN [116]
- Renography provides functional information of the allograft. Improvement of renal function on serial follow-up imaging is helpful to differentiate rejection from ATN. However, even renography cannot differentiate between acute rejection, cyclosporine toxicity, and ATN [119]
- Ultrasound-guided biopsy is recommended for the final diagnosis

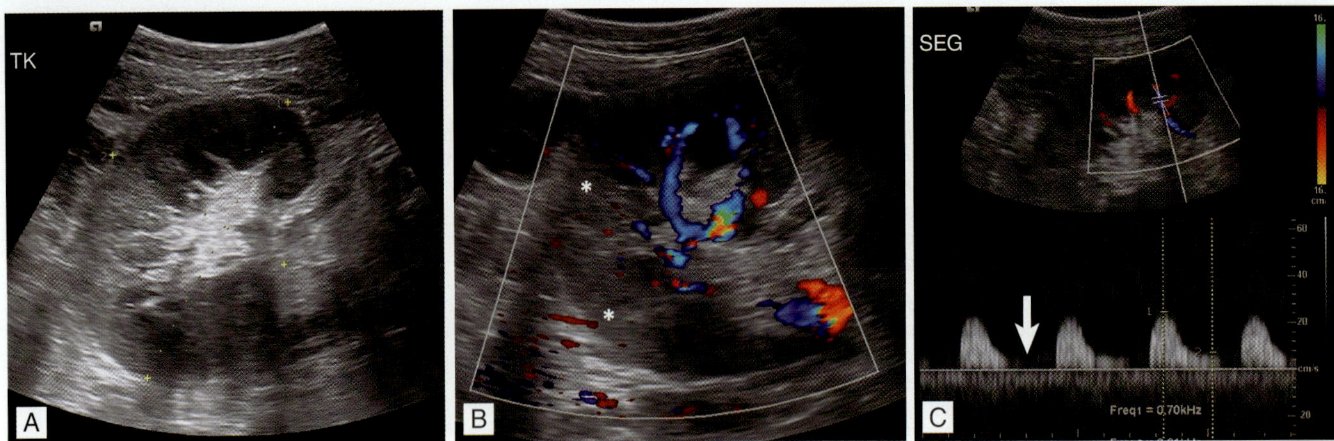

Figure 39.65 Acute tubular necrosis in a transplant kidney. (A) Two-dimensional ultrasound image demonstrates an enlarged kidney. (B) Color Doppler ultrasound image demonstrates a hypoperfused kidney (*white asterisks*). (C) Spectral Doppler waveform demonstrates absent diastolic flow (*white arrow*). (Courtesy: Dr. Rajas Chaubal, radiologist and director, Thane Ultrasound Centre, Thane, Mumbai, Maharashtra, India.)

TABLE 39.24 Various Infections in Postrenal Transplant Patients

	Period	Infections
Early	Postoperative period: up to 1 month	Related to surgery and nosocomial infections Antimicrobial-resistant bacteria: (MRSA) and VRE [16] Donor-related infection less common The incidence of pneumonia, surgical wound infections, and UTI in renal transplant patients is similar to nonimmunocompromised postsurgical patients
Intermediate	2–6 months post-transplant	Opportunistic infections: CMV followed by polyomavirus (BK virus) and EBV Related to a prior donor or recipient infection or susceptibility Immunosuppression of the recipient
Late	After 6 months	Early viral and latent infections risk diminishes after 6 mo CAP and UTI common Continued immunosuppression risk for opportunistic pathogens: Nocardia spp. and fungal organisms such as Aspergillus spp. and Mucor spp.

CAP, community-acquired pneumonia; *CMV,* cytomegalovirus: *EBV,* Epstein-Barr virus; *MRSA,* methicillin-resistant Staphylococcus aureus; *UTI,* urinary tract infection; *VRE,* vancomycin-resistant enterococci.

Delayed Graft Function

Delayed graft function is defined as a post-transplant poor renal function within 1 week of transplantation and requires dialysis [120]. It is seen in around 20–30% of recipients of cadaveric renal transplants. Patients showing DGF eventually show improvement in renal function; however, there is an approximately 41% increased risk of graft loss. Cold ischemia time and other factors such as infarction, ATN, rejection, and fluid collection around the allograft are thought to be common factors for DGF. On imaging, no definitive diagnosis can be made.

On grayscale USG, the transplanted kidney may be normal and may show absence or diminished diastolic blood flow with elevated resistivity index [113].

Infection

Immunosuppression makes the transplant recipient vulnerable to reactivation of latent infections and secondary infections. Additional risk factors include female gender, presence of indwelling urinary catheters, diabetes mellitus, trauma, and history of prior UTIs [121]. They are also susceptible to donor-related infections within the allograft.

Depending on the period from transplantation, various infections can occur in a predictable pattern (Table 39.24), albeit they may be influenced by the state of immunosuppression, prophylactic antimicrobials, and the susceptibility and virulence of the recipient.

Imaging plays an important role in the timely detection of complications as perinephric fluid collections or abscess formation that can be managed with appropriate antimicrobials or percutaneous drainage.

The kidney may be normal on USG in patients with uncomplicated pyelonephritis. The echogenicity of the kidney may be decreased with loss of corticomedullary differentiation with an increase in the size of the kidney during the acute phase. The altered echogenicity of the kidney, a streaky pattern of alternating hypoechoic bands at grayscale, focal wedge-shaped areas of hyperechogenicity, or hypoechogenicity may be seen. On Doppler examination, increased resistivity index in the renal arteries and diminished cortical perfusion on power Doppler may be seen [122].

Perinephric or parenchymal fluid collections with internal echogenic components and peripheral hypervascularity are seen in abscess formation. Echogenic debris or mobile masses indicate pyonephrosis or a fungus ball, respectively [123].

Striated nephrogram, wedge-shaped areas of hypoperfusion, and perinephric fat stranding on contrast-enhanced CT or MRI suggest pyelonephritis (Fig. 39.66). Renal parenchymal and

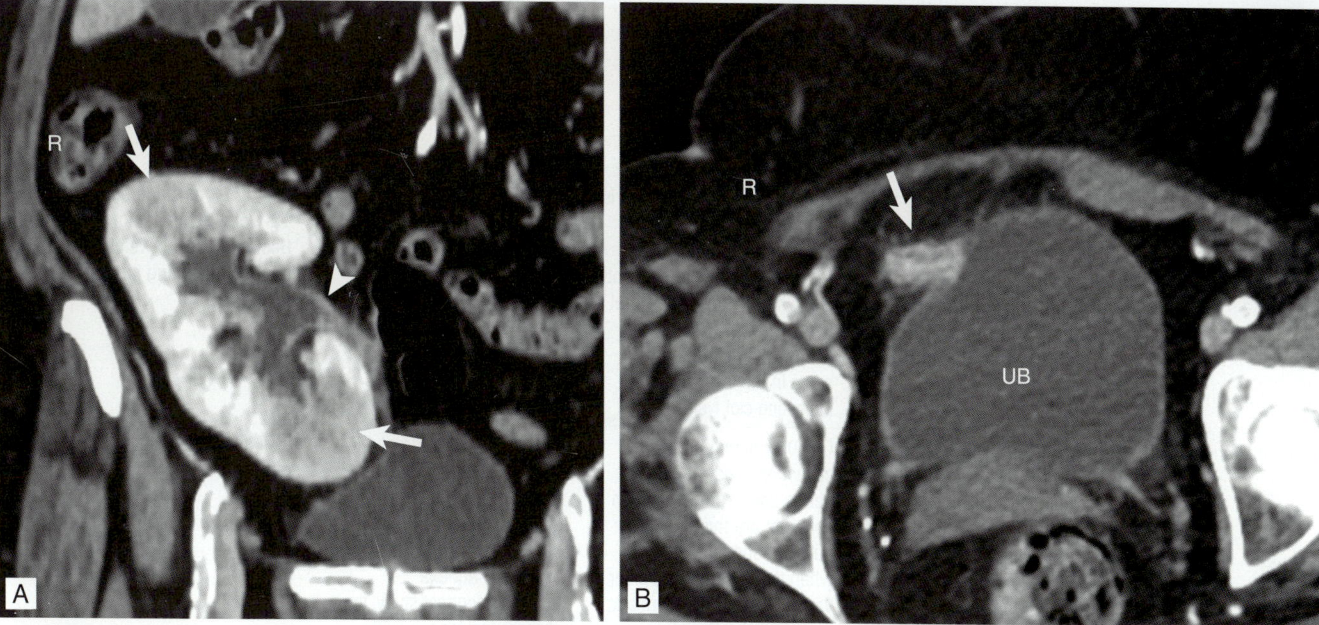

Figure 39.66 Pyelonephritis of a transplant kidney. (A) Contrast-enhanced computed tomography (CT) in the coronal plane during the nephrographic phase of transplant kidney in the right lower quadrant demonstrates a focal poorly enhancing lesion (*white arrows*) in the upper and lower poles involving the corticomedullary region. Hydronephrosis is seen with uroepithelial thickening (*white arrowhead*). (B) Contrast-enhanced CT in the axial plane at the level of the urinary bladder (UB) demonstrates stricture caused by significant uroepithelial thickening (*arrow*) of the juxtavesical ureter at the vesicoureteric junction.

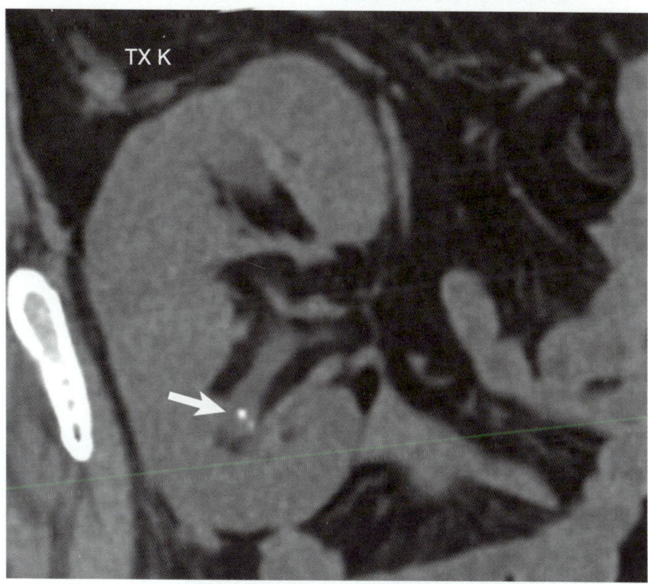

Figure 39.67 Stone in a transplant kidney (TxK). Noncontrast computed tomography of transplant kidney in oblique coronal multiplanar reconstruction demonstrates early calculi formation (*white arrow*) in the lower pole calyx.

perinephric collections and their extent can be better mapped on contrast-enhanced CT or MRI. Air pockets within the collection increase the confidence in diagnosis of infection on CT.

Renal Calculi

Renal calculi may be donor related. Renal recipients are prone to developing renal calculi caused by hypercalcemia associated with vitamin D and calcium metabolism abnormalities. CT is the modality of choice for the detection of size, site, and obstructive uropathy and associated complications (Fig. 39.67). Most calculi formed in transplanted kidneys are calcium oxalate.

TABLE 39.25 Types of Perirenal Collections

Type	Subcapsular Collections	Perinephric Collections
Location	Deeper to the renal capsule; often small	Surrounding the graft; often large
Mechanism	After biopsy or trauma to the graft	
	Resolves of its own if small; if persistent, leads to hypertension because of mass effect	Displaces the kidney Lateral to the graft: venous in origin Medial to the graft: from the anastomotic site
Imaging	Caused by altered renal perfusion; the arterial resistive indices increase	Large collection around the allograft

Perinephric Fluid Collections

Most allografts are placed in the confined extraperitoneal space. Any collection in this space results in a mass effect on the graft with resultant dysfunction. Various types of collections are outlined in Table 39.25. Imaging features of various collections are outlined in Table 39.26.

Hematoma, urinoma, abscess, and lymphoceles are the perinephric collections that occur in descending order concerning the time from transplant [112].

Large collections may lead to hydronephrosis; compression or thrombosis of the renal vein, or compression of femoral vessels and subsequent swelling of the lower extremity or deep vein thrombosis [110] (Fig. 39.68).

The management of the perigraft collection depends on the nature, size, and extent of the fluid collection. The role of imaging is to diagnose the perinephric collection and its size, extent, and mass effect. Ultrasound-guided aspiration is diagnostic.

TABLE 39.26 Imaging Features of Various Collections

		IMAGING		
	Etiology	USG	CT	MRI
Perinephric hematoma	Inadequate surgical hemostasis, coagulopathy, anticoagulation, or complication of biopsy Perinephric hematomas are often large and displace the kidney rather than flattening the contour	Acute hematoma: anechoic and echogenic mobile debris Subacute or chronic hematoma: heterogeneous hyperechoic and subsequently show heterogeneous central hypoechoic or cystic areas with scattered internal thin septa in the late state, indicating clot lysis	Acute hematoma hyperdense (>30–40 HU) Subacute iso to hyperdense on non-contrast CT Chronic hematoma hypodense on plain CT scan	Appearance varies as per the age of hemorrhage on T1- and T2-weighted imaging Best seen on T1-weighted fat images; blooming on gradient images
Perinephric abscesses	Infrequent complication in the first week of transplant; they develop as a result of secondary infection of the graft or perinephric fluid collection or may spread from surrounding abdominopelvic organs or abdominal wall Fever, sepsis, and tenderness at the transplant site Systemic antibiotics and image-guided drainage are the initial lines of treatment; at times surgical drainage may be required	Complex perinephric collections and may show debris and septations when contents are thick and purulent and hypoechoic when the contents are clear. Variable rim of hyperemia is seen on color Doppler.	Pre- and post-contrast CT demonstrates the entire extent of the abscess and involvement of adjacent structures such as the psoas muscle or adnexa In the noncontrast study, the abscess hypodense fluid collections and may show hyperattenuating debris or blood products and peripheral enhancement on contrast-enhanced CT; gas foci are seen within the abscess	DWI shows restriction of diffusion
Lymphocele	Leakage of lymph from recipient lymphatic channels; seen 2 weeks to 6 months post-transplant; mostly asymptomatic; may present with pain over the graft site or scrotal edema; graft dysfunction caused by mass effect or hydronephrosis when there are large lymphoceles	Well-marginated anechoic collections and show septa compared with other collections	Clear fluid collections with a barely perceptible wall	Marked hyperintense on T2-weighted imaging

CD, color Doppler; *CT*, computed tomography; *DWI*, diffusion-weighted imaging; *MRI*, magnetic resonance imaging; *USG*, ultrasonography.

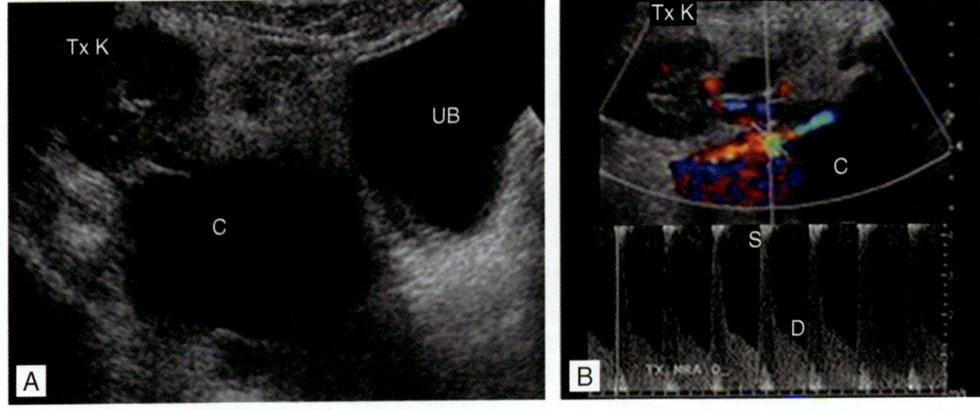

Figure 39.68 Postoperative collection causing compression of the renal artery. (A) Two-dimensional ultrasound image demonstrates a collection (C) adjacent to the hilum of the transplanted kidney (TxK). Note that the collection is separate from the urinary bladder (UB). (B) Color Doppler ultrasound image demonstrates aliasing at the site of compression of the renal artery (*white arrow*). The corresponding spectral Doppler demonstrates high systolic velocity at the site of compression (S). *D*, diastolic velocity. (Courtesy: Dr. Rajas Chaubal, radiologist and director, Thane Ultrasound Centre, Thane, Mumbai, Maharashtra, India.)

Collecting System Complications

The most common complications of the urinary collecting system are urinary leak and stricture formation. The incidence of ureteral complications is declining because of advanced graft harvesting technology, use of shorter ureters, and reduction of steroid dosage. Patients present with increasing serum creatinine and decreasing urine output.

Urinoma

Urinomas are often seen in the first 10 post-transplant days and are often located between the graft and bladder.

Urine Leakage

The incidence of urine leaks is around 1.1–6.5% of transplant recipients [124], and patients present within the first to 4 weeks post-transplant. The leaks are seen in the distal ureter, bladder, and proximal ureter or pelvicalyceal system in descending order. Direct ureteric injuries during the procedure, retransplantation, and ischemia are the common causes.

- USG:
  - Localized or ill-defined hypo to anechoic fluid collections around the graft with or without debris
  - Urinoma: enlarging collection around the allograft; may cause mass effect or secondary infection
- CT: low attenuated collection (HU <10) on noncontrast scans showing peripheral thin-walled enhancement
- CT/ MRI urography using 3D T2-weighted imaging or post-contrast excretory phase images helps detect the location, extent, and site of the leak
- Nuclear medicine studies using Tc^{99m} are performed to identify the site of urine leaks when contrast urography is contraindicated [125]

The role of imaging is to detect the site, extent, and size of the leak which decides the management. Smaller defects are managed conservatively by placing ureteric stents; while large ureteric defects warrant re-implantation, uretero-ureterostomy, or nephrostomy tube placement.

Urinary Obstruction

Ureteral obstruction may present in the first 48 hours post-transplant or late within 6 months with a prevalence of 2–7.5% [126].

Early ureteral obstructions are secondary to kinking, ischemia, or external compression. Ischemic strictures often present around 6 months post-transplant [124]. Ureteric stents are commonly placed to reduce the risk of early obstruction. On grayscale USG, a dilated collecting system can be identified as anechoic relatively tubular communicating structures. The dilated ureter can be traced along its entire course up to the bladder for detection of stricture or compression. Secondary infection of the dilated system may lead to pyonephrosis. On grayscale USG, pyonephrosis shows internal echoes or debris within. Uroepithelial thickening may be evident. The absence of a ureteric jet within the bladder suggests obstruction.

Balloon dilation or endoscopic management of the stricture is prepared. Distal strictures may require reimplantation.

Neoplasms

Renal transplant patients have a three to five times increased risk of malignancies compared with the general population. Longer graft survival, older donors (as well as recipients), more potent immune suppressants [127], and unregulated oncogenic viral infections [128] are the attributed risk factors. According to Sprangers et al. [129], there is an increasing incidence of nonmelanomatous skin cancers, lymphomas, and colon cancer among these patients. There is a six times greater risk of primary renal malignancies in the allograft compared with native kidneys with a higher prevalence of papillary subtype [130]. Patients with BK virus infection are prone to urothelial malignancy [131]. (BK virus is a member of polyomavirus family and an abbreviation of the name of the first patient in whom the virus was isolated.)

Postrenal Transplantation Lymphoproliferative Disorders

Postrenal transplantation lymphoproliferative disorder (PTLD) is common among transplant patients taking higher doses of immunosuppressive drugs. Epstein-Barr virus-related B-lymphocyte proliferation is also associated with PTLD [132]. Among solid organs transplants, kidney transplant has the lowest risk of PTLD, with a bimodal incidence, the first peak in the early post-transplant period, and the second 10–14 years after transplant.

Postrenal transplantation lymphoproliferative disorder (Fig. 39.69) may show a varied spectrum that ranges from a relatively benign lymphoid hyperplasia to aggressive lymphoma. Solitary or multiple low-attenuation masses may be seen involving the transplanted kidney or other solid organs. A mass replacing or encasing the hilum and resultant obstructive uropathy is a common feature [132]. On MRI, these masses display low signal intensity on both T1- and T2-weighted imaging and show restriction of diffusion on DWI images. No significant postcontrast enhancement is seen. Increased fluorodeoxyglucose uptake is usually observed on positron emission tomography/CT. Whereas a reduction of immunosuppressive agents may be sufficient for low-grade disease, chemotherapy is recommended for aggressive lesions [108].

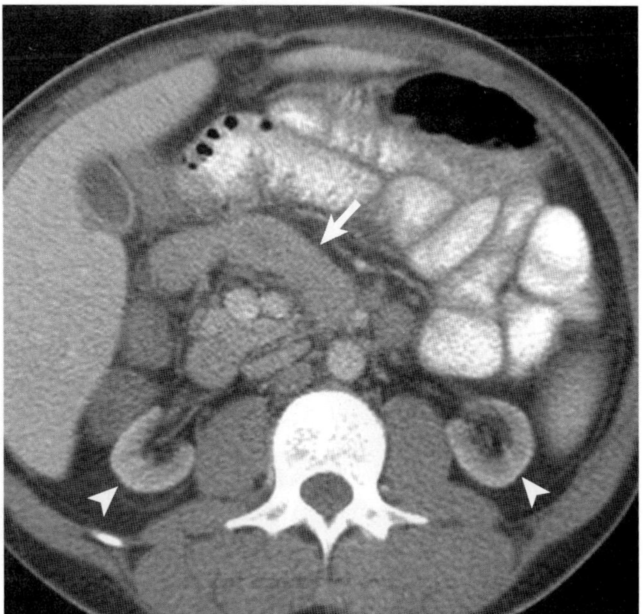

Figure 39.69 Contrast-enhanced computed tomography obtained in the abdomen at the renal level demonstrates small kidneys (*white arrowheads*). There are multiple matted lymph nodes in the small bowel mesentery (*white arrow*).

Genitourinary Trauma

The incidence of trauma to the kidneys and urinary tract is around 8–10% in abdominal trauma cases [133]. Around 89% of cases of all renal injuries occur as a result of blunt trauma [134]. CT is the modality of choice for assessment in hemodynamically stable patients [135].

Renal Trauma

Grading in Renal Injury

Although the grading of renal injuries [136] is described in detail in Chapter 89, examples of various grades are shown in Figs. 39.70–39.74.

Various treatment strategies for different grades of renal trauma are summarized in Table 39.27.

Iatrogenic Renal Trauma

Various surgical and endourologic procedures such as percutaneous renal biopsy, PCNL, and percutaneous nephrostomy can lead to iatrogenic injuries to the kidneys; these injuries are rare in occurrence (Fig. 39.75A).

Retroperitoneal hematoma, AFV, and PSA can be detected with duplex USG. However, multislice CT scanners have increased sensitivity and specificity in identifying renal vascular lesions. On CTA, hemorrhage can be detected in the form of active extravasation of the contrast. AFVs appear as early and simultaneous

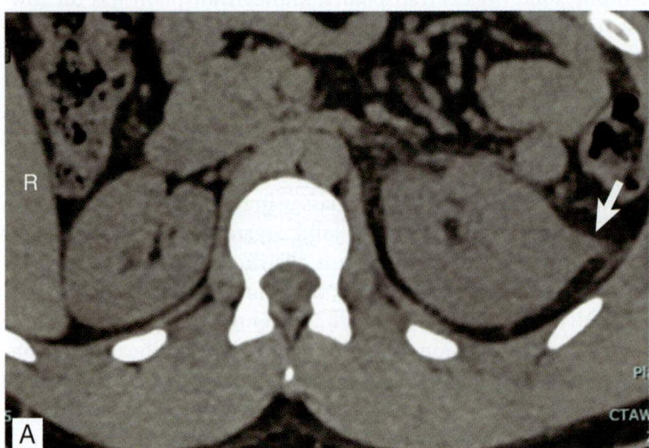

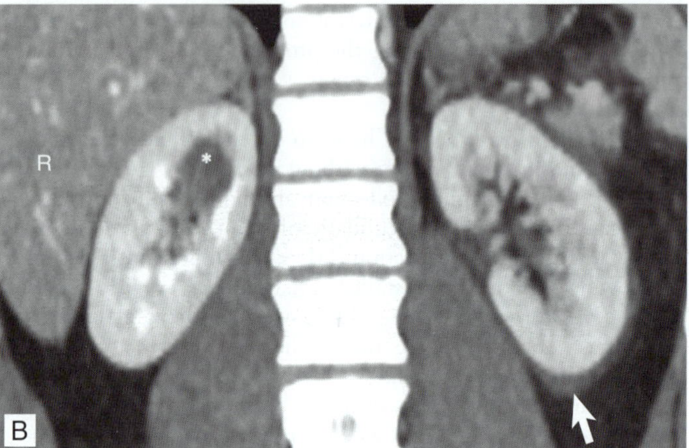

Figure 39.70 Grade I renal injury: renal contusion. (A) Noncontrast computed tomography (CT) in the axial plane demonstrates a bulky left kidney and fluid in the perinephric space (*white arrow*). (B) Postcontrast CT in the coronal plane demonstrates perinephric fluid to be in subcapsular space (*white arrow*). The *white asterisk* is a cyst in the right kidney.

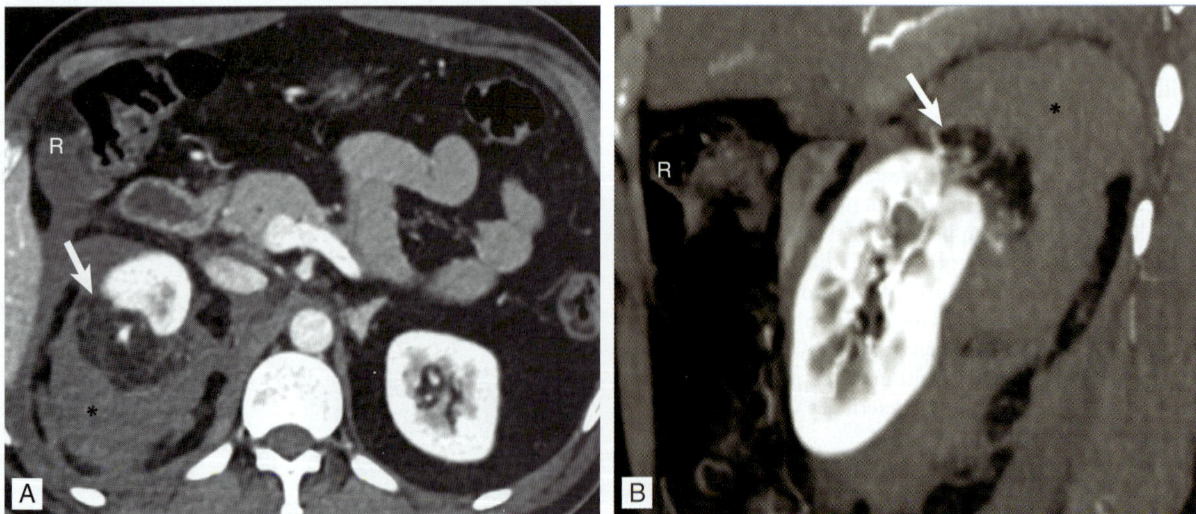

Figure 39.71 Grade II renal injury: perinephric hematoma in a ruptured angiomyolipoma following blunt trauma. (A) Contrast-enhanced computed tomography in the axial plane during the corticomedullary phase demonstrates angiomyolipoma (*white arrow*) arising from the upper pole of the right kidney with perinephric hematoma (*black asterisk*). The kidney demonstrates normal enhancement. (B) Sagittal multiplanar reconstruction demonstrates same findings as image A. *White arrow* is angiomyolipoma and *black asterisk* is hematoma.

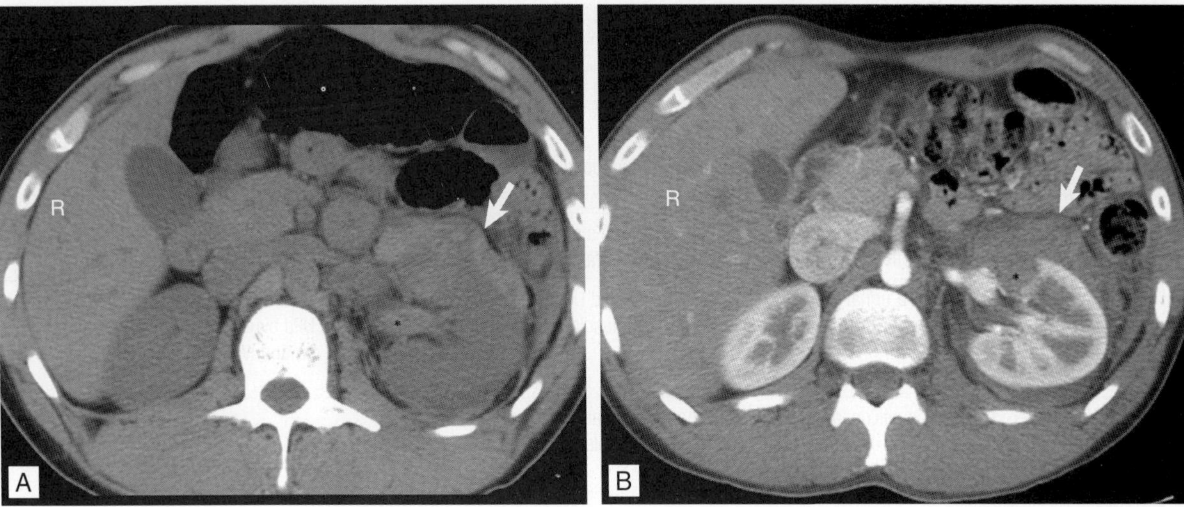

Figure 39.72 Grade III renal injury: renal laceration. (A) Noncontrast computed tomography (CT) in the axial plane demonstrates hyperdense subcapsular hematoma (*white arrow*). The *black asterisk* is hemorrhage in the renal pelvis. (B) Contrast-enhanced CT in the axial plane demonstrates deep cortico-medullary laceration (*black asterisk*) with subcapsular hematoma (*white arrow*).

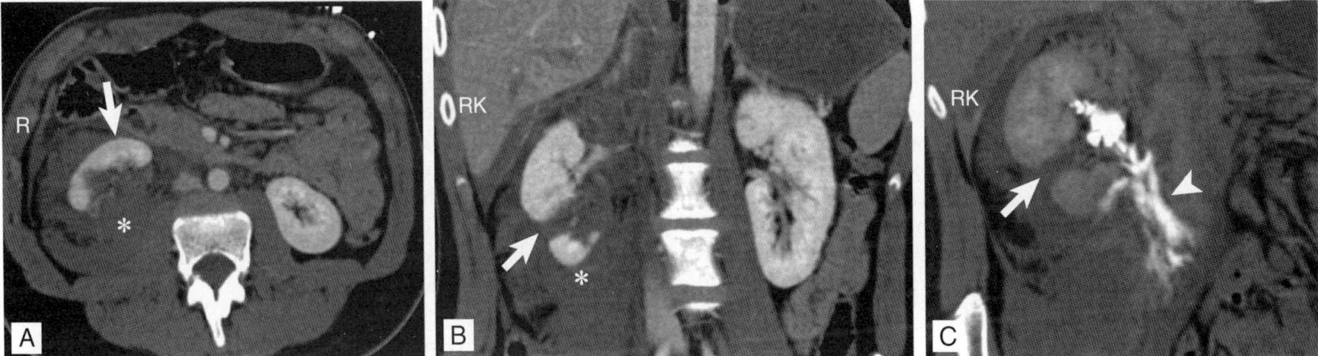

Figure 39.73 Grade IV renal injury: renal laceration and contrast extravasation. (A) Contrast-enhanced computed tomography (CT) in the axial plane during nephrographic phase demonstrates major laceration (*white arrow*) in the right kidney (RK) with perinephric hematoma (*white asterisk*). The rest of the kidney demonstrates enhancement. (B) Contrast-enhanced CT in the coronal plane during the nephrographic phase demonstrates similar findings. (C) Contrast-enhanced CT in the coronal plane during the excretory phase demonstrates contrast leak from the collecting system (*white arrowhead*) with urinoma formation. The *white arrow* is a laceration.

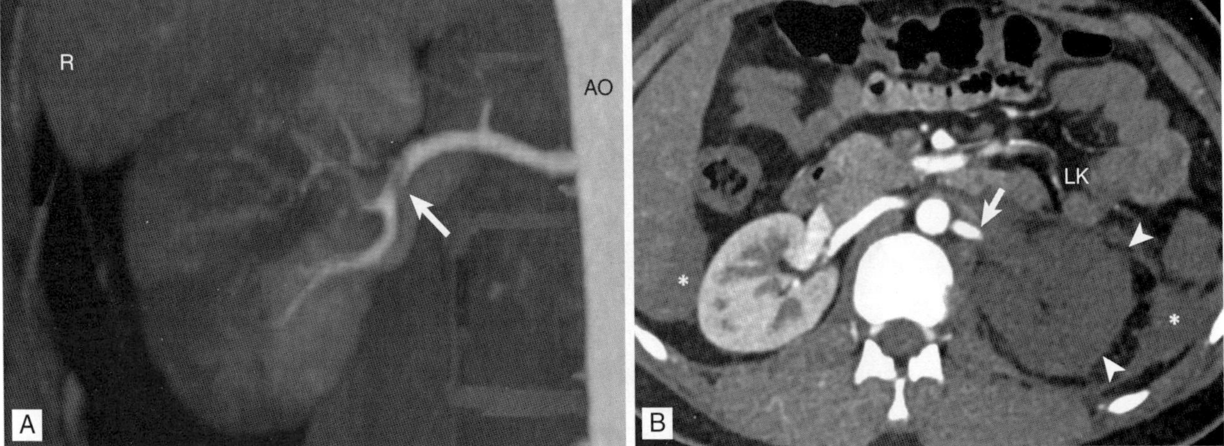

Figure 39.74 Grade V renal injury: renal artery injury. (A) Coronal maximum intensity projection of the computed tomography angiography (CTA) phase of the right renal artery demonstrates dissection in the renal artery at the hilum before bifurcation (*white arrow*). A paucity of intrarenal arterial branches is seen. Geographic areas of ischemia are seen in both kidneys. (B) Contrast-enhanced CT in a different patient during the angiographic phase demonstrates a lack of parenchymal enhancement in the left kidney (LK) (*white arrowheads*) caused by occlusion of the left renal artery (*white arrow*). The *white asterisks* on both sides represent a hematoma. The right kidney demonstrates normal enhancement. *AO,* aorta.

TABLE 39.27 Grades of Renal Injury and Treatment Strategies

Grade of Injury	Features	Treatment Strategies
I	Contusions and subcapsular hematoma	Conservative management
II	Perinephric hematomas and superficial parenchymal lacerations without active hemorrhage	Conservative management
III	Deep lacerations without a urinary leak, development of AVFs and pseudoaneurysms, active bleeding contained within Gerota fascia	Endovascular management for active bleeding, pseudoaneurysms and AVFs
IV	Deep laceration with a urinary leak, injury to renal pelvis and UPJ, segmental vascular injury, active bleeding beyond Gerota fascia	▪ Segmental vascular injuries are considered low risk: no intervention ▪ Renal pelvic injuries and UPJ avulsions: ureteral stenting ▪ Perirenal hematoma >4 cm and IV contrast extravasation: arterial embolization
V	"Shattered" kidney, avulsion, and laceration of the main renal artery or renal vein, and devascularized kidney with active bleeding	Nephrectomy

AVF, arteriovenous fistula; *IV*, intravenous; *UPJ*, ureteropelvic junction.

enhancement of renal arteries and veins involved. A PSA is detected as a rounded or ovoid contrast-enhancing structure communicating with the injured vessel.

Ureteral Trauma

Ureteral trauma caused by external injuries are very rare, accounting for fewer than 1% of all urologic trauma cases [137]. When they happen, they are primarily caused by penetrating injury such as a gunshot wound [138] or are iatrogenic. Ureteric trauma can happen while negotiating a DJ stent. The excretory phase of CT urography is used to visualize the collecting system and the ureter. In the case of ureteral injury, contrast extravasation is seen in the periureteral soft tissues (Fig. 39.75B).

Bladder Trauma

The majority of bladder ruptures have a traumatic cause [139]. Traumatic bladder ruptures can be further classified into extraperitoneal, intraperitoneal, and mixed extraperitoneal and intraperitoneal ruptures. It is paramount to make such a diagnosis because extraperitoneal ruptures (Fig. 39.76) are treated conservatively with catheter drainage, but others are treated surgically.

The types of bladder rupture are summarized in Table 39.28.

- Extraperitoneal ruptures are managed conservatively with 90% of them healing within 10 days [140]
- Intraperitoneal bladder rupture comprises around 10% to 20% of bladder injuries [141]. The mechanism of injury commonly is a direct blow to the lower abdomen with a distended bladder resulting in rupture at the bladder dome
- A mixed pattern of bladder rupture occurs in approximately 5% of bladder injuries [142]

Urethral Trauma

Etiology

The commonest cause of urethral trauma is iatrogenic, and most of these injuries happen during catheterization [143]. The commonest

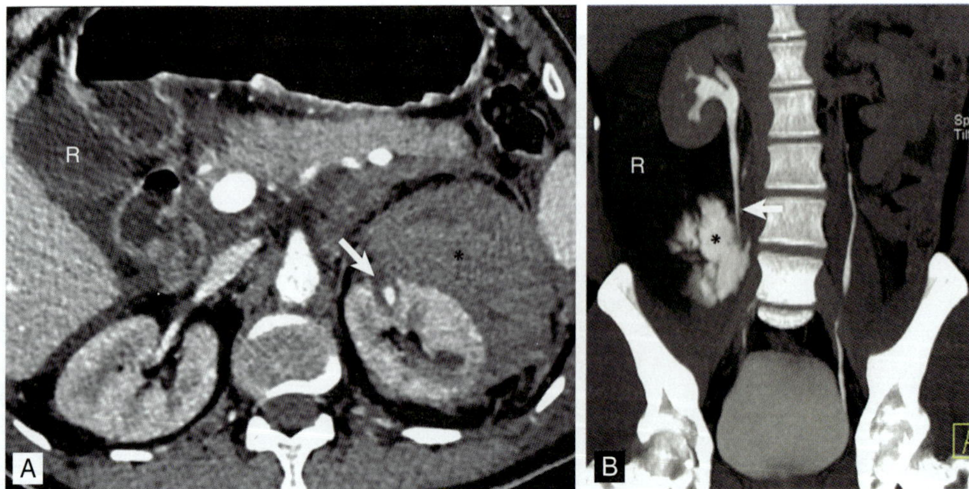

Figure 39.75 Iatrogenic trauma to the kidney and ureter. (A) Contrast-enhanced computed tomography (CT) in the axial plane during the arterial phase demonstrates a focal laceration with pseudoaneurysm (*white arrow*) in the anterior cortex of the left kidney with perinephric hematoma (*black asterisk*) after renal biopsy. The right kidney demonstrates normal enhancement. (B) Contrast-enhanced CT coronal thin maximum intensity projection during excretory phase demonstrates contrast leak and formation of urinoma (*black asterisk*) in relation to the mid right ureter (*white arrow*). This is an iatrogenic injury of the ureter after the removal of a DJ stent.

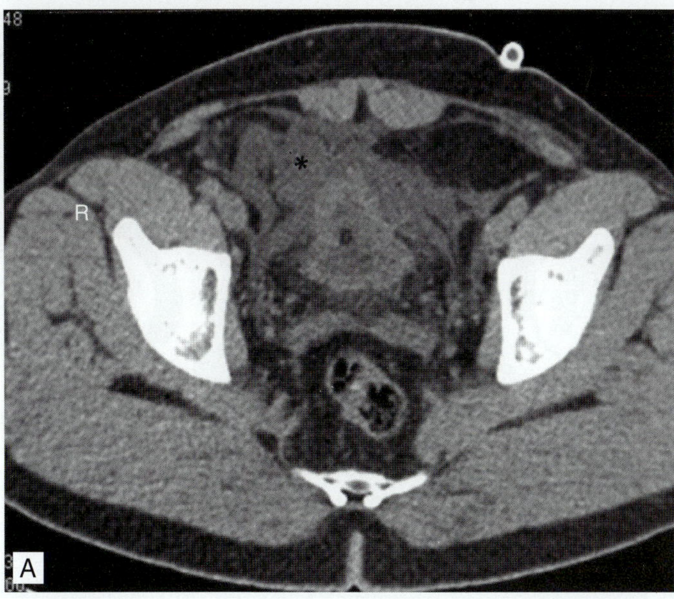

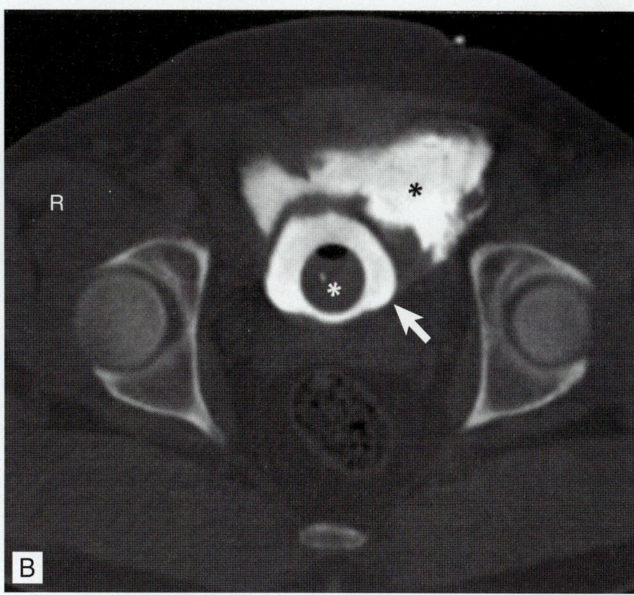

Figure 39.76 Extraperitoneal rupture of the urinary bladder. (A) Noncontrast computed tomography (CT) scan in the axial plain phase demonstrates a collapsed bladder with a Foley catheter and fluid in the extraperitoneal space. (B) Postcontrast CT scan in the axial plain during the excretory phase demonstrates collapsed bladder (*white arrow*) with a Foley catheter (*white asterisk*) and contrast leak in the extraperitoneal space with urinoma formation (*black asterisk*).

traumatic urethral injuries are caused by pelvic fracture-related injuries in the setting of high-velocity accidents. Straddle injuries are less common and result in injury to the bulbar urethra.

Clinical Features

Clinical features include blood at the meatus, difficulty in voiding, pelvic fracture, scrotal or perineal ecchymosis or hematoma, and a high-riding prostate on digital rectal examination. Transurethral catheterization of the bladder is discouraged before ruling out urethral injury.

TABLE 39.28 Types of Bladder Rupture

Type of Bladder Rupture	Imaging Findings in CT Cystography	
Extraperitoneal (Fig. 39.76)	Simple	Extravasation of contrast material limited to the perivesical space
	Complex	Extravasation into the prevesical space, anterior abdominal wall, penis, scrotum, and the thigh region
Intraperitoneal		Contrast extravasates into the peritoneal cavity and is seen surrounding the bowel loops and in the paracolic gutters, in the rectovesical or rectouterine pouch, and between the mesenteric folds
Mixed		Extravasation of the contrast agent into both the intraperitoneal and extraperitoneal compartments

CT, computed tomography.

Imaging

Retrograde urethrography is the best initial study for the evaluation of urethral and periurethral injuries in men [144]. A 16- or 18-Fr Foley catheter is placed into the urethra. After inflation of the balloon, 20–30 mL of 60% iodinated contrast material should be injected under fluoroscopic guidance. Spasm of the external urethral sphincter is common, and slow and gentle pressure is needed. Spot radiographs are taken for confirmation of contrast material flowing into the bladder.

Injuries to the male urethra are broadly classified into injuries to the anterior and posterior urethra because the pathophysiology of both the urethral injuries varies widely.

Posterior Urethral Injuries

These affect around 10% of the men who sustain a fracture of the anterior pelvic arch (Fig. 39.77) with some degree of ligamentous disruption affecting the sacroiliac joints posteriorly [145].

When the bladder cannot be filled in presence of extravasation of contrast, the urethral rupture is assumed to be complete. Complete ruptures have a greater incidence of developing urethral strictures.

Role of Computed Tomography in the Evaluation of Urethral Trauma

Because CT is the accepted front-line imaging modality for blunt abdominopelvic trauma, it may precede retrograde urethrography by hours or even days. Ali et al. [146] have reported the following findings most commonly found in CT:

- Distortion or obscuration of urogenital diaphragm plane
- Hematoma of ischiocavernosus
- Distortion or obscuration of the prostatic contour
- Distortion or obscuration of the bulbocavernosus
- Hematoma of the obturator internus

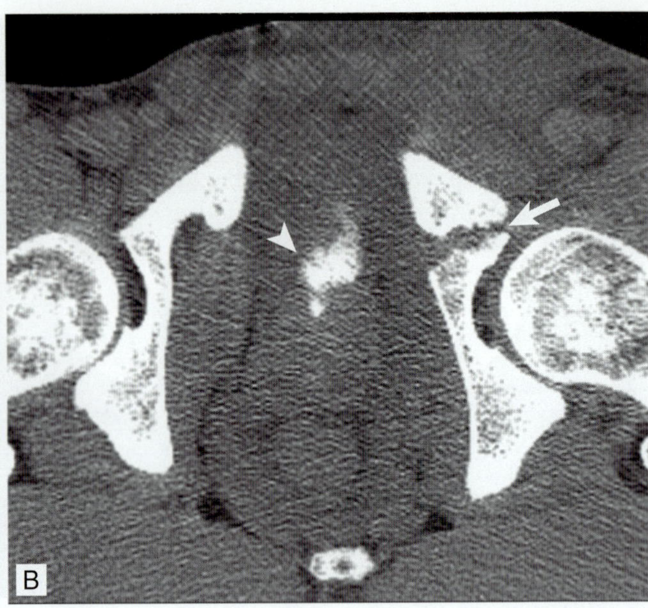

Figure 39.77 Urethral tear after trauma. (A) Retrograde urethrogram done under fluoroscopy demonstrates contrast opacifying the penile urethra. The *small arrow black* is the bulbar urethra and is distended because of pressure injection. Contrast leakage is seen from the junction of the prostatic urethra and penile urethra, tracking to the interpubic region (*black arrowhead*). Note the fracture of the left inferior pubic ramus (*long black arrow*). (B) Contrast-enhanced computed tomography axial section at the level of pubic symphysis during the excretory phase demonstrates diastasis of the pubic symphysis and contrast leak into the soft tissues (*white arrowhead*). The *white arrow* is the fracture of the left superior pubic ramus extending up to the anterior wall of the acetabulum.

Anterior Urethral Injuries

The most common cause of injury to the anterior urethra is iatrogenic [146]. Straddle injuries are the types of injuries in which the corpus spongiosum and bulbar urethra are crushed against the inferior aspect of the pubic bone. Pelvic fractures are uncommon in anterior urethral injuries.

Suggested Readings

- WD Craig, BJ Wagner, MD. Travis, Pyelonephritis: Radiologic-pathologic review, Radiographics 28 (2008) 255–276.
- J Demertzis, CO. Menias, State of the art: imaging of renal infections, Emerg Radiol 14 (2007) 13–22.
- EA Wolin, DS Hartman, JR. Olson, Nephrographic and pyelographic analysis of CT urography: differential diagnosis, Am J Roentgenol 200 (2013) 1197–1203.
- FL Coe, A Evan, E. Worcester, Kidney stone disease, J Clin Invest 115 (2005) 2598–2608.
- D Marin, DT Boll, A Mileto, RC. Nelson, State of the art: dual-energy CT of the abdomen, Radiology 271 (2014) 327–342.
- NP Ghonge, S Gadanayak, V. Rajakumari, MDCT evaluation of potential living renal donor, prior to laparoscopic donor nephrectomy: what the transplant surgeon wants to know? Ind J Radiol Imag 24 (2014) 367.

40

Urinary Tract: Tumors

SUMIT MUKHOPADHYAY, DAYANAND LINGEGOWDA, BHARAT GUPTA

Solid Renal Tumors

Introduction

Renal masses are divided into solid and cystic lesions. With the increased use of cross-sectional imaging, there is an increase in the number of incidentally detected renal masses [1]. *Overall, up to 66% of the small (<4 cm) renal masses are incidentally found and 20% of them are benign [2].*

Renal tumors have been pathologically classified by the World Health Organization (WHO 2016). According to the WHO classification approximately 90% of solid renal masses are renal cell carcinomas (RCCs), and 85% of these are clear cell tumors [3–4]. Apart from clear cell RCCs, solid malignant masses frequently encountered in clinical practice include papillary and chromophobe RCC (crRCC), urothelial carcinoma, lymphoma, and metastasis, whereas the most frequently encountered benign solid renal masses are angiomyolipoma (AML) and oncocytoma. These common benign lesions are occasionally difficult to differentiate from RCC.

The goals of imaging are:

- Differentiate cystic from solid renal masses
- Differentiate between benign and malignant renal masses
- RCC subtyping
- Staging
- Preoperative surgical planning and tumor staging
- Treatment response and follow up

Benign Tumors

Angiomyolipoma

Epidemiology and Pathology

AML is the most common benign tumor encountered in clinical practice. It usually occurs in the fourth to sixth decade with increased incidence in women [5]. AML can occur sporadically (80%) or in association with genetic syndromes like tuberous sclerosis (55–90%) and lymphangioleiomyomatosis (30–50%) [6].

On pathology, AML is a solid tumor composed of varying amounts of three elements: dysmorphic blood vessels, smooth muscle, and mature adipose tissue [7]. Some AMLs contain only a small amount of fat which may not be appreciable on imaging, known as minimal fat AMLs. These account for 4–5% of all histopathological specimens [8]. Minimal fat AML is pathologically described as an AML containing less than 25% fat cells per high-power field [5,9]. Other rare variants include epitheloid AML and AML with epithelial cysts [10]. Most AMLs are asymptomatic and incidentally detected. In a minority of cases, symptoms such as flank pain are produced by mass effect and intratumoral or perirenal hemorrhage. Larger AMLs >4 cm can present as life-threatening spontaneous hemorrhage which is also known as Wunderlich syndrome (Fig. 40.1) [11].

Imaging Features

- Ultrasonography (USG) alone cannot definitively diagnose AML, but is useful in the follow-up of patients with known AML. AMLs are hyperechoic to the renal parenchyma on ultrasonography [12,13]. On contrast-enhanced ultrasonography (CEUS), AML shows heterogeneous enhancement with progressive hypoenhancement (washout compared with renal parenchyma) in the delayed phase [14]
- *Unequivocal demonstration of macroscopic fat by CT (HU <-10) or MR imaging in a renal lesion is a specific finding for the diagnosis of classic AML* (Fig. 40.1). On the contrary, minimal fat AML demonstrates intense enhancement in the corticomedullary phase without demonstrable fat on CT, making it difficult to differentiate it from RCC
- On MR imaging, the fatty component of classic AML follows the signal intensity of subcutaneous and intra-abdominal fat on all sequences, characterized by a hyperintense signal on T1-weighted or T2-weighted (T2W) images, with signal saturation using fat-saturation techniques. On opposed phase (OP) images there is signal dropout at the interface of the lesion with the kidney giving India ink artifact [8,15]. However, minimal fat AML does not show macroscopic fat on imaging. It may show a drop in signal in OP images (Table 40.1)
- A challenging imaging question is to differentiate clear cell RCC from minimal fat AML. Minimal fat AML shows avid enhancement with subsequent washout on contrast-enhanced sequences, similar to clear cell RCC. The degree of washout although tends to be greater in minimal fat AML. The presence of intratumoral necrosis and cystic changes and calcification favors clear cell RCC [16]. *The diagnosis of minimal fat AML should be considered for renal masses with a homogeneous low signal on T2W images* seen as a result of the smooth muscle component of these lesions
- Another simplified vascular parameter, known as arterial/delay enhancement ratio (ADER), defined as the difference in signal intensity between arterial and precontrast phase divided by the difference between delayed and precontrast phase;

$$\text{ADER: [SIart – SIpre]/[SIdel – SIpre])}$$

has been proposed to distinguish *minimal fat AML from RCC, with values greater than 1.5 favoring AML* [17] (Fig. 40.2). However, a percutaneous biopsy should be performed for confirmation of the diagnosis

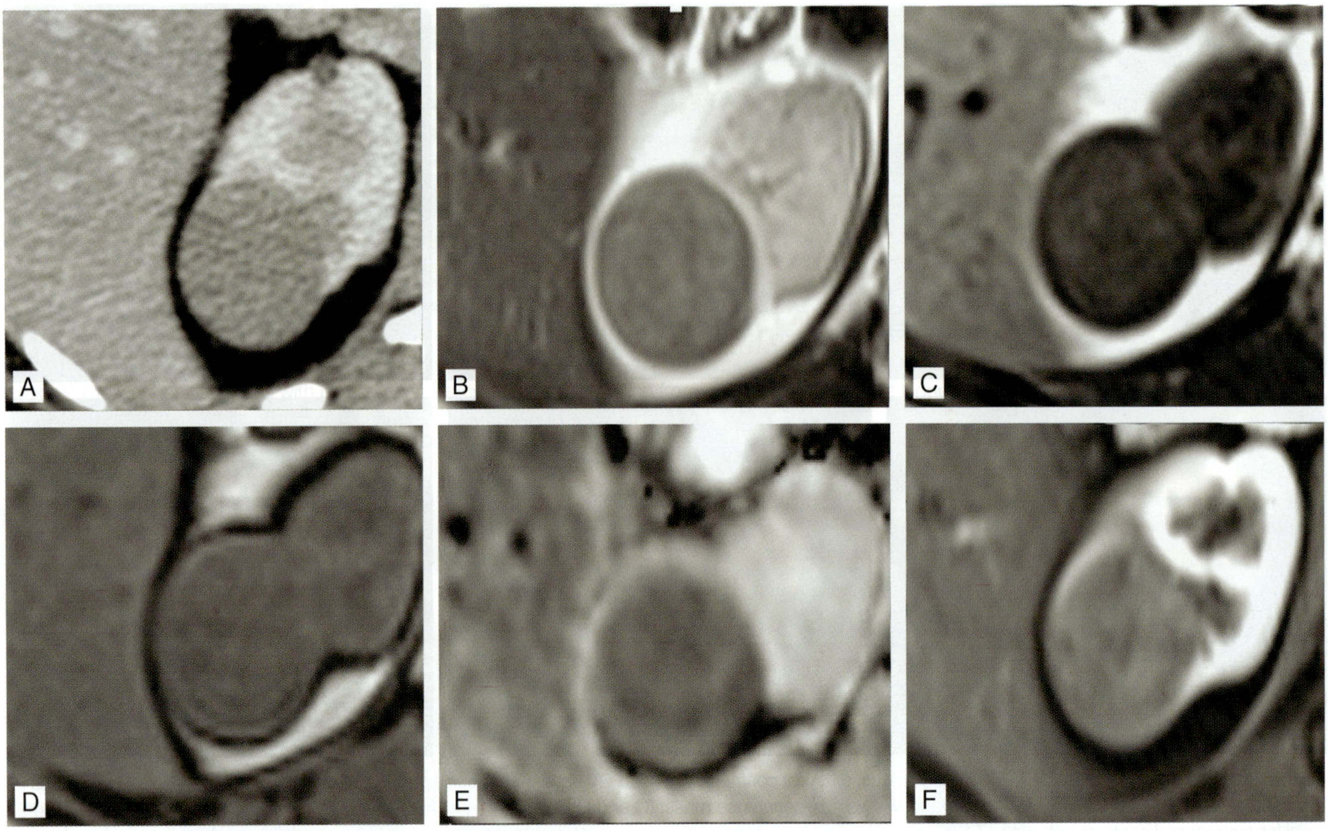

Figure 40.8 Papillary RCC. (A) Axial contrast CT shows a well-defined mildly enhancing hypodense solid mass in the right kidney. (B) Axial T2-weighted MRI image shows a hypointense mass. (C and D) Axial in-phase (C) and out-of-phase (D) T1-weighted images show a drop in signal intensity on the *in-phase* image suggesting intralesional hemosiderin. (E) ADC image shows restricted diffusion. (F) Axial fat-suppressed contrast-enhanced T1-weighted image in corticomedullary phase shows a mildly enhancing mass.

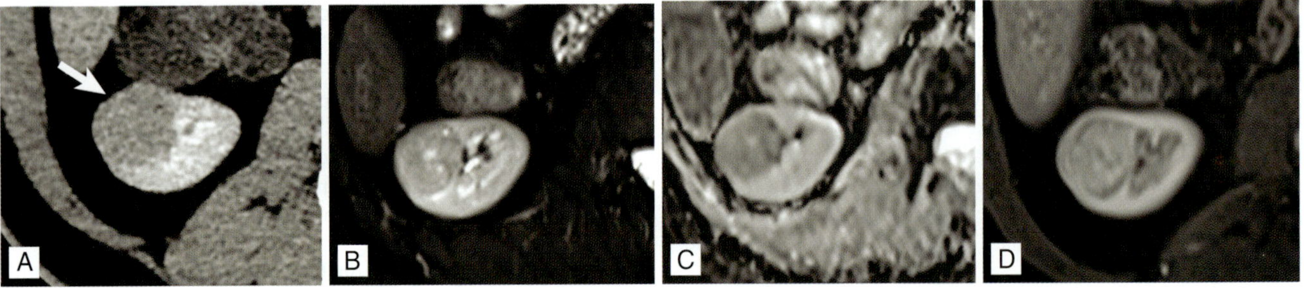

Figure 40.9 Chromophobe RCC. (A) Contrast-enhanced axial CT shows an enhancing mass in the right kidney (*arrow*). (B) Axial T2-weighted fat-suppressed MRI image shows an isointense mass. (C) Axial ADC image shows mild restricted diffusion. (D) Axial fat-suppressed contrast-enhanced T1 weighted.

a male-to-female ratio of approximately 2:1. The age range is 13–83 years (mean age, 55 years). It is characteristically epicenter in the pelvicalyceal system and has an infiltrative growth pattern at imaging. Larger neoplasms present as heterogeneous masses with areas of necrosis, hemorrhage, and calcification, and are indistinguishable from the more common RCC subtypes. Collecting duct carcinoma commonly shows low signal intensity on T2W MR images. They are aggressive tumors with metastatic disease at initial presentation [57].

Renal medullary carcinoma is a rare malignant neoplasm occurring almost exclusively in patients with sickle cell trait. Renal medullary carcinoma is thought to arise from medullary collecting ducts. It is exclusively found in young patients with an age range between 10 and 40 years (mean age, 22 years). The male-to-female ratio is 2:1. They are heterogeneous on imaging owing to hemorrhage and necrosis and associated with caliectasis. Similar to collecting duct carcinoma they appear hypointense on T2W MR images likely due to the presence of by-products of hemorrhage and necrosis [58].

Xp11.2 translocation–TFE3 gene fusion carcinomas account for approximately 20% of RCCs in the pediatric and adolescent age group. Both translocations t(X;17)(p11.2;q25) and t(X;1)(p11.2;q21.2) result in overexpression of transcription factor E3 protein. No specific imaging findings are yet described with Xp translocation carcinomas, with age being the biggest differentiator. Initial clinical data suggest an indolent clinical course despite advanced stage at presentation [59] (Tables 40.3 and 40.4).

TABLE 40.3 Imaging Features of Various Subtypes of RCC

Subtype	Incidence	Origin, Histology	Associations and Predispositions	Biologic Behavior	CT/MRI Precontrast	Postcontrast Imaging
Clear cell	75%	Proximal nephron, tubular epithelium	Von Hippel–Lindau (25–45%), tuberous sclerosis (2%)	Aggressiveness as per stage, ISUP grade and sarcomatoid/rhabdoid transformation. 5-year survival rate: 44–69%	Heterogeneous density/moderate to high T2 signal intensity. May contain fat	Intense to moderate enhancement
Papillary	10%	Distal nephron, tubular epithelium	Hereditary papillary RCC	Aggressiveness as per stage, ISUP grade and sarcomatoid/rhabdoid transformation. Type II have poorer prognosis. 5-year survival rate: 90%	Hypodense, low T2 signal intensity. May contain hemosiderin	Hypovascular/mild enhancement
Chromophobe	5%	Distal nephron, intercalated cells of the distal tubules	Birt–Hogg–Dubé syndrome (in association with oncocytomae)	Low mortality, 5-year survival rate: 78–93%	Isodense, intermediate T2 signal intensity	Moderate enhancement
Collecting ducts (Bellini)	1%	Collecting tubules	Subtle predominance in men	Very aggressive, mortality: 70% in 2 years	Low T2 signal, heterogeneous	Hypovascular
Medullary	1%	Distal nephron	Associated with sickle cell disease	Extremely aggressive	Heterogeneous, infiltrating	Hypovascular
Xp11 translocation	Rare	Distal/proximal nephron, may be similar to papillary or clear cell carcinoma	TFE3 gene involved in the tumor genesis	Indolent	Hypodense, intermediate to low T2 signal intensity	Hypovascular
Mucinous tubular and spindle cell	Rare	Distal nephron, tubular cells	Predominance in women	Slow-growing, rare metastases	Subtle T2 hyperintense signal, central scar may be observed	Hypovascular

TABLE 40.4 Imaging Features of Common Solid Renal Masses

Renal Lesion	Imaging Features
ccRCC	High SI on T2WI + may contain fat + hypervascular
Papillary RCC	Low SI on T2WI + may contain hemosiderin + hypovascular
Chromophobe RCC	Iso to high SI on T2WI + moderate enhancement → diagnosis is on histopathology
Classic AML	Macroscopic fat
Minimal fat AML	Low SI on T2WI + may contain microscopic fat + avid early enhancement
Oncocytoma	Iso to high SI on T2WI + avid/moderate enhancement + may show segmental inversion → diagnosis on histopathology

Staging RCC

Primary Tumor

- Preoperative imaging for staging and anatomic considerations is vital for the surgeon [60]. *As per ACR recommendations both CECT and CEMRI can be used in the staging of the primary tumor* [61]. The size of the primary tumor and degree of local invasion determine the T-stage classification in the AJCC TNM staging system (Table 40.5 and Fig. 40.10A). Tumors confined to the kidneys are staged as T1 or T2, depending on the size
- Extrarenal extension into the perinephric/renal sinus fat/pelvicalyceal system or renal vein is staged as T3a; extension of tumor thrombus into the IVC is staged as T3b (below the diaphragm) or T3c (above the diaphragm/IVC wall invasion) (Figs. 40.10 and 40.11). The extent of venous invasion of tumor is an important factor in the T-stage classification and surgical planning

TABLE 40.5 TNM AJCC 8th Edition for Renal Cell Carcinoma

T Primary Tumor
TX—Primary tumor cannot be assessed
T0—No evidence of primary tumor
T1—Tumor <7 cm or less in greatest dimension, limited to the kidney
T1a—Tumor <4 cm or less
T1b—Tumor more than 4 cm but not more than 7 cm
T2—Tumor more than 7 cm in greatest dimension, limited to the kidney
T2a—Tumor more than 7 cm but not more than 10 cm
T2b—Tumors more than 10 cm, limited to the kidney
T3—Tumor extends into major veins or perinephric tissues but not into the ipsilateral adrenal gland and not beyond the Gerota fascia
T3a—Tumor extends into the renal vein or its segmental branches, or tumor invades the pelvicalyceal system or tumor invades perirenal and/or renal sinus fat (peripelvic fat), but not beyond the Gerota fascia
T3b—Tumor extends into the vena cava below the diaphragm
T3c—Tumor extends into the vena cava above the diaphragm or invades the wall of the vena cava
T4—Tumor invades beyond the Gerota fascia (including contiguous extension into the ipsilateral adrenal gland)
N—Regional Lymph Nodes
NX—Regional lymph nodes cannot be assessed
N0—No regional lymph node metastasis
N1—Metastasis in regional lymph node(s)
M—Distant Metastasis
M0—No distant metastasis
M1—Distant metastasis

- Depending on the level of the IVC thrombus, the surgeon may need to perform more extensive surgery to obtain suprahepatic IVC access or a cardiac bypass for an intracardiac extension
- Transmural invasion of the IVC wall might necessitate a graft placement. IVC wall invasion has been described in up to 23% of cases with tumoral venous extension [62,63]

Both CECT and MRI have equal sensitivity in detecting venous involvement [64]. The invasion of the IVC wall is however better recognized on MRI. The highest sensitivity and specificity in assessing venous involvement is achieved with a gradient-echo sequence [65,66] (Figs. 40.12 and 40.13).

- Mayo classification system for intravascular tumor extent aids in guiding the extent of surgical complexity necessary for tumor resection [67] (Fig. 40.14 and Table 40.6)
- Extension beyond the Gerota fascia (Fig. 40.13C), involvement of the ipsilateral adrenal gland, and adjacent organ involvement is T4 disease [68]. Both CT and MRI have low positive predictive value for differentiating invasion from the abutment [69,70]

Nodes

- Regional lymph nodes extend from the renal hilum to the aortic bifurcation (Fig. 40.10B). Cross-sectional imaging criteria for diagnosing involvement of lymph nodes include a short-axis diameter of >1 cm, disruption of the normal lymph node architecture and shape. Based on these criteria, CT has a false-negative rate of about 10%, but has a high false-positive rate with nearly 50% of enlarged nodes being benign [71]

Metastases

- *The most common sites are lungs, bones, lymph nodes, liver, adrenal gland, and brain in decreasing order* (Figs. 40.15 and 40.16). RCC can however spread virtually anywhere in the body, including pancreas, soft tissues, nasal septum, and gall bladder and present with atypical symptoms. Metastases from RCC are notorious to occur even years after surgical treatment of the primary (Figs. 40.15C and 40.16) [72]. Local recurrence can be in the

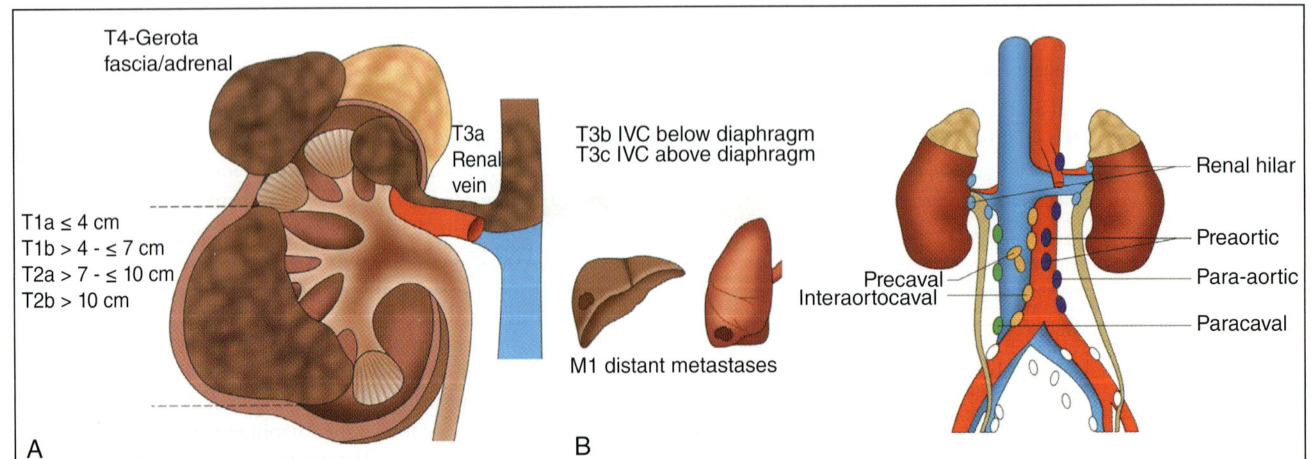

Figure 40.10 AJCC staging. (A) Schematic representation of TNM staging of renal cell cancer according to AJCC 8th edition. (B) Regional nodal stations (AJCC 8th edition). Corticomedullary phase image shows moderate enhancement.

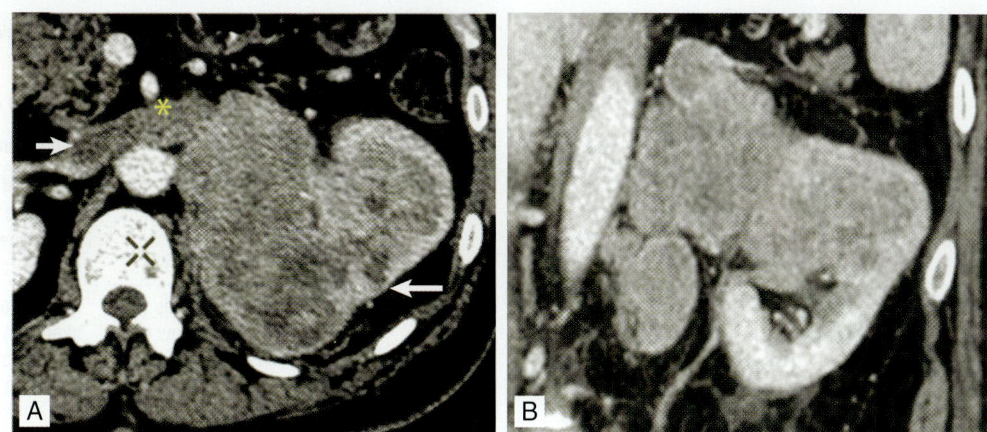

Figure 40.11 Clear cell RCC with sarcomatoid features. Axial and coronal CECT images demonstrate a large mass with epicenter in the interpole of the left kidney. On the axial contrast image (A), the mass (*large arrow*) is showing heterogeneous enhancement. Enhancing thrombus noted in the renal vein suggesting tumor thrombus (*asterisk*) proximally and nonenhancing bland thrombus downstream (*small arrow*). (B) Coronal CT image again shows the extensive soft-tissue component.

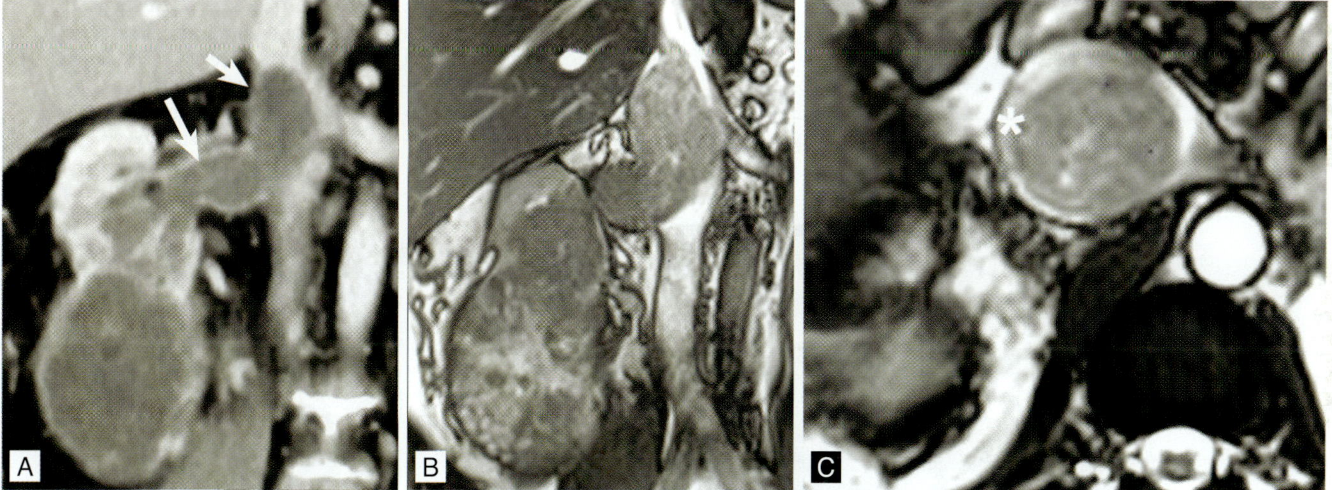

Figure 40.12 RCC with tumor thrombus—T3b. (A) Coronal CT image shows an enhancing heterogeneous hypodense mass arising from lower pole of the right kidney. Tumor thrombus extends into the renal vein (*long arrow*) and IVC (*short arrow*). (B and C) Coronal and axial T2-weighted GRE MR images show a heterogeneous hyperintense mass. The smooth margin of the tumor thrombus can be separately seen from the IVC wall, which is not involved (*asterisk* in C).

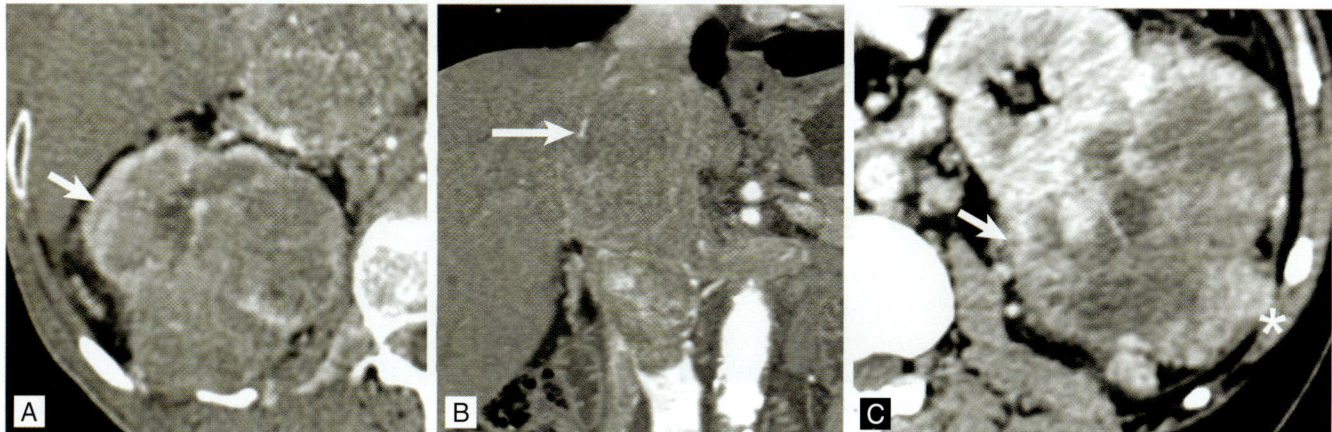

Figure 40.13 (A and B) Axial and coronal contrast-enhanced CT image shows a heterogeneous enhancing mass (*short arrow*) arising from the right kidney. There is a tumor thrombus extending into IVC (*long arrow*) up to the level of the diaphragm, causing IVC expansion with wall invasion—T3c. (C) Axial contrast-enhanced CT of a different patient shows an advanced stage ISUP grade III clear cell RCC (*short arrow*) extending to involve the Gerota's fascia (*asterisk*).

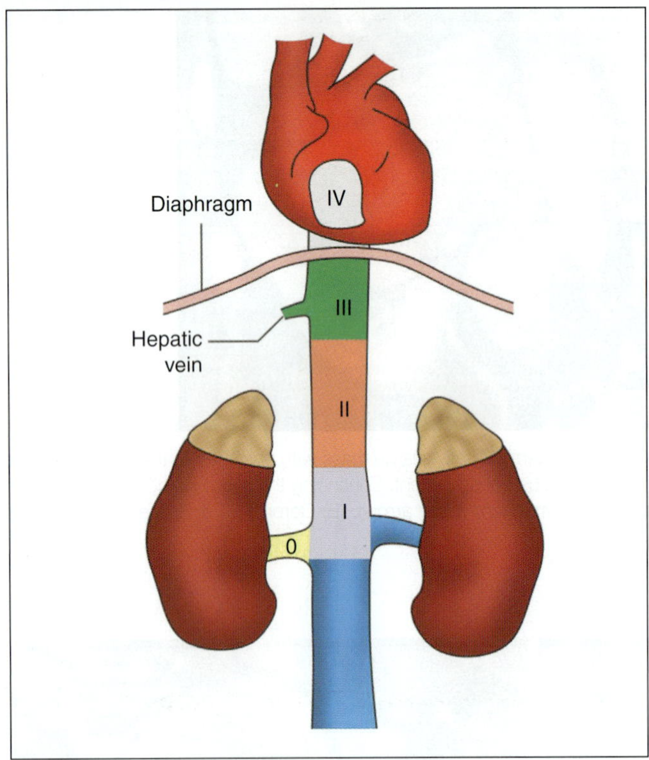

Figure 40.14 Mayo classification of tumor thrombus. Schematic representation of Mayo classification of tumor thrombus.

TABLE 40.6 Mayo Classification of Tumor Thrombus With Surgical Approach

Level	Extension of Thrombus	Surgical Approach
Level 0	Into the renal vein	Renal vein ligation
Level 1	Tumor thrombus is either at the entry of renal vein or extends within the IVC < 2 cm	Milking of IVC tumor thrombus into the renal vein followed by renal vein ligation
Level 2	Tumor thrombus extends within the IVC > 2 cm but below the hepatic veins	Minor mobilization of liver with clamping of intrahepatic IVC, clamping of infrarenal IVC and contralateral renal vein
Level 3	Tumor thrombus involves the intrahepatic IVC/ hepatic vein below the diaphragm	Extensive mobilization of liver including ligation of diaphragmatic attachments, clamping of suprahepatic IVC with adjunctive venovenous or cardiopulmonary bypass
Level 4	Tumor thrombus extends above the diaphragm or into the right atrium	Involvement of cardiothoracic surgery, with potential thoracotomy and open-heart surgery

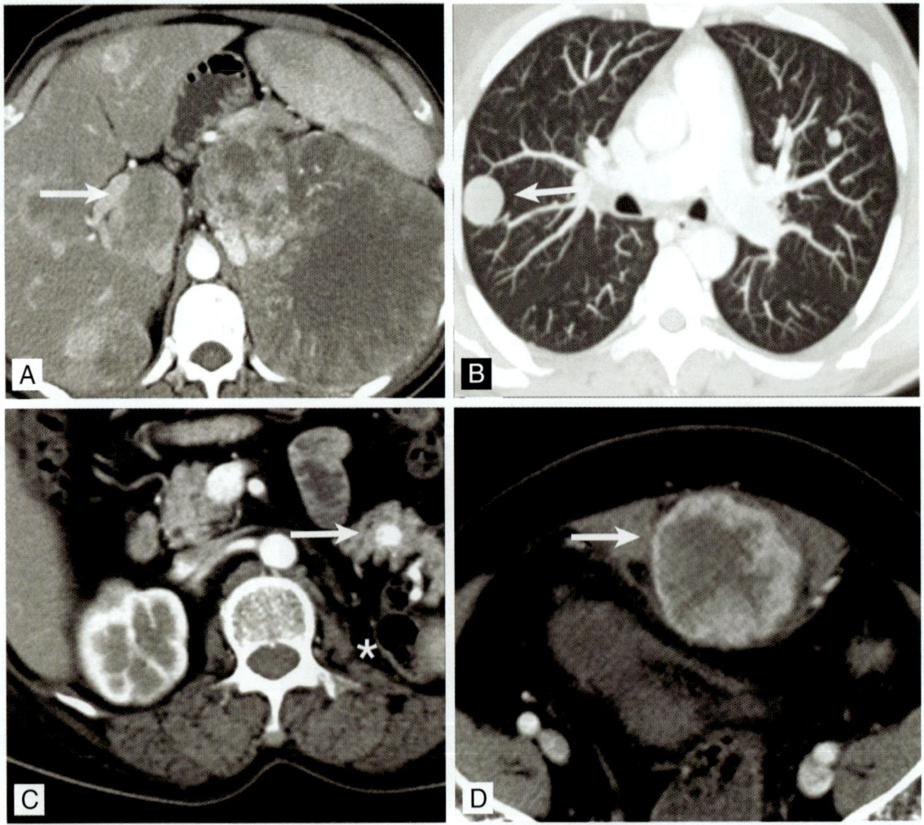

Figure 40.15 (A) Axial contrast-enhanced CT abdomen with large clear cell carcinoma arising from the left kidney. Liver shows multiple hypervascular metastatic lesions (*arrow*). (B) Axial CT thorax of the same patient shows multiple lung metastases (*arrow*). (C) A 45-year-old female 5 years post left nephrectomy for clear cell RCC, on surveillance. There is an avidly enhancing nodule in the tail of pancreas (*arrow*) which was biopsied and proved to be metastasis from renal origin. (D) Another 55-year-old male patient, 1 year after partial nephrectomy (clear cell RCC ISUP grade IV) presented with an enhancing anterior abdominal wall mass (*arrow*), proved on biopsy to be metastatic RCC.

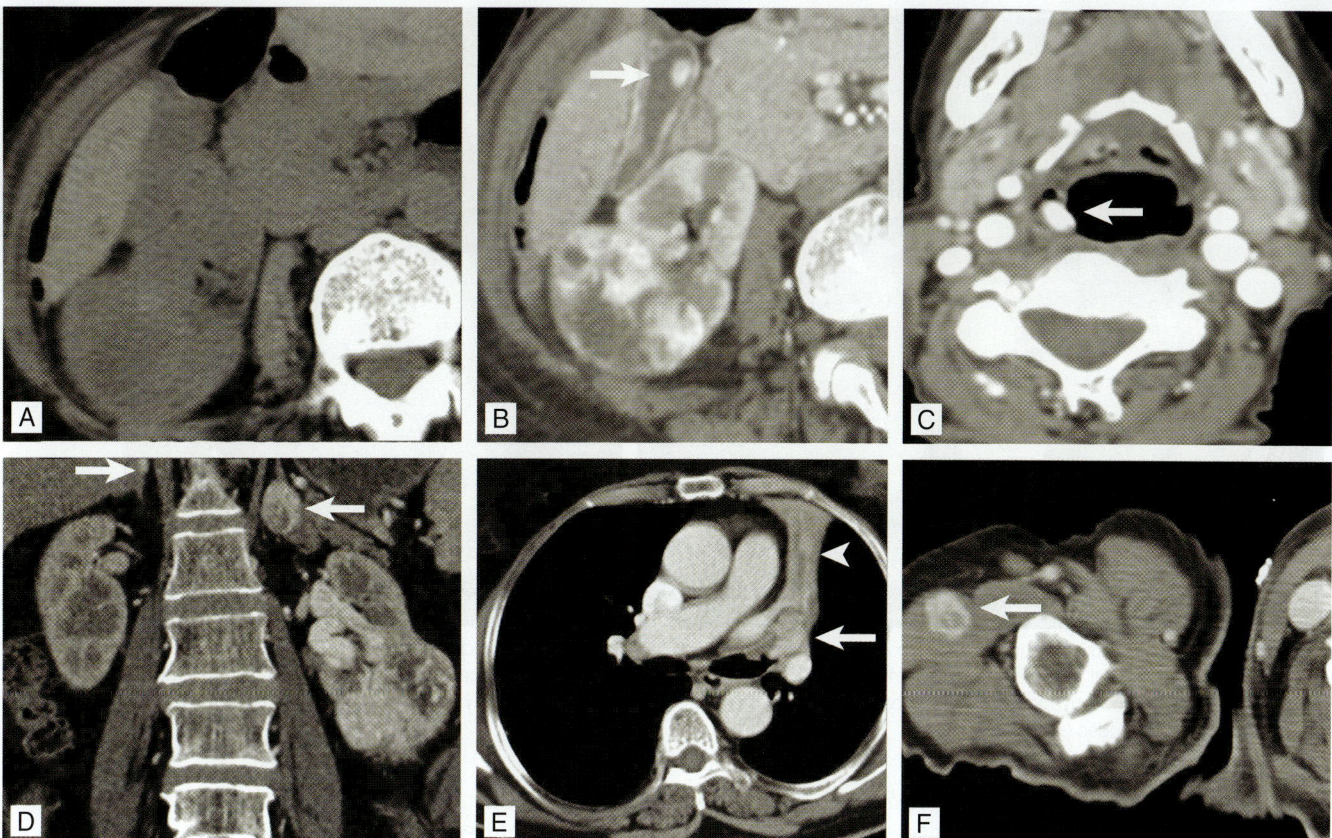

Figure 40.16 Other metastatic sites. (A and B) Axial noncontrast and contrast-enhanced CT images show right renal clear cell RCC with metastatic nodule in the gall bladder (*arrow*). This patient had multiple other sites of metastases with similar enhancement pattern. (C) A 70-year-old male patient presented with bleeding from oral cavity. Contrast-enhanced CT shows an enhancing nodule in the right pharyngeal region (*arrow*). HPE revealed metastases from RCC. Patient had a history of nephrectomy for RCC. (D) Left renal mass with bilateral adrenal metastases (*arrows*). (E) RCC with endobronchial metastases (*arrow*) leading to collapse of lingula of the left lung (*arrowhead*). (F) Hyperenhancing metastatic nodule in the right trapezius muscle (*arrow*) in a known patient of RCC.

form of single or multiple enhancing soft-tissue nodules in the surgical bed along with pancreatic nodules

- Chest CT should be used to detect pulmonary metastasis in patients with large or locally advanced tumors. The risk of pulmonary metastasis increases with the size of the primary tumor, although universally accepted guidelines have not yet been developed on whom to screen with a CT chest [60]. Few series suggest tumor size ≥T1b, N1, and systemic symptoms are associated with higher risk of positive chest CT [73]. In our institution, we perform CT chest in any indeterminate renal mass >T1a lesions. A chest radiograph is a minimum requirement. In patients with suspicion for metastatic disease, other investigations such as an MRI brain and or a bone scan may be performed [60]

Teaching Points

- Clear cell RCC is the most common variant with the majority being sporadic
- The presence of microscopic fat is a common feature of ccRCC
- Papillary RCC has a better prognosis and survival compared with clear cell RCC
- Papillary RCC is hypovascular and shows progressive enhancement. They show hypointense signals on T2-weighted images and signal drop on in-phase chemical shift images
- Chromophobe RCC originates from the intercalated cells of the renal cortex (same as the oncocytomas) and demonstrates an eosinophilic cytoplasm. Approximately 30–40% of cases show central stellate scar. They show segmental enhancement inversion similar to oncocytoma
- Both CT/MRI are accurate in staging and preoperative planning
- Tumor thrombus in renal vein T3a/IVC below the diaphragm T3b/IVC above the diaphragm/wall invasion/T3c
- Gradient echo MR sequences have high sensitivity specificity for IVC wall invasion

Other Malignant Tumors

Lymphoma

Lymphomatous involvement of the kidneys can be primary or secondary with the latter being more common [74,75]. *Primary renal lymphoma is rare accounting for 1% of cases* [76]. *The most common variety being B cell type non-Hodgkin lymphoma.*

Imaging Features

- Renal lymphoma can present as multiple or solitary nodules/masses, retroperitoneal and perinephric space involvement, and diffuse infiltration of one or both kidneys [77] (Fig. 40.17A)

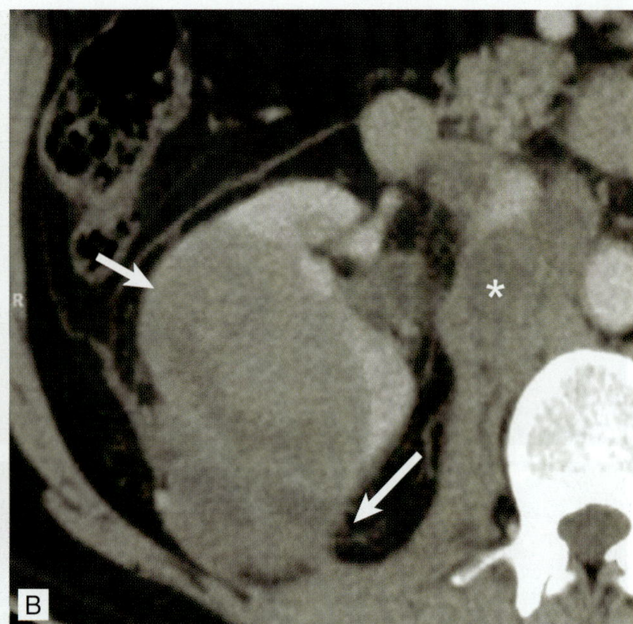

Figure 40.17 Non-Hodgkin lymphoma with secondary renal involvement. (A) Contrast-enhanced CT shows hypodense bilateral renal masses (*short arrow*) with retroperitoneal lymphadenopathy (*long arrow*). (B) Axial contrast-enhanced CT image of another patient presenting with high-grade non-Hodgkin lymphoma shows hypodense mildly enhancing lobulated mass (*arrow*) in the right kidney with perinephric extension (*long arrow*) and enlarged retroperitoneal lymph nodes (*asterisk*).

- *The most common presentation is multiple renal masses* of size 1–3 cm seen in up to 60% of the patients. They have homogeneous hypoattenuation on CT, hyperintense on MR imaging, and hypoenhancing compared with background renal parenchyma [78]
- Contiguous extension to the kidneys or perinephric space from large retroperitoneal masses is the second most common pattern (25–30% of cases). These patients usually have widespread disease with bulky tumors, and many are immunocompromised. At imaging, large retroperitoneal masses are seen invading or displacing the adjacent kidney. Hydronephrosis caused by entrapment of the ureters is common
- Another pattern of involvement is nephromegaly without distortion of the normal shape of the kidneys, resulting from diffuse infiltration of the renal interstitium by malignant lymphocytes. This appearance is more common in Burkitt lymphoma, either disseminated or limited to the kidneys (primary renal lymphoma). Acute renal failure caused by destruction of the normal renal architecture may lead the patient to seek medical attention if both kidneys are extensively infiltrated
- Perirenal lymphomatous involvement, while uncommon, is pathognomonic for lymphoma. It can be secondary to direct extension from retroperitoneal lymphoma or due to renal disease having transcapsular spread, or rarely isolated perirenal soft tissue without renal compression or functional impairment

Another uncommon presentation is as a solitary renal lesion (10%). They are difficult to differentiate from pRCC and need a biopsy for this purpose [79] (Fig. 40.17B). Associated abdominal lymphadenopathy may be present in more than half the cases.

Metastases

Metastases to the kidney are relatively uncommon. The reported incidence of renal metastasis from extrarenal neoplasms is 2–20% [77]. *The most common primary tumor that metastasizes to the kidney is lung carcinoma, breast, female genital tract, head and neck, colon, and prostate are other sites.* Renal metastases occur more commonly at the junction of the renal cortex and medulla, with ill-defined borders and low-level enhancement [80,81].

Differential Diagnosis for Renal Lesions

Developmental renal pseudotumors like prominent columns of Bertin, dromedary humps, persistent fetal lobulations must be differentiated from true renal masses by characterization of normal renal parenchyma imaging features [82] (Table 40.7).

Apart from the benign and malignant neoplasms discussed earlier, the differential diagnosis of a true renal lesion includes infectious, inflammatory, and granulomatous diseases (e.g., pyelonephritis/abscess, xanthogranulomatous pyelonephritis, and IgG4 disease). Focal/multifocal pyelonephritis and abscess are associated with fever, chills, flank pain, and pyuria [83]. Xanthogranulomatous pyelonephritis is seen more commonly in diabetic middle-aged women with renal stones, infection (most common by *Escherichia coli* and Proteus), and/or congenital anomalies. There is destruction of the normal renal architecture, enlarged kidney, contracted pelvis, staghorn calculus, and perinephric inflammatory changes [84,85]. Imaging shows hypoperfused wedge-shaped areas, extending from the papilla to the cortex and associated inflammatory changes.

IgG4-related disease is an uncommon disorder that can affect any organ, but commonly involves pancreas, retroperitoneum, lymph nodes and salivary glands. Renal involvement in IgG4-related disease is observed in 35% patients with autoimmune pancreatitis. A tubulointerstitial nephritis pattern with fibrosis and abundant IgG4-positive plasma cell infiltration is the most common finding on histopathology. Various imaging patterns have been described: *The most common pattern is bilateral round or wedge-shaped peripheral cortical lesions.* Other less common patterns include diffuse patchy involvement, a rim of soft tissue around the kidney, bilateral nodules in the renal sinuses, and diffuse wall thickening of the renal pelvis. Rarely it manifests as a solitary round lesion. The differential diagnosis for the most common pattern includes pyelonephritis, vascular insult, metastases, and lymphoma [86].

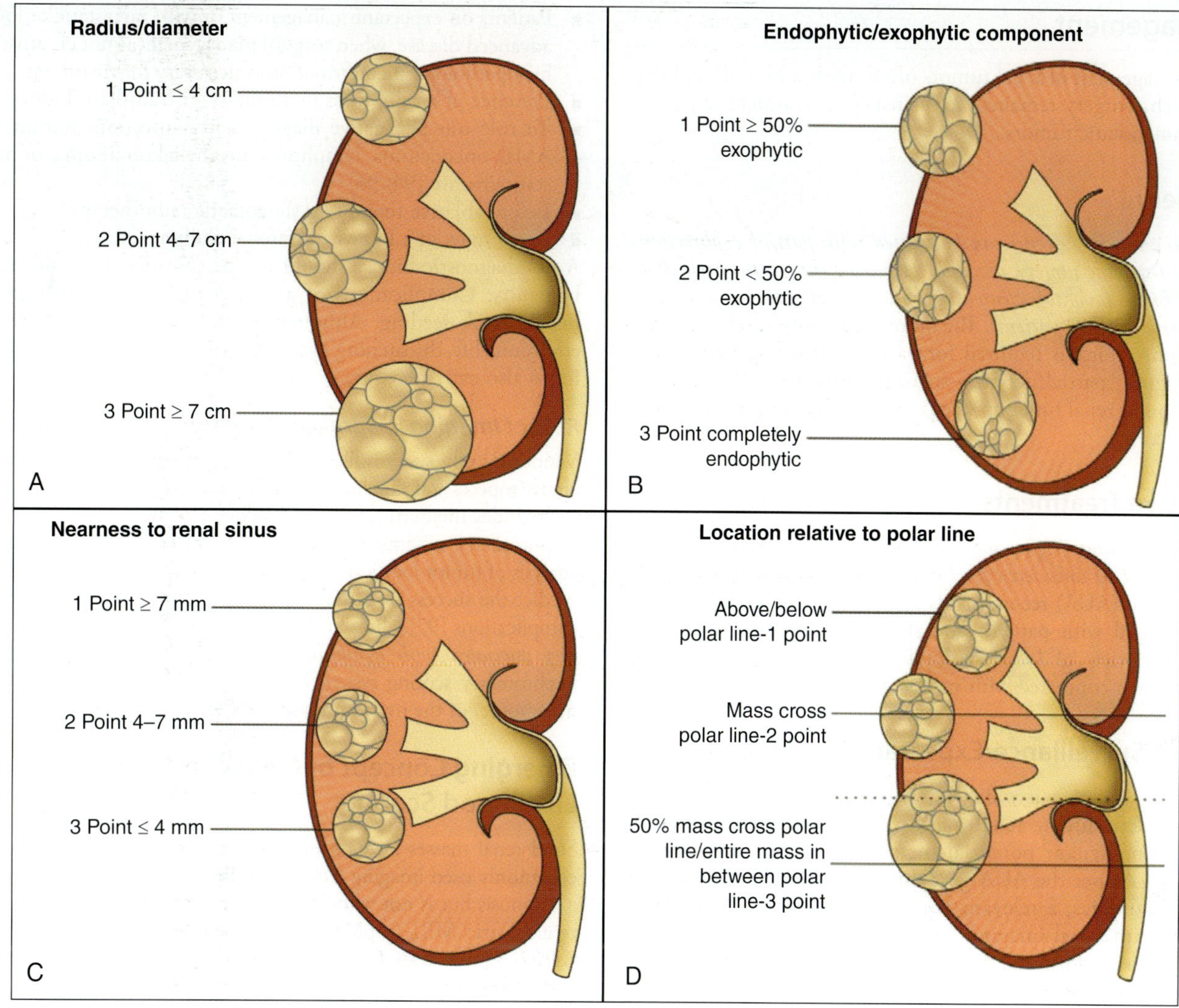

Figure 40.18 Renal nephrometry score.

TABLE 40.7 Differential Diagnosis of Renal Mass

Developmental	
1. Hypertrophic columns of Bertin	USG similar echogenicity of renal parenchyma and smooth contour. CT/MRI have the same enhancement pattern as the kidney.
2. Dromedary hump	Focal bulge on the lateral border of the left kidney. USG shows the same echogenicity as the kidney. CT/MRI shows normal renal parenchyma.
3. Persistent fetal lobulations	Normal variant diagnosed in 4% of children and 10% of the adult population. It consists of an indentation of the renal surface in between the renal pyramids, caused by an incomplete fusion of the renal lobules during early childhood.
Infectious	
1. Abscess	Subacute and chronic forms may lack signs of infection and are difficult to differentiate from a renal malignancy. On CT low-attenuation mass with thick irregular wall. Perinephric fat stranding and fascial thickening.
2. Pyelonephritis	Clinical features—Fever, leucocytosis. Poorly defined interface of lesion with renal parenchyma. Edema in the surrounding renal parenchyma, no overlying bulge on the renal surface and asymmetric perinephric fat stranding.
Inflammatory	
1. Xanthogranulomatous pyelonephritis	Associated with staghorn calculus in 70% cases. More common in diabetics. USG—Single or multiple hypoechoic areas in the parenchyma of an enlarged kidney, with central echogenic foci representing calculi. CT—Multiple low-attenuation areas (lipid-rich xanthogranulomatous tissue) and calcification in the mass.
2. IgG4-related disease	The most common pattern is bilateral round or wedge-shaped peripheral cortical lesions. Other less common patterns are diffuse patchy involvement, a rim of soft tissue around the kidney, bilateral nodules in the renal sinuses, and diffuse wall thickening of the renal pelvis. Differential diagnosis ranges from infection to malignancy.

Management

The management of renal tumors often needs a multidisciplinary approach. Surgery remains the mainstay of treatment, especially in nonmetastatic tumors.

Surgery

Smaller tumors (<4 cm) can be treated with partial nephrectomy/nephron-sparing surgery, which is considered the treatment of choice as it achieves favorable clinical and oncological outcomes and minimizes risk in CKD patients. The more commonly performed radical nephrectomy is required for patients with larger tumors or challenging partial/nephron-sparing surgeries. The baseline background renal function needs to be considered before radical nephrectomy.

Ablative Treatments

Thermal ablation (e.g., microwave ablation or radiofrequency ablation) should be considered for lesions <3 cm. American Urological Association (AUA) recommends ablative therapy options should be discussed with patients and should be preferred in smaller lesions in view of lesser morbidity and potentially equivalent results when compared with surgery [87].

Active Surveillance/Expectant Management

Active surveillance is watchful waiting for the management of small indeterminate renal masses. Many series have reported the low malignant potential for small (<4 cm) renal masses [88–90]. As per the AUA guidelines, in elderly and poor surgical candidates, a relevant approach may be to follow these masses with serial imaging rather than performing surgery as there is no additional benefit on overall survival [91,92]. Intervention can happen if the tumor is growing too rapidly or there are other concerning features which develop while on surveillance.

Table 40.8 lists the factors favoring active surveillance.

Percutaneous Biopsy

Despite the advances in imaging, distinction between various subtypes of RCC may not be possible. Differentiating benign from malignant renal masses can be challenging. Incidentally detected enhancing renal masses pose significant diagnostic dilemmas, necessitating a diagnostic biopsy which can avoid unnecessary surgery [93].

Indications for percutaneous biopsy of renal mass are:

- Confirmation of RCC when the surgical risk is high so as to avoid operating on benign masqueraders
- Patients on expectant management or with metastatic or locally advanced disease, when surgical management is not curative and histopathological confirmation is necessary for treatment
- Presence of a solid mass in a solitary or transplant kidney
- To rule out alternative diagnoses like infection, minimal fat AML, oncocytoma, lymphoma, urothelial carcinoma, or metastatic disease [94–96]
- Before ablative therapy or stereotactic radiotherapy
- Renal mass in a known extrarenal malignancy

A nondiagnostic biopsy should not be considered as evidence of benignity. Complications of a biopsy include hemorrhage and needle track seeding. Although a small amount of bleeding is common, life-threatening events are unusual. Needle track seeding is also extremely rare.

TABLE 40.8 Factors Favoring Active Surveillance

Patient Related	Tumor Related
Elderly	Tumor size <3 cm
Comorbidities (life expectancy <5 years)	Favorable histology
High perioperative risk	Growth rate <5 mm/year
Poor performance status	Noninfiltrative
Patient preference	
Deranged renal function	

Role of Imaging in Surgical Planning

Various scoring systems like RENAL nephrometry, PADUA (preoperative aspects and dimensions used for anatomy), and C-Index (centrality index method) have been developed to guide surgical planning. Nephrometry systems achieve two primary goals: a methodological analysis of tumor location and standardization of reporting. They also predict the success of partial nephrectomy and risk of postoperative complications [97]. *Any score above 10 predicts high complexity in surgery associated with significant postoperative complications.* RENAL nephrometry scoring system is an easy-to-remember acronym (i.e., mnemonic) of the five features scored (Table 40.9, Fig. 40.18).

Emerging Concept of Clear Cell Likelihood Scoring

Solid renal masses have an unknown malignant potential with the commonly used imaging techniques. Biopsy can be used to arrive at a diagnosis but is not without complications. There is scope of multiparametric MRI (mpMRI) to diagnose aggressive histology (i.e., ccRCC vs non-ccRCC) through a clear cell likelihood score (ccLS). It does not intend to replace histopathologic evaluation but focuses only on determination of the probability of ccRCC (or non-ccRCC) to guide management decision-making. ccLS does not differentiate low- versus high-grade ccRCC nor does it differentiate other less common aggressive non-ccRCC malignancies. ccLS provides a five point scale (1–5) which assigns probability of ccRCC. It can help the

TABLE 40.9 Renal Nephrometry Score

Component	1 Point	2 Points	3 Points
R (radius, maximal diameter) (cm)	≤4	>4 but <7	≥7
E (exophytic/endophytic)	≥50% exophytic	<50% exophytic	Completely endophytic
N (nearness to collecting system/renal sinus) (mm)	≥7	>4 but <7	≤4
A (anterior/posterior locator)/no points given			
L (location relative to polar lines)	Entirely below lower polar or above upper polar line	Mass crosses polar line	50% of mass is across polar line or mass is entirely between polar lines or mass crosses axial midline

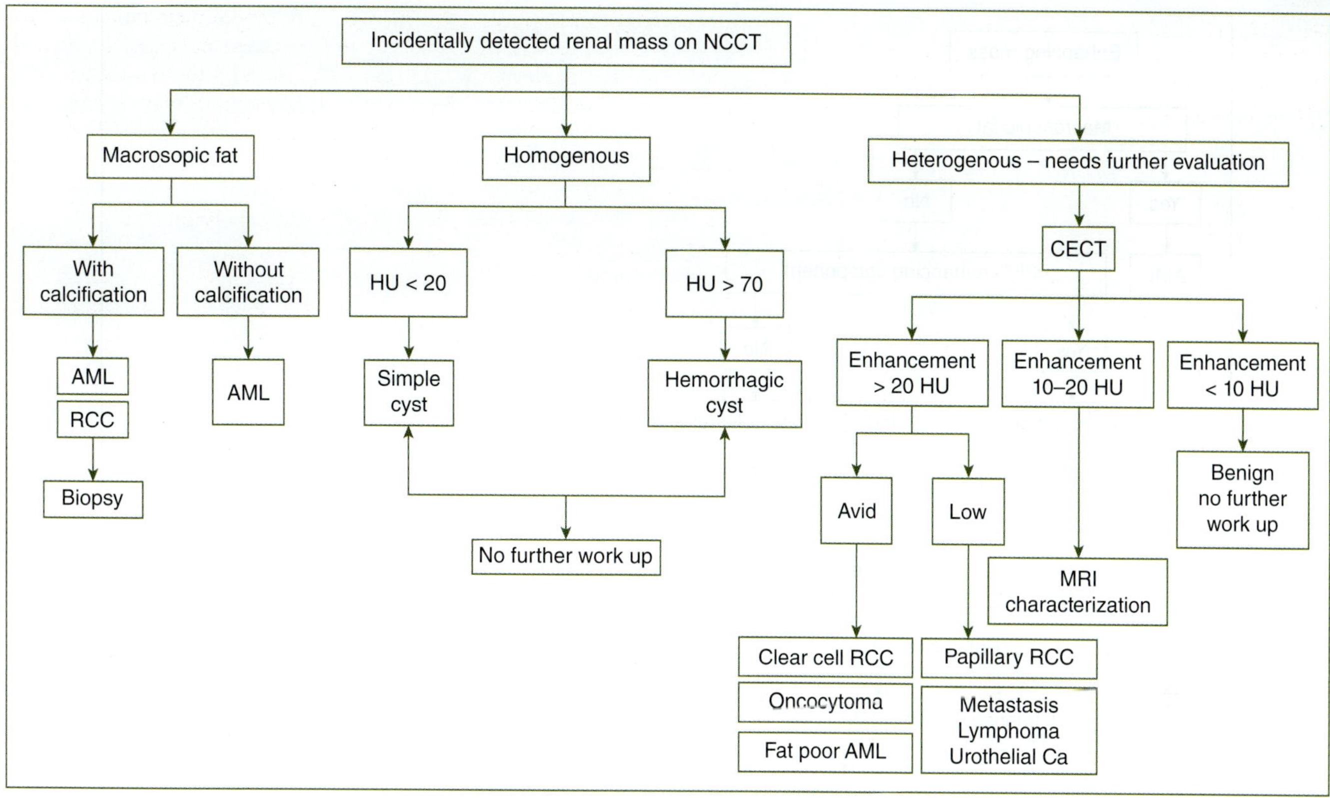

Figure 40.19 Algorithmic approach of diagnosis and workup of renal masses on the CT scan.

patient and treating physician decide between definitive treatment (ccLS ≥ 4), biopsy (ccLS3), or AS (ccLS ≤ 2), depending on other patient factors and shared decision-making. A ccLS is based on a Likert scale (1—very unlikely, 2—unlikely, 3—equivocal, 4—likely, and 5—very likely) for interpretation of mpMRI examinations to noninvasively detect ccRCC [98].

Imaging in Metastatic RCC

Approximately 25–30% of patients with RCC have metastases at presentation [99]. There has been a paradigm shift in management from chemotherapy agents to tyrosine kinase inhibitors, antiangiogenic agents, and immunotherapy, limiting the importance of traditional criteria (RECIST/WHO) for response evaluation. Newer classifications like Choi or modified Choi criteria, and Morphology, Attenuation, Size, and Structure criteria provide better assessment of tumor response to these new therapies, incorporating decrease in tumoral enhancement and attenuation as a marker of response [100].

Using a template/checklist is ideal while reporting solid renal masses. This brings uniformity in reporting and contributes to better overall patient management.

Approach to Renal Masses

An algorithm for an approach to renal masses on CT and MRI is given in Figs. 40.19 and 40.20.

Cystic Masses of the Kidney

Introduction

Cystic renal lesions are commonly encountered at routine imaging. Majority of them are benign simple cysts which can be confirmed on ultrasonography [101]. However, even malignant renal lesions can have a cystic appearance on imaging. The diagnostic challenge is to distinguish them from the more common benign cysts. *The definition of "cystic mass" is a lesion with the solid portion occupying not more than one-fourth (<25%) of the volume* [102]. Cystic renal masses constitute about 15% of all renal masses [103]. The Bosniak classification system introduced in 1986 by Mortan Bosniak is a CT-based classification system which helps robustly categorize cystic renal lesions and guide further management [104]. It initially described four categories, but was later modified to include five categories—namely, I, II, II-F, III, and IV, according to their degree of complexity and likelihood of malignancy.

Although both radiologists and urologists use the Bosniak classification in clinical practice, several studies highlighted important limitations. Inter-observer agreement is low for Bosniak IIF and III masses, in part because the criteria for "thickened" and "multiple" septa were undefined and subjective. Furthermore, approximately half the Bosniak III lesions are benign, and surgical resection is often performed without benefit [105]. To overcome these shortcomings a new Bosniak classification system (version 2019) has been proposed. In the recent version 2019, previously subjective terms, such as "thickened" and "multiple" are objectively defined, and other criteria such as perceived versus measurable enhancement and lesion size, have been removed. It attempts to be more objective and have greater applicability [106]. MRI has been formally incorporated into the classification system. We will discuss the 2019 Bosniak classification system (Fig. 40.21 and Table 40.10).These guidelines have to be followed after infections/inflammatory/vascular lesions have been excluded.

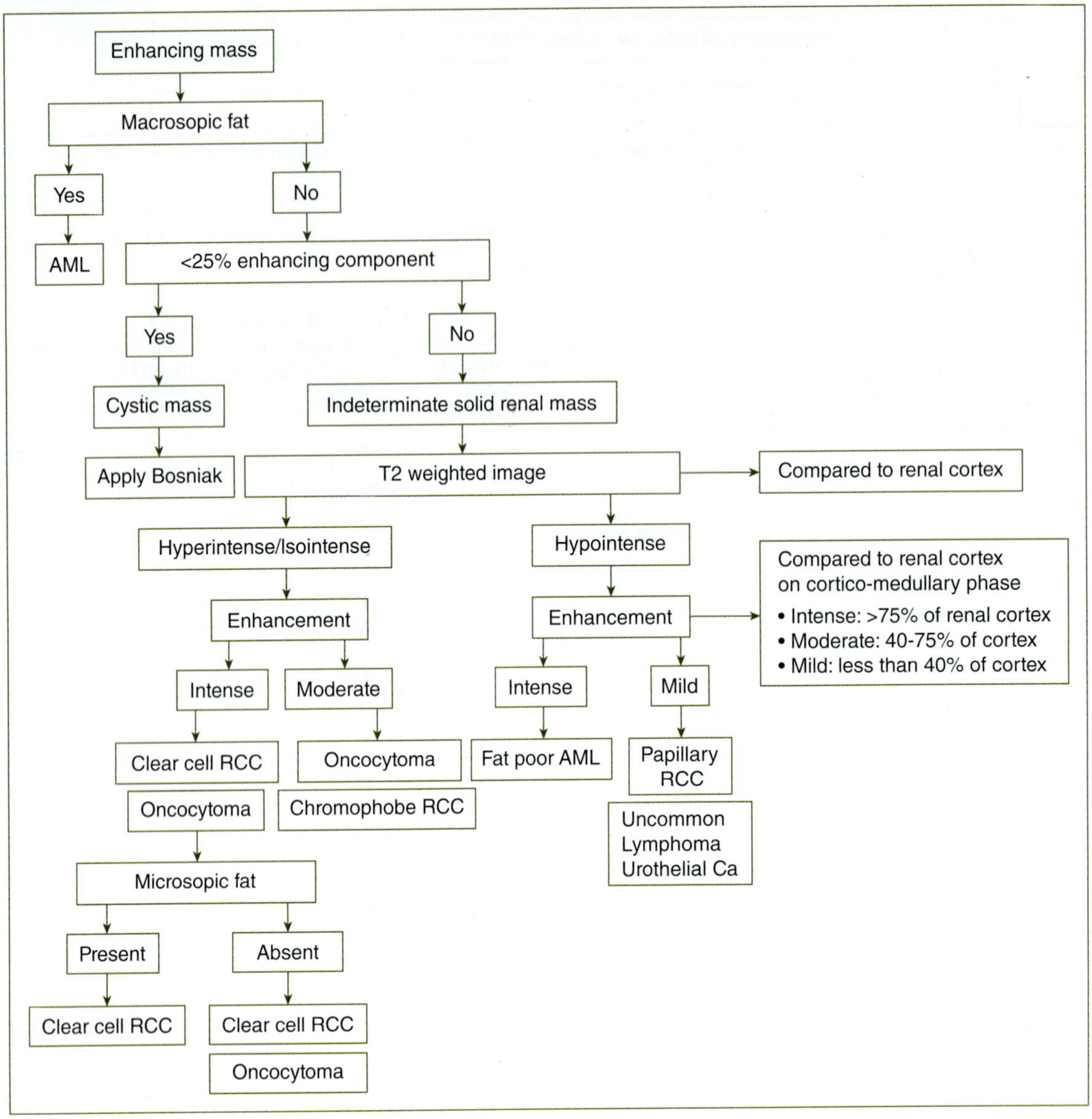

Enhancing mass
Macrosopic fat
- Yes → AML
- No → <25% enhancing component
  - Yes → Cystic mass → Apply Bosniak
  - No → Indeterminate solid renal mass → T2 weighted image (Compared to renal cortex)
    - Hyperintense/Isointense → Enhancement
      - Intense → Clear cell RCC, Oncocytoma → Microsopic fat
        - Present → Clear cell RCC
        - Absent → Clear cell RCC, Oncocytoma
      - Moderate → Oncocytoma, Chromophobe RCC
    - Hypointense → Enhancement
      - Intense → Fat poor AML
      - Mild → Papillary RCC; Uncommon Lymphoma Urothelial Ca

Compared to renal cortex on cortico-medullary phase
- Intense: >75% of renal cortex
- Moderate: 40-75% of cortex
- Mild: less than 40% of cortex

Figure 40.20 Algorithmic approach of diagnosis and workup of renal masses on MRI.

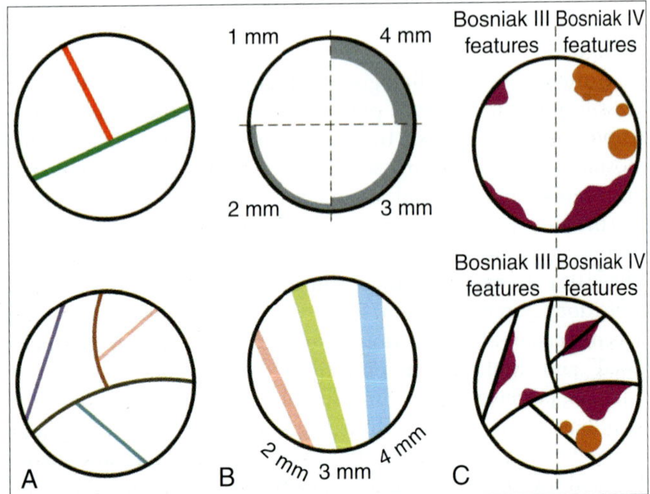

Figure 40.21 (A–C) Schematic representation of cystic renal masses according to Bosniak classification 2019 version.

Imaging Modalities

Ultrasonography

Ultrasonography is the first line of investigation to differentiate between simple and complex renal cysts. When characteristic features of simple cysts (anechoic, well-defined margins and posterior acoustic enhancement) are absent, the lesion is called a complex cyst, warranting further cross-sectional imaging [107]. CEUS with microbubble agents provides real-time evaluation of microvasculature and is emerging as promising modality for differentiating cystic and solid renal lesions, characterizing complex renal cystic and indeterminate renal masses [14,108,109]. Ultrasonography is however not formally incorporated in the Bosniak classification system; hence a formal Bosniak category should not be given on an ultrasonography report.

CT and MRI

CECT/CEMRI are the modality of choice in evaluating cystic renal masses. CEMRI is used when CT is contraindicated (e.g., patients

TABLE 40.10 Bosniak Classification

Bosniak Classification	Wall	Septa	Calcification	Enhancing Nodule	Management	Percentage Malignancy
I	Thin ≤2 mm May enhance Smooth wall	–		–	No follow-up	Nil
II	Thin ≤2 mm May enhance	Thin ≤2 mm Few ≤3	Any type of calcification suggested. MRI if thick and nodular calcification	–	No follow-up	Approaching nil
IIF	Smooth minimal thickening (3 mm) Enhancement present	Many ≥4 thickness – 3 mm Enhancement present	Any type of calcification	–	Observe	5% (0–38%)
III	Thick ≥4 mm Irregular (≤3 mm obtusely marginated convex protrusion) Enhancement present	Thick ≥4 mm Irregular (≤3 mm obtusely marginated convex protrusions) Enhancement present	Any type of calcification	–	Surgery/follow-up	50% (25–100%)
IV	Well defined Enhancement present		Any type of calcification	1) Convex protrusion ≥4mm Obtuse margins 2) Convex protrusion of any size with acute margins	Surgery/follow-up	80%

with allergy to iodinated contrast agent) or as a problem-solving modality. MRI can demonstrate definitive enhancement in those cysts that show equivocal enhancement at CT [110]. Dual-energy CT and MRI subtraction techniques have value in equivocal enhancement to ascertain true versus pseudoenhancement [111]. In cystic renal masses, ACR recommends CT or MRI with and without contrast and CEUS as the initial imaging modality of choice. These procedures are equivalent alternatives [112].

Bosniak Classification

Bosniak Category I

Category I is a simple benign cyst with a thin well-defined wall ≤2 mm and no septa or calcifications. The wall may enhance. On CT they have fluid attenuation with HU values <20. On MRI they have uniform signal intensity similar to CSF.

Bosniak Category II

Bosniak category II cysts are essentially benign.

This category includes:

1. Cysts with 1–3 thin septa, that is, septa ≤2 mm in thickness on CT or MRI. The septa or wall may enhance and have calcification of any type
2. Homogeneous nonenhancing cysts with >20 HU attenuation at renal mass protocol CT; may have calcification of any type
3. Homogeneous lesions of attenuation 21–30 HU at portal venous phase CT or homogeneous lesions of attenuation −9 to 20 HU or ≥70 HU on noncontrast CT
4. Homogeneous low-attenuation lesions that are too small to characterize
5. Homogeneously markedly T2 hyperintense (similar to cerebrospinal fluid) cysts or markedly T1 hyperintense (approximately 2.5 times normal renal parenchymal signal intensity) cysts on noncontrast MRI
6. Cystic lesions with any number of thin (≤2 mm) nonenhancing septa on MRI

These cysts are benign and do not require treatment or radiological follow-up (Fig. 40.22A and B).

Bosniak Category IIF

Cystic masses in this category are more complicated than category II but with less worrisome features than lesions in category III. This category includes cystic lesions with a smooth minimally thickened (3 mm) enhancing wall, or smooth minimal thickening (3 mm) of one or more enhancing septa, or many (≥4) smooth thin enhancing septa. Cystic masses that are heterogeneously hyperintense at unenhanced fat-saturated T1-weighted imaging are also included. Progression in these cysts is generally a strong indicator of malignancy. The development of enhancing soft-tissue component(s) should upgrade the cystic mass and result in surgical treatment.

Malignancy rates for category IIF cysts of up to 5% have been reported [113]. There are no definitive studies determining duration or frequency of follow-up for Bosniak IIF cysts. *ACR white paper recommends first semiannual and then annual follow-up for a minimum of 5 years to allow for morphologic change to be identified* [114] (Fig. 40.22C).

Bosniak Category III

Cystic masses that are more complicated and contain enhancing thick irregular walls and/or septa are included here. This category includes cystic masses with one or more enhancing thick (≥4 mm width) walls or septa, or enhancing irregular (displaying ≤3 mm obtusely marginated convex protrusion/s) on the walls or septa. *Approximately 50% of the Bosniak III masses are malignant* (ranging from 25% to 100%) [115] (Fig. 40.23). *Definitive treatment of lesions in this category is surgery.*

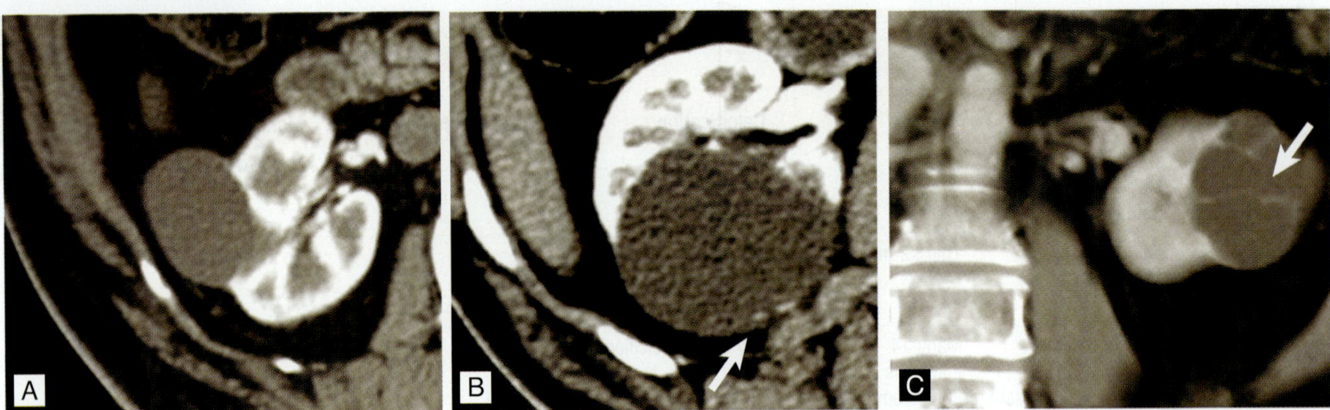

Figure 40.22 Bosniak I, II, IIF cysts. (A) Axial contrast-enhanced CT image shows an exophytic thin walled cyst in the interpolar region of the right kidney (Bosniak I). (B) Axial contrast-enhanced CT shows a thin walled cyst with linear wall calcification (*arrow*), consistent with Bosniak II cyst. (C) Coronal contrast-enhanced CT image shows a cyst (*arrow*) with three septae with smooth minimal thickening (3 mm) of septae in the upper pole of the left kidney, representing a Bosniak IIF cyst according to Bosniak 2019 version.

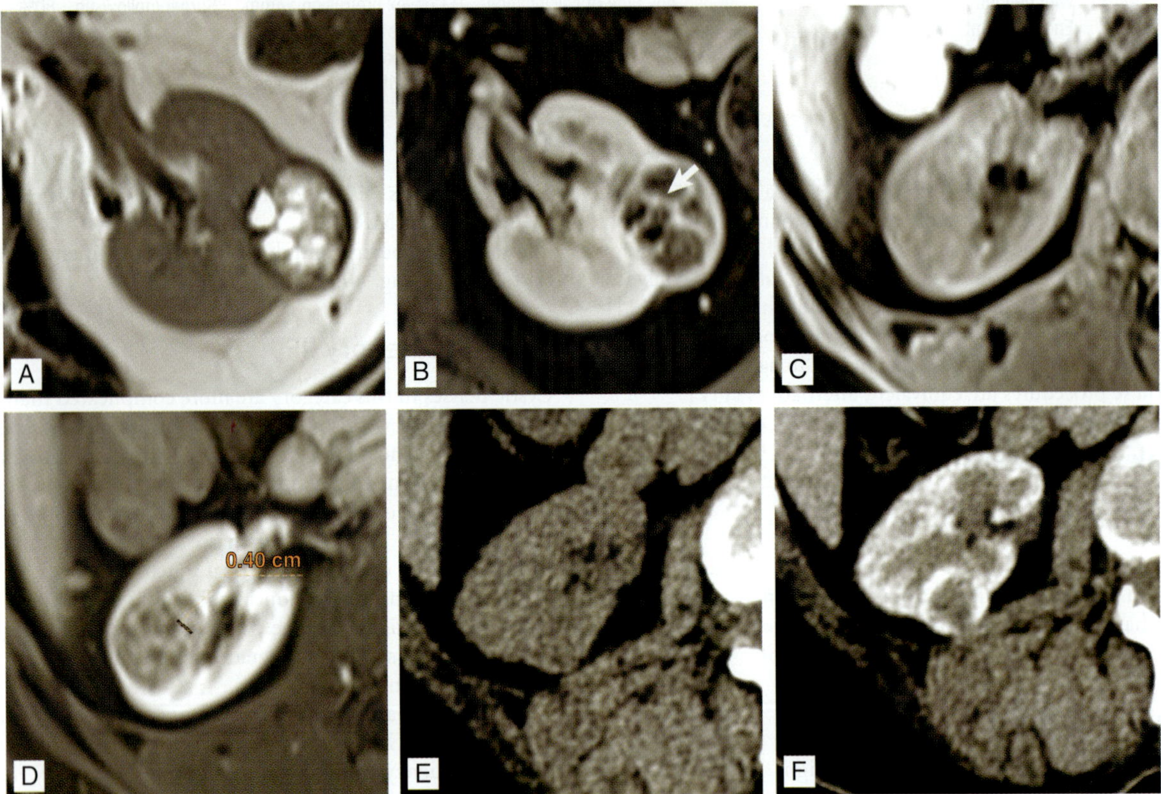

Figure 40.23 Bosniak III. (A and B) A 73-year-old woman incidentally detected left renal lesion. (A) Axial T2-weighted MR image and (B) fat-saturated contrast-enhanced T1-weighted image showing cystic mass with multiple thickened (>3 mm) septa (*arrow*). (C and D) Images in a 54-year-old male with prostate cancer and incidentally detected cystic right renal mass. (C) Axial T1W MR image showing an endophytic isointense renal mass. (D) Axial fat sat contrast-enhanced MR image shows a cystic mass with multiple foci of nodular enhancement and septal thickness of 4 mm. (E and F) Images in 68-year-old man with indeterminate renal mass. (E) Axial noncontrast CT showing an isodense mass in the right kidney. (F) Axial contrast-enhanced CT in the corticomedullary phase showing a cystic mass with thick (4 mm) enhancing wall.

Bosniak Category IV

Bosniak IV cystic masses have an enhancing nodule. The "nodule" is defined as a focal enhancing convex protrusion in the wall or septa that has acute margins (of any size) or a focal enhancing convex protrusion ≥4 mm that has obtuse margins with the wall or septa. An enhancing convex protrusion with obtuse margins that is less than or equal to 3 mm is not considered as a nodule, and is a feature of a Bosniak III mass. *Malignancy rates in this category are approximately 80%* (range 67–100%) [116,117]. *Definitive treatment of these lesions is surgery.* Imaging surveillance is considered an acceptable alternative management approach in patients with a short life expectancy or comorbidities, especially because these lesions tend to be less aggressive than ccRCCs (Fig. 40.24).

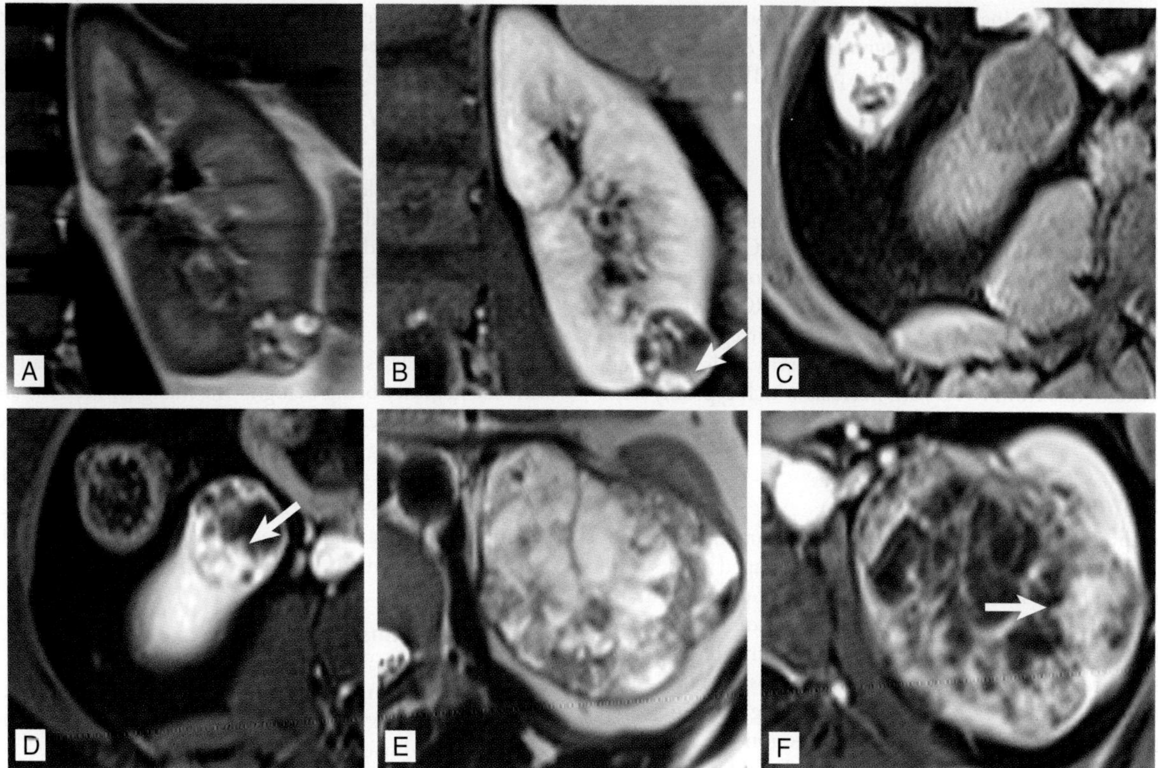

Figure 40.24 Bosniak IV cyst. (A and B) Incidentally detected left renal mass in a known case of adenocarcinoma lung. (A) Axial T2-weighted MR image and (B) fat-saturated contrast-enhanced T1-weighted image show cystic mass with multiple (≥4) thickened (>3 mm) septa and peripheral, enhancing nodule with acute margins (*small arrow*). (C) Renal mass in a patient presented with pain right flank. Axial fat-suppressed noncontrast and contrast-enhanced image shows a right renal cystic mass with multiple septa and (D) an enhancing convex protrusion >4 mm having obtuse margins (*arrow*). (E and F) Axial T2-weighted image shows large cyst with multiple thickened irregular septa and (F) enhancing nodule (*arrow*).

Cystic Renal Masses (Bosniak IIF/III/IV)

Benign lesions

1. Mixed epithelial stromal tumor family (MEST)/adult cystic nephroma
2. AML with epithelial cysts—AMLEC

Malignant lesions

1. Malignant cystic RCC—clear cell and papillary variants
2. Multilocular cystic renal neoplasm of low malignant potential
3. Tubulocystic carcinomas

Evaluation and Management of Cystic Renal Lesions

USG is neither recommended for initial evaluation nor follow-up of cystic renal masses, but is usually the modality which detects these lesions. Simple cysts on ultrasonography do not need further evaluation. CT and MRI both can be used to better assess the more complex appearing cysts and classify them according to the Bosniak system. An MRI is recommended after a CT scan in the following scenarios:

1. Mass with abundant calcifications (thick or nodular)
2. Heterogenous and nonenhancing lesion on CT
3. Hyperattenuating, homogenous, nonenhancing and >3 cm size on CT

Bosniak I and II cysts need no further follow-up and are considered benign. Bosniak IIF lesions need follow-up, while Bosniak III and IV lesions require urological consultation and are usually surgically removed.

Benign Lesion

Adult Cystic Nephroma/Mixed Epithelial and Stromal Tumor

Mixed epithelial and stromal tumor (MEST) and adult cystic nephroma (ACN) or multilocular cystic nephroma are uncommon renal tumors that have historically been described as separate entities in terms of histologic and imaging findings. However, these entities share many epidemiologic, radiologic, and pathologic features. Accordingly, the recent WHO classification considers ACN to be a part of the MEST family of tumors [7]. Note that pediatric cystic nephroma is a distinct entity. These lesions predominantly occur in middle-aged females. Pathologically, *ACNs are more cystic, whereas MESTs have a greater solid ovarian like stromal component* [118].

Imaging features for both entities include a multilocular cystic mass with variable septal enhancement. MEST usually has a solid enhancing component. They often herniate into the renal pelvis causing dilatation of the pelvicalyceal system, more commonly associated with ACN. *These lesions do not undergo malignant transformation.*

AML With Epithelial Cyst

This cystic variant of AML is rare and usually seen in women. There are no specific ultrasonography features. They may present as a Bosniak category 4 mass, mimicking a cystic RCC. The solid part is usually hyperattenuating on CT, homogeneously enhancing, and hypointense on T2WI, which are diagnostic clues. A signal drop on CS-MRI may sometimes occur in this type of AML [8,119].

Malignant Lesions

RCC With Cystic Changes

RCC can undergo cystic changes, more commonly seen with ccRCC. These constitute less than 5% of all RCCs. It demonstrates a male predominance (male-to-female ratio of 2:1), mostly occurring in the sixth to seventh decades. ccRCC with cystic changes is a multiloculated cystic mass with an irregularly thickened wall and areas of enhancing solid nodularity. It is important to differentiate this from RCC with necrosis which typically has a poorer prognosis [120].

Multilocular Cystic Renal Neoplasm of Low Malignant Potential

Multilocular cystic renal cell neoplasm is an uncommon neoplasm [121]. These tumors are seen in middle-aged adults with no gender predilection. They are almost entirely cystic, containing serous fluid. The septa are lined by single or few layers of clear cells without any expansile component. On imaging, they are classified ranging from a Bosniak IIF to Bosniak IV lesion, with the higher Bosniak categories corresponding to an increased degree of vascularized fibrosis within the lesion [122]. It is a low-grade tumor with an excellent prognosis and no reported cases of metastasis.

Tubulocystic RCC

Tubulocystic RCC is another rare tumor. *It is also termed low-grade collecting duct carcinoma and Bellini duct carcinoma, and has overlapping pathologic features with pRCC.* Tubulocystic RCCs occur mostly in men (85% men vs 15% women) in the sixth decade [7,123]. On imaging, the lesions have increased echogenicity and may appear solid on USG, cystic to indeterminate attenuation on CT, and cystic on MRI (Fig. 40.25) [124]. *This pattern of increased echogenicity/solid appearance (due to microcysts) on USG and cystic on CT/MRI indicate the probable diagnosis.* Prognosis is excellent with metastases being rare.

Role of Biopsy in Cystic Renal Lesions

Percutaneous biopsy to differentiate benign from malignant cystic masses is a low yield technique. This is due to the paucity of cells within cystic renal masses that limits a definitive sample and hence a definitive diagnosis [125].

Conclusion

Cystic renal masses are commonly encountered in daily practice, with the majority being benign. The malignant lesions are usually indolent in nature. Therefore, the radiologist must stratify the masses by applying the Bosniak classification to help appropriate management (Fig. 40.26). With increasing recognition that complex cystic masses rarely metastasize or are locally aggressive, patients are increasingly directed toward active surveillance or expectant management.

Teaching Points

- Ultrasonography is the initial modality for differentiating simple and complex cysts. Complex cystic masses on ultrasonography should be further evaluated with cross-sectional imaging
- Contrast-enhanced CT and MR imaging are both recommended modalities for the classification of cystic lesions. CEUS can be used in cases of contraindication to CT and MRI
- Differential diagnosis of Bosniak IIF/III/IV cystic lesions include both benign and malignant conditions
- Management of Bosniak III/IV cystic masses usually require surgical intervention
- Cystic renal malignancies are less aggressive compared with solid renal malignancies

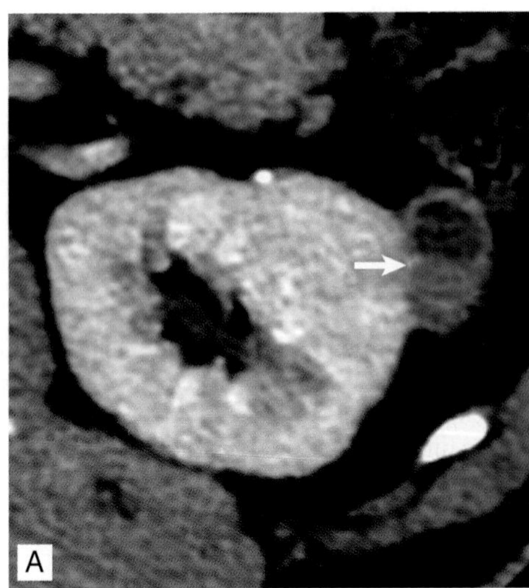

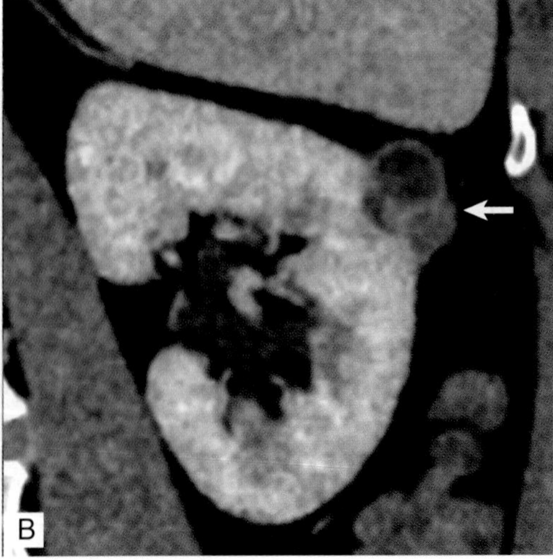

Figure 40.25 Tubulocystic RCC (A and B). Axial and coronal contrast-enhanced CT in nephrographic phase shows an exophytic mass (*arrows*) arising from the interpolar region of the left kidney, having cystic and solid component. The mass surgically removed and histopathological examination showed tubulocystic RCC.

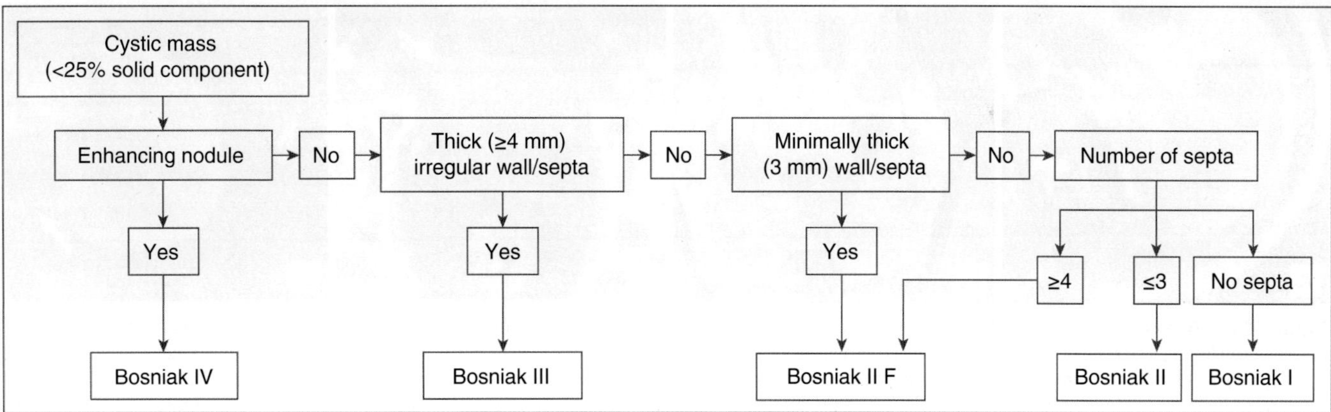

Figure 40.26 Algorithmic approach for stratification of renal cystic masses as per Bosniak 2019 version.

Upper Urinary Tract Tumors

Urothelial carcinoma of the upper urinary tract (renal pelvis and ureters) is an uncommon but lethal malignancy. It has a high incidence of recurrence and is commonly multifocal. Hence long-term rigorous surveillance is warranted [126].

Pathology and Clinical Features

These tumors occur more commonly in men (male-to-female ratio of 2:1), usually in the seventh decade [127]. They comprise 5–10% of all urothelial malignancies. *Renal pelvis is the most common site, with the ureter being less frequently involved (lower more common followed by mid and proximal ureter respectively) [128].* Bilateral ureteric involvement is seen in 2–5% cases [129]. Multifocal and metachronous lesions in the upper urinary tract and urinary bladder are common. Risk factors overlap with that of the urothelial cancer of the urinary bladder (discussed ahead).

Macroscopically two forms of tumors are noted:

- Papillary form (~85%); these present as early-stage tumors with an indolent behavior
- Solid and flat tumors (~15%); these are more aggressive and present at a later stage [130]

Upper urinary tract tumors (UUTC) more commonly spreads by the direct contiguous route and lymphatic involvement as the ureteric wall is thin and drained by rich lymphatics [131].

Patients can present with either genitourinary or systemic symptoms or both. Tumors can also be detected during surveillance for urinary bladder cancer. Hematuria is the most common symptom (60–70%), followed by lumbar or flank pain. No specific systemic symptoms may be present, such as weight loss and anorexia.

Imaging Modalities and Findings

Tumors of the upper urinary tract are usually diagnosed by radiological procedures similar to the tumors of the urinary bladder. Cystoscopy is the diagnostic modality of choice.

Intravenous Urography

It was the most commonly used method for evaluation of hematuria before the advent of CT urogram. The common findings are smooth or irregular, single or multiple filling defects within the renal collecting system. Filling defects may be present in the ureter with or without hydroureteronephrosis.

Ultrasonography

It is one of the most frequently ordered investigations for the evaluation of hematuria. Although its utility is limited in UUTC. On ultrasonography, renal pelvic urothelial tumor may appear as a heterogeneous hypoechoic mass within the echogenic sinus fat. Infundibular tumors may cause focal calyceal dilatation [128].

CT Urogram

- CT urogram is the imaging modality of choice in evaluating patients with hematuria having completely replaced intravenous urography [132]
- The most common pattern of presentation is focal mural thickening. It may be obscured by the renal medulla. However, calyceal dilatation helps in the diagnosis. Viewing images in a wide window and maximum intensity projection settings is recommended
- The tumor may also present as a focal mass or filling defect, typically lower attenuation than a calculus (except indinavir calculi). Dense excreted contrast may obscure small lesions, and wide window settings are recommended to avoid this pitfall. The differential diagnosis for filling defects includes benign entities like blood clots and debris from the sloughed papilla. Usually, these filling defects are totally intraluminal, completely surrounded in contrast and do not show enhancement
- Dual-energy CT with iodine enhancement technique has shown promising results in improving tumor conspicuity, particularly when there are concerns regarding the amount of contrast administration in patients of renal insufficiency [133]
- Infiltrative mass may be seen in some cases, with involvement of the renal sinus fat and adjacent parenchyma with hydronephrosis. Centrally located RCC is a close mimic. Imaging differentiation of the two can be diagnostically challenging but distinction is important as management strategies differ. Certain imaging characteristics point toward diagnosis of central intrarenal TCC's including epicenter in collecting system, filling defect in renal pelvis, preserved renal outline, homogenous enhancement, and extension toward the ureteropelvic junction. Cystic or necrotic change favors RCC
  Other differential diagnosis includes lymphoma and metastasis. Diagnosis is usually confirmed by biopsy (Figs. 40.27 and 40.28)
- Three-dimensional imaging including maximum intensity projection and VR are routinely used while evaluating UUTC

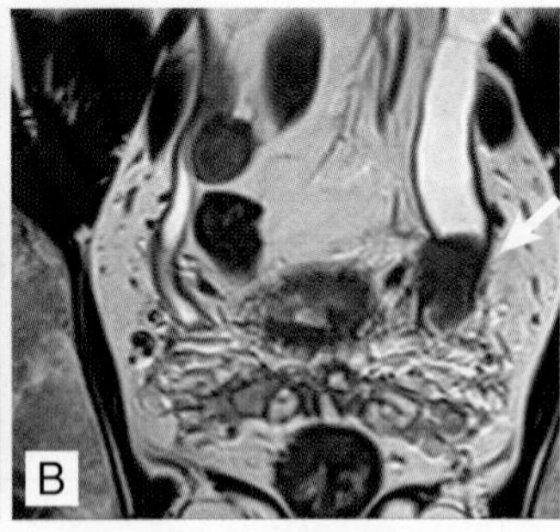
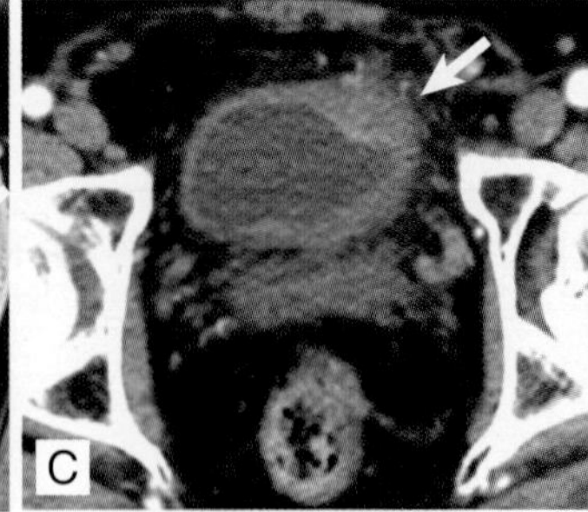
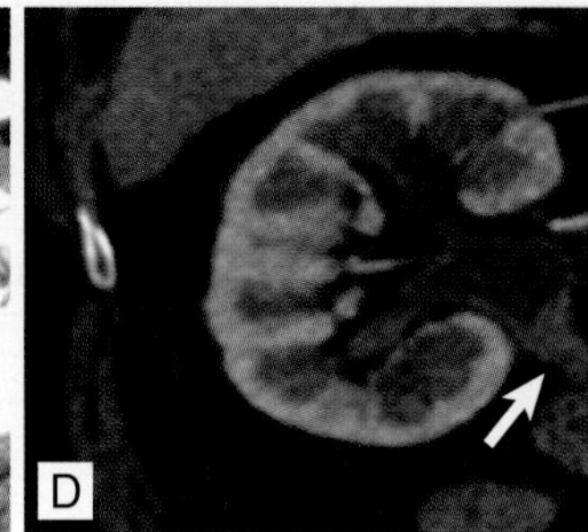

Figure 40.27 (A) Axial T2-weighted image shows an isointense mass (*arrow*) in the right renal pelvis, suggestive of urothelial carcinoma. (B) Coronal T2-weighted image in a patient who presented with hematuria shows a hypointense mass in the left distal ureter (*arrow*). Proximal ureter is dilated. (C and D) An 80-year-old male with hematuria. (C) Axial contrast-enhanced CT image shows enhancing thickening of the urinary bladder wall (*arrow*). (D) Coronal sections of the right kidney shows enhancing mass in the renal pelvis with thickening of upper ureter (*arrow*). This highlights the importance of screening for multifocality of lesions in urothelial carcinoma.

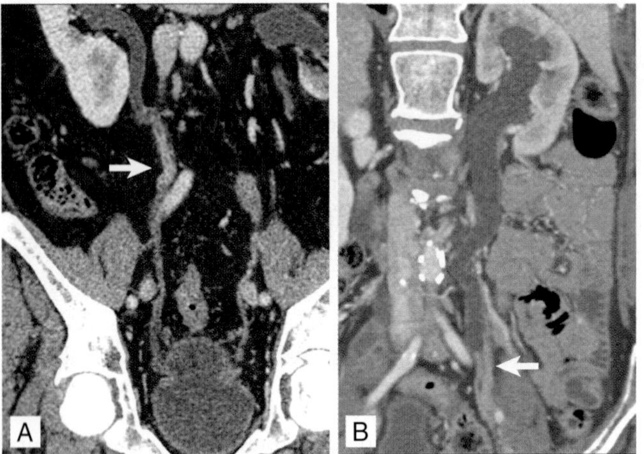

Figure 40.28 (A) Ureteric urothelial carcinoma in a 68-year-old man with hematuria. (A) Coronal reformatted image shows hydronephrosis and proximal hydroureter with an enhancing irregular wall thickening and stricture (*arrow*) along the mid ureter. (B) Lower ureteric TCC in an 80-year-old female. Coronal reformatted CT image shows enhancing irregular wall thickening in the lower ureter (*arrow*) with upstream hydroureteronephrosis.

MR Urogram

- *It is usually used when CTU is contraindicated.* Diagnostic accuracy of CTU is better than MRU, which lacks the spatial resolution of CT. Motion artifacts are also a challenge for optimal imaging in MRU. Imaging features are similar to those in CTU

Management and Surveillance

The management algorithm is shown in Fig. 40.29. Urothelial cancers are notorious for recurrence. Hence strict surveillance is necessary. Invasive methods of surveillance include ureteroscopy and cystoscopy [134]. CTU is the noninvasive imaging method of choice.

Conclusion

UUTC is a lethal and uncommon cancer. The hallmark of urothelial carcinoma is recurrence and multifocality. Imaging plays a key role in diagnosis and management of these lesions. Hence, the radiologist should have a thorough understanding of the imaging finding.

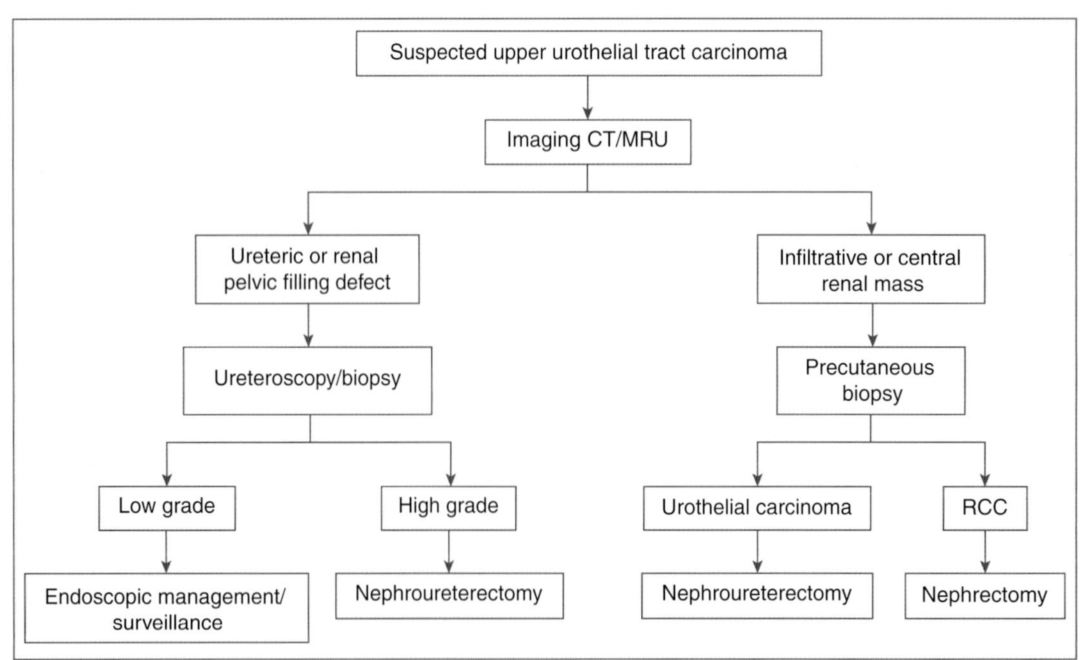

Figure 40.29 Algorithmic approach to the management of UUTC (upper urinary tract cancer).

Imaging of Urinary Bladder Cancer

Epidemiology and Pathology

Urinary bladder cancer is the most common malignancy of the urinary tract and the ninth most common cause of cancer-related deaths in men [135,136]. Bladder cancer occurs more commonly in men between 50 and 70 years, with a male-to-female ratio of 3–4:1 [137]. There is a known causal link between urothelial cancer and smoking or occupational exposure to carcinogens in the dye industry (such as 2-naphthylamine, 4-aminobiphenyl, and benzidine). Other risk factors include chronic infection, irritation, arsenic in drinking water, and stasis of urine in the bladder diverticula [138].

The urinary bladder wall consists of four layers (urothelium, lamina propria, muscularis propria, and adventitial layer). Neoplasms can arise from any of the four bladder layers and are broadly classified as either epithelial or nonepithelial (mesenchymal) (Table 40.11). The term urothelial carcinoma is the preferred terminology over transitional carcinoma for tumors arising from the epithelium.

Squamous cell carcinoma accounts for less than 5% of bladder neoplasms, although in schistosomiasis (bilharziasis) endemic areas, it accounts for more than 50% of bladder cancers in younger age groups. Risk factors include chronic irritation from indwelling catheters, bladder calculi, or chronic infection.

Adenocarcinoma accounts for less than 2% of bladder neoplasms. It can present as primary (two-thirds nonurachal and one-third urachal) or secondary (metastases). The mean age at presentation for nonurachal cancer is 60 years, with urachal cancer occurring a decade earlier.

TABLE 40.11 Classification of Urinary Bladder Tumors

Epithelial Neoplasms (95%)	
Benign neoplasms	Papilloma Papillary urothelial neoplasm of low malignant potential (PUNLMP)
Malignant neoplasms	Urothelial carcinoma Squamous cell carcinoma Adenocarcinoma Metastases Small cell or neuroendocrine carcinoma Carcinoid Melanoma
Nonepithelial Neoplasms (5%)	
Benign neoplasms	Leiomyoma Paraganglioma Fibroma Plasmacytoma Hemangioma Solitary fibrous tumor Neurofibroma Lipoma
Malignant neoplasms	Rhabdomyosarcoma Leiomyosarcoma Lymphoma Osteosarcoma Angiosarcoma Malignant fibrous histiocytoma

Clinical Presentation

The most common presentation of patients with bladder cancer is painless hematuria, which can be either gross hematuria or microhematuria. According to the AUA, *microhematuria is defined as three or more red blood cells per high-power field on microscopic evaluation of the urinary sediment. Hematuria visible to the physician or patient is considered as gross hematuria* [139]. Typically, patients present with macro or gross hematuria warranting further evaluation by cystoscopy and cross-sectional imaging [139]. Microhematuria should be evaluated based on risk stratification after excluding benign gynecological etiology like menstruation, exercise, trauma, and infection [140]. Patients may also experience voiding symptoms such as frequency, dysuria, and pelvic pain and pressure.

Staging

The TNM-AJCC system is widely accepted for staging (Table 40.12) [141].

Clinical management is determined on the basis of distinguishing nonmuscle invasive bladder cancer (NMIBC) versus muscle invasive bladder cancer (MIBC). According to TNM staging NMIBC is defined T1 or lower and MIBC as T2 or higher. At presentation about 70–85% of the bladder tumors are nonmuscle invasive. NMIBC is

TABLE 40.12 AJCC 8th Edition Staging of Urinary Bladder Tumors

Primary Tumor (T)	
TX	Primary tumor cannot be assessed
T0	No evidence of primary tumor
Ta	Noninvasive papillary carcinoma
Tis	Carcinoma in situ: flat tumor
T1	Tumor invades subepithelial connective tissue
T2	Tumor invades muscularis propria pT2a—Tumor invades superficial muscularis propria (inner half) pT2b—Tumor invades deep muscularis propria (outer half)
T3	Tumor invades perivesical tissue pT3a—Microscopically pT3b—Macroscopically (extravesical mass)
T4	Tumor invades any of the following: prostatic stroma, seminal vesicles, uterus, vagina, pelvic wall, abdominal wall T4a—Tumor invades prostatic stroma, uterus, vagina T4b—Tumor invades pelvic wall, abdominal wall
Regional Lymph Nodes (N)	
NX	Lymph nodes cannot be assessed
N0	No lymph node metastasis
N1	Single regional lymph node metastasis in the true pelvis (hypogastric, obturator, external iliac or presacral lymph node)
N2	Multiple regional lymph node metastases in the true pelvis
N3	Lymph node metastasis to the common iliac lymph Nodes
Distant Metastasis (M)	
M0	No distant metastasis
M1	Distant metastasis

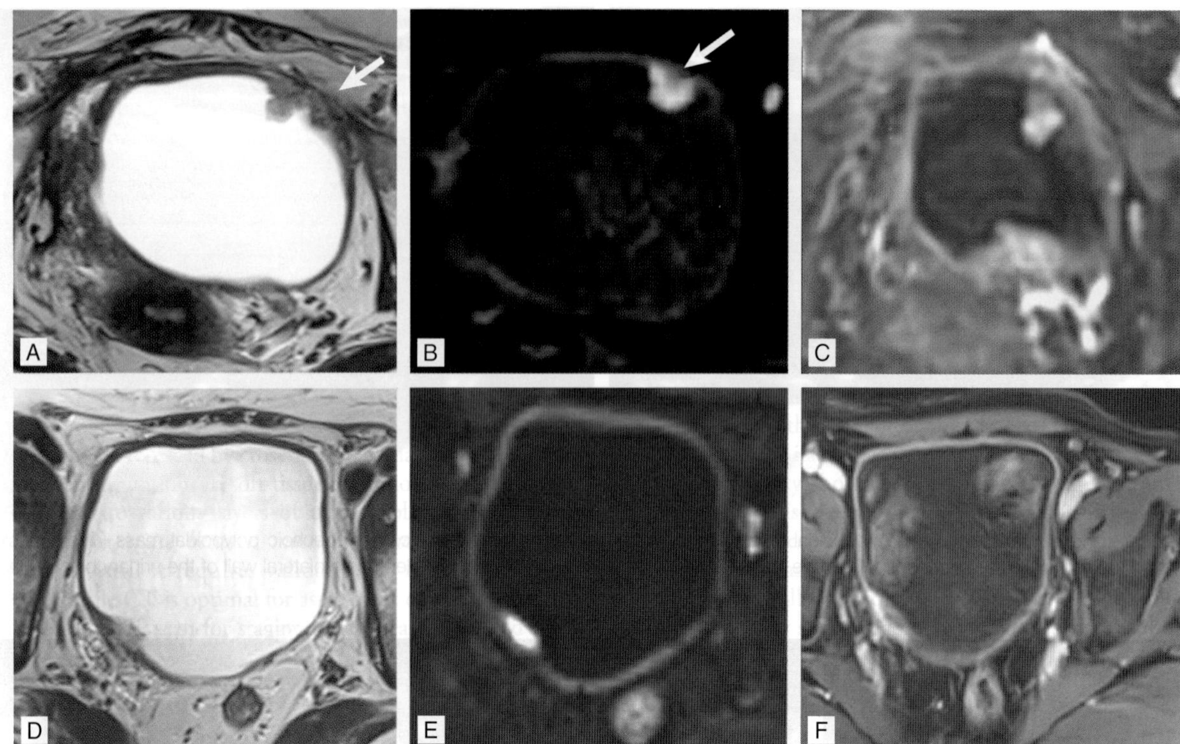

Figure 40.33 (A–C) A 55-year-old male with early bladder tumor. (A) T2-weighted MR image showing nonmuscle invasive category T1 lesion along the dome and lateral wall with uninterrupted submucosal layer (*arrow*). (B) Axial diffusion-weighted image shows classical inchworm sign (*short arrow*). (C) Axial DCE image shows rapid enhancement within the tumor. (D–F) A 65-year-old male with sessile bladder tumor. (D) T2-weighted MR image shows muscle invasive bladder T2 category tumor involving the bladder wall without extravesical extension. (E) Axial diffusion-weighted image shows restricted diffusion. (F) Axial dynamic postcontrast image shows enhancement relative to the bladder wall (*arrow*).

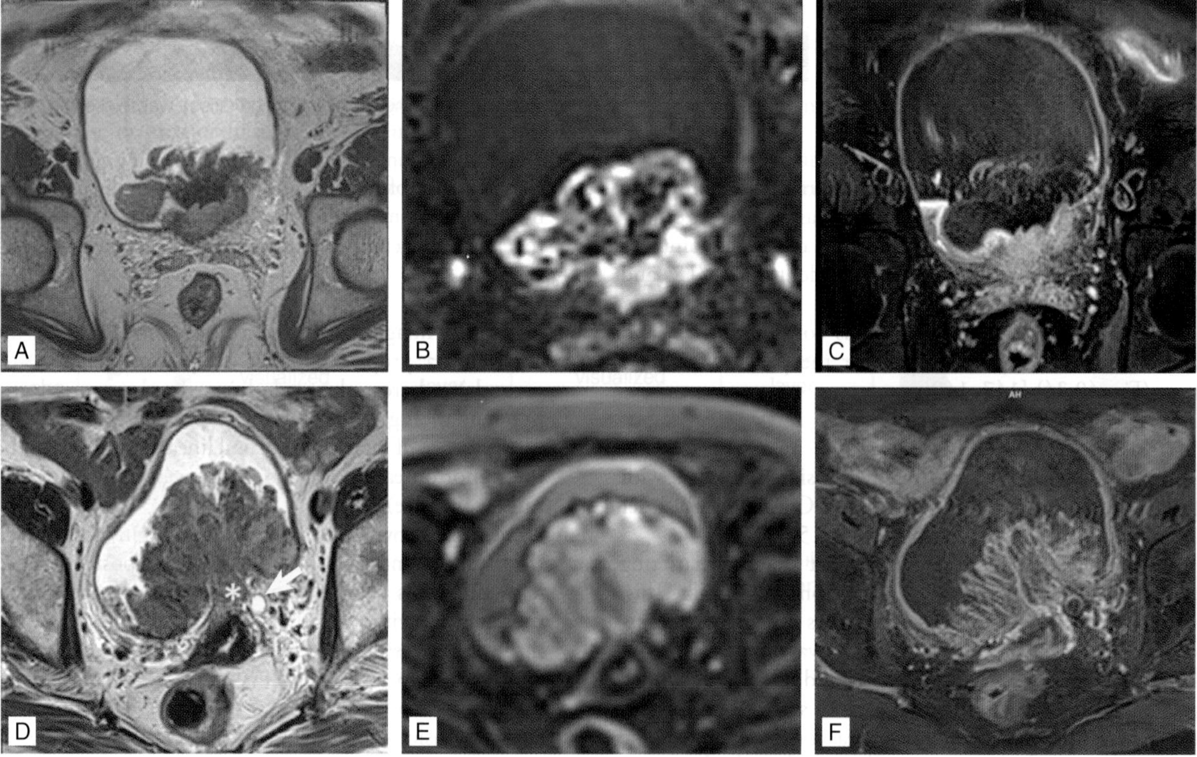

Figure 40.34 (A–C) A 55-year-old male with gross hematuria and T3b disease. (A) Axial T2-weighted image shows an intermediate signal tumor with a hypointense bladder clot and macroscopic perivesicular extension. (B) Axial diffusion-weighted image shows restricted diffusion. (C) Dynamic postcontrast T1-weighted image shows tumoral enhancement and perivesical extension. (D–F) A 65-year-old female with hematuria and T4 disease. (D) Axial T2-weighted image shows T4 tumor involving the cervix (*asterisk*), with a dilated left ureter (*arrow*). (E) Axial diffusion-weighted image shows restricted diffusion. (F) Dynamic postcontrast T1-weighted image shows linear heterogeneous enhancement.

TABLE 40.13 VI-RADS Interpretation

VI-RADS 1 (muscle invasion is highly unlikely)
VI-RADS 2 (muscle invasion is unlikely to be present)
VI-RADS 3 (the presence of muscle invasion is equivocal
VI-RADS 4 (muscle invasion is likely)
VI-RADS 5 (invasion of muscle and beyond the bladder is very likely)

MRI and risk stratification of muscle invasiveness of tumor (NMIBC vs MIBC). mpMRI is useful in patients with early disease, in expediting radical treatment or for determining response to bladder-sparing approaches.

In VI-RADS, appearances in T2W images, DWI, and DCE are taken into consideration to generate a five point VI-RADS score (Fig. 40.35). *The dominant sequences are DWI and DCE.* The second dominant sequence DCE is taken into account if the DWI is suboptimal. The T2 sequence is helpful as a first pass guide for categories 1–3. It is worth noting that VI-RADS is applicable to untreated patients (uVI-RADS scoring) and to patients having received "only" diagnostic TURBT (tVI-RADS) [151].

Virtual Cystoscopy

Virtual cystoscopy is a technique, which reconstructs a three-dimensional model from cross-sectional imaging data (ultrasonography, CT or MRI), to visualize bladder wall abnormalities like cystoscopy [152].

Uncommon Neoplasms of the Urinary Bladder

Squamous cell carcinoma (<5%) and adenocarcinoma (<2%) occur in the setting of chronic bladder infection and irritation [4]. Mesenchymal tumors represent the remaining 5% of bladder tumors. The most common types of mesenchymal tumor are rhabdomyosarcoma in children and leiomyosarcoma in adults. There is a significant imaging overlap in the history and imaging findings of the various bladder tumors, and ultimately they all require biopsy for diagnosis [4]. However, some tumors such as botryoid rhabdomyosarcoma, plexiform neurofibroma, solitary fibrous tumor, leiomyomas, and urachal adenocarcinoma have suggestive clinical and radiological features, which may allow differentiation (Table 40.14 and Fig. 40.36).

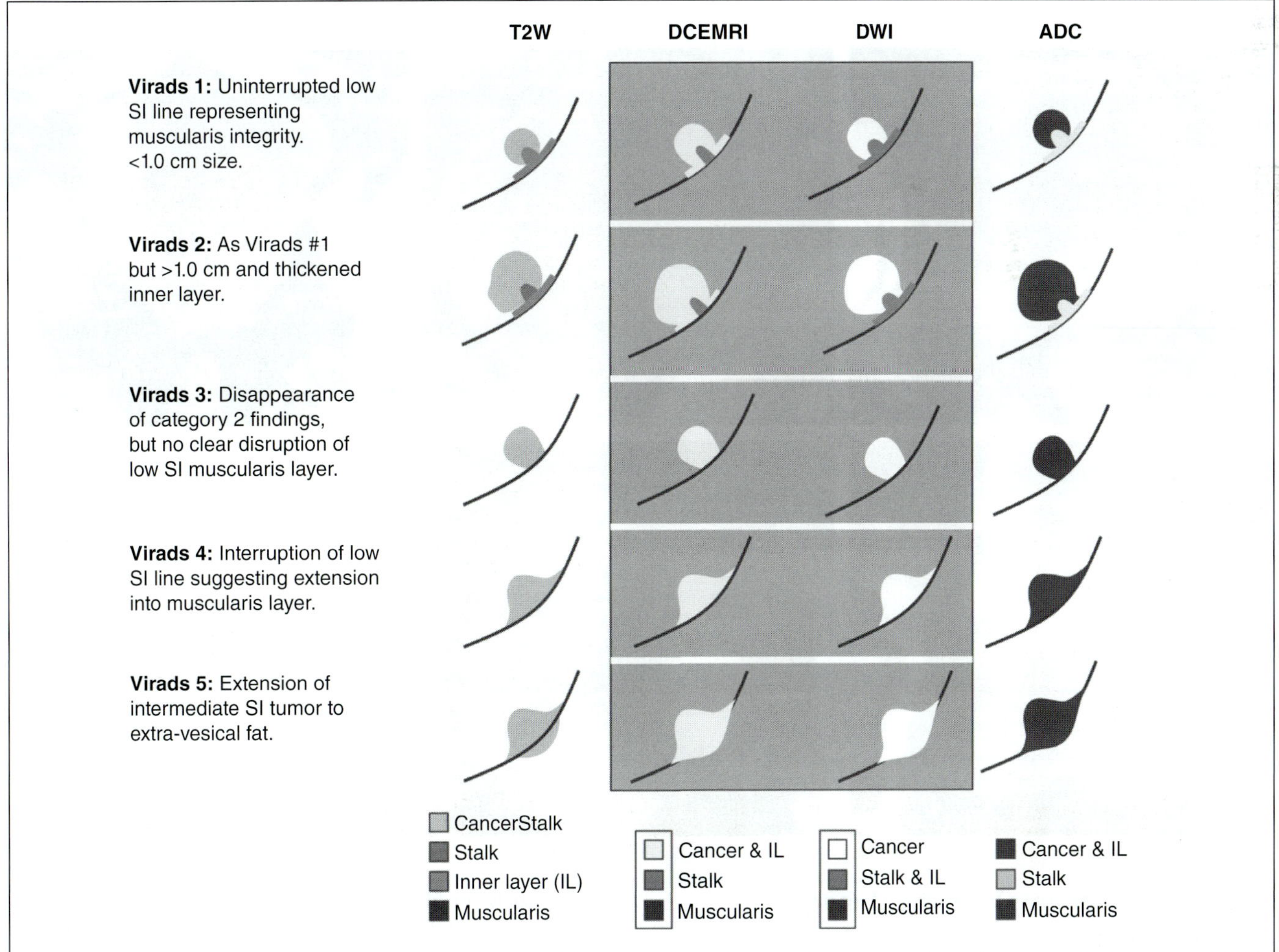

Figure 40.35 Schematic illustration of mpMRI appearance of VI-RADS scores 1–5 using T2, DCE, DWI, ADC-weighted images. *ADC*, apparent diffusion coefficient; *DCE*, dynamic contrast enhancement; *DWI*, diffusion-weighted imaging; *MRI*, magnetic resonance imaging; *mpMRI*, multiparametric MRI; *SI*, signal intensity.

TABLE 40.14 Other Uncommon Urinary Bladder Tumors

	Demography and Clinical Features	Imaging Features
Squamous cell carcinoma	Risk factors: schistosomiasis (bilharziasis), bladder calculi, or chronic infection, cyclophosphamide, smoking and intravesical BCG	■ Appear as a single-enhancing bladder mass or as a diffuse or focal wall thickening ■ Sessile ■ Muscle invasion and extensive extravesical spread common
Adenocarcinoma	Risk factors: associated with the bladder exstrophy and a persistent urachus	Occur close to the dome of the bladder/along the course of the urachus Large, solid, and cystic with calcification
Small cell or neuroendocrine tumor	Rare; smoking is a risk factor	Large and polypoidal or nodular mass with central necrosis with patchy enhancement
Leiomyoma and leiomyosarcoma	Rare; radiation therapy and cyclophosphamide are risk factors	Smooth, solid, homogeneous masses with or without cystic components. Normal mucosa Low signal intensity on T2w images
Rhabdomyosarcoma	Most common bladder tumor in children Presentation: hematuria, dysuria, retention, or urinary tract infection.	Large, polypoid or grape-like nodular masses at bladder base
Paraganglioma	Very rare Risk factors: familial syndromes such as NF, VHL, Sturge–Weber syndrome, tuberous sclerosis, or MEN	Marked enhancement. Ring calcification may be present
Lymphoma	Secondary involvement of the bladder may be present in 10–25% of patients	Mimic urothelial carcinoma

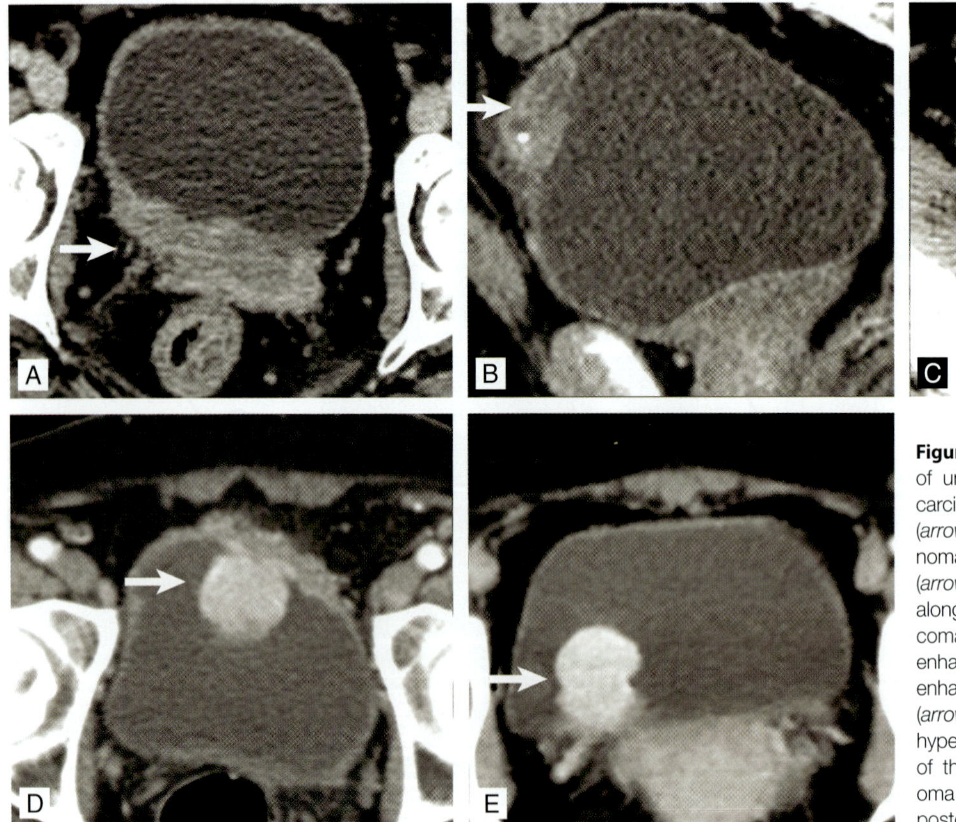

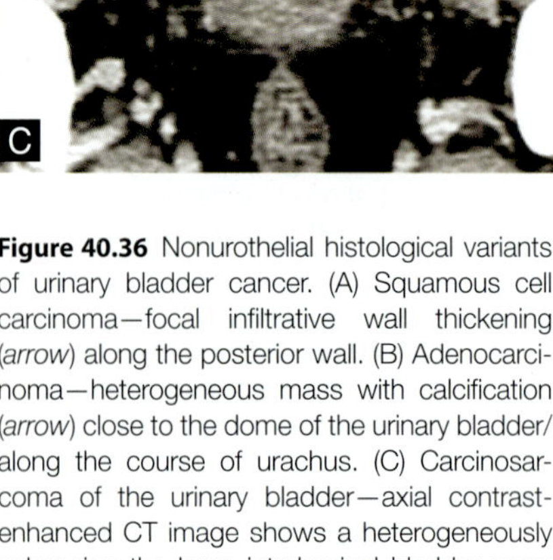

Figure 40.36 Nonurothelial histological variants of urinary bladder cancer. (A) Squamous cell carcinoma—focal infiltrative wall thickening (*arrow*) along the posterior wall. (B) Adenocarcinoma—heterogeneous mass with calcification (*arrow*) close to the dome of the urinary bladder/ along the course of urachus. (C) Carcinosarcoma of the urinary bladder—axial contrast-enhanced CT image shows a heterogeneously enhancing the large intraluminal bladder mass (*arrow*). (D) Small cell carcinoma—nodular hyperenhancing mass along the anterior aspect of the urinary bladder (*arrow*). (E) Paraganglioma—nodular intensely enhancing mass in the posterior wall of the urinary bladder (*arrow*).

Approach to Patients With the Urinary Bladder Lesion

Once a urinary bladder mass is detected, these patients typically undergo evaluation with urine cytology and cystoscopy (Fig. 40.37) [135]. If a tumor is present on cystoscopy, TURBT is performed. Approximately 30–50% of urothelial cancers are clinically understaged even after TURBT [153]. At least one imaging study to evaluate both the upper and lower urinary tracts is, however, essential. The recommended current guidelines include pelvic MRI for local staging [147]. The management decision is based on a combination of histology of the TURBT specimen and imaging findings [135].

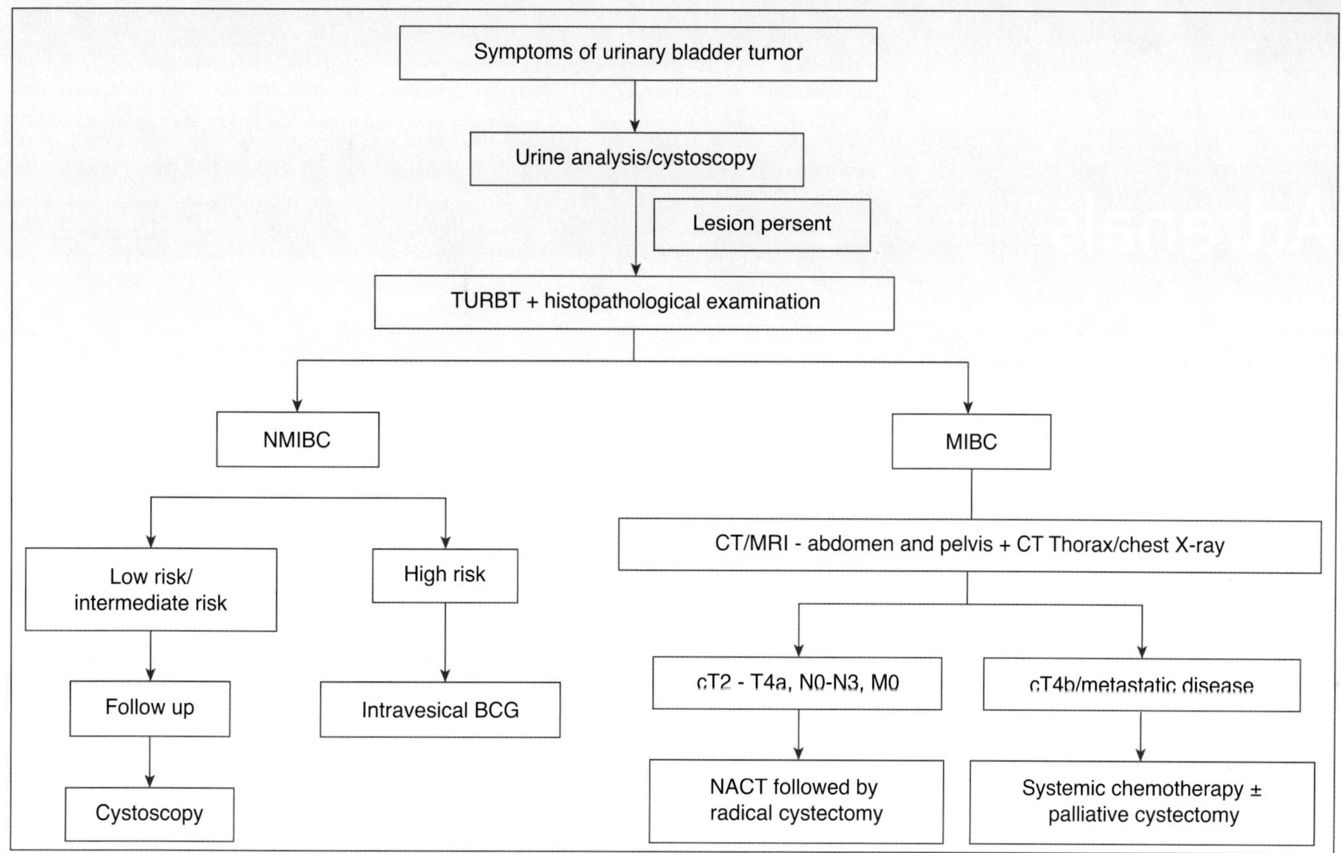

Figure 40.37 Approach to the management of the urinary bladder tumor. *BCG*, Bacille Calmette Guerin; *MIBC*, muscle invasive bladder cancer; *NACT*, neoadjuvant chemotherapy; *NMIBC*, nonmuscle invasive bladder cancer; *TURBT*, transurethral resection of the bladder tumor.

The problem with TURBT is many times it does not include detrusor muscle in the resection specimen, thus understaging the tumor in approximately 30–50% of the cases [154]. In view of these limitations mpMRI is emerging as a valuable tool in accurate preoperative local staging of bladder cancer [155]. For distant staging CT or MRI of abdomen and pelvis with and without IV contrast is preferred.

The aim of pretreatment workup is to classify the bladder lesion into superficial or NMIBC, MIBC, or metastatic disease [143]. *NMIBC is often treated with conservative bladder-sparing techniques (TURBT with or without intravesical chemotherapy)* [147], *while MIBC is treated with neoadjuvant chemotherapy and radical cystectomy.* Metastatic disease is treated by chemotherapy and immunotherapy.

Teaching Points

- Ultrasonography does not play a significant role in the preoperative staging of bladder cancer
- CT plays an important role in the case of muscle invasive tumors to rule out metastatic disease
- Multiparametric MRI is better in local staging of UB tumors compared with CT

Conclusion

Early detection of bladder cancer is important. Conventional CT and MR imaging are only moderately accurate in the diagnosis, local staging and distant spread of bladder cancer. Cystoscopy and pathologic staging remains the pivot for the management of bladder cancer. The role of mpMR imaging in accurate local staging of bladder cancer is evolving.

Suggested Readings

- AM Elkassem, SS Lo, AJ Gunn, BM Shuch, ME Dewitt-Foy, R Abouassaly, Role of imaging in renal cell carcinoma: a multidisciplinary perspective, Radiographics 41 (2021) 1387–1407, doi:10.1148/rg.2021200202.
- SG Silverman, I Pedrosa, JH Ellis, NM Hindman, N Schieda, AD Smith, et al., Bosniak classification of cystic renal masses, version 2019: an update proposal and needs assessment, Radiology 292 (2019) 475–488, doi:10.1148/radiol.2019182646.
- M Pecoraro, M Takeuchi, HA Vargas, VF Muglia, S Cipollari, C Catalano, et al., Overview of VI-RADS in bladder cancer, Am J Roentgenol 214 (2020) 1259–1268, doi:10.2214/AJR.20.22763.

41 Adrenals

SHALINI GOVIL, ANU EAPEN

Despite their small size, the adrenal glands are among the most important and vital organs in the body. Their function was quite unknown until 1855, when Addison first described the syndrome resulting from their destruction. In 1856 Brown-Séquard showed that their removal led to death in animals. The adrenal glands lie just above the kidneys and are composed of a cortex and a medulla. The medulla has a totally different origin to the cortex, and arises with the sympathetic nervous system. Both cortex and medulla secrete hormones. The adrenal cortex secretes three main groups of hormones that are chemically related and have a similar basic chemical structure: glucocorticoids, mineralocorticoids, and androgens. Glucocorticoid secretion is controlled by the pituitary gland through its adrenocorticotrophic hormone (ACTH). The most important glucocorticoid is cortisol, which is normally secreted at the rate of about 20 mg/day. Glucocorticoids stimulate protein breakdown, oppose the action of insulin, and inhibit tissue response to injury. Aldosterone is the most important mineralocorticoid, the secretion of which is mainly controlled by the renin–angiotensin system and by the level of plasma potassium. Aldosterone stimulates the reabsorption of sodium in the distal renal tubules of the kidney in exchange for potassium. Although androgens are produced in relatively large amounts, the adrenal androgens are very weak compared with testosterone. The medulla also secretes hormones, mainly adrenaline (epinephrine) and noradrenaline (norepinephrine).

Introduction

In both children and adults, the adrenal gland is the site of a multitude of pathologies, ranging from infections, hemorrhage, and hyperplasia to benign and malignant tumors. Tumors can function and secrete hormones that result in clinically evident endocrine disease or remain hidden by virtue of their nonfunctional nature, detected incidentally when the patient undergoes an ultrasonography (USG), computed tomography (CT), or magnetic resonance imaging (MRI).

In fact, the widespread use of these techniques has led to the increased detection of adrenal incidentalomas, occurring in about 4% of the CT scans performed across all age groups [1]. Although mostly benign, nonfunctioning adenomas, these lesions can present a challenge when found during an oncology workup and need to be distinguished from metastases or a second malignancy [2]. An array of imaging techniques holds the key to characterizing adrenal lesions with the use of classic appearances and a constellation of signs that enable specific diagnosis. Radiologists have an important role in this clinical setting to avoid the misdiagnosis of malignancy with all its attendant difficulty. With advances in technology, imaging can often arrive at a specific diagnosis without the use of invasive diagnostic procedures.

Due to the retroperitoneal location and small size of the adrenal, USG imaging is impeded by overlying bowel gas and elusive acoustic windows. USG is therefore unable to provide the resolution needed to accurately characterize small adrenal lesions but can classify large lesions as cystic or solid. In neonates, where the gland is large and nearly one-third the size of the kidney, USG has a dominant role to play in the detection and characterization of adrenal hemorrhage.

Speed, spatial resolution, and tissue enhancement make CT the first-line imaging tool when investigating adrenal pathology, while MRI has the advantage of high contrast resolution, multiplanar and multiparametric capabilities, chemical shift MRI (CS-MRI), and the lack of radiation. However, MRI remains expensive and less widely available and despite advances in technology, is still limited by long scan durations, and lower spatial resolution due to motion from respiration, cardiac contraction and bowel peristalsis.

Nuclear scintigraphy is functional imaging that can improve diagnostic specificity when anatomical imaging is equivocal and is especially helpful in determining the functional status of adrenal nodules, the site of extra-adrenal/ectopic functional tumors, and the extent of metastases/recurrences in malignancy. Adrenal cortex scintigraphy is performed with labeled cholesterol analogues, while adrenal medulla scintigraphy is performed with iodine-labeled metaiodobenzylguanidine (^{123}I-mIBG), a norepinephrine precursor analogue. PET-CT provides resolution sufficient to detect 5-mm lesions and accurately differentiate benign from malignant lesions. ^{18}F-fluorodeoxyglucose PET-CT (^{18}FDG PET-CT) is useful in the staging of adrenal cortical carcinoma (ACC), neuroblastoma, locating primary malignancy, and assessing response to treatment in lymphoma [3].

Anatomy and Physiology

The adrenal glands are located within the perinephric space above the kidneys. The right adrenal gland is triangular in shape, lies lateral to the diaphragmatic crus, medial to the liver and abuts the posterior surface of the IVC. The left adrenal gland is crescent-shaped, lies anterior to the upper pole of the kidney and posterior to the splenic vein and pancreas. Left adrenal masses therefore displace the splenic vein anteriorly, while pancreatic or gastric masses displace the splenic vein posteriorly.

The average size of the adrenals varies, with length 3–5 cm, width 2–3 cm, limb thickness 5 mm, and weight 3–5 g with the cortex occupying 90% of the gland. The gland is much larger in infants and small children, where the size is one-third the renal size.

There are three main arteries of supply: inferior adrenal artery arising from the renal artery, middle adrenal artery arising from

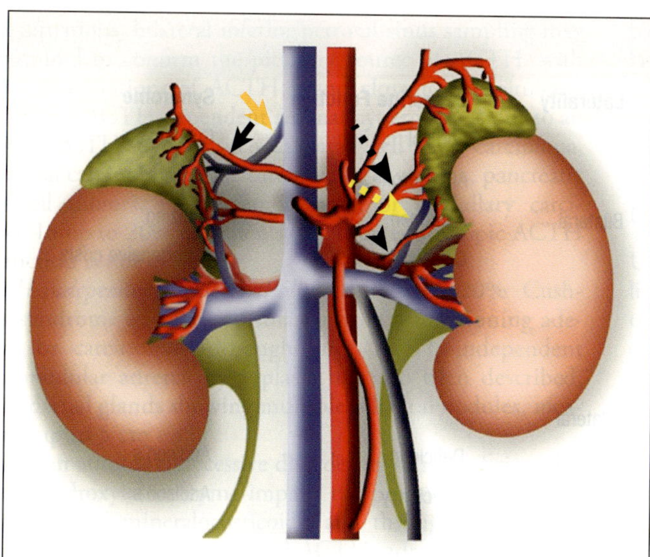

Figure 41.1 Adrenal vasculature. Arteries: inferior adrenal artery arising from the renal artery (*black arrowhead*), middle adrenal artery arising from the aorta (*black dashed arrow*), and superior adrenal artery arising from the inferior phrenic artery (*black arrow*). Veins: right adrenal vein (*solid yellow arrow*) drains into the IVC and the left adrenal vein (*dashed yellow arrow*) drains into the left renal vein. (Courtesy: Dr. B. Karthikumar.)

the aorta, and superior adrenal artery arising from the inferior phrenic artery.

There is usually a fairly large adrenal vein on the left that passes downward and medial to the upper pole of the kidney to join the main left renal vein, lying just lateral to the vertebral border. The right adrenal vein has a very short trunk that passes directly into the posterolateral surface of the IVC at a level just above the upper pole of the right kidney (Fig. 41.1).

The adrenal gland contains two different organs: the adrenal cortex and the adrenal medulla. The adrenal cortex is an endocrine gland that secretes cortisol, aldosterone, and androgenic steroids synthesized from cholesterol esters. Functioning adrenal cortical adenomas are of high lipid content because of these cholesterol esters. The adrenal medulla is from the neural crest and releases epinephrine and norepinephrine in response to stress.

Adrenal physiology is a complex feedback interaction involving the hypothalamus and pituitary. Stress stimulates the release of epinephrine and cytokines that, in turn, stimulates the pituitary to release ACTH, resulting in the adrenal secretion of cortisol. Cortisol and epinephrine are appropriately known as "stress hormones." Cortisol, in a negative feedback interaction, suppresses the hypothalamus and pituitary to reduce the release of ACTH.

Pathology

Adrenal pathology can arise de novo (primary) or as part of a disseminated disease (secondary) [2]. Primary adrenal disease can originate in the cortex or medulla of the gland and can be either functioning or nonfunctioning. Adrenal lesions can be classified based on etiology, cell origin, functional status, and laterality. Laterality is especially of significance since bilateral lesions can present clinically due to the effects of excess or inadequate hormone secretion as Cushing's syndrome, Conn's syndrome, or Addison's disease. Adrenal lesions can also be classified based on benign or malignant biologic behavior (Table 41.1).

Pathophysiology of Endocrine Dysfunction

Cushing's syndrome presents with violaceous abdominal striae, supraclavicular fat pads, truncal obesity, hirsutism, amenorrhea, osteoporosis, fractures, excessive callus formation (Fig. 41.2), proximal muscle weakness, diabetes, and hypertension. The syndrome results from excess, exogenous/endogenous cortisol, or ACTH although exogenous steroid medication is by far the commonest source. Endogenous excess cortisol can arise from an adrenal adenoma, ACTH stimulation from a pituitary adenoma or ectopic, extrapituitary tumor. About 20% of adrenal incidentalomas secrete cortisol. Laboratory proof is based on the disruption of normal adrenal cortical physiology: loss of the normal midnight cortisol nadir resulting in elevated night-time saliva cortisol and loss of HPA negative feedback as demonstrated by the dexamethasone suppression test.

Pituitary adenoma (Cushing disease) is the cause of 80–85% of endogenous Cushing syndrome and results in bilateral adrenal hyperplasia, with added adrenal nodularity in 40% and a lack of any adrenal abnormality in up to 30%.

Conn's syndrome presents with hypertension, hypokalemia, alkalosis, muscle weakness, and cardiac dysfunction and is due to excess aldosterone caused by adenoma (70%), hyperplasia (25%), or carcinoma (rare). Aldosterone-secreting tumors account for 1–3% of incidentalomas, while 5–10% adults with hypertension have primary hyperaldosteronism caused by aldosteronomas or adrenal hyperplasia [2]. All incidentalomas with hypertension and/or unexplained hypokalemia should be screened for hyperaldosteronism, with a sensitive test such as the aldosterone:renin ratio (ARR) >20–30. Conn's syndrome adenomas tend to be small and imaging negative in the setting of elevated aldosterone. CT/MRI may demonstrate unilateral neoplasm but excess aldosterone may be from bilateral secretion or microadenoma within the contralateral gland.

Addison's disease is due to adrenal insufficiency and results in hypotension, weight loss, and altered pigmentation. There is an inadequate secretion of corticosteroids resulting from partial or complete destruction of the adrenal glands. Primary adrenal insufficiency is caused by idiopathic autoimmune adrenalitis in developed countries while TB is the most common cause in developing countries. Other causes include adrenal sarcoidosis, metastases, lymphoma, hemorrhage, necrosis, fungal infections, and AIDS-related opportunistic infections [3]. Central adrenal insufficiency is due to reduced hypothalamic–pituitary ACTH and is diagnosed when cortisol level fails to rise on the ACTH stimulation test.

Slow-onset Addison's disease is caused by autoimmune disorders, TB, metastases, or AIDS, while the abrupt-onset Addisonian crisis is caused by adrenal hemorrhage, steroid withdrawal, or postpartum pituitary necrosis (Sheehan syndrome). Autoimmune disorders are chronic in presentation and cause small, atrophic glands, while small atrophic calcified glands are more likely a result of TB or fungal infection. It is important to consider adrenal insufficiency when imaging reveals bilateral adrenal infection, hemorrhage, or tumors.

Incidentalomas: 15% incidentalomas are hormonally active but often result in asymptomatic or subclinical disease, therefore requiring testing to exclude hypercortisolism and pheochromocytoma [1]. All patients with incidentalomas who have hypertension or hypokalemia require workup for primary aldosteronism, while signs of androgen excess can occur in ACC.

Functioning adenomas present clinically, based on the substance secreted. Nonfunctioning adenomas are commonly detected incidentally and are the commonest cause of "incidentaloma" (75%).

embryogenesis. Hydatid cysts are the main parasitic cysts involving the adrenal glands although they are rarely involved even where the disease is endemic. Adrenal hydatid cyst is usually asymptomatic, unilateral, and secondary to disseminated hydatid disease, being detected incidentally on imaging done for other reasons.

Pseudocysts are thick-walled, contain debris, septations, fluid–fluid levels, blood products, and soft tissue related to previous hemorrhage, all easier to visualize on USG and MRI than CT.

Imaging Investigations

- On x-ray, dense, laminated, and porcelain-like calcification can be seen in calcified hydatid cysts (Fig. 41.21)
- On USG, simple epithelial cysts are well defined, anechoic with an imperceptible wall (Fig. 41.22)
- On CT, they are homogeneous, nonenhancing, and of water density (Fig. 41.22). Cysts can appear hyperdense and septated in the event of hemorrhage or infection and marginal curvilinear or egg-shell calcification may ensue in the wall in 20%. Cystic degeneration can also occur within pheochromocytoma (Fig. 41.23) and adrenal carcinoma
- On MRI, hydatid cysts have characteristic cyst-in-cyst appearance, a low T2 intensity pericyst and rim-like or nodular calcification

When cysts are very large, the organ of origin can be better defined in the coronal and sagittal planes on CT and MRI, while USG can show a lack of relative motion between the cyst and the organ of origin. Incidental, asymptomatic adrenal cysts with no apparent tumor can be treated conservatively. In doubtful cases, fine needle aspiration of the cyst may prove malignancy or confirm old hemorrhage [3,17].

Teaching Points: Adrenal Cyst

- Simple adrenal cyst: scant septation, no enhancement, thin rim Ca+
- Benign endothelial cyst or pseudocyst
- Coronal imaging: organ of origin
- Complicated cyst: high density, thick-enhancing wall, septations
- Complexity: underlying adrenal neoplasm (secondary pseudocyst)

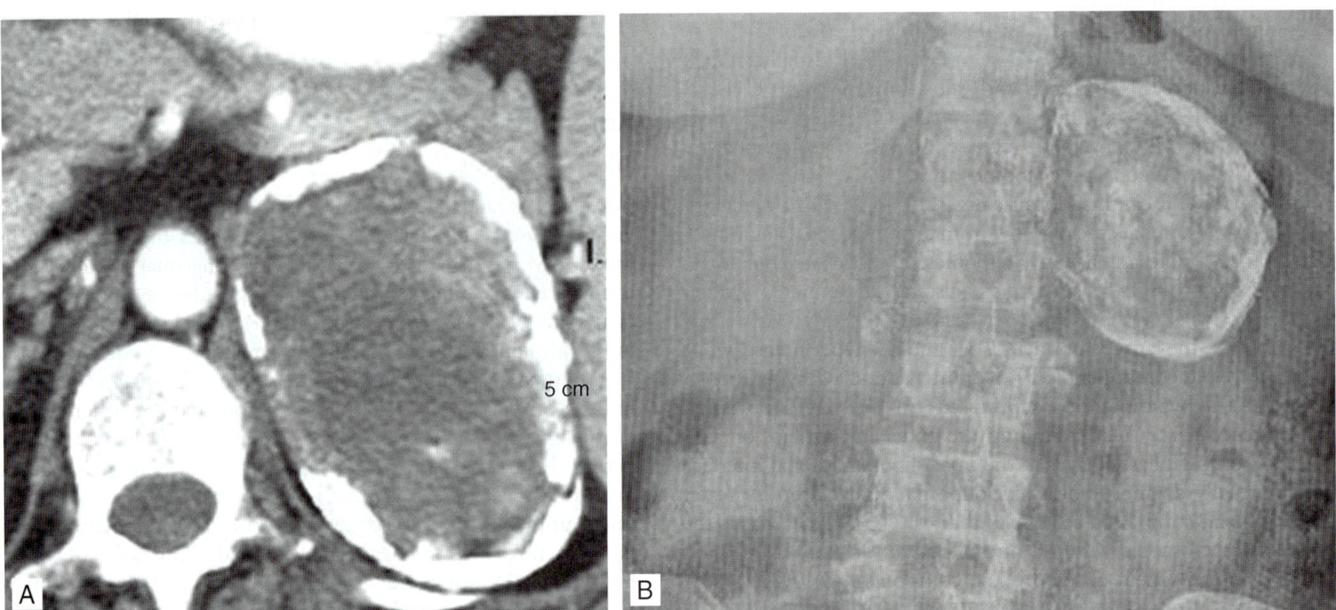

Figure 41.21 Calcified hydatid cyst. (A) Axial CECT and (B) x-ray abdomen. Large, peripherally calcified left adrenal mass with dense, whorled internal contents on CT and porcelain-like calcification in the left suprarenal region on x-ray, inferiorly displacing the left renal shadow.

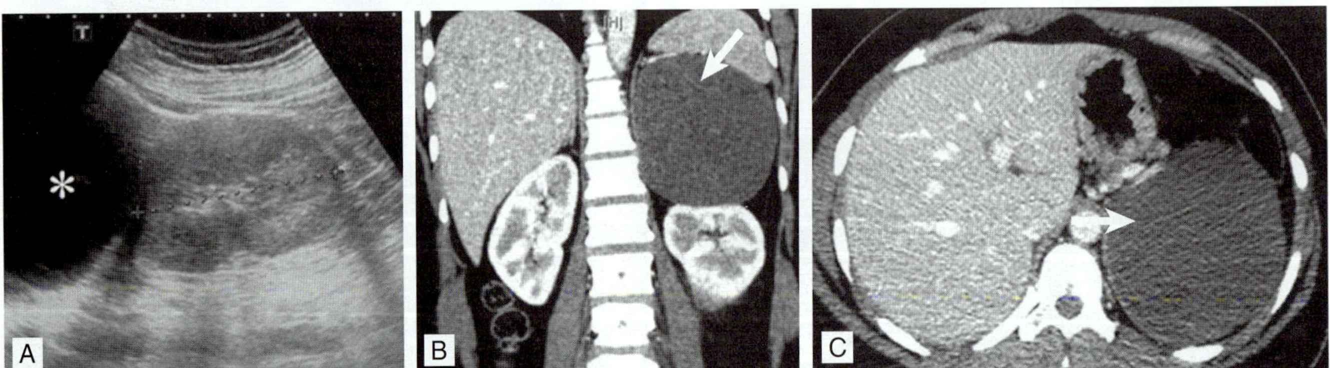

Figure 41.22 Adrenal cyst. (A) Ultrasonography longitudinal left flank, (B) CECT coronal, and (C) CECT axial. Anechoic, round, left suprarenal mass (*asterisk*) with posterior acoustic enhancement, confirmed on CT to be a homogeneous, water-density cyst (*white arrows*) arising from the left adrenal gland, inferiorly displacing the left kidney and contained by an imperceptible wall.

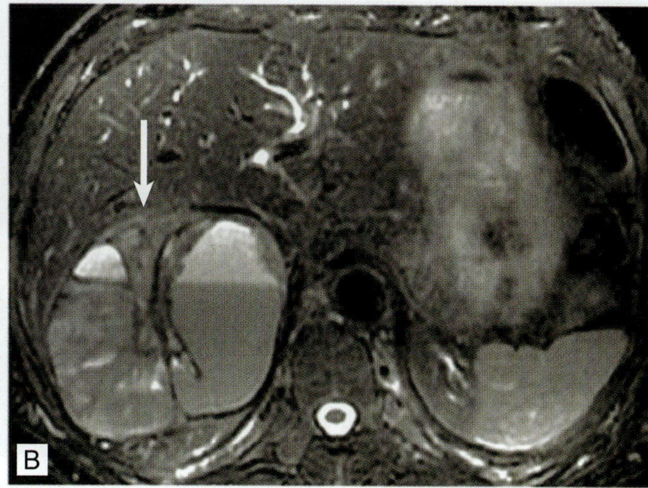

Figure 41.23 Cystic pheochromocytoma. (A) Axial venous phase CECT and (B) T2W MRI. Large, multiloculated, thick-walled, septated right adrenal cyst with internal fluid–fluid levels related to cystic degeneration and hemorrhage within a pheochromocytoma. (Courtesy: Dr. Mukesh Harisinghani.)

Pheochromocytoma

Overview

Pheochromocytomas are rare tumors that arise from adrenal medulla chromaffin cells and produce norepinephrine and epinephrine, causing hypertension in 0.1–0.2%, often without the classic presentation of paroxysmal hypertension, headache, sweating, palpitations, anxiety, and tremor. About 20% of patients present with "silent pheochromocytoma," with normal blood pressure and none of the classic symptoms, suggesting that it would be prudent to screen all patients with adrenal incidentaloma for pheochromocytoma.

Pheochromocytoma "Rule of 10s":
- 10% bilateral
- 10% extra-adrenal
- 10% malignant
- 10% pediatric

Extra-adrenal or ectopic pheochromocytomas are known as paragangliomas. They arise from sympathetic ganglia anywhere in the body, with 90% located below the diaphragm, mostly around or below the kidney, in the pelvis, urinary bladder wall, at the aortic bifurcation or the organ of Zuckerkandl ganglia at the inferior mesenteric artery (IMA) origin. Bladder pheochromocytomas can present with attacks of hypertension brought on by micturition (Fig. 41.24). Other extra-adrenal locations include sympathetic ganglia in the neck, mediastinum, and paravertebral region. Thoracic tumors are usually paravertebral or found in the mediastinum.

Malignant pheochromocytomas are locally infiltrative and metastasize to bone, liver, lymph nodes, lungs, and brain. Although 30% these tumors can be a part of syndromes: MEN-2A, MEN-2B, von Hippel–Lindau (Fig. 41.25), and NF-1, most are sporadic. The Carney triad is the combination of gastric GIST, pulmonary chondroma, and extra-adrenal paraganglioma that can sometimes occur with an additional fourth component: adrenal adenoma (Fig. 41.26) [23].

Adrenal pheochromocytomas secrete catecholamines in 90% of cases, while only 50% of extra-adrenal tumors do so. Raised 24-hour urine vanillylmandelic acid or increased plasma catecholamine levels provide lab confirmation of the diagnosis. Plasma metanephrine test has 99% sensitivity and 89% specificity for levels greater than three to four times the upper limit of normal. Because the values may be affected by position, activity, smoking, and stress, the blood sample is best collected from an indwelling IV cannula after the patient has been supine for 30 minutes and has avoided smoking for 4 hours. Normal plasma metanephrine almost always rules out pheochromocytoma.

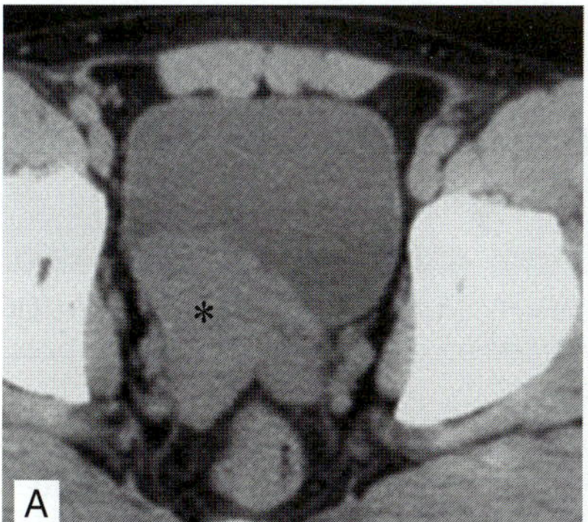

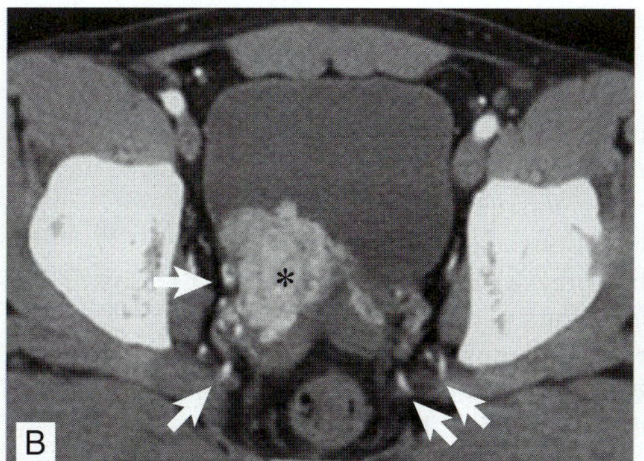

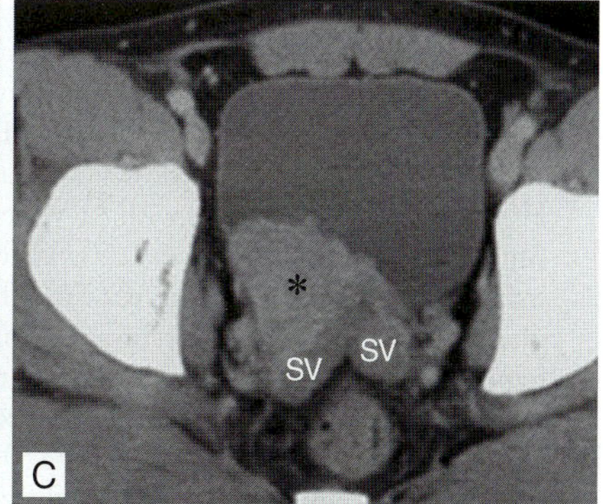

Figure 41.24 Malignant bladder paraganglioma. (A) Noncontrast, (B) arterial phase, and (C) venous phase. Lobulated bladder base mass (*asterisk*) containing punctate calcifications and demonstrating avid arterial enhancement, hypervascularity (*white arrows*), delayed washout, and seminal vesicle (SV) invasion. (Courtesy Dr. Varun S.)

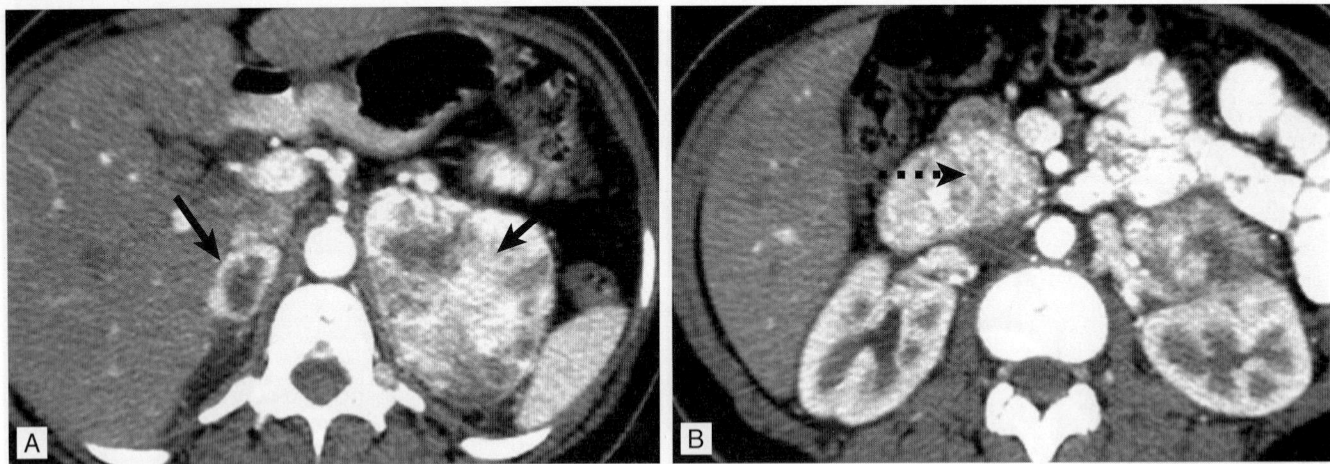

Figure 41.25 Bilateral adrenal pheochromocytomas in von Hippel–Lindau syndrome. CECT arterial phase at level of (A) adrenals and (B) pancreas. Bilateral intensely enhancing adrenal pheochromocytomas (*black arrows*) and an intensely enhancing pancreatic neuroendocrine tumor (*dashed black arrow*).

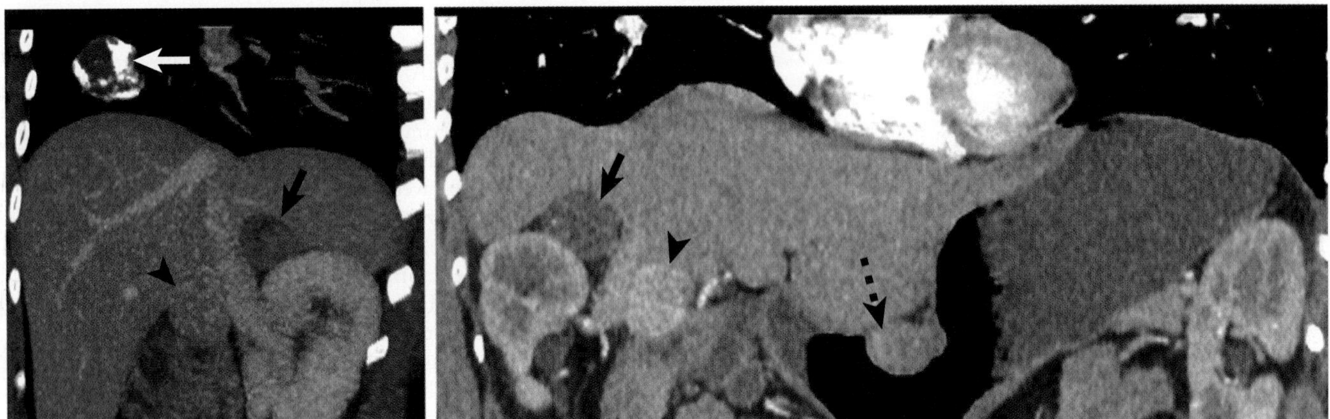

Figure 41.26 Adrenal adenoma: fourth component of the Carney triad. CECT curved MPR reformat. Right adrenal adenoma (*black arrow*) seen with the Carney triad: gastric GIST (*dashed black arrow*), pulmonary chondroma (*white arrow*), and extra-adrenal paraganglioma (*black arrowhead*). (Courtesy: Dr. Suma Jacob.)

Imaging Investigations

The tumor can vary in size from 2 to 20 cm, with a mean size of 5.5 cm and is heterogeneous with foci of necrosis, fibrosis, calcification, cystic and fatty change, mimicking other lesions, and earning the nickname "imaging chameleon." This heterogeneity and hypervascularity is reflected on all imaging techniques.

- On USG, pheochromocytomas are well defined, mixed echogenicity, solid masses with intralesional hypervascularity on color Doppler, and CEUS demonstrating arterial enhancement
- On CT, small tumors are homogeneous while larger tumors are solid and heterogeneous, showing foci of hemorrhage, necrosis, and cystic change. CECT shows avid enhancement similar to HCC and RCC metastases with APW and RPW rapid washout similar to adenomas (Fig. 41.27). Calcifications and venous invasion occur more often in ACC and their presence favors the diagnosis of ACC over pheochromocytoma. There is no risk of hypertensive crisis with iodinated contrast and routine premedication (α and β blockade) is not recommended [24]
- MRI in pheochromocytoma has a 98% sensitivity, being mildly T1 hypointense and T2 brightly hyperintense with no drop in signal on opposed-phase images and can therefore be differentiated from an adenoma, although foci of fatty degeneration can sometimes create a challenge on CS-MRI. DWI is useful in differentiating malignant and benign pheochromocytoma with lower ADC observed in malignant lesions, and is useful in detecting liver and nodal metastases

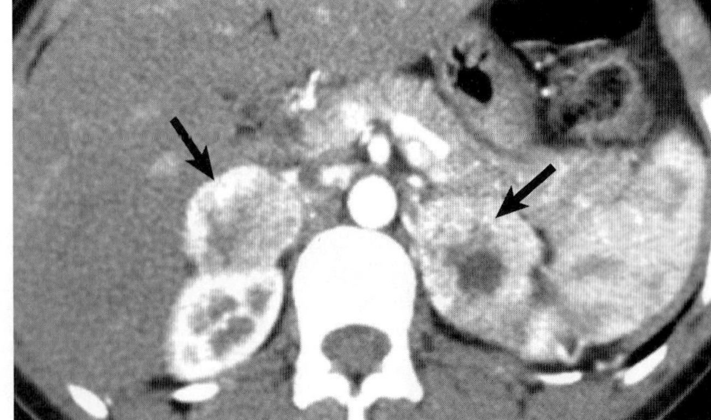

Figure 41.27 Bilateral pheochromocytoma. CECT arterial phase. Bilateral, intensely enhancing, heterogeneous adrenal masses (*black arrows*).

CEMR shows a "salt and pepper" pattern due to tumor hypervascularity with "salt" enhancing parenchyma and "pepper" flow voids of vessels. Fluid–fluid levels related to hemorrhage from

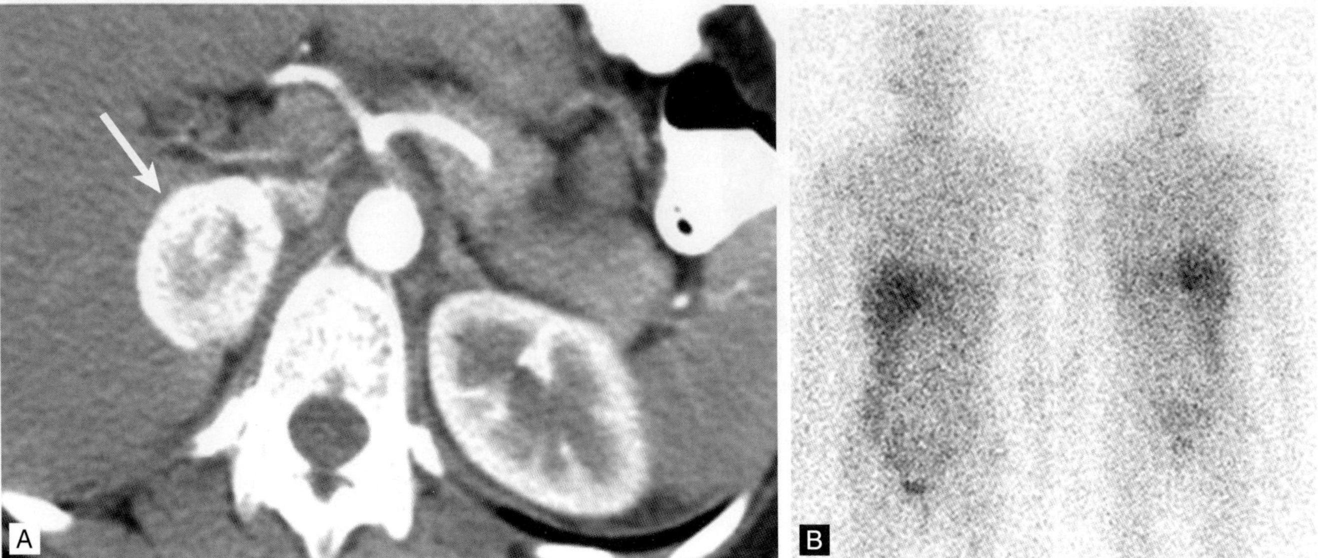

Figure 41.28 Right adrenal pheochromocytoma. (A) CECT arterial phase and (B) mIBG. Well circumscribed, intensely enhancing right adrenal mass (*white arrow*) with increased mIBG tracer uptake.

this hypervascularity are uncommon but well demonstrated on MRI (Fig. 41.23). Although pheochromocytomas show characteristic peaks on MRS due to catecholamines, this method is limited by the location of the adrenal gland near the diaphragm.

Given the higher sensitivity and specificity of CT and MR in the diagnosis of pheochromocytoma, radionuclide imaging is limited mostly to locating elusive extra-adrenal tumors and screening the body for metastatic deposits.

- ^{123}I-mIBG scintigraphy is limited by false negatives related to low spatial resolution, lack of tracer uptake by necrotic and hemorrhagic tumors, and interaction with certain medicines with resulting low specificity and 80% sensitivity. ^{123}I-mIBG uptake in an adrenal nodule is highly suggestive of pheochromocytoma (Fig. 41.28) but uptake outside the adrenal is not as specific since many neuroendocrine tumors also demonstrate uptake with mIBG

Uptake of octreotide-labeled-^{111}In-DTPA occurs in over 70% of tumors due to the expression of somatostatin receptors. Again, uptake by somatostatin receptors at other sites such as the kidney, breasts, liver, spleen, bowel, gallbladder, thyroid gland, salivary glands and within sites of inflammation, reduce the specificity

- 68Ga-DOTANOC PET-CT imaging has been found to have a high accuracy of 92%, superior to mIBG imaging, because of greater lesion-to-background-tissue contrast and higher specificity for pheochromocytoma [1,20,25]

Teaching Points: Adrenal Pheochromocytoma
- Heterogeneous, necrosis, cystic
- Enhance avidly
- T2 hyperintense
- No signal loss out-of-phase

Bilateral Adrenal Disease

Bilateral adrenal disease can be of a benign or malignant origin and can be due to metastases, lymphoma, hemorrhage, or infection from TB or fungal pathogens. Bilateral adrenal hemorrhage can be observed in the setting of trauma or coagulopathy when tumors like neuroblastoma or pheochromocytoma can sometimes bleed. Unfortunately, bilateral adrenal masses are likely to be due to metastases or lymphoma given that both these malignancies tend to be bilateral in 40–50% of cases and tend to cause adrenal insufficiency. Restricted diffusion also favors malignancy while calcification favors granulomatous disease [3].

Adrenal Infection

By usually causing bilateral adrenal disease, tuberculosis continues to be the main cause of adrenal insufficiency in the developing world. In the early stages, on CT and MRI, the adrenal is enlarged without loss of its adreniform shape, accompanied by peripheral enhancement around a central low density or hypointensity related to caseous necrosis. This progresses to bilateral atrophy with diffuse, focal, or scattered punctate calcifications. Caseous necrosis, when treated, heals by enhancing central fibrosis and calcification.

Infections are markedly FDG-avid during the early, acute stage and can mimic metastases, although this does reduce with treatment.

In disseminated histoplasmosis, CT can demonstrate hepatosplenomegaly, enlarged nodes, focal splenic lesions, adrenal enlargement with preserved adreniform shape or peripherally enhancing, centrally hypodense adrenal masses with foci of calcification. In the early stages especially, bilateral adrenal TB also closely resembles bilateral histoplasmosis (Fig. 41.29) and lymphoma, requiring guided needle biopsy for histopathological diagnosis [17].

Teaching Points: Adrenal Infection
- Usually bilateral enlargement with preserved adreniform shape in acute infection
- Adrenal calcification in chronic phase

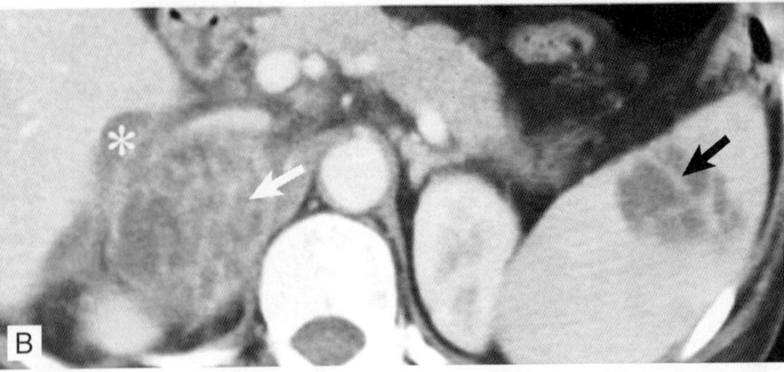

Figure 41.29 Adrenal granuloma. CECT. (A) Histoplasmosis. Bilateral adrenal masses with heterogeneous enhancement and foci of necrosis (*white arrows*). (B) Tuberculosis. Right adrenal mass with necrotic foci, periadrenal fat stranding, and fluid associated with a similar density lesion in the spleen.

Adrenal Lymphoma

Overview

Primary adrenal lymphoma (PAL) is rare and less commonly seen than secondary adrenal NHL. PAL incidence is 1–4% with 50% occurring bilaterally and associated with retroperitoneal lymphadenopathy. The adrenals can appear normal in the early stages, progressing to a subtle, nodular appearance, a diffusely infiltrated gland with a maintained adreniform shape and later an infiltrative soft-tissue mass replacing the adrenal gland. Large retroperitoneal nodal masses can encase the adrenal gland and be difficult to discern separately.

Imaging Investigations

- On USG, lymphoma is solid, homogeneous, and hypoechoic. On CT, lymphoma appears as a mildly enhancing, hypodense mass, without intralesional calcification (Fig. 41.30)
- On MRI, lymphoma is T1 hypointense to isointense and mildly T2 hyperintense

Secondary adrenal lymphoma causes bilateral adrenal enlargement without alteration of the adreniform shape and is more homogeneous than PAL, demonstrating mild enhancement and slow washout. As is true for lymphoma elsewhere, DWI shows restricted diffusion related to a high nuclear-to-cytoplasmic ratio and consequent reduced water diffusion and is FDG-avid on ^{18}FDG PET-CT.

Apart from these few distinctive appearances, adrenal lymphoma has a nonspecific appearance and cannot be easily differentiated from metastases. Secondary adrenal lymphoma may be suspected in patients with NHL but has to be definitively proved with guided needle biopsy. Lymphoma responds well to chemotherapy, unlike metastases, with decreased FDG uptake and resolution to normal.

Immunotherapy-related adrenalitis is a rare complication of immunotherapy that may cause adrenal insufficiency. CT (Fig. 41.31) and MRI show bilateral adrenal enlargement with bilateral mild ^{18}F-FDG-avidity on PET/CT [3,17].

Adrenal Hemorrhage

Overview

Adrenal hemorrhage can occur for a variety of reasons including trauma, anticoagulation, complex pregnancy, sepsis, surgery, or within most adrenal neoplasms other than lymphoma. Adrenal insufficiency occurs when >90% adrenal is destroyed.

Post-traumatic hemorrhage is the most common cause, can be bilateral in 20% of cases, but is usually not accompanied by

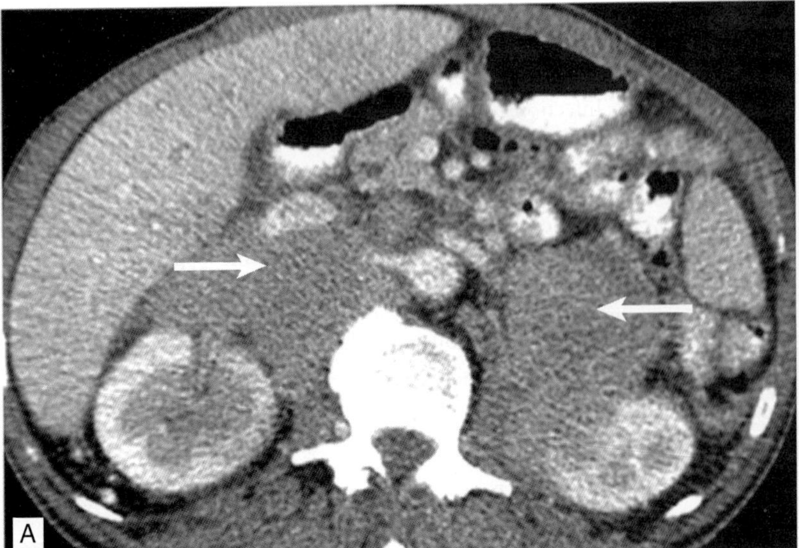

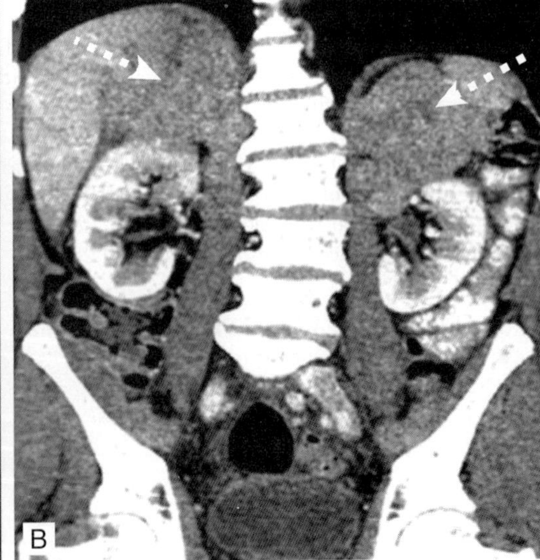

Figure 41.30 Diffuse large B cell lymphoma. CECT (A) axial image and (B) coronal image. Large, homogeneous, mildly enhancing, ill-defined adrenal masses (*white* and *dashed white arrows*).

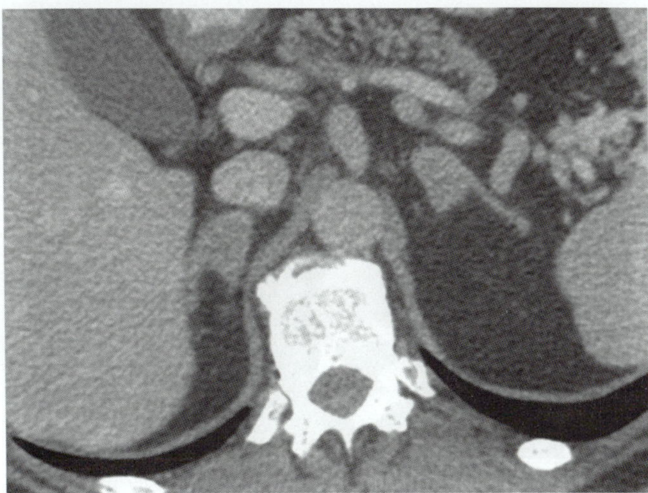

Figure 41.31 Immunotherapy-induced adrenalitis. A 69-year old. CECT. Diffuse bilateral adrenal thickening after immunotherapy. Fine needle aspiration: chronic inflammation with immunotherapy-induced adrenalitis. (Courtesy: Dr. Mukesh Harisinghani.)

adrenal insufficiency. The right adrenal is more prone to hemorrhage during blunt abdominal trauma.

Neonatal adrenal hemorrhage is the most common cause of an adrenal mass in an infant, in the first week of life within the large infantile adrenal (Fig. 41.32). Neonatal hemorrhage may present as an abdominal mass or as bilateral masses which can develop marginal calcification as they regress over several weeks. If clinically suspected, the diagnosis can best be confirmed by USG, which can differentiate hemorrhage from the more solid neuroblastoma.

Nontraumatic intratumoral adrenal hemorrhage occurs in 1% of autopsies, and usually occurs when the patient with underlying pheochromocytoma, myelolipoma, metastasis, or carcinoma is on anticoagulants. Findings that indicate hemorrhage have occurred within an underlying adrenal lesion include the presence of enhancement, calcification, and increased metabolic activity on PET imaging.

Imaging Investigations

- USG is a good first-line imaging in children and the newborn: acute hemorrhage appears as a mixed, mostly echogenic blood clot that liquefies and turns hypoechoic, showing no vascularization
- On CT, acute hemorrhage appears as a hyperdense enlarged gland, and in the setting of trauma, is associated with periadrenal and retroperitoneal hematoma (Fig. 41.33). Acute or subacute hematoma presents as a round or oval mass of high density (50–90 HU) in an asymmetrically enlarged gland, usually homogeneous and nonenhancing with inflammatory periadrenal fat stranding, thickening of diaphragmatic crura, with or without periadrenal hemorrhage. Additionally, traumatic pneumothorax, hydropneumothorax, rib fracture, and contusion of the lung, liver, spleen, or pancreas can be present

Chronic hematoma can liquefy into an adrenal pseudocyst or retract, with or without foci of calcification. Unilateral or bilateral adrenal hematomas may be associated with adrenal or renal vein thrombosis. Or, in the case of nontraumatic hemorrhage, an underlying large adrenal cyst or myelolipoma may be visualized.

- On MRI, within the first week, acute hematoma is T1 isointense to mildly hypointense and T2 hypointense due to deoxyhemoglobin. Between 1 and 7 weeks, subacute hematoma appears T1 and T2 hyperintense due to methemoglobin. After 7 weeks, chronic hematoma shows a hypointense rim on T1 and T2 due to hemosiderin and fibrosis [3,17]

Teaching Points: Adrenal Hemorrhage

- Neonatal USG echogenic > liquefies > hypoechoic, no vascularization
- CT
  - Round or oval, periadrenal fat stranding
  - Acute high density > decreased size, density > resolves
- MRI
  - Acute: isointense T1, hypointense T2 (<1w)
  - Subacute: hyperintense T1, T2 (1w–7w)
  - Chronic: hypointense rim T1, T2 (>7w)
- *Organized adrenal hematoma > calcification/pseudocyst*

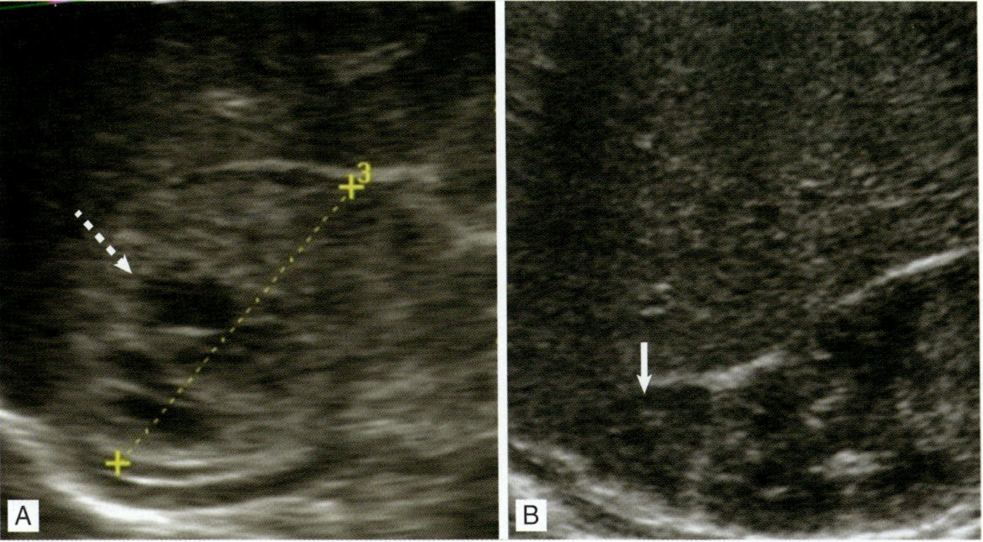

Figure 41.32 Neonatal adrenal hemorrhage. Ultrasonography (A) initial presentation and (B) 2-month follow-up. Heterogeneous, echogenic right adrenal mass with cystic foci (*dashed white arrow*). Two-month follow-up scan shows marked reduction in size, indicating resolution of hemorrhage (*white arrow*).

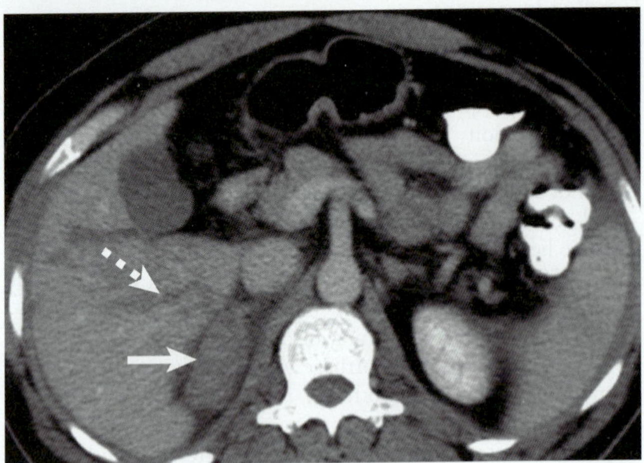

Figure 41.33 Traumatic adrenal hemorrhage. Blunt injury abdomen. CECT. Right adrenal hemorrhage (*white arrow*) and liver laceration (*dashed white arrow*).

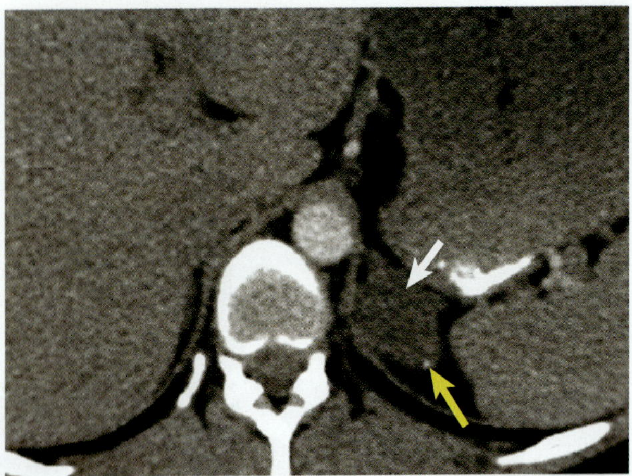

Figure 41.34 Adrenal lymphangioma. CECT. Low-density mass (*white arrow*) in the left adrenal gland with a single punctate calcification (*yellow arrow*). (Courtesy: Dr. Mukesh Harisinghani.)

Unusual Adrenal Tumors

The following tumors are rare but of relevance when atypical features are encountered in an adrenal mass.

Lipomas

Lipomas are well-defined lobules of fat, which in contrast to myelolipomas, show no evidence of soft-tissue and may demonstrate foci of calcification.

Hemangiomas

Hemangiomas may be incidentally discovered in women 40–70 years and are capillary or cavernous in type. NECT may reveal calcified phleboliths or dystrophic calcification at the site of previous bleeds. On MRI, hemangioma T1 hypointense and markedly T2 hyperintense "lightbulb sign," with T2 hypointense foci of calcification. On CECT and CEMR, hemangiomas may exhibit nodular peripheral enhancement, with or without centripetal delayed filling.

Lymphangiomas

Lymphangiomas are asymptomatic, incidental, benign lesions that can present at any age, appearing on CT as a well-defined hypodense, near-water density, septated, enhancing mass with scattered punctate or thick curvilinear calcification (Fig. 41.34). On MRI, lymphangiomas are nonspecific, appearing T1 hypointense and T2 hyperintense.

Schwannoma

Schwannoma is a benign tumor arising from nerve sheaths, usually asymptomatic although hemorrhage can cause abdominal pain. On CT, schwannomas are hypodense and heterogeneously enhancing with larger masses showing hemorrhage, calcification, and cystic areas, T1 isointense, and mildly T2 hyperintense on MRI.

Adenomatoid Tumor

Adenomatoid tumor is a benign, mesothelial, asymptomatic tumor, hypodense, and heterogeneously enhancing on CT with foci of calcification and septations.

Oncocytoma

Oncocytoma is an epithelial tumor, most often benign and nonfunctioning tumor that can be large and affect the left adrenal more often than the right. On CT and MRI, the mass is well defined, encapsulated, and heterogeneously enhancing. Differentiation from cortical carcinoma can be challenging [17].

Adrenal Incidentalomas

Incidentaloma refers to unexpected pathology found in the course of an unrelated imaging investigation. The incidence of incidentalomas has increased with the widespread availability of CT and increases with age, but can present at any age.

When there is a known malignancy, 27% of incidentalomas are metastases but in the absence of known malignancy, an incidentaloma is usually a benign nonfunctioning adenoma, while cysts, myelolipoma, and hemorrhage have characteristic imaging features.

"Rule of Four" in Adrenal Incidentalomas

- 4% CTs across all age groups
- 4% malignant etiology
- 4 cm needs surgical removal
- 4 years follow-up to prove stability

Incidentalomas >4 cm

Size is a major predictor of malignancy in adrenal masses. If the lesion is indeterminate and ≥4 cm in diameter with no primary malignancy consider resection because of the possibility of an adrenocortical carcinoma without biopsy. If there is a malignancy history consider PET-CT or guided needle biopsy.

Although adrenalectomy performed for incidentalomas >4 cm has a low specificity (42%), largely due to the low prevalence of ACC, this highly aggressive cancer still warrants the removal of adrenal lesions >4 cm, especially in younger patients without comorbidities or evidence of extra-adrenal malignancy.

Indeterminate Incidentalomas 1–4 cm

Of indeterminate 1–4 cm lesions, those measuring 1–2 cm in patients without history of malignancy are probably benign and require only a 12-month follow-up.

In those >2 cm indeterminate lesions that fit the criteria for a lipid-poor adenoma on CT, there is no need for follow-up. If

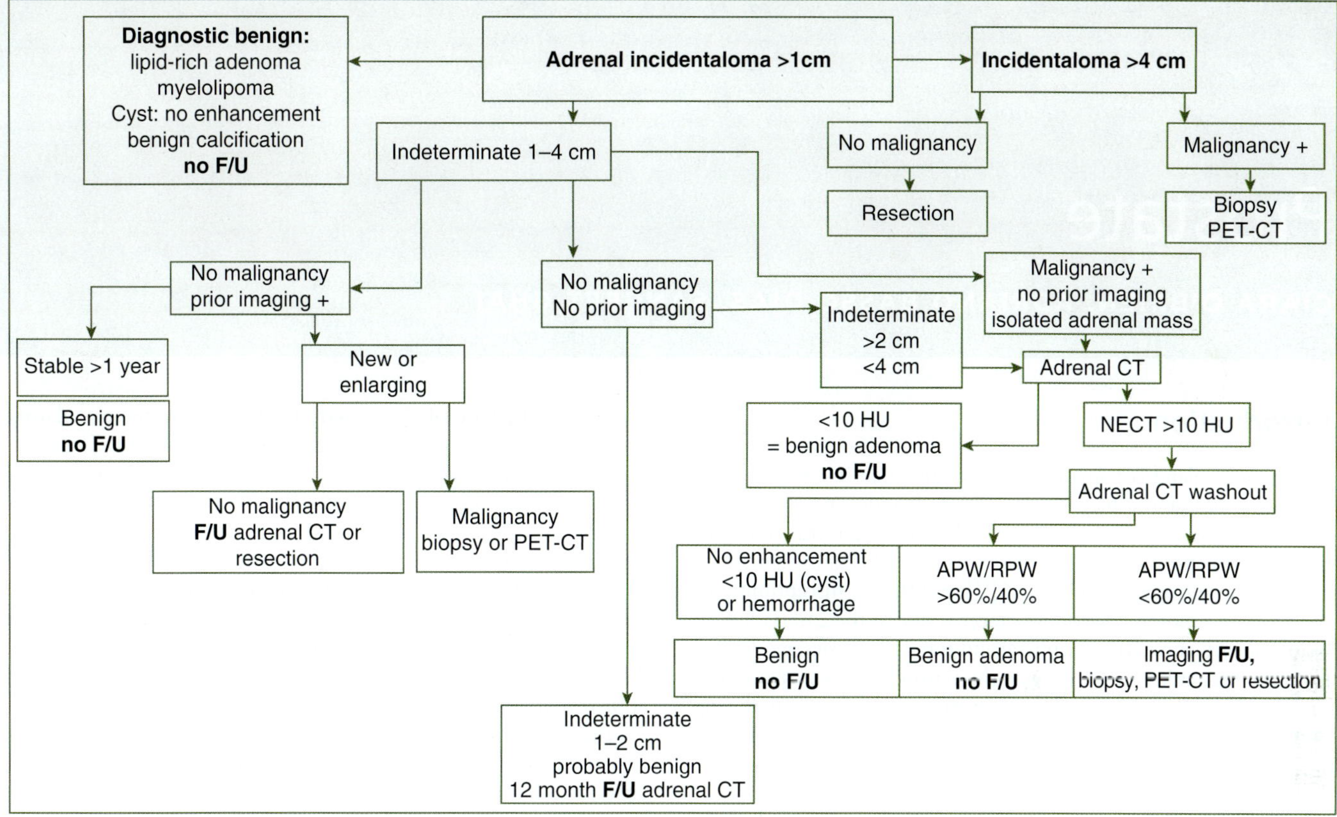

Figure 41.35 Adrenal incidentaloma algorithm. Guidelines for the management of an incidentally discovered adrenal mass.

the lesion is not a lipid-poor adenoma, and the patient has a malignancy history, consider PET-CT or guided needle biopsy. If there is no malignancy history, consider follow-up or resection.

ACR Guidelines for the Management of Incidentalomas [26]

- <1 cm: do nothing
- >1 and <2 cm: benign—optional follow-up 1 year
- >2 but <4 cm: need to confirm benign nature—CT adrenal protocol
- >4 cm: if no known malignancy, proceed to surgical resection as for a presumed ACC

Many adrenal lesions can be categorized as typically benign and need no follow-up:

- Lipid-rich adenoma (NECT <10 HU, signal drop on MRI)
- Myelolipoma (macroscopic fat)
- Cyst (water density, no enhancement)
- Hemorrhage (no enhancement defined as <10 HU difference)
- Lesions with benign calcifications (coarse, curvilinear, septal)
- Unchanged (>12 months) lesions (+ no history of cancer)

Adrenalectomy is reserved for:

- Functional adenomas
- Indeterminate nodules >4 cm
- Myelolipomas >4 cm and
- Suspicion of malignancy (Fig. 41.35) [26–28]

Suggested Readings

- PJ Mazzaglia, J Varghese, MA Habra, Evaluation and management of adrenal neoplasms: endocrinologist and endocrine surgeon perspectives, Abdom Radiol 45 (2020) 1001–1010.
- M Taffel, S Haji-Momenian, P Nikolaidis, FH Miller, Adrenal imaging: a comprehensive review, Radiol Clin North Am 50 (2) (2012 Mar) 219–243.
- TP Johnson, KM Horton, EK Fishman, Adrenal mass imaging with multidetector CT: pathologic conditions, pearls, and pitfalls, Radiographics 29 (5) (2009) 1333–1351.
- SZ Adam, P Nikolaidis, JM Horowitz, H Gabriel, NA Hammond, T Patel, et al., Chemical shift MR imaging of the adrenal gland: principles, pitfalls, and applications, Radiographics 36 (2) (2016) 414–432.
- D Albano, F Agnello, F Midiri, G Pecoraro, A Bruno, P Alongi, et al., Imaging features of adrenal masses, Insights Imaging 10 (1) (2019 Jan 25) 1.

42

Prostate

CIARA O'BRIEN, ADRIANO BASSO DIAS, SANGEET GHAI

Introduction

The prostate gland is a small organ resembling an inverted cone or walnut, it lies at the base of the urinary bladder anterior to the rectum and surrounding the urethra. During the third month of gestation, the prostate gland develops from epithelial invaginations at the posterior urogenital sinus [1]. The differing susceptibility of the prostate zones to developing cancer is due to the embryological origin of each zone. The peripheral and transition zones are derived from the urogenital sinus, whereas the central zone is derived from the Wolffian duct. Morphological prostate changes occur during puberty as the gland enlarges to weigh approximately 20 g by the age of 25–30 years. The function of the prostate is to secrete alkaline fluid that is a component of seminal fluid. Despite the small size of the prostate it is associated with three major morbidities in men: benign prostatic hyperplasia (BPH), prostatitis, and prostate cancer. The anatomy of the prostate gland has been described in the literature since the mid-16th century [2]. Today prostate anatomy is described using zones to delineate the different anatomical areas of the prostate gland. Imaging of the prostate gland is performed using ultrasonography (USG) and magnetic resonance imaging (MRI).

Anatomy

McNeal described the contemporary zonal anatomy of the prostate gland in 1981. The prostate is divided into four glandular zones surrounding the prostatic urethra: the peripheral zone, transition zone, central zone, and anterior fibromuscular zone (Figs. 42.1–42.3). Each prostate zone has a different embryological origin and therefore different susceptibility to disease [3]. The gland has an anterior, posterior, and inferior-lateral surface, it is divided into regions called the apex, mid, and base of the prostate each accounting for approximately one-third of the prostate volume. Blood supply is from the prostaticovesical arteries that arise from the internal iliac arteries. Lymphatic drainage is through the internal iliac lymph nodes. Nerve supply is from the prostatic plexus, this is composed of parasympathetic supply from S2 to S4 sacral nerve roots and sympathetic supply through the hypogastric nerve [1]. The presence of a prostate capsule in contentious, the "real" prostate capsule at the outer layer of the gland is made of fibromuscular tissue composed of predominantly smooth muscle that can be separated from the prostate stroma. This lining surrounds the entire prostate gland and is the landmark for extraprostatic extension of cancer.

The peripheral zone is the largest zone containing approximately 70% of the normal prostate tissue (Fig. 42.4). The peripheral zone surrounds the distal urethra and occupies the posterior, lateral, and apical regions of the gland [1,3]. The peripheral zone includes the area at the base of the urinary bladder where the ejaculatory ducts feed into the urethra, called the verumontanum. The verumontanum is a longitudinal mucosal fold that forms an elliptical segment of the prostatic urethra [1]. The preprostatic sphincter stretches from the base of the bladder to the verumontanum [2]. The peripheral zone is separated from the transition and central zones by a surgical capsule. The peripheral zone is composed of numerous ductal and acinar elements with sparsely interwoven smooth muscle; its composition makes it high signal intensity on T2-weighted MRI sequences. The peripheral zone is the site of approximately 70–75% of prostate cancer [1,3].

The transition zone makes up 5% of the normal prostate and lies superior to the verumontanum. It is made of two small glandular areas straddling the proximal prostatic urethra. The normal transition zone is made up of two types of histologically different tissue: glandular and stromal tissue [4]. The glandular tissue is hyperintense and the stromal tissue is hypointense on T2-weighted MRI sequences. The T2 hypointense appearance of the stromal tissue can mimic cancers making interpretation difficult. Approximately 20–30% of prostate cancer occurs in the transition zone. BPH arises in the transition zone, this is a progressive disease related to age. It is estimated that BPH affects 50% of men over the age of 60 years and 90% of men over the age of 70 years. The transition zone progressively increases in size with age doubling in volume from the age of 40–80 years (5.5–11.1 mL) [5,6].

The central zone (Fig. 42.5) accounts for 25% of the glandular prostate tissue and lies between the peripheral and transition zones at the base of the prostate. The central zone surrounds the ejaculatory ducts and narrows at the verumontanum to form a wedge shape [3]. Prostate carcinoma of the central zone is rare accounting for only 5%. On MRI, the central zone is low signal intensity on T2-weighted sequences [7].

The anterior fibromuscular stroma (AFMS) is a nonglandular thick sheath of the tissue that is continuous with the detrusor muscle of the urinary bladder neck [3]. It forms an apron of the tissue forming the anterior surface of the prostate contacting the urethra at the apex of the gland and forms a crescent shape. The AFMS is low signal on T2-weighted MRI. Prostate cancer does not arise in the AFMS, but peripheral and transition zone cancer can extend into the AFMS and lead to loss of the normal symmetry. Anterior tumors in the prostate account for approximately 21% and are not palpable on digital rectal exam (DRE) [8,9].

The seminal vesicles are paired secretory glands that lie cephalad to the prostate gland. They are extraperitoneal and are located posterior to urinary bladder and anterior to the rectum. Their function is to produce seminal fluid that supports and maintains sperm. Seminal fluid makes up 80% of the ejaculate volume [10]. In the setting of prostate cancer, the seminal vesicles are a frequent site for extraprostatic disease.

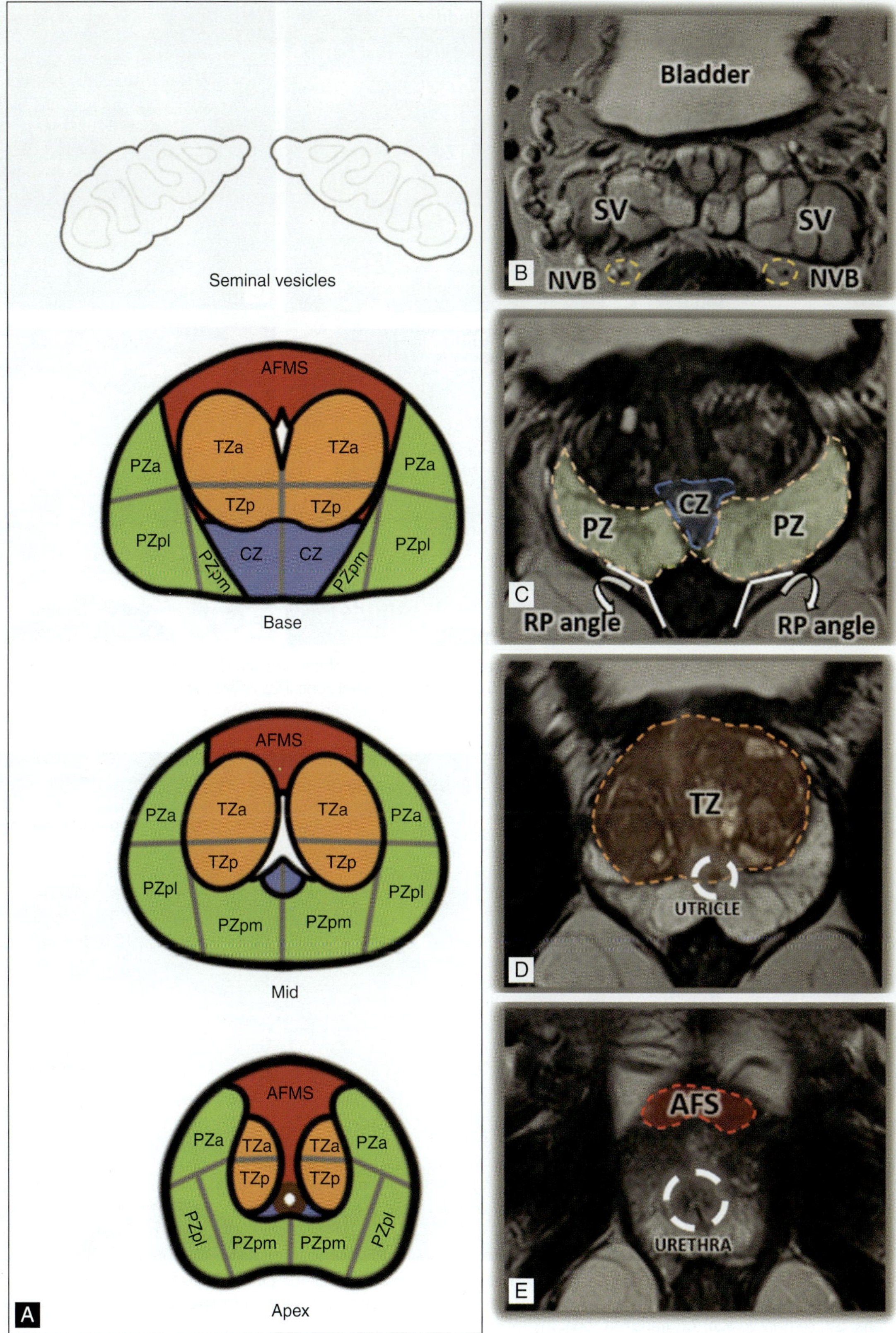

Figure 42.1 Main anatomic concepts of the prostate. The PI-RADS sector map (A) and the corresponding MRI images (T2WI), in the axial plane (B–E). The prostate is divided into three main regions: base (C), midgland (D), and apex (E). The gland is also divided into four zones: anterior fibromuscular stroma (AFMS), transition zone (TZ), central zone (CZ), and peripheral zone (PZ). The neurovascular bundles (NVB) course posterolateral to the prostate bilaterally, usually at the 5 o'clock and 7 o'clock positions. The rectoprostatic angles (RP angles) are depicted posteriorly to the prostate gland. The utricle (the verumontanum) is a small indentation on the posterior wall of the mid prostatic urethra at the site of ejaculatory ducts opening into the prostatic urethra. *AFMS*, anterior fibromuscular stroma; *CZ*, central zone; *NVB*, neurovascular bundle; *PZ*, peripheral zone; *RP*, rectoprostatic; *SV*, seminal vesicles; *TZ*, transition zone. Note: The PI-RADS sector map was adapted from the PI-RADS Version 2.1 document. (Data from: https://www.acr.org/-/media/ACR/Files/RADS/Pi-RADS/PIRADS-V2-1.pdf).

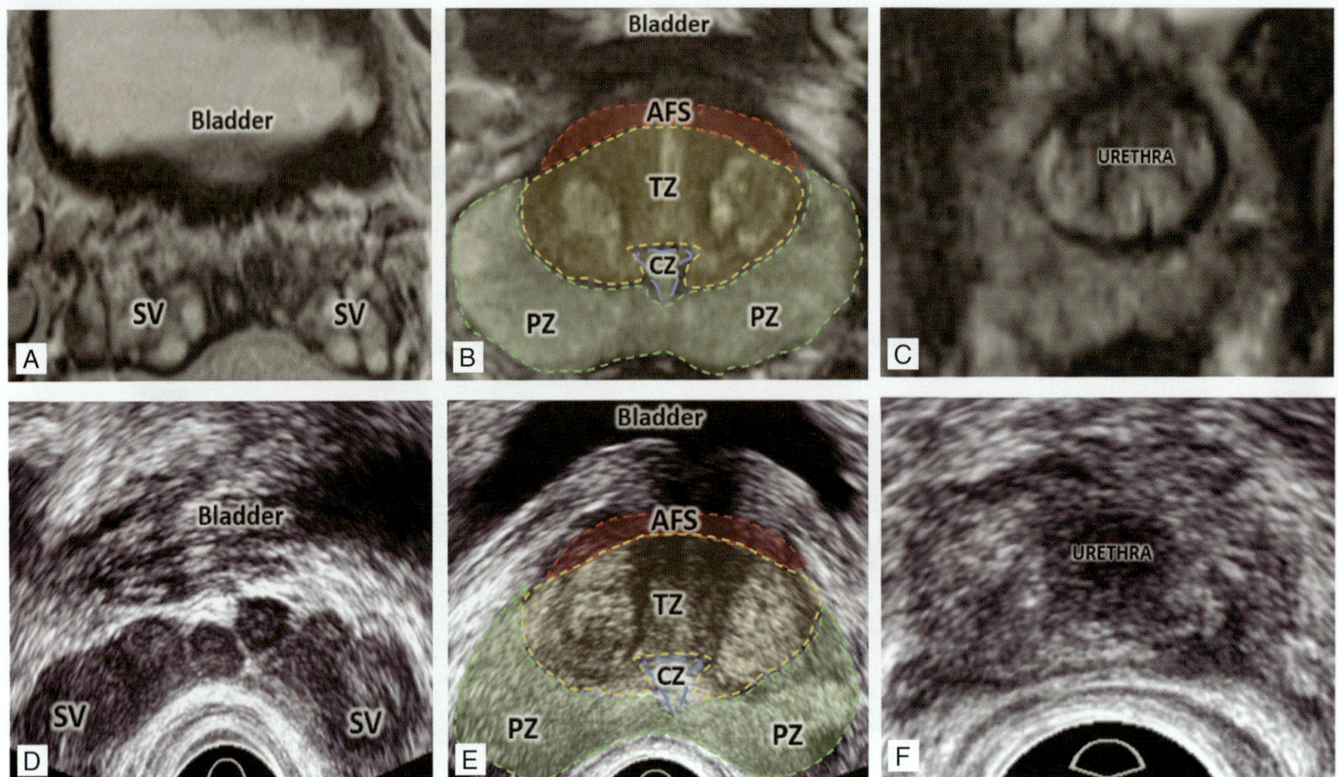

Figure 42.2 Correlation of axial MRI T2W images (A–C) and axial ultrasonography images of the prostate (D–F). The prostate is divided into four zones: anterior fibromuscular stroma (AFMS), transition zone (TZ), central zone (CZ), and peripheral zone (PZ). *AFMS*, anterior fibromuscular stroma; *CZ*, central zone; *PZ*, peripheral zone; *SV*, seminal vesicles; *TZ*, transition zone.

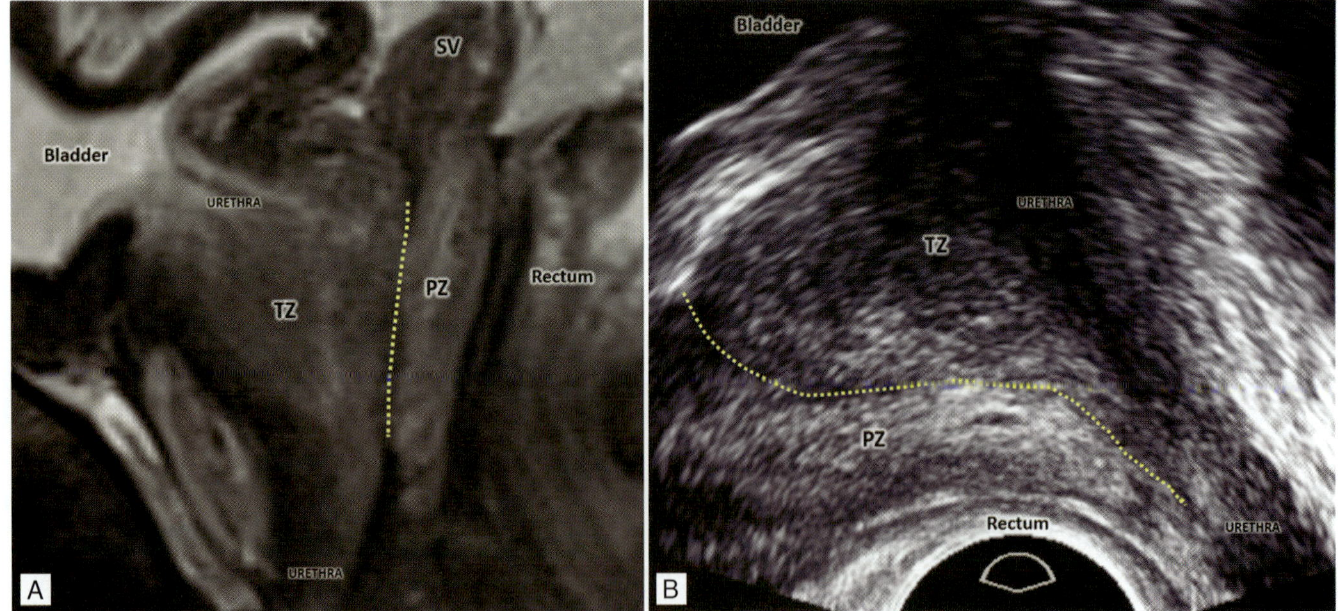

Figure 42.3 Correlation of sagittal MRI T2W image (A) and sagittal ultrasonography image of the prostate (B). Note that the surgical capsule (*yellow dashed line*) separates the transition zone from the peripheral zone. In this midsagittal view of the prostate, the prostatic urethra is entirely seen. *PZ*, peripheral zone; *SV*, seminal vesicle; *TZ*, transition zone.

Diseases

Benign Prostate Cysts

Benign prostate cysts are often identified on USG of the prostate gland; these include Mullerian duct cysts and prostatic utricle cysts.

- Mullerian duct cysts arise from the embryological remnants of the Mullerian duct and can arise anywhere along the path of the Mullerian duct; however, they are commonly seen in the midline of the prostate gland. They range in size and can extend above the prostate gland
- Utricle cysts (Fig. 42.6) arise secondary to dilatation of the prostatic utricle; they are also midline cysts and can be

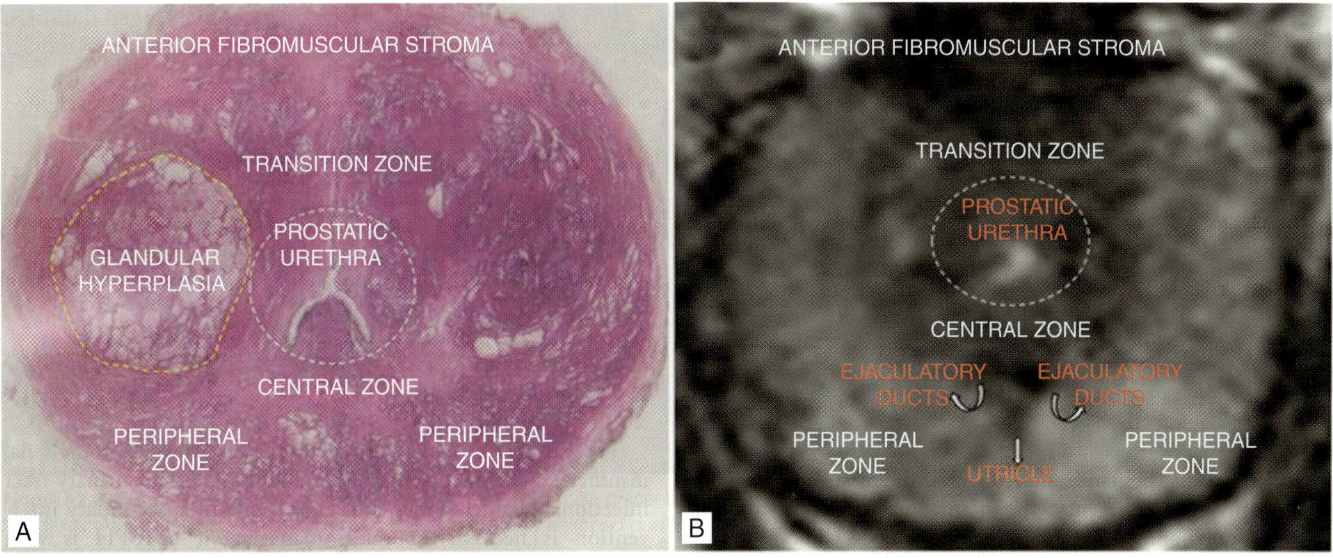

Figure 42.4 Histological concepts (A) and correlation with MRI prostate (T2WI, axial plane) (B). The peripheral zone is separated from the transition and central zones by a surgical capsule and it is composed of numerous ductal and acinar elements with sparsely interwoven smooth muscle, its composition makes it high signal intensity on T2WI (B). The transition zone is made up of two types of histologically different tissue: glandular and stromal tissue. Note that a nodule of benign prostatic hyperplasia, with predominant glandular component (*yellow circle*), is showed in the histology image (A). The central zone surrounds the ejaculatory ducts and narrows at the utricle (or the verumontanum). The utricle is a small indentation on the posterior wall of the mid prostatic urethra at the site of ejaculatory ducts opening into the prostatic urethra. The anterior fibromuscular stroma is a nonglandular thick sheath of the tissue that is continuous with the detrusor muscle of the urinary bladder neck.

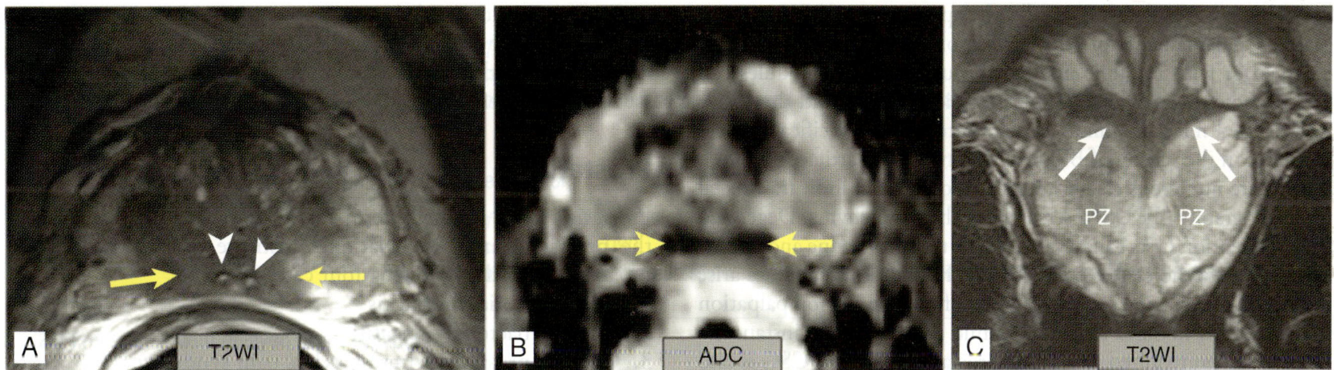

Figure 42.5 Anatomy of the central zone (CZ). Axial images of the prostate base show the normal CZ (*yellow arrows*) visible on T2WI (A) and ADC map (B) as bilaterally symmetric low signal intensity tissue encircling the ejaculatory ducts (*arrowheads*). Coronal image of the posterior prostate (C) illustrates the CZ (*white arrows*) and peripheral zone (PZ). Note that on the coronal plane, the CZ has the shape of an inverted cone with its base oriented toward the base of the gland and is homogeneously hypointense as it contains more stroma than the glandular tissue.

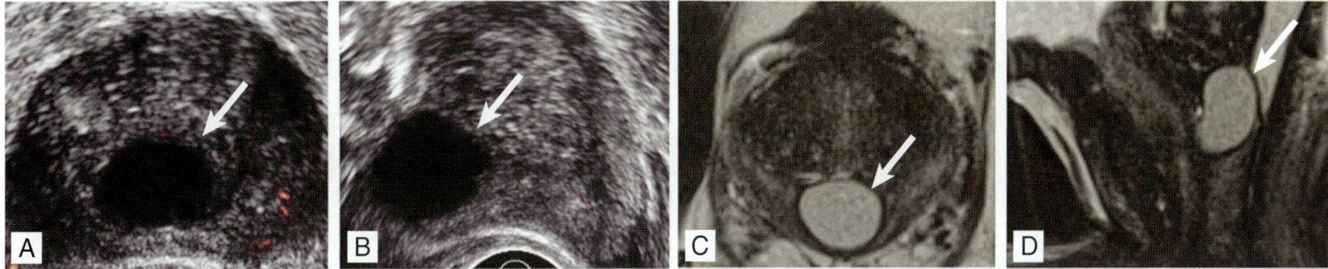

Figure 42.6 Prostatic utricle cyst. Transrectal ultrasonography (axial: A; sagittal: B) and prostate MRI, T2WI (axial: C; sagittal D) show a midline cystic structure in the level of the verumontanum, compatible with a utricle cyst (*arrows*).

indistinguishable from Mullerian duct cysts on imaging. However, utricle cysts are typically smaller and do not extend beyond the prostate

Although both cysts are benign, they can cause obstructive or irritative urinary tract symptoms. Rarely these cysts develop cancers including endometrial, clear cell, or squamous cell carcinoma. Ejaculatory duct cysts are extremely rare and typically asymptomatic [11]. Benign ductal ectasia is a condition of older men in the setting of prostatic atrophy and dilation of the peripheral prostatic ducts.

Figure 42.15 Transrectal ultrasonography (TRUS) images (7.5 MHz) of the prostate—axial plane (grayscale: A; color Doppler: B) demonstrating a hypoechoic lesion in the right peripheral zone (*arrow* in A), with increased vascularity on Doppler (*arrow* in B), suspicious for a malignant lesion.

adjacent smooth tubular structures that can be identified entering the prostate gland at the mid-base becoming the ejaculatory ducts.

The zonal anatomy of the prostate gland may be difficult to delineate on TRUS, the central gland incorporates the transition and central zones, while the peripheral zone is seen as a homogenous outer layer. The anterior aspect is often difficult to appreciate due to its location and the probe orientation. The transition zone is more echogenic than the peripheral zone; these are separated by a thin hypoechoic rim called the "surgical capsule." *The surgical capsule is a frequent site for calcific deposits called corpora amylacea.* The surrounding periprostatic fat creates a plane allowing for delineation of the margins of the prostate gland.

Approximately 40–60% of prostate cancers are not detected by grayscale TRUS, therefore a normal appearance on TRUS does not exclude prostate cancer and systematic biopsy of the prostate gland should be considered if there is clinical suspicion of cancer. When cancer is detected by TRUS in the peripheral zone prostate cancer it classically appears as a hypoechoic nodule (Fig. 42.15) because tumors replace the normal loose glandular tissue of the peripheral zone with a packed mass of tumor cells. Cancer in the peripheral zone may also appear as an ill-defined area of reduced echogenicity compared with the background parenchyma. Occasionally, prostate cancer can also appear hyperechoic on B-mode imaging secondary to a desmoplastic reaction of the tumor.

Prostate cancer often demonstrates neovascularity and increased microvascular density. Color and power Doppler imaging can increase the detection of peripheral zone cancer which is isoechoic on grayscale imaging. When performing Doppler imaging, power Doppler mode is preferred because it is more sensitive to flow, providing a more uniform display of vascular density within the lesion [6,28].

Cancers originating in the transition and central zones are less common and more difficult to detect with TRUS. This is particularly true in the setting of BPH where the background gland is heterogeneous with increased vascularity from the hyperplasia. Transition zone cancers may be detected as asymmetric hypoechoic areas relative to the background parenchyma, there may be asymmetric bulging of the surgical capsule or at the margin of the prostate gland. Tumors at the anterior midline of the prostate are typically not well visualized with TRUS due to their location in the fibromuscular area of the gland anterior to the urethra.

It is also important to further emphasize the pitfalls of TRUS and Doppler imaging—not all cancers are vascular, and some benign inflammatory conditions can mimic hypoechoic tumor and demonstrate increased Doppler flow.

- The initial prostate biopsy typically involves 10–12 samples obtained in a systematic fashion from the prostate gland (Fig. 42.16). If a suspicious area is identified on TRUS, additional samples are obtained from this area first
- Follow-up or extended biopsy protocols are typically performed when the initial biopsy is negative and a high clinical suspicion for cancer remains. An extended biopsy consists of up to 17 systematic samples, which includes sampling of transition zones

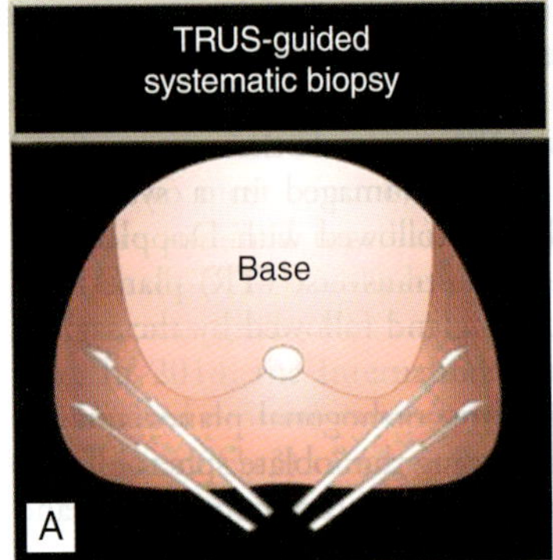

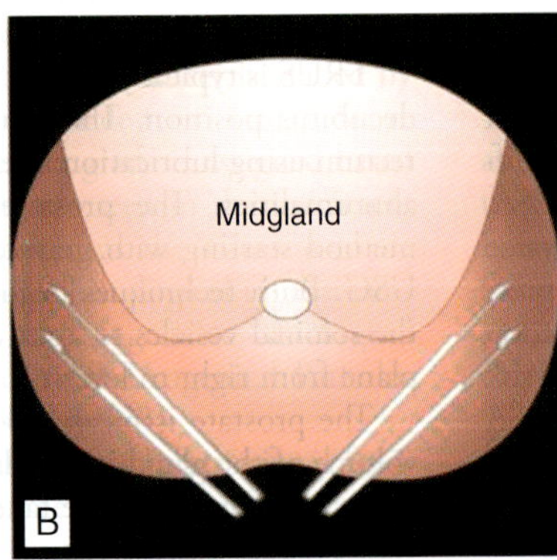

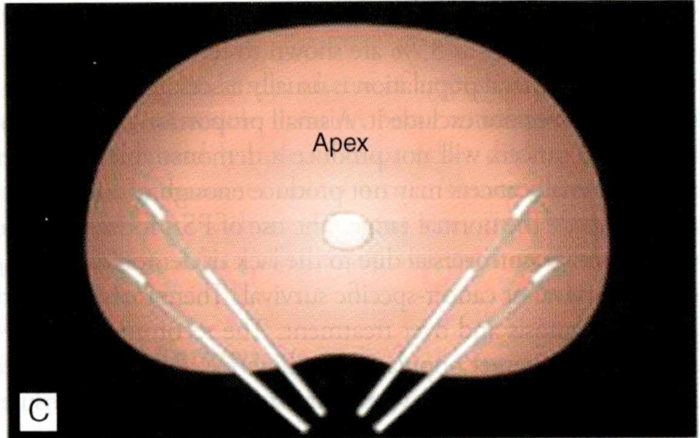

Figure 42.16 Transrectal ultrasonography (TRUS)-guided prostate biopsy scheme. The standard systematic biopsy procedure consists of sampling randomly the parasagittal midline and lateral basal (A), medial (B), and apical (C) regions bilaterally for a total of 12 cores.

(two samples from either side) and from midline gland in addition to repeat extended sextant 12-core sampling

- A saturation biopsy involves >20 core biopsies. These are again, obtained in a systemic fashion from the prostate gland; however, this biopsy is typically performed using a template transperineal approach and traditionally involves sedation or anesthesia for the procedure. The risk of complication from a saturation biopsy is about twice that of a standard 12 core TRUS biopsy [20]

New advances in USG are emerging, which demonstrate greater sensitivity and specificity for the detection of prostate cancer. Nonlinear imaging (tissue harmonic imaging) allows improved contrast resolution and reduced clutter (noise) due to lower USG aberrations from the second harmonic. Spatial compound imaging uses pulses that steer at different angles (typically 3–5 angles) improving structure delineation and identification.

Improvements in the shape and frequency of transducers such as linear array transducers have resulted in improved spatial and contrast resolution, although may lead to increased attenuation of sound. Microconvex arrays require more interpolation to form images and typically provide reduced spatial resolution than linear arrays. The microconvex arrays are located at the tip of the transducer (end-fire probes) or proximal to the tip (biplane probes).

There are ongoing trials examining the latest noninvasive USG techniques both as stand-alone techniques and in combination with other imaging techniques to evaluate their diagnostic accuracy. These techniques include:

- Contrast-enhanced ultrasonography (CEUS)
- Ultrasonography biomicroscopy
- Elastography
- Multiparametric ultrasonography

CEUS is a technique that exploits the increased microvascular density of prostate tumors. The contrast agent used is microbubbles that are blood pool agents and do not enter the interstitial space. They provide improved detection of low-volume blood flow by increasing the signal-to-noise ratio (SNR) and delineating the neovascular anatomy therefore enhancing the signal strength from small vessels. Contrast agents within the vascular lumen are more reflective than blood and improve flow detection with USG while the vibrations from the contrast agents generate higher harmonics in tumors compared with the surrounding tissue. Multiple studies have shown that CEUS provides greater sensitivity and specificity for the diagnosis of prostate cancer compared with conventional TRUS [19,29]. The limitations of CEUS are mainly linked to USG contrast agents and the enhancement pattern of prostate parenchyma/carcinoma. The resonant frequency of most USG contrast agents is close to 2 MHz. A TRUS transducer frequency ranges between 6 and 12 MHz therefore only a limited number of smaller size microbubbles administered intravenously provide the harmonic signals from the resonating microbubbles. Prostate cancer enhancement is transient during the arterial phase and can only be distinguished from surrounding parenchyma for 20 seconds after the bolus injection. It does not exhibit washout and therefore a short wash-in phase is useful in CEUS. BPH is also a limiting factor as the vascularity of the transition zone may overshadow the flow associated with malignancy. Finally, CEUS is dependent on identifying the target on B-mode imaging (single-level technique), having previously identified the target for biopsy on the reference diagnostic method [19].

Ultrasonography elastography is an emerging technique that is reported to improve both prostate cancer detection and characterization of the lesion. This technique is based on the fact that prostate cancer tissue is stiffer than the surrounding normal tissue because it has increased cellular density with associated microvascularization with destruction of the normal glandular architecture. Two techniques have been developed and are utilized in clinical practice: strain elastography and shear-wave elastography.

- Strain elastography assesses the difference in tissue strain produced by freehand manual compression and analyze the deformation generated by the compressive force. A speckle comparison before and after compression produces a color-coded map of local tissue deformation that is overlaid on a B-mode image from TRUS—this is called an elastogram. The limitations of strain elastography are like other techniques, small cancers can be missed, other inflammatory conditions such as prostatitis can produce greater tissue stiffness and the technique requires significant operator training [19,30]
- Shear-wave elastography is a technique based on the measurement of shear-wave speed propagating through the tissues. This technique is impeded by compression on the prostate gland and also requires an experienced operator. This is a multiwave technique combining two different waves, the first is generated by the acoustic radiation force and the second is an ultrasonic wave that captures the propagation of the shear wave. The speed of the shear wave is linked to the stiffness of the analyzed tissue. The shear wave produces a dynamic quantitative map of soft-tissue stiffness in quasi-real-time which is derived from measuring the propagation speed and is color coded for each pixel overlaid on a B-mode TRUS image

Both elastography methods are limited by very large prostate glands, artifacts, and the limitation that not all cancers are stiff and not all stiff lesions are cancers [19,30].

Multiparametric ultrasonography is a concept derived from mp-MRI, it takes advantage of B-mode TRUS and combines it with newer techniques such as elastography and perfusion imaging to generate volumetric imaging of the prostate gland. This method is used in conjunction with mp-MRI to produce a map identifying potential targets for biopsy.

Advances in USG technology have resulted in the development of new and promising high-frequency systems ranging between 14 and 29 MHz (microultrasound) compared with conventional TRUS frequencies between 7 and 9 MHz. Microultrasound allows for spatial resolution to 70 μ, three times higher than conventional platforms, and allows clearer and more defined anatomical evaluation. The resolution of 70 μ allows alterations in ductal anatomy and cellular density to be appreciated. A recent randomized multicenter trial comparing microultrasound to conventional USG showed a 19% improvement in the detection of clinically significant prostate cancer (csPCa) [31].

Subsequently the "prostate risk identification using microultrasound" (PRI-MUS) grading system (Fig. 42.17), analogous to prostate imaging reporting and data system (PI-RADS) (Fig. 42.18), was proposed to allow for more consistent interpretation of prostate images [32]. Multiple studies have also shown sensitivity of microultrasound comparable to that of mp-MRI [33–35]; however it is a new technology and the data are preliminary. The studies are small and there is substantial heterogeneity between the cohorts in the different studies. Therefore, microultrasound requires multicenter trials to establish and cement its role in prostate cancer detection [19,36]. Nonetheless, this technology has a number of potential benefits including lower relative technology costs compared with MRI, convenience for the patient (diagnostic test and biopsy performed in a single setting), ease of use and interpretation, and fewer contraindications.

Multiparametric Magnetic Resonance Imaging

Over the past decade the use of mp-MRI for the diagnosis and staging of prostate cancer has exponentially increased (Fig. 42.19).

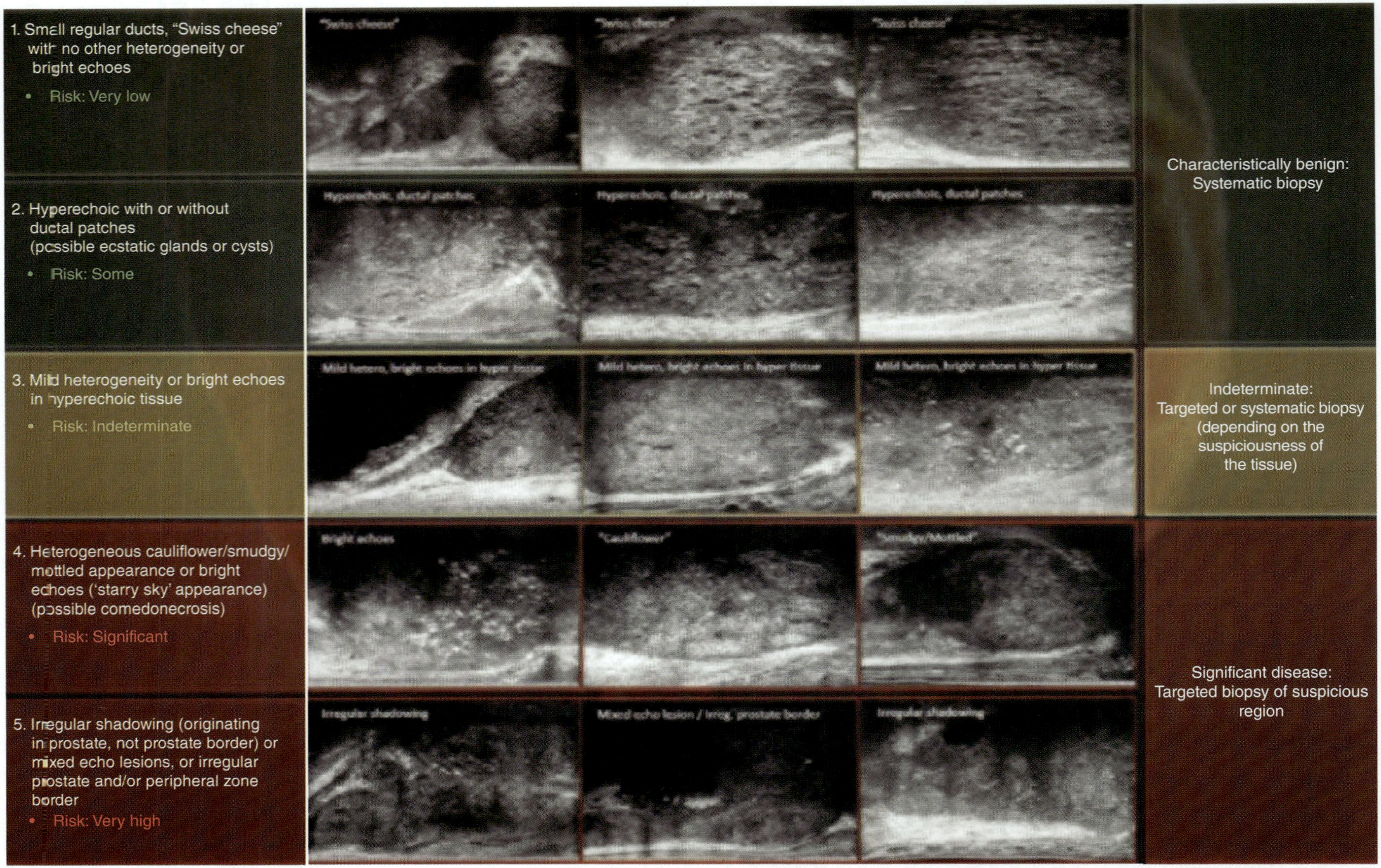

Grade	Image labels	Recommendation
1. Small regular ducts, "Swiss cheese" with no other heterogeneity or bright echoes • Risk: Very low	"Swiss cheese" / "Swiss cheese" / "Swiss cheese"	Characteristically benign: Systematic biopsy
2. Hyperechoic with or without ductal patches (possible ecstatic glands or cysts) • Risk: Some	Hyperechoic, ductal patches / Hyperechoic, ductal patches / Hyperechoic, ductal patches	
3. Mild heterogeneity or bright echoes in hyperechoic tissue • Risk: Indeterminate	Mild hetero, bright echoes in hyper tissue / Mild hetero, bright echoes in hyper tissue / Mild hetero, bright echoes in hyper tissue	Indeterminate: Targeted or systematic biopsy (depending on the suspiciousness of the tissue)
4. Heterogeneous cauliflower/smudgy/mottled appearance or bright echoes ('starry sky' appearance) (possible comedonecrosis) • Risk: Significant	Bright echoes / "Cauliflower" / "Smudgy/Mottled"	Significant disease: Targeted biopsy of suspicious region
5. Irregular shadowing (originating in prostate, not prostate border) or mixed echo lesions, or irregular prostate and/or peripheral zone border • Risk: Very high	Irregular shadowing / Mixed echo lesion / irreg. prostate border / Irregular shadowing	

Figure 42.17 Prostate risk identification using microultrasound (PRI-MUS) grading system.

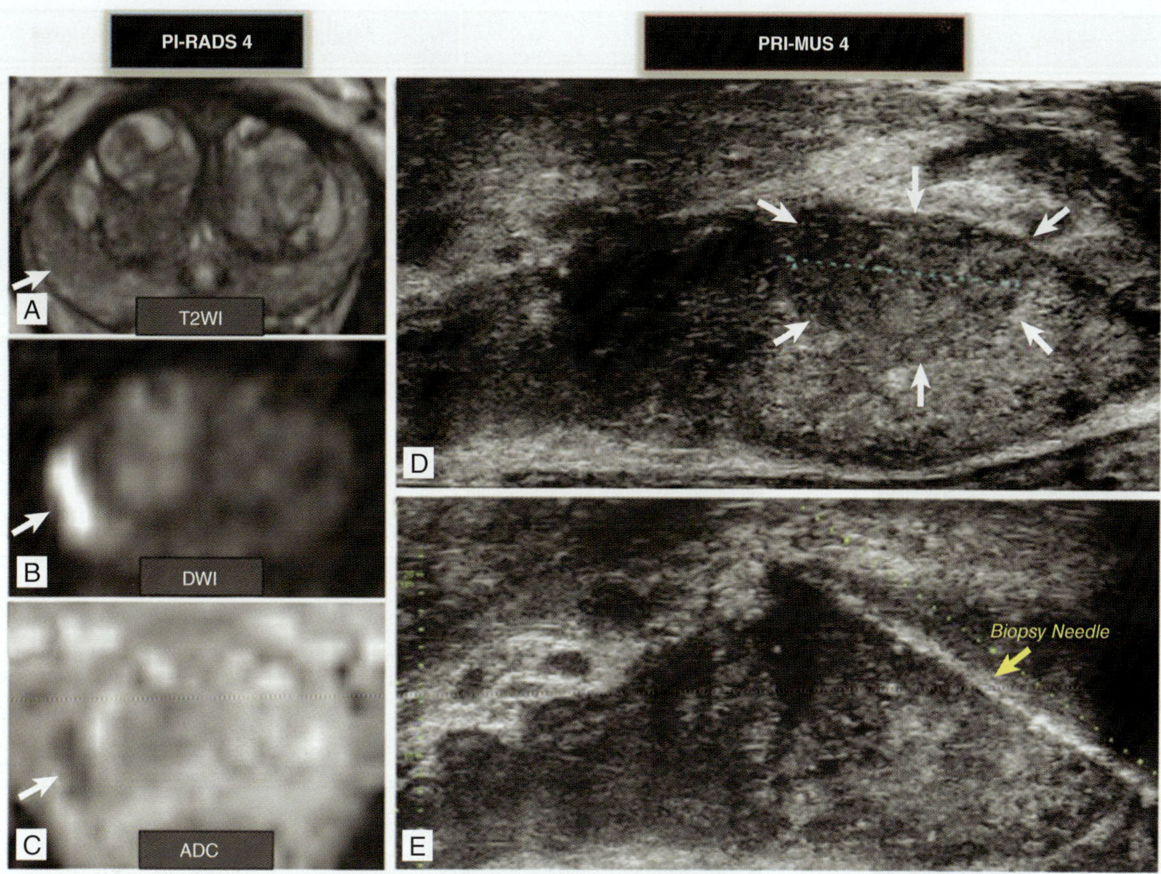

Figure 42.18 Comparative MRI (A, B, C) and microultrasound (D, E) images of index lesion. Axial T2WI (A) shows a hypointense focal abnormality with noncircumscribed margins in the right lateral midgland peripheral zone (*white arrow* in A), without evidence of extraprostatic extension (T2WI score: 3). High *b* value DWI (B) and ADC map (C) show a 1.3-cm lesion that is markedly hyperintense on the DWI (*white arrow* in B) and markedly hypointense on the ADC map (*white arrow* in C) (DWI-ADC score: 4). Therefore, this focal lesion was assigned a PI-RADS assessment category of 4. Parasagittal microultrasound (D) of right lateral edge of prostate shows this hypoechoic index lesion with smudgy/mottled appearance consisted with PRI-MUS 4 score (*white arrows*). Microultrasound-guided biopsy (E) was performed, with pathological result compatible with Gleason 7 (3+4) involving 85% of the core.

Mp-MRI includes high-resolution T2-weighted imaging (T2WI) with functional MRI techniques including diffusion-weighted imaging (DWI), dynamic contrast-enhanced (DCE) perfusion imaging, and spectroscopic imaging (MRSI). MRSI is an MRI technique that utilizes abnormalities of tissue metabolism. The metabolites produce photon peaks on the spectra derived from choline, creatinine, and citrate. In cancer, choline signals are elevated whereas the citrate signals decrease. There are high citrate levels in the peripheral zone which allows for interpretation of the choline plus creatinine-to-citrate ratios as a biomarker for prostate cancer. T1-weighted imaging is of limited use except for ruling out postbiopsy hemorrhage.

Patient Preparation and Clinical Considerations: There are clinical considerations to address before performing MRI including patient preparation and information (Fig. 42.20). Some institutions recommend that men refrain from ejaculation for 3 days before the exam to ensure maximum distention of the seminal vesicles. In institutions where an endorectal coil (ERC) is used stool in the rectum can interfere with coil placement. If an ERC is not used air/stool in the rectum may cause artifact, particularly for DWI. Therefore, patients are given a minimal preparation enema a couple of hours before the MRI. It is worth noting that the enema may promote peristalsis which can also cause artifacts. Antispasmodic agents may be administered to reduce bowel peristalsis; however this increases the cost of the study and can result in adverse drug reactions.

The timing of MRI postbiopsy is important to consider as hemorrhage is hyperintense on T1WI and may confound MRI assessment of the prostate gland and seminal vesicles. This is particularly important in the setting of MRI cancer staging and *it is recommended that the study is postponed for 6 weeks or longer to allow the bleeding and inflammatory changes to settle.* In instances of a recent negative TRUS biopsy, patients may proceed with MRI as the likelihood of a clinically significant cancer at the site of hemorrhage is exceptionally low.

Technical Specifications: MRI is routinely performed at magnetic field strengths of 1.5T and 3T, both provide reliable diagnostic exams when the acquisition parameters are optimized (Fig. 42.20). Magnetic field strength of 3T is often preferred as it has a greater SNR than at 1.5T. The SNR can also be exploited to increase spatial resolution and temporal resolution; however, 3T can be associated with signal heterogeneity and artifacts that are successfully addressed by the new state-of-the-art MRI scanners. Magnetic field strength of 1.5T imaging may be preferred if a patient has an implanted MRI compatible device that will cause artifact or if not rendered safe for 3T.

ERCs are used in some institutions and have the advantage of increasing the SNR in the prostate at any magnetic field strength. The use of ERCs with a 1.5T system is valuable to ensure high spatial resolution providing diagnostic quality studies. Image quality with a 3T system is considered to be comparable to a 1.5T study with an ERC. ERCs are also valuable in larger patients

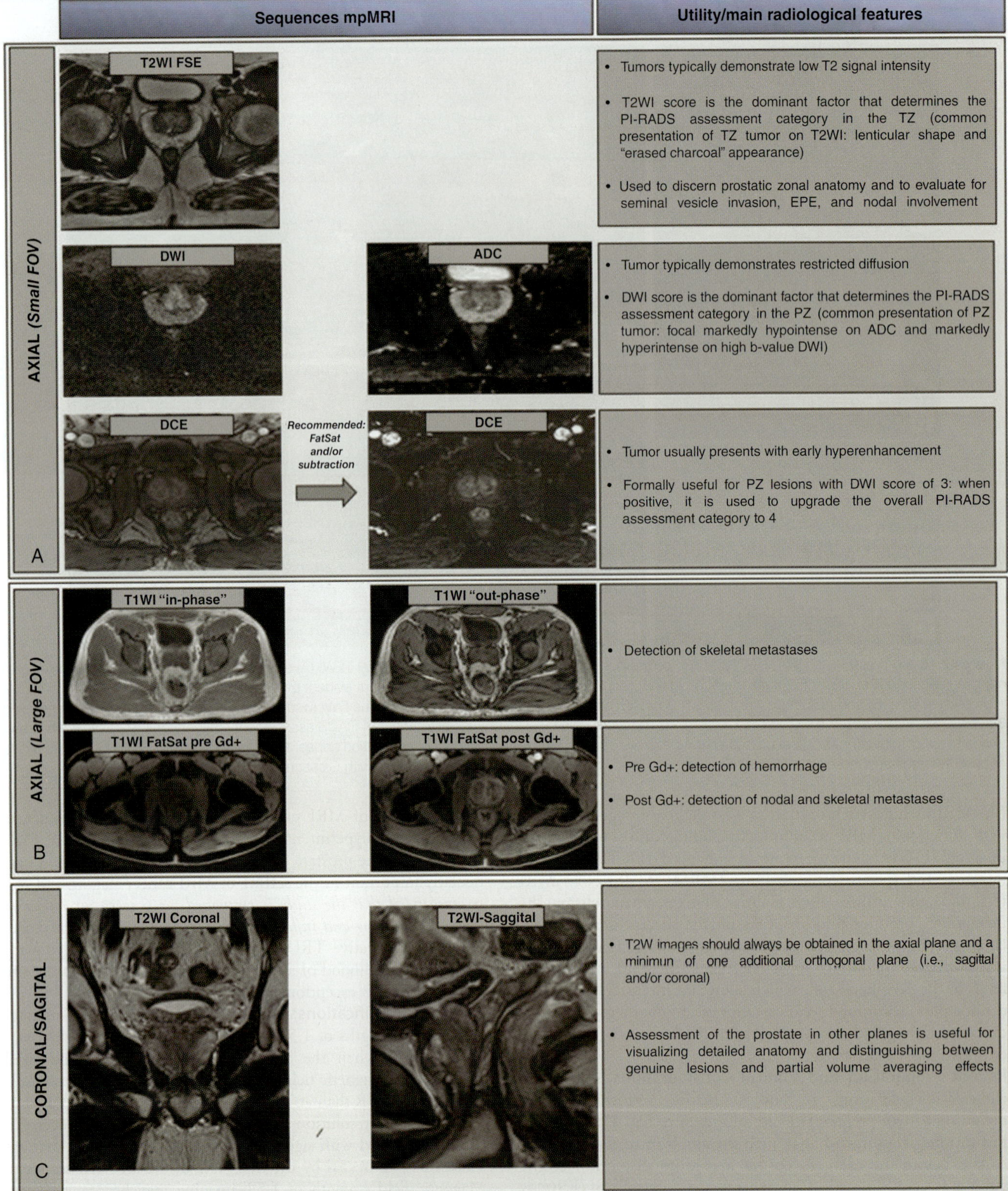

Figure 42.19 Chart shows a proposal of sequences to be acquired in the performance of multiparametric MRI (adapted from PI-RADSv2.1). Chart also describes the clinical utility of these sequences and main radiological features that must be noted in each of them. *ADC*, apparent diffusion coefficient; *DCE*, dynamic contrast enhanced; *DWI*, diffusion-weighted imaging; *EPE*, extraprostatic extension; *FatSat*, fat saturation; *FOV*, field of view; *FSE*, fast spin-echo; *Gd+*, gadolinium; *mp-MRI*, multiparametric magnetic resonance imaging; *PI-RADS*, prostate imaging reporting and data system; *PZ*, peripheral zone; *T1WI*, T1-weighted imaging; *T2WI*, T2-weighted imaging; *TZ*, transition zone.

Recommended	Controversial	Not recommended
▪ Patient information that should be available: - PSA level and PSA history - Date and results of prior prostate biopsy - Other relevant clinical history *(DRE findings, medications, prior prostate infections, pelvic surgery, radiation therapy and family history)*	**▪ Timing of MRI following prostate biopsy: ≥ 6 weeks**	**▪ MR spectroscopy**
▪ Surface coil *(usually recommended for both 1.5T and 3.0T)*	**▪ Refrain from ejaculation for 3 days prior to the MRI exam**	**▪ DCE Time-Curve analysis**
▪ 1.5-3.0T field strength *(preferably 3.0T)*	**▪ Microenema**	
▪ mpMRI*: **T2WI FSE** *(straight axial or oblique axial and a minimum of one additional orthogonal plane)* **▪ DWI and ADC map** **DCE** *(3D T1W GRE is preferred)* **▪ T1WI** *(pre and postcontrast)*	**▪ Antispasmodic agent** **▪ Endorectal coil** *(might still be used for some 1.5T systems, especially older ones, that considered it indispensable for achieving high resolution imaging)* **▪ bpMRI** *(need further studies, reserved for select clinical indications)*	

Figure 42.20 Chart categorizes prostate MRI protocol according to clinical considerations, patient preparation, and technical specifications that are recommended, those that are not recommended and some that are controversial practices, according to PI-RADS v2.1. *3-D*, three dimensional; *ADC*, apparent diffusion coefficient; *bpMRI*, biparametric magnetic resonance imaging; *DCE*, dynamic contrast enhanced; *DRE*, digital rectal exam; *DWI*, diffusion-weighted imaging; *FOV*, field of view; *FSE*, fast spin-echo; *GRE*, gradient echo; *mp-MRI*, multiparametric magnetic resonance imaging; *MR*, magnetic resonance; *PSA*, prostate-specific antigen; *T*, Tesla; *T1WI*, T1-weighted imaging; *T2WI*, T2-weighted imaging.
**At least one pulse sequence should use a FOV that permits evaluation of pelvic lymph nodes to the level of the aortic bifurcation.*

where the SNR of the prostate may be reduced. The disadvantages of ERCs include patient discomfort, added cost, deformity of the prostate gland, and the introduction of artifacts. Adequate images can be obtained with and without ERCs; therefore radiologists are encouraged to use the MRI protocol that achieves the best image quality at their institution.

Mp-MRI Sequences: *T2WI* is used to differentiate the zonal anatomy of the prostate, tumor detection, and local cancer staging (Fig. 42.19). The neurovascular bundles, ejaculatory ducts, seminal vesicles, and AFMS are all identified most clearly on T2WI.

- The peripheral zone is high signal intensity and cancer is low signal on T2WI. However, other benign processes can also appear low signal on T2WI (prostatitis, fibrous scar tissue, postbiopsy hemorrhage, and postirradiation)
- *T2WI is considered the dominant sequence for the detection of transition zone cancers;* these can be more difficult to differentiate in the setting of BPH. Transition zone cancer is typically ill-defined or lenticular in shape, it is low signal intensity and may extend into the peripheral zone or AFMS; the appearance is described as "erased charcoal" or "smudgy fingerprint" [27]. Stromal BPH nodules and transition zone tumors have some imaging overlap as both appear low signal on T2WI; however, stromal nodules are more encapsulated with heterogeneous low T2-weighted signal compared with homogeneously low signal, ill-defined, and lenticular-shaped transition zone cancers [8]

DWI is a functional imaging tool that measures the Brownian motion of water molecules in the tissue to produce image contrast. The ADC on MRI is calculated by acquiring at least two sets of images with differing magnetic field gradient duration and amplitude (*b* value). The degree of diffusion weighting is controlled by the amplitude, duration, and temporal spacing of gradient pulses and expressed in the diffusion *b* value unit (s/mm^2). Higher *b* values allow better tumor detection by suppression of normal benign gland as well as to assess for treatment response. A "high *b* value" is defined between 1000 and 2000 s/mm^2, and a high *b* value of ≥1600 s/mm^2 is recommended (preferably ≥2000 s/mm^2). High *b* values can be obtained by the following two methods:

- the first method is by directly acquiring a high *b* value sequence which adds to scan time and
- the second method is to calculate the *b* value by extrapolating it from the lower *b* value data acquired for the ADC map

The SNR decreases as the *b* value increases. At least two *b* values are required to generate an ADC map, low *b* value (50–100 s/mm^2) and an intermediate *b* value (800–1000 s/mm^2). The maximum recommended b value for ADC calculation is 1000 s/mm^2 to avoid diffusion kurtosis effects described at higher b values [9,37,38].

The hallmark of prostate cancer is low signal intensity on ADC and iso to high signal intensity on the high b value (>1400 s/mm²) [27]. Studies have shown that DWI is the dominant MRI sequence for tumor detection, particularly in the peripheral zone [39]. DWI can also be used as a problem-solving tool to differentiate cancer from benign etiologies such as prostatitis, fibrosis, scar tissue, hemorrhage and postirradiation which will appear low signal on T2WI and ADC.

DCE is a technique that exploits the dynamic uptake and rapid washout of gadolinium chelate. DCE consists of a series of fast T1-weighted (T1WI) sequences covering the entire prostate before and after rapid injection (2–4 mL/s) of a bolus of a low-molecular-weight gadolinium chelate [40]. During DCE-MRI, tumors demonstrate early and high amplitude enhancement followed by rapid washout in some cases compared with normal prostate tissue. DCE sequences should be inspected for focal early enhancement. PI-RADS document describes a positive DCE as having focal, early, or contemporaneous with enhancement of adjacent normal prostate parenchyma corresponding to a finding on T2WI and DWI images. Visual assessment is improved with fat suppression and subtraction techniques. DCE is performed for 2 minutes to detect early enhancing lesions, the temporal resolution should be <15 seconds per acquisition to identify focal early enhancement [9]. There is overlap of the prostate cancer enhancement pattern with benign conditions such as prostatitis and BPH nodules; therefore, DCE is not considered a dominant imaging sequence for cancer assessment in the peripheral or transition zones. DCE is often applied as an adjunct to T2WI and DWI findings [27]. DCE-MRI is a valuable tool for the detection of residual or recurrent tumor after radiation therapy, prostatectomy, and focal therapy.

Spectroscopic MRI (MRSI) (Fig. 42.21) is based on the principle that

- prostate cancer is associated with proportionally lower levels of citrate and higher levels of choline and creatinine compared with those seen in the normal tissue or BPH nodules

MRI spectroscopy can identify the metabolic differences in prostate tissue using a strong magnetic field. MRI spectroscopy has shown promise in assessing the aggressiveness of cancer, detecting recurrence of cancer, and monitoring treatment response. Like all techniques this has limitations such as distortions from hemorrhage, requirement for operator expertise, and adds time to the examination [41]. Because of the previously mentioned reasons, its clinical application is limited and has been dropped in PI-RADS v2 document for the assessment of prostate cancer by mp-MRI.

Benefit of mp-MRI after a negative biopsy is well established in the literature and endorsed by scientific committees. In a meta-analysis of 14 studies, the mean cancer detection rate on MRI-targeted biopsy after a negative biopsy was 37.5% [42]. In another study Hoeks et al. reported cancer detection rates of 25% after mp-MRI in patients with at least one previous negative biopsy [43]. Various studies have also shown upgrading after MRI-targeted biopsy in patients on active surveillance (AS) [44]. At the same time, the absence of a lesion on mp-MRI in AS patients has been suggested as a good prognostic indicator with potential to reduce the number of unnecessary biopsies [45]. Recent publications have described MRI as a helpful tool in stratifying patients suitable for AS [27,44].

In the setting of a biopsy-naïve patient (patients with no previous prostate biopsy), studies have shown detection of more clinically significant tumors in the MRI imaging arm compared with systematic biopsy, although the overall cancer detection rates may be similar [46]. More recently, the PROMIS and PRECISION prospective trials demonstrated that MRI and targeted biopsy led to fewer biopsies and an increase in the number of clinically significant cancers being identified compared with systematic sampling. They also demonstrated a decrease in the number of clinically insignificant cancers being detected [47,48]. In the PRECISION randomized clinical trial, csPCa was detected in 12% more patients in the MRI-targeted biopsy arm compared with the systematic biopsy arm (38% vs 26%) and 28% of patients in the MRI arm avoided a biopsy based on a negative MRI while all patient in the systematic biopsy arm underwent a TRUS-guided biopsy. MRI has recently been shown to have comparable healthcare costs with increased quality of life compared with systematic biopsy. The benefit regarding quality of life derives from a decrease in overdiagnosis and overtreatment in patients who have mp-MRI-targeted versus systematic biopsy [27,47–49].

There is mounting evidence that mp-MRI used in conjunction with PSA and followed by a targeted biopsy in an appropriate clinical context is a better alternative to systematic TRUS-guided biopsy (Fig. 42.22) in the diagnosis of prostate cancer. The greatest benefit is the negative predictive value of mp-MRI resulting in a decrease in the number of unnecessary biopsies and therefore a decrease in overdiagnosis and overtreatment of prostate cancer.

Patients with recent biopsy can have residual hemorrhage within the gland for about 2–3 months postbiopsy because

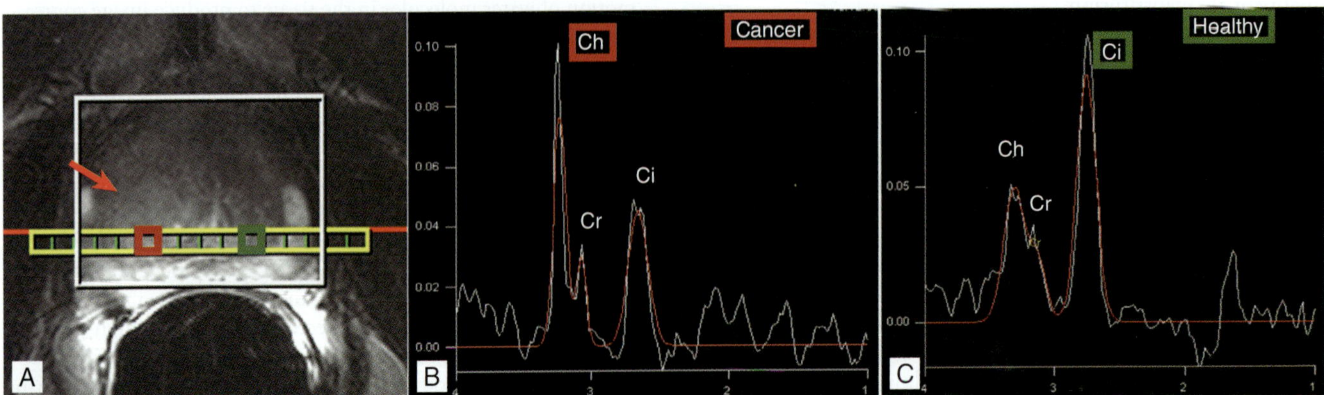

Figure 42.21 Axial T2W (A) shows prostate cancer in right transition zone (*arrow*). MR spectroscopic (MRS) image corresponding to voxel in the tumor location (B) shows increased choline (Ch) + creatine (Cr) to citrate (Ci) ratio (B). MRS image corresponding to voxel in the left transition zone (normal tissue) (C) shows normal Ch+Cr/Ci ratio. MRS is based on the principle that prostate cancer is associated with proportionally lower levels of citrate and higher levels of choline and creatinine compared with those seen in the normal tissue or BPH nodules.

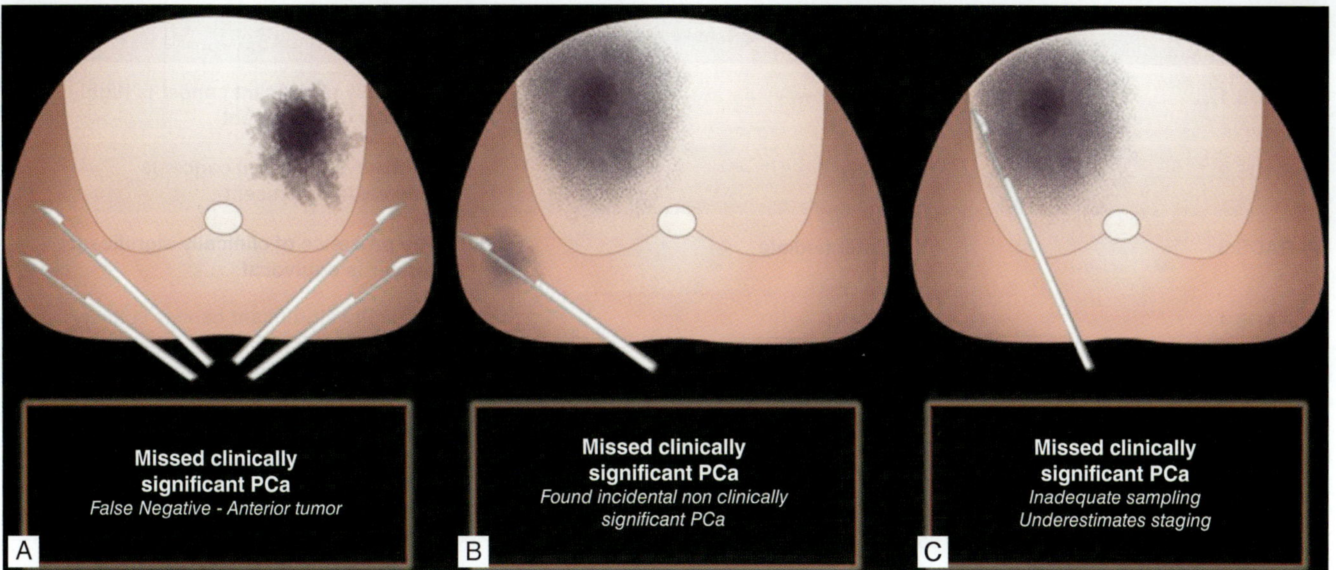

Figure 42.22 Potential errors of the TRUS-guided systematic biopsy in the detection of clinically significant prostate cancer. PCa, prostate cancer.

prostate tissue produces citrate that has an anticoagulant property. Often imaging is postponed or rescheduled to allow the hemorrhage to resolve. However, *the hemorrhagic exclusion sign* has been described whereby prostate tumors are outlined by postbiopsy change on T1-weighted sequences. On T1WI the abnormal prostate tissue will be low signal and outlined by hemorrhage in the adjacent normal prostate tissue. This is based on the pathologic finding that the degree of postbiopsy hemorrhage is significantly less in areas of prostate cancer compared with benign prostate tissue [50] (Fig. 42.23).

Prostate Imaging Reporting and Data System: The role of mpMRI has rapidly expanded since the advent of MR in prostate imaging in 1982. In 2012 experts from the European Society of Urogenital Radiology introduced a structured reporting system for prostate MRI in treatment-naïve prostate glands called the PI-RADS. PI-RADS was developed in a consensus-based process using a combination of published data, and expert observations and opinions. It was developed to standardize image-acquisition techniques and interpretation of prostate MRI. PI-RADS has received rapid and broad international acceptance among radiologists and urologists with implementation in daily practice and research.

PI-RADS v2 was published in 2015 to further standardize the parameters of prostate MRI. Numerous studies have validated the value of PI-RADS; however, some limitations have also been highlighted. The current version is PI-RADS v2 with recent modifications in 2019 creating PI-RADS v2.1. The standardization of prostate MRI is by a scale from 1 to 5, each lesion is assigned a score indicating the likelihood of clinically significant cancer (Fig. 42.24). The volume of the prostate gland should always be reported and can be calculated using an ellipsoid formula, the measurements include maximum AP dimension × maximum longitudinal (L) length × maximum TR dimension. The AP and L dimensions should be obtained on sagittal T2WI and the TR dimension on the axial T2WI (Fig. 42.25).

Prostate cancer can be multifocal; however, PI-RADS recommends that up to four most suspicious lesions should be reported. The minimum requirement for reporting suspicious lesions is to report the largest dimension on the axial image; however, if the largest dimension is on either the sagittal or coronal sequence this should be reported.

DWI is the dominant sequence for the assessment of the peripheral zone (Fig. 42.26); however, the score may be modified by the DCE sequence for lesions with a score of 3. Peripheral zone lesions should be measured on ADC with the image number and series included in the report.

- PI-RADS category 4 (Fig. 42.27) lesions in the peripheral zone are typically described as a well-circumscribed T2 (Table 42.3) hypointense mass measuring <1.5 cm and confined to the prostate

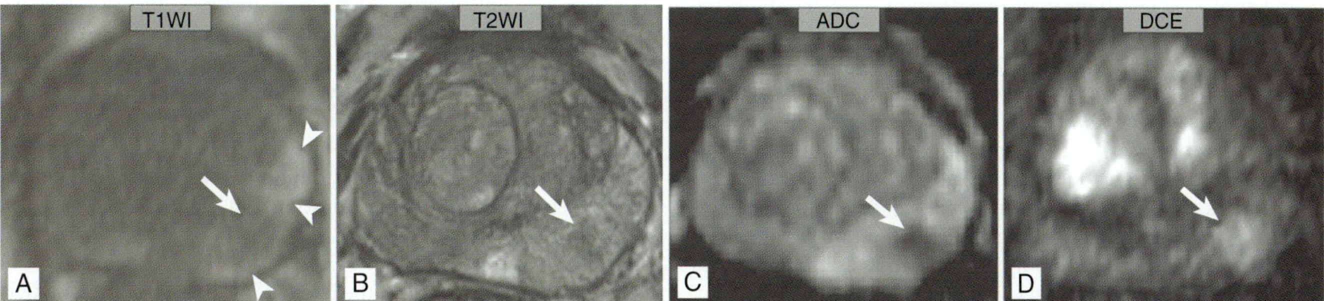

Figure 42.23 Hemorrhage exclusion sign. Focal area in the left peripheral zone (*arrows*) demonstrating low signal on T1WI (A) (absence of blood products), low signal on T2WI (B), low signal on ADC map (C) (restricted diffusion), and early enhancement on DCE (D), categorized as a PI-RADS assessment category of 4 and consistent with biopsy-proved clinically significant prostate cancer. This example illustrates the hemorrhage exclusion sign (*arrows*). The abnormal prostate tissue is outlined by the hemorrhage in the adjacent normal prostate (*arrowheads*). This sign can be a useful MRI finding in the postbiopsy status.

PI-RADS v2.1 Assessment Categories		
PI-RADS 1	Very low	Clinically significant cancer is highly unlikely to be present
PI-RADS 2	Low	Clinically significant cancer is unlikely to be present
PI-RADS 3	Intermediate	The presence of clinically significant cancer is equivocal
PI-RADS 4	High	Clinically significant cancer is likely to be present
PI-RADS 5	Very high	Clinically significant cancer is highly likely to be present

Figure 42.24 Chart shows the PI-RADS v2.1 assessment categories, which uses a five-point scale based on the likelihood (probability) that a combination of mp-MRI findings on T2WI, DWI, and DCE correlates with the presence of a clinically significant cancer for each lesion in the prostate gland. According to PI-RADS v2.1, clinically significant prostate cancer is defined as a tumor with a Gleason score ≥7 (including 3+4 with prominent but not predominant Gleason 4 component), and/or volume >0.5 cc, and/or extraprostatic extension (EPE).

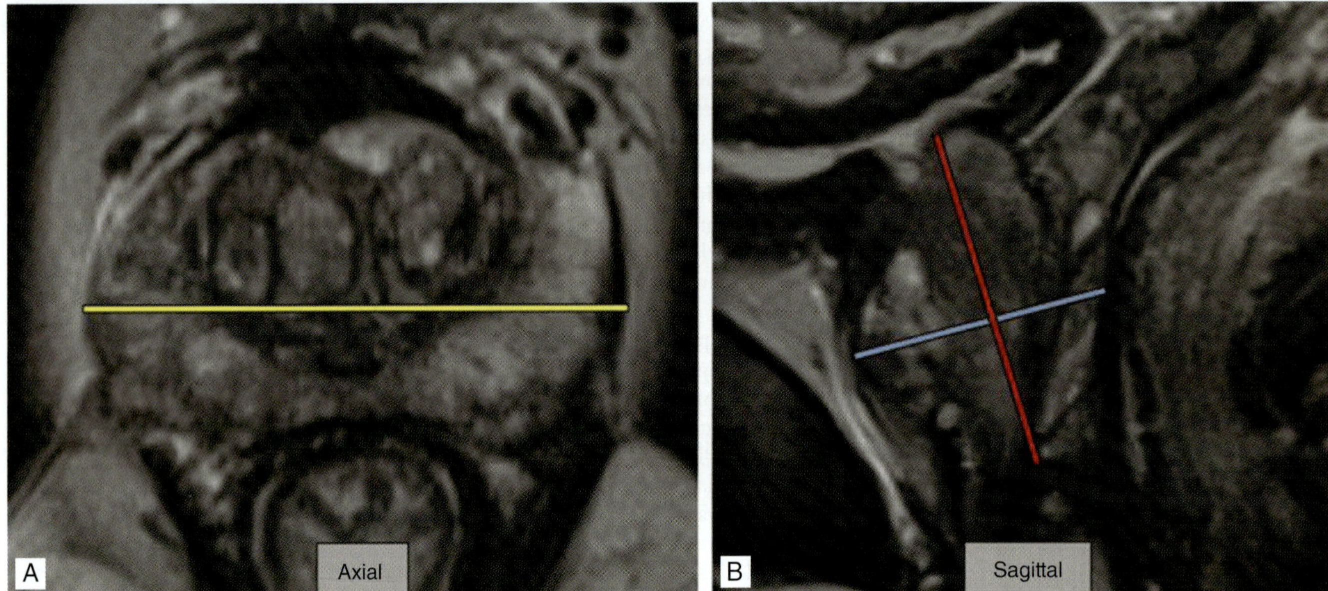

Figure 42.25 Suggested measurements for ellipsoid formula when calculating prostate volume at MRI (T2WI) according to PI-RADS v2.1. Maximum transverse diameter (yellow line) should be measured on axial T2WI (A). Maximum longitudinal diameter (red line) and maximum anteroposterior diameter (blue line) should be measured on mid sagittal T2WI (B).

- PI-RADS category 5 (Fig. 42.28) lesions are the same as 4 but measure ≥1.5 cm in greatest dimension or have definite extraprostatic extension or invasive appearance

On DWI assessment (Table 42.4) PI-RADS category 4 and 5 lesions are markedly hypointense on ADC and markedly hyperintense on high *b* value DWI.

T2WI (Table 42.5) is the dominant sequence for the assessment of the transition zone (Fig. 42.29) and may be modified by appearances on DWI. Transition zone lesions should be measured on T2WI again, including the image number and series. Identification of zonal anatomy is imperative as the dominant sequences differ for the zones. Currently, reliably detecting clinically significant cancer in the transition zone is less than the peripheral zone.

- PI-RADS category 4 lesions in the transition zone are typically lenticular or ill-defined and moderately T2 hypointense measuring <1.5 cm
- PI-RADS category 5 (Figs. 42.30 and 42.31) lesions are the same as 4 but measure ≥1.5 cm in greatest dimension or have definite extraprostatic involvement

On DWI assessment (Table 42.4) PI-RADS category 4 and 5 lesions are markedly hypointense on ADC and markedly hyperintense on high *b* value DWI. PI-RADS does not provide management recommendations as these decisions are made clinically in conjunction with the imaging findings [9]. PI-RADS v2.1 Structured Report Template is demonstrated in Figure 42.32.

Biparametric MRI

There is growing interest in the role of biparametric MRI (bpMRI) for the detection of prostate cancer. The term bpMRI refers to a protocol that includes T2-WI and DWI but excludes DCE.

Although DCE imaging can assist when DWI or T2-WI is degraded, its benefit otherwise is limited. Overall PI-RADS v2.1 assessment category utilizes DCE imaging only for upgrading a

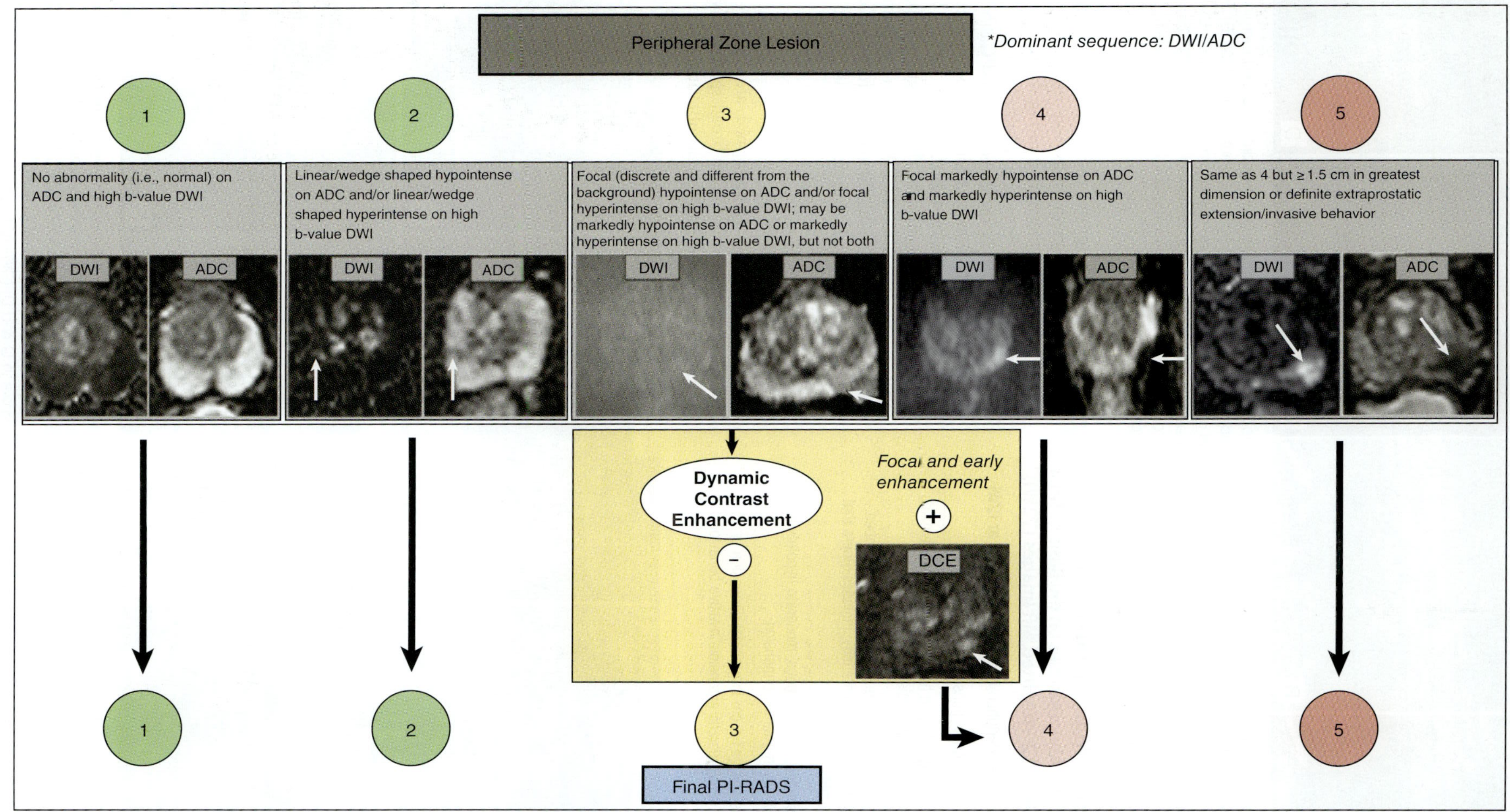

Figure 42.26 Peripheral zone assessment according to PI-RADS v2.1 For peripheral zone lesions, the overall PI-RADS assessment usually follows the DWI score, but a score of 3 can be upgraded by the presence of dynamic contrast enhancement.

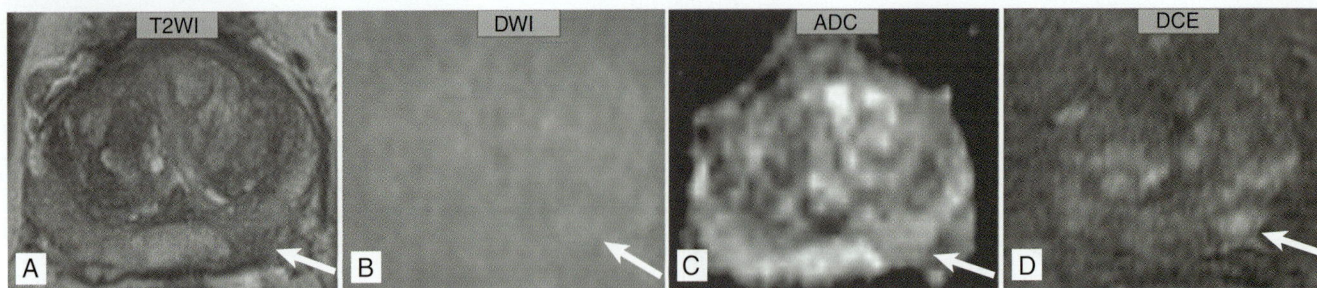

Figure 42.27 Peripheral zone PI-RADS 4 lesion. Axial T2WI (A) shows a hypointense focal abnormality with noncircumscribed margins in the left posterolateral peripheral zone at the base (*arrow* in A), without evidence of extraprostatic extension (T2WI score: 3). High *b* value DWI (B) and ADC map (C) show a 1.1-cm lesion that is mildly hyperintense on the DWI (*arrow* in B) and moderately hypointense on the ADC map (*arrow* in C) (DWI-ADC score: 3). Axial dynamic contrast-enhanced T1WI (D) shows early enhancement of the lesion (*arrow* in D) relative to the rest of the gland (DCE: positive). For peripheral zone lesions, the overall PI-RADS assessment usually follows the DWI-score, but a score of 3 can be upgraded by the presence of dynamic contrast enhancement. Therefore, this focal lesion was assigned a PI-RADS assessment category of 4.

TABLE 42.3 Scoring Scheme Within PI-RADS Version 2.1 for Peripheral Zone Abnormalities on the Basis of Their Appearance on T2-Weighted MR Images (T2WI)

T2WI Score	Appearance of Peripheral Zone Abnormalities at T2WI
1	Uniform high signal intensity (normal)
2	Linear or wedge-shaped hypointensity or diffuse mild hypointensity, usually indistinct margin
3	Heterogeneous signal intensity or noncircumscribed, rounded, moderate hypointensity; includes others that do not qualify as 2, 4, or 5
4	Circumscribed, homogeneous, moderate hypointensity, and <1.5 cm in greatest dimension
5	Same as 4 but ≥1.5 cm in greatest dimension or definite extraprostatic extension/invasive behavior

score of 3–4 in peripheral zone lesions, while multiple studies have shown that benign transition zone nodules often show early enhancement, therefore limiting the role of DCE imaging in transition zone lesions [51]. Multiple studies have supported the value of bpMRI in the detection of csPCa [52–54]. Benefits of bpMRI include reduced scan time, cost, and reduced adverse effects from gadolinium-based contrast agents. DCE imaging, however, remains essential in the evaluation of patients following previous treatment. PI-RADS steering committee recommends that bpMRI should be reserved for select clinical indications and that further multicenter trials is needed to evaluate bpMRI.

Image-Guided Biopsy

TRUS-guided biopsy is performed after a diagnostic TRUS. Before biopsy patients are given broad-spectrum antibiotic cover, typically a quinolone such as ciprofloxacin this is taken on the

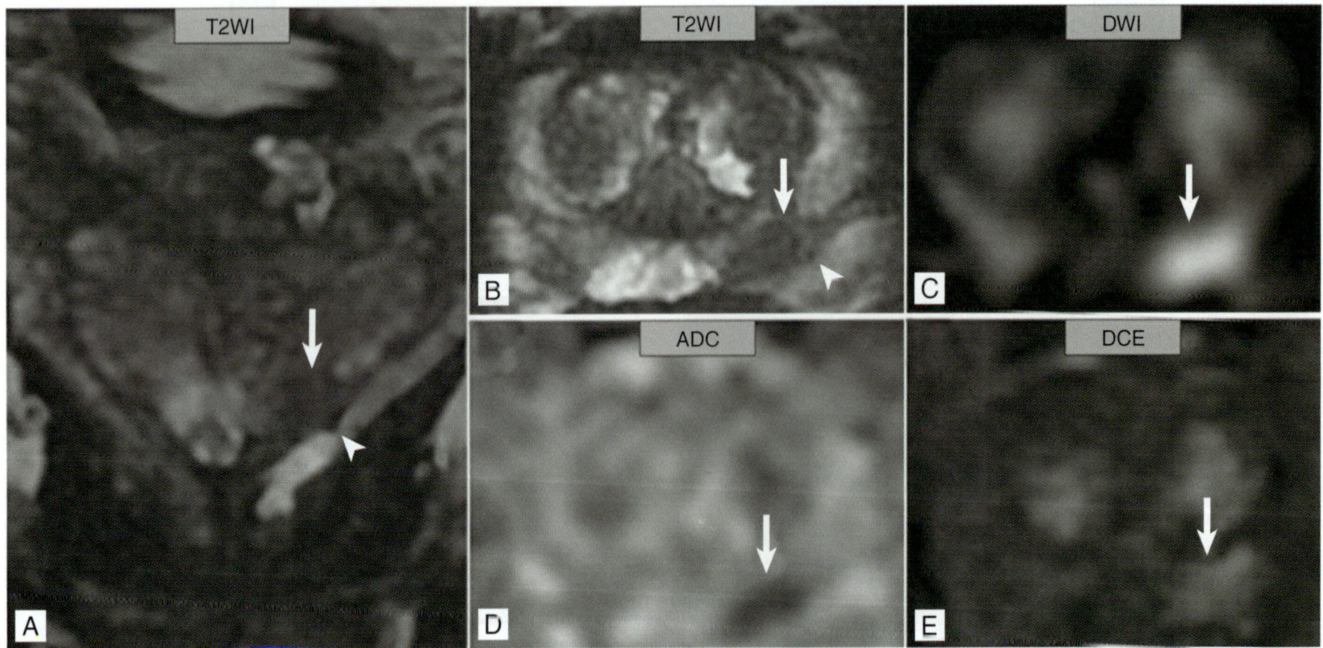

Figure 42.28 Peripheral zone PI-RADS 5 lesion. MRI of a 61-year-old patient with a prostate nodule discovered at digital rectal examination, who had an elevated PSA level (4.7 ng/mL). Coronal T2WI (A) and axial T2WI (B) show a hypointense focal lesion (*arrows* in A and B) in the left posterolateral and posteromedial peripheral zone at the midgland/apex; the lesion has an irregular or spiculated margin (*arrowheads*) and a tumor–capsule interface of more than 1 cm, findings consistent with extraprostatic extension (T2WI score: 5). High *b* value DWI (C) and ADC map (D) show a 1.7-cm lesion that is markedly hyperintense on the DWI and markedly hypointense on the ADC map (*arrows* in C and D) (DWI-ADC score: 5). Axial dynamic contrast-enhanced T1WI (E) shows early enhancement of the lesion (*arrow* in E) relative to the rest of the gland (DCE: positive). Therefore, this focal lesion was assigned a PI-RADS assessment category of 5, consistent with the biopsy-proved clinically significant cancer in this region—Gleason 8 (4+4).

TABLE 42.4 Scoring Scheme Within PI-RADS Version 2.1 for Peripheral Zone and Transition Zone Abnormalities on the Basis of Their Appearance on Apparent Diffusion Coefficient (ADC) Maps and High *b* Value Diffusion-Weighted MR Images (DWI)

DWI-ADC Score	Findings in the Peripheral Zone and Transition Zone at DWI-ADC
1	No abnormality on ADC or high *b* value DWI
2	Linear/wedge-shaped hypointensity on ADC and/or hyperintensity on high *b* value DWI
3	Focal (discrete and different from background), mild/moderate hypointensity on ADC and/or mild/moderate hyperintensity on high *b* value DWI; may be markedly hypointense on ADC or markedly hyperintense on high *b* value DWI, but not both
4	Focal, marked hypointensity on ADC and marked hyperintensity on high *b* value DWI; <1.5 cm in greatest dimension
5	Same as 4 but ≥1.5 cm in greatest dimension or definite extraprostatic extension/invasive behavior

TABLE 42.5 Scoring Scheme Within PI-RADS Version 2.1 for Transition Zone Abnormalities on the Basis of Their Appearance on T2-weighted MR Images (T2WI)

T2WI Score	Appearance of Transition Zone Abnormalities at T2WI
1	Normal appearing transition zone (rare) or a round, completely encapsulated nodule ("typical nodule" of benign prostatic hyperplasia)
2	A mostly encapsulated nodule or a homogeneous circumscribed nodule without encapsulation ("atypical nodule"), or a homogeneous mildly hypointense area between nodules
3	Heterogeneous signal intensity with obscured margins; includes others that do not qualify as 2, 4, or 5
4	Lenticular or noncircumscribed, homogeneous, moderately hypointense, and <1.5 cm in greatest dimension
5	Same as 4, but ≥1.5 cm in greatest dimension or definite extraprostatic extension/invasive behavior

day of biopsy and can be continued up to 3 days postbiopsy. All anticoagulation is stopped before biopsy with local guidelines recommending when patients can restart their medication. Biopsies should be avoided during a urinary tract infection, which predisposes patients to infection. TRUS-guided prostate biopsy can be performed by a transrectal or transperineal approach. Traditionally a transrectal approach is utilized although more recently, transperineal approaches are being adopted because of increased risk of sepsis from TRUS biopsy. TRUS-guided biopsy is performed in a systematic fashion obtaining 12 (extended sextant) (Fig. 42.16) 18-guage core biopsies from the prostate gland using a spring-loaded biopsy gun. If a suspicious area has been identified on TRUS, this area is biopsied first followed by a systematic TRUS-guided biopsy of the gland. The urethra,

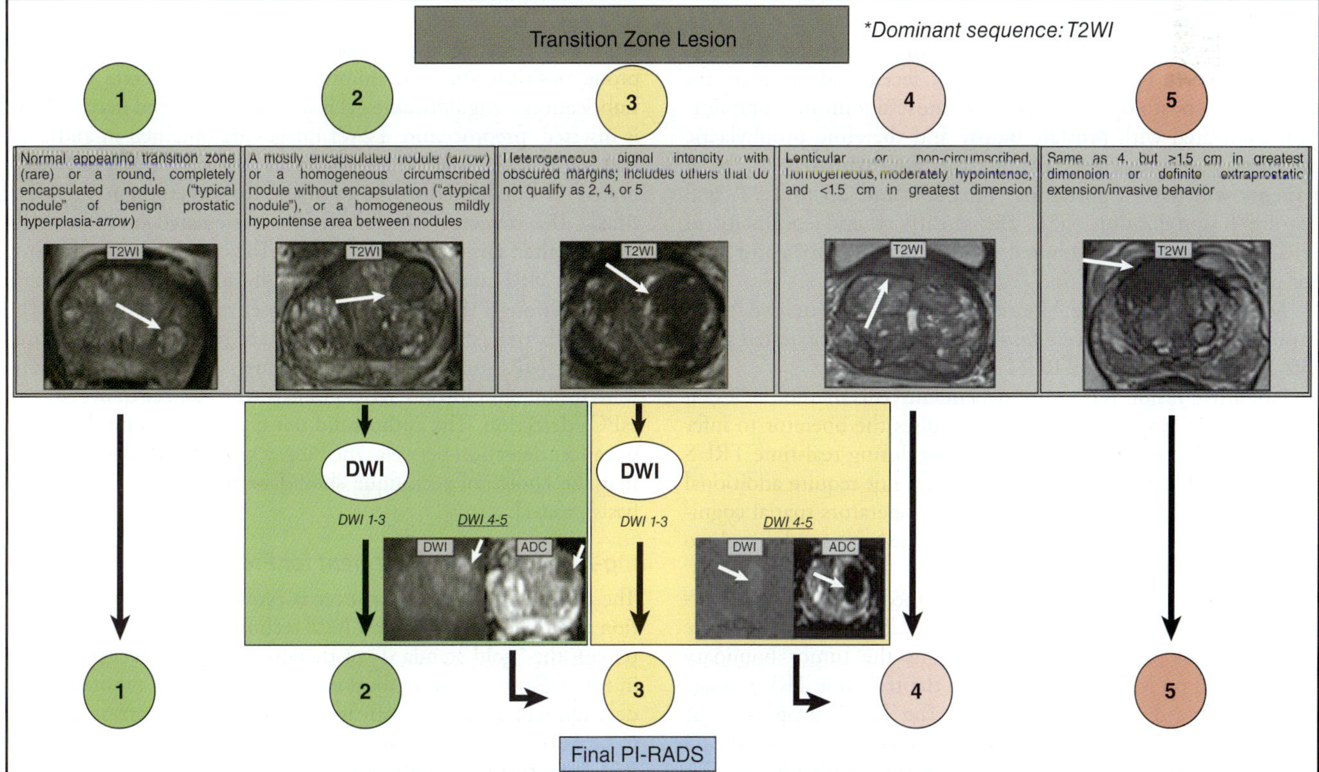

Figure 42.29 Transition zone assessment according to PI-RADS v2.1. For transition zone lesions, the overall PI-RADS assessment usually follows the T2WI score. For transition zone lesions with a T2WI score of 2 or 3, a high DWI score (i.e., 4 or 5) is used to upgrade the overall PI-RADS assessment by one point (i.e., 3 or 4, respectively).

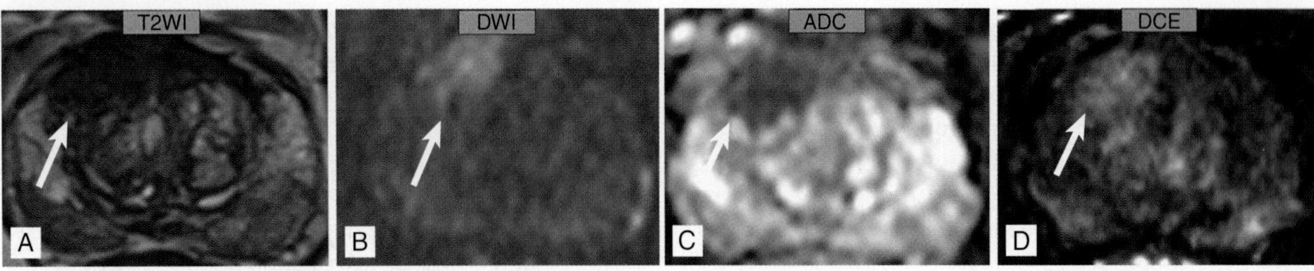

Figure 42.30 Transition zone PI-RADS 5 lesion. MRI of a 60-year-old patient with an elevated PSA level (13.6 ng/mL), who had undergone two previous systematic transrectal ultrasonography (TRUS)-guided biopsies with normal findings. Axial T2WI (A) shows a 2.0-cm low signal intensity lenticular lesion centered in the right anterior transition zone at the midgland (*arrow* in A), extending to the adjacent anterior fibromuscular stroma (T2WI score: 5). High *b* value DWI (B) and ADC map (C) show that the lesion is markedly hyperintense on DWI and hypointense on the ADC map (*arrows* in B and C) (DWI-ADC score: 5). Axial dynamic contrast-enhanced T1WI (D) shows early enhancement of the lesion (*arrow* in D) relative to the rest of the gland (DCE: positive). Therefore, this lesion was assigned a PI-RADS assessment category of 5. The findings at software-based MR imaging/US fusion-guided biopsy of this lesion disclosed prostate adenocarcinoma with a Gleason score of 7 (4+3).

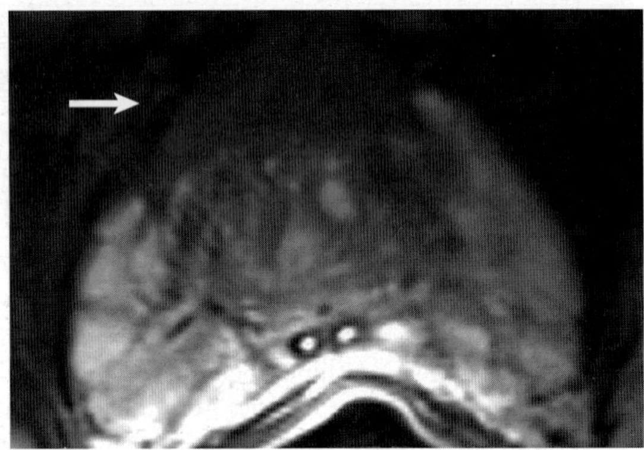

Figure 42.31 Axial T2W image shows a 2.1-cm low signal intensity lenticular lesion centered in the anterior transition zone at the midgland/base (*arrow*), invading the adjacent anterior fibromuscular stroma.

ejaculatory ducts, and internal urethral sphincter are avoided as if biopsied can cause bleeding and stricture postbiopsy. Patients will often have bleeding in the urine, feces, and ejaculate for several days postbiopsy. Sepsis is the most significant complication associated with prostate biopsy and therefore prophylactic antibiotics are prescribed. Despite this approximately 5–7% of patients will have a postbiopsy infection and up to 1.3% will require hospitalization [55]. The sensitivity and specificity of TRUS-guided biopsy is limited ranging between 40% and 50% for prostate cancer detection [19].

MRI-assisted prostate biopsies are performed in two ways; *cognitive fusion* and *software fusion* of a previously acquired prostate MRI with real-time TRUS.

- Cognitive fusion is operator dependent. This method relies on TRUS for biopsy guidance and requires the operator to infer the location of the MRI-target lesion during real-time TRUS imaging. Cognitive fusion biopsy does not require additional software; however, the onus is on the operators spatial cognition to accurately guide the probe to the target and sample to appropriate area
- MRI-TRUS-fused biopsies are performed using software platforms to integrate the MRI data to the USG for more accurate targeted biopsies. The software aligns the tumor boundary identified on MRI as an overlay on the real-time TRUS image to enable a direct targeted biopsy. The TRUS images can be obtained in 3-D using a 3-D TRUS probes or a standard 2-D TRUS probe can be used with affixed tracking hardware. This method reduces the uncertainty of alignment and misregistration of the cross-modality anatomy

Studies of cognitive and software fusion TRUS biopsies have shown higher cancer detection rates than TRUS alone. There are limitations to these techniques including operator training, patient movement, length of time for the procedure, and misregistration of images secondary to gland swelling from the initial biopsies [20,56,57]. The PROFUS trial carried evaluated these two biopsy methods in 2013 and demonstrated that although there was no overall increase in cancer detection rate between cognitive and software-fused biopsies, the use of fusion biopsies results in a likely reduction in over detection of clinically insignificant prostate cancer [58].

In-bore MRI-guided biopsy has been performed in recent years especially for targeted biopsy of suspicious lesions identified at the time of diagnostic mp-MRI. A recent study showed an increase in biopsy yield compared with TRUS in patients with increased PSA and a previous negative biopsy when targeting MRI-identified lesions [59]. In-bore MRI-guided biopsy is not commonly available due to the cost and length of procedure. In-bore MRI-targeted biopsies are performed with the patient in the prone position after the administration of moderate sedation. Lubrication using lidocaine gel is used and the rectal needle sleeve is inserted, preprocedure T2WI images are obtained in and axial and sagittal plane are then obtained. The needle sleeve is calibrated on a dedicated workstation and the target lesions are identified. The trajectory angles are then calculated and the MRI lesion is then targeted for the biopsy. The core biopsy is obtained using an MRI compatible 18-guage fully automatic needle that is guided through the sleeve to the chosen target lesion [60]. The FUTURE trial, a recent multicenter study, compared the three different MRI-guided biopsy techniques (visual cognitive, software fusion, and in-bore MRI guided) with respect to overall and csPCa detection. The authors did not find a significant difference in cancer detection between the biopsy groups and recommended that the choice of technique should be made on a case-by-case basis [56,61].

mp-MRI Following Treatment for Prostate Cancer

The treatment of prostate cancer is evolving from surgical resection and radiotherapy to new focal techniques. Radical treatments remain the "gold standard" of therapy; however, recent advances in mp-MRI to delineate focal areas of cancer have resulted in the development of focal therapy techniques. Focal therapy is reported to be associated with reduced treatment comorbidities compared with surgery and radiotherapy.

After prostatectomy, patients are surveilled by monitoring of PSA levels that should be undetectable or <0.05 ng/mL.

PROSTATE MRI

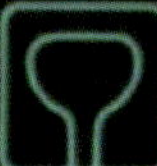

- **INDICATION:** *(including the date and value of serum PSA level and any prior biopsy type- TRUS, FUSION, IN BORE, date and results), prior therapy (Radiation, Hormones)*
- **TECHNIQUE:** *(state it is PI-RADS-compliant; explicit description of field strength, coils used, route and rate of IV contrast administration, and pulse sequence parameters is recommended)*
- **COMPARISON:**
- **FINDINGS:**

Size: *L × W × H cm or V cubic cm (with inclusion of PSA density)*
Quality
Hemorrhage:
Peripheral zone:
Transition zone:

Lesion (s) in rank order of severity (highest score- to lowest score, then by size):

#1:

- Location:
- Size:
- T2:
- DWI:
- DCE:
- Prostate margin: *(no involvement, indeterminate, or definite extraprostatic extension)*

Lesion overall PI-RADS category:

Extra-prostatic extension:

Neurovascular bundles: *(distance from index lesion or any PI-RADS 4/5 lesion to NVB's)*

Seminal vesicles:

Lymph nodes:

Other pelvic organs:

- **IMPRESSION:**

Overall PI-RADS category
(listing of PI-RADS categories)

Figure 42.32 PI-RADS v2.1 Report Template.

TABLE 42.6 Definition of Biochemical Recurrence

Biochemical Recurrence	
Rising serum level of PSA after a curative-intent prostate cancer treatment	
After radical prostatectomy	PSA level above 0.2 ng/mL across two consecutive measures (and rising)
After radiation therapy	PSA level equal to or greater than 2.0 ng/mL above the nadir

Rise in PSA after surgery is an indication of recurrent disease (Table 42.6) [62].

- *The commonest site of local recurrence is at the vesicourethral anastomosis* (Fig. 42.33) and may show as an isointense to mildly hyperintense soft-tissue nodule on T2-WI with early enhancement on DCE imaging [63]
- Other sites to look for recurrent disease include the seminal vesicles (Fig. 42.34), anterolateral surgical margins and the prostate bed

As per the Phoenix Criteria, increase in PSA levels by 2 ng/mL from nadir levels after radiation therapy raises suspicion of recurrent disease. At post-treatment imaging, there is decrease in T2 signal intensity from glandular loss and fibrosis. Recurrent disease is most often seen at the site of the primary tumor before treatment. Restriction diffusion on DWI and especially early enhancement on DCE imaging are variably helpful in detecting recurrent disease on mp-MRI.

Focal therapy for prostate cancer, whereby the part of gland harboring the tumor is treated, leaving the rest of the gland intact, depends on mp-MRI for localization of disease within the prostate gland; these lesions must be reproducibly visualized on imaging for targeted therapy. Multitude of ablative and nonablative energy sources is being investigated for focal therapy of prostate cancer. These include:

- High-intensity focused ultrasonography
- Focal laser ablation
- Irreversible electroporation
- Cryotherapy
- Photodynamic therapy

Studies have shown mp-MRI to be more sensitive than PSA for the assessment of residual or recurrent disease after focal therapy [64]. Post-treatment imaging often shows volume loss in the

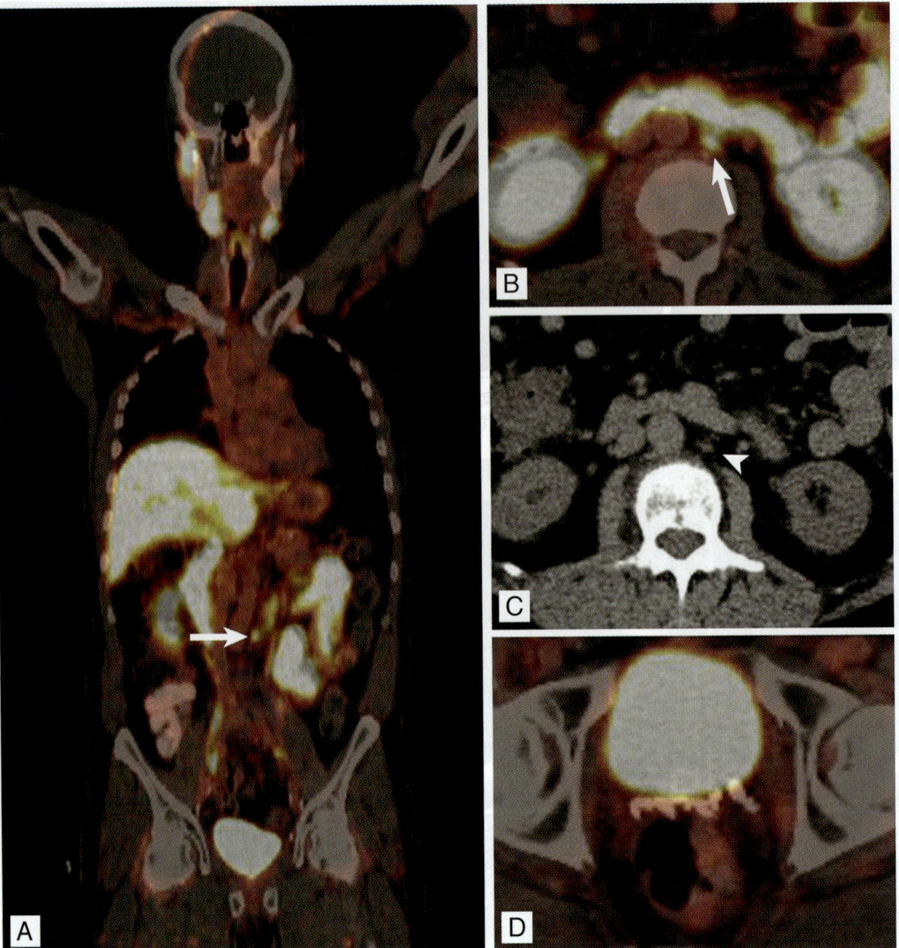

Figure 42.39 Biochemical recurrence (PSA level = 1.29 ng/mL) in a 64-year-old patient 3 years after radical prostatectomy and radiation therapy for Gleason score 9 (4+5) prostate cancer. ^{68}Ga-PSMA PET/CT images (coronal: A, axial: B) show increased uptake (SUV 5.3) (*arrows*) in a small left para-aortic lymph node, measuring <5 mm (axial CT image: C) (*arrowhead*), suspicious for lymph node metastasis (systemic recurrence: M1a, as this is a retroperitoneal lymph node). PET/CT axial image of the pelvis (D) shows no signs of tumor recurrence in the radical prostatectomy bed. This example illustrates the most established role of the PSMA PET in patients with prostate cancer (scenario of biochemical recurrence after a curative-intent prostate cancer treatment).

is a type 2 integral membrane glycoprotein which is highly expressed in prostate cancer. The expression of PSMA increases with tumor aggressiveness, metastatic disease, and disease recurrence.

- The first clinical application of PSMA-PET/CT was for investigation of metastasis in biochemical recurrence of prostate cancer after definitive primary treatment (Fig. 42.39). Classically bone scintigraphy is used to detect bone metastasis in the setting of prostate cancer; however, recent studies have shown that PSMA-PET/CT has greater sensitivity for the detection of metastatic bone disease
- PSMA-PET/CT is also used for the localization and staging of primary disease which has demonstrated the greatest yield for intermediate- to high-risk prostate cancer (Fig. 42.40). Lymph node metastasis represents a significant adverse prognostic marker in prostate cancer staging, PMSA-PET/CT has shown increased sensitivity and specificity for the detection of lymph node metastases before surgery
- The role of PMSA-PET/CT for local detection of prostate cancer is currently being investigated; many studies have shown a benefit when used in conjunction with mp-MRI to localize the tumor and perform targeted biopsies [67–69]

Teaching Points

- The peripheral zone is the site of approximately 70–75% of prostate cancer
- When cancer is detected by TRUS in the peripheral zone, it classically appears as a hypoechoic nodule
- Utricle cysts arise secondary to dilatation of the prostatic utricle (midline cysts)
- BPH is characterized by expansile nodules caused by proliferation of stroma, newly formed glandular structures or a mixture of both
- Prostatitis is a pitfall for cancer diagnosis on MRI and can result in false-positive reports
- Hematospermia can be caused by urogenital infections, trauma, recent instrumentation, calculi, BPH, and urogenital cancer
- The role of mp-MRI has been extensively studied and demonstrated considerable promise in the detection, localization, risk stratification, and staging of prostate cancer
- PI-RADS was developed to standardize image-acquisition techniques and interpretation of prostate MRI. Each lesion is assigned a score from 1 to 5 indicating the likelihood of clinically significant cancer

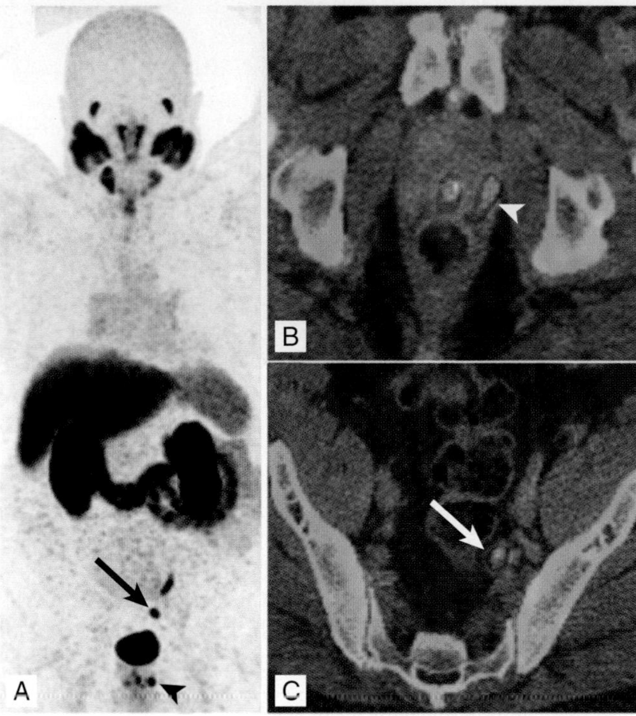

Figure 42.40 Primary staging of a high-risk prostate cancer in a 67-year-old patient. Pelvic MRI (not shown) showed a primary tumor classified as a PI-RADS 5 in the left peripheral zone and no suspicious lymph node. MIP image from ^{68}Ga-PSMA PET (A) and axial PET/CT images (B, C) show increased uptake in the prostate tumor (*arrowheads*) and also in a small (<5 mm) left internal iliac lymph node (*arrows*), suspicious for metastasis (positive regional lymph node: N1).

- DWI is the dominant sequence for the assessment of the peripheral zone
- T2WI is the dominant sequence for the assessment of the transition zone
- Imaging features suggesting ECE include bulging prostatic contour, capsule contact of tumor for >10 mm, capsular breach of low signal intensity tumor to neurovascular bundles, irregular or spiculated margin, obliteration of rectoprostatic angle, or direct extension to adjacent organs (bladder or rectum)
- The commonest site of local recurrence after radical prostatectomy is at the vesicourethral anastomosis
- Restriction diffusion on DWI and early enhancement on DCE imaging are variably helpful in detecting recurrent disease after radical therapy on mp-MRI

- The first clinical application of PMSA-PET/CT was for investigation of metastasis in biochemical recurrence of prostate cancer after definitive primary treatment

Suggested Readings

- European Association of Urology (EUA) guidelines (v.2020).
- https://uroweb.org/guideline/prostate-cancer/.
- American Urological Association (AUA) guidelines.
- https://www.auanet.org/guidelines.
- National Comprehensive Cancer Network (NCCN) guidelines (v2.2020).
- https://www.nccn.org.
- Prostate Imaging Reporting & Data System (PI-RADS) document (v2.1).
- https://www.acr.org/-/media/ACR/Files/RADS/Pi-RADS/PI-RADS -V2-1.pdf.
- B Turkbey, AB Rosenkrantz, MA Haider, et al., Prostate imaging reporting and data system version 2.1: 2019 update of prostate imaging reporting and data system version 2, Eur Urol 76 (3) (2019) 340–351.
- SM Walker, PL Choyke, B Turkbey, What you need to know before reading multiparametric MRI for prostate cancer, AJR Am J Roentgenol 214 (6) (2020) 1211–1219. doi:10.2214/AJR. 19.22751. Epub 2020 Apr 7.
- AB Rosenkrantz, SS Taneja, Radiologist, be aware: ten pitfalls that confound the interpretation of multiparametric prostate MRI, AJR Am J Roentgenol 202 (1) (2014) 109–120. doi:10.2214/AJR.13.10699.
- L Aaron, OE Franco, SW Hayward, Review of prostate anatomy and embryology and the etiology of benign prostatic hyperplasia, Urol Clin North Am 43 (3) (2016) 279–288.
- J Yu, AS Fulcher, SG Winks, MA Turner, RD Clayton, M Brooks, et al., Diagnosis of typical and atypical transition zone prostate cancer and its mimics at multiparametric prostate MRI, Br J Radiol 90 (1073) (2017) 20160693.
- SM Walker, PL Choyke, B Turkbey, What you need to know before reading multiparametric MRI for prostate cancer, Am J Roentgenol 214 (6) (2020) 1211–1219.
- B Turkbey, AB Rosenkrantz, MA Haider, AR Padhani, G Villeirs, KJ Macura, et al., Prostate imaging reporting and data system version 2.1: 2019 update of prostate imaging reporting and data system version 2, Eur Urol 76 (3) (2019) 340–351.
- S Ghai, MA Haider, Multiparametric-MRI in diagnosis of prostate cancer, Indian J Urol 31 (3) (2015) 194–201.
- JP Zawaideh, E Sala, N Shaida, B Koo, AY Warren, L Carmisciano, et al., Diagnostic accuracy of biparametric versus multiparametric prostate MRI: assessment of contrast benefit in clinical practice, Eur Radiol 30 (7) (2020) 4039–4049.

43
Male Genital Tract

ISHA D. ATRE, MUKESH G. HARISINGHANI

Male Urethra

Anatomy

The male urethra is approximately 17.5–20 cm long and runs from the bladder neck to the external meatus. It consists of two portions, anterior and posterior, each of which is divided into two parts (Fig. 43.1).

The posterior portion is about 3.5 cm in length, extends from the bladder neck to the inferior aspect of the urogenital diaphragm (UGD) and is divided into prostatic and membranous urethra.

- Prostatic urethra is normally the widest part of the urethra and has a rounded prominence of smooth muscle—verumontanum, along its posterior wall. At the center of the verumontanum is a small diverticulum (prostatic utricle) which receives the ejaculatory ducts at its lateral margins
- The membranous urethra is the shortest (1–1.5 cm) and least distensible narrow section of the urethra. It is enclosed by the sphincter urethrae (external sphincter), which, along with the deep transverse perineal muscles and their covering fasciae, form the UGD. Cowper glands are two pea sized glands lying on either side of the membranous urethra within the UGD and their ducts open into the proximal portion of the bulbar urethra on either side of the midline. Glands of Littré are the intramural glands of anterior urethra, more numerously found along the dorsal penile aspect

The anterior portion of the urethra is divided into bulbous and penile urethra which relate to the root and body of the penis, respectively.

- The bulbous urethra is located between the inferior margin of the UGD and the penoscrotal junction
- The penile urethra extends from the penoscrotal junction to the external meatus, encased by the corpus spongiosum of the penis. Fossa navicularis is a normal focal small dilatation at the distal end of the penile urethra

Posterior urethra is lined by transitional columnar epithelium while the anterior urethra is lined by pseudostratified columnar epithelium, with its distal most portions lined by squamous epithelium.

Urethral Trauma

Pathophysiology and Clinical Presentation

Traumatic urethral injuries are divided into anterior (penile/bulbar) and posterior (membranous/prostatic) urethral injuries. The frequency of anterior urethral injuries is about one-third that of posterior urethral injuries [1]. In male patients with pelvic trauma, the classic symptoms of a traumatic urethral injury include inability to void, blood at the urethral meatus, or hematuria. The causes are typically divided into blunt (most common) or penetrating trauma and iatrogenic.

a. Posterior Urethral Injuries: Posterior urethral injuries are seen with around 3–25% of pelvic fractures. The common mechanisms of injury are motor vehicle accidents and fall from a height. Around one-fifth of the patients with posterior urethral injuries also have associated bladder injury, which can be evaluated with retrograde urethrography (RGU) [2].

b. Anterior Urethral Injuries: These are mostly isolated injuries with the common mechanisms of trauma being straddle/shearing injuries or during attempted catheterization or instrumentation. Straddle injuries are due to blunt perineal trauma when the bulbar urethra and corpus spongiosum are compressed against the inferior aspect of the anterior pelvic ring (Fig. 43.2). The injury is not usually associated with a fracture. Penetrating urethral injuries are relatively uncommon and more commonly affect the anterior urethra.

"Goldman classification of urethral injuries" is a comprehensive and widely accepted based on the anatomical location of urethral injury [3].

- Type I injury: The posterior urethra is stretched and elongated but intact. The prostate and bladder apex are displaced superiorly due to disruption of the puboprostatic ligaments and the resulting hematoma. In this mildest type of injury, there is only contusion or partial tear of the membranous urethra and

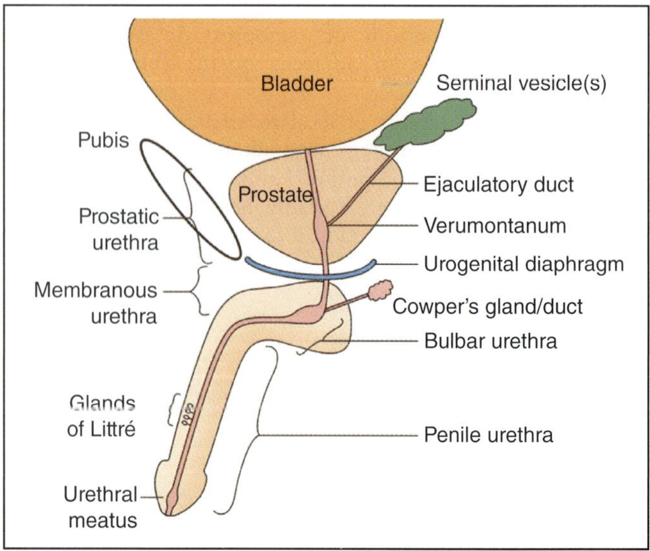

Figure 43.1 Schematic diagram showing normal anatomy of male urethra.

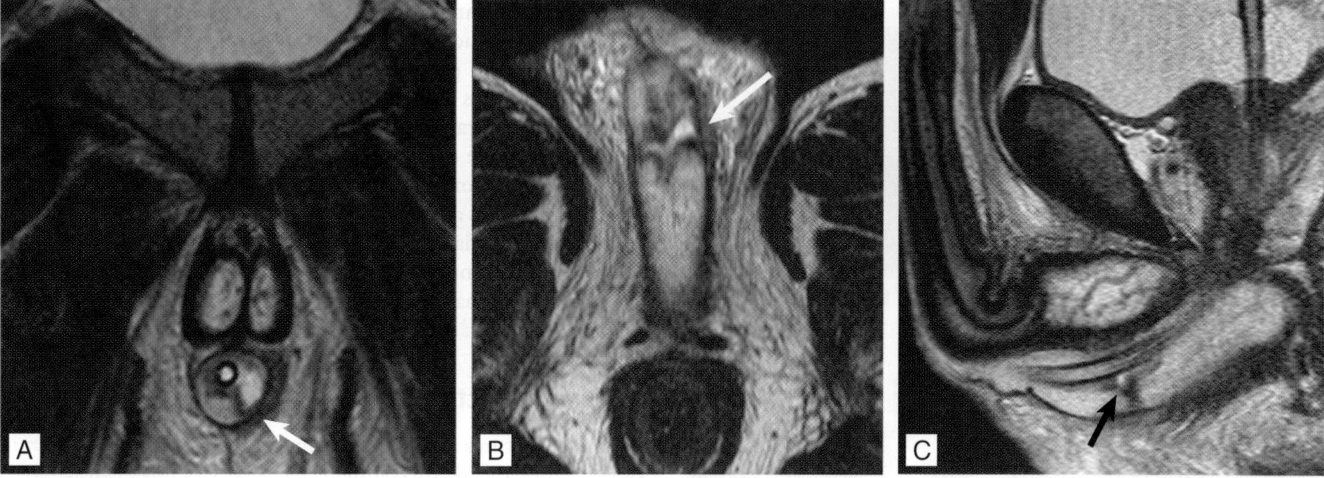

Figure 43.2 MRI T2-weighted coronal (A), axial (B), sagittal (C) images showing bulbar urethral injury (*arrows*) due to perineal trauma.

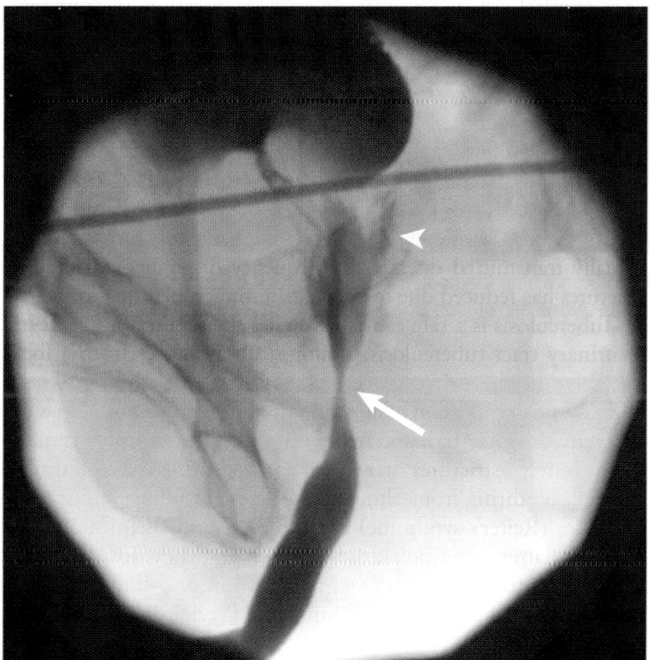

Figure 43.3 Micturating cystourethrography (MCU) showing Type II urethral injury involving posterior urethra evidenced by irregularly narrowed and stretched posterior urethra (*white arrow*) and contained extravasation in the posterior aspect of prostatic urethra (*arrowhead*). No evidence for urethral transection.

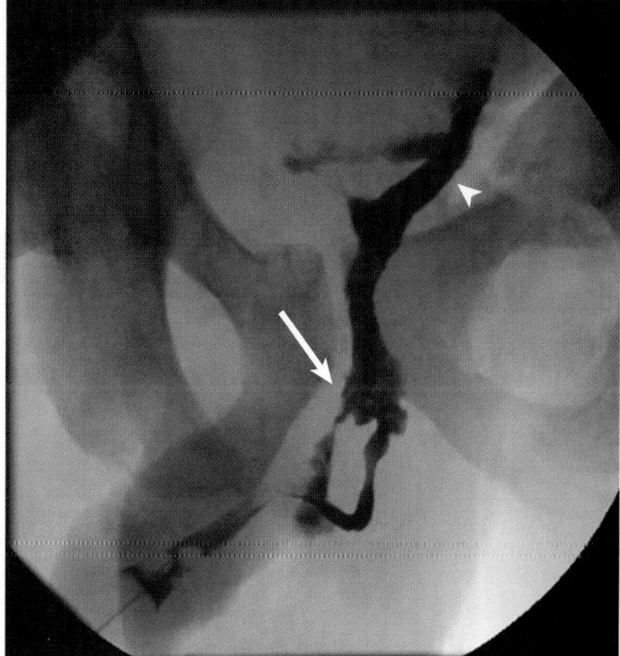

Figure 43.4 Retrograde urethrography in a patient with pelvic trauma showing contrast extravasation (*white arrow*) at the level of the posterior prostatic/membranous urethra, consistent with Type II injury. Linear contrast accumulation in the retropubic space (*arrowhead*) suggestive of urethral injury with consequent urinoma formation in the retropubic space.

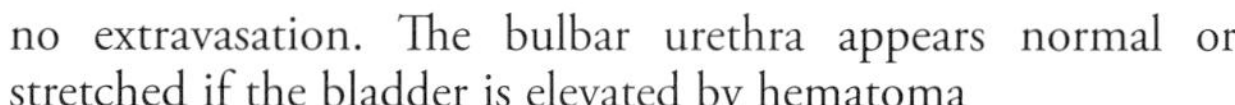

no extravasation. The bulbar urethra appears normal or stretched if the bladder is elevated by hematoma

- Type II injury: Disruption of the urethra occurs above the UGD in the prostatic segment. The membranous urethra is intact (Fig 43.3). This is the commonest injury type of urethral injury, with rupture at the prostatic apex (prostatomembranous junction) immediately above the UGD with sparing of the UGD itself. Extravasation therefore occurs into the retropubic space but cannot extend into the perineum and the bulbar urethra is intact (Fig. 43.4)
- Type III injury: The membranous urethra is disrupted with extension of injury to the proximal bulbous urethra and/or disruption of the UGD

  In the type III injury the membranous urethra ruptures at the bulbomembranous junction below the UGD, which itself is disrupted. The bulbar urethra is often also ruptured. Contrast extravasation is then in the direction of least resistance and into the perineum.
- Type IV injury: Bladder neck injury with extension into the proximal urethra (Fig. 43.5)
- Type IVA injury: Injury of the base of the bladder with periurethral extravasation simulating a true type IV urethral injury
- Type V injury: Partial or complete pure anterior urethral injury (Fig. 43.6)

Around two-thirds of type II injuries involve complete urethral rupture; one-third is partial. Type III injuries are more severe and virtually

- During the voiding phase of cystourethrography, these lesions typically appear as smooth filling defects. On MRI, these lesions demonstrate intermediate signal on T1W images, low to intermediate signal on T2W images, and demonstrate contrast enhancement

Malignant Tumors

- Malignant tumors of male urethra are rare, with usual incidence after 50 years of age. Predisposing factors include chronic inflammation secondary to sexually transmitted infectious urethritis and urethral stricture. The most frequently involved location is the bulbomembranous urethra (60% of cases), followed by penile (30%) and prostatic urethra (10%) [4]
- Over 75–80% are squamous cell carcinomas and majority of the rest (15%) are transitional cell carcinomas. Adenocarcinomas are occasionally encountered and arise from Littré or Cowper's glands
- The salient features of the TNM staging for urethral malignancy are:

  T1—tumor invading subepithelial connective tissue.

  T2—tumor invading any of periurethral muscle, corpus spongiosum, or prostate.

  T3—tumor invading any of bladder neck, corpus cavernosum, or anterior vagina (Fig. 43.15).

  T4—tumor invading any of the other adjacent organs, including the bladder.
- Metastatic spread is virtually always via the lymphatics, the penile urethra metastasizing to the deep inguinal and external iliac lymph nodes, while the bulbar and posterior urethra masses go to the internal iliac and obturator lymph nodes
- Patients usually present with a palpable mass (most common) along the shaft of urethra or in the perineum, or insidious onset of poor urinary stream, hematuria, and serosanguinous discharge
- On urethrography, carcinomas appear as one or more irregular filling defects; may be eccentric or circumferential and may be associated with irregular stricturing
- MRI is the favored modality for staging urethral carcinoma because of its better demonstration of the soft-tissue anatomy of the perineum. It appears as a lesion of low signal intensity on both T1- and T2-weighted imaging, compared to the normal corporal tissue (Fig. 43.16)
- Secondary urethral involvement: due to metastases from a distant primary is rare. The urethra is more commonly involved by direct spread of tumor from adjacent organs, most often carcinoma of the bladder or rectum, and occasionally prostate, vagina, or cervix (Fig. 43.17)

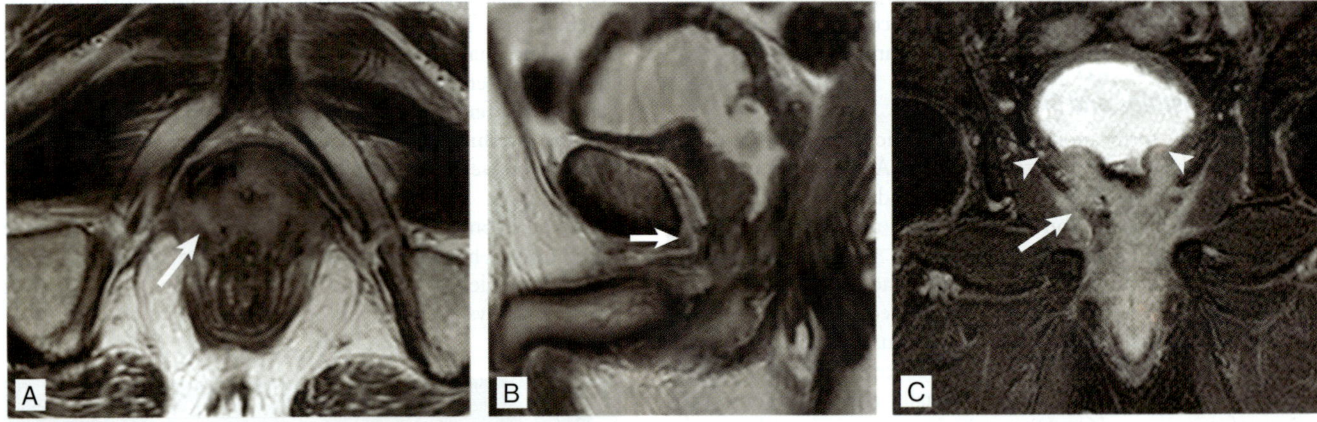

Figure 43.15 MRI T2 axial (A) and sagittal (B) images show an ill-defined heterogenous mass (*white arrow*) centered in the prostatic urethra and extending to the bulbous urethra. (C) shows heterogenous enhancement (*arrow*) extending along the prostate base. There is involvement of the bladder base (*arrowheads* in C).

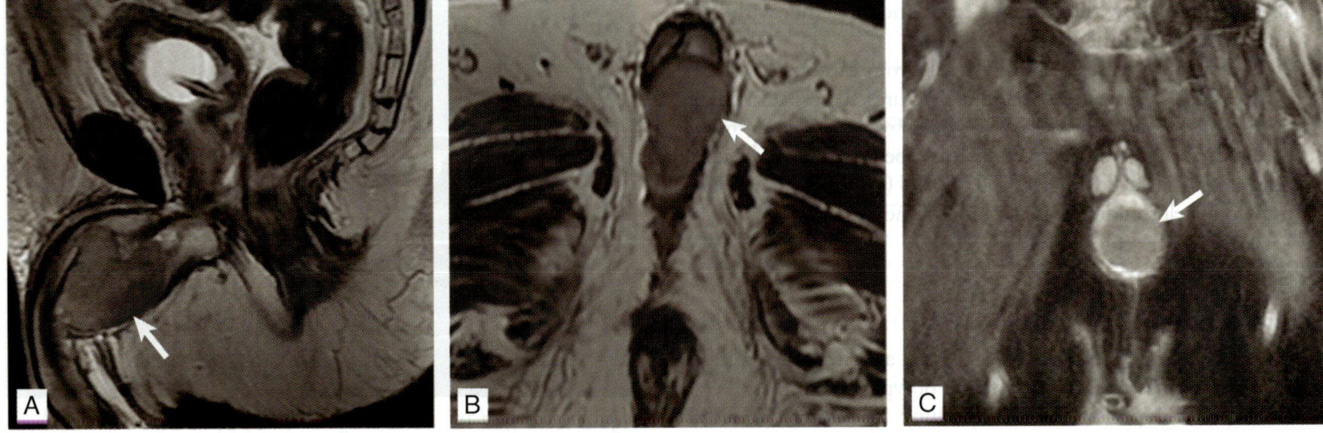

Figure 43.16 MRI T2 sagittal (A) and axial (B) images of the same patient as in Fig. 43.10. There is an irregularly marginated mass (*white arrow*) in the penile urethra showing intermediate signal on T2W images and heterogenous enhancement (*arrow*) on postcontrast sequences (C).

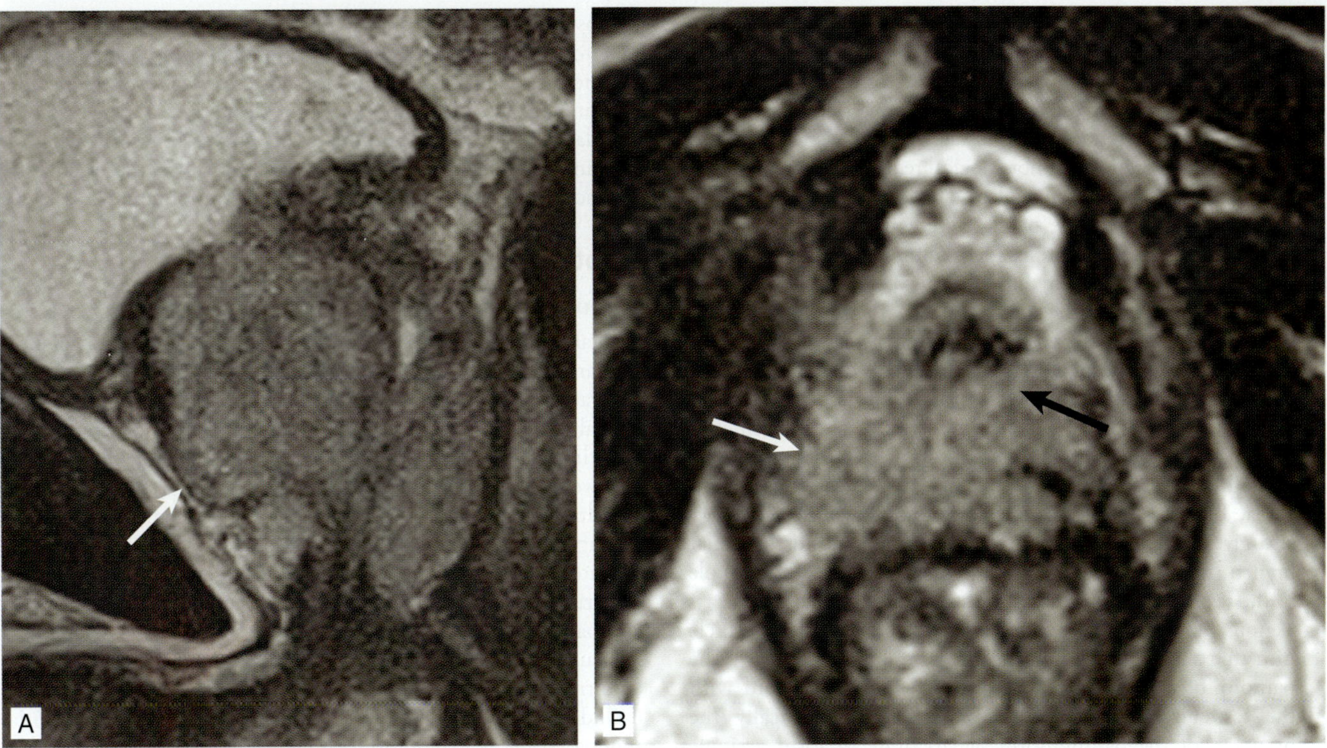

Figure 43.17 MRI T2 sagittal (A) and axial (B) images show an infiltrative heterogenous intermediate signal intensity mass (*white arrows*) in the region of prostate, which was found to be prostate carcinoma on biopsy with invasion of the prostatic urethra (*black arrow*).

Scrotum and Testes

Anatomy

- The scrotum is a pouch of skin that contains the testes, epididymis, and spermatic cord (Fig. 43.18). It has three layers from superficial to deep: skin, dartos muscle, and Colles' fascia (continuous anterosuperiorly with the anterior wall membranous fascia—Scarpa's fascia). It is divided into two compartments by a midline fibrous septum (median raphe). Each compartment contains a testicle, epididymis and proximal spermatic cord

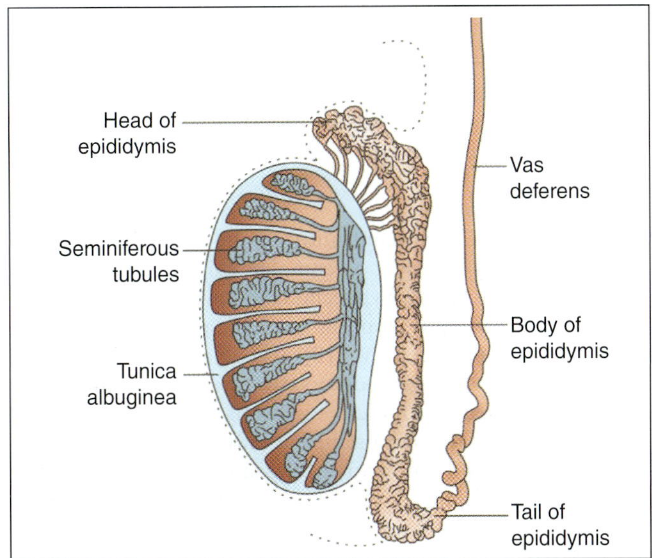

Figure 43.18 Schematic diagram of normal anatomy of testes and epididymis.

- During embryological development, the testicles originate on the posterior abdominal wall around the level of the first lumbar vertebra. They descend retroperitoneally through the abdomen along with their associated neurovascular structures, lymphatics, and ducts, and exit the pelvis via the inguinal canal at around seventh to eighth month of intrauterine life. They are preceded by a peritoneal diverticulum (processus vaginalis), remnants of which may persist into adult life
- As they leave the pelvis, they acquire a covering from each layer of the anterior abdominal wall which surrounds the spermatic cord and the testes. The transversalis fascia gives rise to the internal spermatic fascia, the internal oblique muscles to the cremasteric muscle and fascia and the external oblique aponeurosis to the external spermatic fascia
- Deep to these three layers is the tunica vaginalis. This is a serous membrane (derived from peritoneum) with two layers: parietal, against the internal spermatic fascia, and visceral, which closely invests the testis and the epididymis. The tunica vaginalis envelops the testicle and applies it to the posterior scrotal wall. There is a potential space between these two layers which extends a little way along the spermatic cord and normally may contain up to 1–2 mL of serous fluid. In disease states a more substantial collection may be seen (hydrocele)
- The outermost layer of the testicle is the tunica albuginea, a dense fibrous capsule. Posteriorly there is a vertical linear extension of the tunica albuginea into the testicular parenchyma (mediastinum of the testis). The testicle is divided into 200–400 lobules by numerous trabeculae that extend from the mediastinum. The lobules consist of interstitial tissue (which includes the androgen producing Leydig cells) and 2–4 seminiferous tubules (which include the supporting Sertoli cells) that drain via a common tubule. These converge into a network of tubules at the mediastinum (the rete testis)

that drain via 10–15 efferent tubules out of the testicle into the epididymis

- The epididymis consists of a convoluted common tubule with supporting tissue. Its upper, mid, and lower portions may be referred to as the head, body, and tail. Drainage is from the tail into the vas deferens. An embryological remnant a couple of millimeters long (so-called appendix or hydatid) may be identified related to the upper pole of the epididymis (derived from the mesonephric duct) or the testis (derived from the Mullerian duct)
- The testicle is supplied by an end artery, the testicular artery, which originates from the aorta just below the renal artery. This runs inferiorly along the posterior abdominal wall on the surface of the psoas muscle and enters the scrotum via the inguinal canal within the spermatic cord. At the mediastinum of the testis, the dominant testicular artery (sometimes referred to as the inferior testicular artery) divides into several capsular arteries which run around the testicular parenchyma just deep to the tunica albuginea. Before reaching the mediastinum, the testicular artery also gives rise to the epididymal artery and a minor testicular branch (internal testicular artery), which enters the upper pole of the testicle and contributes to the capsular branches
- Venous blood drains from the posterior border of the testicle into an extensive venous plexus (the pampiniform plexus). The pampiniform plexus ascends within the spermatic cord with the testicular artery and the vas deferens. Classically the branches of the pampiniform plexus unite to form a single testicular vein (the internal spermatic vein) as it enters the abdomen via the inguinal canal. The testicular vein runs superiorly along the posterior abdominal wall in the retroperitoneum and terminates in the renal vein on the left and in the inferior vena cava just below the renal vein on the right. This, however, is extremely variable and often there are multiple collaterals to the renal or retroperitoneal veins, multiple terminal ostia and multiple testicular veins
- The spermatic cord runs from the testicle to the abdominal cavity via the inguinal canal. It contains the vital supply and drainage structures of the testicle surrounded by continuations of the three deep fascial layers of the scrotum (the internal spermatic, cremasteric, and external spermatic fasciae). The contents include the testicular artery, pampiniform plexus, lymphatic vessels, and the vas deferens. The veins are routinely visualized and are normally no more than 1–2 mm maximum diameter
- The lymphatic vessels follow the testicular artery and vein retroperitoneally to terminate in the first—echelon nodes (sometimes referred to as the sentinel lymph nodes) in the upper abdomen. On the left, these are immediately lateral to the para-aortic lymph nodes and medial to the renal lymph nodes around the level of the first to the second lumbar vertebrae, while on the right they are in the para-caval region just below the renal vessels around the level of the first to the third lumbar vertebrae (both potentially into the aortocaval nodes centrally). In a minority, the lymphatics drain directly into nodes at the level of the aortic bifurcation and occasionally directly into the common iliac nodes. Testicular lymph node drainage is usually to the ipsilateral nodes, but bilateral drainage may occur, more often from the right than the left. These considerations are important when staging testicular malignancy
- The vas deferens is a muscular duct responsible for the transport of the sperm from the testicle to the urethra. It originates from the tail of the epididymis and leaves the scrotum in the spermatic cord. After passing through the inguinal canal, it enters the pelvis at the deep inguinal ring, hooks round the lateral aspect of the inferior epigastric artery, and runs posteroinferiorly on the lateral wall of the pelvis (on the obturator internus) to the level of the ischial spine, where it turns inferomedially to run along the posterior aspect of the bladder immediately anterosuperior to the distal ureters. The distal vas dilates to form the ampulla. This curves inferiorly where it joins the duct of the seminal vesicle to form the ejaculatory duct, which joins the urethra at the verumontanum

Scrotal Trauma

Pathophysiology and Clinical Presentation

Scrotal trauma is not very common because of its anatomical location and mobility [7]. However, prompt recognition is helpful for accurate evaluation and triage. The most common mechanism of scrotal injury is blunt trauma followed by penetrating injuries [8]. Sporting activities account for more than half of all the cases followed by motor vehicle accidents (9–17%) [9].

Ultrasound helps in effective triage for medical or surgical management as it can reliably detect intra- and extratesticular hematomas, contusions, tunica albuginea disruptions, and testicular ruptures. The role of imaging depends on the treatment approach. When the conservative approach is adopted for intratesticular abnormality after trauma, follow-up ultrasounds help in confirmation of resolution of the detected abnormality and to exclude underlying any tumor [10]. When there is substantial trauma, surgical exploration approach with drainage of hematoma and repair of testicular tears may enhance the subsequent viability of the testicle.

Imaging Features

Ultrasound is the most appropriate first line imaging modality.

A. Blunt Trauma: Injuries that result from blunt trauma include intratesticular hematoma, disruption of tunica albuginea, testicular rupture, testicular fracture (Fig. 43.19), dislocation, contour abnormality, absence of vascularity, testicular torsion.

1. *Testicular rupture*:

Ultrasound plays a critical role in early detection of testicular rupture helping in prompt surgical management. It is said that if the surgical repair is performed within 72 hours of trauma in testicular rupture, around 80% of ruptured testes can be successfully salvaged [10]. Discontinuity of the echogenic tunica albuginea which indicates disruption of the underlying testicle is critical since it supports the diagnosis of testicular rupture and emergency surgery can salvage the testes. Along-with discontinuity of tunica albuginea, other findings that together suggest testicular rupture include presence of heterogenous echogenicity within the testes, contour abnormality, and absence of vascularity within the testes [10].

2. *Testicular fracture*:

It refers to break or discontinuity in the parenchyma of the testes which may be linear or complex. On ultrasound, it can be identified as a linear hypoechoic and avascular area. Color Doppler is of particular importance in these cases as it helps in guiding further management [10]. if the flow is detected, then the cases can be managed conservatively, otherwise emergency surgery is required as it indicates ischemia [11]. Color flow and Doppler imaging are very useful not only for assessing the testicular viability but also for detecting any vascular injuries like pseudoaneurysms [11].

3. *Testicular torsion*:

Around 5–8% of the cases of torsion are thought to be due to trauma with the most common predisposing abnormality being bell-clapper deformity [12]. Clinical presentation and ultrasound

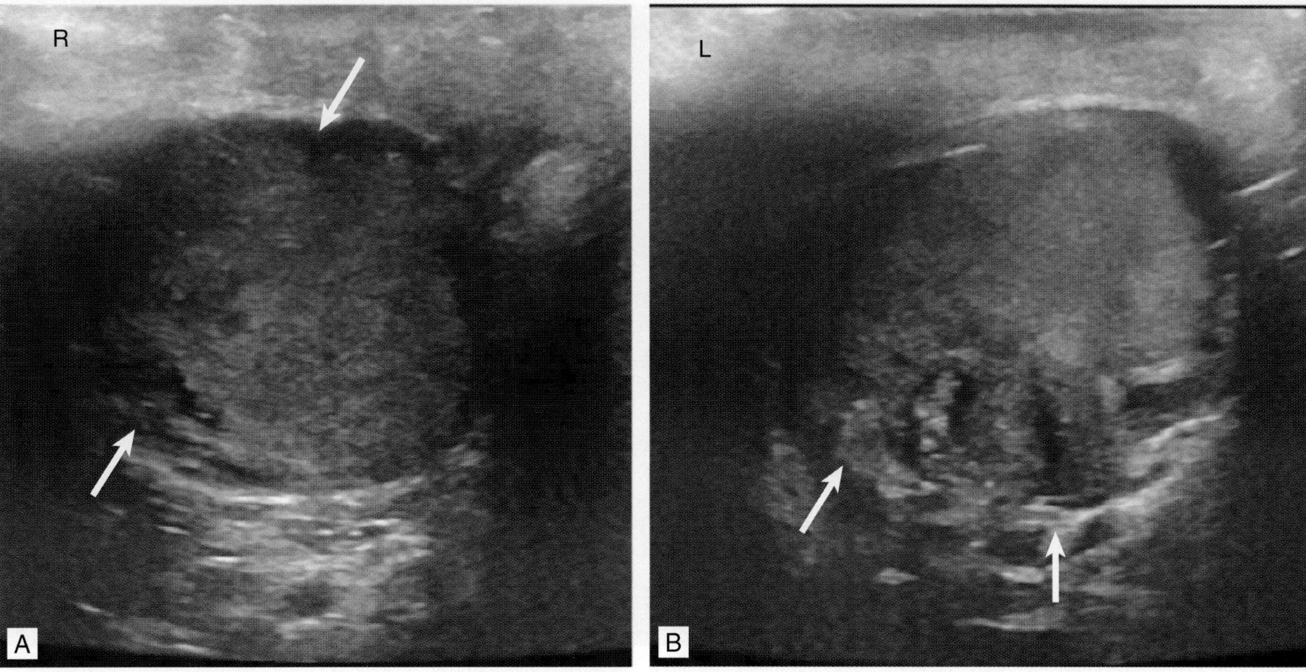

Figure 43.19 Both testes (A and B) appear disorganized and echogenic (*arrows*) consistent with testicular trauma/fracture with surrounding hemorrhage.

appearance of testicular torsion due to trauma are similar to cases that occur without trauma.

4. *Intratesticular hematoma*:

Appearances of testicular hematoma depend upon the time passed between the trauma and evaluation. Hyperacute to acute hematomas can appear isoechoic or may have diffusely heterogenous echogenicity. Follow-up ultrasound after 12–24 hours helps in better delineation and changes in the echogenicity. Chronic hematomas appear more hypoechoic to anechoic and show gradual resolution. Most important aim of ultrasound in these cases is to exclude a possibility of testicular rupture.

5. *Extratesticular hematoma/hematocele*:

This is the most common finding in a blunt injury identified as echogenic collection within the tunica vaginalis on ultrasound. Presence of large hematocele is an indication for urgent surgery because it can compromise blood flow due to large extrinsic pressure and also it may preclude detection of ruptured tunica albuginea.

Scrotal wall hematomas are identified as echogenic focal wall thickening or complex fluid collection and they usually resolve with conservative management or spontaneously, however large hematomas may need surgical management [10].

B. Penetrating Injuries: Penetrating injuries can range from small hematocele to testicular rupture.

Role of ultrasound in this form of injuries is the same as that of blunt injuries, to assess the severity of trauma for effective triage.

Extratesticular Disorders

Hydrocele

Pathophysiology and Clinical Presentation

A hydrocele is the formation of fluid between the two layers (visceral and parietal) of the tunica vaginalis. Ultrasonographically, it is seen as an echo-free area (Fig. 43.20) partly surrounding the testicle (in comparison to cysts, which do not surround the testicle). A hydrocele may develop as a result of infection (epididymo-orchitis), trauma, malignant testicular tumor or infarction (including torsion) or could be congenital. In most cases, however, an underlying cause for the hydrocele cannot be found. Hydroceles most commonly present as painless and progressive scrotal mass.

Imaging Features

- Ultrasound is the commonest modality to evaluate hydrocele It demonstrates fluid surrounding the testis or spermatic cord
- When infection is a cause, there are usually obvious clinical and radiological features of epididymitis. The hydrocele may demonstrate internal echoes (Fig. 43.20), especially on the rare occasions when infection is sufficiently severe for frank pus (pyocele) to develop. The commonest infective organisms are usually bowel-related Gram-negative bacilli, but a variety of other agents may be responsible
- Chronic infective hydrocele (especially tuberculous) may be associated with considerable calcification of the tunica
- Following trauma, a hematocele (hemorrhagic hydrocele) will also exhibit considerable echogenicity

Cysts

Simple cysts are common in the scrotum and are usually found incidentally during ultrasound examination for other pathologies. They may be seen at any age from adolescence onward but are most common in the elderly. The majority are seen in the epididymis, particularly in the upper pole, and they may be single or multiple.

On ultrasound, they show the classic features of cysts elsewhere in the body, being anechoic, showing distal acoustic enhancement and having no appreciable wall thickness (Figs. 43.21A and B).

Hemorrhage or infection may alter the appearance of a preexisting cyst to show some degree of echogenicity, occasionally with a visible fluid level (Fig. 43.21C). Alternatively, infection or trauma

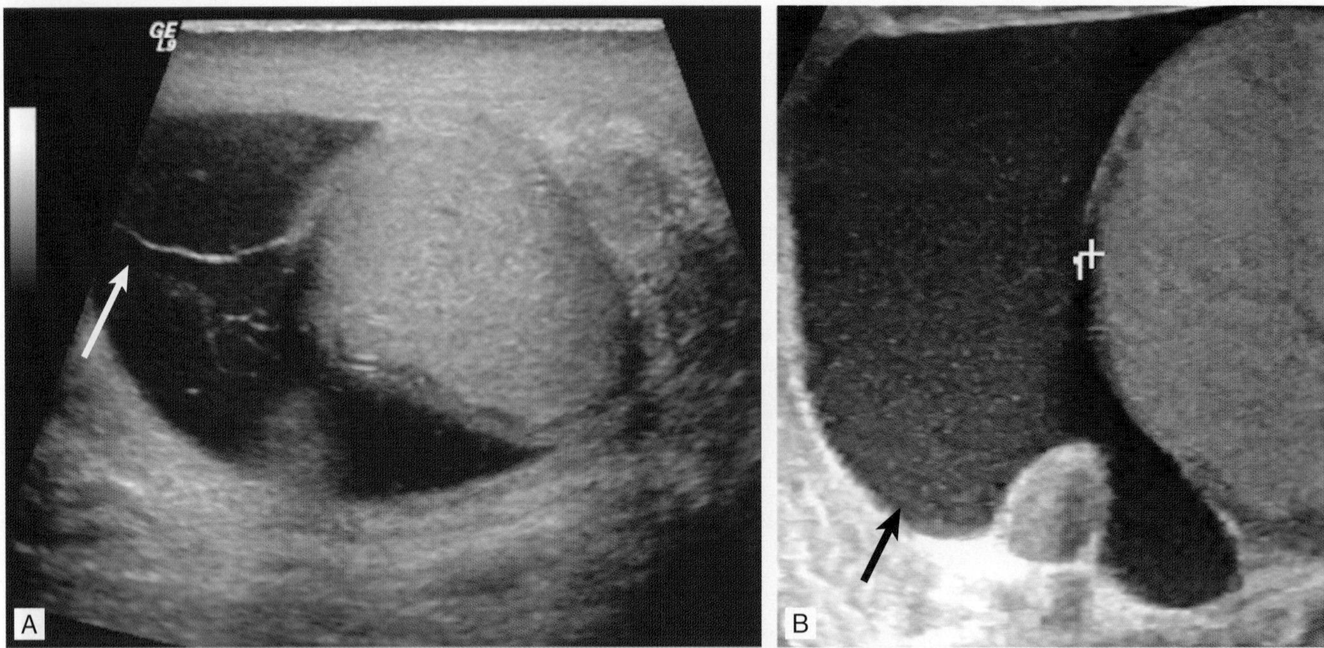

Figure 43.20 Ultrasound images showing hydrocele with septations (A) and echoes (B) consistent with an infected hydrocele (*arrows*).

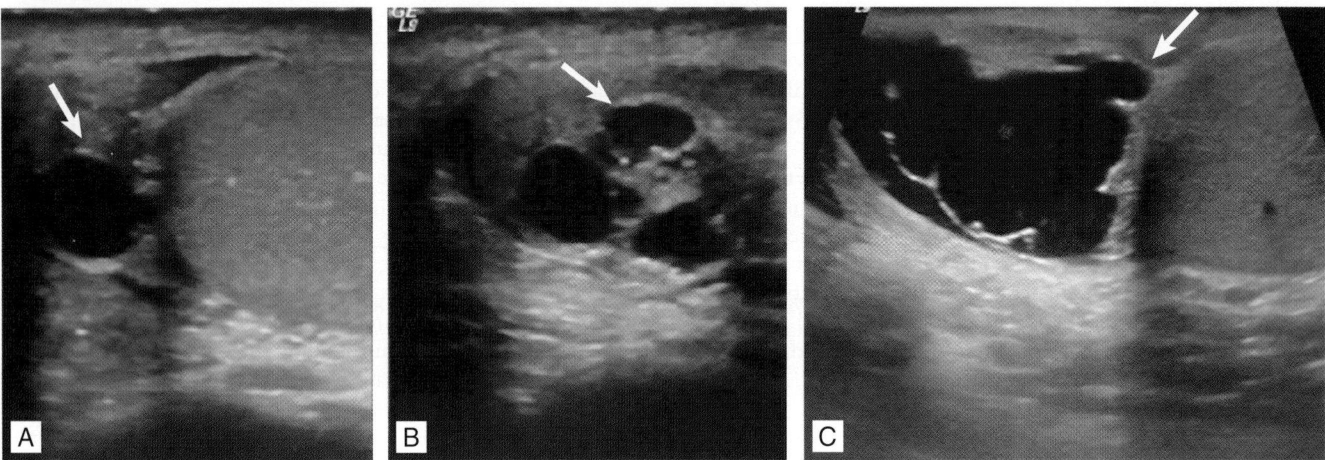

Figure 43.21 Patient with recent onset left-sided testicular pain and nausea (no history of acute trauma). Ultrasound showed bilateral epididymal cysts (images A and B showing cysts on right side and image C on left side). Largest cyst on the left side had thickened irregular walls (*white arrow*) and dependent echoes suggestive of infection in the given clinical settings.

(including vasectomy) may provoke the creation of a cystic lesion with internal echoes, partly due to the presence of spermatozoa. These again are more common in the upper pole of the epididymis.

Ultrasound is used as an adjunct modality after clinical examination and may aid in the diagnosis due to its ability to detect internal characteristics of cysts and can also guide therapeutic options such as USG guided aspiration, percutaneous sclerotherapy based on the origin, and nature of intrascrotal lesions [13,14].

Varicocele

Pathophysiology and Clinical Presentation

Dilatation of the network of veins draining the testicle (pampiniform plexus) found in the spermatic cord is described as a varicocele. They are extremely common (up to 8–16% of the male population), and usually asymptomatic, often being discovered incidentally on clinical or ultrasonographic examination for other conditions.

Two types of varicoceles are identified based on the etiopathogenesis: primary and secondary [15]. Primary varicoceles almost always occur on the left side due to the anatomical nature of the left internal spermatic vein draining into the ipsilateral renal vein at 90° angle leading to backward transmission of endoluminal pressure of the renal vein into the internal spermatic vein. On the right side, the internal spermatic vein drains into the inferior vena cava at an acute angle thus facilitating its drainage [16].

There is a possible association with subfertility, reported in 21–39% of males being investigated for subfertility. They are most frequent between 15 and 25 years of age, and when symptomatic, present with scrotal aching and/or soft scrotal swelling. Classically these symptoms worsen during the day while the patient is upright. Occasionally they present relatively acutely as a manifestation of a renal carcinoma. Treatment may be offered for discomfort or as part of management of subfertility.

Imaging Features

Ultrasound is the diagnostic modality of choice. On ultrasound, varicoceles are seen as a leash of predominantly anechoic serpiginous tubular structures measuring more than 2 mm maximum diameter (Fig. 43.22). Visible flow may be seen within larger varicoceles on conventional ultrasound. Confusion with cysts is unlikely, even when the varicocele is small, but confirmation of their nature can be obtained with slow-flow Doppler ultrasound. Demonstration and evaluation of reflux flow in patients suspected of having varicoceles is the most important part of the Doppler ultrasound study. One of the most essential parameters to be assessed is reflux duration, with reflux lasting >2 seconds considered the most useful parameter for varicocele diagnosis. Grading of varicoceles is not mandatory while reporting; Sarteschi classification on color Doppler ultrasound is preferred if provided (details below) [17,18].

Color Doppler ultrasound classification of varicocele:

Grade	Description
1	Reflux in vessels in the inguinal channel is detected only during the Valsalva maneuver, while scrotal varicosity is not evident in the standard ultrasound study.
2	Small posterior varicosities that extend to the superior pole of the testis. Their diameters increase and venous reflux is seen in the supratesticular region only during the Valsalva maneuver.
3	Vessels appear enlarged at the inferior pole of the testis when the patient is evaluated in a standing position; no enlargement is detected if the patient is examined in a supine position. Reflux observed only under during the Valsalva maneuver.
4	Vessels appear enlarged even when the patient is studied in a supine position; the dilatation is more marked in the upright position and during the Valsalva maneuver. Testicular hypotrophy is common at this stage.
5	Venous ectasia is evident even in the prone decubitus and supine positions. Reflux is observed at rest and does not increase during the Valsalva maneuver.

- The vast majority of varicoceles are described as primary and are presumed to be due to developmental abnormalities of the valves and/or the veins themselves. This is far more likely on the left, where at least 85% are encountered [19]. Testicular growth may be affected by varicocele, hence testicular volume should be measured for asymmetry when evaluated with ultrasound [20]
- A minority occur secondary to a lesion compressing or occluding the testicular vein. The classical cause is a left-sided renal cell carcinoma extending along the renal vein as far as the termination of the testicular vein, but benign (e.g., hydronephrosis) and other malignant conditions (including abdominal lymphadenopathy) can provoke a varicocele on either side. There is a higher risk of an underlying cause, particularly a tumor, if the varicocele is of recent onset with an acute presentation, the patient is older than 40 years, it is right-sided and is unchanged with provocative maneuvers. A unilateral right-sided varicocele should prompt an evaluation of the retroperitoneal region for excluding the possibility of a mass obstructing the testicular vein

Management

Treatment of varicoceles is usually for persistent discomfort or as part of the treatment of subfertility and is by percutaneous embolization or surgery. Direct surgical ligation of the testicular vein (by open operation or laparoscopy) has a low primary failure rate (of the order of 1%) with a recurrence rate around 16%. Surgery, however, is more traumatic than percutaneous embolization and is associated with specific risks not encountered with the alternative procedure, in particular damage to the testicular artery and resultant infarction.

The total failure rate for percutaneous embolization is comparable with that for surgery, although the technical failure rate may be higher (6–12%) and the recurrence rate similar or lower (4–16%). Morbidity is minor and infrequent, with up to 10% experiencing transient discomfort in the loin or scrotum on the side of the varicocele, with few other symptoms.

Postvasectomy Epididymis

Numerous individuals have had a vasectomy and many will undergo subsequent scrotal ultrasound for one reason or other, often unrelated to the vasectomy. In these patients the epididymis often appears thickened and slightly echo-poor. These findings can almost be regarded as variations of normal and are not usually related to any specific symptoms.

Epididymo-Orchitis

Pathophysiology and Clinical Presentation

Inflammation of the epididymis, usually due to ascending infection with Gram-negative bacilli (*E. coli*, etc.), *Chlamydia* or tuberculosis is common. If it is associated with the inflammation extending to testes, the term epididymo-orchitis is used. It is particularly seen in young adult males, with a second peak in late middle age and the elderly, where it may be associated with cystitis and/or prostatitis in association with benign prostatic disease and bladder outflow obstruction. The clinical presentation varies in severity and

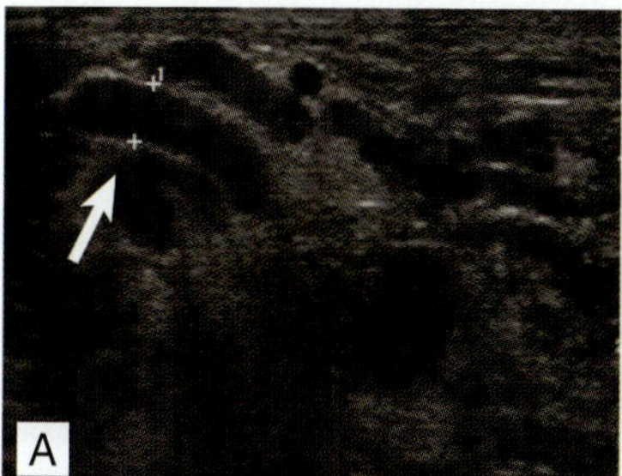

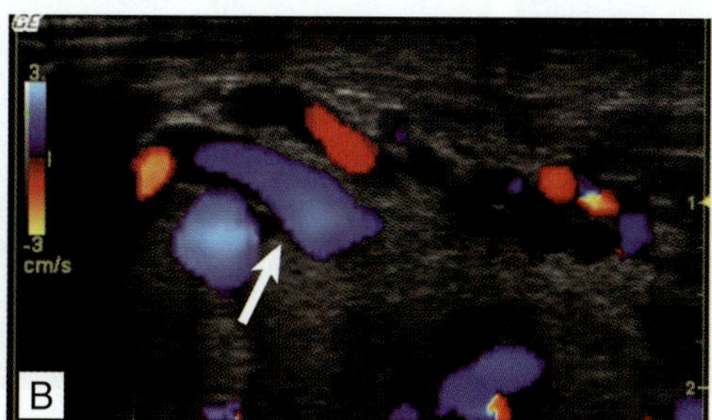

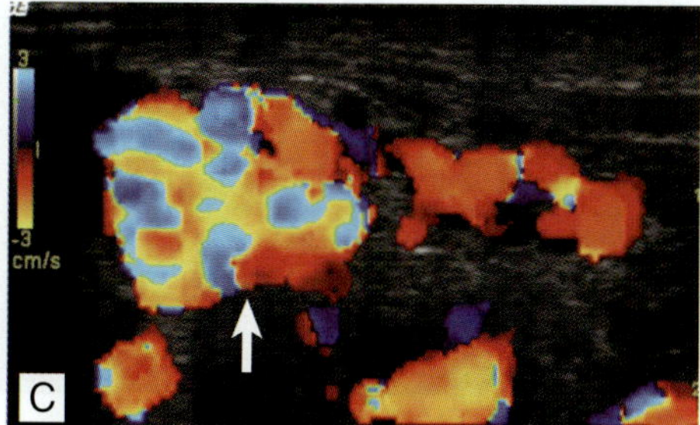

Figure 43.22 Ultrasound images showing dilated tubular anechoic structures >2 mm (*arrows*) in diameter (A) with visible flow (B). Reversal of flow is noted on Valsalva (C). Right-sided hydrocele. Given that isolated right-sided varicoceles are unusual and may represent occult retroperitoneal process, evaluation for possible occult abdominal/retroperitoneal malignancy is advised in such a case.

acuteness from mild pain, tenderness, and scrotal swelling to a severe pyrexial illness with marked scrotal pain and swelling. Although usually unilateral, epididymitis is not uncommonly bilateral.

Imaging Features

- On ultrasound, epididymo-orchitis commonly appears as swollen epididymis, often appearing nodular and particularly affecting the tail region or upper pole (head region). There is often diffuse or patchy reduction in echogenicity, although sometimes the epididymis shows considerable heterogeneity (Fig. 43.23B) and even rarely a diffuse increase in echogenicity. A heterogeneous pattern of predominant increase in echogenicity is more frequently associated with chronic epididymitis
- Doppler ultrasound often demonstrates hypervascularity. It is particularly useful in cases that show clinical findings with normal gray-scale ultrasound findings. Rarely, the condition progresses so that there is demonstrable abscess formation within the testes (Fig. 43.23C)
- There is often an associated hydrocele of variable size, which may be septated and contain echogenic fluid
- Severe cases may be associated with demonstrable edematous thickening of the overlying skin, and there may be coexisting orchitis in up to 20% of cases
- Earlier, scrotal scintigraphy (a nuclear medicine study to predict blood flow to scrotum and its contents) used to be performed when the diagnosis was not clear, especially in acute cases. It can demonstrate increased perfusion of the scrotal contents in epididymo-orchitis and nonperfusion in acute torsion. This procedure is infrequently performed these days. Although the reported accuracy of scintigraphy (95%) exceeds that of ultrasound (88%), choice of diagnostic modality is dictated by easily available ultrasound as compared to nuclear medicine study [21]

Isolated inflammation of testes is rare. It may be seen in systemic viral illness (classically mumps) or in association with bacterial epididymitis. Up to 25% of postpubertal males with mumps will suffer some degree of orchitis, usually 7–10 days after the parotitis. Other viruses implicated include echoviruses, group B arboviruses and the lymphocytic choriomeningitis virus. In the acute phase, ultrasound may show testicular swelling with patchy or diffuse reduction in echogenicity. Following resolution, the testicle may return to normal but in severe orchitis there may be atrophy, with reduction in size and echogenicity, usually apparent within 6 months of the acute insult.

Bacterial orchitis shows similar features of viral orchitis such as testicular swelling with patchy or diffuse reduction in

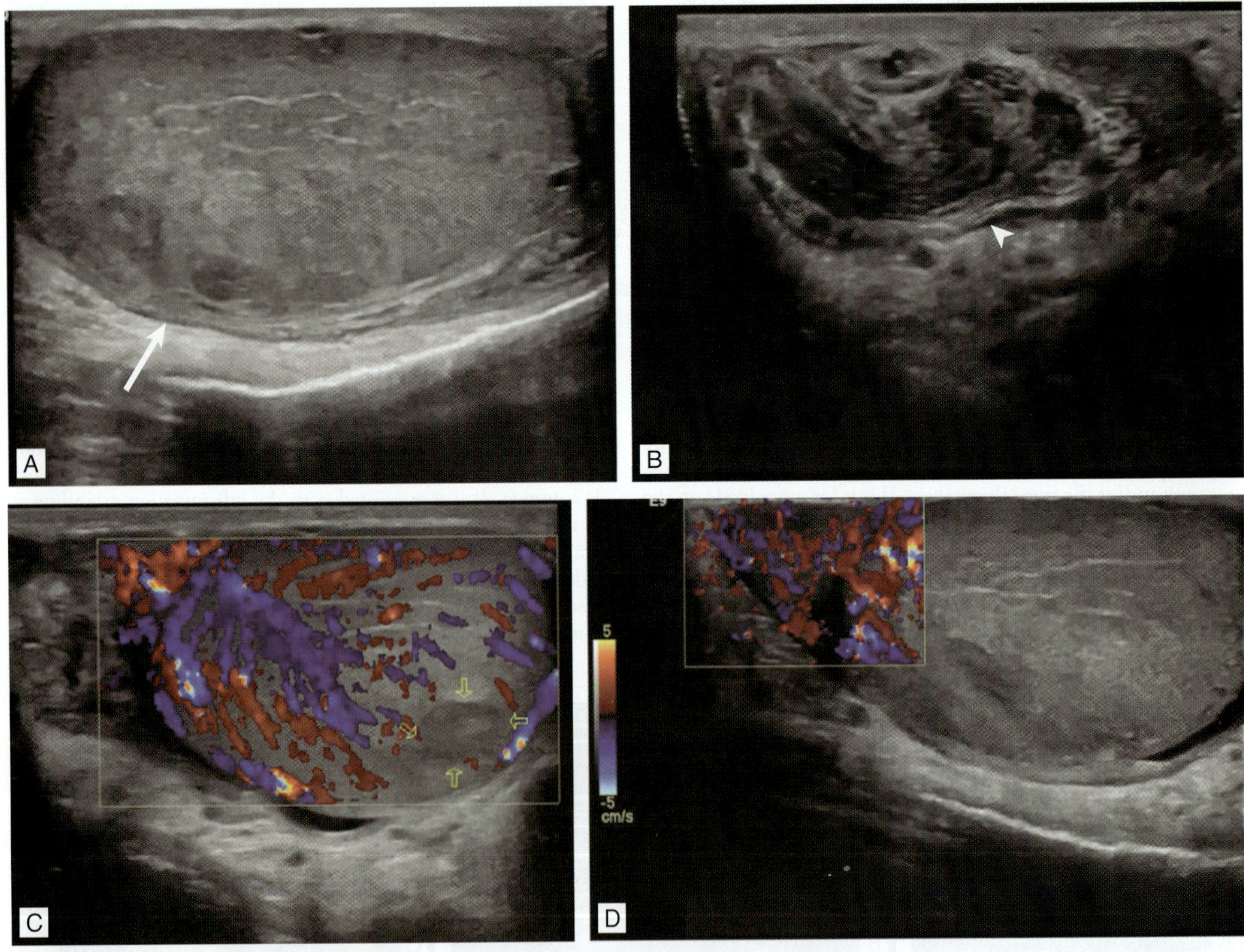

Figure 43.23 Ultrasound images of right testicle (*white arrow*, image A) and right epididymis (*white arrowhead*, image B) are enlarged and hyperemic (C and D). Additionally, there is a well defined hypoechoic focus (*yellow arrows*) within the inferior right testicle that does not demonstrate internal flow (*yellow arrows*). These findings are concerning for epididymitis–orchitis with testicular abscess. Follow-up ultrasounds confirmed progressive evolution of this lesion into abscess.

echogenicity. They are however usually accompanied by marked changes of epididymitis. Doppler ultrasound may show increased vascularity but severe orchitis may be associated with ischemia and infarction with reduced or absent vascularity. In severe orchitis, heterogeneous areas may develop with a potential for intratesticular abscess formation (irregular areas of liquefaction containing debris). There is again a substantial risk of subsequent atrophy leading to a small echo-poor testicle with little or no spermatogenesis. The underlying organisms are usually the same as for epididymitis, although rarely chronic epididymitis, especially with abscess formation, may be due to tuberculosis. Calcific scars may be seen following any form of orchitis. Granulomatous epididymo-orchitis is a condition occurring postpuberty and consists of a granulomatous reaction to sperm or some microorganisms resulting in chronic inflammation [20].

Extratesticular Tumors

These are rare and usually benign. The most common extratesticular tumor is adenomatoid tumor of the epididymis, which is a benign hamartoma most frequently seen in the tail. It varies in size from about 5 to 50 mm and is of similar or slightly increased echogenicity compared with normal testicle.

Others include benign neoplasms, such as mesenchymal tumors (leiomyoma, fibroma, lipoma), adrenal rests, and benign mesothelioma. This latter condition arises from the tunica vaginalis. It produces small paratesticular hyperechoic masses and a disproportionately large hydrocele.

Extratesticular malignancies are extremely rare. Although carcinoma and metastases have been described, sarcoma of the spermatic cord is relatively more common, usually embryonal rhabdomyosarcoma (in younger patients), but sarcomas of other mesenchymal tissues such as liposarcomas are seen occasionally as well.

Cystic Lesions of Scrotum

Epididymal Cysts and Spermatocele

Epididymal cysts are the most common cystic lesions found in scrotum and can be found in around 20–40% of asymptomatic patients undergoing USG study [22]. These are benign lesions which can grow slowly over time to reach larger size and may need medical or surgical attention (sclerotherapy/surgical excision). On USG, these cysts are generally located at the head of epididymis. They can be completely anechoic when small (2–4 mm in diameter) or can have internal septa/material when large [13].

Spermatoceles are a type of epididymal cysts which form from the obstruction and subsequent dilatation of efferent ductal system of epididymis and contain spermatozoa, cellular debris, and lymphocytes. Larger cysts (both epididymal cysts and spermatoceles) may have septations and can look similar to hydrocele. The key differentiation between the two is that cysts displace testes whereas a hydrocele envelops them [23].

Testicular Disorders

Undescended Testicle (Cryptorchidism)

In the majority of prepubertal males, the testes may normally be retractile into the groin because of the cremasteric muscle reflex. If, however, the testicle can never be located within the scrotum, it should be considered undescended. An undescended testicle most commonly lies in the inguinal canal (canalicular). Otherwise, it may lie higher up along the normal line of descent (abdominal testicle) or in a site away from the normal line of descent (ectopic). Most abdominal testicles lie just proximal to the inguinal ring, although they may lie further cranially within the pelvis or retroperitoneum. Ectopic testicles are uncommon and are most often found in the superficial inguinal pouch, occasionally coming to lie in the femoral canal, suprapubic fat pad, the perineum, and the opposite scrotum.

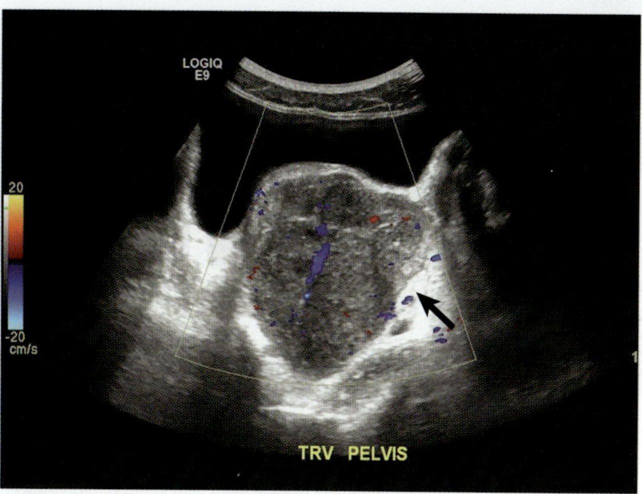

Figure 43.24 Color Doppler image in a patient with undescended testes showing a well-defined heterogenous lesion with vascularity within, suspected to be seminoma, subsequently proven on histology.

Cryptorchidism occurs in 1–3% of full-term and up to 30% of premature male infants and is the most common genitourinary anomaly in male infants [7].

Undescended testes have increased risk of testicular cancer (up to 40 times normal, particularly seminoma) and infertility (Fig. 43.24). To reduce these risks, orchiopexy is recommended at 12 months of age. Other associations of undescended testes include abnormalities of Wolffian duct-derived structures, for example, seminal vesicle cysts and agenesis.

Imaging does not have a role in routine evaluation, but is an important tool in certain clinical scenarios such as in children with ambiguous genitalia or hypospadias and cryptorchidism to locate Mullerian structures [7]. Ultrasound is generally the first investigation performed to locate an undescended testicle, being quick and able to locate the testicle at its commonest sites (within the inguinal canal or just proximal to it) (Fig. 43.25). The testicle may look relatively normal, although the longer it has remained undescended the more likely it is to be small, atrophic, and echo-poor. If the testicle cannot be identified on ultrasound, a more extensive search may be performed with an MRI (Fig. 43.26). The testicle shows a conspicuous high signal on T2-weighted and STIR sequences with distinct hyperintense signal on diffusion-weighted images. Testicular phlebography or arteriography has been employed in the search for undescended testes in the past. If both ultrasound and MRI are negative it is unlikely that these angiographic procedures will detect the missing organ, as it is probably absent or extremely atrophic. This is particularly the case if the patient is above 30 years of age.

Torsion

Pathophysiology and Clinical Presentation

Testicular torsion refers to twisting of the spermatic cord with testicular rotation leading to first venous and later arterial obstruction, producing testicular ischemia. It may occur at any age but is most frequent in the first year of life or in adolescence, when the

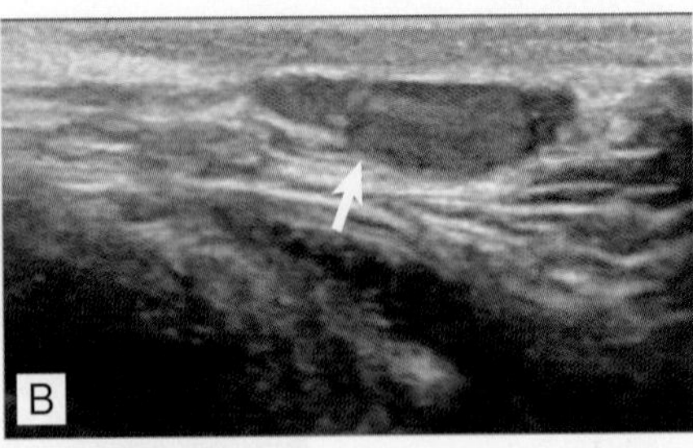

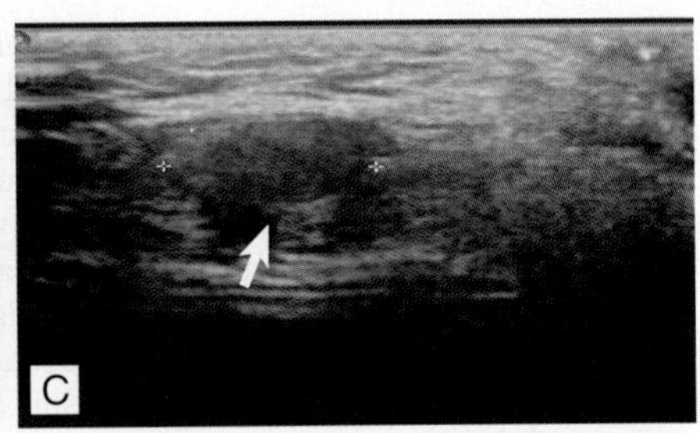

Figure 43.25 USG showing empty scrotum (image A). Both testes (B and C) (*arrows*) are in the inguinal canals, suggestive of bilateral cryptorchidism.

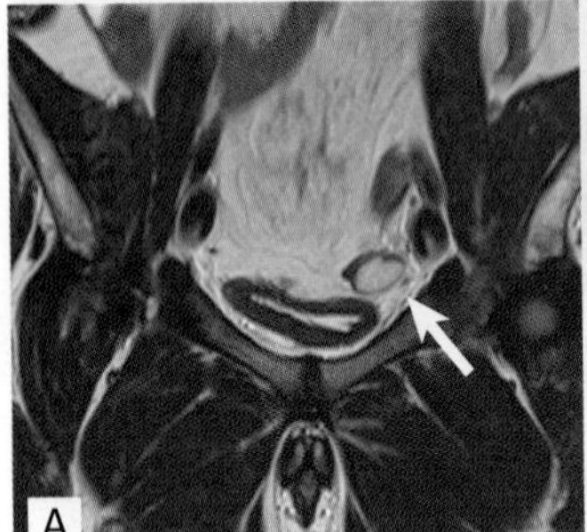

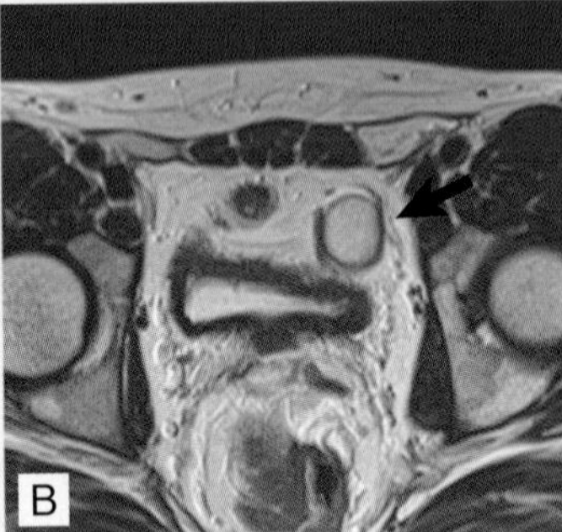

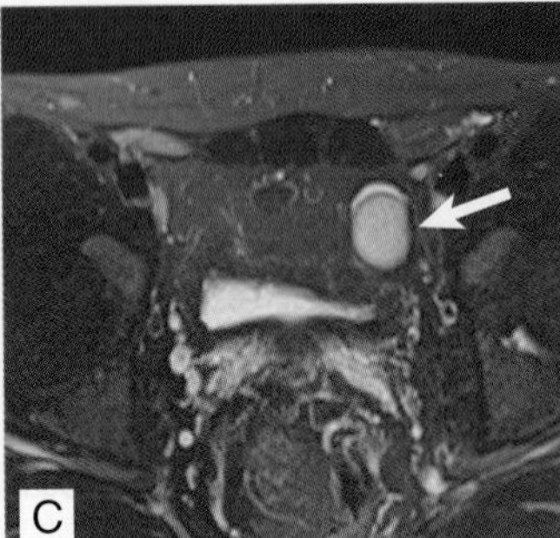

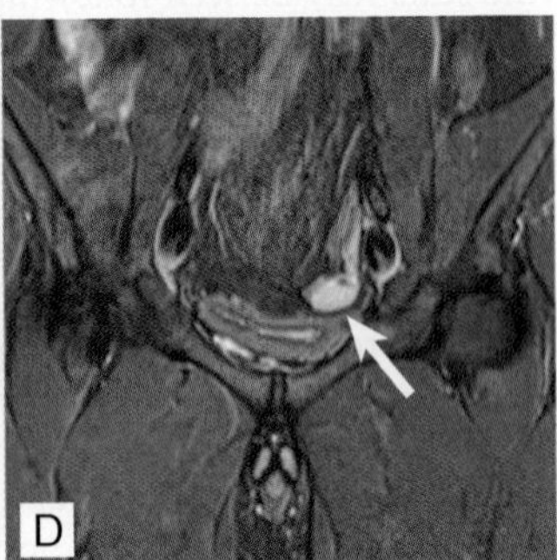

Figure 43.26 MRI in a case of absent left testes in scrotum: T2-weighted (A and B), T2 FS (C), and postcontrast T1-weighted images (D) images show a well-defined hyperintense structure in left side of pelvis (*arrows*) suggestive of undescended testes.

testicle is rapidly enlarging. Different patterns of torsion have been described. The loose attachment of the testicle and spermatic cord to the scrotum in infants and neonates predisposes to torsion of the entire cord above the level of the scrotum (extravaginal torsion). Rotation of the cord within the tunica vaginalis (intravaginal torsion) is the commonest situation in the older age group. This is most often due to high attachment of tunica vaginalis to the spermatic cord which leaves the testis free to rotate. This anatomical situation has been referred to as the bell-and-clapper malformation and it may be bilateral in up to 80% of cases, with simultaneous bilateral torsion in up to 5%. Surgical treatment of testicular torsion should therefore include detorsion of the affected testicle and fixation of the contralateral testicle to prevent subsequent torsion.

Torsion may be complete (i.e., rotation of at least 360°) or incomplete, and spontaneous torsion–detorsion may occur. The degree and duration of torsion determines the severity of the ischemia and the rapidity with which irreversible changes occur within the testicle. Testicular salvage is more likely if patients are treated within 4–6 hours of onset of torsion [20].

Differentiation between torsion and acute epididymo-orchitis is clinically challenging since both entities present with similar symptoms of pain, swelling, and scrotal redness, making imaging extremely important.

Imaging Features

- In the early acute stage, ultrasound may be normal. With progression, a swollen testicle with patchy or diffuse hypoechogenicity is commonly seen (Fig. 43.27). The epididymis may also become swollen and echo-poor
- There may be a reactive hydrocele and the overlying scrotal skin may be thickened and edematous
- Doppler ultrasound has a sensitivity of upward of 85% in the diagnosis of torsion by virtue of reduced vascularity (absence or poor color flow, reduced peak systolic velocities) compared to the unaffected side. Raised testicular arterial resistive index is a finding seen in cases of partial torsion whereas complete absence of flow in testes and epididymis is seen in complete torsion [24]
- False positives (e.g., ischemia associated with severe epididymo-orchitis) and false negatives (due to difficulty in obtaining an adequate color flow, intermittent nature of torsion, etc.) can be encountered and should be kept in mind

Given the importance of operating within a few hours of the onset of symptoms, it remains axiomatic that neither the performance nor interpretation of an ultrasound examination should delay surgical treatment. If there is doubt, the surgeon should operate on clinical grounds.

Appendix Torsion

The testicular appendix (often referred to as the hydatid of Morgagni) and rarely other vestigial scrotal appendices (such as the epididymal appendix) may undergo torsion. This is associated with acute scrotal pain and localized swelling and tenderness. On ultrasound, there is a focal extratesticular soft-tissue mass adjacent to the upper pole of the epididymis which often shows high or mixed echogenicity [20] and an associated hydrocele. On Doppler ultrasound, only peripheral vascularity and no internal vascularity is noted. The lesion may slough off and become calcified, giving rise to mobile highly echogenic shadowing foci between the layers of the tunica vaginalis (scrotoliths or scrotal pearls, Fig. 43.28).

Cysts Within the Testes

Testicular Cyst

As with cysts elsewhere in the body, testicular cysts are well-defined, thin-walled and anechoic on ultrasound, with distal acoustic enhancement. They vary in size from a 1–2 mm to 1–2 cm and lie within the testicular tissue (Fig. 43.29). They are occasionally multiple, are often situated at or close to the

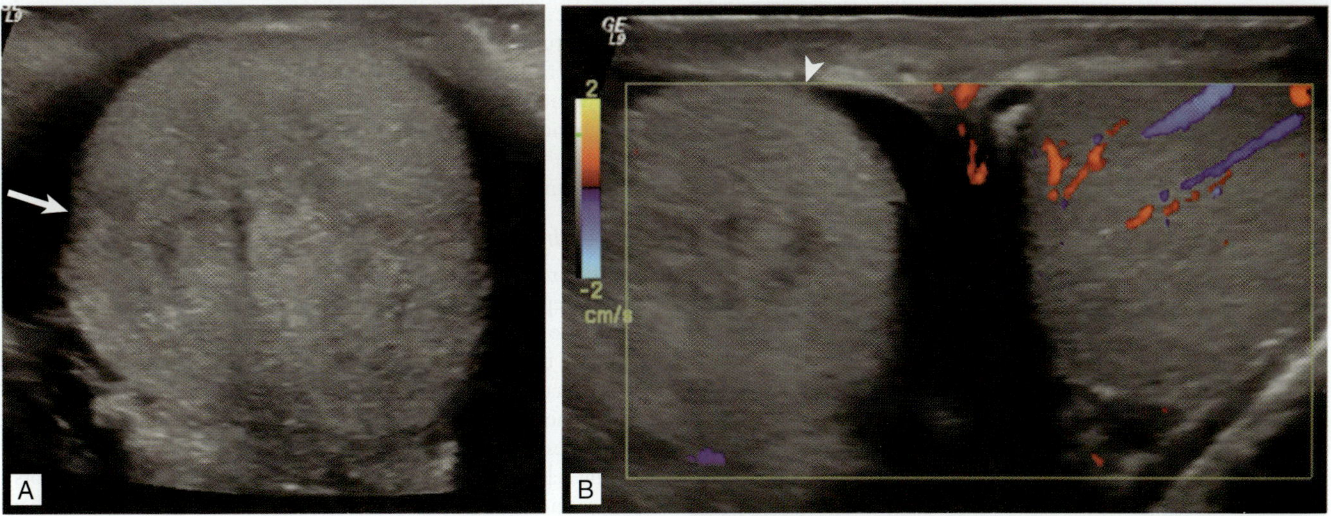

Figure 43.27 A and B: Transverse section ultrasound images of the right testicle showing its enlargement and heterogenous predominantly hyperechoic echotexture (*arrow* in A). It appears edematous and demonstrates no internal vascularity (*arrowhead* in B) suggestive of acute right testicular torsion.

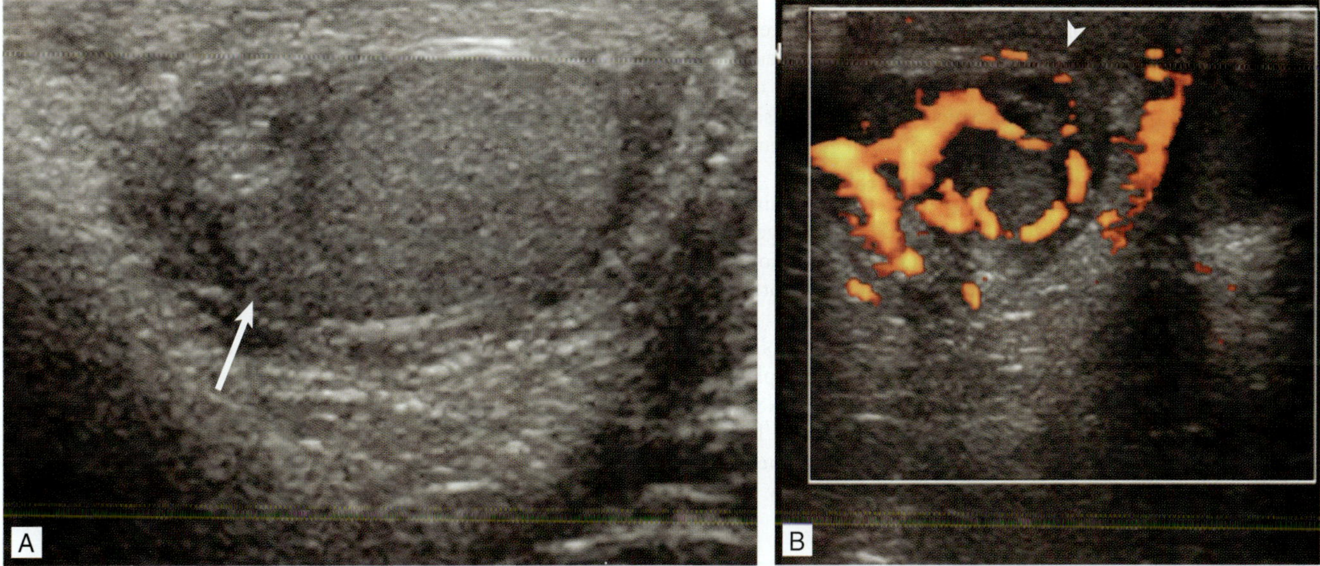

Figure 43.28 USG image shows right testes and epididymis are very hypoechoic (*arrow* in A) with thickening of the appendix testis. The appendix testis is avascular with a surrounding rim of hyperemia (B, *white arrowhead*). This finding suggests a torsion of the appendix testes. The skin around the right testis is thickened.

testicular hilum and may be associated with epididymal cysts. Cysts directly arising from the tunica albuginea have been described with similar ultrasound features and benign nature.

Multiple small cystic areas are not infrequently seen at the testicular hilum. These are often referred to as dilatation of the rete testes and again are often seen with epididymal cysts. All these lesions are entirely benign.

Epidermoid Cyst

These uncommon benign tumors are thought to derive from epithelial rests or inclusions. They consist of layers of keratin within a fibrous capsule lined with squamous epithelium. On ultrasound, these are seen as well-defined avascular rounded well-marginated lesions and may be solitary, multiple, or bilateral. Calcification may be present and adopt a variety of patterns (multiple foci within the cyst, curvilinear along the wall or a target pattern of concentric circles). Otherwise, they are usually diffusely echo-poor. Occasionally, they may appear highly echogenic, presumably if calcification becomes widespread throughout the lesion (Fig. 43.30). If the typical ultrasound features are present, the urologist may be able to perform partial rather than total orchidectomy.

Testicular Malignancies and Related Conditions

Testicular Cancer

Epidemiology and Pathophysiology

Although uncommon (representing approximately 1% of cancers in males), testicular cancer is the commonest malignancy in males between 20 and 40 years of age, with the incidence apparently rising.

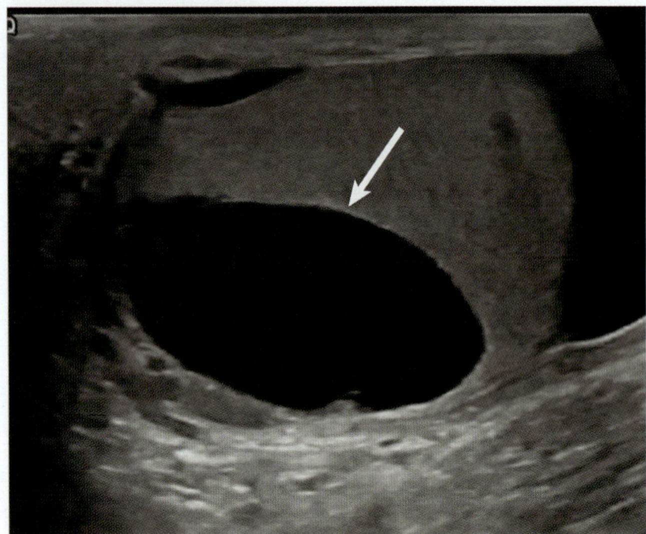

Figure 43.29 USG showing a well-defined anechoic structure (*arrow*) within the testicle suggestive of testicular cyst.

Approximately 95% of testicular neoplasms are of germ cell origin, 4% lymphomas, and 1% are rarities such as metastases, Leydig cell, and Sertoli cell tumors. Approximately 50% of germ cell tumors are pure seminomas, which are less aggressive and present in an older age group (peak 30–45 years). The remaining 50% are classified as nonseminomatous germ cell tumors (NSGCTs), although up to a fifth of these may contain some seminomatous element. They present in the younger age group (peak 15–30 years) and a majority produce one or more biochemical tumor markers (beta-human chorionic gonadotrophin, alpha-fetoprotein, or lactate dehydrogenase).

Subdivision of germ cell tumors into seminoma and NSGCTs is very important since it plays a major role in treatment planning [25]. There are two main histological classifications of NSGCTs, the World Health Organization and the British Testicular Tumour Panel systems, the former being more widely used in the North American literature. The two classifications are broadly similar with the overall categorization into germ cell tumor, sex-cord stromal tumor, and miscellaneous tumors.

Risk factors for the development of testicular malignancy include undescended testes, testicular atrophy, previous testicular malignancy, infantile hernia, low birth weight, and maternal exposure to diethylstilboestrol. There is a weak genetic tendency, with a family history of the disease seen in 2% of patients.

Presenting Symptoms

Testicular cancer most commonly presents as a painless scrotal mass inseparable from the testicle, although the patient may sometimes also complain of a dull ache or sensation of heaviness. Occasionally, the condition presents with widespread pulmonary or abdominal metastases, rarely when the primary is no longer evident. The rare Leydig and Sertoli cell tumors may produce sex hormones, which can provoke premature virilization (especially Leydig cell tumors) or gynecomastia (especially Sertoli cell tumors).

Around 20% of patients have metastatic disease at initial diagnosis and present with complaints of abdominal or backpain, lethargy, and malaise, with bulky retroperitoneal lymphadenopathy detected on imaging. The complete evaluation in such patients (especially in the younger age group) should include a testicular ultrasound along with physical examination [25].

Sometimes a male patient presents with widespread metastases (which may include abdominal, pelvic and mediastinal lymphadenopathy, and pulmonary metastases) that are confirmed histologically to originate from a malignant teratoma, but without a palpable testicular tumor. In some of these patients, the teratoma may have originated outside the testicle. In a proportion, however, a small primary lesion, with the classical echo-poor ultrasound appearances described above, is identified in a testicle on ultrasound. Rarely ultrasound demonstrates a small echogenic area within a testicle (Fig. 43.31), which is believed to represent the scar of a burnt-out primary, a situation that has been described with both seminoma and NSGCT.

Diagnosis

- Scrotal ultrasound is the investigation of choice, with a sensitivity approaching 100% when combined with physical examination [25]

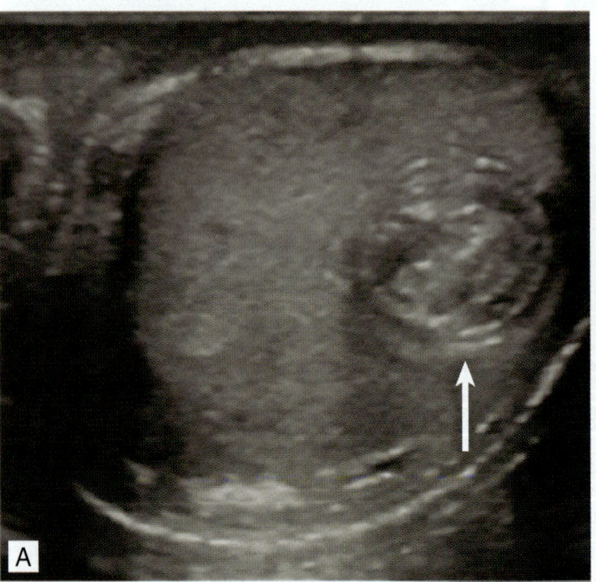

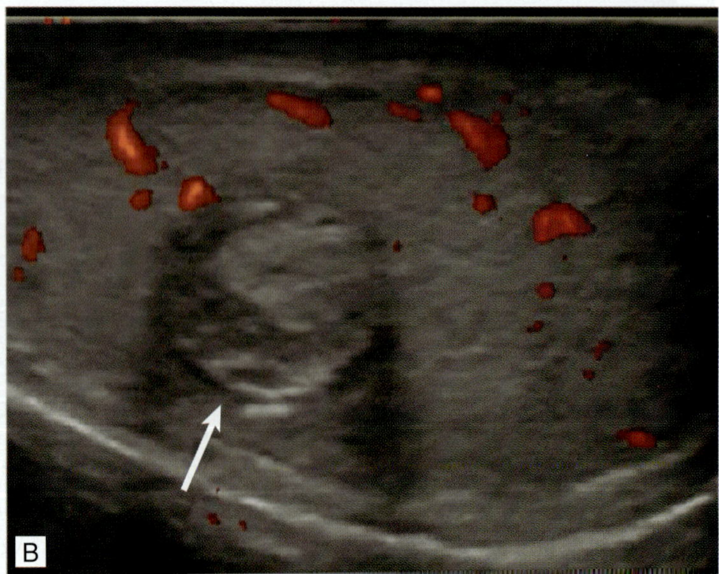

Figure 43.30 (A) USG showing a well-circumscribed, round, heterogeneous lesion within the mid pole of the left testicle laterally (*arrows*). The mass contains multiple rings resulting in a laminated, "onionskin" appearance with no flow on doppler (B). Appearances are characteristic for epidermoid cyst.

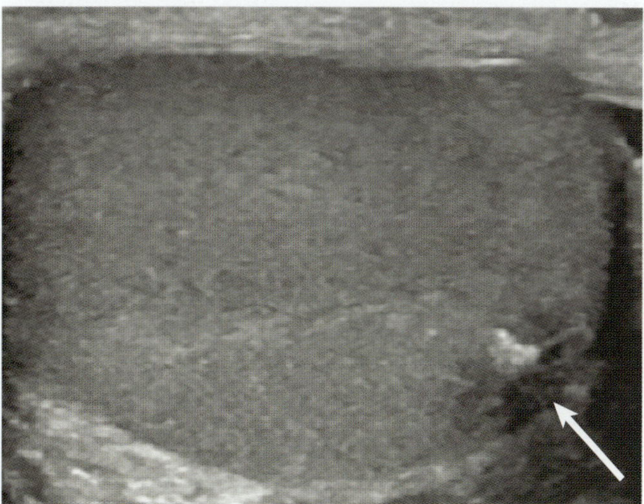

Figure 43.31 Left testicular hypoechoic lesion (*arrow*) containing coarse calcification, in setting of marked retroperitoneal lymphadenopathy favoring a burnt-out testicular neoplasm.

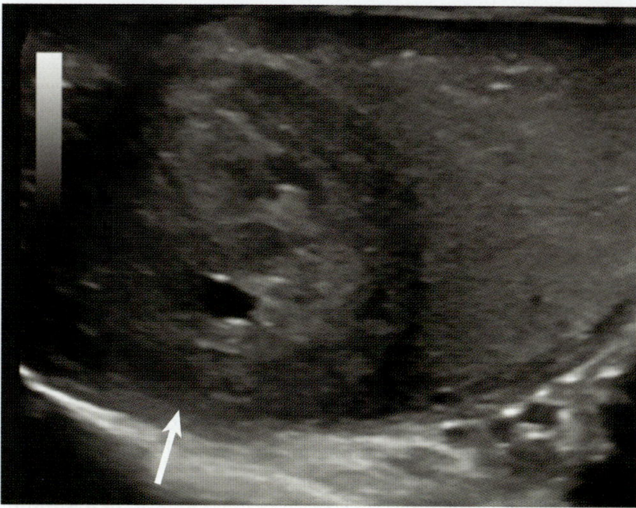

Figure 43.33 USG showing a focal well-defined lesion (*arrow*) with heterogeneity within. Histopathology was suggestive of malignant mixed germ cell tumor.

- Tumors are seen as intratesticular lesions predominantly of low echogenicity, but could be heterogeneous with calcification or cystic changes [25]. Small tumors may show no mass effect, while those larger than 2–3 cm are associated with deformity and expansion of the outline of the testicle. There is an occasional associated hydrocele
- The histology cannot be predicted from the ultrasound appearances, which are usually nonspecific. However, classically, seminomas are well-defined and uniformly modestly echo-poor (Fig. 43.32). NSGCTs on the other hand more often show significant echogenic areas of fibrosis or calcification and echo-free cystic areas (Fig. 43.33)
- Larger tumors (above approximately 1.5 cm) may show increased vascularity on color flow Doppler, while smaller ones are more often hypovascular [26]
- The differential diagnosis includes focal or diffuse acute orchitis, abscess, infarct, and hematoma. The clinical presentation and course usually permits differentiation. It is, however, important to exercise extreme caution, and an echo-poor lesion within the testicle must always be regarded as potentially representing a malignancy. Therefore, if an intratesticular lesion is not showing progressive resolution within a short time (a fortnight or less), consideration of orchidectomy would be recommended and the dilemma should be discussed with the patient

Lymphatic Spread: The management of testicular cancer depends heavily on the detection and treatment of lymph node metastases. The lymphatic vessels from the testes follow the spermatic cord through the inguinal canal, cross the pelvis, and ascend to drain into lymph nodes along the inferior vena cava and aorta in the lumbar region around the L2 level. These retroperitoneal nodes are the most common site for metastatic disease.

Lymph node involvement virtually always starts on the side of the affected testicle. The sentinel nodes for the right-sided tumors are interaortocaval nodes followed by precaval and preaortic nodes, and for left-sided tumors are para-aortic and preaortic lymph nodes followed by the interaortocaval nodes. Bilateral nodal involvement is uncommon when the primary is left-sided but is more often encountered when the disease starts in the right testicle.

Following initial lymphadenopathy, disease may spread cranially and caudally. Iliac and inguinal lymph nodes may be involved by retrograde spread, especially on the right, or directly in circumstances where the tumor gains access to the ilioinguinal lymphatic system via scrotal involvement. Tumor may also extend retrogradely into the mesenteric lymph nodes and antegradely into the retrocrural, mediastinal, and supraclavicular lymph nodes. The nodal spread is almost always sequential, and skip metastatic adenopathy is rare. Drainage into the thoracic duct may occur, with subsequent hematogenous metastases to the lungs and, less

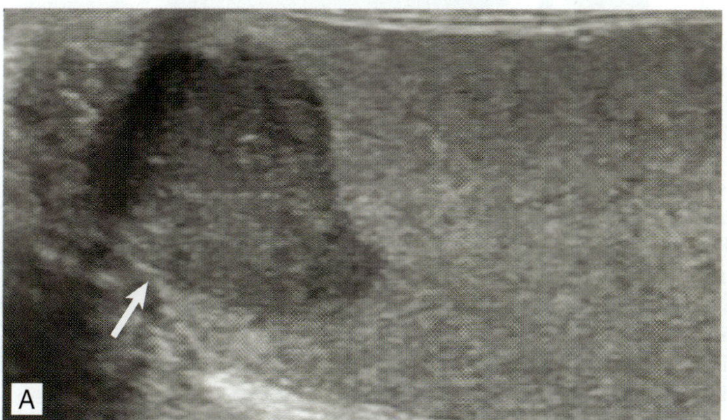

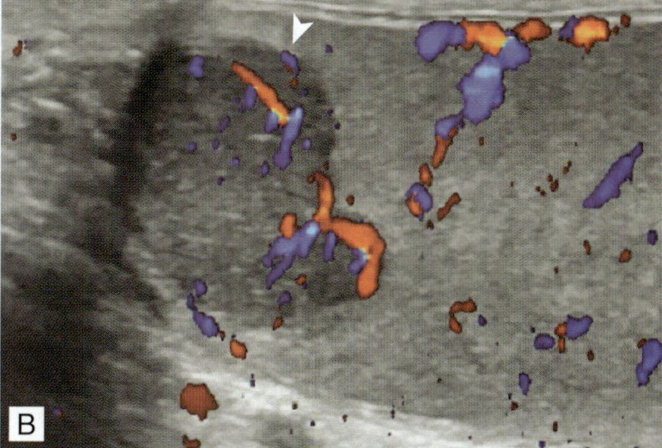

Figure 43.32 A well-defined hypoechoic lesion (*white arrow*) in right testicle on USG showing vascularity on doppler (*white arrowhead*).

often, the liver, brain, and skeleton. Hematogenous spread is rare before lymphatic spread, except with choriocarcinoma. It is generally more common with nonseminomatous tumors.

A thorough understanding of lymphatic drainage is extremely helpful for planning retroperitoneal nodal dissection [25]. Tumor, node, metastasis, serum marker is the commonly used staging system for testicular cancer [26]. It is a comprehensive system that depends upon surgical pathology of the orchiectomy specimen, tumor markers before and after orchiectomy (AFP, HCG, and LDH), chest radiography or chest CT, and CT of the abdomen and pelvis.

The American College of Radiology has outlined recommendations for appropriate radiological procedures to be used for staging testicular tumors [27]. According to these American College of Radiology appropriateness criteria:

- In most cases, diagnosis of testicular tumor can be established with careful physical examination and scrotal ultrasound
- Tumor markers help in determining presence of residual disease
- Cross-sectional studies (CT and MRI) are helpful in determining location of metastases. CT is the most common study for assessment of the retroperitoneum to detect metastatic testicular malignancy. Evidence suggests that MRI is comparable to CT for staging purposes [28]
- ESMO guidelines recommend contrast-enhanced CT in all patients for staging before orchiectomy. PET-CT and MRI are not routinely recommended in all patients for staging [29]. MRI may be helpful for characterization of equivocal CT findings (in liver, bone, and brain) or when CT is contraindicated due to allergy to contrast media. Brain MRI is the modality of choice in patients presenting with CNS symptoms or suspected bone marrow involvement
- Due to inability of FDG-PET to reliably detect disease activity in subcentimeter nodes, it shows no advantage over CT as an imaging modality in clinical stage I disease [30]. It may have a role when CT shows equivocal findings due to its slightly higher sensitivity; alternatively targeted CT can be performed at an interval of 6–8 weeks to reassess the borderline nodes using lower dose of radiation. It is important to be aware of the limitations of FDG-PET as inflammatory lesions can also show FDG avidity on PET [29]

Staging

Broadly, the testicular tumors are classified as stage I if limited to testes, retroperitoneal nodal spread constitutes stage II and distant spread is categorized as stage III.

CT is the reference standard for staging. CT detection of lymph node metastases depends on size since CT cannot differentiate between benign and malignant nodes based on morphology alone. Nodes are considered to be malignant if more than 8–10 mm in short axis diameter, with nodes above 8 mm considered suspicious in high-risk cases such as tumors with a higher proportion of embryonal subtype on pathology, T category >II, or presence of lymphovascular invasion [25].

Metastatic nodal masses may become enormous; in the case of seminomas they usually remain relatively homogeneous on CT, although they do occasionally demonstrate central necrosis. NSGCT deposits, however, often become heterogeneous as they enlarge, with lower density and even cystic elements (Fig. 43.34). These cystic elements often represent teratomatous components and may remain cystic post-treatment and after normalization of tumor markers as these are chemo resistant (note that this residual teratomatous element post-treatment may contain only benign elements). Sometimes these lesions may increase in size during ongoing or after completed chemotherapy with decreasing tumor markers, an entity referred as "Growing Teratoma Syndrome" [31].

Management

Treatment of all testicular cancers initially involves radical inguinal orchiectomy (removal of testicle and spermatic cord). Further management depends on the clinical stage and histology of the tumor, that is, whether the tumor is seminomatous or NSGCT [26].

Further treatment options for seminoma stage I involve three options: surveillance, radiotherapy, or adjuvant chemotherapy. Seminomas are highly radiosensitive. Patients who opt to undergo radiotherapy to the retroperitoneum need less intensive follow-up with CT imaging. For most patients with clinical stage I and pure seminoma, surveillance is the preferred option, because seminomas have a good overall prognosis [32]. Patients with higher clinical stage are offered either radiotherapy to retroperitoneum or chemotherapy. Induction chemotherapy is offered to patients with more extensive metastatic disease.

Patients with stage I NSGCTs are offered three management options: surveillance, adjuvant chemotherapy, and RPLND (retroperitoneal lymph node dissection). Surveillance is the preferred strategy for clinical stage IA (pT1). The rationale behind primary RPLND in clinical stage I is that it offers correct staging, cure of micrometastatic disease, less follow-up requirement and has a significant reduction in the overall lifetime risk of needing chemotherapy [32].

Patients with limited retroperitoneal disease without any metastasis outside are generally offered RPLND or chemotherapy. Those with distant metastatic disease or extensive retroperitoneal disease are offered induction chemotherapy. One important chemotherapy side effect to watch out for on restaging CTs of patients on chemotherapy is bleomycin-induced pneumonitis (Fig. 43.35), which is a potentially fatal side effect in patients treated with bleomycin, etoposide, cisplatin therapy.

Role of Imaging in Surveillance: Surveillance is being increasingly used in stage I seminoma and NSGCT as majority of these patients are cured with radical orchiectomy and do not have disease elsewhere [25]. Most surveillance protocols include serial clinical examinations, serum tumor markers, CXR, and abdominopelvic CT. Follow-up scans are performed relatively frequently (every 3–6 months) for the first 2 years depending on the pathol-

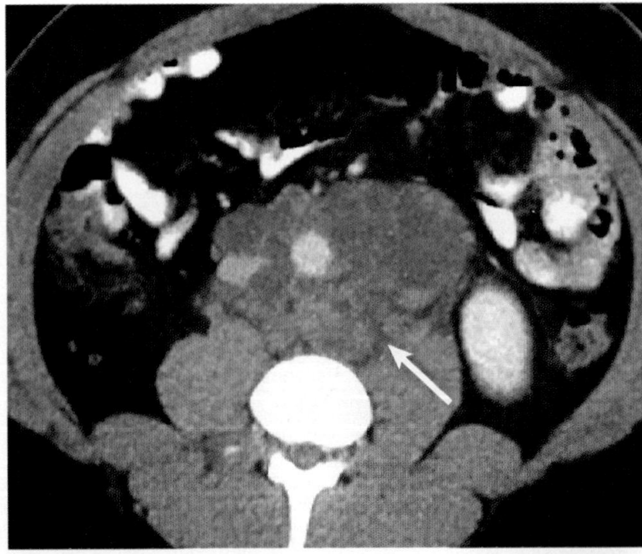

Figure 43.34 Contrast enhanced CT of abdomen showing bulky heterogeneous retroperitoneal lymphadenopathy (*arrow*). Histopathology suggested metastases from malignant nonseminomatous germ cell tumor of testis.

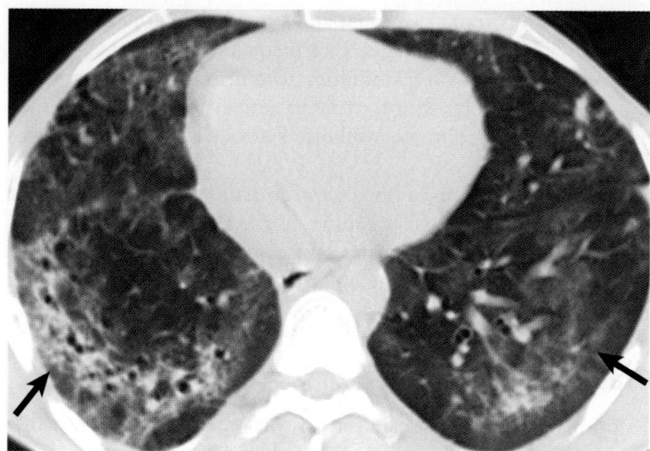

Figure 43.35 Patient with Hodgkin's lymphoma treated with chemotherapy, including Bleomycin. The lungs were clear on the baseline CT scan (not shown). Patient complained of breathlessness while on treatment. CT scan demonstrates bilateral consolidative and ground glass opacities with mild interstitial thickening (*arrows*), consistent with Bleomycin-induced pneumonitis. (Picture Courtesy: Akshay Baheti, Tata Memorial Hospital, Mumbai.)

ogy (seminoma vs. nonseminoma) and stage of the disease, with yearly scanning continued for at least 5 years [33,25,26].

Testicular Metastasis

Metastases to the testicle are rare. The ultrasound appearance is of mixed, often predominantly reduced, echogenicity; they are indistinguishable from primary malignancies except that they generally affect a significantly older age group. The tumors that most commonly metastasize to the testicle are cancers of the prostate, lung, kidney, colon, and melanoma [26]. Other testicular malignancies include lymphoma and leukemia (in childhood, the testicle being a classical sanctuary site for relapse).

Testicular Lymphoma

This condition is rare, accounting for less than 5% of malignancies of the testicle, although it is the commonest testicular tumor in men over the age of 60. It is bilateral in up to 25% and is associated with extranodal disease, especially in the pharynx, skin, and central nervous system. It is virtually always a non-Hodgkin's disease and carries poor prognosis [26]. The ultrasound appearance is of a well-defined mass of low echogenicity (Fig. 43.36). It often extends to involve the epididymis and spermatic cord. The dominant feature of the mass is its homogeneity. Multiple nodules or foci of hemorrhage or necrosis are uncommon.

Testicular Calcification

Coarse areas of calcification (above 3 mm diameter) that are relatively few in number are seen within some malignant testicular tumors, particularly NSGCTs. A solitary substantial focus may be associated with the so-called burnt-out primary tumor (Azzopardi tumor) (Fig. 43.31). Infection, trauma, or infarct may also produce dystrophic calcific areas. They are usually solitary or few in number and vary from 1 to 2 mm in diameter to several millimeters.

Testicular Microlithiasis

Testicular microlithiasis is a condition characterized by calcium deposits in the seminiferous tubules or within the tubular basement membrane components [34]. A definitive explanation of cause of this entity is still unknown.

Ultrasound is the modality of choice for detection.

- Testicular microlithiasis is seen as small (1–3 mm), often uniformly sized nonshadowing hyperechoic foci seen throughout the testicles [35]. It is usually bilateral but may be asymmetric
- Classical testicular microlithiasis has been defined as five or more microliths visible on at least one ultrasound image (Fig. 43.37). More than one but less than five has been referred to as limited testicular microlithiasis
- The frequency of tumor occurrence with microlithiasis and the risk of tumor development remain uncertain. Currently, there is no definite evidence that testicular microlithiasis causes testicular cancer. As per European Society of Urogenital Radiology guideline, follow-up ultrasound is recommended in the patients of testicular microlithiasis if risk factors such as history

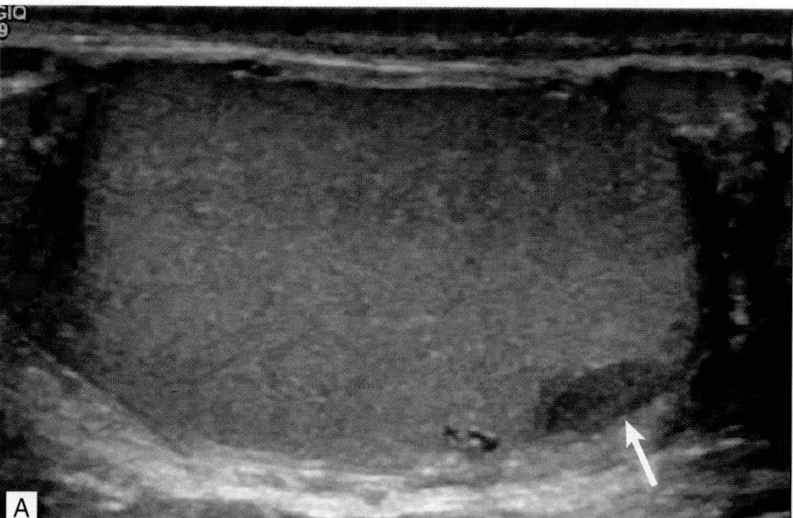

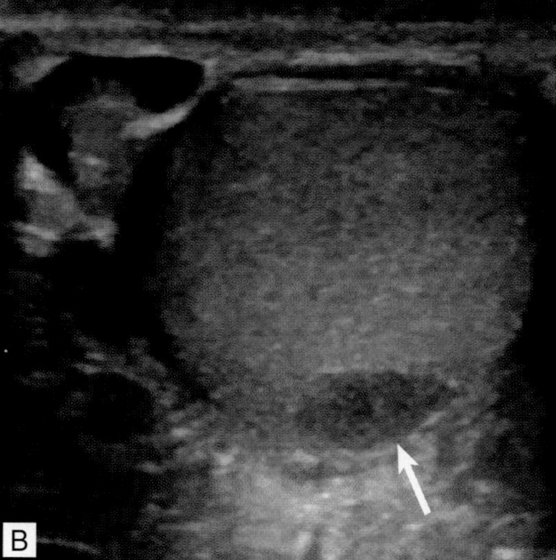

Figure 43.36 USG of scrotum of a 66-year-old patient with suspected central nervous system diffuse large B cell lymphoma. Long axis (A) and short axis (B) images of right testicle show a focal hypoechoic well-defined lesion at the periphery (*white arrows*), which on pathology was proven to be lymphoma.

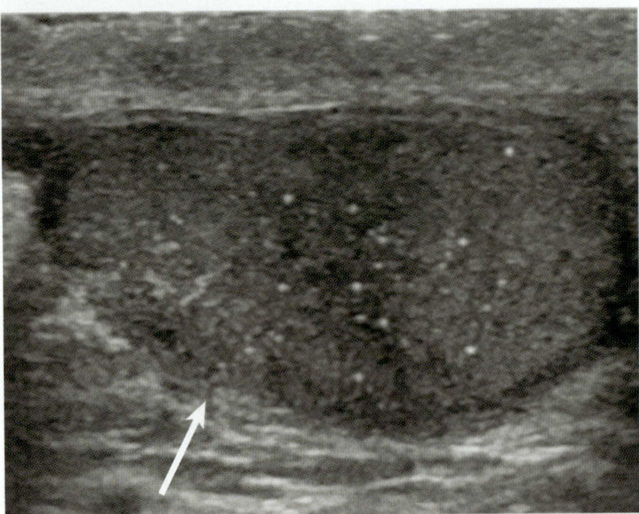

Figure 43.37 USG showing tiny hyperechoic foci (*arrow*) in the testicle representing microlithiasis.

of germ cell tumor, testicular atrophy, infertility, cryptorchidism/orchiopexy are present [34]

- In the absence of these risk factors, the probability of occurrence of testicular cancer in patients of microlithiasis is similar to the general population [36]

Penile Disorders

Normal Anatomy of Penis

The penis consists of paired corpora cavernosa along its dorsal aspect and a midline corpus spongiosum along the ventral aspect. Proximally, paired corpora cavernosa form crura and attach to ischial tuberosity. These are composed of venous sinusoids. Corpus spongiosum surrounds penile urethra and terminates as glans distally. Both corpora cavernosa and spongiosum appear hyperintense on T2-weighted images, intermediate on T1W images, and show enhancement on gadolinium administration. They are surrounded by a strong sheath of fascia known as tunica albuginea which appears hypointense on both T1- and T2-weighted images [37] (Fig. 43.38).

Proper positioning of both scrotum and penis is necessary for scanning. After patient lies supine on the table, a towel is placed between the upper thighs to elevate scrotum and penis dorsiflexed and taped against the anterior abdominal wall to prevent motion [37].

Trauma

Rupture of the tough fascia over the corpora cavernosa (the penile tunica albuginea) is a rare injury, referred to as fracture of the penis. It is usually due to lateral trauma during athletic or unusual sexual activity, generally presenting with a history of a sensation of a snap at the time of injury, with immediate detumescence and marked ecchymosis.

Imaging in cases of penile trauma helps to assess the presence of contusion, hematoma, and urethral injury. The investigation of choice is ultrasound, while retrograde urethrogram is helpful in assessing urethral integrity. In equivocal cases, MRI may be helpful. Penile fracture is seen as a focal discontinuation of the hypointense tunica albuginea on T1- and T2-weighted MR imaging. This manifests as focal high T2 signal across the fascial covering of the corpora, and which may be accompanied by hematoma or deformity [38] (Figs. 43.39A and B). If treated conservatively, it may lead to stricture urethra.

Peyronie's Disease

This is an idiopathic inflammatory condition characterized by focal induration and fibrosis within the tunica albuginea with resultant penile deformity and/or shortening which may be

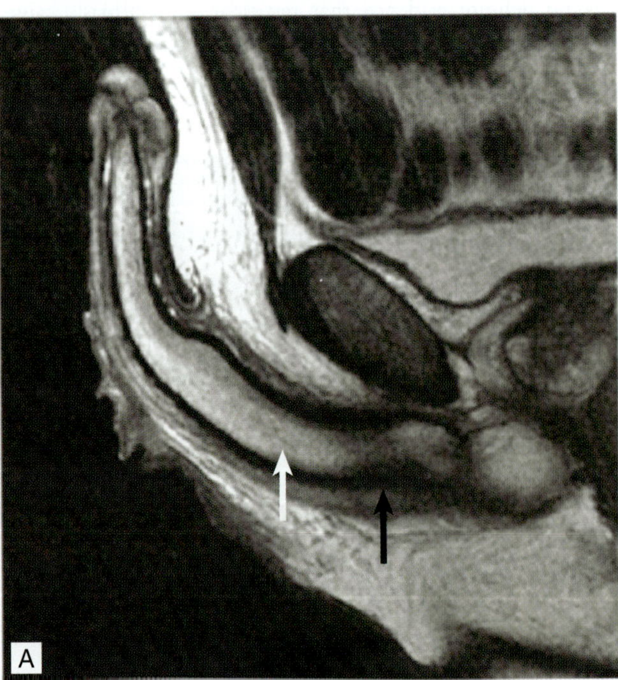

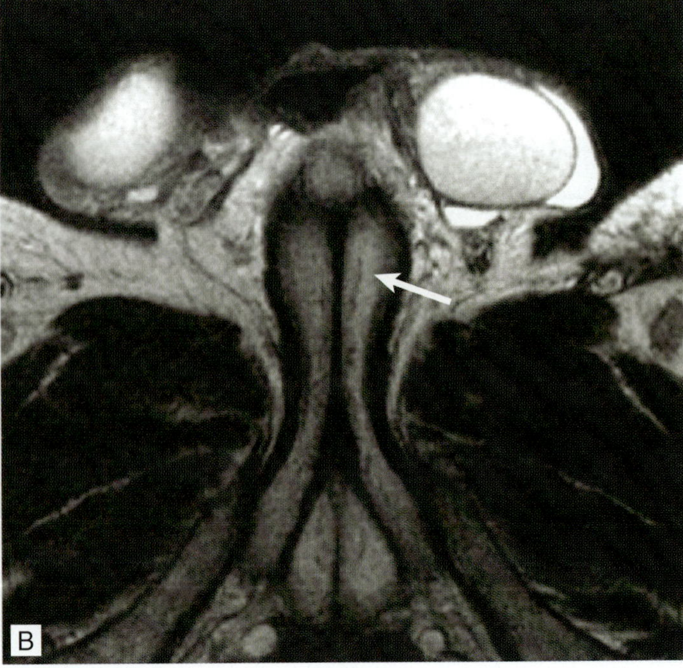

Figure 43.38 Sagittal (A) and axial (B) T2 MR images of penis showing high signal intensity corpora cavernosa (*white arrow*). *Black arrow* points toward tunica albuginea.

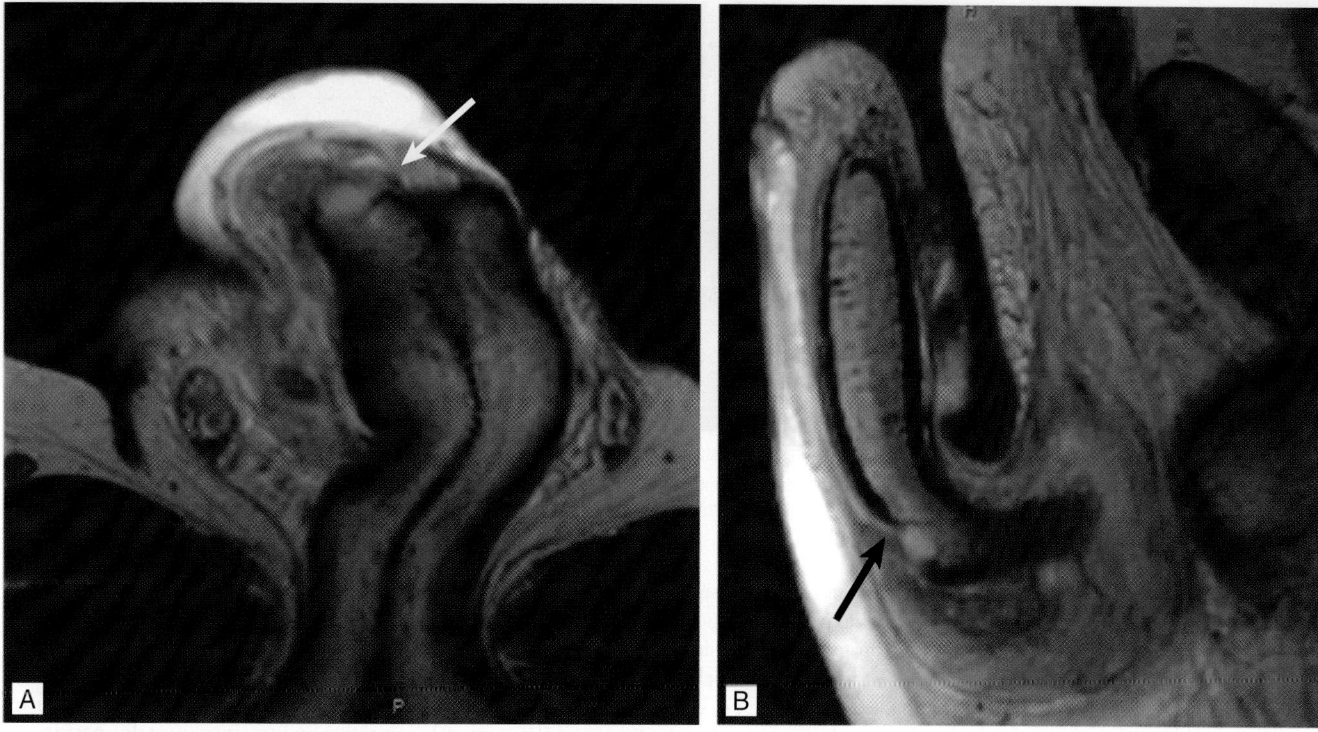

Figure 43.39 MRI T2 axial (image A) and sagittal (image B) showing a focal defect in the tunica albuginea (*arrows*) surrounding the right corpus cavernosa with an associated hematoma which appears contained by Buck's fascia.

painful. Plaques can be localized or diffuse, appear hyperechoic on ultrasound, and are commonly seen along the dorsal surface of the penis. Calcification may develop as the disease stabilizes, leading to distal acoustic shadowing (Fig. 43.40). MRI is helpful for evaluation of plaques in areas that may be difficult to evaluate clinically or with ultrasound such as base of penis [38]. On MR, plaques appear as hypointense thickening of tunica albuginea on T1- and T2-weighted images. Imaging is particularly helpful in assessment of involvement of penile septum, corpora cavernosa, and adjacent neurovascular structures and is manifested as irregular T2 hypointensity.

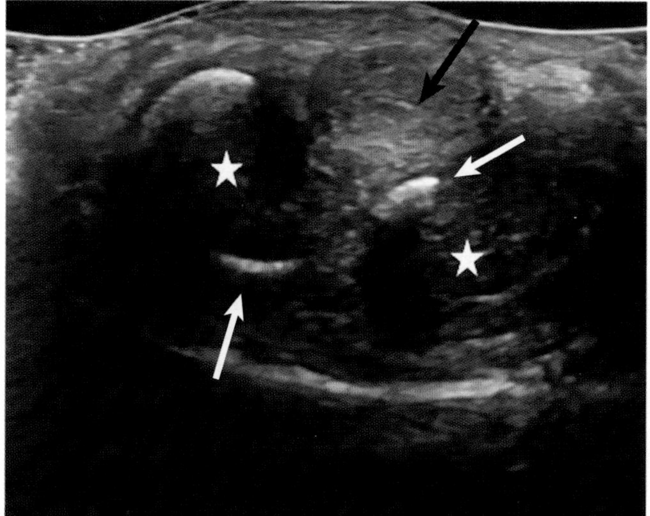

Figure 43.40 USG image showing multiple calcified plaques (*white arrows*) in penis, consistent with Peyronie's disease (paired corpora cavernosa are represented by white star whereas corpora spongiosa is represented by *black arrow*).

Carcinoma of the Penis

Pathophysiology and Clinical Presentation

Squamous cell carcinoma is the most common histology type of primary penile cancer with risks factors such as presence of foreskin, human papilloma virus infection, other sexually transmitted diseases and chronic inflammatory states like balanitis. Superficial lesions are identified clinically as visible palpable lesions. Deeper lesions arising from the urethra or base of penis are better assessed with imaging, preferably MRI.

For staging, it is important to address the status of involvement of the glans/corpora cavernosa and spongiosum, inguinal/pelvic nodes, urethra, neurovascular bundles, as well as the pubic bone, scrotum, and prostate [38]. Lymphatic spread depends on the location of primary tumor. Lymphatics from the skin and prepuce primarily drain into superficial inguinal nodes whereas that from the glans penis drains into the deep inguinal and external iliac nodes. Internal iliac nodes drain the erectile tissue and penile urethra. For N-staging it is important to identify if the nodal involvement is unilateral or bilateral and the number of nodes involved [39].

Imaging Features

- MRI is the investigation of choice for local staging [39]. It helps in local T- and N-staging and in planning the overall surgery
- Squamous cell carcinomas appear hypointense to corpora on T1- and T2-weighted imaging and show hypoenhancement on postcontrast images (Fig. 43.41). Invasion of corpus spongiosum and corpora cavernosa as identified by disruption and irregularity of tunica albuginea constitutes T2 and T3 disease, respectively. T4 disease is identified with invasion of scrotum, prostate, and pubic bone
- MRI is extremely useful for surgical planning. It helps determine factors such as penile shaft length, presence of satellite nodules, and involvement of urethra, and can predict the postsurgical

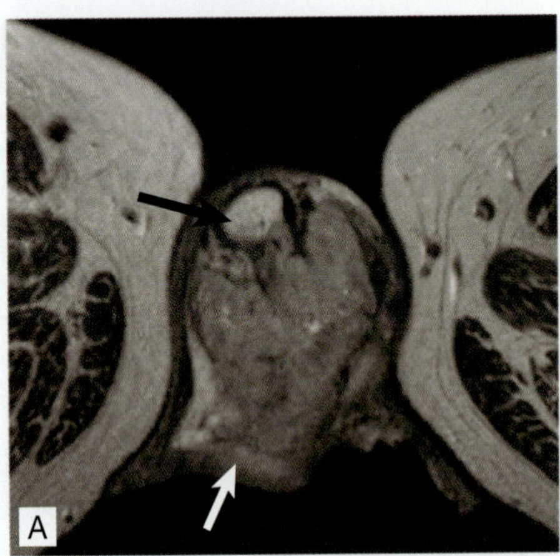

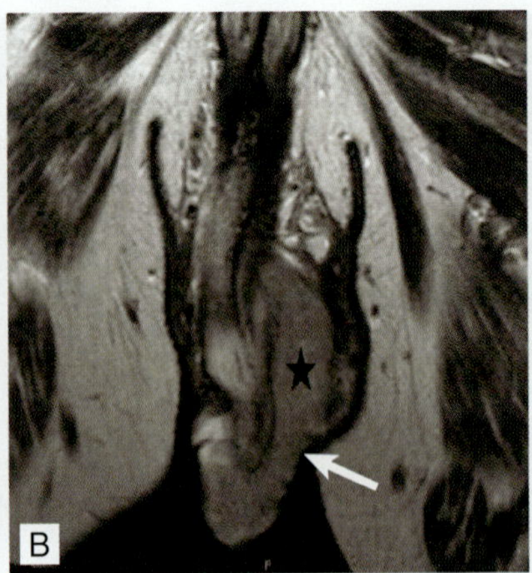

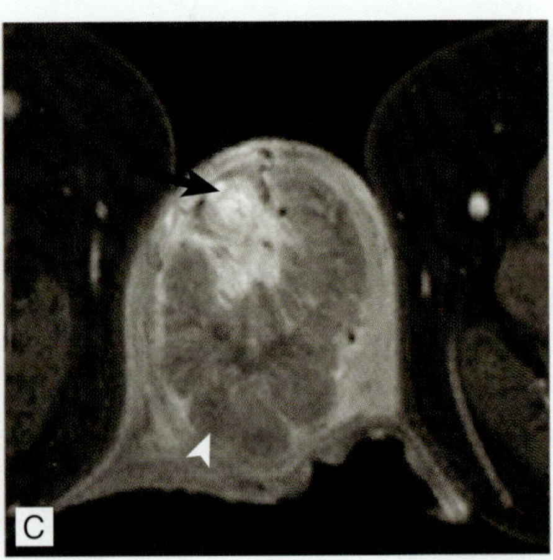

Figure 43.41 A and B (axial T2W) and C (contrast-enhanced T1W FS) MR images showing a T2 intermediate (relatively hypointense to the bright corpus) abnormal soft tissue surrounding the penile shaft (*white arrows*), which is inhomogenously hypoenhancing (*white arrowhead* in C), consistent with penile carcinoma invading both corpora cavernosa, more on the left (*black arrow*—right cavernosa, *black star*—left cavernosa), and the corpus spongiosum.

residual penile length and fat thickness over pubic symphysis, which helps in evaluation of feasibility of partial penectomy

- Nodal involvement is the most important prognostic factor in penile cancer [39]. MR helps in detection of inguinal and pelvic nodal spread and potentially extranodal extension. PET-CT scanning aids in detection of pelvic nodal involvement in difficult cases and helps in identification of distant metastases in patients diagnosed with inguinal lymphadenopathy [40,39]

Radionuclide Imaging of the Testis

Scrotal Scintigraphy

Scintigraphic demonstration of testicular perfusion is used in the setting of acute scrotal pain, it offers a noninvasive approach to distinguish primarily between the ischemia associated with testicular torsion and the hyperemia associated with acute epididymo-orchitis.

A rapid bolus injection of minimum of 185 MBq of 99mTc-pertechnetate is given intravenously, and a rapid sequence of images of the scrotal region is obtained immediately (e.g., one frame per second for 40 seconds). After the initial dynamic series, one or two further spot views with high count density should be obtained, but typically the most informative data are those derived from summating the first-pass frames to a single image.

The scan is interpreted on the basis of assessment of blood flow to the scrotum and its contents [41]. With torsion, the testis appears avascular or severely ischemic. This is manifested on the images as a photon-deficient area, which is often surrounded by a rim of increased activity representing surrounding hyperemia. The line of the spermatic cord also often shows increased activity. The findings depend on the time interval between the onset of event and scan to some extent. Abrupt cutoff of the iliac artery that supplies the affected testicle may be seen, which is known as "nubbin sign" [41].

With acute epididymo-orchitis, activity within the testis itself is usually normal, but the inflammatory response in the epididymis produces a C-shaped margin of markedly increased activity, and in some cases this may appear to extend across the testis as well.

The contralateral normal testis is used as a benchmark to indicate whether the affected side shows increased or reduced activity. In all these cases, it is very important that the interpreting physician is aware of the clinical presentation such as which side of the testes is painful to avoid misinterpretation.

The main value of this test is as a supplement to Doppler ultrasound for the patients presenting acutely with unilateral testicular pain. Easy availability of ultrasound both routinely and after hours makes scrotal scintigraphy an infrequently performed nuclear medicine study for acute scrotal pain nowadays.

Role of Radiology in Andrology Disorders

Imaging in Erectile Dysfunction

Pathophysiology

Erectile dysfunction (ED) is defined as a persistent inability to achieve or maintain penile erections sufficient enough to engage in satisfactory sexual activity. Causes could be psychological or organic or mixed, the organic causes are vascular insufficiency, others being anatomical, neurological, hormonal, or drugs. Imaging is mainly used in the assessment of suspected vascular abnormality, which is believed to be the commonest cause of organic ED. Vascular ED can either be due to dysfunction of penile veno-occlusive mechanism or could be arteriogenic.

ED may result from abnormal penile venous leakage in patients who have a failure of the veno-occlusive mechanism to provide adequate venous resistance during erection. Venous drainage of erectile tissue occurs via the deep dorsal vein, which drains into the periprostatic plexus, and paired cavernosal veins, which drain via the internal pudendal veins. Commonly, incompetence originates in the deep dorsal vein (Fig. 43.42).

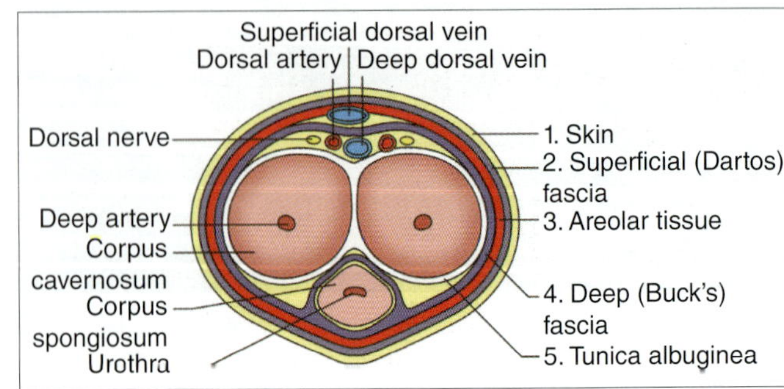

Figure 43.42 Schematic diagram of cross-sectional anatomy of penis.

Arterial blood supply to the penis originates from the internal iliac arteries via the internal pudendal arteries, which divide and form paired cavernosal arteries at the base of the penis. It has been estimated that penile arterial inflow may increase up to 30-fold during tumescence.

For many years, assessment was based upon arteriography and cavernosography, which have now largely been replaced by duplex ultrasonography, duplex ultrasonography of the penis and cavernosal arteries was first described in 1985 and is now the investigation of choice for penile arterial screening, despite some debate regarding protocol and velocity thresholds (particularly for moderate reductions in systolic velocity). It has a more limited role in demonstrating impaired veno-occlusion.

Imaging Technique

- Penile Doppler is the investigation of choice. Tests of penile hemodynamics are performed following intracavernosal injection of a vasoactive agent to induce a pharmacological erection. An adequate response to these agents confirms proper arterial supply and veno-occlusive mechanism
- The ultrasound transducer (7.5 or 10 MHz) is positioned on the ventral surface of the base of the penis
- Paired cavernosal arteries are found close to the septum and are identified as parallel hyperechoic lines. Spectral Doppler wave forms are recorded after intracavernosal injection of a pharmacological agent, commonly alprostadil (a prostaglandin E1 derivative)
- In a stepwise manner, repeated sampling of these waveforms is performed to achieve maximum peak systolic and minimal diastolic velocities. Peak systolic velocity (PSV) and end-diastolic velocity (EDV) are recorded every 5 minute for 30 minutes and measurements are recorded. The PSV is considered normal if the recorded value is >35 cm/s and EDV is normal if the minimal value recorded is close to 0 cm/s
- During the initial phase of erection, both systolic and diastolic flow are increased and continuous, which reflects smooth muscle relaxation. PSV then stabilizes after which intracavernosal pressure increases. The diastolic waveform decreases at an intracavernosal pressure over 40 mm Hg and is reversed at an intracavernosal pressure over 80 mm Hg (Figs. 43.43A and B)
- It is now generally accepted that PSV >35 cm/s predicts normal arterial inflow and that PSV <25 cm/s is a useful predictor of arterial insufficiency. Threshold values for the diagnosis of arterial insufficiency vary in the literature. Validation for these thresholds comes from studies correlating duplex ultrasonography with arteriography in patients with ED. A PSV of <25 cm/s has a correlation with severe arterial disease on arteriographic imaging [42] (Fig. 43.43C)
- The relationship between EDV at duplex ultrasonography and venous incompetence at cavernosometry has also been examined. Although, overall, EDV correlates poorly with venous incompetence, EDV <5 cm/s in association with normal PSV (>35 cm/s) is believed to be an indicator that veno-occlusion is normal and further investigation (e.g., cavernosometry) is unnecessary
- In patients with arterial insufficiency diagnosed by these duplex criteria, confirmation by arteriography is required if surgical intervention is planned (see below). Catheterization of internal pudental artery helps to evaluate arterial supply to penis and document the extent and location of arterial lesion [42]

Cavernosography is a technique used to investigate defects in the veno-occlusive mechanism. In this procedure, both corpora cavernosa are cannulated with 19-gauge needles. A pump injection of 150 strength contrast medium is injected via one of the needles to demonstrate sites of abnormal venous leakage. This is often combined with cavernosometry, to quantify the flow rate required to maintain a pharmacological erection. Synchronous pressure measurements are recorded through the other needle. Although this technique remains the best method of demonstrating venous incompetence as a cause of ED, poor results with venous ligation procedures have reduced their popularity and led to a dramatic reduction in the use of this test.

- MRI may be useful in certain cases where further characterization of a structural abnormality such as Peyronie's disease plaques is required

Imaging in Male Infertility

Azoospermic men with a normal FSH level may be evaluated radiologically in an attempt to discover a treatable, obstructive cause for infertility. Traditionally this has been achieved via vasography; more recently there has been increased interest in the use of TRUS.

When both vasa are clinically palpable in the scrotum, obstruction may be from congenital causes (most commonly midline cysts compressing the ejaculatory ducts) or acquired causes (commonly inflammatory or traumatic stenoses of the ejaculatory ducts or vasa). TRUS is useful in demonstrating distal obstruction at the level of the ejaculatory ducts, typically showing duct dilatation proximal to the obstruction and also congenital cysts, if

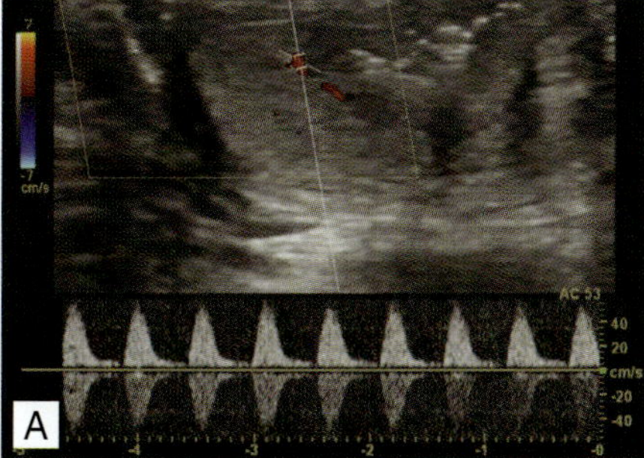

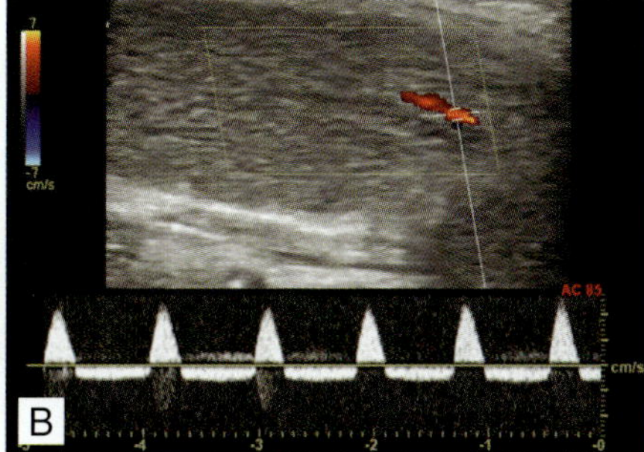

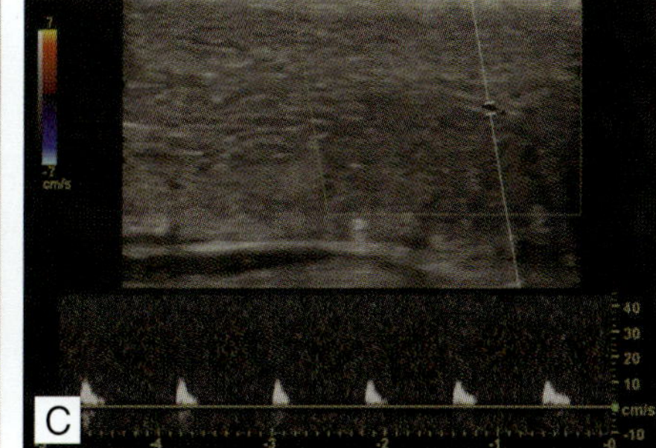

Figure 43.43 Normal penile Doppler (images A and B): 10 minutes (image A) postinstillation of pharmacological agent image shows normal PSV (>35 cm/s) and normal EDV (close to 0 cm/s); 20 minutes (image B) postinstillation image shows normal PSV and reversal of EDV. Arterial insufficiency (image C): 15 minutes postinstillation shows decreased PSV (10 cm/s) with no diastolic flow PSV-Peak systolic velocity; EDV-End diastolic velocity.

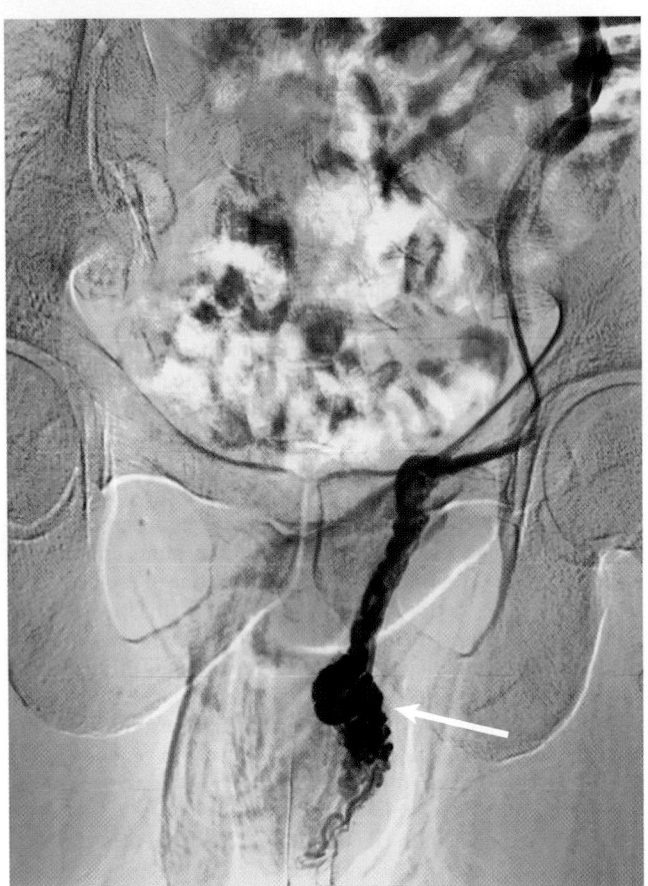

Figure 43.44 Digital subtraction venography demonstrating left varicocele in a case of male infertility (*white arrow*). (Courtesy: Dr. Sagar Tyagi, Max Hospital, New Delhi.)

present. Multifocal stenoses (which occur in up to 20% of obstructed vasa) or proximal stenoses of the vas deferens may be identified by vasography, with the vas cannulated just distal to the inguinal canal. Obstruction may be relieved surgically by epididymovasostomy in some patients.

Although its relevance is debated, the presence of scrotal varicoceles (Fig. 43.44) in association with oligospermia may represent a treatable cause of hypofertility. Treatment of varicoceles for subfertility has been the subject of controversy but at best it has been reported to consistently improve the semen analysis and be associated with demonstrable fertility in up to 40% of treated individuals.

Suggested Readings

- R Nicola, N Carson, VS Dogra, Imaging of traumatic injuries to the scrotum and penis, Am J Roentgenol [Internet] [cited 2020 Oct 4]. Available at: https://www.ajronline.org/doi/full/10.2214/AJR.13.11676.
- D V, B S, Acute painful scrotum, Radiol Clin North Am 42 (2) (2004) 349–363. [Internet] [cited 2021 May 21]. Available at: https://europepmc.org/article/med/15136021.
- RA Parker, CO Menias, R Quazi, AK Hara, S Verma, A Shaaban, et al., MR imaging of the penis and scrotum, RadioGraphics 35 (4) (2015) 1033–1050. [Internet] [cited 2021 May 24]. Available at: http://pubs.rsna.org/doi/10.1148/rg.2015140161.
- S Krishna, K Shanbhogue, N Schieda, F Morbeck, B Hadas, G Kulkarni, et al., Role of MRI in staging of penile cancer, J Magn Reson Imaging 51 (6) (2020) 1612–1629. [Internet] [cited 2020 Oct 14]. Available at: https://onlinelibrary.wiley.com/doi/abs/10.1002/jmri.27060.

44 Uterus and Cervix

ANURADHA CHANDRAMOHAN, SOURAV PANDA

Introduction

The uterus and the cervix are prone to a wide range of congenital, infective, benign, and malignant pathologies. Symptoms pertaining to these diseases are often nonspecific and include vaginal discharge, abnormal uterine bleeding, lower abdominal pain, palpable mass per abdomen, congestive dysmenorrhea, dyspareunia, and postcoital bleeding. Imaging plays a key role in identifying abnormalities; suggesting a specific diagnosis and the need for biopsy; aiding in image-guided interventions; and staging cervicouterine malignancy. The imaging appearance of the female reproductive tract undergoes continuous change throughout the life span owing to the influence of hormones on these organs. It is important to be aware of the imaging appearances related to the physiological changes during the menstrual cycle and those related to age to avoid pitfalls in image interpretation. Commonly, ultrasonography (USG) is the primary and the only imaging modality used in the evaluation of female pelvic conditions including those of the uterus and cervix. In most gynecological practices, USG is almost an extension of clinical examination. Based on the clinical and USG findings, a subset of patients may undergo magnetic resonance imaging (MRI) for better characterization of abnormalities seen on USG and for local staging of biopsy proved cervicouterine malignancy. Computed tomography (CT) and fluorine-18 2-fluro deoxy D-glucose positron emission tomography with CT (F18-FDG PET-CT) are reserved for assessing the extent of extrapelvic disease in known malignancies of the uterus and the cervix.

In this chapter, we will provide an overview of the imaging modalities used in the evaluation of uterine and cervical diseases; normal imaging appearance of the uterus and cervix; imaging appearance of common benign and malignant conditions; potential pitfalls, and challenges in the image interpretation.

Imaging Techniques

Ultrasonography

USG either transabdominal or endovaginal, is the mainstay of imaging of the pelvis. Transabdominal ultrasonography (TAS) is usually performed with a 3–4 MHz sector or convex probe and requires the patient to have a full bladder. The distended bladder displaces the small bowel out of the pelvis, pushes the uterus posteriorly, and the ovaries laterally toward the pelvic sidewalls. The optimally distended bladder projects just beyond the fundus of a normal sized uterus. If the bladder is inadequately distended the pelvic structures may be obscured by bowel gas, but if overdistended the uterus becomes elongated and the ovaries displaced too far laterally. Longitudinal (sagittal) and transverse scans are performed using the bladder as a window. *Transvaginal or Endovaginal scanning (EVS) is best performed with an empty bladder* and utilizes a higher frequency sector/curvilinear probe (typically 5–7 MHz) giving improved resolution of structures close to the probe but a limited field of view. Whereas many patients prefer EVS, it is inappropriate in the very young, the very elderly, and any patient who is virgo intacta. It is, therefore, important to be able to perform both types of scan with confidence. Color Doppler and spectral Doppler are currently available in all USG machines and act as a useful tool for assessing the vascularity of pelvic abnormalities. Three-dimensional ultrasonography (3D USG) involves performing two-dimensional TAS in a usual manner followed by 3D reconstruction of images. The role of 3D USG has been increasing in the evaluation of uterus and now has proved roles in screening for congenital uterine anomalies.

Magnetic Resonance Imaging

MRI is an important technique in the evaluation of pelvic pathology due to its ability to obtain images with a high soft-tissue contrast resolution and discrimination in multiple planes. It is the primary technique of choice for local staging of uterocervical malignancy. MRI also has an important role in the comprehensive evaluation of Mullarian duct abnormalities and other benign conditions such as fibroids and adenomyosis.

The patient should have a partially distended bladder by asking the patient to void 1 hour before the study. An overfull bladder will result in patient being restless during the examination and may falsely obliterated tissue planes leading to overstaging of cervicouterine malignancy. An antiperistaltic agent can be administered to reduce bowel motion artifact. A pelvic phased-array coil should be used for the evaluation of the whole pelvis and abdomen. Followed by sagittal images of the pelvis, oblique transverse and coronal small field of view (typically 20–24 cm) T2-weighted high-resolution images of the pelvis are obtained perpendicular and parallel to the planes of uterus and cervix in uterine and cervical pathologies, respectively. The use of intravenous gadolinium-chelate is not mandatory, but it can be helpful to demonstrate small lesions and the extent of tumor spread through and beyond the uterus and cervix. A T1 fat-suppressed dynamic contrast-enhanced (DCE) technique produces the best results, as malignant masses usually enhance in the early phase following contrast injection and washes out the contrast quickly when compared with the normal structures. This feature is especially useful in the local staging of cervicouterine malignancies especially in the postmenopausal women.

Computed Tomography

The role of CT in the evaluation of gynecological diseases in the pelvis has declined since the advent of EVS and MRI. As a general rule, benign disease should be investigated initially by ultrasonography and then MRI if needed. Staging of malignant disease requires CT or MRI, depending on the site of the primary tumor. MRI is superior to CT for local staging cervical and uterine carcinoma. Currently, CT and MRI have similar capabilities for detecting lymphadenopathy, with MRI being slightly more superior. However, CT is frequently used as an imaging modality in patients with nonspecific lower abdominal symptoms such as pain, or to determine the site of origin of a mass, so it is clearly necessary to be aware of the CT appearances of gynecological conditions. Intravenous contrast administration is essential for evaluating pelvic pathologies. CT is most commonly used in a setting for radiotherapy treatment planning in known cervical malignancy.

F-18-FDG PET-CT

PET-CT is the combination of metabolic information of fluorine-18 2-fluoro deoxy D-glucose (FDG) and exquisite anatomical information from contrast-enhanced CT. This is achieved by first performing low-dose CT along with PET for attenuation correction and coregistration of PET data, which is followed by standard-dose CT with intravenous and oral contrast. PET-CT is superior to CT and MRI in assessing extrapelvic extent of cervicouterine malignancies, both the nodes and distant metastases. PET-CT also has a role in assessing treatment response and recurrence of cervicouterine malignancies [1,2]. Patients with gynecological malignancy are catheterized to prevent bladder activity from overlapping with the activity of the pelvic mass.

Table 44.1 summarizes the indications for the previously mentioned imaging modalities.

Normal Anatomy, Physiology, and Imaging Appearance of the Uterus and Cervix

USG Appearance of the Uterus and Cervix

Size and Shape of the Uterus

The uterus is a pear-shaped structure, which varies in size according to the age and hormonal status of the patient. Due to the influence of maternal hormones, a neonatal uterus is prominent and uniformly hyporeflective, the cervix is bulbous and nearly twice as long as the uterus, the endometrium is seen as a thick echogenic line and there is minimal fluid in the endometrial cavity [3,4]. As the maternal hormones wane, the uterus and cervix become small thin structures with a uterine body-to-cervix ratio of 1:1 and endometrium is seen as pencil-thin

TABLE 44.1 Indications and Use of Different Imaging Modalities for Evaluating Diseases of the Uterus and Cervix

Ultrasonography	Magnetic Resonance Imaging	Computed Tomography	PET-Computed Tomography
Initial investigation of choice for various gynecological complaints	Superior soft-tissue resolution of magnetic resonance imaging allows delineation of anatomy of female genital tract. It is used for better characterization of abnormalities identified on ultrasonography	Contrast-enhanced computed tomography has poor soft-tissue contrast compared with magnetic resonance imaging	Fluorine-18-2-fluoro2-deoxy-D-glucose (FDG)-PET/computed tomography scan is a hybrid imaging technique which provides information both on the anatomy and metabolism
Indications 1. Premenarchal age group ▪ Initial evaluation of congenital genital tract anomalies ▪ Evaluation of delayed menarche ▪ Acute pelvic pain—ovarian torsion, hydrometrocolpos/ hematometrocolpos 2. Reproductive age group ▪ Evaluation of dysmenorrhea, amenorrhea, dysfunctional uterine bleeding, and dyspareunia ▪ Evaluation of infertility ▪ Evaluating the position of intrauterine contraceptive device ▪ Leiomyomas, adenomyosis, endometriosis, PCOD, pelvic inflammatory disease, and malignancies of the cervix and endometrium 3. Postmenopausal age group ▪ Evaluation of postmenopausal bleeding and abnormal vaginal discharge ▪ Initial investigation for gynecological malignancies ▪ Useful for assessing endometrial thickness and endometrial cavity	**Indications** 1. Mullerian duct anomalies 2. Benign conditions ▪ Leiomyomas ▪ Adenomyosis ▪ Endometriosis ▪ Uterine vascular malformations ▪ Pelvic inflammatory disease 3. Gynecologic Malignancies ▪ Modality of choice for local staging of uterocervical malignancies ▪ Evaluation of local response to treatment ▪ Imaging extent of local recurrence	**Indications** 1. Acute gynecological emergencies when ultrasonography findings were equivocal and to exclude other significant abnormalities 2. Staging gynecological malignancies by assessing extrapelvic extent 3. Surveillance for distant recurrence	**Indications** 1. Pretreatment N- and M-staging of uterocervical cancer when available 2. Pretreatment N-staging and M-staging of select patients with type 2 endometrial carcinoma and nonendometroid uterine malignancies 3. Restaging of recurrent disease before extensive surgeries like pelvic exenteration

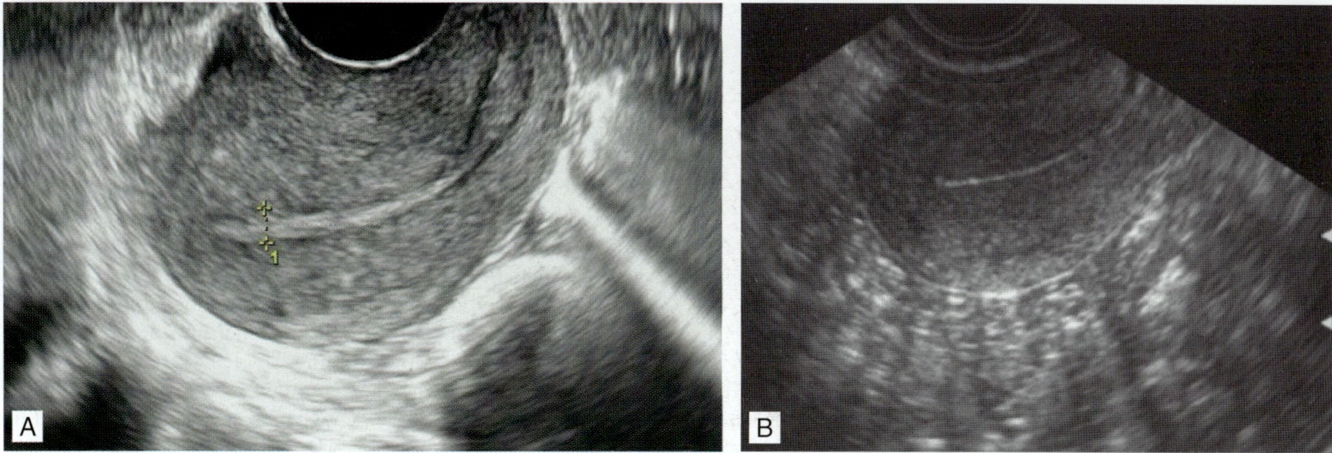

Figure 44.1 Normal ultrasonography appearance of the uterus in the reproductive age and postmenopausal female. (A) Sagittal endovaginal scan (EVS) in a female of reproductive age group showing normal luteal phase endometrium (within the calipers). (B) Sagittal EVS in a postmenopausal female showing pencil-thin endometrial lining.

echogenic line [5,6]. There is subsequent gradual increase in size of the uterus in the prepubertal period till the uterus reaches 5–8 cm in length. After menarche the uterine body increases in size to an overall length of 7–8 cm, uterus becomes pear shaped and uterine body-to-cervix ratio is 1.5–2:1, which is identical to that in women of reproductive age group (Fig. 44.1A). The uterus in childbearing age group measures about 8 cm in length, 5 cm in width, and 4 cm in thickness, with the uterus of a multiparous female being larger than that of a nulliparous by as much as 1 cm in each dimension [7]. After menopause, the uterus and cervix slowly involute to 5–6 cm (Fig. 44.1B). Table 44.2 lists the change in size of the uterus and the utero-cervical ratio with age [8,9].

TABLE 44.2 Change in Size of the Uterus With Age [3–9]

Stage	Uterine Length (in cm)	Uterine Body-to-Cervix Ratio
Neonatal	3.5	1:2
Pediatric	1–3	1:1
Prepubertal	3–4.5	1–1.5:1
Pubertal	5–8	1.5–2:1
Reproductive	8–9	2:1
Postmenopausal	3.5–7.5	1–1.5:1

Myometrium and Cervix

Three layers of myometrium can be identified on ultrasonography—outer, intermediate, and inner layers. The intermediate layer appears homogenous with low to moderate echogenicity and it is the thickest of the three layers forming the major bulk of the myometrium and it is formed by loosely arranged smooth muscle cells. The inner layer of myometrium, which is also called the junctional myometrium appears hypoechoic and surrounds the echogenic endometrium, forming a subendometrial halo (Fig. 44.2A). The junctional myometrium is formed by compactly arranged smooth muscle cells giving its distinct appearance. The

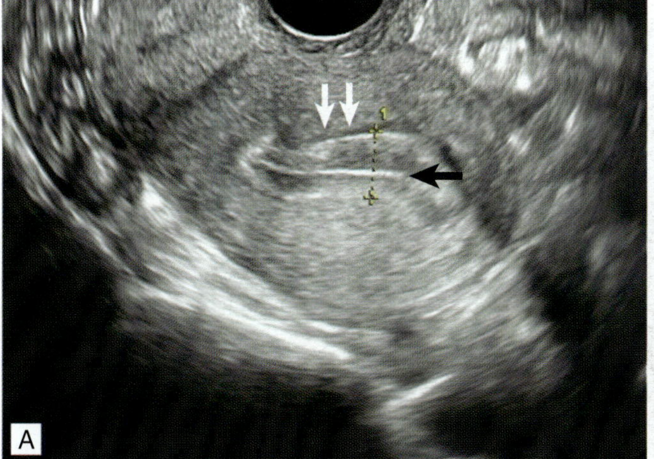

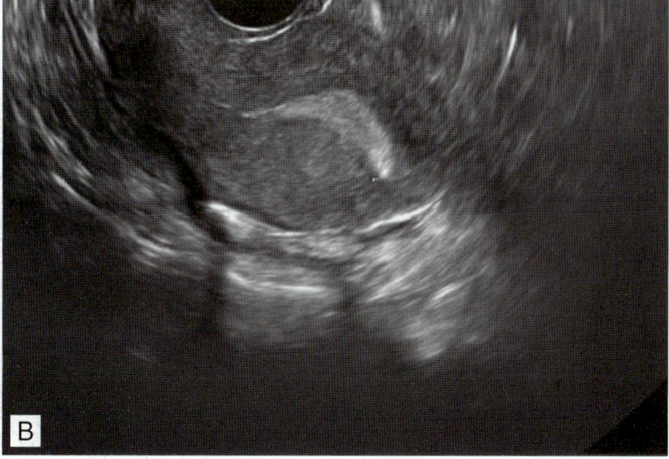

Figure 44.2 EVS showing measurement of the endometrium. (A) Note the laminar appearance of the endometrium in the preovulatory phase of the menstrual cycle and all five layers are included in the measurement but the deeper hypoechoic layer (*white arrows*) is not included since it denotes the junctional zone or the inner layer of the myometrium. The central echogenic line (*black arrow*) is due to the interface of the two layers of endometrium. (B) Homogeneously echogenic luteal phase or secretory phase endometrium. *EVS*, endovaginal scan.

BOX 44.1 Normal Endometrial Thickness and Appearance in Different Phases of the Menstrual Cycle [17,19]

USG appearance of endometrium in different phases of menstrual cycle
- Menstrual phase: Thin echogenic line (<5 mm)
- Proliferative phase: Hypoechoic (4–8 mm)
- Periovulatory phase: Trilaminar appearance (6–10 mm)
- Secretory phase: Diffusely echogenic (7–14 mm)

thin outer layer is slightly less echogenic than the intermediate layer and is separated from it by arcuate vessels. These layers are most conspicuous in the reproductive age group and less distinct in the prepubertal and postmenopausal uterus. The cervix is homogenous in echotexture and similar in echogenicity as the myometrium with a hypoechoic central cervical canal. Nabothian cysts which are mucus retention cysts are commonly seen in women of reproductive and postmenopausal age group and are usually smaller than 2 cm [10].

Endometrium and Its Changes During the Menstrual Cycle

- The normal endometrial cavity appears as a thin echogenic line due to specular reflection from the interface between the opposing surfaces of endometrium (Box 44.1) [11]. Sonographic appearance of the endometrium changes throughout the menstrual cycle under influence of hormones and this has been correlated with histology (Box 44.1) [12–14]
- Endometrium has two layers histologically—the superficial functional layer that thickens throughout the menstrual cycle and is finally shed, and the deep basal layer (stratum basale) which remains intact throughout the cycle
- During the menstrual phase (typically 1–5 days), the endometrium is seen as the thin echogenic line
- In the proliferative phase, under the influence of estrogen, the functional layer increase in thickness. Before ovulation, the endometrium has a layered appearance also called trilaminar appearance (Fig. 44.2), which consists of an echogenic central line or interface, surrounded by a hypoechoic functional layer, and an echogenic deep basal layer. Hypoechoic appearance of the functional layer has been attributed histologically to an orderly increase in the glandular elements
- After ovulation, in the secretory phase, the functional layer changes from low to high echogenicity. Hyperechogenicity of the functional layer is due to increase in mucin and glycogen within the glands as endometrium prepares for a possible implantation. The endometrium appears diffusely hyperechoic toward the end of secretory phase with thickness varying from 7 to 16 mm (Fig. 44.2)
- Endometrial thickness is best measured in midline sagittal scan of uterus by placing the cursors at anterior and posterior endometrial–myometrial interfaces (Fig. 44.2). It should be measured where the endometrium appears widest and that is usually close to the fundus. Care should be taken not to include the hypoechoic junctional myometrium or the subendometrial halo
- The central echogenic line representing the uterine cavity is normally continuous. Discontinuity in the central echogenic line may represent pathologies like endometrial polyps, submucosal fibroids, and adhesions

Normal Appearance in the Postpartum Period

Uterus measures approximately 20 cm in length and weighs around 1 kg immediately after childbirth and undergoes gradual involution throughout the puerperium (6–8 weeks after delivery). Rapid involution occurs within the first few days after delivery with size decreasing by nearly 50% in the first 24–48 hours. After that, the involution is more gradual with the uterus appearing near normal at 6 weeks postpartum. On USG, normal postpartum myometrium appears heterogeneous and has higher echogenicity than the myometrium of nongravid uterus [15,16]. In the absence of abnormal postpartum bleeding, diffuse or focal increase in the vascularity of the myometrium at the placental insertion site is a normal finding [17,18]. Intracavitary fluid, blood products, and gas are commonly seen in asymptomatic women until 3 weeks after vaginal and caesarean delivery and do not indicate postpartum infection [19–21]. After caesarean section, heterogeneity and thinning of myometrium at the site of incision is a normal finding. Similarly, minimal postoperative pelvic and anterior abdominal wall fluid is normal.

Normal Appearance in the Postmenopausal Age Group

- Menopause is the cessation of menstruation and is defined as 12 months of the continuous period of amenorrhea after the last menstrual cycle in a female with an intact uterus. The age of onset varies from 40 to 60 years, with average age between 51 and 53 years in Western countries [22]
- After menopause, there is a gradual decrease in the uterine size. Myometrium appears more heterogeneous in postmenopausal women with or without calcification of the arcuate arteries (Fig. 44.1B)
- Calcification of the arcuate arteries in the superficial myometrium is seen as a circumferential peripheral echogenic reflection with dense acoustic shadowing. This circumferential pattern of calcification helps in differentiating this entity from a calcified fibroid
- Nabothian cysts in the cervix are also common in postmenopausal women. Small amount of anechoic fluid in the pouch of Douglas is normal in early postmenopausal women but it is pathological in late postmenopausal women
- The lack of hormonal influence renders the endometrium atrophic and appears as a thin echogenic line (Fig. 44.1B). Small amount of fluid within the endometrial cavity measuring less than 2 mm in thickness is a normal finding in this age group, which is due to mild cervical stenosis. When present, fluid should not be included in the measurement of endometrial thickness
- Normal transvaginal sonogram (TVS) in postmenopausal women has high negative predictive value and accuracy rates for excluding major disorders of the uterus [23,24]. The risk of missing a significant endometrial abnormality using a single measurement of 4 mm or less at endovaginal USG is very low, with a negative predictive value of 99% for the presence of endometrial cancer [25]. Thus, a cut of 4 mm or more is recommended by the American College of Obstetricians and Gynecologists for determining which symptomatic postmenopausal patients should undergo endometrial biopsy. In asymptomatic postmenopausal women, those with endometrial thickness of ≥11 mm must undergo endometrial biopsy [26]

Position of the Uterus

The uterus is variable in position and may lie straight or obliquely within the pelvis depending on the degree of urinary bladder and rectal distension. Position of the uterus is described either based on the angle between the long axis of uterine body and the long axis of the cervix (flexion) or based on angle between the long axis of

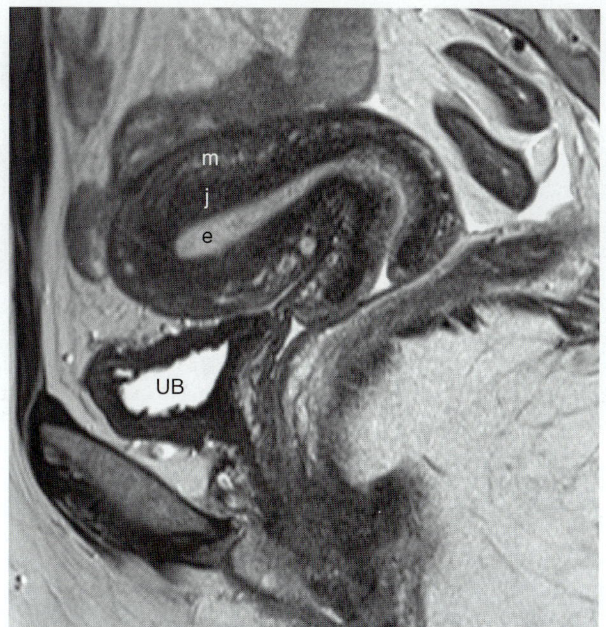

Figure 44.3 Normal uterus on a sagittal T2-weighted spin-echo (TSE 3500/100) MR image with normal zonal anatomy of central high-signal endometrium (e), the junctional zone (j), and the outer myometrium (m). *UB*, urine-filled bladder.

uterine body and the long axis of vagina (version). Most commonly, the uterus is anteflexed and anteverted. When the uterus is retroverted/retroflexed, transabdominal evaluation of the uterus becomes difficult requiring transvaginal ultrasonography evaluation. Also, retroverted uterus can be mistaken for a mass in some cases.

Normal MRI Appearance of the Uterus and Cervix

- MRI clearly depicts the anatomy, morphology, and pathological changes in the uterus and cervix. The zonal anatomy of the uterus and cervix is best depicted on T2-weighted imaging. The innermost layer or the endometrium appears homogenously T2 hyperintense owing to the presence of mucin-rich endometrial glands. As in ultrasonography, the endometrial thickness is best measured in mid-sagittal plane and the thickness varies in different phases of menstrual cycle
- Normal myometrium has inner and outer layers on MRI. The inner layer, also called junctional zone, appears T2 hypointense and surrounds the endometrium (Fig. 44.3). It corresponds to the subendometrial halo seen on ultrasonography. The T2 hypointense signal of the junctional zone is due to the presence of compact smooth muscle cells and less water content. The normal thickness of the junctional zone is between 5 and 8 mm [27–30]; thickness >12 mm is highly suggestive of adenomyosis. The outer myometrium displays intermediate T2 signal due to the presence of less compact smooth muscle cells, increased water content, and vascularity [31]
- A premenarchal and postmenopausal uterus is low to medium in signal intensity with indistinct zonal anatomy. In an unenhanced T1-weighted MRI, the uterus and the cervix appear homogeneously low in signal intensity like that of skeletal muscle, and the zonal anatomy is not apparent. After intravenous gadolinium-chelate, the endometrium and myometrium enhance homogeneously with the delayed enhancement of the junctional zone
- *The cervix* is a cylindrical-shaped structure measuring 2–4 cm in length, connecting with the body of the uterus at the isthmus. The level of the isthmus is approximately at the peritoneal reflection on the bladder
- The cervix has two distinct layers: a hyperintense central zone representing cervical mucus and epithelium, with an outer zone of low signal, like the uterine junctional zone, due to the fibromuscular stroma (Fig. 44.4). A further peripheral layer of the intermediate signal may be seen continuous with the myometrium. The *parametrium* has an intermediate signal on T1-weighted images and high signal on T2-weighted images. After intravenous contrast, the compact cervical stroma retains its low signal, with enhancement of the paracervical tissue and inner cervical epithelium on T1-weighted images

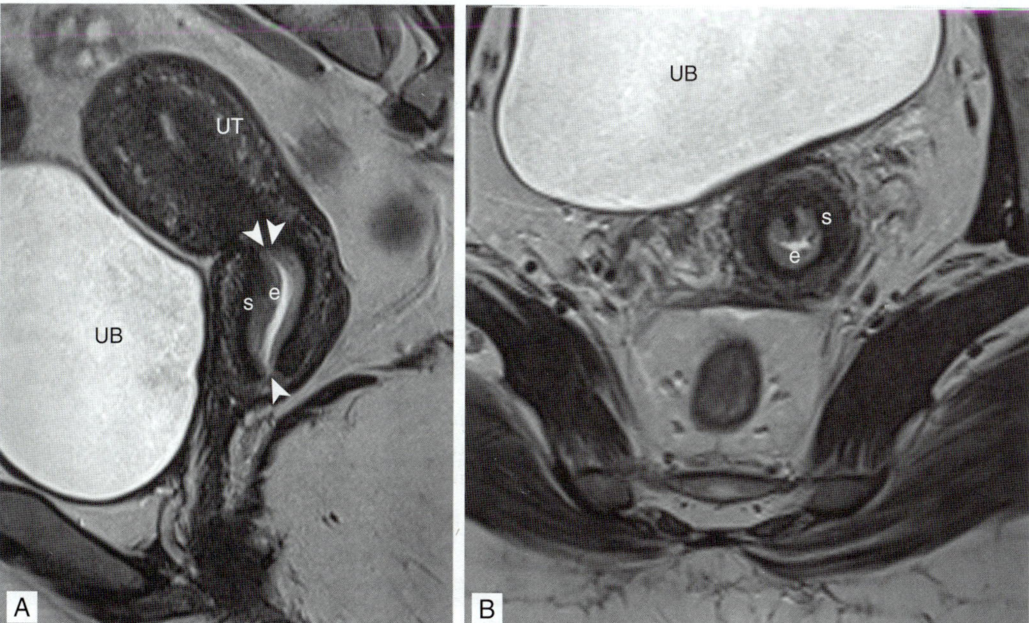

Figure 44.4 Normal zonal anatomy of the cervix on an (A) sagittal and (B) axial T2-weighted spin-echo MR image. *e*, cervical mucus and epithelium; *double arrowhead*, internal os; *s*, cervical stroma; *single arrowhead*, external os; *UB*, bladder; *UT*, uterus.

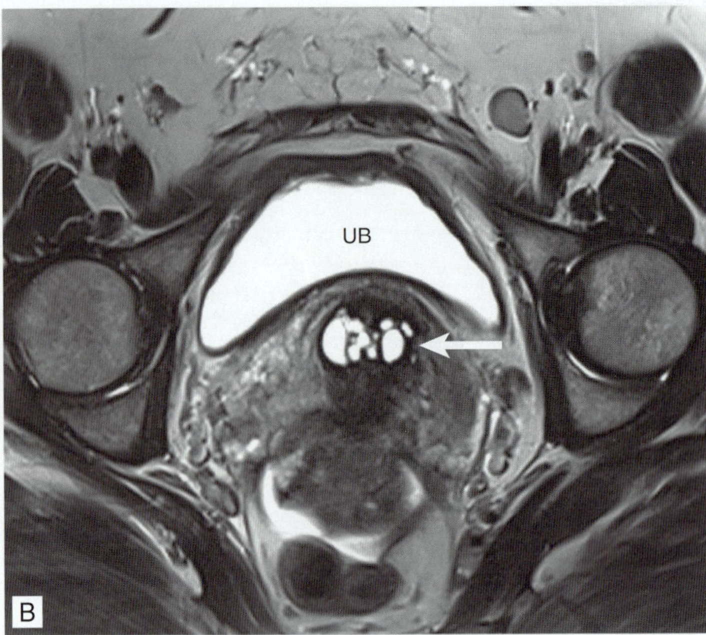

Figure 44.5 Nabothian cysts (*arrow*) within the cervix on (A) sagittal and (B) axial T2-weighted spin-echo MR image. *Arrows*, nabothian cysts; *UB*, bladder; *UT*, uterus.

- There are numerous glands lining the cervical canal and the ducts of these glands when blocked cause retention (Nabothian) cysts (Fig. 44.5). These are commonly seen on MRI of the female pelvis
- *The vagina* can be identified as a T2 high-signal central zone of mucus and epithelium surrounded by a T2 low-signal muscular wall appears H-shaped or butterfly shaped on axial sections [32]. The vagina can be divided into three regions: an upper third is characterized by the lateral vaginal fornices, a middle third is at the level of the bladder base, and a lower third is at the level of the urethra. There is a high-signal venous plexus surrounding the cervix and vagina, best seen on transverse T2-weighted images

Normal CT Appearance and Pitfalls in CT Interpretation

- In view of poor soft-tissue contrast, CT is generally not used as preferred modality of imaging for the evaluation of gynecological disorders. However, radiologists should be aware of certain normal imaging findings which could be misinterpreted as disease on CT scans performed for nongynecological indications
- Depending on the menstrual phase, age, and time following contrast, myometrium may have variable enhancement patterns on contrast-enhanced CT scans. This can range from homogeneous myometrial enhancement, rim of subendometrial and serosal enhancement, heterogeneous enhancement, or poor contrast enhancement (Fig. 44.6) [33,34]
- Normal endometrium enhances less than the myometrium and appears low in density compared with the myometrium. This can be misinterpreted as fluid in uterine cavity. Endometrial thickness cannot be assessed on CT and it is not possible to distinguish fluid or blood in the endometrial cavity from endometrium. Any concern regarding uterine pathology on a CT should be evaluated further using TVS
- Normal cervix shows less enhancement compared with the uterus due to dense fibrous stroma (Fig. 44.7) and this appearance should not be mistaken for a mass lesion [34,35]

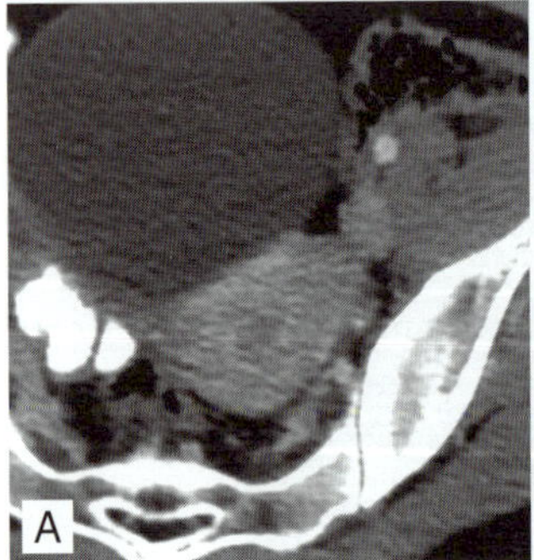

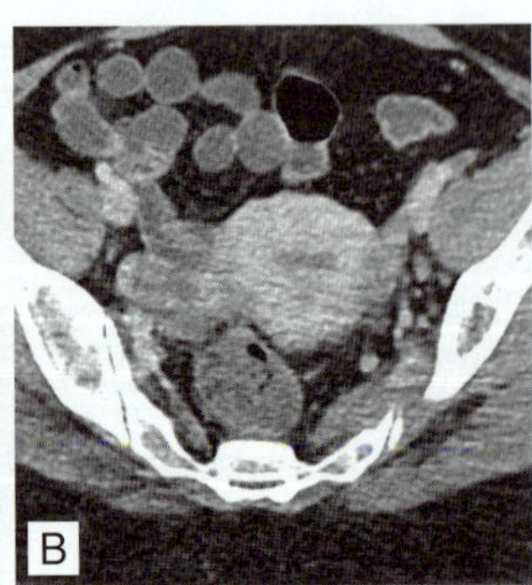

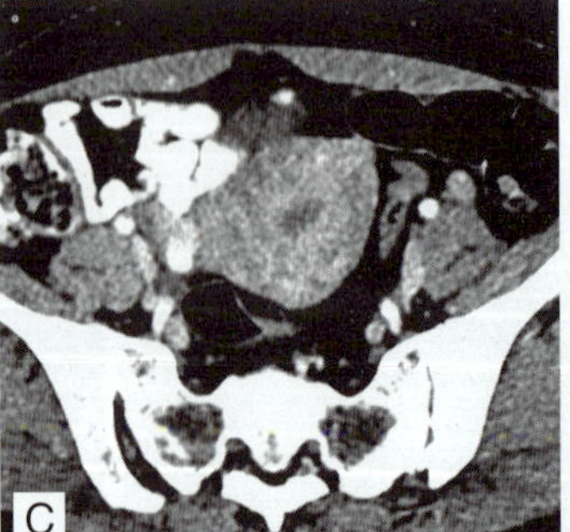

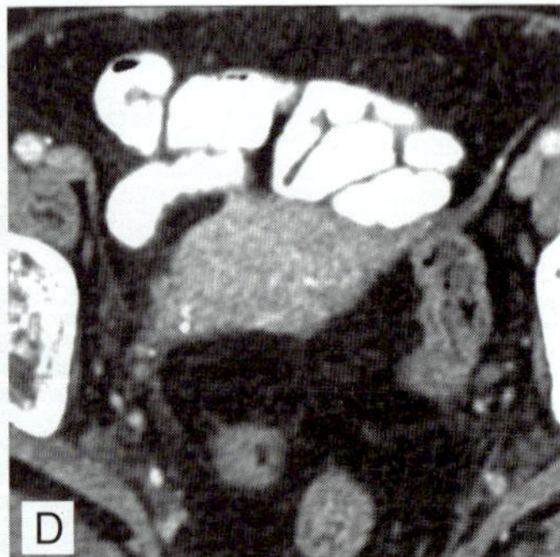

Figure 44.6 Patterns of enhancement of uterine myometrium on contrast-enhanced CT. (A) Subendometrial enhancement, (B) homogeneous myometrial enhancement, (C) heterogeneous enhancement, (D) poor enhancement in postmenopausal uterus with arcuate vessel calcifications. Note that endometrium appears hypodense on CT and must not be mistaken for fluid in the endometrial cavity. *CT*, computed tomography.

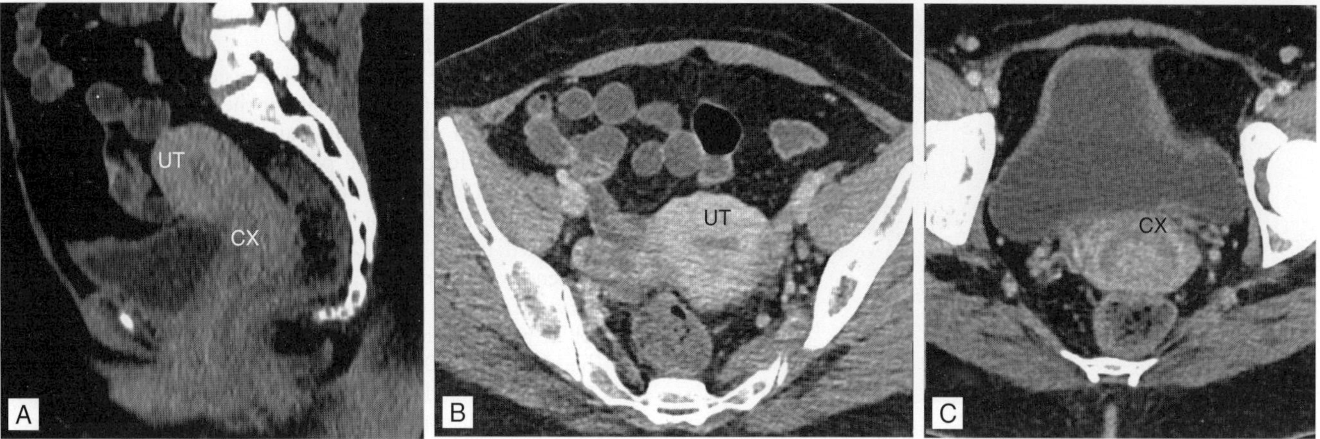

Figure 44.7 CECT (A) sagittal and axial CT through the (B) uterus and (C) cervix shows differential enhancement of the myometrium of the uterus (UT) compared with the cervix (CX). *CT*, computed tomography.

- Similarly, unless recognized as such, retroverted uterus and cervix that is deviated to the left or right of the midline can be misinterpreted as mass

Effect of Hormones

Combined oral contraceptive pill: The uterus and the ovaries are suppressed. The endometrium should be thin and the ovaries small with no evidence of follicular activity.

Progesterone-only pill: The progesterone-only pill does not necessarily inhibit follicular activity but the uterus should look small, with a thin endometrium.

Tamoxifen: Tamoxifen is used in the treatment of breast cancer and has both antiestrogenic and estrogenic effects. Long-term intake of tamoxifen is associated with endometrial hyperplasia, endometrial proliferation, increased risk of endometrial carcinoma (EC), and uterine sarcomas. The uterus of women on tamoxifen can have a characteristic appearance with increased thickness of the cavity with multiple tiny cysts (Fig. 44.8). These patients must be asked to promptly report for further investigations should they develop symptoms such as abnormal vaginal bleeding, vaginal discharge, spotting, or staining. Although postmenopausal women on tamoxifen need close monitoring for these symptoms, premenopausal women on tamoxifen with no known increased risk factor for uterine cancer do not need additional monitoring. Routine endometrial surveillance with ultrasonography is not proved to be effective for early detection of endometrial cancer unless there is a high risk for endometrial cancer as indicated by symptoms. Also, current evidence suggests that the presence of pretamoxifen benign endometrial polyps increases the risk of atypical hyperplasia after tamoxifen. Thus, there may be a role for pretreatment screening of postmenopausal women with TVS to exclude endometrial polyps before initiation of tamoxifen [36].

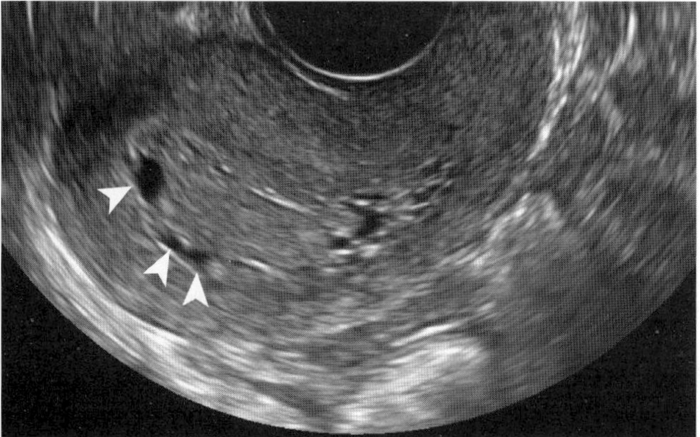

Figure 44.8 EVS showing thickened irregular endometrium due to tamoxifen. Note the small cysts (*arrowheads*) at the myometrial endometrial interface. *EVS*, endovaginal scan.

Hormone replacement therapy (HRT): The effect of HRT on the uterus and ovaries depends on the type of HRT taken. Unopposed estrogen administration causes thickening of the endometrium due to endometrial hyperplasia. This is a precursor to EC; therefore unopposed estrogen regimens are only recommended if the patient has had a hysterectomy. Sequential HRT, that is, estrogens followed by progesterones, is usually prescribed for perimenopausal and early postmenopausal patients who have persistent but unpredictable ovarian function. Most patients have regular monthly bleeds on such a regimen. Thus, they have an endometrium that varies in thickness during the cycle. The maximum thickness should still be less than 8 mm. Any patient found to have a mildly thickened endometrium on sequential HRT should have a repeat scan after a withdrawal bleed. Continuous combined hormone replacement involves taking estrogen and progesterone together continuously and should result in endometrial atrophy within 6 months, that is, endometrial thickness less than 4 mm. Routine screening is not indicated for patients on HRT but should be performed in those with abnormal vaginal bleeding.

Intrauterine Contraceptive Devices

- Intrauterine contraceptive devices (IUCDs) are a common incidental finding in patients who undergo pelvic USG. They are easily visualized as highly echogenic structures with acoustic shadowing and should be entirely within the uterine cavity, not protruding into the myometrium or endocervical canal (Fig. 44.9)
- Large fibroids, particularly if calcified, can occasionally cause difficulty in visualizing the IUCD. Expulsion during menstruation does occur. However, most patients referred with "missing coil" will have the IUCD present normally in the cavity, the threads having retracted into the cervical canal. Complications such as migration of the coil into or through

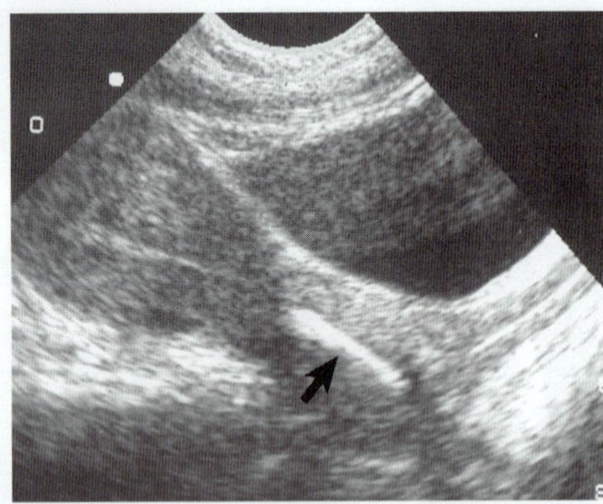

Figure 44.9 TAS. IUCD (*arrow*) in the cervical canal. *IUCD*, intrauterine contraceptive device; *TAS*, transabdominal ultrasonography.

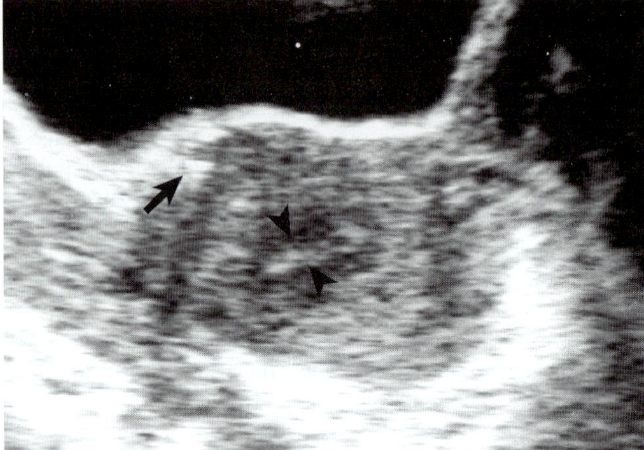

Figure 44.10 TAS. IUCD embedded in the myometrium (*arrow*), well outside the cavity (*arrowheads*). *IUCD*, intrauterine contraceptive device; *TAS*, transabdominal ultrasonography.

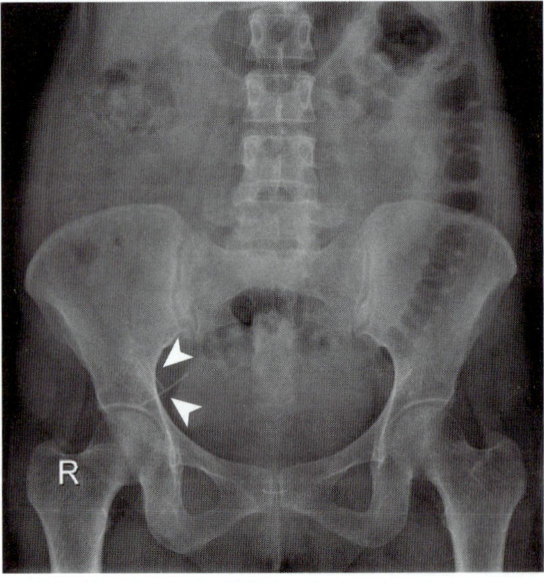

Figure 44.11 Plain radiograph of the abdomen in a female with suspected uterine perforation after IUCD placement shows misplaced IUCD in the right side of pelvis (*arrowheads*). *IUCD*, intrauterine contraceptive device.

the myometrium usually occur at the time of insertion and are associated with pain (Fig. 44.10)

- It is rarely possible to see an IUCD outside the uterus on ultrasonography. If there is doubt about the presence of an IUCD on the USG, a plain abdominal radiograph should be performed to exclude uterine perforation (Fig. 44.11). USG is also indicated to look for causes of difficulty in inserting a coil, for example, large fibroid distorting the cavity or a severely retroflexed uterus. IUCDs are associated with an increased incidence of pelvic infection. In particular, colonization with *Actinomycosis* may occur with long-term use and patients may well be asymptomatic
- The Mirena IUCD contains progestogens and is used for both contraception and to treat dysfunctional uterine bleeding. Although similar in shape to most other coils, the Mirena coil is less echogenic than standard IUCDs and hence it is harder to visualize on ultrasonography, even when performed endovaginally. It is often seen by virtue of its acoustic shadow rather than direct visualization of the coil itself
- IUCDs are safely imaged with MRI, with no adverse heating or torque effects demonstrated. All IUCDs show a signal void on all pulse sequences, the extent of which depends on the type of device in situ (Fig. 44.12). A contraceptive diaphragm will, however, produce a significant signal artifact

Benign Conditions of the Uterus and Cervix

Leiomyoma

Pathophysiology

Leiomyomas (fibroids) are the most common benign neoplasms of the uterus occurring in 20–30% of females over the age of 30 years [37]. Fibroids are smooth muscle tumors that are estrogen dependent and develop in women of reproductive age group. They do not occur before puberty and symptoms become less severe and the size decreases after menopause. Risk factors for the development of fibroids include high estrogenic conditions like early menarche, late menopause, nulliparous women, and HRT [38,39]. Pregnancy and HRT cause increase in size of fibroids.

Based on the location within the uterus, fibroids can be classified as follows.

- *Submucosal fibroids* are least common, project into the endometrial cavity, and may often become pedunculated. These are most likely to cause symptoms like menorrhagia and infertility
- *Intramural fibroids* remain confined to the myometrium and are the most common type
- *Subserosal fibroids* protrude from the peritoneal surface of the uterus
- *Pedunculated fibroids* are attached to the uterus through a pedicle, which measures less than one-third the dimension of its maximum diameter. These are most commonly subserosal or submucosal
- *Cervical fibroids* are rare, that is, less than 5% fibroids

Box 44.2 lists the International Federation of Gynecology and Obstetrics (FIGO) classification of fibroids which is based on the location of the fibroid [40]. This classification helps in better communication and helps the referrer offer the patient a range of treatment options available for fibroids.

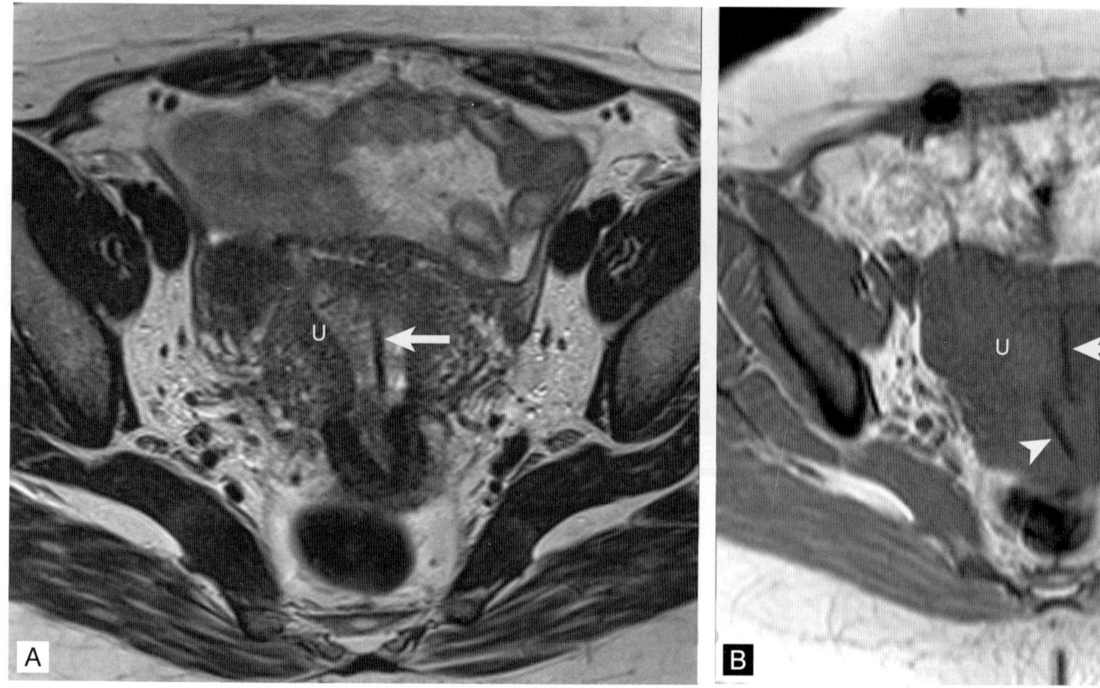

Figure 44.12 An IUCD (*arrow*) (Mirena) within the uterus (U) on a (A) transverse T2-weighted and (B) transverse T1-weighted MR image. Arrows, Mirena device within the endometrial cavity; arrowhead, string of the Mirena device; *IUCD*, intrauterine contraceptive device.

BOX 44.2 FIGO Classification of Fibroids [40]

Submucosal
Type 0: Pedunculated intracavitary fibroid (entirely within the endometrial cavity)
Type 1: <50% of the fibroid is intramural
Type 2: >50% of the fibroid is intramural
Other types
Type 3: Intramural fibroid in contact with endometrium
Type 4: Completely intramural fibroid, not in contact with endometrium or serosa
Type 5: Subserosal fibroid with >50% intramural component
Type 6: Subserosal fibroid with <50% intramural component
Type 7: Pedunculated subserosal fibroids
Type 8: Extrauterine fibroids like cervical or broad ligament fibroids
Hybrid leiomyomas
Fibroids which are in contact with both endometrium and serosa hence are represented by two of the above types

Clinical Presentation

Fibroids are the most common cause of enlargement of the non-gravid uterus. Although frequently asymptomatic, fibroids may cause abnormal menstrual bleeding (menorrhagia and dysmenorrhea), infertility, symptoms due to mass effect on adjacent organs (urinary frequency, constipation, and dyspareunia), and may present as palpable pelvic mass.

Imaging Features

Ultrasonography

- Fibroids have variable appearances on sonography. Classic fibroids are well defined, round to oval hypoechoic masses, often distorting the uterine contour, and the endometrial cavity. However, the presence of calcification, cystic, myxoid, and fatty degeneration of fibroid cause heterogeneity of echotexture
- Leiomyomas demonstrate alternate bands of shadowing and through transmission (venetian blind appearance; Fig. 44.13) due to transitional zones between fibrous and smooth muscle tissues within the fibroid [41]. Calcification is more common in fibroids seen in older women and it is seen as focal areas of increased echogenicity with dense acoustic shadowing
- During rapid growth, fibroids tend to outgrow their blood supply resulting in hemorrhagic degeneration and necrosis, which is seen as areas of low echogenicity or cystic areas within the fibroids. This is red degeneration, which is often seen during pregnancy and affects about 7–8% of pregnant women with fibroids, after HRT and after uterine artery embolization (UAE) [42]
- TVS is useful in diagnosing fundal fibroids in a retroverted uterus. TVS can also be used to demonstrate uterine origin of subserosal and pedunculated fibroids which simulate adnexal masses. However, the small field of view precludes optimal evaluation of large uterine fibroids and broad ligament fibroids. TAS is more appropriate for this purpose
- Three-dimensional ultrasonography is useful for demonstrating the relation of fibroid with endometrium and to assess the extent of intracavitary extension [43]
- Fibroids with greater than 50% extension into the endometrial cavity (FIGO type 1) are resected hysteroscopically [44,45]

MRI

- Box 44.3 gives the indications for MRI in a setting of leiomyoma. T2-weighted MRI is most useful for evaluating the morphology and the anatomy of leiomyomas
- Classic fibroids are well circumscribed, round to oval with homogenous T2 hypointense signal compared with the surrounding myometrium due to uniformly arranged whorls of smooth muscle cells with various amounts of intervening

	Subcategory of adnexal lesion	Features	Graphical representation	Imaging example
1	Unilocular cyst	No septations No solid projections Normal ovarian stroma not classified as solid Large peritoneal inclusion cyst with embedded ovary is classified unilocular.	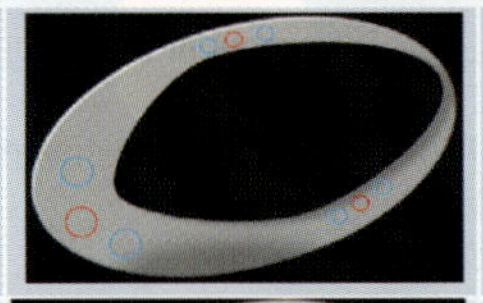	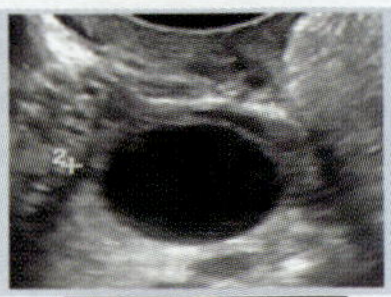
2	Unilocular-solid cyst	No septations Solid component or at least one papillary structure. Hydro or pyosalpinx may be classified in this category.	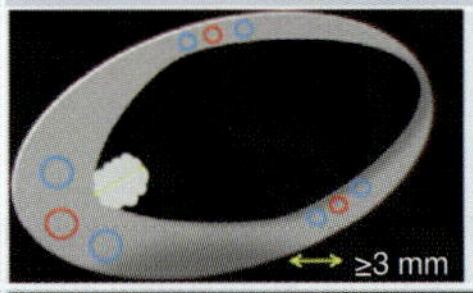 ≥3 mm	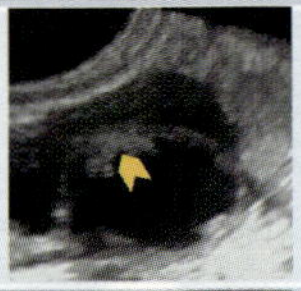
3	Multilocular cyst	At least one complete septum. No solid projections	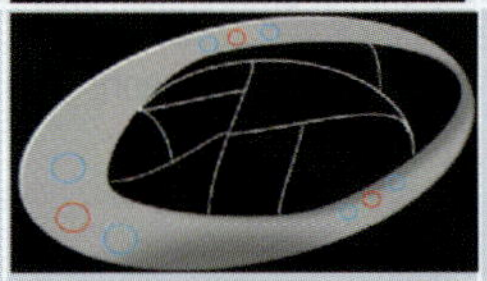	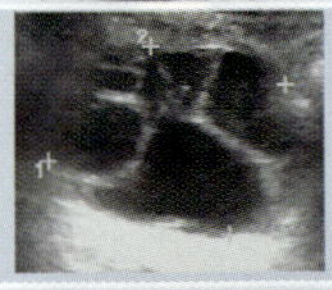
4	Multilocular-solid cyst	At least one complete septum. Solid component or at least one papillary structure.	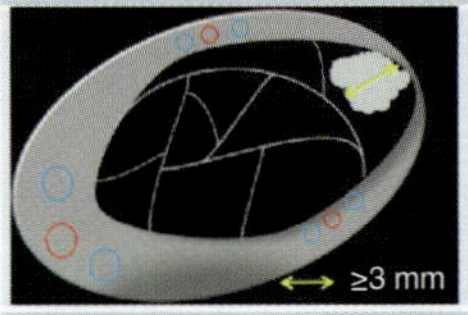 ≥3 mm	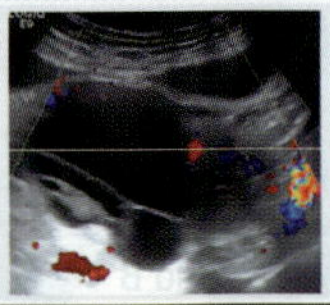
5	Solid	A lesion where solid component comprises > 80% of the lesion. Includes a large papillary projection filling almost the entire cyst.	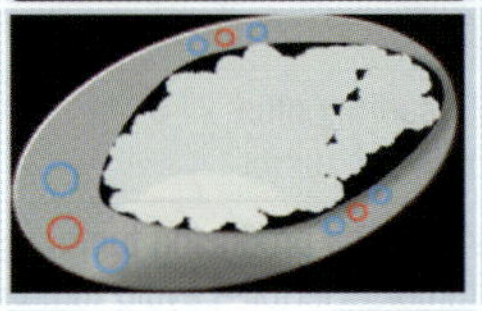	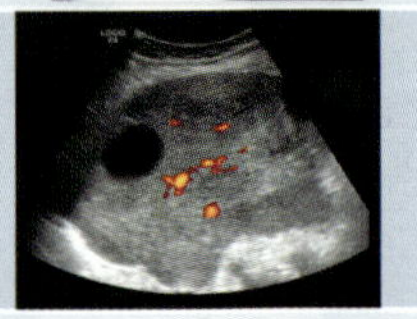
6	Incomplete evaluation	When it cannot be well assessed because of poor acoustic window due to body habitus, shadowing in heavy calcification (like in dermoid), excessive bowel gas etc		

Figure 45.7 Graphical depiction of sonological classification of adnexal lesions.

It is important to note that corpus luteum does not have solid component.

Owing to cyclical changes, larger physiological (functional) cysts are also very commonly encountered in female pelvic imaging, and they may undergo hemorrhagic changes as well. It is important to confidently identify them and label them as such to avoid patient distress and unnecessary investigations.

Simple Cysts: These are defined as round or oval anechoic structures on ultrasound with smooth thin walls, no solid component or septation, no internal color flow, and posterior acoustic enhancement. Extraovarian simple cysts also fall in this category.

On CT/MRI, simple or "benign-appearing" cysts are defined as oval or round unilocular lesions with uniform fluid attenuation/signal, with a regular or imperceptible wall (Fig. 45.9), without solid component or mural nodule, and *<10 cm in size.* In premenopausal women, cysts containing layering hemorrhage can still be considered "benign-appearing" and physiological. Most of these cysts resolve in 8–12 weeks. These vary in size and can still resolve spontaneously.

Accordingly, simple cysts up to 5 cm in premenopausal women and 3 cm in postmenopausal women do not need follow-up imaging [9,13]. Follow-up imaging may be needed to document resolution or stability in larger lesions. In these cases, SRU guidelines [13] recommend a 2–6-month follow-up in premenopausal woman (or 3–6-month follow-up in postmenopausal women) if early characterization of the lesion is desired, versus a 6–12-month follow-up for everyone if assessing growth is the primary goal. In contrast, O-RADS [9] simply recommends an 8–12-week follow-up in premenopausal women and a 1-year follow-up in postmenopausal women. *The cutoff can be raised from 5 cm to 7 cm (premenopausal) and 3–5 cm (postmenopausal) if there is excellent visualization and documentation of the lesion and one is confident of the diagnosis of simple cyst as per the SRU guidelines.* The incidence of malignancy in simple cysts <10 cm is very low.

Ruptured and Hemorrhagic Cysts: Physiologic cysts or corpus luteum can get complicated by rupture or internal hemorrhage. These typically present with pain during the expected time of ovulation, but may be seen incidentally as well.

A ruptured cyst appears as an irregularly shaped cyst with surrounding fluid on ultrasound. A hemorrhagic cyst (Fig. 45.10) can present as:

- Diffuse internal echoes or a clump of solid echoes within due to a clot
- *Reticular pattern of thin fine intersecting strands within the cyst (due to the fibrinous component of the clot); variably called "cob-web," "spider web," "fishnet," or "lacy" appearance: specific sign*
- Echogenic avascular component showing concave, straight, or angular margins: representing the retracted clot
- Internal mobility of the clot can be confirmed by changing the position of patient

TABLE 45.4 Differential Diagnosis of Adnexal Lesions—Morphology Based

Non-Neoplastic	Benign Neoplasms	Malignant Neoplasms	Miscellaneous
Cystic lesions Physiological cysts Hydrosalpinx, pyosalpinx, hematosalpinx Polycystic ovarian syndrome Ovarian hyper stimulation syndrome (OHSS) Peritoneal inclusion cyst Paraovarian cyst Obstructed uterine horn Appendiceal mucocele Bowel duplication cyst Lymphocele/lymphangioma	***Cystic lesions*** Mature cystic teratoma/dermoid cyst Cystadenomas	***Cystic lesions*** Borderline tumors	Ovarian torsion Ovarian vein thrombosis Ruptured ectopic pregnancy Endometriosis
Solid and solid-cystic lesions Pelvic inflammatory disease Broad ligament leiomyoma (fibroid) Adenomyoma Fibromatosis/desmoid tumor Nerve sheath tumors—schwannoma/ neurofibroma	***Solid and solid-cystic lesions*** Fibroma, thecoma, and fibrothecoma Stromal tumors Brenner tumor/transitional cell carcinoma Cystadenofibroma Struma ovarii	***Solid and cystic lesions*** Serous cystadenocarcinoma Mucinous cystadenocarcinoma Clear cell carcinoma Endometroid carcinoma Carcinosarcoma Ovarian metastases Yolk sac tumors Embryonal carcinoma Granulosa cell tumors	
		Solid lesions Dysgerminoma Ovarian metastases Primitive neuroectodermal tumor (PNET) Lymphoma Undifferentiated or unclassified	

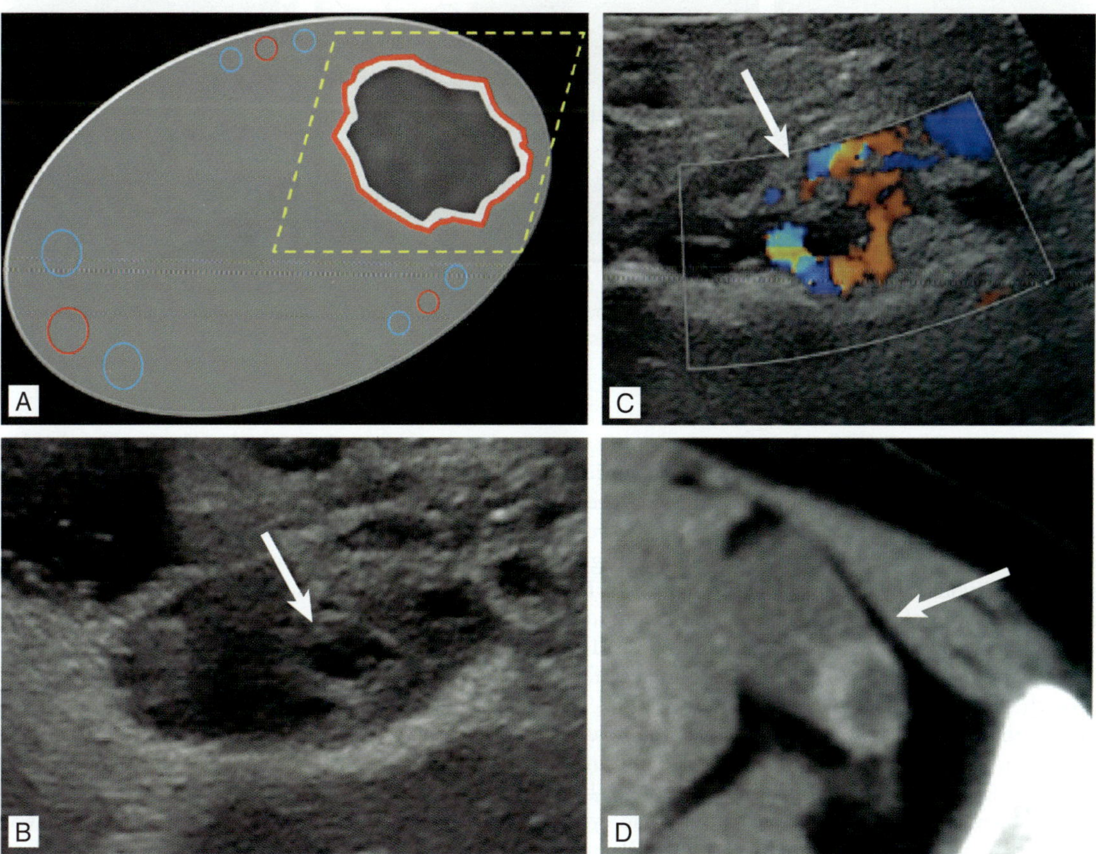

Figure 45.8 Typical appearance of corpus luteal cyst (A) as an irregular cyst with crenulated margins, internal echogenic content (proteinaceous or hemorrhagic), no solid component, with peripheral flow on Doppler—"ring of fire." Corresponding findings are observed on grayscale (B) and Doppler ultrasound (C). Axial CT (D) shows this peripheral vascularity as thick peripheral enhancement, not to be confused for a more sinister pathology.

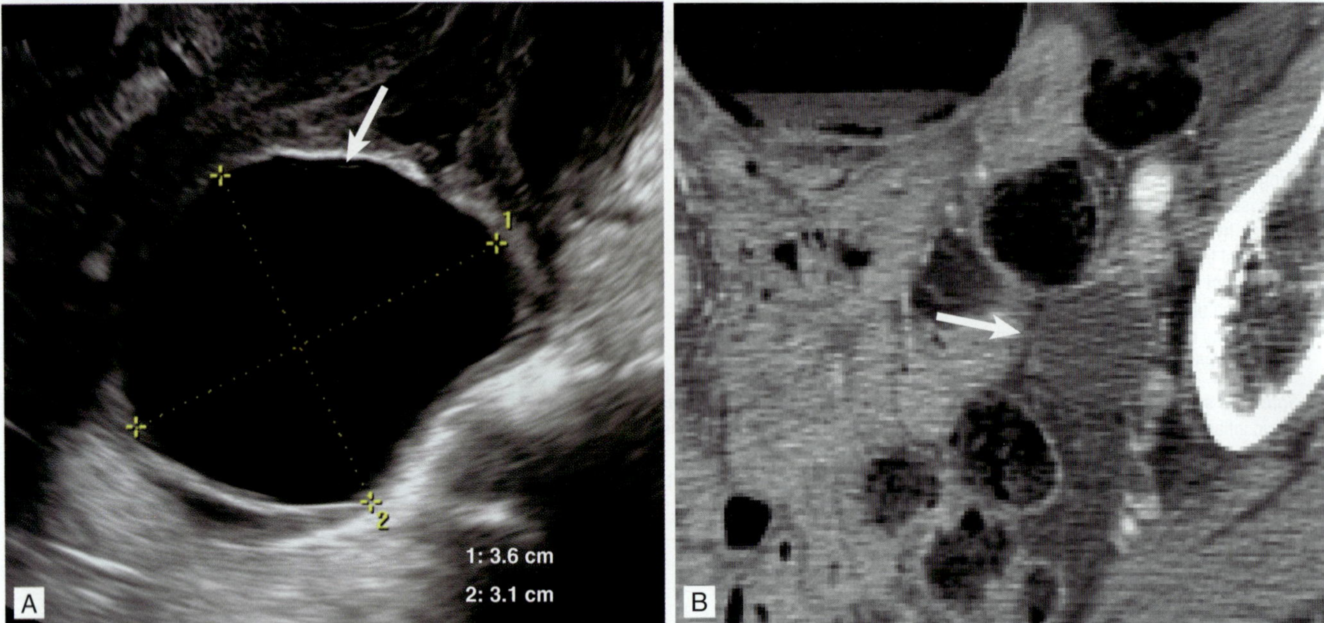

Figure 45.9 Simple adnexal cyst (*arrows*). Ultrasound (A) shows a round anechoic cystic structure with smooth thin walls and postacoustic enhancement. No septations, wall irregularities or solid component present. CT (B) shows a well-defined round unilocular lesion with uniform fluid attenuation, imperceptible wall, without solid component or mural nodule.

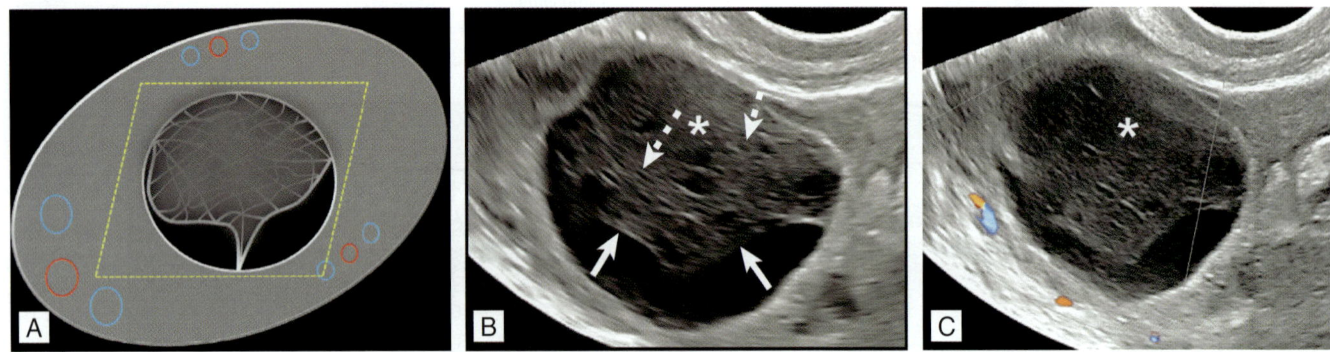

Figure 45.10 Hemorrhagic cyst. Graphical representation shows (A) a retracted echogenic clot with concave margins, with multiple internal septations: a "fishnet" appearance. Grayscale (B) and Doppler (C) ultrasound shows an echogenic retracted clot (*asterisk*) with concave margins (*arrows*) and no internal vascularity. Internal septations give rise to a "mesh-like" appearance (*broken arrows*).

Hemorrhagic cysts are commonly confused with endometrioma and can at times be difficult to differentiate. MRI is more promising in this regard. The T2 shading sign (described subsequently) has been regarded specific as it reflects different stages of bleeding. However, recent studies have showed that it can also be seen in hemorrhagic cysts too [14]. Endometriomas are usually T1 hyperintense due to early and late subacute stages of bleed while hemorrhagic cysts are usually iso to hypointense on T1 due to recent acute bleed. A "T2 dark spot sign" has been described [15] as a specific marker for chronic bleeds with hemosiderin foci in cases of endometrioma.

In cases when the distinguishing is not feasible, follow-up based on O-RADS or SRU guidelines is suitable: cysts measuring 5–10 cm in size should be called for follow-up USG in 8–12 weeks. In postmenopausal women, any sized hemorrhagic cyst should be evaluated by a specialist radiologist and/or MRI and with a gynecology consult.

There are certain physiological cysts and lesions unique to pregnancy. The most common is the theca lutein cysts seen in molar pregnancy; these develop due to high levels of ß-HCG. These are seen as bilateral diffusely bulky ovaries with multiple cysts. The apparent grouping of these cysts results in the so-called "spoke wheel" appearance. These cysts can also be sometimes seen with multiple pregnancies, fetal hydrops, or estrogenic tumors. In this situation, some authors label it hyperreactio luteinalis.

Hydrosalpinx, Pyosalpinx, and Hematosalpinx

The fallopian tubes are not seen routinely on USG but may be visualized as low-signal structures within the high-signal parametrial fat on T1W MRI. After pelvic inflammatory disease, scarring may occur within the fallopian tube causing hydrosalpinx. Two important signs to diagnose hydrosalpinx are the "waist" sign and the "string of bead" sign (Fig. 45.11).

- *The waist sign* refers to indentations along the walls of a tubular structure due to tortuosity resulting in a waist like narrowing and is highly specific for hydrosalpinx [16]

- *The string of beads* signs refers to nodular thickening of mucosal folds along a tubular structure adjacent to a normal ovary. This is also a specific sign for hydrosalpinx

Internal debris may be present in chronic hydrosalpinx. Although readily identified on ultrasound, the serpentine cystic tube adjacent to the ovary can also be demonstrated on MRI. Hematosalpinx and pyosalpinx also show a similar imaging appearance, making imaging distinction difficult. Patient history of ectopic pregnancy or endometriosis (hematosalpinx) versus fever and pain (pyosalpinx) helps (Fig. 45.12). On MRI, the typical SI of hemorrhage may be seen in hematosalpinx (Fig. 45.12), while pyosalpinx may show restriction of DWI.

Polycystic Ovarian Syndrome

Pathophysiology and Clinical Presentation: Approximately 12–21% of women in reproductive age group are affected with polycystic ovarian syndrome (PCOS). *This is a condition with a wide spectrum of clinical features, ranging from asymptomatic patients to the rare Stein–Leventhal syndrome, comprising amenorrhea, obesity, and hirsutism. Insulin resistance is now considered to be pathological basis of this entity.* Many, but not all, patients have measurable hormonal abnormalities, the commonest of which is a raised LH:FSH ratio, thought to cause excess androgen production by the ovaries. Clinical features of polycystic ovaries include:

- Oligomenorrhea and other menstrual disorders including dysmenorrhea and menorrhagia
- Hirsutism (70–80%)
- Acne
- Infertility (the commonest cause of anovulatory infertility)
- Recurrent miscarriage
- Obesity due to insulin resistance and impaired glucose tolerance and type 2 diabetes mellitus
- Endometrial hyperplasia (and rarely endometrial carcinoma)

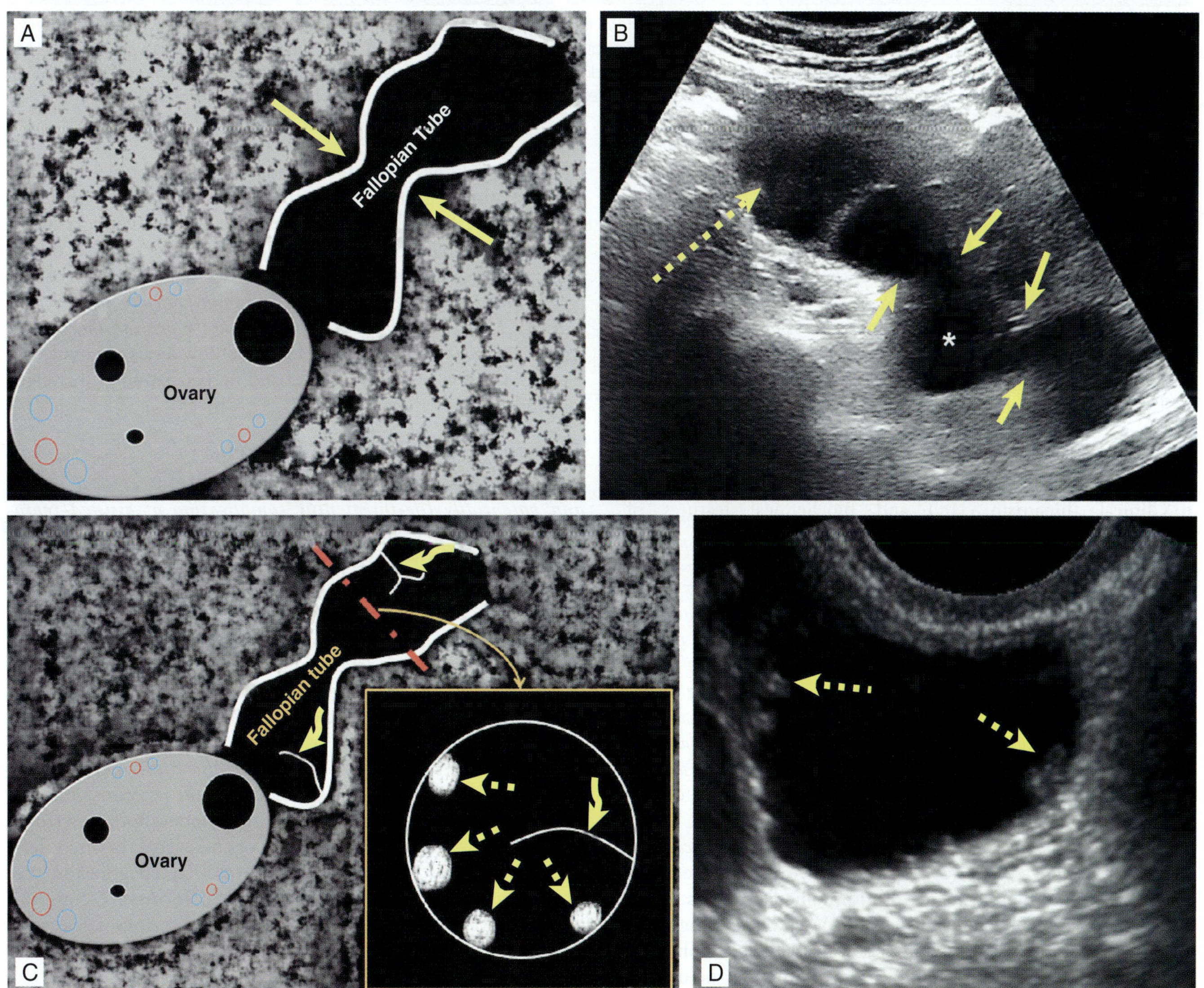

Figure 45.11 Ultrasound signs of hydrosalpinx. (A and B) Waist sign. Graphical (A) and USG (B) images show a dilated and tortuous fallopian tube (*asterisk*). Due to tortuosity, indentations develop along the walls with resultant "waist-like" narrowing (marked with *arrows*). On USG, fallopian tube is seen leading up to a endometriotic cyst (*broken arrow*). (C and D) String of beads sign. Graphical (C) and USG (D) images. Inset in C shows axial cuts through the dilated fallopian tube, demonstrating nodular thickening of mucosal folds (*dashed arrows*). *Curved arrows* depict incomplete septations formed by mucosal folds (D). (Reprinted with permission from: MM Horrow, Ultrasound of pelvic inflammatory disease, Ultrasound Q 20 (4) (2004) 171–179. doi:10.1097/00013644-200412000-00003. Copyright (2007) by Elsevier.)

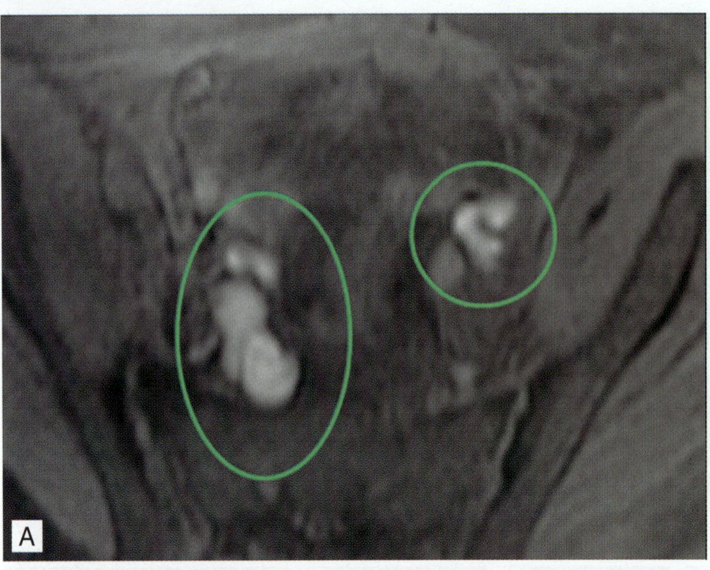

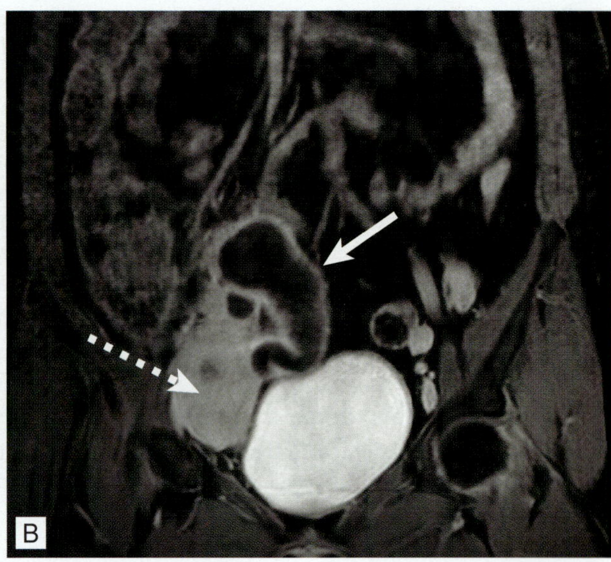

Figure 45.12 (A) Bilateral hematosalpinx in a patient with endometriosis. T1W fat-saturated noncontrast axial MRI (A) shows bilateral hyperintense tubular structures (*encircled*). There was no enhancing solid component on the subtraction images (not shown). (B) Pyosalpinx associated with tubo-ovarian abscess. Coronal postcontrast T1W fat-saturated image shows tortuous and dilated right fallopian tube (*solid arrow*) with thick enhancing walls, appearing adherent to an enlarged and heterogeneous right ovary (*dashed arrow*). (Courtesy for B: Dr. Mukesh Harisinghani, Harvard Medical School, Boston, USA.)

- Dyslipidemia, coronary artery disease, and cerebrovascular accidents
- Hypertension

Normally, multiple follicles are recruited and start growing in ovulatory phase, one of which becomes the dominant follicle and ruptures during ovulation. *PCOS occurs due to (androgen induced) nonprogression of one of these follicles into a dominant follicle, resulting in visualization of multiple possibly peripherally arranged follicles within the ovary, typically measuring 2–9 mm in diameter.*

The clinical, biochemical, and imaging diagnosis of PCOS remains a challenge. The Rotterdam ESHRE/ASRM Sponsored PCOS Consensus Workshop Group laid the criteria for PCOS diagnosis as [17]:

i. Menstrual irregularities: oligomenorrhea or amenorrhea
ii. Clinical (hirsutism, etc.) and biochemical features of hyperandrogenism
iii. USG/MRI showing typical polycystic ovaries

Imaging Features: *Patients with suspect ovulation disorders are ideally imaged between days 3 and 7 of menstrual cycle.* Patients with irregular cycles can be scanned at any time or between 3 and 7 days of hormonal-induced bleeding. The precise definition of polycystic ovaries on imaging is a matter of debate and constant evolution. The definition on USG as per recent consensus guidelines [18] is as follows:

1. One or both ovaries >10 cm^3 in volume. *This volume should be calculated with exclusion of dominant follicles or luteal cysts if present*
2. One or both ovaries showing ≥20 follicles per ovary; follicles are defined as cystic lesions of size 2–9 mm

It is important to note that these guidelines are not applicable to patients with young gynecological age (i.e., <8 years from the age of menarche) due to high incidence of multifollicular ovaries. These measurements are preferably made on TVS. When using older machines or while evaluating transabdominally; where number of follicles may be underestimated, ovarian volume may be used as diagnostic criteria. Typically, the central stoma may appear echogenic with numerous follicles distributed peripherally (Fig. 45.13). However, follicles can be distributed randomly, and peripheral distribution does not constitute a diagnostic criterion.

The Rotterdam group does not mention the utility of MRI. Some studies have shown MRI to be superior to USG in the measurement of ovarian volumes (with USG underestimating the volume) and demonstrating a greater number of follicles compared with USG. MRI may be helpful in certain scenarios such as young patients where transvaginal USG is not feasible. MRI features are like that of USG: enlarged ovaries with multiple follicles within (Fig. 45.14).

An imaging differential of PCOS is multifollicular ovaries [19] (Fig. 45.15), which represent a reversion to the ovarian morphology seen at the menarche. They are a feature of low levels of circulating estrogens and are seen in athletes and in association with weight loss and anorexia nervosa.

Ovarian Hyper Stimulation Syndrome

Pathophysiology and Clinical Presentation: *It is a serious and potentially life-threatening complication of assisted reproductive techniques.* It can occur either in secretory phase of menstrual cycle or in early pregnancy. It is a result of administration of clomiphene citrate, luteinizing hormone, or HCG, which can cause release of vasoactive compounds which increase capillary permeability. Two distinct components are rapid enlargement of developing follicles in both ovaries and sudden movement of fluid from intravascular space into third spaces like pleural and peritoneal spaces, which can cause sudden abdominal distension (ascites) and breathlessness (pleural effusions). The *rapid fluid movement also causes hemoconcentration (hypercoagulable state) and can result in acute thromboembolic episodes* with pulmonary thromboembolism, stroke, hepatic failure, renal failure, etc. When severe, this may lead to hypovolemia, disseminated intravascular coagulation, venous thrombosis, and even death. Mild forms are common and usually self-limiting.

Imaging Features

- Rapid enlargement of follicles: diffusely bulky ovaries (as large as 10 cm) with multiple cysts within (Fig. 45.16)
- Appearance of "spoke wheel" appearance, akin to that of theca lutein cysts
- Ascites and pleural effusions

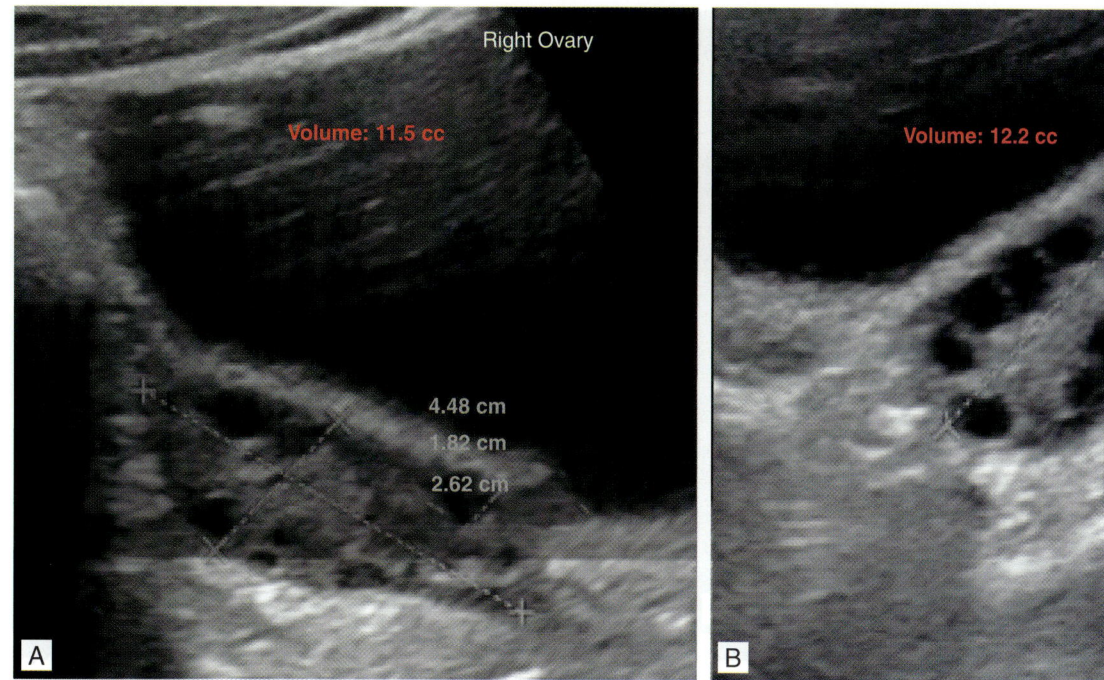

Figure 45.13 PCOS. USG (A shows right ovary and B shows left ovary) shows bilateral ovarian volumes >10 cc with multiple (>20) evenly sized follicles in a peripheral distribution, none >9 mm. The stroma appears echogenic on left. On biochemical examination, there was a raised LH:FSH ratio, consistent with PCOS.

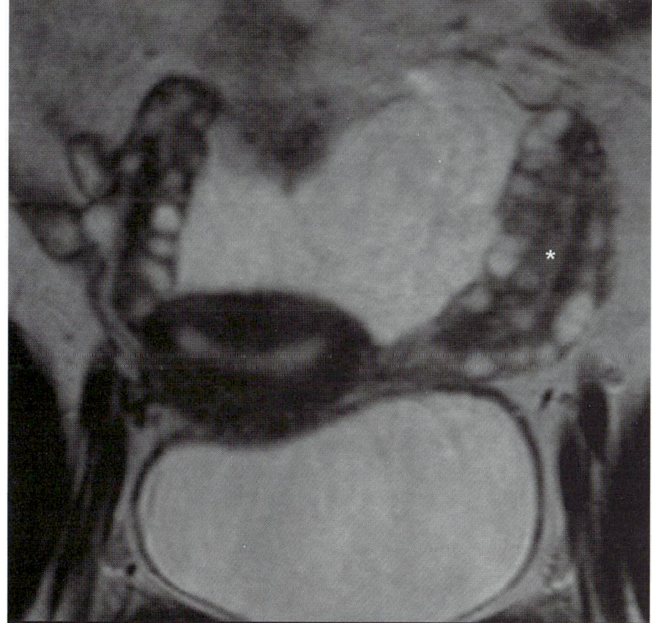

Figure 45.14 Coronal T2W MRI shows bilateral enlarged ovaries with multiple peripherally arranged follicles. Thickening of central stroma present on the left (*asterisk*), which is intermediate to mildly hyperintense. (Courtesy: Dr. Bharat Agarwal, Max Hospital, New Delhi, India.)

Peritoneal Inclusion Cyst

These occur in patients with history of pelvic surgery (most common), endometriosis or infection, due to fluid getting entrapped around the ovary due to adhesions (also called peritoneal pseudocysts). They may be asymptomatic or cause cyclical pain (*entrapped ovary syndrome*).

Peritoneal inclusion cysts have a pathognomonic appearance on ultrasound and MRI:

- Conform to the shape of the pelvic peritoneal cavity or of adjacent pelvic organs
- Do not cause mass effect (Fig. 45.17)
- A morphologically normal ovary present either within the cyst or along its periphery (*embedded ovary appearance*)
- Smooth internal septations may be seen owing to the underlying inflammatory/infective etiology

The classic history and imaging appearance is sufficient for the diagnosis. These are benign and if not causing much distress, can be left alone with follow-up as per recommended guidelines. Large cysts which cause distress or pain can be removed surgically.

Paraovarian Cyst

These are developmental in origin and arise usually *from mesonephric or paramesonephric duct remnants within the broad ligament.* They present as simple cysts on imaging seen separately from an adjacent normal ovary (Fig. 45.18). They may reach a large size but can be separated from the ovary by gentle pressure with the ultrasound probe or external pressure by hands on the lower abdomen. Rare complications include torsion and development of a paraovarian cystadenoma.

Obstructed Uterine Horn

This is with unicornuate uterus with a rudimentary horn. This *rudimentary horn may get obstructed and result in an apparent cystic adnexal lesion, usually containing blood products.* MRI is the investigation of choice.

Lymphocele

Lymphoceles are commonly seen in *postoperative cases of pelvic nodal dissection*, representing collections of lymphatic fluid. They have a fibrous wall with no epithelization. These are seen as *well-defined fluid collections with thin walls which usually do not show peripheral enhancement* (Fig. 45.19). These can be easily diagnosed in the appropriate postsurgical setting.

Other differentials of cystic adnexal lesions include appendicular mucocele, bowel duplication cyst, and a lymphangioma/venolymphatic malformation, discussed elsewhere in the textbook.

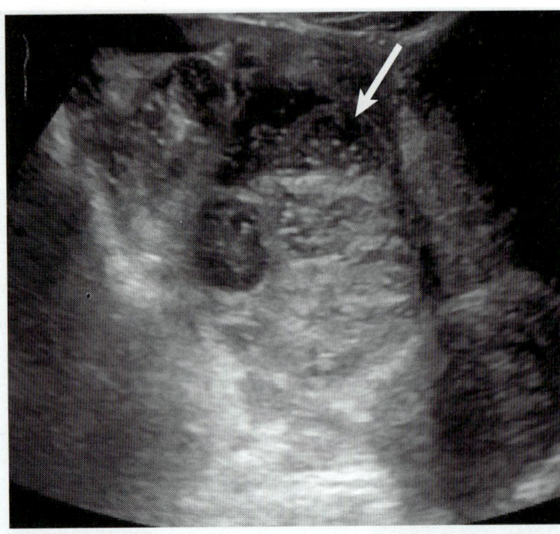

Figure 45.20 A 36-year-old lady with chronic pelvic pain. Axial ultrasound image shows a right adnexal complex cystic lesion, not seen separate from the ovary, along with a serpiginous tubular dilated fallopian tube with debris within (*arrow*). Probe tenderness was present. The patient had tubercular tubo-ovarian abscess. (Courtesy: Dr. Mukesh Harisinghani, Harvard Medical School, Boston, USA.)

- Salpingitis typically shows tubal tortuosity, hydrosalpinx and increased vascularity. The hydrosalpinx may contain internal echoes due to either blood or pus with fluid-debris level. Probe tenderness on transvaginal sonography should arouse a suspicion, although this can also be seen in endometriosis
- Doppler shows low impedance flow due to a surrounding inflammatory reaction with increased vascularity

CT usually shows:

- Free fluid in rectouterine pouch
- Thickening of pelvic soft tissue, particularly the uterosacral ligaments, along with reactive enlarged pelvic and para-aortic nodes
- Fat stranding of pelvic peritoneum. This fat stranding usually renders the normally sharp lateral uterine margins hazy. This is specific for acute PID and seen in up to two-thirds of cases [21]
- Fallopian tube thickening may be encountered
- Rarely, air foci may be encountered in tubo-ovarian abscess

Similar changes are demonstrated on MRI. It is more useful in distinguishing pyosalpinx from hematosalpinx.

Rarely patients present with right hypochondrial pain due to perihepatitis (Curtis–Fitz–Hugh syndrome). Adhesions around the liver have been described on ultrasound but are rare to see on imaging.

A mention needs to be made about pelvic TB, which shows imaging features similar to chronic PID. In general, tubal involvement in TB is most common and is generally bilateral. Hysterosalpingogram findings of genital TB are described elsewhere in the book.

Neoplasms

Epidemiology and Classification

Primary ovarian tumors are classified into three main types, according to their cells of origin: epithelial, sex cord stromal, and Germ cell tumors (GCTs) (Fig. 45.21). In addition, approximately 10% of ovarian tumors are metastatic. The distribution of these tumors

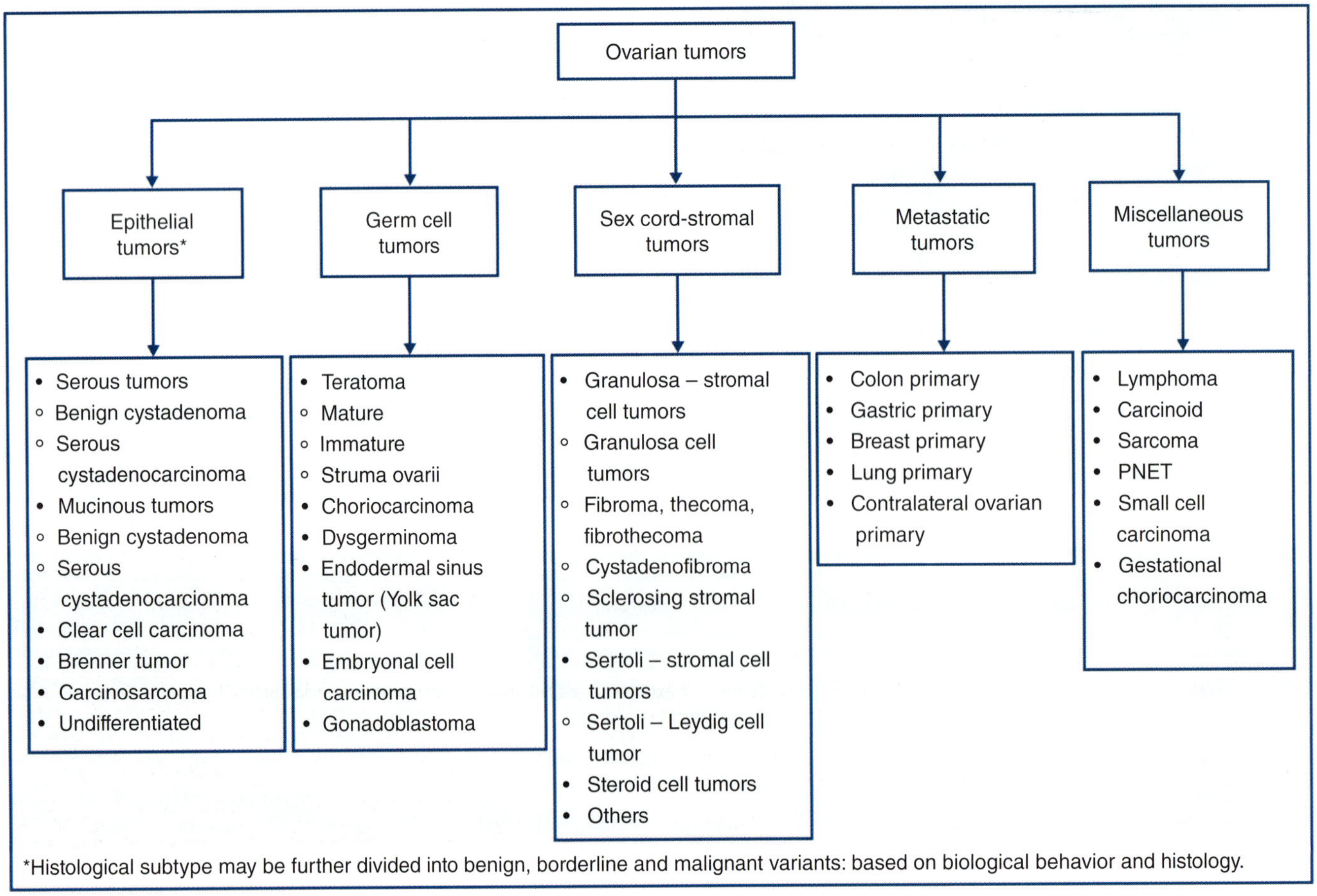

Ovarian tumors

Epithelial tumors*
- Serous tumors
  - Benign cystadenoma
  - Serous cystadenocarcinoma
- Mucinous tumors
  - Benign cystadenoma
  - Serous cystadenocarcionma
- Clear cell carcinoma
- Brenner tumor
- Carcinosarcoma
- Undifferentiated

Germ cell tumors
- Teratoma
  - Mature
  - Immature
  - Struma ovarii
- Choriocarcinoma
- Dysgerminoma
- Endodermal sinus tumor (Yolk sac tumor)
- Embryonal cell carcinoma
- Gonadoblastoma

Sex cord-stromal tumors
- Granulosa – stromal cell tumors
  - Granulosa cell tumors
  - Fibroma, thecoma, fibrothecoma
  - Cystadenofibroma
  - Sclerosing stromal tumor
- Sertoli – stromal cell tumors
  - Sertoli – Leydig cell tumor
- Steroid cell tumors
- Others

Metastatic tumors
- Colon primary
- Gastric primary
- Breast primary
- Lung primary
- Contralateral ovarian primary

Miscellaneous tumors
- Lymphoma
- Carcinoid
- Sarcoma
- PNET
- Small cell carcinoma
- Gestational choriocarcinoma

*Histological subtype may be further divided into benign, borderline and malignant variants: based on biological behavior and histology.

Figure 45.21 Pathological classification of ovarian neoplasms.

varies based on age and geographic distribution. However, *broadly, epithelial neoplasms constitute the most common subtype followed by GCTs*. As in other malignancies, ovarian neoplasms are broadly divided into benign and malignant variants. In addition, some ovarian tumors are classified as borderline, indicating that they have a better prognosis, with a lower risk of local recurrence and metastatic disease compared with malignant tumors.

Malignant ovarian tumors carry the highest mortality among gynecological malignancies in the West, whereas carcinoma cervix carries the highest mortality in south Asia [22]. Ovarian tumors are usually detected at an advanced stage, with extraovarian spread. *The ovary does not have a true capsule and is only covered by visceral peritoneum, making peritoneal spread common.* Lymphatic spread to the draining retroperitoneal nodes is also common.

The role of imaging is to characterize an adnexal mass as benign or malignant, identify the tumor histology, if possible, help guide further management, give a roadmap for surgery, and to assess response to chemotherapy. Although ovarian neoplasms are managed based on histopathology, a morphological approach is necessary for preoperative imaging work-up and risk stratification.

Risk factors for the development of ovarian carcinoma include:

- Family history of ovarian, breast, endometrial, or colorectal carcinoma including syndromes such as Lynch and Peutz–Jeghers
- BRCA1 or BRCA2 mutation—This confers a lifetime risk of 40% and 25%, respectively [23]
- Increased number of episodes of ovulation, for example, nulliparous woman, after treatment with ovulation induction agents, and menopause at late age
- Fertility treatments
- Smoking (particularly for mucinous tumors)

Some protection is conferred by:

- Multiparity
- Breast-feeding
- Use of oral contraceptives
- Tubal ligation
- Posthysterectomy status

Staging

Gynecological tumors are usually surgically staged using the International Federation of Gynecology and Obstetrics (FIGO) staging system (Table 45.5) [24].

Epithelial Neoplasms

Pathophysiology, Presentation, and Current Concepts

Ovarian *epithelial neoplasms* originate from the surface covering (surface epithelium) of ovaries, which is similar to peritoneal cavity lining (mesothelium). These peak in the sixth to seventh decade. Majority are benign, very few are borderline (~5%), and the rest malignant. Morphologically, most epithelial tumors are cystic and malignant variants develop solid components, presenting as solid-cystic masses.

TABLE 45.5 FIGO Staging of Ovarian Cancer

FIGO STAGING			
Stage		**Definition**	
I	IA	■ Confined to *one* ovary/fallopian tube ■ Intact capsule ■ No tumor on surface ■ No tumoral cells in ascites/peritoneal washing	
	IB	■ Involving *both* ovaries. ■ Rest all features of IA	
	IC *One or more ovaries* involved with *peritoneal spread*	IC 1	Tumor spillage intraoperatively
		IC 2	Capsular rupture before surgery (e.g., tumor biopsied), or tumor involving ovary/fallopian tube surface
		IC 3	Ascites or peritoneal washing showing positive cytology
II	IIA	Contiguous extension and/or implantation on uterus and/or fallopian tubes	
	IIB	Involvement of other pelvic intraperitoneal structures	
III	IIIA	III A1	III A1 (i) Metastatic retroperitoneal (RP) node, ≤10 mm
			III A1 (ii) Metastatic RP node, >10 mm
		III A2	Microscopic involvement of extrapelvic peritoneum (peritoneum above pelvic brim), regardless of RP nodal status
	IIIB	Macroscopic involvement of extrapelvic peritoneum (peritoneum above pelvic brim): ≤2 cm. *Hepatic or splenic capsular involvement included*	
	IIIC	Macroscopic involvement of extra-pelvic peritoneum (peritoneum above pelvic brim): >2 cm. *Hepatic or splenic capsular involvement included*	
IV	IVA	Malignant pleural effusion (positive pleural fluid cytology)	
	IVB	Distant parenchymal metastases to the liver, spleen, other abdominal organs, lungs, etc.	

Benign, Borderline, and Malignant Neoplasms

On histopathology, epithelial neoplasms are broadly classified as benign, borderline, and malignant and this determines their biologic behavior. Broadly, nuclear atypia, number of mitoses and presence of infiltrative component determines the nature of these tumors. Radiologically, the differentiation between the three can be challenging.

Borderline epithelial neoplasms are intermediate grade tumors between benign and malignant lesions and have also been described as "semimalignant," "atypical proliferative tumors," or "low malignant potential" tumors by some authors. On pathology, they show features of cellular atypia and high mitosis without infiltration of basement membrane/stromal invasion. *These tumors occur at a younger age compared with their malignant counterparts* (second to fourth decades) with some studies showing these to occur about 20 years earlier than invasive carcinomas [25].

These tumors may also have peritoneal disease in 10% of cases, and up to 25% may show associated regional adenopathy in advanced FIGO stages. *Borderline tumors tend to have an indolent course and much better prognosis than malignant neoplasms.* An important aspect on imaging is the presence of profuse solid papillary projections without any infiltrative or solid component, which can show mild to moderate contrast enhancement.

Table 45.6 lists imaging features which can help differentiate benign and malignant epithelial neoplasms.

In 2014, WHO further classified the malignant tumors into two groups: Group I and group II [26]. These have different pathological, morphological, and molecular abnormalities and biologic behavior (Table 45.7).

Serous and Mucinous Neoplasms

Pathophysiology and Clinical Presentation: These tumors form a spectrum ranging from benign cystadenomas, borderline tumors to malignant cystadenocarcinomas, which can be low grade or high grade.

- Serous tumors are the most common epithelial neoplasms and most common subtype of ovarian neoplasm overall. Among serous tumors, cystadenoma is the commonest variant (30%), whereas serous cystadenocarcinoma is the commonest malignant ovarian neoplasm
- Mucinous neoplasms constitute 10–15% of all epithelial neoplasms with up to 90% being benign or borderline
- Between 60–70% of serous tumors and 5–10% of mucinous tumors are bilateral
- Cystadenomas (serous and mucinous) account for up to half the tumors in the reproductive age and 80% of benign tumors in postmenopausal women

TABLE 45.6 Imaging Differences of Benign and Malignant Epithelial Neoplasms

Feature	Benign Epithelial Tumor	Malignant Epithelial Tumor
Morphology	Cystic with thin septations: can be multilocular	Cystic lesion with irregular thickened walls or septae, enhancing solid component or a large solid mass with cystic/necrotic areas within
Cyst wall	Regular or thin. Smooth mild contrast enhancement may be present	Irregular thickened walls. Both cyst wall and septae may show perceptible enhancement
Solid component/papillary projection	Absent	Present
Free fluid	Reactive mild free fluid may be present in the pouch of Douglas	Ascites usually present
Peritoneal implants	Absent	Can be present
Adenopathy	Absent	Metastatic adenopathy may be present

TABLE 45.7 Two Groups of Malignant Ovarian Epithelial Neoplasms

	Group I	Group II
Examples	▪ Low-grade serous cystadenocarcinoma ▪ Low-grade endometroid carcinoma ▪ Low-grade mucinous cystadenocarcinoma ▪ Low-grade clear cell carcinoma ▪ Malignant Brenner tumor	▪ High-grade serous cystadenocarcinoma ▪ High-grade endometroid carcinoma ▪ High-grade mucinous cystadenocarcinoma ▪ Undifferentiated cancer ▪ Carcinosarcoma
Course	Indolent tumors	Aggressive tumors
Presentation	▪ Detected early: Stage I or II ▪ Confined to ovaries	▪ Detected late: Stage III or IV ▪ Usually have extraovarian spread at presentation
Pathogenesis	▪ 25% of all epithelial malignant neoplasms ▪ Share molecular and morphological similarities with benign counterparts. ▪ Likely develop from benign tumors through intermediate step of borderline tumor	▪ 75% of all epithelial malignant neoplasms ▪ Do not share molecular and morphological similarities with benign counterparts ▪ Likely develop from extraovarian sites (fallopian tubes most commonly) and probably involve the ovaries secondarily ▪ Arise likely de novo rather than from benign counterparts
Prognosis	Usually good	Poor

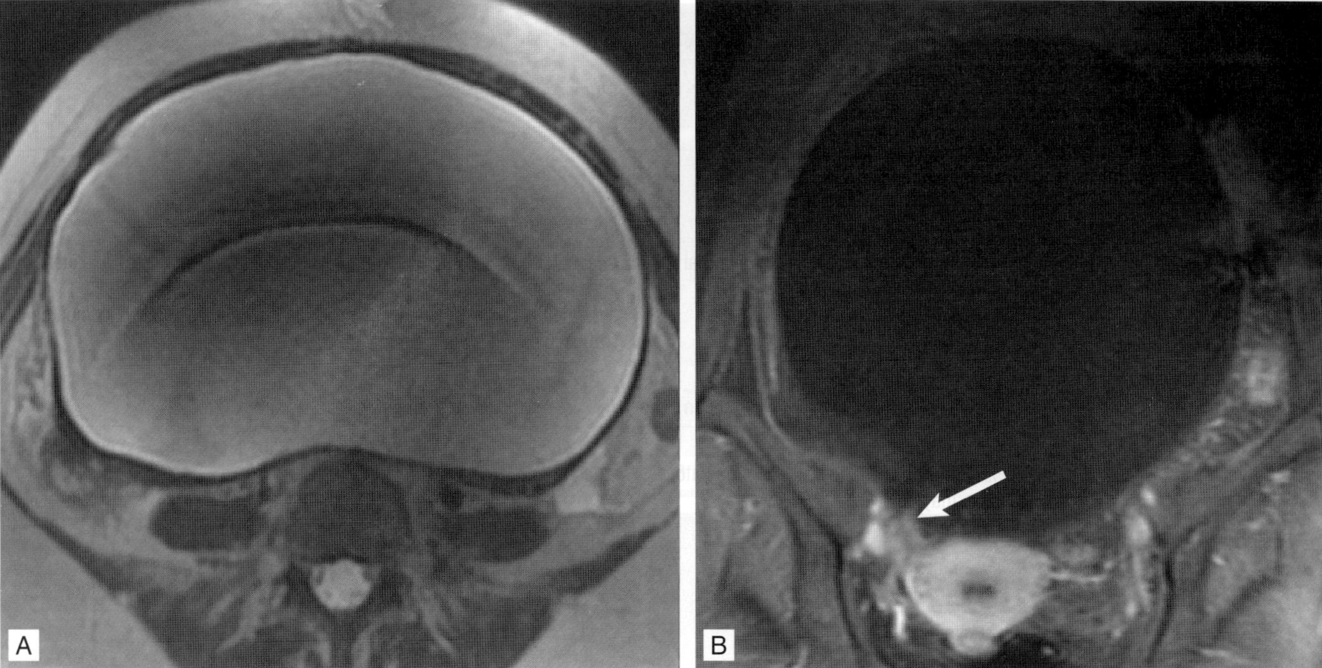

Figure 45.22 Serous cystadenoma. Axial T2 (A) and coronal postcontrast T1WI (B) show a cystic abdominopelvic lesion without any septations or solid component. There is mild smooth wall enhancement, with enhancement of broad ligament structures (*solid arrow*) leading to the cystic lesion, suggestive of right ovarian origin. Note artifacts in A due to dielectric effect.

- Serous tumors contain serous or fluid-like contents and mucinous tumors contain mucin
- Serous tumors' lining resembles those of fallopian tubes' internal lining. Serous cystadenocarcinomas can resemble primary peritoneal carcinomas on pathology
- The lining of mucinous tumors can resemble that of intestinal mucosa (intestinal type) or lining of endocervix (endocervical type)
  - Endocervical variants are usually bilateral, can have coexisting endometriosis and closely resemble serous borderline neoplasms
  - Intestinal type is commonly associated with pseudomyxoma peritonei and may often actually be a metastasis from an appendicular primary
- Borderline mucinous tumors tend to be larger in size compared with serous counterpart (nearly twice the size)

Imaging Features

Serous and Mucinous Cystadenomas

- They have overlapping features on imaging (Figs. 45.22 and 45.23), and essentially present as thin-walled cystic lesions with or without internal septations and echogenic contents. They have no solid component or papillary projections
- Even though they appear benign on imaging, at pathology, these may show small foci of borderline or malignant neoplasm. The imaging differences between serous and mucinous cystadenoma have been summarized in Table 45.8 but distinguishing between them on imaging is often challenging

Malignant Cystadenocarcinomas

- Usually present as cystic lesions with or without solid component with thick enhancing septations, papillary projection or large solid components (Fig. 45.24)

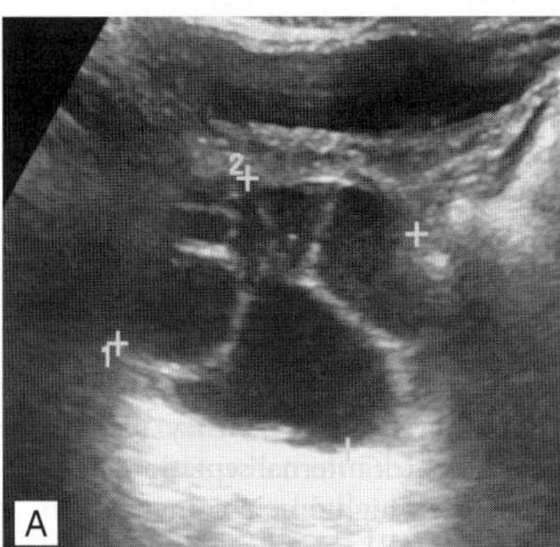

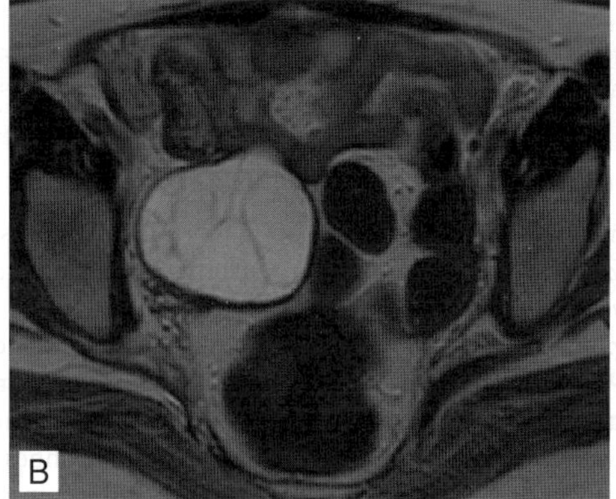

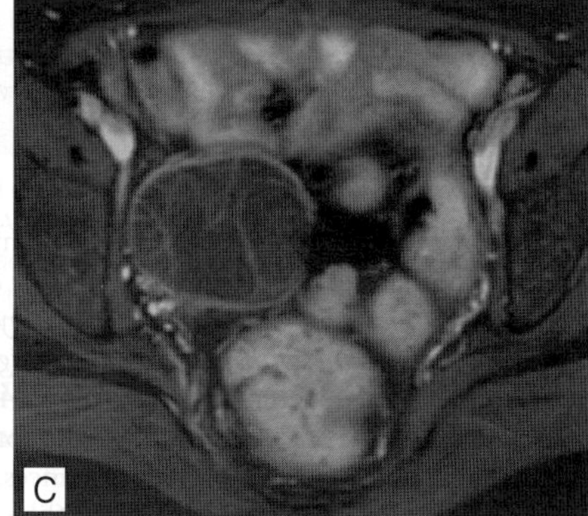

Figure 45.23 Mucinous cystadenoma. Ultrasound (A) shows a multilocular right adnexal cyst with no vascularity on Doppler (image not shown). Axial T2W (B) and postcontrast fat-saturated T1WI (C) show a smooth-walled right adnexal multilocular cystic lesion with multiple thin mildly enhancing internal septations. No solid component present.

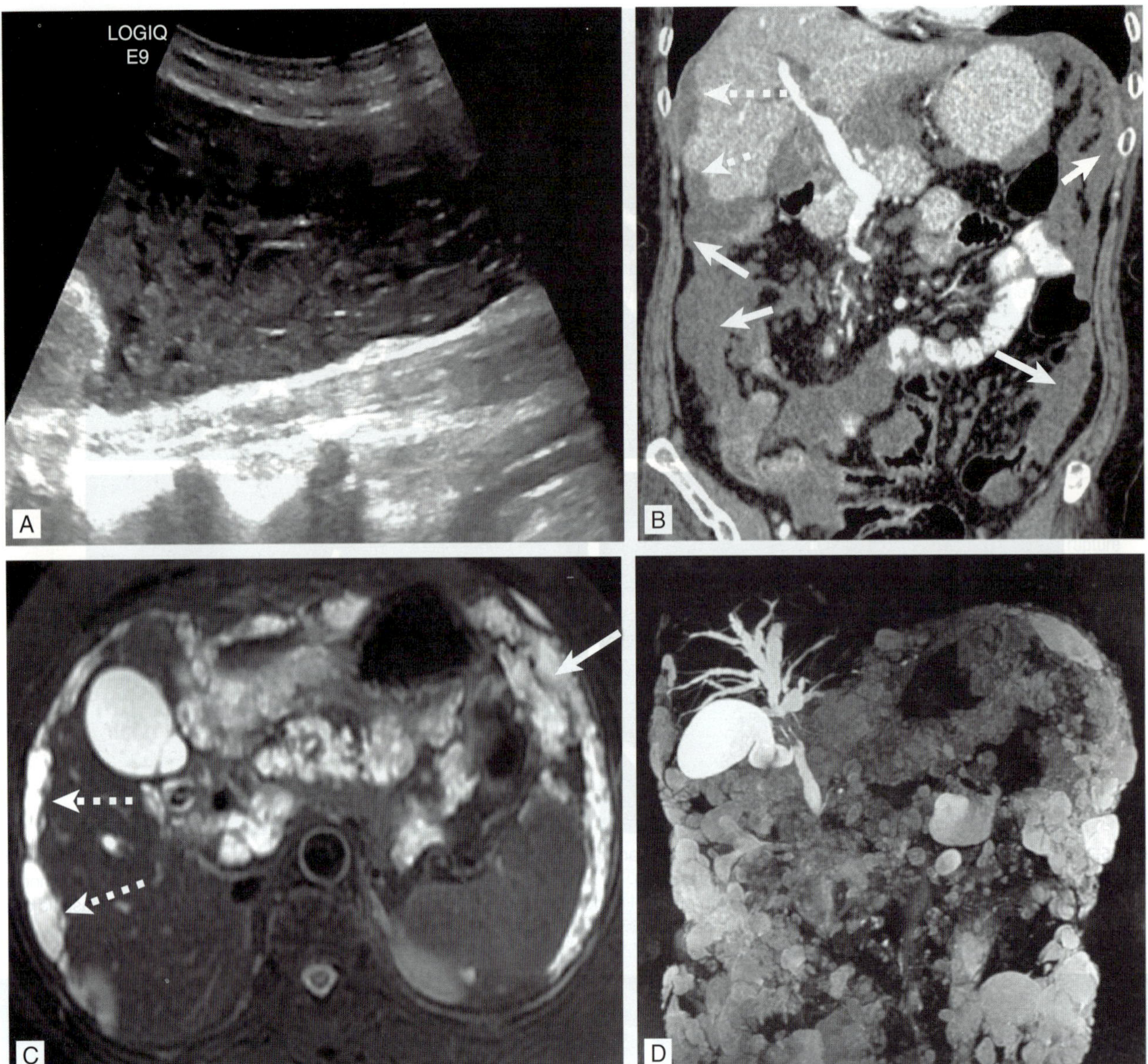

Figure 45.27 Pseudomyxoma peritonei. Right flank ultrasound image (A) shows large volume "ascites" which appears echogenic and "jelly"/"mucinous" like. Coronal CECT (B) shows multiple deposits (*arrows*) showing fluid-like attenuation, with characteristic scalloping of the liver (*dashed arrows*). Axial fat-saturated T2WI (C) shows these mucinous deposits (*arrows*) appearing fluid like. Scalloping of the liver (*broken arrows*) seen again. Coronal heavily T2W maximum intensity projection (MIP) (D) shows the extend of mucinous deposits in the abdominal cavity.

borderline. Most are detected incidentally on resected specimen. These may be associated with synchronous transitional tumor of urinary bladder or with another epithelial ovarian tumor in about 30% cases. Surgical resection is curative.

Imaging Features

- Usually predominantly solid and small but can present as a multilocular cystic lesion with solid component (Fig. 45.29)
- Show amorphous calcifications in more than half the cases
- T2 hypointense on MRI due to their fibrous component, with mild to moderate enhancement, mimicking a fibroma
- Borderline Brenner tumors are usually solid cystic in nature with solid component occurring as polypoidal lesions or papillary projections [27]. These mostly have a biologically benign behavior. Malignant tumors show similar morphology as borderline tumors but may be bilateral
- Ovary confined malignant Brenner tumors have a stage-by-stage better prognosis than malignant serous tumors

Endometroid Carcinoma

Pathophysiology and Clinical Presentation: As the name suggests, these epithelial *tumors resemble uterine endometrium*, and account for 10–15% of all epithelial tumors, with a peak in fifth to sixth decade of life. About half of these are bilateral and up to 30% are associated with endometrial thickening due to endometrial hyperplasia or carcinoma. These are also commonly associated with endometriosis. Although almost always malignant (without a benign or borderline counterpart), they usually present at an early stage (i.e., without peritoneal disease), and have better prognosis.

Imaging Features: Imaging findings are nonspecific (Fig. 45.30).

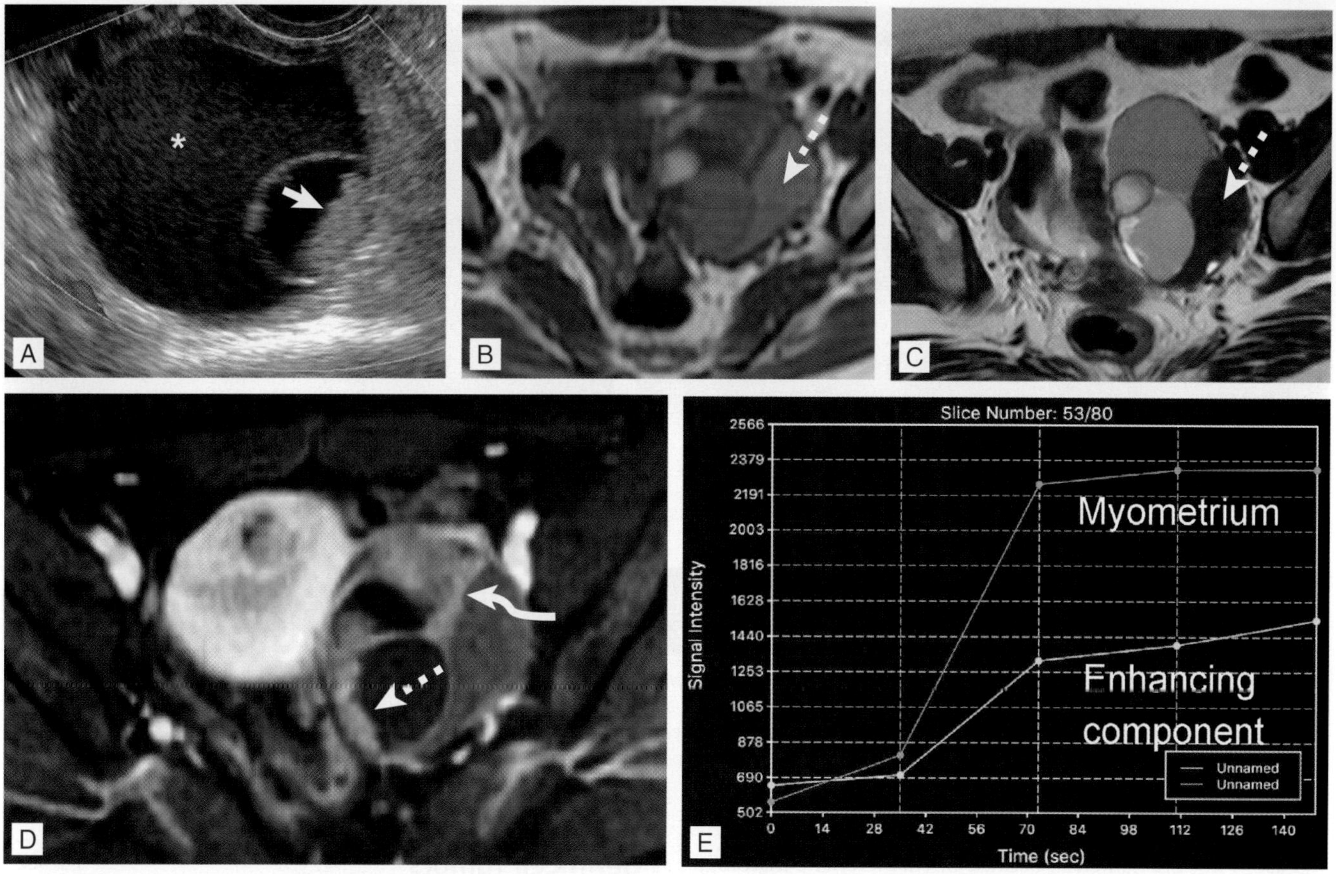

Figure 45.28 Borderline serous neoplasm. Ultrasound (A) shows a multilocular cyst with low level internal echoes (*asterisk*) and papillary projections (*arrow*). Axial T1W and T2W MRI (B and C) show multilocular cyst with areas of hemorrhage/proteinaceous content (*dashed arrows*). Dynamic postcontrast study (D) shows thick moderately enhancing septa (*curved arrow*) and enhancing papillary projections (*dashed arrow*) with a type II curve (E). No infiltrative component or peritoneal implants were seen.

- They usually demonstrate both solid and cystic components; hemorrhagic contents may also be present
- When arising from a pre-existing endometrioma, an enhancing mural nodule may be present in an otherwise classic endometrioma
- Features of endometrial carcinoma or hyperplasia may be seen

Clear Cell Carcinoma

Pathophysiology and Clinical Presentation: These are relatively rare epithelial ovarian neoplasms (5% of the total ovarian epithelial tumors) with a peak in the fifth decade of life. *Nearly three-fourths of patients have pre-existing endometriosis.* Majority of these present at stage I, with 20% having bilateral

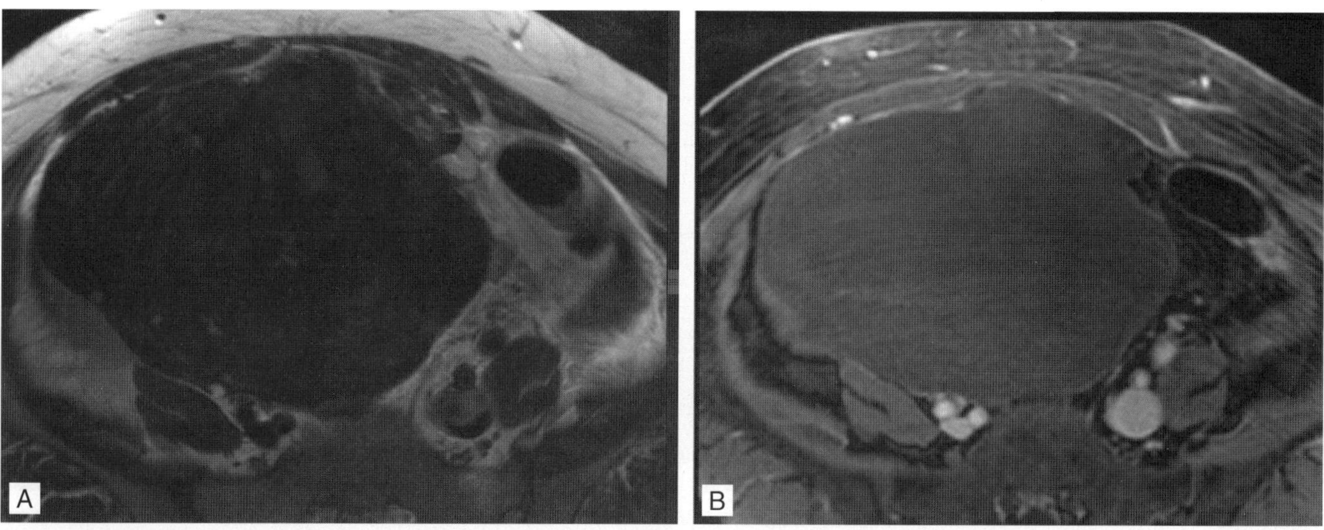

Figure 45.29 Brenner tumor. Axial T2 (A) and contrast-enhanced T1W fat-saturated (B) images show a large lobulated T2 hypointense right adnexal mass with minimal contrast enhancement.

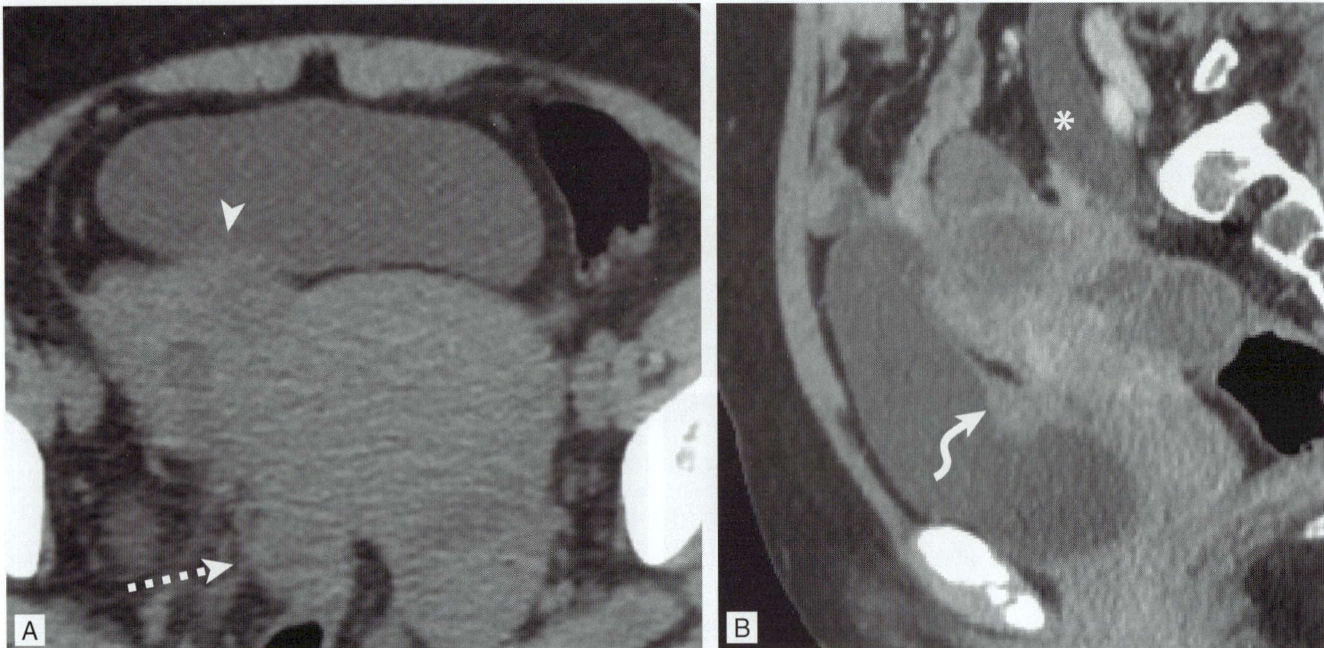

Figure 45.30 A 47-year-old female with known endometriosis presenting with hematuria. Axial noncontrast CT (A) shows classical hyperdense, bilateral ovarian endometriotic cysts, and a deposit along the uterosacral ligament (*dashed arrow*). Note the suspicious infiltration involving the posterior bladder wall (*arrowhead*), better seen on the sagittal postcontrast image (*curved arrow* in B—sagittal CECT image) along with right hydroureter (*asterisk*). A cystoscopic biopsy of the bladder component showed endometrioid carcinoma of the ovary.

disease. They are named so because of characteristic histologic appearance comprising of clear cells (also known as hobnail cells). Benign and borderline variants of clear cell tumors are again rare. They may be associated with thromboembolic events, hypercalcemia (paraneoplastic syndrome), and Lynch syndrome (which is also associated with endometroid carcinoma and endometrial carcinoma).

Imaging Features: They have a nonspecific imaging morphology (Fig. 45.31) ranging from completely solid to solid-cystic to a cystic mass with large internal polypoidal solid component. A typical endometrioma with enhancing solid component should raise suspicion of clear cell or endometroid carcinoma [28].

Germ Cell Tumors

GCTs arise from germ cells within the substance of ovaries, likely from primordial germ cells. These are the female counterparts of testicular GCTs. They secrete various hormones and can be diagnosed based on the tumor markers.

Mature Cystic Teratoma/Dermoid Cyst

Pathophysiology and Clinical Presentation: Dermoid cysts (mature cystic teratomas) are the *most common benign neoplasm in women of reproductive age group, accounting for 20% of all ovarian tumors.* Approximately 10–15% are bilateral. These arise from more than one

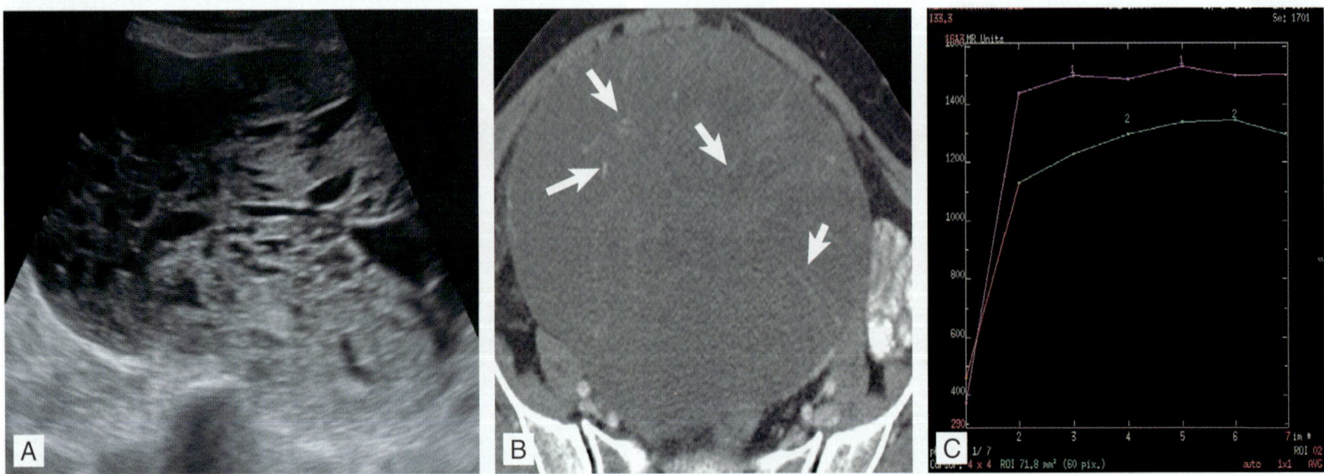

Figure 45.31 A 52-year-old female presenting with pelvic lump. Ultrasound (A) showed a large multilocular pelvic cystic mass with thick mobile internal echoes. CECT (B) showed multiple enhancing septations within (*arrows*) without peritoneal disease. MRI showed type III curve (C), indicating malignancy. Histopathology showed right ovarian clear cell carcinoma.

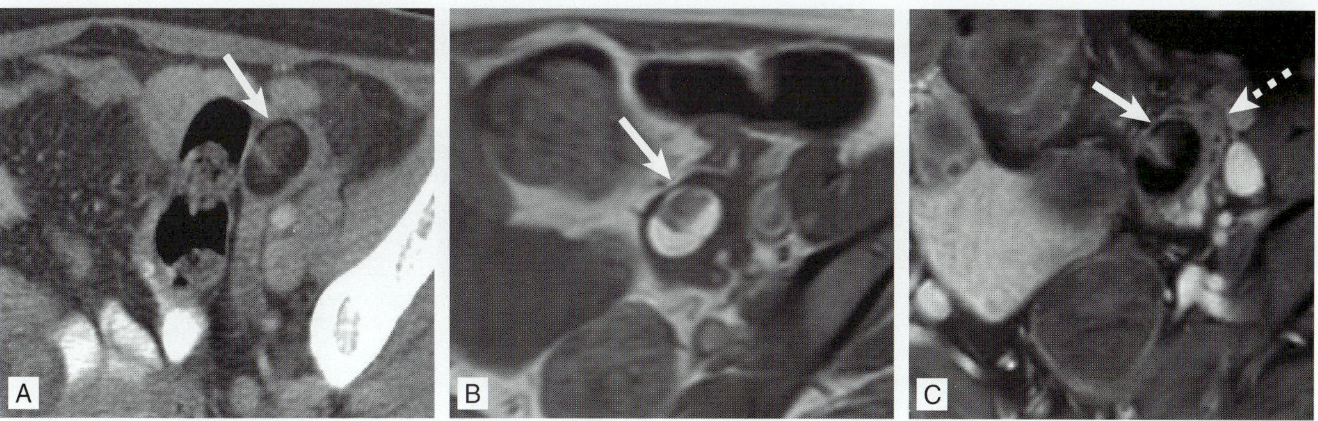

Figure 45.32 Dermoid cyst. Axial CECT (A), axial T1W (B), and axial T1W fat-saturated postcontrast (C) images show a fat containing left adnexal lesion (*solid arrow*), with the fat getting completely suppressed in C. Note the adjacent normal ovarian follicles (*dashed arrow* in C).

of the three embryonic layers (endoderm, mesoderm, and ectoderm). They can be both solid and cystic. If a teratoma contains components from predominantly one of the three layers, they may be referred to as specialized or monodermal (struma ovarii containing thyroid tissue being an example). Almost all dermoid cysts contain lipid material, either sebaceous or adipose tissue, which demonstrates a similar signal to subcutaneous fat. A focal internal protuberance (Rokitansky nodule) containing hair, teeth, muscle, bone, neural tissue, thyroid tissue, cartilage, etc. can be demonstrated. The cyst wall is most commonly lined by squamous epithelium.

Malignant degeneration occurs in less than 2% [28]. Most common malignancies encountered are squamous cell carcinoma and papillary carcinoma of thyroid. Other related complications include rupture (which can lead to chemical peritonitis), ovarian torsion, autoimmune hemolytic anemia, secondary infections, and rarely, anti–N-methyl-D-aspartate receptor encephalitis, a paraneoplastic syndrome.

Imaging Features

These can be confidently diagnosed on imaging by identifying macroscopic fat within the lesion (Fig. 45.32).

Ultrasound: They typically present as a unilocular cystic mass with solid component, with a few showing septae within the cystic component. Majority are 5–15 cm in diameter. The solid components are usually hyperechoic due to fat or calcification. The echogenic nature of the cyst can also make it difficult to differentiate from bowel; hence the size of a dermoid cyst may be underestimated with ultrasound. *Calcification of Rokitansky nodule may demonstrate "twinkling" artifact on Doppler study.* Various descriptors have been recommended to standardize reporting of dermoid cysts (Fig. 45.33).

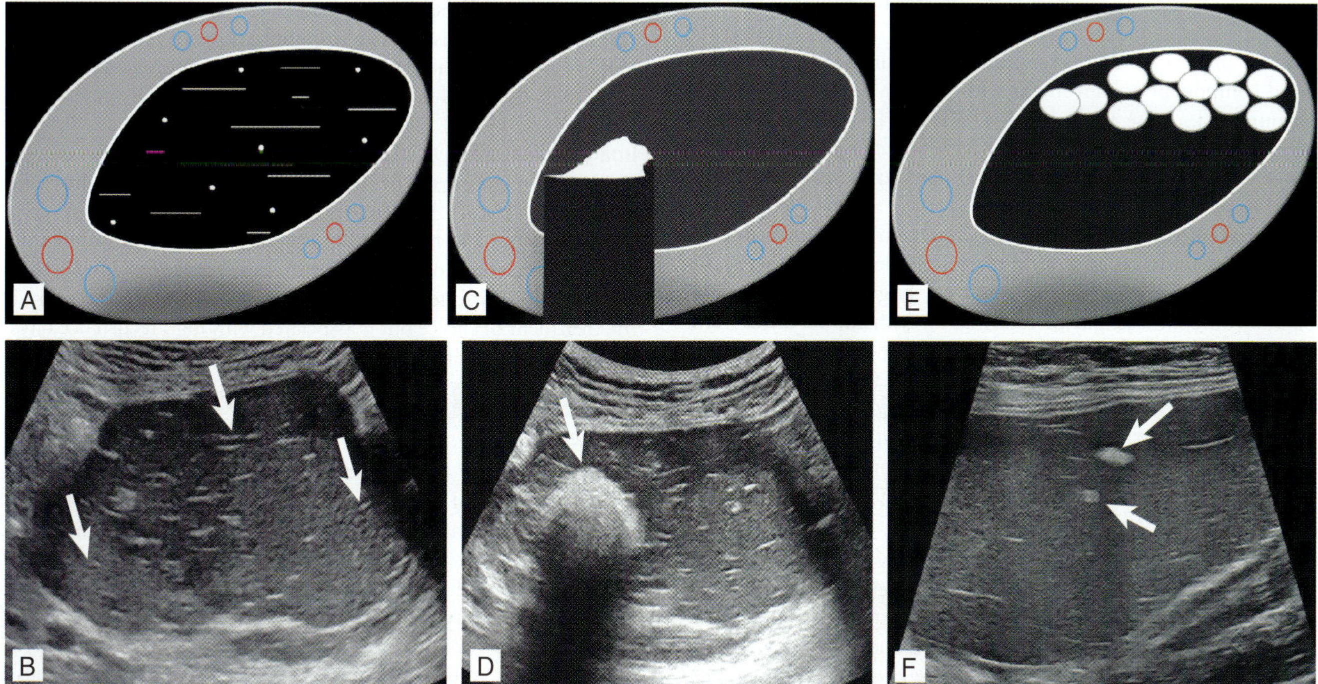

Figure 45.33 Various O-RADS. Ultrasound descriptors of dermoid cyst. (A and B) *Hyperechoic lines and dots*. Represent tufts of hair: lines on longitudinal and dots on transverse sections. Referred by many as *"dermoid mesh"* and *"dot and dash."* Ultrasound image (B) with *arrows* marking the *lines and dots*. (C and D) *Acoustic shadowing from a hyperechoic component*. Commonly referred as "*Tip of the iceberg sign*." The hyperechoic component (*arrow* in D) is commonly referred as "*Rokitansky Nodule*." (E and F) *Floating hyperechoic nondependent spherical structures*. Very specific, rarely seen (*arrows* in F). Commonly referred as "*dermoid balls*."

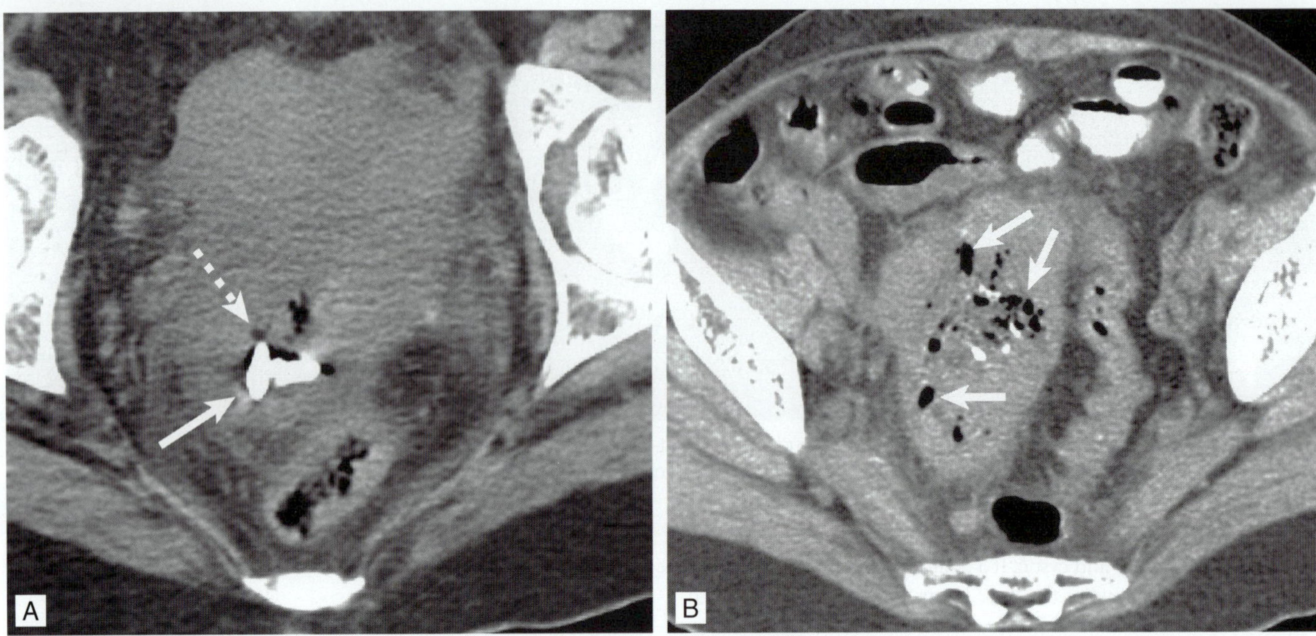

Figure 45.34 Malignant degeneration of dermoid. Axial images show a large pelvic soft-tissue mass with foci of fat (*dashed arrow* in A) and chunky calcification (*solid arrow*) in A, suggestive of teratoma. There is loss of fat plane with the adjacent bowel with air foci within (*solid arrows* in B), suggesting fistulous communication. Final diagnosis was malignant degeneration (to squamous cell carcinoma) in ovarian teratoma.

When confirmation or additional information is required, CT or MRI can be helpful.

CT/MRI: CT shows typical fat containing areas, soft-tissue component, and presence of bone/coarse calcification/tooth within. These can be heterogeneous on MRI, but presence of macroscopic fat is diagnostic. Approximately 15% dermoids have none or very small foci of fat. Such fat-poor dermoids can be identified as chemical shift artifact at the fat-fluid interface and on fat-suppressed sequences [29]. Importantly, diffusion restriction may be present in solid component, even in benign dermoids. Solid component enhancement with rarely type III curve may be encountered. These findings on DWI and DCE should not be confused with malignant transformation. *Capsular penetration is the most important sign to indicate an underlying malignancy* [29] (Fig. 45.34).

Management: Smaller dermoid cysts with typical features can be observed with serial ultrasounds. Larger dermoid cysts in postmenopausal women may be removed surgically. In premenopausal women, these may be followed up with annual ultrasounds if confident of diagnosis. If in doubt, a repeat USG in 8–12 weeks may be performed to confirm stability and then, annually thereafter. In postmenopausal women, when confident of diagnosis of dermoid cyst, these may be followed up with annual USG. If there is a change in size or morphology on follow-up, further evaluation with MRI and gynecological evaluation is warranted.

Struma Ovarii

Struma ovarii is a specialized mature teratoma comprising entirely or predominantly of thyroid tissue (at least 50% of the total tumor volume should be thyroid tissue to label as struma ovarii on pathology) [30]. This *can be a source of ectopic thyroid hormone production* and can present with features of hyperthyroidism (<10% of patients). These have nonspecific imaging features and most commonly present as solid cystic lesions. About 30% of patients can show associated ascites. The *solid component can be hyperdense on plain CT* like thyroid due to accumulated iodine. Transformation to papillary carcinoma of thyroid is a rare complication.

Immature Teratoma

Pathophysiology and Clinical Presentation: Immature teratomas are malignant counterparts of mature cystic teratoma, containing immature or embryonal tissue admixed with mature tissues on histopathology. These may be associated with raised β-hCG or AFP levels due to associated trophoblastic and yolk sac component, respectively. These are rare (<1% of all teratoma), and present in women <20 years of age. They are usually large at presentation (median size 18 cm) [28].

Imaging Features On imaging, they are *larger and more heterogeneous than mature cystic teratomas,* with increased enhancing solid component (Fig. 45.35). They demonstrate smaller and more scattered foci of fat and have smaller irregular calcifications unlike the coarse calcifications of dermoid. Immature teratomas grow rapidly and may demonstrate capsular penetration on imaging. Surgery is the treatment of choice but is associated with high recurrence rates. Peritoneal deposits may be present at presentation or at the time of recurrent disease, with similar imaging features.

Dysgerminoma

Pathophysiology and Clinical Presentation: Dysgerminomas are counterparts of testicular seminomas in females (usually <30 years age) and comprise of primordial germ cells on histopathology. These can be bilateral in up to 20% patients. Many show elevated levels of lactate dehydrogenase, which may be used for post-treatment surveillance to look for residual/recurrent disease [31]. Syncytiotrophoblastic elements may be present in up to 5% of tumors, causing elevated β-hCG levels. Some tumors also show elevated AFP levels. They are typically solid and stage 1 at presentation. Distant spread is commoner through lymphatic route, with retroperitoneal nodes being the first to get involved. Surgical excision is the treatment of choice, although these tumors are also radiosensitive.

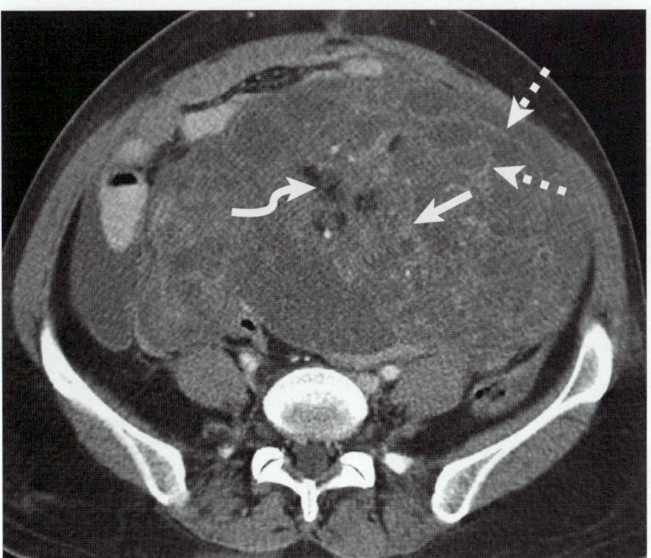

Figure 45.35 Immature teratoma in a 14-year-old girl. Axial CECT shows a large heterogeneous predominantly cystic mass, with enhancing septations (*dashed arrows*) and enhancing solid components (*solid arrow*), with calcifications present along the septae and solid component. Macroscopic fat (*curved arrow*) can also be seen. Compared with mature teratomas, there are scant areas of fat with relatively more septations and solid components.

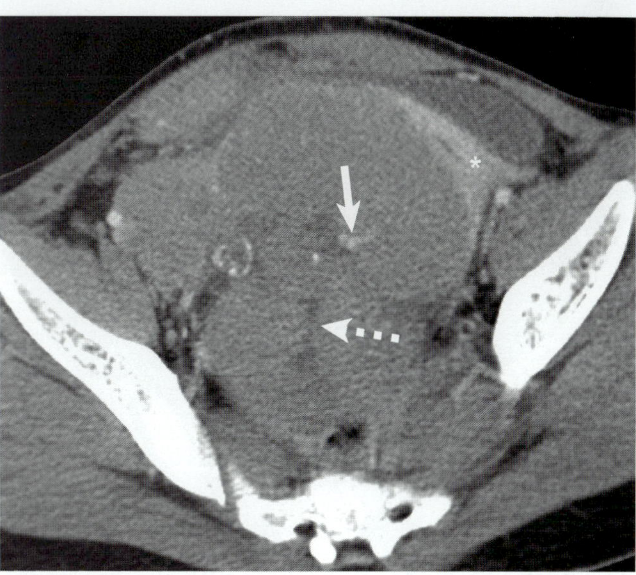

Figure 45.36 Dysgerminoma in a 19-year-old female. CECT shows a large lobulated relatively homogeneous solid pelvic mass with prominent vessels (*solid arrow*) and hypoenhancing septae (*dashed arrow*), indicating the presence of "fibrovascular septae." Uterus is displaced anteriorly and toward left and is compressed (*asterisks*).

Imaging Features: On imaging, they present as unilateral large solid multilobulated tumors with *characteristic enhancing fibrovascular septae* (Fig. 45.36). Unlike other solid ovarian neoplasms like fibromas and Brenner tumors, they demonstrate intermediate SI on T2WI (mildly brighter than muscle). They have relatively homogeneous contrast enhancement, although cystic and hemorrhagic changes may be present. Some tumors may show speckled calcifications.

Yolk Sac Tumor (Endodermal Sinus Tumor)

Pathophysiology and Clinical Presentation: These resemble the yolk sac (vitelline cells), and most commonly affect young women in their second decade of life. They are predominantly unilateral, and involvement of contralateral ovary is considered metastatic rather than synchronous primary. They are very aggressive tumors with early spread, have poor prognosis and are treated with combination of surgery and chemotherapy (usually radio resistant). AFP levels are raised, a useful marker for the diagnosis and surveillance.
Imaging Features: They usually present as a large solid or solid-cystic mass with hemorrhagic areas within, with intense, heterogeneous enhancement. At times, a "*bright dot*" *sign* may be seen representing foci of dilated vessels/small aneurysms within the solid component.

Embryonal Cell Carcinoma

Pathophysiology and Clinical Presentation: These are extremely rare GCTs resembling cells of early embryonal development and are least differentiated of all GCTs. These can have elevated AFP or β-hCG or both. They present slightly earlier than yolk sac tumors in the first and second decades. These are very aggressive in nature with peritoneal disease often present at the time of presentation.
Imaging Features: They again present with nonspecific imaging features as large heterogeneous, predominantly solid unilateral adnexal masses (Fig. 45.37). Involvement of contralateral ovary is considered to be metastatic involvement.

Choriocarcinoma

Pathophysiology and Clinical Presentation: There are two forms of choriocarcinoma: *gestational* and *nongestational*. *Gestational* form is considered to be metastatic involvement of primary uterine choriocarcinomas related to pregnancy [32]. *Nongestational form* usually occurs in the first and second decades and is associated with elevated β-hCG levels. Clinically, they can present with precocious puberty and dysfunctional uterine bleeding. These are aggressive tumors with early lymphatic and hematogenous spread.
Imaging Features: They usually present as unilateral solid masses which may show cystic and hemorrhagic changes (Fig. 45.38). They are hypervascular tumors with postcontrast hyperenhancement. *Prominent arterial feeders may be seen with some cases showing secondary arteriovenous malformations.* Lung metastases must be ruled out on imaging before starting treatment. Choriocarcinomas are chemosensitive tumors and respond well to chemotherapy.

Sex Cord—Stromal Tumors

Sex cord—stromal tumors arise from the mesenchyme or sex cord (coelomic epithelium). These comprise of granulosa cells, theca cells, Sertoli cells, Leydig cells, fibroblasts, etc. Majority of these tumors are benign in nature. Even when malignant, these tend not to have extraovarian spread.

Granulosa Cell Tumors

Pathophysiology and Clinical Presentation: Granulosa cell tumors are the most common malignant ovarian stromal neoplasm, likely arising from the cells surrounding developing follicles which produce estrogen and other androgens. These tumors have two distinct age peaks: one in postmenopausal women (*95%*) and another in younger women and children (*5%*). They are commonly unilateral and confined to the ovaries with good prognosis. They *present with features of hyperestrogenism in up to 25% of patients*, including postmenopausal bleeding, endometrial

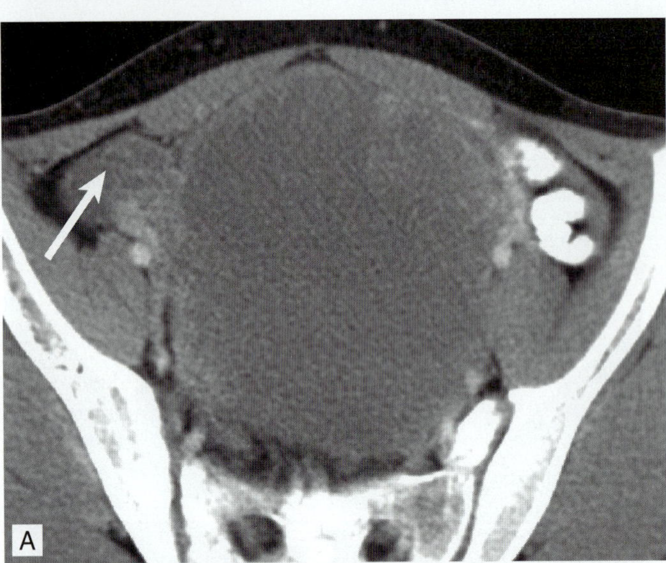

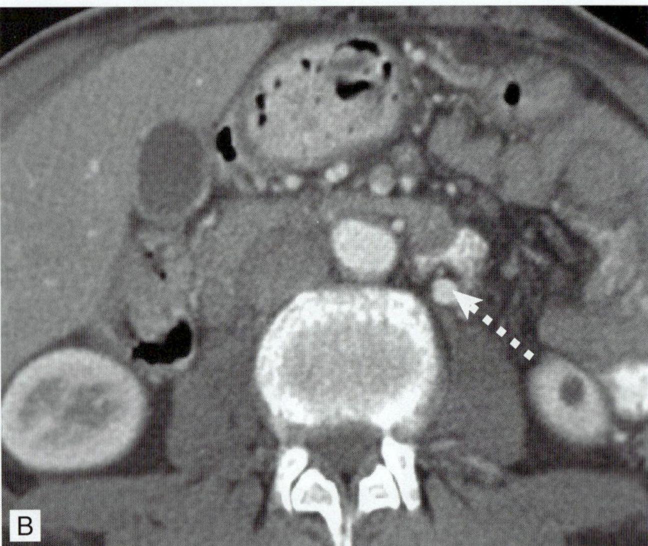

Figure 45.37 A 16-year-old girl with elevated AFP levels and malignant mixed germ cell tumor with embryonal components on pathology. CECT images show a large heterogeneously hypoenhancing pelvic mass (A). The normal right ovary was seen separately (*solid arrow*). In addition, dilated left ovarian vein (*dashed arrow* in B) is present, suggestive of left ovarian origin.

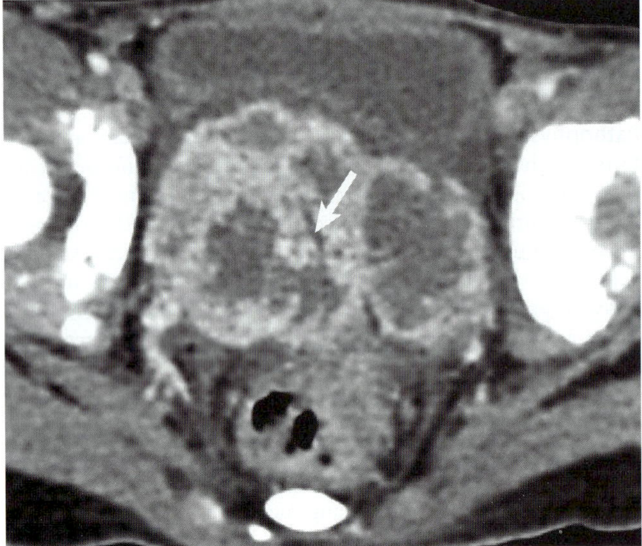

Figure 45.38 Axial CECT of a 11-year-old girl presenting with uterine bleeding. CT shows bilateral heterogeneously enhancing adnexal masses, with few prominent vessels within (*arrows*). She had raised β-HCG levels; choriocarcinoma on histology.

hyperplasia, endometrial polyp, and rarely endometrial carcinoma in postmenopausal women and precocious puberty in adolescents. Overall, they are low-grade tumors with good prognosis, but may recur in the peritoneum or retroperitoneum even decades after surgery (more common in the adult form). *Juvenile forms are known to be associated with enchondromatosis* (Ollier's and Maffucci syndromes) [33].

Imaging Features

- Usually large encapsulated solid cystic masses (Fig. 45.39) but can be completely solid or cystic as well. The solid component can show areas of hemorrhage, infarct, or fibrosis. The cystic component may have hemorrhagic content, manifesting as fluid–fluid or blood–fluid levels on MRI
- Papillary projections (typical of epithelial neoplasms) are not encountered
- *Solid component may demonstrate a "sponge-like" appearance on MRI resembling Swiss cheese, due to microcystic changes*
- Associated endometrial hyperplasia, polyp, or carcinoma may also be seen

Fibroma, Thecoma, Fibrothecoma, and Cystadenofibroma

Pathophysiology and Clinical Presentation: These are a spectrum of benign sex-cord stromal tumors arising from fibroblasts and theca cells interspersed in ovarian stroma, constituting 1–4% of all ovarian neoplasms. These are benign and solid tumors of ovaries, constituting most common benign solid ovarian neoplasms. These may be asymptomatic or detected incidentally.

- *Thecomas* commonly present in postmenopausal women with features of hyperestrogenism (usually postmenopausal bleeding) similar to granulosa cell tumors (which present more commonly with these features). Hence, *estrogen levels are useful tumor markers in thecoma.* On pathology, these tumors are seen to contain microvesicular fat. Surgical resection is curative
- *Fibromas* arise from stromal fibroblasts (spindle cells) of ovarian stroma. Bilateral ovarian fibromas are rare and can be associated with *Gorlin syndrome* (with basal cell nevus). Very rarely, the malignant variant viz. *fibrosarcoma* may be encountered. *Fibroma may rarely present with ascites and pleural effusions* (Meig's syndrome) in about 1% cases
- Fibrothecomas contain both elements of fibroma and thecoma on pathology. These are commoner in middle-aged women (fourth and fifth decades). These are endocrinologically neutral. Surgical resection is curative

Imaging Features

- On USG, these have varied appearance, but most commonly present as a solid homogeneous adnexal mass with or without postacoustic shadowing
- On CT they present as low-density solid masses which can show mild delayed enhancement
- *Fibromas can show dense calcification which may be seen on pelvic radiograph*

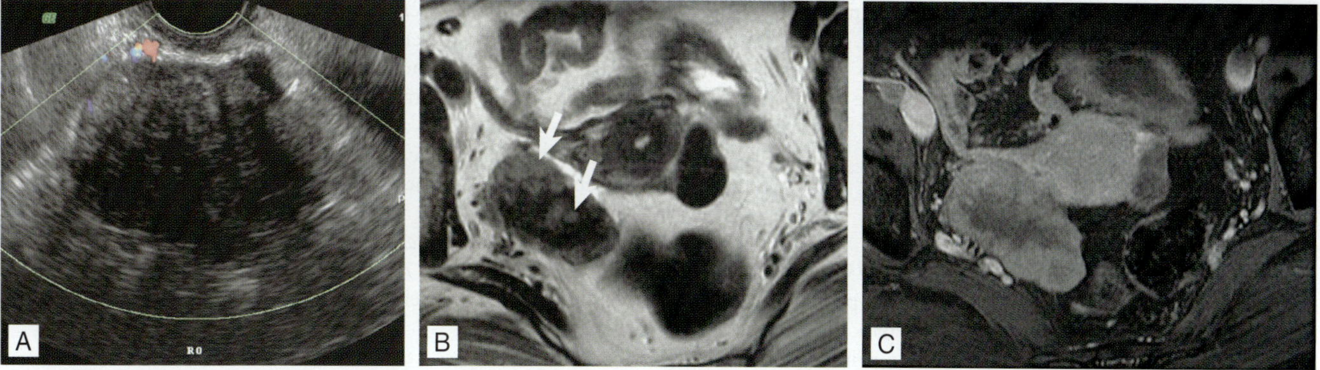

Figure 45.39 Granulosa cell tumor in a postmenopausal woman. Ultrasound Doppler shows a large right adnexal solid mass with minimal internal vascularity (A). Axial T2W (B) and postcontrast (C) MR images show a lobulated T2 hypointense (*arrows* in B), hypoenhancing lesion with associated enhancing T2 intermediate areas. No endometrial hyperplasia is seen in this patient.

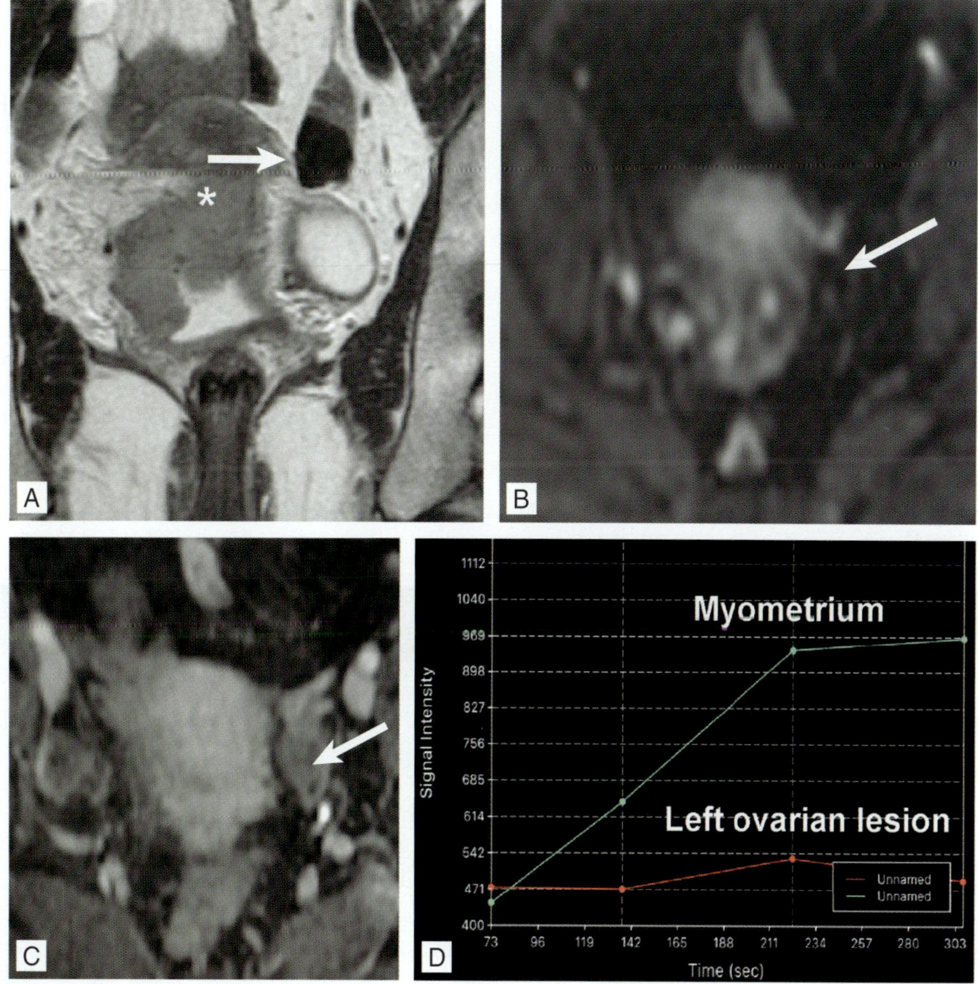

Figure 45.40 Incidentally detected left ovarian fibroma (*solid arrows*) in a case of carcinoma cervix (*asterisk*). Coronal T2W MRI (A) shows the incidental T2W dark left adnexal, without any restriction on DWI (B), and with mild homogeneous contrast enhancement (C). Dynamic postcontrast study (D) shows a Type 1 curve, consistent with benign etiology.

- MRI can be diagnostic (Fig. 45.40): Fibromas appear as well-defined lobulated lesions with smooth margins, hypointense on both T1 and T2WI, with type I curve. They show no restriction on diffusion
- *As per the European Society of Urogenital Radiology (ESUR) guidelines, a T2 hypointense adnexal lesion with no restriction can be confidently called a fibroma without the need to administer contrast*
- Thecomas may also show similar MRI features with depiction of lipid content on opposed phase imaging in some cases. These lesions may demonstrate T2 bright foci due to edema or cystic degeneration

The most important differential is a pedunculated uterine fibroid or broad ligament fibroid, with similar USG, CT, and MRI characteristics. Identifying ovaries separately from the lesion is the most important imaging marker to differentiate between the two. Vascular supply at times may also be useful in differentiating fibroids from fibroma/thecoma.

Ovarian Metastases

Pathophysiology and Clinical Presentation

Ovarian metastases most commonly arise from primary tumors of the stomach, colon and rectum, appendix, pancreas, gall bladder, or breast. Deposit from contralateral ovarian primary is also common. They account for about 10% of all ovarian neoplasms. *The term "Krukenberg's" tumor is ideally reserved for ovarian metastases showing "signet" cells on pathology which secrete mucin, usually stomach and colon malignancies, but is often used interchangeably in clinical practice for any ovarian metastasis.*

Imaging Features

- Ovarian metastases (Fig. 45.41) may be solid, cystic, or solid-cystic ovarian masses. They are frequently bilateral and usually associated with ascites with or without peritoneal disease
- Secondary tumors are less likely to be multilocular than primary ovarian tumors
- Krukenberg's tumors have somewhat more specific imaging features, presenting as bilateral solid/solid-cystic masses which show low attenuation on CECT
- Cystic component if present, can be bright on both T1W and T2W sequences due to mucin

Miscellaneous Tumors

Peritoneal mesothelioma: Benign peritoneal mesothelioma is a slow-growing rare tumor of peritoneum that is difficult to treat because of its propensity to local recurrence. Secondary infiltration of the liver, ovaries, or other solid viscera may be seen. Important differentiating features are identification of ovaries separately and presence of a mass conforming to expected peritoneal lining.

Collision tumor: These are rare tumors characterized by the presence of two histologically distinct tumors involving the ovary, present subjacent to each other but without admixture of the two on pathology and with a clear distinction between two types. *Most commonly, these are associated with cystic teratoma with coexistence of a serous or mucinous tumor.* However, any combination is feasible. Imaging features reflect the underlying histological neoplasms (Fig. 45.42).

Overall Role of Imaging

As per the American College of Radiology appropriateness criteria, *CECT of the abdomen and pelvis (with or without CT chest) is the imaging of choice for initial staging, follow-up, and suspected recurrence of ovarian cancer* [34]. Single phase CECT with oral contrast is generally performed for staging ovarian cancer, with coronal reformats useful in assessing subdiaphragmatic deposits.

Majority of the patients with ovarian cancer present with peritoneal disease, and the diagnosis is straightforward given the imaging findings and raised CA-125 levels. The treatment involves hysterectomy and salpingo-oophorectomy with cytoreductive surgery (CRS) [35]; along with neoadjuvant or adjuvant platinum-based chemotherapy. The extent of CRS is an important prognostic factor; with macroscopic residual disease after CRS being associated with poor outcome [35]. Thus, the primary role of imaging in assessing patients with ovarian cancer is to stage the disease, identify resectability, and give a surgical roadmap for resection. CT is excellent for this purpose, with an accuracy of up to 94% for ovarian cancer staging [34]. It is also very useful for identifying obvious unresectable disease so as to avoid an unnecessary surgery, although small deposits (<5 mm) along serosa, mesentery, or peritoneum may be missed.

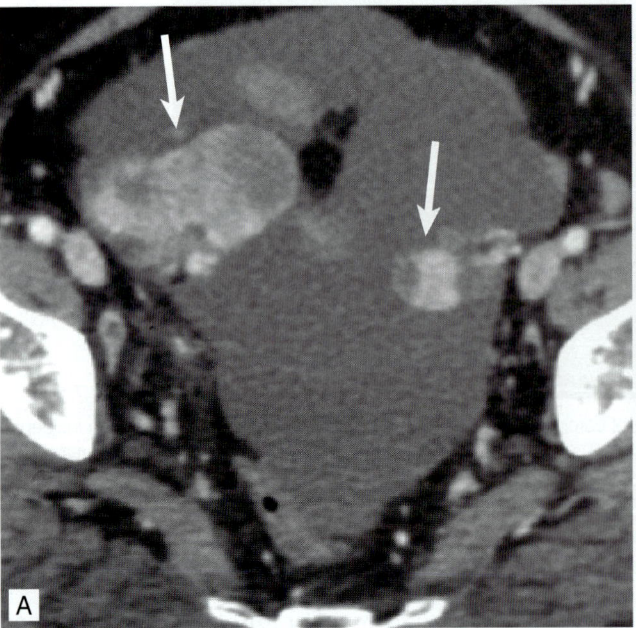

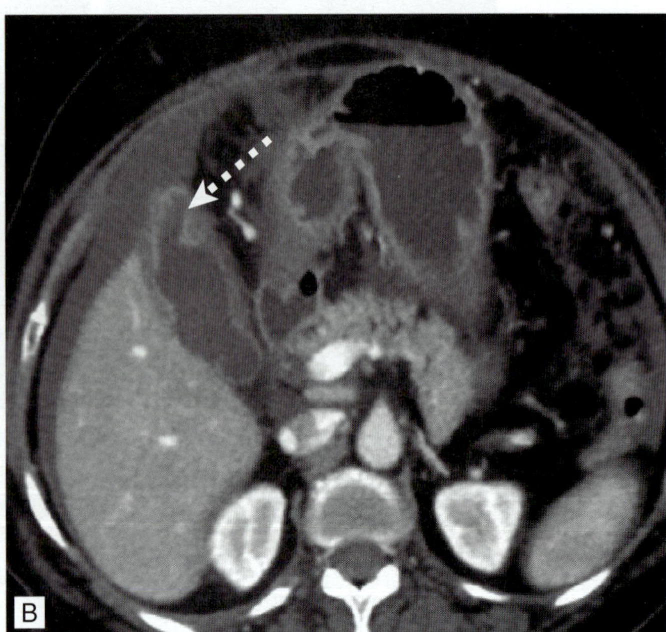

Figure 45.41 A 56 year old female with abdominal distension since 1 month. Axial CECT images show bilateral solid-cystic ovarian masses (*solid arrows* in A) with moderate ascites. There is asymmetric heterogeneous thickening of the fundus of the gall bladder (*dashed arrow* in B). Findings were consistent with bilateral ovarian deposits from gall bladder carcinoma.

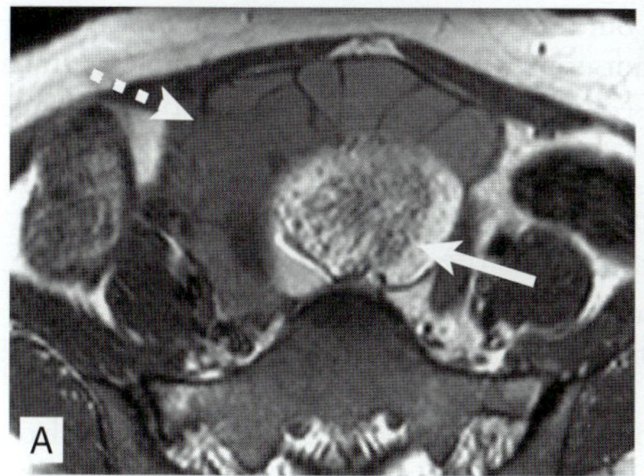
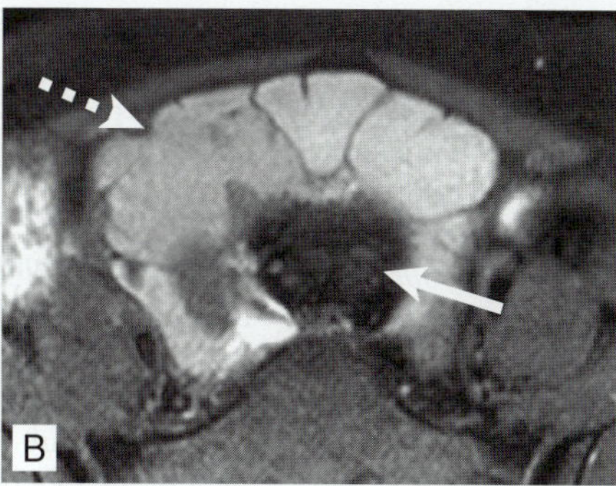
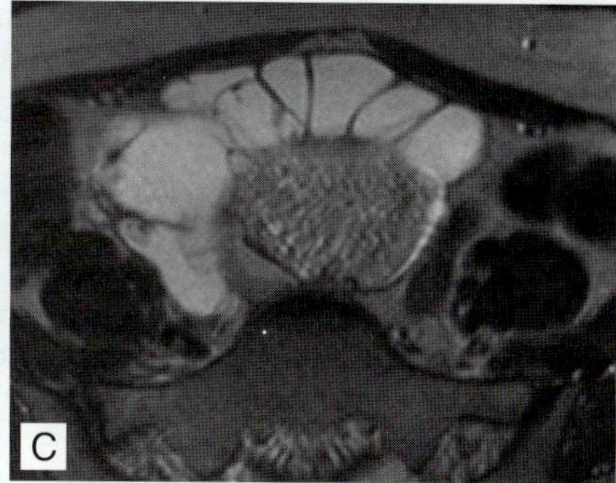

Figure 45.42 Collision tumor (teratoma and mucinous cystadenoma). Axial T1 without and with fat saturation (A and B) and axial T2W (C) images show a large pelvic mass with macroscopic fat along its posterior aspect, which suppresses on fat saturation (*solid arrows* in B). Multiple hypointense linear areas are seen within, reflecting tufts of hair. Additionally, a large multilocular cystic component (*dashed arrows* in A and B) is also present, with T1 and T2 hyperintense contents of varying signal intensity. Histopathology showed mature teratoma with a mucinous cystadenoma.

FDG PET/CT is not recommended technique for initial staging, as although it may catch subtle small deposits, CECT is sufficient to provide the information needed for surgical planning. It may however be performed in select cases of known or suspected recurrent serous ovarian cystadenocarcinoma (Fig. 45.43), especially if CT is indeterminate with high clinical suspicion. MRI is useful for characterizing indeterminate adnexal masses and may be used for staging when the patient cannot be given IV iodinated contrast.

It is also important to understand the role of lesion sampling. *Lesions which are indeterminate or suspicious for malignancy on imaging without any metastatic disease should not be sampled percutaneously to avoid peritoneal seeding;* this upstages an IA or IB tumor to an IC tumor. Sampling is reserved for tumors with definite metastatic disease, or lesions which appear benign such as infections (for culture and sensitivity).

Approach to Reporting an Ovarian Cancer Study

Apart from describing the primary adnexal mass, the assessment of ovarian cancer on imaging should focus on:

i. Identifying sites of metastatic involvement, both peritoneal and extraperitoneal;
ii. Mapping sites of peritoneal involvement and overall peritoneal disease burden; and
iii. Identifying any sites of peritoneal disease which may make surgery difficult or impossible.

Identifying Sites of Metastatic Involvement

Peritoneal Disease: The *most common pattern of peritoneal disease is in the form of moderate–severe ascites along with diffuse omental and peritoneal nodularity and fat stranding;* with plaque-like thickening and omental caking or sheet-like involvement

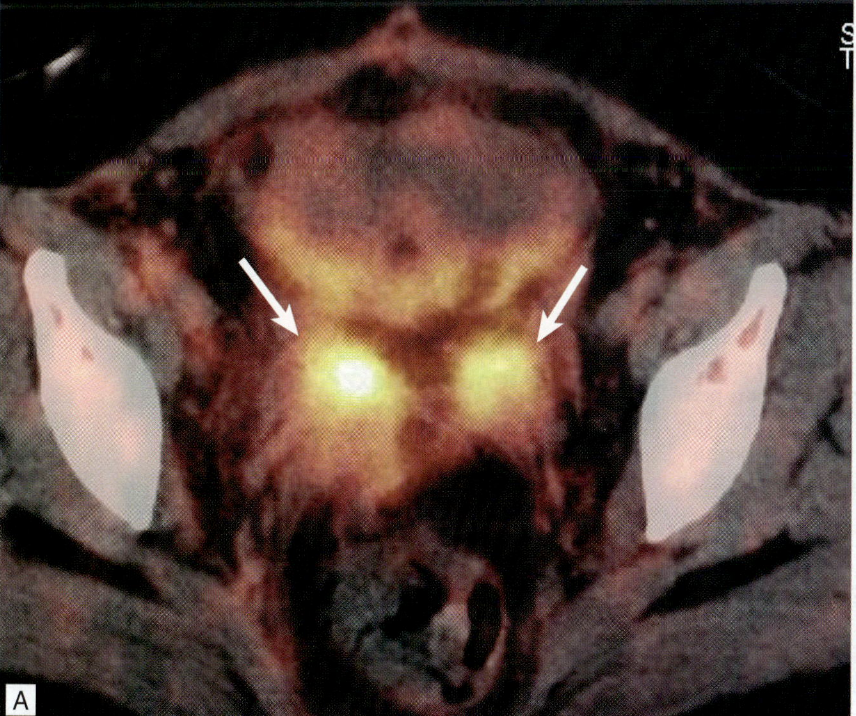
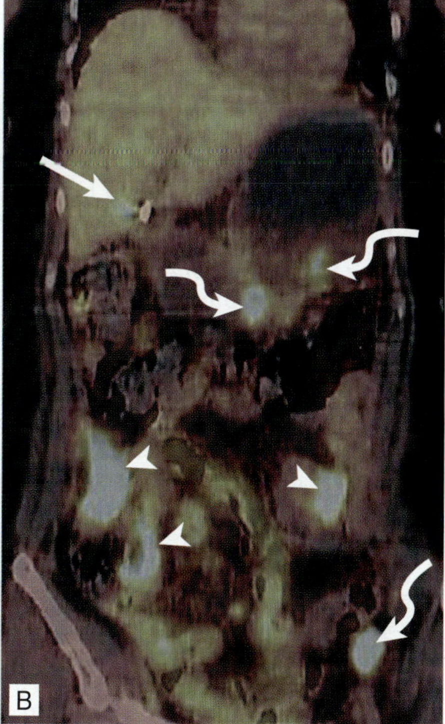

Figure 45.43 Patient with recurrent ovarian carcinoma, status posthysterectomy, and bilateral salpingo-oophorectomy. Axial and coronal fused PET/CT images (A and B) show bilateral avid vault soft tissue (*solid arrows* in A), suggesting vault recurrence. The patient also had FDG avid hepatic subcapsular deposits (*solid arrow* in B), gastric serosal deposits (*curved arrows*), peritoneal and mesenteric deposits (*arrowheads*), and left pelvic side wall adenopathy. (Courtesy: Dr. Bharat Agarwal, Max Hospital, New Delhi, India.)

often present. The deposits are often confluent and nonmeasurable, although well-defined discrete lesions may also be present. *Calcifications may be present in metastases from serous cystadenocarcinomas.* Peritoneal disease may only manifest only as subtle fat stranding or minimal peritoneal thickening or nodularity, especially in the postneoadjuvant treatment setting. Greater omental disease may be further classified as *supramesocolic* and *inframesocolic* (with respect to transverse mesocolon). Although inframesocolic omentum is anyway resected in all cases, presence of supramesocolic diseases should be mentioned as it may not be always resected.

Subdiaphragmatic disease should be evaluated on coronal reformats as well, as the lesions *may masquerade as intrahepatic or intrasplenic deposits on axial images.* Labeling them intrahepatic will falsely upstage the patient from stage III to stage IV disease and should be avoided. Similarly, perihepatic or perisplenic surface deposits may invade the hepatic or splenic parenchyma; this should still be considered as stage III disease and have similar outcomes [36]. They should be specifically mentioned as they may need associated partial hepatic resection or splenectomy (the patient would also need to be vaccinated preoperatively for the latter). Bowel obstruction is particularly common in the recurrent setting, due to a combination of the disease itself along with postoperative adhesions.

Extraperitoneal Disease: *Abdominal wall and nodal involvement are relatively common sites of extraperitoneal disease.* The presence of abdominal wall deposits is not an absolute contraindication for CRS [36]. However, this increases the complexity of the surgery and reconstruction involved.

Nodes which are ≥10 mm in short axis or with altered morphology (heterogeneity or necrosis) or loss of oval shape are considered metastatic on imaging. Pelvic and infrarenal retroperitoneal nodes are most commonly involved and can be resected along with the CRS if not associated with severe vascular encasement or infiltration. Suprarenal retroperitoneal nodes (above the level of renal vessels) are usually unresectable. Epicardiac nodes are often enlarged on imaging, either due to metastatic involvement or reactive to the peritoneal disease (a site of drainage). Although they are not resected, presence of enlarged epicardiac nodes is associated with poorer outcomes [37].

Parenchymal metastases due to hematogenous spread confer poor prognosis, with liver being a common site of involvement.

Mapping Sites of Peritoneal Involvement and Overall Peritoneal Disease Burden

It is crucial to provide an accurate surgical map to the oncosurgeon; The *Peritoneal Carcinomatosis Index (PCI)* is an increasingly used surgical score for mapping and quantifying malignant peritoneal disease of any etiology in a standardized fashion [37]. This helps reduce interobserver variability in defining the disease burden and standardizes treatment protocols for newer therapies like hyperthermic intraperitoneal chemotherapy.

- A total of 13 subsites have to be evaluated to calculate the PCI score: the nine peritoneal quadrants and four small bowel/mesenteric regions (proximal and distal jejunum and ileum respectively with their mesentery)
- The size of the largest deposit in each subsite is recorded and scored from *1 to 3 (1: <0.5 cm, 2: 0.5–5 cm, 3: >5 cm)*
- A total score of 39 can thus be given to every patient of peritoneal disease

Although it remains a surgical score based on laparotomy/laparoscopy findings, the same principle should be used while reporting to scan through all potential sites of disease involvement and quantify the disease burden. *CT- or MRI-based PCI scoring is fairly accurate*; although not usually provided in routine reporting, this may be reported based on the preferences of the referring surgeon and the treatment planned for the patient.

Identifying Sites of Peritoneal Disease Which May Make Surgery Difficult or Impossible

There are no standard guidelines defining optimal CRS. Involvement of an unfavorable site can hinder complete CRS regardless of the overall PCI. There are certain sites within the peritoneal cavity which are considered unresectable. For example, involvement of the root of mesentery or multifocal serosal disease involving the bowel is deemed unresectable as the extensive bowel resection needed for complete resection is not feasible. However, several other sites which are borderline resectable; depend on various patient, surgeon, and institutional factors (Table 45.9), and may require more complex procedures such as Whipple's procedure, splenectomy, segmental bowel resection, or partial excision of urinary bladder wall. These may require surgical inputs of various specialties. Accordingly, these sites should specifically be commented upon if there is disease involvement to allow proper surgical planning.

A useful acronym PAUSE [37] can be used to ensure adequate evaluation of ovarian carcinoma on baseline imaging.

- P: Peritoneal Carcinomatosis Index (PCI) and site and extent of primary tumor
- A: Ascites and abdominal wall involvement
- U: Unfavorable sites of involvement
- S: Small bowel and mesenteric disease
- E: Extraperitoneal disease

Ovarian Cancer Screening

As majority of ovarian cancers are detected at an advanced stage, it is desirable to have a screening test for it. Multiple large studies have however demonstrated no improvement in survival in patients who underwent ultrasound or CA-125 screening, and it is hence not recommended for general population [38]. However, for high-risk patients (BRCA1/BRCA2 mutations, family history of breast or ovarian cancer, known syndromes with high risk of ovarian malignancies), ACR recommends annual TVS screening along with CA-125 levels [38]. Prophylactic bilateral salpingo-oophorectomy improves survival in these patients.

Miscellaneous Adnexal Lesions

Ovarian Vein Thrombosis

Ovarian vein thrombosis is a rare disease affecting postpartum women. The clinical features are similar to puerperal sepsis: fever with chills, lower abdominal pain with raised leucocyte counts. Majority present in first 10 days of the postpartum period. The right ovarian vein is more commonly involved due to its longer course and relatively lesser competent valves. If not detected and treated early, these can lead to septicemia (secondary to septic thrombophlebitis) and pulmonary thromboembolism. It is managed conservatively with anticoagulants and antibiotics. Hence, the imaging diagnosis is essential to prevent unnecessary surgical intervention.

Ultrasonography usually demonstrates a tubular anechoic to hypoechoic structure extending from a level just superior to the ovary to the IVC/left renal vein without any flow on Doppler.

TABLE 45.9 Probably Resectable and Unresectable Peritoneal Disease

Sl No	Subsite	Probably Resectable	Unresectable
1	Omentum/peritoneal cavity	▪ Lesser omentum ▪ Hepatic and splenic surface deposits ▪ Encasement of left gastric artery. ▪ Portocaval region ▪ Gall bladder fossa ▪ Peripancreatic and paraduodenal space ▪ Subdiaphragmatic disease (Fig. 45.44)	
2	Peritoneal ligaments	▪ Falciform ligament (to be differentiated from hepatic parenchymal deposit, Fig. 45.45) ▪ Ligamentum teres ▪ Hepatoduodenal ligament/porta hepatis	▪ Hepatoduodenal ligament deposit with biliary obstruction
3	Pelvic viscera	▪ Deposit along bladder trigone	▪ Presacral disease
4	Retroperitoneum and pelvic side walls	▪ Ureteric encasement with or without hydronephrosis) ▪ Infiltration of iliopsoas or quadratus lumborum ▪ Suprarenal nodal disease	▪ Supraceliac nodal disease ▪ Epiphrenic nodal disease ▪ Pelvic side wall disease with encasement of pelvic vessels
5	Bowel serosa and mesentery	▪ Gastric serosal deposit ▪ Distal small bowel serosal deposit (Fig. 45.46)	▪ Root of mesentery (Fig. 45.46) ▪ Ligament of Trietz/DJ flexure ▪ Proximal small bowel serosal deposit
6	Abdominal solid viscera	–	▪ Liver and splenic parenchymal deposits
7	Miscellaneous	▪ Abdominal wall deposit	

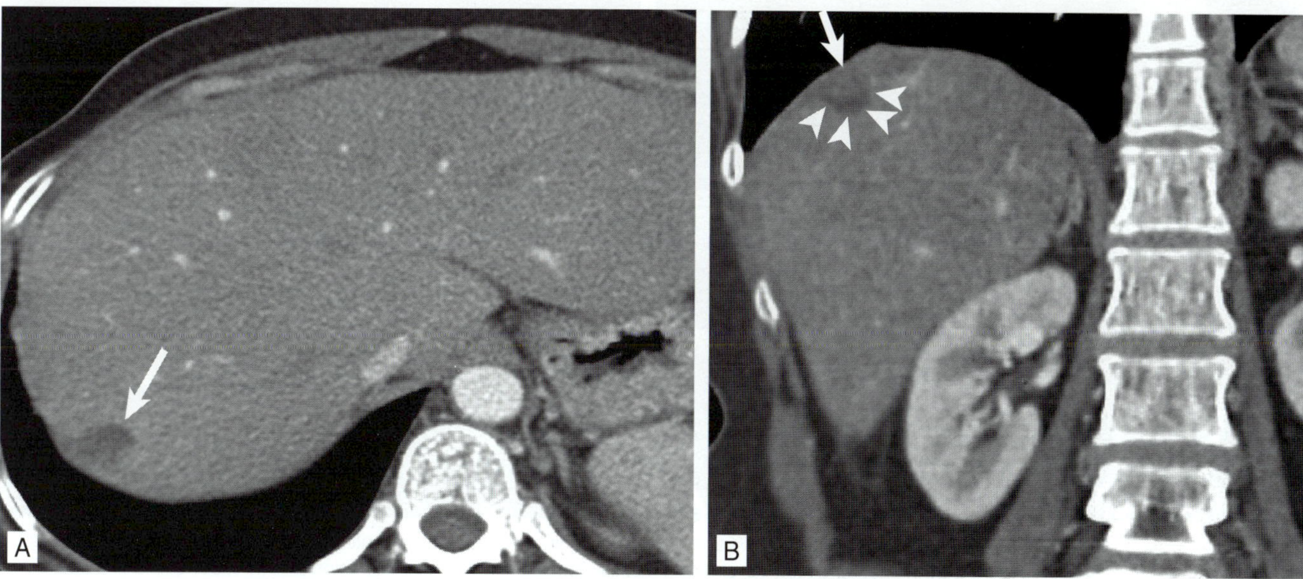

Figure 45.44 Importance of reformats in assessing subdiaphragmatic disease. Axial CECT (A) shows a hypodense subcapsular hepatic lesion (*arrow*) which appears intraparenchymal. Coronal reformat (B) shows the lesion (*solid arrow* in B) to be subdiaphragmatic, causing scalloping of the liver (*arrowheads*).

However, in conditions like excess bowel gas, patient body habitus, ultrasound evaluation be sensitive, and is often diagnosed on CT/MRI (Fig. 45.47). CT demonstrates the thrombosed vein extending from ovaries to IVC/left renal vein.

Ovarian Torsion

Pathophysiology and Clinical Presentation

Ovarian torsion is twisting of the ovary cantered at ovarian vascular pedicle. This causes obstruction of venous outflow and cuts off the arterial supply which can result in rapid ischemic changes within the ovaries. Adnexal torsion is broader term encompassing twisting of ovaries as well as fallopian tubes. Up to two-thirds of torsions are a combination of the ovary as well as fallopian tube. It is most commonly seen in women of reproductive age group, with higher incidence among pregnant women. By far, the commonest cause of ovarian torsion is mature cystic teratoma [39]. Immediately after torsion, the venous and lymphatic outflow is blocked first with reduced forward arterial flow (veins and lymphatic collapse more readily than the more muscular arterial walls). This results in a vicious cycle where inflow is maintained and outflow is blocked,

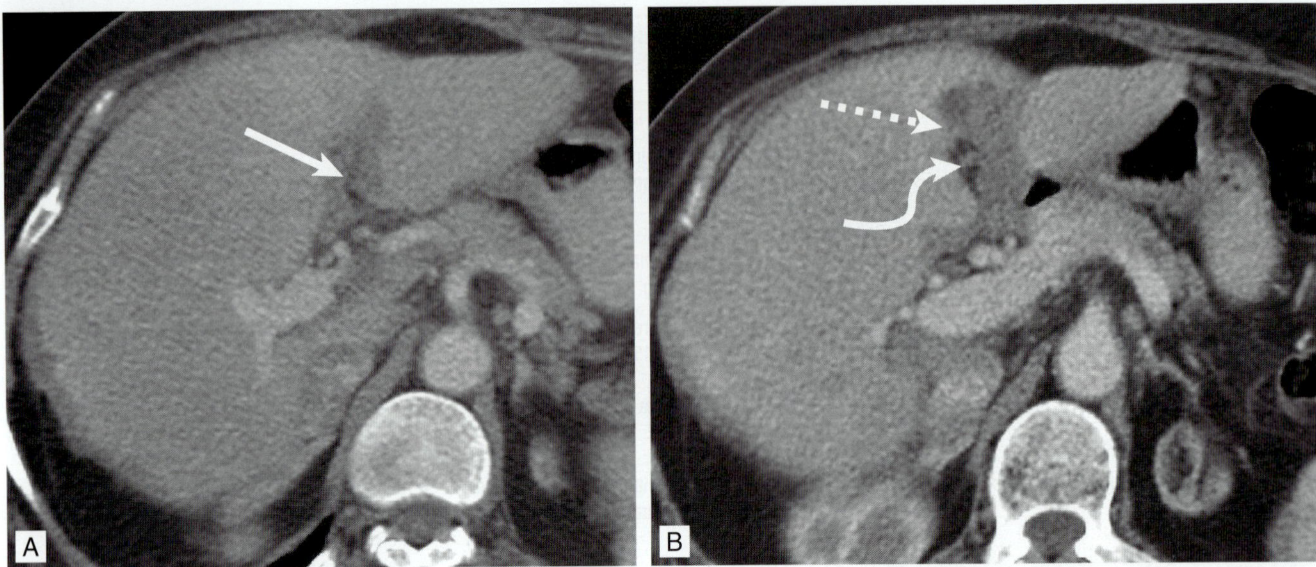

Figure 45.45 Falciform ligament deposit (*arrow* in A) versus parenchymal deposit (*dashed arrow* in B). In B, the lesion is parenchymal as evidenced by the "claw" of normal parenchyma. In addition normal falciform ligament (*curved arrow*) can be seen. Falciform ligament deposit is stage III whereas parenchymal disease is stage IV.

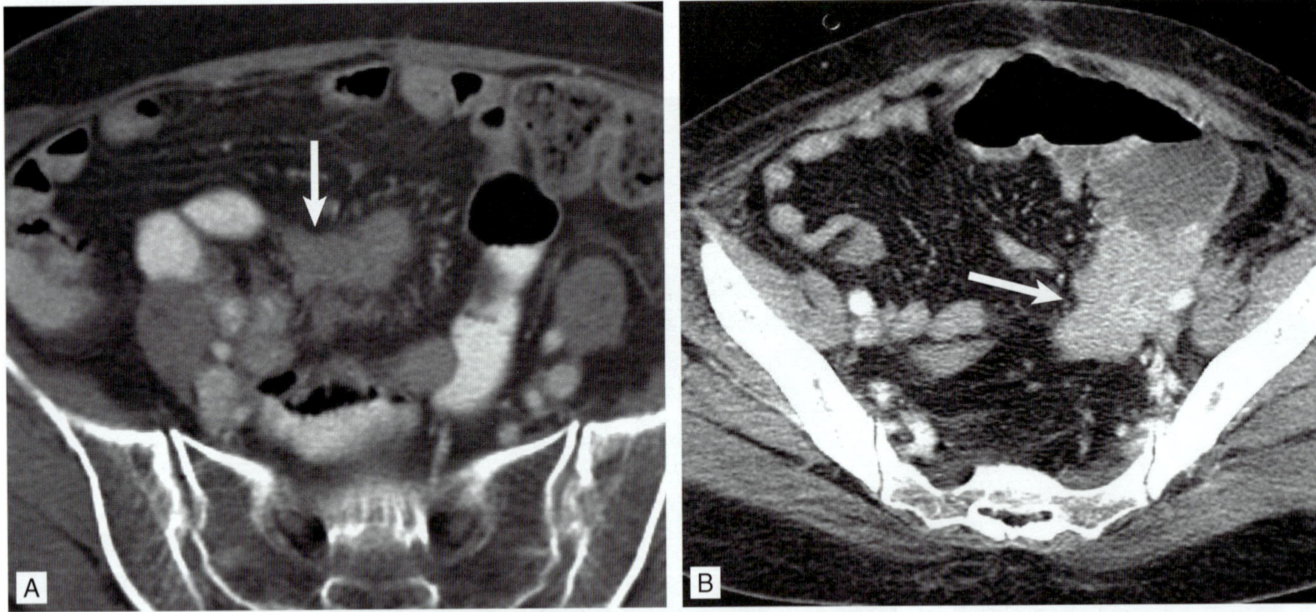

Figure 45.46 Bowel and mesenteric disease. Axial CECT (A) shows a large deposit within the distal ileal mesentery (*solid arrow*); it is potentially resectable with segmental bowel resection. Axial CECT in another patient (B) shows a serosal deposit along the sigmoid colon (*arrow*) causing mild proximal bowel dilatation.

resulting in rapid engorgement, ultimately worsening the twist and eventually cutting off the arterial supply, resulting in an ovarian infarct.

The clinical presentation is usually acute onset lower pelvis or iliac fossa region pain, with tenderness on palpation. Guarding and rigidity can be present, suggestive of peritoneal inflammation.

Imaging Features

- Ultrasound with Doppler evaluation is the primary imaging technique of choice. The most common imaging finding is enlargement of the involved ovary, which may be heterogeneous with edema and hemorrhagic change, especially if long standing. It may be hyper or hypoechoic. A predisposing adnexal mass may be identified
- The follicles are displaced to the periphery with hyperechoic central stroma, with the ovary often being midline in position. The follicles may also demonstrate a hyperechoic margin (follicular ring sign)
- Associated pelvic free fluid is present in over 80% cases
- Probe tenderness can be an important diagnostic clue
- On Doppler, the most common abnormality is reduced or absent venous flow. Absent arterial flow is a poor prognostic feature, while high resistance flow is more commonly observed (Fig. 45.48). Normal Doppler flow however does not rule out

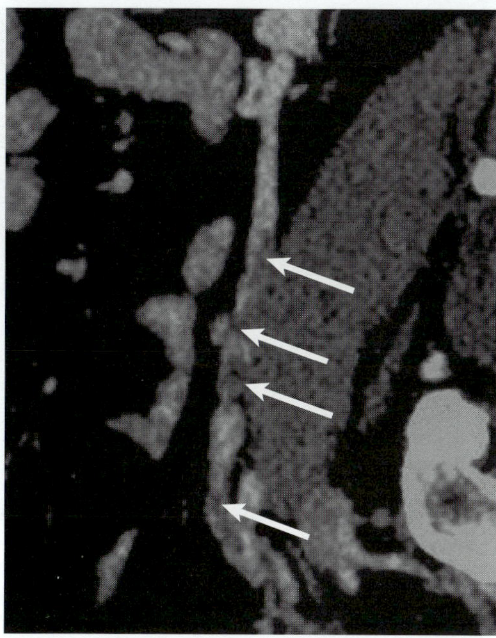

Figure 45.47 Left ovarian thrombosis in a postpartum woman. Oblique sagittal image with narrow window presets shows multiple filling defects within the right ovarian vein (*arrows*).

torsion due to dual supply from both ovarian and uterine arteries. Twisted pedicle with characteristic "whirlpool sign" on Doppler can be seen, specific for the diagnosis

- CT and MRI may be used, and demonstrate the enlarged ovary with ipsilateral uterine deviation. Lack of enhancement may be present if the ovary is infarcted. Associated tubal thickening may be demonstrable as well
- Torsion is a common gynecological emergency requiring urgent surgical management, with detorsion and adnexal preservation usually performed rather than salpingo-oophorectomy in adolescents and children irrespective of the appearance of the ovary [40]

Transposed Ovaries

Certain pelvic malignancies like rectal cancer need to be treated with radiation therapy. In women of reproductive age group, it is desirable to preserve ovarian function in such a situation. At many centers, the ovaries are surgically mobilized off the pelvic cavity and implanted within the peritoneum of lateral and lower abdomen while preserving the vascular pedicle. This procedure is known as ovarian transposition. The transposed ovaries may be found anywhere along the flank region from the level of lowest ribs to iliac fossae. During surgery, transposed ovaries are marked with a surgical clip to enable identification of the transposed

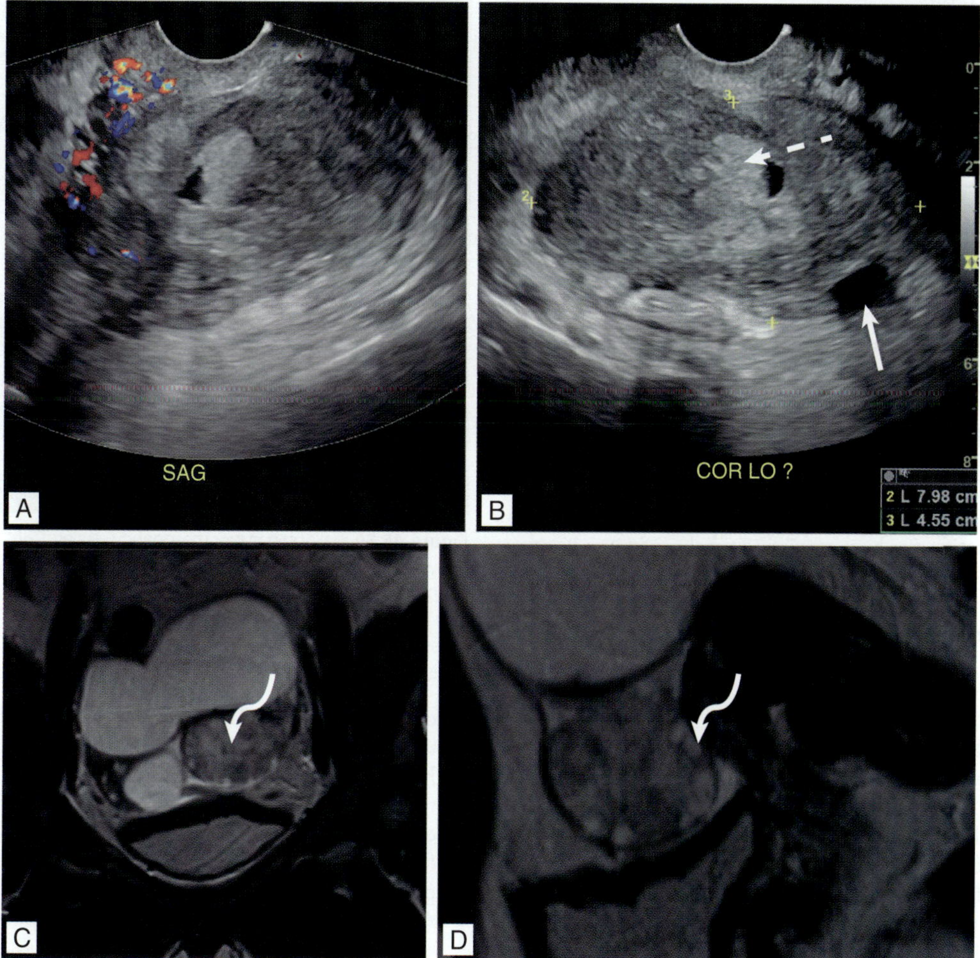

Figure 45.48 Transvaginal ultrasound images of left ovarian torsion (A and B). The left ovary is enlarged with decreased vascularity, with a peripheral follicle present (*arrow* in B). The central part is echogenic (*dashed arrow*). Coronal (C) and sagittal (D) T2WI show the midline position of the left ovary (*curved arrow*) with few peripherally placed follicles (*curved arrow*). The central stroma appears bright, suggesting edema. (Courtesy: Dr. Mukesh Harisinghani, Harvard Medical School, Boston, USA.)

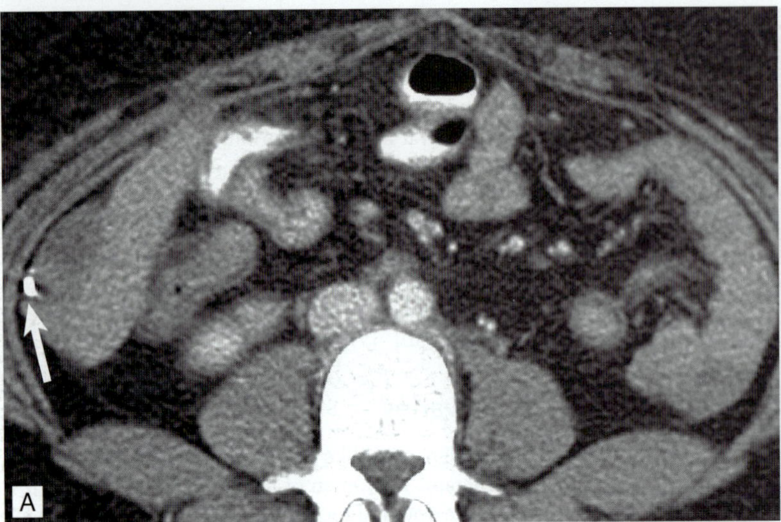

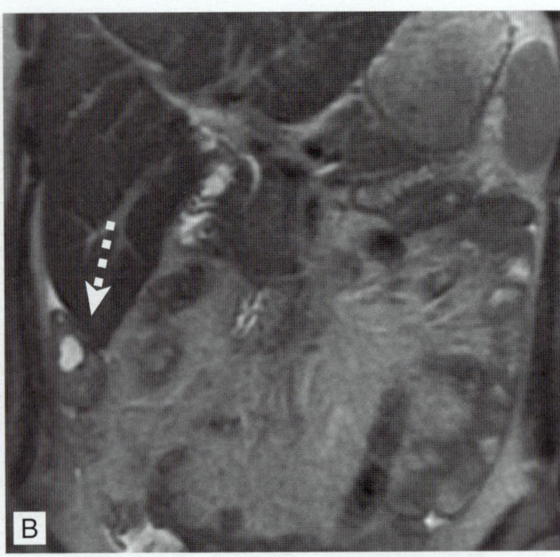

Figure 45.49 Normal transposed ovaries. Case of rectal cancer in a female of reproductive age group who underwent ovarian transposition before pelvic radiation and surgery. Axial CECT (A) shows an ovoid hypodense structure in the right subhepatic region. This should not be confused with a peritoneal deposit; the presence of the surgical clip helps for this (*solid arrow*). Coronal T2W MRI (B) confirms the normal ovary with follicles within (*dashed arrow*).

ovaries on imaging (Fig. 45.49). It is important for radiologists to be aware of the surgical details as they may otherwise be confused with peritoneal deposits.

Normal ovarian cysts are known to be encountered more frequently in transposed ovaries. These can be sites of endometriosis and PID. Rarely, primary ovarian neoplasms or metastasis may develop in transposed ovaries.

Fallopian Tube Malignancies

Pathophysiology and Clinical Presentation

Primary fallopian tube carcinomas (PFTCs) are virtually impossible to distinguish from serous adenocarcinoma of the ovary on pathology. Indeed, the present belief is that primary high-grade ovarian cystadenocarcinomas may arise from the fallopian tube, spilling over to ovarian surfaces where they present subsequently as ovarian masses. This is based on observations on pathology of patients of BRCA1/BRCA2 germline mutations undergoing prophylactic salpingo-oophorectomy, which have shown presence of early carcinoma in situ along fallopian tube mucosal lining rather than on the surface of the ovaries [41]. Other studies have found that cases of pelvic cystadenocarcinomas have coexisting tubal carcinoma in situ, usually involving the fimbrial end.

PFTCs usually present in about sixth and seventh decades with nonspecific features of lower abdominal pain or postmenopausal bleeding. Often, a large adnexal mass is detected incidentally. A classical clinical triad termed "Latzko's Triad" is seen in very few patients [42]:

1. Intermittent large volume serosanguinous vaginal discharge
2. Intermittent pelvic colicky pain relieved by vaginal discharge
3. Abdominal or pelvic mass

As with epithelial ovarian tumors, CA-125 levels may be raised. Treatment protocols are similar to epithelial malignant ovarian neoplasms. The diagnosis of PFTC is usually made on pathology and rarely on pretreatment imaging.

Imaging

- Imaging appearance is dependent on coexisting hydrosalpinx (Fig. 45.50). Tumoral cells secrete fluid which causes distension of fallopian tubes. The hydrosalpinx component may contribute to the cystic component of a solid cystic mass
- Hydrosalpinx with solid mural nodules or papillary projections can be readily seen on sonography. The solid component can show internal vascularity on Doppler, distinguishing it from clots or concretions. The solid component may show punctate calcifications on CT
- A predominantly solid variant may show heterogeneous enhancement. These may be tubular or "sausage" shaped
- Dynamic change due to accumulation and release of tubal fluid is characteristic of PFTC; it may appear solid cystic on initial sonography and appear predominantly solid on subsequent CT/MRI study

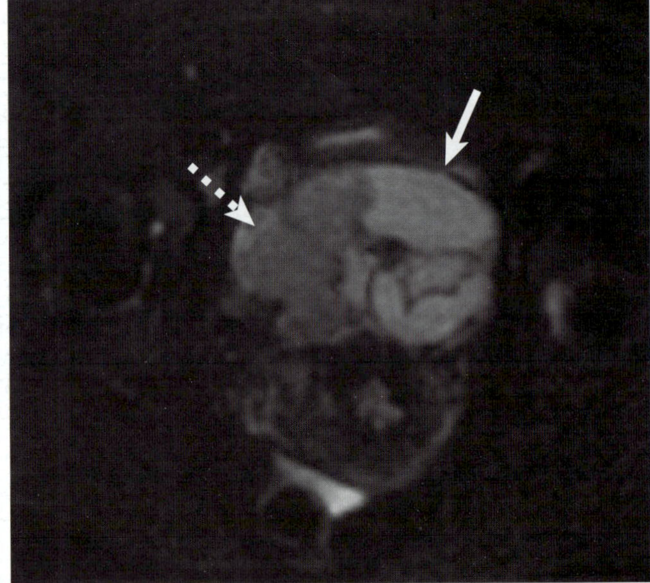

Figure 45.50 Fallopian tube malignancy. Axial T2W fat-saturated image shows a tortuous and tubular structure (*solid arrow*) with an intermediate intensity solid mass filling the medial aspect of the structure (*dashed arrow*). The tubular structure is a fluid-filled fallopian tube with the intermediate solid mass representing primary fallopian tube carcinoma. (Courtesy: Dr. Mukesh Harisinghani, Harvard Medical School, Boston, USA.)

- Visualization of normal ovaries separately is necessary to raise the suspicion of PFTC

Broad Ligament Pathologies

Broad ligament can also be a seat of various adnexal pathologies. The most common of these is a broad ligament fibroid (Fig. 45.51), showing typical morphology of fibroid but without any definite communication with uterine wall. To characterize any lesion to be of broad ligament in origin, it is necessary to identify the lesion to be separated from the uterus and ovaries. After leiomyoma, Müllerian duct tumors are the most common pathologies of this region. Paraovarian cysts (Fig. 45.18) have already been discussed. All variants of epithelial neoplasms of the ovary can involve broad ligament with similar imaging features.

The remnants of Wolffian duct in females, namely, the epoophoron, paroophoran, and the Gartner duct, can also present with tumors which involve the broad ligament, termed as female adnexal tumor of adnexal origin. Majority of these tumors arising are benign but few can be low-grade malignancies. The imaging findings are nonspecific: appearing as solid cystic adnexal lesion with vascularity on Doppler and solid component showing heterogeneous enhancement on CT/MRI. Another tumor of Wolffian ductal origin is papillary cystadenoma of the broad ligament (Fig. 45.52), typically seen in patients with Von Hippel–Lindau (VHL) syndrome. The counterpart of the same involves the epididymis in males (papillary cystadenoma of epididymis). It is a predominantly solid or solid-cystic tumor, visualized separately from the ovaries and the uterus and can be easily diagnosed in a known case of VHL syndrome.

Radiological Approach to Adnexal Lesions

Given the myriad of differential diagnoses for adnexal masses, many of them physiologic or self-limited, a systematic approach is necessary to narrow down the differentials and more importantly, ascertain the probability of malignancy to guide further management.

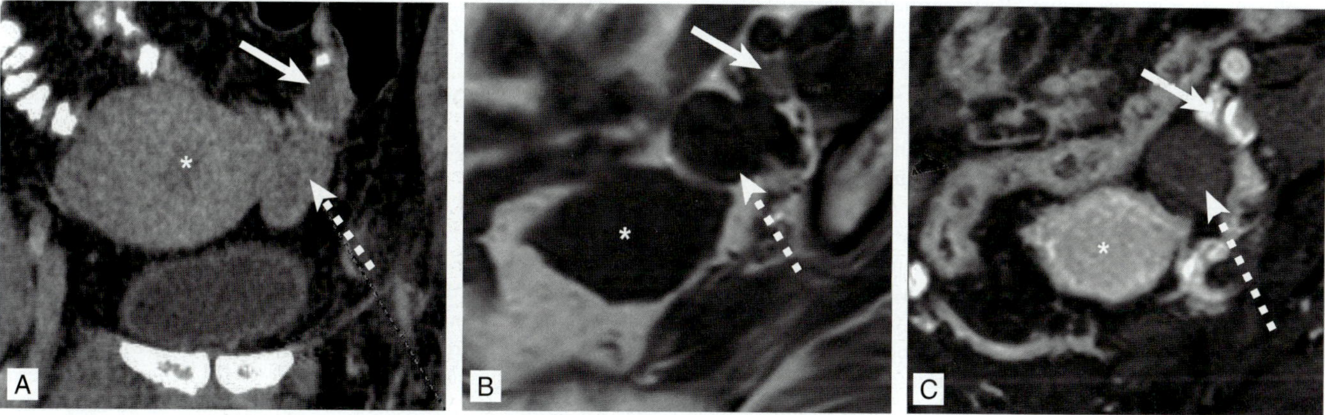

Figure 45.51 CT and MRI of 36-year-old female incidentally detected to have a solid left adnexal mass on ultrasound. (A) Coronal postcontrast CT shows a mildly lobulated homogeneously enhancing left parametrial lesion (*dashed arrow*) (uterus marked with *asterisk*) with a normal left ovary (*solid arrow*) just lateral to it. Axial T2W and contrast-enhanced MR images (B and C) show a mildly enhancing homogeneous hypointense left parametrial soft-tissue lesion (*dashed arrow*), and an adjacent normal left ovary (*solid arrow*). Imaging features are typical of broad ligament fibroid.

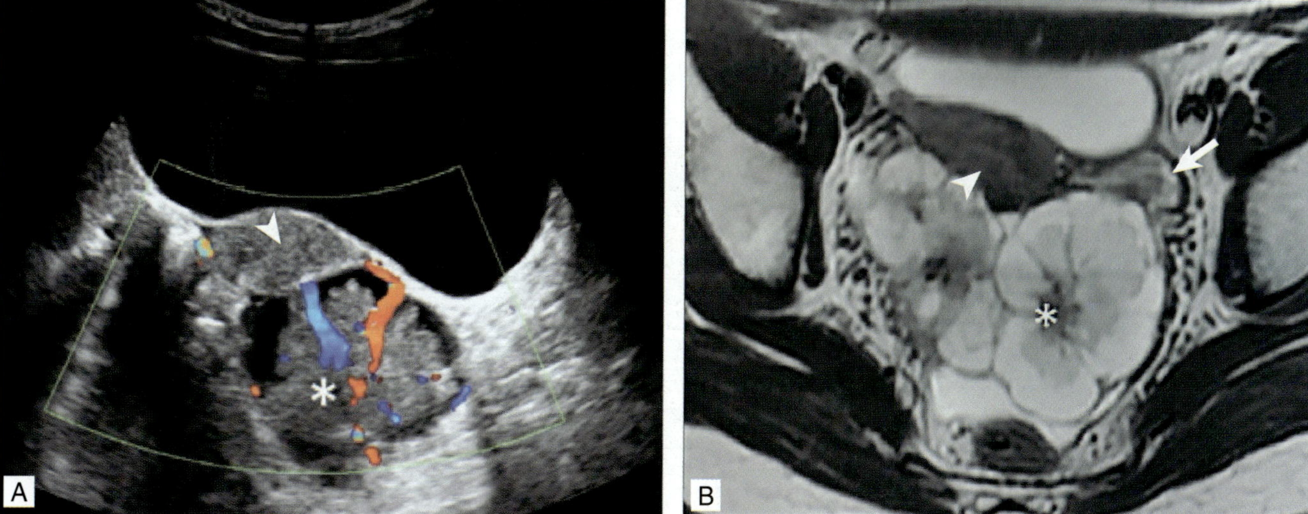

Figure 45.52 Papillary cystadenoma of broad ligament in a known case of VHL syndrome. (A) Transvaginal ultrasound shows a solid cystic lesion posterior and to the left of uterus (*arrowhead*) with internal vascularity. (B) MRI shows heterogeneous T2 hyperintense lesion (*asterisk*) posterolateral to uterus (*arrowhead*). Left ovary (*arrow*) is seen separately. (Reprinted with permission from: JD Oliveira, TM Cunha, A Tereso, Tumors of the broad ligament: what and when to suspect such rare location, Radiol Bras 53 (5) (2020) 349–355. doi:10.1590/0100-3984.2019.0073. Copyright (2020) by SciELO.)

Many patients are detected to have a pelvic or adnexal mass incidentally. Most others present with nonspecific symptoms like lower abdominal pain or fullness or menstrual irregularities, and have an adnexal lesion detected on ultrasound. A systematic approach is helpful in approaching a pelvic/adnexal mass [43].

First, correlate with history, clinical examination, and other laboratory findings.

- *Accurate and detailed history and laboratory parameters are of paramount importance.* Past surgical history is often very useful. If there is a history of oophorectomy, it is important out find out the reason of surgery and surgical pathology. The value of tumor markers is of substantial importance as discussed. History suggestive of hyperestrogenism or hyperandrogenism may sometimes be obtained
- The *age and menstrual status* of the patient is important with different pathologies affecting women in premenopausal, reproductive, and postmenopausal age group. GCTs and stromal tumors are present in young adults or premenopausal patients. PID, endometrioma, fibroid, torsion, ectopic pregnancy, and certain benign ovarian neoplasms present in women of reproductive age group. Postmenopausal women present more often with malignant neoplasms. Certain lesions like dermoid cyst however can present across all age groups
- *Duration and cyclical nature of symptoms* can be helpful
- Any syndromic association must be sought for, such as broad ligament cystadenoma in VHL, or malignant epithelial ovarian tumors in BRCA1/BRCA2 germline mutation carriers

Second, identify the organ or compartment of origin.

- If feasible, it is useful to identify the organ/site of origin: ovarian, extraovarian adnexal, uterine, cervical, pelvic peritoneal, etc. Determining the organ of origin may be easier on MRI than ultrasound. The "claw sign" and "leash of vessels" sign (discussed in detail in the chapter on uterine pathologies) for example help differentiate a pedunculated fibroid from an adnexal lesion
- Identifying normal ovaries is important when dealing with a pelvic/adnexal mass. Normal ovaries are identified by the presence of multiple peripheral-based follicles. Displacement of ureters can also give a clue about origin. The ovaries are located anterior or anteromedial to the pelvic ureters. A pelvic mass displacing the ureters posteriorly or posterior-laterally may be ovarian in origin

Third, ascertain the shape of the mass.

- A cystic lesion conforming to peritoneal reflections is typical of peritoneal inclusion cyst. Similarly, a solid or plaque-like mass conforming to peritoneal reflections may indicate a primary peritoneal tumor such as mesothelioma or diffuse peritoneal metastatic disease
- Well-defined uniform round lesions are generally benign or of low-grade malignant potential
- Ill-defined or irregular masses generally imply malignant or infiltrative lesions
- Irregular masses with desmoplastic changes/spiculations are commonly seen in deep infiltrating endometriosis. They can also be seen in postoperative scars or post-therapy changes
- Elongated tubular cystic lesions usually imply a fallopian tube lesion

Finally, analyze the internal morphology and contents of the mass.

- The differentials of the mass change completely based on the whether it contains simple fluid, fat, mucin, hemorrhage, solid components, etc. MRI is very useful in this characterization. Lack of a solid component essentially rules out a malignant etiology
- Ovarian lesions are accordingly classified using the O-RADS lexicon as unilocular cyst, unilocular-solid cyst, multilocular cyst, multilocular cyst, multilocular-solid cyst, solid tumor, unclassifiable

Approach to Diagnosis

Overall, a radiologist must mentally classify an adnexal lesion into one of three categories—definitely benign (simple cyst, hemorrhagic cyst, dermoid, endometrioma, peritoneal inclusion cyst, and hydrosalpinx), indeterminate, and definitely malignant. Up to 25% lesions can remain indeterminate on ultrasound after initial evaluation. The job of the radiologist in this setting is to classify the lesion as benign or malignant rather than accurately predict tumor histology. A stepwise approach helps in this situation, based on the O-RADS scoring system. An MRI may be performed as well to characterize indeterminate lesions.

The ultrasound-based IOTA Simple Rules were developed based on a prospective study [44] in which they helped give a conclusive result of benign versus malignant in 77% patients and were as accurate as ultrasound by an experienced radiologist (Table 45.10). These have now been incorporated into the more comprehensive Ultrasound O-RADS lexicon by ACR (Table 45.11). O-RADS is more comprehensive in nature as it is applicable to both surgical and non-surgical lesions, and

TABLE 45.10 IOTA USG-Based Rules for Adnexal Lesions

	Features Favoring Malignancy (M-Rules)		Features Favoring Benignity (B-Rules)
M1	Solid irregular lesion	B1	Unilocular
M2	Ascites	B2	Solid component present but largest solid component measuring <7 mm
M3	At least four papillary structures	B3	Acoustic shadows present
M4	Irregular multilocular solid tumor with largest dimension >100 mm	B4	Smooth multilocular tumor with largest dimension <100 mm
M5	Very strong blood flow (CS 4)	B5	No blood flow (CS 1)
Rule 1	One or more M findings with no B findings—malignant		
Rule 2	One or more B findings with no M findings—benign		
Rule 3	Both M and B findings—lesion cannot be classified/indeterminate		
Rule 4	Neither M nor B findings—lesion cannot be classified		

TABLE 45.11 Ultrasound O-RADS

Score	Category	Descriptor		RECOMMENDATION: Premenopausal	RECOMMENDATION: Postmenopausal
1	Normal	Simple cyst ≤3 cm (follicle)		None	—
		Corpus luteal cyst ≤3 cm			
2	Almost certainly benign (<1% probability of malignancy)	Simple cyst	≤3 cm	None	None
			3–5 cm	None	Follow-up in 1 year*
			5–10 cm in greatest dimension	Follow-up USG in 8–12 weeks	
		Classic benign lesions	Typical hemorrhagic cyst	None if less <5 cm 5–10 cm: follow-up USG in 8–12 weeks *If persistent, manage as per postmenopausal guidelines*	Ultrasound by specialist and/or MRI, gynecological evaluation
			Typical dermoid cyst (<10 cm)	If diagnosis confident: follow-up in 8–12 weeks	Ultrasound by specialist and/or MRI, gynecological evaluation, then annual USG if not operated
			Typical endometrioma (<10 cm)	Annual USG follow-up if not operated	
			Simple paraovarian cyst (any size)	None If any atypical features: manage as per ovarian cystic lesion	Follow-up USG in 1 year (optional)
			Typical peritoneal inclusion cyst or hydrosalpinx of any size	Gynecological evaluation	Gynecological evaluation
		Nonsimple unilocular cyst with smooth inner margin	≤3 cm	None	Follow-up USG in 1 year*
			3–10 cm	Follow-up USG in 8–12 weeks	Ultrasound by specialist and/ or MRI
3	Low risk (1–10%) of malignancy	Unilocular cyst ≥10 cm (both simple and nonsimple) or typical dermoid, endometrioma or hemorrhagic cyst ≥10 cm		Ultrasound by specialist and/or MRI, gynecological evaluation	
		Unilocular cyst with irregular inner wall, <3 mm in height			
		Multilocular cyst ≤10 cm with smooth inner wall and CS of 1–3			
		Smooth solid lesion with CS of 1			
4	Intermediate risk (10–50%) of malignancy	Multilocular cyst without solid component	>10 cm with smooth inner wall and CS 1–3	Ultrasound by specialist and/or MRI Specialist gynecological oncologist consultation/management	
			Any size with smooth wall with CS of 4		
			Any cyst showing irregular inner wall thickening or septae		
		Unilocular cyst with solid component	0–3 papillary projections		
		Multilocular cyst with a solid component	Any size with CS 1–2		
		Solid	Any size with smooth outer margins and CS 2–3		

Continued

TABLE 45.11 Ultrasound O-RADS—cont'd

			RECOMMENDATION	
Score	Category	Descriptor	Premenopausal	Postmenopausal
5	High risk (>50%) of malignancy	Unilocular cyst with ≥4 papillary projections	Specialist gynecological oncologist consultation/management	
		Multilocular cyst with solid component and CS 3–4		
		Smooth solid mass with CS 4		
		Irregular solid mass with any CS		
		Presence of ascites and/or peritoneal implants#		

* = At least 1-year follow-up showing stability or decrease in size is recommended with consideration of annual follow-up of up to 5 years, if stable. However, there is currently a paucity of evidence for defining optimal duration or interval of timing for surveillance.
# = Presence of ascites with category 1–2 lesion, must consider other malignant or nonmalignant etiologies of ascites.
CS, color score.
Adapted, with permission, from the American College of Radiology.

TABLE 45.12 O-RADS MR Scoring System [45]

Score	Risk Category	PPV for Malignancy	Lexicon Description
1	Normal ovaries	Not applicable	▪ No mass
2	Almost certainly benign	~0.5%	▪ Unilocular cyst without solid component: Any type of fluid content and no enhancing wall ▪ Unilocular cyst without solid component with smooth enhancing wall: Simple or endometriotic content ▪ Lesion with lipid content ▪ Lesion with 'dark T2 dark DWI' solid tissue: homogeneously hypointense on T2WI and DWI ▪ Dilated Fallopian tube with simple fluid content and no solid component; thin smooth wall/folds with enhancement ▪ Parovarian cyst without solid component with any type of fluid; with or without smooth enhancing wall
3	Low risk	~5%	▪ Unilocular cyst without solid component with smooth enhancing wall – hemorrhagic, proteinaceous or mucinous content ▪ Multilocular cyst without solid component with any type of fluid; no fat; smooth wall or septal enhancement ▪ Solid lesion (excepting dark T2 dark DWI lesion) with low risk time intensity curve on DCE MRI ▪ Dilated Fallopian tube without solid component; non-simple fluid content or thick smooth wall/folds
4	Intermediate risk	~50%	▪ Lesions with solid tissue and intermediate risk time intensity curve on DCE MRI. If DCE MRI not performed, solid tissue which enhances ≤ myometrium at 30–40 sec ▪ Lesion with lipid content and large volume enhancing solid tissue
5	High risk	~90%	▪ Lesion with solid tissue with high risk time intensity curve on DCE MRI. If DCE MRI not performed, solid tissue which enhances > myometrium at 30–40 sect ▪ Peritoneal, omental or mesenteric nodularity or irregular thickening

DCE, dynamic contrast-enhanced; *DWI*, diffusion weighted imaging.

incorporates management guidelines, including the use of MRI and referral to a general gynecologist or a specialist gynecologic oncosurgeon. It must be noted that the management is ultimately decided on a case-to-case basis.

MRI Risk Stratification

O-RADS MR scoring system has been tabulated in Table 45.12 [45]. The readers are directed to the algorithmic ESUR for MR imaging of sonographically indeterminate adnexal lesions for understanding the approach to these lesions on MRI [46] and to the ACR MR O-RADS article for understanding application of O-RADS [45]. Descriptors are relatively similar to ultrasound O-RADS. The key concept to remember is that lack of solid component rules out malignancy. If a solid component is present, DCE MRI can be utilized to characterize the lesion based on time intensity curves. Note that solid tissue on MRI is defined as a component that demonstrates contrast enhancement along with one of the following morphologic characteristics: papillary projections, mural nodules, irregular septations or walls, and larger solid portion. Nonsolid tissue is defined as components that do not fit the definition of solid tissue, and includes thin or thick smooth septations or walls, blood clot, nonenhancing debris, fibrin strands, and fat; these indicate benign etiology.

Suggested Readings

- C Reinhold, A Rockall, EA Sadowski, ES Siegelman, KE Maturen, HA Vargas, et al., Ovarian-adnexal reporting lexicon for MRI: a white paper of the ACR Ovarian-Adnexal Reporting and Data Systems MRI Committee, J Am Coll Radiol 18 (5) (2021) 713–729.
- D Levine, MD Patel, EJ Suh-Burgmann, RF Andreotti, BR Benacerraf, CB Benson, WR Brewster, BG Coleman, et al., Simple adnexal cysts: SRU consensus conference update on follow-up and reporting, Radiology 293 (2) (2019) 359–371.
- JA Spencer, R Forstner, TM Cunha, K Kinkel, ESUR Female Imaging Sub-Committee. ESUR guidelines for MR imaging of the sonographically indeterminate adnexal mass: an algorithmic approach, Eur Radiol 20 (1) (2010) 25–35.
- EC Taylor, L Irshaid, M Mathur, Multimodality imaging approach to ovarian neoplasms with pathologic correlation, Radiographics 41 (1) (2021) 289–315.
- RF Andreotti, D Timmerman, BR Benacerraf, et al., Ovarian-Adnexal Reporting Lexicon for Ultrasound: A White Paper of the ACR Ovarian-Adnexal Reporting and Data System Committee, J Am Coll Radiol 15 (2018) 1415–1429.
- RF Andreotti, D Timmerman, LM Strachowski, W Froyman, BR Benacerraf, GL Bennett, et al., O-RADS US Risk Stratification and Management System: A Consensus Guideline from the ACR Ovarian-Adnexal Reporting and Data System Committee, Radiol 294 (2020) 168–185.
- EA Sadowski, I Thomassin-Naggara, A Rockall, et al., O-RADS MRI Risk Stratification System: Guide for Assessing Adnexal Lesions from the ACR O-RADS Committee, Radiol 303 (2022) 35–47.

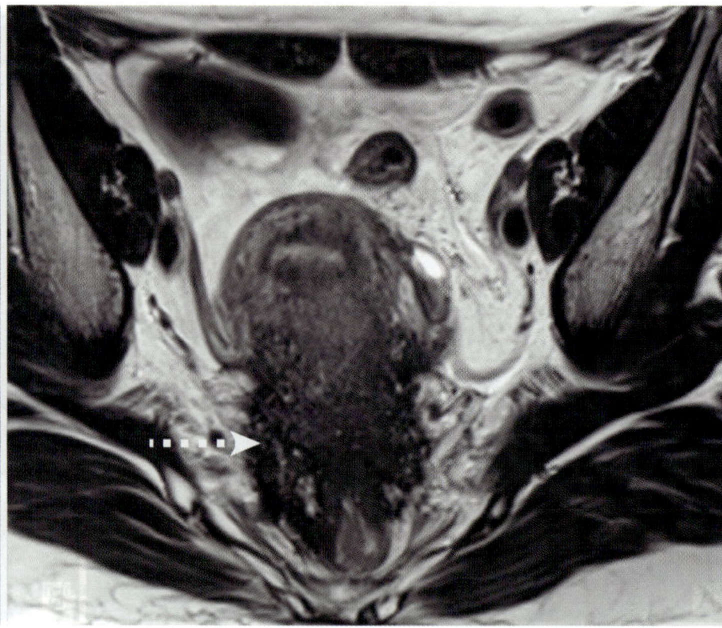

Figure 46.11A Rectouterine endometriosis. Sagittal and axial T2-weighted MR images show bulky hypointense deposits in rectouterine space (*white arrow* on sagittal), involving posterior serosal surface of uterus with mild retroversion. Focal obliteration of the rectouterine space (*dashed white arrow*) is seen on axial image.

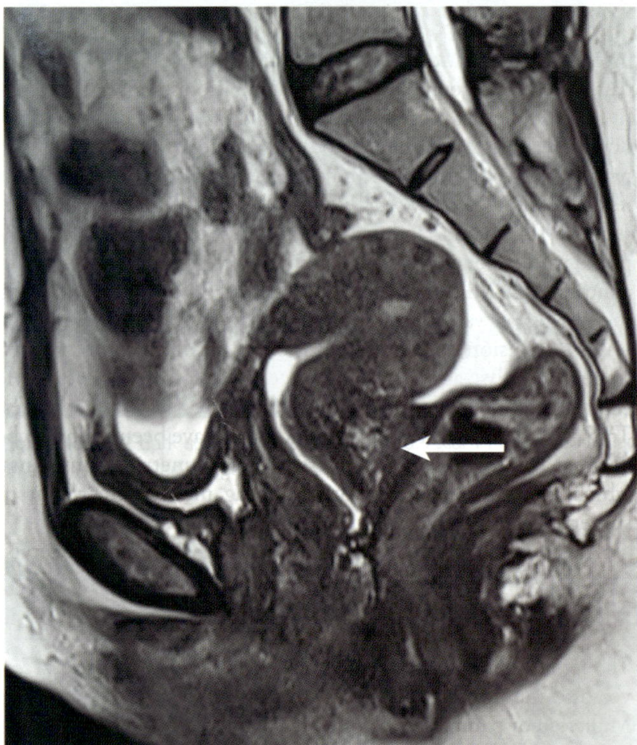

Figure 46.11B Retrocervical space endometriosis. Sagittal T2-weighted MR image shows thickened hypointense deposits in the retrocervical region (*white arrow*) with retroversion of the uterus.

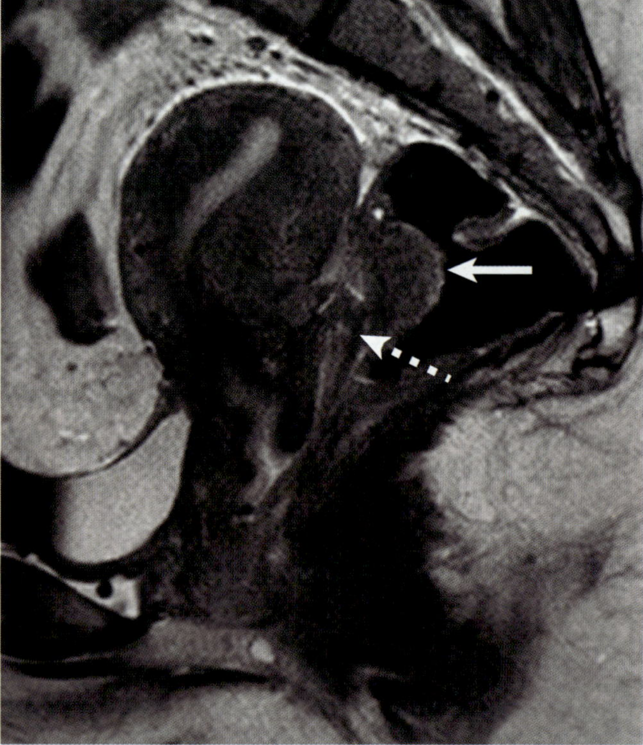

Figure 46.11C Rectal endometriosis with mushroom cap sign. Sagittal T2-weighted MR image shows focal nodular, hypointense thickening of rectal wall with a relatively hyperintense layer of mucosa and submucosa (*white arrow*), known as mushroom cap sign. Retraction and elevation of posterior vaginal fornix by endometriotic deposit is seen (*dashed white arrow*) with retroversion of uterus.

production of Mullerian inhibiting substance (MIS) by Sertoli cells of testes, the Wolfian duct involutes and the Mullerian duct develops into uterus, fallopian tubes, and upper vagina. The lower one-third of the vagina develops from the urogenital sinus [39].

The Mullerian ducts grow in a bidirectional manner, the upper ends open to the peritoneal cavity and the lower ends are closed. Between 8 and 12 weeks of embryologic development, the Mullerian ducts grow caudally to reach the urogenital sinus. The inferior part of the Mullerian ducts gives rise to uterus, cervix, and upper two-thirds of the vagina. The fallopian tubes develop from the superior part of the Mullerian ducts [40]. The Mullerian ducts fuse in the midline and this is followed by resorption of the septum (Figs. 46.13A–C Adapted from Ref [41]).

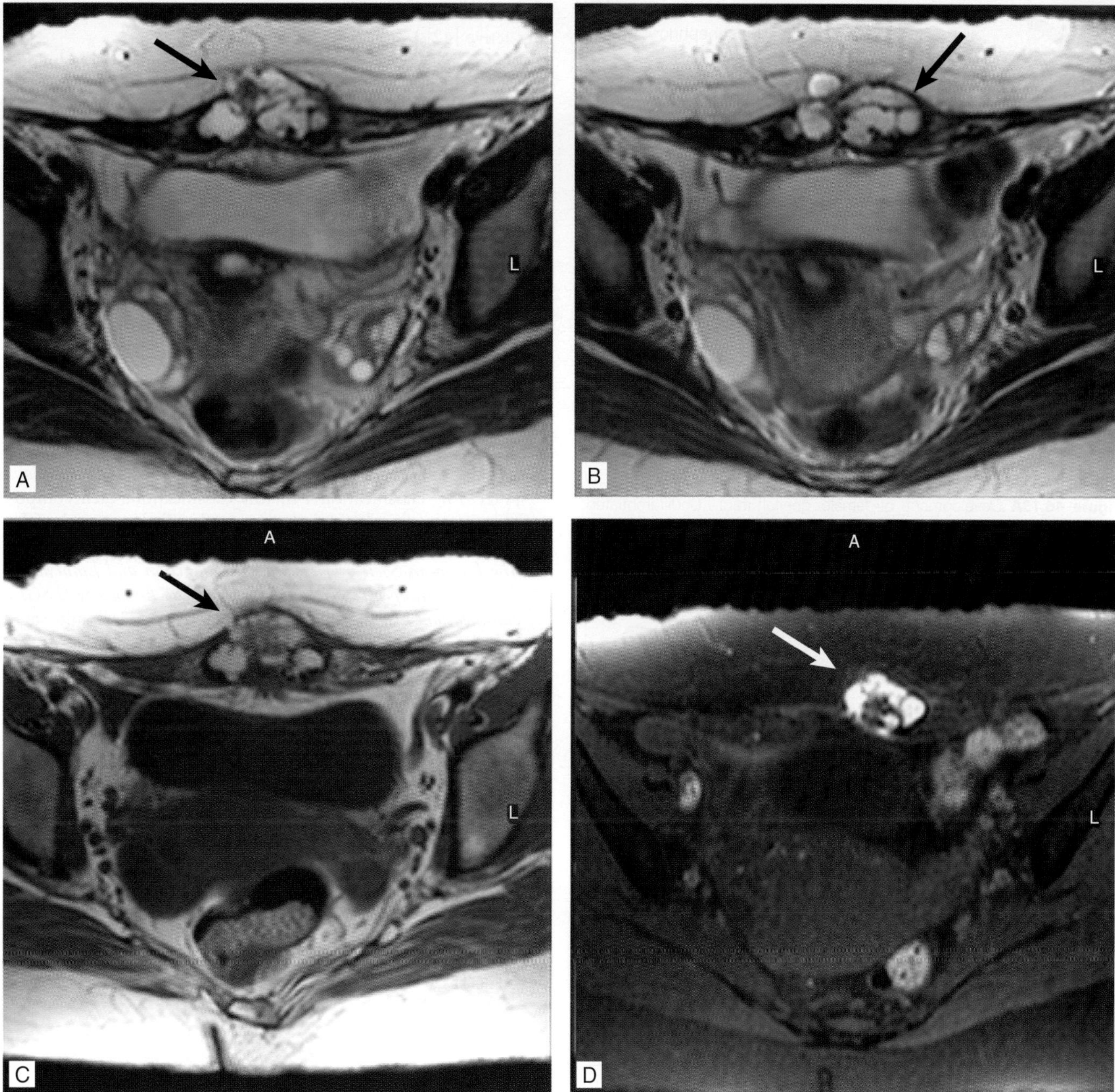

Figure 46.12 (A–D) Scar endometriosis. Axial T2 (A and B) T1-weighted (C) and T2 fat-suppressed (D) MR images show a mixed signal intensity lesion with hyperintense and hypointense foci on all images, in the lower part of rectus sheath in the midline (*arrows*).

- Failure of organogenesis of both or one of the Mullerian ducts results in agenesis/hypoplasia or the unicornuate uterus.
- Failure of fusion of the ducts results in bicornuate uterus or uterus didelphys and failure of septal resorption causes septate or arcuate uterus [35].
- T-shaped uterus is an abnormality of the uterine cavity attributed to diethyl stilbestrol (DES).

Imaging Modalities

USG

It is easily available, affordable, and free of radiation. TVS with 3D technique is particularly useful to evaluate the external uterine fundal contour as also the endometrial cavity [40]. It can thus help in the diagnosis and accurate classification of MDA.

MRI

It is the considered the gold standard investigation for the evaluation of MDA [40]. T2-weighted images best delineate the uterine zonal anatomy with hyperintense endometrial cavity, hypointense junctional zone, and intermediate signal intensity myometrium adjacent to the junctional zone [40]. The coronal oblique plane (along the long axis of the corpus) is useful to delineate the external uterine fundal contour. T1W fat-suppressed images are useful to detect blood products when there is obstruction. Other associated anomalies such as renal anomalies can be also be detected on MRI. MRI is particularly useful in the

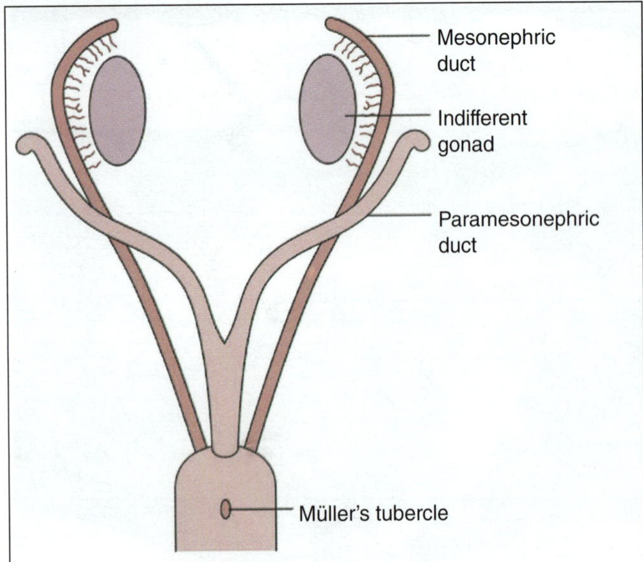

Figure 46.13A Development of female genital tract. Undifferentiated gonad with two pairs of ducts, the Mullerian (paramesonephric) and Wolfian (mesonephric) ducts.

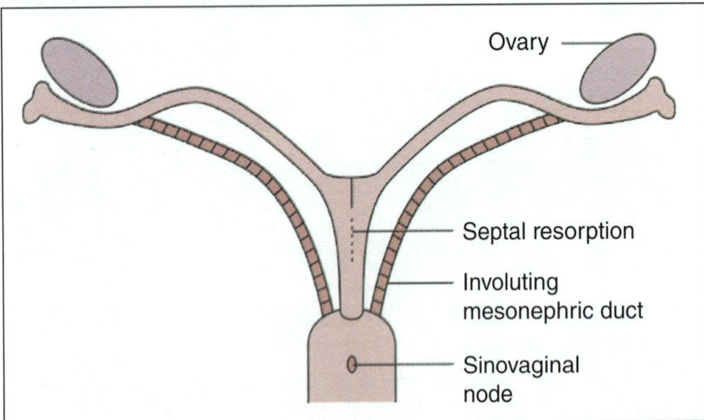

Figure 46.13B Development of female genital tract. Wolfian (mesonephric) ducts involute and the Mullerian (paramesonephric) ducts develop into uterus, upper vagina, and fallopian tube. The medial portion of the Mullerian ducts fuse in the midline, followed by resorption of the septum.

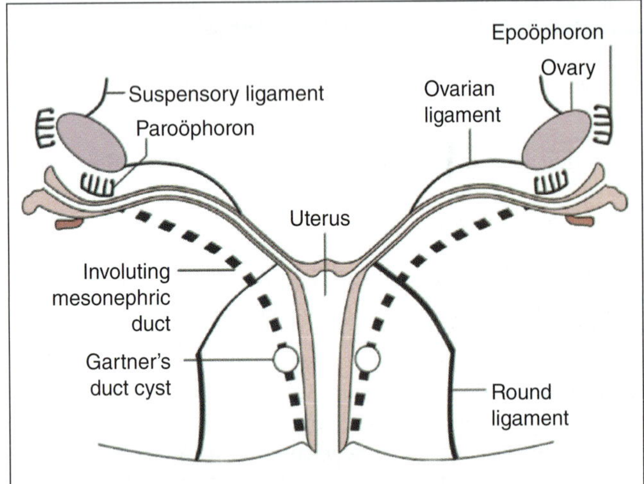

Figure 46.13C Female internal genitalia after its development, at 5 months of embryonic life.

evaluation of MDA in children and adolescents who are not sexually active [42].

Hysterosalpingography (HSG)—This is not the preferred technique for the evaluation of MDA since it does not provide information about the myometrium and external uterine fundal contour. However, it is used to evaluate tubal patency and endometrial cavity [40].

Classification of Mullerian Duct Anomalies

There are several classification systems.

1. *The American Society for Reproductive Medicine (ASRM)* classification, based on the stage of failure of Mullerian duct development, is the most widely accepted classification (Table 46.1). It divides MDA into seven major anatomic uterine types with subtypes. This classification system has some drawbacks. Complex Mullerian anomalies with features of more than one ASRM category are difficult to classify. In addition, the focus of this classification system is on the uterine abnormality and it does not include an approach to obstructive vaginal anomalies [40,43].
2. *Vagina, cervix, uterus, adnexa, and associated malformations (VCUAM)* classification—In this classification, each component of the female genital tract is classified separately. The main drawback of this system is its complexity [40].
3. *The European Society of Human Reproduction and Embryology (ESHRE)/European Society for Gynaecologic Endoscopy (ESGE) classification*—In this classification, uterus, cervical, and vaginal abnormalities are classified independently (Table 46.2). The main classes include deviations of uterine anatomy which are of the same embryological origin with further subclasses

TABLE 46.1 ASRM Classification of MDA (Adapted From Reference [43])

Class	Uterine Abnormality
Class 1: Mullerian agenesis or hypoplasia a. Vaginal b. Cervical c. Fundal d. Tubal e. Combined	Agenesis or hypoplasia of the paired Mullerian ducts
Class 2: Unicornuate uterus a. Rudimentary horn with a communicating cavity b. Rudimentary horn without a communicating cavity c. Rudimentary horn without a cavity d. Complete absence of one horn	Agenesis or hypoplasia of one of the paired Mullerian ducts
Class 3: Uterus didelphys	Failure of fusion of the Mullerian ducts
Class 4: Bicornuate uterus a. Complete b. Partial	Incomplete fusion of the Mullerian ducts at the level of body and fundus
Class 5: Septate uterus a. Complete b. Partial	Incomplete or absent resorption of the uterovaginal septum
Class 6: Arcuate uterus	Normal variant, near complete resorption of the uterovaginal septum
Class 7: Diethylstilbestrol related uterine hypoplasia	T-shaped uterine cavity with shortened upper uterus

TABLE 46.2 ESHRE/ESGE Classification of Cervical and Vaginal Anomalies (Reference [44])

Cervical/Vaginal Anomaly	
C0	Normal cervix
C1	Septate cervix
C2	Double "normal" cervix
C3	Unilateral cervical aplasia
C4	Cervical aplasia
V0	Normal vagina
V1	Longitudinal nonobstructing vaginal septum
V2	Longitudinal obstructing vaginal septum
V3	Transverse vaginal septum and/or imperforate hymen
V4	Vaginal aplasia

[40,44]. Some of the drawbacks mentioned in other classifications are not seen with ESHRE classification.

ASRM Classification of MDA (adapted from reference [43])

Class 1—Mullerian Hypoplasia/Agenesis

This is the most severe form of MDA, resulting from an early failure of paramesonephric ducts to develop, at around 5 weeks gestation [41,45]. It accounts for 5–10% of MDA [40]. The most common form is the Mayer–Rokitansky–Kuster–Hauser syndrome with complete agenesis of the vagina, and in 90% of cases with complete agenesis of the cervix and uterus. A rudimentary uterus is seen in 10% of cases which could have a functioning endometrium [46]. Normal ovaries are usually present.

Clinically, these patients have a normal phenotype due to the presence of normal functioning ovaries. They present at puberty with primary amenorrhea. If a functional uterine remnant is present, the patient may have severe cyclical abdominal pain [46].

Imaging

USG

- It is the initial imaging modality.
- Rudimentary uterine bud may be difficult to identify on USG.
- Normal morphology of ovaries seen on USG.

MRI

- Best imaging modality to confirm agenesis or hypoplasia of vagina and uterus (Fig. 46.14).
- T2 sagittal images are particularly useful to confirm uterine agenesis.
- They also help to locate the rudimentary uterine bud, if present.
- Rudimentary uterine bud is seen as a low signal intensity structure with or without a zonal anatomy.
- T2 axial images are useful to identify vaginal agenesis [46].

Class 2—Unicornuate Uterus

This occurs when there is failure of development, either complete or partial, of one of the paired Mullerian ducts. This accounts for 20% of all MDAs [40,42]. This anomaly has four subtypes; rudimentary horn with a communicating cavity, rudimentary horn with a noncommunicating cavity, rudimentary horn without a cavity, and complete absence of one horn. A rudimentary horn with endometrial tissue is called a functional rudimentary horn [46]. A higher incidence of renal anomalies is seen with unicornuate uterus (up to 40% of cases), the most common being renal agenesis ipsilateral to the rudimentary horn [40,42]. Unicornuate uterus is also seen more often in the right side of the pelvis [40].

Clinically, in the absence of a noncommunicating, functional rudimentary horn, unicornuate uterus causes no symptoms and is often incidentally discovered. When there is a rudimentary noncommunicating functional horn, retrograde menstruation from obstructed horn can cause endometriosis and symptoms of chronic pelvic pain as a symptom [35,46]. There is also a risk of ectopic pregnancy, preterm labor, miscarriage, and uterine rupture [35].

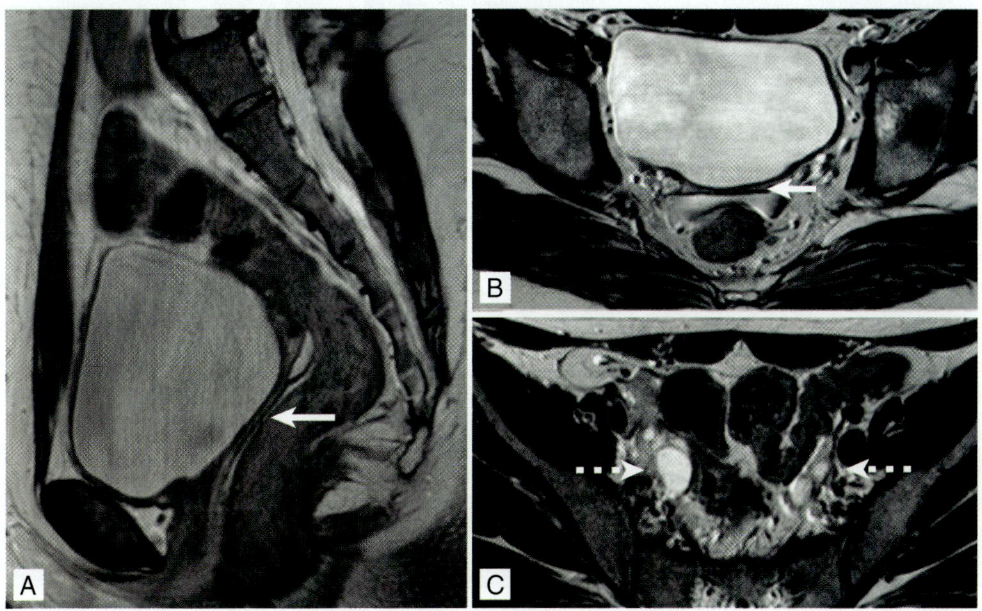

Figure 46.14 Mayer–Rokitansky–Küster–Hauser syndrome. Sagittal (A) and axial (B, C) T2-weighted MR images show absent uterus posterior to bladder (*white arrows* in A, B) and presence of normal ovaries bilaterally (*dashed white arrows* in C).

Imaging

USG

- Shows the uterus deviated off midline to one side of the pelvic cavity.

HSG

- There is contrast opacification of a fusiform-shaped uterine cavity deviated to one side of the pelvis with a single fallopian tube.
- A noncommunicating rudimentary horn cannot be identified at HSG (Fig. 46.15A).

MRI

- This reveals an elongated, banana-shaped uterus off the midline, to one side of the pelvic cavity.
- This is best seen on T2-weighted axial images [40,46].
- The myometrium and zonal anatomy is normal [35].
- The endometrium is narrow with tapering at the apex [46].
- MRI is useful to identify the rudimentary horn, presence of an obstructed horn, and to look for associated renal abnormalities [40,43] (Fig. 46.15B).

Class 3—Uterus Didelphys

This results from complete failure of fusion of the Mullerian ducts at the ninth week of gestation [46]. This accounts for 5% of all MDA [40,42]. The two ducts which are fully developed form two noncommunicating uterine cavities with normal zonal anatomy and two cervices. About 75% of cases have a longitudinal vaginal septum [40]. In some patients, an obstructing hemivaginal transverse septum maybe present, causing hematometrocolpos [35,40]. Majority of patients with obstructed hemivagina also have ipsilateral renal agenesis (OHVIRA syndrome - obstructed hemivagina and ipsilateral renal agenesis, or the Herlyn–Werner–Wunderlich syndrome).

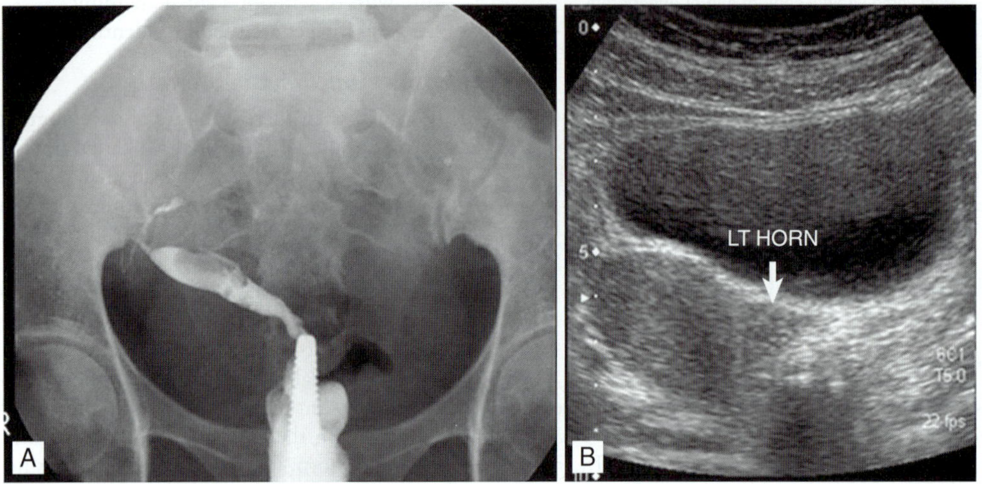

Figure 46.15A Unicornuate uterus. HSG spot radiograph (A) shows fusiform-shaped uterine cavity deviated to the right side of the pelvis with single fallopian tube. USG images of same patient shows a rudimentary noncommunicating horn (*white arrow* in B), not seen on HSG.

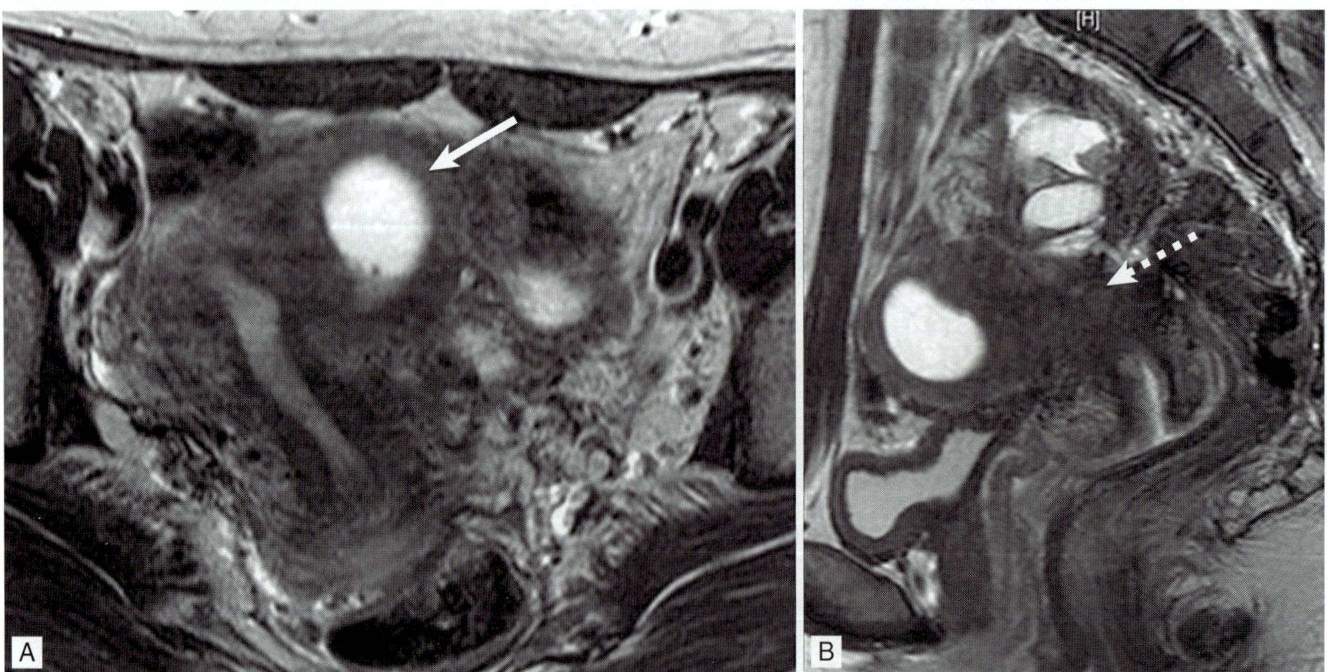

Figure 46.15B Unicornuate uterus. Axial and sagittal T2 weighted MR images of another patient with unicornuate uterus show uterus deviated to one side of the pelvis with a noncommunicating cavity in the rudimentary horn (*white arrow* in A). T2 hypointense nodular deposits (*dashed white arrow* in B) and cysts in adnexa indicate secondary changes of endometriosis.

Clinically, patients with uterus didelphys are symptomatic only in the presence of hemivaginal obstruction. Retrograde menstruation and endometriosis may cause cyclical pelvic pain [46].

Imaging

USG

- This reveals two widely divergent, noncommunicating uterine cavities with two separate cervices.

HSG

- There is contrast opacification of two separate cervical canals and uterine cavities which leads to a fallopian tube on each side (Fig. 46.16A).
- Only one cavity will be opacified in the presence of a hemivaginal septum [35].

MRI

- This will show two widely divergent uterine cavities with two separate cervices and a deep fundal cleft.
- Majority of patients also have a longitudinal vaginal septum (Fig. 46.16B).
- The endometrial-myometrial ratio and zonal anatomy of both uterine horns are normal [35,46].
- In the presence of an obstructing hemivaginal septum, hematometrocolpos will be seen with blood signal intensity in the obstructed uterine horn (Fig. 46.17).
- Treatment is directed at removal of obstructing vaginal septum.

Class 4—Bicornuate Uterus

This occurs when there is incomplete fusion of the Mullerian ducts at the ninth week of gestation [46] and accounts for 10% of all MDA [40,42]. A fundal cleft of more than 10 mm depth is typically seen with bicornuate uterus [42].

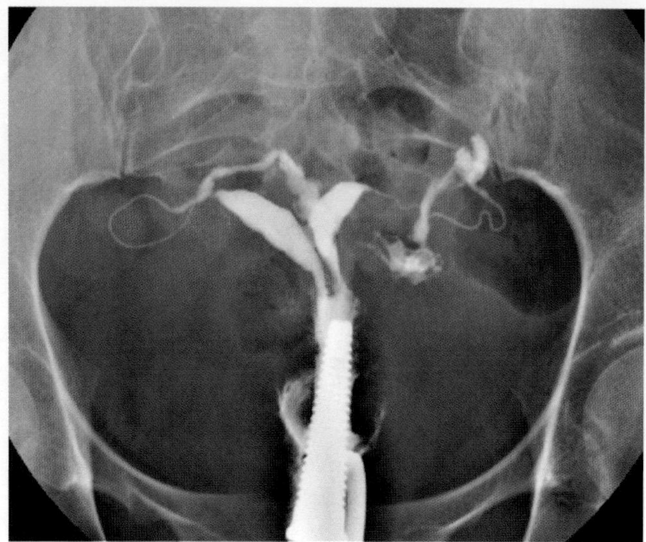

Figure 46.16A Uterus didelphys. HSG spot radiograph shows two separate cervical canals and uterine cavities which lead to a fallopian tube on each side.

If fusion of the ducts occurs at the level of the internal cervical os, the uterus is termed bicornuate unicollis and if fusion occurs at the external os with two cervices, it is known as bicornuate bicollis [40,42]. About 25% of patients with bicornuate uterus may have longitudinal vaginal septum [40]. Thus, it may be difficult to differentiate bicornuate bicollis uterus from uterus didelphys [35].

Clinically, these patients are largely asymptomatic but with higher prevalence of pregnancy loss in the presence of vaginal septum and uterus bicornis bicollis [46].

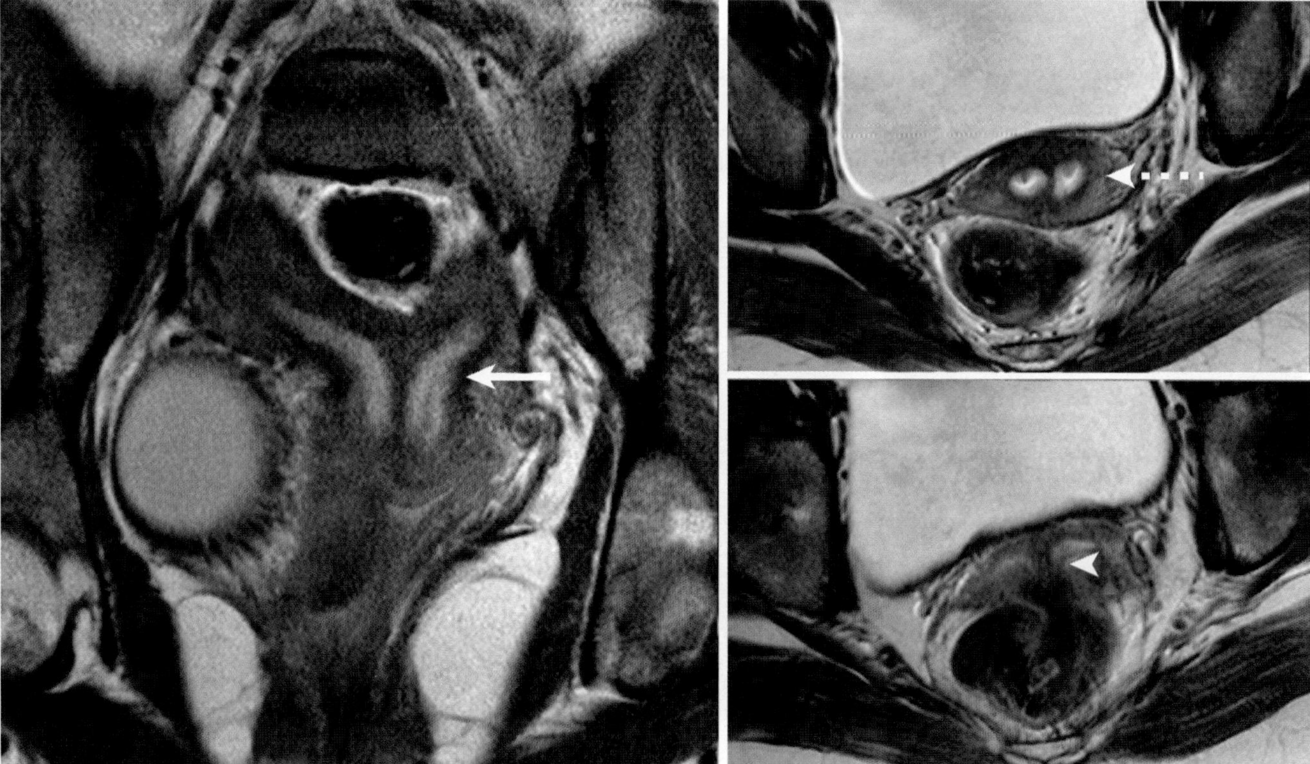

Figure 46.16B Uterus didelphys. Coronal and axial T2-weighted MR images show two divergent uterine cavities (*white arrow*), two separate cervices (*dashed white arrow*), and a midline vaginal septum (*white arrowhead*).

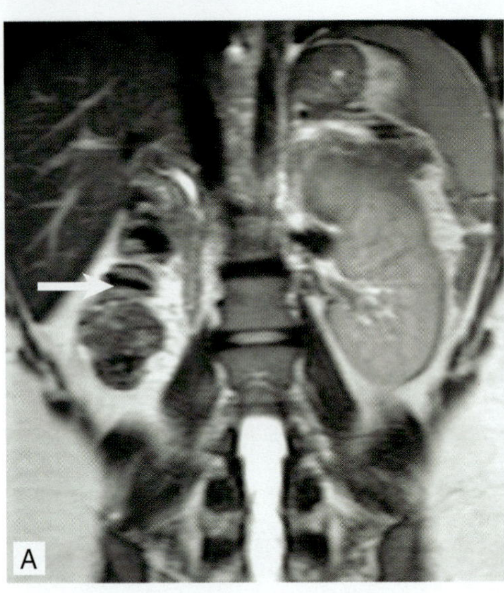

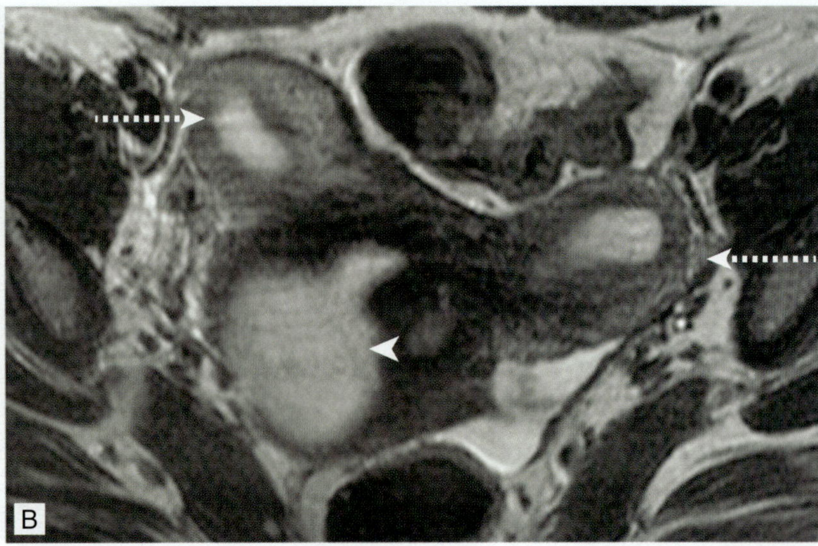

Figure 46.17 OHVIRA syndrome. Coronal and axial T2-weighted MR images show absent right kidney (*white arrow* in A), two divergent uterine cavities (*dashed white arrows* in B), and a distended fluid filled right hemivagina (*white arrowhead* in B) adjacent to collapsed left hemivagina.

Imaging

USG

- This will reveal two divergent uterine horns with echogenic endometrium and a deep fundal cleft [35,46].

HSG

- There is contrast opacification of two widely divergent uterine cavities with intercornual angle historically exceeding 105 degrees [35] (Fig. 46.18A).
- A single cervical canal is seen with uterus bicornuate unicollis and two cervical canals with uterus bicornuate bicollis.

MRI

- This reveals diverging uterine horns with a fundal cleft more than 10 mm in depth [35].
- The endometrial-myometrial ratio and zonal anatomy are normal.
- Uterine morphology can be bicornuate unicollis or bicornuate bicollis (Fig. 46.18B–C).
- The presence of smaller uterine horns and some communication between the two cervical canals in the former will help to differentiate bicornuate bicollis uterus from uterus didelphys [43]. The presence of longitudinal vaginal septum with two vaginal cavities in approximately 75% of cases of uterus dildelphys [40] (Fig. 46.18D).

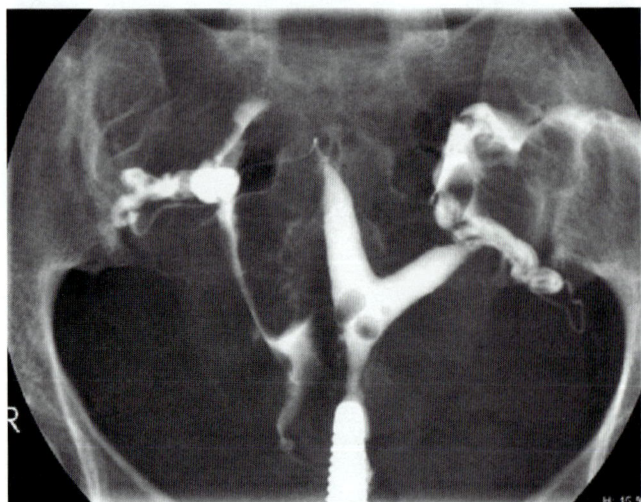

Figure 46.18A Bicornuate uterus. HSG spot radiograph shows two widely divergent uterine cavities and a single cervix indicating uterus bicornuate unicollis.

Class 5—Septate Uterus

This results from complete or partial failure of reabsorption of the uterovaginal septum by the 12th week of gestation [46]. It the most common MDA and accounts for 55% of cases [35,40]. The septum is fibrous or fibromuscular and maybe complete or partial. A complete septum extends up to level of external cervical os while a partial septum can be of varying length [40]. This anomaly has the highest association with poor reproductive outcome and pregnancy loss.

Imaging

USG

- USG, particularly 3D USG, is useful to evaluate the external fundal contour.
- In septate uterus, the apex of the external fundal contour is more than 5 mm above a line drawn between uterine ostia.
- This differentiates it from anomalies of Mullerian duct fusion.
- The septum can be visualized on USG with varied echogenicity in the muscular and fibrous portions of septum [46].

HSG

- Typically an angle of less than 75 degrees between the two uterine cavities favors a septate uterus over a bicornuate uterus [35] (Fig. 46.19A).

MRI

- This shows the external fundal contour to be convex, flat, or mildly concave with less than 10 mm indentation.
- Septum can be partial or complete (Figs. 46.19B–C).
- On T2W images, the higher signal intensity of the muscular portion of septum near the fundus resembling uterine myometrium can be differentiated from the low signal intensity fibrous septum [35,46].
- Treatment involves resection of the septum with better reproductive outcome.

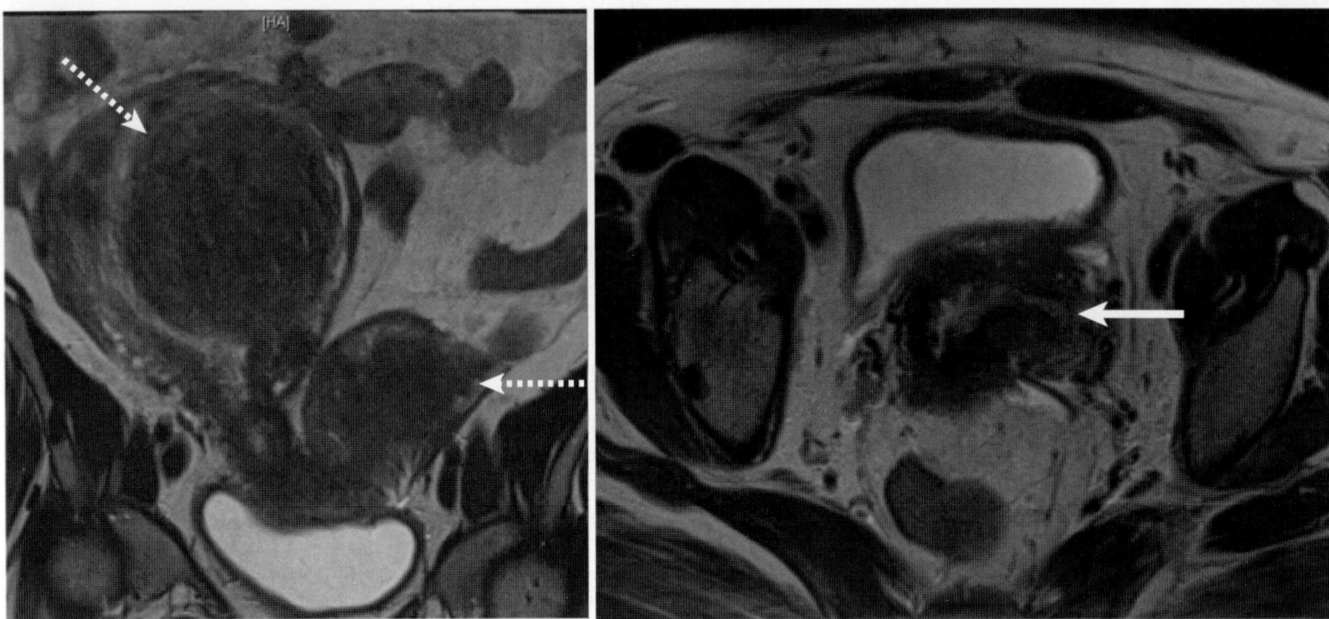

Figure 46.18B Bicornuate unicollis uterus. Coronal and axial T2-weighted MR images show two divergent uterine horns with fibroids seen as hypointense lesions (*dashed white arrow*) and a single cervix (*white arrow*).

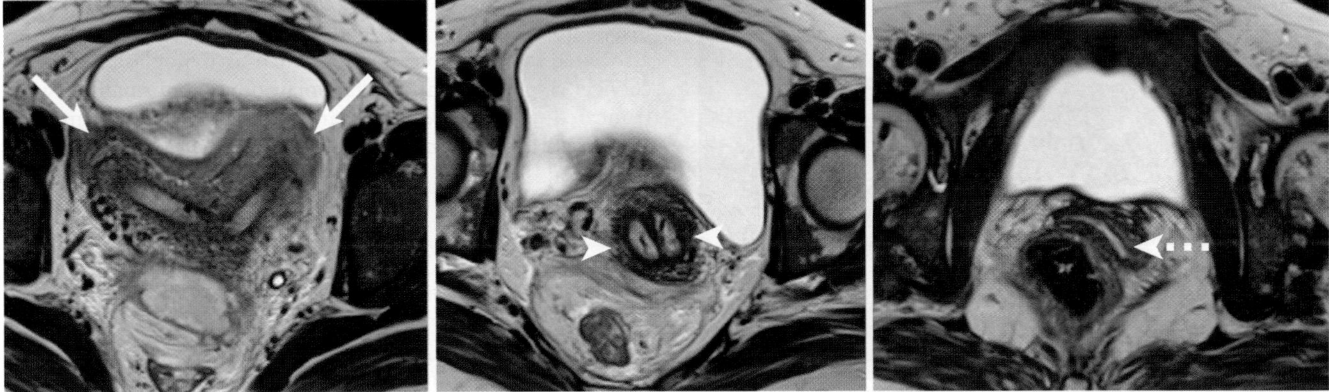

Figure 46.18C Bicornuate bicollis uterus. Axial T2-weighted MR images show two divergent uterine horns (*white arrows*), two cervical canals (*white arrowheads*), and single vagina (*dashed white arrow*).

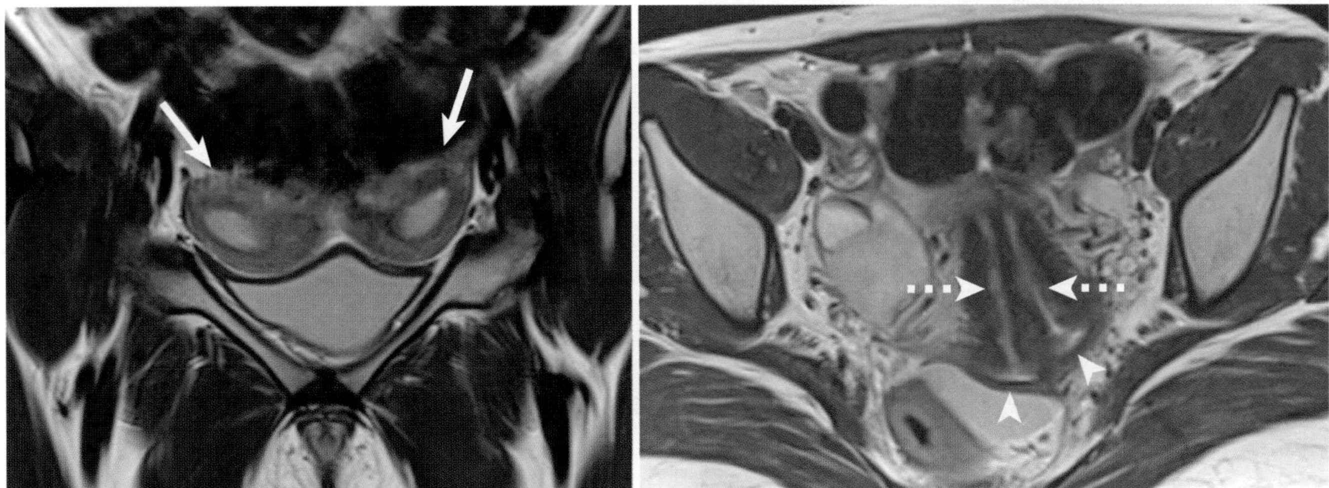

Figure 46.18D Uterus didelphys .The presence of longitudinal vaginal septum seen in 75% of cases of uterus didelphys with two vaginal cavities (*white arrowheads*) can help to differentiate this from bicornuate bicollis uterus. *White arrows* demarcate divergent uterine horns and *dashed white arrows*, the cervical canals.

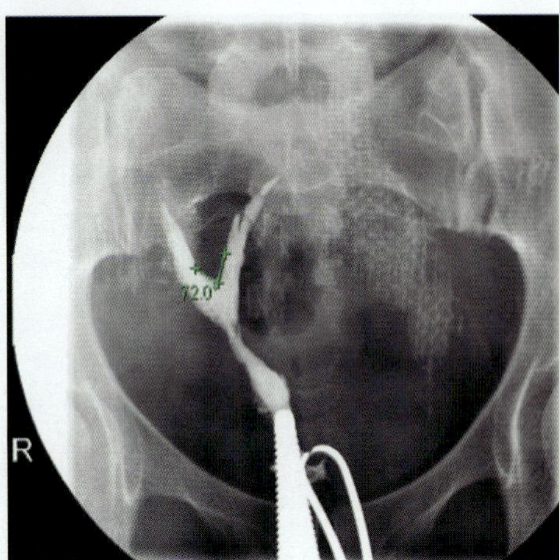

Figure 46.19A Septate uterus. HSG spot radiograph shows a narrow angle of less than 75 degrees between the two uterine cavities and single cervix indicating partial septate uterus.

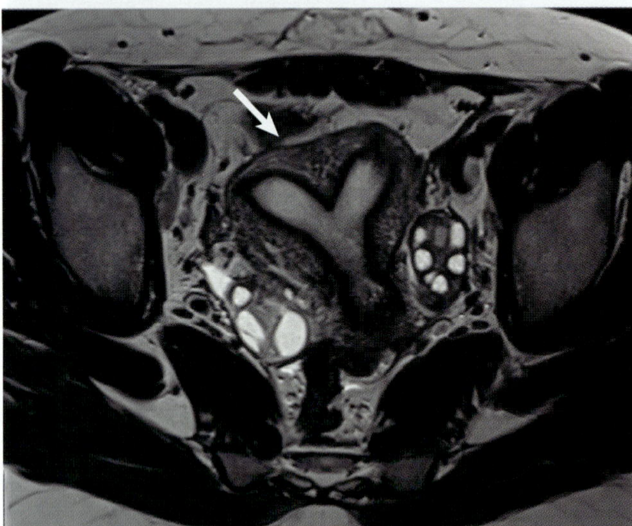

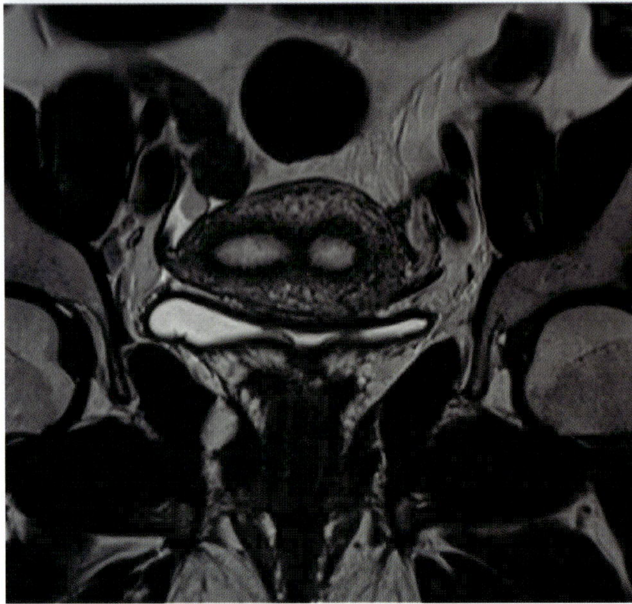

Figure 46.19B Partial septate uterus. Axial and coronal T2-weighted MR images show a flat external uterine fundal contour (*white arrow*) with two uterine cavities and a single cervical canal.

Class 6—Arcuate Uterus

It is often considered a normal variant, results from near complete reabsorption of the uterovaginal septum with focal myometrial thickening at the fundus [40,42].

Imaging

USG

- USG reveals a convex external fundal contour.
- Mild indentation on the endometrial canal at fundus, due to focally thickened myometrium.

HSG

- There is a broad indentation on the endometrial cavity at the fundus [35] (Fig. 46.20).

MRI

- This confirms a convex external fundal contour.
- There is thickening of fundal myometrium which is isointense to the rest of the uterine myometrium [40,42].

Class 7—DES Uterus

It is associated with diethylstilbestrol, a nonsteroidal estrogen historically used in women at high risk for miscarriage or poor reproductive outcome. Its use was discontinued after discovery of an increased risk of vaginal malignancy and uterine malformations using this drug. It is typically associated with a T-shaped uterine cavity which has a widened lower uterine cavity, narrowed endometrial canal at fundus, a small hypoplastic uterus and irregular endometrial margins. There may be associated cervical abnormalities such as hypoplasia, anterior cervical ridge or collar and fallopian tubes abnormalities with truncated appearance, saccular outpouchings, and fimbrial abnormalities. This can occur rarely in the absence of DES exposure [35].

Imaging

HSG

- This shows the classical T-shaped cavity is seen with truncated and irregular fallopian tubes (Fig. 46.21).

MRI

- This also demonstrates a hypoplastic uterus, T-shaped endometrial cavity and constriction bands due to focal thickening of junctional zone, resulting in narrow and irregular cavity [35].

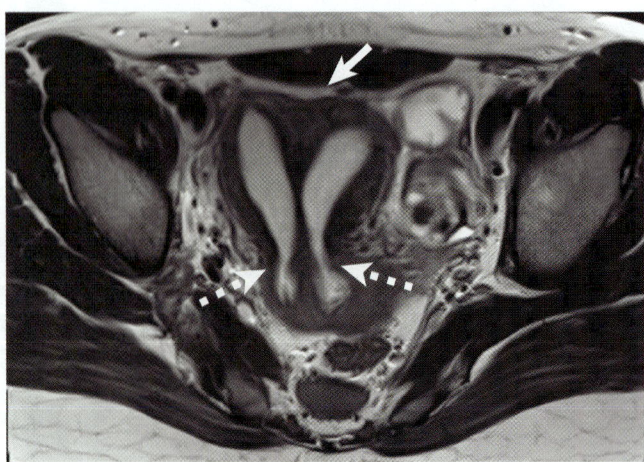

Figure 46.19C Complete septate uterus: axial T2 weighted MR image shows almost flat external fundal contour (*white arrow*) with two uterine cavities and two cervical canals (*dashed white arrows*).

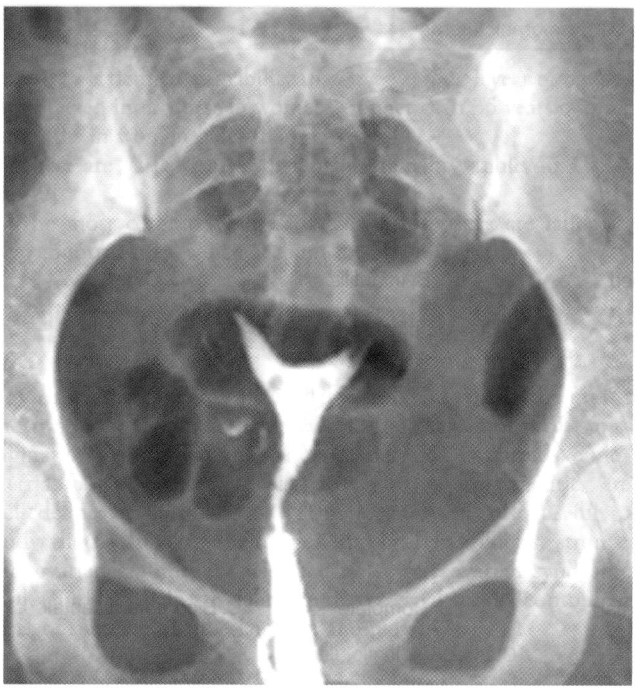

Figure 46.20 Arcuate uterus. HSG spot radiograph shows broad indentation on the endometrial cavity at the fundus.

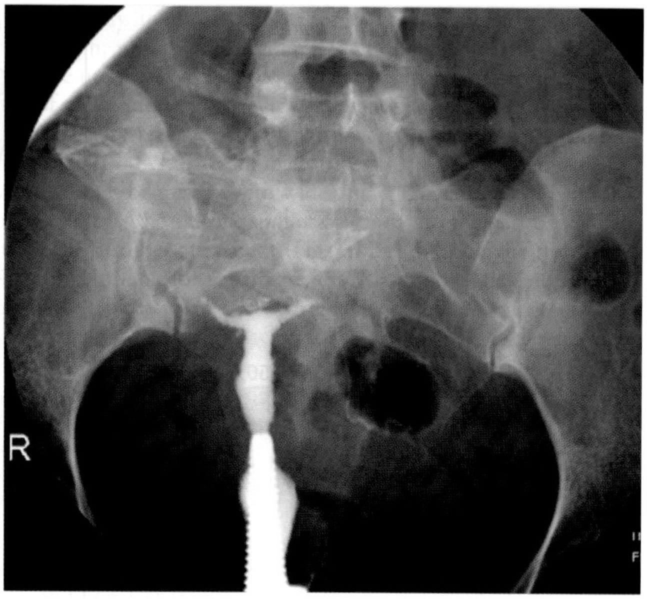

Figure 46.21 T-shaped uterus. HSG spot radiograph shows a T-shaped uterus, classically described with DES exposure.

The European Society of Human Reproduction and Embryology (ESHRE)/European Society for Gynecologic Endoscopy (ESGE) Classification

In this classification, each group has deviations of uterine anatomy, which are of same embryological origin with further subclasses. In each of the classes or subclasses, deviations of uterine anatomy are placed in order of increasing severity with the more severe variants placed at the end and less severe ones in the beginning. Cervical and vaginal abnormalities are classified separately in supplementary subclasses [44] (Fig. 46.22).

Class U0 Normal uterus with a straight or curved interostial line with an internal indentation on fundus not more than 50% of myometrial thickness.

Class U1—This group includes all cases with an abnormal shape of uterine cavity except septa but with a normal uterine outline. It has three categories.

Class U1a—T-shaped uterus with thickened lateral walls causing a narrow uterine cavity with two-thirds uterine corpus and one-third cervix.

Class U1b—Uterus infantilis with narrow cavity, no lateral wall thickening and one-third uterine corpus and two-thirds cervix.

Class U1c—Others. This group comprises all minor deformities of uterine cavity including an inner fundal indentation of less than 50%.

Class U2—Septate uterus in which there is normal fusion but a failure of resorption of midline septum. It is characterized by normal uterine outline, but an internal fundal indentation which is more than 50% of wall thickness. It may be complete or partial.

Class U2a—Partial septate uterus with septum partially dividing uterine cavity above level of internal cervical os.

Class U2b—Complete septate uterus with septum dividing uterine cavity up to level of internal cervical os.

Class U3—Bicorporeal uterus which includes all anomalies of fusion. The uterine fundal outline is abnormal with an external fundal indentation more than 50% of wall thickness [44]. It has three subclasses.

Class U3a—Partial bicorporeal uterus with partial division of uterine corpus above the cervix by an external fundal indentation.

Class U3b—Complete bicorporeal uterus with complete division of uterine corpus up to cervix by an external fundal indentation. There may be associated cervical and vaginal defects.

Class U3c—Bicorporeal septate uterus with a resorption defect in addition to the main fusion defect. The width of fundal indentation is more than 150% the uterine wall thickness.

Class U4—Hemiuterus which is a formation defect characterized by unilateral uterine development and incompletely developed or absent contralateral portion. It is divided into two subclasses.

Class U4a—Hemiuterus with a rudimentary, functional contralateral horn which may be communicating or noncommunicating.

Class U4b—Hemiuterus without rudimentary, functional contralateral horn. This includes aplasia of contralateral horn or nonfunctional contralateral horn.

Class U5—Aplasia of uterus is a formation defect and includes all cases of uterine aplasia. There may be associated rudimentary horn with or without cavity and other defects. It is divided into two subclasses.

Class U5a—Aplastic uterus with a rudimentary, functional cavity, unilateral or bilateral.

Class U5b—Aplastic uterus without rudimentary, functional cavity and includes complete aplasia or rudimentary, nonfunctional remnants.

Class 6—Unclassified anomalies are included in this group [44].

Mullerian duct anomalies thus includes a wide range of developmental anomalies of uterus, cervix, and vagina (Fig. 46.23). USG with 3D techniques and MRI are the best imaging modalities for accurate characterization of these anomalies, before planning treatment and to identify associated anomalies.

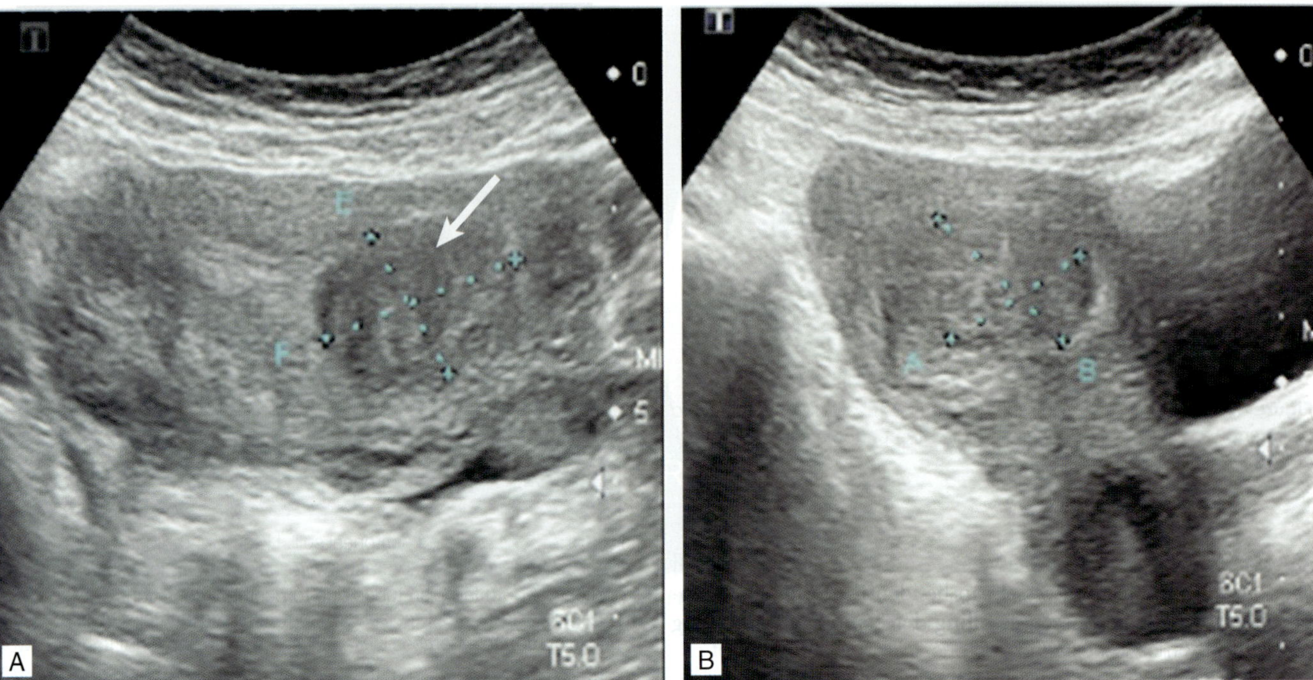

Figure 46.30 Submucosal fibroid. Transabdominal USG images show a well-circumscribed hypoechoic lesion (*white arrow* in A) protruding into endometrial cavity, surgically confirmed to be submucosal fibroid.

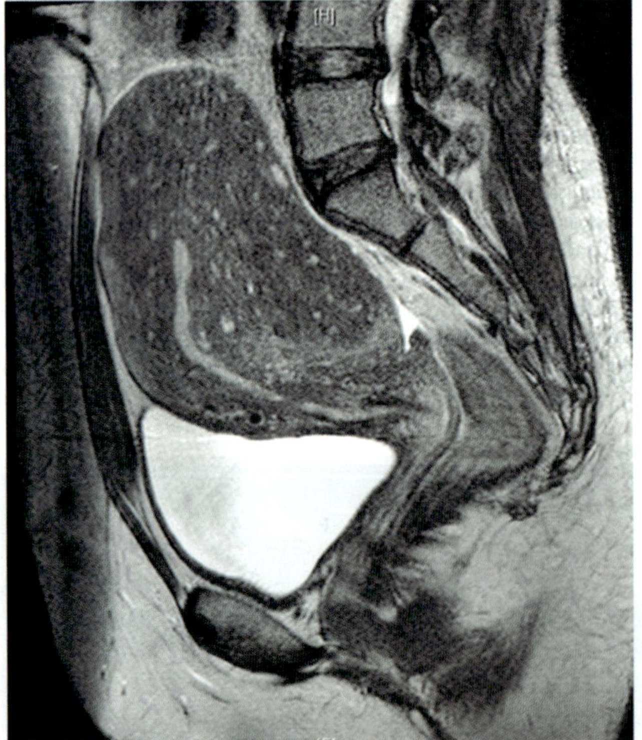

Figure 46.31 Diffuse adenomyosis. Sagittal T2-weighted MR images show an enlarged uterus with thickened junctional zone and multiple small T2 hyperintense foci within the myometrium.

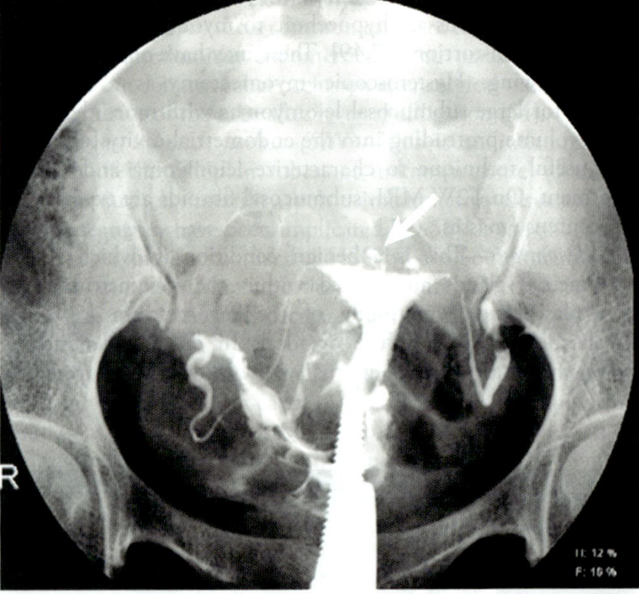

Figure 46.32 Adenomyosis. HSG spot radiograph shows few small contrast filled outpouchings protruding beyond margins of endometrial cavity (*white arrow*).

partial loss of the uterine cavity. On HSG, synechiae are seen as irregular or linear fixed filling defects in the uterine cavity [47,50] (Fig. 46.33). Complete or partial obliteration of the endometrial cavity maybe another feature. Sonohysterography is also useful to delineate uterine synechiae and the size of endometrial cavity. Infertility resulting from uterine synechiae is called Asherman's syndrome.

Endometriosis and congenital uterine anomalies are associated with infertility. These have been described in detail elsewhere in this chapter.

Cervical Causes of Infertility

Cervical stenosis is defined as narrowing which does not allow a 2.5 mm or thinner dilator into the cervical canal [49,50]. Cervical

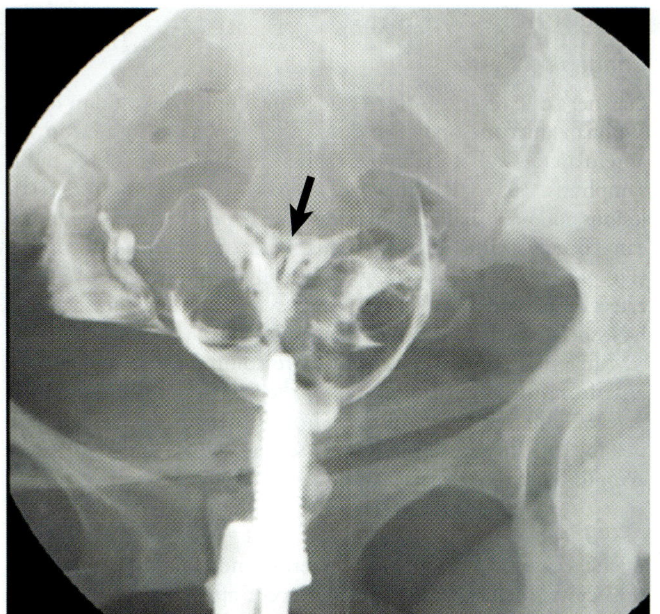

Figure 46.33 Uterine synechiae. HSG spot radiograph shows multiple linear fixed filling defects in the uterine cavity (*black arrow*).

stenosis maybe congenital or due to infection or trauma related to biopsy, cryotherapy, or laser treatment. Severe degree of stenosis can cause symptoms of amenorrhea, dysmenorrhea, and also infertility related to decreased sperm entry. On HSG, there may be narrowing of the cervical canal or complete stenosis, which prevents insertion of HSG catheter. Hematometra secondary to cervical stenosis can be seen on USG or MRI [49,50].

Ovarian Causes of Infertility

Polycystic ovarian syndrome is a common cause of female infertility, characterized by elevated androgens and serum levels of luteinizing hormone, oligo or anovulation, and polycystic ovaries. Clinically, patients present with obesity, hirsutism, and oligoamenorrhea.

Pelvic USG and MRI help to characterize polycystic ovaries, which are typically enlarged with ovarian volumes more than 20 ml, increased echogenicity of ovarian stroma, and increased number of small peripherally located cysts, usually more than 12 in number (Fig. 46.34). However, polycystic ovaries may be seen in 20–30% of normal women with no clinical features of polycystic ovarian syndrome [47,49,58].

Gonadal dysgenesis—This condition is characterized by streak gonads which are replaced by fibrous stroma and absent germ cells. This is classically seen in Turner's syndrome (45XO). Streak gonads are best identified on MRI although they are seen in only 40–65% of cases and appear as T1W iso to mildly hypointense small linear structures [50].

Female infertility is thus multifactorial with congenital or acquired causes which may involve uterus, fallopian tubes, and ovaries. Role of imaging is to identify the cause, before initiating therapy. The initial investigation is usually HSG to look for tubal patency. Findings on HSG may help to decide on further imaging which could be USG (which could include SIS) or MRI in the presence of other uterine abnormalities, such as contour defects. Imaging helps in planning before surgery and a multimodality approach is useful to investigate female infertility.

Benign and Malignant Conditions of Vagina and Vulva

Anatomy of the Vagina

The vagina is a fibromuscular tube that extends from the uterus to the vulva and has a H-shaped configuration on axial imaging. It is divided into thirds with the upper third corresponding to the lateral vaginal fornices, the middle third is at the level of the bladder base and the lower third is below the bladder base. Lymphatic drainage from the upper vagina is to the external and internal iliac nodes, the middle third drains to the internal iliac nodes and the lower third into the superficial inguinal nodes.

Table 46.4. The differential diagnosis of vaginal lesions (References [59,60]).

Imaging Modalities

Vaginal anatomy is well depicted on MRI, which is the technique of choice. The main role of imaging would be to localize and characterize the lesion and in assessment of malignant tumors, including staging, treatment response, and in the accurate diagnosis of disease recurrence. Endovaginal USG gel can be used to distend the cavity allowing for accurate staging of small/early malignancies. The routine sequences include T2W imaging in axial, coronal and sagittal

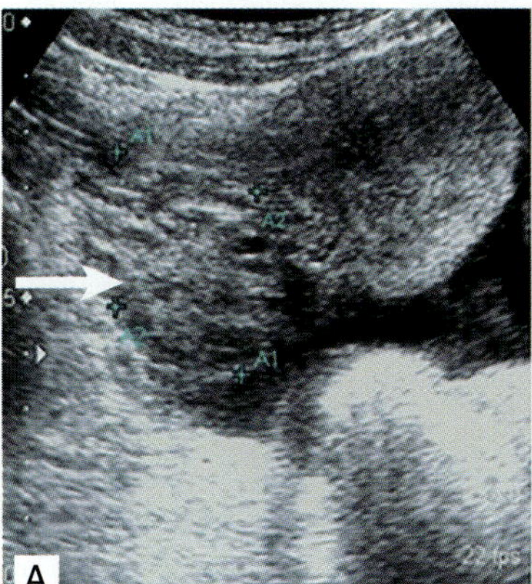

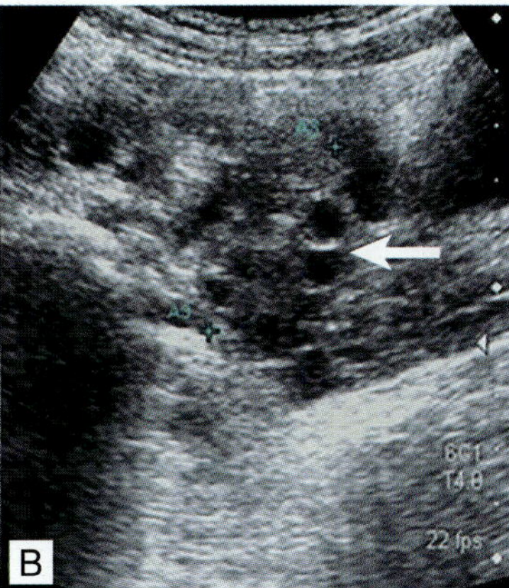

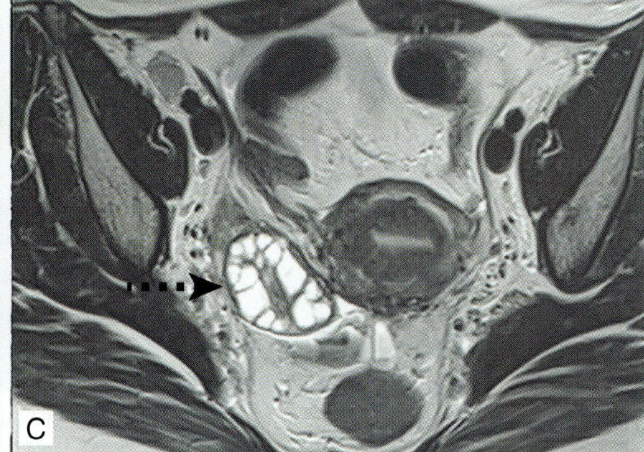

Figure 46.34 Polycystic ovarian syndrome. USG images shows enlarged ovaries with increased echogenic stroma and multiple small peripherally placed cysts (*white arrows* in A, B). Axial T2- weighted MR image shows enlarged right ovary with multiple small peripherally placed cysts (*dashed black arrow* in C).

- Stage 1 tumors are confined to the vagina with disruption of the vaginal mucosa;
- In stage 2 disease the tumor extends to the paravaginal fat with abnormal tumor signal extending into the fat;
- Stage 3 tumors involve the pelvic side wall; and
- Stage 4 tumors infiltrate the bladder, rectum or extend out of the pelvis.

Contrast-enhanced study will show enhancement of the tumor and can be used in follow-up as well. These lesions will show early enhancement on postcontrast T1W imaging.

The treatment of vaginal malignancies depends on the stage of the lesion. In very early lesions, surgical resection with radiation can be done. However, in most patients and in more advanced stages, radiation therapy is the mainstay of treatment. It must be remembered that T2 hyperintense signal may be present for up to 6 months after pelvic radiation due to edema, which can obscure small residual and recurrent lesions.

Adenocarcinoma of the vagina occurs in younger age group. Clear cell variant of adenocarcinoma is associated with in utero exposure to diethylstilbestrol.

Secondary Vaginal Malignancy: Ninety percent of vaginal tumors are from direct extension of adjacent malignancies. Metastatic tumor deposits can also occur and have similar imaging appearance to the primary tumors.

Anatomy of Vulva

The vulva includes the mon pubis, which extends posteriorly to the labia majora. The labia minora fuse anteriorly at the level of the clitoris. The vestibule is medial to the labia minora and contains the vaginal orifice, external urethral meatus, vestibular bulb, and vestibular glands (Skene glands and Bartholin glands). The lymphatic drainage is to the medial group of inguinal nodes.

Imaging Modalities

MRI is the technique of choice for imaging of the vulva due to excellent soft-tissue resolution. On T1W imaging the vulva demonstrates low to intermediate signal intensity and shows slightly higher signal on T2W imaging. CT is indicated in vulval malignancies, to assess for metastatic pelvic nodes and also metastases to other organs.

Table 46.5 enumerates the lists the differential of vulval lesions ([59,63]).

TABLE 46.5 The Differential Diagnosis of Vulval Lesions [59,63]

Congenital
Vascular malformations
Hydrocele of the canal of Nuck
Benign
Bartholin's cyst
Fibroma
Lipoma
Leiomyomas
Aggressive angiomyxoma
Malignant
Squamous cell carcinoma
Adenocarcinoma
Melanoma
Basal cell carcinoma
Paget's disease of the vulva
Bartholin's gland cancer
Sarcoma

Congenital Anomalies

Hydrocele of the canal of Nuck: The canal of Nuck is a peritoneal fold that extends along the round ligament up to its attachment with the labia majora. Normally, it obliterates during the first year of life, failure of which results in a hydrocele in the inguinolabial region [68].

Benign

Bartholin's Cyst: These are the most common type of vulval cyst and they arise from Bartholin's gland due to obstruction of the duct [60]. They are typically seen in the distal vagina, medial to the labia minora. On MRI the lesions are hyperintense on T2W imaging with variable signal on T1 depending on the content (Fig. 46.38). There is wall thickening and enhancement in case of associated inflammation. The presence of mural nodules should alert the radiologist to the rare Bartholin's gland carcinoma.

Bartholin's cyst may be difficult to differentiate from Skene duct cyst which are lateral to the external urethral meatus and are caused by obstruction to the paraurethral glands (Fig. 46.38).

Tumors: Benign tumors that involve the vulva are uncommon and include fibroma, lipoma, and leiomyoma (Fig. 46.39). These tumors show signal intensity similar to those found elsewhere.

Aggressive angiomyxoma: This is a benign mesenchymal tumor which occurs in women of reproductive age. It has a high recurrence rate due to its infiltrating nature and is hence termed "aggressive." Given the presence of myxoid stroma, the tumor is hyperintense on T2W imaging and demonstrates enhancement. It is isohypointense to muscle on T1W sequences. The lesion shows a characteristic appearance with "swirled" linear low signal intensity on both T1 and T2W imaging which allows for a definite diagnosis (Fig. 46.40) [69].

Malignant

Primary Vulval Carcinoma: Squamous cell carcinoma is again the most common accounting for 90% [66]. Other rare neoplasms include adenocarcinoma, melanoma, basal cell carcinoma, Paget's disease of the vulva, Bartholin's gland cancer, and sarcoma.

Squamous cell carcinoma affects the older age group; however, those associated with human papilloma virus tend to affect younger patients. Vulval malignancy most commonly involves the labia with other sites including the clitoris and the perineum. Sometimes the disease is extensive and the primary site cannot be determined. Tumors which are laterally located drain into the ipsilateral inguinal nodes, whereas tumors in the midline or within 1 cm of the midline can drain bilaterally [70].

MRI can be done for assessment of local staging of the disease, including invasion into adjacent structures and also to detect lymphadenopathy. The tumor shows intermediate to high signal intensity on T2W imaging and is hypointense on T1W imaging (Fig. 46.41). Diffusion-weighted imaging is also helpful for delineation of the tumor. Postcontrast study does not add value during initial staging of the disease but may be helpful for detecting a small recurrent lesions [71].

Superficial inguinal nodes more than 10 mm in short-axis diameter had a sensitivity of 40% and specificity of 97% and deep inguinal nodes more than 8 mm also in short-axis diameter had a sensitivity of 50% and specificity of 100% [72].

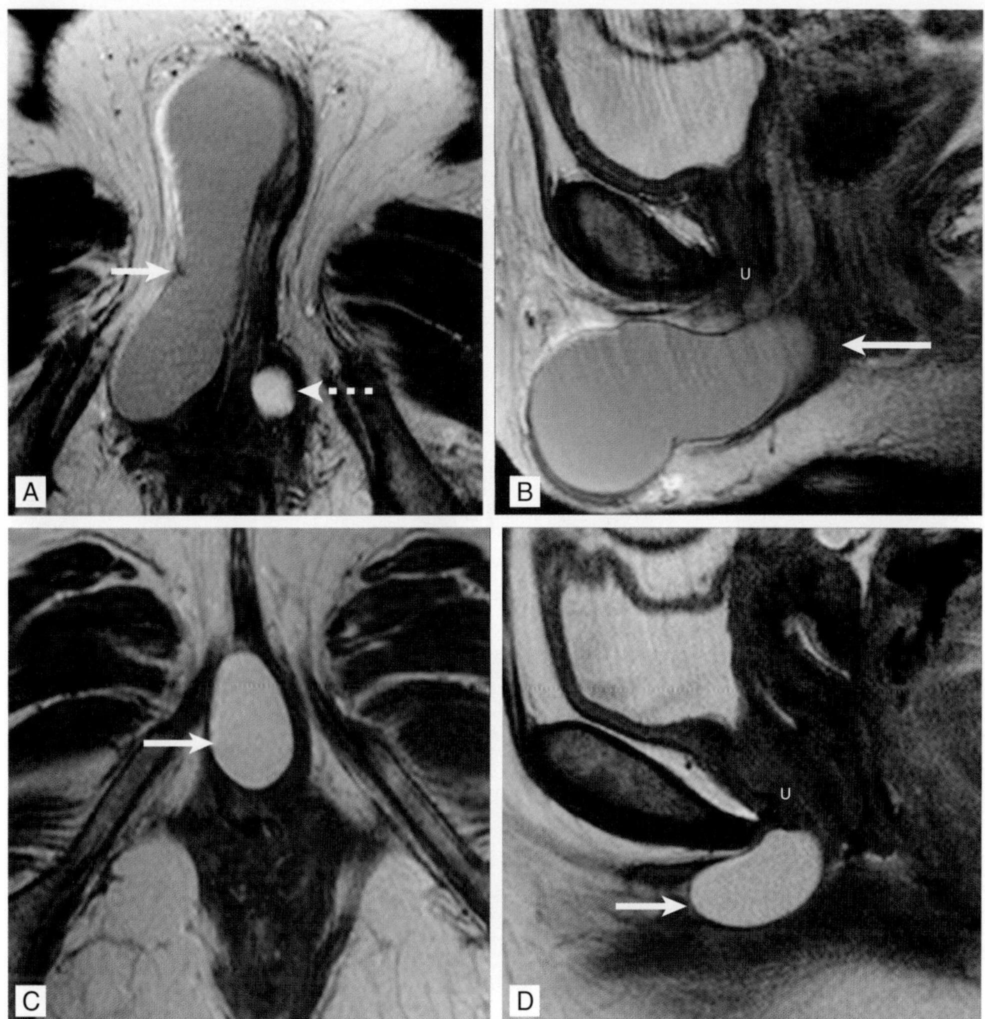

Figure 46.38 Bartholin's cyst (A and B). T2-weighted axial image (A) shows a well-defined tubular hyperintense cystic lesion in the right side of the labia (*arrow* in A) and another smaller cystic lesion on the left side (*dashed white arrow* in A). T2 sagittal image (B) shows the cystic lesion anterioinferior to the distal vagina. Skene duct cyst (C and D). T2-weighted axial image (C) shows a well-defined hyperintense cystic lesion (*arrow* in C) in the anterior periurethral region. T2 sagittal image (D) shows the cystic lesion (*arrow* in D) anterior to the distal urethra and the external urethral meatus. Urethra marked as U.

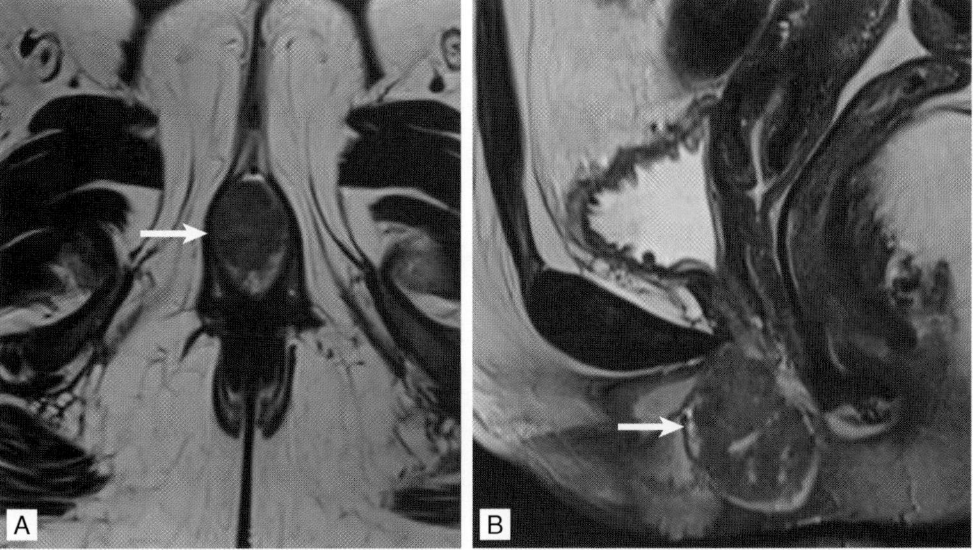

Figure 46.39 Vulval leiomyoma. T2-weighted axial image (A) shows a well-defined hypointense lesion (*arrow*) in the vestibule of the vulva. T2W sagittal image (B) shows the elongated T2 hypointense lesion just distal to the external urethral meatus (*arrow*).

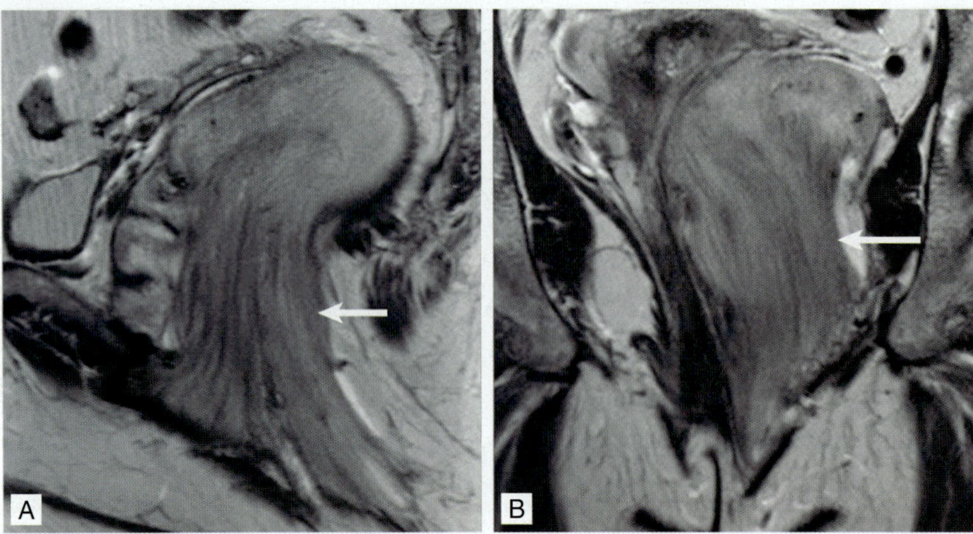

Figure 46.40 Aggressive angiomyxoma. T2-weighted sagittal image (A) shows a well-defined T2 hyperintense lesion (*arrow*) with T2 hypointense bands resulting in a swirled or laminated appearance. T2-weighted coronal images (B) show the characteristic translevator extension of the lesion (*arrow*).

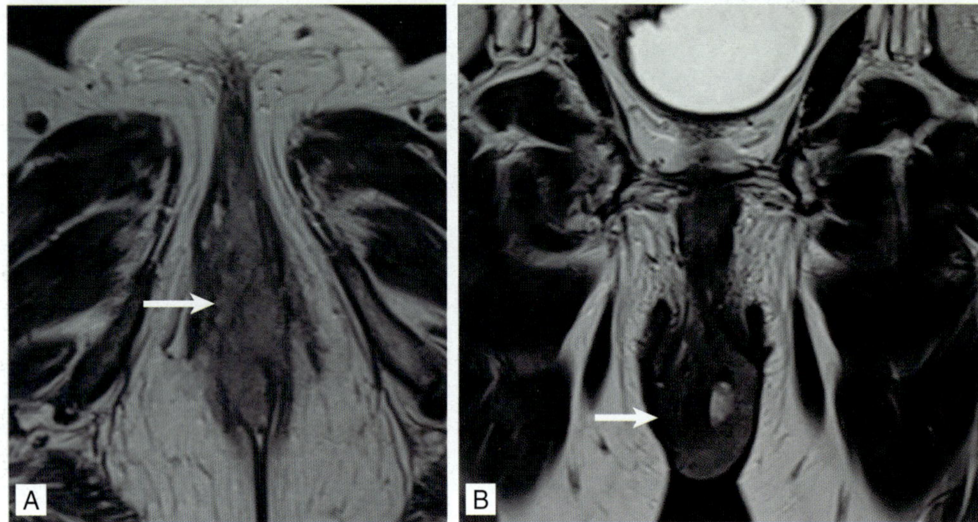

Figure 46.41 Vulval squamous cell carcinoma. T2-weighted axial image (A) shows an irregular intermediate signal intensity mass (*arrow*) involving the labia. Squamous cell carcinoma in a 70-year-old lady. T2-weighted coronal image (B) shows an exophytic tumor (*arrow*) involving the labia. The labia is the most common site of primary vulvar malignancy.

Suggested Readings

- P Jha, M Sakala, LP Chamie, M Feldman, N Hindman, C Huang, et al., Endometriosis MRI lexicon: consensus statement from the society of abdominal radiology endometriosis disease-focused panel, Abdom Radiol (NY) 45 (6) (2020) 1552–1568.
- M Bazot, N Bharwani, C Huchon, K Kinkel, TM Cunha, A Guerra, et al., European Society of Urogenital Radiology (ESUR) guidelines: MR imaging of pelvic endometriosis, Eur Radiol 27 (7) (2017) 2765–2775.
- JK Son, S Ali, N Al Khori, EY Lee, MR imaging evaluation of pediatric genital disorders: MR technologic overview and interpretation, Magn Reson Imaging Clin N Am 27 (2) (2019) 301–321.
- K Kaproth-Joslin, V Dogra, Imaging of female infertility: a pictorial guide to the hysterosalpingography, ultrasonography, and magnetic resonance imaging findings of the congenital and acquired causes of female infertility, Radiol Clin North Am 51 (6) (2013) 967–981.
- K Hosseinzadeh, MT Heller, G Houshmand, Imaging of the female perineum in adults, RadioGraphics 32 (4) (2012) E129–E168.

47

Obstetrics: First Trimester

NITIN CHAUBAL, MRUDULA BAPAT, ANUPAM BAM

Introduction

The first trimester is the period beginning from conception to completion of 13 weeks + 6 days. It is a period of rapid changes in the conceptus that begins with fertilization; and proceeds through the germinal period (from conception to the second week), embryonic period (third to eighth week), and the early fetal stage (ninth to twelfth week). Ultrasonography (USG) examination plays a key role during this period in diagnosis, evaluation, surveillance, and management of various pathologies in utero. Therefore, a sonologist must be well versed with different USG techniques adopted during this period and guidelines for the diagnosis of various conditions. From a sonologist's perspective, the first trimester can be divided into early and late parts. The early first trimester, which spans up to 10 weeks + 6 days, is primarily concerned with establishing fetal viability and documenting the normal sequential developmental events. Certain fetal features such as limbs and cranial ossification appear later in the later first trimester, which is a period between 11 and 14 weeks of gestation. This is a period when a detailed study of various fetal structures can be undertaken.

First-Trimester USG

Sonographic evaluation of the conceptus during the first trimester allows evaluating gestation for potential risks, and to detect anomalies early on. It is important for various reasons:

- Confirmation of intrauterine pregnancy (IUP) by visualizing gestational sac, evaluation of certain characteristics of the sac and its contents
- Dating of pregnancy by measurement of crown-rump length (CRL)
- Visualization of embryo and confirmation of its viability
- Documentation of multiple gestations
- Establishment of chorionicity and amnionicity in multifetal gestations
- Evaluation of first-trimester bleeding
- Examination of the uterus and adnexa for the presence of fibroids, ovarian cysts, and other masses
- Follow-up scan to assess normal structural development during embryogenesis, and to rule out congenital anomalies, especially in the late first trimester, which begins at 11 weeks
- Measurement of nuchal translucency (NT) along with other ultrasonography markers like nasal bone, ductus venosus flow, tricuspid flow, and a detailed structural survey of the fetal head, thorax, abdomen, spine and limbs between the beginning of the 11th week and 13 weeks 6 days
- Screening for preeclampsia

Early First-Trimester Fetal Evaluation

Confirmation and Dating of Pregnancy

The first trimester is a period of rapid morphogenesis. Fertilization in the ampulla of the fallopian tube results in the formation of a zygote, which undergoes rapid cell division as it traverses the tube. It converts into "morula" at about day 17 (after the last menstrual period or LMP), when it enters the uterine cavity. At day 20, the morula becomes "blastocyst." Blastocyst implantation inside decidua basalis is completed by day 23. The amniotic cavity forms within the inner cell mass soon after, while the blastocystic cavity gives rise to the primary yolk sac, along with the emergence of a bilaminar embryonic disc. Later on, a part of the primary yolk sac is extruded while its remaining part forms the secondary yolk sac (which can be located on USG), as extraembryonic coelom develops around it (Fig. 47.1). The latter eventually becomes the chorionic cavity. At this time, the conceptus is a two-to-three millimeter anechoic structure surrounded by a hyperechoic ring, which can be detected by state-of-the-art vaginal transducers. This is the *earliest sonographic sign of an intrauterine pregnancy* that can be identified as "gestational sac" between 4 and 5 weeks of gestation [1]. The presence of "double decidual sac sign" (Fig. 47.2) around this time, differentiates a gestational sac from a simple fluid collection within the endometrial cavity (pseudo-gestational sac). In it, decidua capsularis and decidua parietalis form two concentric rings around an anechoic gestational sac. Another early sonographic sign of pregnancy is "intradecidual sac sign" (Fig. 47.3), which describes the gestational sac as a tiny cystic structure embedded in the leaf of the decidualized endometrium adjacent to the collapsed endometrial cavity. Around 35% of IUPs do not show these early signs [2]. *The appearance of the yolk sac within the gestational sac establishes the diagnosis of an IUP*. It is the first structure to be identified within the gestational sac at around 5–6 weeks. It is readily visible on transvaginal USG (TVU) as a ring-like rounded structure within the gestational sac (Fig. 47.4), varying between 3 and 5 mm in size [3]. It provides nutrition to the developing embryo and is a site of early hematopoiesis. It grows at a rate of 0.1 mm per mm of mean sac diameter (MSD)

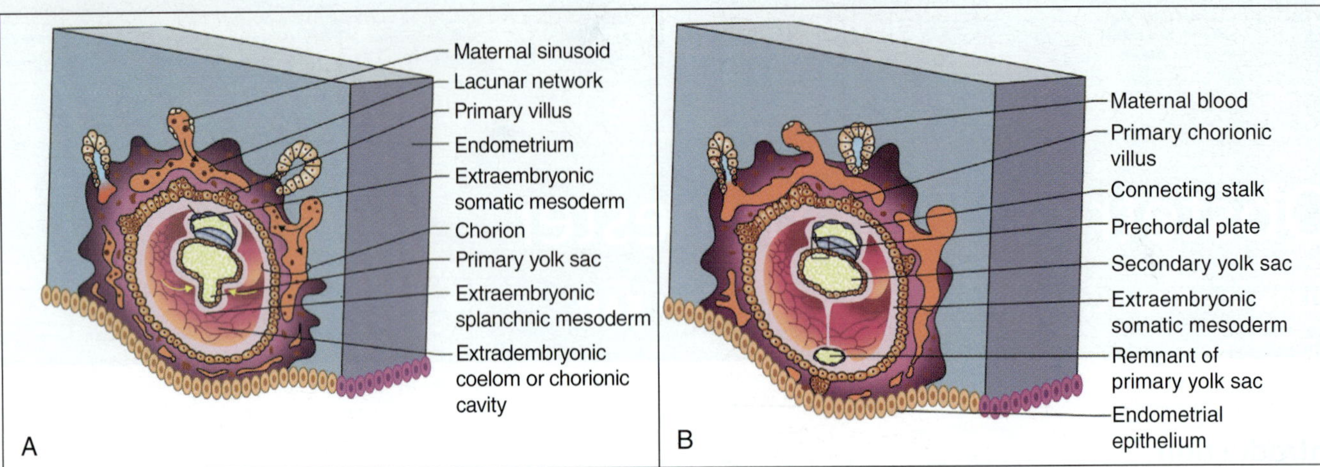

Figure 47.1 A schematic diagram of the early embryo. (A) A completely implanted blastocyst at about the 23rd days of gestation. (B) Formation of the secondary yolk sac around the 26th day of gestation. The primary yolk sac is being extruded.

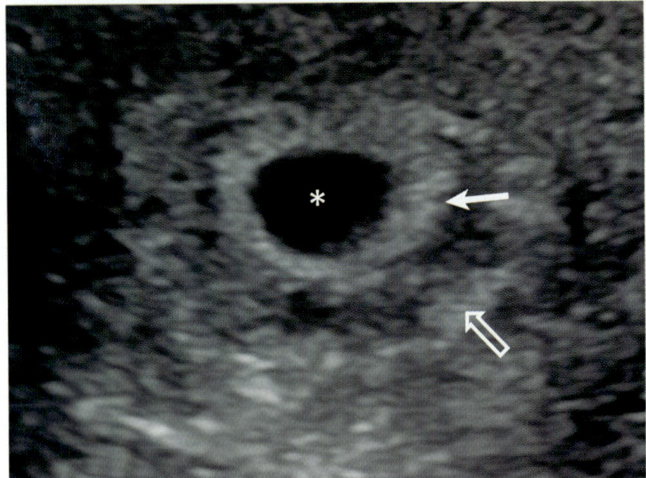

Figure 47.2 Double decidual sac sign. B-mode USG image of a gravid uterus showing two distinct echogenic rings representing decidua capsularis (*white arrow*) and decidua parietalis (*white block arrow*) surrounding the gestational sac (*white asterisk*). The yolk sac is absent at this early stage.

[4]. It reaches the size of 5.5 mm between 5 and 10 weeks, after which it gradually disappears [5].

"Embryonic pole" can be visualized as a juxta-yolk sac thickening measuring 1–2 mm by 5–6 weeks of gestation (Fig. 47.5). *Crown-rump length (CRL), the length of embryo measured from its cranial to caudal end, is the most accurate measurement for pregnancy dating during this period.* This is especially important given the fact that many women have irregular menstrual cycles, which along with an increased rate of conception with assisted reproductive techniques makes it impractical to use the last menstrual period (LMP) as a reliable criterion for dating. Amnion becomes easily distinguishable at around 7 weeks of gestation (Fig. 47.6). The embryo reveals cardiac pulsations as early as 5–6 weeks, however, the appearance of cardiac activity may be delayed in a few normal pregnancies [6].

Table 47.1 summarizes various normal fetal USG findings observed in the early first trimester.

Evaluation of Fetal Viability

Once a gestational sac is seen on USG, the next step is to confirm its viability. For that, certain criteria have been laid down

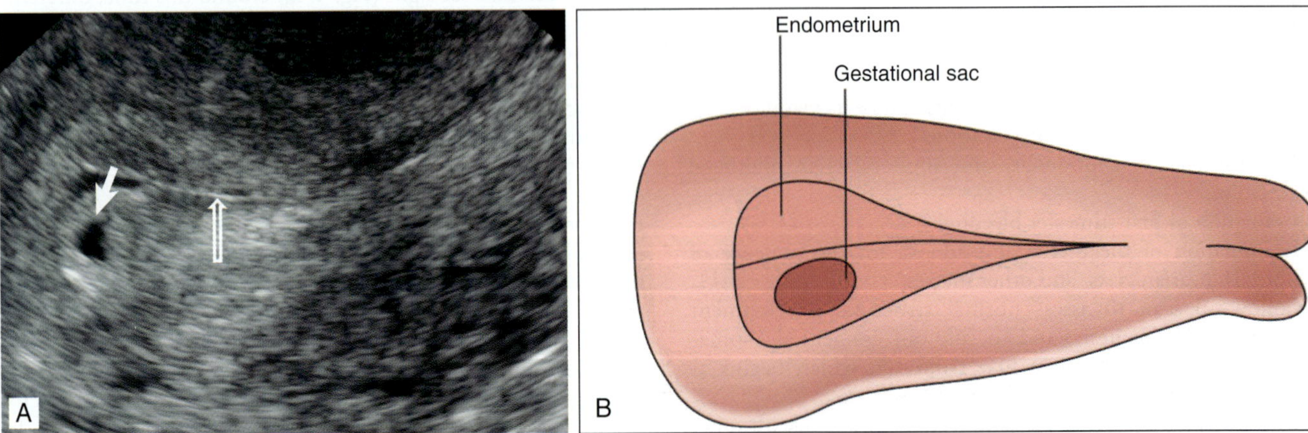

Figure 47.3 Intradecidual sac sign. (A) B-mode USG image of a gravid uterus showing a gestational sac (*white arrow*) implanted eccentrically in one of the two leaves of the endometrium. The *white block arrow* points to the collapsed endometrial cavity. (B) A schematic diagram of the same sign.

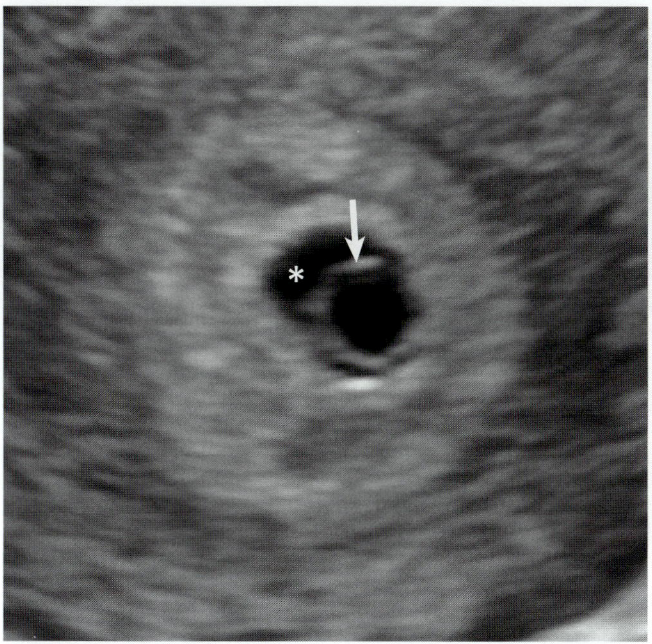

Figure 47.4 B-mode USG image of a yolk sac, which is seen as a ring-like rounded structure (*white arrow*) within the gestational sac (*white asterisk*).

TABLE 47.1 Normal USG Findings in the Fetus During the Early First Trimester in Chronological Order

Gestational Age	USG Findings
3–5 weeks	The gestational sac appears giving rise to the "double decidual sac sign" and the "intradecidual sac sign."
5 weeks	A tiny echogenic structure appears adjacent to the yolk sac with or without cardiac pulsations.
6–7 weeks	Featureless disc-like structure with discrete cardiac pulsations. Absent cardiac pulsations may be normal in an embryo less than CRL of 7 mm. In such a situation follow up is warranted before calling it nonviable. Cardiac pulsations at 6 weeks of around 100 beats per minute may be considered normal.
7–8 weeks	The cranial end of the embryo is more definable with the appearance of a vesicle in the cranial end (rhombencephalon).
8–9 weeks	Clear demarcation of the cranial end with tiny limb buds visible. By this time the yolk sac is extra amniotic
9–10 weeks	A more human type of morphology is visible with developing limbs seen, the vitelline duct is visible clearly.
10–11 weeks	Some amount of cranial ossification is seen and the human form is definable.

by the Society of Radiologists in Ultrasonography 2012 Consensus Panel [1]. *The aim of every early pregnancy USG must be to prevent any inadvertent termination of a potentially viable pregnancy.*

Mean Sac Diameter

Mean sac diameter (MSD) is an important USG parameter to confirm failed gestation in the first trimester. It is the average of the sagittal, transverse, and anteroposterior diameters of the gestational sac. *An MSD of 16–24 mm without visible embryo warrants a follow-up to prevent termination of a potentially viable IUP, while the absence of an embryo at MSD of 25 mm or more is a sure sign of nonviable gestation.*

Crown-Rump Length

Crown-rump length (CRL) is the most accurate method of pregnancy dating. If a 5 mm embryo does not show cardiac pulsations, it is advisable to follow-up before labeling it as a nonviable gestation. *The absence of fetal cardiac activity above a CRL of 7 mm is a definitive sign of nonviability (Fig. 47.7).*

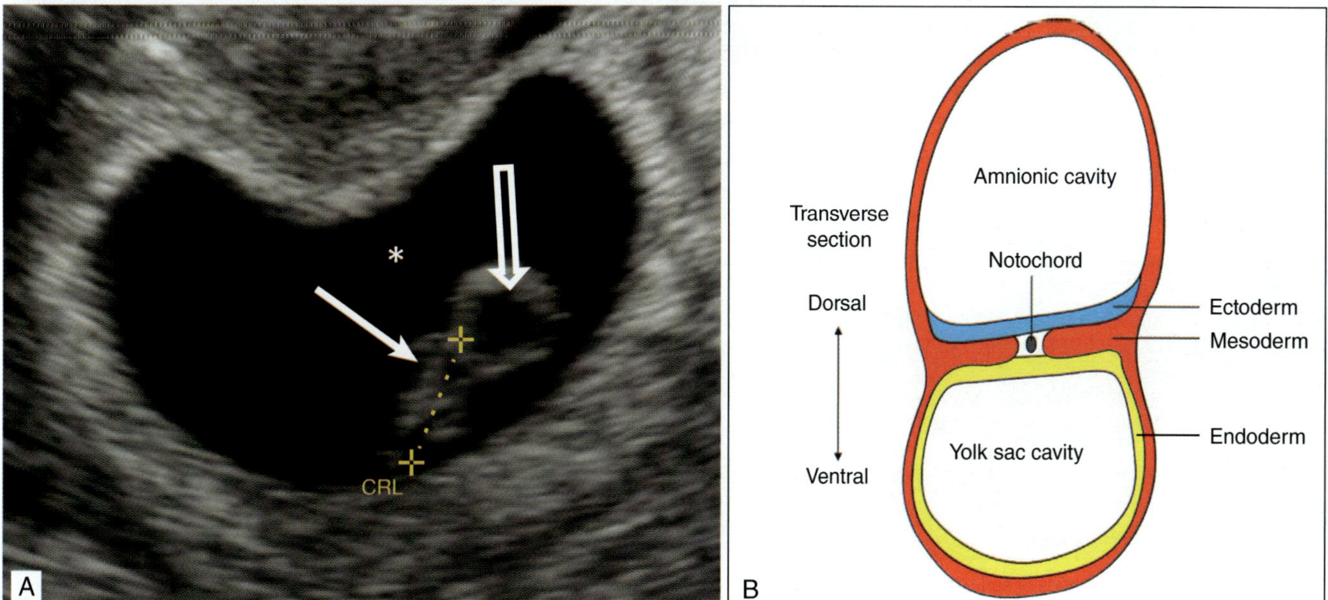

Figure 47.5 Embryonic pole. (A) B-mode USG image of an early embryo. The embryo (*white arrow*) is seen in close approximation with the yolk sac (*white block arrow*). The crown-rump length (*marked by the yellow callipers*) corresponds to 6 weeks. *White asterisk*: extraembryonic coelom/chorionic cavity. (B) A schematic showing various embryological structures at this stage as seen in the embryonic cross section.

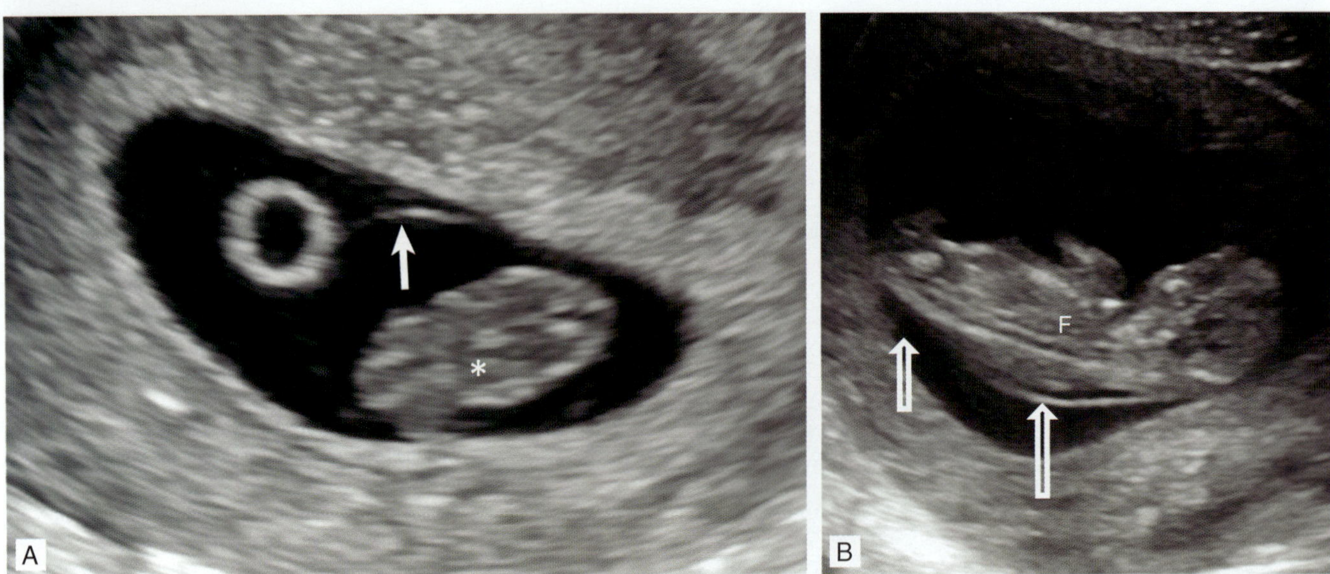

Figure 47.6 B-mode USG images of the amnion. (A) An 8 weeks embryo (*white asterisk*) surrounded by its amnion (*white arrow*), which is seen as a reflective membrane. (B) A 13 weeks fetus (F) with its amnion (*white block arrows*).

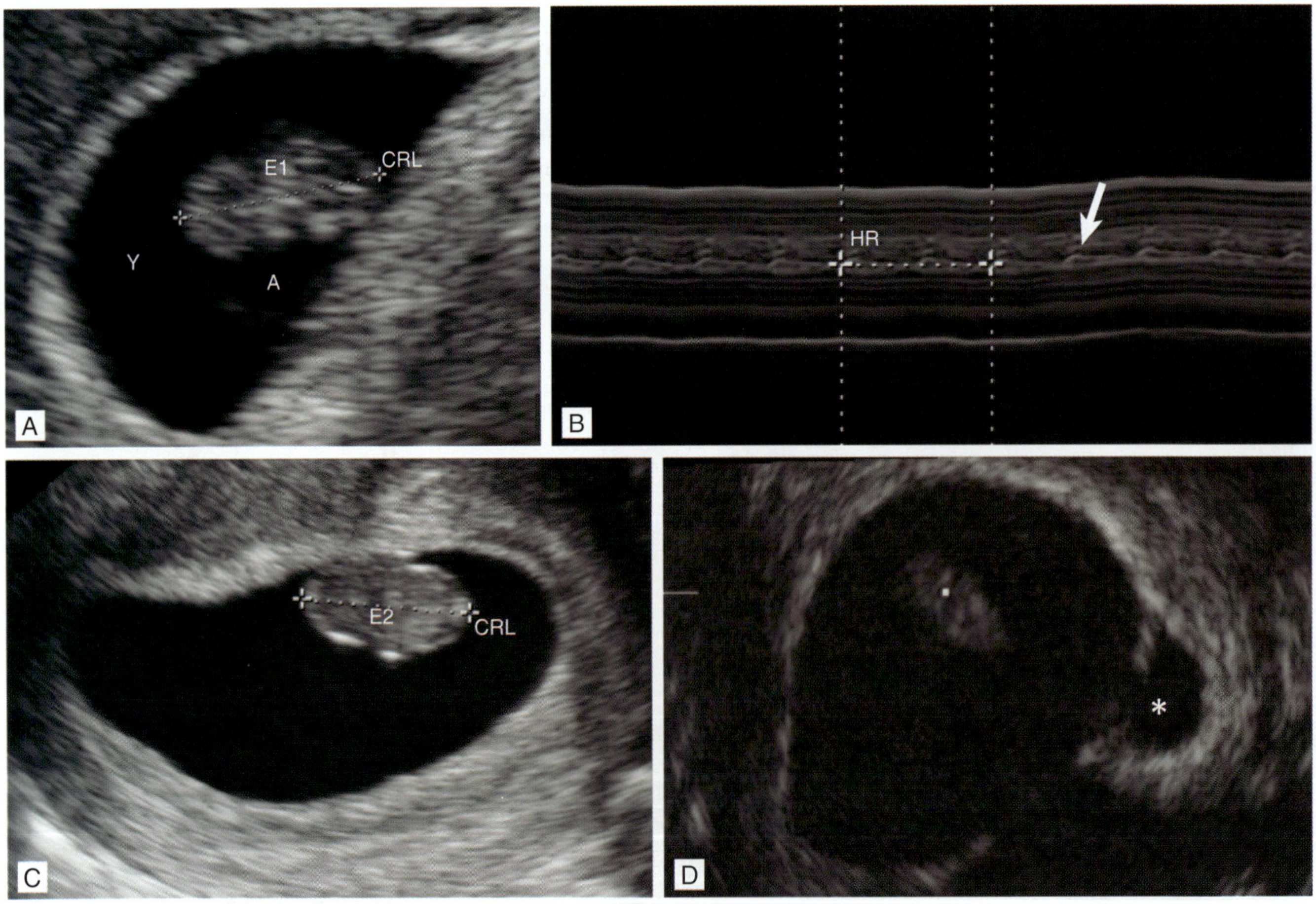

Figure 47.7 B-mode USG images of early-stage embryos. (A) A 6 weeks old embryo (E1), which is seen as a featureless disc-like structure, with a crown-rump length of 7.2 mm. (B) M-mode image of the embryo showing cardiac pulsations (heart rate of 158 beats per minute, *white arrow*), which establishes its viability. (C) Another embryo (E2) has a crown-rump length of 14 mm without visible cardiac pulsations, establishing the diagnosis of nonviable gestation. (D) A small subchorionic hemorrhage (*white asterisk*) is identified on the reconstructed coronal image of the same embryo, which is sometimes associated with a nonviable gestation. *Y*, yolk sac; *A*, amnion.

Follow-Up Scan

A follow-up scan is necessary for two situations during the early first trimester.

- In the first, the absence of a yolk sac and embryo in the gestational sac at the very first USG necessitates a follow-up scan at least 2 weeks later. If the follow-up scan fails to demonstrate the above, a diagnosis of failed pregnancy is established
- In contrast, if the first scan reveals only a yolk sac and a follow-up scan obtained at least 11 days later does not reveal an embryo, it should be diagnosed as a failed pregnancy [3]

Thus, the follow-up scan helps avoid an inadvertent termination of a potentially viable pregnancy.

Embryonic Cardiac Pulsations

Normal first-trimester fetal cardiac pulsations begin at about the sixth week of gestation and have a rate of 100 beats per minute or more. They can become apparent in embryos as small as 1–2 mm in size.

Yolk Sac

Abnormalities of the yolk sac size and appearance are reliable predictors of early pregnancy outcome. A normal yolk sac measures less than 5.6 mm between 5 and 10 weeks of gestation in singleton pregnancies. A yolk sac less than 2 mm, or pregnancies without a defined yolk sac are associated with a poor outcome [7]. Similarly, a yolk sac more than 5.6 mm indicates a likely presence of chromosomal abnormalities in the fetus and may be associated with embryonic demise (Fig. 47.8). Yolk sac calcifications, which are visible as hyperechoic structures with posterior shadowing, may indicate a dead embryo. The presence of an embryo with visible cardiac pulsations without a yolk sac, observed on a careful endovaginal scan, warranties a follow-up scan as such embryos frequently turn out to be nonviable.

Amnion

Amnion is seen as a thin echogenic membrane around embryo by 7 weeks of gestation. It is seen as a separate membrane up to about 14 weeks. After that, it fuses with the chorionic cavity and ceases to be distinctly visible on USG. Visualization of amnion in the absence of an embryo is termed as the "empty amnion sign," which has a poor prognosis.

TABLE 47.2 Fetal Viability Evaluation With USG [1]

USG Finding	Further Action/Conclusion
22 mm ≤ MSD < 25 mm without visible embryo	Follow-up scan
MSD ≥ 25 mm without visible embryo	Nonviable gestation
5 mm ≤ CRL < 7 mm without cardiac pulsations	Follow-up scan
CRL ≥7 mm without cardiac pulsations	Nonviable gestation
Absence of yolk sac and embryo at first scan	Follow-up scan after 2 weeks
Absence of yolk sac and embryo at 2 weeks follow-up scan	Nonviable gestation
Absence of embryo but the presence of yolk sac at first scan	Follow-up scan after 11 days
Absence of embryo at 11 days follow-up scan	Nonviable gestation
Yolk sac absent or <2 mm in size	Poor prognosis, follow-up viability scan after a week
Yolk sac >5.6 mm	Weekly follow-up scan
Yolk sac calcifications	Probable fetal demise, confirm with embryonic cardiac activity
Presence of amnion without embryo	Poor prognosis, follow-up scan to confirm the presence of a viable embryo

CRL, crown-rump length; *MSD*, mean sac diameter.

Table 47.2 and Figure 47.9 summarize the criteria needed to establish the diagnosis of a failed pregnancy.

Multifetal Gestation

The incidence of multifetal gestation is increasing with assisted reproductive techniques like in vitro fertilization (IVF). Other risk factors for the same include family history, race, and increased parity. *The early first trimester is the best time to determine the*

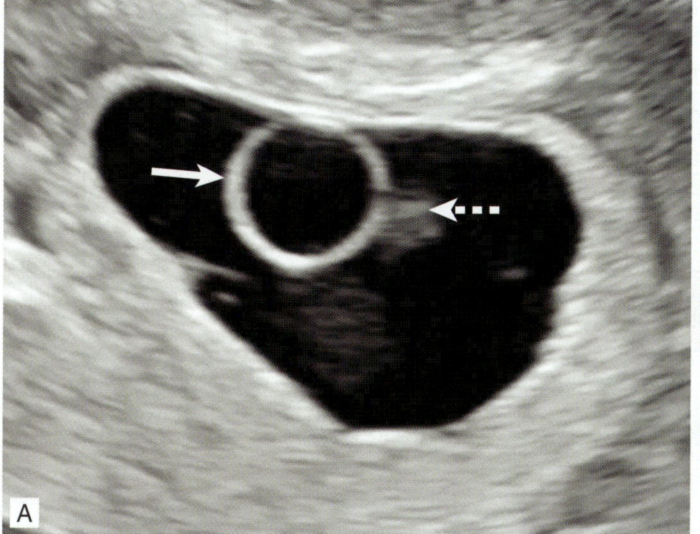

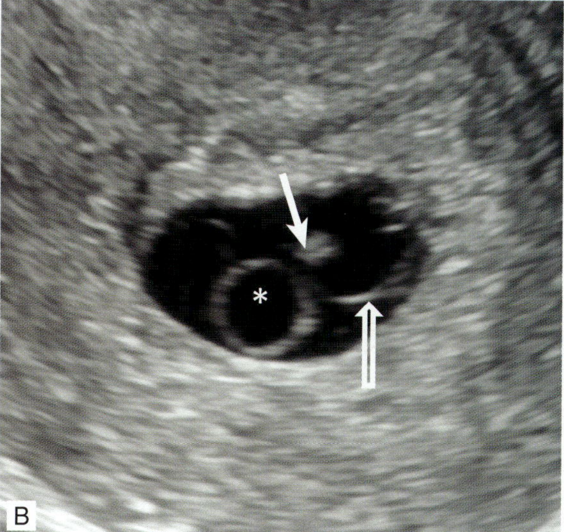

Figure 47.8 B-mode USG images showing yolk sac abnormalities. (A) A large (6.4 mm) yolk sac (*white arrow*) with a small embryonic pole (*white dashed arrow*) is seen. The lady presented after 2 days with heavy vaginal bleeding and a pregnancy loss was confirmed on the follow-up ultrasonography. (B) A large yolk sac (*white asterisk*) measuring 5.8 mm with a small embryonic pole (*white arrow*) and a thick amnion (*white block arrow*) are visible. The follow-up USG revealed no embryonic growth and the absence of cardiac pulsations.

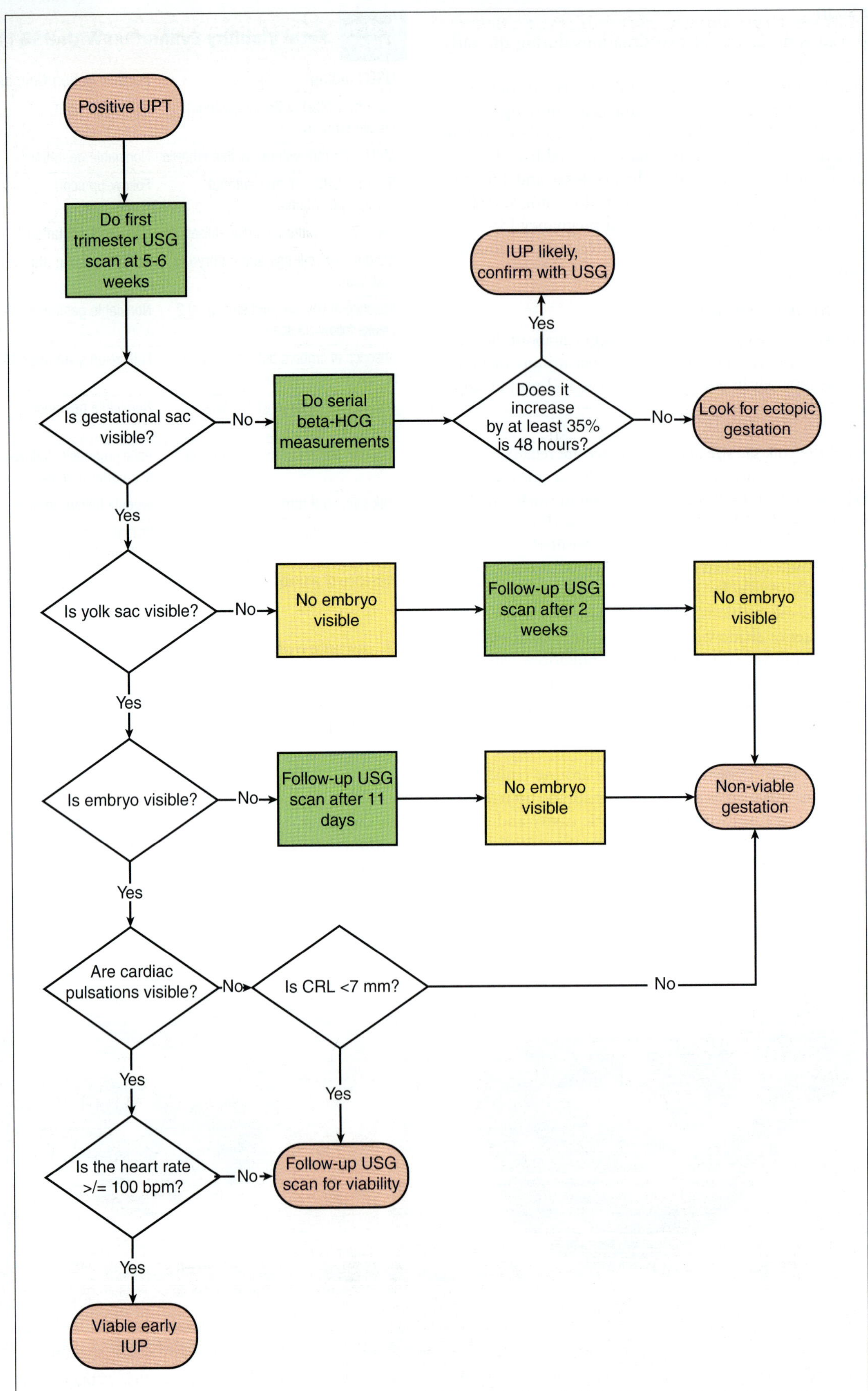

Figure 47.9 Early first-trimester evaluation of gestation. *Peach oval*, starting point/conclusion; *green rectangle*, action point; *white kite*, decision node; *yellow rectangle*, observation.

TABLE 47.3 Different Types of Multifetal Gestation Based on the Placental Status

Type of Multifetal Gestation	Placental Status
Dizygotic (fraternal) twins	Dichorionic–diamniotic
Monozygotic twins—cleavage before blastocyst stage (<4 days)	Dichorionic–diamniotic
Monozygotic twins—cleavage between day 4 and day 7, after blastocyst is formed but before amnion is formed	Monochorionic–diamniotic
Monozygotic twins—cleavage between day 8 and day 12, both amnion and blastocyst have formed	Monochorionic–monoamniotic
Incomplete cleavage after day 12	Conjoined twins

placental status in multifetal gestations. The concepts of zygosity and chorionicity are important in this regard.

Zygosity

Zygosity pertains to the source zygote/s of different members of multifetal gestation. It influences the extent of similarity in the genetic makeup of the members. Fertilization of two separate sperms with two individual oocytes results in two zygotes giving rise to dizygotic twins. Each member of such twins has a separate chorion as well as a separate amnion. Monozygotic twins arise from fertilization of one oocyte with one sperm forming a single zygote, which cleaves at the blastocyst stage to develop into separate embryos.

Chorionicity

Chorionicity refers to the membrane status of the placenta, which depends upon the timing of cleavage of the early conceptus in the case of monozygotic twins, while dizygotic twins are always dichorionic (Table 47.3).

- Cleavage before 4 days from fertilization, that is, before the formation of the blastocyst, results in two blastocysts. Each resulting embryo has a separate placenta and develops into a dichorionic-diamniotic pregnancy
- Cleavage occurring between 4 and 7 days after fertilization results in the division of the inner cell mass forming two embryos having two separate amnions. Thus, it develops as a monochorionic-diamniotic pregnancy
- Cleavage occurring between day 8 and day 12 after fertilization results in a monochorionic-monoamniotic gestation, as both chorion and amnion develop before that time
- Incomplete cleavage after day 12 results in conjoined twins (Fig. 47.10) which is an aberration in the process

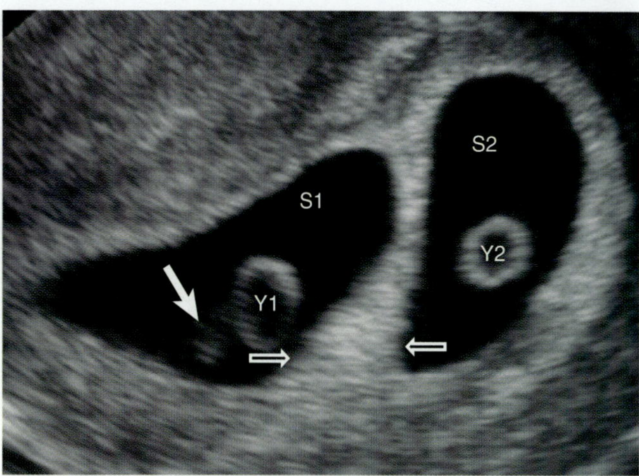

Figure 47.11 B-mode USG images of a 5 weeks old dichorionic–diamniotic twin gestation. A thick chorionic plate (*twin-peak sign, white block arrows*) can be seen separating the two gestational sacs (S1 and S2). *Y1* and *Y2*, yolk sacs; *white arrow*, embryonic pole.

USG Diagnosis of Multifetal Gestations

Chorionicity and amnionicity can be established with great accuracy using USG in the early first trimester between 6 and 9 weeks.

Dichorionic–diamniotic gestation appears as two gestational sacs separated by a thick chorionic membrane. This membrane is best appreciated in the early first trimester. With advancing gestation, if two separate placentae are visualized, there is no ambiguity in establishing the chorionicity. The "twin-peak sign" helps establish dichorionicity; it is seen as a continuation of chorionic tissue into the intertwin membrane (Fig. 47.11). It, however, may not be present in a dichorionic gestation in the late second or the third trimester.

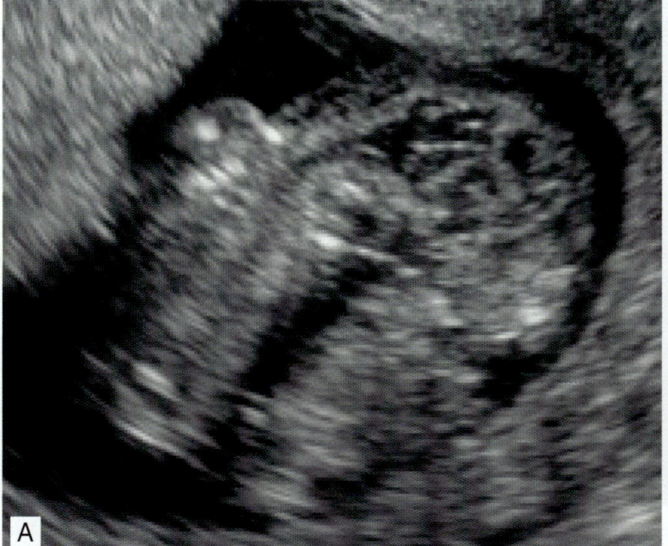

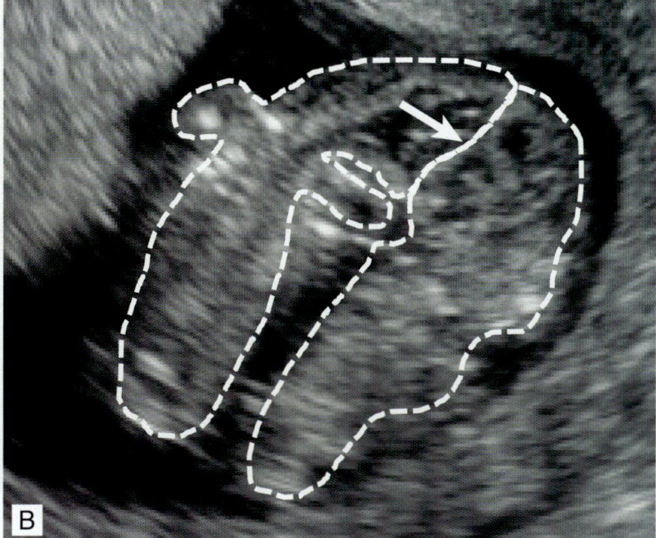

Figure 47.10 (A) B-mode USG image of a conjoined twin gestation. (B) The same image highlighting how the twins (*white outlines*) are fused to each other at their cranial ends (craniopagus twins, *white arrow*).

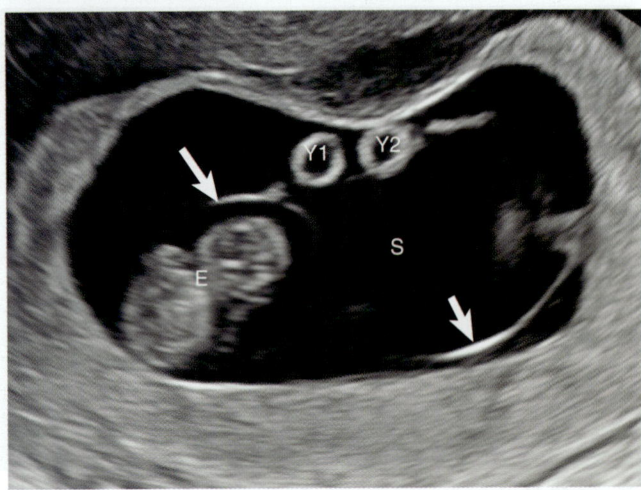

Figure 47.12 B-mode USG images of a 8 weeks old monochorionic–diamniotic twin gestation showing two yolk sacs (Y1 and Y2) and two separate amnions (*white arrows*) within a single gestational sac (S). One of the two embryos (E) is also visible in this section.

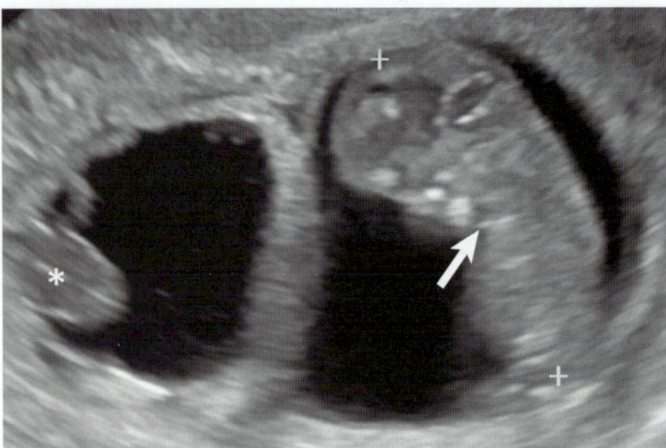

Figure 47.14 Vanishing twin. B-mode USG image of the gravid uterus in a 29-year-old primigravida lady, who conceived after in vitro fertilization resulting in a dichorionic-diamniotic twin gestation. At about 9 weeks of gestation, the fetus on the right (*white arrow*) is showing a normal growth (a crown-rump length (CRL) corresponding to 9 weeks and 5 days), while the one on the left shows a nonviable embryo (*white asterisk*, *CRL* corresponding to 7 weeks and 1 day). On a follow-up scan, the sac with the nonviable gestation disappeared.

In a monochorionic–diamniotic twin gestation, a thin membrane is visible between the embryos with the presence of two yolk sacs (Fig. 47.12). Twin peak sign is not seen in a monochorionic gestation.

If two embryos and only one yolk sac is seen inside a gestational sac, it is a monochorionic-monoamniotic gestation.

Three-dimensional reconstruction of B-mode images (Fig. 47.13) better demonstrates the chorionicity in an early multifetal gestation. It is also a great tool for patient education.

Vanishing Twin

In approximately 10–20% of twin pregnancies, a follow-up USG reveals the loss of one embryo with the absence of cardiac pulsations, continuing as a singleton pregnancy (Fig. 47.14). The other nonviable sac slowly shrinks in size and is eventually resorbed. This, however, does not affect the outcome of the viable twin at this early stage.

Evaluation of Anatomic Features

During the early embryonic period from 5 to 7 weeks, the embryo appears as a featureless disc showing cardiac pulsations. As the gestation advances, it develops certain anatomical features, which can be detected on USG. At the beginning of the eighth week, the precursor of the fourth ventricle of the brain—rhombencephalon—appears as a cystic structure at the cranial end (Fig. 47.15). At 9–10 weeks, the lateral ventricles can be identified as two more small cystic structures. They become

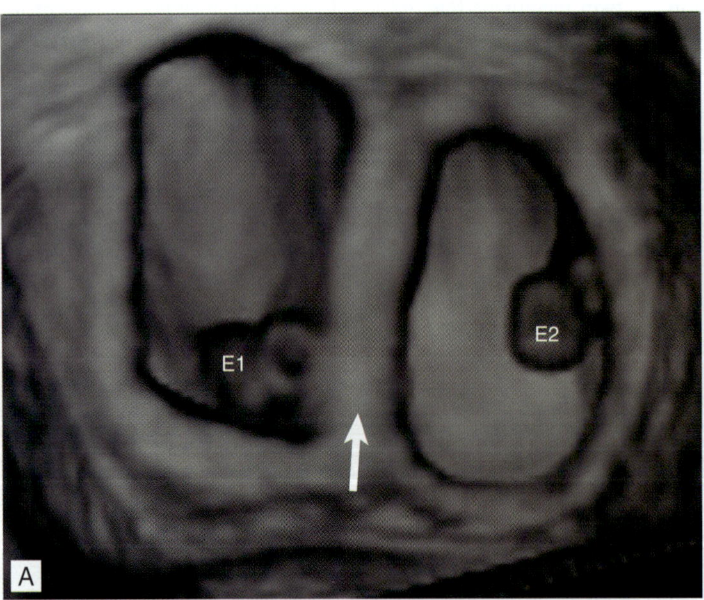

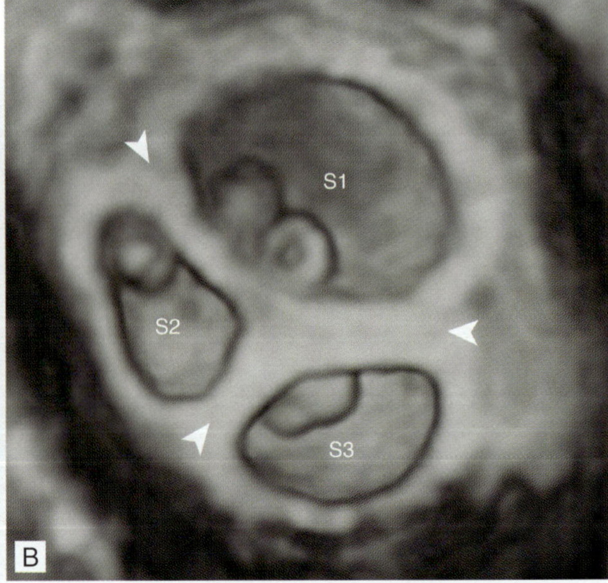

Figure 47.13 Use of three-dimensional USG in the diagnosis of multifetal gestation. (A) A dichorionic–diamniotic gestation at 6 weeks showing a thick chorionic plate (*white arrow*) separating the two embryos (E1 and E2). (B) A trichorionic–triamniotic gestation showing three distinct sacs (S1, S2, S3) separated by their respective chorions (*white arrowheads*).

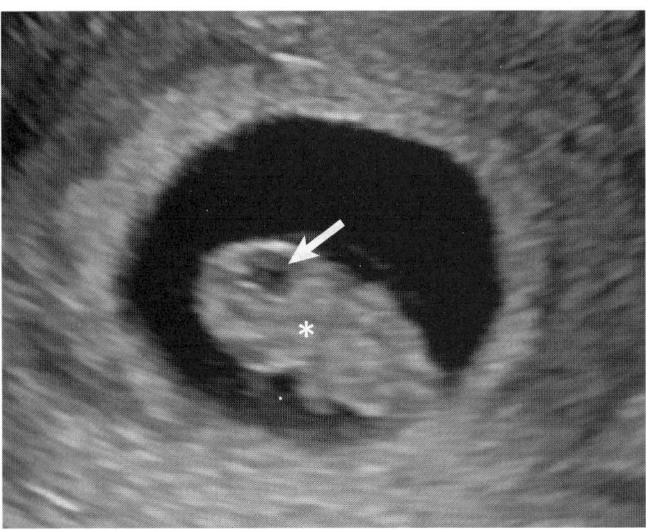

Figure 47.15 Rhombencephalon. B-mode USG image of a 8 weeks old embryo (*white asterisk*) showing a cystic vesicle at its cranial end (*white arrow*).

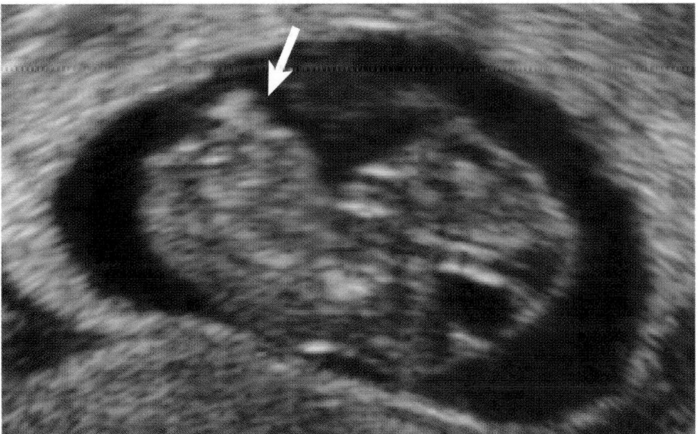

Figure 47.16 Physiological gut herniation. B-mode USG image of a 9 weeks embryo showing an echogenic thickening (*white arrow*) inside the umbilical cord.

more evident at 13 weeks when the choroid plexus fills them. Limb buds appear at 9–10 weeks.

Physiologic Anterior Abdominal Wall Herniation

Herniation of the midgut into the umbilical cord begins at 8 weeks, which may be seen as a small echogenic structure protruding into the cord, measuring 6–9 mm in size (Fig. 47.16). It rotates 90 degrees counterclockwise and returns to the abdominal cavity by 12th week. Thus, it gradually decreases in size as the gestation advances and completely disappears by 12 weeks. In some pregnancies, it may persist beyond 12 weeks, which is suggestive of exomphalos/omphalocele (Fig. 47.17A)—an abdominal wall defect in the midline through which the bowels herniate. This can be associated with aneuploidies, mainly trisomy 13 and 18.

Evaluation of Uterus and Ovaries

It is necessary to conduct a detailed sonographic evaluation of the uterus and its adnexa after establishing an intrauterine pregnancy, to identify comorbidities, if any.

- Uterine fibroids are a common coexisting pathology. Sometimes, they enlarge and undergo necrosis, giving rise to pelvic pain. The size and site of fibroids must be documented for ease of comparison during follow-up scans. Large and complicated fibroids may contribute to early pregnancy loss
- Corpus luteal cyst is the most common ovarian mass seen in the early first trimester. It secretes progesterone to support the pregnancy. It is visualized in 98% of pregnancies and is usually less than 5 cm in size (Fig. 47.18) [19]. It usually regresses as the gestation advances. Luteal cysts which increase in size must be followed up, as larger cysts pose a risk of torsion
- Hemorrhagic cysts are also commonly seen during early pregnancy. They occasionally give rise to pelvic pain. They show no internal vascularity on USG and may show a hyperechoic retracted clot that resolves with advancing gestation
- Malignant lesions are rare during pregnancy. They typically show solid papillary components with a central anechoic area due to necrosis. The solid components show low impedance blood flow on Doppler USG

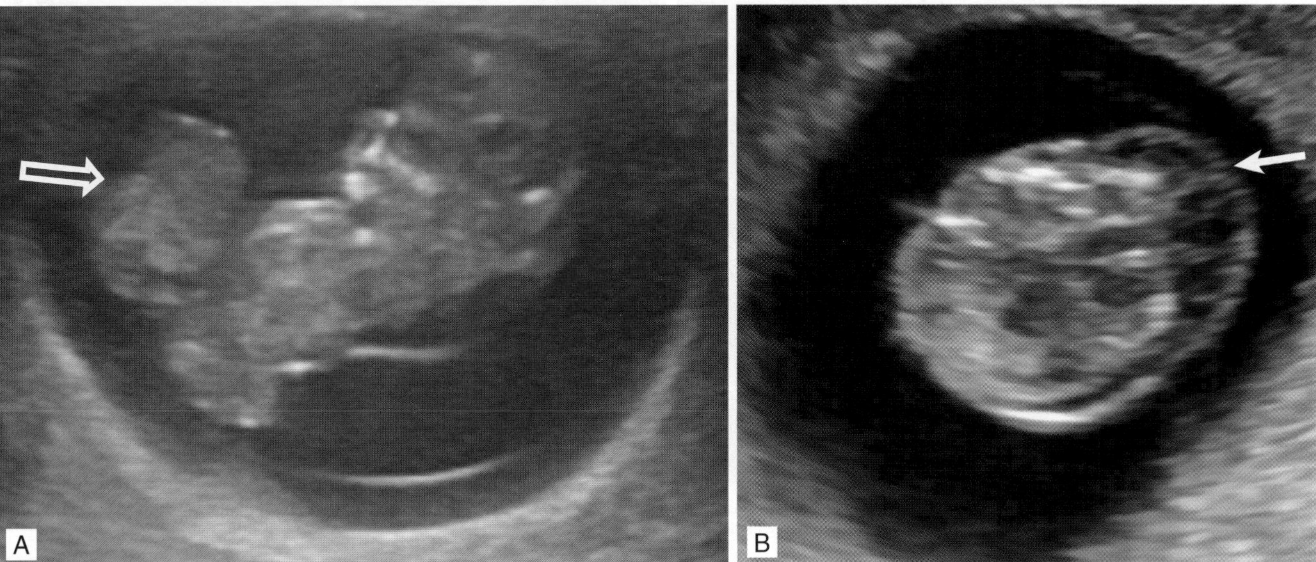

Figure 47.17 B-mode USG evaluation of an embryo in a 35-year-old primigravida. The presence of (A) an omphalocele (*white block arrow*) and of (B) an increased nuchal translucency (seen in a cross section of the fetal head, *white arrow*) is highly suggestive of the presence of a genetic anomaly. Subsequent karyotyping revealed trisomy 18.

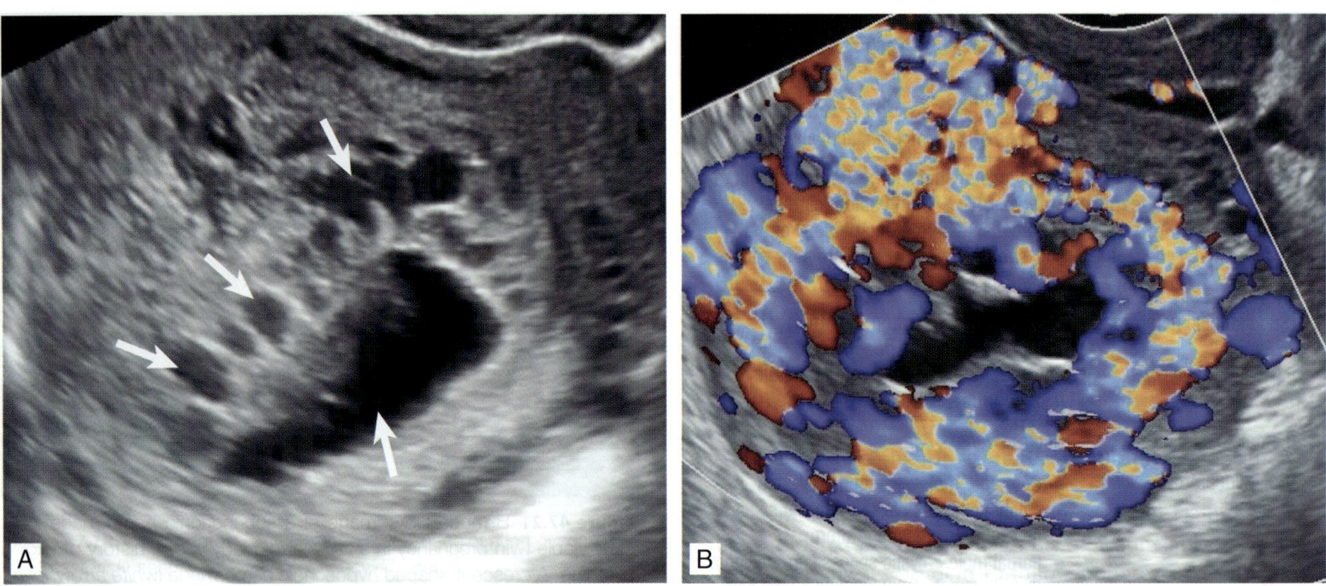

Figure 47.22 A complete hydatidiform mole in a 30-year-old primigravida lady with history of passing grape-like vesicles per vaginam. (A) Transvaginal B-mode USG shows multiple intrauterine cystic vesicles (*white arrows*) with no evidence of a viable fetus. (B) Color Doppler USG of the same pathology showing extreme vascularity.

TABLE 47.5 USG Features in Ectopic Gestation

Type of Ectopic Gestation	USG Features
Tubal	▪ Adnexal mass separate from ovaries ▪ Presence of yolk sac and/or embryo inside the mass is diagnostic ▪ The embryo may demonstrate cardiac pulsations ▪ Tubal ring sign – reflective ring surrounding gestational sac ▪ Ring of fire sign – the presence of low impedance vascularity around the lesion on Doppler USG (less specific) ▪ Centrally located fluid collection in the endometrial cavity, known as "pseudogestational sac"—can be present with any type of ectopic gestation ▪ Absent intradecidual sac sign
Interstitial	▪ Eccentrically placed gestational sac with a thin myometrial layer around, less than 5 mm in size ▪ Interstitial line sign—reflective line bordering the intramural gestational sac
Cornual	▪ Gestational sac surrounded by a thin myometrial layer ▪ 3D coronal reconstruction is helpful in documentation
Ovarian	▪ Gestational sac with surrounding hyperechoic ring within the ovary
Cervical	▪ Hourglass appearance of the cervix due to an expanding sac inside the cervical canal ▪ Bimanual sliding sign to rule out an impending abortion—sac should not move on bimanual pressure ▪ Vascularity surrounding sac on color Doppler
Scar	▪ Empty uterus ▪ Gestational sac implanted at or very near the scar line of previous lower segment cesarian section
Intra-abdominal	▪ Intra-abdominal fetus with an unusual orientation ▪ No defined myometrium ▪ Poorly defined placenta ▪ Bowel loops may be seen around the fetus

collection in the endometrial cavity, known as "pseudogestational sac." It is located centrally in the endometrial cavity, whereas a true gestational sac is situated eccentrically in the endometrium. The absence of the "intradecidual sac sign" is another distinguishing feature of a pseudogestational sac.

Interstitial Pregnancy

Interstitial pregnancies occur in the interstitial portion of the fallopian tube and are relatively rare. This is the intramyometrial portion of the tube, which has more distensibility. Hence, such ectopic gestations may be detected as late as the 16th week of gestation. Rupture of such gestations can lead to life-threatening hemorrhage due to proximity with the uterine artery. USG findings include an eccentrically placed gestational sac with a thin myometrial layer around (Figs. 47.23A and 47.26), often less than 5 mm in thickness. The "interstitial line sign" presents as a reflective line bordering the intramural gestational sac, which extends into the uterus.

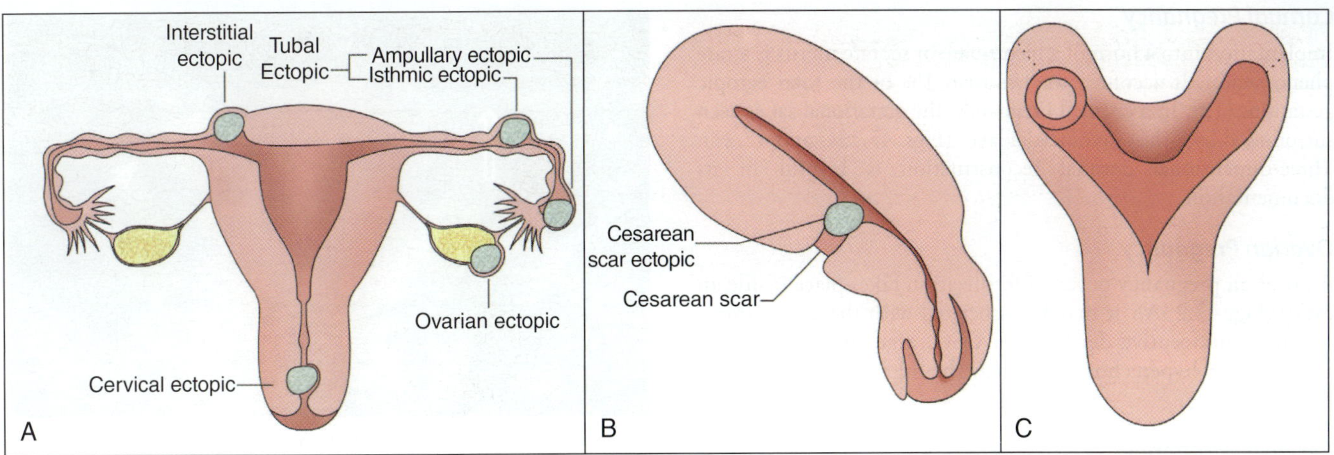

Figure 47.23 Schematic of ectopic gestation (TS, use the provided redraw images). (A) Coronal view of uterus showing tubal, interstitial, ovarian, and cervical pregnancies. (B) Sagittal view of uterus depicting a scar pregnancy. (C) Coronal view of a bicornuate uterus with a cornual pregnancy.

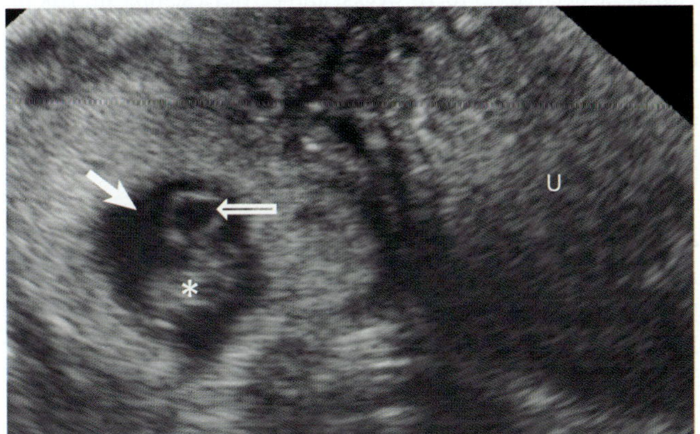

Figure 47.24 B-mode USG image of a tubal ectopic gestation. The extrauterine adnexal sac (*white arrow*) shows the presence of a yolk sac (*white block arrow*) and an embryo (*white asterisk*). *U*, uterus.

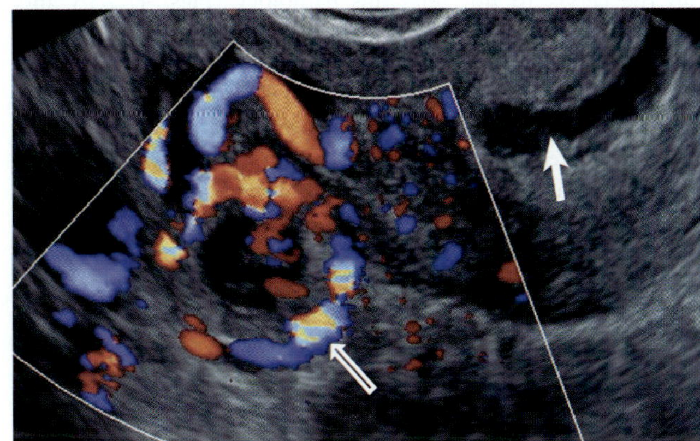

Figure 47.25 Ring of fire sign. Color Doppler image showing a ring-like signal (*white block arrow*) around an ectopic gestational sac. *White arrow*, endometrial cavity.

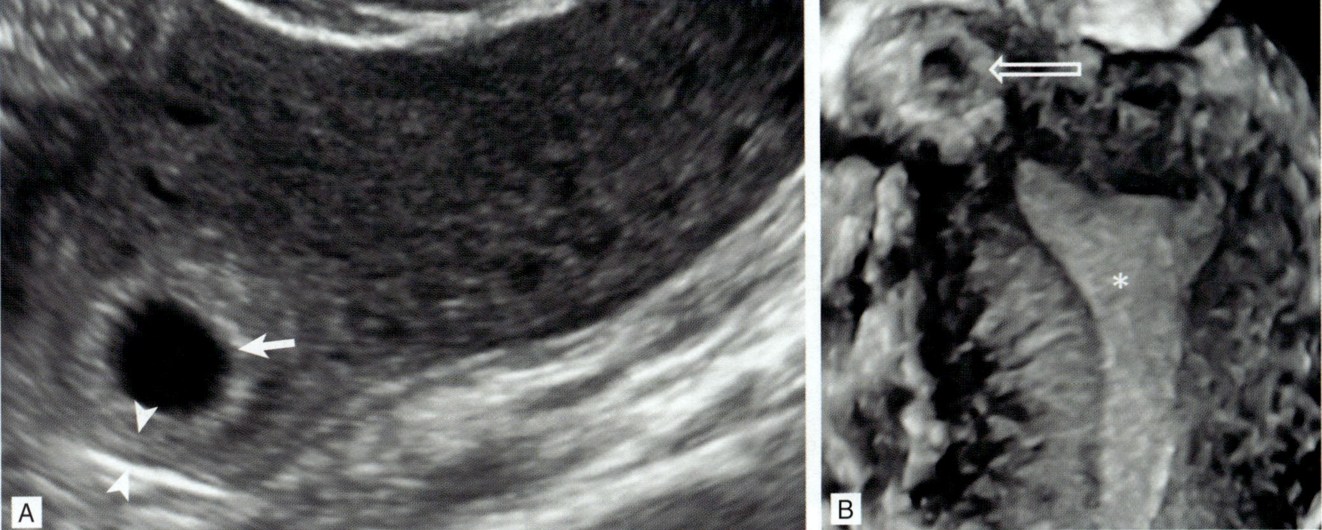

Figure 47.26 Interstitial gestation. (A) B-mode USG image showing the gestational sac (*white arrow*) implanted in the interstitial portion of the fallopian tube. A very thin rim of surrounding myometrium can be noted (*white arrowheads*). (B) Three-dimensional coronal image showing an ectopic implantation of the sac in the interstitial portion of the fallopian tube (*white block arrow*). *White asterisk*, endometrial cavity.

Cornual Pregnancy

Implantation into a horn of a bicornuate or septate uterus is a rare phenomenon. It accounts for less than 1% of the total ectopic gestations [12]. In a cornual pregnancy, the gestational sac is seen surrounded by a thin myometrial layer (Figs. 47.23C and 47.27). Three-dimensional coronal reconstruction is helpful in its documentation.

Ovarian Pregnancy

An ovarian pregnancy occurs if fertilization takes place inside an ovary (Fig. 47.23A). It may be associated with the use of intrauterine contraceptive devices. On USG, a gestational sac with surrounding hyperechoic ring may be identified within the ovary.

Cervical Pregnancy

Implantation within the cervical canal is rare, but its incidence is rising with an increasing number of assisted reproductive techniques. An expanding sac inside the canal gives it an hourglass appearance. During a pelvic scan, it is important to thoroughly scan the cervix to not miss this pathology (Figs. 47.23A and 47.28). It is also important to rule out an aborting sac with the "bimanual sliding sign." This is accomplished by applying bimanual pressure on the uterus while doing TVU. If the sac moves on the maneuver, it is likely an aborting sac. Otherwise, it can be safely considered to be adherent to the cervical canal. Vascularity arising due to decidual reaction surrounding the sac is usually visible on color Doppler.

Scar Pregnancy

Implantation occurring within the scar of a previous cesarean section is known as a scar pregnancy, in which the blastocyst is surrounded by myometrium and fibrous tissue of the scar. The pregnancy may present with vaginal bleeding as early as 6 weeks or may be delayed up to 16 weeks, and carries a significant risk of rupture. On USG, a scar pregnancy shows an empty uterus, while the gestational sac is seen implanted at or very near the scar line of a previous LSCS (Figs. 47.23B and 47.29A). A thin myometrial interface between the conceptus and urinary bladder wall may be appreciated. It can be treated with USG-guided methotrexate injections within the sac (Fig. 47.29B).

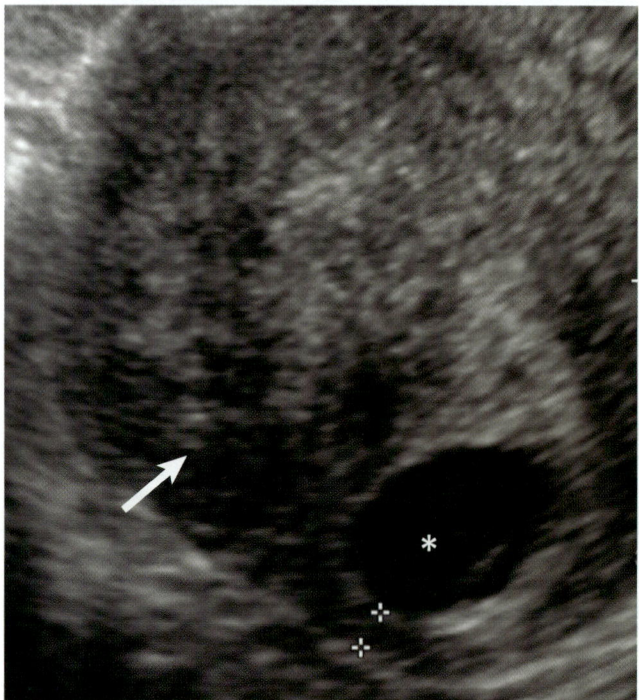

Figure 47.27 B-mode USG image of a cornual ectopic gestation. The implantation occurred inside the left cornu (*white arrow*) of the uterus. Note a thin myometrial layer (*marked by a pair of calipers*) surrounding the sac (*white asterisk*).

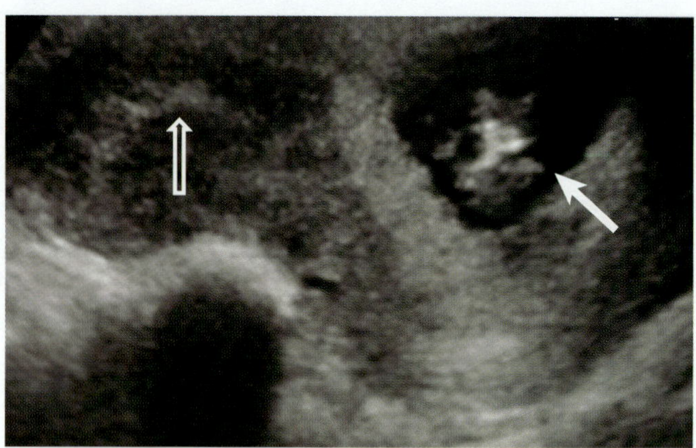

Figure 47.28 B-mode USG image in a 29-year-old lady with a positive urine pregnancy test, showing a cervical implantation (*white arrow*). Note that the uterine cavity is empty (*white block arrow*).

Intra-Abdominal Pregnancy

Intra-abdominal pregnancy is a rare condition (~1% of all ectopic pregnancies) [13] in which implantation occurs inside the peritoneal cavity excluding tubal, ovarian, and intraligamentous sites. It carries a risk of life-threatening hemorrhage. USG is the first-line diagnostic imaging, which shows an empty uterine cavity. The intraabdominal fetus reveals an unusual orientation without definable myometrium around it, with a poorly defined placenta. Additionally, bowel loops may be identified around the fetus.

Management of Ectopic Gestation

Once the diagnosis of ectopic gestation is established, a thorough USG evaluation should be carried out to decide whether a surgical, medical or combined management is best suited. *Factors that contribute to the decision include the size of the ectopic gestation, presence of embryo with cardiac pulsations, presence of hemoperitoneum with signs of tubal rupture, and hemodynamic condition of the patient.* If the patient's condition is stable without any hemoperitoneum, medical management with systemic methotrexate can be initiated. Serum β-HCG level above 10,000 mIU/mL is a contraindication to medical management [14]. For surgical management, minimally invasive methods (such as laparoscopy) are preferred to preserve fertility. USG-guided direct injection of methotrexate or potassium chloride into the ectopic sac is another therapeutic option that has been successfully used [15,16]. It is a relatively safe procedure except for some pelvic pain complained by a few patients after the procedure. This approach is especially beneficial to patients with a cervical or cornual ectopic pregnancy in whom surgery can be associated with significant morbidity and blood loss. It requires a follow-up scan after about 2 months to detect any complications; and to record the resolution of the ectopic gestation (in the form of serum β-HCG to becoming negative), which takes up to 54–60 days [15].

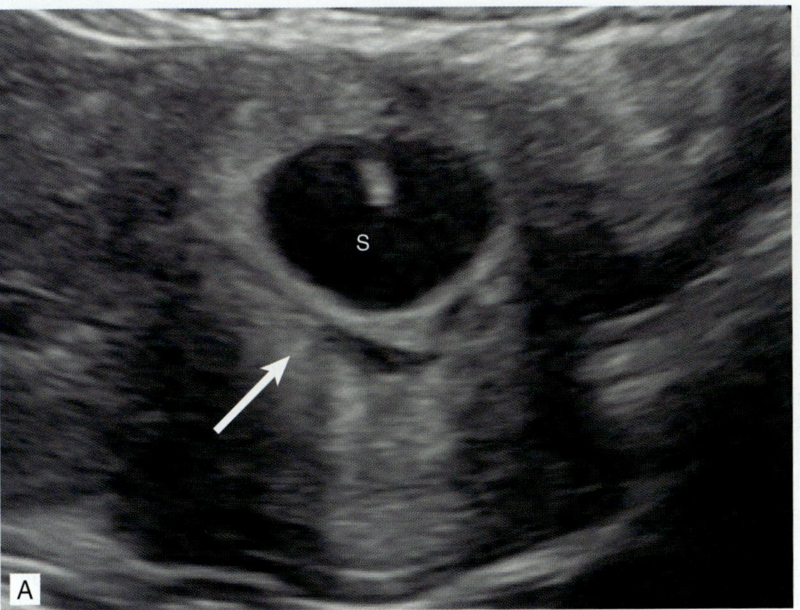

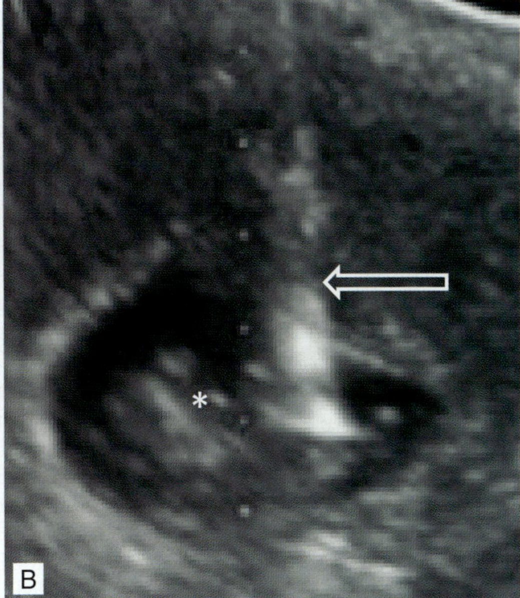

Figure 47.29 B-mode USG image of scar pregnancy. (A) A gestational sac (S) implanted along a previous LSCS scar (*white arrow*). (B) USG-guided therapeutic injection of methotrexate into the sac of a scar pregnancy (*white asterisk*). The echogenic needle track is well visualized (*white block arrow*) in this image.

Heterotopic Pregnancy

The simultaneous presence of intrauterine and extrauterine pregnancies is referred to as heterotopic pregnancy. Its incidence has risen due to more women undergoing assisted reproductive techniques, especially when multiple embryos are transferred. A careful evaluation of the adnexa is necessary while performing an early trimester USG to suspect the presence of heterotopic pregnancy. Patients diagnosed with heterotopic pregnancy can undergo USG-guided ablation of the extrauterine gestation, to allow the intrauterine gestation to grow. Laparoscopic removal of the extrauterine gestation can also be done.

Pregnancy of Unknown Location

Pregnancy of unknown location represents a transient stage where there is no definite IUP detected on TVU, and there is no sign of an ectopic gestation as well. In such cases, maternal serum β-HCG level plays a crucial role in management. β-HCG level around 1000–2000 mIU/mL without an intrauterine gestational sac on TVU raises suspicion of an ectopic gestation [17]. In such cases, serial β-HCG values must be obtained along with follow-up USG scans. A rise of at least 35% in β-HCG level over 48 hours is highly suggestive of a viable IUP, whereas smaller rise points toward an ectopic gestation [18].

Late First-Trimester Fetal Evaluation

The USG evaluation between 11 and 14 gestational weeks plays a vital role in the early detection of multiple anomalies. It includes documentation of certain markers for chromosomal abnormalities like nuchal translucency, nasal bone, the flow in the ductus venosus, flow across the tricuspid valve; and a structural survey of the fetal anatomy. Table 47.6 describes the normal findings observed during the late first trimester.

TABLE 47.6 Normal USG Findings in the Late First Trimester

- Nuchal translucency lies within a certain range for a given crown-rump-length value
- The nasal bone can be identified as a part of the "equal sign" or the "three-line sign"
- Ductus venosus shows a continuous forward flow on color Doppler
- Fetal cranium shows definite ossification, the falx cerebri is visible, the choroid plexus is seen as a butterfly-shaped symmetric hyperechoic structure, the posterior fossa shows a translucent fourth ventricle, the brain stem is well delineated
- Fetal heart structure and cardiac pulsations can be visualized
- Multiple fetal internal organs such as stomach, kidneys, umbilical arteries, and urinary bladder become visible
- Fetal spine and limb segments can be identified

Screening for aneuploidy forms a major part of this evaluation. Fetuses with chromosomal abnormalities tend to have abnormal flow in the ductus venosus and the presence of tricuspid regurgitation. Fetuses with Down's syndrome are known to have thicker nuchal translucency. This finding becomes commoner with advanced maternal age due to a higher incidence of Down's syndrome. Fetuses with trisomy 13 and 18 tend to show gross abnormalities in the NT, and their placentae tend to secrete lower levels of both β-HCG and pregnancy-associated plasma protein-A (Papp-A). Inclusion of other markers such as fetal nasal bone increases the detection rate for these anomalies to about 97% [20].

Evaluation of the Markers for Chromosomal Abnormalities

Nuchal Translucency

Trisomy 21 or Down's syndrome is the commonest aneuploidy associated with mental retardation. Fetuses with trisomy 21 have an excess subcutaneous fluid collection in the posterior cervical region, which appears as increased lucency on USG. This is labeled as increased nuchal translucency (NT) or increased nuchal fold thickness (Figs. 47.17B and 47.30A). It occurs due to abnormal lymphatic drainage and abnormalities of the extracellular matrix. Evaluation of NT is part of a standard protocol for fetal screening for chromosomal abnormalities. Other components of the screening include maternal age and biochemical assessment (free β-HCG and Papp–A). *The placenta is known to secrete higher amounts of free β-HCG and lower amounts of Papp–A in Down's fetuses.*

NT progressively increases as the gestation advances and its value is closely related to the CRL value. For a given CRL, the NT measurement represents a likelihood ratio (LR). This LR, when multiplied by the a priori maternal and gestational age-related risk, gives a new risk specific for each case. The smaller the measurement of NT, smaller is the LR and the posterior risk is thus lower. The minimum CRL required to measure and document NT is 45 mm and the maximum CRL up to which NT can be measured is 84 mm [21]. Hence it is important that the gestational age and CRL are taken into account when interpreting the NT measurements. Online calculators for determining the acceptable values of NT for a given CRL value are useful tools in this regard [21].

The accurate assessment of NT requires a specialized technique. The measurement of NT must be preceded by a good CRL measurement with the fetus in a neutral position. The Fetal Medicine Foundation [21] has laid down the following criteria for USG imaging of NT:

- Acquire an image in the mid-sagittal section
- Include only the fetal head and upper thorax in the image
- Keep the magnification at the highest possible value, such that a slight movement of the caliper should not produce changes of more than 0.1 mm
- The fetal head should be in a neutral position (the distance between the chin and chest should be the same as the thickness of the palate); hyperextension can increase NT value by up to 0.6 mm, while hyperflexion can cause erroneously low measurements
- It is important to differentiate between the amnion and fetal skin, as both appear echogenic (Fig. 47.30B). For this, a simple trick is to give a gentle tap to the maternal abdomen to stimulate fetal movement toward the probe. This makes it easy to reliably identify the amnion separately for accurate measurement of NT
- Correct placement of calipers is important for the accurate measurement of NT. The commonly practiced technique is called "on to on" in which the inner border of the horizontal crossbar of the calipers and the inner border of the two retronuchal lines perfectly superimpose (Fig. 47.31)
- Measure the maximum thickness of the subcutaneous translucency between the skin and the soft tissue overlying the cervical spine

Nasal Bone

The process of nasal bone formation through intramembranous ossification is delayed or absent in some genetic syndromes and chromosomal abnormalities like trisomy 21. As a result, around 65% of Down's fetuses show the absence of the nasal bone [22]. Incorporation of this feature in the screening for fetal anomalies (along with NT scan and serum levels of free β-HCG and Papp–A) improves the overall detection rate for Down's syndrome.

A good technique of evaluation of the nasal bone involves:

- Obtaining a mid-sagittal section
- Tilting the probe side-to-side to ensure adequate visualization of the nasal bone
- *Demonstration of "equal sign"—the upper line represents the skin of the nose, while the parallel line below is the nasal bone (Fig. 47.30A). A third echogenic line may be observed, which represents the tip of the nose*

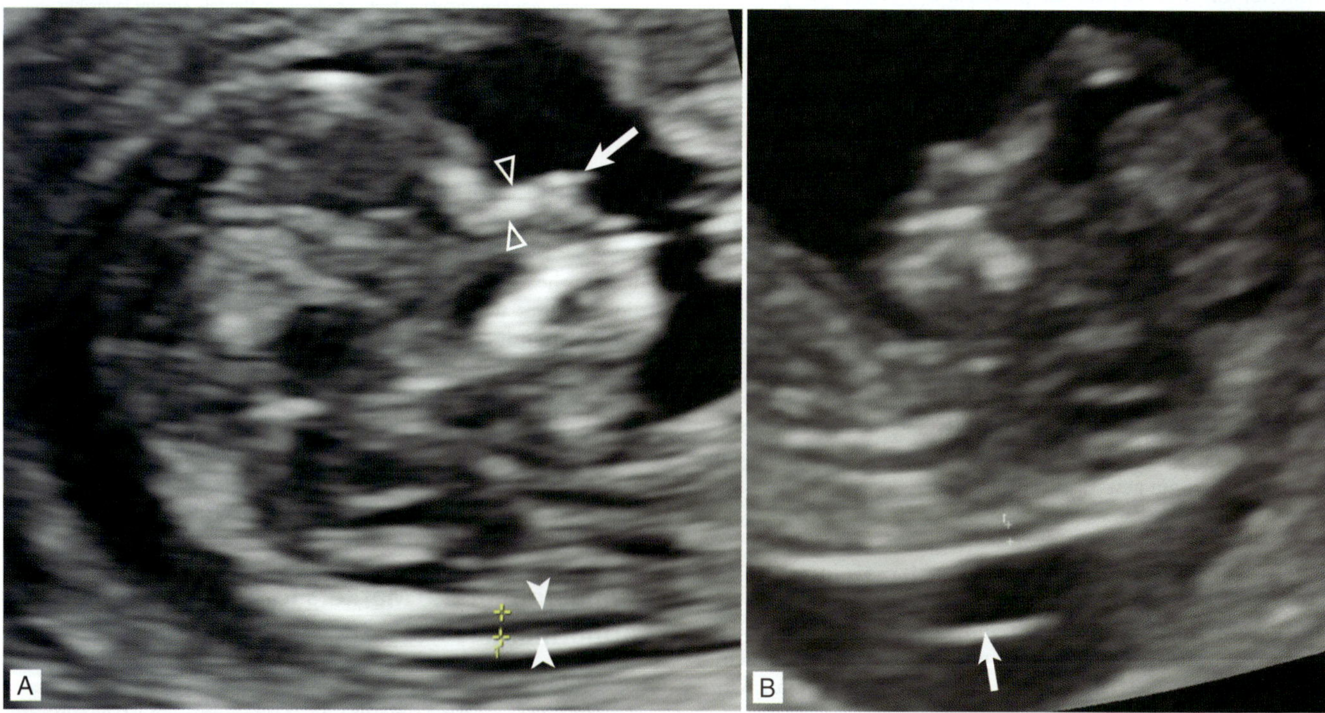

Figure 47.30 B-mode USG images of the mid-sagittal view of a fetal head (NT scan) as per the Fetal Medicine Foundation guidelines. (Source: The Fetal Medicine Foundation. Certificates of competence—Nuchal translucency scan [Internet] [cited 2020 Sep 2]. Available from: https://fetalmedicine.org/fmf-certification/certificates-of-competence/nuchal-translucency-scan). (A) Nuchal translucency (NT) is the hypoechoic region bounded by two linear hyperechoicities representing the fetal skin and the soft tissue overlying its cervical spine (*white arrowheads*). Fetal nasal bone (inferior) and the skin (superior) are seen forming the "equal sign" (*white block arrowheads*), while the inclusion of the nasal tip constitutes the "three-line sign." (B) The hyperechoic line below the fetal nuchal skin (*white arrow*) represents the amnion.

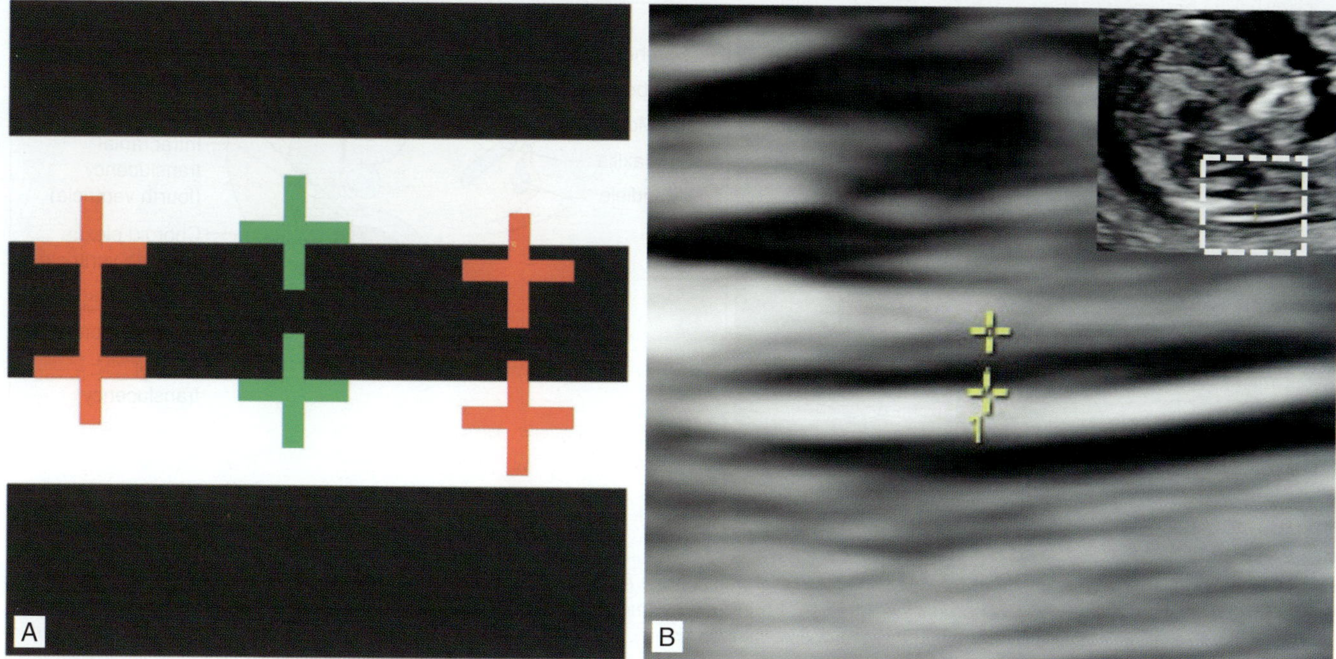

Figure 47.31 The "on to on" placement of the calipers for the measurement of the nuchal translucency. (A) The *green calipers* represent the correct position, while the *red* ones are incorrect. (B) B-mode image showing the correct placement of the calipers. Inset: the area of the entire image highlighted for the demonstration.

Ductus Venosus

Ductus venosus is an important structure in the fetal circulation that shunts blood from the umbilical vein to the right atrium bypassing the hepatic circulation. It has a triphasic forward flow—the "S" wave represents systole, "D" wave represents early diastole, and the "A" wave represents atrial contraction. "A" wave reversal is seen in chromosomally abnormal fetuses (Fig. 47.32).

An appropriate technique for the evaluation of ductus venosus includes:

- Obtaining a mid-sagittal section, fetus facing the probe. The fetal thorax and abdomen should occupy the whole screen for adequate visualization of the ductus venosus
- Setting the pulse repetition frequency to a low value, which induces aliasing and helps identify the tiny vessel
- Placing the pulsed Doppler sampling window with a small sample width (0.5 mm) at the area of aliasing—a triphasic flow pattern is obtained as described earlier

Tricuspid Regurgitation

Tricuspid regurgitation (TR) is an adjunct first-trimester sign of aneuploidies. This measurement is obtained by spectral Doppler of the fetal tricuspid valve in the apical four-chamber view. To diagnose TR, it must be present over at least half of the systole with a velocity of 60–80 cm/s [23]. Significant TR has been reported in 74% of Down's syndrome fetuses compared with 6.9% of normal fetuses in a study [24]. Thus, the addition of TR to the first-trimester screening increases the detection rate of Down's syndrome.

The essential components of the USG scan between 11 and 14 weeks include NT, fetal nasal bone, ductus venosus, and TR as described earlier. Despite the current state-of-the-art USG machines, rigorous training is required for the performance of this scan, because the results are highly influenced by operator expertise. A meticulous USG evaluation as per the guidelines is essential for accurate risk stratification. The Fetal Medicine Foundation through its online training course grooms fetal

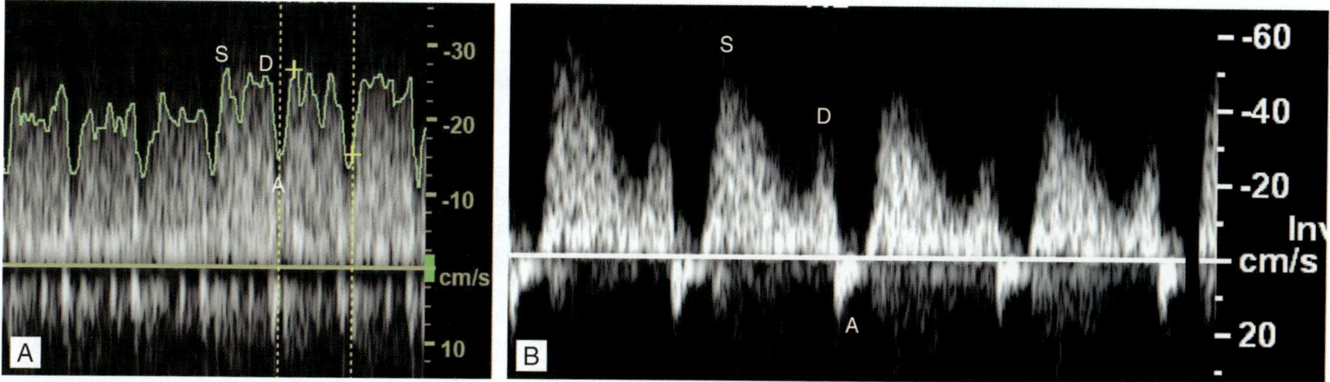

Figure 47.32 Spectral Doppler USG image of ductus venosus. (A) Normal spectrum showing S-wave (S), D-wave (D), and A-wave (A). (B) A-wave reversal seen in a case of Down's syndrome.

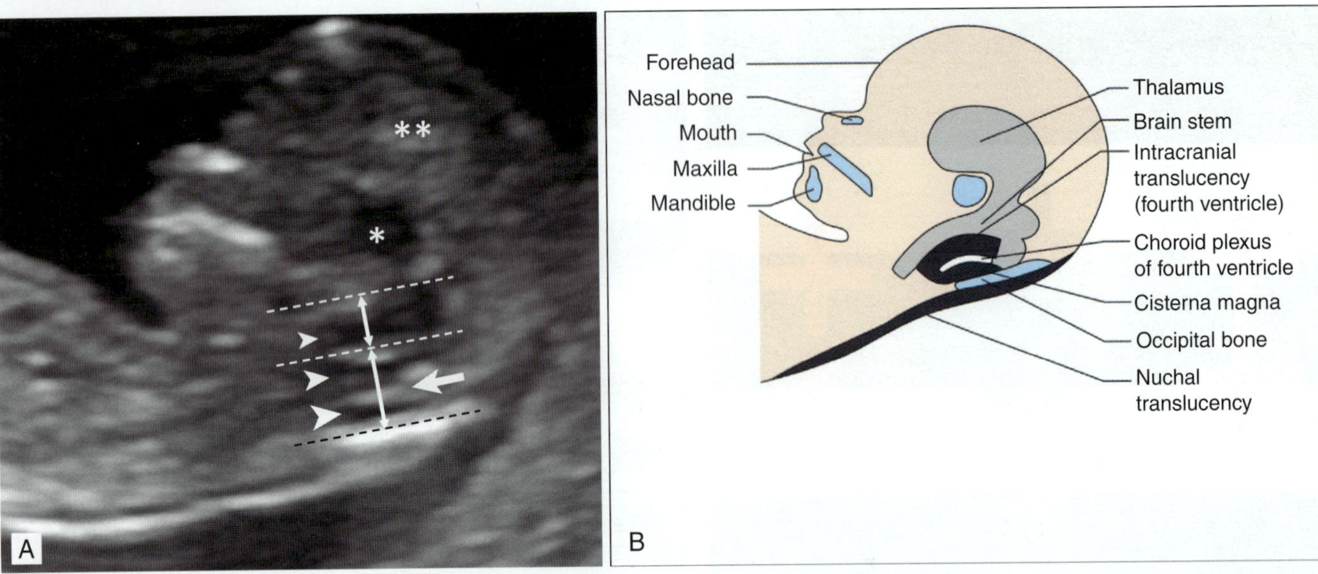

Figure 47.33 (A) B-mode USG image of the mid-sagittal view of a fetal head showing falx cerebri (*double white asterisk*), thalamus (*white asterisk*), brainstem (*small white arrowhead*), fourth ventricle/intracranial translucency (*midsized white arrowhead*), cisterna manga (*large arrowhead*), choroid plexus (*white arrow*), brainstem diameter (*shorter white double-headed arrow*), and brainstem-occipital bone distance (*longer white double-headed arrow*). (B) A schematic diagram depicting the same structures.

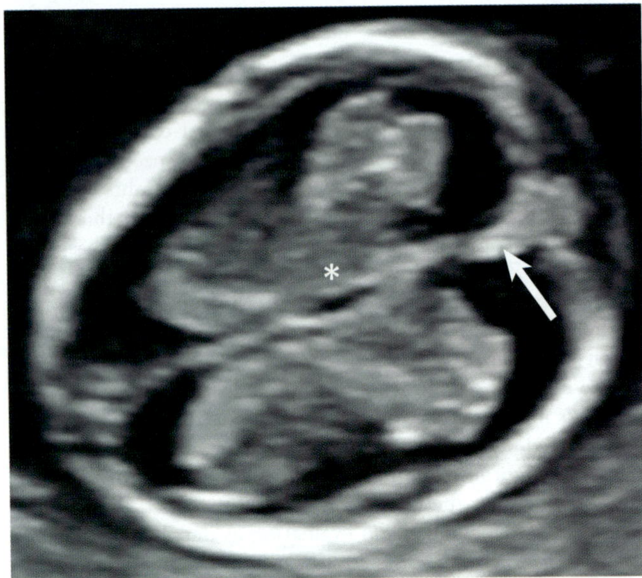

Figure 47.34 Fetal choroid plexus. B-mode USG image of a transverse section through a normal fetal head at 13 weeks showing the characteristic "butterfly" appearance of the bright choroid plexus (*white asterisk*). The midline falx cerebri is also well seen (*white arrow*).

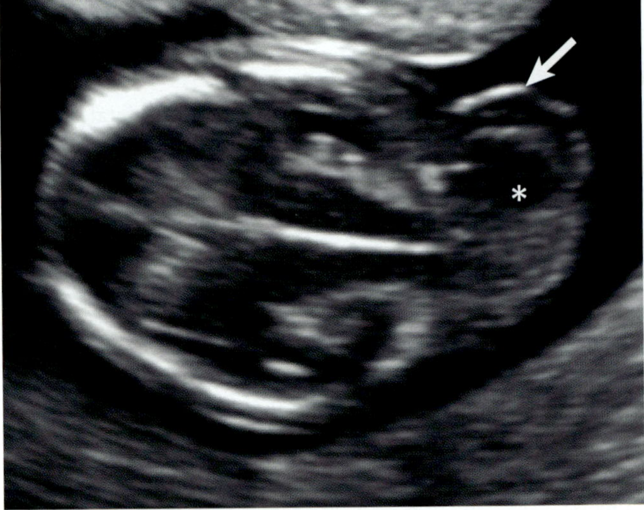

Figure 47.35 Occipital encephalocele. B-mode USG image of a transverse section through a fetal head showing a hypoechoic mass (*white asterisk*) emerging through a defect in the cranial bones (*white arrow*).

medicine experts, sonographers, and radiologists worldwide for a proper combined risk assessment for aneuploidies in the first trimester.

Fetal Structural Survey

Fetal Head

Fig. 47.33 depicts the structures visible in the mid-sagittal section of normal fetal head around 11 weeks of gestation. At this time, the fetal cranium shows definite ossification, while the falx cerebri can also be visualized. At the same time, choroid plexus fills the ventricles and is seen as a butterfly-shaped symmetric hyperechoic structure (Fig. 47.34). The posterior fossa shows an intracranial translucency that represents the fourth ventricle. The brain stem is well delineated, which makes it easier to calculate the brain stem to brainstem–occipital bone distance (BS/BSOB) ratio. This ratio normally increases with CRL. Nomograms for the 5th and 95th percentile reference ranges enable the assessment to detect and follow-up abnormalities like open spina bifida.

An encephalocele can be identified in the first trimester as a hypoechoic brain tissue protruding through a defect in the cranial vault (Fig. 47.35). The absence of an ossified cranial vault with distortion of the underlying brain are hallmarks of acrania (Fig. 47.36). Continuous exposure of the fetal brain to the amniotic fluid in these fetuses causes cerebral degeneration giving rise to anencephaly which is generally observed in the second trimester. Complete or partial absence of the falx cerebri, which is seen in alobar and semilobar holoprosencephaly, can be easily detected at 11 weeks (Fig. 47.37).

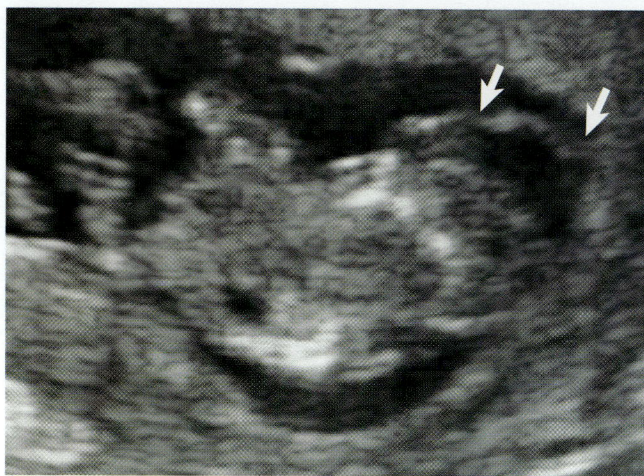

Figure 47.36 Acrania. B-mode USG image of a sagittal section through a fetal head showing the absence of the cranial vault ossification and distortion of the underlying brain (*white arrows*).

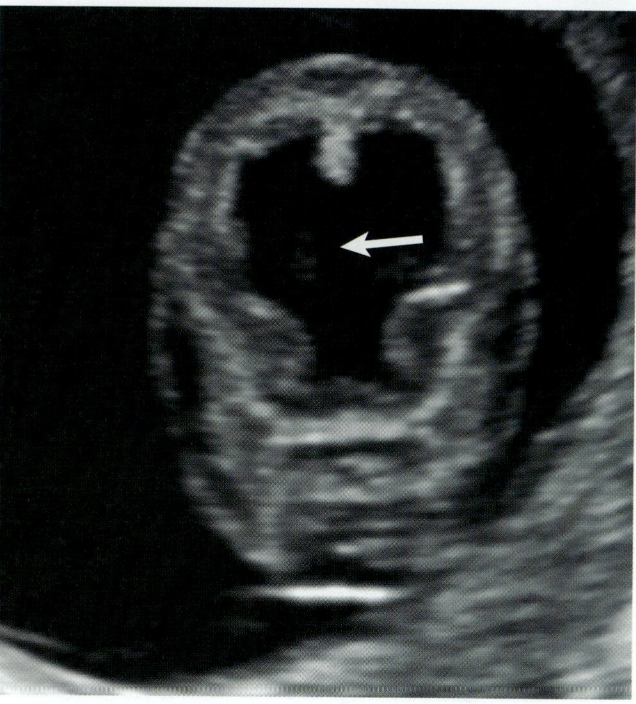

Figure 47.37 Holoprosencephaly. B-mode USG showing a fetal head at 13 weeks. The midline cleavage defect in the falx cerebri (*white arrow*) can be easily seen.

Fetal Thorax

A combination of transvaginal and transabdominal sonography helps to visualize fetal cardiac and pulmonary structures as early as 12 weeks of gestation. Cardiac apex and the four-chamber view (Fig. 47.38) can be identified in the majority of fetuses in an axial section through the thorax. This is easier in the case of mothers with lean body habitus. It is important to visualize and document two equal-sized atria and ventricles, the outflow tracts, and continuity of the ventricular septum with the anterior wall of the aorta; and of the anterior mitral leaflet with the posterior wall of the aorta. The "x" (crossover of the major arteries) and "y" (pulmonary artery and aorta)signs must be demonstrated at this stage. This early evaluation of the fetal heart can detect 70% of fetal cardiac anomalies [18]. The detection of congenital heart disease (CHD) in the first trimester is challenging. It largely depends on the type of the cardiac anomaly. The four-chamber anomalies like hypoplastic left heart, atrioventricular septal defect (AVSD), and ventricular septal defect (VSD) have a higher detection rate in the first trimester. The three vessel view or outlet abnormalities like transposition of great vessels and tetralogy of Fallot are relatively difficult to diagnose at this stage. The detection rate of these anomalies can be improved by following structured protocols like inclusion of both transabdominal and transvaginal USG particularly in high-risk pregnancies.

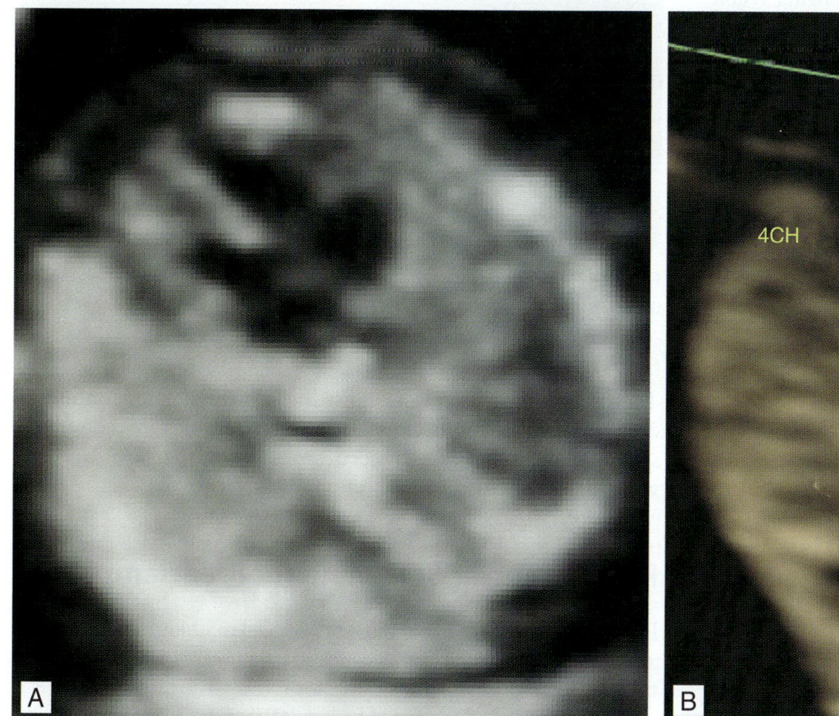

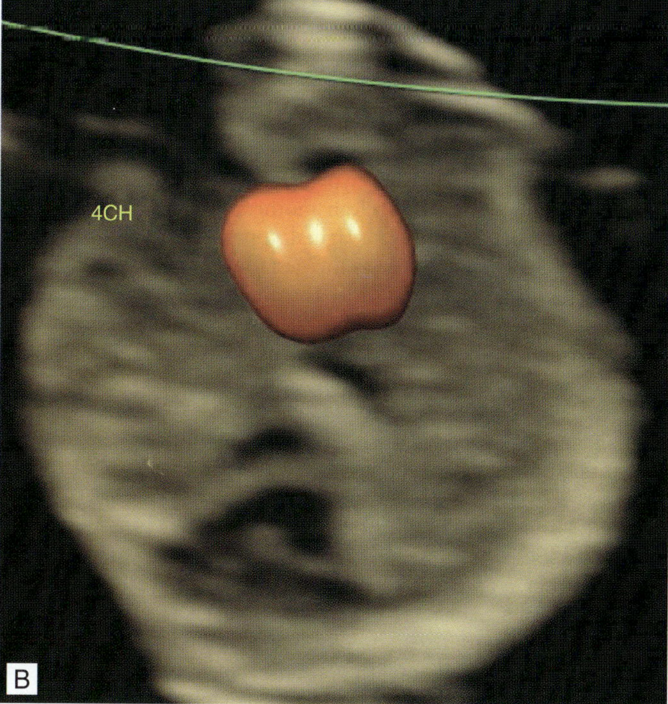

Figure 47.38 The four-chamber view of fetal heart. (A) B-mode USG image and (B) color Doppler image showing the atrioventricular inflows.

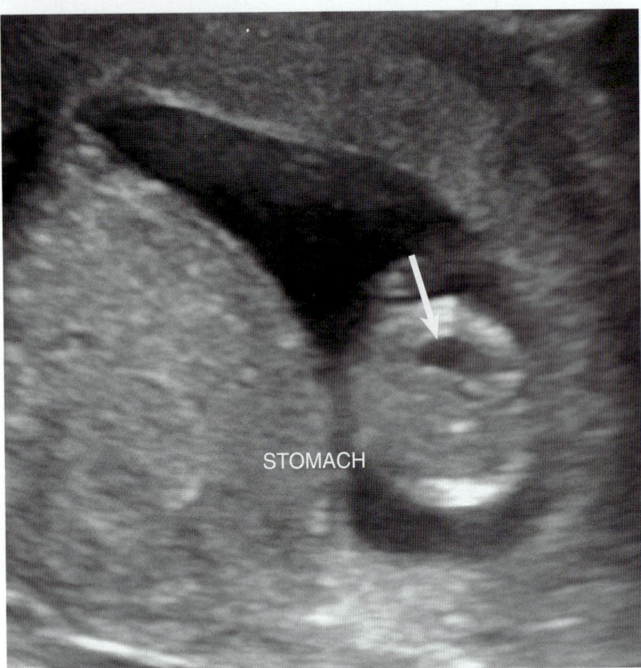

Figure 47.39 B-mode USG image of a fetal abdomen at 13 weeks of gestation showing the fetal stomach as a small, round anechoic structure (*white arrow*).

Fetal lungs are seen as homogeneous structures on either side of the heart without the presence of any cystic or solid masses.

Fetal Abdomen

Evaluation of the ventral wall of the fetus reveals several important findings. As mentioned earlier, the physiologic herniation of midgut seen as early as 7–8 weeks lasts till about 12 weeks of gestation, which makes it possible to document the insertion of the umbilical cord into the abdomen at that time [25]. Color Doppler can be reliably used to ascertain the presence of two umbilical arteries around the fetal bladder; the latter being visible in 93–100% fetuses between 11 and 14 weeks [26,27]. The stomach is identified in 99% of fetuses between 11 and 14 weeks as a rounded anechoic structure with a slightly reflective rim on the left side of the upper fetal abdomen (Fig. 47.39) [26]. Fetal stomach whenever visible must be documented during the first-trimester scan, as its visualization helps establish a situs. Fetal kidneys may be identified as relatively hyperechoic structures on either side of the spine, especially in lean mothers. In mothers with a thick abdominal wall, the transvaginal approach may be better suited. This is, however, easier as the gestation progresses toward 13–14 weeks. Fetal urinary bladder is seen as a tiny cystic round structure in the midline in the pelvis. It is visualized in almost all the fetuses by 13–14 weeks. Megacystis is defined as a fetal urinary bladder more than 7 mm in longitudinal diameter in the first trimester (Fig. 47.40). It carries a 25% risk of a chromosomal anomaly in the affected fetus [28]. The fetal umbilical arteries can be identified using color Doppler, when traced at the cord insertion (Fig. 47.41).

Fetal Spine

Fetal evaluation in the first trimester is incomplete without the evaluation of fetal spine. Although it is difficult to diagnose spinal dysraphism in the first trimester, major body stalk anomalies can be detected with relative ease. Evaluation of the spine for abnormal curvatures can sometimes reveal rare anomalies like iniencephaly, which involves a fixed hyperextension of the fetal spine (Fig. 47.42).

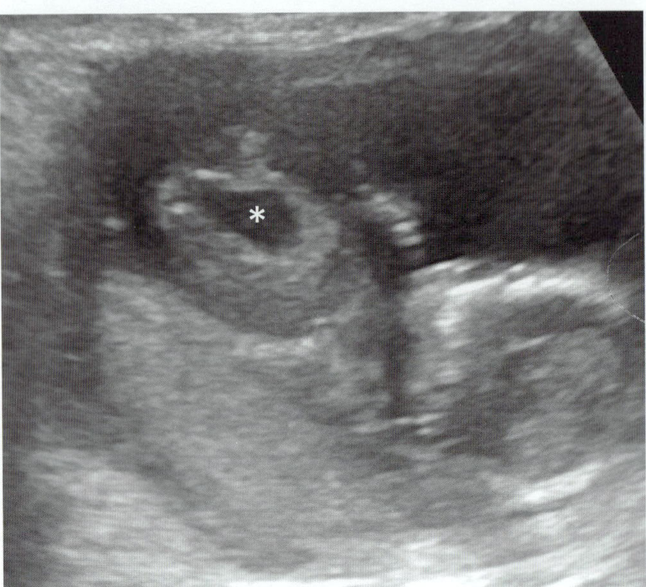

Figure 47.40 Megacystis. B-mode USG image showing a fetal urinary bladder (*white asterisk*) measuring 9 mm longitudinally. The fetus also showed an absent nasal bone and a single umbilical artery. Karyotyping revealed trisomy 21.

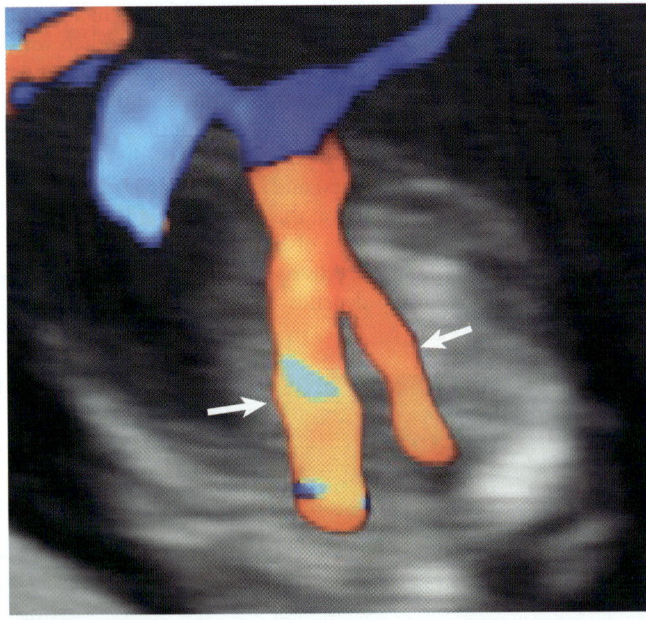

Figure 47.41 Color Doppler image showing the two fetal umbilical arteries (*white arrows*).

Fetal Limbs

The late first-trimester scan must include the documentation of each segment of the upper and lower extremities in the sagittal section (Fig. 47.43). Both sided limbs should be seen together, with all 3 segments in axial section of the fetus.

First-Trimester Screening for Preeclampsia

Preeclampsia (PE) is a major cause of perinatal morbidity and mortality affecting about 2–8% of pregnancies [29]. Impaired placentation is thought to be primarily responsible for it [30]. The first trimester is a good time for early detection of high-risk factors for PE, and for taking appropriate measures to prevent further impairment of placentation. A

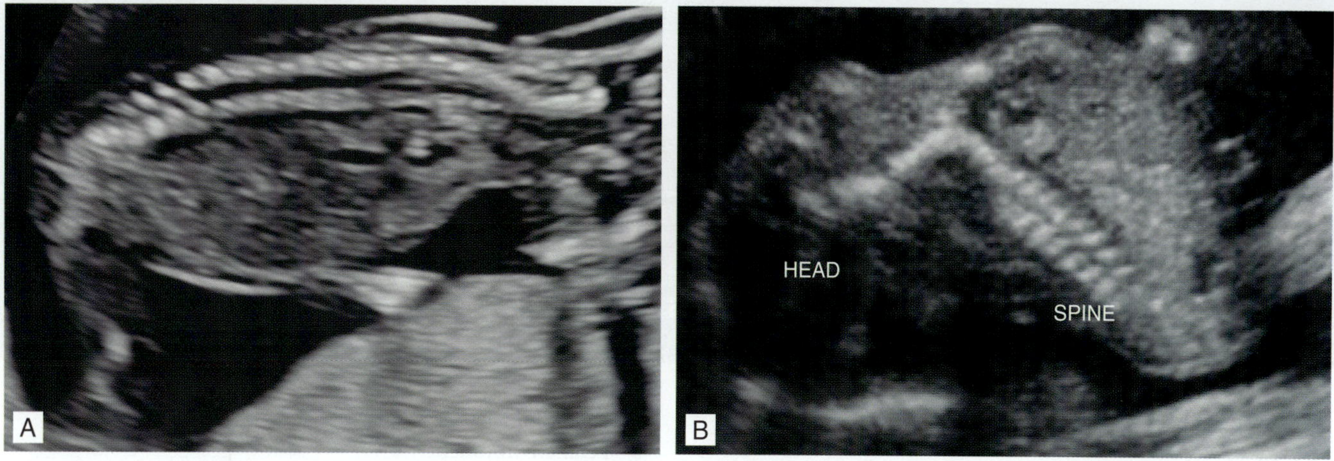

Figure 47.42 Iniencephaly. B-mode USG images of sagittal views of fetuses in the first trimester showing (A) a normal fetal spine and (B) a fixed hyper-extension of the head.

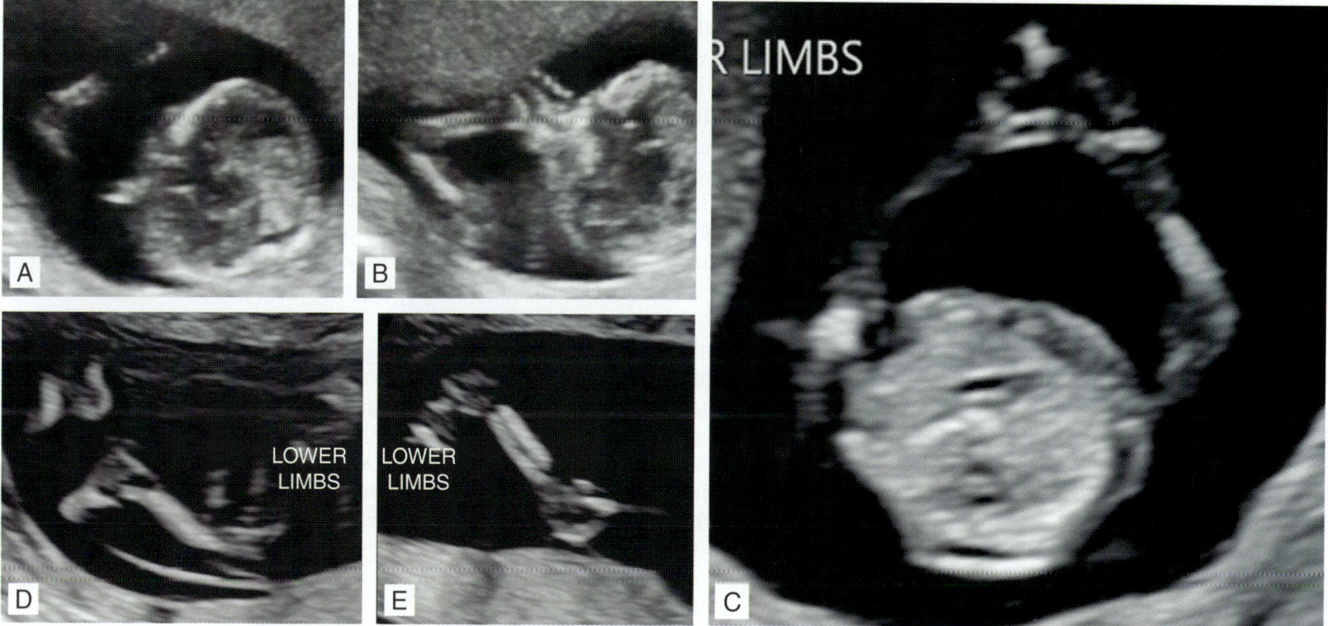

Figure 47.43 Normal fetal limbs. B-mode USG images showing sagittal (A, B, D, and E) and transverse (C) sections of a fetus in the first trimester. A and B show all the three segments of the left and right upper extremities while D and E depict the three segments of the left and right lower extremities. C axial scan shows both the upper limbs emphasizing the importance of documenting fetal limbs bilaterally.

combination of maternal history, maternal serum Papp-A and placental growth factor (PlGF), maternal mean arterial pressure (MAP), and mean uterine artery pulsatility index (PI) at 11–13 weeks of gestation can successfully disclose a significant proportion of high-risk pregnancies. Low serum Papp-A is often associated with impaired placentation, and hence is a good predictor of PE [31]. PlGF, which is synthesized by villous and extravillous cytotrophoblast, is a pro-angiogenesis agent. Its levels are often reduced preceding the development of PE [30], making its estimation important for the detection of PE. Regular monitoring of maternal blood pressure as a part of antenatal care similarly helps to catch PE early on [30]. MAP should be measured by automated devices, while a patient is in a sitting position, with her back supported and legs uncrossed. The average value of four such measurements should then be considered for analysis [32]. Uterine artery Doppler provides a noninvasive method for the evaluation of uteroplacental circulation. The addition of increased mean PI of the right and left uterine arteries as a risk of PE to maternal serum screening improves the overall detection rate of PE [30].

Suggested Readings

- SK Rodgers, C Chang, JT DeBardeleben, MM Horrow, Normal and abnormal US findings in early first-trimester pregnancy: review of the society of radiologists in ultrasound 2012 consensus panel recommendations, Radiographics 35 (7) (2015) 2135–2148.
- R Lee, C Dupuis, B Chen, A Smith, YH Kim, Diagnosing ectopic pregnancy in the emergency setting, Ultrasonography 37 (1) (2018) 78.
- PM Doubilet, CB Benson, T Bourne, M Blaivas, Diagnostic criteria for nonviable pregnancy early in the first trimester, N Engl J Med 369 (15) (2013) 1443–1451.
- EP Lin, S Bhatt, VS Dogra, Diagnostic clues to ectopic pregnancy, Radiographics 28 (6) (2008) 1661–1671.
- BR Murthy, Imaging of Fetal Brain and Spine: An Atlas and Guide, Springer, 2019.

48

Obstetrics: Second Trimester

NITIN CHAUBAL, RAJAS CHAUBAL, AVINASH BANSAL

Introduction

The second trimester sonography is a very important scan in several aspects [1]. Besides screening for anomalies, this period also provides an opportunity to establish gestational age, if not done earlier and look at early growth related problems. Evaluation of amount of liquor, placental morphology, and cervix can be easily done during this period. Uterine artery Doppler can be added to predict risk of pre-eclampsia.

Major congenital anomalies have a significant effect on the life expectancy of a fetus and occur in 2–3% of all live births and 20–30% of stillbirths [2,3]. Congenital disabilities are also emerging as the most common cause of neonatal mortality [4]. The principal objectives of prenatal diagnosis are to provide in-depth and proactive information to pregnant women and healthcare providers to make informed decisions [5].

Ultrasonography (USG) is the cornerstone for detecting congenital anomalies. The steady evolution of machines, transducers, and research has helped USG to remain the preferred technique for visualizing embryonic and early fetal anatomy. Mid-trimester USG imaging (18–24 weeks) forms a crucial part of every pregnancy.

The incidence of detection of congenital anomalies varies between 16% and 85%. Hence, following a stepwise approach to imaging and prescribed guidelines for mid-trimester scan is essential.

It is suggested that ultrasonography performed between the 22nd and 24th weeks of pregnancy can detect majority of congenital anomalies, as structurally complex organs such as the fetal heart and components of the central nervous system can be examined with sufficient clarity to allow the detection of significant developmental abnormalities [6]. Worldwide, routine mid-trimester ultrasonography is often performed between 18th and 22nd weeks of gestation [7,8]. *In countries where pregnancy termination by law is restricted by gestational age, optimal timing of a scan is established, considering the time needed for counseling, additional investigation, and necessary intervention within the legal time frame.*

For assessing the biometric parameters and detecting congenital malformations, it is necessary to follow a systematic approach. For this purpose, one of the most frequently used guidelines is the ISUOG (International Society of Ultrasonography in Obstetrics and Gynecology) guidelines.

Ultrasonography Techniques and General Considerations

The three critical components of the second-trimester scan are:
- Detailed evaluation of fetal anatomy
- Fetal biometry
- Fetal environment

The sonographic parameters that can be used to estimate gestational age and fetal size assessment are given in Table 48.1 [9].

Estimated Fetal Weight

Hadlock et al. [11] presented the most commonly used mathematical formula for deriving the estimated fetal weight (EFW) using the four biometric parameters described in Table 48.1. The second-trimester scan provides a more accurate EFW than the third trimester. However, EFW is clinically relevant in the third trimester when it can provide vital information to detect fetal growth restriction or macrosomia [12]. The obtained EFW is compared with the general population reference fetal weight percentile chart by week using the gestational age obtained from an earlier scan.

Amniotic Fluid Assessment

Amniotic fluid volume is assessed subjectively or using a quantitative measurement such as the deepest vertical pocket or amniotic fluid index, although the single pocket is most relevant at this stage [13]. Deviation from the typical values should warrant a detailed anatomical assessment and a follow-up examination.

Fetal Movements

Normal fetuses show relaxed and regular movements, without any specific pattern at this stage of pregnancy. Abnormal positioning and unusually restricted or absent fetal movements should be monitored.

Anatomical Survey

The minimum requisites as per ISUOG guidelines 2011 for performing a primary fetal anatomical survey during the mid-trimester of pregnancy are compiled in Table 48.2.

Skull

- Four aspects of the fetal skull should be evaluated: size, shape, integrity, and bone density

Brain

- Two axial planes, the transventricular plane and the transthalamic plane (Fig. 48.1A) allow imaging of cerebral structures to assess the anatomical integrity of the brain
- Axial transcerebellar plane (Fig. 48.1B) imaging enables the examiner to evaluate structures in the posterior cranial fossa

TABLE 48.1 Sonographic Parameters for the Estimation of Gestational Age and Fetal Size [7,10]

Biometry	Anatomical Considerations While Scanning (Sonographic Landmarks)	Caliper Placements	Diagram
1. Biparietal diameter (BPD)	▪ Cross-sectional view of the fetal head at the level of thalami ▪ The ideal angle of insonation should be 90 degrees to the midline echoes ▪ The symmetrical appearance of both hemispheres ▪ Continuous midline echo (falx cerebri) broken in the middle by the cavum septum pellucidum and thalamus ▪ No cerebellum visualized	From the outer edge to the outer edge. (Comment: Cephalic index—Ratio of maximum head width to maximum length. This can be used to characterize head shape.)	
2. Head circumference (HC)	Similar to the biparietal diameter	**Method 1:** Place the ellipse around the skull bone echoes. **Method 2:** When the ellipse option is not available, occipitofrontal diameter can be measured by placing the calipers in the middle of the bone echo at occipital and frontal skull bones. Head circumference can be calculated using the following formula: HC = 1.62 × (BPD + OFD).	
3. Abdominal circumference (AC)	▪ Transverse section of the fetal abdomen ▪ Umbilical vein at the level of portal sinus ▪ Stomach bubble visualized ▪ Kidneys should not be visible	Measured at the outer surface of the skin line, either directly with ellipse calipers or calculated from linear measurements perpendicular to each other, namely anteroposterior abdominal diameter (APAD) and transverse abdominal diameter (TAD). Abdominal circumference = 1.57 × (APAD + TAD).	
4. Femur diaphysis length (FL)	▪ Both ends of ossified metaphysis should be imaged ▪ The longest axis of the ossified diaphysis is measured ▪ The angle of insonation between 45 and 90 degrees is ideal	At each end of the ossified diaphysis. It should exclude triangular spur artifacts that can falsely extend the diaphysis length.	

Face

- Midsagittal view for a facial profile (Fig. 48.2A), orbits and lens, hard palate, premaxillary triangle (Fig. 48.2B), and nose and lips (Fig. 48.2C) should be evaluated

Neck

- Cylindrical structure with no masses, protuberances, or fluid collections is normal ultrasonography findings; any deviation from these should be evaluated carefully

Thorax

- Ribs should have a normal curvature without deformities
- The shape of the thorax should be regular, with a smooth transition to the abdomen
- Both lungs should appear homogeneous and without any evidence of mediastinal shift or masses
- The diaphragm is seen as a hypoechoic line between thoracic and abdominal contents

Heart

An essential examination of the heart should include an evaluation of the four chamber heart and 3 vessel view. A detailed description of cardiac imaging is addressed in the "Fetal Echocardiography" chapter. The following features should be noted while performing the second-trimester scan:

- The heart should be located in the left side of the chest
- The heart should not occupy more than one-third of the area of the chest
- The normal axis of the heart (45° ± 20° (±2 SD))
- Four-chamber view of the fetal heart to assess size and morphology of chambers
- No pericardial effusion

TABLE 48.2 Recommended Checklist for Basic Mid-Trimester Fetal Anatomical Survey

Organs/Systems	Particulars to be Emphasized Upon While Performing USG
Head	■ Intact cranium ■ Cavum septi pellucidi ■ Midline falx ■ Thalami ■ Cerebral ventricles ■ Cerebellum ■ Cisterna magna
Face	■ Both orbits present ■ Median facial profile (optional) ■ Mouth present ■ Upper lip intact
Neck	■ Absence of masses (e.g., cystic hygroma)
Chest/heart	■ Normal-appearing shape/size of chest and lungs ■ Heart activity present ■ Four-chamber and 3 vessel views of the heart in normal position ■ Aortic and pulmonary outflow tracts (optional) ■ No evidence of diaphragmatic hernia
Abdomen	■ Stomach in normal position ■ Bowel not dilated ■ Both kidneys present ■ Cord insertion site
Skeletal	■ No spinal defects or masses (transverse and sagittal views) ■ Arms and hands present, normal relations ■ Legs and feet present normal relations
Placenta	■ Position ■ No masses present ■ Accessory lobe
Umbilical cord	■ Three-vessel cord (optional)
Genitalia	■ Gender determination as per local laws

- Heart rate (normal range 120–160 beats/min)
- Three-vessel view and three-vessel trachea view to assess the great vessels
- Visualization of the aortic and pulmonary outflow tracts to detect major cardiac malformations
- Great vessels are typically near identical and should cross each other immediately after leaving the respective ventricular chamber [14]

Abdomen

- Identification of the stomach bubble
- The abdominal situs should be determined, and anomalies recognized if present [15]
- The bowel should be contained within the abdominal wall
- The cord should be inserted into the intact abdominal wall
- Cystic lesions in the abdomen should be examined
- Bowel dilatation should be looked for

Kidneys and Bladder

- The fetal bladder and both kidneys should be identified
- If either bladder or renal pelvis appears enlarged, it should be documented
- Filling and emptying of the urinary bladder should be documented

Spine

- It should be imaged in two planes; sagittal (Fig. 48.3A) and axial (Fig. 48.3B), at all levels of the spine
- The sacral tip should be imaged
- The contour of the spine should be checked

Limbs and Extremities

- All three segments of all four limbs should be imaged
- Observe flexion and extension movements
- Counting fingers or toes are not a part of a routine mid-trimester scan but should be conducted when there is suspicion of a syndrome or an anomaly

Placenta

- The location and relation to internal os should be documented

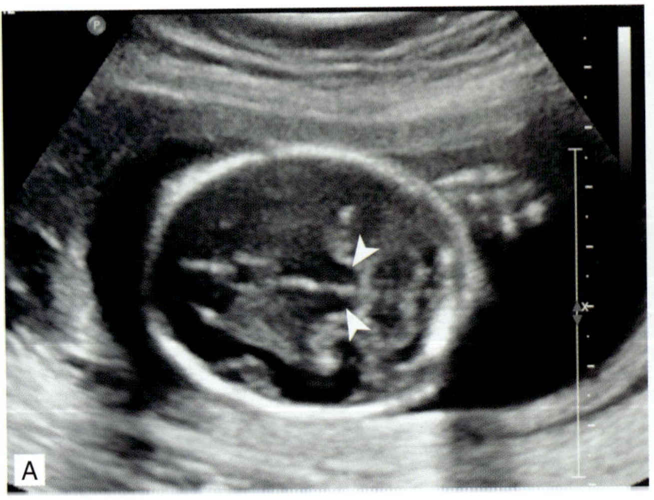

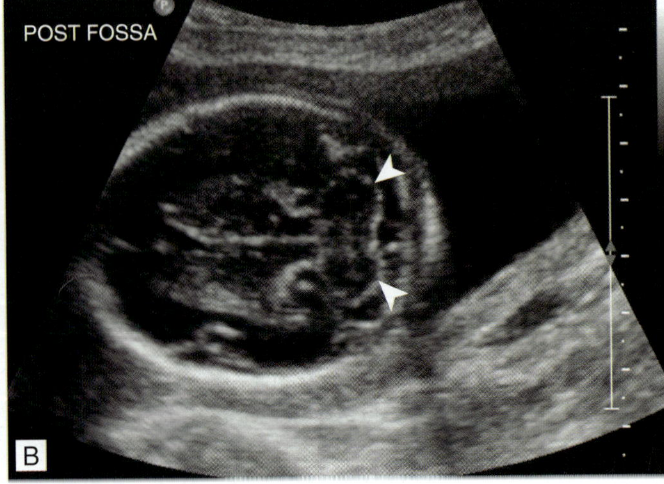

Figure 48.1 (A) Transthalamic view showing the thalami (*white arrowheads*). (B) Transcerebellar view showing the cerebellar hemispheres (*white arrowheads*).

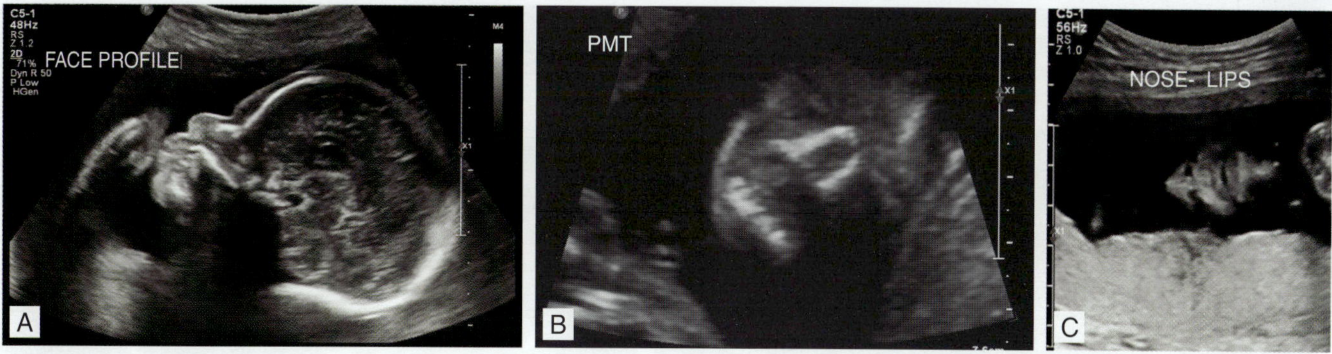

Figure 48.2 (A) Midsagittal view of the face profile with nasal bone. (B) Coronal view of the face demonstrating pre maxillary triangle. (C) Coronal view of the face demonstrating nose and lips.

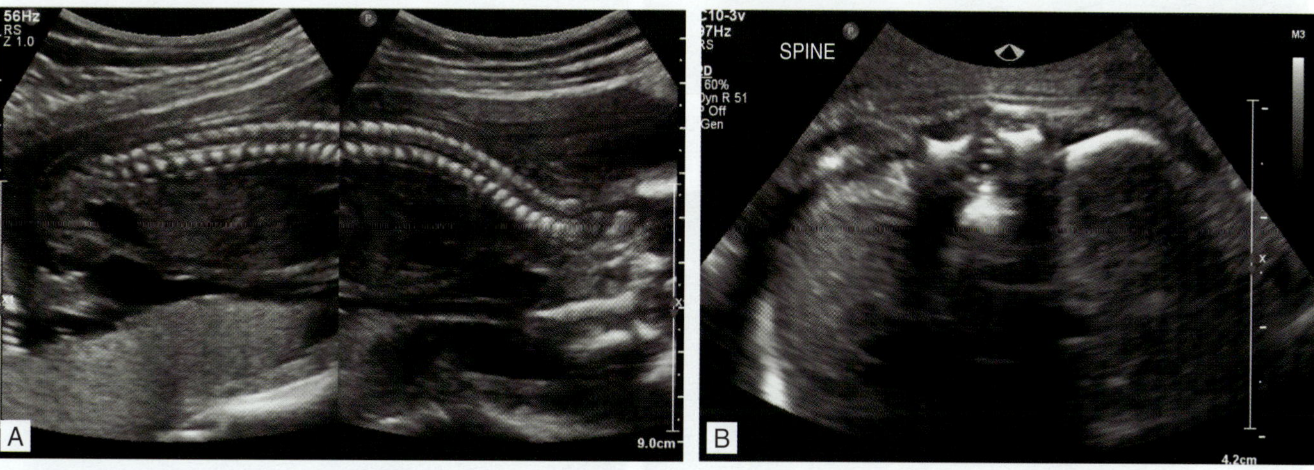

Figure 48.3 (A) Sagittal view of the spine. (B) Transverse view of the spine.

- Women with a history of uterine surgery and low anterior placenta or placenta praevia are at risk of placental attachment disorders
- The placenta should be examined for the following features:
  - Presence of multiple irregular placental lacunae that show arterial or mixed flow
  - Abnormal appearance of the uterine wall and bladder wall interface

Maternal Cervix, Uterine Anomalies, Adnexal Masses, and Uterine Artery Doppler

- A transvaginal scan of the cervix helps to predict preterm birth
- Uterine fibroids and adnexal masses should be documented
- Uterine artery Doppler—a pulsatility index of more than 1.35 can be indicative of a potential risk of the female developing preeclampsia in the later part of pregnancy

Central Nervous System Anomalies

Midline Defects

Corpus Callosum Dysgenesis/Agenesis

Various conditions, including chromosomal and metabolic disorders, as well as intrauterine exposure to teratogens and infection that disrupt early cerebral development, can cause corpus callosum developmental anomalies in their spectrum of manifestations. Corpus callosum agenesis affects approximately 1.4 per 10,000 live births [16]. The most extreme form of developmental malformation of the corpus callosum is agenesis (agenesis of the corpus callosum). Partial agenesis of the corpus is also referred to as dysgenesis and typically involves the posterior portion of the corpus callosum [17].

Diagnosis: Embryological development of the corpus callosum progresses from the anterior to the posterior direction and the last part of development is the rostrum. Although the corpus callosum is visualized in the midsagittal view by 18 weeks of gestation, it is best visualized at about 22 weeks.

Direct features: The midsagittal view is essential for the diagnosis of the corpus callosum agenesis/dysgenesis (Fig. 48.4A). The corpus callosum can also be visualized in the coronal section. The diagnosis is more difficult in the cases of partial agenesis, where the findings tend to be subtle. In the cases of partial agenesis, the corpus callosum appears shorter than average and does not arch over the third ventricle [18].

Indirect features: Obtaining the midsagittal views in all cases may be difficult, and the ultrasonologist may have to rely on the indirect signs for ascertaining the diagnosis. This includes the following:

- Axial view demonstrating the absent septum cavum pellucidum (Fig. 48.5A)
- Axial view showing dilatation of the occipital horns of the lateral ventricles (colpocephaly/teardrop shape) (Fig. 48.5B)
- Alteration in the course of the pericallosal artery seen in the sagittal view (Fig. 48.4B)
- Separation of the frontal horns (comma shape) is appreciated in the coronal view

Prognosis: Up to 11% of the children develop severe mental retardation and neurological abnormalities.

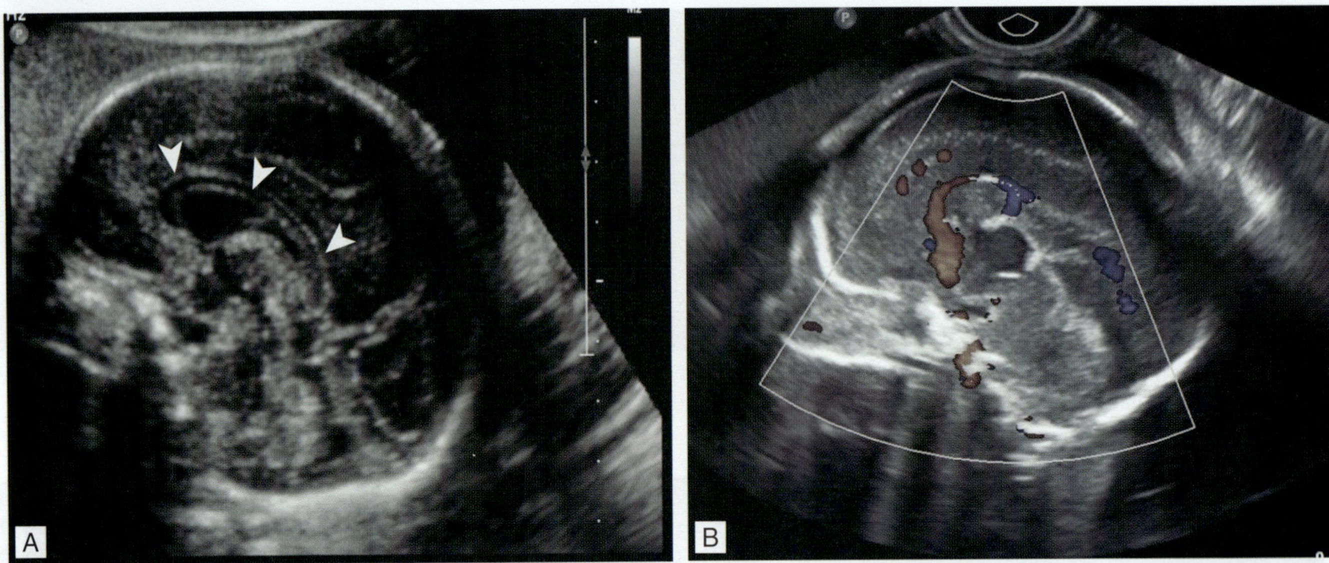

Figure 48.4 (A) Normal corpus callosum—Midline sagittal view showing a normal corpus callosum (*white arrowheads*). (B) Corpus callosum agenesis—Midline sagittal view shows absent corpus callosum with aberrant course of pericallosal artery.

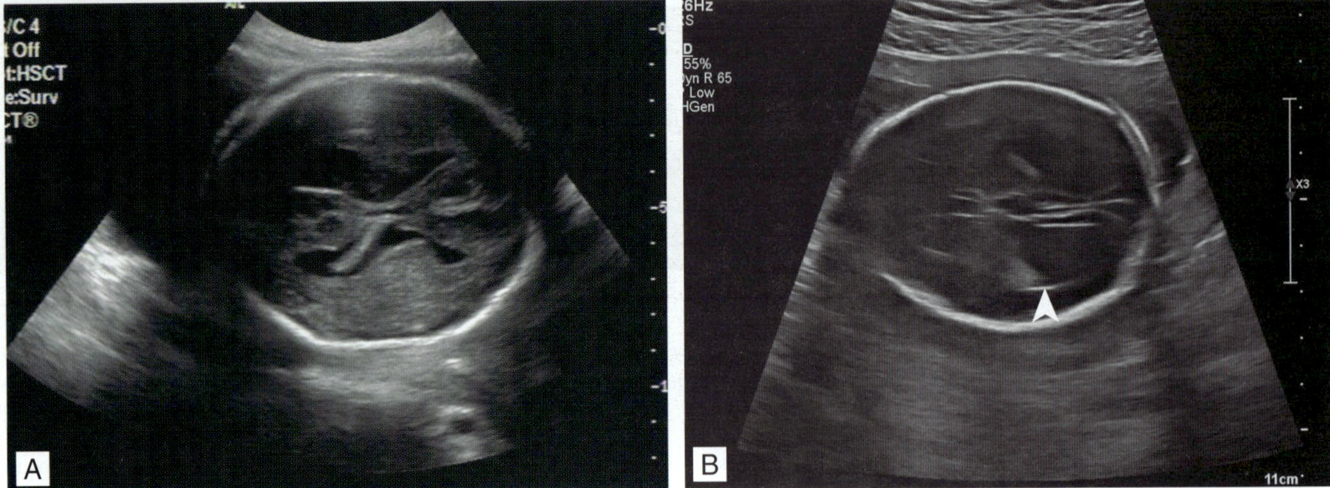

Figure 48.5 (A) Axial view demonstrating the absence of septum cavum pellucidum. (B) Axial view showing dilatation of the occipital horn in the case of corpus callosum agenesis (*white arrowhead*).

This can be associated with Trisomy 13, Trisomy 18, Aicardi syndrome, Apert syndrome, Fryns syndrome, and Gorlin syndrome. Other commonly seen CNS malformations are Chiari II malformation, Dandy–Walker malformation, interhemispheric cysts, intracranial lipoma, holoprosencephaly, polymicrogyria, gray matter heterotopia, septo-optic dysplasia, and schizencephaly [19].

Dandy–Walker Malformation

The classical Dandy–Walker malformation includes a cystic dilatation of the posterior fossa, agenesis of the cerebellar vermis, and upward displacement of the trocula/tentorium [19]. Theories suggest that it is a more global developmental defect affecting the roof of the rhombencephalon leading to the vermian hypoplasia to a varying extent and variable fenestration of the fourth ventricular outlet foramina [20]. The use of the term Dandy–Walker variant has been superseded by the term Vermian agenesis or hypoplasia [21].

The incidence of Dandy–Walker malformation is approximately 1 in 30,000 [22]. Most cases tend to be isolated; however, there is a chance of recurrence of about 1–5%.

Ultrasonography Diagnosis: USG can help identify approximately 90% of the cases antenatally. The midsagittal plane is the most important for the diagnosis. Although the cerebellar vermis can be seen as early as the 17th week, one needs to be cautious before making a diagnosis before the 20th week [23].

Features seen on USG:

- Grossly enlarged fourth ventricle communicating with cisterna magna. (Fig. 48.6A)
- Hypoplastic or absent vermis
- Elevation of the tentorium (Fig. 48.6B)
- Occasional hydrocephalus

Associations: Dandy–Walker malformation has a 75% probability of association with other neural anomalies, including corpus callosum agenesis, holoprosencephaly, and other midline anomalies. It is also associated with chromosomal aberrations such as Trisomy 13, 18, and Turner syndrome in up to 30% of the cases. Additional associations include syndromes like Walker–Warburg, Meckel–Gruber, and Acardi syndrome [24].

Prognosis: With a 24% mortality rate the prognosis for the Dandy–Walker malformation is poor, especially when associated

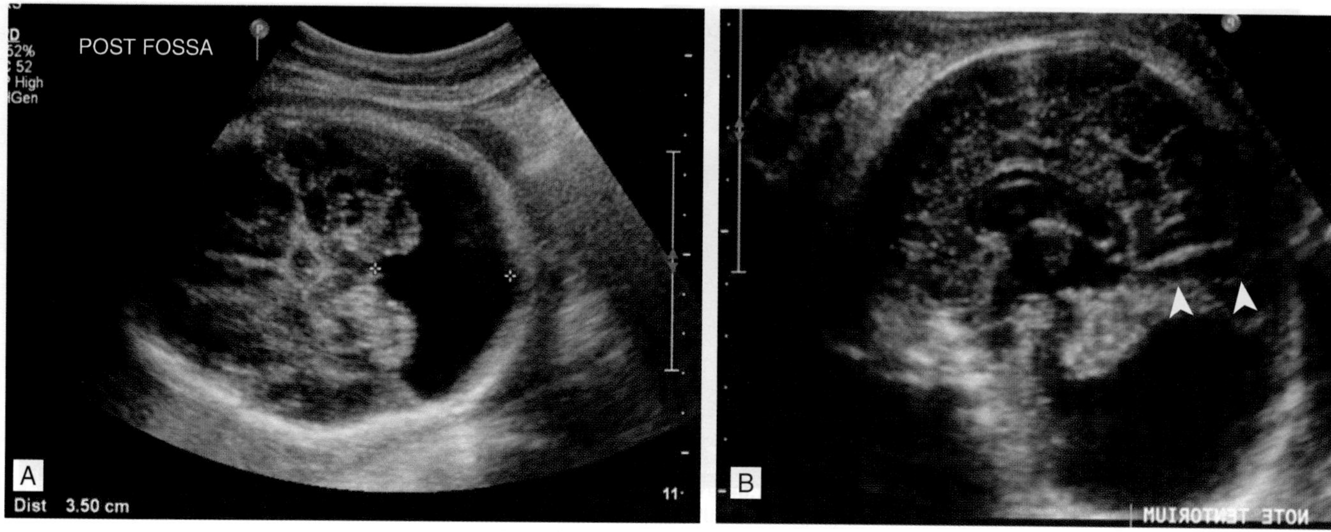

Figure 48.6 (A) Dandy–Walker malformation—Axial view demonstrating large cyst in the posterior fossa and hypoplastic vermis. (B) Dandy–Walker malformation—Sagittal view shows elevation of tentorium (*white arrowheads*).

with other anomalies. The prognosis is less severe if isolated. The differential diagnosis includes megacisterna magna, Blake's pouch cyst and vermian hypoplasia.

Choroid Plexus Cyst

The cystic structure in the choroid plexus of lateral ventricles is formed by infolding of the neuroepithelium. The incidence rate is ~2% of pregnancies at 20 weeks of gestation. They generally resolve between the 26th and 28th weeks [25].

Ultrasonography Findings

- Single or multiple cystic areas in one or both choroid plexuses of lateral ventricles (at the level of atrium) (Fig. 48.7)

Associated Abnormalities: Choroid plexus cyst is a soft marker of aneuploidy and if seen as an isolated finding, is not significant. A screening test to rule out Trisomy 18 can be carried out.

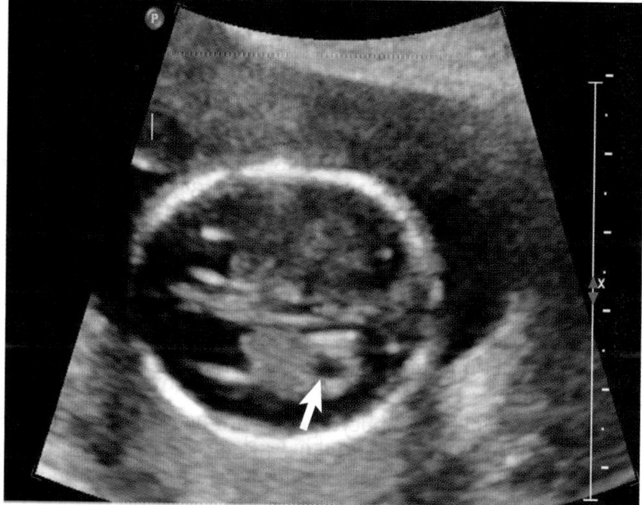

Figure 48.7 Choroid plexus cyst—Cystic area within the choroid plexus (*white arrow*).

Arachnoid Cysts

Arachnoid cysts are extra axial cysts with regular walls, filled with cerebrospinal fluid and are usually not connected to the subarachnoid space. They represent about 1% of all intracranial masses [26].

Ultrasonography Findings

- The cysts usually are unilocular, an avascular structure that does not communicate with the ventricular system
- 50–60% are found in the middle cranial fossa
- 10% of the cases are seen in the posterior fossa
- Arachnoid cysts tend to be variable in size, and their shape is adapted to surrounding structures

Associated Anomalies, Follow-Up, and Prognosis: Arachnoid cysts are usually found isolated. Follow-up should be done every 4 weeks to monitor the size of the cyst and progression toward secondary hydrocephalus (when the large cyst blocks foramen of Monro or aqueduct of Sylvius). When the cyst is large and symptomatic, surgery may be required to prevent long-term neurological sequelae [27]. There is no recurrence risk associated with arachnoid cysts.

Ventriculomegaly

Mild ventriculomegaly is seen in 1% of fetuses. The incidence of severe VM is about 1:1000 new-borns [28].

Ultrasonography Findings

- Dilatation of lateral ventricle measuring ≥10 mm in axial trans ventricular plane at the level of parieto-occipital fissure
- A measurement of 10–12 mm is commonly referred to as mild ventriculomegaly, whereas measurement of 12–15 mm and above 15 mm are defined as moderate and severe ventriculomegaly respectively. (Fig. 48.8) [29,30]

Associated Anomalies: Ventriculomegaly may be isolated or associated with other abnormalities such as infections, chromosomal aberrations, genetic syndromes, and other congenital anomalies (such as Dandy–Walker malformation, agenesis of corpus callosum, Chiari II malformation) [31].

Follow-Up: Follow-up should be conducted every 4 weeks to reassess whether they are static, progressed, or regressed in size. The following investigations should be done for every case of ventriculomegaly:

- Detailed neurosonography
- TORCH testing for fetal infections
- Direct/invasive testing such as amniocentesis to rule out underlying chromosomal/genetic disorders
- Maternal blood testing for antiplatelet antibodies (in cases of a brain hemorrhage)

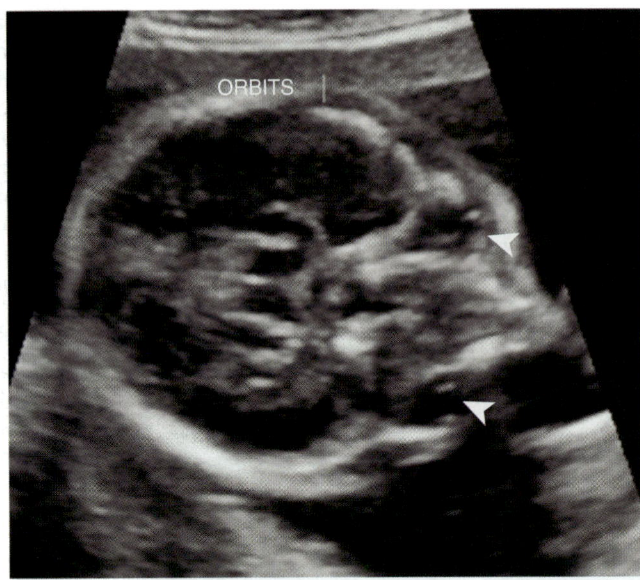

Figure 48.16 Microopthalmia—Axial view showing the presence of small orbits (*white arrowheads*).

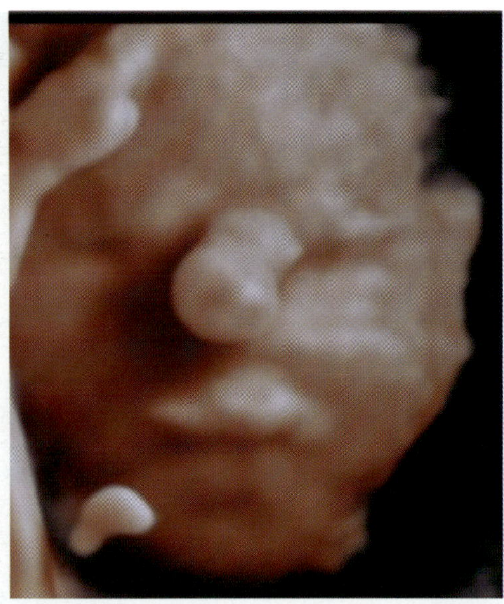

Figure 48.17 3D image of the face showing Cyclops.

The Jaw index is measured to define the small size of the mandible. A value less than 21 has nearly 100% specificity and positive predictive value for micrognathia [46].

Anophthalmia/Microphthalmia

This is characterized by a complete absence or severe hypoplasia of one or both bony orbits and eye bulbs. It is often associated with chromosomal and nonchromosomal syndromes. It can also be a result of an infection or exposure to a teratogen.

Ultrasonography Diagnosis: In anophthalmia and severe microphthalmia, an axial view at the level of the orbits shows a hypoplastic bony orbital cavity with absent or extremely small ocular globe (Fig. 48.16). In mild and moderate cases of microphthalmia, diagnosis is established using normogram for the given gestational age. They are often associated with aphakia or cataract.

Hypertelorism

Hypertelorism is the increased interocular distance (>95th percentile). It can be a developmental defect due to partial arrest of the migration process of orbits from lateral to medial. It can also be secondary to any space occupying lesion in the midline, such as the anterior cephalocele.

Ultrasonography Diagnosis: On the axial view at the level of the orbits, the increased distance between two orbits is defined by an increased binocular and interocular distance (>95 percentile for the gestational age).

Hypotelorism and Cyclopia

Hypotelorism is the decreased interocular distance (<5th percentile). It is almost always associated with the migrational defects and holoprosencephaly.

Ultrasonography Diagnosis: On the axial view, at the level of orbits, severe cases of hypotelorism are straightforward with very closely placed orbits. Mild and moderate cases are diagnosed by decreased binocular and interocular distance (<5th percentile for the gestational age). Cyclopia typically presents with a median single eye or a partially divided eye in a single orbit, absent nose, and a proboscis above the eye (Fig. 48.17).

Proboscis

A proboscis is a trunk like appendage with either one or two internal openings, usually associated with the absence of a nose. A single midline appendix of soft tissues (can have a bony skeleton as well) departing from the nasal root area is seen with the midsagittal plane of the fetal profile.

Chest

Congenital Diaphragmatic Hernia

Congenital diaphragmatic hernia (CDH) is a result of increased intra-abdominal pressure and the presence of a diaphragmatic defect. CDH is classified into three categories based on the site of the defect [47]:

- 85% involve the left posterolateral area (Bochdalek type)
- 10% of the cases involve the right hemidiaphragm
- 5% of the cases are bilateral

CDH can be considered as an "evolving" lesion, which results in prenatal diagnosis of only 50–60% of CDHs.

The incidence rate for CDH is 1 in 4000 births [48].

Ultrasonography Findings

- **Indirect signs**: These include abnormal intrathoracic position of the stomach and/or the other migrated viscera and the displacement of the heart and the mediastinum. This can be observed on the four-chamber view
- **Left posterolateral CDH**: On the four-chamber view, the stomach is either found in the left hemithorax or in the mediastinal area (~90%) (Fig. 48.18). A few ileal loops can be found near the stomach, while the heart and the mediastinum are displaced contralaterally. On rare occasions, the spleen and/or the left liver lobe may migrate as well
- Additional signs that may confirm the existence of the hernia are as follows:
    - Tortuous appearance of inferior vena cava
    - Absence of the hypoechoic contour of the diaphragm
    - Paradoxical movement of diaphragm
    - Upturned superior mesenteric artery

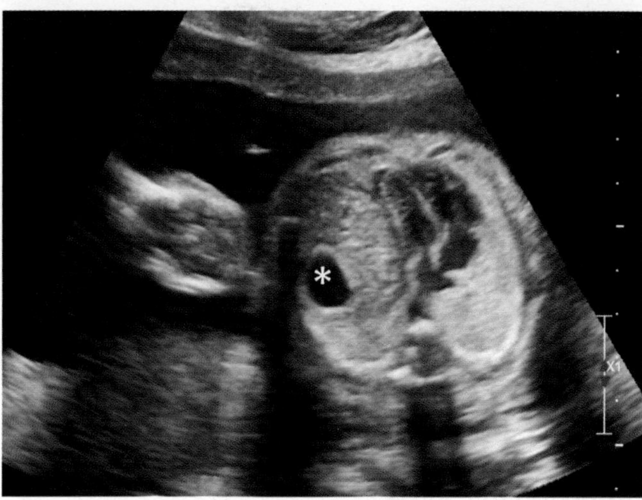

Figure 48.18 Left-sided congenital diaphragmatic hernia—Stomach (*asterisk*) is seen within the thorax with shift of mediastinum to the right.

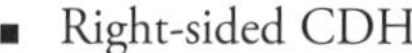

- Right-sided CDH
  - Extreme leftward rotation of the heart, because of abnormal increase in the cardiac axis
  - Upward displacement of the right hepatic lobe
  - Hepatic vessels in the thorax

In most cases, polyhydramnios at ≥26 weeks is thought to be either due to esophageal compression, kinking of the stomach or reduced absorption of fluid by the hypoplastic lungs.

Follow-Up and Prognosis

USG scans should be done every 4 weeks to monitor lung growth and amniotic fluid volume. Amniodrainage may be necessary if there is polyhydramnios and cervical shortening. The risk of fetal death is about 5%. Long-term compression of the lungs results in pulmonary damage, involving alveolar hypoplasia. The association of pulmonary hypoplasia with pulmonary hypertension represents the main determinant of death in neonates with nonsyndromic CDH.

Prognosis is very poor if it is associated with aneuploidy or nonchromosomal syndromes. For left-sided CDH, survival rates range between 30% and 80%. The quality of life is generally good, once the primary closure of the defect has been achieved.

Lung-to-head ratio (LHR) can be estimated on antenatal scans and is calculated as the observed LHR/expected LHR (O/E LHR). LHR is calculated by multiplying the two orthogonal diameters of the right lung, located between the rib cage and the heart in the right hemithorax, and dividing the result by the head circumference. The LHR value indicates the survival rate:

- LHR ≤1, Poor prognosis (despite ECMO)
- LHR >1.4, Improved prognosis

  LHR between 1 and 1.4 were associated with 38% survival and in the majority of cases required ECMO [49].

Antenatal cases diagnosed before 24 weeks have worse prognosis with mortality as high as 60–80% due to pulmonary hypoplasia. Another poor prognostic indicator that has recently been reported in the literature, is a formerly increased nuchal translucency (NT) [50].

Recurrence Risk

- Isolated: No increased risk
- Part of trisomy's: 1% risk
- Part of syndromes: 25% risk

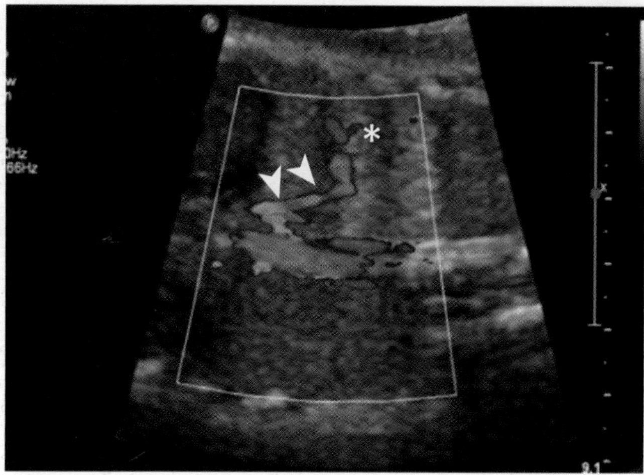

Figure 48.19 Bronchopulmonary sequestration—Presence of an echogenic area in the lung (*asterisk*) with a feeding vessel arising from the aorta (*white arrowheads*).

Bronchopulmonary Sequestration

Pulmonary sequestration (PS) consists of a segment of the lung parenchyma that does not communicate with the bronchial tree and is supplied by the systemic circulation. There are two types of sequestration: *intralobar and extralobar.* The extralobar variant is further subdivided into a supradiaphragmatic (90%) and subdiaphragmatic subtype (10%). The lesion is unilateral and involves the left lower lobe in 90% of the cases. In general, PS shows a roughly triangular shape, with the apex pointing toward the mediastinum. Typically, extralobar sequestrations present a feeding artery branching off from the descending thoracic or abdominal aorta.

The exact etiology of PS is unknown, although it has been suggested that it might share the same pathogenesis as CPAM. The two lesions are frequently associated. The incidence of PS is 1 in 15,000 births [51].

Ultrasonography Findings

- **Four-chamber view**: A well-defined homogeneously hyperechoic, roughly triangular mass, often involving the lower part of the left lung is observed
- **Sagittal views**
  - Caudal extension of mass is visible
  - Detection and characterization of subdiaphragmatic extralobar sequestrations
  - Recognition of the feeding artery branching off the descending aorta, on power or color Doppler (Fig. 48.19)

Differential Diagnosis

- **Solid microcystic variant of CPAM:** PS lesions are described in the D/D section

Follow-Up and Prognosis

USG scans should be done every 4 weeks to monitor growth of the sequestration and hydrothorax or hydrops. In >30% of the cases there is regression or disappearance during the third trimester.

Presence of hydrops is a poor prognostic indicator. The survival rate of prenatally detected cases is very high (>95%). Active prenatal management (by drainage and thoracoamniotic shunt placement) of cases associated with hydrops contributes significantly to the extremely good survival rates.

Postnatal Therapy

The sequestrated lung can be removed by endoscopic surgery or selective embolization of the feeding artery may also be done.

Congenital Pulmonary Airway Malformation

Congenital pulmonary airway malformation (CPAM) is a developmental anomaly of the lung characterized by a mass of disordered pulmonary parenchyma with proliferation of terminal respiratory bronchioles and a lack of normal alveoli, thought to represent a hamartomatous lesions. It is unilateral in 97% of the cases.

Histologically, classification depending on the size of cysts is as follows:

- Type I: Large cysts (2–10 cm)
- Type II: Small cysts (0.5–2 cm)
- Type III: Solid or microcystic (<0.5 cm)

The etiology of CPAM is unknown. This lesion represents a developmental anomaly. CPAM is found to be associated with pulmonary sequestration or segmentary bronchial atresia. The incidence of CPAM is 1 in 4000 births [51].

Ultrasonography Findings

Hyperechogenic tumor in the fetal chest, usually presenting at ≥16 weeks' gestation. It can be further divided into the following:

- Solid or microcystic,
- Macrocystic with one or more large cysts (>2 cm) (Fig. 48.20), and
- Mixed with areas that are solid intermixed with areas containing multiple cysts <2 cm in diameter.

The lesion usually involves one lobe or segment of the lung. Hydrops is found in <10% of the cases. Polyhydramnios, due to a compressed and obstructed esophagus, may present at ≥26 week's gestation.

CPAM is frequently seen with PS. Other pulmonary or thoracic anomalies, such as CDH, duplication cysts, tracheoesophageal fistulas, and pulmonary artery branching abnormalities.

Follow-Up and Prognosis

USG scans should be done every 4 weeks to monitor growth of lung lesion and amniotic fluid volume. During the early third trimester >80% of the microcystic lesions resolve, but in >80% of these cases this is not a true resolution but purely an inability to detect the lesion by USG as the normal lungs also become echogenic. The lesion can only be detected postnatally by the CT scan.

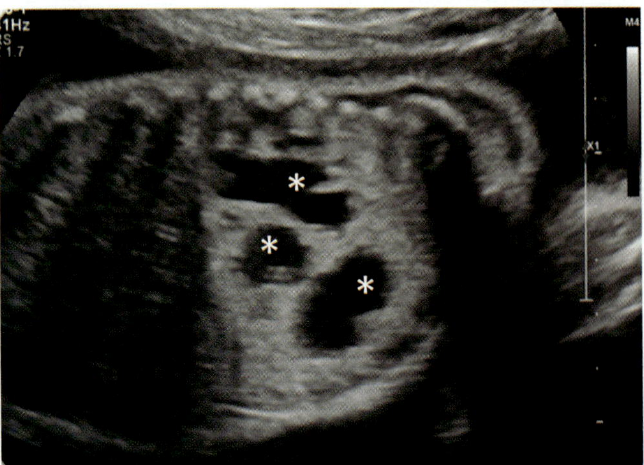

Figure 48.20 Congenital pulmonary airway malformation—Lung is echogenic with macrocystic changes (*asterisk*).

CPAM is an evolving lesion and displays rapid growth between 20 and 26 weeks of gestation, after which the volume of the mass plateaus. If there is no hydrops by 26 weeks, then it is highly unlikely that this will develop afterward. About 10–20% of the cases regress almost completely during the third trimester of pregnancy.

CAM volume ratio (CVR) is a good prognostic indicator. This parameter is calculated by dividing the volume of the CPAM lesion by the circumference of the head, just as with LHR in CDH. The incidence of hydrops is 75% for CVR >1.6 and 17% for CVR <1.7. Hydrops frequently results in perinatal demise and is more likely to occur if there is a dominant cyst. If there is no hydrops the chances of survival are >95%.

Bronchogenic Cysts

Bronchogenic cysts result from an anomalous development of the ventral foregut. They can occur along the whole tracheoesophageal course, but with a predilection for the area around the carina. These cysts form because of abnormal budding of the bronchial tree during embryogenesis (between fourth and sixth weeks).

Ultrasonography Findings

- Well-defined unilocular cystic lesions within the mediastinum or lung parenchyma
- Cystic in nature and adjacent to the mediastinum
- Usually, single
- No mediastinal shift, polyhydramnios, or fetal hydrops present
- Compression of the adjacent lung can give rise to pulmonary hypoplasia
- The cyst usually increases in size with advancing gestation
- Rarely, bronchogenic cysts appeared prenatally as hyperechoic lesions

USG scans should be done every 4 weeks to monitor the evolution of the lesion. Bronchogenic cysts may remain asymptomatic for years.

Congenital High Airway Obstruction Syndrome

Congenital high airway obstruction syndrome (CHAOS) is defined as a complete or partial obstruction of the fetal upper airways. CHAOS is usually caused by atresia or stenosis of the larynx or trachea. Laryngeal and tracheal atresias are not distinguishable on US and are detected based on the unmistakable intrathoracic signs.

Etiology and Pathogenesis

The most accepted theory is an impaired blood supply during embryogenesis, which prevents the development of the trachea/larynx during the 10th week of gestation. Obstruction in the tracheobronchial tree leads to accumulation of fetal lung fluid resulting in the increase of the intratracheal pressure leading to the enlargement of the lungs. This in turn causes compression of the heart and great veins. Due to the compression, the heart is located centrally and becomes small and dysfunctional. The decreased venous return and dysfunctional cardiovascular system ends in ascites and hydrops. The diaphragm flattens or inverts according to the severity of the process.

Other rare underlying causes of CHAOS are laryngeal agenesis, subglottic stenosis or atresia, and laryngeal webs or cysts.

Compression of the esophagus by dilated airways may lead to polyhydramnios, due to the disruption of fetal swallowing.

Ultrasonography Findings

- USG features become evident in ≥16 weeks of gestation
- Bilaterally enlarged hyperechoic lungs
- Dilated airways: Trachea appears as a small round sonolucent area behind the heart which is squeezed in between the lungs, and appears smaller due to the degree of pulmonary enlargement (Fig. 48.21A)
- On coronal view of the fetal thorax: Flattened or inverted diaphragms are the typical findings (Fig. 48.21B)
- Fetal ascites and nonimmune hydrops
- Compression of the esophagus by dilated airways may lead to polyhydramnios and cause disruption of fetal fluid swallowing

Follow-Up and Prognosis

If the pregnancy continues, serial scans should be carried out to define the best time for delivery based on the evolution of the hydrops. CHAOS is invariably a lethal condition and usually results in stillbirth or death shortly after delivery. In current clinical practice, an EXIT procedure (ex utero intrapartum treatment) can be offered to patients if CHAOS is diagnosed in the late second or third trimester and if severe hydrops has not occurred.

Gastrointestinal Tract

Esophagus

The normal esophagus is a collapsed structure that is not routinely imaged. It is possible to see the esophagus after 19 weeks, however this is not part of a routine sonography. The presence of a patent esophagus is indirectly confirmed by noting fluid in the fetal stomach.

Esophageal Atresia

Esophageal atresia (EA) occurs due to improper development of the mid portion of the esophagus. It is frequently associated with an abnormal communication with the trachea. The reported incidence rate is 2.4 per 10,000 pregnancies [52]. EA almost always leads to a disruption in the continuity of the esophagus and depending on whether there is a communication (tracheoesophageal fistula) between the proximal or distal esophageal pouches with the trachea, the EA is grossly classified into the following categories [53].

- Type A: EA with no fistula (7%)
- Type B: EA with proximal TEF (2%)
- Type C: EA with distal TEF (86%)
- Type D: EA with proximal and distal TEF (1%)
- Type E: TEF without concomitant EA (4%)

Ultrasonography Features

- Polyhydramnios
- Fetal stomach
  - **Failure to visualize a fluid-filled stomach:** The failure to refill in a 30-minute period is suggestive of some obstruction to swallowing. The combination of polyhydramnios and failure to visualize the fetal stomach is virtually diagnostic of EA
  - A **persistently small stomach is also suspicious for EA**
- **The most reliable predictor is the presence of** a blind ending pouch in the fetal neck or upper mediastinum called a "Pouch sign" (Fig. 48.22)

There are other causes of persistently small/absent stomachs, summarized in Table 48.3.

EA is associated with many chromosomal and nonchromosomal syndromes. The most common associations are [52] as follows:

- Chromosomal aneuploidy
  - Trisomy 18 (6%)
  - Down's syndrome (2%)
- Genetic syndromes
  - Coloboma, heart defect, choanal atresia, retarded growth and development, genital hypoplasia, ear anomalies (CHARGE) (1%)
  - Vertebral defects, anal atresia, cardiac defects, tracheoesophageal fistula, renal anomalies, and limb abnormalities (VACTERL) (10%)

Prognosis: Association with other major anomalies, which is a fairly common occurrence, represents the most important sign for poor prognosis. The frequent occurrence of a low birth weight, as a result of FGR, may render the outcome even more guarded. The

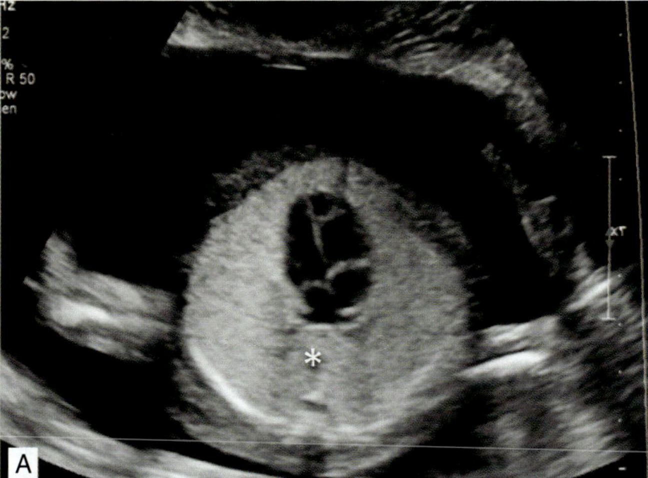

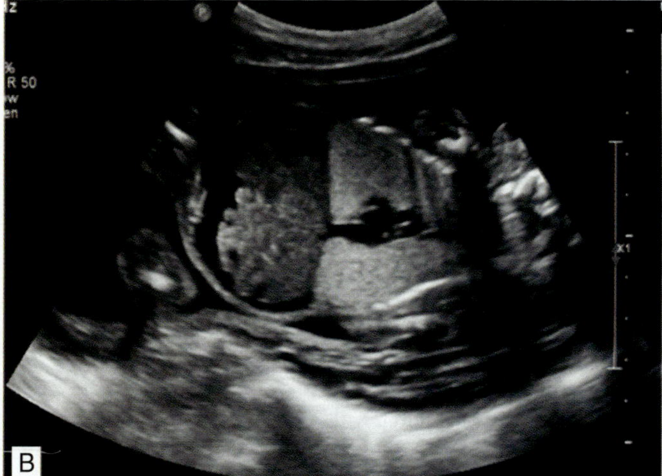

Figure 48.21 (A) Congenital high airway obstruction syndrome—Axial image with both lungs appearing hyperechoic with mid posed heart and trachea behind the heart (*asterisk*). (B) Congenital high airway obstruction syndrome—Coronal image of the same fetus showing hyperinflated thorax with an altered diaphragmatic contour.

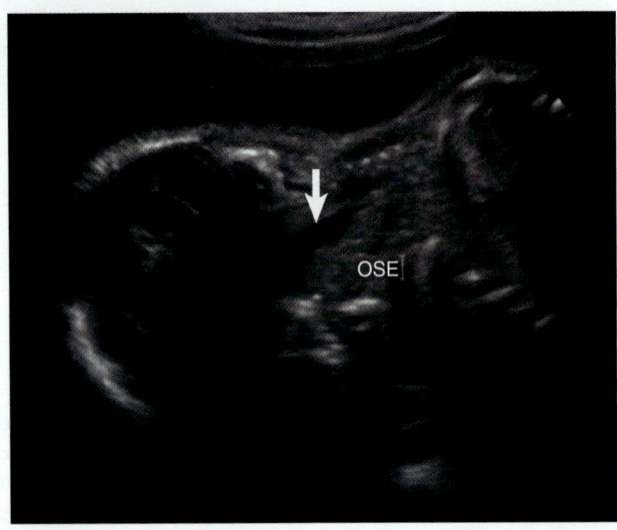

Figure 48.22 Pouch sign in esophageal atresia—presence of a blind ending pouch in the fetal neck (*arrow*). This is the most reliable sign of esophageal atresia.

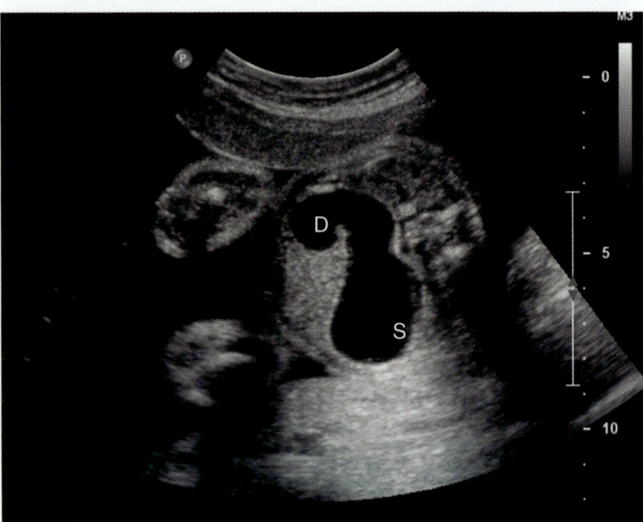

Figure 48.23 Double bubble sign in duodenal obstruction—enlarged stomach (ST) and duodenum (D); documentation of communication between two bubbles crossing midline is important to confirm the diagnosis.

TABLE 48.3 Pathological Causes for Persistently Small or Absent Stomach Bubble in the Fetus

Oligohydramnios due to any cause (e.g., preterm premature rupture of membranes, bilateral renal disease) that leads to less fluid to swallow resulting in inadequate filling of the stomach
Neuromuscular disorder which impairs active swallowing and is caused by conditions that are associated with hypokinesia and/or arthrogryposis
Abnormalities of the face or neck that can interfere with active swallowing such as micrognathia, facial cleft, neck masses (teratoma, large goiter)
Esophageal atresia with or without tracheoesophageal fistula

survival rate of the EA–TE fistula repair in a full term baby with no associated anomalies is about 95% [55].

Duodenal Atresia

In duodenal atresia, the tract between the proximal and distal portions of the duodenum is atretic. In up to 80% of the cases, the obstruction is due to complete atresia and is caudal to the ampulla of Vater. In the remaining 20% of the cases, the obstruction can be due to a diaphragm or membrane located within the lumen of the duodenum, and it can be complete or partial (stenosis) [56].

The prevalence of duodenal obstruction is about 1.8 per 10,000 births [57].

Ultrasonography Features

- A "double bubble" sign as a result of an enlarged stomach and duodenal cap is observed and is usually found at >24 weeks of gestation. Care should be taken in demonstrating a communication between the two anechoic bubbles, crossing the midline to obtain confirmation that the second bubble is actually the dilated proximal duodenum [58] (Fig. 48.23)
- Polyhydramnios is mostly seen after 24 weeks' gestation

Up to one half of children with duodenal obstruction also have Down's syndrome [59]. Duodenal atresia can be associated with different anomalies [60] such as:

- Vertebral anomalies: one-third of duodenal atresia cases
- Cardiac anomalies: one-third of duodenal atresia cases
- Gastrointestinal anomalies: one-fourth of duodenal atresia cases
- Association with EA: 5% (frequently with Trisomy 21 and 18)
- Malrotation of the bowel (commonly mesenteric)
- Anorectal malformation
- Renal anomalies: 8%

Prognosis

The frequent association with other anomalies represents the main poor prognostic sign. The final outcome of fetuses diagnosed with duodenal atresia is generally good, except for the cases in which severe biliary tract anomalies are present. About 90% of neonates with isolated duodenal atresia survive [61].

Small Bowel Atresia

In fetal life small bowel loops are usually collapsed. During the third trimester, minimal fluid can be seen within the bowel lumen. Fetal bowel dilatation is diagnosed when fluid-filled intestinal loops measure at least 15 mm in length or 7 mm in diameter [62].

Ultrasonography Features

- The hallmark of small bowel obstruction on the USG is dilated small bowel loops and polyhydramnios, often seen in the third trimester (Fig. 48.24)
- Ascites may be an initial clue to the identification of frank obstruction at a later stage
- Small bowel atresia maybe observed at the jejunal or ileal level and it is not always possible to detect the level of obstruction on USG

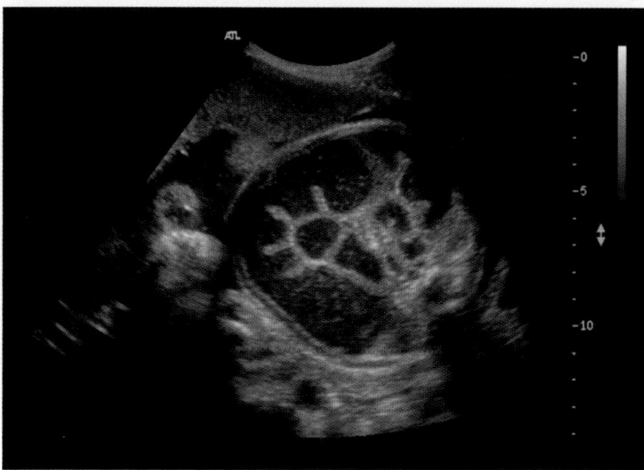

Figure 48.24 Small bowel obstruction—abdominal section in a 28 weeks fetus showing multiple dilated small bowel loops.

Prognosis

The prognosis depends on the bowel condition and hence it is important to mention the following points in the USG report:

- Presence of peristalsis: Normal peristalsis in distal segment indicates healthy bowel
- Thickness of the dilated bowel: Echogenic thick wall indicates possibility of necrotic/gangrenous bowel
- Clear fluid (healthy bowel) versus echogenic material within dilated bowel (possibility of necrotic gangrenous bowel)
- Presence of free fluid, encysted fluid collection (possibility of bowel perforation)

Meconium Peritonitis

Fetal meconium peritonitis is a sterile chemical peritonitis resulting from the extrusion of bowel content into the abdominal cavity through a bowel perforation. The etiology of the perforation can be varied, such as intestinal atresia, volvulus, intussusception, or vascular compromise; and the cause cannot be determined in utero [63].

Detection of abdominal calcifications and ascites arouses suspicion of meconium peritonitis. Extraluminal calcifications are seen along the peritoneum, often on the surface of the liver, and appear as linear echogenic densities (Fig. 48.25). Ascites may be observed initially but resolves over time. A meconium pseudocyst occurs when extravasated intestinal contents become walled off. It typically appears as a complex round intra-abdominal cystic collection with an echogenic wall.

Anorectal Malformation

Anorectal malformations (ARMs) represent a spectrum of abnormalities ranging from mild anal anomalies to complex cloacal malformations (also referred to as urorectal septal malformation). The incidence rate for ARM is approximately 4 in 10,000 births [64].

Ultrasonography Features

- Overdistention of the rectum and sigmoid colon in the second and third trimester (Fig. 48.26A and B)
- Intraluminal meconium calcification or enterolith is secondary to mixing of meconium and urine. Hence it indicates fistulous communication between the bowel and urinary systems
- Persistent cloaca is the most severe form of ARM and is seen only in females. The distal portion of the urinary tract, vagina, and rectum, join to form a single common structure which opens onto the perineum. Hydrocolpos develops as a result of the passage of urine and meconium into the vagina, and is seen as a midline cystic mass in the pelvis, posterior to the bladder. Hydrocolpos is frequently associated with urinary tract obstruction; hydronephrosis and oligohydramnios. Ascites is seen in a minority of cases

A wide variety of additional findings are present in the majority of cases and include VACTERL, chromosomal abnormalities,

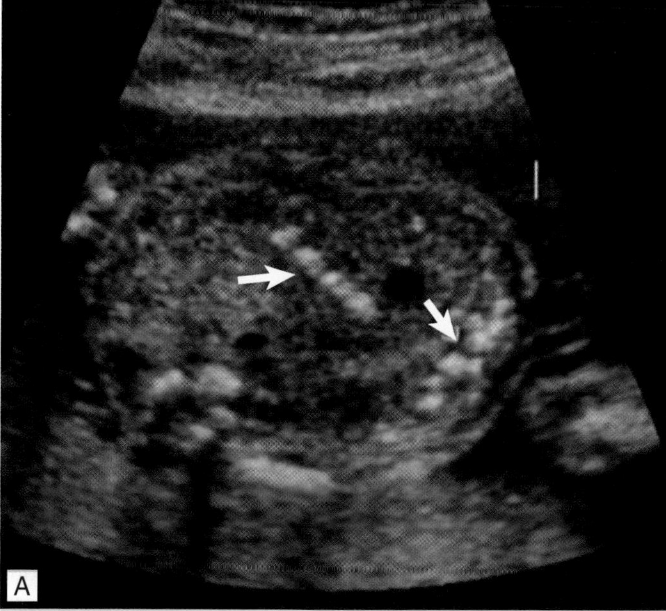

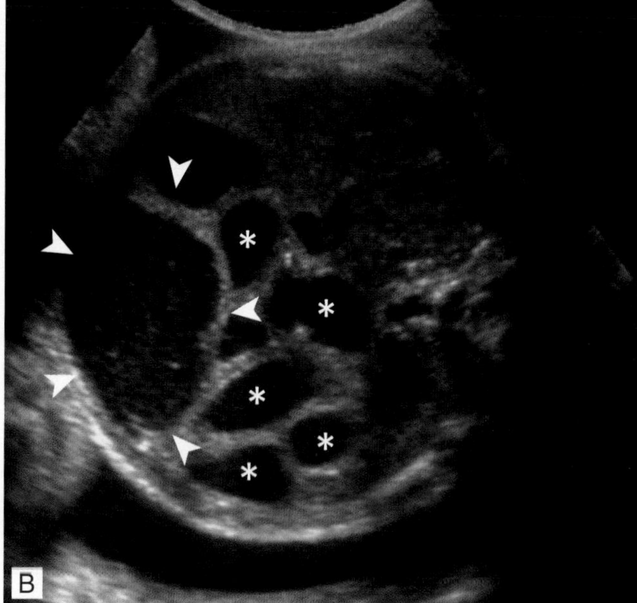

Figure 48.25 (A) Meconium peritonitis—multiple calcific foci (*white arrows*) noted in fetal abdomen; (B) abdominal section in a different fetus showing intra-abdominal cystic collection with an echogenic wall suggestive of meconium pseudocyst (*white arrowheads*) and dilated small bowel loops (*asterisks*).

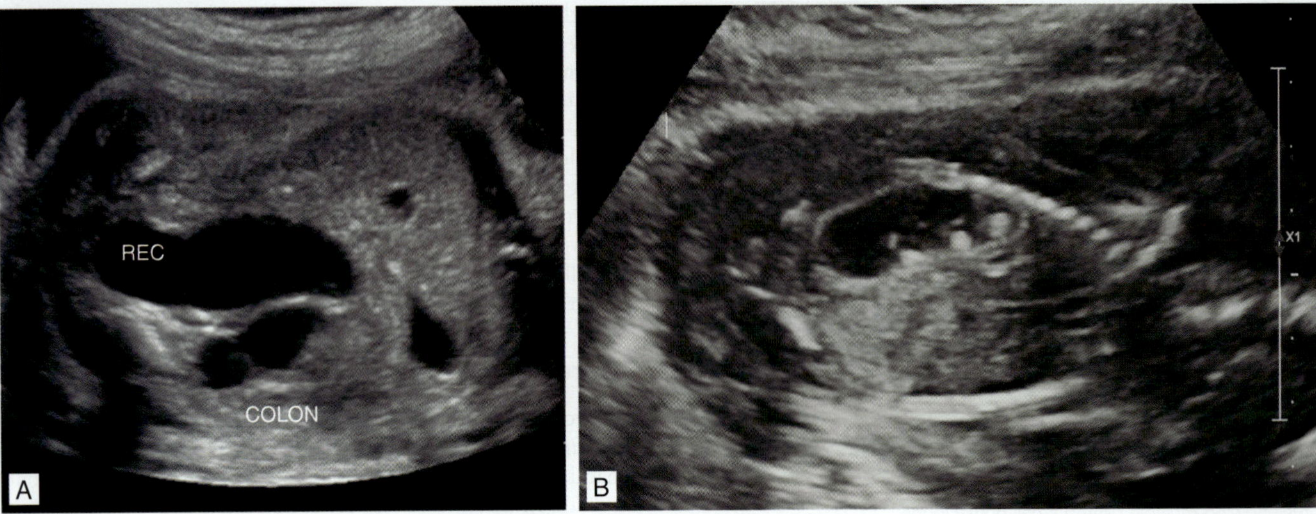

Figure 48.26 (A) Dilated rectum (REC) seen as elongated cystic structure at 24 weeks gestation (B) cloacal malformation with intraluminal enteroliths at 18 weeks gestation.

nonchromosomal syndromes, and multiple anomalies involving the genital system, central nervous system, face, limbs, and musculoskeletal system [65].

Echogenic Bowel

In the second trimester, the fetal liver, small intestine, and bone demonstrate an increasing echogenicity in that order. *When the echogenicity of the fetal bowel is similar or higher than the adjacent fetal bone it is termed as echogenic bowel.* The iliac bones are used as reference points. There are no standardized criteria for the sonographic diagnosis of an echogenic small intestine and it remains a subjective USG observation. The prevalence of echogenic small intestine in routine second-trimester sonograms ranges from 0.2% to 1.8% [66].

There are many conditions known to be associated with the finding of an echogenic bowel like Down's syndrome, cystic fibrosis, congenital infections, and fetal growth restriction. Hence a detailed evaluation of the fetus is warranted, such as:

- Targeted anomaly scan—to look for other markers of aneuploidy and signs of congenital infections
- Genetic work-up for aneuploidy and cystic fibrosis
- TORCH titer
- Follow-up for the assessment of growth

Fetal Ascites

Ascites is an excess amount of free intraperitoneal fluid in the fetal abdomen. Ascites may be an early manifestation of fetal hydrops, both immune and nonimmune. Sonographically detectable causes of fetal ascites are summarized in Table 48.4.

Once ascites is detected it is important to do a detailed anomaly scan including fetal echo. To rule out fetal anemia, the measurement of Middle Cerebral Artery-Peak Systolic Velocity is important.

TABLE 48.4 Sonographically Detectable Causes of Ascites

Hydrops
Congenital infections
GI causes: meconium peritonitis secondary to bowel perforation
Thoracic space occupying lesions
Cardiac anomalies causing cardiac failure (arrhythmia, cardiomyopathy)
Ovarian cyst rupture
Persistent cloaca
Urinary tract obstruction causing urinary ascites

Intra-Abdominal Cysts

The list of differential diagnosis of abdominal cysts is exhaustive and is enumerated in Table 48.5. The detection of a cystic lesion mandates a hunt for the location of the cyst. Cystic lesions located posteriorly, near the spine are of renal origin. The cysts found in the pelvis are usually of an ovarian origin, hydrocolpos, and rarely anterior sacral meningocele. Upper abdominal cysts are choledochal cysts, cysts of bowel origin. Mid abdominal cystic lesions can be mesenteric and enteric duplication cysts. Enteric duplication cysts can show double wall (gut signature) indicating its bowel etiology. Color Doppler aids in the diagnosis of the umbilical vein varix.

Ventral Wall Defects

Omphalocele and gastroschisis are the most frequently encountered congenital ventral wall defects. The majority of cases of omphalocele are associated with other serious structural defects and chromosomal abnormalities. In contrast, gastroschisis is usually an isolated lesion and is not associated with other structural defects and abnormal karyotype.

Omphalocele

Omphalocele is a midline abdominal wall defect with herniation of the abdominal content into the base of the umbilical cord. Omphalocele has to be differentiated from the physiologic bowel herniation which is seen from the 8th to 11th week of gestation. This is considered a normal sonographic finding and presents as a

TABLE 48.5 Fetal Abdominal Cystic Lesions

- Ovarian cyst
- Choledochal cyst
- Meconium pseudocyst
- Mesenteric cyst
- Intestinal obstruction
- Renal anomalies such as hydronephrosis especially dilated pelvis in PUJ obstruction, renal cyst, perinephric urinoma
- Adrenal hemorrhage
- Umbilical vein varix
- Anterior sacral meningocele
- Hydrocolpos
- Enteric duplication cyst

mass at umbilical cord insertion. Physiological midgut herniation never contains a herniated liver and is usually smaller than 7 mm in diameter. This disappears before 12 weeks of gestation.

The prevalence of omphalocele among live births, stillbirths, and induced abortions is about 2.0–2.6 per 10,000 [67,68]. It appears to be more common in pregnant women of extreme reproductive ages (less than 20 and more than 40 years old) [69].

Ultrasonography Features (Fig. 48.27)

- Smooth midline protruding mass covered by membranes
- Umbilical cord insertion onto the membrane of the mass
- Mass contains mainly small intestine and liver. There can be other organs protruding into the omphalocele such as large intestine, bladder, stomach, spleen
- Increased volume of the amniotic fluid

Trisomy 13 and 18 are the most common aneuploidies associated with omphalocele. It is also associated with the Beckwith–Wiedemann syndrome.

Gastroschisis

Gastroschisis is a congenital malformation characterized by visceral herniation through a right-sided abdominal wall defect adjacent to an intact umbilical cord and not covered by a membrane. The prevalence is inversely related with maternal age, that is, >60 times more common in women younger than 20 years of age, compared with women older than 35 [70].

Ultrasonography Features (Fig. 48.28)

- Extra abdominal bowel loops with no covering membrane
- Defect usually on the right side from the umbilical cord insertion
- Normal umbilical cord insertion
- Dilation of the bowel loops
- Thickened, echogenic bowel wall
- Malposition of the stomach

Increased dilation of the bowel loops suggests poor prognosis. The bowel wall is directly exposed to the amniotic fluid which causes chemical peritonitis. As a result of this chemical irritation, the bowel wall thickens and becomes echogenic and nodular. The stomach is often moved from the typical location. Intrauterine growth restriction and decreased amount of the amniotic fluid is also a common finding.

Abnormalities of the gastrointestinal tract such as atresia, stenosis, necrosis, perforation, malrotation, and volvulus may be seen with gastroschisis. The incidence of growth restriction, fetal demise, and spontaneous preterm delivery is increased.

The differentiating features of different ventral wall defects are summarized in Table 48.6.

Genitourinary System

Ultrasonography Anatomy

Kidneys

Kidneys can be assessed anatomically in two scanning planes: *axial and longitudinal.* In the axial view, the kidneys appear as two round paravertebral structures with the pelvis oriented medially. In the longitudinal or sagittal view, they appear elliptical. The adrenal glands are located just cranial to the kidneys.

The fetal kidneys can be visualized on USG by the 11th–12th weeks, where they are seen as two echogenic paravertebral structures. In the second trimester, they appear isoechoic with an anechoic area medially which is the renal

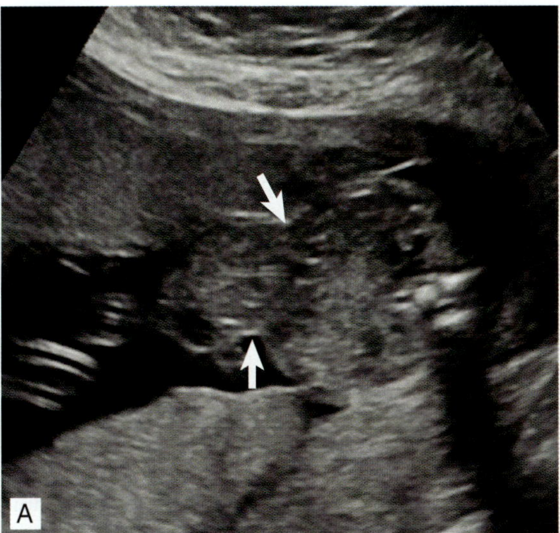

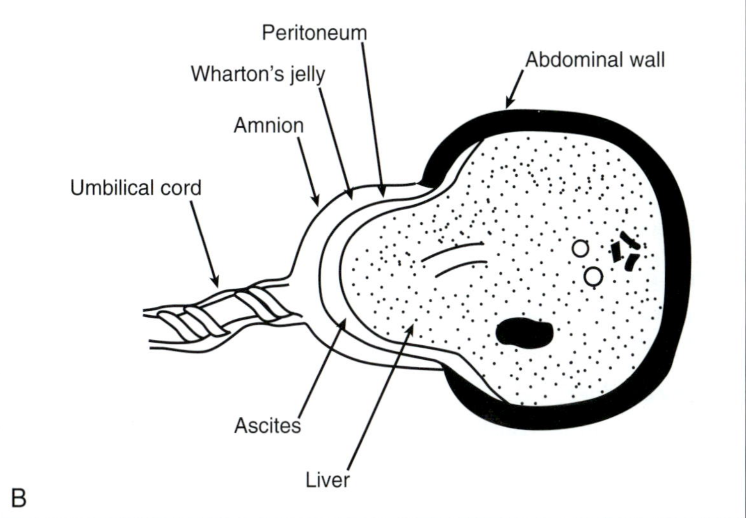

Figure 48.27 Omphalocele— (A) Midline protruding mass covered by membranes (*arrows*) with umbilical cord insertion onto the membranes. (B) Diagrammatic representation of the same.

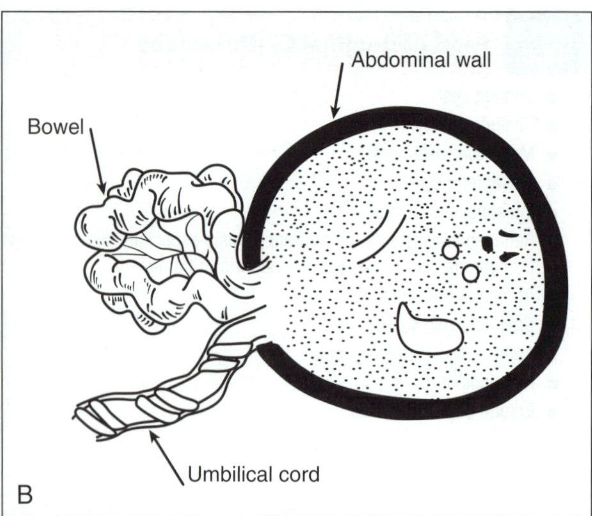

Figure 48.28 (A) Gastroschisis—presence of extra abdominal bowel loops with no covering membranes noted. (B) Gastroschisis—Diagrammatic representation showing extra-abdominal bowel loops and normal insertion of the umbilical cord over the anterior abdominal wall.

TABLE 48.6 Differentiating Features of Ventral Wall Defects

Type of Defect	Description	USG Findings	Other Anomalies
Gastroschisis	Para umbilical defect	Typically, only bowel is eviscerated; occasionally other organs but never liver	Uncommon, little to no risk of aneuploidy, high chance of bowel-related complications
Omphalocele	Midline defect, contained by membrane	With liver outside large mass With liver inside small mass	High risk of other anomalies and /or aneuploidy
Pentalogy of cantrell	1. Omphalocele 2. Anterior diaphragmatic hernia 3. Partial sternal defect 4. Pericardial defect 5. Cardiac anomalies	High omphalocele, pleural effusion Diaphragmatic hernia Heart partially or completely outside thorax	
Bladder extrophy	Eviscerated urinary bladder	Nonvisualization of bladder, soft-tissue mass over the abdominal wall	Increased risk of aneuploidy
Limb-body wall complex	Multiple anomaly condition	Bizarre complex defect with ventral wall defect, cranial defects, scoliosis	100% lethal but no risk of aneuploidy

pelvis. By the third trimester, it is possible to distinguish between the cortex and medulla, and the renal pyramids appear hypoechoic. The cortex is peripheral to the medulla and seems slightly more echogenic. The pelvis size in axial sections should not exceed 4 mm before the 32nd week and 7 mm from the 33rd week until term [71].

Ureters and Urethra

The ureters and urethra are not visible antenatally, except in cases of any pathology.

Urinary Bladder

The bladder can be visualized around 10 weeks of gestation as soon as urine production begins. On USG, the bladder is always visualized by 12 weeks in the middle of the fetal pelvis as a circular cystic structure with echogenic walls. Clinicians should look for the filling and emptying of the urinary bladder in every scan.

Renal Agenesis

Renal agenesis is defined as the complete absence of one or both kidneys in their anatomical or ectopic locations (unilateral or bilateral renal agenesis). Its incidence is 1–2 per 1000 births for the unilateral form and 1 per 3000–4000 births for the bilateral condition [72]. This anomaly is due to the developmental failure of the ureteric bud or interaction with the metanephric blastema.

Unilateral Renal Agenesis

Ultrasonography Findings

- **Second trimester:** Diagnosis of unilateral renal agenesis include, (1) an absent kidney in renal fossa or ectopic locations, (2) an absent unilateral renal artery on color Doppler, (3) enlarged contralateral kidney, (4) standard amniotic fluid index, and (5) normal bladder (Fig. 48.29A and B)

Indirect sign includes the presence of an enlarged adrenal gland in the ipsilateral renal fossa and before arriving at a definitive

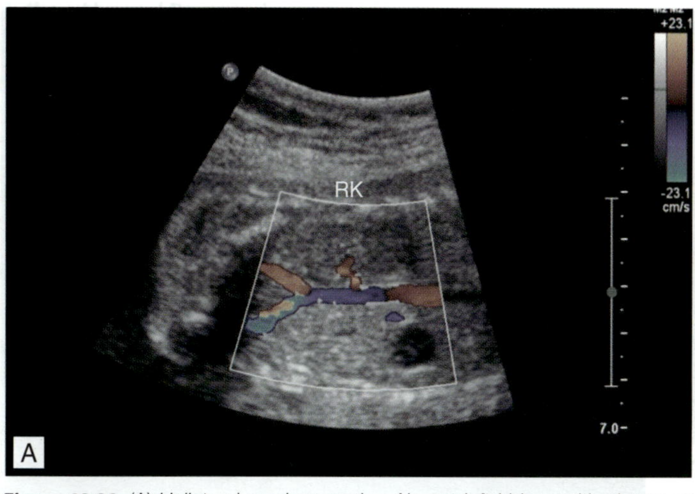

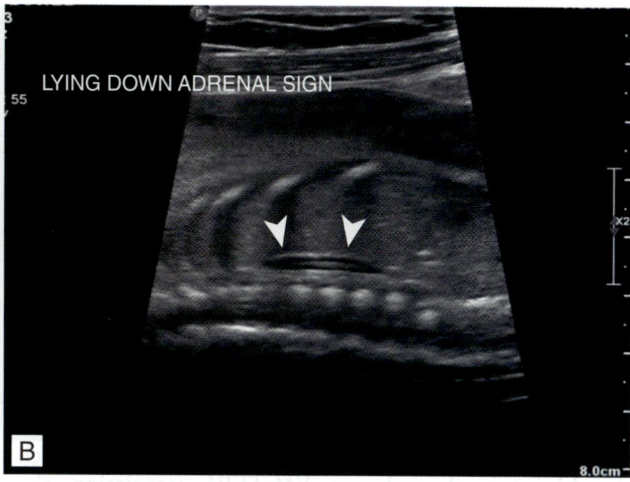

Figure 48.29 (A) Unilateral renal agenesis—Absent left kidney with absent renal artery. (B) Unilateral renal agenesis—Absent kidney with absent renal artery with "lying down adrenal" sign (*white arrowheads*).

diagnosis of unilateral renal agenesis, care should be taken to rule out ectopic kidney or hypoplastic kidney.

Abnormalities of the contralateral kidney have been described in up to 90% of patients. The most common abnormality is vesicoureteric reflux (VUR). Others include renal ectopia and malrotation, pelviureteric junction (PUJ) obstruction, duplication, and multicystic dysplasia.

The prognosis is good with a normal survival rate and quality of life. Females with unilateral renal agenesis should undergo a pelvic USG postnatally to look for associated Mullerian anomalies.

Bilateral Renal Agenesis

It is usually associated with the oligohydramnios sequence. It was synonymous with Potter syndrome previously. Bilateral renal agenesis is generally sporadic in occurrence, but in 20–36% of cases, a familial recurrence (possibly autosomal dominant with incomplete penetrance and variable expression) is likely.

- **Direct signs of bilateral renal agenesis**: Nonvisualization of kidneys in their anatomical or ectopic locations
- **Indirect signs**: Nonvisualization of the bladder and absence of renal arteries on color, and power Doppler

These are associated with severe oligohydramnios after the 16th week. Additionally, the adrenal glands may be mistaken for the kidneys since the glands appear rounder than usual and fill the renal fossa ("lying down" adrenal sign). The combination of renal agenesis, small chest, oligohydramnios, club feet, low set ears, and facial deformation is known as "Potter syndrome."

Prognosis: Bilateral renal agenesis is always fatal due to associated severe pulmonary hypoplasia.

The risk of nonchromosomal syndromes is high (20–25%). Renal agenesis can be the main sign of more than 40 different syndromes. The most common syndromes and associations are Fraser syndrome, VACTERL, and caudal regression syndrome.

Ectopic Kidney

When a kidney is not seen in its anatomic position, that is, the renal fossa, but is located in an abnormal position, it is called an ectopic kidney. In most cases, the kidney is located in the fetal pelvis. Other locations are below the aortic bifurcation, at the midline in the presacral area.

Ectopic kidney results from the arrested cephalic migration of the kidney in the typical retroperitoneal region. The aortoiliac vessels supply the arrested ectopic kidney rather than the renal artery. There are two types of ectopic kidneys; simple pelvic ectopic and complex ectopic kidneys such as the horseshoe kidney or cross fused ectopic kidney.

Ultrasonography Findings

- Empty renal fossa, along with the visualization of the kidney in the pelvis adjacent to the urinary bladder, usually below the level of the aortic bifurcation, is diagnostic of a simple pelvic ectopic kidney. Amniotic fluid as well as the filling and emptying of the urinary bladder appear normal
- Horseshoe kidneys are suspected when the axis of the lower poles is oriented more obliquely toward the midline. The lower poles are fused into the midline, with a thin strip of renal parenchyma seen in the midline

Follow-Up and Prognosis

A serial follow-up scan every 4 weeks is recommended to detect possible late-onset hydronephrosis. In isolated forms, the prognosis is good. Vesicoureteric reflux and ureteropelvic junction obstruction may occur.

Cystic Renal Diseases

Cystic renal diseases have a wide range of outcomes depending on whether they are: (1) unilateral or bilateral, (2) have any organ involvement apart from kidneys, and (3) the extent of kidney damage determined by characteristics of the particular syndrome complex.

Ultrasonography Findings

The echogenicity of the kidney can have two patterns in the context of cystic renal diseases: *cysts and renal hyperechogenicity*. The cysts may vary from a subcentimeter to a large size and can develop anywhere in the kidney.

A detailed renal sonogram measures the following:

- renal size
- echogenicity of the cortex (hyperechoic, isoechoic, hypoechoic compared with the liver and spleen) and medulla (hypoechoic, anechoic, hyperechoic)
- Corticomedullary differentiation (present, absent)
- Cysts (number, size, location) and calcifications
- Pelvicalyceal system

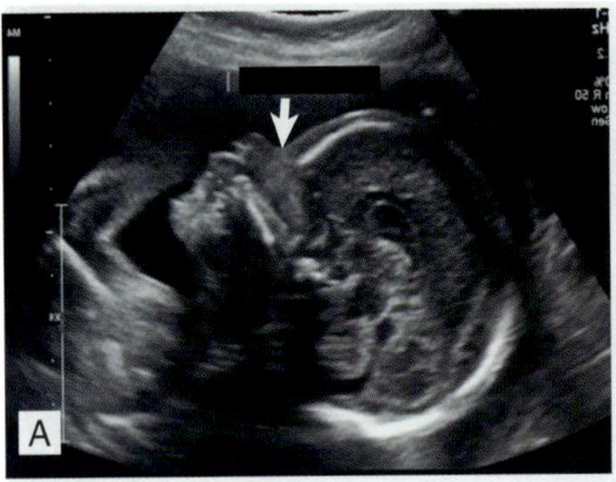
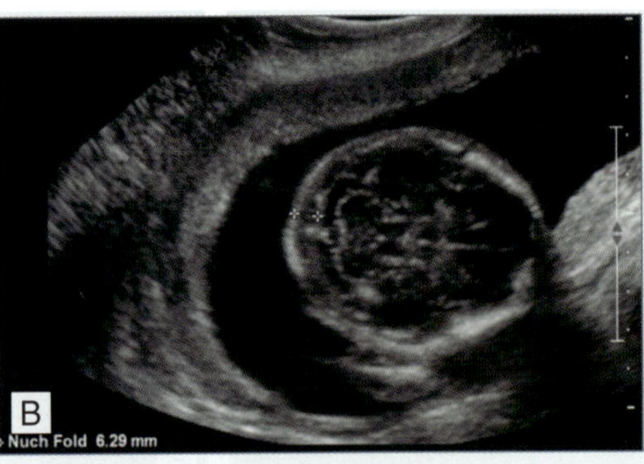

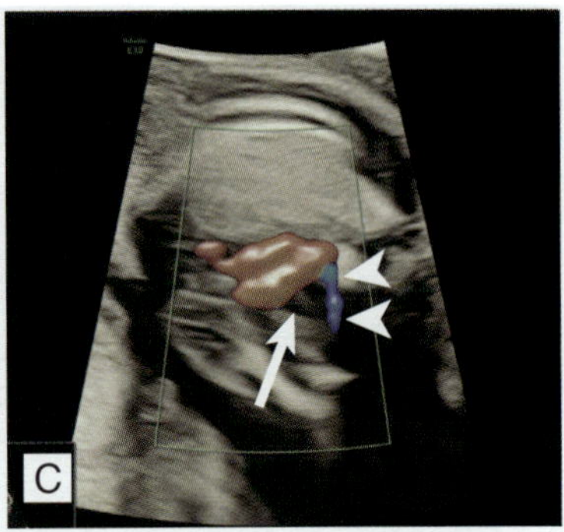

Figure 48.39 (A) Nonossified nasal bone—Sagittal view of the face demonstrating nonvisualization of nasal bone (*white arrow*). (B) Thickened nuchal fold—Axial transcerebellar view of an 18-week fetus showing an increase in the nuchal fold thickness (*calipers*). (C) Aberrant right subclavian artery (ARSA)—3VT view demonstrating a vessel traversing on the right side (*white arrowhead*) behind the trachea (*white arrow*).

- lateral cerebral ventriculomegaly,
- absent or hypoplastic nasal bone (Fig. 48.39A),
- increased nuchal fold thickness (Fig. 48.39B),
- intracardiac hyperechogenic focus,
- aberrant right subclavian artery (Fig. 48.39B),
- hyperechogenic bowel,
- mild hydronephrosis, and
- shortening of the femur or humerus.

Each of these markers has a positive LR (likelihood ratio) and a negative LR based on the validity of that marker in several studies. The pretest odds derived from the maternal age second-trimester serum biochemical testing or first-trimester combined testing, is multiplied by the positive LR of each present marker and the negative LR of each undetected marker to get a post-test odds ratio for Trisomy 21. This can be done using on-line calculators (e.g., Perinatology.com).

For example, if a mother is 25 years old and assuming no previous biochemical tests have been done, her apriori risk would be 1 in 1030 (low risk). Assuming she has abnormal nuchal fold (>6 mm), the LR of NF is 17. Assuming all other markers are negative, her posterior probability would be 1 in 61.5 (high risk). An invasive test (amniocentesis) would now be advised.

Noninvasive Prenatal Test

Noninvasive prenatal test (NIPT) or cell-free DNA test is a blood test done to determine a fetus's risk of having chromosomal disorders, including Down's syndrome. Some of the fetal DNA circulates in the maternal blood during pregnancy, and NIPT analyses these tiny fragments of DNA. The test is considered noninvasive since only the maternal blood is taken and does not pose any risk to the fetus.

In addition to chromosomal anomalies, NIPT is also able to identify several microdeletions including DiGeorge syndrome, Van der Woude syndrome, Cat-eye syndrome, Cornelia de Lange syndrome, Cowden syndrome, and Jacobsen syndrome.

If the NIPT test result is "high risk," it must be confirmed with an invasive test (amniocentesis/chorionic villus sampling).

Invasive Testing

Invasive testing including amniocentesis and chorion villus sampling can be carried out in the case of a positive result in the screening test. These procedures have been explained in detail in the chapter on fetal interventions.

Suggested Readings

- EC Toy, AC Fleischer, FA Manning, J Abramowicz, L Goncalves, I Timor-Tritsch, et al., Fleischer's Sonography in Obstetrics & Gynecology, eighth ed., McGraw-Hill Education, 2017.
- ME Norton, PW Callen, Callen's Ultrasonography in Obstetrics and Gynecology, sixth ed., Elsevier, 2016.
- BS Rama Murthy, Imaging of Fetal Brain and Spine: An Atlas and Guide, Springer Singapore, 2019.

49

Obstetrics: Third Trimester

NITIN CHAUBAL, ALPANA JOSHI

Introduction

A third-trimester ultrasonography (USG) scan is important for the assessment of fetal growth and well-being. It encompasses fetal biometric measurements, assessment of fetal presentation and lie, amniotic fluid (AF) estimation, detection of the abnormalities of the placenta and umbilical cord that might alter the mode of delivery, Doppler interrogation, and the assessment of fetal movements.

Fetal growth restriction (FGR) is the commonest condition associated with stillbirth [1]. The third trimester is a critical period to diagnose FGR to avoid adverse perinatal outcomes. Certain B-mode and Doppler USG findings highly suggestive of FGR facilitate protocol-based management of FGR fetuses. The fetal environment has a strong influence on the pregnancy outcome. Therefore, it is equally important to study the pathologies of the placenta, umbilical cord, AF, and cervix during this period. Multifetal gestations are known to develop unique complications in the late second and third trimesters, which also warrant a thorough USG assessment.

Fetal Growth Restriction

FGR is the failure of a fetus to reach its biologic growth potential as a consequence of pathological environmental influence. Poor uteroplacental perfusion as a result of abnormal placentation is its most common placental etiology. As fetal oxygen demand increases with advancing gestational age, oxygen delivery to the fetal circulation may fall below a critical point. This leads to a compensatory redistribution of fetal blood away from its body to its brain, adrenal glands, and heart; resulting in stunted growth.

Common causes of FGR are mentioned in Table 49.1.

TABLE 49.1 Common Causes of FGR [2]

Maternal causes	Advanced maternal age
	Preeclampsia
	Chronic medical diseases
	  Hypertension
	  Cardiovascular diseases
	  Diabetes mellitus
	  Chronic nephropathy
	  Collagen vascular diseases
	  Thrombophilia
	Inadequate nutrition, malabsorption, poor weight gain

Fetal causes	Chromosomal and genetic anomalies Multiple gestations TORCH infection
Placental causes	Single umbilical artery Abnormal cord insertions (velamentous, marginal) Bilobed or circumvallate placenta Small placenta
Medications	Phenytoin (Dilantin) Trimethadione
Drug abuse	Alcohol Cocaine Smoking

Evaluation of Fetal Growth

Early detection of FGR is important as such fetuses are prone to poor perinatal outcomes. There is growing evidence demonstrating how being born small has important implications on the quality of health during adulthood [3].

It is a routine practice to do a USG scan at 18–22 weeks of gestation for the detection of congenital anomalies. As growth is an ongoing process, assessment of growth requires a comparison between two scans with an appropriate time interval in between. Hence, a second scan between 26 and 30 weeks (called "growth scan" or "well-being scan") is done for the assessment of the interval growth. During this scan, the following fetal biometric parameters are measured and compared with standard growth charts [4]:

- Biparietal diameter
- Head circumference (HC)
- Abdominal circumference (AC)
- Femur diaphysis length (FL)
- Estimated fetal weight (EFW)

Accurate estimation of gestational age is a prerequisite for the determination of fetal growth. Nuchal translucency (NT) scan between 11 + 0 to 13 + 6 weeks is most reliable for dating.

Based on the values of the biometric parameters mentioned earlier, fetal growth falls under one of the following:

- Appropriate for gestational age (AGA)—AGA fetuses have individual biometric parameters between the 10th and 90th percentile for gestational age
- Small for gestational age (SGA)—SGA fetuses have EFW or AC below the 10th percentile for gestational age
- Large for gestational Age (LGA)—LGA fetuses have EFW or AC above 90th percentile for gestational age

Role of Fetal Doppler

Doppler USG examination of the placental circulation plays an important role in screening for impaired placentation and its complications—preeclampsia, FGR, and perinatal death. It can

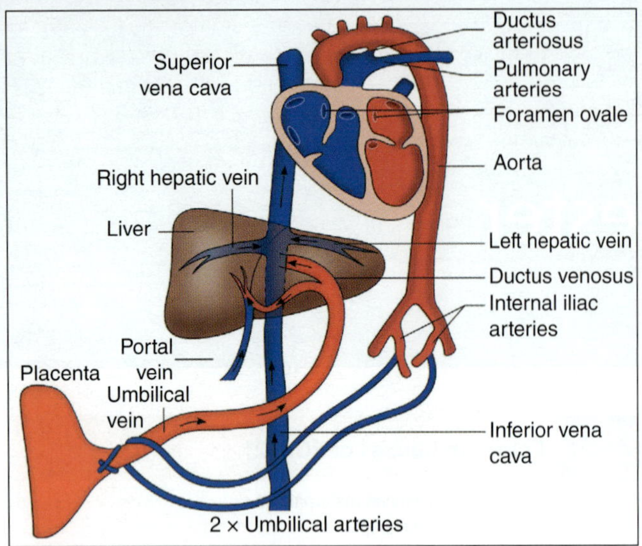

Figure 49.1 Schematic diagram of fetal circulation.

be used to assess blood flow waveform patterns in various vascular beds in the maternal, fetal, and placental circulations. It also aids in differentiating between SGA and FGR fetuses. It is good to be conversant with the salient features of fetal circulation when discussing fetal Doppler.

Fetal Circulation

Fetal circulation differs from postnatal circulation in many ways. The former consists of two parallel blood flow pathways and three vascular shunts (Fig. 49.1).

The supply of oxygen and nutrients to a fetus comes from its placenta. Oxygenated blood from the placenta passes through a single umbilical vein and enters the fetal liver. About 30% of umbilical venous blood bypasses the liver in this manner and enters the right atrium through ductus venosus (DV) and inferior vena cava (IVC) [5].

On reaching the right atrium, fetal blood is effectively divided into two streams. The larger stream (oxygenated blood coming from DV) is shunted to the left atrium through the foramen ovale. The smaller stream passes into the right ventricle through the tricuspid valve, where it is joined by blood from the superior vena cava. Thus, it has a lesser oxygen concentration. Blood entering the left atrium passes into the left ventricle through the mitral valve, then empties into the ascending aorta. This relatively oxygen-rich blood passes predominantly to the head and upper extremities.

Because of high pulmonary arterial pressure in fetal lungs, only a small portion of blood from the right ventricle passes through the pulmonary circulation through pulmonary arteries and reaches the left atrium through pulmonary veins. A substantially larger portion flows through the ductus arteriosus into the systemic circulation through the descending aorta. Deoxygenated fetal blood is returned to the placenta through two umbilical arteries that arise from internal iliac arteries.

Optimization of Spectral Doppler Tracing

It is essential to obtain a crisp, interpretable spectral tracing for accurate assessment of Doppler parameters. Here are some guidelines about how to obtain an optimum image [6]:

- Adequately zoom in on the region of interest
- Identify the vessel of interest by placing a narrow color box over it
- Start with a relatively wide Doppler gate (sample volume) to ensure the recording of maximum velocities during the entire pulse
- Keep the insonation angle as close to zero as possible. This ensures the best conditions for assessing absolute velocities and waveforms
- Set the vessel wall filter as low as possible (≤60 Hz) to eliminate the low-frequency noise from the vessel wall motion
- Obtain spectral Doppler tracing during the phase of quiescence, that is, in the absence of fetal breathing and body movements to ensure recording a uniform waveform (Fig. 49.2A and B). If necessary, instruct the mother to hold her breath temporarily
- Adjust the horizontal sweep speed to obtain 4 to 6 (no more than 10) separate successive waveforms (Fig. 49.2C)
- Adjust the pulse repetition frequency according to the vessel being studied
- Use the autotracing tool only when the waveform is uniform. Else, manual tracing is advised (Fig. 49.2D and E)

Interpretation of Doppler Waveforms

Absolute velocity measures from a Doppler spectrum, such as peak systolic velocity (PSV) and end-diastolic velocity (EDV), are dependent on the angle of insonation. Indices such as systolic/diastolic (S/D) ratio, pulsatility index (PI), and resistivity index (RI) that are independent of the angle of insonation better reflect the true information about vascular blood flow and resistance (Table 49.2). Of the three indices, S/D and RI have limitations when the diastolic flow approaches zero. Hence, PI is the best index for fetal Doppler evaluation. It is important to report the percentile PI for a given gestational age for the stage-based management of FGR (described later), in addition to its absolute value. One can easily get the percentile values from online calculators such as the one on the website of Fetal Medicine Barcelona [7].

Doppler Features of Various Vessels

During the third trimester, the following vessels are examined with Doppler USG:

- Umbilical artery (UA)
- Middle cerebral artery (MCA)
- Uterine artery
- Ductus venosus
- Aortic isthmus (AoI)
- Fetal venous circulation

Various normal and pathological Doppler features in these vascular structures are summarized in Table 49.3.

TABLE 49.2 Insonation Angle-Independent Doppler Indices

Name of Index	Meaning of Index
Systolic-to-diastolic (S/D) ratio	= PSV/EDV
Resistivity index (RI)	= (PSV – EDV)/PSV
Pulsatility index (PI)	= (PSV – EDV)/mean velocity

EDV, end-diastolic velocity; *PSV*, peak systolic velocity.

Umbilical Artery

UA has been widely accepted as the standard subject of the Doppler examination to identify FGR for almost two decades. The assessment of UA blood flow provides information on the perfusion of the fetoplacental unit and helps to improve perinatal outcome in FGR fetuses [8].

Practical tips: It is recommended to insonate a free loop of the umbilical cord for documenting a Doppler tracing. However, in some cases it is not feasible. For example, in oligohydramnios and twin pregnancy. In the latter, sometimes it is difficult to assign a free loop to the correct fetus. In such cases, it is better to sample the UA just distal to the abdominal insertion of the umbilical cord.

Normal findings: UA waveform changes with advancing gestation. In the first trimester, the end-diastolic flow (EDF) is often absent. From the second trimester on, the artery shows forward diastolic flow (Fig. 49.3A), which increases with progressing gestation because of decreasing placental vascular resistance leading to a fall in the PI.

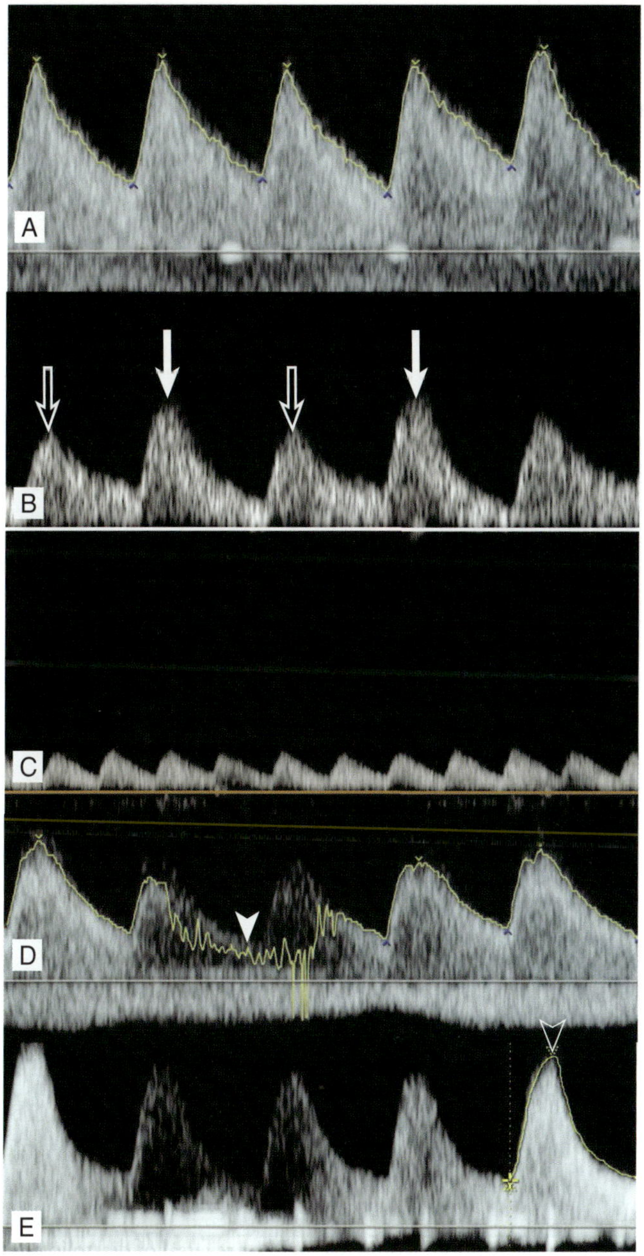

Figure 49.2 Optimization of spectral Doppler tracing. (A) An appropriate waveform obtained during fetal apnea with uniformly displayed spectrum. (B) An uneven waveform obtained during fetal breathing movements with some waves (*white arrows*) being taller than the others (*white block arrows*). (C) An inappropriate waveform with too many crowded and small waves. This happens as a result of high pulse repetition frequency and low sweep speed. (D) A nonuniform spectral waveform due to fetal breathing. Auto-tracing can lead to incorrect results (*white arrowhead*) in such cases. (E) In a nonuniform spectral waveform, manual tracing of adequately displayed waves (*white block arrowhead*) gives correct values of the indices.

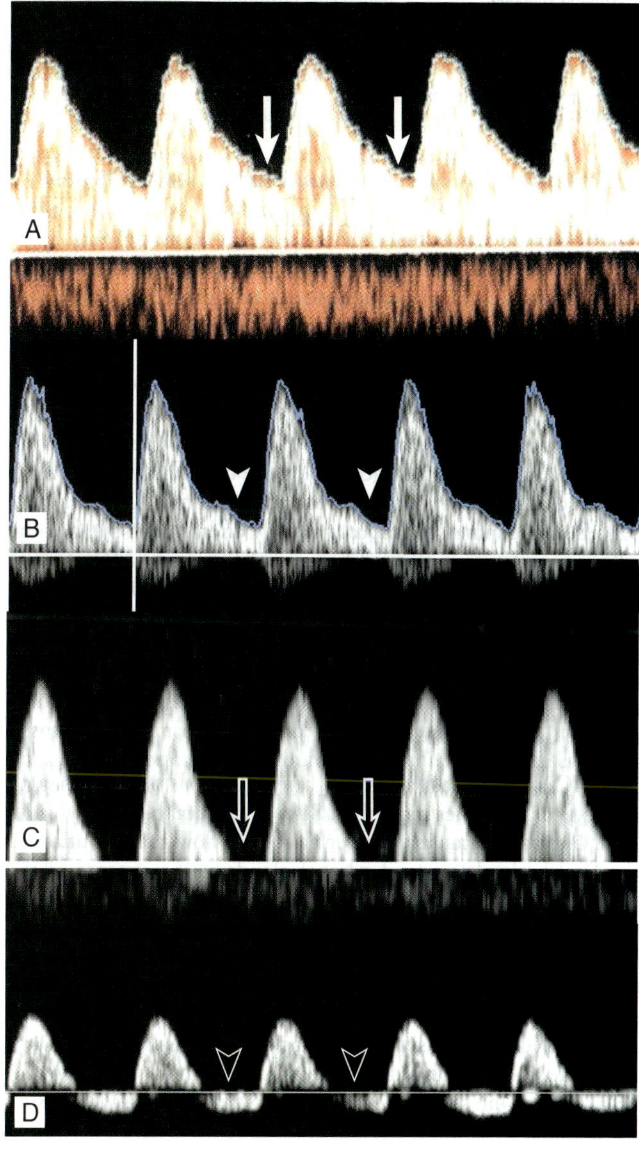

Figure 49.3 Spectral Doppler tracing of umbilical artery. (A) Normal waveform showing a forward diastolic flow (*white arrows*). The pulsatility index (PI) value is 1.0, which is within the normal range. (B) Reduced forward diastolic flow with high PI of 1.8. It corresponds to underperfusion of about 30% villous vessels. (C) Absent end diastolic velocity (*white block arrows*), seen typically when about 50% villous vessels are underperfused. (D) Reverse end diastolic velocity (*white block arrowheads*) indicates underperfusion of about 70% villous vessels (Data from: JR Duncan, ML Cock, R Harding, SM Rees, Relation between damage to the placenta and the fetal brain after late-gestation placental embolization and fetal growth restriction in sheep, Am J Obstet Gynecol 183 (4) (2000) 1013–1022.

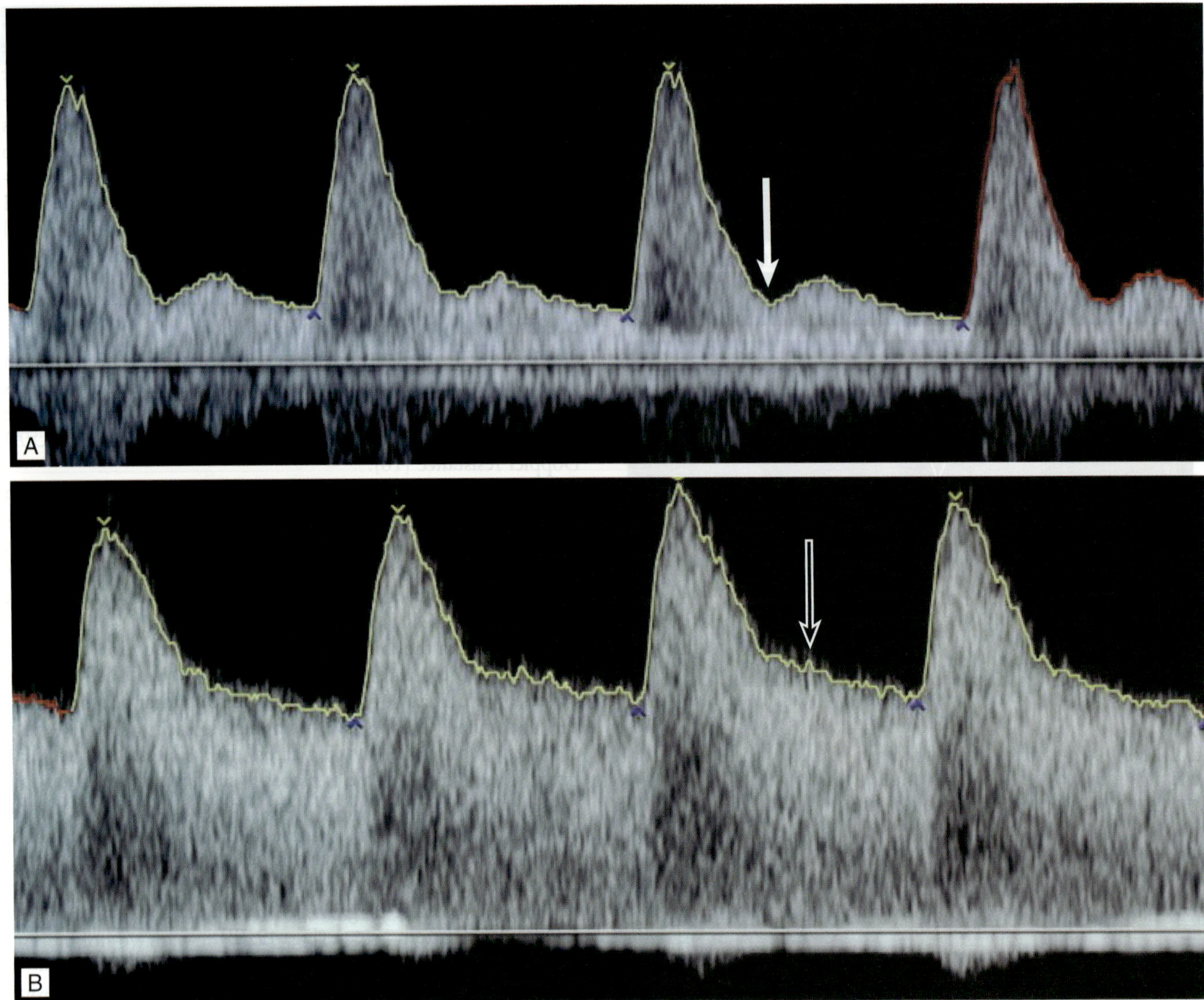

Figure 49.7 Spectral Doppler image of uterine artery. (A) First trimester waveform showing a prediastolic notch (*white arrow*). (B) Third trimester waveform where the prediastolic notch has been replaced by a high diastolic flow pattern (*white block arrow*).

Increasing right ventricular afterload is reflected in a progressive decrease in the A-wave velocities, which eventually may get reversed (Fig. 49.9B and C). DV-PI increases as a result [22]. A-wave reversal is associated with increased perinatal mortality independent of the gestational age at delivery. Hence, this finding is considered sufficient to recommend delivery after steroid administration at any gestational age. DV-PI more than 95th percentile for gestational age is associated with higher risks of fetal acidosis.

Aortic Isthmus

AoI is a small vascular segment of the aortic arch located between the origin of the left subclavian artery and the opening of the ductus arteriosus. It acts as an arterial watershed between the subdiaphragmatic (including placental) and the brachiocephalic (including cerebral) fetal circulations, orchestrating a fine balance between these two circulatory systems [23].

Practical tips: AoI can be imaged in two different sonographic planes of the aortic arch. In the longitudinal aortic arch view, the spectral gate is placed a few millimeters beyond the origin of the left subclavian artery (Fig. 49.10A and B). This view is quite difficult to obtain in the third trimester owing to the shadowing from the vertebral column. The easier approach is to insonate AoI in the three-vessel trachea (3VT) view (Fig. 49.10C and D). The characteristic V-shape shows the convergence of AoI and the arterial duct, making it easy to identify [24]. The color scale should be adjusted to avoid aliasing and the insonation angle should always be less than 30°. Nomograms for the PI values at different gestational ages [25] and online calculators for the same [7] come in handy to assign percentiles to the acquired values.

Normal findings: AoI normally shows a forward flow both in systole and diastole, because of the low placental vascular impedance (Fig. 49.11A).

Abnormal findings: Decreased forward diastolic flow, reflected as high AoI-PI (more than 95th percentile), and retrograde diastolic flow in AoI are abnormal findings. In the initial stages of decreased oxygen delivery to a fetus, it can still maintain adequate cerebral oxygenation because of adaptive mechanisms such as brain sparing. The defense against cerebral hypoxia, however, eventually gets overwhelmed pushing the fetus into the phase of decompensation. Abnormal AoI Doppler findings help to identify the fetus whose defense mechanisms are about to fail. Additionally, retrograde AoI diastolic flow has a strong association with

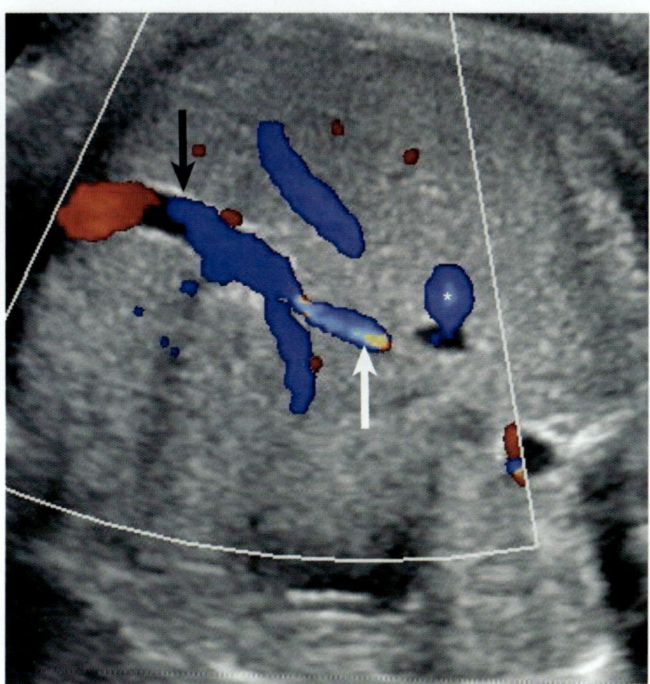

Figure 49.8 Color Doppler image of a slight oblique section of fetal abdomen showing ductus venosus (DV, *white arrow*) connecting umbilical vein (*black arrow*) and inferior vena cava (*white asterisk*). Note the aliasing within DV.

both adverse perinatal [26] and neurological outcomes. The reversal of flow in the AoI (Fig. 49.11B) generally precedes DV abnormalities by a week [27].

Fetal Venous Circulation

Fetal arterial Doppler provides information about the downstream distribution of cardiac output. Fetal venous Doppler obtained from the venous circulation (umbilical vein, IVC, and DV); in contrast; reflects right ventricular preload, myocardial compliance, and fetal cardiac function. Thus, it improves the detection of fetal compromise.

Practical tips: The umbilical vein is sampled in a free loop of the umbilical cord. IVC Doppler waveforms can be obtained from a coronal plane of the fetal chest and abdomen. In this view, IVC can be imaged as it enters into the right atrium.

Normal findings: After 15 weeks of gestation, the umbilical vein normally shows a continuous flow without any pulsations (Fig. 49.12A). In contrast, IVC shows a triphasic spectrum (Fig. 49.13), with the first peak corresponding to ventricular systole, the second peak to early diastole, and the third phase to the atrial kick (small reverse "A" wave). Its flow may be anterograde throughout the cardiac cycle or there can be a brief reversal of flow during the atrial systole.

Abnormal findings: The presence of umbilical venous pulsations (Fig. 49.12B) is the ultimate sign of increased central venous pressure in progressive cardiac dysfunction [28]. Marked reversal of the A-wave in IVC also suggests impaired cardiac function.

Approach to Diagnosis and Management

To ensure consistency and quality, it is recommended to follow a stepwise approach in the overall management of FGR. The first step is the identification of small fetuses using USG. Next, it is important to differentiate between an FGR fetus and a constitutionally small fetus. Close monitoring of FGR pregnancies for fetal well-being and appropriate timing of delivery largely influence the delivery outcome and long-term health in postnatal life. Distinguishing between early- and late-onset FGR helps in deciding the appropriate delivery timing.

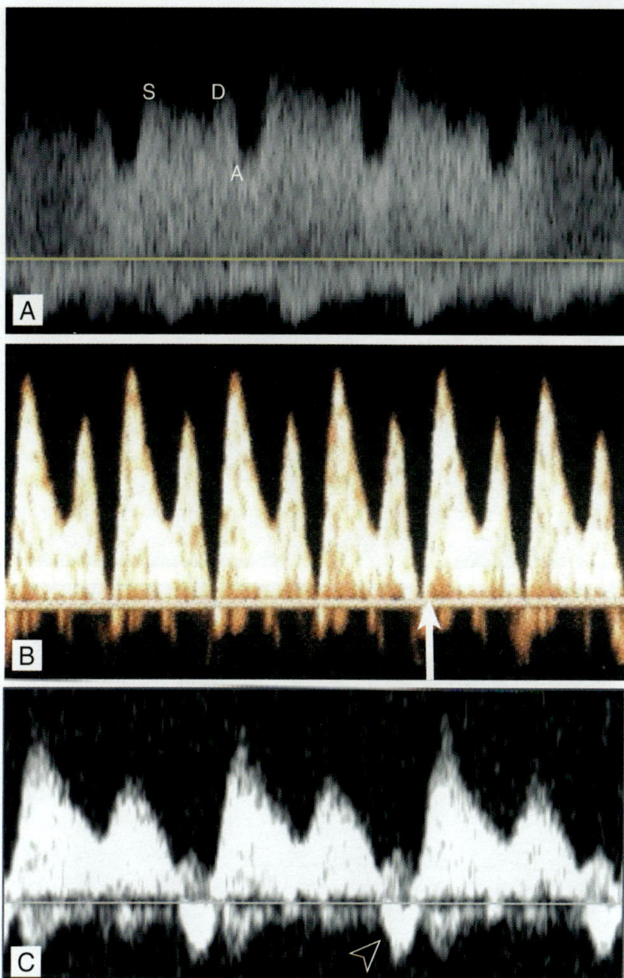

Figure 49.9 Spectral Doppler image of ductus venosus. (A) Normal spectrum showing S-wave (S), D-wave (D), and A-wave (A). (B) Increased right ventricular afterload reflected as decrease in A-wave velocity (*white arrow*). The pulsatility index is more than 95th percentile. (C) Reversed A-wave (*white arrowhead*) in a case of severe cardiac compromise.

Step 1: Identify Small Fetus

A small fetus is identified with the help of fetal biometric parameters. Any fetus whose EFW/AC is below the 10th percentile for gestational age is termed as a small-sized fetus. This finding should alert any sonologist for further evaluation.

Step 2: Differentiate Between FGR and SGA

The next clinically relevant step is to decide if the smallness is physiological or pathological. Almost 70% of small fetuses are SGA, which are constitutionally small with normal growth trajectory [29]. The remaining are growth-restricted fetuses secondary to an underlying pathology.

FGR fetuses are at a higher risk of fetal deterioration, stillbirth, and overall poor perinatal outcomes. They are associated with Doppler signs suggesting hemodynamic redistribution and hypoxia, histological and biochemical signs of placental disease, and a higher incidence of preeclampsia. There is no effective treatment for FGR. Timely detection, optimal surveillance, and timely

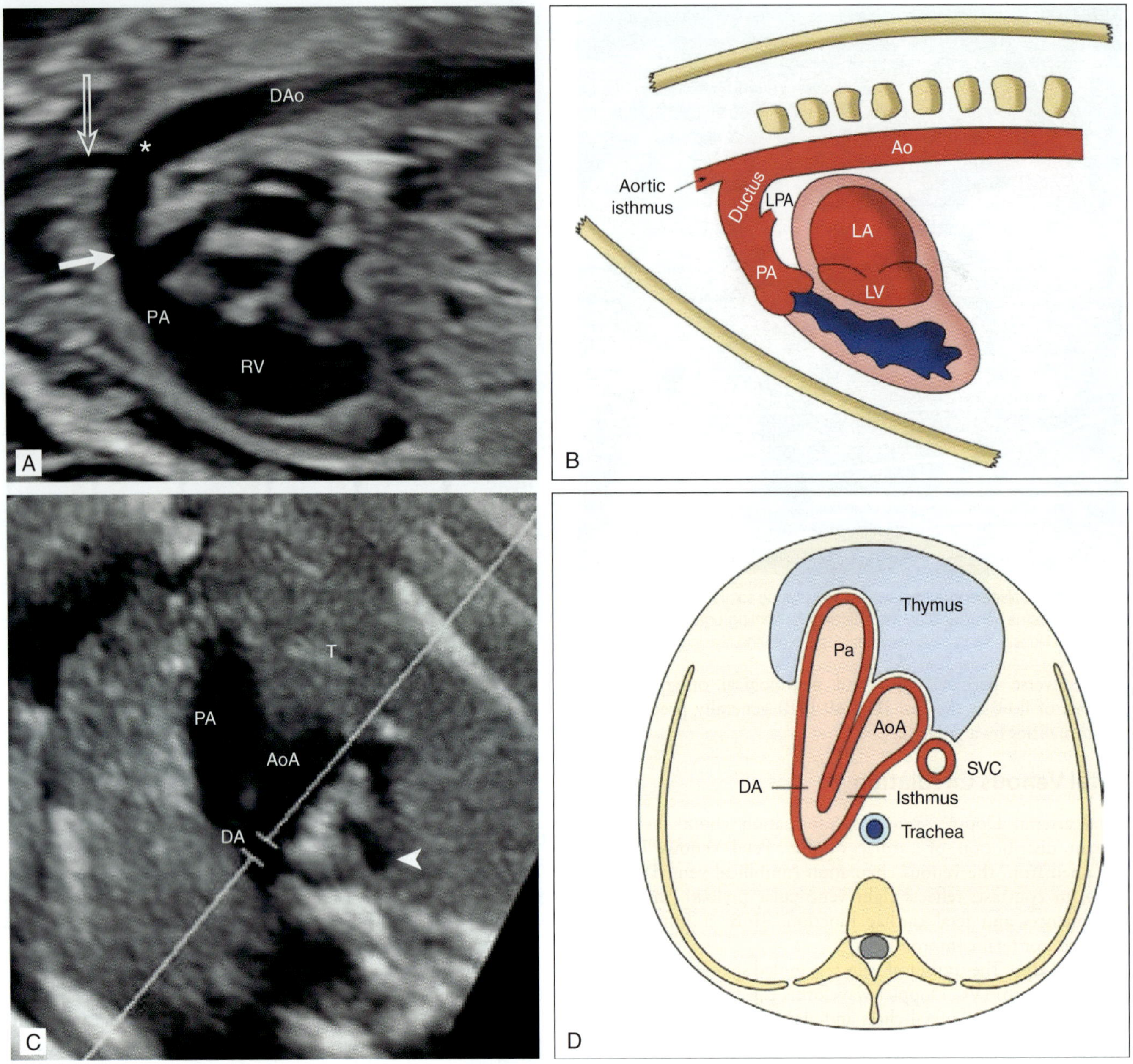

Figure 49.10 B-mode USG techniques to visualize the aortic isthmus. (A) The longitudinal aortic arch view showing the ductus arteriosus (DA, *white arrow*) originating from the pulmonary artery (PA), which in turn is arising from the right ventricle (RV). The further course of the DA before it opens into the aortic arch (AoA) is out of the plane of the image, hence not visible. The narrow portion of the AoA between the left subclavian artery (*white block arrow*) and the DA is the aortic isthmus (*white asterisk*). (C) The three-vessel trachea view at the level of the upper mediastinum demonstrating PA, DA, AoA, and the trachea (*white arrowhead*). (B and D) are the schematics of the corresponding two views. *DAo*, descending aorta, *LV*, left ventricle, *LA*, left atrium, *LPA*, left pulmonary artery, *SVC*, superior vena cava, *T*, thymus.

intervention are crucial to improving the perinatal outcome in these pregnancies. SGA fetuses, in contrast, do not present these challenges and show perinatal outcomes similar to normally growing fetuses.

FGR fetuses can be differentiated from SGA fetuses based on any one of the following:

- *Absolute biometric measurements*—Severe smallness defined as AC or EFW being less than the third centile is sufficient as a solitary parameter to diagnose FGR. In fetuses whose biometry falls between the 3rd and 10th centiles, diagnosis of FGR should be considered only when associated with other criteria
- *Sequential USG measurements focusing on declining growth centiles*—Assessment of serial biometric measurements can depict fetal well-being better than a single measurement. When the biometric parameters remain between the 10th and 90th percentile, it is possible to miss a potential FGR fetus. In such cases, it is important to consider the trend in the centile values over multiple scans (growth velocity) in addition to absolute values. A drop of more than two quartiles (or 50 centiles) confirms the diagnosis of FGR (Fig. 49.14) [30]
- *Functional parameters*—Several Doppler parameters reveal the impaired placental function responsible for FGR and the

hemodynamic adaptation by the fetus to it. These parameters have already been described in the previous sections and include:

- UA-PI more than 95th percentile/absent EDV/reversed EDV
- MCA-PI less than fifth percentile
- CPR less than fifth percentile
- UtA-PI more than 95th percentile

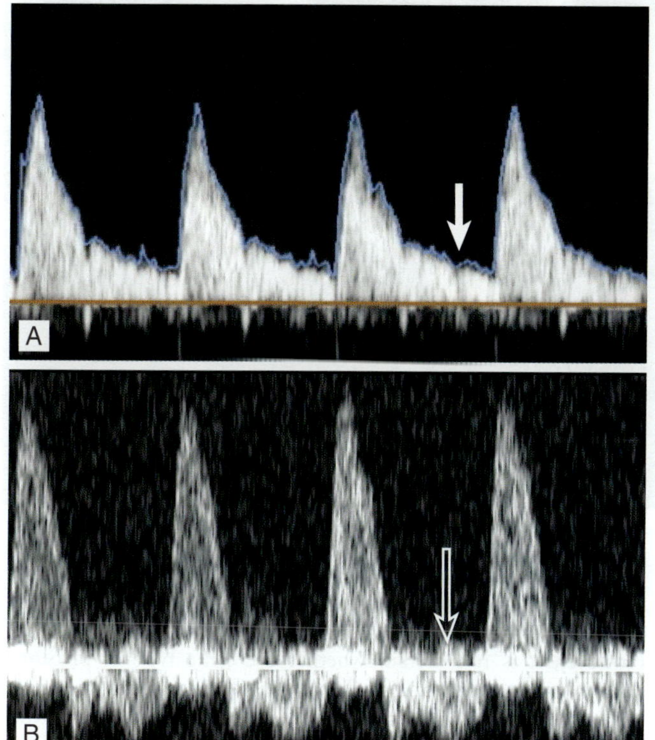

Figure 49.11 Spectral Doppler image of the aortic isthmus. (A) Normal waveform shows continuous forward diastolic flow (*white arrow*) (B) Reversed diastolic flow (*white block arrow*) suggesting severe fetal hypoxia.

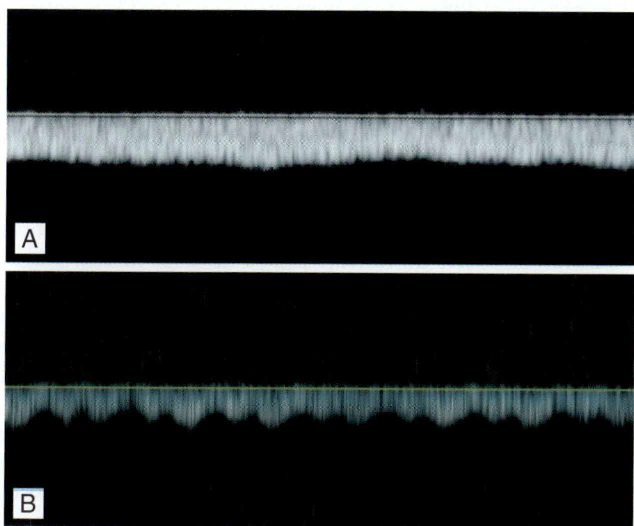

Figure 49.12 Spectral Doppler image of the umbilical vein. (A) Normal continuous flow. (B) Pulsatile waveform.

Diagnostic and Prognostic Parameters

Certain Doppler parameters are useful in the diagnosis of FGR, and differentiation between FGR and SGA. Some Doppler features correlate with acute changes occurring in the advanced stages of fetal compromise secondary to severe hypoxia and metabolic acidosis. These changes usually precede fetal death by a few days. Hence such features are called prognostic markers. These Doppler parameters have been covered in detail in the previous sections.

Umbilical artery: UA Doppler provides both diagnostic and prognostic information for the management of FGR. Increased UA-PI identifies FGR, while the progression of UA Doppler patterns to absent or reversed EDF correlates with the risks of injury or death [10].

Middle cerebral artery: MCA Doppler informs about the existence of cerebral vasodilation, which is a surrogate marker of hypoxia. There is an association between abnormal MCA-PI and adverse neurological outcomes, but it does not help in timing delivery. Thus it is only a diagnostic parameter.

Cerebroplacental ratio: CPR is primarily a diagnostic index. In the late-onset FGR, abnormal CPR is associated with a higher risk of adverse outcomes at the induction of labor.

Uterine artery: UtA Doppler is of diagnostic value mainly in the first and second trimesters. It has limited diagnostic usefulness in the third trimester.

Ductus venosus: DV flow waveforms become abnormal only in the advanced stages of fetal compromise. Hence, it is an important prognostic parameter for FGR [31]. The absent or reversed velocities during atrial contraction are associated with perinatal mortality and are considered sufficient to recommend delivery at any gestational age, after administration of steroids [32].

Aortic isthmus: Reversed AoI flow is a sign of advanced deterioration. It is a prognostic marker that necessitates delivery.

Fetal venous circulation: As the venous changes occur in the advanced stages of cardiac decompensation, the venous parameters only help in prognostication.

Table 49.4 summarizes the clinical significance of the above fetal Doppler parameters.

TABLE 49.4 Clinical Significance of Various Fetal Doppler Parameters

Fetal Vascular Structures	Doppler Parameters With Clinical Significance
Umbilical artery	UA-PI—diagnostic A/R-UA-EDF—prognostic
Middle cerebral artery	MCA-PI—diagnostic
	CPR—diagnostic
Uterine artery	UtA-PI—diagnostic mainly in the first two trimesters
Fetal venous circulation (including ductus venosus)	DV-PI, UV pulsations, reversed A-wave in DV/IVC—prognostic
Aortic isthmus	AoI-RDF—prognostic

AoI-RDF, aortic isthmus reversed diastolic flow; *A/R-UA-EDF*, absent/reversed umbilical artery end-diastolic flow; *CPR*, cerebroplacental ratio; *DV-PI*, ductus venosus pulsatility index; *IVC*, inferior vena cava; *MCA-PI*, middle cerebral artery pulsatility index; *UA-PI*, umbilical artery pulsatility index; *UtA-PI*, uterine artery pulsatility index; *UV*, umbilical vein.

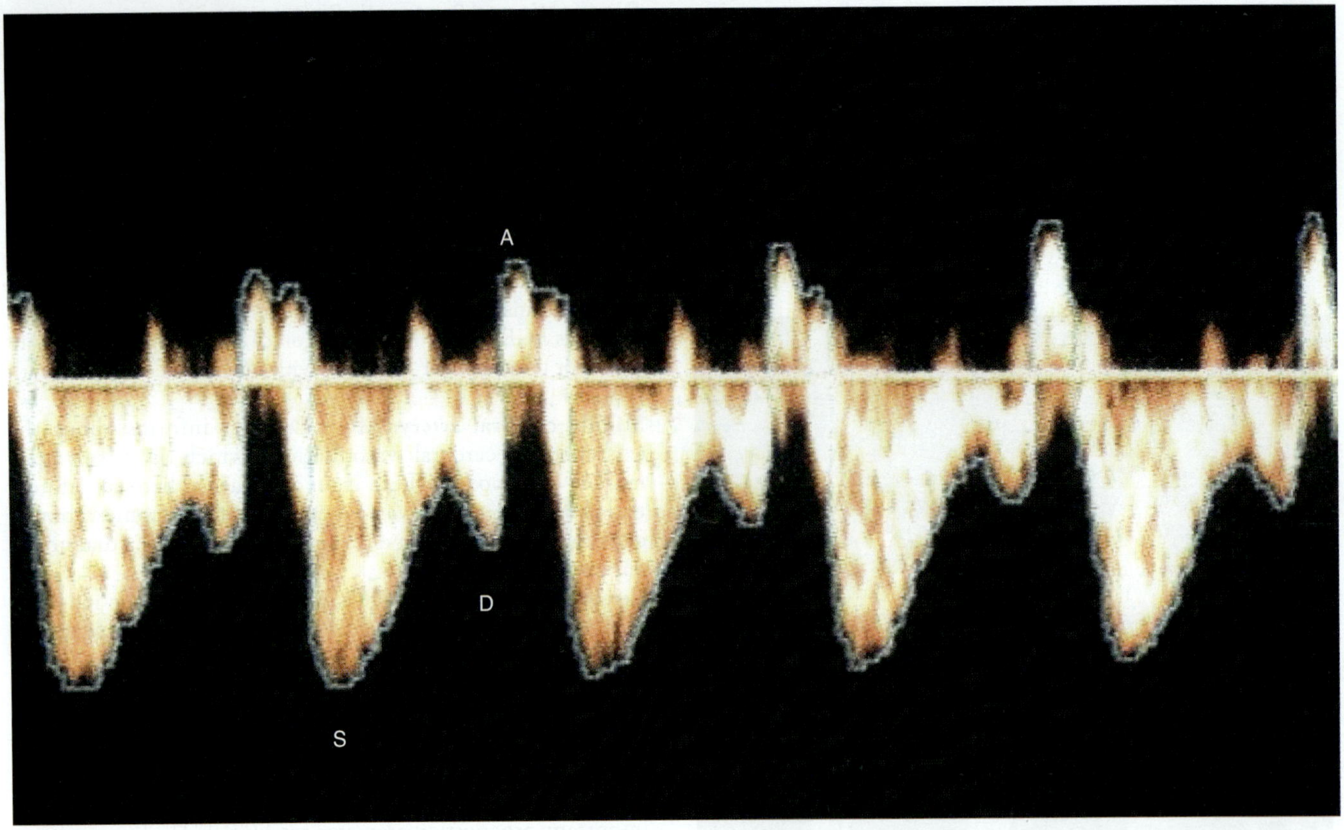

Figure 49.13 Spectral Doppler image showing normal triphasic flow in inferior vena cava. *S*, ventricular systole; *D*, ventricular diastole; *A*, atrial systole.

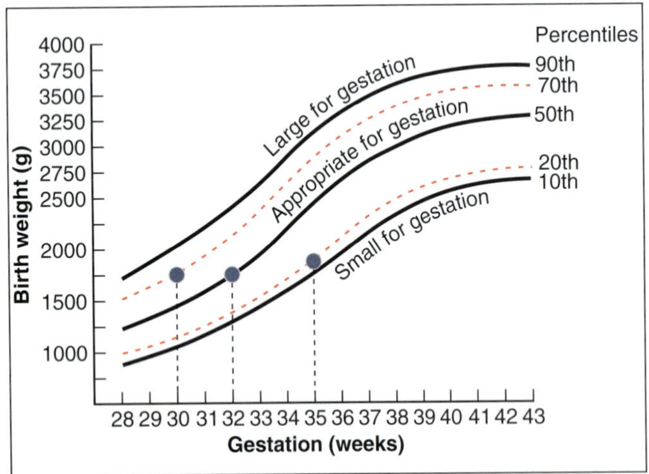

Figure 49.14 Diagnosis of fetal growth restriction (FGR) with the help of serial measurements of estimated fetal weight (EFW). All the three EFW measurements taken between the 30th and 35th weeks of gestation fell within the normal range (10th–90th percentile). However, there was a fall of nearly 50 percentiles (from 70th to 20th centile) between the two extreme readings, cementing the diagnosis of FGR.

Step 3: Define Early-Onset Versus Late-Onset FGR

FGR presents as two separate phenotypes depending on the timing of its onset during gestation. It is labeled as early-onset FGR if it occurs up to 32 weeks of gestation, else it is called late-onset FGR. Both types are believed to be caused by placental disease. However, it is not certain whether the same type of placental disease leads to each one of them. The placental insufficiency in early-onset FGR is associated with histological signs of abnormal early implantation. Late-onset FGR could be a milder manifestation of the same phenomenon or could be superimposed placental damage occurring during the second half of pregnancy.

Early-Onset FGR: Early-onset FGR, which represents 20–30% of all FGR cases [33], is often associated with severe placental insufficiency and chronic fetal hypoxia. It is commonly accompanied by preeclampsia and a typical deteriorating UA Doppler pattern: reduced forward flow > absent forward flow > reversal of diastolic flow on sequential USG scans. A similar worsening pattern is observed on DV Doppler. This allows monitoring of the progression of fetal deterioration to decide about the timing of elective delivery.

Management of early-onset FGR is quite challenging. The goal should be to achieve a balance between the risks associated with leaving fetuses in utero versus the complications of prematurity. If the condition is left untreated, acidosis develops in later stages, which is detrimental to neonatal health.

Late-Onset FGR: In contrast, late-onset FGR, accounting for nearly 70–80% of FGR cases [33], is associated with a milder degree of placental dysfunction. It is also less likely to be associated with preeclampsia and changes in UA Doppler.

Doppler findings typically observed in the late-onset FGR are as follows:

- Brain vasodilation suggesting chronic hypoxia, as reflected by an MCA PI less than the fifth percentile

- CPR less than the fifth centile
- Advanced signs of fetal deterioration with changes in DV are seldom observed
- The pattern of sequential fetal deterioration described in early-onset FGR does not occur

Once a diagnosis of late-onset FGR is established, its management is straightforward as the decision to deliver these fetuses can be taken at this time of gestation. However, there is a risk of acute fetal deterioration before labor and a high association with intrapartum fetal distress and neonatal acidosis. Thus, it lacks a "natural history" and may lead to severe injury or death without the late-stage signs seen in the early-onset FGR. Consequently, late-onset FGR contributes to a large share of late pregnancy stillbirths.

Table 49.5 discusses the differences between the two types of FGR.

Step 4: Decide Follow-Up Intervals and Delivery Timing

Once a diagnosis of FGR is established, it is important to decide follow-up intervals and timing of delivery as there is no definitive treatment of FGR. The management depends upon fetal Doppler parameters and gestational age. Delay in delivering an FGR fetus increases its exposure to hypoxia and the potential risk of acidosis, which can affect fetal brain development. In contrast, early delivery carries the risk of neonatal comorbidities due to prematurity. According to the latest International Society of Obstetrics & Gynecology (ISUOG) guidelines [35], monitoring and management options differ in early-onset FGR and late-onset FGR.

Monitoring in Early-Onset FGR: An early FGR pregnancy should be monitored and managed in a tertiary care center. At every visit, Doppler parameters are closely monitored for progressive deterioration. If they are normal, biweekly follow-up is advised. If UA parameters show progressive deterioration, or when absent or reversed UA-EDF is observed, intensive monitoring every 2–3 days is recommended [36]. The majority of women with early FGR develop hypertensive disorders of pregnancy. Therefore, regular blood-pressure documentation, monitoring of urinary protein, and baseline renal and hepatic function testing are necessary for such patients. Besides, corticosteroid prophylaxis is recommended, if delivery is planned before 34 weeks of gestation, to prevent neonatal respiratory distress syndrome [35].

Mode and Timing of Delivery: Considering the strong association with severe placental insufficiency and fetal hypoxia, a planned cesarean section is indicated in the majority of early-onset cases of FGR. It should be timed according to the following recommendations [35]:

- Delivery is indicated at any gestational age based on maternal indications if the continuation of the pregnancy is likely to adversely affect maternal health
- Between 26 + 0 and 29 + 6 weeks: Delivery is recommended if DV A-wave is at or below the baseline
- Between 30 + 0 and 31 + 6 weeks: Delivery is recommended if reversed UA-EDF is documented
- After 32 + 0 weeks: Delivery is recommended if absent UA-EDF is documented

Monitoring in Late-Onset FGR: Late-onset FGR is characterized by milder placental disease. Hence alterations in UA and venous Doppler are rare and fail to identify the vast majority of these cases. CPR may improve the prediction of adverse perinatal outcomes in late-onset FGR fetuses. If UA-PI is more than the 95th percentile or CPR is less than the fifth percentile, monitoring at least once or twice a week is indicated.

Mode and Timing of Delivery: In the absence of contraindications, induction of labor is preferred in the case of late-onset FGR. Continuous fetal heart rate monitoring is advisable during labor. One may follow the following guidelines about the timing of delivery to ensure the best outcome [35]:

- Delivery is indicated at any gestational age based on maternal indications if the continuation of the pregnancy is likely to adversely affect maternal health
- Between 34 + 0 and 35 + 6 weeks: Delivery is recommended if UA-EDF is absent or reversed
- Between 36 + 0 and 37 + 6 weeks: Delivery is recommended if UA-PI is more than 95th percentile or AC/EFW is less than third percentile
- Between 38 + 0 and 39 + 0 weeks: Delivery is recommended if there is evidence of cerebral blood-flow redistribution or any other features of FGR

TABLE 49.5 Differences Between Early and Late-Onset FGR [30,34]

	Early-Onset FGR	Late-Onset FGR
Onset	Up to 32 weeks of gestation	After 32 weeks of gestation
Diagnostic criteria	AC/EFW <3rd centile or UA-AEDF OR a. AC/EFW <10th centile along with b. UtA-PI >95th centile and/or c. UA-PI >95th centile	AC/EFW <3rd centile OR at least two of three of the following: a. AC/EFW <10th centile b. AC/EFW reducing by >2 quartiles c. CPR <5th centile or UA-PI >95th centile
Pathophysiology	Hypoxia++/ systemic cardiovascular adaptation	Hypoxia ± central cardiovascular adaptation
Placental disease	Severe; abnormal UA Doppler, preeclampsia	Mild; normal UA Doppler, low association with preeclampsia
Main challenge	Management	Detection and diagnosis
Clinical outcome	High mortality and morbidity	Lower mortality, but common cause of stillbirth; poor long-term outcome

AC, abdominal circumference; *AEDF*, absent end-diastolic flow; *CPR*, cerebroplacental ratio; *EFW*, estimated fetal weight; *UA*, umbilical artery; *UtA*, uterine artery.

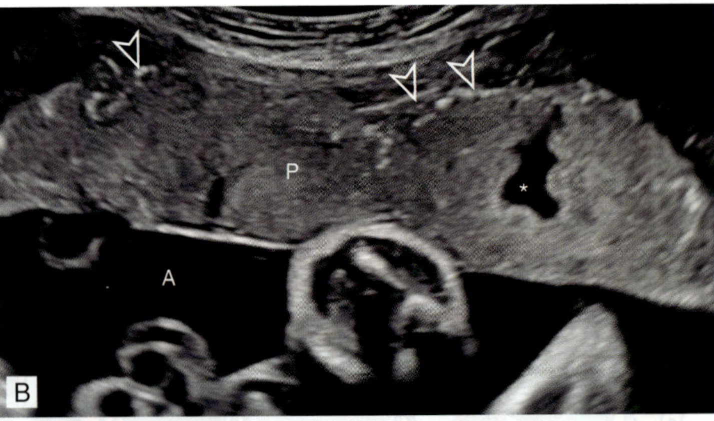

Figure 49.16 B-mode USG images of normal placenta. (A) At 20 weeks, the placenta (P) is homogenously echogenic. The retroplacental complex is seen as a hypoechoic zone behind the placenta (*white arrowheads*). The placental thickness is being measured at the midpoint of the placenta (*white dashed arrow*) where the umbilical cord inserts (*white arrow*) excluding the adjacent myometrium. (B) In the third trimester, the placenta (P) becomes inhomogeneous and shows linear calcifications along the maternal surface (*white block arrowheads*). *White asterisk*, a placental lake, *A*, amniotic fluid.

Abnormal Placental Location

Placental location can be reliably assessed with a routine transabdominal scan (TAS) by 16 weeks of gestation. It should be always mentioned in the USG report. Transvaginal sonography (TVS) is considered the gold standard for the examination of the placenta. It can reliably detect placenta regardless of placental location, even in the presence of bleeding. Translabial sonography is not commonly done but is useful when TAS is inadequate and patient compliance is poor for TVS.

Low-lying placenta: In a low-lying placenta, the inferior placental edge lies above the internal os within 2 cm of the latter. TVS is better than TAS in visualizing the lower placental edge more accurately.

Placenta previa: Derived from the Latin term *previa*, meaning "coming before, in the way," placenta previa is a condition wherein the placenta is the presenting part rather than the fetus. It is an important cause of painless vaginal bleeding in the second and third trimesters. Risk factors for this condition include previous cesarean delivery, older maternal age, multiparity, multifetal gestation, and cigarette smoking [42].

Traditionally, three types of placenta previa are described (Fig. 49.17A):

- In a complete placenta previa, the placenta completely covers the internal os
- Partial placenta previa indicates that the placenta partially covers the internal os
- In a marginal placenta previa, the placental edge just reaches the margin of the internal os

As per the new guidelines, the diagnosis of placenta previa is made when the placenta covers or just reaches the internal os (Fig. 49.17B and C); avoiding the terms "complete," "partial," and "marginal" [43].

Placental migration: Many times, low-lying placenta or placenta previa detected in the second trimester convert to normal placental location by the third trimester. This apparent migration of the placenta with advancing gestational age is well documented. The later in the gestation that a low-lying placenta or placenta previa is identified, the higher is the likelihood that it will persist until delivery. About 90% of cases of placenta previa diagnosed before 20 weeks resolve before delivery; those identified after 24 weeks continue long after in approximately 50% of the cases; whereas those identified around 32 weeks persist in nearly 75% of the cases [44]. Thus, it is important to confirm a second-trimester finding of low-lying placenta or placenta previa in the third trimester by TVS, to define the final location of the placental margin.

TABLE 49.8 Grannum Grading of Placental Maturity [40]

Placental Grade	Gestational Age During Which Normally Observed	B-Mode USG Features
Grade 0	10–17 weeks	Uniform moderate echogenicity, smooth chorionic plate without indentations
Grade I	18–29 weeks	Subtle indentations of the chorionic plate; small, diffuse calcifications randomly dispersed in the substance of the placenta
Grade II	30 weeks to term	Larger indentations along the chorionic plate; larger calcifications in a "dot-dash" configuration along the basal plate
Grade III	39 weeks onward	Complete indentations of the chorionic plate through to the basilar plate creating "cotyledons"; more irregular calcifications with substantial acoustic shadowing

TABLE 49.9 Placental Pathologies

Abnormal placental location	■ Low lying placenta ■ Placenta previa
Abnormal placental thickness	■ Thin placenta ■ Thick placenta
Abnormal placental morphology	■ Bilobed placenta ■ Succenturiate lobe ■ Circumvallate placenta ■ Circummarginate placenta ■ Placenta membranacea
Abnormal placental adherence	■ Placenta accreta ■ Placenta increta ■ Placenta percreta
Placental hematoma	■ Marginal hematoma ■ Preplacental hematoma ■ Intraplacental hematoma ■ Retroplacental hematoma
Vascular pathologies	■ Venous lakes, ■ Intervillous thrombi ■ Placental infarction
Placental masses	■ Cysts ■ Tumors (chorioangioma, teratoma)
Gestational trophoblastic disease	■ Hydatidiform mole ■ Invasive mole ■ Choriocarcinoma ■ Placental site trophoblastic tumor

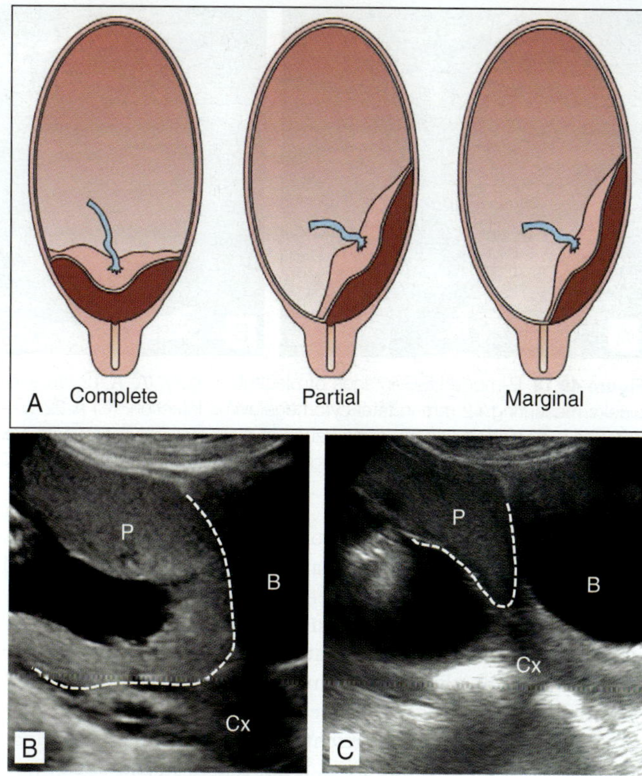

Figure 49.17 Placenta previa. (A) A schematic showing the traditional three types of placenta previa—complete, partial, and marginal. Transabdominal B-mode USG images depicting (B) the placenta completely covering the internal os and (C) the lower edge of the placenta touching the internal os. The placenta has been outlined in both the images for clarity. *P*, placenta, *Cx*, cervix, *B*, urinary bladder.

Abnormal Placental Thickness

Placentomegaly (thick placenta) can be diagnosed when the placental thickness exceeds 4 cm (the second trimester) or 6 cm (the third trimester) [38]. It is a result of various pathological processes (Table 49.10) such as certain chromosomal anomalies (e.g., triploidy, Fig. 49.18A); intrauterine infections with cytomegalovirus (Fig. 49.18B) and parvovirus, and gestational trophoblastic disease. Placentomegaly is also a component of hydrops fetalis, both immune and nonimmune types. A thick "jelly-like" placenta (also known as hyperinflated placenta, Fig. 49.18C), with mobile uniformly suspended internal echoes, is associated with an increased risk of FGR [39]. A careful fetal growth assessment and evaluation for anomalies are required once a thickened placenta is identified on prenatal sonography.

Placental thinning is rare and is generally indicative of preeclampsia or FGR. Focal placental attenuation may occur if a hematoma develops and subsequently resolves. Severe polyhydramnios tends to compress the placenta creating an illusion of a thin placenta.

TABLE 49.10 Causes of Placentomegaly

- Maternal diabetes mellitus
- Maternal/fetal anemia
- Hydrops fetalis
- Placental hemorrhage
- Intrauterine infections
- Beckwith–Wiedemann syndrome
- Hydatidiform mole (partial mole)
- Chromosomal abnormalities (e.g., triploidy)
- Confined placental mosaicism
- Placental hyperinflation
- Placental mesenchymal dysplasia (PMD)

Abnormal Placental Morphology

A *bilobed placenta* arises when a placenta develops as two separate disks of nearly equal size. The umbilical cord usually inserts between the two placental lobes into the intervening membranes (velamentous insertion) in such cases. This condition is also called "placenta duplex" or "bipartite placenta." A placenta with more than two equivalently sized lobes is termed a multilobate placenta, which is a very rare condition.

The *succenturiate lobe* is an accessory placental lobe that develops away from the main placental disk. The umbilical cord inserts into the main placenta, from which blood vessels course to the succenturiate lobe along the intervening membranes. On USG, two separate placental components are seen. The cord is usually seen inserting into the main placental lobe (Fig. 49.19). A myometrial contraction can simulate a succenturiate lobe on USG. It usually disappears on a repeat USG scan when the uterus relaxes. An undetected accessory lobe can be retained inside the uterus

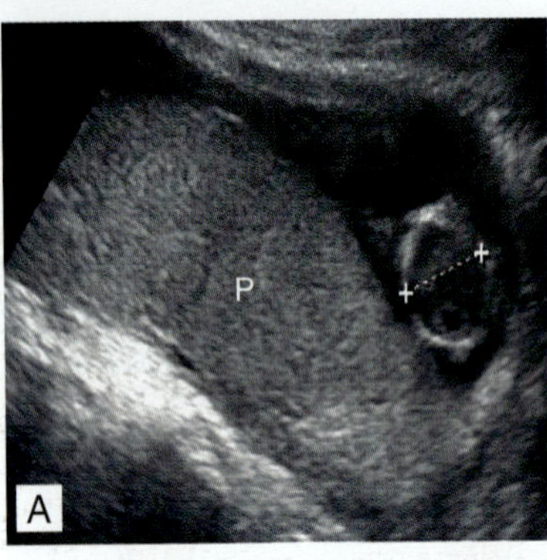

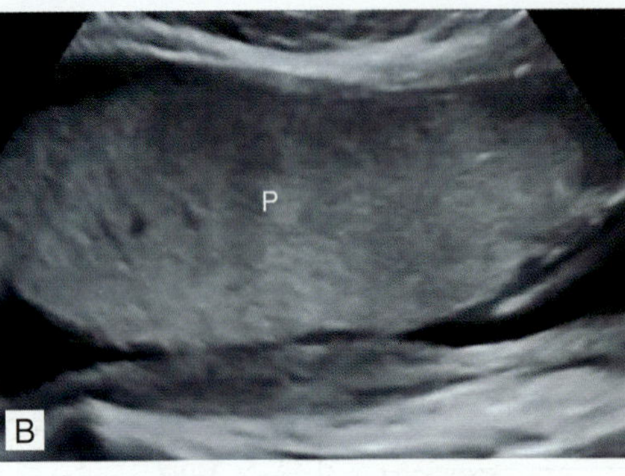

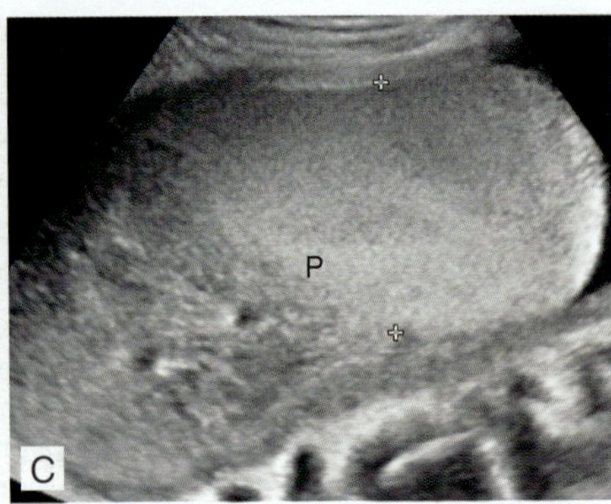

Figure 49.18 B-mode USG images of placentomegaly. (A) A 12-week-old placenta with thickness of 37 mm in a case of triploidy. (B) Placenta at 19 weeks measuring 42 mm in fetal cytomegalovirus infection. (C) A 22-week-old gestation with a hyperinflated placenta measuring 53 mm in thickness; note the hyperechoic uniform appearance of placenta. This represents areas deficient in placental villi and contain maternal blood that on real-time imaging can be seen moving slowly around the basal plate. *P*, placenta.

after delivery, which can cause postpartum complications. There is an increased incidence of vasa previa and velamentous cord insertion in the cases of the succenturiate placenta.

Circumvallate placenta is a rare embryologic abnormality in which the chorionic plate is unusually smaller than the basal plate. As a result, the amniotic membrane inserts medial to the placental edge. As it is predisposed to premature separation, the circumvallate placenta can present with second-trimester vaginal bleeding [45]. On B-mode USG, it appears as a band of elevated membranes near the placental edge, described as the "marginal shelf" (Fig. 49.20A and B).

Circummarginate placenta is an uncommon variation in placental morphology. The chorionic membranes are inserted inward from the margin of the placental edge, similar to the circumvallate placenta, but unlike the latter, the placental edge is not rolled up (Fig. 49.20C).

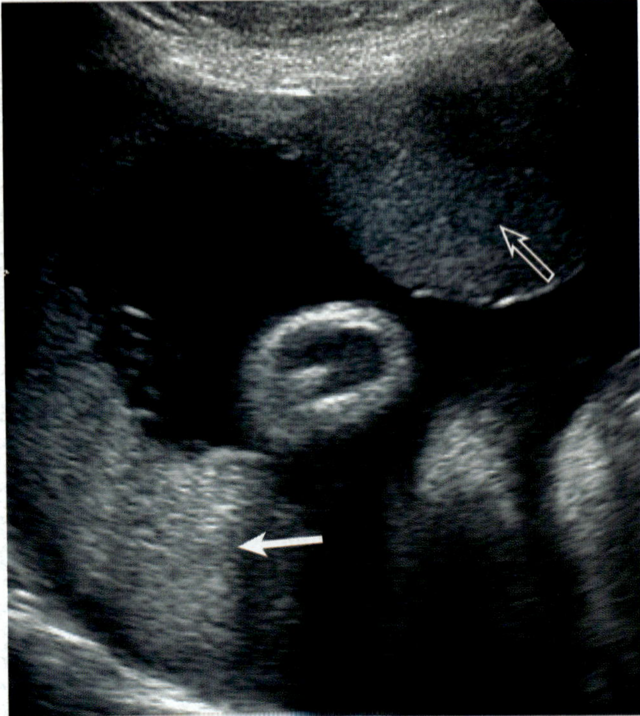

Figure 49.19 B-mode USG image of a placenta (posterior, *white arrow*) having a succenturiate lobe (anterior, *white block arrow*).

Placenta membranacea, also known as *placenta diffusa*, is another rare morphologic variation in which the placenta develops as a thin membranous structure occupying the entire periphery of the chorion.

Abnormal Placental Adherence

A morbidly adherent placenta (MAP) or abnormally invasive placenta (AIP) results from trophoblast invasion beyond the decidua basalis. In this condition, a defect in the decidua basalis allows the chorionic villi to attach directly to or to invade the myometrium. This gives rise to a high possibility of incomplete expulsion of the placenta at the time of delivery. The two most important risk factors for MAP are the previous cesarean section and placenta previa. The incidence of MAP is rising primarily as a result of an increase in cesarean deliveries. Other procedures such as myomectomy, dilation and curettage, lysis of adhesions for Asherman syndrome, and uterus septum removal also increase its risk (Table 49.11).

MAP is classified according to the depth of placental invasion into the uterine wall (Fig. 49.21) into:

- Placenta Accreta—Chorionic villi are Attached to the myometrium but do not invade into it
- Placenta Increta—Chorionic villi Invade the myometrium
- Placenta Percreta—Chorionic villi Penetrate through the entire myometrium and beyond

US features: USG is the primary diagnostic tool for MAP, with an overall sensitivity of 90.72% and specificity of 96.94% [46]. The presence of multiple vascular lacunae within the placenta (Swiss-

TABLE 49.11 Risk Factors for MAP

- Previous C-section
- Placenta previa
- Other previous uterine surgeries
- Advanced maternal age
- Multiparity
- Uterine irradiation
- Endometrial ablation
- Asherman syndrome
- Uterine leiomyoma
- Uterine anomalies
- Hypertensive disorders of pregnancy
- Smoking

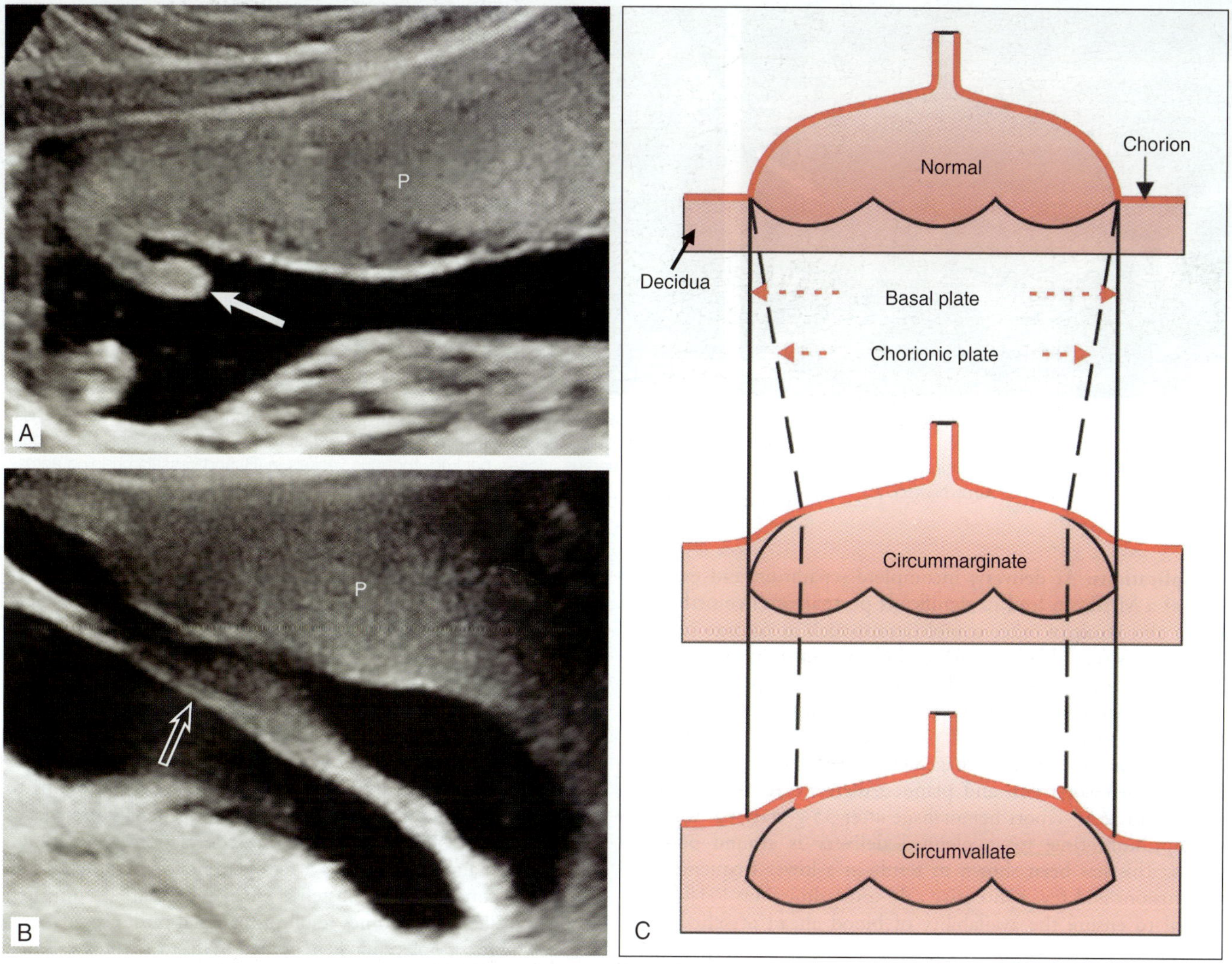

Figure 49.20 Abnormal placental morphology. (A) B-mode USG image of a longitudinal section of a circumvallate placenta showing the rolled up edge (marginal shelf, *white arrow*). (B) A transverse section image of the same placenta revealing the shelf as a thick continuous band (*white block arrow*). (C) A schematic depicting the placental morphology in a normal, circummarginate, and circumvallate placenta. *P*, placenta.

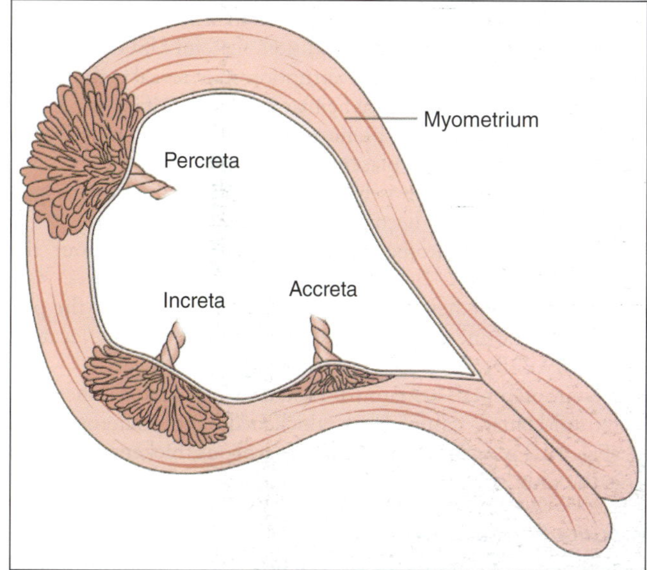

Figure 49.21 A schematic depicting the three grades of morbidly adherent placenta.

cheese appearance) on the B-mode USG is the hallmark of MAP. This finding has high sensitivity and positive predictive value for MAP in the second trimester [47], and it continues to be present in the third trimester. Additionally, the myometrial thickness is reduced to less than 1 mm leading to reduction or even complete loss of the retroplacental clear zone (Fig. 49.22A). Another finding in the third trimester is an abnormal uterine serosa-bladder interface [48]. Normally, this interface is a thin smooth line without irregularities or vascular signals. In MAP, there can be an interruption, thickening, or irregularity in the line; or increased vascularity at the interface. On color Doppler USG, turbulent lacunar blood flow is the most common finding associated with MAP (Fig. 49.22B). Other Doppler findings include increased subplacental vascularity and the appearance of vessels crossing the placenta-myometrium interface into the surrounding organs, often running perpendicular to the myometrium (Fig. 49.22C) [49].

MRI features: MRI findings suggestive of MAP are the presence of uterine bulging, heterogeneous signal intensity within the placenta, abnormal placental vascularity, focal interruptions in the myometrial wall, dark intraplacental bands on T2-weighted images, and tenting of the bladder [50]. MRI should be reserved for difficult cases in which USG is nondiagnostic, such as in obese patients.

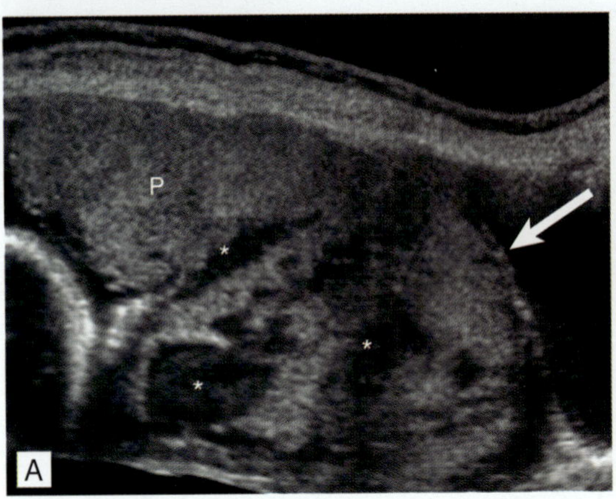

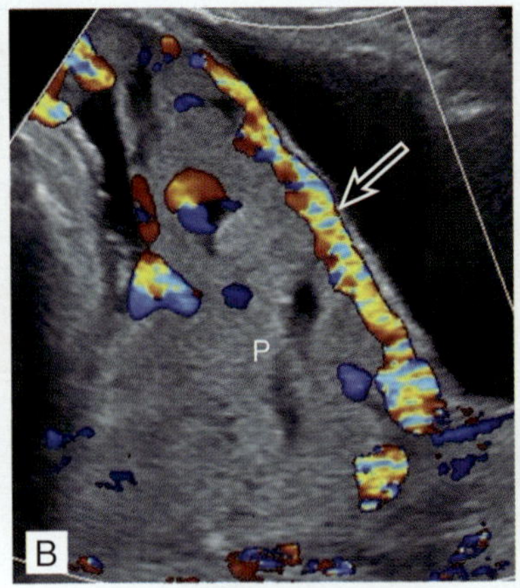

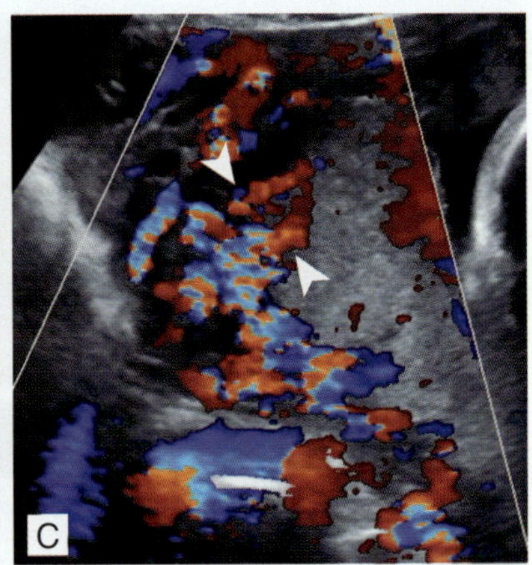

Figure 49.22 Morbidly adherent placenta. (A) B-mode USG image of a placenta increta (P) showing numerous lacunae and focal outpouching (Swiss-cheese appearance, *white asterisks*), and a thinned out myometrium with absent clear zone (*white arrow*). (B and C) Color Doppler images showing an intense aliasing signal in the placental bed (*white block arrow*) indicating numerous, closely packed, tortuous vessels in (B) and vessels bridging across the myometrium in (C) (*white arrowheads*). *P*, placenta.

Complications: At delivery, incomplete separation and expulsion of a MAP can lead to significant postpartum hemorrhage. It can also result in other complications such as damage to the local organs (e.g., bladder), AF embolism, consumptive coagulopathy, acute respiratory distress syndrome, postoperative thromboembolism, infectious morbidities, multisystem organ failure, and maternal death.

Management: Successful management of MAP is dependent on its prenatal recognition and planned delivery. As 93% of patients with MAP report hemorrhage after 35 gestational weeks, the optimum time for a planned delivery is around 34–35 weeks. This has been shown to result in a lower frequency of transfusions and fewer intensive care unit admissions [51]. It is crucial to ensure the availability of blood ahead of scheduled surgery. USG is useful for the intraoperative localization of the placenta before making a uterine incision to avoid entry through the placenta. This minimizes bleeding while delivering the fetus. If necessary, a cesarean hysterectomy may be performed while keeping the placenta attached to the uterine wall. It is a good practice to obtain patient consent in advance keeping this possibility in mind. In cases of uncontrolled peripartum pelvic hemorrhage, hypogastric artery ligation, or embolization can help minimize the blood loss.

Conservative management of MAP that involves leaving behind the leftover placenta inside the uterine cavity has been found to give promising results in terms of spontaneous resorption of the placenta in about 75% of cases [52]. However, as large-scale data supporting this finding is lacking, conservative management is generally not recommended.

Placental Hematoma

Hematoma can be found on USG at various locations within and around the placenta (Fig. 49.23A). Such patients often present with vaginal bleeding.

- Subchorionic (or marginal) hematoma is the most common presentation. It results from the rupture of the uteroplacental veins near the placental margin. It extends between the chorioamniotic membranes and the placenta proper
- Subamniotic (or preplacental) hematoma is a rare form that remains confined between the amnion and chorion
- Intraplacental hematoma is a collection of blood within the substance of the placenta
- Retroplacental hematoma occurs due to a partial or complete detachment of the placenta from the uterine wall with a hematoma confined behind the placenta

Placental Abruption

Placental abruption is the premature separation of a normally implanted placenta after 20 weeks of gestation and before the third stage of labor. It results from hemorrhage into the decidua basalis probably due to the rupture of spiral arterioles, which tends to detach the placenta from the uterine wall. It generally presents as painful vaginal bleeding with uterine contractions. Sometimes, bleeding remains concealed as a retroplacental hematoma. Acute abruption constitutes an obstetric emergency that can threaten fetal survival and sometimes result in maternal cardiovascular collapse. A large retroplacental hematoma can decrease transplacental perfusion and lead to fetal demise. Maternal risk factors for abruption include hypertension, preeclampsia, cocaine abuse, cigarette smoking, alcohol use, and advanced maternal age [53].

USG features: Placental abruption is primarily a clinical diagnosis. USG has low sensitivity and negative predictive value (24% and 53%, respectively) [54] for its detection. Therefore, a normal sonogram cannot exclude the condition. Careful USG evaluation in clinically suspected cases of abruption may reveal a thickened heterogeneous placenta. If a hematoma is identified on USG, there is an increased risk of preterm delivery. The following are the classic USG features of a placental hematoma:

- An acute hemorrhage is hyperechoic to isoechoic to the placental tissue, which becomes hypoechoic a week after
- A resolving hematoma appears sonolucent after about the second week
- A subchorionic hematoma is found at the margins of the placenta as the membranes are easily separable at this location (Fig. 49.23B)
- A retroplacental hematoma should be suspected when the retroplacental complex is thickened and heterogeneous (Fig. 49.23C). Sometimes, a heterogeneous thickened placenta is the only clue to arrive at the diagnosis

Vascular Pathologies

Sometimes, multiple hypo or anechoic focal lesions (placental sonolucencies) may be observed on USG within the placenta (Fig. 49.24A). They mostly represent a condition called *placental*

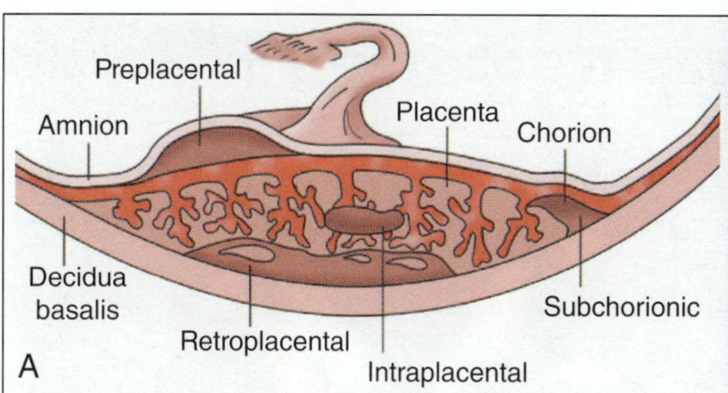

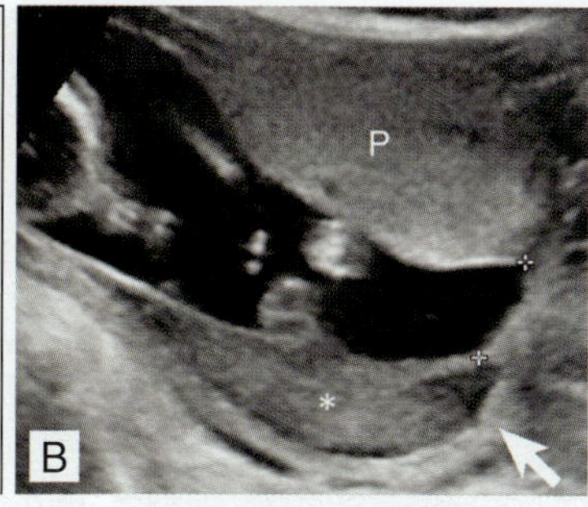

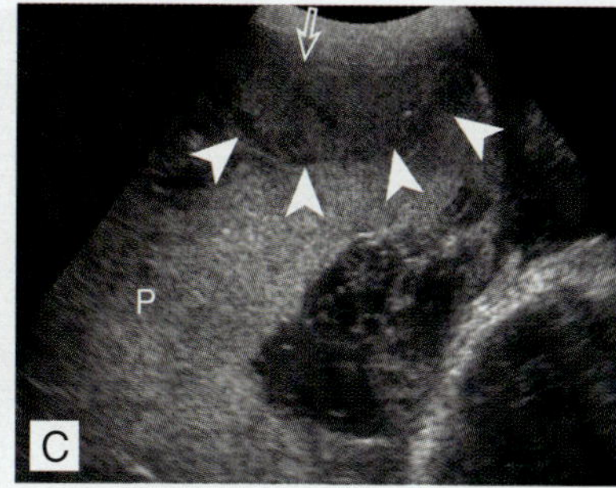

Figure 49.23 Placental hematoma. (A) A schematic showing the morphological types. B-mode USG images showing (B) a subchorionic hematoma (*white asterisk*) seen as a homogeneous isoechoic fluid collection extending from the margin of the placenta (P) tracking along the uterine wall (*white arrow*) and (C) a retroplacental hematoma visible as a large heterogeneous hypoechoic lesion separating the bulky placenta (P) from the myometrium (*white block arrow*).

venous lakes, which are enlarged intervillous spaces. It is generally considered a normal finding. In it, internal swirling echoes may be detected due to flowing blood, which can be better seen on the higher gain settings. Occasionally, the lakes get thrombosed (intervillous thrombi), which also appears hypoechoic on the B-mode USG. Color Doppler USG can distinguish the latter from the former by the absence of any color flow (Fig. 49.24B). Venous lakes may also be confused with chronic small intraplacental hematomas that appear as anechoic lesions. Other differential diagnoses include molar pregnancy, chorioangioma, and spontaneous abortion with hydropic placental changes.

Placental infarction refers to a localized area of villous ischemic necrosis. It can occur in pregnancy-induced hypertension, placental abruption, and toxoplasmosis, rubella, cytomegalovirus, herpes simplex (TORCH) infections. On USG, it appears as a hyperechoic mass or placental thickening.

Placental Masses

Placental masses appear either as anechoic cystic lesions or as solid appearing lesions on USG. Solid appearing lesions are divided into trophoblastic and nontrophoblastic tumors. The latter include chorioangiomas, teratomas, hemangiomas, and metastases. Placental infarctions may also have a mass-like appearance.

Placental cysts may occur under the fetal plate (subchorionic) or within the placental tissue (septal). They are usually benign and do not alter obstetric management. On USG, they appear as anechoic thin-walled structures along the placental surface without any vascularity.

Placental chorioangioma is the most common benign tumor of the placenta. It is a hamartoma that arises as a malformation of the placental primitive angioblastic tissue. It is most commonly located on the fetal side of the placenta near the cord insertion point. Lesions greater than 5 cm can lead to polyhydramnios [55], while smaller lesions have no clinical significance. On USG, it appears as a well-defined, encapsulated, and hypoechoic intraplacental lesion with or without calcification. Doppler examination sometimes reveals a feeder vessel (Fig. 49.25). Chorioangiomas, with an extremely elevated flow, are commonly associated with adverse perinatal outcomes. Such pregnancies warrant a close follow-up, as well as surveillance for polyhydramnios and other signs of fetal hydrops [56].

Placental teratoma is a rare benign tumor. On USG, it appears as a soft tissue placental mass with variable echogenicity. Calcifications are almost always seen within the mass, which is a characteristic feature.

Placental metastases are very rare. They mostly originate from melanomas. On USG, they appear as hyperechoic or hypoechoic masses. A multiplicity of lesions favors their diagnosis. However, a history of a primary malignancy is essential before making the diagnosis.

Gestational Trophoblastic Disease

Gestational trophoblastic disease is a heterogeneous group of lesions arising from the placental trophoblastic tissue. It includes partial and complete hydatidiform mole, invasive mole, choriocarcinoma, and placental site trophoblastic tumor. This condition should be suspected when a greater than appropriate level of serum HCG is detected.

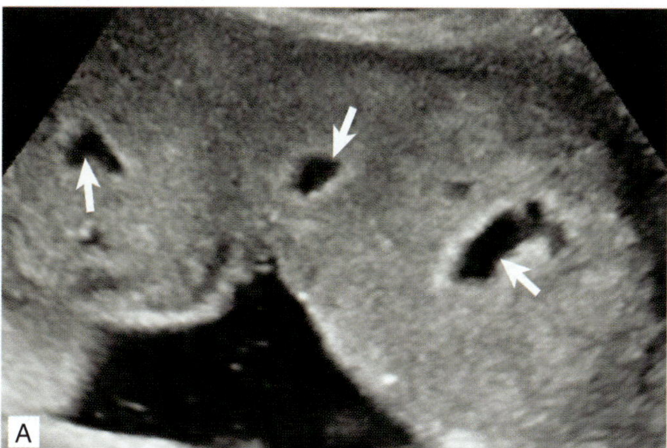

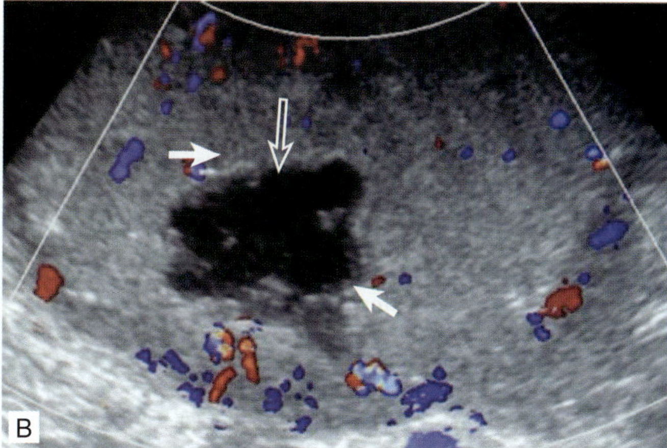

Figure 49.24 Placental sonolucency. (A) B-mode USG image of a 26 weeks' placenta showing multiple well-defined hypoechoic lesions (*white arrows*). (B) Color Doppler image showing a lack of flow within a thrombosed sonolucency (*white block arrow*).

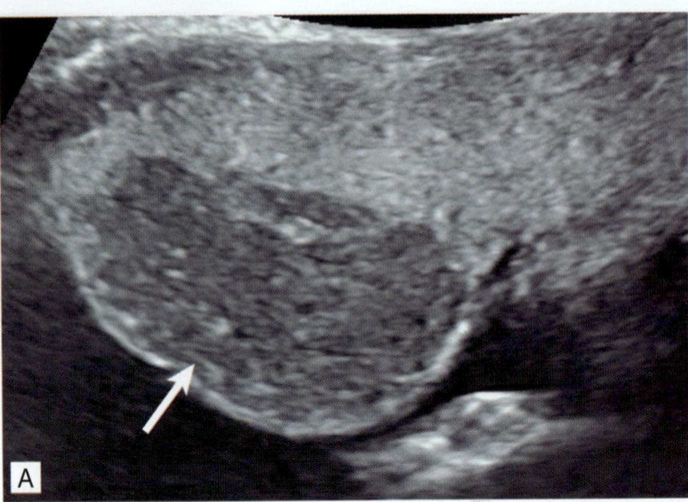

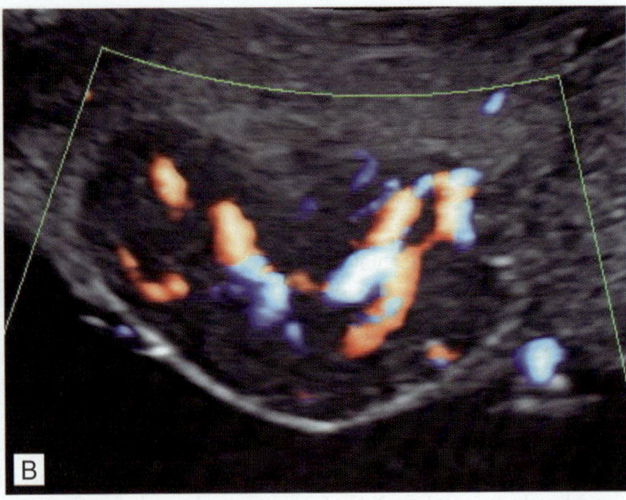

Figure 49.25 Placental chorioangioma (A) B-mode USG image showing an inhomogeneous hypoechoic well-defined ovoid mass (*white arrow*) within the placenta (P). (B) On color Doppler, hypervascularity was noted within the lesion.

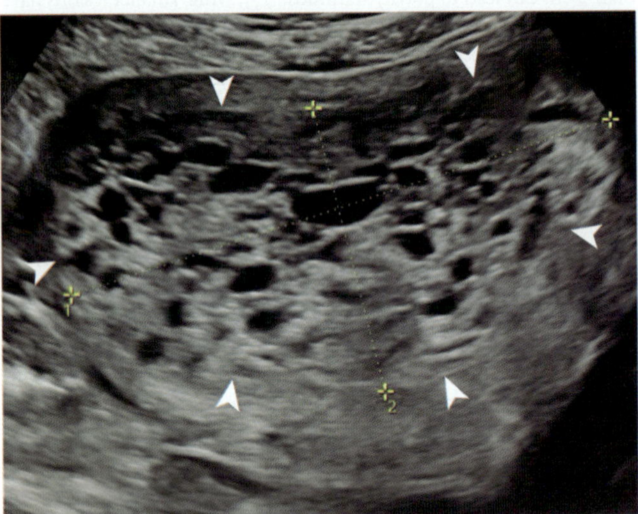

Figure 49.26 Complete hydatidiform mole. A B-mode USG image showing a large heterogeneous lesion (*white arrowheads*) within the endometrial cavity showing multiple variable size cysts.

A partial hydatidiform mole shows the presence of fetal parts, unlike a complete mole. A complete molar pregnancy in the first trimester exhibits an enlarged uterus and the endometrial cavity is filled with heterogeneous vascular hyperechoic tissue with small cysts on USG (Fig. 49.26). The appearance of an echogenic mass containing multiple anechoic spaces is described as the "Swiss cheese" or "snowstorm" appearance. Doppler USG shows high velocity and low resistance flow within the lesion. The ovaries may contain bilateral theca lutein cysts. Coexistent mole and pregnancy may be seen in a dizygotic twin pregnancy. Hydatidiform mole is a benign entity. However, it can differentiate into an invasive mole, placental site trophoblastic disease, or choriocarcinoma (the latter three are collectively known as "gestational trophoblastic neoplasia)."

Invasive mole and choriocarcinoma are manifestations of persistent trophoblastic proliferation. High levels of HCG after the treatment or abortion of a molar pregnancy suggests a persistent trophoblastic process. USG is the initial examination of choice in such cases. Doppler USG demonstrates a mass invading into the myometrium with a high-velocity, low-impedance flow [57]. Cross-sectional imaging is always advised in these conditions for the accurate assessment of local and distant spread.

Placental Membranes: In early pregnancy, the amnion and chorion are separated by the exocoelomic cavity. These layers later fuse and line the entire uterine cavity as the chorioamnion. Any alterations in this relationship create abnormal structures that are sometimes identified as bands on USG. These structures can be mistaken for other common sonologic findings such as the thick dividing membrane of dichorionic (DC) twin gestation, the linear echoes overlying a resorbed placental hematoma, the curled peripheral edge of a circumvallate placenta, uterine septum, or the membranes from vanishing twins.

Amniotic Sheet: Uterine synechiae are linear bands of scar tissue within the uterus, which commonly develop secondary to previous uterine surgery such as curettage. During pregnancy, the chorioamnion covers the synechiae like a sheet; which appears as a thick, linear echogenic structure with a broad base attached to the placental margin; extending from one wall of the uterine cavity across to the other (Fig. 49.27). It does not generally hamper the fetal movements and does not cause any fetal damage.

Amniotic Bands: Amniotic bands are theorized to develop due to an early rupture of the amnion, which gives rise to these "sticky" mesodermal bands from the underlying chorion entangling various fetal structures. These bands cut across, constrict, or amputate fetal parts leading to various fetal malformations ranging from minor defects such as limb abnormalities, amputation of extremities, to more complex body wall defects, craniofacial defects, and sometimes gross defects noncompatible with life [58]. Amputation of digits is common, and fetal hands are involved more often than the feet [59]. An amniotic band typically appears as a wispy thin strand extending from the uterine wall and tethering the fetal parts (Fig. 49.28). A short and straight umbilical cord is a common accompaniment to this finding.

Umbilical Cord

The mature umbilical cord contains two umbilical arteries and one umbilical vein embedded in the Wharton jelly. The cord plays a critical role in normal fetal development and well-being and requires careful USG assessment. The three-vessel cord is best examined at the level of urinary bladder on color Doppler USG (Fig. 49.29). Its insertion over the placenta and the fetal abdomen should be always documented at 20 weeks. Some cord abnormalities are associated with other fetal structural and chromosomal anomalies. If such anomalies are diagnosed, a thorough fetal USG

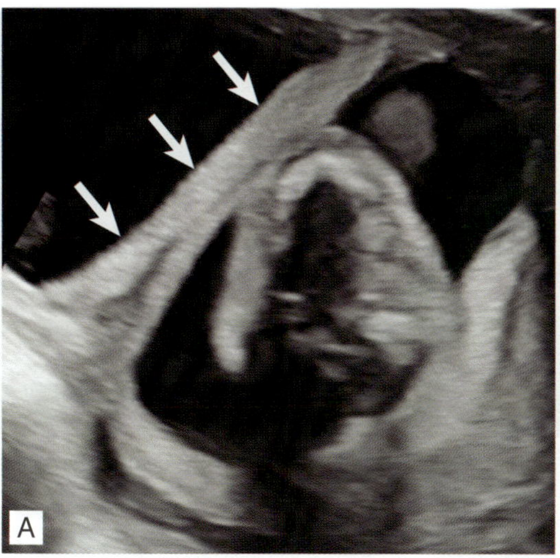

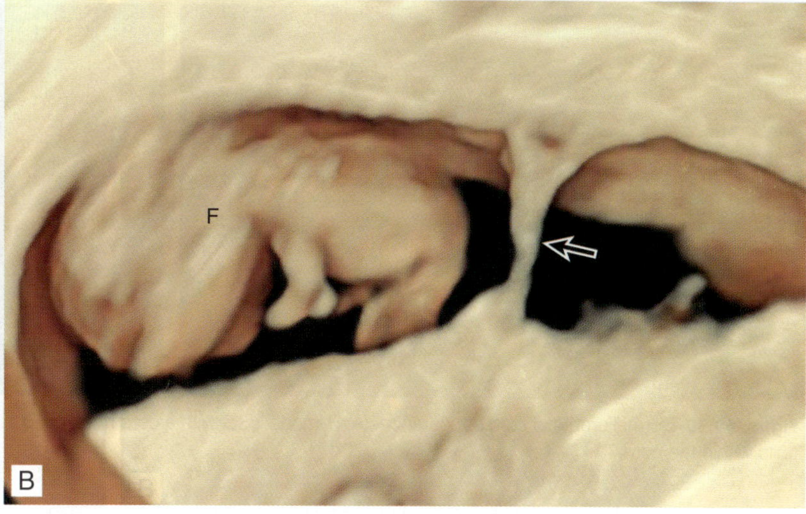

Figure 49.27 Amniotic sheet. (A) B-mode USG image showing a linear, echogenic tissue (*white arrows*) that appears to project into the amniotic cavity, although it is extra-amniotic in location. (B) 3-D-USG image showing an amniotic sheet (*white block arrow*) in a different patient. *F*, fetus.

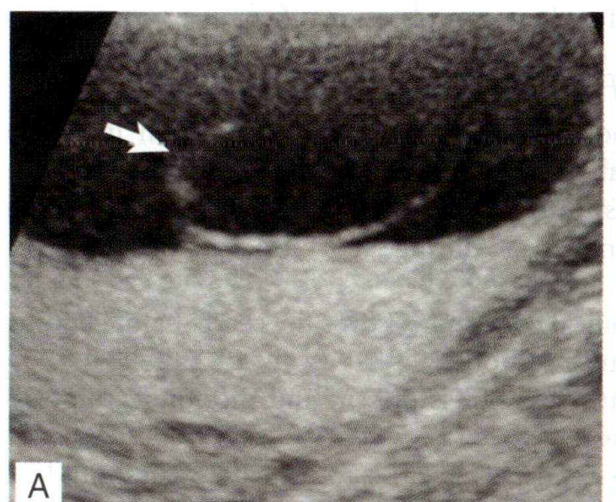

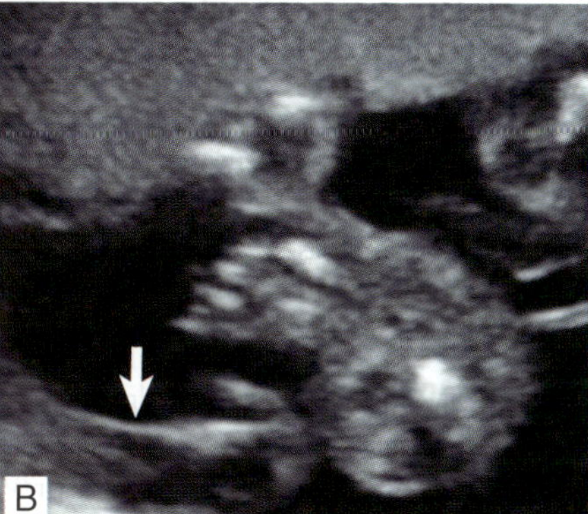

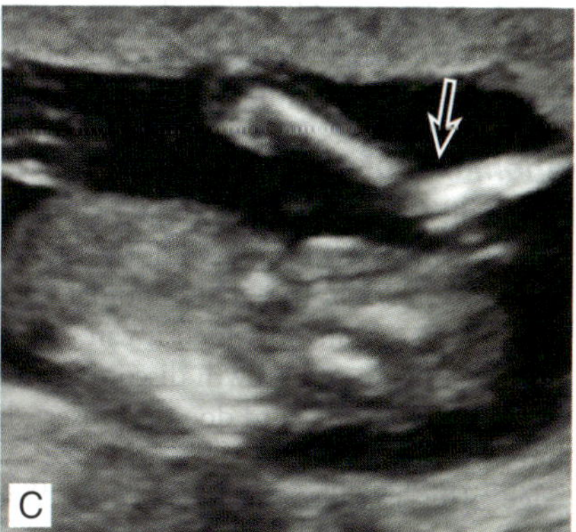

Figure 49.28 B-mode USG images depicting amniotic bands. (A and B) Seen as subtle thin linear structures (*white arrows*). (C) Abnormal position of the upper extremity (*white block arrow*) is a clue to actively search for the amniotic bands.

TABLE 49.12 Umbilical Cord Anomalies

Type of Anomaly	Examples
Morphologic anomalies	Shorter or longer cord, hyper- or hypocoiling, increased or decreased thickness
Anomalies of cord insertion	Marginal insertion, velamentous insertion
Abnormal cord presentation	Vasa previa
In utero distortion	Cord knot, cord entanglement
Vascular anomalies	SUA, PRUV, umbilical vein varix
Cord tumors	Cysts, hemangioma, angiomyxoma, teratoma, hamartoma

PRUV, persistent right umbilical vein; *SUA*, single umbilical artery.

anatomic survey is necessary. Various cord anomalies are discussed later and summarized in Table 49.12.

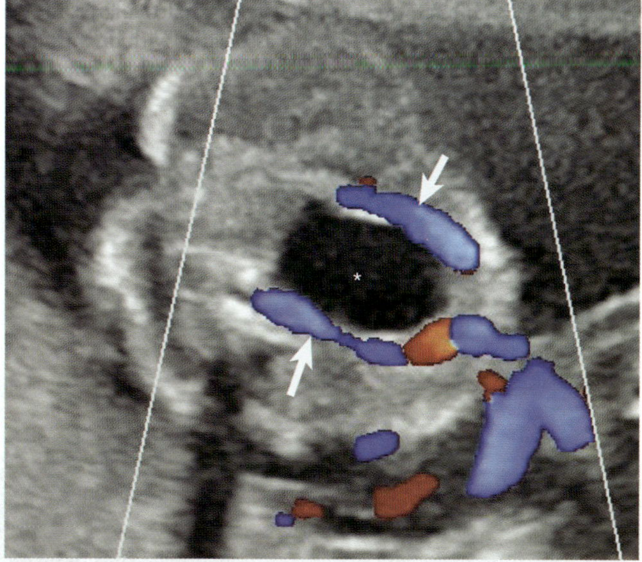

Figure 49.29 Color Doppler USG demonstrating the two umbilical arteries (*white arrows*) encircling the fetal bladder (*white asterisk*).

Morphologic Anomalies

A normal umbilical cord is less than 2 cm in diameter (Fig. 49.30) [60] and measures between 40 and 70 cm in length. It contains up to 40 helical turns (i.e., one coil per 5 cm, or an umbilical coiling index of 0.20–0.24 coils per cm) [61]. A thinner cord is associated with an increased prevalence of FGR, oligohydramnios, and fetal distress during delivery [60]. A thicker cord is seen in mothers with diabetes and fetuses with aneuploidy [62]. However, measurement of cord thickness on USG is not indicated as a routine procedure

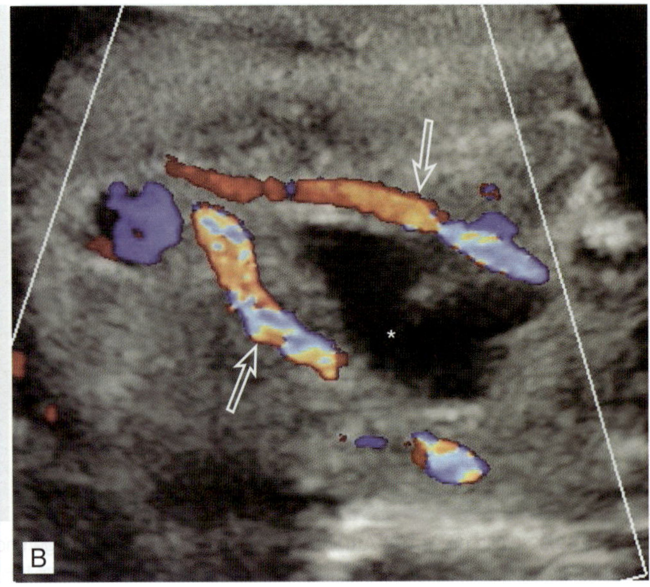

Figure 49.34 Single umbilical artery. (A) Color Doppler USG showing the absence of one of the two umbilical arteries (*white arrow*). (B) A normal color Doppler USG for comparison showing two umbilical arteries (*white block arrows*) traversing around the urinary bladder (*white asterisk*).

should be pursued. Demonstration of the absent intra-abdominal segment of the missing UA at the level of the urinary bladder on color Doppler is the best USG technique to diagnose this condition (Fig. 49.34).

Occasionally, the *right umbilical vein persists* and the left one atrophies. This can be associated with cardiovascular and renal anomalies [73]. In the transverse section USG of the fetal abdomen, the vein is seen curving to the left toward the stomach and connecting to the right portal vein instead of the left. The gall bladder and stomach are seen on the same side of the vein (Fig. 49.35).

Normally, the diameter of the intra-abdominal portion of the fetal umbilical vein measures approximately 3 mm at 15 weeks of gestation and 8 mm at term [74]. In an *umbilical vein varix*, which is a focal dilatation of the umbilical vein, the dilated intra-abdominal extrahepatic portion of the vein has a diameter of more than 9 mm. Also, it is at least 50% larger than the intrahepatic portion (Fig. 49.36). There is an increased risk of aneuploidies, fetal hydrops, anemia, and intra uterine growth restriction [75]; which necessitates targeted sonographic evaluation. Generally, the pregnancy outcome is favorable when it is an isolated finding. Rarely, a thrombus in the dilated segment blocks fetal venous circulation causing fetal death [76].

Cord Tumors

Cord cysts are an isolated finding appearing as an anechoic lesion on USG. True cysts originate from embryonic remnants such as allantois and omphalomesenteric duct and are internally lined by epithelial. Pseudocysts are without an epithelial lining and appear secondary to local degeneration of the Wharton jelly. The former are detected roughly in 4% of the first-trimester pregnancies of which 20% persist in the second trimester. They have no clinical significance [77].

Solid tumors of the cord include hemangioma, angiomyxoma, hamartoma, and teratoma. On USG, hemangiomas appear as either echogenic or multicystic. Demonstration of flow with color Doppler helps to differentiate them from other cord tumors [78]. Teratomas appear heterogeneous due to the presence of both solid and cystic components.

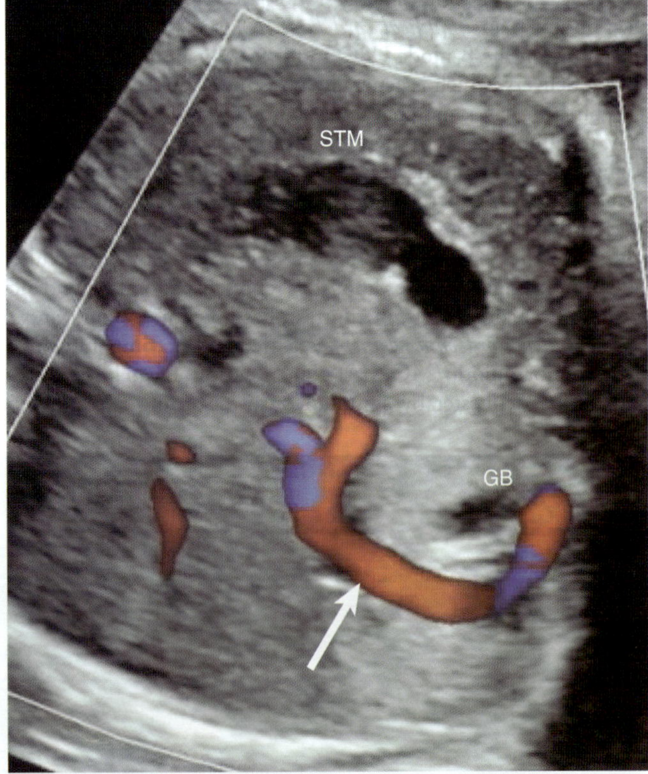

Figure 49.35 Persistent right umbilical vein. B-mode USG image with color Doppler showing the abdominal course of the right umbilical vein (*white arrow*) that is seen curving with its concavity to the left toward the stomach (STM). The stomach and the gall bladder (GB) are seen on the same side of the umbilical vein.

Amniotic Fluid

AF is essential for a developing fetus. It protects the fetus from trauma, provides a source of water, allows normal fetal movements that are important for musculoskeletal development, and contribute to fetal lung maturation. Hence, the estimation of the

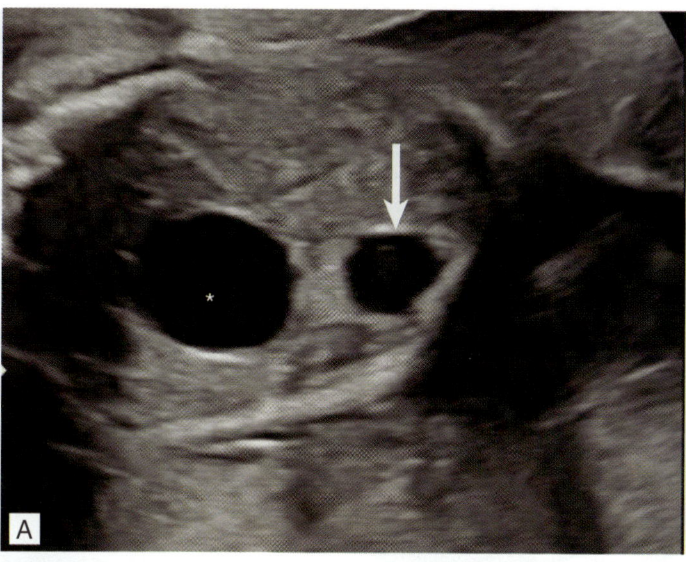

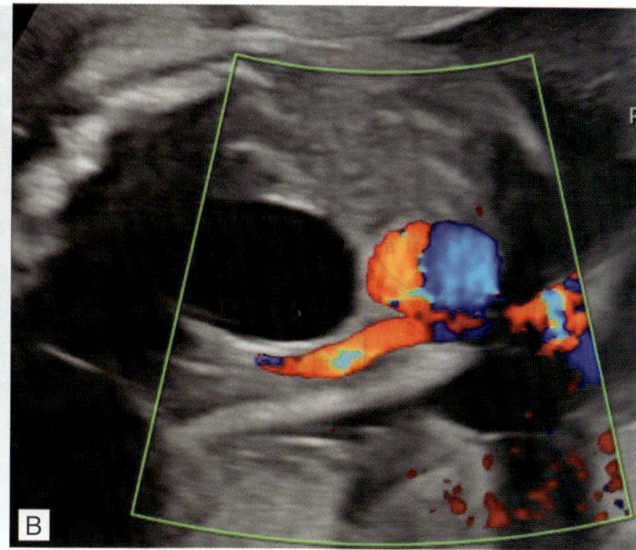

Figure 49.36 Umbilical vein varix. (A) B-mode USG image showing a cystic structure (*white arrow*) in the lower fetal abdomen adjacent to the urinary bladder (*white asterisk*). (B) On color Doppler examination, the lesion showed a color flow and was seen in continuation with umbilical vein.

AF volume (AFV) is an essential component of every prenatal USG examination.

AF Dynamics

Several fetal factors influence AF dynamics. They include fetal urine production, fetal swallowing, fetal lung fluid production, the intramembranous pathway (movement of water and solutes between the AF and the placenta), the transmembranous pathway (movement of water and solutes across the surface area of the chorioamnion), secretions by the fetal oronasal cavities, and movement of fluid across the fetal skin during early gestation [79].

Determination of AFV

The true AFV can be determined with the dye dilution technique using amniocentesis or at the time of cesarean delivery [80]. As this technique is not feasible routinely, AFV can be estimated using alternative subjective and objective techniques.

Subjective Assessment: A quick real-time eyeballing method of estimating AFV consists of comparing the anechoic AF with the space occupied by the fetus and placenta, which is based on the sonologist's experience. Using this technique, AF volume can be graded as decreased, increased, or normal. The disadvantages of subjective assessment are operator dependency and difficulty in assessment on follow-up scans.

Objective Assessment

The quantitative assessment of AF volume can be carried out using either the AF index (AFI) [81] or the deepest vertical pocket (DVP) method [82].

AF index: For the measurement of the AFI, a USG transducer is kept in the maternal sagittal plane while the patient is lying supine. The maternal abdomen is divided into four quadrants with the help of the transverse line at the umbilicus and the midsagittal line (Fig. 49.37A). The DVP of AF, not containing any fetal parts and umbilical cord, is measured in each quadrant (Fig. 49.37B) and the four measurements are added together to obtain the AFI. AFI of 8–24 cm is considered normal depending on the gestational age. It increases exponentially from the early gestation up to 30 weeks. It plateaus between 30 and 36 weeks and decreases thereafter [83]. AFI nomograms according to the gestational age are available. A value of 5 cm or less is associated with the markers of increased risk of adverse pregnancy and neonatal outcomes; such as nonreactive nonstress tests (NST), fetal heart rate decelerations, meconium staining, cesarean delivery for labor intolerance, and low Apgar score [84].

Deepest vertical pocket: DVP, alternatively known as the maximum vertical pocket, is the largest single vertical pocket of AF that is at least 1 cm in width not containing the fetal parts and umbilical cord. Color Doppler can be particularly useful to rule out the presence of umbilical cord coils within an AF pocket that may not be appreciated on B-mode images [85].

AFV grading based on AFI and DPV is summarized in Table 49.13.

Oligohydramnios

Oligohydramnios is suspected clinically when the fundal height is less than expected for the gestational age, or if the patient complains of leaking vaginal fluid. It is diagnosed on USG when AFI is less than or equal to 5 cm or DVP is less than 2 cm. Once oligohydramnios is detected, one should follow the checklist mentioned in Table 49.14. Various causes contributing to oligohydramnios are discussed in Table 49.15.

Prolonged oligohydramnios from any cause increases the risk of fetal pulmonary hypoplasia [87]. Severe oligohydramnios may result in deformation syndromes such as craniofacial deformities and positional deformation of fetal hands and feet

TABLE 49.13 AFV Grading Based on AFI and DVP [86]

AFI-Based Grading	DVP-Based Grading
Normal: AFI between 8 and 24 cm	Oligohydramnios: DVP <2 cm
Marginal oligohydramnios: AFI between 5 and 8 cm	Polyhydramnios: DVP ≥8 cm
Oligohydramnios: AFI ≤5 cm	
Anhydramnios: the absence of any detectable AF	
Polyhydramnios: AFI ≥24 cm	

AF, amniotic fluid; *AFI*, amniotic fluid index; *AFV*, amniotic fluid volume; *DVP*, deepest vertical pocket.

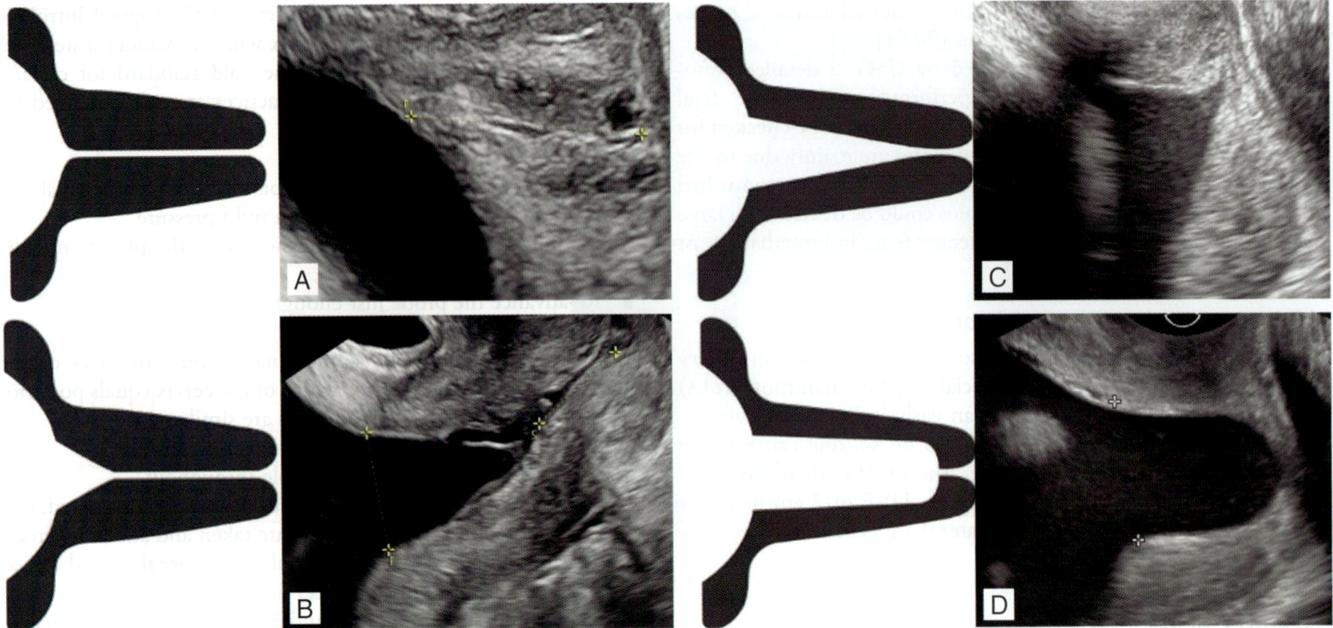

Figure 49.39 Stages of cervical incompetence (schematic along with associated B-mode images). (A) T-shaped cervix, (B) Y-shaped cervix, (C) V-shaped cervix, and (D) U-shaped cervix.

- Y-shaped cervix wherein the internal os starts opening up and the vertical arm of "Y" represents the closed cervical length,
- V-shaped cervix in which no measurable closed cervical length can be observed, and
- U-shaped cervix has a rounded shape at the external os in addition to the absence of a measurable closed cervical length.

In the case of funneling, the open portion of the cervix (funnel length) and the internal os diameter (funnel width) should be measured. The percentage of funneling is calculated as the funnel length divided by the total cervical length. Functional or closed cervical length is a good prognostic marker. When it is less than 10 mm, the pregnancy outcome tends to be poor [96]. The U-shaped funneling is more likely to be associated with preterm birth compared with the V-shaped funneling [97].

Twins

The incidence of multifetal gestation has increased dramatically in recent decades due to the increased use of assisted reproductive technologies. USG plays a central role in the assessment of multiple gestations. It not only helps diagnose the condition, but it is also quite useful in determining the number of fetuses and the placental status early in the gestation. This allows the counseling of parents about the potential risks associated with the pregnancy, timely screening for these risks, and the institution of treatment if required.

Embryology

Fertilization of one ovum by one sperm with subsequent division into two embryos gives rise to monozygotic or identical twins. Dizygotic or fraternal twins, in contrast, arise due to the fertilization of two individual ova by two sperms (Fig. 49.40). Zygosity refers to the genetic constitution of a twin pregnancy, while chorionicity and amnionicity describe the placentation and membrane composition of pregnancy. A DC pregnancy exists with two separate placental disks (two chorions), whereas in an MC pregnancy the twins share a single placental disk (one chorion). MC twins are at an increased risk of adverse outcomes. Similarly, a pregnancy with two different amniotic cavities is described as DA, while one with a single amniotic cavity is called MA. A dizygotic pregnancy is always DC–DA.

The effect of the timing of cleavage of the early conceptus in monozygotic twins on the type of placentation is described in chapter "Obstetrics (first trimester)." DC placentation is present in approximately one-third of monozygotic twins while MC placentation occurs in about two-third of the cases. MA pregnancies are much less common in occurrence.

Sonographic Evaluation of Chorionicity

During the first trimester, TVS is accurate at revealing the chorionicity of a twin gestation (Table 49.16). At that time, the

TABLE 49.16 Sonographic Determination of the Type of Twinning in the First Trimester

Type of Twinning	Number of Gestation Sacs	Number of Yolk Sacs	Number of Embryos Per Sac	Number of Amniotic Cavities
Dichorionic-diamniotic	2	2	1	2
Monochorionic-diamniotic	1	2	2	2
Monochorionic-monoamniotic	1	1	2	1

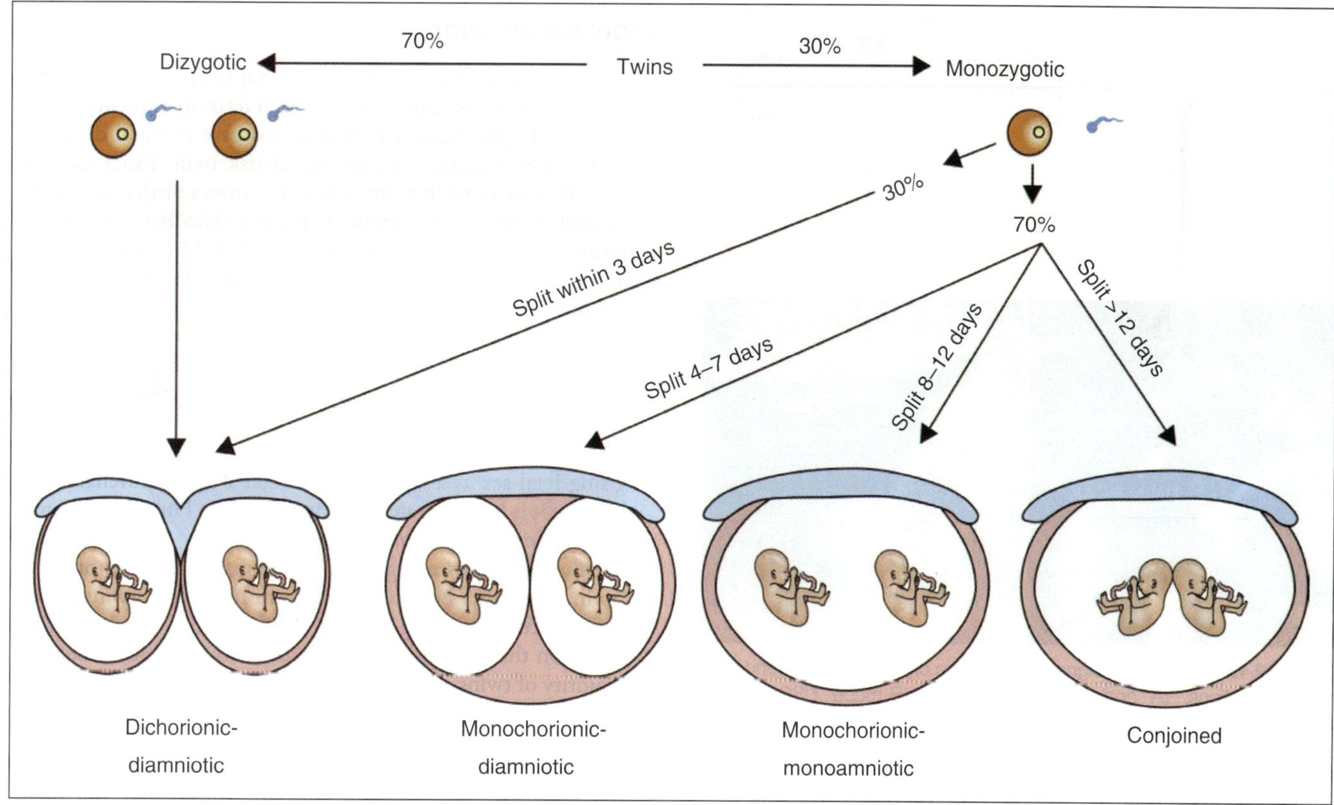

Figure 49.40 Embryology of twin gestation.

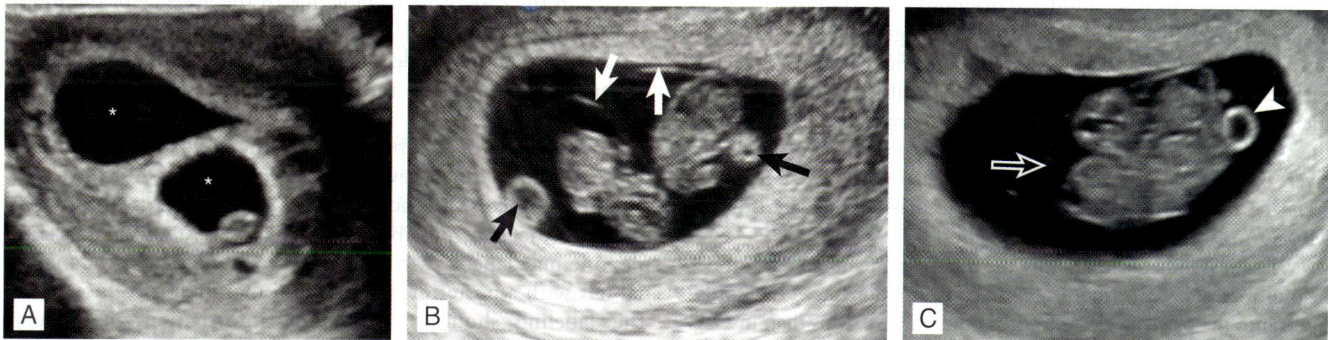

Figure 49.41 First trimester B-mode USG images of multiple gestations. (A) A dichorionic-diamniotic twin with two separate gestational sacs (*white asterisks*). (B) A monochorionic-diamniotic gestation having single gestational sac but two yolk sacs (*black arrows*) and two amnions (*white arrows*). (C) A monochorionic-monoamniotic twin showing a single gestational sac, yolk sac (*white arrowhead*), and amnion (*white block arrow*).

number of gestational sacs equals the number of chorions (Fig. 49.41), while the presence of two yolk sacs confirms the presence of two amnions.

After the first trimester, the placenta becomes visible on USG. Visualization of two separate placentas generally indicates dichorionicity.

During this period, various sonographic signs assist in distinguishing between DC and MC twins (Table 49.17). The separating membrane tends to be thicker in DC twins as it is composed of two layers of amnion and chorion each, compared with only two layers of amnion in MC twins. Membrane thickness of 2 mm has traditionally been considered as a threshold, but it lacks reliability as a

TABLE 49.17 Ultrasonography Features of Placentation After the First Trimester

Type of Placentation	Number of Placentas	Intertwin Membrane	Umbilical Cord Insertion	Fetal Genders
Dichorionic-diamniotic	2	Thick (lambda sign)	Far apart	Discordant or concordant
Monochorionic-diamniotic	1	Thin (T sign)	Closer	Concordant
Monochorionic-monoamniotic	1	None	Closer	Concordant

TABLE 49.20 Morphologic Features Present in Twin–Twin Transfusion Syndrome

Feature	Recipient Twin	Donor Twin
Size	Large	Small
Amniotic fluid	Increased	Decreased
Mobility	Increased	Restricted
Urinary bladder	Distended	Small/empty
Umbilical cord	Enlarged	Small to normal
Blood volume	Increased	Decreased
Complications	Cardiomyopathy, hydrops, death	Stuck twin phenomenon, FGR, hypoxia, death

FGR, fetal growth restriction.

- Artery-to-artery (A–A) connections; which are superficial, bidirectional, and protective against TTTS
- Artery-to-vein (A–V) connections; which are deep, unidirectional, unbalanced connections associated with TTTS
- Vein-to-vein (V–V) connections; which are superficial, bidirectional, and of less clinical significance

Thus, the predominance of A–V connections in TTTS leads to an imbalance of blood exchange wherein one fetus receives more blood (the recipient) than the other (the donor). As a result, the recipient twin becomes polyuric and polycythemic, while the donor becomes oliguric and anemic. Eventually, the donor develops a classic growth restriction sequence whereas the recipient may develop high output cardiac failure with severe hydrops. The onset of these events in TTTS is unpredictable. Table 49.20 summarizes various features of the recipient and donor twins (Fig. 49.46).

The pathognomonic USG features of TTTS include:

- Oligohydramnios in the donor sac, defined as DVP of ≤2 cm
- Polyhydramnios in the recipient sac, defined as DVP of ≥8 cm
- An oliguric donor twin with a small or empty bladder
- A polyuric recipient twin with a persistently distended bladder

Sometimes it is difficult to detect the intertwin membrane on USG as it is wrapped closely around the donor or "stuck" twin (Fig. 49.47). Care should be taken not to falsely label such MC–DA twins as MC–MA twins, and the membrane should be actively searched for around the fetal limbs, especially during fetal movements. Once a diagnosis of TTTS is made, Doppler should always be done for the staging of TTTS. A staging system by Quintero [112] is described in Table 49.21.

Screening for TTTS: In an MC twin pregnancy, screening for TTTS should start at 16 weeks' gestation, with scans repeated every 2 weeks thereafter. At every scan, one should look for the evidence of membrane folding carefully, and measure the DVP for each fetus along with biometry for EFW assessment. If there is just an AF discordance with no signs of TTTS then further follow-up scans should be done every week to exclude the progression to TTTS. When TTTS is diagnosed, the patient should be referred to a tertiary care center.

Management: A timely diagnosis of TTTS is crucial, as more advanced stages tend to have a worse prognosis. Without treatment, the perinatal mortality rate in advanced TTTS is 70–100%, while it reduces to 50–70% following intervention with laser therapy [113]. When severe TTTS is detected before 16 gestational weeks,

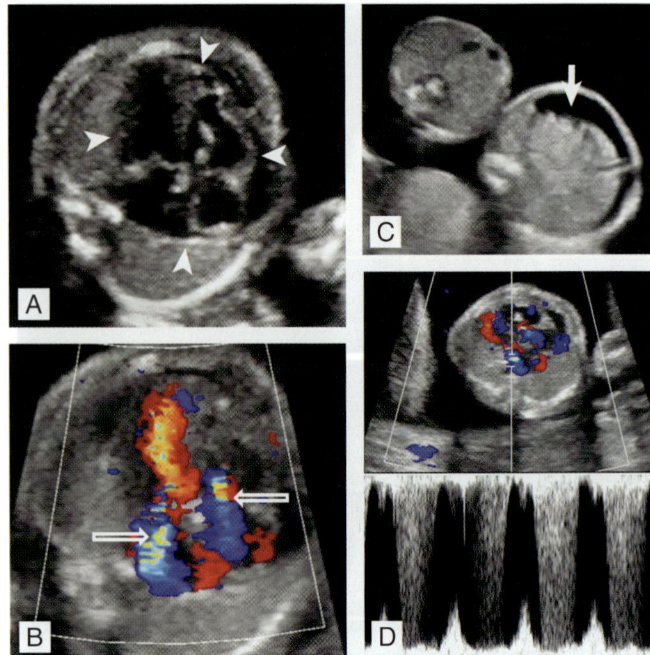

Figure 49.46 Complications associated with twin–twin transfusion syndrome. (A) B-mode USG image of a recipient twin showing cardiomegaly (*white arrowheads*). (B) Color Doppler image of the same fetus showing mitral and tricuspid regurgitations (*white block arrows*). (C) B-mode USG image of monochorionic-diamniotic twins showing the presence of ascites (hydrops fetalis, *white arrow*) in the recipient twin). (D) Color and spectral Doppler images of a recipient twin showing mitral regurgitation.

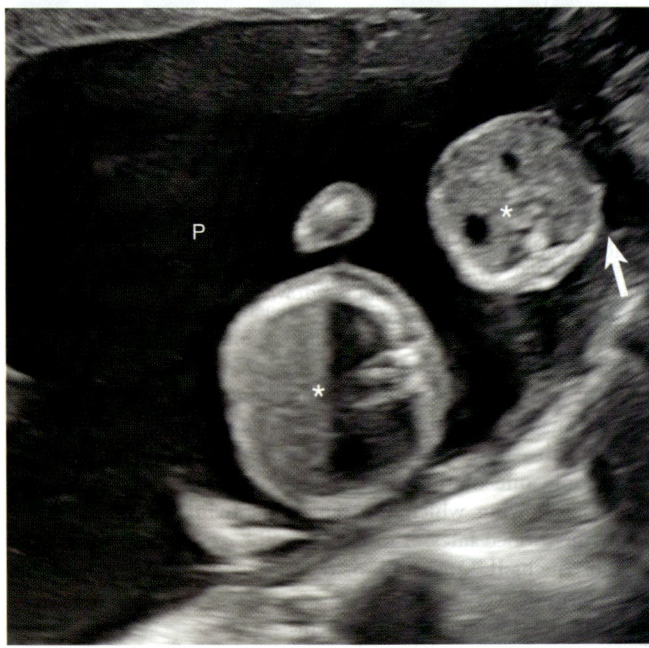

Figure 49.47 Twin–twin transfusion syndrome. B-mode USG image of a monochorionic-diamniotic twin gestation showing discordant growth (abdominal circumference discrepancy, *white asterisks*). The larger fetus has polyhydramnios (P) while the smaller one has an extreme oligohydramnios. The smaller twin appears to be affixed to the periphery of the gestational sac (stuck twin) with the intertwin membrane being almost invisibly wrapped around it (*white arrow*).

TABLE 49.21 Quintero Staging of Twin–Twin Transfusion Syndrome [112]

Stage	Feature
I	Polyhydramnios in the recipient twin sac and oligohydramnios in the donor twin sac with a visible bladder in the donor
II	Same as stage I without a visible bladder in the donor twin
III	Same as stage II plus abnormal Doppler flow—an absent or reversed UA diastolic flow, reversed DV a-wave flow, pulsatile umbilical venous flow in either twin
IV	Same as stage III plus hydrops in either twin
V	The fetal demise of one or both twins

DV, ductus venosus; *UA*, umbilical artery.

the pregnancy may be terminated considering the poor prognosis. In other cases, one of the undermentioned therapies can be resorted to (details presented in the chapter "Obstetric Interventions and Fetal Echo"). These therapies target either the unequal fluid between the twin sacs or interrupt the vascular communications between the twins.

- *Reduction amniocentesis*: In this procedure, the excess AF is aspirated from the polyhydramniotic sac in milder cases of TTTS as a temporary measure to postpone delivery to 30–32 weeks. As the fluid generally refills spontaneously, the procedure needs to be repeated frequently
- *Selective laser ablation of the placental anastomotic vessels*: It is the treatment of choice for TTTS stages II and above
- *Selective cord occlusion*: This procedure is reserved for saving one of the twins when the other twin shows signs of impending death

Twin Anemia Polycythemia Sequence

TAPS is a condition wherein one of the twins suffers from fetal anemia while the other twin is polycythemic. It is believed to that the presence of minute arteriovenous anastomoses, which allows slow transfusion of blood from the donor to the recipient, leads to highly discordant hemoglobin concentrations at birth. Spontaneous TAPS occurs in up to 5% of MC-DA twins, whereas up to 13% of cases of TTTS develop this condition following laser ablation [114].

USG findings: Antenatal diagnosis of TAPS is primarily based on discordant MCA-PSV measurements. MCA-PSV MoM of 1.5 or more in the donor twin suggests fetal anemia, while a value of less than 1.0 MoM in the recipient twin indicates fetal polycythemia. A staging scheme for TAPS based on MCA-PSV is described in Table 49.22. Additional USG findings include differences in the placental echogenicity and thickness—the donor usually has a bright thickened placenta and the recipient has an echolucent thin placenta.

Screening for TAPS: To screen for TAPS, the MCA-PSV should be measured from 20 weeks onward in both the fetuses of an MC-DA pregnancy, especially during the follow-up scans for all the cases treated for TTTS.

Management: The management options include early delivery, laser ablation or intrauterine blood transfusion (IUT) for the anemic twin, and combined IUT for the anemic twin—partial exchange transfusion to dilute the blood of the polycythemic twin [116].

TABLE 49.22 Antenatal Staging of Twin Anemia-Polycythemia Sequence. Adapted From [115]

Stage	Doppler Ultrasonography Findings
1	Donor MCA-PSV more than 1.5 MoM and recipient MCA-PSV less than 1.0 MoM, without other signs of fetal compromise
2	Donor MCA-PSV more than 1.7 MoM and recipient MCA-PSV less than 0.8 MoM, without other signs of fetal compromise
3	Stage 1 or 2 changes plus cardiac compromise in the donor (A/R UA-EDF, UV pulsatile flow, or DV increased or reversed flow)
4	Hydrops in the donor twin
5	Death of one or both fetuses

A/R, absent/reversed; *DV*, ductus venosus; *EDF*, end-diastolic flow; *MCA*, middle cerebral artery; *MoM*, multiples of the median; *PSV*, peak systolic velocity; *UA*, umbilical artery; *UV*, umbilical vein.

Twin Reversed Arterial Perfusion Sequence

Twin reversed arterial perfusion (TRAP) sequence is a rare complication of MC twin pregnancy wherein one twin is essentially normal while the other develops incompletely and is nonviable. The normal "pump" twin supplies the entire blood supply to the underdeveloped "acardiac" twin, which lacks a functioning heart, through an abnormal vascular connection. This puts the normal twin at high risk for high-output cardiac failure. Therefore, more than 50% of the pump twins die in utero in the absence of intervention [117]. The larger the recipient twin grows, the poorer is the prognosis for the donor twin. Table 49.23 describes the morphologic types of the acardiac twin.

USG findings: An acardiac twin can appear as an amorphous, edematous mass; or as a partially formed fetus with a poorly developed upper body and small or absent head, and often absent or underdeveloped upper extremities. If the head develops, it is usually inflicted with holoprosencephaly or other severe brain malformations. Diffuse fetal edema and cystic hygroma are frequently present. Cardiac pulsations are generally absent; their presence does not exclude the diagnosis. Doppler USG demonstrates a reversed flow in the UA toward the acardiac fetus (Fig. 49.48).

TABLE 49.23 Morphologic Types of the Acardiac Twin

Type of Acardiac Twin	Morphologic Features
Acephalic	Cephalic structures are absent (most common variety)
Anceps	Some cranial structures and/or neural tissue are present
Acormus	Cephalic structures are present but the truncal structures are absent (the rarest variety)
Amorphus	No discernible cephalic or truncal structures

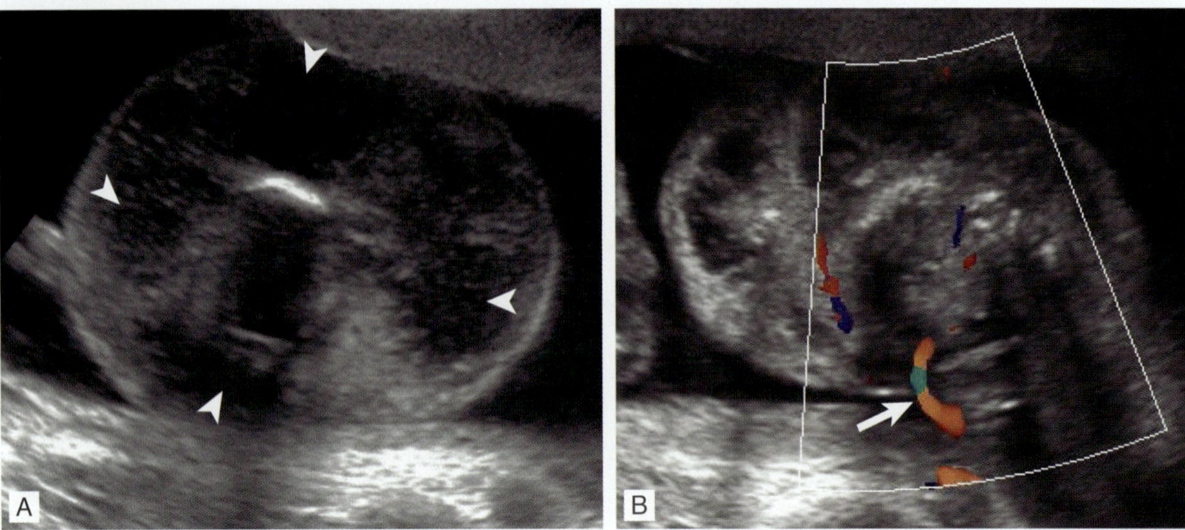

Figure 49.48 Acardiac twin. (A) B-mode USG image showing severe edema (*white arrows*). (B) Color Doppler USG image in the same twin revealed a reversed arterial flow directed toward the acardiac fetus (*white arrow*).

Management: Considering its overall poor outcome, if TRAP is diagnosed early in pregnancy, termination of the twin pregnancy can be offered. Different techniques such as cord coagulation, cord ligation, and radiofrequency ablation are good options to prevent the demise of the pump twin [118].

Conjoint Twins

Conjoint twinning is a rare phenomenon, observed in less than 1% of monozygotic twin pairs [119]. The potential for surgical separation and postnatal survival of the twins largely depends on the location and extent of fusion between the twins. Table 49.24 summarizes the various morphological variants of conjoint twins.

USG findings: The following USG findings should raise a suspicion of the presence of conjoint twins (Fig. 49.49):

- The bifid appearance of the first-trimester fetal pole ("V/Y" shaped twin pregnancy)
- The absence of the intertwin membrane
- Permanent position of the fetus relative one to another
- The appearance of the heads and bodies of both the twins at the same level
- Unusual extension of the spines

TABLE 49.24 Common Morphological Variants of Conjoint Twins

Type of Conjoint Twins	Morphologic Features
Thoracopagus	Ventrally joined from the thorax to upper abdomen
Parapagus	Laterally joined and share the pelvis
Cephalopagus	Laterally joined from the top of the head to the umbilicus
Omphalopagus	Ventrally joined from the abdomen to the lower thorax; never involves the heart
Fetus-in-fetu	A parasitic fetus develops inside the abdomen of its twin
Craniopagus	Fused skulls with shared meninges; separate faces and trunks

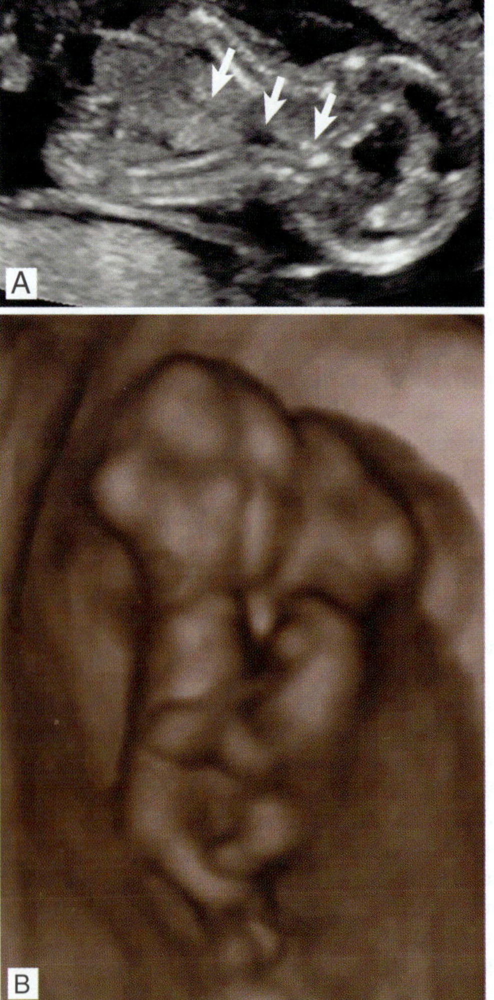

Figure 49.49 Conjoint twin. (A) B-mode USG image of a conjoint twin at 13 weeks showing the twins joint at thorax and abdomen (*white arrows*). (B) Three-dimensional reconstruction of the different twins showing two heads and fusion at the level of abdomen.

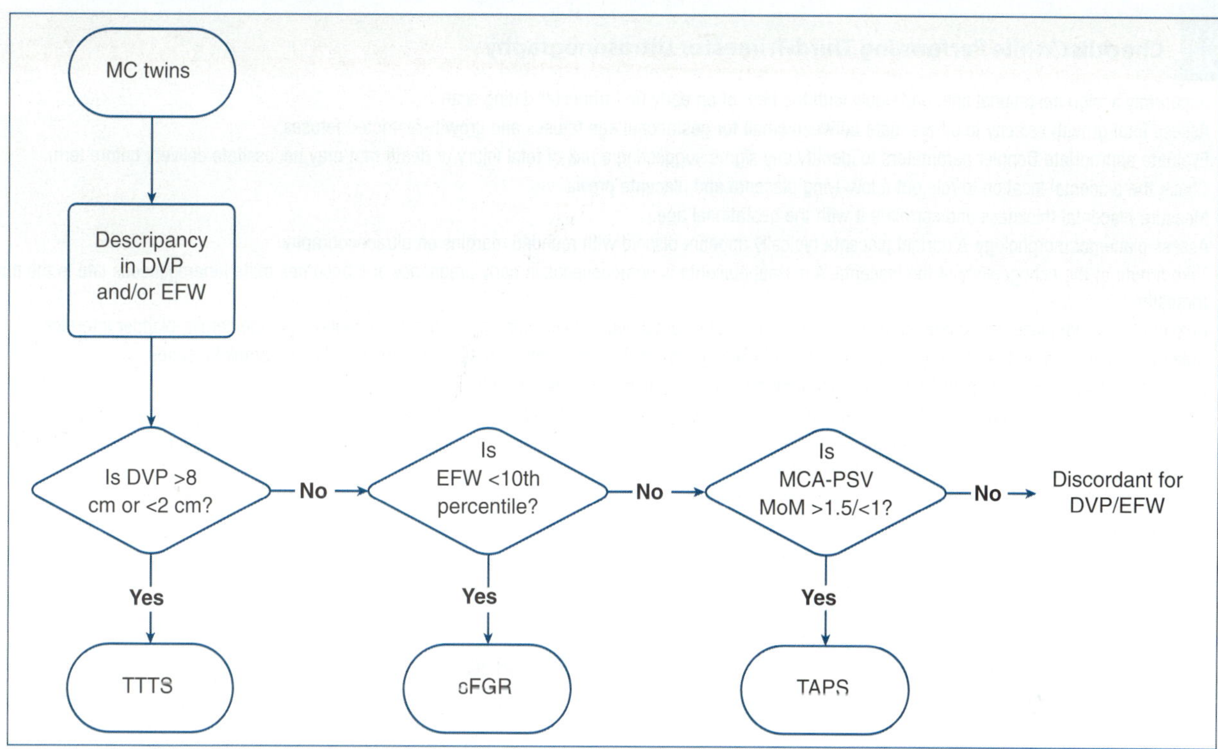

Figure 49.50 Clinical decision workflow for differentiating between the different complications of monochorionic twins. If all the known complications are ruled out, a discordant DVP/EFW warranties further regular follow-up scans. *DVP*, deepest vertical pocket; *EFW*, expected fetal weight; *MC*, monochorionic; *MCA*, middle cerebral artery; *MoM*, multiples of the median; *PSV*, peak systolic velocity; *sFGR*, selective fetal growth restriction; *TAPS*, twin anemia-polycythemia sequence; *TTTS*, twin–twin transfusion syndrome.

- Unusual proximity of the extremities
- The presence of a single heart

In all MC–MA pregnancies, it is mandatory to document that the body structures of both the twins are well apart and are moving independently.

Management: When conjoined twinning is detected early in pregnancy, termination is advised because of the grave prognosis. It can be technically very difficult beyond the first trimester, while cesarean delivery is often necessary for maternal safety in the third trimester.

Fig. 49.50 depicts the clinical decision flow for differentiating between the various complications of MC twins.

Summary

Early diagnosis, adequate monitoring, and timely delivery of an FGR pregnancy are crucial to ensure favorable perinatal outcomes. A single biometric parameter is not sufficient to diagnose FGR; except AC/EFW < third percentile, which denotes an extremely small fetal size. Additional evaluation with Doppler is needed in every FGR fetus to track its progression. There are two phenotypes of FGR, early-onset, and late-onset. At present, the most recognized criteria to define early and late FGR are those derived from an international Delphi survey with an international panel of experts on FGR [30].

Early-onset FGR is more strongly associated with the risk of perinatal mortality and morbidity. Hence, such pregnancies should be managed in multidisciplinary tertiary care units. Despite the severity of the pathological process, the cascade of Doppler abnormalities seen in this type of FGR is quite predictable. Therefore, monitoring such pregnancies and delivering them according to the set protocols can result in favorable perinatal outcomes.

Late-onset FGR has a milder clinical presentation. It is not plagued by the problems of prematurity. Yet, it can be associated with significant morbidity. Its diagnosis and management, especially near term, is challenging. Assessment of MCA-PI and CPR plays a significant role in its identification.

Assessment of the placenta and umbilical cord is an important component of obstetric USG in the second and third trimesters. Familiarity with their normal and abnormal imaging appearances enables radiologists to alert clinicians for prompt management decisions. It decreases the chances of fetal and maternal morbidity and mortality in conditions such as MAP, placenta previa, and vasa previa. AF status is a surrogate marker for fetal well-being. Hence, one cannot afford to skip AFV evaluation during the third-trimester obstetric scan. Short cervical length is an important predictor of preterm birth. TVS is the best technique for accurate measurement of the cervical length.

Many of the indications for a USG scan in multiple pregnancies are similar to those for singleton pregnancies. Similar to the latter case; pregnancy dating, NT assessment, structural anatomic survey, and use of Doppler USG to plan management strategies are standard practices in multiple gestations. Besides, they warrant careful sonographic evaluation of chorionicity, cervical length assessment to predict preterm births, and frequent USG scans for the evaluation of fetal growth. MC pregnancies require meticulous sonographic surveillance for a multitude of unique potential complications.

Table 49.25 is a checklist of things to remember while undertaking a third trimester USG scan.

TABLE 49.25 Checklist While Performing Third-Trimester Ultrasonography

- Accurately assign gestational age, preferably with the help of an early first trimester dating scan.
- Assess fetal growth velocity to differentiate between small for gestational age fetuses and growth-restricted fetuses.
- Evaluate appropriate Doppler parameters to identify any sign/s suggesting a risk of fetal injury or death that may necessitate delivery before term.
- Check the placental location to rule out a low-lying placenta and placenta previa.
- Measure placental thickness and correlate it with the gestational age.
- Assess placental morphology. A normal placenta typically appears discoid with rounded margins on ultrasonography.
- Take a note of the echogenicity of the placenta. A normal placenta is homogeneous in early pregnancy and becomes quite heterogeneous late in the third trimester.
- Rule out abnormal placental adherence by noting a clear retroplacental hypoechoic zone and a smooth echogenic uterine serosa-bladder interface.
- Rule out placental hematomas, masses, vascular pathologies, gestational trophoblastic disease, amniotic sheets, and amniotic bands.
- Look for the three-vessel umbilical cord and document the cord insertion site on the placenta.
- Rule out umbilical cord anomalies. Assess the fetal heart thoroughly if vascular anomalies are detected.
- Determine the amniotic fluid volume. In the case of decreased or increased amniotic fluid in the second trimester, rule out fetal anomalies and infections. Always measure the amniotic fluid index in the third trimester.
- Measure the cervical length preferably by transvaginal sonography. Perform a careful assessment of the closed cervical length in case of cervical incompetence.
- Additional things to remember in case of multiple gestations:
  - Determine the chorionicity and amnionicity
  - Ensure appropriate pregnancy dating and labeling of the twins
  - Screen for congenital anomalies and risk of preterm birth
  - Perform frequent surveillance for timely detection of complications specific for monochorionic twins

Suggested Readings

- A Bhide, G Acharya, CM Bilardo, C Brezinka, D Cafici, E Hernandez-Andrade, et al., ISUOG practice guidelines: use of Doppler ultrasonography in obstetrics, Ultrasound Obstet Gynecol 41 (2) (2013) 233.
- F Figueras, E Gratacos, Update on the diagnosis and classification of FGR and proposal of a stage-based management protocol, Fetal Diagn Ther 36 (2) (2014) 86–98.
- CC Lees, T Stampalija, A Baschat, F da Silva Costa, E Ferrazzi, F Figueras, et al., ISUOG practice guidelines: diagnosis and management of small-for-gestational-age fetus and FGR, Ultrasound Obstet Gynecol 56 (2) (2020) 298–312.
- SF Zaidi, M Moshiri, S Osman, TJ Robinson, JR Siebert, P Bhargava, DS Katz, Comprehensive imaging review of abnormalities of the placenta, Ultrasound Quart 32 (1) (2016) 25–42.
- S Fadl, M Moshiri, CL Fligner, DS Katz, M Dighe, Placental imaging: normal appearance with review of pathologic findings, Radiographics 37 (3) (2017) 979–998.
- M Moshiri, SF Zaidi, TJ Robinson, P Bhargava, JR Siebert, TJ Dubinsky, DS Katz, Comprehensive imaging review of abnormalities of the umbilical cord, Radiographics 34 (1) (2014) 179–196.
- A Khalil, M Rodgers, A Baschat, A Bhide, E Gratacos, K Hecher, et al., ISUOG practice guidelines: role of ultrasound in twin pregnancy, Ultrasound Obstet Gynecol, 47 (2) (2016) 247–263.

50

Obstetrics: Fetal Echocardiography and Interventions

NITIN CHAUBAL, POOJA PUNJANI VYAS, RAJAS CHAUBAL, SWATI GAREKAR

Section 1: Fetal Echocardiography

Introduction

Congenital heart disease (CHD) represents one of the major congenital anomalies, with a global incidence of 8–12 per 1000 live births [1]. In utero detection of cardiac anomalies goes a long way in making it possible to take timely clinical decisions. The first-trimester scan can pick up certain cardiac anomalies making it easier for parents to understand the impact of anomaly on fetus and possible survival rate and quality of life postnatally. Potentially fatal anomalies can be diagnosed early and parents can be offered termination for the same. In selected cases, genetic workup can be done on time. The time, mode, and place of delivery can be predetermined. Timely intervention and medication (such as prostaglandin) in duct-dependent anomalies can reduce neonatal morbidity and mortality.

Screening of Fetal Heart and Fetal Echocardiography

Screening of the fetal heart can be done during any stage of gestation but is typically done in the first trimester (11–14 weeks) and during an anomaly scan between 18 and 22 weeks [2]. Generally, the International Society of Ultrasound in Obstetrics and Gynecology (ISUOG) guidelines are followed for the screening of the fetal heart. In selected indications described later, the screening examination is converted into a fetal echocardiography examination [3]. American Institute of Ultrasound in Medicine (AIUM) has developed guidelines for the same [4].

Indications for Fetal Echocardiography

Fetal echocardiography is warranted in a variety of conditions, some of maternal origin, while others of fetal origin [4].

Maternal/Familial Indications: There are various maternal indications for fetal echocardiography. Some of the common ones include:

- History of CHD or syndromes associated with CHD in first degree relatives
- Gestational diabetes mellitus
- History of metabolic disease—pregestational diabetes mellitus [5], phenylketonuria [6]
- Presence of autoimmune antibodies or connective tissue disease
- Presence of maternal infection with a risk of fetal myocarditis
- History of teratogenic drug exposure like anticonvulsants, ACE inhibitors, NSAIDs, alcohol, lithium, etc.
- Use of assisted reproduction technology as a means of conception [7]
- History of rubella or parvovirus infection in the first trimester

Fetal Indications: There are situations when an abnormal finding during the screening of fetal heart requires further evaluation by performing fetal echocardiography. Few of the common situations are:

- Abnormal cardiac or extracardiac finding suspected on routine obstetric ultrasonography (USG)
- Fetal arrhythmias
- Increased nuchal translucency [8]
- "A" wave reversal of ductus venosus or tricuspid regurgitation in the first-trimester scan
- Fetal hydrops or effusion
- Monochorionic twins
- Single umbilical artery and systemic venous anomaly such as persistent right umbilical vein [9], left superior vena cava (SVC) [10], or absent ductus venosus

Guidelines for Screening of Fetal Heart

The ISUOG formulated guidelines in 2013 for the screening of fetal heart between 18 and 22 weeks of gestation. These guidelines are useful for evaluating low-risk fetuses as a part of routine prenatal care, which enables the detection of the majority of fetal cardiac anomalies [2].

As per the guidelines, screening of fetal heart should include the following views in both grey scale and color Doppler:

- Upper abdomen view
- Four-chamber view
- Outflow tracts view
- Three-vessel view (pulmonary artery, ascending aorta, and SVC)
- Three-vessel trachea view (pulmonary artery, ductal arch, the transverse aortic arch in relation to the trachea)

Fetal Heart Imaging Techniques for Screening

Transverse Sweep Technique

This is the simplest technique to screen fetal cardiac anomalies in one sweep. A cephalad sweep is performed starting from the fetal abdomen (section of abdominal circumference); going up to the four-chamber view, outflow tracts view (left and right ventricular), three-vessel view, and three-vessel trachea view [11] (Fig. 50.1).

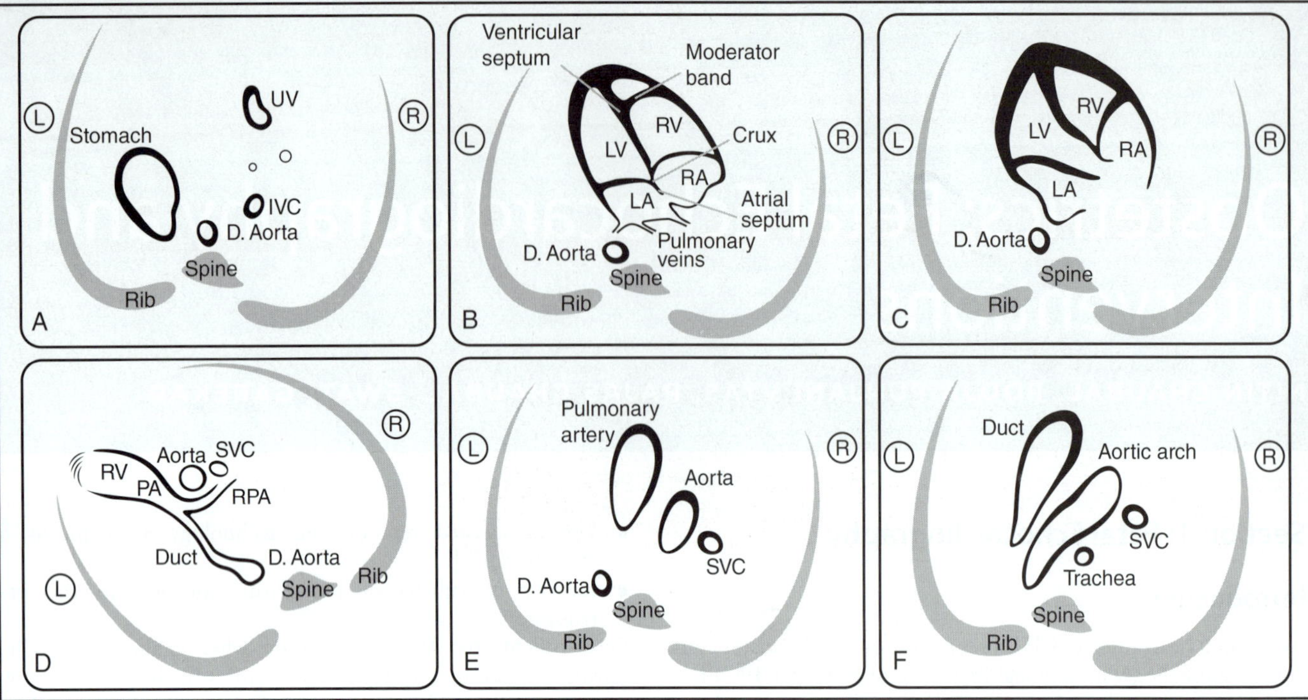

Figure 50.1 Technique for fetal heart screening (ISUOG practice guidelines 2013). (A) Fetal abdomen (section of abdominal circumference). (B) Four-chamber view. (C) Left ventricular outflow tract. (D) Right ventricular outflow tract. (E) Three-vessel view. (F) Three-vessel trachea view. *D. aorta*, descending aorta; *Duct*, ductus arteriosus; *IVC*, inferior vena cava; *ISUOG*, International Society of Ultrasound in Obstetrics and Gynecology; *LA*, left atrium; *LV*, left ventricle; *PA*, pulmonary artery; *RA*, right atrium; *RPA*, right PA-pulmonary artery; *RV*, right ventricle; *SVC*, superior vena cava; *UV*, umbilical vein.

Rotational Technique

This technique is used to evaluate the outflow tracts including the entire ascending aorta [12]. From the four-chamber view, the transducer is rotated toward the fetal right shoulder to visualize the left ventricular outflow tract (LVOT). After that, the transducer is angled cephalad to view the pulmonary artery (direction being almost perpendicular to that of aorta) (Fig. 50.2). This helps to obtain the right ventricular outflow tract (RVOT).

Guidelines for Fetal Echocardiography

Detailed fetal echocardiography includes color Doppler, pulsed Doppler, and M-mode, apart from screening protocol for further assessment as per AIUM guidelines [4] (Figs. 50.3–50.7).

The components of fetal echocardiography as per AIUM guidelines are given in Table 50.1.

Grayscale imaging or B-mode imaging provides useful diagnostic information about the fetal heart and includes the following planes:

- Four-chamber view
- Left ventricular outflow tract
- Right ventricular outflow tract
- Three-vessel trachea view
- Short-axis view ("low" for ventricles and "high" for outflow tracts)
- Long-axis view
- Aortic arch view
- Ductal arch view
- Superior and inferior vena cava view (bicaval view)—"Hammock sign"

Color Doppler should be used to evaluate the following structures for flow disturbances:

- Systemic veins (including SVC, IVC, and ductus venosus)
- Pulmonary veins
- Foramen ovale
- Atrioventricular valves
- Atrial and ventricular septa
- Semilunar valves
- Ductal arch
- Aortic arch
- Right subclavian artery—to look for normal or aberrant right subclavian artery (Fig. 50.8)

Pulsed Doppler should be used as an adjunct to evaluate the following:

- Atrioventricular valves
- Semilunar valves
- Ductus venosus (Fig. 50.9).
- Cardiac rhythm disturbance
- Any structure in which an abnormality on color Doppler is noted

Common Anomalies of the Fetal Heart

Ventricular Septal Defect

Ventricular septal defects (VSDs) are the most common defects seen in infancy and on fetal echocardiography [13]. They are diagnosed in the second and third trimesters. They are not reliably diagnosed in the first trimester. Defects more than 2–3 mm can be diagnosed on USG. For defects smaller than these, use of color Doppler may be useful in the diagnosis occasionally. These are of four types of VSD as discussed in Table 50.2 (Fig. 50.10).

Associated Anomalies: VSD is associated with various cardiac and chromosomal anomalies [14]. It is a part of some cardiac anomalies such as atrioventricular septal defect (AVSD), tetralogy of Fallot (TOF), absent pulmonary valve syndrome, common arterial trunk, double outlet right ventricle (DORV), interrupted aortic arch, tricuspid atresia with VSD, mitral atresia with VSD, pulmonary atresia with VSD. It may be occasionally seen in D-TGA, cTGA, and coarctation of aorta.

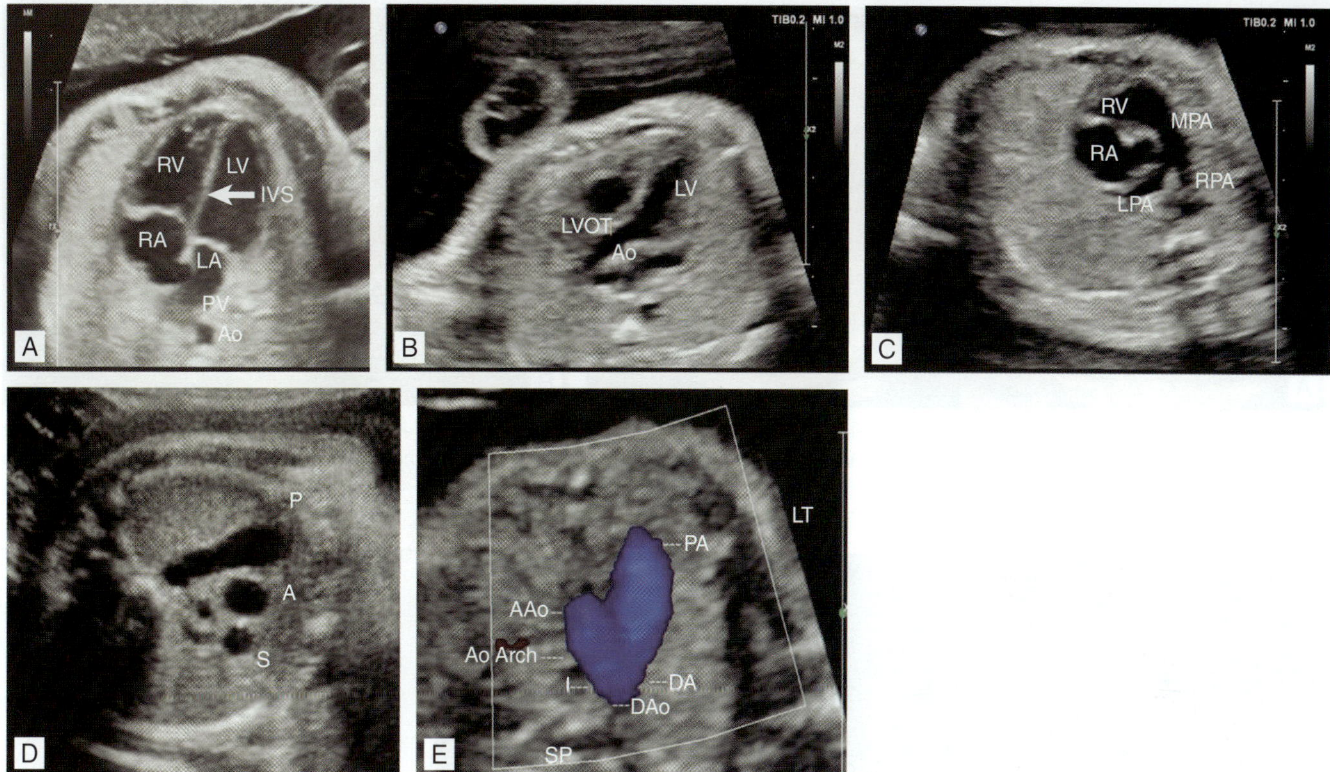

Figure 50.2 (A) Normal four-chamber view of the heart. It shows normal axis, two atria of same size, pulmonary veins (PV) entering left atrium, two ventricles of same size, moderator band in right ventricle, intact interventricular septum (IVS), intact crux, differential offsetting of the atrioventricular valves. (B) LVOT view showing septoaortic continuity. (C) RVOT view obtained by moving cephalad from LVOT. (D) Three-vessel view. It is showing pulmonary artery in longitudinal plane (P), aorta (A), and superior vena cava (S) in transverse plane from left to right. Pulmonary artery is anterior and to the left. (E) Three-vessel view. It is showing pulmonary artery, ductal arch, transverse aortic arch. *Ao Arch*, aortic arch; *Ao*, aorta; *AAo*, ascending aorta; *DA*, ductus arteriosus; *DAo*, descending aorta; *I*, aortic isthmus; *IVS*, interventricular septum; *LA*, left atrium; *LPA*, left pulmonary artery; *LV*, left ventricle; *LVOT*, left ventricular outflow tract; *MPA*, main pulmonary artery; *PA*, pulmonary artery; *PV*, pulmonary veins; *RA*, right atrium; *RPA*, right pulmonary artery; *RV*, right ventricle; *RVOT*, right ventricular outflow tract; *SP*, spine.

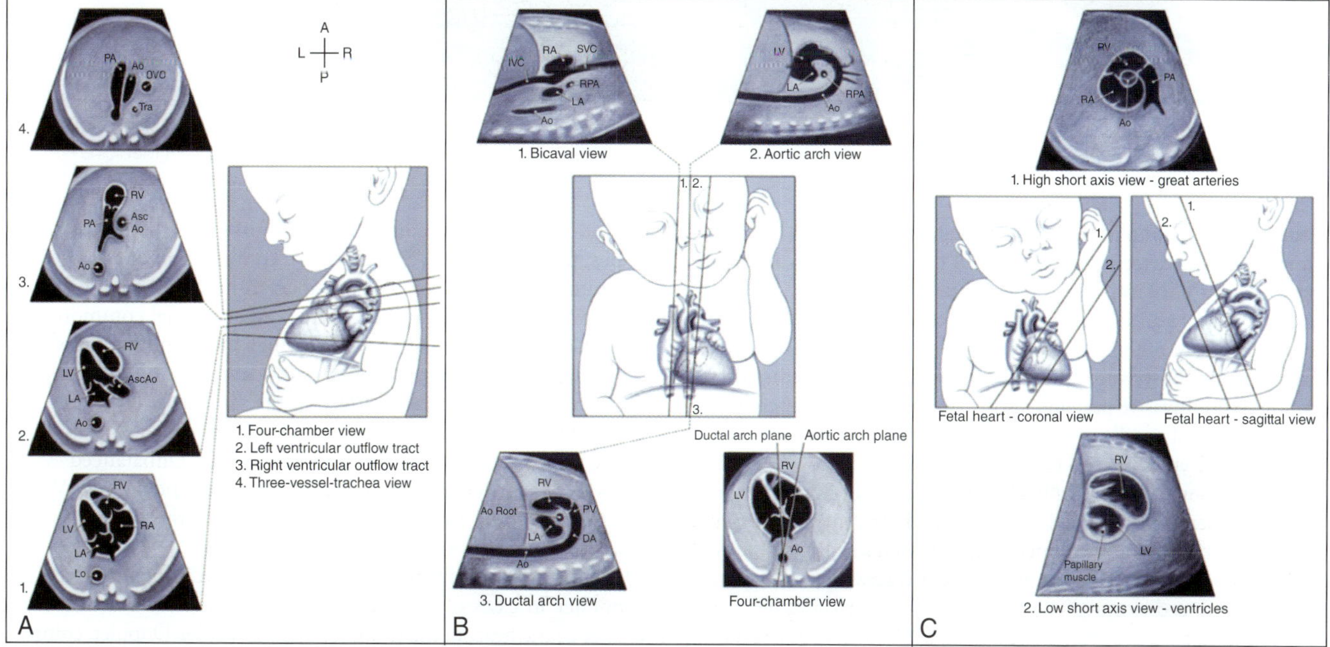

Figure 50.3 (A) Standardized transverse scanning planes. (B) Sagittal views. (C) Low and high short-axis views, for fetal echocardiography (as recommended in the guidelines of the American Institute of Ultrasound in Medicine—AIUM). *Ao*, aorta; *Asc Ao*, ascending aorta; *DA*, ductus arteriosus; *IVC*, inferior vena cava; *LA*, left atrium; *LPA*, left pulmonary artery; *LV*, left ventricle; *MPA*, main pulmonary artery; *PA*, pulmonary artery; *RA*, right atrium; *RPA*, right pulmonary artery; *RV*, right ventricle; *SVC*, superior vena cava.

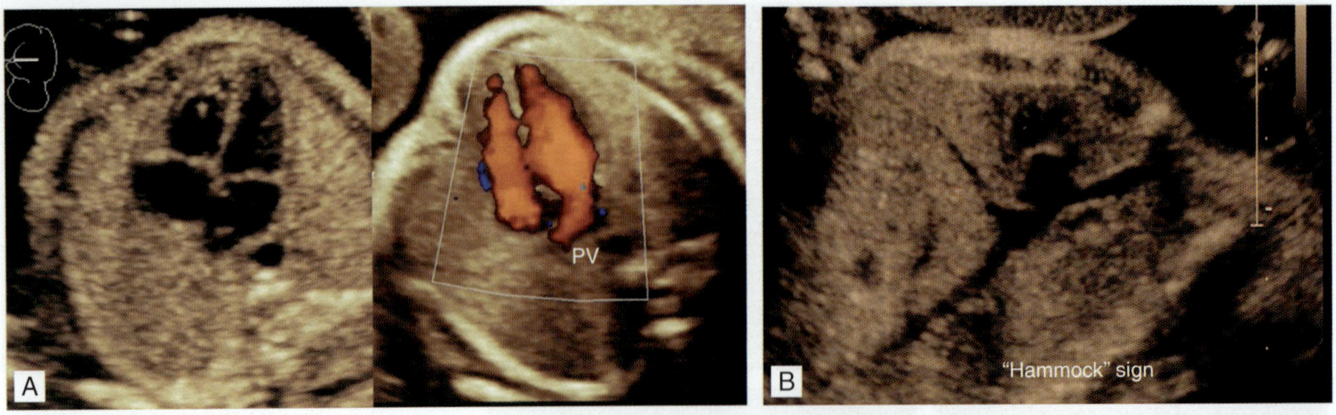

Figure 50.4 (A) Four-chamber view on B-mode and power Doppler showing two inflows in four-chamber view and pulmonary veins (PV) draining into left atrium. (B) "Hammock sign"—SVC and IVC draining into right atrium (as recommended in the Guidelines of the American Institute of Ultrasound in Medicine—AIUM).

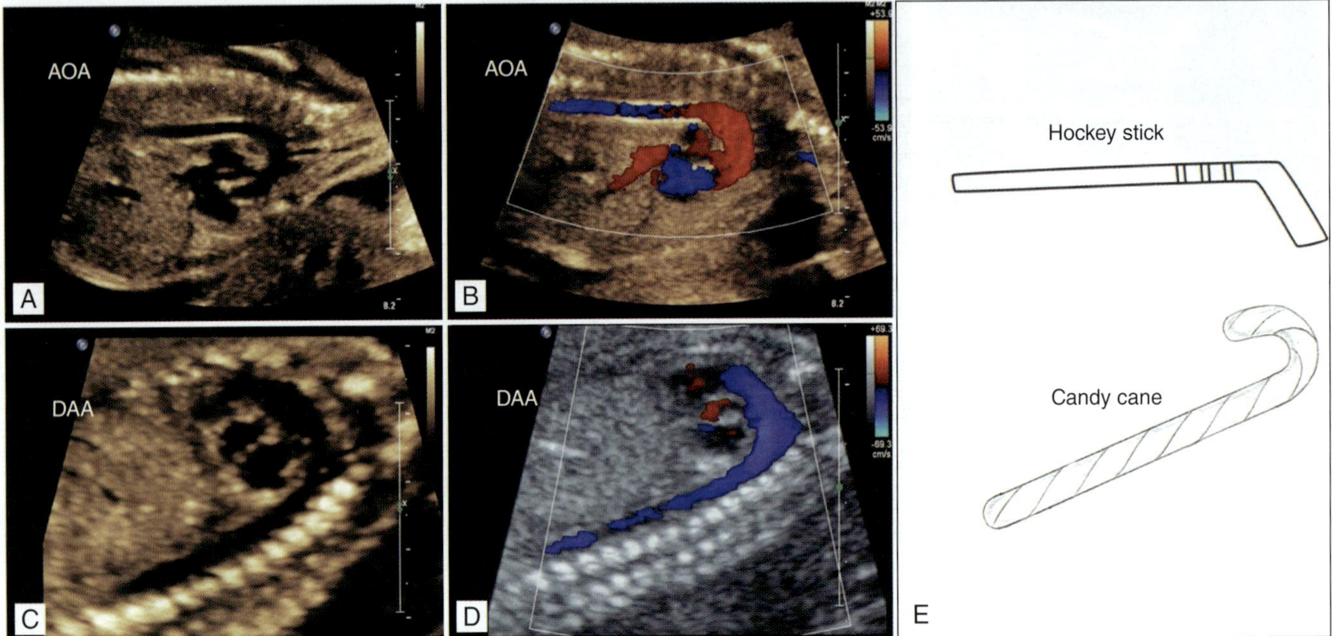

Figure 50.5 B-mode and color Doppler. (A and B) Aortic arch (AoA)—(candy cane appearance). (C and D) Ductal arch (DAA)—(hockey stick appearance). (E) Schematic drawing of hockey stick and candy cane (as recommended in the guidelines of the American Institute of Ultrasound in Medicine—AIUM).

Prognosis: The implication of antenatal detection of a VSD differs from postnatal detection. Antenatally, there is a concern that the presence of a VSD implies presence of significant genetic mutations and/or extracardiac anomalies. Studies show that fetuses with VSDs where there are other sonographic anomalies (noncardiac), have a higher chance of having abnormal genetic screening results (karyotyping or noninvasive prenatal testing or chromosomal microarray). Almost 80% of small muscular VSDs close spontaneously before birth or by 2 years of life [13–15]. An isolated large VSD (whichever type) should be surgically closed at the age of 3 months postnatally. If there are associated defects in the heart, then those can be addressed in one combined operation. It is vital to keep a child with a small/moderate unoperated VSD under follow-up until spontaneous or induced closure.

Atrioventricular Septal Defect

It is also known as AV canal defect or endocardial cushion defect (Fig. 50.11A–D). This is caused due to failure of the endocardial cushions to fuse. It accounts for 4–5% of CHD [27]. It is of two types: (a) Complete AVSD which is a combination of atrial septum primum defect and an inlet VSD apart from the presence of a common AV valve annulus. Thus, there is an abnormal common atrioventricular valve. (b) Partial AVSD which is a combination of atrial septum primum defect and a cleft in the mitral valve. In these cases, both atrioventricular valves attach at the same level [16].

AVSD can also be classified into (a) Balanced AVSD in which there is no ventricular disproportion and (b) Unbalanced AVSD in which ventricular disproportion arises secondary to AV connection draining predominantly into one of the ventricles. It is usually associated with heterotaxy syndromes.

Ultrasonography Findings: AVSD can be diagnosed in the first trimester in cases of complete AVSD. It is seen as a defect in the center of the heart in the region of crux. On color Doppler, common valve regurgitation maybe noted.

In the second and third trimester of gestation, the diagnosis of AVSD can be made easily. Both AV valves are inserted at the same level

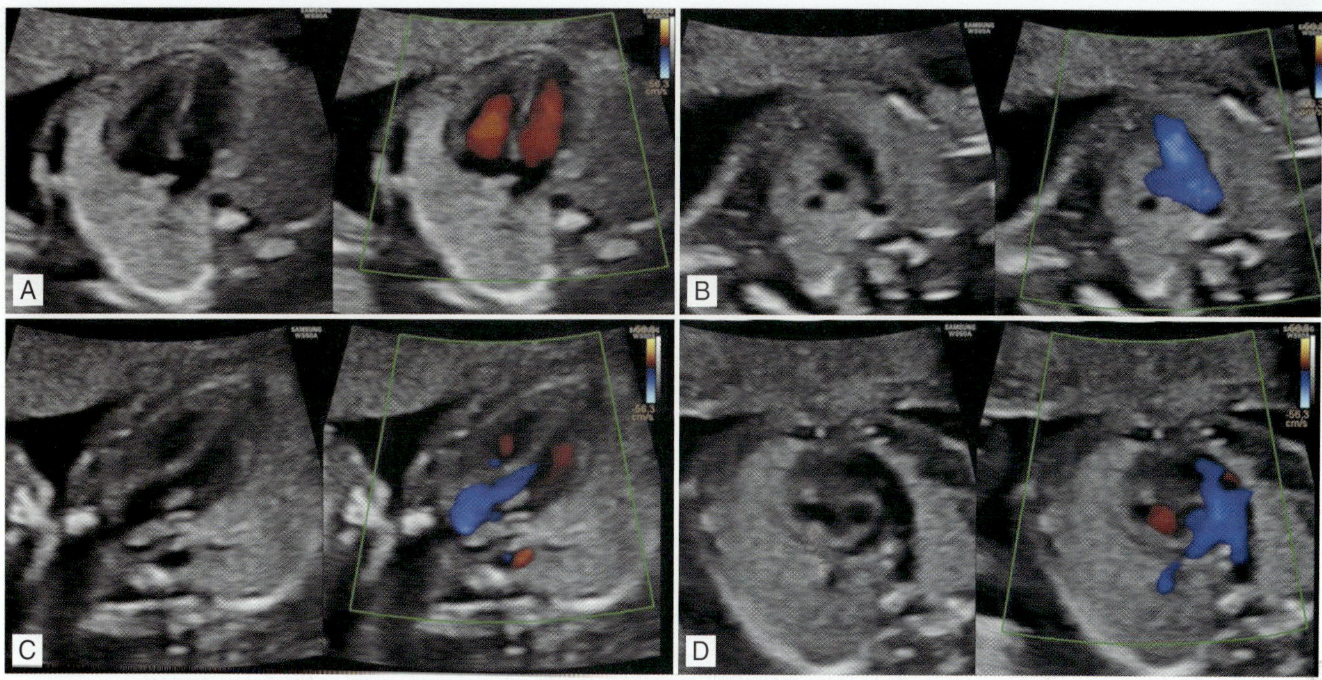

Figure 50.6 Color Doppler. (A) Four-chamber view. (B) Three-vessel view. (C) Left ventricular outflow tract (LVOT). (D) Right ventricular outflow tract (RVOT) (as recommended in the guidelines of the American Institute of Ultrasound in Medicine—AIUM).

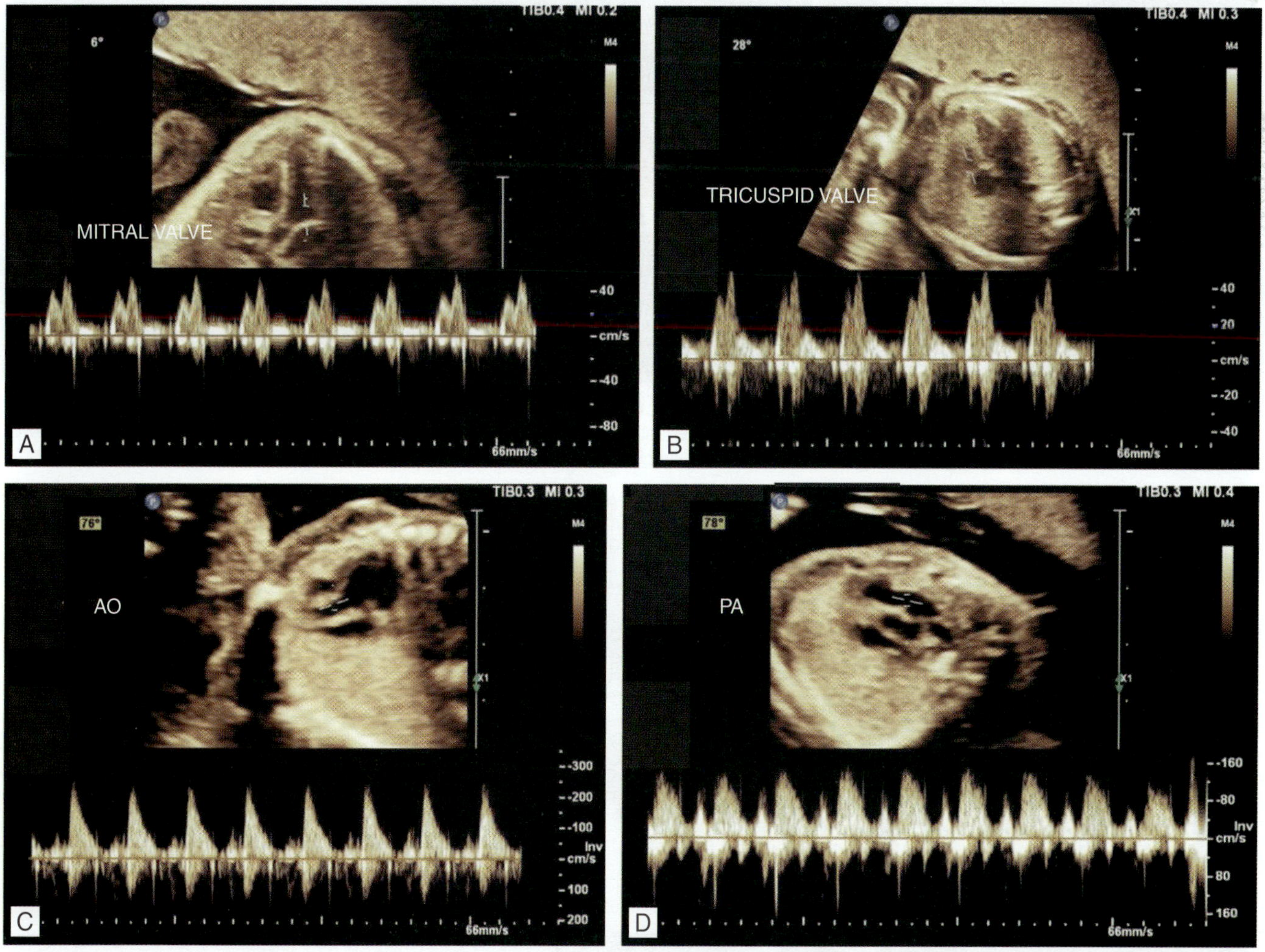

Figure 50.7 Pulse Doppler across (A) mitral valve, (B) tricuspid valve, (C) aortic valve, (D) pulmonary valve. *AO*, aorta; *PA*, pulmonary artery.

TABLE 50.1 Components of Fetal Echocardiography

Component	Features to be Evaluated
Visceral/abdominal situs	■ Stomach position, portal vein, descending aorta, and inferior vena cava in axial section ■ Cardiac apex position and axis
Atria	■ Situs ■ Systemic and pulmonary venous connections ■ Venous anatomy (systemic and pulmonary) ■ Atrial anatomy (including septum, foramen ovale, and septum primum)
Ventricles	■ Position ■ Atrial connections ■ Ventricular anatomy (including septum) ■ Relative and absolute size ■ Function ■ Pericardium
Great arteries ■ Aorta ■ Main pulmonary arteries and branches ■ Ductus arteriosus	■ Position relative to trachea ■ Ventricular connections ■ Vessel size, patency, and flow (both direction and velocity) ■ Relative and absolute size of aortic isthmus and ductus arteriosus ■ Pulmonary artery bifurcation ■ Position of transverse arch and ductus arteriosus relative to trachea
Connections to be evaluated in addition to a segmental analysis	■ Atrioventricular junction: anatomy, size, and function of atrioventricular valves ■ Ventriculoarterial junction: anatomy, size, and function of semilunar valves including assessment of subpulmonary and subaortic regions

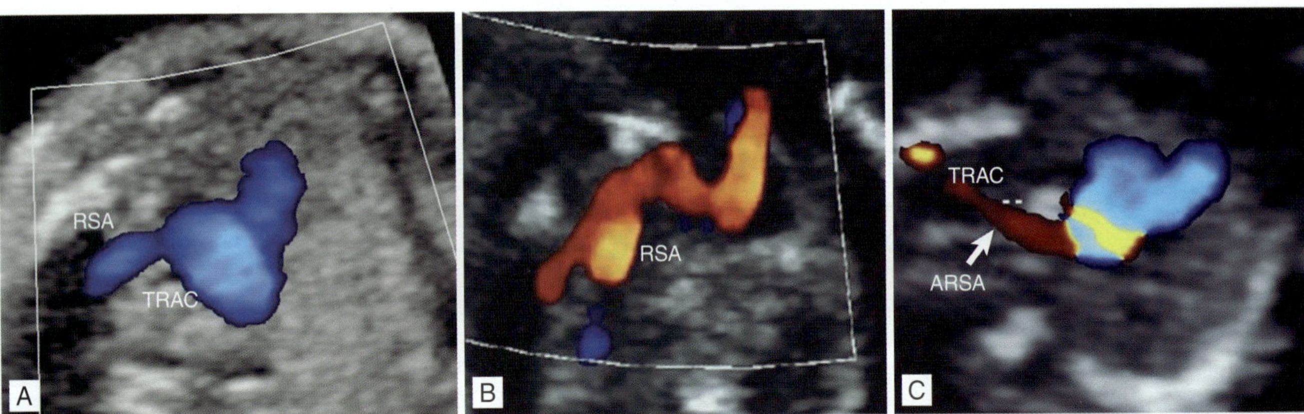

Figure 50.8 Right subclavian artery and aberrant right subclavian artery. (A and B) Normal Right subclavian artery (NRSA)—seen arising in front of the trachea and following a sinuous course at the level of clavicle. (C) Aberrant right subclavian artery (ARSA)—seen arising behind the trachea and following a straight course. *ARSA*, aberrant right subclavian artery; *RSA*, right subclavian artery; *TRAC*, trachea.

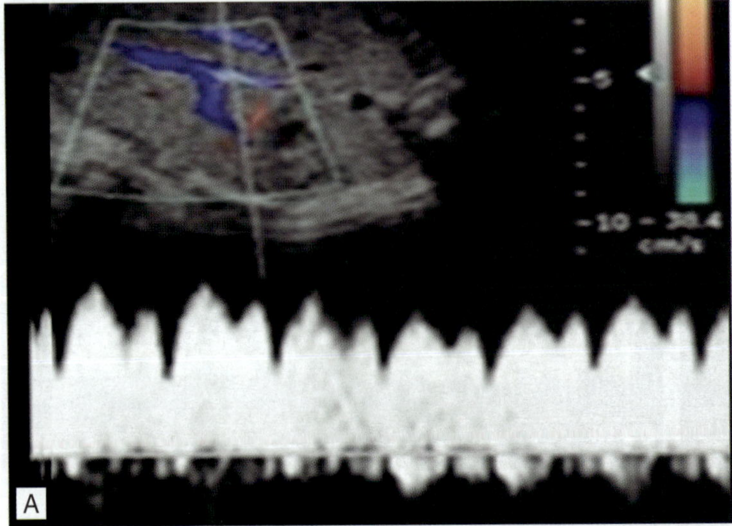

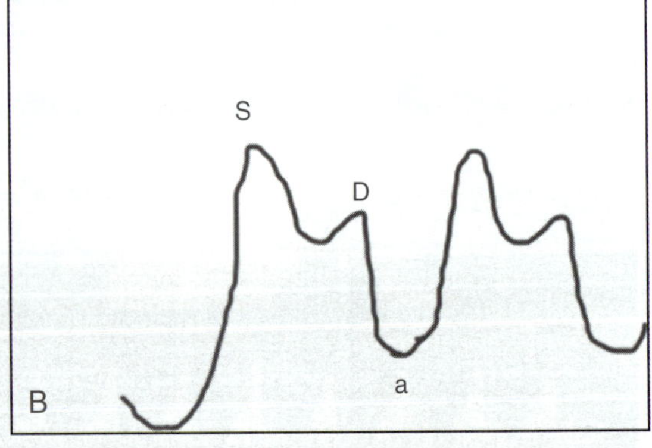

Figure 50.9 (A) Normal ductus venosus waveform. (B) Schematic diagram showing components of ductus venosus waveform—"S" wave, "D" wave, and "a" wave. *a*, atrial systole; *D*, ventricular end diastole; *S*, ventricular systole.

TABLE 50.2 Ultrasonography (USG) Findings of Different Types of VSD

Type of VSD	Location	USG Findings
Inlet type	Posterior to septal leaflet of tricuspid valve	■ Seen in the apical four-chamber view in the region of atrioventricular (AV) valves ■ Can be confirmed in lateral view to reduce false-positive cases or "echo drop outs" (artifact when the ultrasonography beam is parallel to ventricular septum)
Outlet/subpulmonary/ doubly committed type	Under the pulmonary valve	■ Seen in right ventricular outflow tract (RVOT) view ■ Very rarely seen
Muscular type	Apical, mid-muscular or multiple ("Swiss cheese appearance")	■ Seen in the four-chamber view or the transverse view ■ Borders appear echogenic ■ Bidirectional flow is noted on color Doppler
Perimembranous type	In the outflow tract under the aortic valve	■ Seen in five-chamber view ■ Breach in the continuity of ventricular septum and medial wall of ascending aorta (septoaortic discontinuity)

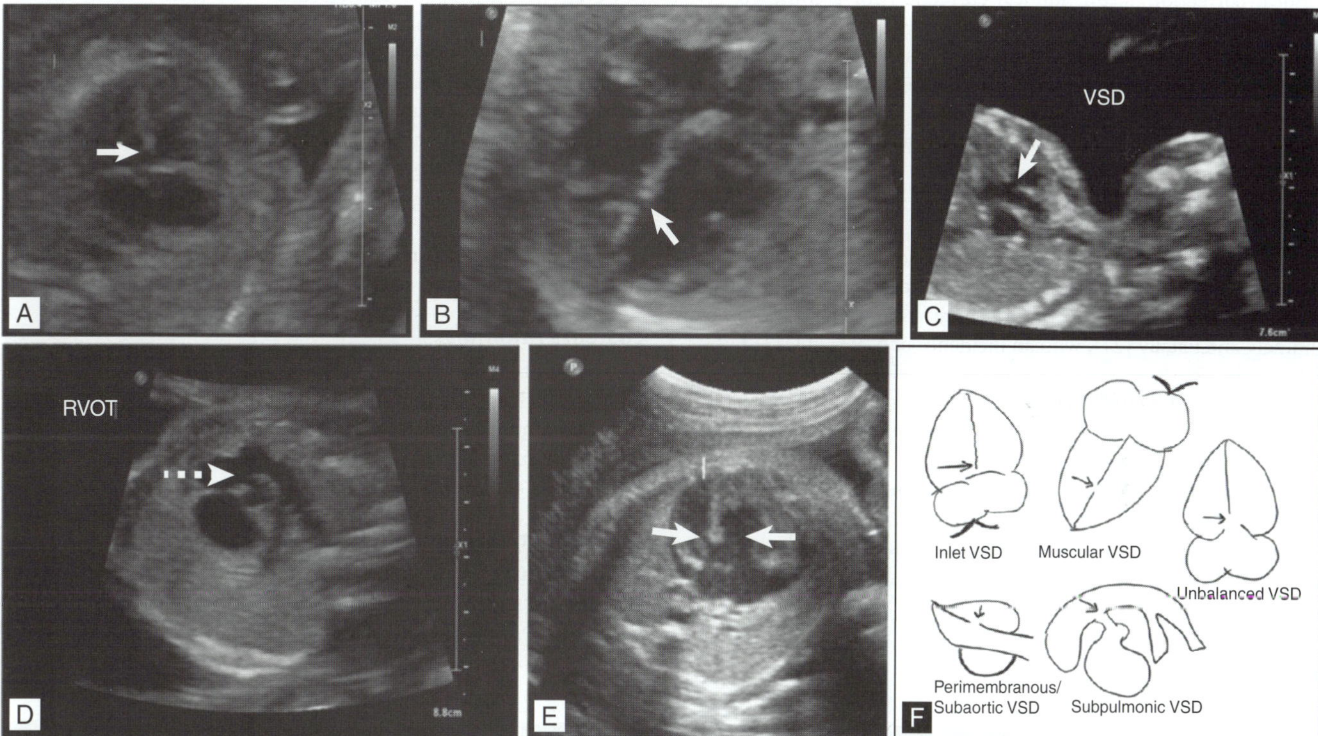

Figure 50.10 Types of VSD. (A) Inlet—four-chamber view showing a defect in the interventricular septum in the region of atrioventricular valves. (B) Muscular—four-chamber view showing discontinuity in the mid-muscular portion of interventricular septum (*arrow*). (C) Perimembranous/subaortic—LVOT view showing septoaortic discontinuity. (D) Subpulmonary—RVOT view showing subpulmonary VSD (*dotted arrow*). (E) Unbalanced—ventricular disproportion (RV > LV) and a common AV valve. (F) Schematic diagram of types of VSD. *LV*, left ventricle; *LVOT*, left ventricular outflow tract; *RV*, right ventricle; *RVOT*, right ventricular outflow tract; *VSD*, ventricular septal defect.

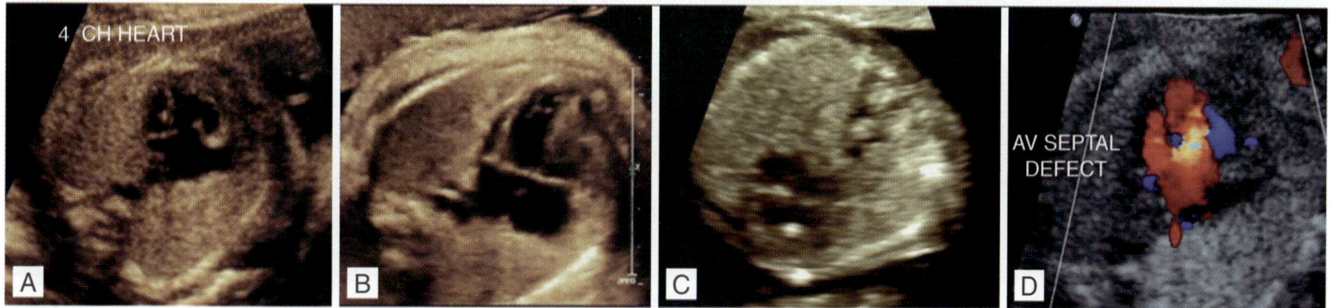

Figure 50.11 AVSD. (A) Complete/unbalanced AVSD—ventricular disproportion with combination of atrial septum primum defect and inlet VSD. (B) Partial/balanced AVSD—linear insertion of AV valves. (C) First-trimester AVSD. (D) Color Doppler—common valve regurgitation.

in partial AVSD. A defect in the crux region is visible during diastole in cases of complete AVSD. There is evidence of common valve regurgitation during systole in a majority of complete AVSD cases.

Atrioventricular length ratio is increased to >0.6 compared with normal fetuses (normal–0.5), since the atrial length increases in AVSD [17]. This helps to detect 83% cases with false-positive rate of 5.7% [17].

Associated Anomalies: Various cardiac anomalies associated with AVSD are TOF, double outlet ventricle, right-sided aortic arch, pulmonary atresia, ventricular disproportion, and coarctation of aorta.

It is estimated that 58% of patients with Down syndrome have isolated AVSD [18]. It may also be associated with heterotaxy and CHARGE syndrome [19]. Association of other chromosomal abnormalities and nonchromosomal syndromes is also known. Serial follow-up is required for any deterioration and cardiac failure.

Prognosis: Isolated cases of AVSD have an excellent long-term outcome (20-year survival rate is 95%; mortality rate <2% postsurgical correction) [20]. Surgical correction for a complete AV septal defect is ideally undertaken at age 3 months postnatally. The common AV valve is divided into two separate valves and the regurgitant valve leaflets are repaired. The ASD/VSD is patch closed at the same time. When AVSD is associated with other cardiac and extracardiac malformations, the survival and prognosis depend on associated anomalies.

Hypoplastic Left Heart Syndrome

It is characterized by sequential underdevelopment of the LVOT (severe aortic stenosis or atresia) and left ventricle (severe mitral stenosis or atresia). It is one of the more commonly seen cardiac anomaly antenatally [21], with an incidence of 5–9% of CHD [27].

Ultrasonography Findings

First trimester: Hypoplastic left heart syndrome (HLHS) can be diagnosed in the first-trimester scan. Cases of mitral and aortic atresia are easily picked up in early gestation with the advent of higher resolution machines and transvaginal USG in the first-trimester scan. However, it is important to keep in mind that a normal four-chamber scan in the first trimester does not rule out HLHS as it is an evolving anomaly.

Second and third trimesters

Four-chamber view: The left ventricle appears small with an echogenic wall in most cases, but may be dilated and globular in some cases. Apex is formed by the right ventricle. No color flow is appreciated in the left ventricle through the atretic mitral valve on color Doppler. Flap of the foramen ovale is seen to open from left to right atrium. Spectral trace of pulmonary vein reveals end-diastolic reversal of A-wave due to increased left atrial pressure [22].

Outflow tracts: The aortic outflow is not well visualized since it is hypoplastic. Two vessels are seen (dilated pulmonary artery adjacent to SVC) in the three-vessel view. Aorta is not seen since it is hypoplastic. In three-vessel trachea view, anterograde flow is seen in the ductal arch with reversal of flow in the transverse aortic arch. This often clinches the diagnosis of HLHS (Fig. 50.12).

Associated Anomalies: HLHS is associated with chromosomal anomalies in about 4–5% of cases [21,23]: Turner syndrome, trisomy 13, 18, and 22q11 microdeletions are known.

Prognosis: Over the years, prognosis has been considered bad, however, in experienced centers and with timely interventions and surgeries, better outcomes can be expected.

No treatment is feasible that will convert the heart to a normal biventricular heart. Instead, three-staged palliative surgeries are performed. The end result of the surgeries is that the heart is used to pump blood to the (newly constructed) aorta while the SVC and IVC are connected (stages 2 and 3 of palliative surgery) to the pulmonary arteries by surgical sutures. Post the final stage, the child can be expected to have a fair quality of life. Major long-term concerns remain heart failure, protein losing enteropathy, plastic bronchitis, liver disease, and sustaining a pregnancy postsurgery.

Ebstein's Anomaly

Incidence of Ebstein's anomaly is less than 1% of all CHDs [27]. Characteristically, there is displacement of the septal and posterior leaflets of the tricuspid valve into the right ventricle leading to a part of the right ventricle being incorporated into the right atrium (atrialized right ventricle).

Ultrasonography Findings

First trimester: Only tricuspid regurgitation can be seen in the 11–14 weeks scan. Other cardiac findings are seen in the second

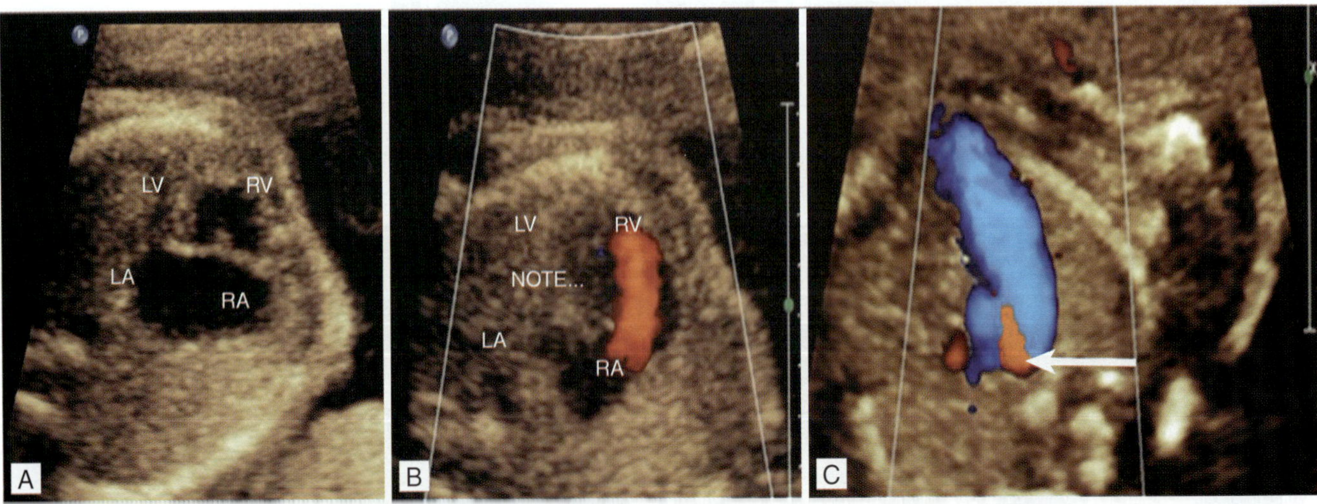

Figure 50.12 Hypoplastic left heart syndrome with (A) Hypoplastic left ventricle on B-mode. (B) No color flow in the left ventricle on color Doppler. (C) Anterograde flow in the ductal arch with reversal of flow in the aortic arch (*white arrow*). *LA*, left atrium; *LV*, left ventricle; *RA*, right atrium; *RV*, right ventricle.

and third trimester. It may be associated with increased nuchal translucency and hydrops in severe cases.

Second and third trimesters:

Four-chamber view: Classical findings on four-chamber view include dilated right atrium, low attachment of septal and posterior leaflets of tricuspid valve to the ventricular wall, and severe holosystolic tricuspid regurgitation (>200 cm/s) seen on color Doppler. The systolic jet is seen from the middle of the right ventricle.

Cardiothoracic ratio is increased on B-mode indicative of cardiomegaly [24].

In severe cases, large atrialized right ventricle, paradoxical movements of ventricular septum, cardiomegaly, cardiac failure, and hydrops may be seen.

The common condition with tricuspid regurgitation apart from Ebstein's anomaly includes tricuspid dysplasia which is characterized by moderate to severe TR at the level of tricuspid annulus, thickened tricuspid valve, cardiomegaly, and right atrial dilation. Pulmonary stenosis and pulmonary atresia with intact ventricular septum are also associated with TR.

Outflow tracts: If pulmonary stenosis or atresia is present, the pulmonary artery is narrow compared with ascending aorta. The RVOT on color Doppler shows reversal of flow in cases of pulmonary atresia.

Associated Anomalies: Most cases are sporadic, although familial conditions have been reported. Associated anomalies are uncommon but developing pulmonary atresia [25] and restricted growth of functional lung tissue worsen prognosis.

Tricuspid Atresia With Ventricular Septal Defect

Tricuspid atresia is a relatively rare anomaly with an incidence of less than 0.5 per 1000 live births [28]. The tricuspid valve is atretic resulting in no communication between right atrium and right ventricle, resulting in a small right ventricle [29]. This is a common variety of heart disease designated as "single ventricle" as no surgical treatment is possible for them. Rather, stage palliative surgery is done (see later), which enables them to lead a fair to good quality of life postsurgery.

Ultrasonography Findings

First trimester: Findings such as increased nuchal translucency, "a" wave reversal in ductus venosus may be seen in cases of tricuspid atresia [30,90].

Second and third trimesters

Four-chamber view: The right ventricle appears hypoplastic (size of ventricle is dependent on the size of VSD) along with inlet type VSD. Right atrioventricular junction appears thickened and echogenic. Foramen ovale is widely patent, with a redundant flap valve. There is delayed filling of the right ventricle in the diastole through VSD (Fig. 50.13).

Due to increased preload in the right atrium, "a" wave reversal of the ductus venosus is seen [30].

Outflow tracts: In Type 1, there is normal orientation of aorta and pulmonary arteries. Types 2 and 3 are associated with malposed vessels. Type 2 is associated with D-TGA and Type 3 is associated with L-TGA [31].

Associated Anomalies: Describing these has less significance as the primary determinant of the surgical strategy for tricuspid atresia is the atretic tricuspid valve. An atretic AV valve precludes a normal anatomy of the heart post surgery. So, in a constellation of heart defects present along with tricuspid atresia, whether it is D or L malposition of the great arteries, or the VSD or status of the pulmonary outflow tract, the atretic tricuspid valve alone determines the direction of surgical pathway chosen. It is helpful to determine whether or not pulmonary blood flow is reduced, as this will determine which and when the first stage of surgery will be.

Prognosis: A two- or three-staged palliative set of surgeries are carried out namely PA band or Blalock–Taussig shunt in the first stage, bidirectional Glenn shunt in the second stage and Fontan completion surgery in the final stage. The prognosis following this palliative set of surgeries is fair to good. Survival rates of 80% after 1 year following intervention have been reported [32]. The top three long-term concerns are heart failure, protein losing enteropathy, and plastic bronchitis.

Tetralogy of Fallot

TOF constitutes about 4–9% of patients with CHD [27].

It is caused because of incomplete rotation and faulty partitioning of conotruncus during septation.

Components of TOF antenatally include:

- Subaortic (mal-aligned) VSD
- Overriding of aorta
- Pulmonary stenosis

The fourth component, right ventricular hypertrophy is seen postnatally.

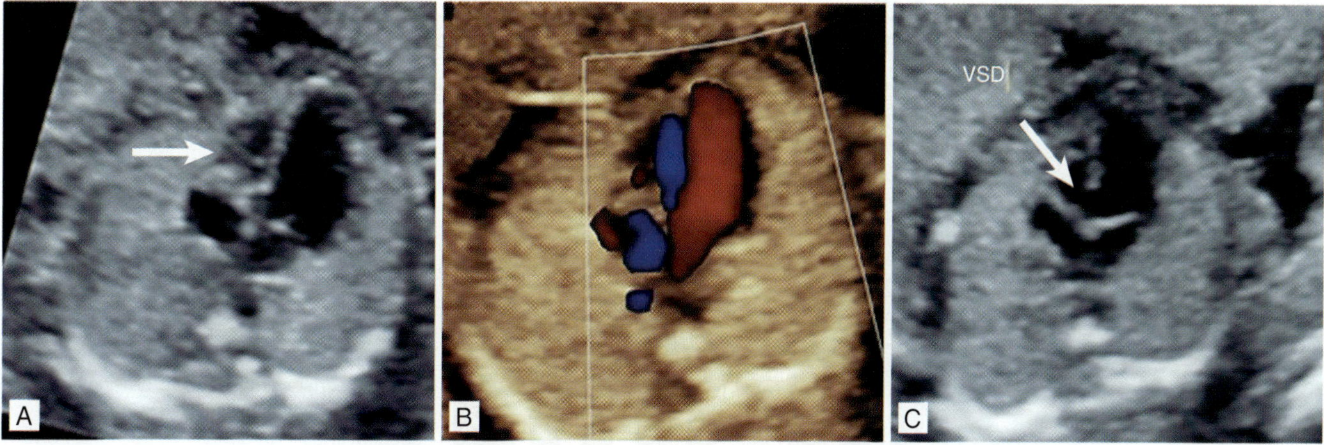

Figure 50.13 Tricuspid atresia with ventricular septal defect (VSD). (A and B) Hypoplastic right ventricle (*white arrow*) with no flow on color Doppler. (C) Hypoplastic right ventricle with inlet VSD (*white arrow*).

Ultrasonography Findings

First trimester: Increased cardiac axis is the first clue in the early gestation. A prominent aorta with narrow pulmonary artery often gives rise to the "Y" sign in the first trimester [35]. There is a strong association with increased nuchal translucency in cases of TOF [36].

Second and third trimesters

Four-chamber view: Usually the four-chamber view is normal. There may be left axis deviation.

Outflow tracts: Subaortic VSD with aortic override is seen classically in left ventricular outflow view [33]. Three-vessel view shows narrow pulmonary artery showing anterograde flow along with dilated aorta. Aorta becomes prominent, tortuous, and tends to come anterior. This often gives rise to question "?" mark appearance on three-vessel trachea view [34].

Ductus arteriosus shows anterograde flow on three-vessel trachea view (pink TOF); however, the flow may be reversed in cases of pulmonary atresia (blue TOF).

Besides the classical presentation, TOF can also occur with pulmonary atresia or TOF with absent pulmonary valve syndrome (Fig. 50.14A–E).

The steps for evaluation of suspected TOF are described in Fig. 50.15.

Associated Anomalies: Besides chromosomal abnormalities like trisomy 21, 18, and 13, which form 30% of cases [36], there is an increased incidence of single gene disorder like 22q11.2 deletion (DiGeorge syndrome) [37].

Almost 50% of fetuses have extracardiac anomalies which could affect any system [36]. There is a small risk of siblings and offspring being affected by the same.

Prognosis: In a minority of babies with TOF, a Blalock–Taussig shunt is required if there is profound cyanosis postnatally or life-threatening cyanotic spells before the age of 4 months. Complete intracardiac repair of TOF is ideally carried out between the ages of 6 and 12 months. The quality and quantity of life post-TOF repair is excellent when repair is done at the correct age.

Transposition of Great Arteries

In this condition, both great arteries (i.e., aorta and pulmonary artery) are parallel to each other.

There are two types of transposition of great arteries (TGAs):

a. Complete TGA or D-TGA: atrioventricular concordance with ventriculoarterial discordance
b. Congenitally corrected TGA or L-TGA: atrioventricular and ventriculoarterial discordance

D-TGA: D-TGA accounts for 5–7% of congenital cardiac anomalies [38]. This results from abnormalities of the development of subaortic and subpulmonary infundibulum.

Ultrasonography Findings

First trimester: Complete TGA can be diagnosed as early as in the first-trimester scan. The four-chamber view appears normal except abnormal cardiac axis in some cases. In the three-vessel trachea view, there is reverse curvature of the RVOT known as the "reverse boomerang sign" [40]. There is an association of increased nuchal translucency and D-TGA in chromosomally normal fetuses [41].

Second and third trimesters:

Four-chamber view: Usually it appears normal except in cases with associated VSD.

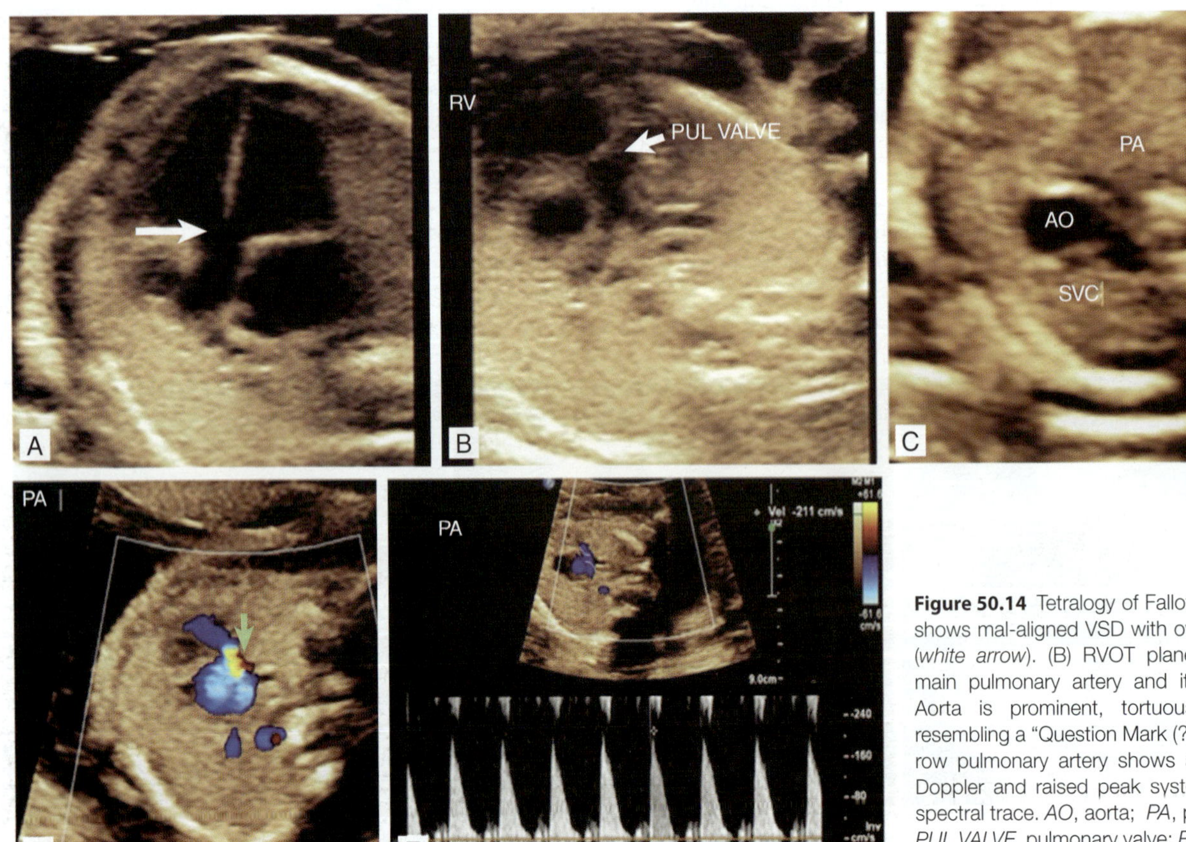

Figure 50.14 Tetralogy of Fallot. (A) LVOT plane shows mal-aligned VSD with overriding of aorta (*white arrow*). (B) RVOT plane shows narrow main pulmonary artery and its branches. (C) Aorta is prominent, tortuous, and anterior resembling a "Question Mark (?)". (D and E) Narrow pulmonary artery shows aliasing on color Doppler and raised peak systolic velocities on spectral trace. *AO*, aorta; *PA*, pulmonary artery; *PUL VALVE*, pulmonary valve; *RV*, right ventricle; *SVC*, superior vena cava.

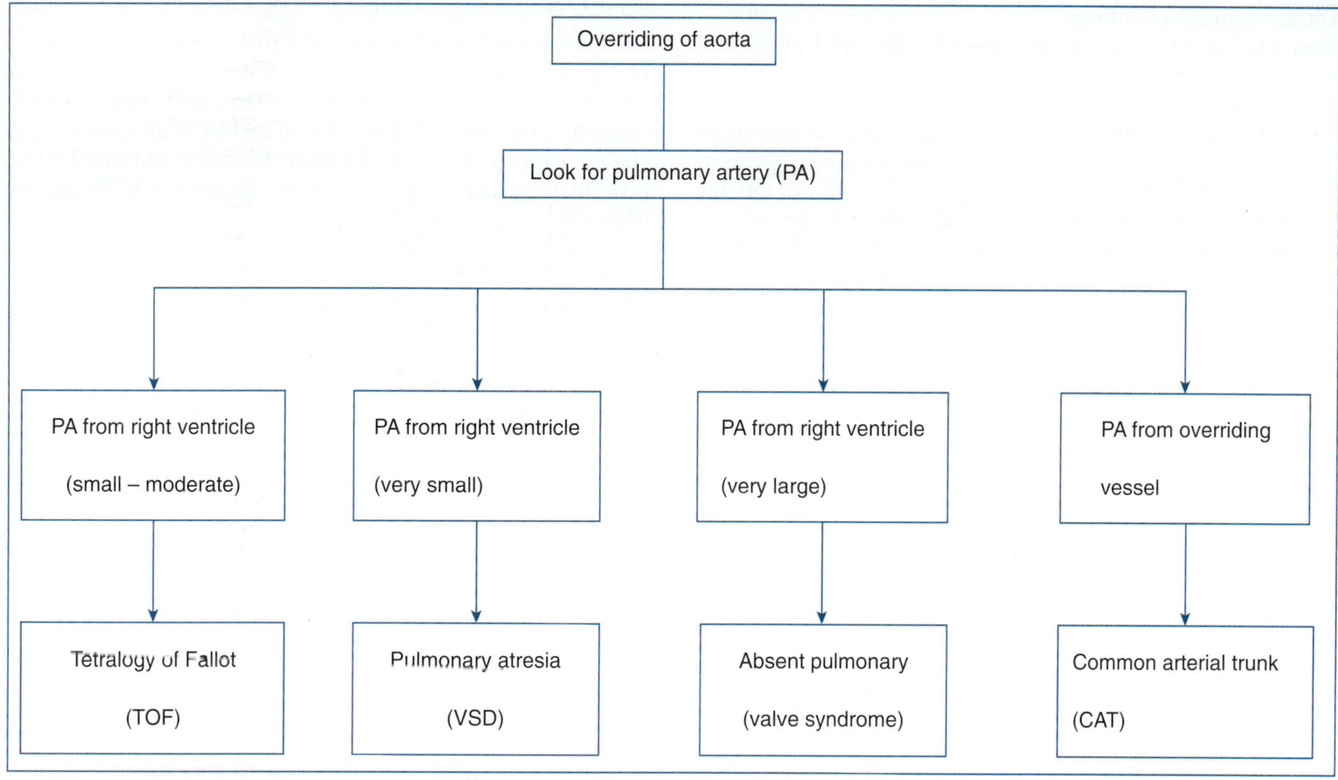

Figure 50.15 Tetralogy of Fallot. Steps for evaluation in a case suspected of TOF.

Outflow tracts: As we take a sweep cranially from abdomen, the first vessel to arise is a branching pulmonary artery from the left ventricle instead of the normal aorta. This is followed by aorta which arises from anterior right ventricle and arches toward right. In D-TGA, the LVOT view is always abnormal as it shows branching. Once the branching is noted, the oblique view is taken to check for the orientation of the great vessels.

In the oblique longitudinal view, the aorta appears parallel to the pulmonary artery. Aorta is anterior, superior, and to the right of pulmonary artery; hence it superimposes the pulmonary artery on three-vessel trachea view and only one artery is visualized in this view, with its convexity toward SVC. This is often referred to as an "I" sign [39]. This is similar to the "reverse boomerang" sign in the first trimester [40] (Fig. 50.16).

Associated Anomalies: D-TGA is associated with VSD in 40% cases, with pulmonary stenosis in 30% cases [38], and with DiGeorge syndrome when situs abnormalities are present. Overall association of extracardiac abnormalities is less compared with other cardiac abnormalities.

Prognosis: A corrective arterial switch surgery is performed in the neonate (TGA with intact ventricular septum) or at age 1 month (TGA with VSD). The outcome is excellent when diagnosed prenatally and the child is born in a tertiary center with pediatric cardiac setup [42]. When there is premature closure of the ductus arteriosus or restricted foramen ovale in TGA intact ventricular septum subset, it may lead to worsening neonatal outcome.

Congenitally Corrected Transposition of Great Arteries (L-TGA): This is a rare cardiac anomaly with an incidence of 0.03 per 1000 live births [43]. There is atrioventricular and ventriculoarterial discordance. Due to this dual discordance, there is hemodynamic compensation since the venous blood from systemic circulation goes to the pulmonary artery and the venous blood from the pulmonary circulation goes to the aorta. Hence, this type of transposition is called "corrected."

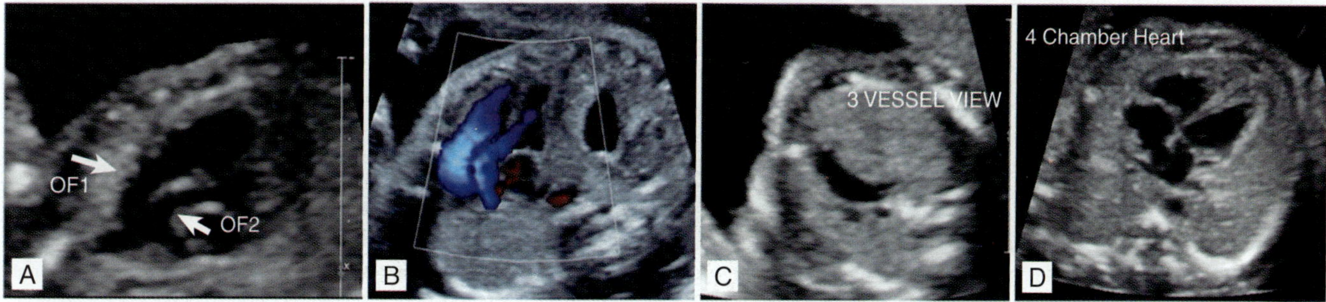

Figure 50.16 D-TGA. (A/B) The oblique view showing parallel orientation of both the outflow tracts (OF) in B-mode and color Doppler. (C) Three-vessel view—two vessels seen. Aorta is seen with its convexity toward SVC ("I" sign). (D) Four-chamber view—normal. *SVC*, superior vena cava.

Ultrasonography Findings

First trimester: It is usually diagnosed by abnormal origin and orientation of the aorta and pulmonary artery.

Second and third trimesters

Four-chamber view: The morphological right ventricle (characterized by the presence of moderator band and apical attachment of atrioventricular valve) is connected to the left atrium and the morphological left ventricle is connected to the right atrium.

Outflow tracts: As we take a sweep cranially, the first vessel to arise is the pulmonary artery from the morphological left ventricle and then the aorta is seen to arise from the morphological right ventricle. The aorta is anterior and to the left of the pulmonary artery.

In oblique longitudinal view, both great vessels are parallel. In three-vessel trachea view, a single vessel is seen (aorta) with its convexity away from SVC.

Associated anomalies: Extracardiac anomalies are rare but several intrinsic cardiac anomalies are known including tricuspid valve dysplasia, VSD, pulmonary stenosis, mesocardia, arch anomalies, and heart block [44].

Prognosis: Prognosis depends largely on associated cardiac anomalies. Surgical options include pulmonary artery banding, tricuspid valve repair, or heart transplantation. The presence of complex cardiac anomalies such severe tricuspid valve dysplasia, atresia of great vessels, or functional univentricular heart worsen prognosis [45].

Although it is referred to as "corrected," the right ventricle is not built to take care of systemic circulation. Tertiary level cardiac centers perform a double switch to correct the double discordances in the heart in carefully selected patients.

Double Outlet Right Ventricle

The Congenital Heart Surgery and Database Project has defined DORV as "type of ventriculoarterial connection in which both great vessels arise either entirely or predominantly from the right ventricle" [46]. This condition has an incidence of about 0.1 per 1000 live births [47]. It is important to understand that DORV is of different types, depending upon the type of VSD and the relationship of great arteries.

Ultrasonography Findings

First trimester: Abnormal cardiac axis may be seen in the four-chamber view. When four-chamber view is normal, the diagnosis of DORV is tricky and relies on the abnormal three-vessel trachea view. There may be either a single vessel seen or parallel vessels on 3VT view.

Second and third trimesters:

Four-chamber view: Usually, it appears normal, except in some cases large VSD may be present. Chamber discrepancy may be seen with a relatively prominent right ventricle and smaller left ventricle.

Outflow tracts: VSD is seen mainly in the LVOT view. The location and position of VSD in relation to great arteries should be noted. VSD can be subaortic, subpulmonary, doubly committed, or remote. When the transducer is angled between LVOT and three-vessel trachea view, parallel orientation of pulmonary artery and aorta is noted.

Outflow tract obstruction like stenosis or atresia should be looked for. Pulmonary stenosis is associated in approximately 70% cases [48].

There are four types of DORV (Fig. 50.17) depending on the anatomic relation of great arteries [49]:

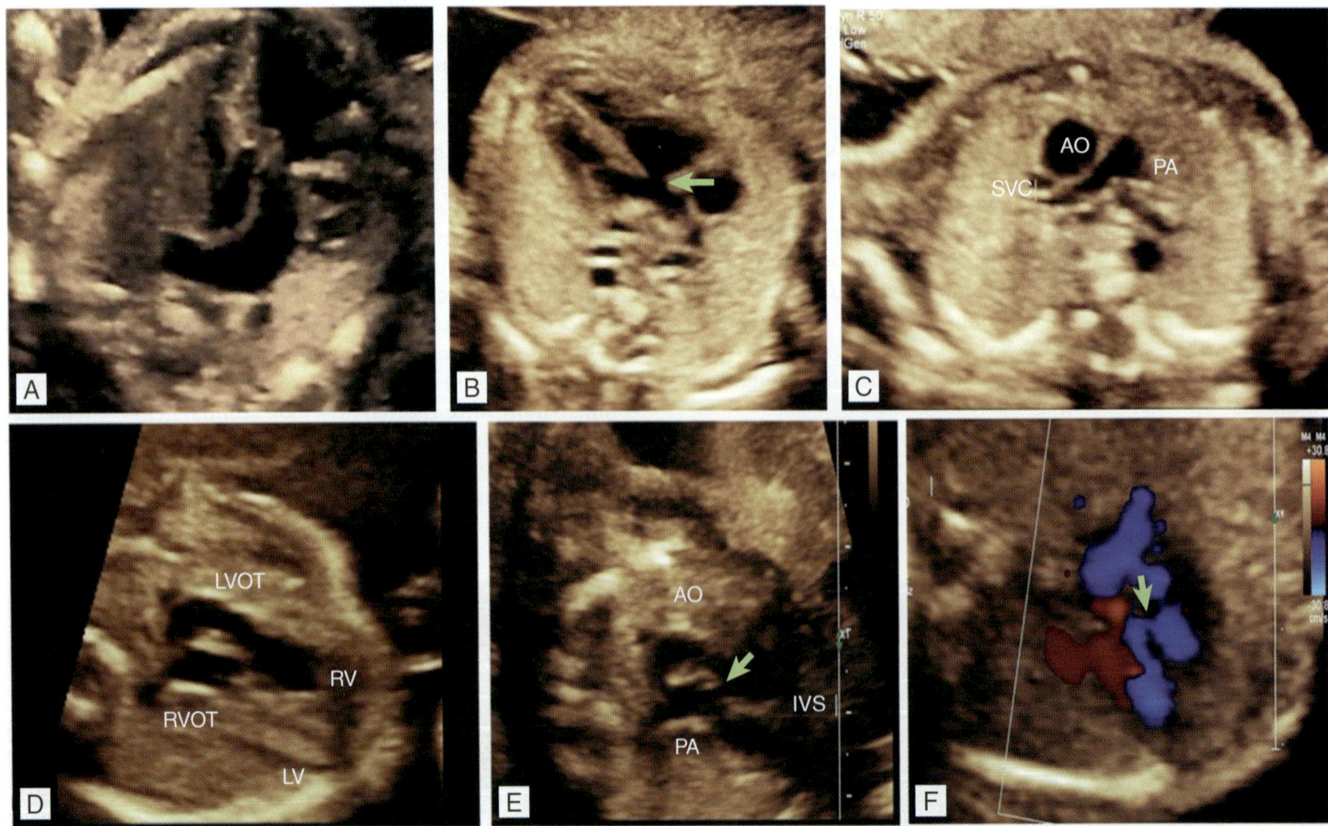

Figure 50.17 DORV (side to side type). (A) Aortic and pulmonary artery seen arising from right ventricle. (B) Subaortic VSD seen. (C) Aorta is to the right of the pulmonary artery, DORV (D-transposition type). (D) Aortic and pulmonary artery seen arising from right ventricle. (E) Subpulmonary VSD seen (*green arrow*) on B-mode. (F) Color Doppler shows bidirectional flow across the VSD. *AO*, aorta; *IVS*, interventricular septum; *LV*, left ventricle; *LVOT*, left ventricular outflow tract; *PA*, pulmonary artery; *RV*, right ventricle; *RVOT*, right ventricular outflow tract.

1. Side by side type DORV: aorta is seen to the right of pulmonary artery, subaortic VSD is seen.
2. D-transposition type DORV: aorta is right and anterior to pulmonary artery, subaortic, or subpulmonary VSD is seen.
3. TOF type DORV: aorta is posterior and right to pulmonary artery.
4. L-transposition type DORV: aorta is seen to the left, subaortic, or subpulmonary type VSD is seen.

Associated Anomalies: DORV is most commonly associated with pulmonary stenosis (70% cases) [48]. Other associated anomalies are mitral atresia, AVSDs, persistent left SVC, coarctation of aorta, etc. It may be associated with trisomy 13, 18, and deletion of 22q11 (DiGeorge syndrome) in 12–40% cases [50].

Prognosis: DORV has variable prognosis depending on its association with other anomalies. Prognosis is poor when it is associated with pulmonary atresia, AVSD, mitral atresia, aortic arch hypoplasia, hypoplastic left ventricle, single ventricle, or situs abnormalities. Infants operated for DORV with subaortic VSD have a good long-term prognosis [51] as well as patients with TOF or TGA type.

Coarctation of Aorta

It is characterized by narrowing of an aortic arch in the isthmus region (between ductus arteriosus and left subclavian artery). It is seen in about 8% of newborns and infants [52]. Left-sided obstructive lesions account for about 14% of CHDs.

Ultrasonography Findings

First trimester: Coarctation of aorta can be suspected in the first-trimester scan when findings such as ventricular discrepancy in four-chamber view and narrowing of aortic arch in the three-vessel view are seen. It is difficult to be sure of a diagnosis of coarctation of aorta in the first trimester but suspicion can definitely be raised. When it is suspected along with other features such as cystic hygroma, hydrops, or growth restriction, possibility of trisomy 13 should be ruled out.

Second and third trimesters

Four-chamber view: Ventricular disproportion (left ventricle appears narrow in width) is seen. Ratio of right ventricle width to left ventricle width is >1.69 in coarctation of aorta [53]. Normally it is around 1.0. Left ventricle shows normal contractility and length. Unlike HLHS, the apex of the heart is formed by the left ventricle and the mitral valve is normal. When associated with persistent left SVC, coronary sinus appears dilated.

Outflow tracts: The LVOT view shows normal ascending aorta. Diameter of the transverse aortic arch is narrower compared with the main pulmonary artery on three-vessel trachea view. Isthmus/ductal ratio is <0.74. Normally, it is about 1 or 0.9 [54].

When it is associated with persistent left superior vena, four vessels are seen in the three-vessel view (the fourth vessel is anterior and to the left of pulmonary artery). In the absence of right SVC, the left parasagittal view of the thorax shows the left SVC draining into coronary sinus ("tobacco pipe" sign) [91].

The longitudinal plane of the aortic arch reveals narrowing of the isthmus region ("posterior shelf/reverse 3 sign") [55]. There may be displacement of the left subclavian artery.

Three novel aortic arch measurements which are useful in the diagnosis of coarctation of aorta are:

1. Distance between left common carotid artery and left subclavian artery.
2. Angle between ascending aorta and descending aorta.
3. Angle between transverse aortic arch and descending aorta.

In coarctation of aorta, there is increased distance (>4.5 mm) between the left common carotid artery and left subclavian artery. Angle between ascending aorta and descending aorta is more acute (≤20.3°) and angle between transverse aortic arch and descending aorta is more obtuse (≥96.1°) [56].

Serial scans every 4–6 weeks should be done once coarctation of aorta is confirmed to look for progression. Occasionally severe ventricular dysfunction may develop (Fig. 50.18).

Associated Anomalies: Various anomalies are associated with coarctation of aorta. Persistent left SVC is the most common [57]. Others include VSDs [58], bicuspid aortic valve, aortic stenosis, mitral stenosis, corrected TGAs, DORV, and unbalanced AVSD. Multiple left-sided obstructive lesions with coarctation giving rise to tubular hypoplasia of aorta are referred to as Shone complex [59].

Turner's syndrome is the most common chromosomal abnormality [60], but trisomy 13 and 18 are also known to be associated.

Prognosis: Overall, the prognosis is excellent. In cases of prenatally diagnosed coarctation of aorta, delivery should take place in a tertiary care pediatric cardiac center. Prostaglandin should be kept ready for SOS infusion after birth to ensure patency of duct. Neonatal surgical coarctoplasty has better outcome (less chance of recurrence) compared with balloon angioplasty in the cath lab. Long-term concerns after repair of coarctation of aorta are

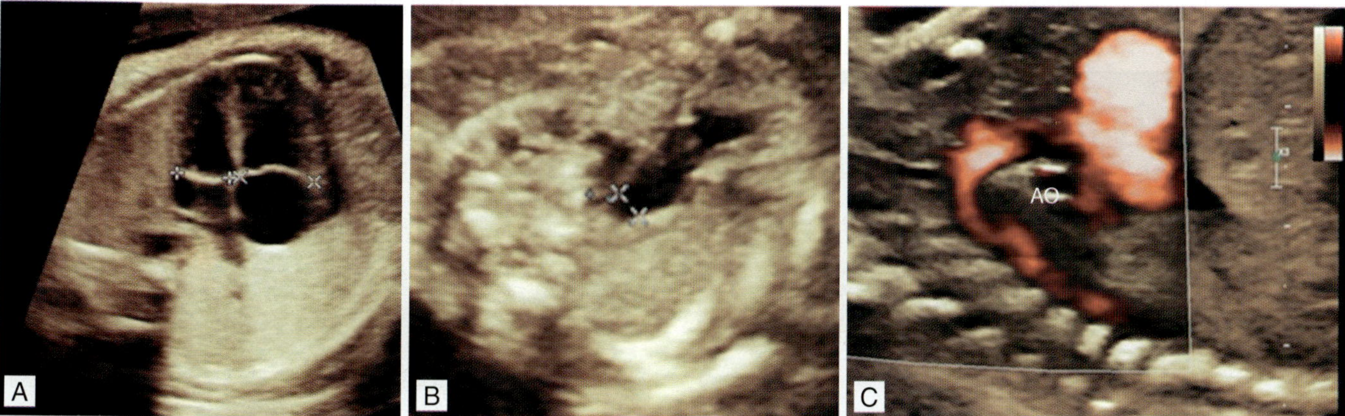

Figure 50.18 Coarctation of aorta. (A) Four-chamber view showing ventricular disproportion (left ventricle < right ventricle). (B) Three-vessel trachea view shows normal ductal arch with narrow transverse aortic arch. (C) Longitudinal section of the aortic arch shows narrowing at the level of aortic isthmus ("reverse 3 sign"/shelf sign). *AO*, aorta.

TABLE 51.3 Differential Diagnosis of Some Types of Lesions

Type of Lesion	Common Differentials
Spiculated mass	▪ Invasive carcinoma ▪ Ductal carcinoma in situ ▪ Surgical scar ▪ Complex sclerosing lesion or radial scar ▪ Rare: fibromatosis and granular cell tumor
Circumscribed mass	▪ Fat density: lipoma, oil cyst, galactocele ▪ Mixed density: hamartoma, galactocele, hematoma ▪ Soft tissue density or high density: cyst, fibroepithelial lesions, abscess, hematoma, papillary lesion, invasive carcinomas, sarcoma, metastases, and lymphoma
Architectural distortion	▪ Surgical scar ▪ Carcinoma, especially lobular ▪ Complex sclerosing lesion ▪ Mastitis and fat necrosis

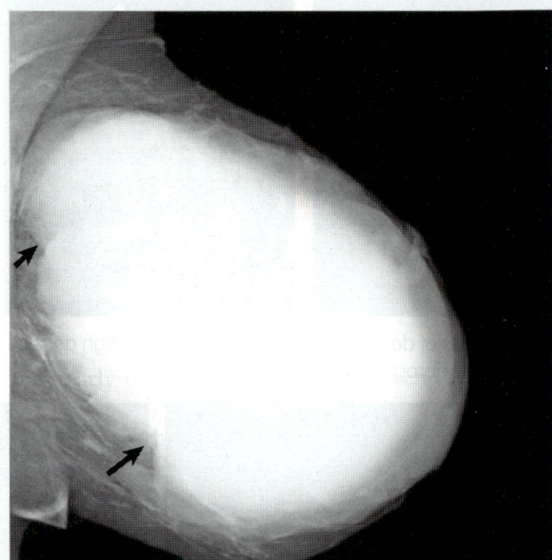

Figure 51.23 Large high-density mass (*arrows*) with a macrolobulated shape, which is now called oval.

assessment. Masses with microlobulated, indistinct, and spiculated margins and masses with irregular shape are also worrisome for cancer and should be further evaluated with USG and biopsy. The other shapes (round and oval) and density (nonfat) are not very useful by themselves (e.g., although most malignant masses are high density, fibroadenomas and cysts can also be of high density, and on the other hand, some special types of cancer, namely, mucinous or colloid, can be low density). Hence, a constellation of findings is more useful.

Architectural Distortion (AD)

AD is a disturbance in normal architecture of breast that results in pulling of structures toward its center. Hence, it is often seen as spiculations without a definite central abnormality, and sometimes it is seen only as distortion of parenchymal edge when the breasts are dense. Usually, AD can get compressed differentially in two projections; hence, it does not retain its form or shape [24]. It can be associated with microcalcifications.

The most common causes of AD are surgical scars, complex sclerosing lesion (CSL) or radial scar, malignancy, and infective or inflammatory conditions.

Surgical scar (Fig. 51.24) can be diagnosed from the appropriate clinical history and physical examination showing that the position of the scar corresponds to the position of the stellate lesion, and if necessary, by carrying out mammograms with skin markers on the scar. Having excluded surgical scars, 50–60% of ADs are caused by carcinoma (Fig. 51.25), often of a special type, such as lobular or tubular or caused by CSL (Fig. 51.26). It is not possible using imaging features alone to distinguish those caused by carcinoma from those caused by CSL, although radiologic and clinical features may indicate which is the most likely diagnosis. A benign CSL is usually not associated with a palpable mass even though the mammographic abnormality may be 4–5 cm in diameter. Both benign and malignant causes of AD may be associated with microcalcification, either within or near the periphery of the lesion.

Localized areas of AD, with the exception of those caused by surgical scars, require a histologic diagnosis. This may be obtained by image-guided needle core biopsy or diagnostic surgical excision. In most malignant cases, a positive diagnosis will be obtained using core biopsy to allow planning of definitive surgery. For cases in which a benign core biopsy of CSL or radial scar is obtained, diagnostic surgical excision with radiologic localization is recommended because of the risk of invasive or in situ malignancy at the periphery of the lesion.

Asymmetry

Asymmetry is the difference in the mirror image appearance of the breast. It is most commonly caused by islands of normal fibroglandular parenchyma but sometimes by an underlying mass that is obscured because of dense breast tissue (Fig. 51.27). When seen on a single view only, it is called just "asymmetry." More than 80% of these are summation

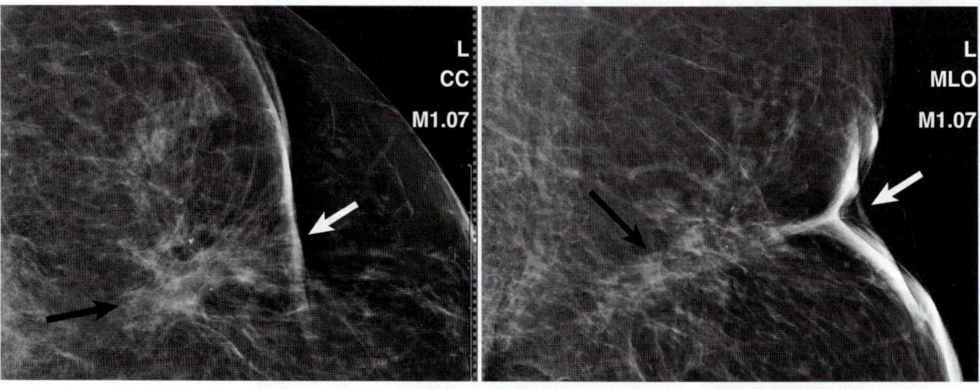

Figure 51.24 Surgical scar after breast-conserving surgery in the form of architectural distortion (*black arrows*); overlying skin thickening and retraction (*white arrows*) are also noted.

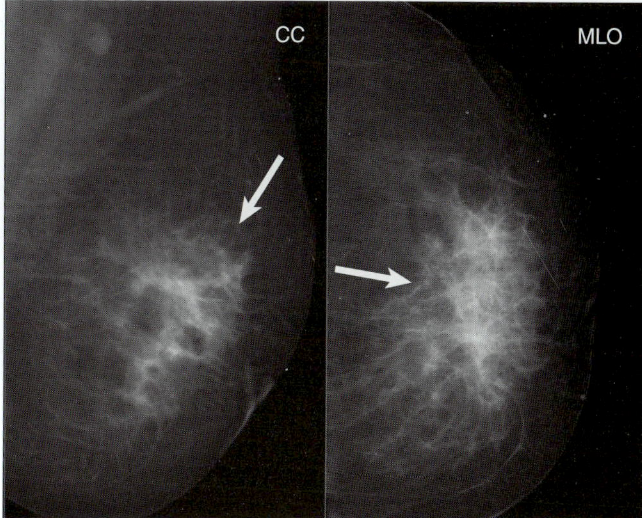

Figure 51.25 Mediolateral oblique (MLO) and craniocaudal (CC) views show a large area of architectural distortion (*arrows*) caused by an invasive lobular carcinoma.

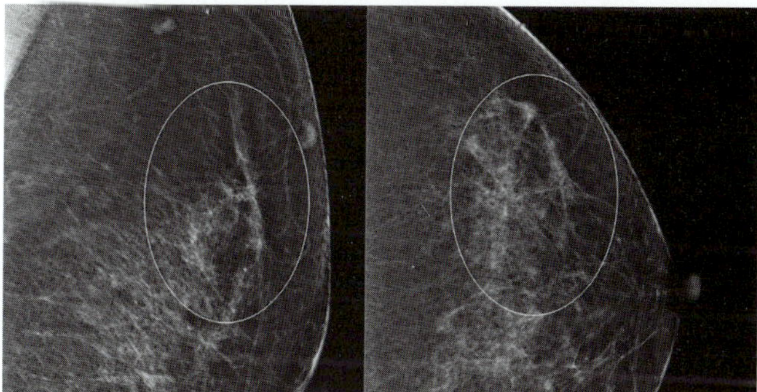

Figure 51.26 Mediolateral oblique and craniocaudal views show an area of architectural distortion caused by a complex sclerosing lesion with a radial scar (*encircled*). Notice how the appearance looks different on two projections, and there is no central mass.

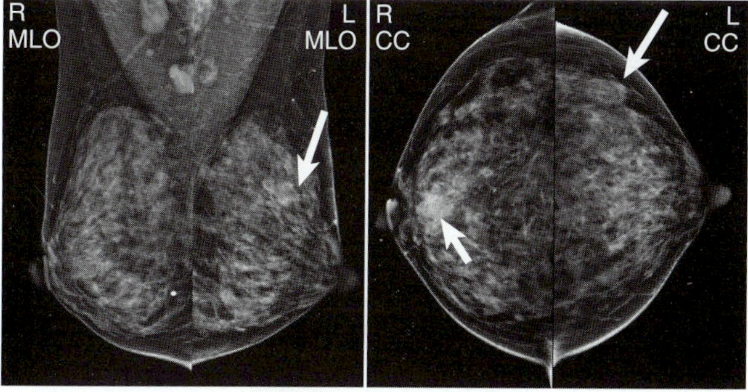

Figure 51.27 Focal asymmetry in the upper outer quadrant of the left breast (*long arrows*) revealed a hypoechoic solid mass on ultrasonography (USG; not shown). Asymmetry is also seen in the retroareolar region on craniocaudal view only of the right breast (*short arrow*) without any correlate on USG or tomosynthesis slices caused by a summation shadow.

artifacts. However, when additional views confirm this to be a true finding, it can be classified as *focal asymmetry, global asymmetry, or developing asymmetry,* according to the BI-RADS guidelines [24]. Prior studies are extremely valuable in assessing asymmetry as shown in Fig. 51.28.

An asymmetry becomes a suspicious finding when it is seen in two projections, is denser than the normal breast parenchyma or denser in the center than its periphery, or is palpable on CBE and requires ultrasound correlation [1]. *Neodensity* or *developing density* is the term used for a focal asymmetry that was not seen on prior studies and is a suspicious finding (Fig. 51.29). If the asymmetry is global or long standing it could be developmental or caused by prior surgery on the opposite side. A larger or diffuse area of increasing density is also a worrisome finding that needs further workup to rule out cancer, especially ILC.

Calcifications

Calcifications in the breast can be caused by a variety of conditions. Pattern reading is useful in assessing calcifications, especially the benign ones, as mentioned in Table 51.4. No further workup is required in such calcifications [24].

Microcalcifications are calcifications measuring less than 1 mm. They are often caused by epithelial proliferative changes such as fibrocystic changes, sclerosing adenosis, atypical ductal hyperplasia (ADH), or malignancy. Based on their size, microcalcifications can be further classified as *fine* when measuring less than 0.5 mm or *coarse* when measuring 0.5 to 1 mm.

Based on their morphologic appearance, microcalcifications are categorized further into four types as per BI-RADS [24]: *amorphous* (no distinct morphology), *coarse heterogeneous (0.5–1 mm and heterogenous in appearance), fine pleomorphic* (<0.5 mm and heterogeneous in appearance, i.e., all of them do not show similar size, shape, or density), and *fine linear or linear branching* (Table 51.5). The fine pleomorphic and fine linear or linear branching microcalcifications are suspicious for malignancy. The other calcifications can be caused by epithelial proliferative conditions mentioned earlier or DCIS, and imaging fails to distinguish them.

The *distribution* of calcification is also useful in deciding the suspicion of malignancy, especially when the morphology is not distinctive (Fig. 51.30). The calcifications can be called *grouped* (previously called as clustered) when there are five calcifications within 1 cm of each other or more numerous calcifications in less than 2 cm of each other, *linear* when they appear oriented in a line, *segmental* when they appear to involve a lobule or two of the breast, *regional* when they are spread over more than 2 cm but not in linear or segmental fashion or involve very large areas but not the entire breast, and *diffuse* when they scattered throughout the breast parenchyma.

Diffuse and especially bilateral calcifications are generally benign (e.g., punctate [<0.1 mm] and amorphous calcifications in this distribution), but similar calcifications in a linear, segmental, or grouped distribution are suspicious. Similarly, coarse heterogeneous calcifications in a single group are worrisome. Segmental and linear distributions are worrisome for malignancy unless the morphology is characteristically benign, and regional distribution can be benign unless the morphology is worrisome.

An Intramammary Lymph Node

An *intramammary lymph node* is an extremely common benign finding in routine practice. Typically, these are small, well-defined, low-density, reniform lesions that most commonly lie in the upper outer quadrant. When this typical appearance is not seen, the lesion can be worked up with review of prior studies, spot compression views, and/or USG (which should show a hilum in a node).

A Solitary Dilated Duct

A solitary dilated duct may be seen as a tubular structure extending from the retroareolar region. Usually, an ultrasound correlation is needed for assessing this lesion further, but effort must be made to look for microcalcifications within.

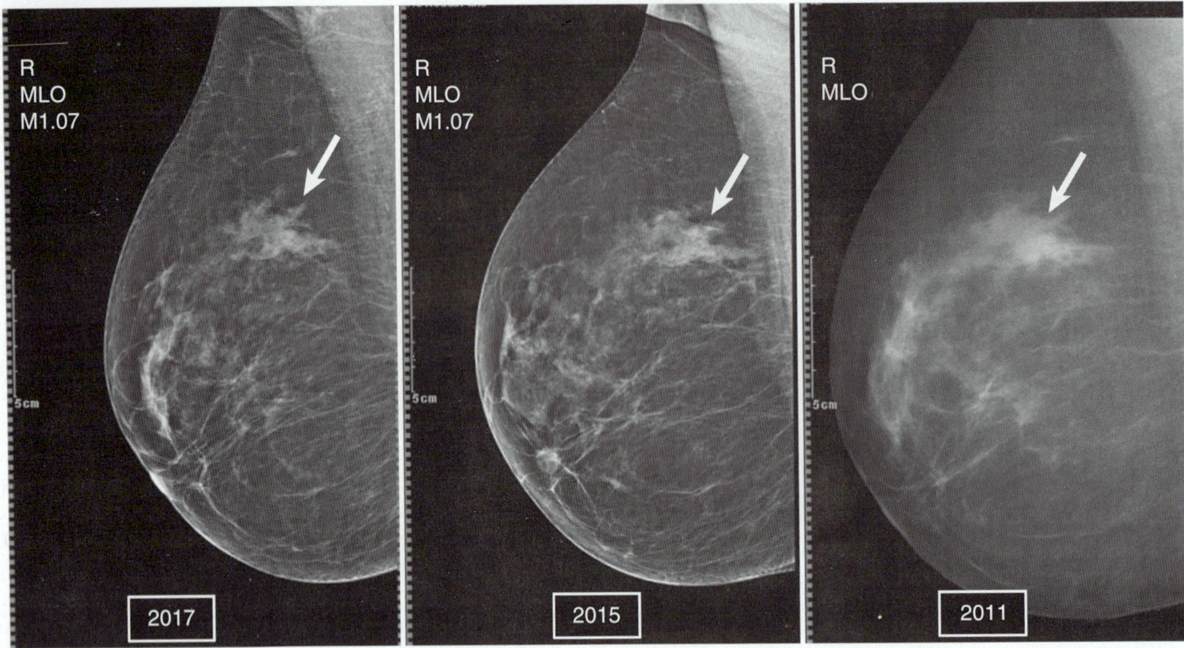

Figure 51.28 Stable focal asymmetry in the upper aspect (*white arrows*) shows stability over a period of time and can be regarded as benign based on comparison. *MLO,* mediolateral oblique.

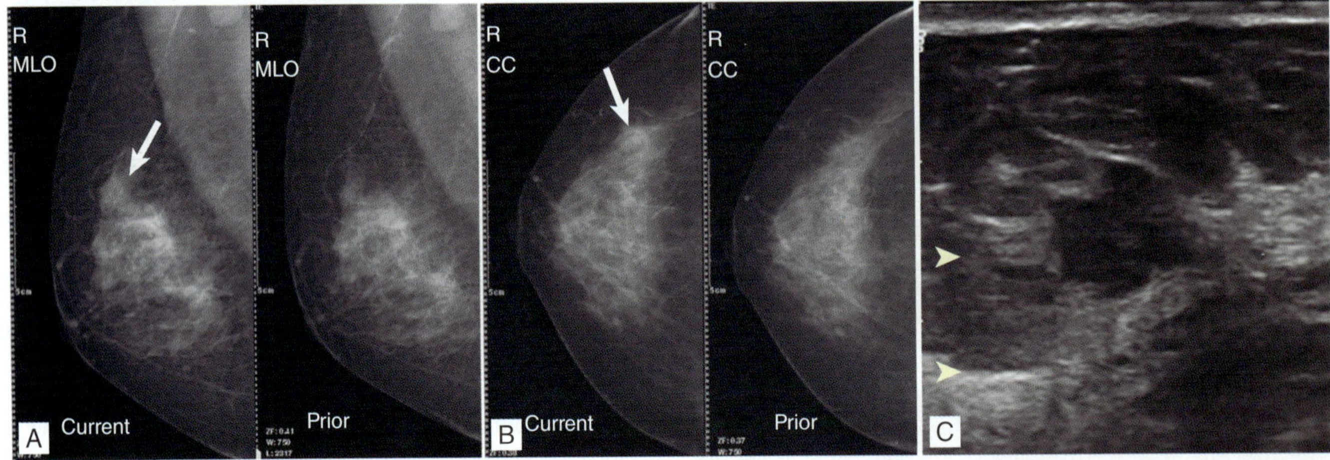

Figure 51.29 Developing asymmetric density in the upper outer quadrant of the right breast (*arrows* in A and B) corresponding to a hypoechoic solid irregular mass (*arrowheads*) as seen on ultrasonography (USG) (C). Also notice how the location matches along the anterior junctional line in mammography and USG. *CC,* craniocaudal; *MLO,* mediolateral obliquo.

Skin

Skin and underlying trabeculae assessment is important. Skin of the breast is thin and symmetric and can get thickened (>2 mm) because of multiple causes such as primary cutaneous disease processes, underlying inflammatory, infective and cancerous conditions of the breast, lymphatic or venous obstruction, or systemic causes of edema such as cardiac failure (Fig. 51.31) [1]. The edema along the Cooper ligament manifests as trabecular thickening when seen tangentially and diffuse increase in density when seen en face.

Nipple–Areola Abnormality

Nipple–areola abnormality may be seen in the form of thickening and retraction and can help in detecting a retroareolar lesion, which otherwise may be hard to see (Fig. 51.32). Nipple inversion is usually a long-standing finding and is considered be benign if stable. It can be bilateral.

Axillary Lymph Nodes

Axillary lymph nodes are common incidental findings, and mammography is not useful in further characterization unless the nodes are grossly enlarged, or they show microcalcifications within (Fig. 51.33). Bilateral adenopathy may represent a systemic disease condition or hematolymphoid disease, which may be correlated with history of any such disease. USG may be more useful for characterizing the nodes.

Breast Ultrasonography

Indications for Breast Ultrasonography

Ultrasonography (USG) complements both the clinical examination and mammography. It is especially valuable in mammographic dense breast; for detecting occult lesions; and in characterizing

TABLE 51.4 Breast Imaging Reporting and Data System Benign Calcifications [15,24]

Type of Calcification	Associated Pathology	Example
Skin	Calcifications in skin glands; commonly seen in axilla, near cleavage, or in inframammary fold	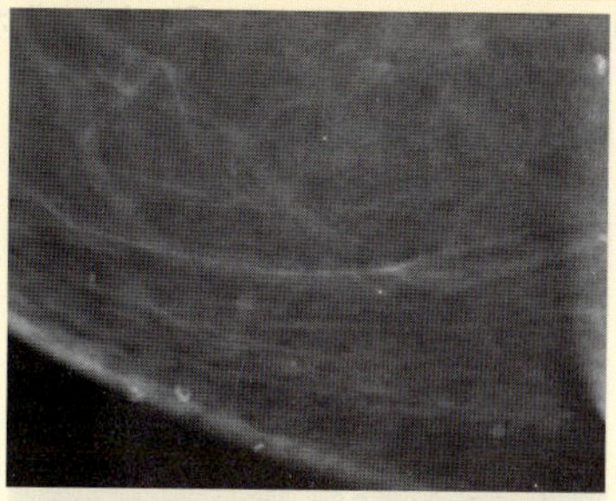
Vascular	Arterial wall calcification, increased incidence in patients with diabetes	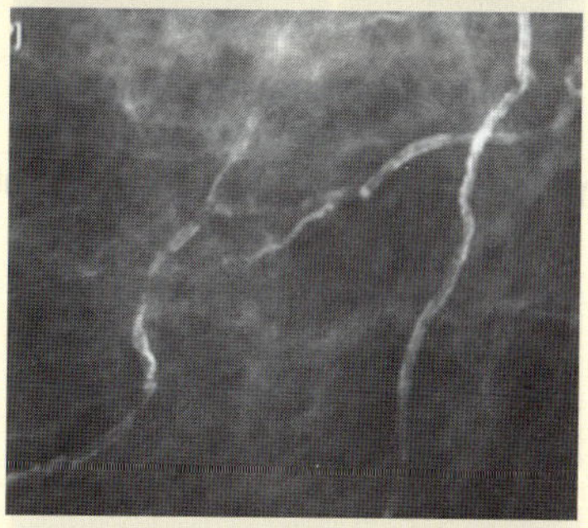
Popcorn	Involuting fibroadenoma	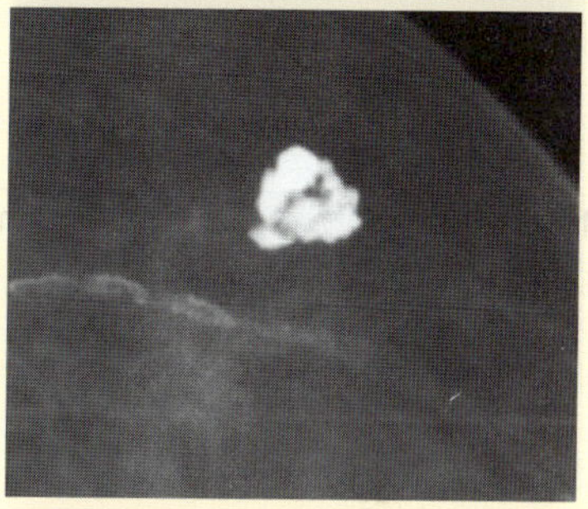
Large rodlike	Secretory calcifications in normal ducts	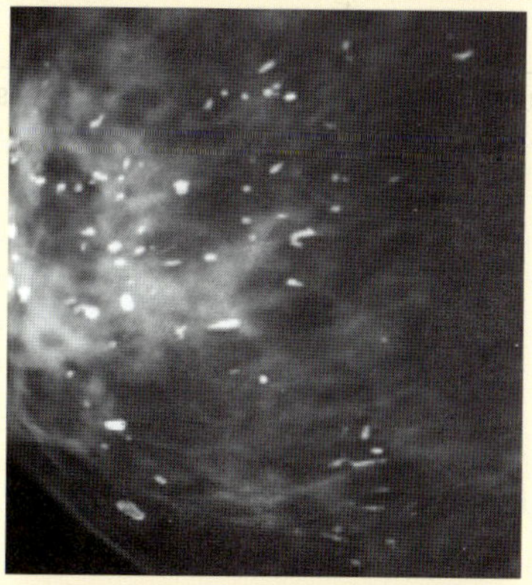
Round	Normal acinar calcification	

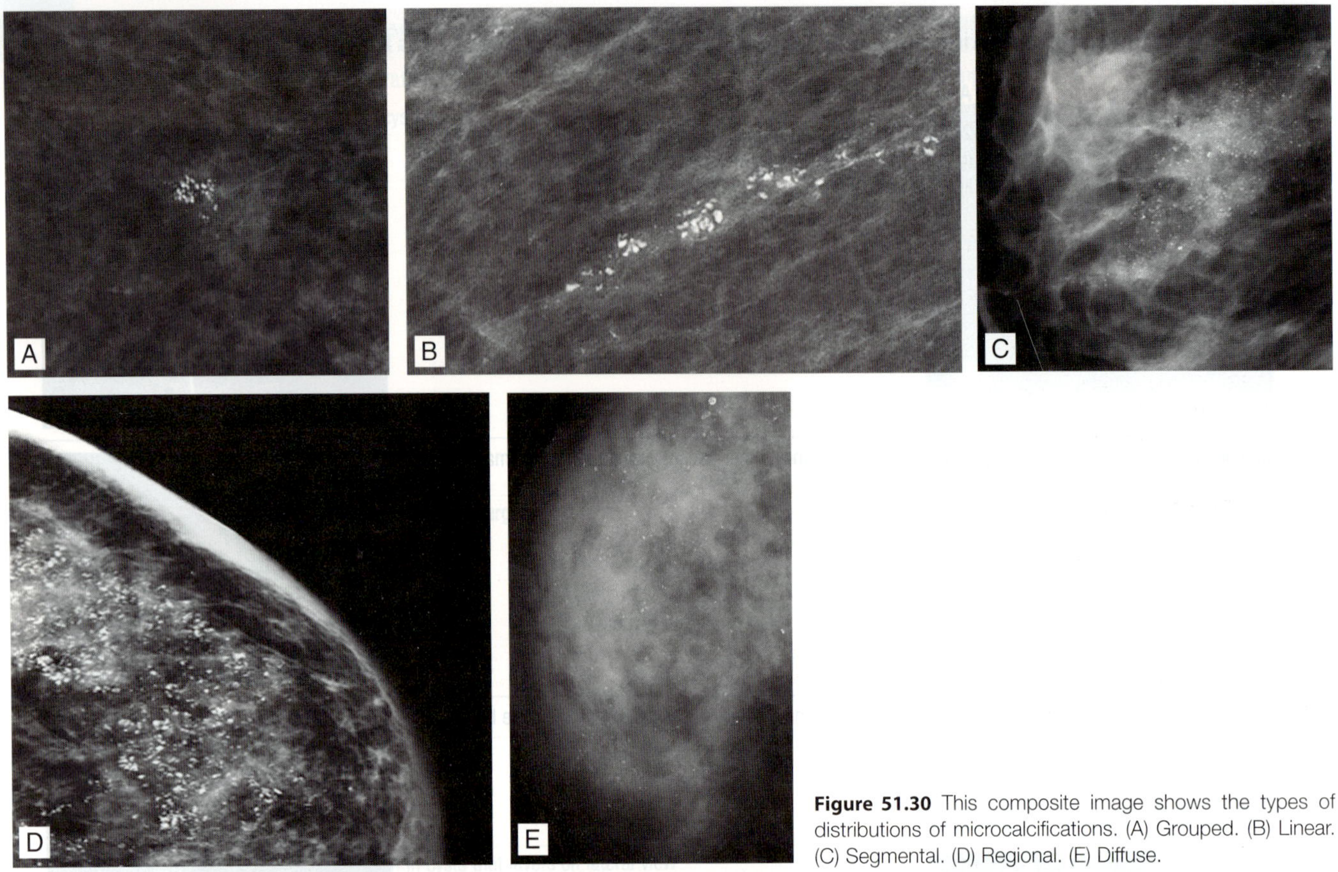

Figure 51.30 This composite image shows the types of distributions of microcalcifications. (A) Grouped. (B) Linear. (C) Segmental. (D) Regional. (E) Diffuse.

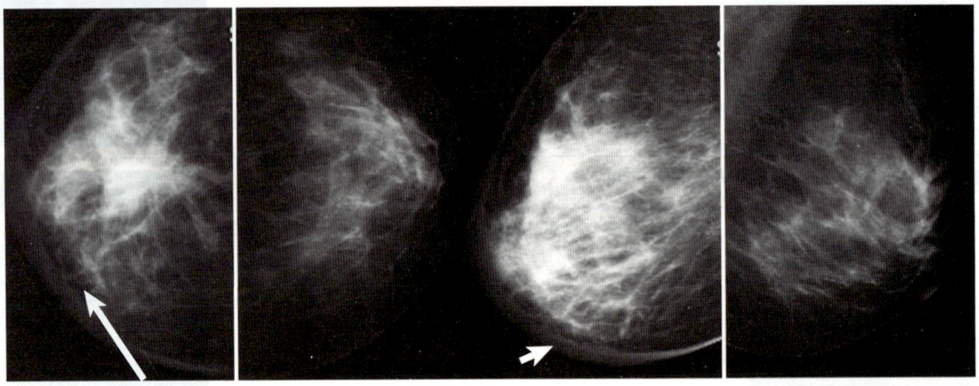

Figure 51.31 Diffuse edematous changes are seen in the right breast in the form of a diffuse increase in density and trabeculae (*long arrow*) and skin (*short arrow*) thickening caused by radiation therapy in this case.

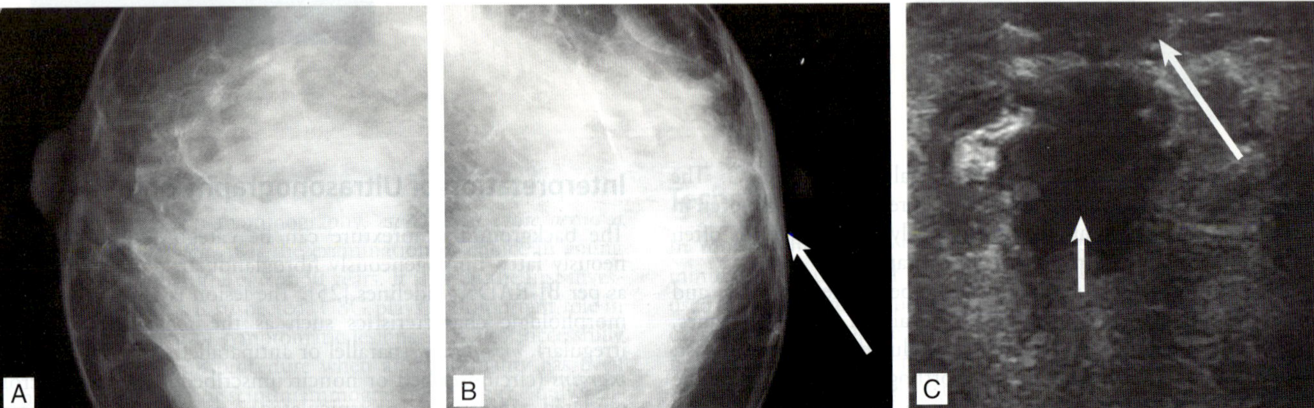

Figure 51.32 Thickening of the left nipple–areola complex is seen on the left side (*long arrows*) with a malignant retroareolar mass seen on ultrasonography (*short arrow*). This mass is difficult to perceive on mammograms.

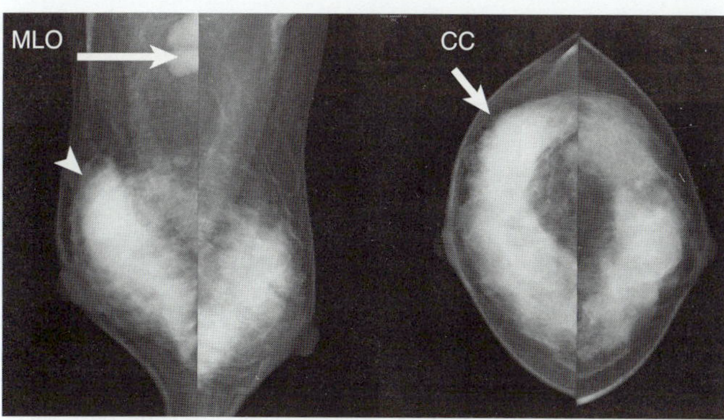

Figure 51.33 Enlarged nodes in the right axilla (*long arrow*) with a subtle mass on mammography seen in the form of asymmetric density (mediolateral oblique view [MLO]; *arrowhead*) and contour abnormality (craniocaudal view [CC]; *short arrow*) in the upper outer quadrant.

enhancement, shadowing, or combined) (Figs. 51.34 and 51.35) (Table 51.6). In the fifth edition of ACR BI-RADS, border (abrupt, echogenic halo) has been dropped, and any mass with echogenic halo is now called *noncircumscribed—indistinct margin*. One can also look for calcifications, vascularity, any associated features, and elastography characteristics [25].

The main use of USG is to distinguish between cyst and all others—solid or complex solid–cystic lesions (Fig. 51.36) [1]. Stavros et al. [26] have reported criteria that can be used to categorize solid masses into benign, indeterminate, and malignant types with 99.5% negative predictive value and 98.4% sensitivity for malignancy. It is, however, important to be aware of the shortcomings and limitations of relying purely on morphologic appearances. The presence of posterior acoustic enhancement and well-defined margins that occurs with benign masses such as fibroadenomas (Fig. 51.37A) is also associated with high-grade

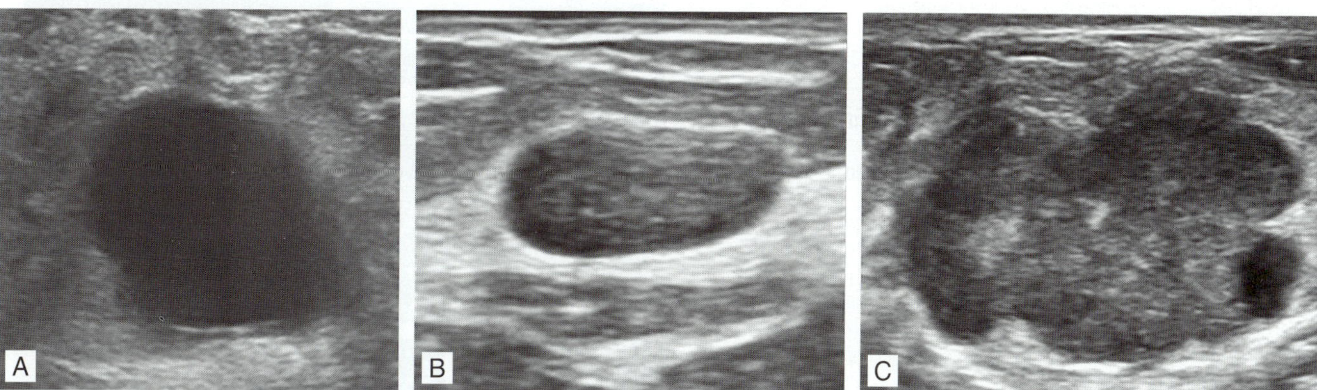

Figure 51.34 Types of shapes and orientation for breast masses on USG. (A) Round. (B) Oval with parallel orientation. (C) Irregular with antiparallel orientation.

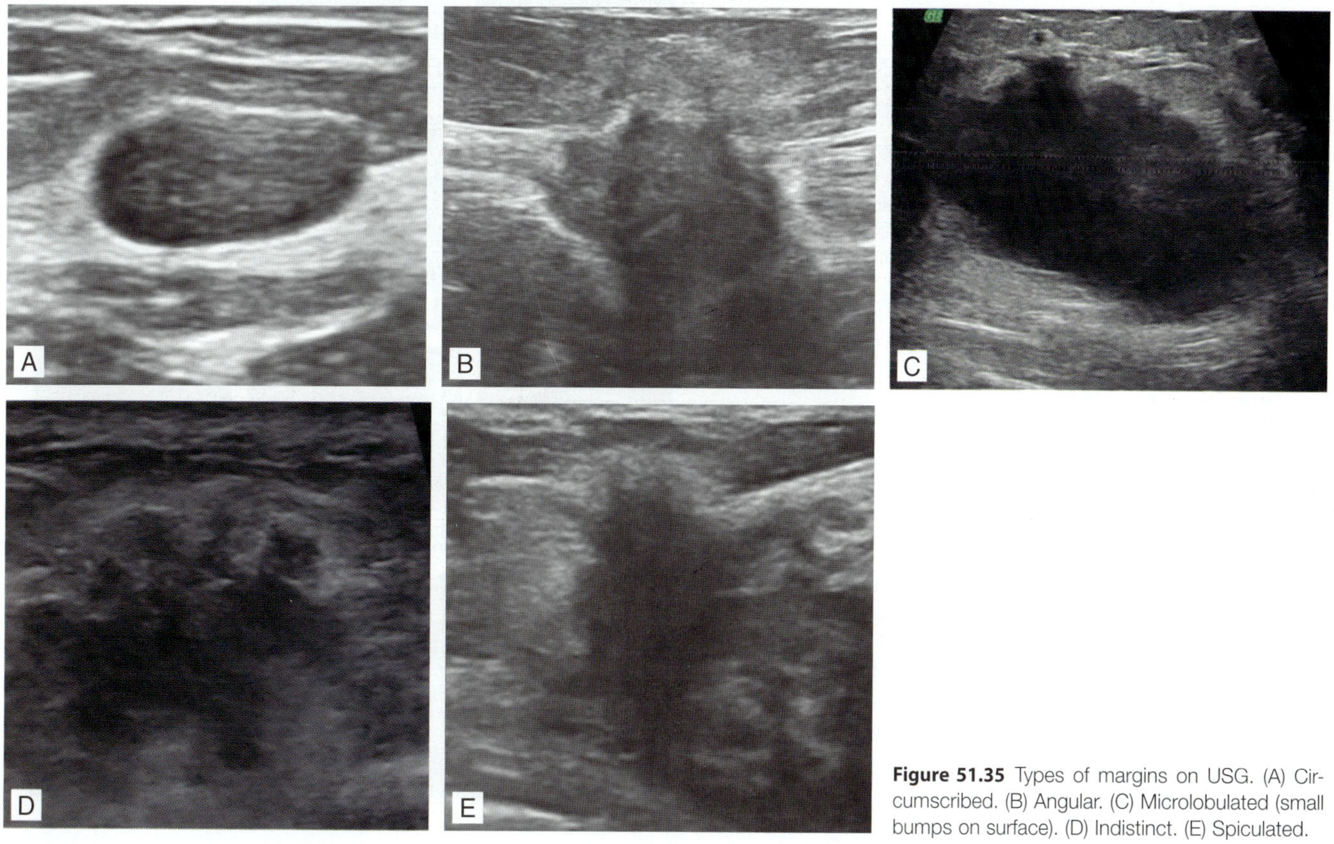

Figure 51.35 Types of margins on USG. (A) Circumscribed. (B) Angular. (C) Microlobulated (small bumps on surface). (D) Indistinct. (E) Spiculated.

TABLE 51.6 Breast Imaging Reporting and Data System Ultrasonography Descriptors for Masses [15,25]

Descriptor	Categories	Images
Shape (Fig. 51.34)	A. Round B. Oval C. Irregular	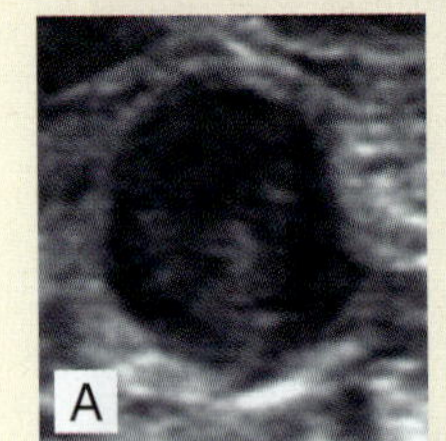 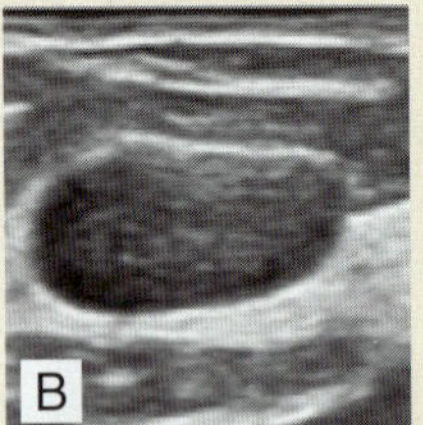 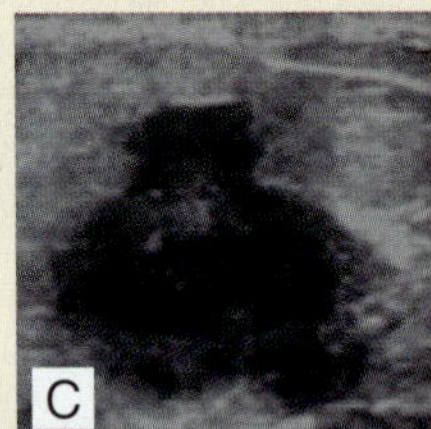
Orientation (Fig. 51.34)	A. Parallel to chest wall B. Not parallel	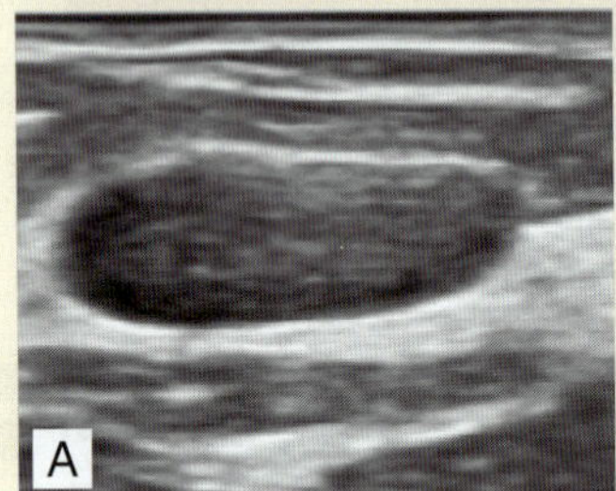 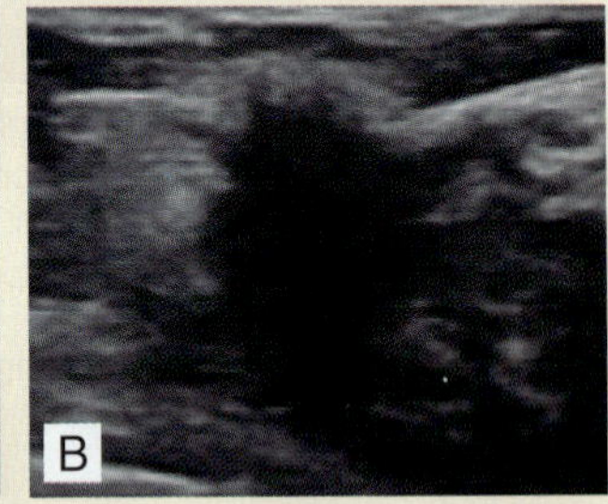
Margins (Fig. 51.35)	A. Circumscribed B. Angular C. Microlobulated D. Indistinct E. Spiculated	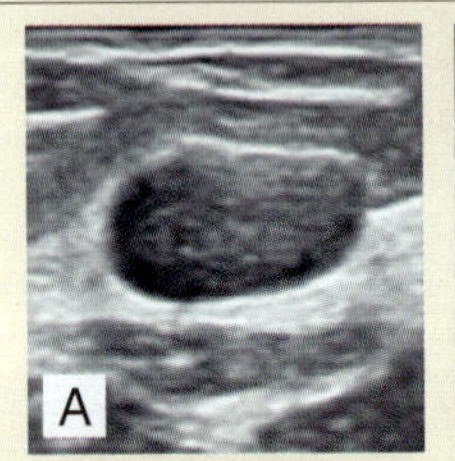 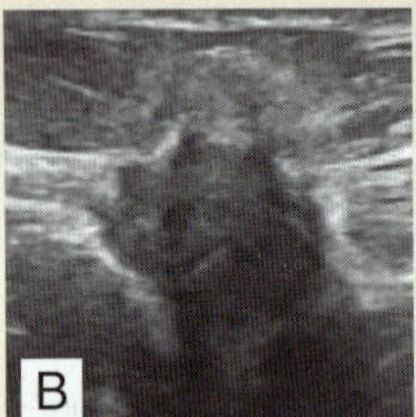 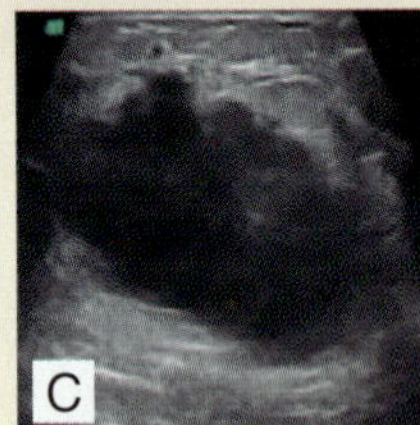 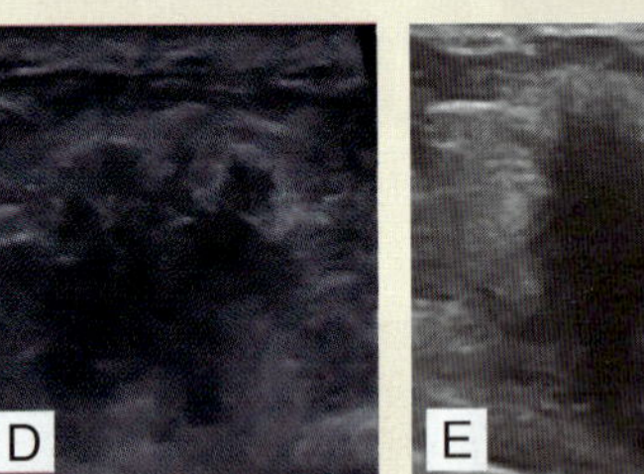
Echogenicity	A. Anechoic B. Hypoechoic C. Isoechoic D. Hyperechoic E. Heterogeneous F. Solid-cystic	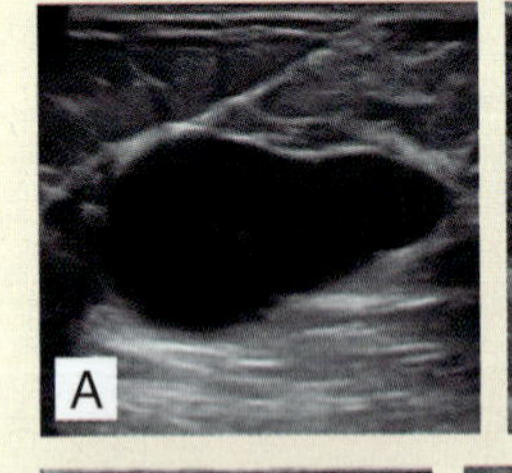 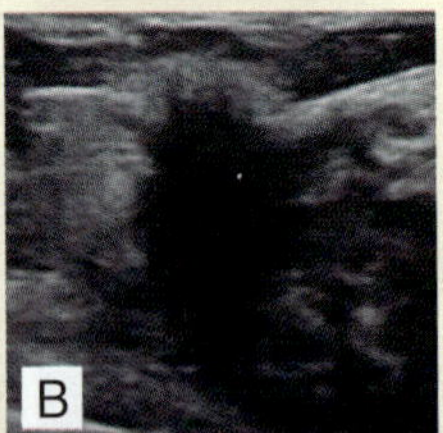 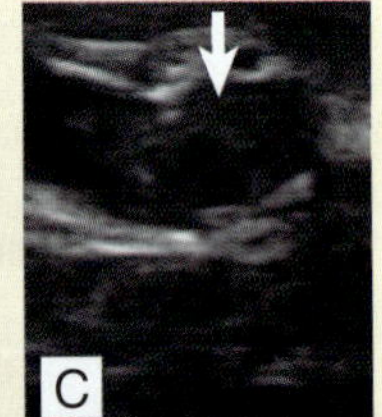 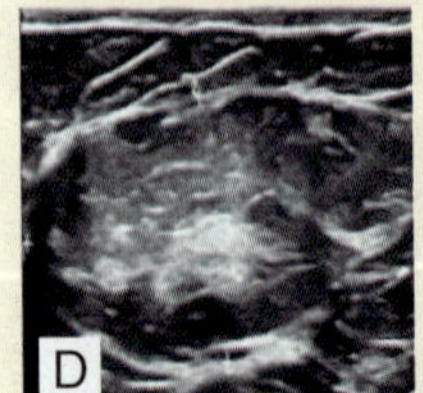 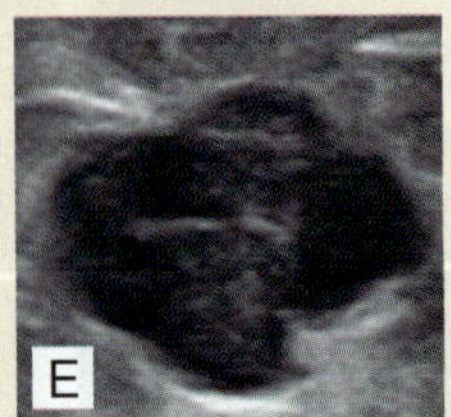 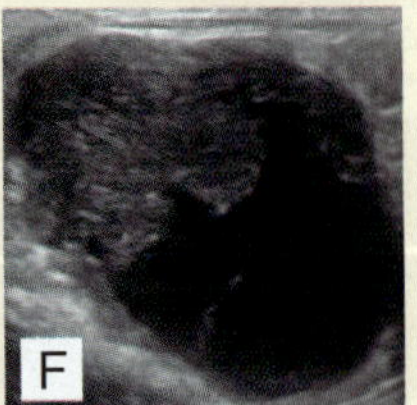
Postacoustic features	A. No postacoustic features B. Enhancement C. Shadowing	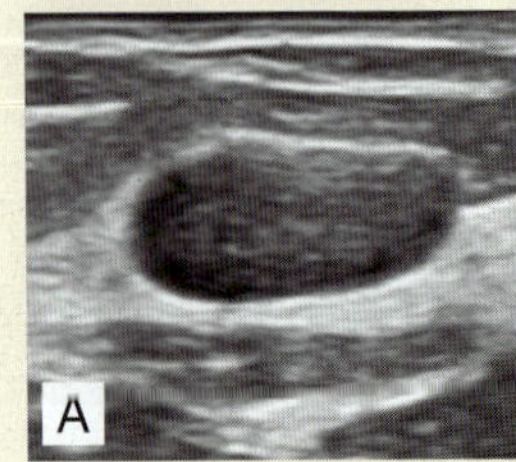 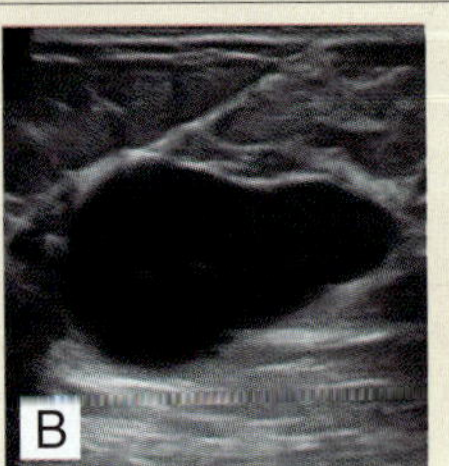 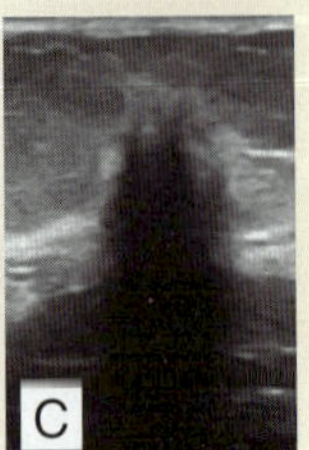

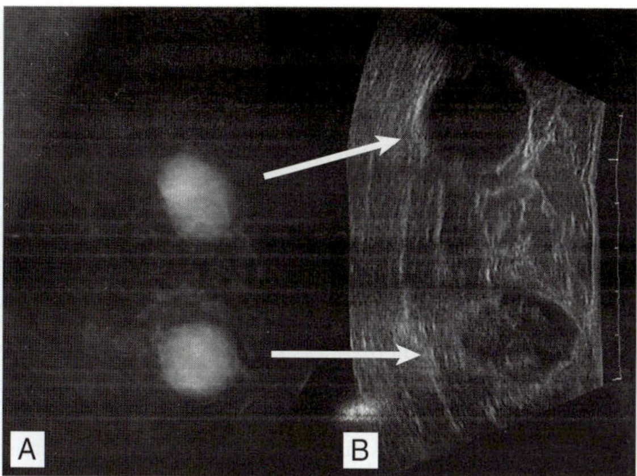

Figure 51.36 Two identical-looking masses on mammography (A). On ultrasonography (B), the superior (as indicated by *arrow*) is cystic and other (as indicated by *arrow*) is solid-cystic.

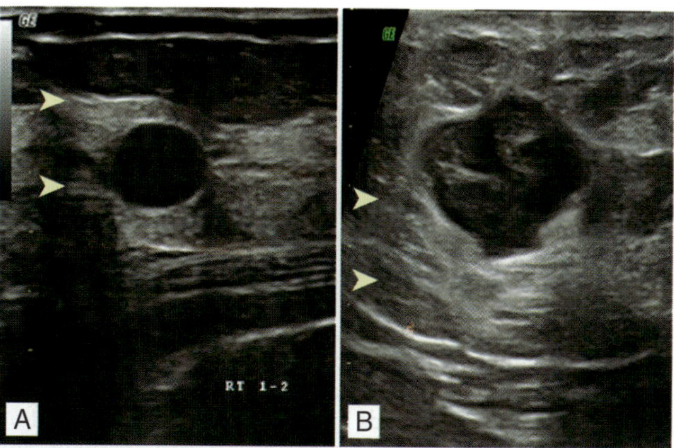

Figure 51.37 Well-defined margins and post acoustic enhancement in a benign cyst (A) and malignant mass (B) on ultrasonography.

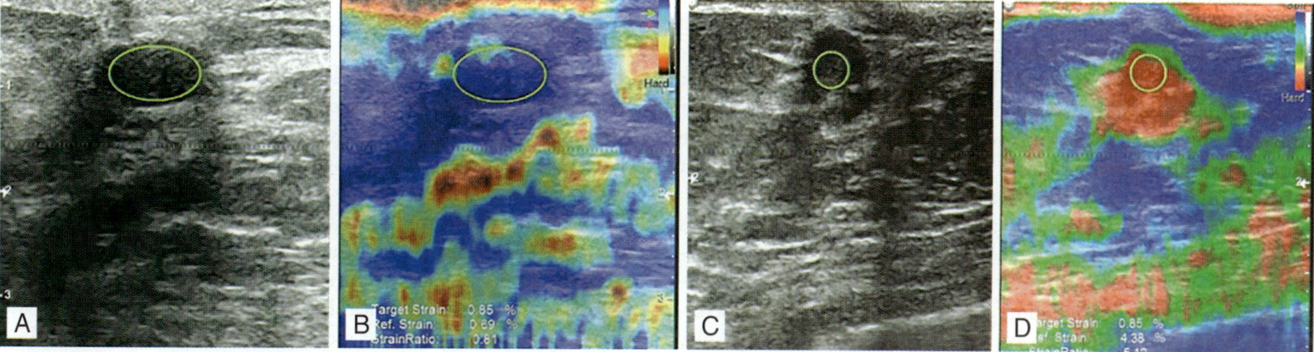

Figure 51.38 Strain-wave elastography shows a well-circumscribed lesion (A) with a low strain ratio (B) consistent with a benign lesion and an irregular lesion (C) with a high strain ratio (D) consistent with a suspicious lesion. (Courtesy of Dr. Richa Bansal, principal consultant in radiology, Max Superspecialty Hospital, Saket, New Delhi, India.)

malignancy, especially triple-negative breast cancers as well as mucinous and medullary carcinoma (Fig. 51.37B). Conversely, hypoechoic attenuating lesions with irregular margins typical of malignant disease can also be demonstrated in benign pathology such as fat necrosis, scarring, or fibrosis. In practice, needle biopsy should be performed as part of triple assessment in the presence of a discrete solid mass. Not all breast pathology presents as a discrete lesion. Inflammatory or lobular cancers may present as areas of scattered indeterminate attenuation. There may be other associated secondary signs such as increased hyperechogenicity of the intramammary fat, lymphatic dilation, or skin thickening. The use of color and power Doppler has also been exploited in aiding the benign versus malignant differentiation of solid masses. In general, malignant masses tend to show an increased number of vessels that penetrate deep into the tumor with a branching morphology. Both shear-wave and strain-wave elastography have been evaluated for breast lesions (Fig. 51.38). Cancers are more commonly stiff, noncompressible lesions. Strain-wave elastography can be used to quantify the stiffness. Hence, elastography can increase diagnostic confidence and accuracy; however, when equivocal, it is better to evaluate the lesion with biopsy [27].

Axillary lymph nodes are also better assessed on USG. A normal node has a reniform shape with a thin cortex and fatty hilum. The pathological nodes can show focal cortical thickening (>3 mm cortex), focal hypoechoic areas in cortex, rounded shape with loss of fatty hilum, or completely replaced hypoechoic node; however, fine-needle aspiration cytology (FNAC) or biopsy is often sought for confirmation.

Breast Magnetic Resonance Imaging

Breast MRI as a technology has been available for a very long time. However, establishing its use in breast clinics has taken a while. Initially, it suffered from a lack of robust data because there was no uniformity in assessment (the European researchers focused on temporal characteristics and the Americans on spatial features) until the technology allowed both to be of optimal quality at the same time. This was followed by standardization of protocols and reporting and building up of evidence to support its use. The difference between standard mammography and MRI is that administration of contrast allows us to explore neoangiogenesis that occurs when the rapidly multiplying cancer cells are outgrowing the oxygen supply and hence creating a network of new abnormal vessels [28]. It is a well-known fact that breast MRI has the highest sensitivity for detection of cancer among all methods of evaluation, the criticized downside, however, being lack of specificity because lesions other than cancers can enhance. Using it for the appropriate indications with the right technique and combining it with mammography and USG yields the best results.

Technique

Breast MRI needs a magnet strength of 1.5 or 3 T. The requirement for high-resolution scans with an adequate signal-to-noise and contrast-to-noise ratio necessitates the use of high-quality dedicated surface coils, capable of imaging both breasts at the same time. The patient is positioned prone with the breasts

"Chromophere" refers to any molecule in biologic tissue that can interact with light, namely, by absorption and scattering [46]. Using external source of light targeting the region of interest, excitation of endogenous or exogenous chromophores occurs with resulting emission of energy [46]. This release of energy can be as delayed emission of light, called *autofluorescence*, or as nonradiating heat to surroundings [48–50]. This heat produces a pressure wave via thermal expansion, in the form of detectable USG, which is called *photoacoustics* [51,52]. This is the basic principle of optical imaging. The common chromophores are hemoglobin (both oxygenated and deoxygenated), water, and lipids [46]. The various techniques of optical imaging used in practice are diffuse optical spectroscopy, diffuse optical imaging, diffuse optical tomography, fluorescence optical tomography, photoacoustic imaging, multiparametric infrared imaging, and hybrid techniques. Descriptions of each technique are out of the scope of this textbook and can be read in detail in an article by Leo et al. [46]. Studies for the detection of lesions and characteristics, as well as for monitoring of tumor response to neoadjuvant therapy, by use of optimal imaging have as yet not revealed clinically useful results [46]. This technique lacks the ability to localize a suspicious lesion, and thus its practical use would still be as an adjunct to mammography, USG, or MRI [46].

Breast-Specific Gamma Imaging

Breast-specific gamma imaging (BSGI) uses the same principles applicable to other nuclear medicine techniques, with the difference being in the use of a breast specific gamma camera. The radiopharmaceutical commonly used is technetium-99m (dose of ~110 MBq), with the imaging performed 10 minutes after injection. Multiple views with slight compression of the breasts similar to mammography are done. This study is based on the principle of increased radiotracer uptake by malignant tissue by virtue of neoangiogenesis and increased mitochondrial activity. When compared with MRI, BSGI is advantageous in that it is less expensive, and it can be done easily in patients with obesity, claustrophobia, metal implants, and other relative contraindications to MRI [53,54]. Studies have mainly evaluated the utility of this technique in the characterization of BI-RADS 4 lesions and lesion detection in dense breasts [55].

Positron Emission Mammography

Positron emission mammography (PEM) is a molecular imaging technique based on the principle of fluorine-18-fluorodeoxyglucose (^{18}F-FDG) uptake in the breasts and generation of high-resolution tomographic slice images, with total radiation dose much less than whole-body PET imaging using standard CC and MLO projections and compression analogous to mammography [56]. PEM can be used in the initial staging evaluation of patients with newly diagnosed cancer (i.e., determining extent of disease but not including axillary node staging because it does not cover the axilla completely), distinguishing recurrent carcinoma from scar or restaging, and monitoring response to neoadjuvant chemotherapy [57]. Studies have shown that PEM has a sensitivity of 90% and specificity of 86% in evaluating known breast cancer or suspicious lesions [56]. It has high sensitivity in the detection of both ductal carcinoma in situ and ILC [58,59]. PEM has also been found to be a useful alternative to MRI in women who have contraindications to or cannot tolerate MRI [58].

Cone-Beam Computed Tomography

Cone-beam computed tomography (CBCT) consists of an x-ray tube, a full-field flat-panel detector, and a design motor-driven rotating table to provide high-quality images and real-time 3D visualization of the breast [60,61]. It can be performed both with and without contrast. Studies have shown that breast coverage and radiation dose using CBCT is similar to that required for conventional diagnostic MG, and thus this technique has the potential to further characterize high-risk breast lesions that have been identified in screening by mammography or USG [61]. Because cone-beam CT does not need breast compression, it scores over mammography in causing much less patient discomfort and anxiety. The 3D images aid in positioning biopsy or radiotherapy, radiofrequency ablation techniques, and especially localizing clinically nonpalpable breast lesions more accurately and precisely [60]. Also, CBCT allows for evaluation of the mass, calcification, and vascularity [61]. This ability to detect and characterize calcifications scores over MRI and has thus proved CBCT to be useful in conjunct to mammography [61].

Common Conditions and Diseases of the Breast With Clinical Radiology–Pathology Correlation

Infective and Inflammatory Conditions

Breast abscess or mastitis often presents in a lactating breast and can be diagnosed clinically. It is more common in the breastfeeding period of the first pregnancy and responds to antibiotics. The most common cause is *Staphylococcus* spp. Breastfeeding should be encouraged and antibiotics safe for the newborn should be used for treatment [62,63]. Ultrasound assessment is done to assess if there is any drainable collection. Infective mastitis manifests as altered echotexture with edematous changes in the subcutaneous fat and erythematous skin thickening. When an ill-defined hypoechoic area with or without moving echoes is seen within, it is evolving into an abscess that can be drained under ultrasound guidance (Fig. 51.46). A fully formed abscess has a necrotic center and thick wall with vascularity.

A *hematoma* can show a similar appearance, but the clinical presentation and history help establish the diagnosis. Sometimes older women develop peripheral abscesses that show similar imaging characteristics and respond to antibiotics.

Galactoceles develop during lactation and are usually 2 to 3 cm in diameter. They are more often mixed density lesions rather than pure radiolucent and can have low level echoes on USG (Fig. 51.47). The differential diagnosis includes lactational abscess,

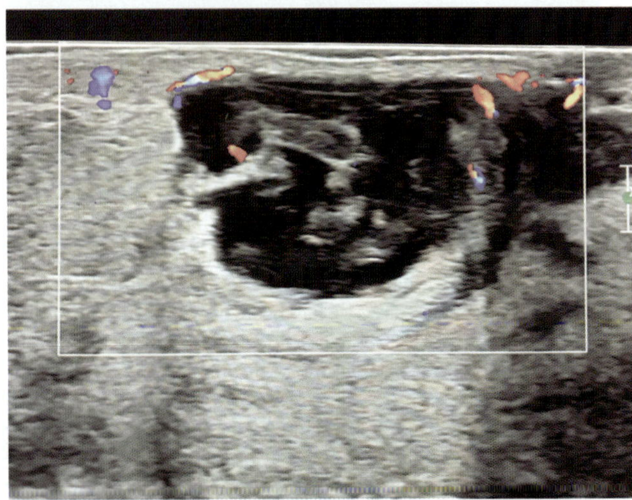

Figure 51.46 Ultrasonography image shows a heteroechoic lesion with anechoic areas of liquefaction with peripheral vascularity in a lactating woman, suggestive of an abscess.

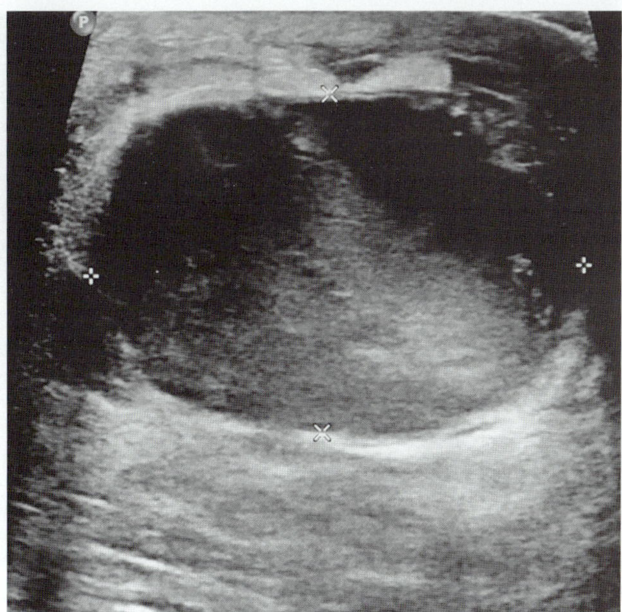
Figure 51.47 Ultrasonography image shows a homogeneous cystic lesion with low-level internal echoes in a lactating woman suggestive of galactocele.

adenoma, and very rarely pregnancy-associated cancer. The yield of aspiration is often thick milky fluid.

Zuska disease, a recurrent painful subareolar abscesses with fistula, is another inflammatory condition seen more commonly in smokers (Fig. 51.48). The lactiferous ducts develop squamous metaplasia, which can produce keratin. This keratin can block the ducts, which then balloon up and rupture, producing a granulomatous inflammatory reaction [64]. It can mimic a carcinoma on

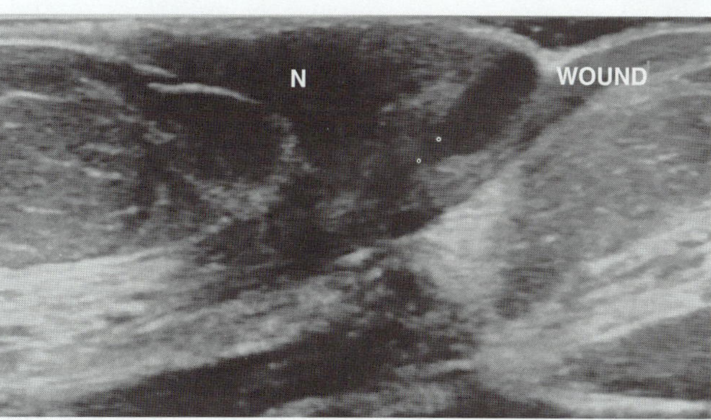

Figure 51.48 Ultrasonography image shows periareolar sinus, labeled as a wound, in a woman with recurrent retroareolar abscess suggestive of Zuska disease. *N,* nipple.

imaging, and if there is any clinical concern of malignancy, a biopsy is recommended.

Lobular granulomatous mastitis is an idiopathic condition that affects multiparous women. Clinically, it mimics cancer. There are no characteristic mammographic features, although focal asymmetric density is seen more commonly than a mass; however, an ultrasound appearance of multiple contiguous hypoechoic tubular lesions can be considered suggestive of the disease (Fig. 51.49) [65]. Biopsy confirmation is recommended, which reveals noncaseating nonvasculitic granulomas and helps to rule out secondary causes of granulomatous mastitis, which can be seen in tuberculosis, sarcoidosis, and other conditions.

Diabetic mastopathy manifests clinically as a large, painless, hard breast mass that is usually indistinguishable from breast cancer. It is a form of lymphocytic mastitis and stromal fibrosis that occurs in patients with uncontrolled insulin-dependent diabetes. It can present

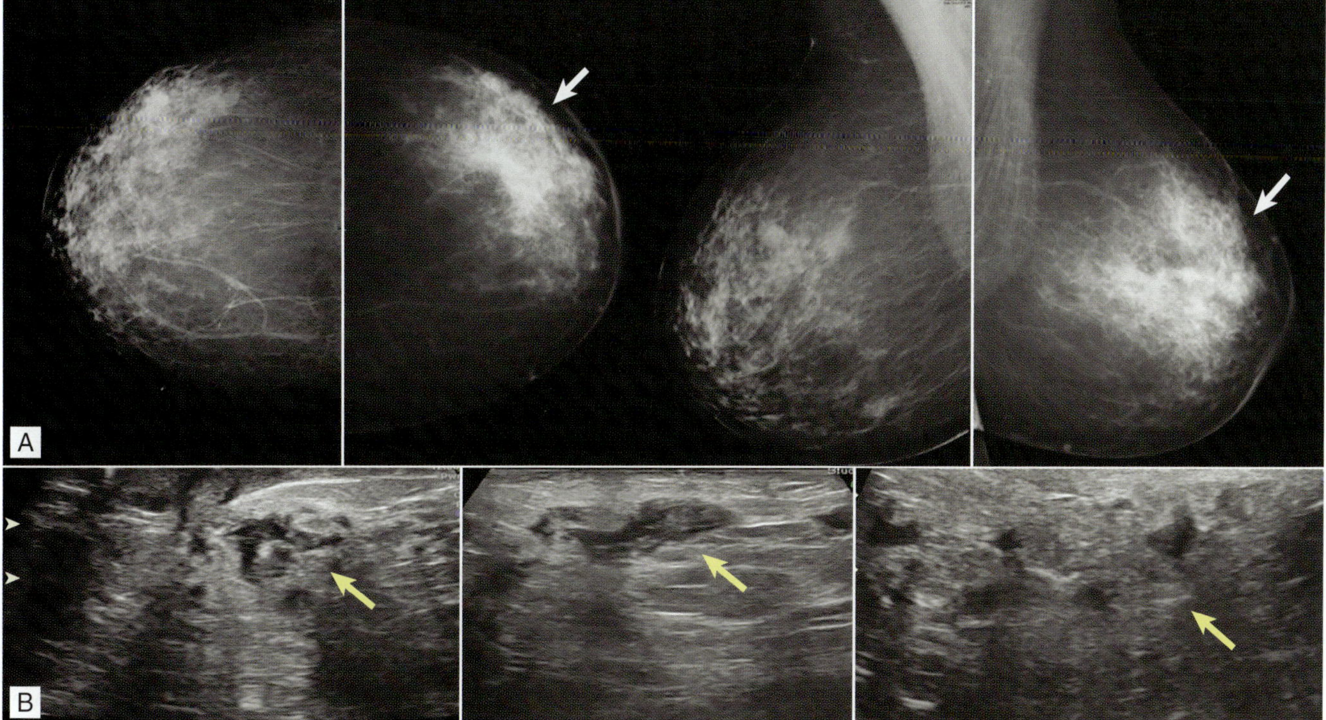

Figure 51.49 Mammogram (A) of a 42-year multiparous woman with a painless lumpish feel in the left breast. There is an asymmetric density (*white arrows*) in the left breast over a large area in the outer central region without any discrete mass or microcalcifications. On ultrasonography (B), tubular hypoechoic lesions are seen in the breast (*yellow arrows*). Again, no discrete mass was seen. On biopsy, this was proven to be granulomatous mastitis.

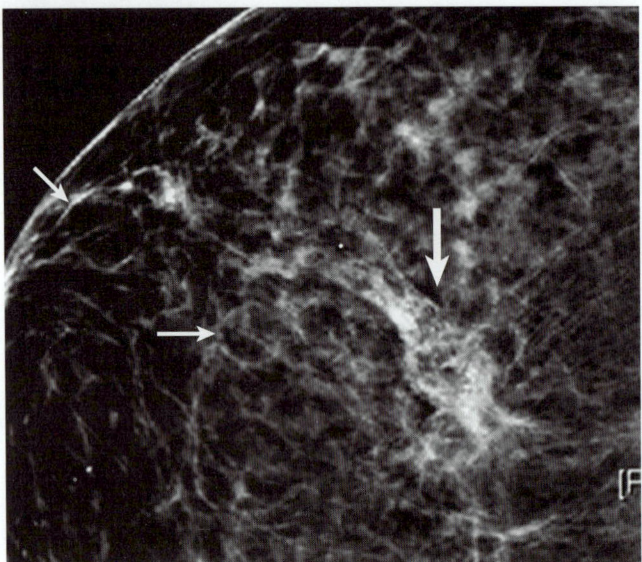

Figure 51.50 Post-BCT mammographic image shows few circumscribed fat density rounded lesions, which are oil cysts (*thin arrows*) and oil cyst with dystrophic calcification and architectural distortion in the deeper scar site (*thick arrow*).

as asymmetric density or masses on mammography, which on USG shows ill-defined hypoechoic lesion with marked postacoustic shadowing, mimicking cancer [66]. On MRI, nonspecific delayed stromal enhancement has been reported, keeping in line with fibrosis at any other site in body. Core biopsy is recommended for confirmation.

Fat necrosis can be seen after trauma or surgery. An encapsulated fat density lesion (an oil cyst in the setting of trauma) is pathognomonic of fat necrosis; however, AD, irregular lesion and calcification can be a manifestation of the same, causing potential confusion with malignancy. In such cases, a biopsy is advisable (Figs. 51.50 and 51.51). Over time, the oil cysts develop peripheral curvilinear calcification, which can mimic recurrent microcalcifications in a setting of treated cancer; however, the key is to look at prior images, which often show lucent oil cysts at that site. Gradually, a complete ring is formed, giving rise to the known classic benign rim calcification. On MRI, demonstration of a fat-containing cyst (suppresses on fat-saturated images and bright on T1-weighted images) that often shows rim enhancement is considered diagnostic. However, as on mammography, sometimes lesions with no obvious fat density may be seen in the form of focal or diffuse enhancement, AD, or irregular masses with variable enhancement kinetics [67], and again biopsy should be advised if there is any suspicion of malignancy.

Cystic Diseases of the Breast

Cysts are lesions formed as a consequence of excessive secretion into a lobule, which leads to its abnormal distension. These lobules can coalesce to form larger cysts. Unopened cysts show brown or blue color (blue dome cyst) on gross pathology [2]. The cyst wall can be lined by atrophic epithelium or with cells showing apocrine metaplasia, basically nonproliferative lesions that can be considered as disorder of normal involution, in the spectrum of aberrations in normal development and involution (ANDI) lesions [68]. They can occur anywhere in the breast and are more commonly seen in women in their fourth decade of life or later. These are well-defined circumscribed masses (often multiple) on mammography, and USG is considered diagnostic when it shows an anechoic lesion with smooth thin walls with postacoustic enhancement suggestive of a benign *simple cyst* (Fig. 51.52). They need to be aspirated only if symptomatic.

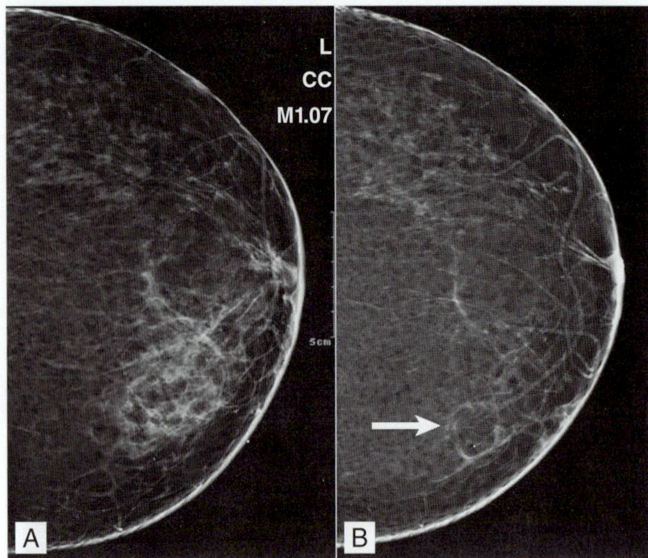

Figure 51.51 A 43-year-old woman who presented with a lumpish feel. (A) Architectural distortion with lucent areas within. On further interrogation, there was history of injury with a ball few days earlier. This was suspected fat necrosis. On follow-up imaging 6 weeks later (B), there is near complete resolution with formation of an oil cyst (*arrow*). *CC,* craniocaudal.

Sometimes the cyst can get complicated with pericystic inflammation, and their contents can be low-level echoes (Fig. 51.53). Such cysts in the right clinical context can be called *complicated cysts* and can be assigned a "probably benign" category and followed up accordingly. The incidence of malignancy in them is less

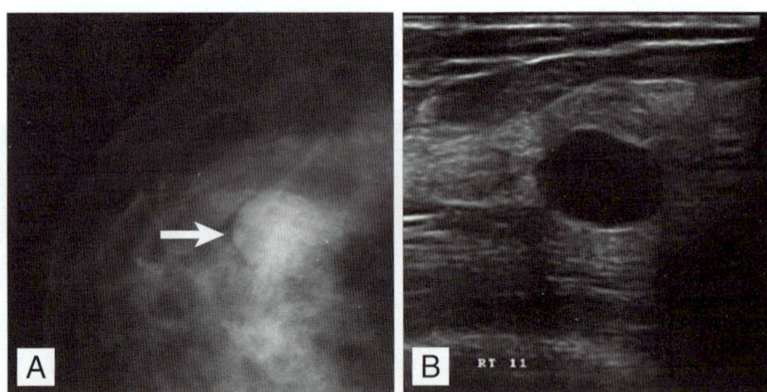

Figure 51.52 An isodense lesion is seen on mammography (*arrow* in A) that corresponds to a well-defined oval anechoic lesion with thin walls, edge shadowing, and postacoustic enhancement on ultrasonography (B).

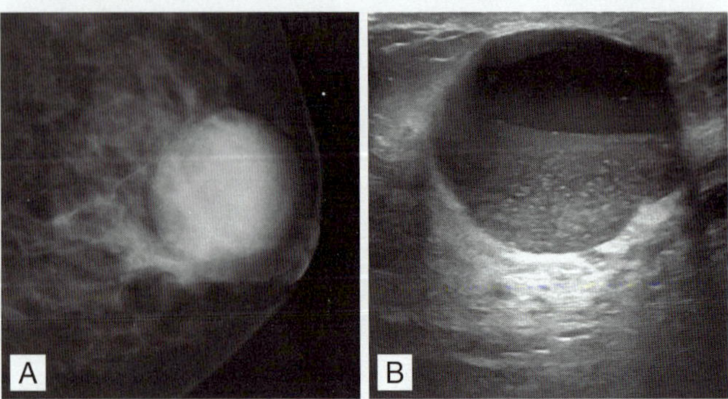

Figure 51.53 A high-density well-circumscribed lesion on mammography (A) that correlates to a slightly thick-walled cystic lesion with a fluid-debris level that was moving on real-time ultrasonography (B) without any solid component suggestive of a complicated cyst. Aspirate was serosanguinous paucicellular aspirate with no atypical cells.

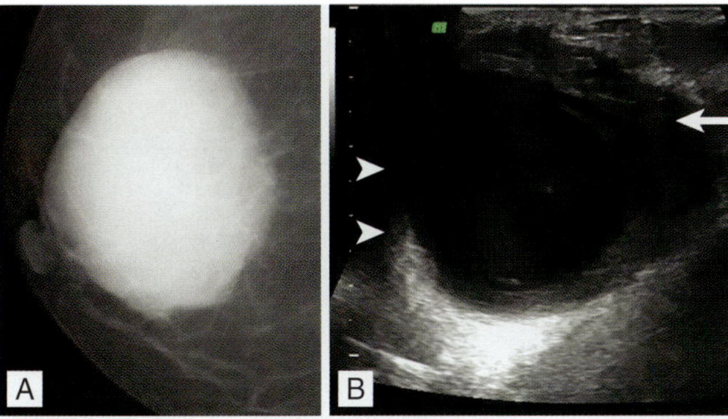

Figure 51.54 A high-density well-circumscribed lesion on mammography (A) correlates to a solid-cystic lesion on ultrasonography (B) with a thick solid wall (*arrow*).

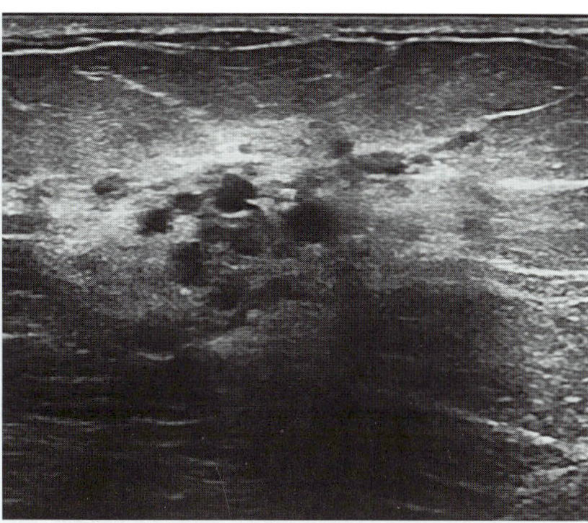

Figure 51.55 Ultrasonography shows clustered microcysts without any solid component.

than 2% [69,70]. However, some radiologists choose to aspirate them, which is easily doable under ultrasound guidance.

Occasionally, the cysts can show thickened walls or solid component within, which can be benign or malignant (Fig. 51.54). Such lesions were previously called *complex cysts* and can now be called *solid-cystic* and need diagnostic needle aspiration, core biopsy, or both. Surgical excision may also be considered if there is any uncertainty.

On MRI, simple cysts are T2 hyperintense lesions with nonenhancing, thin walls. The cyst walls can show enhancement in a complicated cyst. When the contents appear bright on T1-weighted images because of hemorrhagic or proteinaceous contents, it points toward a complicated cyst, but an intracystic enhancing component is suggestive of a solid lesion within.

Clustered microcysts are cysts measuring less than 5 mm in a cluster (Fig. 51.55). On mammography, they can correlate to small oval lesions and on histology can show fibrocystic change or apocrine metaplasia. They can be observed with serial USG because they have a low risk of malignancy [25].

Diseases Associated With Ducts

Papillary lesions, especially papilloma, are rarely visible on mammography because they lie within a duct or sometimes within a cyst (Figs. 51.56 and 51.57). Uncommonly, they can present as grouped microcalcification (Fig. 51.58). They can be identified on USG, especially when the duct is dilated and the solid hypoechoic lesion shows a fibrovascular stalk. They more commonly occur in the central ducts than peripherally [1]. Peripheral papillomas can be multiple and associated with atypia or DCIS [51]. During earlier times, ductography was performed, which showed the lesion as a filling defect in contrast opacified duct (Fig. 51.59). However, today, if a papilloma is strongly suspected and not visualized on routine imaging, some prefer the use of MRI. On MRI, it appears as an enhancing lesion within a dilated duct. The distinction between benign and malignant papillary lesions cannot be made on imaging, so histopathology is often sought [71]. Clinically, a woman with papilloma is likely to present with a single duct and spontaneous serous or bloody nipple discharge and uncommonly with a palpable mass.

Solitary dilated duct can be seen on USG without a papillary lesion within. If this is seen in an asymptomatic and clinically normal woman, it can be observed, although there are anecdotal case reports of cancer in such ducts [1].

Ductal ectasia (ducts >3 mm in diameter) is often seen as an incidental finding in the retroareolar region, often bilaterally. It can be

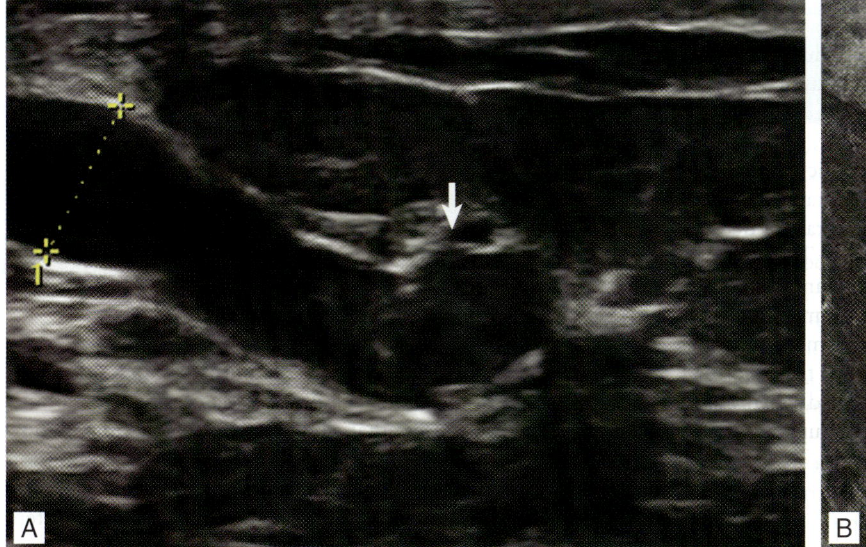

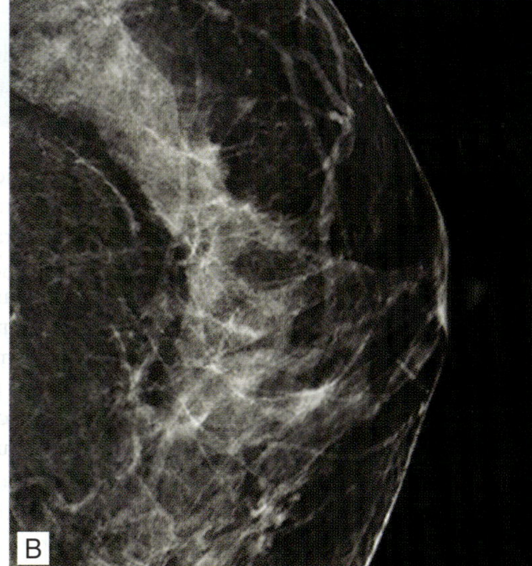

Figure 51.56 A dilated duct with a solid lesion (*arrow*) within suggestive of an intraductal papillary lesion within on ultrasonography of a woman presenting with single-duct blood-stained nipple discharge (A). The corresponding mammogram (B) revealed no abnormality.

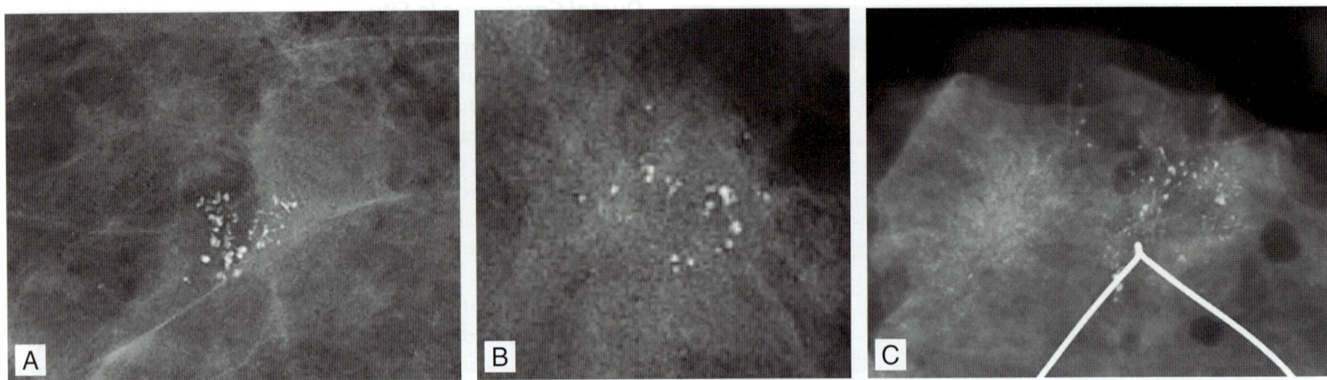

Figure 51.70 Grouped fine pleomorphic clusters on mammograms. (A) A high-grade ductal carcinoma in situ (DCIS) without necrosis. (B) Fibrocystic change. (C) Sclerosing adenosis with fibrocystic change (no DCIS or atypia).

mammography (suggesting that not all DCISs show calcification but can produce NME), whereas mammography would identify a greater number of low-grade DCIS than MRI [76].

Invasive Breast Cancers

As mentioned earlier in the pathology section, IBC-NST is the most common type of breast cancer followed by invasive lobular cancer and other special types. IBC can also be classified into three grades of increasing severity (I, II, and III) based on tubule formation, nuclear pleomorphism, and mitotic index (Nottingham histologic score). On immunohistochemistry, IBC shows a variable expression of hormone receptors (HR)—estrogen (ER) and progesterone (PR)—and expression of erythroblastic oncogene 2 (ERBB2) (previously called Her-2), which not only has prognostic value but also guides treatment, with endocrine therapy given for HR-positive tumors and targeted therapy with monoclonal antibodies such as trastuzumab offered for tumors overexpressing ERBB2 [2].

Apart from histologic subtypes, breast cancer can be classified into *genomic/molecular subtypes*, the common ones being luminal type A, luminal type B, Her-2 enriched, and basal-like, using newer gene profiling tests [77]. The luminal type A tumors are often HR-positive, Her-2–negative tumors with low Ki-67; the luminal type B are HR and Her-2–positive tumors; the Her-2–enriched tumors are HR-negative Her-2–positive tumors; and the basal cell–like tumors are often triple-negative (ER, PR, and Her-2 negative) breast cancer (TNBC).

IBC-NST most commonly present as masses on imaging. These masses are commonly spiculated but can have indistinct, microlobulated, or even circumscribed margins. They can also be associated with microcalcifications. On USG, they are often hypoechoic or heterogeneous masses with noncircumscribed margins and variable postacoustic features. Similarly, on MRI, IBC commonly present as masses that are T2 iso- to hypointense compared with parenchyma, with noncircumscribed margins and heterogenous or peripheral thick rim enhancement. Progressive centripetal enhancement has also been described. It is important to remember that variations do exist; although most cancers are T2 iso- to hypointense, mucinous/colloid carcinoma contains extracellular mucin and can be hyperintense on T2-weighted images. Masses can also be associated with NME when there is DCIS adjacent to invasive cancer, just like mass with microcalcifications on mammography (see Fig. 51.43).

If we were to correlate the morphologic features to molecular subtypes, we would find that the luminal cancers (both A and B) commonly present as spiculated masses, but Her-2–enriched masses are ill defined with microcalcifications, and basal-like/TNBC present as well-circumscribed masses. However, there is an overlap, and imaging is not reliable to distinguish these subtypes (Figs. 51.71 to 51.73) [78,79].

Imaging of Some Special Types of Invasive Breast Cancer

Invasive lobular carcinoma can have variable appearances on mammography. It can present as a mass (most commonly as a spiculated lesion that is isodense to the breast), AD, or asymmetric density that can be difficult to detect on conventional imaging (see Fig. 51.25). MRI is recommended in ILC for ruling out multifocal and bilateral tumors, which may occur because of loss of the E-cadherin gene, leading to a lack of cohesiveness of cells (previously discussed in the

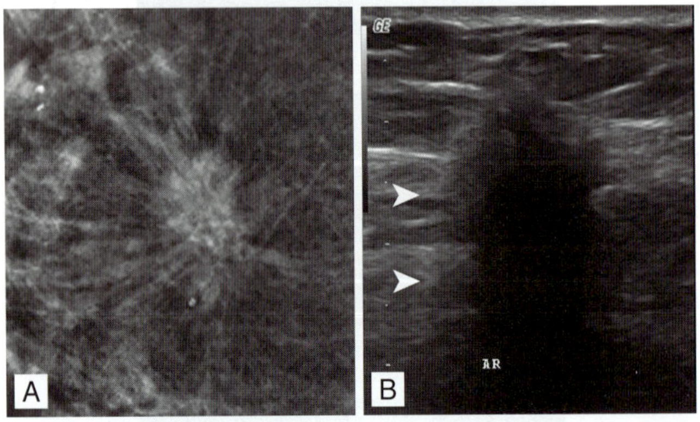

Figure 51.71 Spiculated mass with irregular shape seen on mammogram (A), which appears solid and hypoechoic and causes postacoustic shadowing on ultrasonography (B). A hormonal receptor–positive ERBB2-negative breast cancer (luminal A).

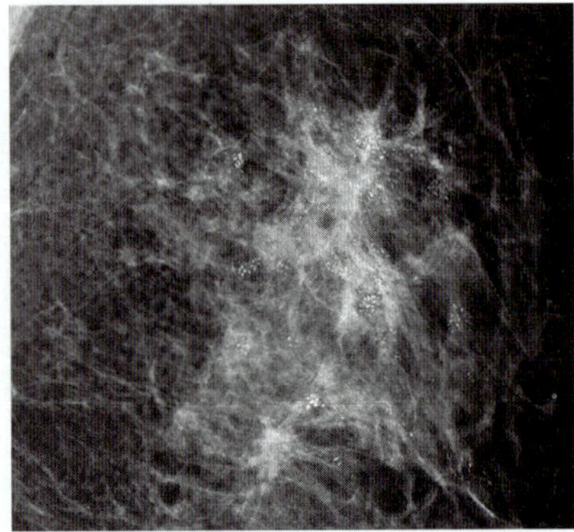

Figure 51.72 Parenchymal edge distortion by asymmetric density, an ill-defined mass, and microcalcification in the anterior aspect of the lesion in the left breast is caused by a Her-2–positive tumor.

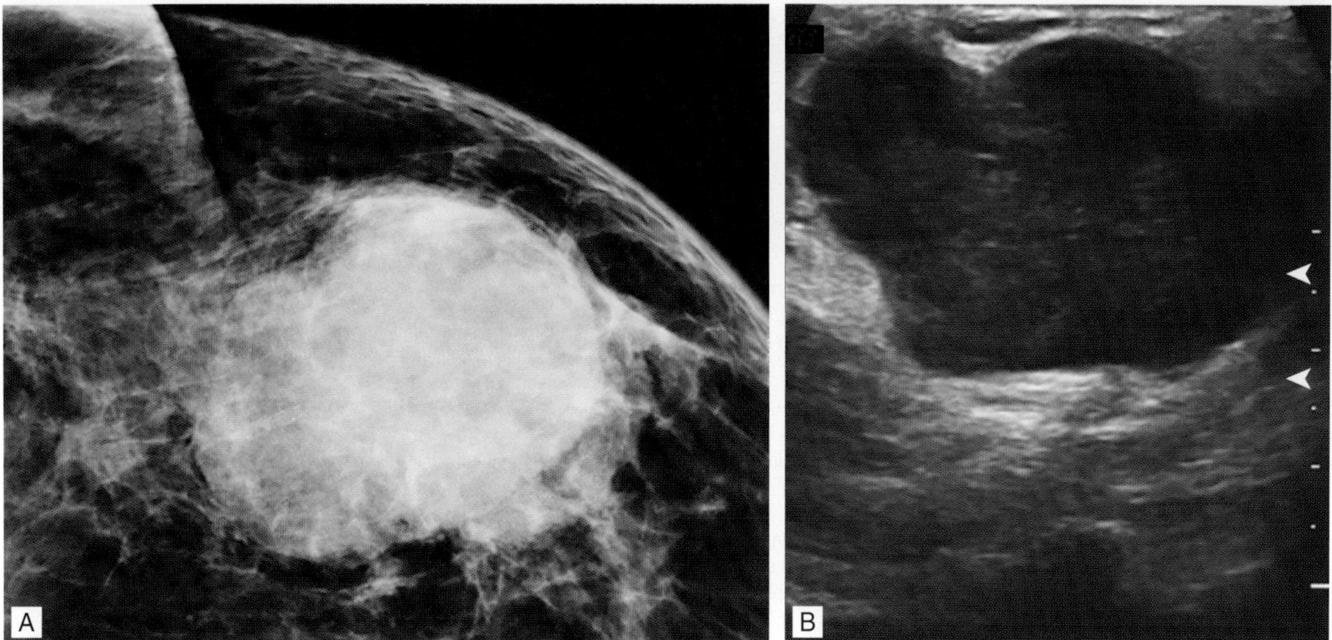

Figure 51.73 An oval mass with circumscribed margins on mammography (A) that appears hypoechoic solid with associated postacoustic enhancement on ultrasonography (B). This was a triple-negative breast cancer.

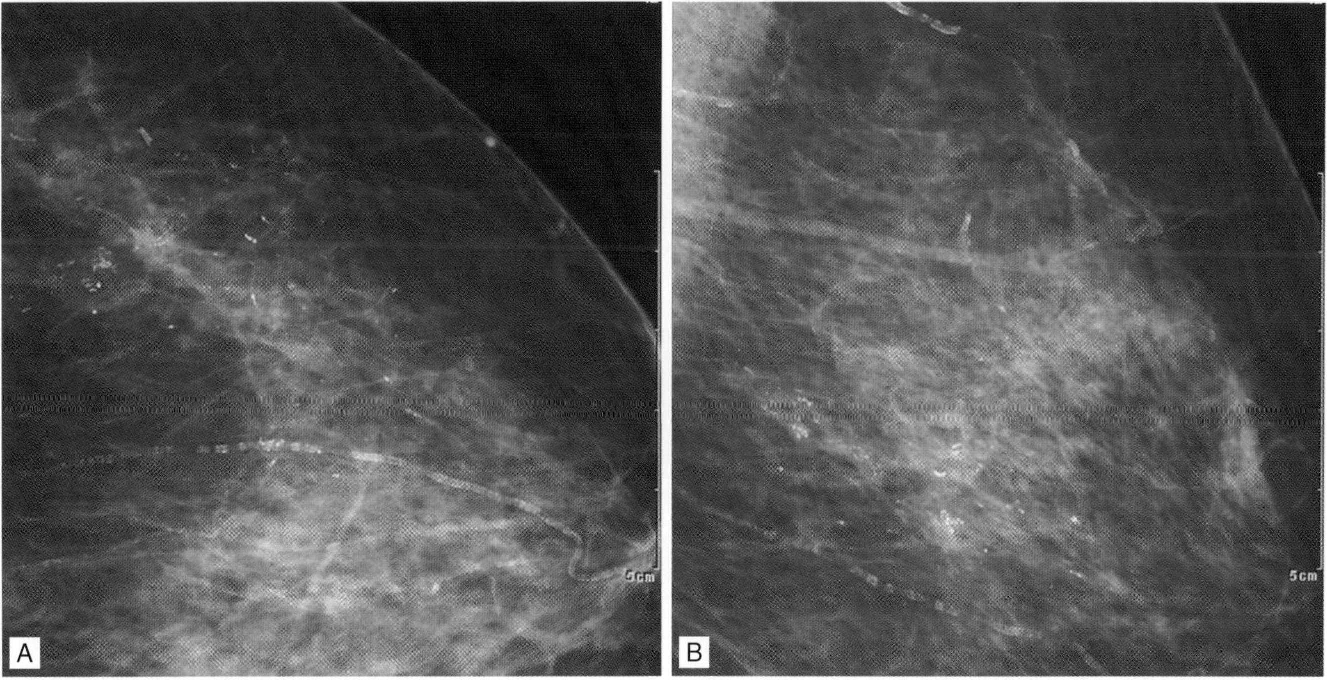

Figure 51.74 Mammograms (A-craniocaudal and B-mediolateral oblique views) in a 55-year-old woman with nipple excoriation but otherwise normal breast examination show segmental fine linear microcalcifications, which was Paget disease with ductal carcinoma in situ.

pathology section). On MRI, ILC can present as an irregular mass-like lesion, a mass lesion with multiple foci adjacent to it with AD, or as clumped segmental NME [80]. It may not show washout kinetics. ILCs are usually not associated with microcalcifications on mammography, and when seen, a histologic variant such as pleomorphic lobular carcinoma is more likely [81].

With regards to other special types, the mucinous tumors often present as ovoid masses with circumscribed or microlobulated margins. They are homogeneous on USG when pure mucinous but can be mammographically occult in about 21% of cases [82]. Papillary carcinoma often presents as a round or oval retroareolar mass with circumscribed or focally indistinct margins. It can appear hypoechoic solid, complex solid-cystic, or intracystic mural nodule on USG [71]. The tubular cancers present as small spiculated masses with a dense center [1].

Paget disease clinically presents as excoriation of the nipple and is characterized by infiltration of the nipple epidermis by adenocarcinoma cells. It is believed that carcinomatous cells from the central lactiferous ducts creep into the epithelium of NAC, and hence more than 90% of the cases are associated with DCIS or IBC in the breast [1,2]. On mammography, one has to carefully look for microcalcifications, which are often central (Fig. 51.74).

TABLE 51.8 T Staging-TNM

T Staging		
T1	<2 cm tumor size	Tumor size measured in greatest dimension
T2	2–5 cm tumor size	
T3	>5 cm tumor size	
T4	Tumor of any size with;	
a	Chest wall involvement i.e. ribs, intercostal muscles and serratus anterior. Note that the involvement of the pectoralis is not a criterion in T staging.	
b	Edema (including peau d' orange of the skin), or ulceration of the skin of the breast, or satellite nodules confined to the same breast. These do not meet the criteria of inflammatory carcinoma.	
c	Combination of a & b	
d	Inflammatory carcinoma defined as diffuse erythema and edema (peau d'orange) involving approximately a third or more of the skin of the breast, with demonstration of tumor emboli in dermal lymphatics.	

Adapted from AJCC Cancer staging manual 8th edition.

When mammogram findings are negative, MRI is recommended before surgery [83,84].

Staging of Breast Cancer

The eighth edition of American Joint Committee on Cancer (AJCC) breast cancer staging has an anatomical TNM staging system and a prognostic staging system that incorporates the histology and molecular profile of the tumor [3,85].

Local Staging of Breast Cancer

When a mass is seen on mammography, its size, any associated findings such as adjacent AD, calcifications within or outside, and any skin or nipple changes must be reported. Often, an adjunct USG is performed to look for additional lesions, especially in a dense breast. The current status of MRI for newly diagnosed breast cancer has been discussed in the MRI section.

T staging is briefly summarized in Table 51.8, and readers are referred to the AJCC manual for greater details on TNM classification [3]. T staging is summarized in Table 51.8. When additional tumors are within the equivalent of one quadrant, the disease is called multifocal, and if in more than one quadrant, it is multicentric. Chest wall infiltration is considered as T4a disease, with the ribs, intercostal muscles, and serratus anterior constituting the chest wall and not the pectoralis [3]. T4b is skin infiltration or skin nodules, T4c is a combination of T4a and b, and T4d is inflammatory breast cancer with demonstration of tumor emboli in dermal lymphatics [3,85].

Lymph Node Evaluation

Nodal stations have been described in the anatomy section. The routine use of axillary USG in clinically node negative axilla is of uncertain clinical significance [85]. However, if the patient has palpable nodes, then imaging is warranted to evaluate the level III axillary nodes, internal mammary nodes, and supraclavicular lymph nodes [85]. Essentially, it is important to look carefully at the axillary, retropectoral, supraclavicular, and internal mammary nodes while reporting any cross-sectional imaging of a patient with breast cancer (Table 51.9).

TABLE 51.9 N Staging TNM

N Staging (Clinical)		
N1	Movable ipsilateral level I & II axillary lymph nodes	Axillary nodal levels: Level I (low-axilla): lymph nodes lateral to the lateral border of pectoralis minor muscle. Level II (mid-axilla): lymph nodes between the medial and lateral borders of the pectoralis minor muscle and the interpectoral (Rotter's) lymph nodes. Level III (apical axilla): lymph nodes medial to the medial margin of the pectoralis minor muscle and inferior to the clavicle.
N2		
a	Matted Ipsilateral level I, II axillary lymph nodes fixed to one another	
b	Clinically detected ipsilateral internal mammary nodes and in the absence of clinically evident level I, II axillary lymph node metastasis	
N3		
a	Ipsilateral infraclavicular (level III axillary) lymph node(s) with or without level I, II axillary lymph node involvement	
b	Clinically detected ipsilateral internal mammary lymph node(s) and clinically evident axillary lymph node(s)	
c	Ipsilateral supraclavicular lymph node(s) with or without axillary or internal mammary lymph node involvement	

Adapted from AJCC Cancer staging manual 8th edition.

Metastatic Disease Status

Invasive breast cancer can spread to the bones, liver, lung, and brain; there is a predilection for sternal metastasis in advanced cases. The metastatic workup in clinical stage I to IIB should be guided based on the patient's symptoms (e.g., chest CT if the patient is breathless). For stages III and IV, a combination of CT chest, CT and MRI of the abdomen and pelvis, bone scan or sodium fluoride scan (for bone metastasis), or whole-body FDG PET/CT can be performed [3,85].

Other Uncommon Malignant Masses of the Breast

Metastases to the breast are unusual and may be single or multiple. They are well defined on mammography, with the most common primary sites being melanoma, the lung, and the ovary (Fig. 51.75). *Lymphoma* in the breast may show the same features as metastases. Lymphoma characteristically lacks calcifications and AD. For B-cell lymphoma, diffuse or ill-defined increases in breast density representing irregular infiltrating processes may be observed [86]. *Mesenchymal tumors* arising from extralobular stroma include benign lesions such as hemangioma; granular cell tumor; nerve sheath tumors; and malignant lesions such as angiosarcoma, rhabdomyosarcoma, and osteogenic sarcoma (Fig. 51.76) [73].

The Male Breast

A normal male breast has a small areola and nipple with undeveloped minimal subareolar ducts. When there is an increase in ducts, it is called *gynecomastia*. Generally, there is no lobule formation. It can be physiological, such as with senile gynecomastia,

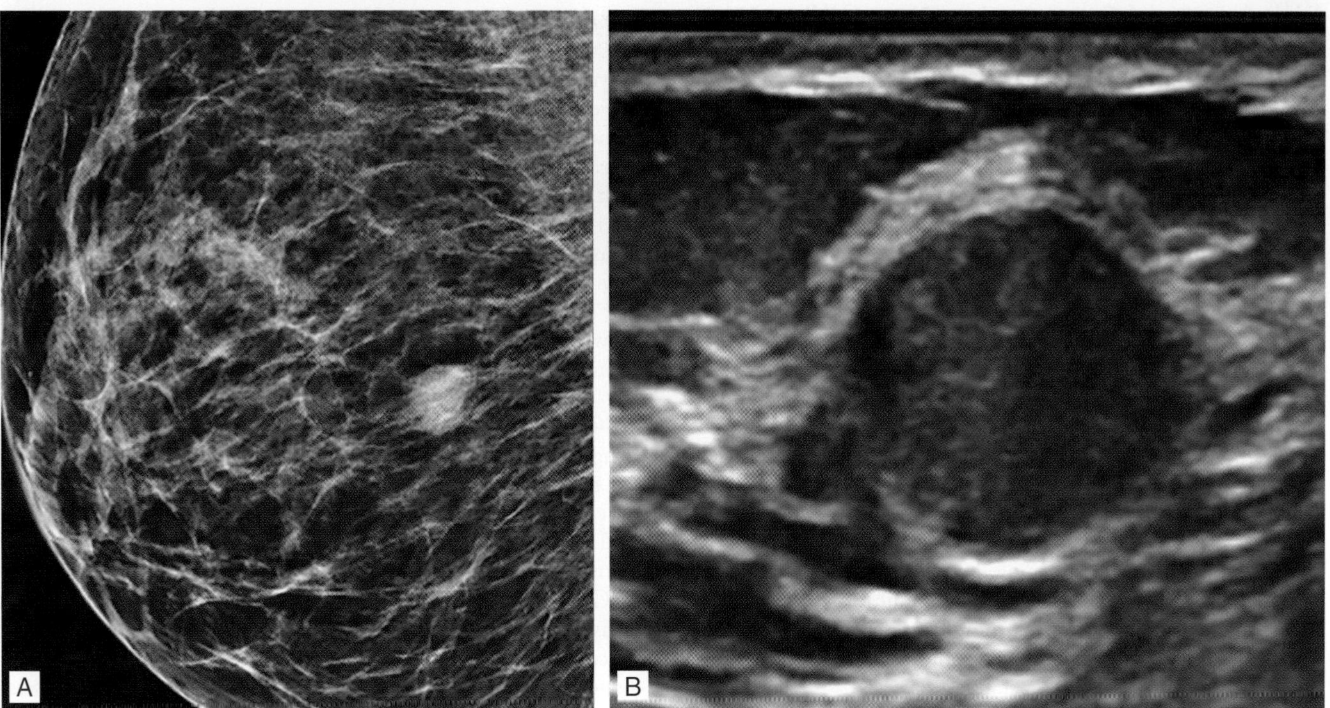

Figure 51.75 High-density oval mass on mammography (A) that on ultrasonography (B) appears solid with circumscribed margins mimicking a fibroadenoma but is a metastatic lesion to the breast from a known neuroendocrine tumor of the small bowel.

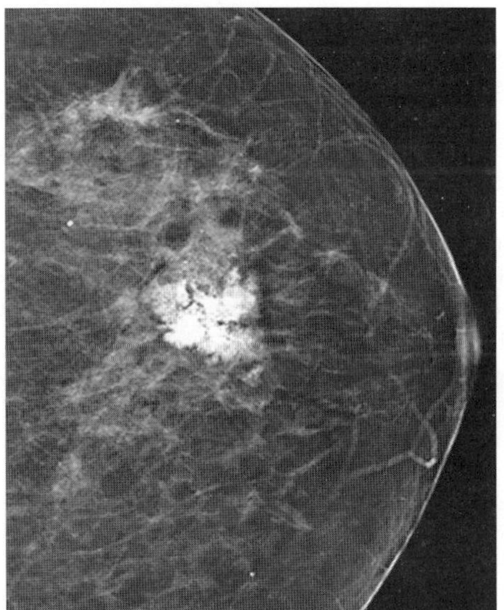

Figure 51.76 Ossifying irregular lesion in the breast in a histologically proven osteogenic sarcoma arising from mesenchymal tumor of the interlobular stroma.

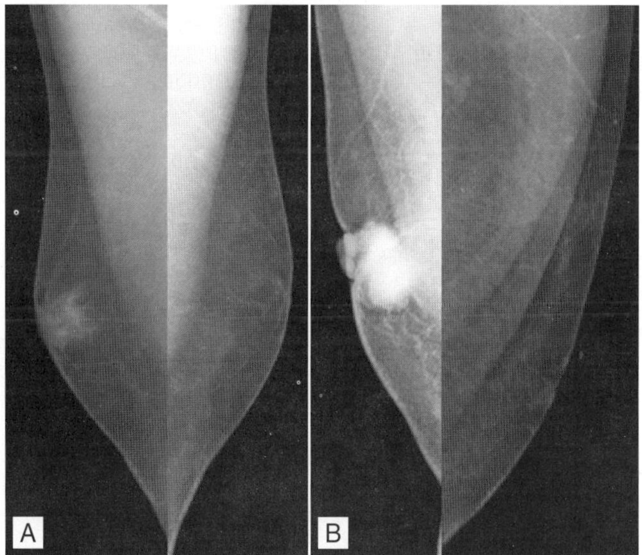

Figure 51.77 Male breast imaging, mediolateral oblique view. (A) Gynecomastia in the right breast with normal appearance of the left breast. (B) A mass in the right breast with normal appearance of the left breast.

secondary to pathologies causing eseferic or antiandrogenic effects (e.g., Sertoli Leydig cell tumor of the testes, adrenal neoplasia, hepatic cirrhosis, other conditions), drug induced (e.g., spironolactone, thiazides, cimetidine and haloperidol), or idiopathic [87]. On imaging, gynecomastia presents as flame-shaped densities radiating from the subareolar region or occasionally can be dendritic or discoid (Fig. 51.77A). Male breast cancer shows imaging characteristics like the female breast cancer, often forming a lobulated or irregular mass (Fig. 51.77B). Benign lesions such as cysts can be seen occasionally, with rare occurrence of stromal tumors such as fibroadenoma or phyllodes because there is generally no lobule formation in male breasts [88].

In routine practice, the most common reason for imaging of a male breast is asymmetric thickening or nodularity, and the most common cause of this is gynecomastia, which is often bilateral but asymmetric on imaging (even if unilateral clinically). Other common causes include pseudogynecomastia (just fatty enlargement without fibroglandular tissue), benign conditions such as lipoma, or rarely breast cancer [89]. Mammography with USG often establishes the diagnosis for the latter, which can be confirmed by biopsy.

Triple Assessment: Symptomatic or Abnormal Breast

In women with symptomatic breast disease, imaging is most effectively used if the clinical findings are fully taken into account. This is extremely important because although mammography is the most sensitive examination available for detecting small breast carcinomas, the false-negative rate for mammography in the detection of symptomatic breast carcinoma is 5% to 15% [1]. A delay in the diagnosis of symptomatic breast carcinomas with negative mammograms can be avoided if radiologists ensure that their clinical colleagues who areefering women for mammography are fully aware of the false-negative rate and will therefore continue the investigation of patients with suspicious clinical findings.

The correct diagnosis in both symptomatic women and in women with screening-detected abnormalities is most likely to be achieved by adopting a combined multidisciplinary approach, popularly known as *triple assessment: clinical history and examination, imaging (mammography, USG, or both), and needle biopsy (FNAC or core biopsy)* [90].

The combination of imaging investigations used (standard views, localized compression views, magnification views, USG) should be chosen according to the clinical findings and age of patient. Supplementary mammographic views are obtained if indicated from the findings on standard views.

Imaging in the Follow-Up of Patients With Breast Cancer

Patients who have been treated for breast cancer may develop locally recurrent tumors and are at an increased risk of developing second primary breast cancer [2]. The aim of the follow-up is to detect recurrence or new primary tumors as early as possible, when the tumors are likely to have a better prognosis. It is important that radiologists are familiar with expected posttreatment changes such as AD because of scar, fluid collections such as seroma, increased breast density, trabecular and skin thickening caused by edema, oil cysts, and dystrophic calcifications caused by fat necrosis and their evolution (see Fig. 51.50). Changes in the mammographic appearance after stabilization should raise suspicions for tumor recurrence [91] (Fig. 51.78). Local tumor recurrence is more common in young patients and in those with cancer showing poor prognostic features. It may be expected to affect 5% of women in the first 5 years, and 10% to 15% of women within 10 years of breast-conserving treatment. Routine mammographic surveillance imaging of the breast after breast-conserving treatment and of the contralateral breast is recommended every 1 to 2 years after treatment and should be carried out in conjunction with clinical examination. The duration of follow-up should consider that the majority of recurrences and 80% of contralateral breast cancers arise within 10 years of the primary diagnosis. Any abnormality detected on routine surveillance should be further assessed using the triple diagnostic approach. MRI has been shown to be useful in cases when the results of the triple approach are not diagnostic.

Breast After Augmentation

Imaging is carried out after insertion of breast prostheses to rule out implant-related complications such as intra- or extracapsular rupture, evaluate symptoms, and screen for cancer.

The Eklund view has been described in positioning section of mammography and is useful to evaluate the native breast tissue. USG is particularly helpful in the examination of augmented breasts because areas of breast tissue that may be partially obscured by the implant on mammography can be satisfactorily demonstrated. MRI is the most sensitive technique for the assessment of implants and should be used if mammography and USG are nondiagnostic or equivocal.

Calcification overlying the surface of the implant is also commonly seen. Features of internal and external implant rupture may be demonstrated. External rupture with siliconoma formation may cause a firm palpable lump and shows a characteristic appearance on mammography and USG; mammography shows a soft tissue opacity with multiple 3 to 4 mm diameter round nodules associated with it due to granuloma formation in response to the presence of silicone. USG shows dense acoustic shadowing.

On MRI, the appearance of an implant depends on the nature of the contents and whether it is a single- or double-lumen implant. Saline and silicon are high signal on T2-weighted sequences, but silicon is higher signal than saline on T1-weighted sequences. The

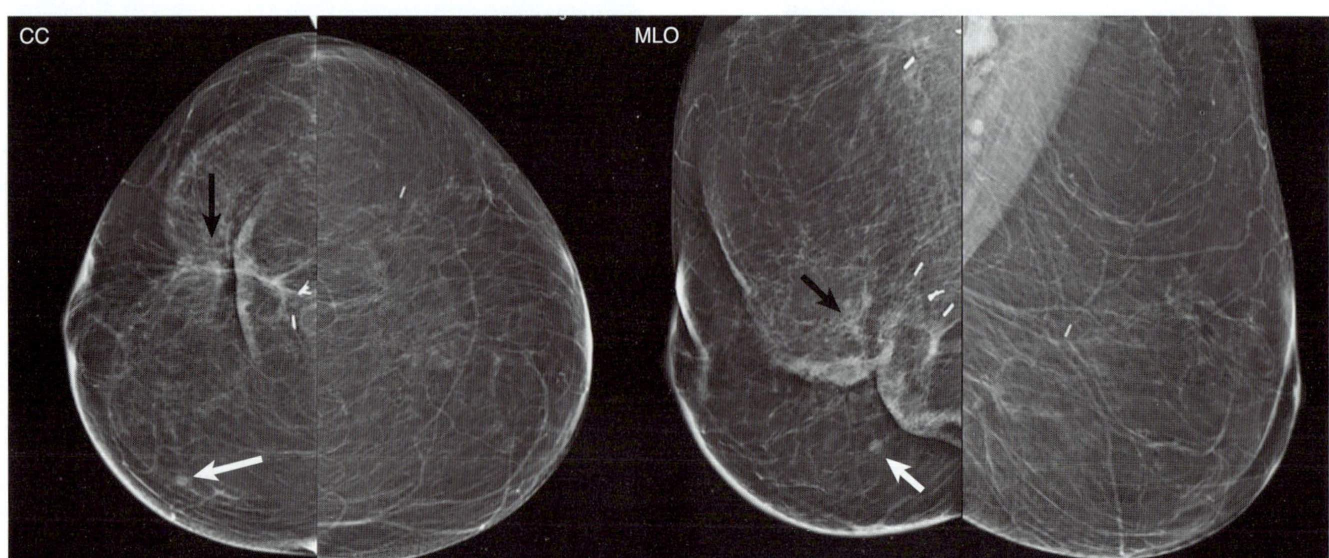

Figure 51.78 Five years after BCT on follow-up. The *black arrows* depict the post-BCT scar (architectural distortion) and associated skin thickening and retraction; surgical staples (*short radiodense white lines*) are also noted. The *white arrows* show a neodensity suspicious for a metachronous lesion. *CC*, craniocaudal; *MLO*, mediolateral oblique.

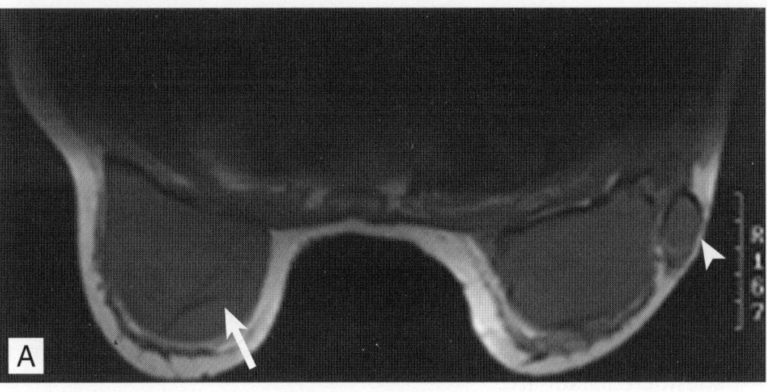
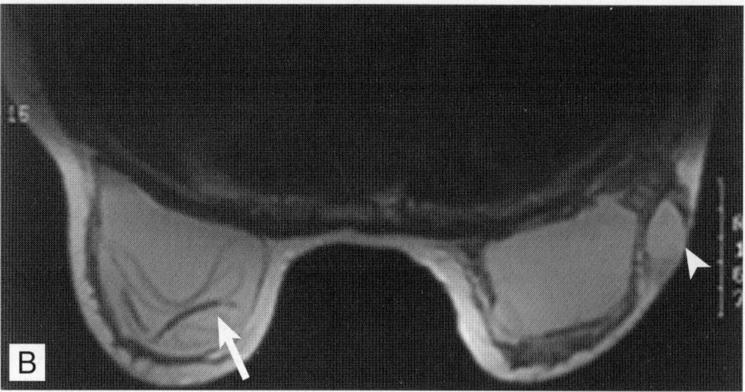

Figure 51.79 T1- (A) and T2-weighted (B) images show an intracapsular implant with linguine sign in the left breast (*arrows*) and an extracapsular rupture (*arrowheads*) with silicon in the outer half of the right breast.

surrounding capsule is low signal intensity on all sequences. Radial folds, normal infoldings of the implant envelope, are seen as thin low-signal folds invaginated into the implant contents. In patients with implants, the presence of a collapsed infolded silicon shell lying within the implant contents (the linguine sign) is diagnostic of intracapsular rupture (Fig. 51.79), whereas collections of silicon lying outside the ruptured fibrous capsule indicate extracapsular rupture [92].

Recently, there have been increasing number of reports of *breast implant-associated anaplastic large cell lymphoma (BIA-ALCL),* which is a rare T-cell lymphoma that manifests as a delayed, noninfective fluid collection around a textured breast implant or residual fibrous scar capsule. The mean age of presentation is 47 years, with an average time frame of 7.5 years after breast implantation. Radiologists should identify this fluid collection as abnormal and recommend cytologic evaluation [93].

Breast Cancer Screening for Average-Risk Women

Pros of Screening: Breast cancer meets the *Wilson-Jungner criteria* for screening: breast cancer is the most common cancer affecting women and it is amenable for early detection in preclinical or latent phase. The efficacy of screening mammography has been shown in several randomized controlled trials: women 50 to 69 years of age who were invited to attend mammographic screening (but not necessarily underwent the test) had a *23% reduction in the risk of death* from breast cancer, and women who actually attended mammographic screening had a higher reduction in risk, estimated at about 40% [94]. *Apart from mortality reduction, screening often detects tumors that are less than 15 mm or node negative, which improves the treatment outcomes and reduces morbidity in women.* Breast-conserving therapy is as successful as mastectomy in early cancer in terms of overall survival and provides a woman with a good quality of life even after the diagnosis of breast cancer. The treatment is affordable and deliverable, and early detection has prognostic benefit. Hence, screening with mammography is recommended by most national guidelines and implemented in high-income countries such as the United States of America, United Kingdom, Canada, Australia, and several European countries. Several other developing nations also support breast cancer screening through national societies and recommend opportunistic screening even though formal screening programs may not be in place. *Opportunistic screening* means referring of patients for screening by healthcare providers or women undergoing the test because of general awareness of cancer. Some nations have other major preventable illnesses, such as communicable diseases and malnutrition, that get more priority, and hence mass screening is not purely a scientific decision but also involves economic and societal concerns.

Guidelines and Recommendations for Screening: According to the recommendations, the most common age at which screening is recommended is from 50 to 69 years. The evidence in support of benefit of screening women between 40 and 50 years is limited, and hence several guidelines recommend sharing of information about the benefits and harms of screening (discussed later) and allow for an informed choice by the woman. The most common screening interval is 2 years, although guidelines vary. The ACR and Society of Breast Imaging recommend annual screening interval for women starting at the age of 40 years and recommends stopping it when the life expectancy is less than 5 to 7 years or comorbidities would not allow dealing with abnormal results of screening [95]. The United Kingdom recommendations are for screening every 3 years, starting at the age of 50 up to 70 years [96].

Organization of Screening: Women as per the country's recommendations are *invited* to the screening program. In most programs, two views (CC and MLO) per breast are considered as standard for *basic screening.* The overall diagnostic accuracy of digital and film–screen mammography for screening is similar, but digital mammography has a better performance [97,98]. The use of dedicated CR systems in mammography is not preferred or encouraged, but they remain to be in use contingent on meeting quality standards. These mammograms are then batch read by at least two radiologists. Double reading is recommended because it improves cancer detection rate by 5% and 15% [1]. After an abnormal screen, prompt referral for *assessment* is mandatory. The assessment clinic is a *multidisciplinary clinic* where facilities are available for clinical examination, standard and supplementary mammography views, USG needle biopsy (FNAC and core biopsy), and counseling. The combination of tests in a particular case is chosen according to the type of abnormality present. The triple assessment (CBE, imaging, and biopsy or FNAC) is used to confirm the diagnosis in women with breast cancer so that treatment can be planned together with appropriate counseling. Women who are found to have normal breasts or benign change are reassured and discharged until their next routine screening examination. Women who have a suspicious lesion in whom a definitive diagnosis cannot be achieved using the triple diagnostic approach are advised to undergo diagnostic surgical excision. This includes cases in which atypical ductal hyperplasia has been diagnosed on image-guided core biopsy because of the risk of associated invasive or in situ carcinoma being found at surgical excision. Women who have a low suspicion lesion, in whom a definitive diagnosis cannot be made using the triple diagnostic approach, may be followed by repeating mammography earlier than the routine recall (e.g., early recall at 6 months).

Quality Assurance: Each country running mass screening programs has to have national standards or quality assurance programs in place that not only ensure high-quality service but also keep a check on *cancer detection rates* (number of DCIS and invasive, size of the tumor, and node-negative cancers), *recall rates, and interval cancer incidence.* Interval cancers in screening programs are cancers that are diagnosed in the interval between a negative screen and the next routine screen. Some of these are truly new fast-growing cancers, but some are "missed cancers." Analysis of the number and type of interval cancers provides an important indication of the effectiveness of the screening service, and review of their mammographic features has enabled film readers to improve their ability to detect small cancers with subtle mammographic features. Interval cancers are an inevitable part of any screening program, but their number should be kept as low as possible.

Cons of Screening: Despite the aforementioned benefits, screening remains a controversial topic. One school of thought is that the reduction in mortality rates is not purely attributable to early detection but also to advances in treatment of breast cancer over past few decades. Some groups highlight the harms of *false positives, overdiagnosis, and overtreatment.* Screening mammogram is said to be a false positive when an abnormality is seen on screening that on further evaluation, whether is its additional views, targeted USG, or biopsy, is not cancer. This rate has been reported variably from 1% to 57%, commonly about 25% to 30% [99]. Of these, 80% of cases get solved without invasive biopsy. However, they do contribute to anxiety in women being recalled and have an impact on the success of a screening program. Of the 20% who end up having a biopsy, about 30% to 50% have cancer. Not all of these cancers would have ended up being lethal in the lifetime of the woman harboring it, particularly when the detected cancer is DCIS. This attributes to overdiagnosis and overtreatment. Unfortunately, as of now, there is no technology that can differentiate between the DCIS that is doomed to become cancer or otherwise. The approximate incidence of this overdiagnosis is about 10% to 11% [100,101].

Mammography, like any other diagnostic test, also suffers from *false-negative rates*, namely, cancers not visible on mammograms. This is largely because of dense breast tissue; subtle finding on mammogram; or the nature of the tumor, as in in lobular cancers. Mammography can miss up to 10% of cancers that are clinically felt or symptomatic. This brings up the role of *supplementary imaging* in screening of breast cancer. A systematic review and metaanalysis of studies using USG as an adjunct modality to mammography reveals that USG can yield an additional 3.8 screen-detected cases per 1000 mammography-negative women; however, this is at a cost of high false positives. Around 50 per 1000 women would be subjected to biopsy based on abnormal USG findings to yield these cancers. The additional costs and resources involved need to be accounted for as well [102]. A large prospective study (American College of Radiology Imaging Network 6666) on asymptomatic women with heterogeneously dense or extremely dense breast tissue and at least one other risk factor for breast cancer (that was a part of the metaanalysis) revealed that USG can identify 5.3 to 3.7 cancers per 1000 women-screens with a PPV of biopsy after mammography plus USG being 11% for the first round of screening and 16% for the second and third rounds. With addition of MRI, in a subset of women, 14.7 per 1000 women-screens were detected with 19% PPV for malignancy [103]. The yield of additional cancers and the PPV is likely to be lower in women with no risk factors for breast cancer. Hence, adjunct screening with USG or MRI is not routinely recommended.

Status of Digital Breast Tomosynthesis in Screening: With regards to the use of DBT in screening, several studies have shown that the yield of cancer increased by 1.2 to 2.7 per 1000 women screened, and more important, the recall rates reduced, ranging from 15% to 37%, but the benefit in reduction of mortality rate is not known [104]. Hence, currently, 2D mammography is considered standard.

Breast Cancer Screening in Women With High Risk: Some of the *high-risk factors* are proven *BRCA1* or *BRCA2* mutation; history of radiation to the mediastinum before age 30 years; personal history of biopsy showing DCIS, LCIS, or ADH; personal history of breast cancer; two first-degree relatives with premenopausal breast cancer; and dense breasts on mammograms. All of these risk factors have different relative risks for breast cancer [105]. Various risk tools or models are available for calculating lifetime risk for a woman. There is more uniformity in recommendations for screening in women at *elevated risk of breast cancer* that is more than 15% to 20% lifetime risk. *Most guidelines recommend annual mammography and MRI starting as early as 30 years.* MRI and mammography can be done at 6-month intervals. This is an acceptable alternative to women with *BRCA1* or *BRCA2* mutations along with other risk-reducing measures such as ovarian suppression and prophylactic mastectomy [37]. For women with elevated but less than 15% to 20% lifetime risk, there is no clear evidence for or against the use of MRI.

Image-Guided Procedures

Imaging is used to ensure accurate needle positioning for the various diagnostic and therapeutic procedures, including

- Simple cyst aspiration (therapeutic)
- Complex cyst aspiration (diagnostic)
- Abscess aspiration
- FNAC
- Core biopsy or wide-bore needle biopsy
- Vacuum-assisted core biopsy
- Preoperative localization of nonpalpable lesions

The type of imaging chosen depends principally on which method (USG or mammography) shows the lesion clearly. Whereas USG is used for cysts and most soft tissue lesions, mammography is used for microcalcification and for soft tissue lesions, particularly distortions, which are not sufficiently well-visualized on USG.

USG-Guided Procedures

For aspiration of complicated cysts or abscess, a 16- to 22-gauge needle can be used, depending on the expected thickness of the contents. For FNAC, a 21- to 23-gauge needle is used to obtain an aspirate containing cellular material, which is analyzed to provide a cytologic diagnosis. Two or three separate passes are made to increase the chance of obtaining a cellular aspirate. Visualization of the needle in relation to the lesion is easiest if the needle is introduced as parallel to the surface of the probe as possible so that the long axis of the needle is perpendicular to the direction of the ultrasound beam. The needle is moved to

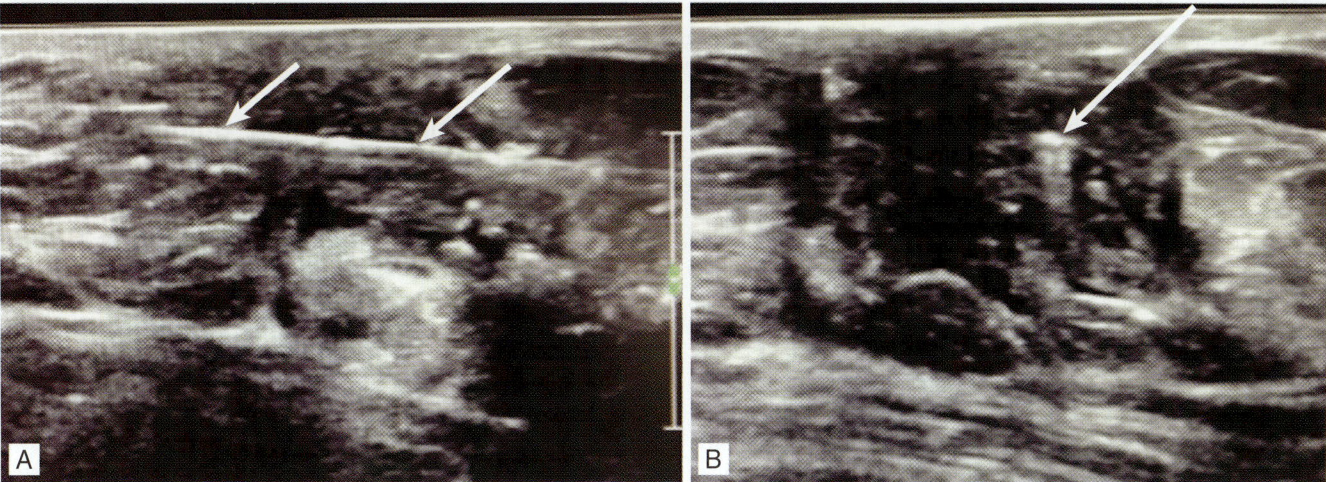

Figure 51.80 USG-guided core biopsy. *Arrows* show the needle within the mass in two planes (A and B).

and fro within the lesion with simultaneous rotation and with negative pressure applied. The negative pressure is most easily applied by an assistant using a syringe connected to the needle by a short extension tube. Aspiration is continued until material is seen within the hub of the needle; the aspirate is then delivered onto slides, and dry and wet preparations are made in accordance with instructions from the local cytopathologist. If local circumstances allow, it may be helpful to have the cellularity of the specimens checked by a cytology technician immediately after the procedure.

Small solid lesions can also be effectively biopsied using ultrasound guidance for core biopsy (Fig. 51.80). A 14- to 16-gauge needle is used together with an automated biopsy device. The biopsy device rapidly advances the central trochar through the lesion; the outer cutting sheath of the needle is then rapidly advanced over the central portion of the needle, cutting a core of tissue that lies within a 17-mm biopsy "port." The needle is withdrawn, and the core of tissue is delivered into formal saline. This procedure is carried out under local anesthetic, and a small 3- to 4-mm skin incision is necessary to allow easy passage of the needle. The biopsy needle should be introduced as parallel as possible both to the ultrasound probe to optimize visualization of the needle and to the chest wall to prevent any risk of the needle tip passing posteriorly into the chest. The 22-mm "throw" of the needle tip on firing must be considered when deciding whether the needle is satisfactorily positioned. The tip of the needle should be positioned just proximal to the edge of the lesion. Maneuvering the needle into the correct position for biopsy is easiest if the needle is passed through the breast tissue in a radial direction in relation to the nipple; in this way, fewer tissue planes need to be traversed. The needle can be observed passing through the lesion during the biopsy (see Fig. 51.80). Several passes are carried out through the same skin incision to ensure that representative material has been obtained. After the procedure, firm pressure should be applied to the area for at least 5 minutes to prevent hematoma formation.

Mammography-Guided Procedures

Stereotactic-Guided Core Biopsy

Conventional mammography apparatus with add-on stereotactic equipment and analogue imaging can be used for stereotactic core biopsy, but more accurate results have been obtained using either add-on digital imaging or dedicated prone stereotactic biopsy equipment with digital imaging. Using this equipment, the patient lies in the prone or prone oblique position, and the breast passes through an aperture in the table. The direction of the x-ray beam is horizontal, and stereotactic views are obtained by rotating the tube 15 degrees either side of the central position. The digital x-ray images obtained are displayed on a computer screen within approximately 5 seconds of exposure, and the computer offers rapid contrast adjustment and zoom facilities. Target areas for biopsy are selected on the computer screen, and the position and angulation of the biopsy needle and gun holder are adjusted automatically. A 14-gauge needle is used; after insertion under local anesthetic, check films are taken to ensure correct positioning. Check films can also be taken after firing the biopsy gun to ensure that the lesion has been traversed by the needle. Five or more core biopsies are usually obtained. Core biopsy specimen radiographs are taken when sampling areas of microcalcification to ensure that representative tissue has been obtained. Problems that may occur with 14-gauge core biopsy include

- Suspicious core biopsy result: The pathologist is unable to make a specific diagnosis on the material provided or ADH is found. At surgical excision, 40% to 50% of such cases will prove to be malignant.
- Underdiagnosis of invasive cancer: A small focus of invasive cancer within an area of malignant microcalcification may not be sampled.
- Targeting of small lesions: Accurate sampling of very small 2- to 3-mm-diameter clusters of microcalcification may be difficult.

Vacuum-Assisted Core Biopsy

Vacuum-assisted core biopsy allows a larger tissue sample to be obtained and overcomes some of the problems of 14-gauge core biopsy, particularly targeting of very small lesions. An 11-gauge probe with a biopsy port attached to a vacuum-producing device is inserted into the breast under local anesthetic and stereotactic guidance. Tissue from the target area is sucked into the biopsy port by the vacuum and is then separated from the surrounding breast by a rotating cutting cylinder that passes down within the probe. The tissue sample is then delivered by withdrawing the cutting cylinder; the probe is left in position in the breast and is rotated so that the biopsy port is aligned with the next site for sampling. In this way, multiple samples are taken, and small clusters of microcalcification are usually completely removed. If the mammographic marker is removed, a small metal clip is deployed at the site of the biopsy to allow accurate localization if subsequent surgical excision is necessary. Vacuum-assisted core biopsy has also been used under ultrasound guidance for sampling of soft tissue lesions and under MRI guidance for lesions that are not visible using either mammography or USG.

Preoperative Localization of Nonpalpable Lesions

Before surgical excision of nonpalpable lesions, information from the combined imaging and needle biopsy workup is used to determine whether the surgery is to be therapeutic, in cases in which a diagnosis of malignancy has been confirmed, or diagnostic, for cases in which the diagnosis remains uncertain. The position of the lesion in the breast is marked using a wire with a hook or barb on the end to prevent movement of the wire within the breast. The wire is contained within a needle that is inserted into the breast under local anesthetic using either x-ray or USG guidance. When x-ray guidance is used, a simple perforated compression plate or aperture compression plate is satisfactory, and stereotaxis is not usually required. When the tip of the needle has been shown to be satisfactorily positioned within 10 mm of the lesion, the needle sheath is withdrawn, leaving the wire in situ. Check CC and lateral views are obtained to show the final position of the wire in relation to the lesion. Peroperative specimen radiography is mandatory to ensure that the excised breast tissue contains the mammographic abnormality.

Ductography

Ductography may be performed in the investigation of patients with unilateral blood-stained nipple discharge to identify the site of pathology within the duct (see Fig. 51.59). The duct orifice from which the discharge is occurring is identified by squeezing the breast tissue to express the discharge. The duct orifice is then cannulated using a fine 30-gauge cannula (e.g., sialogram cannula), the tip of which is passed into the lactiferous sinus. Approximately 3 mL of water-soluble contrast is then injected, the cannula is taped to the nipple, and lateral and CC views are obtained. Ductal filling defects may be caused by papilloma or carcinoma in situ.

Magnetic Resonance Imaging–Guided Interventions

When a suspicious lesion is identified on MR, second-look USG is done for further characterization and localization. If, however, USG is unable to visualize the lesion, MRI-guided breast biopsy is indicated. MRI-guided breast biopsy is, however, performed at very few centers and requires experienced staff and specific equipment [84]. The contradictions to MRI and biopsy are applicable here, and if the lesion is inaccessible, for example, the lesion is close to chest wall or nipple, or the breast implant is at risk of rupture because of proximity with the lesion, the procedure is contraindicated [106]. As described earlier, the vacuum-assisted technique is used. However, if biopsy is technically not feasible, MRI can still be used for preoperative localization, similar to stereotactic or ultrasound guidance, wherein a guidewire or a marker clip is deployed [106]. Unlike stereotactic- and ultrasound-guided procedures however, a contrast-enhanced scan is imperative for MR guidance for procedures [106].

Suggested Readings

- LR Greene, D Wilkinson, The role of general nuclear medicine in breast cancer, J Med Radiat Sci 62 (1) (2015) 54–65. doi:10.1002/jmrs.97.
- D Kopans, Textbook of Breast Imaging, Lippincott Williams & Wilkins, Philadelphia, PA, 2005.
- W Berg, J Leung, Diagnostic Imaging Breast, Elsevier.
- E Morris, L Libermann, Breast MRI: diagnosis and intervention, Springer.

Index

A

Note: Page number followed by *f*, *t* and *b* indicates figure, table and box respectively.